HURST'S

THE HEART

VOLUME 2

HURST'S
THE HEART

ELEVENTH EDITION

Editors

VALENTIN FUSTER, MD, PhD

Director, The Zena and Michael A. Wiener
    Cardiovascular Institute and The Marie-Josée and
    Henry R. Kravis Center for Cardiovascular Health
    Richard Gorlin, MD/Heart Research Foundation,
    Professor of Cardiology, The Mount Sinai Medical
    Center and School of Medicine
New York, New York

**R. WAYNE ALEXANDER,
MD, PhD**

R. Bruce Logue Professor and Chair
Department of Medicine
Emory University School of Medicine
Atlanta, Georgia

ROBERT A. O'ROURKE, MD

Charles Conrad Brown Distinguished Professor
    in Cardiovascular Disease
University of Texas Health Science Center at
    San Antonio
San Antonio, Texas

Associate Editors

ROBERT ROBERTS, MD

Professor of Medicine
President and CEO
University of Ottawa Heart Institute
Ottawa, Ontario, Canada

SPENCER B. KING III, MD

Fuqua Chair of Interventional Cardiology
    The Fuqua Heart Center at Piedmont Hospital
Co-Director, American Cardiovascular Research Institute
    Clinical Professor of Medicine
    Emory University School of Medicine
Atlanta, Georgia

IRA S. NASH, MD

Associate Professor of Medicine
    Mount Sinai School of Medicine
Associate Director, The Zena and Michael A. Wiener
    Cardiovascular Institute and The Marie-Josée and
    Henry R. Kravis Center for Cardiovascular Health
Mount Sinai Medical Center
New York, New York

ERIC N. PRYSTOWSKY, MD

Director, Clinical Electrophysiology Laboratory
St. Vincent Hospital
Indianapolis, Indiana
Consulting Professor of Medicine
Duke University Medical Center
Durham, North Carolina

McGRAW-HILL
Medical Publishing Division

New York   Chicago   San Francisco   Lisbon   London   Madrid   Mexico City
Milan   New Delhi   San Juan   Seoul   Singapore   Sydney   Toronto

Hurst's
THE HEART
Eleventh Edition

1234567890 DOWDOW 0987654

ISBN 0-07-142264-1 (Single vol. ed.)
       0-07-142265-X (2-vol. set ed.)
       0-07-143224-8 (Vol. 1)
       0-07-143225-6 (Vol. 2)

This book was set in Times Roman by *The GTS Companies*/York, PA Campus.
The editors were Darlene B. Cooke, Marc Strauss, Marsha Loeb,
and Lester A. Sheinis.
The production supervisor was Richard C. Ruzycka.
The text designer was Marsha Cohen / Parallelogram Graphics.
The cover designer was Aimee Nordin.
The indexer was Alexandra Nickerson.
RR Donnelley was printer and binder.

This book is printed on acid-free paper.

Library of Congress Cataloging-in-Publication Data

Hurst's the heart / edited by Valentin Fuster ... [et al.].—11th ed.
         p. ; cm.
Includes bibliographical references and index.
ISBN 0-07-142264-1 (single vol.)—ISBN 0-07-142265-X (2-vol. set)
       1. Cardiovascular system—Diseases. 2. Heart—Diseases. I. Title: Heart.
    II. Fuster, Valentin.
       [DNLM: 1. Cardiovascular Diseases. WG 100 H9662 2004]
RC667.H88 2004
616.1—dc22
                                                                                2003059615

CONTENTS

Part 16

SOCIAL ISSUES AND CARDIOVASCULAR DISEASE

CONTRIBUTORS

FADI G. AKAR, PhD
Post Doctoral Fellow
School of Medicine
Division of Cardiology
Johns Hopkins University
Baltimore, Maryland
Chapter 10

MASOOD AKHTAR, MD, FACC, FACP
Clinical Professor of Medicine
University of Wisconsin School of Medicine
Cardiology Department
Milwaukee Clinical Campus
Aurora Sinai Medical Center and St. Luke's
Medical Center
Milwaukee, Wisconsin
Chapter 34

R. WAYNE ALEXANDER, MD, PhD
R. Bruce Logue Professor and Chair
Department of Medicine
Emory University School of Medicine
Atlanta, Georgia
Chapters 7 and 52

SUHAIL ALLAQABAND, MD
Clinical Assistant Professor
Department of Cardiology
University of Wisconsin Medical
School–Milwaukee Clinical Campus
Consultant Interventional Cardiologist
Aurora Sinai Medical Center and St. Luke's
Medical Center
Milwaukee, Wisconsin
Chapter 103

JEFFREY L. ANDERSON, MD
Associate Chief of Cardiology
Professor of Internal Medicine
University of Utah School of Medicine
Salt Lake City, Utah
Chapter 81

JUAN JOSE BADIMON, PhD
Professor of Medicine
Director
Cardiovascular Biology Reserch Laboratory
Mount Sinai School of Medicine
New York, New York
Chapter 45

LINA BADIMON, PhD
Professor and Director
Cardiovascular Institute
High Council for Scientific Research
Director
Catalan Institute for Cardiovascular
Sciences
Hospital de la Santa Creu I Sant Pau
Barcelona, Spain
Chapter 45

JAMES M. BAILEY, MD
Department of Anesthesiology
North East Georgia Diagnostic Hospital
Gainesville, Georgia
Chapter 59

STEVEN R. BAILEY, MD
Professor of Medicine and Radiology,
Director
Interventional Cardiology
Director
Cardiac Catheterization Laboratory
University of Texas Health Science Center
San Antonio
San Antonio, Texas
Chapter 68

TANVIR K. BAJWA, MD
Associate Professor of Medicine
University of Wisconsin Medical
School–Milwaukee Clinical Campus
Director
Cardiac Catheterization Laboratory
Director
Interventional Cardiology Fellowship
Aurora Sinai Medical Center and
St. Luke's Medical Center
Milwaukee, Wisconsin
Chapter 103

GEORGE L. BAKRIS, MD, FACP
Professor of Preventive Medicine and
Internal Medicine
RUSH Medical College of RUSH University
at RUSH-Presbyterian-St. Luke's
Medical Center
Vice-Chairman
Department of Preventive Medicine
Director
Section of Clinical Research
Department of Preventive Medicine
Chicago, Illinois
Chapter 61

EMELIA J. BENJAMIN, MD, ScM
Clinical Associate Professor
Department of Medicine
Boston University School of Medicine
Boston, Massachusetts
Director
Echocardiography Laboratory
Framingham Heart Study
Framingham, Massachusetts
Staff Cardiologist
Boston Medical Center
Cardiology Department
Boston, Massachusetts
Chapter 2

DANIEL S. BERMAN, MD
Professor of Medicine
Department of Nuclear Cardiology
Director
Cardiac Imaging
Cedars-Sinai Medical Center
Los Angeles, California
Chapter 19

GERALD J. BERRY, MD
Associate Professor of Pathology
Director of Cardiac Pathology
Stanford University School of Medicine
Stanford University Medical Center
Stanford, California
Chapter 26

ALAN L. BISNO, MD

Professor of Medicine
Department of Medicine
University of Miami School of Medicine
Medical Service
VA Medical Center
Medical Service
Miami, Florida
Chapter 65

HENRY R. BLACK, MD

The Charles J. and Margaret Roberts
Professor of Preventive Medicine
Professor of Internal Medicine and
Pharmacology
Associate Dean for Research
RUSH Medical College of RUSH University
at RUSH-Presbyterian-St. Luke's
Medical Center
Chicago, Illinois
Chapter 61

DANIEL G. BLANCHARD, MD

Professor of Medicine
Department of Medicine (Cardiology)
University of California
San Diego School of Medicine
Director
Cardiac Noninvasive Laboratory
University of California San Diego Medical
Center
San Diego, California
Chapter 15

ROB A. BLEASDALE, MD

Lecturer
Wales Heart Institute
Heath Park, Cardiff, United Kingdom
Chapter 38

TERESA BOHLMEYER, MD

Division of Cardiology
University of Colorado Health Sciences
Center
Denver, Colorado
Chapter 76

WENDY M. BOOK, MD

Assistant Professor of Medicine
Emory University School of Medicine
Director
Emory Adult Congenital Program
Division of Cardiology
Emory Hospital
Atlanta, Georgia
Chapter 89

HARISIOS BOUDOULAS, MD

Emeritus Professor of Medicine
Cardiology
Ohio State University College of Medicine
and Public Health
Columbus Ohio
Director
Clinical Research Center
Foundation of Biomedical Research
Academy of Athens
Athens, Greece
Chapter 40

KENNETH L. BRIGHAM, MD

Vice Chair for Research
Department of Medicine
Emory University School of Medicine
Atlanta, Georgia
Chapter 64

MICHAEL R. BRISTOW, MD, PhD

Division of Cardiology
University of Colorado Health Sciences
Center
Denver, Colorado
Chapter 76

BRUCE R. BRODIE, MD

Clinical Professor of Medicine
University of North Carolina Teaching
Service
Moses H. Cone Heart and Vascular Center
Greensboro, North Carolina
Chapter 56

RAMON BRUGADA, MD, FACC

Masonic Medical Research Laboratory
Molecular Genetics Department
Director
Molecular Genetics Program
Utica, New York
Chapter 72

ALLEN P. BURKE, MD

Adjunct Professor of Pathology
Georgetown University
Associate Chair
Department of Cardiovascular Pathology
Armed Forces Institute of Pathology
Washington, District of Columbia
Chapter 49

HUGH CALKINS, MD

Professor of Medicine
Divison of Cardiac Electrophysiology
John Hopkins School of Medicine
Johns Hopkins Hospital
Baltimore, Maryland
Chapter 30

LOUIS R. CAPLAN, MD

Professor of Neurology
Harvard Medical School
Chief
Cerebrovascular Disease
Beth Israel Deaconess Medical Center
Boston, Massachusetts
Chapter 99

AGUSTIN CASTELLANOS, MD,
FACC, FAHA

Professor of Medicine
Director
Clinical Electrophysiology
Division of Cardiology
Jackson Memorial Medical Center
University of Miami School of Medicine
Miami, Florida
Chapter 13

SIMON CHAKKO, MD

Chief
Cardiology Section
University of Miami School of Medicine
Veterans Affairs Medical Center
Professor of Medicine
University of Miami School of Medicine
Miami, Florida
Chapter 65

NISHA CHANDRA-STROBOS,
MD

Professor of Medicine
Johns Hopkins University School of
Medicine
Director
Coronary Care Unit
Johns Hopkins Bayview Medical Center
Baltimore, Maryland
Chapter 42

PAMELA CHARNEY, MD, FACP

Clinical Professor of Medicine
Albert Einstein College of Medicine
New York, New York
Program Director
Internal Medicine Residency
Norwalk Hospital
Norwalk, Connecticut
Chapter 97

MELVIN D. CHEITLIN, MD

Emeritus Professor of Medicine
University of California San Francisco
Former Chief of Cardiology
San Francisco General Hospital
Cardiology Service
San Francisco, California
Chapter 88

JAMES T. T. CHEN, MD

Professor Emeritus of Radiology
Duke Medical Center
Durham, North Carolina
Chapter 14

DOMENICO CIANFLONE, MD, FESC

Director Coronary Care Unit
San Raffaele University Hospital
Milan, Italy
Chapter 46

MICHAEL CLARK, MD, FACC

Senior Vice President
Chief Medical Director
Swiss RE Life & Health
Medical Department
Armonk, New York
Chapter 105

STEPHEN D. CLEMENTS JR., MD

Professor of Medicine
Cardiology
Emory University School of Medicine
Atlanta, Georgia
Chapter 59

LYNN CLEMOW, MD

Behavioral Cardiovascular Health and
Hypertension Program
Columbia Presbyterian Medical Center
New York, New York
Chapter 107

STEFANO COLI, MD

Coronary Care Unit
San Raffaele University Hospital
Milan, Italy
Chapter 46

DENTON A. COOLEY, MD

Clinical Professor of Surgery
University of Texas Medical School
Houston, Texas
Chapter 85

ROBERTO CORTI, MD

Consultant
Division of Cardiology
University Hospital
Zurich University
Zurich, Switzerland
Chapter 45

RALPH B. D'AGOSTINO, PhD

Professor of Mathematics
Statistics and Public Health
Mathematics and Statistics Department
Boston University
Boston, Massachusetts
Director of Data Management and
Statistical Analysis
Framingham Heart Study
Framingham, Massachusetts
Chapter 2

KARINA W. DAVIDSON, PhD

Behavioral Cardiovascular Health and
Hypertension Program
Columbia Presbyterian Medical Center
New York, New York
Chapter 107

JOHN E. DEANFIELD, MB, FACC

Cardiothoracic Unit
Great Ormond Street Hospital for Children
Professor of Cardiology
Cardiac Unit
Institute of Child Health
London, United Kingdom
Chapter 74

LOUIS J. DELL'ITALIA, MD

University of Alabama at Birmingham
Birmingham, Alabama
Chapter 67

ANTHONY N. DEMARIA, MD

Judith and Jack White Chair in Cardiology
Professor of Medicine
Chief
Division of Cardiology
University of California at San Diego
San Diego, California
Chapter 15

HOWARD V. DINH, MD

Cardiology Fellow
Division of Cardiology
David Geffen School of Medicine at UCLA
UCLA Medical Center
Los Angeles, California
Chapter 21

THOMAS F. DODSON, MD

Associate Professor of Surgery
Vice Chairman for Education
Program Director for General Surgery
Residency Program
Emory University School of Medicine and
the Emory Clinic
Atlanta, Georgia
Chapter 102

JOHN S. DOUGLAS JR., MD

Professor of Medicine
Emory University Hospital School of
Medicine
Director of Interventional Cardiology
Emory University Hospital
Atlanta, Georgia
Chapters 17, 55, 57

W. LANE DUVALL, MD

Cardiovascular Fellow
Mount Sinai School of Medicine
The Zena and Michael A. Wiener
Cardiovascular Institute and The Marie-Josée
and Henry R. Kravis Center for
Cardiovascular Health
Mount Sinai Medical Center
New York, New York
Chapter 54

VICTOR J. DZAU, MD

Chairman
Department of Medicine
Brigham and Women's Hospital
Hershey Professor of the Practice and
Theory of Medicine
Harvard University
Medical School
Boston, Massachusetts
Chapter 11

KIM A. EAGLE, MD

Albion Walter Hewlett Professor of
Internal Medicine
Clinical Director
Cardiovascular Center
University of Michigan Health System
Ann Arbor, Michigan
Chapter 82

WILLIAM D. EDWARDS, MD

Professor of Pathology
Mayo Medical School and Mayo Graduate
School of Medicine
Consultant in Anatomic Pathology
Mayo Clinic and Mayo Foundation
Rochester, Minnesota
Chapter 3

KENNETH ELLENBOGEN, MD

Kontos Professor of Medicine
Director
Cardiac Electrophysiology and Pacemaker
Laboratory
Medical College of Virginia at Virginia
Commonwealth University
Richmond, Virginia
Chapter 32

WILLIAM J. ELLIOTT, MD, PhD

Professor of Preventive Medicine
Internal Medicine and Pharmacology
RUSH Medical College of RUSH University
at RUSH-Presbyterian-St. Luke's
Medical Center
Chicago, Illinois
Chapter 61

DOMIEN J. ENGELEN, MD

Diakonessen Hospital
Utrecht, The Netherlands
Chapter 53

GREGORY ENGLE, MD

Chief Fellow
Cardiovascular Medicine
Cardiovascular Medicine Division
Stanford University School of Medicine
Stanford, California
Chapter 16

ERLING FALK, MD, PhD

Professor of Experimental Cardiovascular
Pathology
Department of Cardiology
Aarhus University Hospital (Skejby)
Aarhus, Denmark
Chapter 44

MICHAEL E. FARKOUH, MD

Associate Professor of Medicine
NYU School of Medicine
Director, Cardiac Care Unit
NYU Medical Center
New York, New York
Chapter 86

MICHAEL D. FAULX, MD

Cardiology Fellow
Case Western Reserve University
University Hospitals of Cleveland
Cleveland, Ohio
Chapter 80

ZAHI A. FAYAD, PhD

Imaging Science Laboratories
Departments of Radiology and Medicine
(Cardiology)
The Zena and Michael A. Wiener
Cardiovascular Institute
The Marie-Josée and Henry R. Kravis
Cardiovascular Health Center
Mount Sinai School of Medicine
New York, New York
Chapter 22

MAKSIN A. FEDARU, MD

Research Fellow
Department of Internal Medicine/Cardiology
University of Michigan
Research Fellow
Division of Cardiovascular Medicine
University of Michigan Health System
Ann Arbor, Michigan
Chapter 50

GERALD F. FLETCHER, MD

Professor of Medicine
Mayo Clinic College of Medicine
Rochester, Minnesota
Director
Preventive Cardiology
Mayo Clinic
Jacksonville, Florida
Chapter 95

THOMAS R. FLIPSE, MD

Consultant
Cardiovascular Diseases and Internal
Medicine
Mayo Clinic
Jacksonville, Florida
Chapter 95

RICHARD I. FOGEL, MD

The Heart Center of Indiana
The Care Group
Indianapolis, Indiana
Chapter 28

ROBERT H. FRANCH, MD

Professor of Medicine
Emeritus (Cardiology)
Emeritus Staff Emory University Hospital
Egleston Children's Hospital
Grady Memorial Hospital
Department of Cardiology
Emory University Medical School
Atlanta, Georgia
Chapter 17

GARY S. FRANCIS, MD, FACC

Professor of Medicine and Director
Coronary Intensive Care Unit
Cleveland Clinic Lerner College of
Medicine at Case Western Reserve
University
Cleveland Clinic Foundation
Cardiology Department
Cleveland, Ohio
Chapter 24

O. HOWARD FRAZIER, MD

Professor of Surgery
University of Texas Health Science Center
Clinical Professor, Department of Surgery
Baylor College of Medicine
St. Luke's Episcopal Hospital
Chief, Transplant Service
Director, Cardiovascular Surgical Research
Houston, Texas
Chapter 85

MICHAEL D. FREED, MD

Associate Professor of Pediatrics
Harvard Medical School
Senior Associate in Cardiology
Children's Hospital
Boston, Massachusetts
Chapter 73

WILLIAM T. FRIEDEWALD, MD

Clinical Professor
Departments of Medicine, Epidemiology,
and Biostatistics
Columbia University School of Medicine
New York, New York
Chapter 105

WILLIAM H. FRISHMAN, MD,
MACP

Professor and Chair
Department of Medicine
New York Medical College
Westchester Medical Center
Valhalla, New York
Chapters 25 and 90

VICTOR F. FROELICHER, MD

Professor of Medicine
Director
ECG and Exercise Testing
Division of Cardiovascular Medicine
Stanford University School of Medicine
Palo Alto, California
Chapter 16

DAVID R. FULTON, MD

Associate Professor of Pediatrics
Harvard Medical School
Senior Associate in Cardiology
Chief
Cardiology Outpatient Services
Department of Cardiology
Children's Hospital at Boston
Boston, Massachusetts
Chapter 73

VALENTIN FUSTER, MD, PhD

Director, The Zena and Michael A. Wiener
Cardiovascular Institute and The Marie-Josée
and Henry R. Kravis Center for
Cardiovascular Health
Richard Gorlin, MD/Heart Research
Foundation, Professor of Cardiology,
The Mount Sinai Medical Center and
School of Medicine
New York, New York
Chapters 21, 22, 44, 45, 48, 54, 86

WILLIAM GERIN, MD

Behavioral Cardiovascular Health and
Hypertension Program
Columbia Presbyterian Medical Center
New York, New York
Chapter 107

GUIDO GERMANO, PhD

Professor of Medicine and Radiological
Sciences
UCLA School of Medicine
Director
Artificial Intelligence Program
Cedars-Sinai Medical Center
Los Angeles, California
Chapter 19

GARY GERSTENBLITH, MD

Johns Hopkins University School of
Medicine
Department of Medicine
Division of Cardiology
Baltimore, Maryland
Chapter 96

EDWARD M. GILBERT, MD

University of Utah Health Sciences Center
Salt Lake City, Utah
Chapter 76

ANTON P. GORGELS, MD,
PhD

Associate Professor of Cardiology
Cardiovascular Research Institute Maastricht
University Maastricht
Cardiologist
University Hospital Maastricht
Department of Cardiology
Maastricht, The Netherlands
Chapter 53

KATHY K. GRIENDLING, PhD

Professor of Medicine
Division of Cardiology
Emory University School of Medicine
Atlanta, Georgia
Chapter 7

SCOTT M. GRUNDY, MD, PhD

Center for Human Nutrition
University of Texas Southwestern Medical
Center at Dallas
Dallas, Texas
Chapter 43

GARY L. GRUNKEMEIER, MD

Director
Medical Data Research Center
Providence Health Systems
Portland, Oregon
Chapter 70

PATRICIA A. GUM, MD

Staff
Department of Cardiovascular Medicine
Cleveland Clinic Foundation
Cleveland, Ohio
Chapter 100

RORY HACHAMOVITCH,
MD, MSc

Associate Professor of Medicine
Division of Cardiovascular Medicine
Keck School of Medicine
University of Southern California
Los Angeles, California
Chapter 19

ROBERT J. HALL, MD

Director
Cardiac Education
St. Luke's Episcopal Hospital and Texas
Heart Institute
Clinical Professor of Medicine
Baylor College of Medicine and University
of Texas Medical School at Houston,
St. Luke's Episcopal Hospital
Houston, Texas
Chapter 85

JONATHAN L. HALPERIN, MD

Director of Clinical Sevices,
The Zena and Michael A. Wiener
Cardiovascular Institute and
The Marie-Josée and Henry R. Kravis
Center for Cardiovascular Health
Mount Sinai Medical Center
Robert and Harriet Heilbrenner Professor
of Medicine
Mount Sinai School of Medicine
New York, New York
Chapter 98

DAVID G. HARRISON, MD
Director
Division of Cardiology
Bernard Marcus Professor of Medicine
Emory University School of Medicine
Emory Clinic
Atlanta, Georgia
Chapter 7

SEAN HAYES, MD
Cedars-Sinai Medical Center
Los Angeles, California
Chapter 19

BRIAN D. HOIT, MD
Professor of Medicine
Director
Echocardiography
Case Western Reserve University
Cleveland, Ohio
Chapters 78 and 80

J. WILLIS HURST, MD, MACP
Active Consultant to the Division of
Cardiology
Candler Professor and Chairman
Department of Medicine Emeritus
Emory University School of Medicine
Atlanta, Georgia
Foreword

JULIA H. INDIK, MD
Assistant Professor of Medicine
Section of Cardiology
Department of Internal Medicine
University of Arizona
Tucson, Arizona
Chapter 35

ALBERTO INTERIAN JR., MD
Professor of Medicine
Associate Chief
Division of Cardiology
Director of Electrophysiology
University of Miami School of Medicine
Miami, Florida
Chapter 13

VINOD K. S. JAYAM, MD
Senior Clinical Fellow
Division of Cardiac Electrophysiology
Johns Hopkins Hospital
Johns Hopkins University
Baltimore, Maryland
Chapter 30

MARK E. JOSEPHSON, MD
Chief
Cardiovascular Division
Director
Harvard Thorndike Electrophysiology
Institute and Arrhythmia Services
Electrophysiology Institute
Beth Israel Deaconess Medical Center
Cardiology
Boston, Massachusetts
Chapter 41

RONALD J. KANTER, MD
Associate Professor of Pediatrics
Director of Pediatric Electrophysiology
Department of Pediatrics
Duke University School of Medicine
Duke University Medical Center
Durham, North Carolina
Chapter 39

SAMIR KAPADIA, MD
Staff
Cardiovascular Medicine
Cleveland Clinic Foundation
Cleveland, Ohio
Chapter 100

JOEL A. KAPLAN, MD
Executive Vice President
Chancellor, Health Sciences Center
Professor of Anesthesiology
University of Louisville
Department of Anesthesia
University of Louisville Hospital
Louisville, Kentucky
Chapter 83

MARINKA KARTALIJA, MD
Department of Medicine
University of Utah
Salt Lake City, Utah
Alaska Native Medical Center
Anchorage, Alaska
Chapter 81

G. NEAL KAY, MD
Professor of Medicine
Division of Cardiovascular Disease
University of Alabama at Birmingham
Birmingham, Alabama
Chapter 29

BRADLEY B. KELLER, MD
Professor of Pediatrics
University of Pittsburgh
Chief
Pediatric Cardiology
Children's Hospital of Pittsburgh
Pittsburgh, Pennsylvania
Chapter 8

RICHARD E. KERBER, MD
Professor of Medicine
Department of Internal Medicine
University of Iowa
Staff Physician
Department of Internal Medicine
University of Iowa Hospitals and Clinics
Iowa City, Iowa
Chapter 37

MORTON J. KERN, MD
Professor
St. Louis University
Director
Catheterization Lab
St. Louis University Hospital
St. Louis, Missouri
Chapter 17

MICHAEL C. KIM, MD
Assistant Professor of Medicine
Mount Sinai School of Medicine
New York, New York
Chapter 48

SPENCER B. KING III, MD
Fuqua Chair of Interventional Cardiology
The Fuqua Heart Center at Piedmont Hospital
Co-Director, American Cardiovascular
Research Institute, Clinical Professor
of Medicine
Emory University School of Medicine
Atlanta, Georgia
Chapters 17 and 55

ANNAPOORNA S. KINI, MD
Assistant Professor of Medicine
Mount Sinai School of Medicine
New York, New York
Chapter 48

TIMOTHY KNILANS, MD

Associate Professor of Clinical Pediatrics
Department of Pediatrics
University of Cincinnati
Cincinnati Children's Hospital Medical
Center
Division of Cardiology
Director
Clinical Cardiac Electrophysiology and
Pacing
Cincinnati, Ohio
Chapter 39

MITCHELL W. KRUCOFF, MD,
FACC, FCCP

Associate Professor of Medicine
Cardiology
Duke University Medical Center
Durham, North Carolina
Chapter 108

HARLAN KRUMHOLZ, MD, MSc

Professor of Medicine
Cardiology
Epidemiology and Public Health
Department of Internal Medicine
Yale University of Medicine
New Haven, Connecticut
Chapter 104

NILS KUCHER, MD

Venous Thromboembolism Research Group
Cardiovascular Division
Brigham and Women's Hospital
Harvard Medical School
Boston, Massachusetts
Chapter 63

EDWARD G. LAKATTA, MD

Professor of Medicine
Johns Hopkins School of Medicine
Johns Hopkins University
Adjunct Professor of Physiology
University of Maryland
School of Medicine
Baltimore, Maryland
Chapter 96

GAETANO ANTONIO LANZA,
MD, FESC

Institute of Cardiology
Universita Cattolica del Sacro Cuore
Roma, Italy
Chapter 46

E. CLINTON LAWRENCE, MD

Augustus J. McKelvey Professor of Medicine
Director
Andrew J. McKelvey Lung Transplantation
Center
Medical Director of Lung Transplantation
Emory University School of Medicine
Emory University Hospital
Atlanta, Georgia
Chapter 64

MEGAN C. LEARY, MD

Instructor in Neurology
Harvard Medical School
Beth Israel Deaconess Medical Center
Boston, Massachusetts
Chapter 99

THIERRY H. LEJEMTEL, MD

Professor of Medicine
Department of Medicine
Albert Einstein College of Medicine
Montefiore Medical Center
Bronx, New York
Chapter 25

MARTIN M. LEWINTER, MD

Professor of Medicine and Molecular
Physiology and Biophysics
University of Vermont College of Medicine
Director
Heart Failure Program
Fletcher Allen Health Care
Burlington, Vermont
Chapter 4

RICHARD P. LEWIS, MD

Professor Emeritus, Attending Physician
Cardiovascular Medicine
Ohio State University Hospitals
Columbus, Ohio
Chapter 40

RICHARD LIEBOWITZ, MD

Assistant Professor of Clinical Medicine
Duke University
Executive Medical Director
Center for Living
Duke University
Durham, North Carolina
Chapter 108

RICHARD P. LIFTON, MD

Chairman
Department of Genetics
Professor of Genetics
Internal Medicine and Molecular Biophysics
and Biochemistry
Yale University School of Medicine
Associate Investigator
Howard Hughes Medical Institute
Yale University
New Haven, Connecticut
Chapter 9

BRUCE WHITNEY LYTLE, MD

Department of Thoracic and Cardiovascular
Surgery
The Cleveland Clinic Foundation
Cleveland, Ohio
Chapter 58

JOHN J. MAHMARIAN, MD

Professor of Medicine
Section of Cardiology
Department of Medicine
Baylor College of Medicine
Medical Director
Nuclear Cardiology Laboratory
Methodist DeBakey Heart Center
The Methodist Hospital
Houston, Texas
Chapter 20

JOSEPH F. MALOUF, MD

Consultant
Division of Cardiovascular Disease
Mayo Clinic
Rochester, Minnesota
Chapter 3

DONNA MANCINI, MD

Associate Professor
Columbia University
New York, New York
Chapter 79

ALI J. MARIAN, MD

Associate Professor
Baylor College of Medicine
Cardiologist
Baylor Heart Clinic
The Methodist Hospital
Houston, Texas
Chapter 72

DANIEL MARK, MD, MPH
Director
Outcomes Research
Duke Clinical Research Institute
Professor of Medicine
Department of Medicine
Duke University Medical Center
Durham, North Carolina
Chapter 108

ROGER R. MARKWALD, PhD
Professor and Chairman
Department of Cell Biology and Anatomy
Medical University of South Carolina
Charleston, South Carolina
Chapter 8

DAVID J. MARON, MD
Associate Professor of Medicine
Division of Cardiovascular Medicine
Vanderbilt University Medical Center
Nashville, Tennessee
Chapter 43

ATTILIO MASERI, MD, FACC, FESC
Professor of Cardiology
Director Cardio-Thoracic and Vascular Department
San Raffaele University Hospital
Milan, Italy
Chapter 46

JAY W. MASON, MD
Adjunct Professor of Medicine
University of Utah
Salt Lake City, Utah
Professor of Medicine
University of Kentucky
Lexington, Kentucky
Medical Director
Covenance Central Diagnostics
Reno, Nevada
Chapter 75

TAHSIN MASUD, MD
Assistant Professor of Medicine
Renal Division
Emory University School of Medicine
Atlanta, Georgia
Chapter 94

HUGH A. MCALLISTER JR., MD
Clinical Professor
Department of Pathology
Baylor College of Medicine
Clinical Professor
Department of Pathology
University of Texas Medical School
Houston, Texas
Chapter 85

JOHN H. MCANULTY, MD
Professor of Medicine
Oregon Health and Science University
Portland, Oregon
Chapters 71 and 92

WILLIAM M. MCDONALD, MD
J.B. Fuqua Chair of Late-Life Depression
Associate Professor of Psychiatry and Behavioral Sciences
Emory University School of Medicine
Wesley Woods Geriatric Hospital
Atlanta, Georgia
Chapter 91

DONOGH F. MCKEOGH, MD
Assistant Professor
Division of Cardiology
Department of Medicine
Oregon Health and Science University
Portland, Oregon
Chapter 71

LUISA MESTRONI, MD
Associate Professor of Medicine
Department of Cardiology
Director, Molecular Genetics Program
University of Colorado Cardiovascular Institute
University of Colorado
Denver, Colorado
Chapter 76

JAMES METCALFE, MD
Professor Emeritus of Medicine
Oregon Health Sciences University
School of Medicine
Portland, Oregon
Chapter 92

DARRYL MILLER, MD
Cardiology Fellow
Case Western Reserve University
University Hospitals of Cleveland
Cleveland, Ohio
Chapter 78

WILLIAM E. MITCH, MD
Edward Randall Distinguished Chair in Internal Medicine
Chair of Medicine
Department of Medicine
University of Texas at Galveston
Galveston, Texas
Chapter 94

ALEXANDER MITTNACHT, MD
Instructor
Anesthesiology
Clinical Assistant Attending
Department of Anesthesiology
Mount Sinai School of Medicine
New York, New York
Chapter 83

SUSAN D. MOFFATT, MD
Department of Cardiothoracic Surgery
Stanford University School of Medicine
Stanford, California
Chapter 26

DOUGLAS C. MORRIS, MD
J. Willis Hurst Professor of Medicine
Emory University School of Medicine
Vice Chairman of Medicine for Clinical Affairs
Emory Clinic
Atlanta, Georgia
Chapter 59

JOSEPH B. MUHLESTEIN, MD
Department of Cardiology
LDS Hospital
Salt Lake City, Utah
Chapter 81

DEBABRATA MUKHERJEE, MD
Assistant Professor
Division of Cardiology
University of Michigan
Ann Arbor, Michigan
Chapter 82

DOMINIQUE L. MUSSELMAN, MD, MS

Associate Professor
Department of Psychiatry and Behavioral Sciences
Emory University School of Medicine
Atlanta, Georgia
Chapter 91

ROBERT J. MYERBURG, MD

Lemberg Professor of Medicine and Physiology
Director
Division of Cardiology
Department of Medicine
American Heart Association Chair in Cardiovascular Research
University of Miami School of Medicine
Miami, Florida
Chapter 13

ELIZABETH G. NABEL, MD

Scientific Director
Clinical Research
National Heart, Lung, and Blood Institute
National Institute of Health
Bethesda, Maryland
Chapter 11

YOSHIFUMI NAKA, MD

Mechanical Circulatory Support Program
New York–Presbyterian Hospital
Chapter 50

IRA S. NASH, MD

Associate Professor of Medicine
Mount Sinai School of Medicine
Associate Director
The Zena and Michael A. Wiener Cardiovascular Institute and The Marie-Josée and Henry R. Kravis Center for Cardiovascular Health
Mount Sinai Medical Center
New York, New York
Chapter 106

STEVEN D. NELSON, MD

Associate Professor of Medicine
The Ohio State University
Director
Clinical Cardiac Electrophysiology
Division of Cardiology
Department of Internal Medicine
Columbus, Ohio
Chapter 40

CHARLES B. NEMEROFF, MD, PhD

Reunette W. Harris Professor and Chairman
Department of Psychiatry and Behavioral Sciences
Emory University School of Medicine
Atlanta, Georgia
Chapter 91

KONSTANTIN NIKOLAOU, MD

Department of Clinical Radiology
University of Munich
Grosshadern, Germany
Chapter 22

RICK A. NISHIMURA, MD

Judd and Mary Morris Leighton Professor of Medicine
Mayo Clinic College of Medicine
Rochester, Minnesota
Chapter 77

STEVEN E. NISSEN, MD

Professor of Medicine
Cleveland Clinic Lerner College of Medicine
Medical Director
Cleveland Clinic CV Coordinating CTR
Cleveland, Ohio
Chapter 18

R. JOE NOBLE, MD, FACC

Clinical Professor of Medicine
Indiana University School of Medicine
The Heart Center of Indiana
St. Vincent's Hospital
Indianapolis, Indiana
Chapter 33

PETER A. O'CALLAGHAN, MD

Consultant Electrophysiologist
Clinical Teacher
University of Wales College of Medicine
Consultant Electrophysiologist
Department of Cardiology
University Hospital of Wales
Heath Park, Cardiff, United Kingdom
Chapter 38

PATRICK O'GARA, MD

Associate Professor of Medicine
Harvard Medical School
Director, Clinical Cardiology
Vice Chairman, Clinical Affairs
Department of Medicine
Brigham and Women's Hospital
Boston, Massachusetts
Chapter 57

KEITH R. OKEN, MD

Consultant
Cardiovascular Diseases
Mayo Clinic, Florida
Assistant Professor of Medicine
Mayo College of Medicine
Jacksonville, Florida
Chapter 95

JEFFREY W. OLIN, DO

Professor of Medicine
Mount Sinai Medical School of Medicine
Director, Vascular Medicine, The Zena and Michael A. Wiener Cardiovascular Institute and The Marie-Josée and Henry R. Kravis Center for Cardiovascular Health
Mount Sinai Medical Center
New York, New York
Chapter 98

STEVEN R. OMMEN, MD

Assistant Professor of Medicine
Mayo Clinic College of Medicine
Consultant
Division of Cardiovascular Disease and Internal Medicine
Department of Internal Medicine
Rochester, Minnesota
Chapter 77

WILLIAM W. O'NEILL, MD, FACC

Corporate Chairman of Cardiology
William Beaumont Hospital System
Royal Oak and Troy, Michigan
Chapter 56

LIONEL OPIE, MD, DPhil, FRCP
Director
Hatter Institute
Cape Heart Centre and Department of
Medicine
University of Cape Town
Senior Consultant
Hypertension Clinic
Groote Schuur Hospital
Cape Town, South Africa
Chapter 90

ROBERT A. O'ROURKE, MD
Charles Conrad Brown Distinguished
Professor in Cardiovascular Disease
University of Texas Health Sciences Center
San Antonio, Texas
Chapters 12, 14, 51, 57, 68, 69, 84, 85

GEORGE OSOL, PhD
Professor and Director of Research
Department of OB/GYN
University of Vermont College of Medicine
Burlington, Vermont
Chapter 4

RICHARD L. PAGE, MD
Robert A. Bruce Professor
Head
Division of Cardiology
Department of Medicine
University of Washington School of Medicine
Seattle, Washington
Chapter 31

EUGEN C. PALMA, MD
Assistant Professor of Medicine
Arrhythmia Service
Albert Einstein College of Medicine
Montefiore Medical Center
Bronx, New York
Chapter 36

THOMAS A. PEARSON, MD,
MPH, PhD, FACC
Albert D. Kaiser Professor and Chair
Community and Preventative Medicine
Professor of Medicine
University of Rochester School of Medicine
and Dentistry
Attending Physician
Department of Medicine
Director
Preventative Cardiology Clinic
Co-Director
Stony Heart Program
University of Rochester Medical Center
Rochester, New York
Chapter 43

THOMAS G. PICKERING, MD,
DPhil
Director
Behavioral Cardiovascular Health and
Hypertension Program
Columbia Presbyterian Hospital
New York, New York
Chapter 107

SEAN P. PINNEY, MD
Instructor of Medicine
Department of Internal Medicine
Columbia University–College of Physicians
and Surgeons
Attending Physician
Department of Medicine
Division of Circulatory Physiology
New York Presbyterian Hospital
New York, New York
Chapter 79

DAVID J. PINSKY, MD, FACC
Division Chief
Cardiovascular Medicine
Professor
Cardiovascular Medicine
Scientific Director
Cardiovascular Center
Internal Medicine
Cardiology
University of Michigan
Ann Arbor, Michigan
Chapter 50

DUANE S. PINTO, MD
Instructor of Medicine
Harvard Medical School
Program Director
Fellowship Training Program
Cardiovascular Division
Beth Israel Deaconess Medical Center
Boston, Massachusetts
Chapter 41

VANCE J. PLUMB, MD
Professor of Medicine
Division of Cardiovascular Disease
Department of Medicine
University of Alabama at Birmingham
School of Medicine
Birmingham, Alabama
Chapter 29

MICHAEL POON, MD
Associate Professor of Medicine
(Cardiology)
Mount Sinai School of Medicine
Director of Clinical Cardiac MR/CT
Imaging Program and Pulmonary
Hypertension Program
Director of Cardiology
Cabrini Medical Center
New York, New York
Chapter 22

CRAIG M. PRATT, MD
Professor of Medicine
Baylor College of Medicine
Director of Research
DeBakey Heart Center
Director, Coronary Care Unit
The Methodist Hospital
Houston, Texas
Chapter 52

JOHN O. PRIOR, MD
David Geffen School of Medicine at UCLA
Visiting Associate Professor
Department of Molecular and Medical
Pharmacology
University of California at Los Angeles
Los Angeles, California
Chapter 23

ERIC N. PRYSTOWSKY, MD
Director
Clinical Electrophysiology Laboratory
St. Vincent Hospital
Indianapolis, Indiana
Consulting Professor of Medicine
Duke University Medical Center
Durham, North Carolina
Chapters 28 and 33

SHAHBUDIN H. RAHIMTOOLA,
MB, FRCP, MACP, MACC,
DSc(Hon),
Distinguished Professor
University of Southern California
G. C. Griffith Professor of Cardiology
Professor of Medicine
Keck School of Medicine
LAC and USC Medical Center
Los Angeles, California
Chapters 66, 67, 70, 71

ELLIOT J. RAYFIELD, MD
Clinical Professor of Medicine
Attending Physician
Mount Sinai School of Medicine
New York, New York
Chapter 86

DAVID L. REICH, MD
Professor of Anesthesiology
Mount Sinai School of Medicine
Vice-Chair for Academic Affairs
Department of Anesthesia
Mount Sinai Medical Center
New York, New York
Chapter 83

ROBERT W. RHO, MD
Assistant Professor of Medicine
University of Washington
School of Medicine
Seattle, Washington
Chapter 31

PAUL M. RIDKER, MD
Eugene Braunwald Professor of Medicine
Harvard Medical School
Director
Center for Cardiovascular Disease
Prevention
Division of Preventive Medicine
Brigham and Women's Hospital
Boston, Massachusetts
Chapter 43

ROBERT C. ROBBINS, MD
Associate Professor
Department of Cardiac Surgery
Stanford University
Stanford, California
Chapter 26

ROBERT ROBERTS, MD
Professor of Medicine
President and CEO
University of Ottawa Heart Institute
Ottawa, Ontario, Canada
Chapters 5, 9, 52, 72

WILLIAM C. ROBERTS, MD
Director
Baylor Heart and Vascular Institute
Baylor University Medical Center
Dallas, Texas
Chapter 84

JOSE F. ROLDAN, MD
Resident
Department of Rheumatology
University of Texas Health
Science Center
San Antonio, Texas
Chapter 84

THOM W. ROOKE, MD
Professor of Medicine
Department of Internal Medicine
Division of Cardiovascular Diseases
Mayo Graduate School of Medical
Education
Rochester, Minnesota
Chapter 101

LEWIS J. RUBIN, MD
Professor of Medicine
Pulmonary and Critical Care Medicine
University of California at San Diego
School of Medicine
La Jolla, California
Chapter 62

BRUCE RUDISCH, MD
Resident in Psychiatry
Department of Psychiatry and Behavioral
Sciences
Emory University School of Medicine
Atlanta, Georgia
Chapter 91

JEREMY N. RUSKIN, MD
Director
Cardiac Arrhythmia Service
Massachusetts General Hospital
Associate Professor of Medicine
Harvard Medical School
Boston, Massachusetts
Chapter 38

THOMAS J. RYAN, MD
Professor of Medicine
Boston University School of Medicine
Senior Consultant in Cardiology and Chief
of Cardiology Emeritus
Boston University Medical Center
Boston, Massachusetts
Chapter 52

MERLE A. SANDE, MD
Professor of Medicine
Department of Medicine
University of Utah School of Medicine
Salt Lake City, Utah
Chapter 81

STEPHEN F. SCHAAL, MD
Professor of Medicine
Ohio State University
College of Medicine and Public Health
Columbus, Ohio
Chapter 40

MELVIN M. SCHEINMAN, MD
Professor of Medicine
Shorenstein Chair in Cardiology
University of California at San Francisco
San Francisco, California
Chapter 36

HEINRICH R. SCHELBERT, MD,
PhD
Geroge V. Taplin Professor
Division of Nuclear Medicine
Department of Molecular and Medical
Pharmacology
UCLA School of Medicine
Los Angeles, California
Chapter 23

JOHN S. SCHROEDER, MD

Professor of Medicine
Department of Cardiology
Stanford University School of Medicine
Stanford Medical Center
Stanford, California
Chapter 26

STEVEN P. SCHULMAN, MD

Associate Professor of Medicine
Director of Coronary Care Unit
Johns Hopkins University School of
Medicine
Baltimore, Maryland
Chapter 96

JAMES B. SEWARD, MD

Professor of Medicine and Pediatrics
Director
Echo Lab
Consultant
CV Diseases
Mayo Clinic
Rochester, Minnesota
Chapter 3

PREDIMAN K. SHAH, MD

Shapell and Webb Chair and Director
Division of Cardiology and Atherosclerosis
Research Center
Cedars Sinai Medical Center
Professor of Medicine
David Geffen School of Medicine at UCLA
Los Angeles, California
Chapter 44

JAMES A. SHAVER, MD

Professor of Medicine
Cardiovascular Institute
University of Pittsburgh
Director of Cardiovascular Fellowship
Program
University of Pittsburgh Medical Center
Presbyterian University Hospital
Pittsburgh, Pennsylvania
Chapter 12

LESLEE J. SHAW, PhD

Associate Professor
Department of Medicine
Duke University
Durham, North Carolina
Director
Outcomes Research
Atlanta Cardiovascular Research Institute
Atlanta, Georgia
Chapter 19

DOMENIC A. SICA, MD

Professor of Medicine and Pharmacology
Chairman
Section of Clinical Pharmacology and
Hypertension
Division of Nephrology
Medical College of Virginia
Virginia Commonwealth University
Richmond, Virginia
Chapter 90

MARK E. SILVERMAN, MD, MACP, FRCP, FACC

Professor of Medicine
Cardiology
Emory University School of Medicine
Chief of Cardiology
The Fuqua Heart Center
Piedmont Hospital
Atlanta, Georgia
Chapters 1 and 12

ANDREW L. SMITH, MD

Associate Professor of Medicine
Emory University School of Medicine
Medical Director
Heart Failure and Transplantation
Division of Cardiology
Emory Hospital
Atlanta, Georgia
Chapter 89

ROBERT B. SMITH III, MD

John E. Skandalakis Professor of Surgery
Emeritus
Emory University School of Medicine
Medical Director
Emory University Hospital
Associate Chairman
Department of Surgery
Emory University School of Medicine
Atlanta, Georgia
Chapter 102

EDMUND H. SONNENBLICK, MD, FACC

Edward J. Safra Professor of Medicine
Albert Einstein College of Medicine
Weiler Hospital/Montefiore Medical Center
Bronx, New York
Chapters 24 and 25

ALBERT STARR, MD

Professor of Surgery
Oregon Health Sciences University
Director
Heart and Vascular Institute
Providence St. Vincent's Hospital
Portland, Oregon
Chapter 70

LISA M. SULLIVAN, MD

Associate Professor of Biostatistics,
Mathematics and Statistics
Assistant Dean for Undergraduate Education
in Public Health
Boston University
Boston, Massachusetts
Chapter 2

H. ROBERT SUPERKO, MD, FACC, FAHA, FACSM

Director
Cholesterol, Genetics and Heart Disease
Institute
Portola Valley, California
Director
Advanced Cardiovascular Disease
Prevention
Fuqua Heart Center/Piedmont Hospital
Atlanta, Georgia
Director of Research
Berkeley HeartLab, Inc.
Burlingame, California
Chapter 87

PANAGIOTIS N. SYMBAS, MD

Professor of Cardiothoracic Surgery
Emory University School of Medicine
Emory Affiliated Hospitals
Atlanta, Georgia
Chapter 93

A. JAMIL TAJIK, MD

Thomas J. Watson, Jr., Professor
Professor of Medicine and Pediatrics
Mayo Clinic
Consultant
Division of Cardiovascular Diseases
Mayo Clinic
Rochester, New York
Chapters 3 and 77

W. H. WILSON TANG, MD

Assistant Professor of Cardiovascular
Medicine
Cleveland Clinic Lerner College at Medicine
at Case Western Reserve University
Staff Physician
Kaufman Center for Heart Failure
Department of Cardiovascular Medicine
Cleveland Clinic Foundation
Cleveland, Ohio
Chapter 24

VICTOR F. TAPSON, MD

Associate Professor of Medicine
Pulmonary and Critical Care Medicine
Duke University Medical Center
Durham, North Carolina
Chapter 63

THOMAS T. TERRAMANI, MD

Vascular Surgery and Endovascular Therapy
San Diego, California
Chapter 102

GORDON F. TOMASELLI, MD

Professor of Medicine
Johns Hopkins School of Medicine
Johns Hopkins University
Baltimore, Maryland
Chapter 10

KENT UELAND, MD

Professor Emeritus
Department of OB/GYN
Stanford University School of Medicine
Stanford, California
Chapter 92

RAMACHANDRAN S. VASAN, MD

Clinical Associate Professor
Department of Medicine
Boston University School of Medicine
Boston, Massachusetts
Assistant Director
Echocardiography Laboratory
Framingham Heart Study
Framingham, Massachusetts
Chapter 2

PUGAZHENDHI VIJAYARAMAN, MD

Assistant Professor of Medicine
Medical College of Virginia
Virginia Commonwealth University
Co-Director
Cardiac Electrophysiology Section
McGuire Veterans Affairs Medical Center
Richmond, Virginia
Chapter 32

RENU VIRMANI, MD

Chairman
Department of Cardiovascular Pathology
Armed Forces Institute of Pathology
Washington, District of Columbia
Chapter 49

JOHN H. K. VOGEL, MD

Chairman
Cardiology
Santa Barbara Cottage Hospital
Santa Barbara, California
Chapter 108

DAVID A. VORCHHEIMER, MD

Assistant Professor of Medicine
Mount Sinai School of Medicine
Director
Coronary Care Unit
The Zena and Michael A. Wiener
Cardiovascular Institute
Mount Sinai Medical Center
New York, New York
Chapter 54

ALBERT WALDO, MD

Walter H. Pritchard Professor of Cardiology
Professor of Medicine
Professor of Biomedical Engineering
Case Western Reserve University
Cleveland, Ohio
Chapter 27

BRUCE F. WALLER, MD

Clinical Professor of Medicine and Pathology
Indiana University School of Medicine
Director
Cardiovascular Pathology Registry
St. Vincent's Hospital
Cardiologist
The Care Group
Medical Director
The Care Group Laboratory
Indianapolis, Indiana
Chapter 47

RICHARD A. WALSH, MD

John H. Hord Professor and Chairman
Department of Medicine
Case Western Reserve University
Physician-in-Chief
University Hospitals of Cleveland
Department of Medicine
Case Western University/University
Hospitals of Cleveland
Cleveland, Ohio
Chapter 6

CAROLE A. WARNES, MD, MRCP, FACC

Professor of Medicine
Mayo Medical School
Consultant in CV Diseases
Internal Medicine and Pediatric Cardiology
Mayo Clinic
Rochester, Minnesota
Chapter 74

WILLIAM S. WEINTRAUB, MD

Professor of Medicine
Cardiology
Emory University School of Medicine
Director
Cardiovascular Epidemiology
Emory Healthcare
Atlanta, Georgia
Chapter 104

MYRON L. WEISFELDT, MD

Chair of Medicine
Johns Hopkins University School of
Medicine
Johns Hopkins Hospital
Baltimore, Maryland
Chapter 42

HEIN J. J. WELLENS, MD

Professor of Cardiology
University of Maastricht
Chairman
Department of Cardiology
University Hospital Maastricht
Maastricht, The Netherlands
Chapter 53

NANETTE K. WENGER, MD

Professor of Medicine
Cardiology
Emory University School of Medicine
Chief of Cardiology
Grady Memorial Hospital
Atlanta, Georgia
Chapter 60

PAUL W. WENNBERG, MD

Associate Professor of Medicine
Department of Internal Medicine
Division of Cardiovascular Diseases
Mayo Graduate School of Medical
Education
Rochester, Minnesota
Chapter 101

ANDY WESSELS, PhD

Associate Professor
Department of Cell Biology and Anatomy
Medical University of South Carolina
Charleston, South Carolina
Chapter 8

ANDREW L. WIT, PhD

Professor of Pharmacology
College of Physicians and Surgeons of
Columbia University
New York, New York
Chapter 27

CHARLES F. WOOLEY, MD

Department of Cardiovascular Medicine
Ohio State University Medical Center
Columbus, Ohio
Chapter 1

RAYMOND L. WOOSLEY, MD, PhD

Vice President for Health Sciences
University of Arizona
College of Medicine
Tucson, Arizona
Chapter 35

JAY S. YADAV, MD

Director
Vascular Intervention
Department of Cardiovascular Medicine
Cleveland Clinic Foundation
Department of Cardiology
Cleveland, Ohio
Chapter 100

FOREWORD

The very personal story you are about to read is offered here at the request of the editors of the eleventh edition of *Hurst's The Heart*. They wanted a historical account of the conception, birth, and development of the book, *Hurst's The Heart*. I am honored to tell the story that, to a major degree, consumed many of my waking hours during several decades of my life.

There were two factors involved in the original creation of the book: the *mind-set* that was clearly present and the *trigger* that initiated the action.

The *mind-set* gradually evolved in the late forties and fifties. I completed my cardiology fellowship with Dr. Paul Dudley White at the Massachusetts General Hospital in Boston in 1949. His scholarly work inspired me to take care of people with heart disease, engage in clinical research, teach, and write. His book, *Heart Disease,* was my constant companion. I was pleased beyond description when he asked me to contribute a few pages on spatial vector electrocardiography to the fourth edition of his masterpiece.

I joined Dr. Bruce Logue in Dr. Paul Beeson's department of medicine at Emory University in Atlanta, Georgia, in 1950. Bruce was a walking encyclopedia, a remarkable clinician, a rapid decision maker, and the leading cardiologist in Atlanta. We worked side by side and wrote several articles together. I was beginning to appreciate that writing improved my teaching and that both improved my knowledge base, which in turn improved my diagnostic and therapeutic skills. My work with Dr. Robert Grant, who was also at Emory, in electrocardiography led me to write my first book, *Atlas of Spatial Vector Electocardiography*. I began work on the book when I was 29 years old; it was published by Blakiston, a division of the McGraw-Hill Company, 3 years later in 1952. This event showed me that I could put a book together. Bruce Logue had worked with Meakins at McGill and was asked to write the section on the heart in the new edition of *Meakins' Textbook of Medicine;* Bruce passed this task and opportunity along to me. I organized the section and wrote much of it but asked several people to write various chapters in the section. These events led me to conclude that the time was right for a multiauthored book on the heart, arteries, and veins. However, I was in my early thirties and realized not only that there were several good books on these subjects already available but also that I was perhaps a bit young to dream such a dream. I realized too that I did not have the resources required for such an endeavor. Meanwhile, I was asked to become chairman of the department of medicine at Emory in late 1956 and began work there in January 1957. This gave me more resources. By then, I was a few years older and had edited and written part of a small multiauthored book on cardiac resuscitation.

The *trigger* that stimulated me to act came in 1962. I invited the internationally famous Dr. Paul Wood to visit my department at Emory in 1962. His book *Diseases of the Heart and Circulation* had become a classic, along with White's *Heart Disease* and Friedberg's *Diseases of the Heart*. Wood's reputation preceded him. He was known to be uninhibited in making vitriolic remarks to others regarding their competence. He was said to be pedantic and intolerant of anything short of perfection. Despite this, he was considered a genius who rarely made a diagnostic error. I showed him patients with the most difficult problems and waited for his caustic attacks. The hospital auditorium was filled to capacity with house officers, clinical faculty, and practicing physicians. Like the expert swordsman who always hits the right spot, he never missed. Surprisingly, there were no caustic remarks. However, he seemed to be somewhat aloof and obviously frustrated. I asked him, in my own way, to state his problem, hoping that I might make his visit more pleasant. He answered, "I realize that I can't complete the next edition of my book *Diseases of the Heart and Circulation*. By the time I write the last chapter, the first chapter will be out of date." That was the *trigger*. I reasoned then and there that if Paul Wood could not write a single-authored book on the heart, no one could. As I walked and talked with him, he did not complain of chest discomfort. He died in London of a myocardial infarction about 2 weeks after visiting us.

Paul White had already decided not to write a fifth edition of his book, *Heart Disease*. Dr. Charles Friedberg's excellent book was the only remaining established complete treatise on the heart then available. I sensed that he too would have trouble continuing to write a single-authored book. This was obviously true, because cardiovascular research was beginning to bring many new insights to every area of cardiology and no single person could hope to master them all.

The book that was later titled *Hurst's The Heart* was conceived during Paul Wood's visit to Emory. I asked Dr. Logue to join me as co-editor and asked my colleagues Dr. Robert Schlant and Dr. Nanette Wenger to be assistant editors. I also asked Ruth Strange, who was my secretary for many years, to help us keep order. Ruth was unusually gifted and could have served as the chief operating officer of a modern company.

The editorial managers of the Blakiston Division of McGraw-Hill, which published my book on vector electrocardiography in 1952, expressed their interest in the creation of a complete treatise on the heart. This was the beginning of my long and pleasant relationship with the McGraw-Hill Company.

The goals for the book were established as follows: It would be a complete treatise on the heart, arteries, and veins. The Emory staff would write a large part of the book, but authors from elsewhere would be asked to contribute chapters as well. These latter authors would be chosen because they had taught their subjects through their writing and were considered to be experts in their fields. Most importantly, we chose authors with whom we agreed. We were delighted when no one turned down the invitation to write for the new book.

I have always believed that there are two types of reading. The *quick read* is used by physicians who wish to look up information that is needed immediately. Reading about the criteria required to diagnose hypertrophic cardiomyopathy is an example of the *quick read*. The *long read* is used when physicians want to understand certain aspects of a disease process. This type of reading is done in a more leisurely fashion without a feeling of urgency. Reading about and understanding the evolution of an atherosclerotic plaque is an example of the *long read*.

The book I planned would serve clinicians whose professional purpose in life was to take care of patients with heart disease but who also wanted to understand the etiology, pathology, and altered physiology of the disease that produced the clinical problems they identified in their patients. This book, I felt, had to be a rich source for a *quick read* and an excellent source for a *long read*.

In order to create a book, it is necessary to visualize the finished product before the first words are written. This initial step is fortunately relatively easy for me. I created a grid listing the *parts* of the book as well as the *chapters,* showing the authors' names and the dates on which their chapters were due. The grid was placed on the door of my office. It covered the door from top to bottom. I studied it many times each day and could, at a glance, follow the flow of the work in progress.

Dr. Logue and I spent several hours every Thursday morning for more than a year reviewing every sentence of every manuscript before it was sent to the publisher. The authors reviewed every sentence of every page of galley proof and I reviewed every sentence of the page proof before signing off on the project.

The naming of the book was an interesting experience. The choice of names was limited and most names had already been used by the creators of other books. Two gentlemen from McGraw-Hill came to Atlanta from New York to discuss the matter with Dr. Logue and me. The night we named the book was like a scene from an old movie. Dr. Logue and I were seated in a small room of an Atlanta hotel while the two gentlemen from McGraw-Hill walked the floor. We each tossed out names and they would shake their heads. I suggested the name *The Heart*. They stood still—stretched out their hands—changed their facial expressions, and said, "That's it—that's it!" The words *Arteries and Veins* were to be added in smaller print in order to emphasize the book's comprehensive nature.

The authors delivered their manuscripts to us on time and the first edition of *Hurst's The Heart* appeared in 1966.

Having lived with the book night and day for 4 years, we waited for the reactions of readers and book reviewers. We were more than pleased with their responses. The prompt worldwide acceptance of *The Heart* led to its translation into other languages. Eventually, it appeared in French, Spanish, Portuguese, Japanese, Chinese, and Greek editions.

Dr. Charles Friedberg congratulated me and stated how much he liked the book. He was a great man. As stated earlier, Dr. White had decided not to write the fifth edition of his book, but he was well pleased with the first edition of *Hurst's The Heart*. Dr. Paul Wood had died and Dr. Friedberg unfortunately died a few years later as the result of an automobile accident. In my mind's eye, I do remember that other books became available about the time *The Heart* was published. Luisada created a huge three-volume, multiauthored treatise

on the heart and circulation, but, perhaps because of its great size, there was only one edition. Another new, multiauthored, comprehensive treatise on the heart was published before or after *The Heart* appeared, but it too did not reappear after the first edition. Accordingly, *Hurst's The Heart* stood alone for many years and I am happy to say gained a strong foothold throughout most of the world. Now, of course, the book *Hurst's The Heart* has many playmates, because most large publishing houses believe that they must have a heart book.

The second edition of *Hurst's The Heart* was published 4 years after the first. It was somewhat obese, but it too was well received. One reader said it was a bit heavy and that he had his first episode of angina while carrying it! I learned from the second edition the problem we would face in future editions—that is, to control the book's size. The problem was the antithesis of Paul Wood's problem. He realized that a single author could not master the details of the progress being generated in the world's many research laboratories. On the other hand, the multiple authors of *Hurst's The Heart* could, to some degree, do that. So, the authors of *Hurst's The Heart* needed to cover more pages, but chapters had to be shortened, references decreased in number, and many lovely sentences omitted.

Dr. Logue's workday became so crowded that he could not continue as coeditor after the third edition of *Hurst's The Heart,* and I became the sole editor-in-chief. Dr. Logue continued to provide valuable help as an associate editor through the sixth edition.

Ruth Strange died of leukemia in 1972. Thereafter, Carol Miller became responsible for keeping order, typing manuscripts, writing to authors, and so on. She too was a genius and a healthy perfectionist.

The book thrived through its childhood over the next few editions. After that, it entered and left the adolescent period and came to maturity in the sixth edition, which was published in 1986. It was at this time that I gave up the chairmanship of the department of medicine at Emory University. I had held that position for 30 years and was then 66 years old. I was asked to continue my teaching, patient care, clinical investigation, and writing. Although I enjoyed being chairman, I also relished the opportunity to relinquish the shackles of administrative work. I planned to complete the seventh edition of *Hurst's The Heart,* but I thought that after it was on the shelf, it would be wise to relinquish my role as editor-in-chief so that I could help the next editor-in-chief to make a smooth transition in his effort to create the eighth edition. I urged the selection of my friend and associate Dr. Robert Schlant to succeed me. I also asked that Dr. Wayne Alexander, who was at the time director of the division of cardiology at Emory, be added to the editorial staff.

McGraw-Hill officials honored me by naming the book *Hurst's The Heart* in deference to my role in the creation of the book and its nurturance to maturity.

As I close, may I offer a prediction? The future editors of *Hurst's The Heart,* and any other similar book, will find their task to be increasingly difficult for the following reason. When the first edition of *Hurst's The Heart* was created in the early sixties, there were only a few drugs and only a few procedures to consider. A consensus of opinion regarding their use was easy to achieve. With the plethora of new information generated by the explosion of research, there is now often legitimate disagreement as to what would be best for the patient. For example, there is a debate regarding the definition of proper diet and an argument about the value or harm that may result from the use of estrogens in postmenopausal women. Should the editors of a book insist on a single view, or should the physician reading the book be given various options from which to choose? I have no doubt that the smart editors now on the editorial board will address such problems and continue to create an excellent single-source book for all physicians who wish to learn more about the heart. But it will not be easy.

I am especially pleased to have the chance to thank once again all the individuals who helped me to create *Hurst's The Heart*. The dedicated workers of centuries ago set the stage for modern authors (see Chapter 1). They, in turn, passed the baton to the splendid authors who have contributed chapters to the present book and its earlier editions. I thank them all from every cardiac myocyte in my body.

Nelie, my wife, tolerated the transformation of our home into a library filled with manuscripts and books. She deserves much credit, because a stable, secure, and happy home is needed in order to remain focused on any creative act. So I say once again "No Nelie—no book."

Now, as I rush, with a smile of anticipation, to meet the students, house staff, and cardiology fellows at Emory University, please join me and the trainees as we search in the eleventh edition of *Hurst's The Heart* for answers to the questions we are certain to raise. Because of the competence of Fuster, Alexander, who is now chairman of the department of medicine at Emory University, O'Rourke, King, Roberts, Nash, Prystowsky, and numerous other splendid authors who spearheaded the creation of this edition of *Hurst's The Heart*—I can properly say, without timidity, "It is a great book."

J. Willis Hurst, MD, MACP
Emory University
Atlanta, Georgia

PREFACE

The first edition of *The Heart,* published in 1966, was the first multi-authored and comprehensive textbook on cardiovascular disease. The history of the book and its subsequent development are elucidated by its editor J. Willis Hurst in his Foreword to this 11th edition (pages xxv to xxvii). This 11th edition of *Hurst's The Heart,* with 108 chapters written by outstanding and highly recognized experts in each of the examined fields, has several unique features that distinguish it from previous editions.

1. Each chapter of the 11th edition will be updated on an ongoing basis on the website, including the incorporation of "late breaking" clinical trials. Thus, the 11th edition of *Hurst's The Heart* and its continually evolving website will keep you abreast of the latest developments in cardiovascular medicine.

2. Forty percent of the chapters have been modified extensively, particularly those concerned with electrophysiology and with the diagnosis and treatment of acute coronary syndromes.

   Ten new chapters have been added spanning the latest exciting developments concerning the human genome and the genetic basis of many diseases, "high" and "low" risk coronary and noncoronary atherothrombotic plaques, evolving imaging technology for the assessment of coronary and noncoronary atherosclerotic disease and plaque characterization, and the most recent advances in the pathophysiology and treatment of pulmonary hypertension and heart failure. The many major advances in interventional cardiology are discussed in detail.

3. Three revised chapters focus on the new therapeutic challenges and socioeconomic issues affecting medicine in general and cardiovascular medicine in particular: a discussion of alternative and complementary medicine in the treatment of cardiovascular disease, the importance of behavioral modification as the basis of risk factor modification, and the cost-effectiveness of various noninvasive and interventional diagnostic methods and forms of treatment.

4. The ACC/AHA Clinical Practice Guidelines are emphasized throughout the text as well as in a special chapter concerning the use of Clinical Practice Guidelines. Each table utilizing ACC/AHA recommendations is clearly identified.

5. The 11th edition of *Hurst's The Heart* includes hundreds of new references including many that were still in press at the time of publication. The book has been shortened by reducing the number of references and eliminating duplication. The quality of the text paper, the illustrations, and the print size have been made more "reader friendly."

The editors are grateful to the outstanding group of authors who participated in the 11th edition of *Hurst's The Heart* for their extraordinary and timely contributions. As in the previous 10th edition, from the moment that the group of authors accepted to participate in this 11th edition of *Hurst's The Heart* to the moment of the book appearing on the shelves has only taken 15 months. Again, this is an absolute record for a textbook of this size and complexity. Such an approach represents the highest tribute and acknowledgment to our authors.

We thank J. Willis Hurst, the editor of the first seven editions and the author of the Foreword of this 11th edition for his continuous and enthusiastic support.

Finally we wish to thank our families for their support and for the many sacrifices they made to make this volume possible. We especially thank our wives for their strength, love, and support: Maria Fuster, Jane W. Alexander, Suzann O' Rourke, Donna Roberts, Gail King, Beth Nash, and Bonnie Prystowsky.

THE EDITORS
Valentin Fuster, MD, PhD
R. Wayne Alexander, MD, PhD
Robert A. O' Rourke, MD
Robert Roberts, MD
Spencer B. King III, MD
Ira S. Nash, MD
Eric N. Prystowsky, MD

HURST'S
THE HEART

THROMBOGENESIS AND ANTITHROMBOTIC THERAPY

W. Lane Duvall / David A. Vorchheimer / Valentin Fuster

PLAQUE FORMATION AND THROMBOSIS

Coronary heart disease is the leading cause of death in the United States and the industrialized world. While the majority of morbidity and mortality comes from first myocardial infarctions (MIs), a substantial portion also stems from reinfarction. While there have been numerous advances in the treatment of acute coronary syndrome (ACS), which have significantly reduced morbidity and mortality in the acute setting, secondary prevention remains important in decreasing the overall morbidity and mortality of coronary heart disease.

Rupture or erosion of an atherosclerotic plaque with superimposed nonocclusive thrombus is by far the most common cause of acute coronary syndromes (see also Chaps. 44 and 45). However, the atherosclerotic process, which itself underlies all acute coronary syndromes, is a silent process that usually commences 20 to 30 years prior to a patient's presentation with a clinical syndrome.[1,2] Hypercholesterolemia, smoking, hypertension, diabetes, and other coronary risk factors damage the endothelium and initiate the atherosclerotic process. When the endothelium is dysfunctional, macrophages bind to endothelial adhesion molecules and can infiltrate the endothelial cell. Low-density-lipoprotein (LDL) molecules are able to penetrate the vessel wall, and the macrophages digest the LDL, becoming foam cells, which thereby create a lipid-filled atherosclerotic plaque. Oxidized LDL may also have a direct toxic effect on the endothelium and smooth muscle cells, contributing to instability of the atherosclerotic plaque. Such plaques, which are usually lesions with less than 50 percent stenosis, are more prone to rupture.[3,4]

Then, multiple factors contribute to plaque rupture, including endothelial dysfunction, plaque lipid content,[5] local inflammation causing breakdown of the thin shoulder of the plaque,[6] coronary vasoconstriction, local shear stress forces, platelet activation, and the status of the coagulation system (i.e., a potentially prothrombotic state),[7] all of which culminate in the formation of a platelet-rich thrombus on the disrupted plaque.[8,9]

It should be noted however, that more than 95 percent of all plaque ruptures are clinically silent.[10,11] Angiographic studies have shown that many high-grade lesions often appear in segments of the coronary artery that were previously normal.[12] The erratic and unpredictable growth of plaques is caused by plaque disruption or fissuring and intracoronary mural thrombosis. The mural thrombus then undergoes fibrous organization and contributes, often asymptomatically, to the progression of the disease.[1,2] Thus, this process of plaque disruption and local thrombosis is ongoing in patients with clinically "stable" coronary artery disease, a point that reemphasizes the importance of long-term antithrombotic therapy in patients with coronary artery disease.

Atherothrombosis

STAGES OF ATHEROSCLEROSIS

Atherosclerosis is a progressive disease process of the large arteries that involves the gradual accumulation of lipids, inflammatory cells, and fibrous elements in plaques in the vessel walls. The pathogenesis appears to be far more complex than a single causative element; it is, instead, a multifactorial process that involves environmental, dietary, genetic, hemodynamic, metabolic, inflammatory, infectious, and other factors in its development.

The process begins decades earlier than it is clinically evident as "fatty streak" lesions, first described in autopsy studies of young soldiers killed in Korea in the 1950s.[13] These early atherosclerotic lesions, consisting of subendothelial accumulations of cholesterol-laden macrophages, or "foam cells," first appear in the aorta in the first decade of life, in the coronaries in the second decade, and in the cerebral circulation in the third or fourth decade.[14] The more advanced lesions that evolve from these precursors are characterized by a necrotic, lipid-rich core covered by a fibrous cap and can become clinically significant if they grow large enough to obstruct blood flow or if plaque rupture or the formation of overlying thrombosis causes myocardial infarction (MI) or stroke.

The primary initiating event in the generation of an atherosclerotic lesion is the deposition and accumulation of lipoproteins in the intima of the vessel wall. Low-density lipoprotein (LDL) deposition is greater when circulating levels of LDL are higher and both the transport and retention of lipoprotein are increased at predisposed sites in the vasculature. LDL diffuses passively across the endothelium through endothelial cell junctions or is transported by small vesicular carriers.[15] Interactions between the lipoprotein and matrix proteoglycans determine if LDL is either trapped in the intimal matrix or passes through the internal elastic lamina to move into the media. The accumulation of LDL in the intima stimulates the adherence of monocytes to the endothelium and their subsequent transmigration into the intima, where they proliferate and differentiate into macrophages. These macrophages can subsequently become activated to take up the deposited lipoproteins. In normal subendothelial matrix, lipoproteins are degraded and metabolized by smooth muscle cells, scavenged, and "reverse transported" back to the liver by HDL or taken up by macrophages. In the pathologic process of atherogenesis, this normal homeostatic process is altered when the trapped LDL becomes "modified"—through oxidation, lipolysis, proteolysis, and aggregation—which promote inflammation and uptake by macrophages. Under these circumstances macrophages take up oxidized LDL via their scavenger receptors rapidly enough to become foam cells, which eventually die, contributing their contents to the necrotic lipid core of the plaque. Atherosclerosis can thus be conceptualized as a "response to injury," with oxidized LDL being the final common agent but with many factors leading to that point.

As the lipid core of an atherosclerotic plaque grows with the accumulation of lipoproteins and macrophages, smooth muscle cells migrate in from the media. These cells produce fibrous elements of extracellular matrix that both form the fibrous cap and cause the overall size of the lesion to increase. The plaque does not initially narrow the vessel lumen by ingrowth directly; instead, the entire vessel diameter enlarges, compensating for the plaque. The bulging outward of the vessel is caused by the plaque, with associated thinning of the media and outer vessel wall layers. Plaque growth is in this manner directed toward the adventitia until a point is reached when compensatory enlargement is no longer possible. Plaque expansion is then directed toward the intima, and the vessel lumen begins to be

compromised (Fig. 54-1). The majority of acute cardiovascular events are not caused by gradual luminal narrowing but, instead, by plaque complications that acutely occlude the vessel lumen. Events such as plaque rupture, ulceration, hemorrhage, and thrombosis will all acutely disrupt blood flow and result in an ischemic event.

The American Heart Association (AHA) has classified atherosclerotic plaques into six types of lesions of increasing severity (Fig. 54-2).[16–18] The classification scheme labels type I and II as early lesions, type III as intermediate, and types IV through VI as advanced. Early lesions differ from advanced in that advanced plaques cause fundamental deformity of the vessel wall and are prone to the complications causing clinically manifest disease. Type I or initial lesions are not necessarily visible to the naked eye and are composed of microscopic intimal accumulation of foam cells. Type II plaques show increased numbers of macrophages that form adjacent layers; smooth muscle cells containing lipids also appear. In a type III intermediate lesion there is an increase in extracellular lipids with a progression from droplets to pools among the smooth muscle cells. The atheroma or type IV lesion is the first to display a lipid core, usually without narrowing of the vessel lumen. Type V lesions differ from the previous because of prominent new fibrous tissue formation. Finally, type VI plaques are complicated lesions with hemorrhage, thrombus, or plaque rupture.

ENDOTHELIAL DYSFUNCTION

Until recently, the vascular endothelium was considered an inert lining of the blood vessel separating the vascular space from tissues. However, it is now known that the endothelium is actively involved in a wide variety of physiologic and pathologic processes that mediate inflammation within the vascular wall, plaque stability, thrombus formation, and vasomotor tone.[19] The early experiments by Furchgott and Zawadski demonstrated the essential role of the endothelium in regulating vasodilatation via endothelium-derived relaxing factor, which was later identified to be nitric oxide (NO).[20] The endothelium is a single-celled lining covering the internal surface of blood vessels, giving it a strategic location to sense changes in hemodynamic forces and blood-borne signals and respond to them by releasing vasoactive substances. The endothelium thereby plays a key role in maintaining vascular homeostasis by balancing endothelium-derived relaxing and contracting factors.

The term *endothelial dysfunction* has been used to refer to a number of pathologic conditions involving the vascular endothelium. It has been used to describe altered anticoagulant, antithrombotic, and anti-inflammatory properties of the endothelium, impaired modulation of vascular growth, and dysregulation of vascular remodeling.[21] Much of the current literature now uses this term to refer to an impairment of endothelium-dependent vasorelaxation caused by a loss of NO activity in the vessel wall, resulting in impairment in the regulation of vascular homeostasis. This impairment can lead to the development of atherosclerosis and to the aggravation of myocardial ischemia in the setting of preexisting coronary disease. Clinical studies have shown that traditional risk factors for atherosclerosis predispose to endothelial dysfunction[22] and that impaired endothelium-dependent vasodilatation in the coronary circulation predicts adverse cardiovascular events and long-term outcome.[23] This decline in the bioavailability of NO may be caused by a number of different mechanisms: decreased expression of the endothelial cell NO synthase (eNOS), a lack of substrate or cofactors for eNOS, alterations of cellular signaling such that eNOS is not appropriately activated, and accelerated NO degradation by reactive oxygen species (ROS).[21]

NO is the key endothelium-derived relaxing factor that plays a pivotal role in vascular tone and reactivity.[24] NO is generated in the

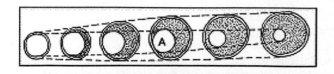

FIGURE 54-1 Compensatory enlargement of arteries. A = transsectional luminal area. (From Kadar and Glasz.[15] With permission.)

endothelial cell by eNOS which converts the amino acid L-arginine to NO and L-citrulline (Fig. 54-3). NO diffuses from the endothelial cell to the vascular smooth muscle and increases cyclic guanosine monophosphate, to cause relaxation of smooth muscle and dilation of the artery. Luminal diffusion of NO and its uptake into circulating platelets inhibits platelet adhesion and, to a lesser extent, suppresses platelet aggregation. NO can also influence gene transcription, leading to differential expression of cell surface adhesion molecules, which influence leukocyte activation, adhesion, and migration.

The endothelium also performs a myriad of functions.[25] It further controls vascular tone by secreting prostacyclin, another potent vasodilator, and also the potent vasoconstrictor peptide endothelin-1 (ET-1). It affects coagulation through the secretion of tissue-type plasminogen activator, and it regulates endothelial permeability to lipoproteins and other plasma constituents (Fig. 54-4).

The traditional risk factors for coronary artery disease (CAD)—including hyperlipidemia, smoking, diabetes, and hypertension—are also associated with coronary endothelial dysfunction.[26] In fact, the total number of coronary risk factors is related to the reduction in endothelium-dependent vasodilator function.[26] It is hypothesized that endothelial dysfunction may initiate the formation of atherosclerotic plaques,[27] which typically form at arterial bifurcations and other sites of disturbed blood flow. The endothelium is uniquely situated to sense these flow disturbances at the interface of the arterial wall and circulating blood. If it is dysfunctional, the endothelium potentiates flow disturbances due to improper vasoreactivity and even initiates the inflammatory response by secreting proinflammatory cytokines and chemokines. These, in turn, encourage leukocyte activation, promote the expression of leukocyte adhesion molecules, and facilitate entry of activated leukocytes and LDL into the subintimal space (Fig. 54-5).[27] Furthermore, endothelial dysfunction also permits smooth muscle proliferation to proceed unchecked in the media and subintima. These processes are accelerated by the presence of risk factors and are central to the more advanced stages of atherosclerosis, characterized by inflammation and a

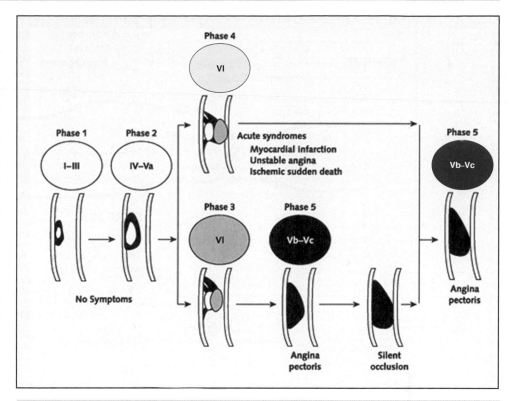

FIGURE 54-2 An early lesion (phase 1) can become an atheromatous or fibrolipid plaque (phase 2). Phase 2 can progress into an acute phase (phase 3 or 4). Formation of thrombosis or hematoma may cause angina pectoris (phase 3) or an acute coronary syndrome due to occlusive thrombus (phase 4). Phase 3 and 4 lesions can evolve into a fibrotic phase (phase 5) characterized by more stenotic plaques that may progress to occlusive lesions. Stenosis and myocardial ischemia can induce the growth of collateral vessels. Patients may have angina or silent vessel occlusion in phase 5. White indicates lipid accumulation, gray indicates thrombosis and hemorrhage, and black indicates fibrous tissue. Roman numerals indicate the lesion types: I-III = early lesions with isolated macrophage-foam cells (I), multiple foam-cell layers (II), or isolated extracellular lipids (III); IV-Va = advanced lesions—atheromatous or fibrolipid plaques with confluent extracellular lipid pools (atheroma) (IV), or fibromuscular tissue layers and atheroma (Va); VI = advanced lesions – complicated plaques with surface defects, hemorrhage, or thrombi deposition; Vb-Vc = advanced lesions with calcifications (Vb) or fibrous tissue (Vc). (From Rauch et al.[393] With permission.)

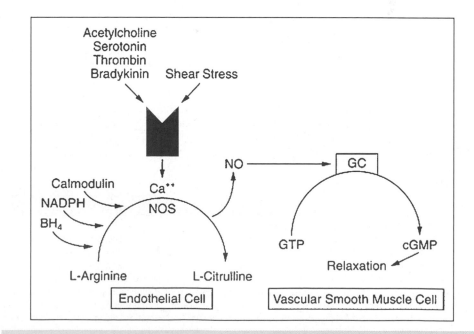

FIGURE 54-3 The nitric oxide pathway. BH_4 = tetrahydrobiopterin; Ca^{2+} = calcium ion; cGMP = cyclic guanosine monophosphate; GC = guanylate cyclase; GTP = guanosine triphosphate; NADPH = nicotinamide-adenine dinucleotide phosphate; NO = nitric oxide; NOS = nitric oxide synthase. (From Kinlay and Ganz.[19] With permission.)

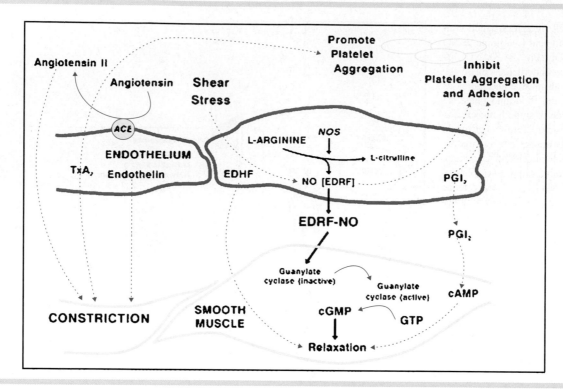

FIGURE 54-4 Endothelium-derived dilating and constricting factors. ACE = angiotensin converting enzyme; camp = cyclic adenosine monophosphate; cGMP cyclic guanosine monophosphate; EDHF = endothelium-derived hyper-polarizing factor; EDRF = endothelium-derived relaxing factor; GTP = guanosine triphosphate; NO = nitric oxide; NOS = nitric oxide synthase; PGI$_2$ = prostacyclin; TXA$_2$ = thromboxane A$_2$. (From Quyyumi.[394] With permission.)

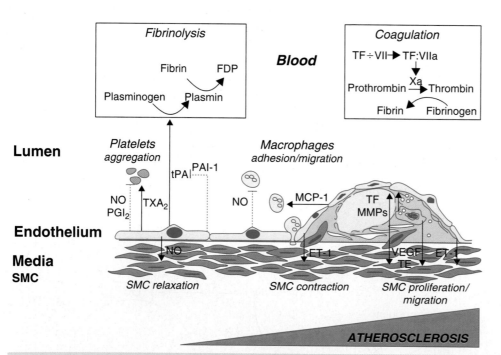

FIGURE 54-5 The endothelium affects vascular homeostasis by regulating vascular tone, thrombogenicity, platlet function, proliferation and migration of smooth muscle cells (SMC), and vasomotion. Normal functioning endothe-lium (*left*) produces several substances that maintain normal shear conditions by balancing the production of va-sodilators (nitric oxide, NO) and vasoconstrictors (endothelin 1, ET-1), avoiding excessive platelet aggregation (NO and prostacyclin I$_2$, PGI$_2$), and balancing the coagulation system by controlling fibrin production (tissue factor path-way inhibitor/tissue factor), and fibrinolysis (tissue plasminogen activator, t-PA/plasminogen activator inhibitor-1, PAI-1). Dysfunctional endothelium (*right*) favors macrophage adhesion and migration (monocyte chemotactic pro-tein 1, MCP-1), and plaque growth, and induces vasoconstriction. Solid line = stimulation; dotted lines = inhibition; FDP = fibrin-degradation product; MMP = matrix metalloproteinase; TXA$_2$ = thromboxane A$_2$; VEGF = vascular endothelial growth factor. (From Corti et al.[395] With permission.)

vulnerable plaque. Finally, impaired endothelium-dependent vasodilatation in coronary arteries with established atherosclerosis results in paradoxical vasoconstriction, which may result in worsened myocardial ischemia during acute coronary syndromes.

Pathogenesis of the Acute Coronary Syndrome

PLAQUE PROGRESSION AND RUPTURE

Coronary lesions of less than 50 percent stenosis may account for as many as two-thirds of the lesions causing ACS and may be associated with acute pro-gression to severe stenosis or total oc-clusion.[11] The degree of plaque disrup-tion (ulceration, fissure, or erosion) or substrate exposure is a key factor in de-termining the severity of the thrombo-genicity at the local arterial site. This unpredictable and episodic progression is most probably caused by disruption of lipid-rich type IV and V plaques, with subsequent thrombus formation. This disruption changes plaque geometry, re-sulting in progression of the plaque type, and leads to acute symptomatic, occlusive coronary syndromes. Plaque

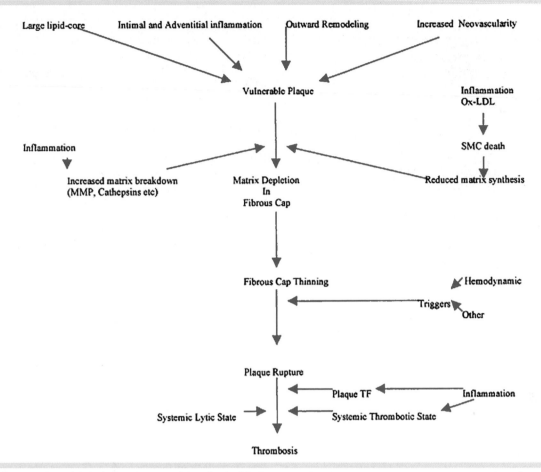

FIGURE 54-6 Conceptual model depicting the potential pathophysiologic mechanisms of plaque vulnerability, rupture, and thrombosis. Ox-LDL = oxidized low-density lipoprotein; MMP = matrix degrading metalloproteinases; SMC = smooth muscle cell; TF = tissue factor (From Shah.[396] With permission.)

disruption seems to depend on both passive and active processes (Fig. 54-6). Passive plaque disruption is related to physical forces, and it occurs most frequently where the fibrous cap is the weakest. This is often where it is thinnest and most heavily infiltrated by foam cells, which, for eccentric plaques, is commonly the shoulder or between the plaque and the adjacent vessel wall. Inflammation plays a more active role in plaque disruption via the macrophages' ability to degrade the extracellular matrix by secreting proteolytic enzymes such as matrix metalloproteinases (MMPs) (collagenases, gelatinases, stromelysins, and others). Tissue factor, a low-molecular-weight glycoprotein that initiates the extrinsic coagulation cascade, has been found to colocalize with macrophages in culprit coronary atherosclerotic lesions, suggesting a mechanism of cell-mediated thrombogenicity.[6]

THROMBOSIS

Thrombosis comprises two interrelated stages: primary and secondary hemostasis. The first stage of hemostasis is initiated by platelets as they adhere to damaged vessels and form a platelet plug (Fig. 54-7). The second phase involves activation of the coagulation system, which comprises a series of inactive proteins (zymogens), are activated by proteolytic cleavage into active enzymes that ultimately cleave fibrinogen to fibrin to form a hemostatic clot (Fig. 54-8). These two phases are dynamically interactive, however, since activated platelets can provide a surface for coagulation enzymes, and the ultimate enzyme of coagulation, thrombin, is a potent platelet activator.

Platelet Activation and Aggregation Platelets play a key role in the transformation of a stable atherosclerotic plaque to an unstable lesion.[28,29] With rupture or ulceration of an atherosclerotic plaque, the subendothelial matrix (e.g., collagen and tissue factor) is exposed to the circulating blood. Platelets mediate "primary hemostasis" at the site of a ruptured plaque: the first step is platelet adhesion via the glycoprotein Ib (GP Ib) receptor as well as von Willebrand factor. This is followed by platelet activation, which leads to (1) a change in the platelet's shape (from a smooth, discoid shape to a spiculated form, which increases the surface area on which thrombin generation can occur); (2) degranulation of the alpha and dense granules, thereby releasing thromboxane A$_2$ (TXA$_2$), serotonin, and other platelet aggregatory and chemoattractant agents; and (3) expression of GP IIb/IIIa receptors on the platelet surface with activation of the receptor, such that it can bind fibrinogen. The final step is platelet aggregation, i.e., the formation of the platelet plug. Fibrinogen (or von Willebrand factor) binds to the activated GP IIb/IIIa receptors of two platelets, thereby creating a growing platelet aggregate (Fig. 54-7).

The platelet's exterior coat, the glycocalyx, contains many distinct glycoproteins that are important for platelet function. They include integrins and leucine-rich glycoproteins. These surface glycoproteins mediate platelet adhesion and aggregation as receptors for adhesive proteins and agonists. The platelets contain dense bodies, alpha granules, actin filaments, microtubules, and an open canalicular system, all of which have their respective functions in the formation of a hemostatic plug.

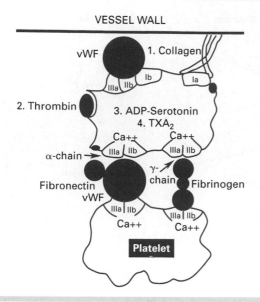

FIGURE 54-7 Interactions among platelet membrane receptors (glycoprotein Ia, Ib, and IIb/IIIa), adhesive macromolecules, and the disrupted vessel wall. Pathways of platelet activation are dependent on (1) collagen, (2) thrombin, (3) ADP and serotonin, and (4) thromboxane A$_2$ (TXA$_2$).

In normal conditions, platelets are quiescent and circulate freely in the blood because they do not attach to a normally functioning endothelium. Vessel injury, however, exposes subendothelial connective tissue to various elements to which platelets can adhere. This

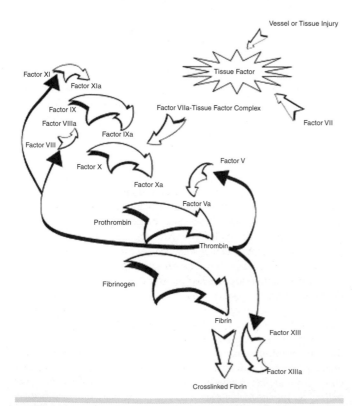

FIGURE 54-8 The coagulation cascade. Intrinsic and extrinsic pathways. (From Cohen.[397] With permission.)

phenomenon, platelet adhesion, is the initial event and one of the most crucial steps in platelet plug formation. The adhesive proteins collagen and fibronectin (and, to a lesser extent, laminin, microfibrils, and thrombospondin) are present in subendothelium and interact readily with von Willebrand factor, whereby this large protein changes its conformation. This allows platelets to bind to von Willebrand factor via their surface GP Ia/IIa and Ic/IIa receptors. Particularly collagen, a ubiquitous structural component of the vessel wall, is important and may provide scaffolding on which other adhesive proteins assemble. Von Willebrand factor, which has two collagen-binding sites, is an absolute requirement for platelet adhesion but only at high shear rates, whereas fibronectin plays a significant role in platelet adhesion at lower shear rates.

After adhesion, platelets lose their discoid shape, form extended pseudopods, and spread out over the injured surface. Through the action of activators such as collagen and eventually thrombin and norepinephrine, the adhered platelets soon become activated, whereby other platelet receptors are expressed and several mediators stored in platelet granules are released. This release reaction seems to be initiated by contraction of a circumferential band of microtubules. Stored granules are discharged through the open canalicular system after fusion of the granular membrane with the membranes of the open canalicular system. Among the granular agents released are adenosine diphosphate (ADP), serotonin, β-thromboglobulin, platelet factor 4, platelet growth factor, and TXA$_2$.

These released substances, particularly ADP and TXA$_2$, induce binding of platelets to one another, a phenomenon called *platelet aggregation*. This process increases the size of the hemostatic plug at the site of injury and, by recruiting additional circulating platelets, transforms the initial monolayer of platelets into an aggregate. The GP IIb/IIIa on the platelet surface undergo a conformational change in the aggregation process so that they can interact with plasma fibrinogen and other adhesive proteins as fibronectin and endothelial thrombospondin, which serve to link platelets together into a tighter aggregate.

Blood Coagulation   Simultaneously with formation of the platelet plug, the plasma coagulation system is activated. Traditionally, the coagulation cascade has been divided into two pathways: the extrinsic or contact system and the intrinsic system (Fig. 54-8). The extrinsic pathway, initiated by the release of tissue factor, is now felt to be the predominant mechanism of initiating hemostasis.[30] Ultimately, factor X is activated and leads to formation of thrombin, which in turn cleaves fibrinogen to fibrin.

Thrombin plays a central role in arterial thrombosis: (1) it converts fibrinogen to fibrin in the final common pathway for clot formation, (2) it is a powerful stimulus for platelet aggregation, and (3) it activates factor XIII, which leads to cross linking and stabilization of the fibrin clot. Thrombin molecules are incorporated into coronary thrombi and can form the nidus of rethrombosis (i.e., reocclusion or reinfarction) as the thrombus undergoes fibrinolysis.

Coagulation factors interact mainly on the membrane of activated platelets and other stimulated cells and tissue factor. Because of the low concentration of these factors in plasma and the abundant presence of circulating inhibitors, the interaction of procoagulants and their subsequent activation can proceed only slowly in the fluid phase of blood. Activated platelets are essential in providing a microenvironment that enhances the acceleration of fibrin formation at the site of injury by rearranging their surface lipoproteins so that phospholipids, on which coagulation factors can concentrate, are now exposed to the bloodstream. This is accompanied by the exposure of high-affinity binding sites for the activated factors V, VIII, IX, and X.

Coagulation factors are activated one by one, mainly through limited proteolysis. When the letter "a" accompanies a Roman numeral (e.g., factor VIIa), this indicates that the factor is in its activated form rather than in its naturally occurring precursor form (e.g., factor X). All activated factors are serine proteases: they split arginyl bonds in their specific substrate, and the latter then becomes another activated coagulation factor ("waterfall" or "cascade" sequence of events). In contrast, factors V and VIII, tissue factor, and high-molecular-weight (HMW) kininogen are not proenzymes but function rather as cofactors. They can thus be considered as regulatory proteins (cofactors) that influence the reaction rate. These cofactors (except tissue factor) still require activation by minor proteolysis, while tissue factor X, present in extravascular spaces, must make contact with blood to function. The traditional coagulation scheme distinguishes an intrinsic from an extrinsic activation pathway.[31]

The Intrinsic Pathway of the Coagulation System: Activation of Factors XII, XI, X, and IX All factors participating in the intrinsic pathway are present in circulating blood, and the reaction sequence is initiated by contact of platelets and/or coagulation components with a subendothelial tissue. This initial contact phase involves the interaction of factor XII (Hageman factor), factor XI, prekallikrein, and HMW kininogen with a foreign surface (a surface other than normal endothelium or blood cells).

Factor XI and prekallikrein exist in plasma as equimolar complexes with HMW kininogen, and these complexes are bound to initiating surfaces via the HMW kininogen moiety. HMW kininogen transports both factor XI and prekallikrein to an appropriate surface. Surface binding is assumed to serve to bring factor XII, prekallikrein, and factor XI to a close spatial orientation. Binding of factor XII to a negatively charged surface also makes the molecule more susceptible to proteolytic cleavage. Initially, traces of factor XIIa presumably generate traces of kallikrein from prekallikrein by the splitting of a single peptide bond. Kallikrein will now activate factor XII more rapidly in a feedback loop, which, in turn, will generate more kallikrein; the reciprocal activation of these two surface-bound molecules continues until the substrates are locally exhausted.

In vitro, factor XIIa converts the next factor of the coagulation cascade, factor XI, from its zymogen form to its enzymatic constellation. Factor XI also circulates in plasma complexed with HMW kininogen; the latter protein thus serves as helper protein, carrying factors XII and XI in the blood.

Factor XIa bound to the surfaces by HMW kininogen interacts upon activation with factor IX in a calcium-dependent two-step reaction. Each light chain of factor XIa contains a catalytic site, while its heavy chain has the binding site for factor IX and HMW kininogen. Binding of calcium ions to factor IX (a vitamin K–dependent protein) induces a conformational change in the molecule, which facilitates its binding to the heavy chain of factor XIa, which is essential for the optimal rate of factor IX activation. Activated factor IX, thrombin-modified factor VIII, negatively charged phospholipid (e.g., activated platelets), and calcium ions form a multimolecular complex called *tenase* because it directly activates factor X (ten).

The Extrinsic (Tissue Factor) Pathway of the Coagulation System: Activation of Factors VII and X In the extrinsic system, membrane-bound tissue factor starts off the chain of events by forming a complex with factor VII in the presence of calcium ions. Tissue factor is a dimer composed of two identical subunits with interacting enzyme-

binding sites.[32] It is present on nonvascular cell surfaces and on microvesicles shed from cell surfaces. Tissue factor is an integral membrane protein composed of protein and phospholipid components, both of which are required for its procoagulant activity. Factor VII is a single-chain protein that, in this form, already has some enzymatic activity and can complex with tissue factor. By cleavage of an Arg-Ile bond, however, the molecule of factor VII splits into a light chain and a heavy chain (containing the active site) linked by two disulfide bonds. This activation increases the coagulant activity of factor VII about 100-fold. However, the activation of factor VII occurs only after it has bound to tissue factor. The tissue factor–factor VIIa complex then combines with the substrate (factor X), producing a further conformational change in factor VIIa, so that it binds still more tightly to tissue factor, precluding dissociation of factor VIIa from tissue factor. The tissue factor–factor VIIa complex activates primarily factor X but also factors IX and XI, which interconnect the intrinsic and extrinsic activation pathways and play a "prima ballerina" role in the activation of coagulation. Tissue factor accelerates these reactions as a cofactor, apparently by inducing a conformational change in factor VIIa.

The Pathway in Common: Prothrombinase, Prothrombin to Thrombin Factor X stands at the crossroad of the extrinsic and intrinsic activation pathways. This means that factor X can be activated either by the tenase complex (IXa, phospholipid, VIIIa, and Ca ions) or by the tissue factor–factor VIIa complex. In both instances, activation of factor X results from the cleavage of a single peptide bond, releasing an activation peptide and unmasking an active site on the heavy chain. This is brought about by the enzymatic activity residing in factor IXa, which is part of the tenase complex. The presence of proteolytically modified factor VIII—whether by thrombin, factor Xa, or factor IXa—by separation of factor VIII from von Willebrand factor enhances 10,000-fold the rate of activation of factor X by factor IXa. Factor VIIIa has no enzymatic activity and is thus a helper protein (a cofactor), which, to exert its function, binds to phospholipid vesicles provided that phosphatidylserine is available on the platelet membrane. In fact, specific binding sites are available on activated platelets for factor VIII that are distinct from the binding sites for factor V expressed during stimulation of platelets.

To be fully active, factor Xa has to form a stoichiometric 1:1 complex with factor Va; the latter molecule enhances the activation of prothrombin by factor Xa 300,000-fold. Normal plasma contains factor V in an inactive state; its activation requires three specific enzymatic cleavages, which can be brought about by thrombin or less efficiently by factor Xa. The association of factor Va with factor Xa on an anionic phospholipid is termed *prothrombinase*. Factor Va increases the turnover (k_{cat}) 1000-fold, which means that the number of thrombin molecules generated by the enzyme upon saturation by the substrate is multiplied by a factor of approximately 1000.

The multimolecular complex prothrombinase initially cleaves one amino acid bond in the prothrombin molecule, producing meizothrombin. This intermediate molecule remains membrane bound but lacks procoagulant properties. To become fully active, another amino acid bond has to be cleaved, yielding alpha-thrombin, which is released from the cell surface.

Thrombin represents the culmination of the coagulation cascade; its action on fibrinogen is most dramatic, because thrombus formation is a visible process. Thrombin itself is responsible for its own nonlinear generation caused by positive feedback activation, whereby thrombin enhances neoformation of thrombin (Fig. 54-9). In addition, thrombin is a pivotal molecule for numerous other

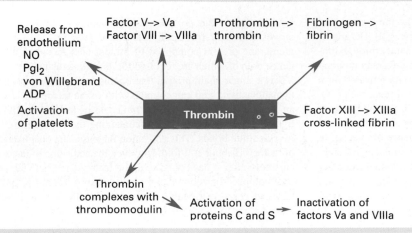

FIGURE 54-9 Thrombin is the pivotal enzyme in coagulation, being responsible for positive feedback activation, rapid activation of platelets and endothelial cells, and indirectly, via thrombomodulin, for its activation. ADP = adenosine diphosphate; PGI$_2$ = prostaglandin I$_2$.

functions. The action of thrombin on platelets results in the release of platelet factor V exteriorization and in the transbilayer movement of its inner membrane surface (flip-flop reaction). Thrombin activates three of the four cofactor or helper proteins (factors V and VIII and thrombomodulin but not tissue factor). Thrombin furthermore activates factor XIII, which increases the strength of fibrin and renders it more resistant to thrombolysis. Thrombin can increase the production and release of prostacyclin, NO, ADP, and plasminogen activator inhibitor 1 (PAI-1) from the normal endothelium, protecting the microcirculation against thrombosis. Thrombin inhibits its own production by a negative feedback mechanism via the thrombomodulin–protein C and S system. Thrombin is also involved in other biological effects, such as chemotaxis and mitogenesis. It also elicits a potent mitogenic response in fibroblasts and macrophages, thereby modulating inflammatory reactions at the site of vascular injury.

The Conversion of Fibrinogen to Fibrin Fibrinogen is a large paired molecule held together by disulfide bridges. Thrombin splits this molecule so that each molecule releases in sequence two small aminopeptides A (FPA) and two small fibrinopeptides B (FPB) from fibrinogen and thus converts this molecule to fibrin monomers that are still soluble. The FPA release exposes a polymerization site in the central region of the fibrinogen molecule (E domain), which subsequently aligns with a complementary site in the outer region (D domain) of another fibrin monomer to form staggered, overlapping two-stranded fibrils. The slower FPB release exposes an independent site for noncovalent intermolecular interaction, resulting in complementary alignment of fibrin monomers. Subsequently, lateral association of fibrin monomers occurs, and the network becomes thicker and branched, still through a nonenzymatic process. These coupled monomers of fibrin, called *polymers*, are still soluble unless they become too large and precipitate; the resulting gel of fibrin forms the skeleton of a thrombus and traps red and white cells.

The structural stability of the fibrin network is achieved through covalent cross-linking. Thrombin activates factor XIII (fibrin-stabilizing factor), a transglutaminase that, in the presence of calcium, forms peptide bonds between side chains of suitable lysine (donor) and Gla (acceptor) residues. The result of such a lysine cross linkage is that the thrombus becomes firmer and more resistant to thrombolysis. It should be noted that fibrin-bound thrombin (approximately 40

percent of the thrombin generated) retains its coagulant and platelet-activating properties and is protected from inactivation by circulating heparin-antithrombin III. During thrombolysis, fibrin-bound thrombin is released and can cause rethrombosis. Of note, two other plasma proteins (fibronectin and α_2-plasmin inhibitor) are also covalently cross-linked to fibrin by factor XIIIa and are incorporated in the fibrin mesh.

FIBRINOLYTIC SYSTEM

The fibrinolytic system is essential for removing excess fibrin deposits to preserve vascular patency; its main components are plasminogen, plasmin, and plasminogen activators. Plasminogen, a single-chain glycoprotein, is organized in seven structural domains. It is converted to a two-chain serine protease called *plasmin* by cleavage of a single peptide bond in between. Plasmin digests a number of proteins—including fibrin, fibrinogen, and factors V and VIII—as well as a number of esters and amides.

Plasminogen may be converted to plasmin by a number of agents called *plasminogen activators*. The principal circulating plasminogen activator in humans is tissue-type plasminogen activator (t-PA). This is a 70-kDa serine proteinase, which in its native form consists of a single polypeptide chain. The distinct domains in t-PA are involved in several functions of the enzyme, including its binding to fibrin, fibrin-specific plasminogen activation, rapid clearance in vivo, and binding to endothelial cell receptors. The presence of fibrin markedly enhances the plasminogen-activating property of t-PA, as it not only binds t-PA and plasminogen but also greatly increases the affinity of t-PA for plasminogen. Thus, fibrin appears to concentrate both t-PA and plasminogen on its surface and to enhance their interaction. Plasmin so formed on fibrin surfaces has its lysine-binding and active sites occupied and is relatively protected from the inhibitory action of α_2-antiplasmin.

FIBRINOLYTICS

All fibrinolytic drugs are plasminogen activators, which act to convert plasminogen to plasmin; some are natural activators endogenous to the human fibrinolytic system (e.g., t-PA) and others are not (e.g., streptokinase) (Fig. 54-10). In the late 1980s and early 1990s, the era of reperfusion with fibrinolytics began, with several studies demonstrating improved mortality in patients with acute ST-elevation MI treated with streptokinase.[33] Since that time, the paradigm of fibrinolytic therapy has been that earlier reperfusion leads to improved survival (Fig. 54-11). This realization—that time is a critical factor in saving jeopardized myocardium and reducing mortality—has led to advances and further study in the area of fibrinolytics. The development of faster and simpler bolus fibrinolytic regimens may shorten door-to-needle time, reduce medication errors, and make possible prehospital fibrinolysis. Combination therapy with GP IIb/IIIa inhibitors and the use of reduced-dose fibrinolytics attacking both components of the thrombus is yet another potentially faster and

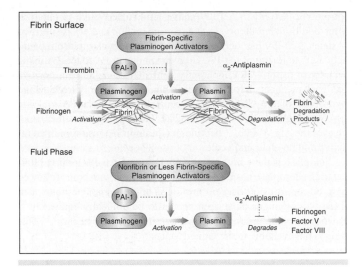

FIGURE 54-10 Components of the fibrinolytic system. Plasminogen is converted by either intrinsic or extrinsic activators to plasmin, which in turn degrades fibrin. More fibrin-specific activators preferentially activate plasminogen at the fibrin surface, whereas nonfibrin or less specific plasminogen activators induce extensive systemic plasminogen activation, with degradation of several plasma proteins including fibrinogen, factor V, and factor VIII. Plasminogen activator inhibitor (PAI) and α_2-antiplasmin are serine protease inhibitors that are the main inhibitors of plasminogen activators and plasmin, respectively, in plasma. (From Llevadot et al.[398] With permission.)

more effective way to open occluded arteries. Finally, facilitated percutaneous coronary intervention (PCI), which combines pharmacologic and interventional reperfusion strategies, holds the potential to achieve earlier and more complete reperfusion, thereby limiting infarct size and improving outcome.

Streptokinase

Streptokinase is a nonenzymatic protein produced by several strains of hemolytic streptococci; it consists of a single polypeptide chain of 414 amino acids with a molecular weight of about 50,000 Da.[34] Streptokinase cannot directly cleave peptide bonds, but it activates plasminogen to plasmin indirectly via a three-step mechanism. First, streptokinase forms a 1:1 complex with plasminogen, which undergoes a conformational change, resulting in the exposure of an active site in the plasminogen moiety. In the second step, this active site catalyzes the activation of plasminogen to plasmin. Finally, plasminogen-streptokinase molecules are converted to plasmin-streptokinase complexes.[35] The active-site residues in the plasmin-streptokinase complex are the same as those in the plasmin molecule, but plasmin is unable to activate plasminogen, whereas the plasmin(ogen)-streptokinase complex is not inhibited by α_2-antiplasmin.

Most individuals have measurable circulating streptokinase-neutralizing antibodies, which may result from previous infections with β-hemolytic streptococci. Therefore, during fibrinolytic therapy, sufficient dose of streptokinase must be infused to neutralize these antibodies. A few days after streptokinase administration, the antistreptokinase titer rises to 50 to 100 times the preinfusion value and remains high for 4 to 6 months.[36] Antibodies can be detected for as long as 4 years after treatment; thus retreatment during with streptokinase is not recommended.[37]

Clinical trials have shown intravenous streptokinase, administered as an infusion of 1.5 million units over 1 h, leads to a significant reduction in mortality rate compared to no fibrinolytic agent. In the GISSI-I trial, for patients with acute MI within 12 h, there was a 19 percent reduction in mortality rate.[38] In ISIS-2, there was a 25 percent reduction in mortality rate.[39] In the ISIS-3 trial, streptokinase was found to have an identical mortality rate as the 3-h regimen of t-PA with either subcutaneous or no heparin.[40] In the Global Use of Strategies to Open Occluded Coronary Arteries (GUSTO)-I trial, however, streptokinase was inferior to t-PA when the latter was

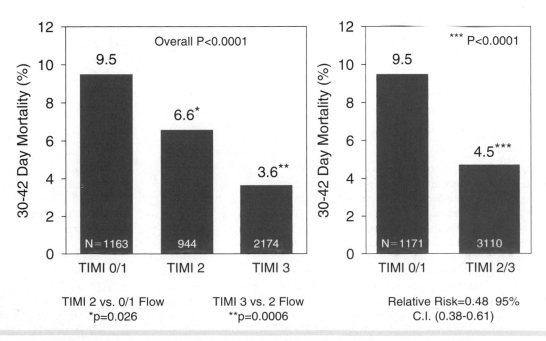

FIGURE 54-11 Relation of TIMI flow grade at 90 min to mortality rate. Overview of > 4000 patients from 13 trials. (From Cannon.[399] With permission.)

administered as an accelerated 90-min bolus and infusion with concomitant intravenous heparin.[41]

Anistreplase (Anisoylated Plasminogen-Streptokinase Activator Complex)

APSAC (anistreplase) was constructed with the aim of controlling the enzymatic activity of the plasmin(ogen)-streptokinase complex by a specific reversible chemical protection of its catalytic center (i.e., by adding a *p*-anisoyl group).[42] Anistreplase is an equimolar, noncovalent complex between streptokinase and human Lys-plasminogen. It has a catalytic center located in the carboxy-terminal region of the molecule. The plasmin(ogen)-streptokinase complex is an efficient activator of plasminogen. Deacylation of anistreplase uncovers the catalytic center, which can then convert plasminogen to plasmin. Deacylation of anistreplase does, however, occur both in the circulation and at the fibrin surface, and the fibrin specificity of anistreplase is only marginal at best. Its plasma half-life is 70 min, compared with 25 min for the plasminogen-streptokinase complex formed in vivo after administration of streptokinase.[43] Because anistreplase is based on streptokinase, patients with high antistreptokinase antibody titers do not respond to it, and anistreplase causes a marked increase in the streptokinase antibody titer within 2 to 3 weeks.

In one large trial (AIMS), anistreplase reduced mortality compared with placebo.[44] In the Thrombolysis in Myocardial Infarction (TIMI)-4 trial, TIMI grade 3 flow at 60 and 90 min was inferior to accelerated t-PA, as were overall clinical outcomes.[45] Because it is a bolus drug (administered as 30 U over 2 to 5 min), anistreplase was used in several trials of prehospital thrombolysis, which showed benefit compared with hospital-based treatment.[46,47] Due to its high cost (approaching that of t-PA) and its inferior patency profile compared with t-PA, its use has waned greatly.

Urokinase

Two-chain urokinase-type plasminogen activator (tcu-PA), is a trypsin-like serine proteinase composed of two polypeptide chains (20,000 and 34,000 Da).[48] It activates plasminogen directly following Michaelis-Menten kinetics but has no specific affinity for fibrin, and it activates fibrin-bound and circulating plasminogen relatively indiscriminately. Extensive plasminogen activation and depletion of α_2-antiplasmin may occur following treatment with tcu-PA, leading to degradation of several plasma proteins, including fibrinogen, factor V, and factor VIII.

Prourokinase

Single-chain urokinase-type plasminogen activator (scu-PA, prourokinase) is a naturally occurring human protein first isolated from natural sources and then produced through recombinant DNA technology.[49] The glycosylated natural scu-PA is a single-chain glycoprotein with a molecular weight of 54,000 Da and containing 411 amino acid residues. The N-terminal domain has a homology with the growth factor domain of other proteins, followed by a "kringle" domain, homologous to plasminogen, t-PA, and other proteins involved in coagulation.[50] However, the single-disulfide-bonded kringle domain of scu-PA does not contain a lysine-binding site, and it does not confer fibrin-binding properties to the enzyme.

The scu-PA is the native zymogenic precursor of urokinase. Limited hydrolysis by plasmin or kallikrein of the Lys[158]-Ile[159] peptide bond converts the molecule to its two-chain form (tcu-PA, urokinase), which is held together by one disulfide bond essential for the fibrinolytic activity.[51] A fully active tcu-PA derivative is obtained after additional proteolysis at position Lys[135]-Lys[136]. In purified systems, scu-PA has only 1 percent of the intrinsic plasminogen-activating potential of tcu-PA. Conversion of scu-PA to tcu-PA in the vicinity of a fibrin clot apparently constitutes a significant positive feedback mechanism for clot lysis in human plasma in vitro. Specific hydrolysis of the Glu[143]-Leu[144] peptide bond in scu-PA yields a LMW scu-PA of 32,000 (scu-PA-32 k). Thrombin, on the other hand, cleaves the Arg[156]-Phe[157] peptide bond in scu-PA, resulting in an inactive double-chain molecule.

Saruplase is the commercial preparation of scu-PA used in clinical trials. Saruplase has been administered as a 20-mg bolus followed by a 60-mg infusion over 60 min or as an 80-mg single bolus, and these two regimens have been shown to be clinically equivalent.[52] Patency rates are improved with coadministration of heparin.[53] This drug is not available in the United States.

t-PA—Tissue-Type Plasminogen Activator

Native t-PA is a serine proteinase with a molecular weight of about 70,000 Da; it is composed of one polypeptide chain containing 527 amino acids.[54] t-PA is converted by plasmin to a two-chain form by hydrolysis of the Arg[275]-Ile[276] peptide bond. The two-chain form is held together by one interchain disulfide bond. t-PA for clinical use is presently produced by recombinant DNA technology and consists mainly of the single-chain form.

The NH2-terminal region of t-PA is composed of four domains with homologies to other proteins: residues 4 to 50 (F domain) are homologous to the "finger domains" in fibronectin; residues 50 to 87 (E domain) are homologous to human epidermal growth factor; and two regions, comprising residues 87 to 176 and 176 to 262 (K1 and K2 domains), are both homologous to the five kringle loop structures of plasminogen (Fig. 54-12). The region comprising residues 276 to

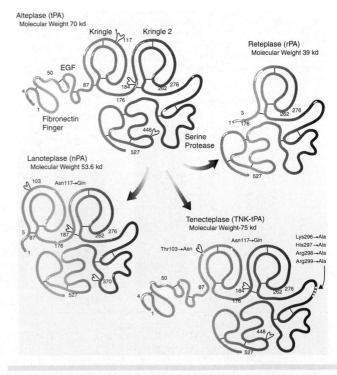

FIGURE 54-12 Structure of tissue-type plasminogen activator (t-PA) and mutants reteplase (rt-PA), lanoteplase (nPA), and tenecteplase (TNK-t-PA). (From Llevadot et al.[398] With permission.)

527 is homologous to that of other serine proteinases and contains the catalytic site, which is composed of His[322], Asp[371], and Ser[478]. t-PA has a specific affinity for fibrin, which is mediated by the finger domain and the second kringle region of the A chain. A lysine-binding site is involved in the interaction of K2 domain with fibrin but not in the interaction of the finger domain with fibrin. The structures required for the enzymatic activity of t-PA are fully contained within the B chain.

The activation of plasminogen by t-PA, both in the presence and in the absence of fibrin, follows Michaelis-Menten kinetics.[55] The presence of fibrin enhances the efficiency of plasminogen activation by t-PA by two to three orders of magnitude. Fibrin provides a surface to which t-PA and plasminogen adsorbs in a sequential and ordered way, yielding a cyclic ternary complex. Fibrin essentially increases the local plasminogen concentration by creating an additional interaction between t-PA and its substrate. The high affinity of t-PA for plasminogen in the presence of fibrin thus allows efficient activation on the fibrin clot, while no efficient plasminogen activation by t-PA occurs in plasma. Plasmin formed on the fibrin surface has both its lysine-binding sites and active site occupied and is thus only slowly inactivated by α_2-antiplasmin (a half-life of about 10 to 100 s); in contrast, free plasmin, when formed, is rapidly inhibited by α_2-antiplasmin (a half-life of about 0.1 s). The fibrinolytic process thus seems to be triggered by and confined to fibrin.

PILOT STUDIES: DOSE RANGING AND SAFETY

After an initial pilot study of t-PA,[56] t-PA was compared with intravenous streptokinase in the TIMI-1 trial, in which 290 patients with acute MI underwent baseline coronary angiography and were then treated with either streptokinase or t-PA and adjunctive heparin.[57,58] The primary endpoint, reperfusion of initially occluded coronary arteries after 90 min, was achieved in 62 percent of t-PA–treated patients, compared with 31 percent of streptokinase-treated patients ($p < 0.001$). The patency rate at 90 min, independent of findings on the baseline arteriogram, was 70 percent for t-PA and 43 percent for streptokinase ($p < 0.001$). Nearly identical results were observed in the European study.[59] In a review of the numerous angiographic trials, the 3-h dosing regimen of t-PA had superior patency and TIMI grade 3 flow at both 60 and 90 min compared with streptokinase or anistreplase.[60] Subsequently, Neuhaus et al. developed the accelerated 90-min dosing regimen,[61] which was found to achieve even higher rates of early reperfusion compared with the 3-h t-PA dosing regimen,[62] anistreplase,[45,63] or streptokinase.[64] Given the impor-

tance of rapid reperfusion, it was assumed that a higher rate of early infarct-related patency achieved with t-PA would translate into a lower mortality rate. This hypothesis was called into question following the results of GISSI-2/International Study[65,66] and ISIS-3.[40] In these trials, no difference in mortality rates was observed between the 3-h regimen of t-PA and streptokinase with either subcutaneous heparin or no adjunctive heparin.

CLINICAL TRIALS: MORTALITY STUDIES

GUSTO-1 The GUSTO-I trial evaluated the accelerated 90-min dosing regimen of t-PA in conjunction with intravenous heparin.[41] As shown in Table 54-1, the mortality rate at 30 days was significantly lower in the front-loaded t-PA arm as compared with each of the three other arms. The improvement in mortality with t-PA was seen after only 24 h, establishing a link between early reperfusion and improved survival. In addition, other major complications—such as cardiogenic shock, congestive heart failure, and ventricular arrhythmia—were decreased by t-PA. Similar benefits of t-PA in patency and overall clinical outcome were observed in the TIMI-4 trial.[45]

The explanation of the benefit of t-PA in the GUSTO and TIMI-4 trials and the lack of benefit in GISSI-2 and ISIS-3 is based on two factors: (1) the use of the front-loaded t-PA regimen achieved a higher rate of early patency compared with the older 3-h regimen[60] and (2) the use of early intravenous heparin improved late infarct-related artery patency.[67–69] In contrast, the GISSI-2 and ISIS-3 trials used the slower 3 h infusion regimen of t-PA and either no heparin or delayed, subcutaneous heparin, which does not elevate the aPTT until approximately 24 h after the start of treatment. Because the initial 24 h hold the highest risk of reocclusion of an open infarct-related artery (which is associated with a threefold increase in mortality), the subcutaneous heparin regimen is inadequate at preventing this important complication.

Intracranial hemorrhage (ICH) is the most feared complication of thrombolysis, although it is fortunately a rare complication despite aggressive regimens of thrombolysis, aspirin, and heparin. For each of these streptokinase arms, 0.5 percent of patients suffered an ICH as compared with 0.7 percent of patients treated with front-loaded t-PA and 0.9 percent of patients treated with combination thrombolytic therapy. To put their results in full perspective, the GUSTO investigators developed the concept of net clinical benefit—i.e., the occurrence of either death or a disabling stroke. In comparing the net clinical benefit between the accelerated t-PA and streptokinase-only

TABLE 54-1 Results from the GUSTO Trial

Outcome	SK and sq Heparin	SK and IV Heparin	Front-Loaded t-PA and IV Heparin	t-PA and SK and IV Heparin	*p*. Value t-PA vs. Both SK Regiments
No. of patients	9796	10,377	10,344	10,328	
30-Day mortality (%)	7.2	7.4	6.3	7.0	0.005
Net clinical benefit (death or disabling stroke) (%)	7.7	7.9	6.9	7.6	0.006
24-h Mortality (%)	2.8	2.9	2.3	2.8	0.005
Intracranial hemorrhage	0.5	0.5	0.7	0.9	0.03
Congestive heart failure	17.5	16.8	15.2	16.8	<0.001
Cardiogenic shock	6.9	6.3	5.1	6.1	<0.001

ABBREVIATIONS: IV = intravenous; SK = streptokinase; t-PA = tissue-type plasminogen activator; sq = subcutaneous.
SOURCE: Data from the GUSTO Investigators.[41,64]

regimens, t-PA had a significantly lower rate of the combined endpoint at 6.9 percent, compared with 7.8 percent for streptokinase ($p = 0.006$).

DOUBLE-BOLUS TISSUE-TYPE PLASMINOGEN ACTIVATOR

Initial interest in a double-bolus regimen of t-PA came from a series of patients to whom two 50 mg boluses of t-PA were administered 30 min apart; TIMI grade 3 flow was observed in 88 percent of these patients.[70] However, in a subsequent randomized, blinded trial, double-bolus t-PA achieved a nonsignificantly lower 58 percent TIMI grade 3 flow, compared with 66 percent for the accelerated 90-min infusion of t-PA.[71] The Continuous Infusion Versus Double-Bolus Administration of Alteplase (COBALT) trial compared double-bolus t-PA with the accelerated infusion of t-PA but was terminated prematurely because of concern about the safety of the double-bolus regimen.[72] The 30-day mortality rate was nonsignificantly higher in the double-bolus group than in the accelerated-infusion group: 7.98 percent as compared with 7.53 percent. Rates of hemorrhagic stroke were also higher: 1.12 percent after double-bolus t-PA as compared with 0.81 percent for accelerated t-PA ($p = 0.23$). This trial found that, statistically, double-bolus t-PA was not equivalent to t-PA; therefore double-bolus t-PA is not recommended for general clinical use.

The reason that this double-bolus regimen had worse outcomes may relate to the "plasminogen steal" phenomenon.[73] It is hypothesized that very low systemic levels of plasminogen lead to the diffusion of plasminogen out of the coronary thrombus, thereby depleting the substrate and decreasing the amount of plasmin generated on the clot surface, thus ultimately decreasing clot lysis. Because the double-bolus regimen was associated with a more than 80 percent depletion of systemic plasminogen, it was hypothesized that plasminogen steal may have reduced the efficacy of this regimen.

rt-PA—Tissue-Type Plasminogen Activator (Reteplase)

Reteplase is a single-chain nonglycosylated deletion variant of t-PA consisting of only the second kringle and the protease domains (Fig. 54-12). Because the active sites of the protease domains of reteplase and t-PA are similar, their plasminogenolytic activity in the absence of a stimulator do not differ. However, the plasminogenolytic activity of reteplase in the presence of fragments of fibrinogen is fourfold lower than that of t-PA, and the binding of reteplase to fibrin is five times lower. Reteplase and t-PA are inhibited by PAI-1 to a similar degree, but the affinity of reteplase for binding to endothelial cells and monocytes is reduced, probably as a consequence of deletion of the finger and epidermal growth factor domains in reteplase, which seem to be involved in the interaction with endothelial cell receptors. Investigations into the clot penetration and binding of reteplase compared to t-PA found that reteplase penetrates fibrin clots and binds less tightly to them than does t-PA.[74] An initial half-life of 14 to 18 min was also observed with reteplase in healthy human volunteers[75] and in patients with acute MI.[76] The long half-life of reteplase allows it to be administered as a double-bolus rather than a continuous infusion.

PILOT STUDIES: DOSE RANGING AND SAFETY

Dose-ranging studies of bolus reteplase in acute MI performed in a multicenter trial found that a single dose of 10 U of reteplase achieved TIMI grade 3 flow in 46 percent of patients at 30 min, in 48 percent at 60 min, in 52 percent at 90 min, and in 88 percent at 24 to 48 h. With 15 U, slightly higher rates were observed (38, 58, 69,

and 85 percent, respectively). Because there was a 12 to 20 percent reocclusion rate between the 30- and 90-min angiograms, the administration of a second smaller bolus of reteplase (5 U) 30 min after the initial bolus (10 U) was investigated in an open, uncontrolled study and found to have similar patency and a lower reocclusion rate of 2 percent.[77]

In the Reteplase versus Alteplase Infusion in Acute Myocardial Infarction (RAPID-I) trial involving 605 patients with acute MI, single- and double-bolus doses of reteplase (a single dose of 15 U, 10 U plus 5 U, and 10 U plus 10 U given 30 min later) were compared with the 3-h dose regimen of t-PA.[78] TIMI-3 patency rates at 90 min were obtained with the given reteplase regimen in 42.7, 45.4, and 62.9 percent, respectively, and in 47.6 percent of patients treated with t-PA. The difference between the 10 U + 10 U reteplase and t-PA arms was significant ($p = 0.01$) and was the basis of the next clinical trial.

The RAPID-II trial was a randomized, open-label angiographic study of 324 patients with acute MI within 12 h that compared the 10 U + 10 U regimen of reteplase with that of accelerated t-PA (100 mg over 90 min).[79] All patients received aspirin and heparin consisting of a 5000-U bolus followed by an infusion of 1000 U/h for at least 24 h. TIMI grade 3 flow rates of the infarct-related artery at 90 min were significantly higher with reteplase relative to the t-PA control (83.4 vs. 73.3 percent, $p < 0.05$). At 60 min, both the TIMI grade 2 or 3 patency and the TIMI grade 3 flow rates were significantly higher for reteplase than for t-PA. Reteplase-treated patients required significantly fewer additional coronary interventions within the first 6 h of treatment (13.3 vs. 26.5 percent). As expected in a trial of this size, there were no significant differences between the reteplase and alteplase groups with respect to 35-day mortality (4.1 vs. 8.4 percent) and hemorrhagic stroke (1.2 vs. 1.8 percent).

CLINICAL TRIALS: MORTALITY STUDIES

INJECT The International Joint Efficacy Comparison of Thrombolytics (INJECT) study was designed to determine whether reteplase was at least as effective in mortality reduction as streptokinase.[80] In this double-blind study, 6010 patients with acute MI within 12 h were randomized to either double boluses of 10 U + 10 U of reteplase 30 min apart or 1.5 MU of streptokinase over 60 min. All patients received daily aspirin and intravenous heparin for at least 24 h. The 35-day mortality rate was 9.0 percent in the reteplase group and 9.5 percent in the streptokinase group (95 percent CI 0.96 to 1.98), which met the predefined criteria for equivalence. The incidence of recurrent MI was similar in the two groups. At 6 months, mortality rates were 11.0 percent for reteplase and 12.0 percent for streptokinase. Bleeding events were similar in the two groups (0.7 percent for reteplase and 1.0 percent for streptokinase), and the in-hospital stroke rates were 1.23 and 1.0 percent, respectively.

GUSTO-III In the GUSTO-III trial, reteplase as a 10 U + 10 U double bolus regimen was compared to front-loaded t-PA in 15,059 patients treated within 6 h of symptoms of acute MI.[81] Clinical outcomes between the two treatments were very similar, including mortality (7.47 vs. 7.24 percent), ICH (0.91 vs. 0.87 percent), and net clinical benefit (death or disabling stroke, 7.9 percent in each group) for reteplase versus t-PA. In applying post hoc criteria for equivalence (evaluating the upper boundary of the 95 percent CI), reteplase is statistically equivalent for death or disabling stroke when a 1 percent absolute boundary is used (derived from the difference observed between streptokinase and t-PA), although the mortality difference CI did cross unity. Even though the trial was not configured to statistically prove equivalence, given that all of the outcomes measured were similar, the simpler double-bolus regimen of reteplase is generally considered to be clinically equivalent to accelerated t-PA.

TNK—Tissue-Type Plasminogen Activator (Tenecteplase)

TNK–t-PA (tenecteplase) is a genetically engineered variant of t-PA (Fig. 54-12). TNK–t-PA is similar to wild-type t-PA but has amino acid substitutions at three sites, which give it its name: a threonine (T) is replaced by asparagine, which adds a glycosylation site to position 103; an asparagine (N) is replaced by a glutamine, thereby removing a glycosylation site from site 117; and four amino acids—lysine (K), histidine, arginine, and arginine—are replaced by four alanines at the third site. Together, these substitutions lead to a longer half-life of the molecule, increased fibrin specificity, and increased resistance to inhibition by PAI-1.[82-84]

PILOT STUDIES: DOSE RANGING AND SAFETY

TIMI 10A and B The first trial of TNK–t-PA was TIMI-10A, which compared doses ranging from 5 to 50 mg in 113 patients with ST-elevation MI presenting within 12 h of symptom onset to accelerated t-PA.[82] TIMI-10B utilized essentially the same protocol but with a greater number of subjects, 886, and with a refined dosing of TNK–t-PA (30 to 50 mg).[85] TNK–t-PA was demonstrated to have a prolonged plasma half-life of elimination, from 11 to 20 min, compared with 3.5 min as previously reported for t-PA.[86] TNK–t-PA demonstrated more fibrin specificity than t-PA, which is itself more fibrin-specific than streptokinase or reteplase. Systemic fibrinogen and plasminogen levels fell by only 5 to 15 percent over the first 6 h with the 30- to 50-mg doses of TNK–t-PA, compared with 40 to 50 percent drops following t-PA. Also α_2-antiplasmin consumption, the fluid-phase inhibitor of plasmin, and the resultant increase in plasmin–α_2-antiplasmin complexes was four to five times greater with t-PA than with TNK–t-PA. The prolonged plasma half-life, the high level of fibrin specificity, and the fact that TNK–t-PA does not induce the plasminogen steal phenomenon[73] explain this agent's efficacy when it is administered as a 5- to 10-s bolus. Furthermore, these benefits in preserving the systemic coagulation factors appeared to translate into lower rates of major bleeding in the large phase III trial (see below).

In TIMI-10A, the rate of TIMI-3 flow at 90 min was achieved in 57 to 64 percent of patients with the 30- to 50-mg TNK–t-PA doses, which was significantly higher than in patients treated with the lower doses ($p = 0.032$). In TIMI-10B, the 50-mg dose was discontinued after the first 78 patients due to increased ICH and replaced with a 40-mg dose of TNK–t-PA. This dose produced a rate of TIMI-3 flow at 90 min similar to that of t-PA (both 63 percent). The 30-mg dose TNK–t-PA produced a significantly lower rate of TIMI-3 flow at 90 min than t-PA (54.3 percent, $p = 0.035$), whereas the flow produced by the 50-mg dose was not significantly higher (65.8 percent). In TIMI-10B and the parallel safety trial, Assessment of the Safety of a New Thrombolytic (ASSENT)-I, a prespecified weight-based analysis was carried out.[87,88] The rate of TIMI grade 3 flow was 62 to 63 percent for doses of TNK–t-PA of approximately 0.5 mg/kg and higher, but it was 51 to 54 percent at lower doses ($p = 0.028$ across quintiles). Further analysis of the degree of perfusion achieved revealed that, in stratifying dose/weight into tertiles, the median corrected TIMI frame count was significantly lower (i.e., faster flow) in patients who received the highest "weight corrected" dose.[87]

The safety analysis of TIMI-10B and the subsequent dosing of TNK–t-PA with concomitant heparin was influenced by the initial phase of the trial, in which there were three ICHs among the 78 patients (3.8 percent, 95 percent CI = 0.8 to 10.8 percent) treated with the 50-mg TNK–t-PA dose. Due to safety concerns, clinical trials proceeded with the lower 40-mg dose. At the same time, the heparin dose, which was initially at the discretion of the treating physicians, was reduced by a protocol amendment mandating that patients receive the following dose of heparin: for patients weighing more than 67 kg, a 5000-U bolus and 1000-U/h infusion, and for patients weighing 67 kg or less, a 4000-U bolus and 800-U/h infusion. In addition, adjustment of the heparin dose according to the nomogram was mandated to begin with the 6-h aPTT. Further analysis demonstrated that the concomitant heparin may have played a larger role than the dose of TNK–t-PA in defining the rate of ICH.

Following amendment of the protocol, the rates of both ICH and serious bleeding were lower; for 30 mg of TNK–t-PA, the ICH rate fell from 2.2 to 0 percent ($p = 0.047$), and for t-PA, the rate fell from 2.8 to 1.2 percent ($p = 0.29$, overall combined $p = 0.04$).[85] Similar observations and statistically significant reductions in ICH rate were observed in the overall TNK–t-PA combined experience of the TIMI-10B and ASSENT-I trials.[89] Severe bleeding rates also decreased with the reduced heparin dosing: from 3 to 0 percent ($p = 0.02$) for 30 mg TNK–t-PA and from 8 to 2 percent ($p = 0.01$) for t-PA (combined $p = .001$). Lower rates of serious bleeding requiring transfusion were noted with TNK–t-PA (1.0 percent for the 30-mg dose and 1.3 percent for the 40-mg dose) compared to t-PA (7.0 percent, $p < 0.01$).[90] Thus, there appeared to be early evidence that the very fibrin-specific agent TNK–t-PA might be associated with lower rates of bleeding than t-PA.

ASSENT-1 ASSENT-1 was a randomized trial of three doses of TNK–t-PA, the primary goal being to determine the rate of ICH of the three doses and to assist in determining the appropriate dose for a large phase III trial.[88] A total of 3235 patients with acute MI were randomized to receive either 30 mg ($n = 1705$), 40 mg ($n = 1457$), or 50 mg ($n = 73$) of TNK–t-PA. As noted previously, the 50-mg dose was discontinued and replaced by 40 mg because of the increased bleeding observed in the TIMI-10B study but not in ASSENT-1. ICH occurred in 0.77 percent of patients overall: 0.94 percent in the 30-mg arm, 0.62 percent in the 40-mg arm, and 0.0 percent in the 50-mg arm. Death, nonfatal stroke, or severe bleeding complications occurred in a low proportion of patients: 6.4, 7.4, and 2.8 percent in the 30-, 40-, and 50-mg-dose groups, respectively, without significant differences among the treatment groups.

CLINICAL TRIALS: MORTALITY STUDIES

ASSENT-2 In ASSENT-2, TNK–t-PA was compared with accelerated t-PA in a large mortality trial of patients with acute ST-elevation MI presenting within 6 h of the onset of pain.[91] This trial enrolled 16,950 patients in 1021 hospitals worldwide. TNK–t-PA was administered as a weight-adjusted dose of 0.53 mg/kg given in 5-mg increments, ranging from 30 to 50 mg.

Overall mortality was essentially identical between the two agents: 6.18 percent for TNK–t-PA and 6.15 percent for t-PA ($p = $ NS). This trial was designed as an equivalence trial[92] and, using its predefined criteria, TNK–t-PA was shown to be equivalent to t-PA (relative risk = 1.00; 90 percent CI 0.91 to 1.10; p value for equivalence = 0.028). The equivalence of TNK–t-PA to t-PA in reducing mortality was shown in nearly every subgroup tested. Of note, a superior outcome was seen for patients treated more than 4 h after the onset of chest pain with TNK–t-PA compared with t-PA (RR 0.77, 95 percent CI 0.62 to 0.95, $p = 0.018$). This benefit may relate to the greater fibrin specificity of TNK–t-PA. The first observation of the benefit of greater fibrin specificity in later-treated patients came from the TIMI-1 trial, in which 90-min patency was preserved in patients treated with t-PA over various times to treatment, whereas in those treated with streptokinase, patency was significantly worse if time to treatment was more than 4 h.[57,58] Similar findings were seen in an analysis of the German angiographic thrombolytic trials.[93] Finally, in the GUSTO-III trial, t-PA was associated with significantly lower mortality than reteplase, a less fibrin-specific agent, in patients treated more than 4 h after the onset of pain.[81] It is hypothesized that the longer the thrombus has been able to mature, the more resistant it may be; therefore the greater fibrin specificity of a fibrinolytic agent may enhance that agent's ability to lyse the clot.

Safety Observations In ASSENT-2, the rate of ICH was also identical for TNK–t-PA and t-PA (0.93 vs. 0.94 percent, $p =$ NS). Total stroke was also similar (1.78 percent for TNK–t-PA vs. 1.66 percent for t-PA, $p =$ NS). However, there was an intriguingly lower rate (albeit not statistically significant) of ICH in patients above 75 years of age treated with TNK–t-PA (1.7 vs. 2.6 percent for those treated with t-PA). Further analysis found that the highest-risk group for ICH comprised elderly female patients weighing 67 kg or less,[94] similar to two previous multivariate analyses of risk for ICH.[95,96] Most encouragingly, the rates of ICH in this high-risk group were only 1.1 percent for TNK–t-PA versus 3.0 percent for t-PA (OR 0.30, 95 percent CI 0.09 to 0.98, $p < 0.05$). In all other patients, the rates of ICH were similar between the two thrombolytic groups.

Equally important, the study found significantly lower rates of major (noncerebral) bleeding. The rates of major bleeding were 4.7 percent for TNK–t-PA and 5.9 percent for t-PA ($p = 0.0002$), and overall bleeding episodes were also lower in patients ($p = 0.0003$) treated with TNK–t-PA. Similarly, the rate of bleeding episodes requiring transfusion was significantly lower with TNK–t-PA. Independent risk factors for major bleeding were older age, female gender, lower body weight, enrollment in the United States, and a diastolic blood pressure <70 mmHg. The lower rates of major bleeding may also be potentially related to the greater fibrin-specificity of TNK–t-PA.[97]

ASSENT-3 In the ASSENT-3 trial TNK–t-PA was studied in conjunction with LMWH and GP IIb/IIIa inhibitors.[98] In total, 6095 patients were randomized to one of three regimens: full-dose TNK–t-PA and enoxaparin, half-dose TNK–t-PA with unfractionated heparin (UFH) and abciximab, or full-dose TNK–t-PA with UFH. The study found that there was a significant reduction in the primary endpoints of mortality, reinfarction, or refractory ischemia at 30 days in the enoxaparin and abciximab groups (11.4 vs. 11.1 vs. 15.4 percent, respectively). This improvement in clinical efficacy came at the price of an increased rate of major bleeding (3.0 vs. 4.4 vs. 2.2 percent, respectively, $p = 0.0005$).

nPA—Tissue-Type Plasminogen Activator (Lanoteplase)

Lanoteplase is a deletion mutant of t-PA in which the fibronectin fingerlike and epidermal growth factor domains are removed and Asn[117] is substituted by Gln[117].[99] (Fig. 54-12). The resulting compound has a prolonged plasma half-life of 37 min allowing for single bolus administration, a 10-fold increased thrombolytic patency, and lesser fibrin specificity compared to native t-PA.[100,101]

PILOT STUDIES: DOSE RANGING AND SAFETY

InTIME-1 The Intravenous nPA for Infarcting Myocardium Early (InTIME)-1 trial evaluated four weight-based doses of nPA (15, 30, 60, or 120 kU/kg) given as a single bolus injection compared to accelerated rt-PA in 602 patients presenting within 6 h of the onset of ST-elevation MI.[101] nPA demonstrated a dose-response in TIMI-3 flow rates at 60 min, with 23.6 percent TIMI-3 flow with 15 kU/kg and 47.1 percent TIMI-3 flow with 120 kU/kg ($p < 0.001$). Similar results were seen with the combination of TIMI-2 and -3 flow at 90 min (54.1 to 83.0 percent, $p < 0.001$). In comparison, accelerated rt-PA achieved comparable TIMI-3 flow rates at 60 min (37.4 percent, $p =$ NS) but slightly inferior combined TIMI-2 and -3 flow at 90 min (71.4 percent, 95 percent CI 60 to 82 percent). The highest dose of nPA produced a fibrinogen consumption comparable to that of rt-PA.[102] Clinical outcomes—including death, major bleeding, intracranial hemorrhage, or any adverse event—were similar between nPA and rt-PA.

CLINICAL TRIALS: MORTALITY STUDIES

InTIME-2 The 120 kU/kg single-bolus dose was chosen for the large phase 3 study, InTIME-2, in which 15,078 patients with ST-elevation MIs within 6 h of symptom onset were randomized to nPA (120 kU/kg) or rt-PA (100-mg accelerated dose) in a 2:1 ratio.[103] Patients were followed for the primary endpoint of all-cause mortality at 30 days and also received aspirin and heparin [70-U/kg bolus (max 4000U) and 15-U/kg/h infusion max 1000 U]. At 30 days, nPA was found to be equivalent to rt-PA, with mortality rates of 6.75 and 6.61 percent, respectively. While the overall stroke rates were similar (1.87 vs. 1.53 percent) between nPA and rt-PA, the rate of intracerebral hemorrhage was significantly higher with nPA (1.12 percent) compared to rt-PA (0.64 percent, $p = 0.004$). Major and moderate bleeding events were similar between the two groups, but there were more minor bleeding episodes with nPA (19.7 vs. 14.8 percent, $p < 0.0001$). This excessive bleeding seen with nPA may have been explained by the lesser fibrin specificity of nPA, an excessive dose of nPA, or an overly aggressive heparin dosing strategy not customized to the particular agent. In fact, the bolus heparin dosing strategy resulted in higher early aPTT times in the nPA group compared to the rt-PA group. Analysis of the open-label registry InTIME-2b for nPA administered without a heparin bolus found an absence of the early aPTT spike from the InTIME-2 study and a lower intracerebral hemorrhage rate (0.50 percent, 95 percent CI 0.20 to 1.02 percent).[89,104] Even though the trial found that nPA was equivalent to front-loaded rt-PA, the increased incidence of bleeding resulted in cessation of further commercial development of this agent.

Tissue-Type Plasminogen Activator (Monteplase)

Monteplase is another mutant of t-PA that has a substitution of one amino acid in the epidermal growth factor domain (Cys[84] -> Ser).[99] This substitution results in a prolonged half-life of 23 min, as compared to 4 min for t-PA, allowing for single bolus administration. In addition, it provides high thrombolytic potency and enhanced resistance to PAI-1 compared to rt-PA. Up to now, only dose-ranging and patency trials have been conducted, and there have not as yet been any large-scale trials with clinical endpoints of monteplase. An early study among acute myocardial infarction patients in Japan, monteplase (0.22 mg/kg) was associated with recanalization rates of 78 percent TIMI-2 flow and 69 percent TIMI-3 flow at 60-min.[105] In a randomized, double-blind study of 199 patients presenting within 6 h of ST-elevation MI, monteplase (0.22 mg/kg over 2 min) was compared to t-PA (tisokinase, 14.4 million units over 60 min).[106] The study found a shorter time to reperfusion in the monteplase group than in the native t-PA group when vessel patency at 15, 30, 45, and 60 min was measured (37, 62, 74, and 79 percent for monteplase vs. 14, 32, 50, and 65 percent for t-PA, $p = 0.032$ at 60 min). Although total events were few, there was no significant difference between groups in major or minor bleeding. However, as the dose of t-PA (tisokinase) used in Japan is lower than that usually used in Europe and the United States, it is difficult to extrapolate the results of these studies. Three small patency trials of monteplase followed by planned rescue angioplasty including approximately 500 subjects have been reported.[107–109] These trials randomized patients presenting with ST-elevation MI within 12 h of symptom onset to one of two strategies: half-dose monteplase followed by angioplasty or primary angioplasty alone[107,108] or monteplase and angioplasty versus t-PA and angioplasty.[109] TIMI-3 flow was significantly better at the initial angiogram with monteplase compared to t-PA (60 vs. 32 percent, $p = 0.005$) and with monteplase compared to placebo.

Tissue-Type Plasminogen Activator (Pamiteplase)

Pamiteplase is a modified t-PA with a deletion of the kringle-1 domain and a point mutation at the cleavage site of single-chain t-PA (Arg^{274} -> Glu).[99] These changes render pamiteplase resistant to cleavage by plasmin and result in a half-life of 30 to 47 min after a single bolus injection.[110] Only a single dose-finding and a single patency study have been performed with this fibrinolytic agent. The dose-finding study of 157 patients with acute MI evaluated doses of 0.05 mg/kg, 0.1 mg/kg, 0.2 mg/kg, and 0.3 mg/kg.[111] TIMI-3 flow rates were achieved in over half of the patients receiving the two highest doses, but adverse events occurred in 7 and 17 percent of those receiving 0.2 and 0.3 mg/kg, respectively. In a randomized, double-blind patency trial, bolus pamiteplase (0.1 mg/kg) was compared to t-PA (tisokinase 14.4 million units over 60 min) in patients with ST-elevation MI.[112] TIMI-3 flow rates with pamiteplase and t-PA were 25 and 16 percent at 30 min and 50 and 48 percent at 60 min. However, as the dose of t-PA (tisokinase) used in Japan is lower than that usually used in Europe and the United States, it is difficult to extrapolate the results of these studies.

Staphylokinase

Mature staphylokinase consists of 136 amino acids in a single polypeptide chain without disulfide bridges. Staphylokinase, like streptokinase, is not an enzyme but forms a 1:1 stoichiometric complex with plasmin(ogen) that activates other plasminogen molecules. Streptokinase and plasminogen produce a complex that exposes the active site in the plasminogen molecule without proteolytic cleavage, whereas the generation of plasmin is required for exposure of the active site in the complex with staphylokinase.[113,114] Staphylokinase does not bind to fibrin, and fibrin stimulates the initial rate of plasminogen activation by staphylokinase only fourfold as compared with twofold by streptokinase. In purified systems α_2-antiplasmin rapidly inhibits the plasmin-staphylokinase complex, although it does not inhibit the plasmin(ogen)-streptokinase complex. Interestingly the addition of 6-aminohexanoic acid or of fibrin-like substances (e.g., CNBr-digested fibrinogen) induces a more than a hundredfold reduction of the inhibition rates of the plasmin-staphylokinase complex by α_2-antiplasmin. Rapid inhibition by α_2-antiplasmin, indeed, requires the availability of the lysine-binding sites in the plasminogen moiety of the complex. More detailed studies on the interaction between staphylokinase, plasmin(ogen), and α_2-antiplasmin have shown that neutralization of the plasmin-staphylokinase complex by α_2-antiplasmin results in dissociation of functionally active staphylokinase from the complex, followed by its recycling to other plasminogen molecules.[113]

The result of these kinetics is that in plasma, the conversion of plasminogen-staphylokinase to plasmin-staphylokinase complex does not occur at a significant rate because it is prevented by α_2-antiplasmin; without plasmin-staphylokinase complex, no significant plasminogen activation occurs. However, in the presence of fibrin, generation of the plasmin(ogen)-staphylokinase complex is facilitated, and inhibition of plasmin-staphylokinase by α_2-antiplasmin at the clot surface is delayed. Recycling of staphylokinase to fibrin-bound plasminogen, after neutralization of the complex, will result in more efficient generation of the active complex. This mechanism is mediated via the lysine-binding sites of plasminogen and results in significantly enhanced plasminogen activation at the fibrin surface. Thus, the fibrin specificity of staphylokinase is due to rapid inhibition of generated plasmin-staphylokinase complex by α_2-antiplasmin and by a more than hundredfold reduced inhibition rate at the fibrin surface.[113,115]

PILOT STUDIES: DOSE RANGING AND SAFETY

These encouraging results have formed the basis for the evaluation, on a pilot scale, of the pharmacokinetic, thrombolytic, and immunogenic properties of staphylokinase in patients with acute MI. In 4 of 5 patients with acute MI, 10 mg of staphylokinase given intravenously over 30 min was found to induce angiographically documented coronary artery recanalization within 40 min.[116] Plasma fibrinogen and α_2-antiplasmin levels were unaffected, and allergic reactions were not observed. In a second series of 5 patients with acute coronary occlusion, intravenous administration of 10 mg of staphylokinase over 30 min induced recanalization in all patients within 20 min without associated fibrinogen degradation.[117] A third series of 12 patients evaluated bolus therapy and found that a 20 mg infusion of staphylokinase over 5 min resulted in TIMI-3 flow in 7 subjects at 60 min.[118] An additional dose of 10 mg resulted in TIMI-3 flow in 3 of 5 suboptimal patients at 90 min. In all of these patients, however, neutralizing antibodies were consistently demonstrable in plasma at 14 to 35 days. Thus, with respect to immunogenicity, the initial observations in humans are not as encouraging as the experience in baboons.

A subsequent larger trial in 100 patients with MI of less than 6 h duration randomized patients to either accelerated and weight-adjusted rt-PA over 90 min (52 patients) or to staphylokinase (the first 25 patients to 10 mg and the next 23 patients to 20 mg given intravenously over 30 min).[119] All patients received aspirin and intravenous heparin. TIMI-3 flow grade at 90 min was achieved in 58 percent of rt-PA patients versus 50 percent of 10 mg staphylokinase subjects (RR 0.86, 95 percent CI = 0.54 to 1.4 vs. rt-PA) and 74 percent of 20 mg staphylokinase patients (RR 1.3, 95 percent CI 0.90 to 1.2 vs. rt-PA). Residual fibrinogen levels at 90 min were 118 ± 47 percent of baseline with staphylokinase and 68 ± 42 percent with rt-PA ($p < 0.0005$). Staphylokinase therapy was not associated with an excess mortality rate or electrical, hemorrhagic, mechanical, or allergic complications, but patients developed antibody-mediated staphylokinase-neutralizing activity 2 weeks after staphylokinase treatment. An alternative staphylokinase dosing regimen was compared to accelerated rt-PA in another group of 102 patients with evolving MI in an otherwise identical study.[120] In this trial, staphylokinase was given as two 15-mg boluses 30 min apart (50 patients). At 90 min, TIMI-3 flow was achieved in 68 percent (95 percent CI 55 to 81 percent) of patients treated with staphylokinase and in 57 percent (95 percent CI 43 to 72 percent) of rt-PA treated subjects (p = NS). In patients not undergoing coronary intervention, TIMI-3 flow at 24 h was 100 percent after staphylokinase administration and 79 percent after rt-PA (p = 0.005). Double-bolus staphylokinase was significantly more fibrin-specific than rt-PA; residual fibrinogen levels at 90 min were 105 ± 4.1 percent of baseline with staphylokinase and 68 ± 7.5 percent with rt-PA (p < 0.0001). In-hospital adverse events did not significantly differ between the groups, but again 73 percent of patients receiving staphylokinase developed antistaphylokinase IgG antibodies after 2 weeks. Finally, a bolus and 30-min infusion of staphylokinase (SAK42D variant) was evaluated in 82 patients with acute ST-elevation MI. Total doses of 15 to 45 mg of drug resulted in TIMI-3 flow rates at 90 min of 62 to 65 percent without any significant dose-response. There was no significant reduction in plasma fibrinogen and plasminogen levels at 45 min, but a dose-related change in α_2-antiplasmin of borderline significance was observed.

The neutralizing antibodies that develop to staphylokinase are felt to be derived from three non-overlapping immunodominant epitopes, two of which could be eliminated and still retain thrombolytic activity.[121] A variant of staphylokinase with 12 amino acid substitutions and a single linear polyethylene glycol linked to a cystein residue in position 3 has been of interest because of its reduced plasma clearance and reduced immunogenicity. In an early dose-ranging trial, 29 patients with acute ST-elevation MIs were treated with a reduced-dose, single-bolus injection.[122] A 5-mg bolus restored vessel patency in 14 of 18 patients (78 percent) and a 2.5-mg bolus achieved TIMI-3 flow in 7 of 11 subjects (63 percent). The immunogenicity of the variant was roughly half that of the wild type at 3 to 4 weeks (p < 0.002).

BB-10153

In contrast to current agents, BB-10153 is a recombinant variant of human plasminogen that has been genetically modified so that it is activated to plasmin by thrombin rather than by plasminogen activator enzymes. Because thrombin is the key enzyme involved in thrombus formation and thrombin activity is localized at the site of thrombus formation, intravenous administration of BB-10153 results in site-selective production of plasmin. Consequently, thrombus dissolution may be achieved without systemic destruction of hemostatic proteins, thus reducing the potential risk of hemorrhage. The potential advantages of this agent include retention of the fibrin binding of the parent molecule yet still being thrombus-selective; the ability to act only on newly forming thrombi, which may reduce the risk of hemorrhage; and a long half-life (3 h), which allows for single-bolus infusions and may be associated with a lower risk of reocclusion. This new agent is currently being studied in the phase II patency and safety TIMI-31 trial.

Desmodus Salivary Plasminogen Activator

The subsistence of vampire bats on a diet of fresh blood is apparently contingent on their ability to interfere with the hemostatic system of the blood donor. The saliva of vampire bats contains a variety of factors that presumably satisfy two essential requirements: to maintain prolonged bleeding from the wound and to preserve blood fluidity following ingestion of a meal.[123] Different molecular forms of the *Desmodus* salivary plasminogen activator (DSPA) have been purified, characterized, cloned, and expressed. The two HMW forms exhibit a specific activity in vitro equal to or greater than that of t-PA, a

relative PAI-1 resistance, and a greatly enhanced fibrin specificity with a strict requirement for polymeric fibrin as a cofactor.[124]

ZK152387 is recombinant DSPAα1 produced in mammalian cell culture; its amino acid sequence is identical to that of its natural counterpart.[125] DSPAα1 may be suitable for bolus administration; its long half-life and high specific activity may allow a marked reduction of the absolute dose of drug required for effective thrombolysis as compared with t-PA.

Conclusions/Recommendations

The use of fibrinolytic agents for the treatment of acute ST-elevation MI is a highest-level recommendation from both the American College of Cardiology and the American Heart Association (ACC/AHA)[37] and the American College of Chest Physicians (ACCP).[126] Fibrinolytic therapy is recommended for patients with ischemic symptoms characteristic of acute MI for ≤ 12 h who have ST elevation (greater than 0.1 mV in two or more contiguous leads) or left bundle-branch block. For patients with contraindications to fibrinolytics (see also Table 52-7) or those presenting to facilities where primary percutaneous coronary intervention (PCI) is available, direct PCI is a preferred option. In light of emerging evidence that PCI is superior to fibrinolytics even if transfer to a tertiary medical facility is needed,[127] the ongoing role of fibrinolytics continues to evolve.

ANTIPLATELET THERAPY

Primary Prevention

ASPIRIN

Acetylsalicylic acid, or aspirin, was first introduced in the 1890s as treatment for a variety of inflammatory conditions, but it was not until almost 70 years later that its antiplatelet activity was recognized and later still that it was studied for the treatment of CAD.[128] Aspirin exerts its antiplatelet effect by irreversibly acetylating the enzyme cyclooxygenase (COX), thereby inhibiting the production of cyclic prostanoids including TXA$_2$, a potent promoter of platelet aggregation (Fig. 54-13). Platelet production of TXA$_2$ in response to a variety of platelet activation stimuli results in the amplification of platelet aggregation and in vasoconstriction.[129] Aspirin's major antithrombotic effects and clinical utility derive from decreasing the amount of TXA$_2$ released, which decreases overall platelet aggregation at the site of the thrombus. COX exists as two isoforms, COX-1 and COX-2, with a single amino acid substitution in the catalytic site of the enzyme distinguishing the two.[130] COX-1 is constitutively expressed in most cells and is responsible for the synthesis of homeostatic prostaglandins responsible for normal cellular functions.[131] COX-2 is not routinely present but is induced by inflammatory stimuli and is responsible for the production of inflammatory prostaglandins.[132] Aspirin's inhibition of COX is permanent; thus its antiplatelet effects last for the lifetime of the platelets, on the order of 7 to 10 days. While aspirin selectively inhibits platelet aggregation induced by TXA$_2$ formation, it only partially impedes platelet aggregation induced by other stimuli such as ADP, collagen, and low concentrations of thrombin.[133]

There have been two large randomized studies examining the use of aspirin in the primary prevention of MI, both enrolling male physicians without prior MI (Table 54-2). In the U.S. Physicians' Health Study, 22,071 male physicians between the ages of 40 and 84 were randomized to receive 325 mg of aspirin every other day or placebo.[134] The study was stopped prematurely after an average follow-up of 5 years due to a 44 percent relative reduction in MI in the aspirin-treated group (0.26 vs. 0.44 percent per year). This effect was limited to those above 50 years of age, and no decrease in cardiovascular mortality was found. Additionally, there was a nonsignificant increase in hemorrhagic stroke (RR 2.14) and a significant increase in gastrointestinal bleeding requiring transfusion. In the British Physicians' study of 5139 patients, two-thirds were randomized to receive 500 mg/day of aspirin, and one-third were advised to use no aspirin.[135] After 6 years, there was no difference in the rate of MI but a significant increase in disabling strokes. Due to a large number of protocol crossovers (both physicians stopping aspirin in the aspirin group and physicians taking aspirin in the placebo group), the power of the study to show a significant difference in cardiovascular events was diluted. Two combined analyses of these trials have been performed, which demonstrated a significant reduction in nonfatal MIs and a marginally significant increase in hemorrhagic stroke.[136,137] Hennekins et al. combined the data from the U.S. and British studies and found a significant 33 percent reduction in nonfatal MIs ($p < 0.0002$) and a nonsignificant 5 percent reduction in vascular deaths ($p = 0.7$). However they also found a nonsignificant increase in the overall rate of stroke. The 1994 Antiplatelet Trialists' Collaboration reviewed the approximately 28,000 low-risk patients allocated to just over 5 years of therapy and found a reduction of 5 per 1000 in nonfatal MIs ($2p < 0.0005$), no significant difference in vascular deaths (1.9 percent for aspirin vs. 2.0 percent for placebo), a nonsignificant increase of 2 per 1000 in nonfatal strokes ($p = NS$), and a small, marginally significant increase in hemorrhagic strokes ($2p < 0.05$).

Another primary prevention study by the Collaborative Group of the Primary Prevention Project randomized 4495 patients in a 2x2 design to aspirin (300 mg daily), vitamin E, both, or placebo and followed them for an average of 3.6 years before the study was terminated early due to the reports of aspirin's benefit from other trials.[138] Patients were free of known CAD but had one or more of the following: hypertension, hypercholesterolemia, diabetes, obesity, family history of premature MI, or advanced age. Aspirin-treated patients had a lower incidence of cardiovascular death (from 1.4 to 0.8 percent; RR 0.56, 95 percent CI 0.31 to 0.99) and total cardiovascular events—cardiovascular death, nonfatal MI, nonfatal stroke, angina, transient ischemic attack (TIA), peripheral-artery disease, or revascularization procedure (from 8.2 to 6.3 percent; RR 0.77, 0.62 to 0.95). However, there was no significant reduction in overall mortality, MI, angina, stroke, or TIA. Unfortunately, severe bleeding occurred more frequently in the aspirin group than in the placebo group (1.1 vs. 0.3 percent, $p < 0.0008$).

Individuals at a higher risk for cardiovascular events based on their risk factor profile were enrolled in the Thrombosis Prevention Trial.[139] A total of 5085 patients were randomized to aspirin (75 mg daily), warfarin, both, or placebo and followed for 6 years. Aspirin-treated patients experienced a 20 percent reduction ($p = 0.04$) in ischemic heart disease events, cardiac death, or MI, which was almost entirely attributable to a 32 percent reduction in nonfatal MI, as there was no significant effect on mortality. The rate of all strokes

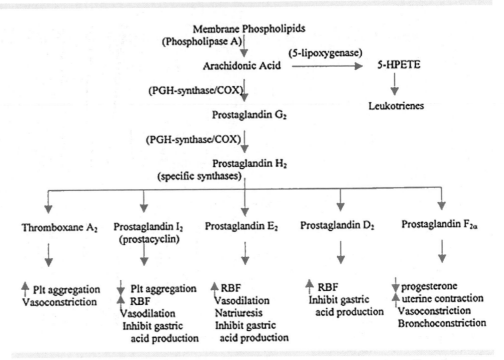

FIGURE 54-13 The production of prostaglandins from arachidonic acid and their physiologic effects. (From Awtry and Loscalzo.[128] With permission.)

TABLE 54-2 Studies of Aspirin for Primary Prevention of Cardiovascular Events

Reference	No. of Patients	Dose, mg	Length of Follow-up	Total Mortality, RR (95% CI)	Nonfatal MI, RR (95% CI)	Stroke, RR (95% CI)[a]
Physicians' Health Study[134]	22,071	325	5 y	0.96 (0.80–1.14)	0.59 (0.47–0.74)	1.22 (0.93–1.60)
Peto et al[135]	5139	500	6 y	0.89[b]	0.97[b]	1.15 (0.75–1.50)
Thrombosis Prevention Trial[139]	5085	75	6.4 y	1.06 (0.88–1.28)	0.68 (0.52–0.88)	0.98 (0.65–1.45)
Manson et al[c139a]	87,678	Varied	5.4 y	0.86 (0.72–1.03)	0.68 (0.49–0.93)	0.99 (0.71–1.36)

[a]RR is for aspirin vs. nonaspirin groups.
[b]Result not statistically significant; CIs not available.
[c]RRs for subgroup taking up to 6 aspirin per week vs. nonaspirin group.
SOURCE: From Awtry and Loscalzo.[128] With permission.

TABLE 54-3 Estimate of Benefits and Risks of Aspirin Given for 5 Years to 1000 People with Various Levels of Baseline Risk for Coronary Artery Disease[a]

BENEFITS AND HARMS	BASELINE RISK FOR CORONARY HEART DISEASE OVER 5 YEARS[b]		
	1%	3%	5%
Total mortality	No effect	No effect	No effect
Coronary heart disease events, n	1–4 avoided	4–12 avoided	6–20 avoided
Hemorrhagic strokes, n[c]	0–2 caused	0–2 caused	0–2 caused
Major gastrointestinal bleeding events, n[d]	2–4 caused	2–4 caused	2–4 caused

[a]Estimates are based on a relative risk reduction of 28% for coronary heart disease events in aspirin-treated patients and assume that risk reductions do not vary significantly by age.
[b]Nonfatal acute myocardial infarction and fatal coronary heart disease. Five-year risks of 1, 3, and 5% are equivalent to 10-year risks of 2, 6, and 10%, respectively.
[c]Data from secondary prevention trials suggest that increases in hemorrhagic stroke may be offset by reduction in other types of stroke in patients at very high risk for cardiovascular disease ($\geq$10% 5-year risk).
[d]Rates may be two to three times higher in persons older than 70 years of age.
SOURCE: From U.S. Preventive Services Task Force.[143]

was nonsignificantly decreased by 3 percent with aspirin use and the rate of major bleeding with aspirin was not significantly increased compared to placebo.

Finally, the Hypertension Optimal Treatment (HOT) Trial was a trial involving 19,193 intermediate-risk subjects that was primarily designed to assess the optimum target diastolic blood pressure in those patients with hypertension, but it also randomized patients to 75 mg of aspirin daily or placebo in a second arm of the study.[140] After a mean follow-up of 3.8 years, there was a 36 percent reduction in MIs in the aspirin-treated group compared to placebo (95 percent CI, 0.49 to 0.85, $p = 0.002$) and also a 15 percent reduction in major cardiovascular events (MIs, strokes, and cardiovascular deaths) (95 percent CI, 0.73 to 0.99, $p = 0.03$). There was no significant difference in total mortality, cardiovascular mortality, total stroke, and hemorrhagic stroke between the two groups. There was, however, an increase in nonfatal major bleeding and minor bleeding with aspirin therapy compared to placebo.

Conclusions/Recommendations

The AHA, ACCP, and U.S. Preventive Services Task Force (USP-STF) all recommend the use of aspirin therapy for the primary prevention of cardiovascular disease when the benefits of cardiovascular risk reduction outweigh the risks of gastrointestinal bleeding and he-

morrhagic stroke. The AHA guidelines for the primary prevention of cardiovascular disease recommend the use of low-dose aspirin (75 to 160 mg daily) in persons at increased risk for CAD, especially those with a 10-year risk of $\geq$ 10 percent.[141] The ACCP recommends that aspirin be considered in men and women > 50 years of age who have at least one major risk factor for CAD and who are free from contraindications to aspirin.[142] (The ACCP further suggests aggressive blood pressure control if antithrombotic agents are used due to the increased risk of serious bleeding with uncontrolled hypertension.) The USPSTF recommends that physicians discuss the potential benefits and harms of aspirin therapy with all adults who are at increased risk for CAD.[143] The USPSTF concluded that the balance of benefits and harms is most favorable in patients at high risk for CAD, defined as those with a 5 year risk $\geq$ 3 percent (Table 54-3).

Non-ST-Elevation Myocardial Infarction

ASPIRIN

Several major studies have demonstrated clear beneficial effects of aspirin in patients with unstable angina and non-ST-elevation MI, with an approximately 50 percent reduction in the risk of death or MI in patients presenting with unstable angina or non-Q-wave MI (Table 54-4).[144–148] Despite employing various doses of aspirin (75 to 1300

TABLE 54-4 The Benefit of Aspirin in Unstable Angina

Reference	No. of Patients	Dose, mg	Duration of Treatment	% DEATH OR NONFATAL MI			% MORTALITY		
				Aspirin	Control	% Reduction (P)	Aspirin	Control	% Reduction (P)
VA Cooperative Study[144]	1266	325 QD	12 wk	5.0	10.1	51 (0.0005)	1.6	3.3	51 (0.054)
Canadian Multicenter Trial[145]	555	325 QID	24 mo	8.6	17.0	51 (0.008)	3.0	11.7	71 (0.004)
Théroux et al[146]	479	325 BID	6 d	3.3	12.0	72 (0.01)	0.0	1.7	...
RISC[147][a]	796	75 QD	5 d	2.5	5.8	57 (0.033)	0.25	0.25	0 (NS)
			6 mo	8.9	19.0	53 (<0.0001)	2.0	3.8	47 (NS)
			12 mo	11.0	21.4	49 (0.0001)	2.8	4.5	38 (NS)

[a]Included patients with unstable angina and non-Q-wave infarctions. Results were similar in both groups.
SOURCE: From Awtry and Loscalzo.[128] With permission.

mg daily) and initiating therapy at different times after initial presentation with symptoms (< 24 h to < 8 days), these trials have consistently demonstrated a benefit to aspirin therapy. The first study from the Veterans Administration (VA) Cooperative Study Group documented a 51 percent reduction in the risk of death or MI in patients presenting with unstable angina, and the overall benefits of aspirin were maintained during the 1-year follow-up period.[144] The Canadian multicenter trial confirmed the large risk reduction by aspirin for the development of death or MI among patients with unstable angina/non-ST-elevation MI.[145] The Montreal Heart Institute study demonstrated the effectiveness of both aspirin and heparin in reducing the incidence of death or MI.[146] A more recent study by the Research on Instability in Coronary Artery Disease (RISC)

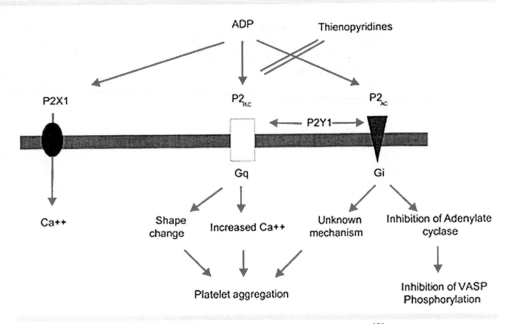

FIGURE 54-14 Platelet ADP receptors and their actions. (From Quinn and Fitzgerald.[151] With permission.)

Group extended these observations to all patients with acute coronary syndromes, showing an approximately 70 percent reduction by aspirin in subsequent risk of death or MI in patients with either unstable angina or non-ST-elevation MI.[147] A review of 12 trials of antiplatelet therapy in unstable angina by the Antithrombotic Trialists' Collaboration found a statistically significant absolute reduction of 5.3 percent in the occurrence of unstable angina in patients treated with antiplatelet therapy (8.0 percent for antiplatelet therapy vs. 13.3 percent for control), given a 46 percent odds reduction.[148]

THIENOPYRIDINES

The thienopyridines, ticlopidine and its chemical analogue clopidogrel, are antiplatelet agents that are noncompetitive but selective antagonists of adenosine diphosphate (ADP)-induced platelet aggregation (Fig. 54-14). Both agents require metabolism by the hepatic cytochrome P450-1A enzyme system to acquire activity.[149] The two agents are postulated to act by selectively and irreversibly inhibiting one of a family of membrane-bound nucleotide receptors (the P2 receptors) on the platelet surface, thereby inhibiting the binding of ADP to its platelet receptor.[150,151] While two types of ADP receptors, the P2X ligand-gated ion-channel receptors and the P2Y G-protein-linked receptors, have thus far been identified, there is good evidence to indicate the presence of a third as yet unidentified receptor.[151] Through their interaction with these receptors, the thienopyridines (1) inhibit ADP-induced inhibition of adenylate cyclase,[152] (2) prevent the ADP-induced inhibition of the cytoskeleton-associated protein VASP (vasodilator-stimulated phosphoprotein) phosphorylation,[153] and (3) prevent the association of labeled G proteins with the platelet membrane.[154] One of their net effects on the platelet is to block GP IIb/IIIa complex activation, the final common pathway for platelet aggregation, via interference with a specific ADP-dependent step and thus ultimately to impair thrombus formation. In summary, although the thienopyridines appear to act through the ADP receptor, the precise mechanism(s) of action of ticlopidine and clopidogrel are still not fully characterized.

Both agents have been studied in clinical trials in patients with atherosclerotic disease, but clopidogrel has essentially replaced ticlopidine in clinical practice. Clopidogrel is approximately six times as potent as ticlopidine in the inhibition of the ADP-induced aggrega-

tion of platelets. The use of ticlopidine is limited by its potential to cause severe neutropenia in about 1 percent of patients, which necessitates close monitoring of blood counts at regular intervals.[155] Both ticlopidine[156] and, to a lesser extent, clopidogrel[157] have been very rarely associated with thrombotic thrombocytopenic purpura. In addition, while the full antiplatelet action of ticlopidine is delayed for several days, the full effects of clopidogrel are evident several hours after a 300-mg bolus dose, making it useful in both acute and chronic settings.[158]

Ticlopidine There has only been one study of ticlopidine in unstable angina, which came from the Studio della Ticlopidina nell'Angina Instabile Group.[159] A total of 652 patients were enrolled on an open-label basis and given either ticlopidine (250 mg twice daily) or no antiplatelet therapy. At 6 months, there was a 46 percent relative reduction in the combined endpoint of vascular death and nonfatal MI with ticlopidine therapy (13.6 percent vs. 7.3 percent, $p = 0.009$). Of note, there was no difference in the number of events over the first 10 days, consistent with the delayed onset of the antiplatelet effect of ticlopidine. These results are difficult to place in clinical context given the lack of a placebo arm, but the effect is similar to that achieved with aspirin therapy in unstable angina.[148]

Clopidogrel The Clopidogrel in Unstable Angina to Prevent Recurrent Events (CURE) trial studied the combination of clopidogrel plus aspirin as the primary antiplatelet therapy of non-ST-elevation MIs.[160] The study randomized 12,562 patients who presented within 24 h of the onset of chest pain with either ECG changes or elevated cardiac enzymes to either clopidogrel (300-mg load then 75 mg daily) or placebo in addition to aspirin (75 to 325 mg daily). Patients were treated for a mean duration of 9 months and followed for a primary outcome of a composite of cardiovascular death, MI, or stroke. During hospitalization, there were significant reductions in severe ischemia, recurrent angina, and congestive heart failure with clopidogrel; at 30 days, there was a 21 percent relative risk reduction (95 percent CI 8 to 33 percent) in the composite endpoint, which persisted at 1 year (RRR 20 percent; 95 percent CI 0.10 to 0.28, $p < 0.001$). There were significantly more patients with major (3.7 vs. 2.7 percent) and minor (5.1 vs. 2.4 percent) bleeding in the clopidogrel group than the placebo group, and a retrospective analysis showed that the risk of major or life-threatening bleeding was dependent on the aspirin dose.[161] The major limitation to the universal applicability of this approach was the trial's setting in a mostly European environment of noninvasive management, in which only 5.9 to 7.2 percent of patients received glycoprotein IIb/IIIa inhibitors and only about 20 percent underwent a revascularization procedure during hospitalization. This conservative management environment differs from the strategy of early catheterization and revascularization that is prevalent in North America.

A nonrandomized, observational substudy of the CURE study, PCI-CURE, involved 2658 patients presenting with non-ST-elevation acute coronary syndrome who underwent PCI during the CURE study.[162] Patients were pretreated with a median of 10 days of study therapy, received 2 to 4 weeks of open-label thienopyridine following PCI and continued with the study drug for a mean of 8 months. At 30 days, there was a significant 30 percent (95 percent CI 3 to 50 percent, $p = 0.03$) relative risk reduction in the primary composite endpoint of cardiovascular death, MI, or urgent target vessel revascularization with clopidogrel plus aspirin pretreatment versus aspirin alone. There continued to be a reduction in cardiovascular deaths or MIs from PCI to the end of follow-up (RRR 25 percent, 95 percent CI 0 to 44 percent, $p = 0.047$) and over the entire length of the study (RRR 31 percent, 95 percent CI 13 to 46 percent, $p = 0.002$). There was no difference in major bleeding between the groups at 30 days or 8 months, even in patients who received GP IIb/IIIa inhibitors.

The Clopidogrel for the Reduction of Events During Observation (CREDO) trial was not specifically a trial of acute coronary syndromes, but it did enroll a patient population that included 53 percent with unstable angina and 13 percent with recent MIs.[163] The study investigated both pretreatment and long-term clopidogrel combined with aspirin to prevent cardiovascular events in 2116 subjects undergoing elective percutaneous intervention. Patients were randomized to 300 mg of clopidogrel 3 to 24 h prior to intervention versus placebo. All patients received clopidogrel for 28 days following PCI. At 28 days, clopidogrel loading did not result in a significant reduction in the composite primary endpoint of death, MI, or urgent target vessel revascularization (18.5 percent RR, $p = 0.23$). However, in the prespecified subgroup of patients who received the loading dose at least 6 h before intervention, there was a 38.6 percent ($p = 0.051$) reduction in events. At day 28, a second randomization compared clopidogrel (75 mg daily) to placebo from days 29 to 365 with all subjects receiving daily aspirin (81 to 325 mg). At 1 year, there was a 26.9 percent relative risk reduction (95 percent CI 3.9 to 44.4 percent, $p = 0.02$) in the composite endpoint of death, MI, and stroke. The benefit occurred beyond the standard 28-day period of treatment, as there was a 37.4 percent (95 CI 1.8 to 60.1 percent, $p = 0.04$) relative risk reduction from 4 weeks to 1 year. There was a trend toward an increase in major bleeding in the clopidogrel group (8.8 vs. 6.7 percent, $p = 0.7$), with approximately two-thirds of all major bleeds occurring in patients undergoing coronary artery bypass grafting (CABG).

GLYCOPROTEIN IIB/IIIA INHIBITORS

The surface of a resting platelet contains 50,000 to 80,000 copies of the glycoprotein (GP) IIb/IIIa receptor, which consists of two noncovalently linked α (α_{IIb}) and β (β_3) subunits (Fig. 54-15).[164] Each subunit contains a large extracellular domain, a single transmembrane region, and a short cytoplasmic tail. The α_{IIb} subunit consists of a heavy chain and a light chain, while the β_3 subunit is a single polypeptide chain. The GP IIb/IIIa receptor has many divalent cation binding sites that are required for both heterodimer assembly in

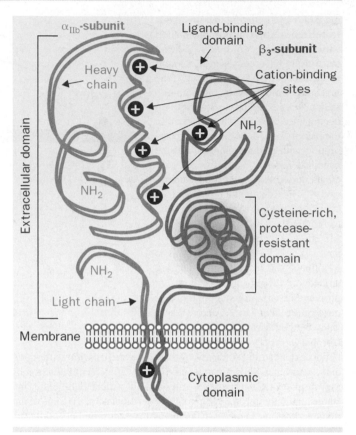

FIGURE 54-15 The GP IIb/IIIa receptor. (From Topol et al.[165] With permission.)

megakaryocytes and binding of adhesive ligands.[165] There are two binding sites on GP IIb/IIIa: one that recognizes the amino acid sequence Arg-Gly-Asp (arginine-glycine-aspartic acid, or RGD) and another that recognizes Lys-Gln-Ala-Gly-Asp-Val.[166] Fibrinogen is the most important ligand for GP IIb/IIIa, although other RGD-containing ligands include fibronectin, vitronectin, and von Willebrand factor. The cytoplasmic tail of GP IIb/IIIa is involved in transmembrane and intracellular signaling and interaction with cytoskeletal components.

Under normal conditions, platelets circulate freely without interacting with the vessel wall, soluble ligands, or each other. Once vascular injury prompts platelet activation via platelet agonists such as ADP, thrombin, and epinephrine, "inside-to-outside" signals trigger a conformational change in the GP IIb/IIIa receptor from the resting to the active state.[167] In the resting state, the affinity of the GP IIb/IIIa receptor for fibrinogen is low, and minimal occupancy occurs despite high levels of fibrinogen in the blood.[168] The activated receptor has a markedly increased affinity for fibrinogen, and a substantial increase in receptor occupancy ensues (Fig. 54-16). Receptor binding by fibrinogen and von Willebrand factor leads not only to platelet aggregation but also to the generation of "outside-to-inside" signals. These signals perform multiple functions, including modifying membrane fluidity and cytoskeletal activity, mobilizing intracellular calcium, and inducing new receptor binding sites (ligand-induced binding sites, LIBS).[169] The GP IIb/IIIa receptor is thereby linked to important platelet functions other than aggregation, such as granule secretion, P-selectin expression, and clot retraction.

GP IIb/IIIa receptor antagonists block the binding of fibrinogen to the membrane GP IIb/IIIa receptors, thus preventing platelet aggregation induced by various platelet agonists. Whereas platelet activation is produced by a wide variety of stimuli, the final common step

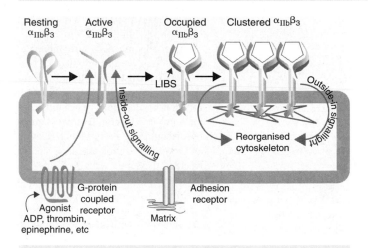

FIGURE 54-16 The Activated GP IIb/IIIa receptor. On nonstimulated platelets, the GP IIb/IIIa receptor exists in a resting conformation and does not bind ligands. Inside-out signaling culminates in conversion of the GP IIb/IIIa receptor to an active form, in which it can bind soluble ligands. The occupied receptor undergoes further transformations to express ligand induced binding sites (LIBS), and clustering of the occupied receptors leads to outside-in signaling that causing reorganization of the cytoskeleton. (From Topol et al.[165] With permission.)

to platelet aggregation is fibrinogen binding. Thus, no matter what stimuli there are for platelet activation, the platelet is inhibited by the GP IIb/IIIa inhibitor, making it an order of magnitude more effective than aspirin or the thienopyridines at inhibiting platelet aggregation. When platelet aggregation is tested in the laboratory, aspirin inhibits ADP-induced platelet aggregation by approximately 5 to 10 percent, ticlopidine and clopidogrel by approximately 30 percent, and parenteral GP IIb/IIIa inhibitors by approximately 80 to 90 percent.

Parenteral Glycoprotein IIb/IIIa Inhibitors The first GP IIb/IIIa antagonist for clinical investigation, the murine monoclonal antibody m7E3, was developed in the early 1980s by Coller and associates.[170] Abciximab is a human-murine chimeric monoclonal Fab fragment that retains the mouse-derived variable portion of m7E3 joined to the constant region of human IgG Fab. Abciximab has high binding affinity for the GP IIb/IIIa receptor and a slow dissociation rate for it in either the active or inactive state.[171] Abciximab is cleared rapidly from the plasma but is detectable bound to circulating platelets for at least 21 days.[172] Thus, the antiplatelet effect lasts much longer than the infusion period—a potential benefit for improving efficacy. On the other hand, if bleeding has occurred, stopping the drug will not reverse the antiplatelet effect immediately; transfusion of platelets, however, will allow the antibodies to redistribute among all the platelets, thereby reducing the level of platelet inhibition. While abciximab has equal affinity for the vitronectin receptor ($\alpha_V\beta_3$)— which plays a role in cell adhesion, migration, and proliferation—it is not clear if this has any therapeutic benefit. Also, it has been shown to inhibit thrombin generation by tissue factor due to its blockade of GP IIb/IIIa and $\alpha_V\beta_3$,[173] and it may inhibit the MAC-1 receptor ($\alpha_M\beta_3$), which is found on granulocytes and monocytes.[174]

A second class of compounds targeting the GP IIb/IIIa receptor are the peptide and peptidomimetic competitive inhibitors. Synthetic peptide compounds were designed based on the disintegrins, a class of RGD proteins found in snake venoms, which interfere with the binding of RGD-containing adhesive proteins to cellular integrins. The cyclic heptapeptide eptifibatide is based on the Lys-Gly-Asp

(KGD) amino acid sequence found in the peptide barbourin, which has unique specificity for GP IIb/IIIa compared with RGD-based peptides and provided a template for this synthetic peptide antagonist.[175] The other approach has been to mimic the charge and spatial conformation of the RGD sequence using nuclear magnetic resonance studies to develop engineered synthetic and semisynthetic compounds. The tyrosine-derivative nonpeptide mimetic tirofiban, the peptidomimetic agent lamifiban, and the entire class of oral agents were all developed in this fashion. These synthetic agents bind to the active and inactive forms of the GP IIb/IIIa receptor and so bind to both stimulated and nonstimulated platelets. Compared with abciximab, these small-molecule agents demonstrate exclusive specificity for GP IIb/IIIa; they have less binding affinity and shorter durations of biologic effect and predominantly undergo renal excretion. Since the level of platelet inhibition is directly related to the drug level in the blood, these short-acting agents require the ratio of drug molecules to GP IIb/IIIa receptors to be greater than 250, whereas for the "tight-binding" agent abciximab, the ratio is only 2 to achieve the same level of inhibition. The short half-lives also mean that when the drug infusion is stopped, the antiplatelet activity reverses after a few hours, which is a potential benefit for avoiding bleeding complications. On the other hand, for prolonged antiplatelet effect, the drug must be given intravenously for a longer period.

Eptifibatide PURSUIT The Platelet Glycoprotein IIb/IIIa in Unstable Angina: Receptor Suppression Using Integrilin Therapy (PURSUIT) trial was the largest of the non-ST-segment-elevation acute coronary syndrome studies.[176] The study enrolled 10,948 patients who presented with chest pain at rest within 24 h and either ECG changes or positive cardiac enzymes and randomized them to either placebo or eptifibatide for 72 to 96 h. The study protocol recommended that all patients receive aspirin and heparin, but cardiac catheterization and revascularization were performed at the discretion of the treating physician. Treatment resulted in a statistically significant 10 percent reduction in the composite endpoint of death or MI at 30 days (15.7 percent vs. 14.2 percent, $p = 0.04$). This absolute benefit of 1.2 to 1.5 percent was apparent by 96 h and persisted up to 6 months.[177] Among the four predefined geographic regions involved in the trial, the greatest treatment benefit (and greatest use of percutaneous intervention) was observed among the 4358 North American patients (11.7 vs. 15.0 percent). There was a 1.5 percent increase in the rate of major bleeding ($p = 0.02$) in the eptifibatide group but no difference in the rate of thrombocytopenia.

Tirofiban PRISM AND PRISM-PLUS The Platelet Receptor Inhibition for Ischemic Syndrome Management (PRISM) trial was the first of two studies evaluating tirofiban in ACS (Fig. 54-17).[178] This study enrolled 3232 patients who were somewhat lower risk than in other trials. They had chest pain at rest or with minimal exertion within 24 h, with either ECG changes, positive cardiac enzymes, or a history of CAD. Patients were randomized to either tirofiban or heparin for 48 h, and a conservative strategy was encouraged, as catheterization and revascularization during study drug infusion were discouraged. Treatment with tirofiban reduced the composite endpoint of death, MI, and refractory ischemia at 48 h by 32 percent (5.6 vs. 3.8 percent, $p = 0.01$). However, at 30 days, this benefit was no longer present. In a retrospective analysis of the data looking at troponin-positive patients, treatment with tirofiban demonstrated a significant reduction in death and MI over heparin at both 48 h (3.4 vs. 0.3 percent) and at 30 days (13.0 vs. 4.3 percent, $p < 0.001$).[179] The second trial—Platelet Receptor Inhibition for Ischemic Syndrome Management in Patients Limited by Unstable Signs and

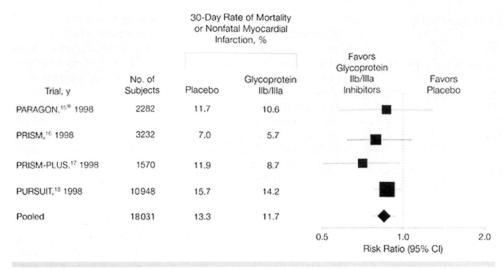

FIGURE 54-17 Pooled analysis of the 30-day rate of mortality or nonfatal MI for GP IIb/IIIa inhibitors in unstable angina and non-ST-elevation MI in the "4 P" trials. (From Bhatt and Topol.[400] With permission.)

patients who presented with anginal symptoms within 24 h with either a positive troponin or ST–segment depression and were randomized to either abciximab bolus plus 48-h infusion, abciximab bolus plus 24-h infusion, or placebo.[185] The study protocol espoused a conservative strategy by discouraging early catheterization and revascularization unless severe refractory ischemia occurred. At 30 days, the composite endpoint of death or MI was not statistically different across the three groups; even among the subgroup with positive troponin, there was no clinical benefit with abciximab. The results of this study demonstrate that abciximab is not appropriate therapy for patients with ACS who are not undergoing PCI.

Symptoms (PRISM-PLUS)—randomized 1915 patients, who were at higher risk than in PRISM, with chest pain at rest or with minimal exertion within 12 h with either ECG changes or positive cardiac enzymes to heparin, tirofiban, or both (Fig. 54-17).[180] An early invasive strategy was encouraged, consisting of a 48-h study drug pretreatment period followed by catheterization and revascularization if possible. Compared with heparin only, treatment with tirofiban plus heparin resulted in a 32 percent risk reduction in the composite of death, MI, and refractory ischemia at 7 days (17.9 vs. 12.9 percent, p = 0.004), which was maintained at 30 days and 6 months. The tirofiban monotherapy arm was terminated prematurely after interim analysis due to excessive mortality at 7 days compared to heparin (4.6 percent vs. 1.1 percent, p = 0.012), a treatment effect not seen in PRISM.

Lamifiban PARAGON A AND B The Platelet IIb/IIIa Antagonism for the Reduction of Acute Coronary Syndromes in a Global Organization Network (PARAGON) A trial was a dose-ranging precursor to the larger B trial, which represent the major research work on the small molecule lamifiban in non-ST-segment elevation ACS (Fig. 54-17). PARAGON A enrolled 2282 patients who had chest pain at rest within 12 h with ECG changes and randomly assigned them to 72 h of one of five strategies: high- or low-dose lamifiban with or without heparin or heparin alone.[181] Catheterization and revascularization were discouraged within the first 48 h. The study found no significant differences in the primary endpoint of death or MI at 30 days in any of the groups and, compared to heparin, high-dose lamifiban significantly increased hemorrhagic events. PARAGON B enrolled 5225 patients who were randomized to lamifiban with a dose tailored to their creatinine clearance or placebo, with the thought that the renally excreted lamifiban ad to be more accurately dosed to be effective (Fig. 54-17).[182,183] There was only a nonsignificant trend toward benefit in the lamifiban group compared to heparin at 30 days. The one positive finding was that in the subgroup of troponin-positive patients, there was a 43 percent reduction in death, MI, and severe recurrent ischemia at 30 days (19.4 vs. 11.0 percent) in those who received lamifiban.[184]

Abciximab GUSTO-IV The Global Use of Strategies To Open Occluded Coronary Arteries (GUSTO)-IV ACS trial enrolled 7800

Conclusions/Recommendations

Current 2002 ACC/AHA guidelines for antithrombotic therapy during non-ST-elevation MI reflect the concept that antithrombotic therapy depends on the reperfusion strategy employed (Table 54-5).[186] The one generalization that can be made is that an initial aspirin dose of at least 325 mg should be given to all patients who do not have a hypersensitivity reaction. In fact, the ACC/AHA guidelines establish aspirin therapy as level of evidence A and recommend that aspirin be administered as soon as possible after presentation and continued indefinitely.[186] For patients in whom early percutaneous intervention is planned, GP IIb/IIIa inhibition with either a small molecule started upstream in the emergency department or abciximab started in the catheterization lab is recommended (Table 54-5). Aspirin and clopidogrel should be used for at least 1 year following percutaneous intervention. Given the increased risk of bleeding during CABG with combination aspirin and clopidogrel seen in PCI-CURE[162] and CREDO[163] and the lack of incremental benefit with a clopidogrel loading dose in CREDO, clopidogrel may be delayed until after the diagnostic catheterization is completed and CABG is excluded as a revascularization alternative. In patients for whom a conservative, noninterventional approach is planned, aspirin plus clopidogrel initially and continued for at least 9 months would be the treatment of choice. The benefit of GP IIb/IIIa blockade is proportional to the patient's risk and eventual use of percutaneous intervention,[187] and as such the choice of using GP IIb/IIIa inhibitor should be individualized depending on patient risk.

ST-Elevation Myocardial Infarction

TREATED WITH FIBRINOLYTICS

Aspirin Multiple clinical trials over the past 15 years have established aspirin as not only critical to the treatment of ST-elevation MI but also one of the most cost-effective therapies for acute MI. In a metanalysis of 32 angiographic trials of acute ST-elevation MI, aspirin decreased the rate of reocclusion by over 50 percent.[188]

The Second International Study of Infarct Survival (ISIS-2) trial unequivocally established the efficacy of aspirin in reducing cardiovascular events during and immediately after acute MI.[39] A total of

TABLE 54-5 ACC/AHA Guidelines for Antiplatelet Therapy in Unstable Angina and Non-Q-Wave Myocardial Infarction

Class I

1. Antiplatelet therapy should be initiated promptly. ASA should be administered as soon as possible after presentation and continued indefinitely. (Level of Evidence: A)
2. Clopidogrel should be administered to hospitalized patients who are unable to take ASA because of hypersensitivity or major gastrointestinal intolerance. (Level of Evidence: A)
3. In hospitalized patients in whom an early noninterventional approach is planned, clopidogrel should be added to ASA as soon as possible on admission and administered for at least 1 month (Level of Evidence: A), and for up to 9 months. (Level of Evidence: B)[a]
4. A platelet GP IIb/IIIa antagonist should be administered, in addition to ASA and heparin, to patients in whom catheterization and PCI are planned. The GP IIb/IIIa antagonist may also be administered just prior to PCI. (Level of Evidence: A)[a]
5. In patients for whom a PCI is planned and who are not at high risk for bleeding, clopidogrel should be started and continued for at least 1 month (Level of Evidence: A) and for up to 9 months. (Level of Evidence: B)[a]
6. In patients taking clopidogrel in whom elective CABG is planned, the drug should be withheld for 5 to 7 days. (Level of Evidence: B)

Class IIa

1. Eptifibatide or tirofiban should be administered, in addition to ASA and LMWH or UFH, to patients with continuing ischemia, an elevated troponin, or with other high-risk features in whom an invasive management strategy is not planned. (Level of Evidence: A)[a]
2. A platelet GP IIb/ IIIa antagonist should be administered to patients already receiving heparin, ASA, and clopidogrel in whom catheterization and PCI are planned. The GP IIb/IIIa antagonist may also be administered just prior to PCI. (Level of Evidence: B)[a]

Class IIb

1. Ptifibatide or tirofiban, in addition to ASA and LMWH or UFH, to patients without continuing ischemia who have no other high-risk features and in whom PCI is not planned. (Level of Evidence: A)[a]

Class III

1. Intravenous fibrinolytic therapy in patients without acute ST-segment elevation, a true posterior MI, or a presumed new left bundle-branch block. (Level of Evidence: A)
2. Abciximab administration in patients in whom PCI is not planned. (Level of Evidence: A)[a]

[a]New indication, not included in September 2000 guidelines.
SOURCE: From Braunwald et al.[186] With permission.

17,187 patients presenting within 24 h of the onset of acute MI were randomized to receive either streptokinase, aspirin (160mg/day for 1 month), both, or neither. At the end of 5 weeks follow-up, patients receiving aspirin therapy had a 23 percent reduction in vascular mortality ($p < 0.0001$), 21 percent reduction in overall mortality ($p < 0.001$), a 36 percent reduction in stroke ($p < 0.01$), and a 44 percent reduction in reinfarction ($p < 0.00001$) compared to placebo. The study found no differences in the rates of major bleeding or cerebral hemorrhage between the two groups (0.4 vs. 0.4 percent). Aspirin was effective at all time points studied in the trial: when given in the first 4 h after MI (mortality reduction 25 percent), after 12 h (mortality reduction 21 percent), or after 12 to 24 h (mortality reduction 21 percent). These reductions translate into preventing 26 deaths and 10 to 15 nonfatal reinfarctions or strokes for every 1000 patients treated with aspirin for 1 month. While the 5-week vascular mortality rate was reduced by 25 percent in those treated with streptokinase alone, the addition of aspirin to streptokinase resulted in a 42 percent reduction in vascular mortality. At 10-year follow-up, the mortality benefit seen with aspirin was maintained.[189]

The Antithrombotic Trialists' Collaboration reviewed 15 trials of 19,288 patients with suspected acute MI, nearly all of whom were in the ISIS-2 trial.[148] Treatment with antiplatelet therapy, mostly aspirin 160 mg daily, for a mean of duration 1 month resulted in 38 fewer serious vascular events, 13 fewer reinfarctions ($p < 0.0001$), 23 fewer vascular deaths ($p < 0.0001$), and 2 fewer strokes ($p = 0.02$) per 1000 patients treated. These benefits were far in excess of the risk of major extracranial bleeds, which was estimated to be about one or two additional bleeds per 1000 patients treated with aspirin.

Parenteral Glycoprotein IIb/IIIa Inhibitors Although thrombolytic therapy has proved to be a major advance in the treatment of patients with acute MI, current thrombolytic regimens have several limitations: (1) failure of initial reperfusion,[190] (2) inadequate perfusion with delayed flow (TIMI grade 2 flow),[190] (3) imperfect myocardial perfusion,[191] and (4) infarct-related artery reocclusion/reinfarction in a significant percentage of patients.[192] Because platelets play a central role in coronary thrombosis—especially failed reperfusion, reocclusion, and reinfarction—attention has turned to the GP IIb/IIIa inhibitors as a means of improving current reperfusion regimens.[193] Treatment directed at both the thrombus with a fibrinolytic agent and the platelet aggregate with a GP IIb/IIIa inhibitor might achieve more rapid, complete, and sustained coronary reperfusion.

Lack of initial reperfusion, which could be termed *thrombolytic resistance*, appears to be due to several mechanisms:

1. Fibrinolytic agents act only on the fibrin portion of the thrombus, leaving activated platelets as a source of rethrombosis.
2. Platelets elaborate PAI-1, which inhibits the action of the thrombolytic agent; platelets also release other agents, such as TXA_2, which causes local vasoconstriction.[194]
3. Lysis of clot-bound fibrin exposes clot-bound thrombin, which remains catalytically active and can cleave fibrinogen to fibrin, facilitating rethrombosis.[195] In addition, thrombosis can stimulate further thrombin production and activation of platelets.[196]
4. Thrombolytic therapy also has a direct platelet-activating effect, leading to increased levels of TXA_2 and platelet-activating factor. The presence of aspirin does not abolish the platelet-activating effect of fibrinolytic therapy.[194]

Thus, thrombolysis promotes platelet activation and therefore actually creates an environment that may lead to subsequent rethrombosis and/or reocclusion.

Abciximab Several dose-ranging patency pilot studies established the prospect of improved outcomes with abciximab combination therapy. The Strategies for Patency Enhancement in the Emergency Department (SPEED)[197] enrolled 530 patients and the Thrombolysis in Myocardial Infarction (TIMI)-14 trial[198] evaluated 888 patients with ST-elevation MI. In the two trials, regimens of abciximab alone, abciximab plus various doses of reteplase, standard-dose reteplase, accelerated-dose alteplase, or abciximab plus reduced doses of alteplase or streptokinase were all studied. In SPEED, TIMI 3 flow at 90 min was significantly improved with the best combination of abciximab, reteplase, and heparin over controls (61 percent combination vs. 47 percent reteplase vs. 27 percent abciximab). In TIMI-14, the most promising regimen involved reduced-dose alteplase plus abciximab, which resulted in TIMI 3 flow at 90 min in 77 percent of subjects. There was no significant increase in hemorrhagic complications in the combined therapy group. These pilot studies were not powered to detect differences in clinical outcomes, but based on data from GUSTO-1, a 23 percent improvement in TIMI 3 flow at 90 min would be associated with a 1 percent decrease in mortality.[41,64]

The Global Use of Strategies To Open Occluded Coronary Arteries (GUSTO) V trial enrolled 16,588 patients with ST-elevation MI of less than 6 h duration and randomly assigned them to either standard-dose reteplase or half-dose reteplase plus full-dose abciximab.[199] At 30 days, the reteplase-plus-abciximab arm had a nonsignificant 0.3 percent absolute (5.9 vs. 5.6 percent) and 5 percent relative reduction in the primary endpoint of mortality and nonsignificant reductions in most secondary endpoints. The secondary endpoint that did reach statistical significance was a 34 percent reduction (2.3 vs. 3.5 percent, $p < 0.0001$) in reinfarction at 7 days. This benefit was achieved at a cost of statistically significant increases in mild and severe bleeding (overall 13.7 percent vs. 24.6 percent) and blood transfusions in the combination group (Fig. 54-1). Although there was no difference in mortality between the two treatment groups at 1 year of follow-up, patients who experienced reinfarction had a significant increase in 1-year mortality (22.6 vs. 8.0 percent, $p < 0.001$).[200]

The Assessment of the Safety and Efficacy of a New Thrombolytic Regimen (ASSENT)-3 trial examined abciximab in combination with another fibrinolytic agent, tenecteplase.[98] In the two arms of the study evaluating abciximab, 4065 patients with ST-elevation MI of less than 6 h duration were randomized to either standard-dose tenecteplase or half-dose tenecteplase plus abciximab. The half-dose tenecteplase–plus-abciximab group was found to have a 28 percent reduction in the primary endpoint (a composite of death, in-hospital reinfarction, or in-hospital refractory ischemia at 30 days) compared to the standard-dose group (11.1 vs. 15.4 percent, $p = 0.0001$). The majority of the benefit was derived from a reduction in reinfarction and refractory ischemia, as there was no statistically significant difference in mortality. While there were no differences in the rate of ICH, there was a significant increase in the rate of major bleeding in the abciximab arm (4.4 vs. 2.2 percent, $p = 0.0005$).

Eptifibatide The small-molecule GP IIb/IIIa inhibitor eptifibatide has been studied in conjunction with fibrinolytics in somewhat less detail than abciximab. The Integrilin to Minimize Platelet Aggregation and Prevent Coronary Thrombosis in Acute Myocardial Infarction (IMPACT-AMI) trial[201] and the Integrilin and Low-Dose Thrombolysis in Acute Myocardial Infarction (INTRO-AMI) trial[202] studied 180 patients and 649 patients respectively with ST-elevation MI of less than 6 h duration. The most promising dose combinations in both studies demonstrated significantly increased rates of TIMI 3 flow at 60 or 90 min with t-PA plus eptifibatide compared to t-PA alone (66 vs. 39 percent, $p = 0.006$ for IMPACT-AMI and 56 vs. 40 percent, $p = 0.04$ for INTRO-AMI). There was no statistically significant increase in major bleeding with combination therapy in either study. In contrast, another dose-ranging study with streptokinase of 181 patients by Ronner et al.[203] showed no statistically significant improvement in TIMI 3 flow at 90 min, and there was a significant increase in major and minor bleeding and transfusion requirements with eptifibatide.

The as yet unpublished INTEGRITI trial studied the effects of reduced-dose tenecteplase for the treatment of acute ST-elevation MI in 350 patients. INTEGRITI is the first trial of eptifibatide combined with fibrinolytics with clinical endpoints. This study showed that combination therapy improved ST-segment recovery, TIMI flow, and TIMI frame count compared to fibrinolytic alone.[204–207]

Lamifiban Lamifiban, another small-molecule GP IIb/IIIa inhibitor, has been studied in conjunction with fibrinolytics only in a single small dose-ranging study. Lamifiban was evaluated in 353 subjects with ST-elevation MIs treated with streptokinase or t-PA in the Platelet Aggregation Receptor Antagonist Dose Investigation and Reperfusion Gain in Myocardial Infarction (PARADIGM) trial.[208] While the study was not powered to detect clinical differences between the groups, it did demonstrate improvement in the speed and stability of ST-segment resolution as measured by continuous ECG monitoring, but at the cost of an increase in major bleeding episodes.

PERCUTANEOUS CORONARY INTERVENTION AS THE PRIMARY STRATEGY

Aspirin Percutaneous coronary interventions result in local vascular trauma with damage to the vascular endothelium and exposure of the subendothelium, creating a highly thrombogenic milieu. Antiplatelet therapy is therefore essential to prevent intraluminal thrombus development and either acute or subacute thrombosis of the vessel. Several studies have demonstrated decreases in acute complications of angioplasty using combination therapy of aspirin and dipyridamole, although the combination provides little additional advantage over aspirin alone.[209,210] In patients undergoing coronary stenting compared to aspirin alone or aspirin plus warfarin, the combination of aspirin (325 mg daily) and ticlopidine (500 mg daily) significantly reduced the 30-day combined endpoint of death, target vessel revascularization, angiographic thrombosis, or MI (RR 0.15 for combined therapy

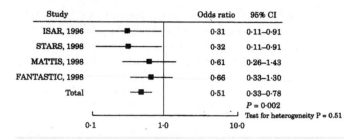

FIGURE 54-18 Death or myocardial infarction in trials of aspirin plus ticlopidine versus aspirin plus oral anticoagulation after coronary stenting. (From the Cure Study Investigators.[158] With permission.)

vs. aspirin alone).[211] This benefit was seen in both low[211] and high-risk[212] patients.

Thienopyridines TICLOPIDINE A number of randomized studies have examined the combination of ticlopidine plus aspirin compared to either aspirin alone or oral anticoagulation in the context of intracoronary stenting (Figs. 54-18 and 54-19). The Intracoronary Stenting and Antithrombotic Regimen (ISAR) study randomized 517 patients to combined antiplatelet or anticoagulant therapy,[213] Hall et al. randomized 226 patients after intravascular ultrasound-guided stent placement to ticlopidine plus aspirin or aspirin alone,[214] the Multicenter Aspirin and Ticlopidine Trial after Intracoronary Stenting (MATTIS) study allocated 350 high-risk patients to combined antiplatelet or anticoagulant therapy,[212] the Full Anticoagulation versus Aspirin and Ticlopidine (FANTASTIC) trial randomized 485 intermediate-risk subjects to the same therapy,[215] and the Stent Anticoagulation Restenosis Study (STARS) compared all three treatment strategies in 1653 low-risk subjects.[211] A metanalysis of these trials demonstrated a marked benefit of aspirin plus ticlopidine in reducing death or MI compared with aspirin alone (OR 0.23, 95 percent CI 0.11 to 0.49, $p = 0.0001$) or compared with aspirin plus warfarin (OR 0.51, 95 percent CI 0.33 to 0.78, $p = 0.002$). Due to safety considerations, a 1 percent incidence of severe pancytopenia, clopidogrel has largely supplanted ticlopidine's role in this setting.

CLOPIDOGREL Several studies have compared the combination of clopidogrel and aspirin with ticlopidine and aspirin after coronary stenting. Moussa et al. compared 1406 patients receiving ticlopidine and aspirin with 283 patients taking clopidogrel and aspirin.[216] Berger et al. reviewed 500 patients treated with clopidogrel and aspirin and 827 patients given ticlopidine and aspirin,[217] Muller et al. studied 700 patients randomized to either therapy,[218] the Clopidogrel Aspirin International Cooperative Study (CLASSICS) randomized 1020 subjects into two clopidogrel groups and one ticlopidine

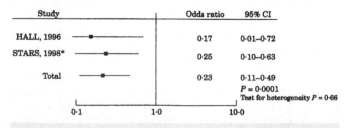

FIGURE 54-19 Death or myocardial infarction in trials of aspirin plus ticlopidine versus aspirin plus oral anticoagulation after coronary stenting. (From the Cure Study Investigators.[158] With permission.)

group,[219] and Mishkel et al. examined a prospective database of 875 patients treated with one of the two agents.[220] The study on which current practice is based was CLASSICS, which compared three treatment regimens: a 28-day regimen of either (1) 300 mg clopidogrel loading dose and 325 mg aspirin on day 1, followed by 75 mg of clopidogrel and 325 mg of aspirin daily; (2) 75 mg of clopidogrel and 325 mg of aspirin daily; or (3) 500 mg of ticlopidine and 325 mg of aspirin daily.[219] Major adverse cardiac events (cardiac death, MI, or target lesion revascularization) were low overall and not significantly different among the groups (0.9 percent with ticlopidine, 1.5 percent with 75 mg/day clopidogrel, 1.2 percent with the clopidogrel loading dose, $p = NS$). The primary endpoint was a combined safety endpoint that occurred in 9.1 percent of patients in the ticlopidine group and 4.6 percent of patients in the combined clopidogrel group (RR 0.50, 95 percent CI 0.31 to 0.81, $p = 0.005$). As a whole, these trials suggest that the combination of aspirin and clopidogrel is better tolerated and at least as safe and effective as aspirin and ticlopidine.

PARENTERAL GLYCOPROTEIN IIB/IIIA INHIBITORS
Abciximab is the GP IIb/IIIa inhibitor that has been most thoroughly evaluated for use in conjunction with percutaneous intervention in the setting of acute MI, while eptifibatide is beginning to accumulate data in this setting.

Abciximab RAPPORT The ReoPro in Acute Myocardial Infarction and Primary PTCA Organization and Randomized Trial (RAPPORT) study was the first to look at the use of GP IIb/IIIa inhibitors in this setting.[221] The trial randomized 483 patients who presented for primary angioplasty with acute ST-elevation MI of less than 12 h duration to abciximab bolus plus 12-h infusion or placebo. By intention-to-treat analysis, there was no significant difference between the two groups in the composite endpoint of death, reinfarction, or target-vessel revascularization at 6 months, 7 days, and 30 days. However, there was a trend toward benefit with abciximab treatment, which became even more apparent in the treated-patient analysis. Abciximab provided most of its benefit by significantly reducing the need for urgent target vessel revascularization by 78 percent at 7 days, 74 percent at 30 days, and 62 percent at 6 months—also by reducing the need for "unplanned bailout" stenting by 42 percent. Unfortunately, there was a near doubling of major bleeding (16.6 vs. 9.5 percent) and transfusion requirements (13.7 vs. 7.9 percent) in the abciximab group, which may have been related to the heparin dose and late sheath removal.

Several small studies have also been performed looking at alternative endpoints. In the Intracoronary Stenting and Antithrombotic Regimen-2 (ISAR-2) trial 401 patients presenting for stent placement within 48 h of ST-elevation MI were randomized to abciximab or heparin and followed to assess for restenosis at 6 months.[222] Although no difference was found in rates of restenosis, the abciximab group showed statistical benefit in reducing the composite endpoint of death, reinfarction, and target lesion revascularization by 52 percent (5.0 vs. 10.5 percent) at 30 days. At 1 year, the absolute difference was still 5.7 percent, but it was no longer statistically significant. The Glycoprotein Receptor Antagonist Patency Evaluation (GRAPE) study enrolled 60 patients presenting for primary PTCA within 6 h of onset of symptoms of ST-elevation MI who were given a bolus and infusion of abciximab prior to catheterization and were then assessed for angiographic vessel patency.[223] Catheterization at 45 min after drug administration found TIMI 2 or 3 flow in 40 percent, with TIMI 3 flow in 18 percent compared to 27 percent and 8 percent in controls who received aspirin and heparin only. And in a study of 200 patients undergoing stenting within 48 h of ST-elevation

MI randomized to abciximab or placebo by Neumann et al.,[224] myocardial flow rates and changes in left ventricular function were assessed at 14 days. Statistically significant improvement was seen in both flow velocities and overall ejection fraction in the abciximab group. In addition the composite clinical endpoint of death, reinfarction, and target vessel revascularization was significantly reduced with abciximab at 30 days. The Stent versus Thrombolysis for Occluded Coronary Arteries in Patients with Acute Myocardial Infarction (STOPAMI-1) trial reconfirmed that mechanical reperfusion with abciximab is a reasonable approach for acute MI.[225] The study randomized 140 patients with ST-elevation MI of less than 12 h duration to either stent plus abciximab or alteplase. The stent-plus-abciximab group was found to have improved myocardial salvage (primary endpoint) as determined by serial scintigraphic studies and also an improvement of 63 percent in a secondary composite endpoint of death, reinfarction, and stroke at 6 months (8.5 vs. 23.2 percent).

ADMIRAL   The Abciximab before Direct Angioplasty and Stenting in Myocardial Infarction Regarding Acute and Long-Term Follow-up (ADMIRAL) trial randomized 300 patients with ST-elevation MI scheduled to undergo primary intracoronary stenting to either abciximab or placebo.[226] The primary composite endpoint of death, reinfarction, or urgent target-vessel revascularization was reduced by 59 percent in the abciximab group (6.0 vs. 14.6 percent, $p = 0.01$) at 30 days and the benefit persisted to the 6-month follow-up. The clinical outcome was linked to the incidence of angiographic TIMI 3 flow, which was significantly higher in the abciximab group before the procedure, immediately afterwards, and at 6 months. Diabetics who received abciximab had a statistically significant reduction in mortality (0 vs. 16.7 percent, $p = 0.02$) and in the composite of death, reinfarction, and any revascularization (20.7 vs. 50.0 percent, $p = 0.02$) at 6 months.

CADILLAC   The Controlled Abciximab and Device Investigation to Lower Late Angioplasty Complications (CADILLAC) study enrolled 2082 patients presenting with ST-elevation MI and followed them for 6 months for the occurrence of the primary endpoint of death, reinfarction, urgent target-vessel revascularization, and stroke.[227] Patients were randomized using a 2×2 factorial design: stent plus abciximab, PTCA plus abciximab, stent plus placebo, and PTCA plus placebo. At 6 months, the major finding was that the composite endpoint was roughly halved with stent placement compared to PTCA (20.0 percent with PTCA, 16.5 percent with PTCA plus abciximab, 11.5 percent with stenting, and 10.2 percent with stenting plus abciximab), as was angiographically determined restenosis (40.8 vs. 22.2 percent). The reduction in primary endpoint was due entirely to differences in rates of target-vessel revascularization, not to reductions in death, reinfarction, or even TIMI 3 flow. Only stenting compared to PTCA demonstrated any statistical benefit in this study, as the comparison of abciximab versus placebo showed only trends toward benefit. This decreased efficacy of abciximab compared to the ADMIRAL study has been partially attributed to the low-risk population enrolled, as reflected by the much lower mortality rate when compared to other primary PCI trials.

Eptifibatide   Limited data involving eptifibatide consist mostly of substudies and pilot studies. The RAPIER trial was a pilot study of 60 patients presenting with ST-elevation MI to be treated with primary angioplasty randomized to either eptifibatide pretreatment or routine care.[228] Pretreatment resulted in TIMI 2 or 3 flow in 57 percent of patients, compared with 13 percent in the control group ($p = 0.001$), and a reduced time from angiography to balloon inflation (10 vs. 22 min). A substudy of 333 patients in the INTRO-AMI trial involved immediate PCI in patients presenting with ST-elevation MI treated with eptifibatide plus reduced-dose t-PA.[229] The corrected TIMI frame count was significantly lower in patients after PCI facilitated by eptifibatide plus t-PA and compared to t-PA alone (17.8 vs. 23.5 percent, $p = 0.0001$). The corrected frame count was also lower following PCI in the group pretreated with eptifibatide plus t-PA (17.8 vs. 20.0 percent, $p = 0.02$), and procedural success was higher if the artery was open at the time of intervention (86 vs. 68 percent, $p = 0.002$). The INTEGRITI trial included 153 patients who underwent facilitated PCI for ST-elevation MI after eptifibatide and reduced-dose tenecteplase.[205] Facilitated intervention was associated with a high rate of vessel patency (TIMI 3 flow 91 percent and TIMI 2 flow 9 percent) and myocardial tissue reperfusion (82 percent complete ST resolution 90 min later).

Conclusions/Recommendations

The current ACC/AHA and ACCP guidelines recommend the routine use of aspirin (160 to 325 mg) on presentation with acute ST-elevation MI.[37,126] Both guidelines also suggest that aspirin be given at the time of primary PCI for acute MI, as aspirin reduces the frequency of ischemic complications after coronary angioplasty.[230,231] Although the minimum effective aspirin dosage in the setting of coronary angioplasty has not been established, a dose of 80 to 325 mg given at least 2 h before PCI is recommended. Only the thienopyridine derivatives, ticlopidine and clopidogrel, have been routinely used as alternative antiplatelet agents in aspirin-sensitive patients during coronary angioplasty. Again both the ACC/AHA and ACCP guidelines further suggest that if a coronary stent is implanted, clopidogrel as a 300-mg loading dose and then 75 mg/day should be given in conjunction with the aspirin and in the place of ticlopidine, which has important side effects.

At the current time, the role of GP IIb/IIIa inhibitors in conjunction with reduced-dose fibrinolytics is still being studied, but current trials demonstrate certain reproducible findings. Combination therapy consistently results in less reinfarction without corresponding reductions in mortality, but at the expense of increased bleeding. Future studies will need to address the issues of why decreased rates of reinfarction do not translate into decreased mortality, why there appears to be a difference in efficacy with the fibrinolytic agent used, and how to use this combination in an aging population at increased risk for bleeding complications. Whether this reperfusion strategy will play a role in the future without being incorporated into a facilitated PCI framework remains to be seen.

Currently, the role of GP IIb/IIIa inhibitors in the setting of ST-elevation MI treated primarily by PCI is still the subject of ongoing studies. Numerous studies have proven the superiority of primary PCI over fibrinolytics, even in the setting of delaying therapy while awaiting transfer to a facility that can perform PCIs.[232] This practice of direct intervention as the primary reperfusion strategy replacing fibrinolytics is likely to progress as the population ages (increased bleeding risks with fibrinolytics will pose contraindication to lysis for greater proportions of MI patients) and as more data emerge for performing PCI in centers without surgical backup.[127] Currently GP IIb/IIIa inhibition is integral to the practice of PCI, especially in high-risk patient cohorts. Unresolved issues include whether to start the GP IIb/IIIa inhibitor early at presentation or instead wait until the intervention is to be performed. At present, abciximab would seem to be the preferred agent as it has the strongest body of evidence in its favor, while eptifibatide is currently being studied in more depth.

Secondary Prevention

While there are over 1.1 million MIs annually in the United States, 450,000 of these represent reinfarctions.[233] Furthermore, there are over 7.5 million people alive with a history of MI, and they have a 15 to 20 percent risk of dying or having a reinfarction in the 2 to 5 years following their initial infarction.[233] Secondary prevention is therefore of utmost importance in decreasing the overall morbidity and mortality of coronary heart disease.

ASPIRIN

As previously described, the ISIS-2 trial was a landmark study responsible for establishing the efficacy of aspirin in reducing cardiovascular events during and after acute MI.[39] Patients were treated for a total duration of 1 month of aspirin (160 mg/day) and experienced a reduction in vascular mortality of 23 percent ($p < 0.0001$) that was maintained over 10 years of follow-up.[189] In addition, there were also significant reductions in all-cause mortality, stroke, and reinfarction without increases in major bleeding or cerebral hemorrhage during aspirin therapy.

The Antithrombotic Trialists' Collaboration analyzed data from 12 trials involving 18,788 patients with a history of MI treated with aspirin or other platelet inhibitors (the majority received aspirin) who received therapy for a mean duration of 27 months.[148] Treatment resulted in 36 fewer serious vascular events per 1000 patients treated, which reflects significant reductions in reinfarction (18 per 1000), vascular death (14 per 1000), and nonfatal stroke (5 per 1000). The Collaboration also reviewed 195 trials examining the long-term use of antiplatelet therapy (again mostly aspirin) in 135,640 patients at high-risk to develop occlusive arterial disease. Among these high-risk patients, antiplatelet therapy reduced the risk of serious vascular events by 19 percent, nonfatal MI by 34 percent, the risk of stroke by 25 percent, and the risk of vascular death by 15 percent ($p < 0.0001$).

Recent data from metanalysis indicate that high-dose (500- to 1500-mg) aspirin is no more effective at reducing cardiovascular events than medium- (160- to 325-mg) or low-dose (75- to 150-mg) aspirin during long-term chronic administration (Fig. 54-20).[148] Among trials comparing varying doses of aspirin to placebo, the proportional reduction in vascular events was 19 percent with 500 to 1500 mg, 26 percent with 160 to 325 mg, and 32 percent with 75 to 160 mg. Higher-dose aspirin has been associated with increased gastrotoxicity.[128] Thus, the available evidence supports a daily dose of 75 to 160 mg for secondary prevention and a loading dose of 160 to 325 mg in acute clinical situations when an immediate effect is required. Very low doses of aspirin (<75 mg/day) have been less widely assessed than low-dose aspirin, but the available data suggest that very low doses are less effective (13 percent reduction in events).[148]

The risks associated with aspirin administration in patients with vascular disease are small but real and include mainly bleeding complications such as gastrointestinal toxicity and hemorrhagic stroke. The ACCP Consensus Conference on Antithrombotic Therapy reports that the absolute excess of ICH with aspirin therapy is < 1 per 1000 in high-risk trials,[234] and a metanalysis of 16 trials comprising 55,462 patients demonstrated an increased relative risk of 1.84.[235] Gastrointestinal side effects have also been shown to be increased with aspirin therapy, with an incidence of minor gastrointestinal symptoms of 5.2 to 40 percent in aspirin users compared to 0.7 to 34 percent of patients taking placebo, peptic ulcers in 0.8 to 2.6 vs. 0 to 1.2 percent, and major gastrointestinal bleeding in <1 percent in both groups.[128] A metanalysis of 24 aspirin therapy trials and almost 66,000 participants found that gastrointestinal bleeding occurred in 2.47 percent of patients taking aspirin versus 1.42 percent of those taking placebo, corresponding to an odds ratio of 1.68.[236] While this metanalysis did not support a statistically significant reduction in bleeding with reduced aspirin dose (1.5 percent relative risk reduction per 100 mg reduction of aspirin dose), a previous overview found that gastrointestinal toxicity was dose-related with daily doses between 30 and 1300 mg.[237] The United Kingdom Transient Ischemic Attack (UK-TIA) trial supported this dose response relationship, finding that gastrointestinal symptoms were significantly

Category of trial	No of trials with data	No (%) of vascular events Allocated antiplatelet	No (%) of vascular events Adjusted control	Observed-expected	Variance	Odds ratio (CI) Antiplatelet : control	% Odds reduction (SE)
Aspirin alone (mg daily):							
500-1500	34	1621/11 215 (14.5)	1930/11 236 (17.2)	-147.1	707.8		19 (3)
160-325	19	1526/13 240 (11.5)	1963/13 273 (14.8)	-219.9	742.6		26 (3)
75-150	12	366/3370 (10.9)	517/3406 (15.2)	-72.0	183.8		32 (6)
<75	3	316/1827 (17.3)	354/1828 (19.4)	-18.9	136.5		13 (8)
Any aspirin*	65	3829/29 652 (12.9)	4764/29 743 (16.0)	-452.3	1717.0		23 (2)

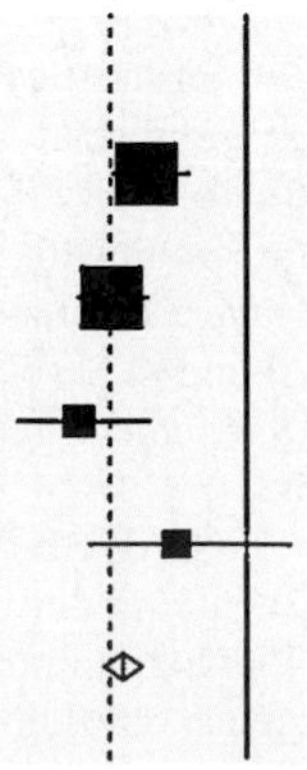

FIGURE 54-20 Data from the Antithrombotic Trialists' Collaboration indicate that high-dose (500–1500 mg) aspirin is no more effective at reducing cardiovascular events than medium (160–325 mg) or low dose (75–150 mg) during long-term chronic administration. (From the Antithrombotic Trialists' Collaboration.[148] With permission.)

more frequent in the high-dose (1200 mg/day) group than in the low-dose (300 mg/day) group.[238] A recent analysis looked at the risks and benefits of aspirin therapy for secondary prevention of vascular events and found that the number needed to treat with aspirin to prevent one death from any cause was 67, while 100 patients would need to be treated to detect one nonfatal gastrointestinal tract hemorrhage.[239]

While aspirin reduces the risk of cardiovascular events and death by 25 percent, it appears that aspirin's antiplatelet effect may not be uniform in all patients, as 10 to 20 percent of those treated with aspirin have recurrent vascular events.[240] Clinical aspirin resistance includes patients who, despite being on therapeutic doses of aspirin, experience thrombotic or embolic vascular events. Measurements of platelet aggregation, platelet reactivity, bleeding time, and TXA_2 production have confirmed the variable effect of aspirin on individual patients.[241] Previous studies have estimated that between 8 and 45 percent of the population are aspirin-resistant[241]; current explanations include the fact that platelet can be activated by pathways not blocked by aspirin, that higher doses of aspirin may be necessary to achieve optimal antithrombotic effect in some patients, and that certain patients can generate TXA_2 despite usual therapeutic doses of aspirin.

THIENOPYRIDINES

Clopidogrel CLOPIDOGREL VERSUS ASPIRIN The Clopidogrel versus Aspirin in Patients at Risk of Ischaemic Events (CAPRIE) trial was designed to assess the efficacy of clopidogrel compared to aspirin in preventing cardiovascular events in patients with known atherosclerotic vascular disease.[242] Over 19,000 patients with either recent ischemic stroke (within the previous 6 months), recent MI (within the previous 35 days), or symptomatic peripheral vascular disease were randomized to either clopidogrel (75 mg/day) or aspirin (325 mg/day) and were followed for an average of 1.9 years for the occurrence of the composite endpoint of ischemic stroke, MI, or vascular death. The intention-to-treat analysis demonstrated a relative risk reduction of 8.7 percent (95 percent CI 0.3 to 16.5 percent, $p = 0.043$) in favor of clopidogrel, with an on-treatment analysis yielding a relative risk reduction of 9.4 percent. The reduction in the composite endpoint was driven mostly by a 16 percent reduction in nonfatal MIs and a 22 percent reduction in fatal MIs. There were no major differences in side effects, with aspirin showing an increase in gastrointestinal hemorrhage (2.66 vs. 1.99 percent), gastrointestinal intolerance (17.59 vs. 15.01 percent), and neutropenia (0.17 vs. 0.10 percent) and clopidogrel having an increase in rash (6.02 vs. 4.61 percent). Interestingly, there was a nonstatistically significant trend toward lack of benefit of clopidogrel in the MI subgroup (event rate of 5.03 vs. 4.84 percent, $p = 0.66$). To clarify this issue, all patients with a previous history of MI in the group with ischemic stroke and peripheral vascular disease (2144) were combined with the patients in the group with MI (6302) and found to have a nonsignificant 7.4 percent (95 percent CI to 5.2 to 18.6 percent) relative risk reduction in the composite primary endpoint.

Another secondary analysis of the CAPRIE data was undertaken in the 617 patients who developed acute MI during the follow-up period.[243] The analysis found that clopidogrel imparted a 19.2 percent relative risk reduction in the occurrence of MI, that the risk of infarction was lower for clopidogrel in all risk categories, and that the benefit was consistent across all subgroups. The combined event rates for the 1480 patients with a history of CABG were also reviewed in a secondary analysis.[244] There was a 36.3 percent relative risk reduction (95 percent CI 13.4 to 53.1 percent, $p = 0.004$) in the CAPRIE

composite endpoint of vascular death, MI, and ischemic stroke. As a result of the CAPRIE study, clopidogrel was approved for the reduction of atherosclerotic events in patients with recent strokes, MIs, or established peripheral vascular disease.

CLOPIDOGREL PLUS ASPIRIN The Clopidogrel in Unstable Angina to Prevent Recurrent Events (CURE) trial examined the use of clopidogrel plus aspirin in acute coronary syndromes and their continued use for secondary prevention of MI.[160] The study randomized 12,562 patients who presented within 24 h of onset of symptoms with ECG changes or elevated cardiac enzymes to either clopidogrel (300 mg load followed by 75 mg/day) or placebo in addition to aspirin (75 to 325 mg/day). Patients were treated for a mean duration of 9 months and followed for a primary outcome of a composite of cardiovascular death, MI, or stroke. After a year of follow-up, there was a 20 percent relative risk reduction with clopidogrel (95 percent CI 0.10 to 0.28, $p < 0.001$). Event reductions were seen during the acute phase in the first 30 days (21 percent relative risk reduction) and also during the chronic phase of prevention from 30 days to the end of the study (18 percent relative risk reduction). There were significantly more patients with major (3.7 vs. 2.7 percent) and minor (5.1 vs. 2.4 percent) bleeding in the clopidogrel group than the placebo group, but there was no significant increase in life-threatening bleeding or hemorrhagic stroke. In a retrospective analysis of bleeding events in the CURE study, it was found that the major and life-threatening bleeding risks with the combination of clopidogrel and aspirin were dose-dependent, while there was no increase in efficacy with increasing aspirin doses.[161] Integration of the results of the CURE study into current practice has been limited, since the trial was conducted in a mostly European environment of conservative, noninvasive management in which only 5.9 to 7.2 percent of patients received GP IIb/IIIa inhibitors and only about 20 percent underwent a revascularization procedure during their hospitalization. This practice was quite different from the more aggressive, invasive North American style and has limited the applicability of the trial findings. Although not strictly a secondary prevention study, CURE suggests that there is benefit to the chronic addition of clopidogrel to aspirin after MI, but at the cost of increased bleeding.

The Clopidogrel for the Reduction of Events During Observation (CREDO) trial investigated the use of long-term clopidogrel combined with aspirin to prevent cardiovascular events after PCI.[163] Although CREDO was not specifically designed as a secondary prevention study as patients were enrolled after elective PCI, 13 percent of subjects had a history of a prior MI and over 50 percent were enrolled with unstable angina. However, the second part of the study randomized 2116 subjects treated with clopidogrel for the standard 28 days to either further clopidogrel (75 mg/day) or placebo, with all subjects taking daily aspirin (81 to 325 mg). At 1 year there was a 26.9 percent relative risk reduction (95 percent CI 3.9 to 44.4 percent, $p = 0.02$) in the composite primary endpoint of death, MI, and stroke. The benefit occurred beyond the standard 28-day period of treatment, as there was a 37.4 percent (95 percent CI 1.8 to 60.1 percent, $p = 0.04$) relative risk reduction from 4 weeks to 1 year (see also Chap. 58). There was a trend toward an increase in major bleeding in the clopidogrel group (8.8 vs. 6.7 percent, $p = 0.7$) with approximately two-thirds of all major bleeds occurring in patients undergoing CABG. In the recently reported CRUSADE registry, 62 percent of ACS patients underwent diagnostic cardiac angiography and 36 percent underwent PCI.[245] As the routine invasive approach to patients with ACS continues to emerge as the predominant strategy, combination clopidogrel and aspirin is likely to be adopted as standard care for secondary prevention after PCI.

ORAL GLYCOPROTEIN IIB/IIIA INHIBITORS

Platelet activation and aggregation is a major component of coronary thrombosis and ACS. While platelets can be activated via several different mechanisms, the final common pathway of platelet aggregation involves the GP IIb/IIIa receptor. The effectiveness of the intravenous GP IIb/IIIa inhibitors for the medical treatment of acute coronary syndromes and as adjunctive therapy for PCI have been well established.[246,247] In ACS, most of the benefit of these agents occurs during infusion, with little benefit accruing after treatment. After episodes of ACS, heightened platelet activity persists and correlates with ongoing ischemia and mortality.[248] Ongoing platelet activity thereby plays an integral role in the pathophysiology of recurrent ischemic events. The secondary prevention benefits of aspirin and the thienopyridines are well established, as they provide a 25 to 30 percent relative risk reduction in vascular events despite being only relatively weak platelet antagonists.[148] Therefore the oral GP IIb/IIIa inhibitors, which have more effective platelet inhibition than these agents, promise to have increased clinical benefit.

Oral GP IIb/IIIa inhibitors are peptidomimetic agents that are competitive inhibitors of the GP IIb/IIIa receptor. They are usually prodrugs, which are absorbed and then converted to active compounds in the blood.[249–255] The oral agents all have longer half-lives, such that they can be given once, twice, or three times daily to achieve relatively steady levels of GP IIb/IIIa inhibition. With oral dosing, long-term therapy (i.e., longer than 1 year) is possible. As with the intravenous compounds, two major groups of drugs exist in the oral class: those with competitive inhibition and short "off time" from the receptor (where a high drug level is critical to achieving high levels of platelet inhibition) and those that have "tight" binding to the platelet (similar to abciximab), with the majority of the drug circulating bound to platelets.

Promising results were seen in phase II pilot studies of all of the oral GP IIb/IIIa inhibitors subsequently brought to larger phase III clinical trials.[250,252,253,255] In the pilot studies, these agents achieved effective, dose-related chronic platelet inhibition ranging from the levels attained by placebo to near complete inhibition as measured by 20 μmol/L ADP-induced platelet aggregation at 4 weeks, but at the expense of a relatively high incidence of minor bleeding, usually bruising or mucocutaneous.

Sibrafiban SYMPHONY-I The first Sibrafiban Versus Aspirin to Yield Maximum Protection from Ischemic Heart Events Post-acute Coronary Syndromes (SYMPHONY) trial was a randomized, double-blind, aspirin-controlled trial of two regimens of sibrafiban for the treatment of patients following an ACS.[256] A total of 9233 patients with either AMI or high-risk unstable angina (with ST deviation of 0.5 mm or more) who were stabilized for at least 12 h were randomized to receive either aspirin (80 mg every 12 h) or high-dose or low-dose sibrafiban (without aspirin) every 12 h for a total of 3 months. The dose of sibrafiban was either 3, 4.5, or 6 mg, based on body weight and renal function. The primary efficacy endpoint was a composite of death, MI, and severe recurrent ischemia. There was no difference in the primary endpoint between aspirin (9.8 percent), low-dose sibrafiban (10.1 percent), and high-dose sibrafiban (10.1 percent). Similarly, there were no differences in mortality alone, MI, or recurrent ischemia. Major bleeding was significantly more common with the two sibrafiban groups, high-dose (5.7 percent) and low-dose (5.2 percent), compared with aspirin (3.9 percent).

SYMPHONY-II The second SYMPHONY trial, which was terminated early at the time the SYMPHONY-I results were available, studied the combination of low-dose sibrafiban plus aspirin, high-dose sibrafiban, and aspirin alone on the composite endpoint of death, MI, or severe recurrent ischemia.[257] A total of 6671 patients with stabilized ACS were randomized prior to termination and followed up for an average of 90 days. The primary efficacy endpoint was not significantly different among the three groups, occurring in 10.5 percent of the high-dose sibrafiban group, 9.3 percent of the aspirin-alone group, and in 9.2 percent of the low-dose sibrafiban-plus-aspirin group. While secondary endpoints did not differ significantly between the aspirin and low-dose sibrafiban-plus-aspirin groups, mortality occurred significantly more often in the high-dose sibrafiban group (OR 1.83, 95 percent CI 1.17 to 2.88), as did MI (OR 1.32, 95 percent CI 1.03 to 1.69). Major bleeding was more common in the two sibrafiban groups, 4.6 percent with high-dose sibrafiban compared with 4.0 percent for aspirin and 5.7 percent for low-dose sibrafiban plus aspirin.

Xemilofiban EXCITE The Evaluation of Oral Xemilofiban in Controlling Thrombotic Events (EXCITE) trial studied the agent xemilofiban in 7232 patients undergoing elective PCI (angioplasty or stent) without adjunctive intravenous GP IIb/IIIa inhibition.[258] Patients were randomized to 6 months of therapy in a double-blind fashion to receive one of three regimens: a single 20-mg dose 30 to 90 min prior to PCI and a maintenance dose of 20 mg given three times daily, a single 20 mg dose 30 to 90 min prior to PCI and a maintenance dose of 10 mg three times daily, or placebo for both. All patients received 80 to 325 mg of aspirin, and those patients in the placebo group in whom stents were implanted also received 250 mg of ticlopidine twice a day for 14 to 28 days. The primary endpoint of death, MI, or urgent revascularization at 6 months occurred in 13.6 percent of patients in the placebo group, 13.9 percent of patients in the 10-mg xemilofiban group, and 12.7 percent of patients in the 20-mg xemilofiban group (p = NS). With respect to individual endpoints, there was increased mortality in the 10-mg xemilofiban group compared to placebo at 30 days (0.8 vs. 0.3 percent, p = 0.02), at 6 months (1.7 vs. 1.0 percent, p = 0.04), and at 7 months (1.9 vs. 1.0 percent, p = 0.02). Moderate or severe bleeding episodes, transfusion requirement, any bleeding, and thrombocytopenia were all significantly more common among the xemilofiban-treated patients.

Orbofiban OPUS-TIMI-16 The Orbofiban in Patients with Unstable Coronary Syndromes (OPUS–TIMI-16) trial involved 10,288 (out of a planned 12,000) patients randomized at 888 hospitals in 28 countries worldwide.[259] Patients with ACS—defined as rest ischemic pain within 72 h lasting at least 5 min associated with either ECG changes, positive cardiac markers, or a prior history of vascular disease—were treated with 150 to 162 mg of aspirin and were randomized, in a double-blind fashion to one of two dosing strategies of orbofiban or to placebo and followed for the primary endpoint, which was a composite of death, MI, recurrent ischemia leading to rehospitalization or urgent revascularization, or stroke. In one arm, orbofiban was given as 50 mg twice daily throughout the trial (50/50 group); in the other (50/30 group), the dose of 50 mg twice daily was given for the first 30 days (the highest-risk period) and then reduced to 30 mg twice daily (50/30 group). The trial was terminated prematurely after an unexpectedly increased mortality rate at 30 days was observed in the 50/30 orbofiban group. While there were no significant differences in the primary composite endpoint at 30 days, the mortality rate was 1.4 percent in the placebo group, 2.3 percent in the 50/30 group, and 1.6 percent in the 50/50 group (p = 0.003 for 50/30 vs. placebo). And through 10 months of follow-up, mortality remained significantly higher in the 50/30 group (5.1 vs. 3.7 percent, p = 0.009), while the composite endpoint remained comparable. The rates of major or severe bleeding and thrombocytopenia were significantly greater in both orbofiban groups than in those taking aspirin.

Lotrafiban BRAVO Blockage of the Glycoprotein IIb/IIIa Receptor to Avoid Vascular Occlusion (BRAVO) study was to be the phase III trial for lotrafiban at doses of 30 to 50 mg twice a day but was terminated early by its data and safety monitoring committee due to concerns about its safety and efficacy.[260] The target enrollment was to be 9200 patients from over 700 centers in 30 countries who had experienced recent unstable angina, MI, TIA, or ischemic stroke or who had "double bed" vascular disease, defined as peripheral vascular disease with coexisting cardiovascular or cerebrovascular disease. Patients were to be followed for 6 months to 2 years for the composite primary endpoint of death, MI, stroke, recurrent ischemia requiring hospitalization, or urgent revascularization. At the time the trial was terminated, 9198 patients had been enrolled, and lotrafiban was found to be associated with an increased mortality versus placebo (2.7 vs. 2.0 percent, $p = 0.022$), an increased incidence of serious thrombocytopenia versus placebo (2.2 vs. 0.5 percent), and with more major bleeding than placebo (4.2 vs. 1.3 percent), respectively ($p < 0.0001$).[261]

Other Agents Two agents to date have been evaluated as both intravenous and oral compounds: Klerval (RPR 109891) and (le)fradafiban. The combined TIMI-15A&B trial was a phase II dose-ranging trial of both intravenous and oral Kerval in 233 patients with non-ST-elevation ACS; it demonstrated a dose-dependent inhibition of platelet aggregation, with the intravenous form achieving a higher degree of platelet inhibition at steady state than the oral form.[249] Unfortunately there were trends for increased major hemorrhage and thrombocytopenia with intravenous plus oral Kerval compared to placebo. Lefradafiban (oral) but not fradafiban (intravenous) was evaluated in the phase II Fibrinogen Receptor Occupancy Study (FROST), in which 532 patients with either unstable angina or non-ST-elevation MI were randomized to one of three doses of lefradafiban for 30 days.[254] While there was an intriguing dose-dependent trend in reduction in composite clinical events among patients with a positive troponin I at baseline (50 percent in the placebo, 42.1 percent in the 20-mg group, and 35.7 percent in the 30-mg group), which is similar to the findings seen with the intravenous GP IIb/IIIa inhibitors, there was also a dose-dependent increase in the risk of bleeding, such that the study involving the highest-dose group had to be stopped early.

Two longer-acting agents have also been evaluated. It is felt that prolonged antiplatelet effect would avoid the possibility of "on-off" proaggregatory effects of the drug binding to the GP IIb/IIIa inhibitor, which may have explained some of the findings from previous trials with oral GP IIb/IIIa inhibitors. Roxifiban binds tightly to platelet receptors and is slow to dissociate, giving it a long half-life and very stable antiplatelet effects over time (i.e., a low peak-to-trough level of platelet inhibition).[251,262] Roxifiban's tight binding is similar to that of abciximab, and its half-life of dissociation is 7 min, more than 40 times longer than that of the short-acting molecules like tirofiban (approximately 10 to 20 s).[262] Another agent, cromafiban, also has a very long half-life and thus may have more predictable and stable levels of platelet inhibition, but it has not yet been extensively studied.

Metanalysis Two metanalyses have pooled data from the 33,326 patients enrolled in the four published large phase III multicenter randomized trials (SYMPHONY 1 and 2, EXCITE, OPUS-TIMI-16) in an attempt to better understand why oral GP IIb/IIIa inhibitors have not enjoyed the same success as their intravenous counterparts in the treatment of ACS (Table 54-6).[263,264] Both analyses revealed a consistent and statistically significant increase in mortality with oral GP IIb/IIIa inhibitors of 31 to 37 percent (Fig. 54-21). This increase in mortality was evident regardless of the coadministration of aspirin (38 to 44 percent) or lack thereof (34 to 37 percent). A similar detrimental effect was also seen with low-dose (32 percent) or high-dose therapy (40 percent). A statistically significant increase in bleeding was observed in each individual trial, and the pooled analyses confirmed this, with a 74 percent increase in major bleeding (OR 1.74, 95 percent CI 1.52 to 2.0, $p < 0.001$). While the pooled analysis of Chew et al. did not demonstrate a significant increase in MIs at 30 days (OR 1.04, 95 percent CI 0.93 to 1.16), the metanalysis of Newby et al. found an increase in MIs when data from beyond 30 days were included (OR 1.16, 95 percent CI 1.03 to 1.29).

In-depth analyses of both the individual trials and the pooled data do not suggest a single explanation for the failure of these agents but instead imply a multifactorial cause. A number of putative mechanisms have been suggested to try to explain the paradoxical dissociation between strong inhibition of platelet aggregation, as evidenced by the increased bleeding rate, and the lack of clinical efficacy, as seen in the increased mortality rates.

Pharmacokinetics and Pharmacodynamics The pharmacokinetic and pharmacodynamic properties of these oral agents have been widely felt to be responsible for their clinical failure. The most basic and important question regarding their use, the correct target level of platelet inhibition during chronic therapy, is unknown. Hindering clarification of this issue is the availability of a rapid, convenient assay to monitor the level of platelet inhibition. Previous clinical studies have suggested that the maximum benefit of GP IIb/IIIa inhibition in the acute setting of ACS or PCI occurs when the degree of platelet inhibition is greater than 80 percent.[265,266] Currently, it is not clear whether lower levels of platelet inhibition are also beneficial. For chronic therapy, the profound inhibition of platelet aggregation achieved with intravenous administration employed in ACS and PCI was not tolerated due to the higher incidence of bleeding; thus a better-tolerated, lower level of inhibition was chosen. However, inadequate plasma levels between these lower oral doses may have resulted in subtherapeutic platelet inhibition for a large proportion of the treatment period. The oral administration, low bioavailability, short half-lives, and rapid "off-rates" of these agents as well as reversible inhibition result in these fluctuations in plasma concentrations and in antiplatelet effect.[264] A "rebound effect" during drug troughs may leave activated GP IIb/IIIa receptors vulnerable to fibrinogen binding and may be responsible for the increases in platelet activation and aggregation seen at low levels of platelet inhibition.[267] The Chew et al. metanalysis attempted to address this issue and found that there was no significant difference between low- and high-dose therapy. Therefore the conclusion was that increased dosing cannot necessarily be expected to deliver superior clinical efficacy.

Concurrent Aspirin and Platelet Activation Lack of concurrent aspirin therapy was thought to be responsible for the negative outcomes of initial oral GP IIb/IIIa inhibitor trials, specifically the first SYMPHONY study. The benefit of the combination of aspirin and an oral GP IIb/IIIa inhibitor is suggested by the synergism in the degree of platelet inhibition with concurrent therapy[268] and the continuous antiplatelet effects provided by aspirin, smoothing the troughs in GP IIb/IIIa blockade that may occur between doses. However, the addition of aspirin to low-dose sibrafiban in the second SYMPHONY study did not improve efficacy but instead increased bleeding rates.

TABLE 54-6 Summary of Phase 3 Studies of Oral Glycoprotein IIb/IIIa Receptor Antagonists

Study (Reference)	Patients Randomly Assigned to Treatment	Patients Included in Efficacy Analysis	Agent and Dose[a]	Indication	Enrollment	Target Effect[b] (%)	Treatment Duration	Primary Endpoint
EXCITE[258]	7232	7232	xemilofiban 10 mg three times daily; 20 mg three times daily	Elective perutaneous coronary intervention	30–90 minutes before coronary intervention	40–70 60–90	6 months	Death, myocardial infarction, revascularization
OPUS-TIMI 16[259]	10,302	10,288	orbofiban 50/30[c] 50/50[d]	Post-acute coronary syndrome	Within 72 hours	45–65 55–80	Planned 1 year	Death, myocardial infarction, urgent revascularization, rehospitalization, stroke[e]
SYMPHONY[256]	9233	9169	sibrafiban low dose[f]; high dose[g]	Post-acute coronary syndrome	12 hours to 7 days	≥25 ≥50	90 days	Death, myocardial infarction, severe recurrent ischemia
2nd SYMPHONY[257]	6671	6637	sibrafiban low dose; high dose	Post-acute coronary syndrome	12 hours to 7 days	≥25 ≥50	Planned 12–18 months	Death, myocardial infarction, severe recurrent ischemia[h]
BRAVO[260]	9198	Not available	lotrafiban	Secondary prevention	>14 days (myocardial infarction) >30 days (stroke)	60–70	Event driven; ≥6 months	Death, myocardial infarction, stroke, recurrent ischemia, urgent revascularization

[a]Background aspirin in all studies except SYMPHONY; only in low-dose arm of 2nd SYMPHONY.
[b]Platelet aggregation inhibition with 20 μM adenosine diphosphate.
[c]50 mg twice daily for 30 days, then 30 mg twice daily.
[d]50 mg twice daily for 30 days, then 50 mg twice daily.
[e]Reported at 30 days and 10 months.
[f]3 mg, 4.5 mg, or 6 mg twice daily, based on weight and serum creatinine to achieve target antiplatelet effect.
[g]3 mg, 4.5 mg, or 6 mg twice daily, based on weight and serum creatinine to achieve target antiplatelet effect.
[h]Time to event analysis.
[i]Study terminated early by Data and Safety Monitoring Committee.
ABBREVIATIONS: BRAVO = Blockade of the Receptor Against Vascular Occlusion; EXCITE = Evaluation of Xemilofiban in Controlling Thrombotic Events; OPUS-TIMI = Orbofiban in Patients with Unstable Angina-Thrombolysis in Myocardial Infarction; SYMPHONY = Sibrafiban versus aspirin to Yield Maximum Protection from ischemic Heart events post-acute cOroNary sYndromes.
SOURCE: From Newby et al.[264] With permission.

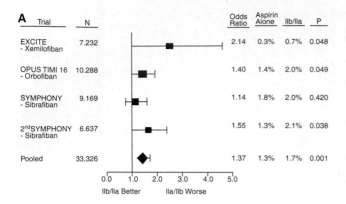

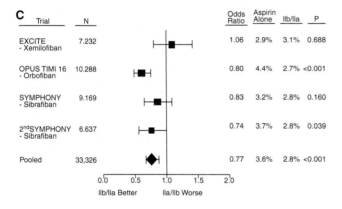

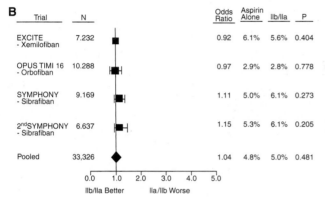

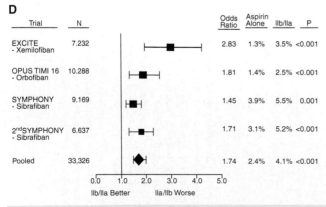

FIGURE 54-21 Odds Ratios and 95% confidence intervals for risk of death (*A*), MI (*B*), urgent revascularization (*C*), and major bleeding (*D*) beyond 30 days in patients treated with oral GP IIb/IIIa inhibitors. (From Chew et al.[263] With permission.)

The results of both metanalyses confirm lack of efficacy for oral GP IIb/IIIa agents with and without aspirin therapy, suggesting that drug–drug interactions are unlikely to account for the negative outcomes.

Potentially the most important aspect of concomitant aspirin therapy is that aspirin works by decreasing the synthesis of TXA_2 by the platelet, which decreases platelet activation, a step proximal to platelet aggregation. GP IIb/IIIa receptor blockers function to inhibit the final common pathway of platelet aggregation but have no effect on platelet activation. Platelet aggregation is only one end product of platelet activation. Another major end product involves platelet degranulation, which releases procoagulants, mediators of vasoreactivity, and growth factors. Activation also results in the expression of inflammatory mediators that are important in thrombosis and atherogenesis. Aspirin and clopidogrel, which are weak platelet aggregation inhibitors, both irreversibly inhibit one of many platelet activation pathways and, in-turn, result in a well-documented reduction in mortality. Thus, aspirin and GP IIb/IIIa inhibitors inhibit different steps in the formation of a platelet thrombus. Suppression of either platelet activation or aggregation may be more critical at different times—i.e., acutely during episodes of acute coronary syndromes or chronically with secondary prevention.

Prothrombotic Effect A prothrombotic effect of oral GP IIb/IIIa inhibitors has been proposed as a mechanism for the increased mortality associated with the use of these agents. The two metanalyses differ as to whether this possible prothrombotic effect translated into clinically apparent ischemic events. While the Chew et al. analysis found no significant increase in the rate of MI, Newby et al. found that if the analysis was extended past 30 days, this increase became apparent. Several potential prothrombotic mechanisms have been postulated. First, while binding of GP IIb/IIIa receptor blockers to the GP IIb/IIIa receptor effectively inhibits platelet aggregation, other platelet functions such as secretion, procoagulant activity, and platelet-leukocyte interactions might actually be potentiated.[269] Binding of the GP IIb/IIIa receptor by endogenous ligands causes a conformational change that results in an "outside-to-inside" signal through the receptor–cell membrane complex, which influences platelet function,[168] and also the generation of new epitopes (ligand-induced binding sites) that, in-turn, may affect platelet function. These synthetic agents can bind to various epitopes on the GP IIb/IIIa receptor and may generate various secondary signals that could be prothrombotic. This paradoxical platelet activation and procoagulant activity has been demonstrated by the measurement of enhanced fibrinogen binding and enhanced alpha-granule release.[267,270–273] Second, data with abciximab suggest that, at the low receptor antagonist concentrations and the low levels of platelet inhibition achieved with oral GP IIb/IIIa inhibitors, increased agonist-induced platelet aggregation is seen, leading to an increased potential for thrombosis.[267,274] Supporting this view are substudies from OPUS–TIMI-16 demonstrating that orbofiban led to increases in platelet reactivity and measures of platelet activation, such as levels of P-selectin.[271,275]

Toxic Effect The RGD (arginine-glycine-aspartic acid) sequence or binding site targeted by the oral GP IIb/IIIa inhibitors is found on many proteins and may become an unintentional target of these agents.[14] Direct toxic effects of the oral agents have been proposed and are supported by observations from animal studies suggesting that this inadvertent binding may cause cell death.[276] Procaspase-3, which when activated to caspase-3 regulates programmed cell death, has a binding site compatible with the oral GP IIb/IIIa inhibitors. Animal studies have demonstrated increases in caspase-3 expression and cardiomyocyte apoptosis when cells are incubated with xemilofiban or orbofiban.[276]

Dipyridamole Dipyridamole is a pyrimidopyrimidine compound whose antithrombotic action is not well understood. It is felt to decrease platelet aggregability and also platelet adhesion to prosthetic valves, to increase platelet survival, and to decrease red blood cell deformability.[277]

Dipyridamole alone and in combination with aspirin has been evaluated in a handful of relatively small studies. With regard to monotherapy, no benefit was found in a small study of dipyridamole versus placebo in the month after MI.[278] The two Persantine-Aspirin Reinfarction Studies evaluated aspirin, aspirin plus dipyridamole, and placebo in over 5000 patients after MI and found reductions of 25 percent in the composite of coronary death and reinfarction and of 20 to 37 percent in reinfarction with aspirin plus dipyridamole versus placebo.[279,280] Finally, in both European Stroke Prevention Studies, patients with a previous cerebrovascular event had a reduction in MIs when treated with aspirin plus dipyridamole compared to placebo.[281,282] However, this reduction reached statistical significance only in the first European Stroke Prevention Study, with a relative risk reduction of 38.9 percent ($p < 0.01$).

Conclusions/Recommendations

Aspirin has been the "gold standard" for antiplatelet therapy for the secondary prevention of MI ever since the ISIS-2 trial[39]; but with new data available from the CREDO trial,[163] the new standard moves to the combination of aspirin and clopidogrel for at least 1 year following the initial coronary event. Although currently no data are available, it would seem prudent to reassess a patient's risk at 1 year, and if the patient is felt to have a high annual risk of repeated cardiac events, clopidogrel in addition to aspirin would be continued for life. Aspirin at a dose of 80 to 325 mg/day is recommended by both the ACC/AHA [37,186,230] and the ACCP,[126,142,231] and doses at the lower end of this range have been shown to be just as effective as higher doses but with fewer bleeding complications.[148]

As for the oral GP IIb/IIIa inhibitors, testing to date has resulted in initial disappointment. Numerous obstacles remain. Since the optimal level of platelet inhibition is unknown, it is unclear how efficacy and safety can best be balanced, whether other adjunctive agents are needed, and whether monitoring of platelet function will assist in the use of these agents. Moreover, recent data demonstrating the benefit of long-term treatment with clopidogrel after PCI or ACS would likely require the combination of aspirin and clopidogrel in the control arm of any future study. Given the consistency of risk seen in the previous trials, it seems unlikely that future large-scale trials of new oral GP IIb/IIIa inhibitors will take place in the absence of breakthroughs in antiplatelet or antithrombotic therapy outside the field of GP IIb/IIIa inhibition.

ANTITHROMBIN THERAPY

Non-ST-Segment-Elevation Myocardial Infarction

UNFRACTIONATED HEPARIN
Unfractionated heparin (UFH) refers not to a single molecule but rather to a family of glycosaminoglycan chains of varying lengths and composition. UFH consists of a heterogeneous mixture of saccharides with molecular weights ranging from approximately 3000 to 30,000 Da (mean molecular weights of approximately 15,000 Da)

and only about one-third of these molecules are anticoagulantly active.[283] UFH by itself has no anticoagulant property but rather is a cofactor to antithrombin (formerly referred to as antithrombin III), a naturally occurring plasma inhibitor of thrombin and activated factors X, IX, XI, and XII. UFH accelerates the action of antithrombin III, increasing its ability to bind to and neutralize thrombin and other activated clotting factors, by forming a 1:1 stoichiometric complex. UFH contains a unique pentasaccharide that binds to the heparin-binding site on antithrombin III (Fig. 54-22), which, interestingly, is present on only one-third of UFH molecules. At very high doses, UFH can also bind to heparin cofactor II, which acts only on thrombin decay; the unique pentasaccharide is not required for this binding.

Thrombin and Factor Xa bound to thrombus, platelets, fibrin degradation products, or the endothelium are protected from inactivation by the heparin-antithrombin III complex.[195,284] Because of this, 20 times greater plasma concentrations of UFH are needed to inactivate fibrin-bound thrombin than to inactivate free thrombin. After parenteral administration, heparin binds to endothelial cells, mononuclear macrophages, and numerous plasma proteins. Some of these neutralize UFH's anticoagulant activity, notably platelet factor 4 and vitronectin, and different levels of these heparin-binding proteins explain the variability of individual UFH dosing to achieve the same antithrombotic effect. The pharmacokinetics of UFH are complicated by disproportionate increases in the anticoagulant response as the dose increases. This variability and complexity explain why the anticoagulant effect of heparin has to be closely monitored.

Unfractionated heparin along with aspirin are current mainstays of therapy in unstable angina and non-ST-segment elevation MI. Several early studies established the superiority of heparin over placebo[146,147,285,286] and over aspirin,[146,147,287,288] but they are no longer clinically relevant as combination therapy with aspirin as the current clinical standard.

To determine the incremental clinical benefit of adding heparin to aspirin in unstable angina and non-ST-segment-elevation MI, several trials compared continuous intravenous heparin added to aspirin

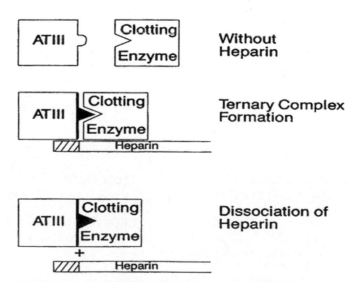

FIGURE 54-22 Inactivation of clotting enzymes by heparin. *Top.* AT-III is a slow inhibitor without heparin. *Middle.* Heparin binds to AT-III through high-affinity pentasaccharide and induces a conformational change in AT-III, thereby converting AT-III from a slow to a very rapid inhibitor. *Bottom.* AT-III binds covalently to the clotting enzyme, and the heparin dissociates from the complex and can be reutilized. (From Hirsh et al.[295] With permission.)

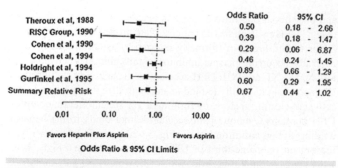

FIGURE 54-23 Metanalysis of trials comparing UFH plus aspirin to aspirin alone in unstable angina and non-Q-wave MI. (From Oler et al.[294] With permission.)

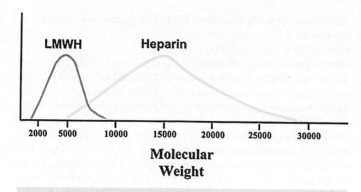

FIGURE 54-24 Molecular weight distributions of LMWHs and UFH. (From Hirsh et al.[295] With permission.)

therapy to aspirin alone. The Canadian aspirin-heparin trial randomized 479 patients with unstable angina to aspirin (325 mg twice daily), heparin (1000 U/h), or both and found, at a mean follow-up of 6 days, a nonsignificant reduction in MI (1.6 vs. 3.3 percent, RR 0.49, 95 percent CI 0.09 to 2.72, $p = 0.4$) and in refractory angina (10.7 vs. 16.5 percent, RR 0.60, 95 percent CI 0.28 to 1.27, $p = 0.18$) in the combination patients compared to aspirin-only subjects.[146] The combination of aspirin and heparin was associated with slightly more serious bleeding (3.3 vs. 1.7 percent). The RISC Group studied 796 patients with unstable angina or non-Q-wave MI treated with aspirin (75 mg/day), intravenous heparin, both, or neither and found no significant difference between the aspirin arm and the combination group in the combined endpoint of MI and death at 5 days, 30 days, and 90 days.[147] Cohen et al., in a pilot study for the Antithrombotic Therapy in the Acute Coronary Syndromes (ATACS) study, compared three different antithrombotic regimens (325 mg of aspirin daily vs. heparin followed by warfarin vs. 80 mg of aspirin daily plus heparin and then warfarin) in 93 patients with unstable angina or non-Q-wave MI.[289] At 3 months, no significant difference in endpoints was found, as the study was insufficiently powered to discriminate between them, especially since only 25 percent of patients enrolled were discharged on trial therapy. The larger ATACS trial randomized 214 patients to aspirin (162.5 mg/day) or a combination of aspirin and heparin followed by aspirin and warfarin (INR 2 to 3).[290] There was a significant reduction in ischemic events (recurrent angina, infarction, or death) with combination therapy at 2

weeks (10.5 vs. 27 percent, $p = 0.004$) and at 12 weeks (13 vs. 25 percent, $p = 0.06$). There was no difference in response between patients with unstable angina and those with non-Q-wave MI.[291] A study by Holdright et al. randomized 285 patients to UFH plus aspirin (150 mg/day) or aspirin alone and showed a trend to benefit in the incidence of MI or death with heparin plus aspirin compared to aspirin alone (27.2 vs. 30.5 percent, $p = NS$).[292] Gurfinkel et al. randomized 219 patients to aspirin (200 mg/day), aspirin plus UFH, or aspirin plus LMWH and found a nonsignificant increase in total ischemic events (63 vs. 59 percent), recurrent angina (44 vs. 37 percent), and major bleeding (3 vs. 0 percent) with UFH plus aspirin compared to aspirin alone.[293]

Data from these individual trials were inconclusive regarding benefit of combination heparin plus aspirin over aspirin alone. In 1996 a metanalysis of six studies was performed in an attempt to overcome the limitations of the smaller studies.[294] A 33 percent reduction in MI or death during the drug treatment period was found in the pooled analysis, but with confidence intervals that crossed unity (95 percent CI 2 to 56 percent) (Fig. 54-23). Although this difference is not statistically significant, these are the data that support the use of UFH and aspirin in non-ST-segment-elevation MI.

LOW-MOLECULAR-WEIGHT HEPARIN

Low-molecular-weight heparins (LMWHs) are derived from UFH by chemical or enzymatic depolymerization, yielding fragments approximately one-third the size of UFH (Fig. 54-24). Since the various commercially available LMWHs are prepared by different methods of depolymerization, they differ to some extent in their pharmacokinetic properties and anticoagulant profile and may not be clinically equivalent. LMWHs have a mean molecular weight of 4500 to 5000 Da, with a distribution of 1000 to 10,000 Da.[295] LMWHs have several advantages over standard, UFH: they have a more predictable anticoagulant effect as well as longer and more stable anticoagulation, provide a simpler route of administration, require no monitoring of anticoagulation, are resistant to inhibition by activated platelets, are associated with less platelet activation, and have a lower incidence of heparin-induced thrombocytopenia (Table 54-7).[296]

TABLE 54-7 Clinical Features of the Low-Molecular-Weight Heparins Compared to Standard Unfractionated Heparin

	UFH	LMWH
Mean molecular weight (Do)	12,000–15,000	4,000–6,500
Anti-Xa:anti-IIa activity	1:1	2 to 4:1
Bioavailability	Less	Higher
Protein binding	HRGP, PF 4	—
Dose adjustments	Frequent, following aPTT	Weight-adjusted, fixed
Platelet inhibition and interaction	++++	++
Risk of HIT	More	Less
Renal clearance	++	++++
Route of administration (common)	Intravenous	Subcutaneous
Half-life	30–60 min	120–180 min

ABBREVIATIONS: aPTT = activated partial thromboplastin time; HIT = hemogglutination inhibition test; HRGP = histidine-rich glycoprotein; PF 4 = platelet factor 4.
SOURCE: From Monrad.[296] With permission.

Most of the pharmacologic benefits of LMWHs are the result of a lower level of nonspecific binding to serum and cellular proteins compared to UFH. As with UFH, LMWH exerts its anticoagulant effect through the activation of antithrombin III via binding of the high-affinity pentasaccharide sequence on LMWH to the heparin binding site (Fig. 54-25). While inhibition of factor Xa occurs through direct binding of the activated antithrombin III, inhibition of thrombin calls for the formation of a complex of thrombin, antithrombin III, and heparin, which requires a minimum heparin chain length (Fig. 54-26).[297] Since only one-quarter to one-half of LMWH is long enough to form this complex, LMWH has reduced antifactor IIa activity relative to antifactor Xa activity. Factor Xa has been shown to contribute more to the procoagulant activity of thrombus in situ than thrombin[298]; therefore the inhibition of factor Xa may be the more important step in ACS.

Currently, enoxaparin and dalteparin are the two LMWHs approved by the U.S. Food and Drug Administration for the treatment of unstable angina and non-ST-segment-elevation MI. Other LMWHs available include tinzaparin, nadroparin, and ardeparin. Fondaparinux, a synthetic pentasaccharide, is a new addition to the LMWH family that is currently under clinical investigation.[299] Fondaparinux has pharmacologic profiles similar to those of other LMWHs but also has selective antifactor Xa activity with no antifactor IIa activity. Two large-scale clinical trials have established the superiority of enoxaparin over unfractionated heparin in unstable angina and non-Q-wave MI, while the results of trials involving dalteparin and nadroparin have been less definitive (Fig. 54-27).[300]

Enoxaparin ESSENCE The Efficacy and Safety of Subcutaneous Enoxaparin in Non-Q-Wave Coronary Events Study (ESSENCE) randomized 3171 patients with ischemic chest pain at rest within 24 h and either ST-segment depression or previously documented history of CAD to either enoxaparin (1 mg/kg twice daily) or standard UFH for 2 to 8 days.[301] At 48 h there was no difference in the composite endpoint of death, MI, or recurrent angina. However, by 14 days, the enoxaparin group demonstrated a 16.2 percent risk reduction in the composite endpoint, with a 16.6 percent event rate, compared to 19.8 percent in the UFH group ($p = 0.019$), and there continued to be a significant reduction at 30 days (15 percent, $p = 0.016$) and even at 1 year follow-up (10 percent, $p = 0.022$).[302] The reduction in the composite endpoint was powered by statistically significant reductions in MI and recurrent angina at the different time points. There was a nonsignificant trend toward a reduction in major bleeding in the enoxaparin group (6.5 vs. 7.0 percent) but an increase in minor bleeding, due mainly to ecchymosis at the injection site. An economic assessment of the 936 patients randomized in the United States showed a cumulative cost savings of $1172 for enoxaparin therapy over UFH at the end of 30 days.[181] While the analysis found that there was a minimal $75 increase in the cost of a course of enoxaparin therapy versus UFH with aPTT measurements, decreased major resource utilization

FIGURE 54-25 Inhibition of thrombin requires simultaneous binding of heparin to AT-III through the unique pentasaccharide sequence and binding to thrombin through a minimum of 13 additional saccharide units. Inhibition of factor Xa requires binding heparin to AT-III through the unique pentasaccharide without the additional requirements for binding to Xa. 5 = unique high affinity pentasaccharide sequence; 13 = additional saccharide units. (From Hirsh et al.[295] With permission.)

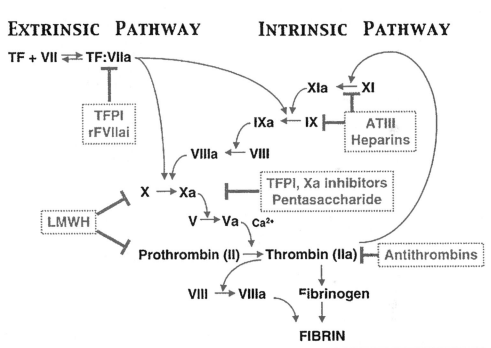

FIGURE 54-26 Tissue factor activation of the coagulation cascade with superimposed sites of drug inhibition. (From Corti et al.[395] With permission.)

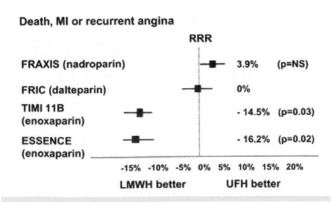

FIGURE 54-27 Metanalysis of LMWH trials in unstable angina/non-ST-elevation MI. (From Cohen.[397] With permission.)

in the enoxaparin group during the initial hospitalization resulted in the overall cost savings. At 30 days, the rates of diagnostic catheterization (57 vs. 63 percent, $p = 0.04$) and coronary angioplasty (18 vs. 22 percent, $p = 0.08$) were lower in patients treated with enoxaparin compared to UFH. Thus, both improved outcomes and lower costs were observed with enoxaparin in the ESSENCE trial.

TIMI-11 The TIMI-11A was an open-label dose-finding study of enoxaparin designed to determine the appropriate dose for treatment of unstable angina for the upcoming phase III TIMI-11B.[303] A total of 630 patients were assigned to either 1.0 mg/kg subcutaneously twice daily, the dose used in venous thrombosis, or a higher 1.25 mg/kg twice daily. The higher dose was associated with a 4.5 percent increase in the rate of major hemorrhage at 14 days (6.5 vs. 1.9 percent). As no difference in the rate of recurrent ischemic events between doses was observed, the lower 1.0 mg/kg dose was chosen.

The TIMI-11B trial studied 3910 patients who had experienced ischemic pain at rest within the previous 24 h and a history of either CAD, ST-segment depression, or elevated cardiac enzymes; these patients were randomized to enoxaparin or UFH for 3 to 8 days while hospitalized and then to either continued enoxaparin (40 or 60 mg twice daily) or placebo as outpatients through day 43.[304] At 8 days, the enoxaparin group demonstrated a 14.6 percent risk reduction ($p = 0.048$) in the composite endpoint of death, MI, or urgent revascularization; at 43 days, there was a 12.3 percent reduction ($p = 0.048$). Again, there were no differences in the rates of major hemorrhage during initial hospitalization between the two groups, but during the outpatient phase, enoxaparin did show an increase compared to placebo (2.9 vs. 1.5 percent, $p = 0.021$).

Metanalysis Two metanalyses of the ESSENCE and TIMI 11B data[305,306] found that there were statistically significant reductions in the composite endpoints of death and MI and death, MI, and urgent revascularization at days 8, 14, and 43. At 1 year, however, the only benefit that persisted was a reduction in death, MI, and urgent revascularization (Fig. 54-28).

Dalteparin FRIC AND FRISC The Fragmin in Unstable Coronary Artery Disease (FRIC) study[307] and the Low-Molecular-Weight Heparin (Fragmin) During Instability in Coronary Artery Disease (FRISC) trial[308] both compared dalteparin (120 U/kg twice daily) to UFH for the acute treatment of unstable angina and non-Q-wave MI. FRIC randomized 1482 patients while FRISC enrolled 1506 subjects with chest pain within 72 h and ECG evidence of ischemia to compare the two agents during the first 5 to 7 days following hospitalization and then dalteparin (7500 U SQ daily) to aspirin alone during the following 35 to 45 days. The FRIC investigators did not find any significant advantage to dalteparin during either time period, while the FRISC group found that dalteparin was superior at both 6 days and 40 days. After 6 days there was a significant 64 percent relative risk reduction ($p = 0.001$) in the primary endpoint of death or MI with dalteparin therapy; this lost statistical significance at 40 days (25 percent RRR, $p = 0.07$) and 5 months. Again, there was no difference in major bleeding, even during the outpatient period, and an increase in minor bleeding due to ecchymosis.

Fraxiparine/Nadroparin FRAXIS The FRAXiparine in Ischaemic Syndrome (FRAXIS) study evaluated the LMWH nadroparin in 3468 patients with unstable angina or non-Q-wave MIs defined as chest pain within 48 h and characteristic ECG changes.[309] Subjects were randomized to either UFH, nadroparin (86 IU/kg twice daily) for 6 days, or nadroparin for 14 days. At day 14 there were no statistically significant differences between the groups in the primary endpoint of cardiac death, MI, or refractory/recurrent angina. While there was no difference in major bleeding rates between the patients treated with LMWH versus UFH for a 6-day course, increased bleeding was seen among patients treated for 14 days.

Tinzaparin EVET The Enoxaparin Versus Tinzaparin in the Management of Unstable Coronary Artery Disease (EVET) trial directly compared these two LMWHs in 438 patients with unstable angina or non-Q-wave MI.[310] Patients were randomized to receive either tinzaparin 175 IU/kg subcutaneously once daily or enoxaparin 100 IU/kg subcutaneously twice daily for 7 days and were followed for the primary endpoints of death, MI, refractory angina, and recurrence of unstable angina at 30 days. While tinzaparin demonstrated similar rates of death, MI, and refractory angina, enoxaparin was associated with significantly lower rates of recurrent angina at 7 days (10.9 vs. 18.8 percent, $p = 0.029$) and lower rates of revascularization at 30 days (16.4 vs. 26.1 percent, $p = 0.019$). Thus, tinzaparin was found to be inferior to enoxaparin for the treatment of unstable angina or non-Q-wave MI in this study.

Fondaparinux PENTUA The Pentasaccharide in Unstable Angina (PENTUA) study was a phase II dose-ranging trial of the synthetic factor Xa inhibitor fondaparinux in patients presenting with non-ST-segment-elevation MI.[311] A total of 1147 patients were randomized to enoxaparin or one of four doses of fondaparinux for a mean treatment duration of 5 days. The composite endpoint of death, MI, and recurrent ischemia at day 9 occurred in 37 percent of the fondaparinux-treated patients and in 40 percent of the enoxaparin-treated

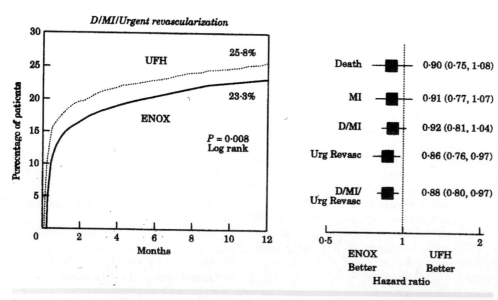

FIGURE 54-28 Metanalysis of ESSENCE and TIMI 11B results at 1-year of follow-up. (From Antman et al.[305] With permission.)

patients, with the fewest events occurring in the lowest-dose fondaparinux group (30 percent, $p < 0.05$, compared to all other arms). The lowest fondaparinux dose was also associated with the fewest occurrences of the combined endpoint at 30 days (33.8 vs. 43.6 percent for enoxaparin and 38 vs. 45 percent for the other fondaparinux doses). The overall bleeding rates were similar in all of the treatment groups, with no episodes of major bleeding occurring in the lowest-dose fondaparinux arm or the enoxaparin arm.

DIRECT THROMBIN INHIBITORS

The direct thrombin inhibitors represent another group of antithrombotic agents that have potential mechanistic advantages over heparin when used as therapy for ACS (Table 54-8). Both UFH and LMWH indirectly inhibit thrombin through an antithrombin III–dependent process, but an important limitation of heparin is its inability to inhibit clot-bound thrombin (Fig. 54-29). Fibrin-bound thrombin is protected from inactivation by heparin but remains enzymatically active, amplifying its own generation through a positive feedback loop via coagulation factors V and VIII and thereby promoting further thrombus formation.[195] Biological and pharmacologic advantages of direct thrombin inhibitors over heparin include the direct thrombin inhibitor's ability to neutralize both fluid-phase and clot-bound thrombin, their more predictable anticoagulant response (since they are not inactivated by plasma proteins or platelet factor 4), their lack of required cofactors, and their inhibition of thrombin-induced platelet activation.[283,312,313]

The prototype direct thrombin inhibitor is hirudin, a 65–amino acid polypeptide derived from the medicinal leech *Hirudo medicinalis*, which is now available through recombinant DNA technology.[314] Hirudin is a potent, selective, and almost irreversible inhibitor of thrombin that binds to thrombin at two sites: the active catalytic site and the substrate recognition exosite (Fig. 54-30).[315] The carboxyl terminus of hirudin binds to the substrate recognition site, the domain of thrombin that recognizes fibrinogen or platelets; the amino terminus of hirudin binds to the catalytic site of thrombin. Hirudin has a plasma half-life of approximately 60 min after intravenous administration and is primarily excreted by the kidneys.[313]

Bivalirudin is a synthetic 20–amino acid polypeptide analogue of hirudin. Bivalirudin contains three domains: a 12–amino acid carboxyl terminus derived from hirudin, a 4–amino acid sequence that binds to the catalytic site of thrombin, and a linker region optimized to facilitate binding to both sites.[316] As a result, bivalirudin, like hirudin, is able to form a bivalent complex with thrombin, blocking both the active site and the substrate recognition exosite (Fig. 54-30). While hirudin is long-acting and essentially irreversible due to an extremely slow dissociation rate, bivalirudin has a shorter plasma half-life of 20 to 25 min because of cleavage by thrombin of the active site-binding peptide.[313] This shorter half-life may give it a potential safety advantage over hirudin by permitting hemostasis to occur, thereby reducing bleeding.

Both hirudin and bivalirudin have been studied in the setting of unstable angina and non-ST-segment-elevation MIs.

TABLE 54-8 Clinical Features of Direct Thrombin Inhibitors Compared to Low-Molecular-Weight Heparin and Standard Unfractionated Heparin

	Unfractionated Heparin	Low-Molecular-Weight Heparin	Direct Thrombin Inhibitor
Pharmacokinetic			
Plasma protein/endothelial binding	Yes	Partial	No
Inactivated by heparinases	Yes	Partial	No
Biologic Effects			
Anticoagulant effects	Xa = IIa	Xa ≫ IIa	IIa
Antithrombin-dependent	Yes	Yes	No
Inactivates clot-bound thrombin	No	No	Yes
Inhibits platelet function	Yes (paradoxical activation?)	Limited	Yes, thrombin-induced only
Vascular permeability	Increased	Not increased	Not increased
Thrombocytopenia	Yes	Rare	No
Liver toxicity (enzyme rise)	Common	Uncommon	No

SOURCE: From Eikelboom et al.[313] With permission.

Hirudin OASIS In the Organization to Assess Strategies for Ischemic Syndromes (OASIS) pilot study, 909 patients with unstable angina or non-ST-segment-elevation MI were randomized to UFH or two doses of hirudin and followed for the occurrence of cardiovascular death, MI, or refractory angina at 7 days.[317] At 7 days, 6.5 percent of patients in the heparin group, 4.4 percent in the low-dose hirudin group, and 3.0 percent in the medium-dose hirudin group experienced the composite endpoint ($p = 0.267$ low-dose and $p = 0.047$

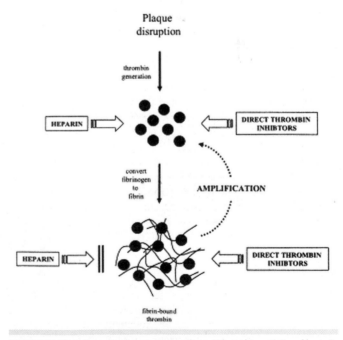

FIGURE 54-29 Schematic demonstrating the antithrombin activity of heparin compared with direct thrombin inhibitors. Both heparin and direct thrombin inhibitors block circulating thrombin, but only direct thrombin inhibitors block tissue-bound thrombin. Tissue bound thrombin remains enzymatically active, promoting further platelet and coagulation activation and thrombin generation. (From Eikelboom et al.[313] With permission.)

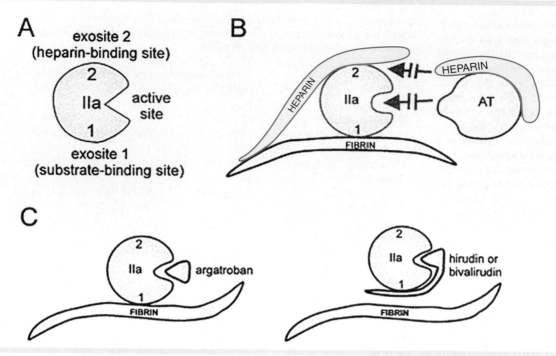

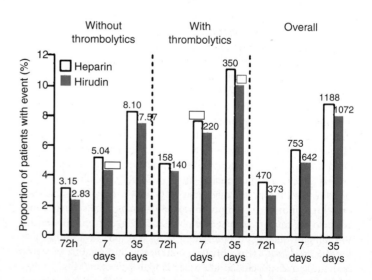

FIGURE 54-30 Thrombin (IIa) and direct thrombin inhibitor interactions. A. Thrombin possesses an active site and two positively charged exosites. Exosite 1 serves as the substrate (fibrin) binding site while exosite 2 binds heparin. B. With simultaneous binding of both heparin and fibrin to thrombin, antithrombin (AT)-bound heparin cannot bind to thrombin to form a ternary heparin/thrombin/AT complex thus demonstrating heparin's inability to inhibit clot-bound thrombin. C. Univalent inhibitors, such as argatroban, inhibit fibrin-bound thrombin without displacing thrombin from fibrin. Bivalent inhibitors, such as hirudin and bivalrudin, displace thrombin from fibrin during the inactivation process. (From Weitz and Buller.[401] With permission.)

medium-dose). OASIS-2 then randomized over 10,000 patients to medium-dose hirudin and observed them for the primary outcome of cardiovascular death or MI at 7 days.[318] There was only a nonsignificant trend toward benefit with hirudin for the primary endpoint (3.6 vs. 4.2 percent, $p = 0.077$); but once refractory angina was added to the composite endpoint, this trend became significant (6.7 vs. 5.6 percent, $p = 0.0125$). There was, however, an increase in major bleeding with hirudin (1.2 vs. 0.7 percent, $p = 0.01$).

GUSTO IIB GUSTO IIb examined 8011 patients with non-ST-segment-elevation MI out of a total of 12,142 enrolled.[319] At 30 days, there was no difference between the groups in the occurrence of death or MI with hirudin versus UFH (8.3 vs. 9.1 percent, $p = 0.22$). There were significant increases in major and moderate bleeding with hirudin in these patients with non-ST-segment-elevation MI. A combined analysis by the OASIS investigators of hirudin versus UFH used without fibrinolytics (OASIS, OASIS-2, GUSTO IIb) found a 28 percent relative risk reduction of cardiac events at 72 h ($p = 0.0002$), 17 percent at 7 days ($p = 0.004$), and 10 percent at 35 days ($p = 0.057$) with hirudin (Fig. 54-31).[318]

Bivalirudin The clinical development of bivalirudin (formerly hirulog) has been interrupted due to termination at one point of the clinical development and testing of the agent by the sponsor due to perceptions that there was insufficient evidence of an advantage over UFH to warrant the cost of further development of the drug.[320]

TIMI-7 was the dose-ranging phase II trial of bivalirudin that enrolled 410 patients with unstable angina and randomized them to aspirin (325 mg/day) and one of four doses of intravenous bivalirudin given for 72 h.[321] While the primary endpoint of "unsatisfactory outcome"—a composite of death, MI, rapid clinical deterioration, or recurrent ischemia—was not significantly different between groups,

the secondary endpoint of death or MI was significantly higher in the lowest-dose group compared to the groups receiving the three higher doses. Major hemorrhage occurred in only 0.5 percent of patients.

The large phase III TIMI-8 trial, which compared a 72 h infusion of bivalirudin to UFH in patients with non-ST-segment-elevation MI,

	Without thrombolytics			With thrombolytics			Overall		
	72h	7 days	35 days	72h	7 days	35 days	72h	7 days	35 days
Relative risk	0.72	0.83	0.90	0.89	0.88	0.86	0.76	0.84	0.80
P		0.0002	0.004	0.051	0.34	0.10	0.13	0.0004	0.002	0.018

FIGURE 54-31 Pooled analysis of all large trials of hirudin versus heparin in acute coronary syndromes. (From the OASIS Investigators.[402] With permission.)

enrolled only 133 patients out of a planned 5320 before it was terminated by the sponsors for "business" reasons.[320] At the time of termination, there was a highly promising reduction in the risk of death or MI with bivalirudin compared to UFH at 14 days (2.9 vs. 9.2 percent).

The six randomized trials of bivalirudin compromising 5674 patients with unstable angina, non-ST-segment-elevation MI, or PCI were reviewed in a metanalysis.[322] In total, bivalirudin was associated with a significant reduction in the composite of death or infarction (OR 0.73, 95 percent CI 0.57 to 0.95, $p = 0.02$) at 30 to 50 days, or 14 fewer events per 1000 patients treated. There also was a significant reduction in major hemorrhage for the same trials (OR 0.41, 95 percent CI 0.32 to 0.52, $p \leq 0.001$, or 58 fewer events per 1000 patients treated).

TABLE 54-9 Direct Thrombin Inhibitors Compared with Heparin in Patients with Acute Coronary Syndrome with or without ST-Segment Elevation at 30 Days

Outcomes	DTI (n = 15,866)	Heparin (n = 14,651)	OR (95% CI)
Death or MI			
ACS	1,288 (8.1%)	1,285 (8.8%)	0.92 (0.85–1.00)
ACS with ST-segment elevation	506 (9.8%)	489 (10.2%)	0.96 (0.84–1.10)
ACS without ST-segment elevation	782 (7.3%)	796 (8.1%)	0.90 (0.81–0.99)
Death			
ACS	672 (4.2%)	629 (4.3%)	0.99 (0.88–1.10)
ACS with ST-segment elevation	317 (6.2%)	271 (5.6%)	1.10 (0.93–1.30)
ACS without ST-segment elevation	355 (3.3%)	358 (3.6%)	0.91 (0.78–1.05)
MI			
ACS	771 (4.9%)	800 (5.5%)	0.88 (0.80–0.98)
ACS with ST-segment elevation	228 (4.4%)	254 (5.3%)	0.83 (0.69–1.00)
ACS without ST-segment elevation	543 (5.1%)	546 (5.5%)	0.91 (0.81–1.03)

ABBREVIATIONS: ACS = acute coronary syndrome; CI = confidence interval; DTI = direct thrombin inhibitors; MI = myocardial infarction; OR = odds ratio.
SOURCE: From Eikelboom et al.[313] With permission.

Univalent Direct Thrombin Inhibitors   Several other synthetic univalent direct thrombin inhibitors have been developed and have been the subject of ongoing phase 1 and 2 clinical trials. These agents block only the active site of thrombin, have a short half-life, and appear to be stronger inhibitors of fibrin-bound thrombin than the bivalent inhibitors.[313] They represent a potential trend toward future therapy and drug development but are not approved for ACS therapy at this time.

Only two of the univalent direct thrombin inhibitors have been studied in the setting of unstable angina and non-ST segment MI. Five doses of efegatran were studied in 432 patients presenting with unstable angina and no benefit was seen with regard to continuous ECG ischemia monitoring or clinical outcomes such as death, MI, recurrent angina, or coronary revascularization when compared to UFH.[323] The largest dose-ranging study involved inogatran, a low-molecular-weight selective thrombin inhibitor, in 1209 patients presenting with unstable angina or non-Q-wave MIs in the Thrombin Inhibition in Myocardial Ischaemia (TRIM) study.[324] Patients were randomized to receive one of three doses of inogatran or UFH for 3 days. The study showed no benefit of inogatran over UFH at 30 days; in fact, UFH was superior to inogatran at 3 and 7 days.

Metanalysis   To better assess the clinical benefit of direct thrombin inhibitors compared with UFH in ACS, determine whether early treatment benefits are maintained long-term, and establish whether excess bleeding offsets any benefit of these agents, the Direct Thrombin Inhibitors Trialists' Collaboration conducted a metanalysis of the major randomized trials of direct thrombin inhibitors. This metanalysis included 11 randomized trials and almost 36,000 patients with both ST-segment-elevation and non-ST-segment-elevation MI and PCI who were treated with bivalent and univalent inhibitors.[325] Overall, direct thrombin inhibitors were found to be associated with a significant 15 percent reduction in death of MI at the end of drug treatment (4.3 vs. 5.1 percent) and a 9 percent reduction at 30 days (7.4 vs. 8.2 percent). In the subgroup of patients presenting with non-ST-segment-elevation ACS, there was a significant 20 percent reduction in death or MI (3.7 vs. 4.6 percent; OR 0.80, 95 percent CI 0.70

to 0.92), a significant 18 percent reduction in MI, and a nonsignificant 18 percent reduction in death at the end of treatment. At 30 days there remained a statistically significant 10 percent reduction in death or MI (7.3 vs. 8.1 percent; OR 0.90, 95 percent CI 0.81 to 0.99) but the 9 percent reductions in the individual endpoints of death or MI were no longer statistically significant (Table 54-9). Individual analysis of hirudin, bivalirudin, and univalent inhibitors found that there was a similar reduction in death or MI with hirudin and bivalirudin compared to UFH, but there was a slight excess of death or MI with the univalent inhibitors. While as a group there was a significant 25 percent reduction in major bleeding during treatment with direct thrombin inhibitors compared to UFH, individually bivalirudin (OR 0.44, 95 percent CI 0.34 to 0.56) and univalent inhibitors (OR 0.55, 95 percent CI 0.25 to 1.20) were associated with lower rates of major bleeding, while hirudin (OR 1.28, 95 percent CI 1.06 to 1.55) was associated with excess bleeding compared to UFH.

Conclusions/Recommendations

Current ACC/AHA and ACCP guidelines for the treatment of unstable angina and non-ST-segment elevation MI recommend that subcutaneous LMWH or intravenous UFH be added to antiplatelet therapy as a class I recommendation (Table 54-10).[142,186] Because of the compelling results of the ESSENCE and TIMI 11B trials, the ACC/AHA guidelines state in a class IIa recommendation that enoxaparin is preferable to UFH in the absence of renal failure and unless CABG is planned within 24 h. Emerging data now supports the safety and efficacy of LMWH with GP IIb/IIIa inhibitors[326–329] and with PCI,[330–333] which had previously hindered the use LMWH in this situation. Given its ease of use and its clinical superiority, LMWH should replace UFH in non-ST-segment-elevation MI and unstable angina.

At this time, although the direct thrombin inhibitors appear to have greater clinical efficacy, this comes at the cost of increased bleeding; therefore these agents have not been approved for use in this setting. Currently the only compelling clinical data for direct thrombin inhibitors are limited to the catheterization laboratory.[334]

TABLE 54-10 ACC/AHA Guidelines for Anticoagulant Therapy in Unstable Angina and Non-Q-Wave Myocardial Infarction

Class I

1. Anticoagulation with subcutaneous LMWH or intravenous UFH should be added to antiplatelet therapy with ASA and/or clopidogrel. (Level of Evidence: A)[a]

Class IIa

1. Enoxaparin is preferable to UFH as an anticoagulant in patients with UA/NSTEMI, in the absence of renal failure and unless CABG is planned within 24 hours. (Level of Evidence: A)[a]

[a]New indication, not included in the September 2000 guidelines.
SOURCE: From Braunwald et al.[186] With permission.

It is unknown whether the direct thrombin inhibitors will prove to have any advantage over the already proven LMWHs exclusive of the cath lab.

ST-Segment-Elevation Myocardial Infarction

ANTITHROMBOTIC THERAPY WITH FIBRINOLYTICS AS THE PRIMARY STRATEGY

Unfractionated Heparin Although heparin has been studied in numerous trials in conjunction with fibrinolytic therapy, its role and dosing are still being debated. Taken together, the studies of heparin therapy in conjunction with fibrinolytic therapy in patients who did not routinely receive aspirin therapy have shown a benefit to heparin administration.[335] However, it is no longer clinically relevant to discuss fibrinolytic therapy in the absence of aspirin, so the question that remains is in the setting of fibrinolytic therapy is whether heparin should be added to aspirin and, if so, how should it be given.

While the ISIS-2 trial was designed to study the benefits of aspirin and fibrinolytic therapy in the setting of ST-segment-elevation MI, the protocol did not mandate or specify the use of heparin. Therefore approximately two-thirds of patients received some form of heparin in a nonrandomized manner in addition to aspirin and streptokinase, which resulted in a 5-week mortality of 9.8 percent in those who received no heparin, 7.6 percent in those treated with subcutaneous heparin, and 6.4 percent in those who received intravenous heparin.[39]

Subcutaneous Heparin The large-scale GISSI-2/International t-PA versus Streptokinase Mortality Trial[66,281] with 20,891 patients and the ISIS-3 trial[40] with 41,299 subjects were designed to specifically address the issue of the coadministration of subcutaneous heparin with fibrinolytics in the setting of acute ST-segment-elevation MI. In the GISSI-2/International Study, patients were randomized to streptokinase or alteplase (t-PA) and also subcutaneous heparin (12,500 U every 12 h) beginning 12 h after the infusion of the thrombolytic agent or usual therapy. All patients were routinely treated with atenolol and aspirin. There was a non-statistically-significant trend toward a decrease in mortality rate seen in those subjects treated with streptokinase and subcutaneous heparin compared with those who received streptokinase alone (7.9 vs. 9.2 percent). The mortality rate

for those receiving t-PA was similar whether or not heparin was added to the regimen (9.2 vs. 8.7 percent). In ISIS-3, patients were randomized to either streptokinase, duteplase (t-PA), or anistreplase and half of the patients were given subcutaneous heparin (12,500 U every 12 h) starting 4 h after the start of thrombolytic therapy. All patients also received aspirin. At 35 days, there was no significant difference in the mortality rates between patients who received heparin with their fibrinolytic and those who did not (10.3 vs. 10.6 percent). There was a slight decrease in hospital reinfarction rate in the heparin group during the heparin treatment period compared to the control group (2.39 vs. 2.81 percent, $p < 0.01$). However, this early benefit was lost when the primary endpoint of 35 days was reached.

Subcutaneous heparin was associated with significantly increased rates of major hemorrhage in each of these large trials. In the GISSI-2/International Study, heparin treatment resulted in a relative risk increase of 1.79 (1.0 vs. 0.5 percent, 95 percent CI 1.31 to 2.45). However, there was no corresponding increase in intracerebral hemorrhage (0.3 vs. 0.4 percent). In ISIS-3, heparin was associated with a very small excess of major bleeding (0.2 percent of patients: 1.0 percent compared with 0.8 percent for no heparin, $p < 0.01$). Intracerebral hemorrhage also seemed very slightly increased (0.056 vs. 0.40 percent, $p < 0.05$).

A pooled analysis of GISSI-2 and ISIS-3 showed a mortality at 35 days of 10.6 percent without heparin and 10.2 percent with heparin (ISIS-3).[40] The overall failure to find significant benefit from heparin was thought to result from subtherapeutic anticoagulation due to suboptimal heparin regimens. The dose administered in the trials was relatively conservative; the subcutaneous route resulted in delayed onset of therapeutic effect and was initiated relatively late (4 h in ISIS-3 and 12 h in the GISSI-2/International Study.

Intravenous Heparin This is an important adjunctive agent in decreasing reocclusion following t-PA for acute ST-segment-elevation MI.[64] Infarct-related artery patency has been studied in four angiographic trials evaluating whether heparin improves patency. No difference in patency was seen at 90 min.[336] Between 18 h and 5 days, however, there was higher patency among patients randomized to receive intravenous heparin.[67–69] Since early patency was similar, the benefit of heparin is felt to be due largely to decreased reocclusion. All clinical trials with novel variants of t-PA (r-PA and TNK–t-PA) have used adjunctive heparin. Following streptokinase or anistreplase, the role of heparin is less clear. One study with APSAC found no difference in coronary artery patency in those receiving heparin plus aspirin versus aspirin alone.[337]

The Global Use of Strategies to Open Occluded Coronary Arteries (GUSTO)-1 trial was partially designed to answer the question regarding subcutaneous heparin, intravenous heparin, or neither in conjunction with fibrinolytics.[41] Of the 41,021 patients enrolled in GUSTO-1, a total of 20,251 were randomized to streptokinase plus aspirin with either subcutaneous heparin (12,500 U twice daily starting 4 h after the start of fibrinolytics) or intravenous heparin (5000 U followed by 1000 U/h started immediately). The intravenous or subcutaneous heparin groups had similar infarct-related artery patency at 90 min and 24 h, but those receiving intravenous heparin had significantly higher patency at 5 to 7 days (84 vs. 72 percent, $p = 0.04$).[64] However, the 30-day mortality and rate of disabling stroke were not significantly different, being 7.2 and 0.5 percent with subcutaneous heparin and 7.4 percent and 0.5 percent with intravenous heparin ($p = NS$). It should be noted, however, that patients randomized to the subcutaneous arm did receive intravenous heparin when recurrent ischemia developed. All 10,396 patients receiving t-PA and aspirin were treated with intravenous heparin and had a 30-day mortality and rate of disabling stroke of 6.3 and 0.6 percent, respectively. GUSTO-1 did not find a significant difference in severe or life-threatening bleeding among any of the groups (0.3 percent for streptokinase and subcutaneous heparin, 0.5 percent for streptokinase and intravenous heparin, and 0.4 percent for t-PA). This study found that there was no benefit of intravenous heparin over subcutaneous heparin when streptokinase and aspirin was used and that there was even a trend toward increased bleeding with intravenous heparin.

TABLE 54-11 Effect of Heparin with or without Aspirin in 26 Randomized Trials of Coronary Fibrinolysis Demonstrating the Clear Advantage of the Addition of Aspirin to Heparin as Adjunctive Therapy to Fibrinolytics[a]

Variables	No Aspirin (n = 5,459)	p Value	Aspirin (n = 68,090)	p Value
Death	35	0.002	5	0.03
Reinfarction	15	0.08	3	0.04
Stroke	10	0.01	1	0.01
Major bleeding	10 more	0.01	3 more	<0.001

[a]Data are presented as reduction per 1000 patients assigned heparin.
SOURCE: From Hirsh et al.[295] With permission.

Metanalysis Two overviews attempted to pool data from multiple studies to clarify the role of heparin in acute MI treated with fibrinolytics because while the incremental value of aspirin is clear, that of heparin is not (Table 54-11). Mahaffey et al. analyzed six randomized trials of fibrinolytic therapy (streptokinase, t-PA, and APSAC) involving 1735 patients treated with intravenous heparin versus placebo.[338] They found a nonsignificant difference in in-hospital mortality of 5.1 percent with heparin versus 5.6 percent with placebo (OR 0.91, 95 percent CI 0.59 to 1.39). No significant difference was found with streptokinase versus t-PA or with or without aspirin therapy. While there was no significant reduction in reinfarction or recurrent ischemia, there was a trend toward increased risk of intracranial bleeding and a clear increase in overall bleeding (OR 1.55, 95 percent CI 1.21 to 1.98) with intravenous heparin. Because of these adverse consequences and the absolute benefit of only 5 deaths per 1000 patients treated, the authors concluded that there were not enough data to support or refute the routine use of intravenous heparin. The overview by Collins et al. pooled data from 26 studies of heparin versus placebo, the majority of patients coming from GISSI-2 and ISIS-3.[339] They found that in the absence of aspirin, heparin reduced mortality by 25 percent (95 percent CI 10 to 38 percent, p = 0.002), while in the presence of aspirin, mortality was reduced by only 6 percent (95 percent CI 0 to 10 percent, p = 0.03). No difference was found between subcutaneous and intravenous heparin and there was again a nonsignificant increase in stroke and a clear increase in major bleeding. These authors concluded that the current evidence from trials does not justify the routine addition of heparin to aspirin with fibrinolytic therapy.

Analysis of almost 30,000 patients from the GUSTO I study revealed a relationship between the activated partial thromboplastin time (aPTT) and clinical outcomes in patients treated with fibrinolytic (t-PA and streptokinase) and intravenous heparin.[340] At 12 h, the

aPTT associated with the lowest 30-day mortality, stroke, and bleeding rates was 50 to 70 s; aPTTs higher than 70 s were found to be associated with a higher likelihood of mortality, stroke, bleeding, and reinfarction (Fig. 54-32).

Low-Molecular-Weight Heparin LMWH has only recently been studied in combination with fibrinolytics and aspirin. With its greater inhibition of thrombin generation, simpler route of administration, more predictable anticoagulant effect, and lack of monitoring requirements, LMWH might be superior to UFH after fibrinolytics.[341] Enoxaparin is currently the only LMWH with consistently positive large-scale trial data supporting its use in this context, but dalteparin is also starting to accumulate results from smaller clinical trials.

Enoxaparin PATENCY STUDIES The Second Trial of Heparin and Aspirin Reperfusion Therapy (HART II) was the initial patency trial enrolling 400 patients undergoing fibrinolytic therapy (t-PA) to either enoxaparin or UFH.[342] Enoxaparin was found not to be inferior to UFH overall, with a trend toward benefit in 90-min patency rates (80.1 vs. 75.1 percent) and in reocclusion rates at 5 to 7 days

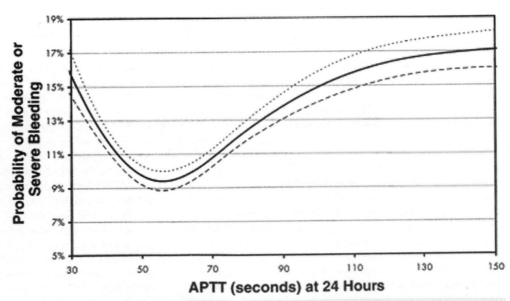

FIGURE 54-32 Activated partial thromboplastin time versus probability of bleeding at 24 h with 95 percent confidence intervals marked from the GUSTO 1 trial.[24](From Granger et al.[340] With permission.)

(5.9 vs. 9.8 percent). No increase in bleeding was seen with enoxaparin therapy.

The AMI-SK study examined enoxaparin in combination with streptokinase in 496 patients with ST-segment-elevation MI.[343] Treatment with enoxaparin (30 mg intravenous bolus followed by 1 mg/kg every 12 h) resulted in improved TIMI 3 flow rates at 8 days (70 vs. 58 percent, $p = 0.01$), improved ST-segment resolution at 180 min, and improved composite clinical endpoint of death, reinfarction, and recurrent angina at 30 days (13 vs. 21 percent, $p = 0.03$).

The Enoxaparin and TNK–t-PA With or Without GP-IIb/IIIa Inhibitor as Reperfusion Strategy in ST Elevation MI (ENTIRE)–TIMI 23 evaluated enoxaparin versus UFH in the setting of either full-tenecteplase or half-dose tenecteplase plus abciximab.[344] In the 483 patients enrolled, there was similar TIMI 3 flow rates at 60 min (51 vs. 50 percent) with enoxaparin and UFH; but at 30 days of follow-up, there was a significant reduction in death and MI in the enoxaparin group (10.7 vs. 5.0 percent, $p = 0.012$). There was a nonsignificant increase in major hemorrhage with enoxaparin (5.2 vs. 3.8 percent).

In a small clinical outcomes trial of 300 patients receiving fibrinolysis (streptokinase, anistreplase, or t-PA) for acute ST-segment-elevation MI, subjects were randomized to enoxaparin or UFH for 4 days.[345] At 90 days there was approximately a 10 percent absolute reduction in the composite endpoint of death, reinfarction, or unstable angina (36.4 vs. 25.5 percent, $p = 0.04$), with no significant differences in major bleeding. There was a suggestion that a "rebound" increase in clinical events was reduced by enoxaparin, with a rate of reinfarction from days 4 to 6 at 6.6 percent for heparin vs. 2.2 percent for enoxaparin ($p = 0.05$).

CLINICAL STUDIES   The Assessment of the Safety and Efficacy of a New Thrombolytic Regimen (ASSENT) –3 trial included the first large-scale trial of enoxaparin compared to UFH in patients with acute MI presenting within 6 h of symptom onset who were treated with tenecteplase and aspirin.[98] Over 2000 patients were randomized to each group and followed for the composite primary endpoint of 30-day mortality, in-hospital reinfarction, and in-hospital refractory ischemia in addition to safety endpoints. The study found a significant 26 percent relative risk reduction (95 percent CI 13 to 37 percent, $p = 0.0002$) with enoxaparin, which was driven by significant reductions in reinfarction and refractory ischemia. While there was also a significant reduction (19 percent, $p = 0.0081$) in the combined efficacy and safety endpoints, the enoxaparin group had a greater incidence of major bleeding than the UFH group (3.0 vs. 2.2 percent, $p = 0.0005$). Interestingly, the relative risk reduction in efficacy plus safety endpoints achieved with enoxaparin was greater than that achieved with half-dose tenecteplase plus abciximab (19 vs. 16 percent).

Dalteparin   Dalteparin has been evaluated in three small pilot studies with rather equivocal results. The first and largest study was the Fragmin in Acute Myocardial Infarction (FRAMI) trial, which randomized 776 patients treated with streptokinase for ST-segment-elevation MI to dalteparin versus placebo.[346] Although the trial's primary endpoint was the occurrence of thrombus formation and arterial embolism, not coronary events, secondary analysis revealed no significant differences in reinfarction or mortality rates between the groups. Safety analysis, however, revealed an increased risk of major (2.9 vs. 0.3 percent, $p = 0.006$) and minor bleeding (14.8 vs. 1.8 percent, $p < 0.001$) with dalteparin compared to placebo. The Biochemical Markers in Acute Coronary Syndromes (BIOMACS II) study

randomized 101 patients treated with streptokinase to placebo or two doses of dalteparin and found a nonsignificant trend toward improved TIMI 3 flow and ischemic events by ST-segment monitoring at 24 h.[318] Finally, the ASSENT-PLUS trial examined 434 patients treated with reteplase and given either dalteparin or UFH as adjuvant therapy.[347] TIMI 3 flow at 4 to 7 days demonstrated a trend toward improvement with dalteparin as compared to UFH without a significant increase in bleeding. Furthermore, dalteparin significantly reduced the occurrence of reinfarction compared to UFH.

Fondaparinux   PENTALYSE   The synthetic pentasaccharide factor Xa inhibitor fondaparinux was evaluated in 333 patients with ST-segment-elevation MI treated with alteplase in this phase II patency trial.[348] The PENTALYSE randomized patients to UFH for 48 to 72 h or low-, medium-, or high-dose fondaparinux for 5 to 7 days. The study demonstrated similar TIMI flow rates at 90 min (64 vs. 68 percent, $p = NS$) and a trend toward improved patency at 5 to 7 days (0.9 vs. 7.0 percent, $p = 0.065$). There were fewer revascularizations during 30 days of follow-up with fondaparinux than with heparin (39 vs. 51 percent, $p = 0.054$) and there was no difference with regard to ICH or blood transfusions.

DIRECT THROMBIN INHIBITORS

Hirudin   Early dose-ranging pilot studies such as TIMI-5 (hirudin with t-PA)[349] and TIMI-6 (hirudin with streptokinase) returned promising[350] results, with improved angiographic findings and low rates of adverse events.

Following the preliminary observations of the TIMI-9a[351] and GUSTO-IIa,[352] trials were designed to examine the role of hirudin in ST-segment-elevation MI treated with fibrinolytics. Both studies used a high dose of hirudin based on TIMI-5 data and an aggressive weight-based heparin dosing scheme and, as a result, experienced an excess of intracranial bleeding in both groups, causing both studies to be terminated prematurely by their data and safety monitoring committees. Both studies were reconfigured and resumed with lower doses of hirudin and heparin as TIMI-9b and GUSTO IIb. TIMI-9b[353] studied 3002 patients, while the 4131 patients among the over 12,000 subjects enrolled in GUSTO-IIb[319] who received either t-PA or streptokinase within 12 h of symptom onset were randomized to either hirudin or UFH. At 30 days, the primary endpoint (death, recurrent MI, congestive heart failure, or cardiogenic shock) in TIMI-9b was reached in 11.9 percent of the heparin-treated patients and 12.9 percent of the hirudin-treated patients ($p = NS$); in GUSTO-IIb, the primary endpoint (death and MI) occurred in 11.3 percent of the heparin group and 9.9 percent of the hirudin group ($p = 0.13$). The occurrence of major bleeding episodes was not significantly different between the two agents.

Hirudin was also studied concurrently on a smaller scale in the Hirudin for the Improvement of Thrombolysis (HIT) trials. HIT-I[354] and HIT-II[355] were dose-ranging patency studies that established the efficacy and safety of hirudin in about 200 patients. HIT-III[356] was similar to TIMI-9a and GUSTO IIa in that it was terminated early due to an increased incidence of intracranial bleeding after only 302 patients of a planned 7000 were enrolled. Finally, HIT-4 studied 1208 patients treated with streptokinase within 6 h of symptom onset and found no significant differences in the 30-day occurrence of death, stroke, MI, or their composite.[357]

Bivalirudin   The initial patency trial of bivalirudin in conjunction with streptokinase and aspirin in patients with acute ST-segment-elevation MI was conducted by Theroux et al.[358] Sixty-eight patients were randomized to one of two doses of bivalirudin or UFH and TIMI flow grade was assessed at 90 and 120 min. Bivalirudin was found to have significantly better TIMI flow rates than UFH at both time points, with the lower-dose bivalirudin group yielding higher patency rates that the higher-dose group.

The Hirulog Early Reperfusion/Occlusion (HERO) trial was a dose-ranging pilot study of bivalirudin in patients with ST-segment-elevation MI treated with streptokinase.[359] A total of 412 patients were randomly assigned to receive either UFH or two doses of bivalirudin. Superior patency rates were achieved with bivalirudin, as TIMI 3 flow was 35 percent (95 percent CI, 28 to 44 percent) with heparin, 46 percent (95 percent CI, 38 to 55 percent) with low-dose bivalirudin and 48 percent (95 percent CI, 40 to 57 percent) with high-dose bivalirudin (heparin vs. bivalirudin, $p = 0.023$; heparin vs. high-dose bivalirudin, $p = 0.03$). These results led to the larger HERO-2 study, which randomized 17,073 patients with acute ST-segment-elevation MI presenting within 6 h of symptoms and treated with streptokinase to either UFH or bivalirudin.[360] The primary endpoint of 30-day mortality was reached in 10.8 percent of the bivalirudin group and 10.9 percent of the heparin group ($p = $ NS). There were fewer reinfarctions at 96 h with bivalirudin (1.6 vs. 2.3 percent, $p = 0.001$), which was a prespecified secondary endpoint of the study. Again, the rates of major bleeding were similar between groups, but the rate of minor bleeding was increased with bivalirudin.

Metanalysis A pooled analysis by the OASIS investigators of hirudin versus UFH with fibrinolytic therapy found a nonsignificant relative risk reduction of 11 to 12 percent at 72 h, 7 days, and 35 days ($p = $ NS) (Fig. 54-31).[318] The Direct Thrombin Inhibitors Trialists' Collaboration conducted a metanalysis of the major randomized trials of direct thrombin inhibitors including 11 randomized trials and almost 36,000 patients.[325] Overall, direct thrombin inhibitors were found to be associated with a significantly lower risk of death or MI at the end of treatment and at 30 days. In the subgroup of patients presenting with ST-segment-elevation ACS, there was a nonsignificant 9 percent reduction in death or MI (6.3 vs. 6.9 percent; OR 0.91, 95 percent CI 0.77 to 1.06), a significant 25 percent reduction in MI (OR 0.75, 95 percent CI 0.59 to 0.94), and a nonsignificant 7 percent increase in death (OR 1.07, 95 percent CI 0.88 to 1.31) at the end of treatment. At 30 days, there were no statistically significant differences in any of the composite endpoints, although the previous trends persisted (Table 54-9).

Univalent Inhibitors Argatroban, a synthetic nonpeptide arginine derivative, has been studied in several dose-ranging pilot patency studies. In the ARGAMI study, a total of 162 patients being treated for ST-segment-elevation MI with alteplase were treated with either argatroban or UFH, and both agents were found to have similar safety and efficacy profiles.[361] In the Myocardial Infarction with Novastan and tPA (MINT) study, 125 patients treated with t-PA were randomized to argatroban or UFH; improved TIMI grade 3 flow rates were found in the high-dose argatroban group versus heparin (57.1 vs. 20.0 percent, $p = 0.03$), while major bleeding and combined clinical endpoints were also nonsignificantly reduced.[362,363] Efegatran, another synthetic arginine derivative, has also been evaluated in two small trials. The ESCALAT trial analyzed 245 patients in a dose-ranging patency trial comparing efegatran and streptokinase to UFH and t-PA; no improvement was found in TIMI flow, clinical outcomes, or safety with efegatran.[364] The Promotion of Reperfusion in Myocardial Infarction Evolution (PRIME) trial also looked at 336 patients with ST-segment-elevation MIs treated with alteplase and found no clear advantage of efegatran over UFH.[365]

Conclusions/Recommendations

The current recommendations from the ACC/AHA on the use of heparin in patients with acute MI undergoing reperfusion therapy with fibrinolytics (class IIa and IIb) vary depending on the type of fibrinolytic—selective or nonselective (Table 54-12).[37] The following is recommended in patients treated with a selective agent such as t-PA: intravenous heparin as an initial bolus of 60 U/kg and subsequent maintenance infusion of 12 U/kg/h (with a maximum of 4000-U bolus and 1000-U/h infusion in patients weighing > 70 kg) adjusted to maintain the aPTT at 50 to 70 s. This regimen is recommended for 48 h, with consideration of longer therapy in patients at high risk for thromboembolism. For nonselective agents such as streptokinase, intravenous heparin adjusted to maintain the aPTT at 50 to 70 s is recommended in patients at high risk for systemic emboli. Heparin should be withheld for 6 h following fibrinolytic and not started until the aPTT falls to < 70. In patients not at high risk, subcutaneous heparin at doses of 7500 to 12,500 U twice a day is recommended until the patient is ambulatory. The ACCP also recommends the use of intravenous UFH for 48 h in patients receiving t-PA, rt-PA, or TNK–t-PA and subcutaneous UFH in patients receiving streptokinase unless they are at high risk of systemic or venous thromboembolism.[126]

Although still under investigation and without recommendations from any major society, the combination of LMWH with fibrinolytics seems extremely promising. In addition to simplifying therapy by obviating the need to monitor anticoagulation, LMWH reduces reinfarction and recurrent ischemia, with only a small increase in bleeding. Currently, the only agent to show reproducible and significant benefit in this area has been enoxaparin. At this time, there is no evidence to suggest that the benefits seen with enoxaparin are generalizable to the remainder of the LMWH class. Given the concern regarding potential hemorrhagic complications whenever any antithrombotic is combined with a fibrinolytic, the clinical data would suggest that enoxaparin would be the LMWH to be used in combination with lytics.

Despite their superior thrombin inhibition, the direct thrombin inhibitors have not shown marked improvements over UFH in clinical trials. The majority of these direct thrombin inhibitors have been employed in conjunction with streptokinase, which is not used as extensively in the United States as it is in Canada and Europe, and there are less compelling data regarding its use with t-PA. As a result, hirudin and bivalirudin are not recommended or approved for use as antithrombotic therapy with fibrinolytics. However, the ACCP does present as a class 2A recommendation that patients with known or suspected heparin-induced thrombocytopenia or thrombosis who receive fibrinolytic therapy should be treated with a direct thrombin inhibitor as their antithrombotic therapy.[126]

ANTITHROMBOTIC THERAPY WITH PERCUTANEOUS CORONARY INTERVENTION AS THE PRIMARY STRATEGY

Unfractionated Heparin Heparin is an important therapeutic component of PCI, as therapeutic levels of anticoagulation with heparin are roughly correlated with therapeutic efficacy in the reduction of complications during coronary angioplasty. The 2001 ACC/AHA guidelines for PCI recommend that, in those patients who do not receive GP IIb/IIIa inhibitors, sufficient UFH be given during coronary angioplasty to achieve an activated clotting time (ACT) of 250 to 300 s with the HemoTec device and 300 to 350 s with the Hemochron device. The UFH bolus should be reduced to 50 to 70 U/kg when GP IIb/IIIa inhibitors are given in order to achieve a target ACT of 200 s using either the HemoTec or Hemochron device.[230]

TABLE 54-12 ACC/AHA Guidelines for Heparin Therapy in Patients with Acute ST-Segment-Elevation Myocardial Infarction Treated with Fibrinolytics

Class I

1. Patients undergoing percutaneous or surgical revascularization.

Class IIa

1. Intravenously in patients undergoing reperfusion therapy with alteplase. *Comment: The recommended regimen is 60 U/kg as a bolus at initiation of alteplase infusion, then an initial maintenance dose of 12 U/kg per hour (with a maximum of 4000 U bolus and 1000 U/h infusion for patients weighing >70 kg), adjusted to maintain aPTT at 1.5 to 2.0 times control (50 to 70 s) for 48 h. Continuation of heparin infusion beyond 48 h should be considered in patients at high risk for systemic or venous thromboembolism.*

2. Intravenous unfractionated heparin (UFH) or low-molecular-weight heparin (LMWH) subcutaneously for patients with non-ST-elevation MI.

3. Subcutaneous UFH (e.g., 7500 U bid) or LMWH (e.g., enoxaparin 1 mg/kg bid) in all patients not treated with thrombolytic therapy who do not have a contraindication to heparin. In patients who are at high risk for systemic emboli (large or anterior MI, AF, previous embolus, or known LV thrombus), intravenous heparin is preferred.

4. Intravenously in patients treated with nonselective thrombolytic agents (streptokinase, anistreplase, urokinase) who are at high risk for systemic emboli (large or anterior MI, AF, previous embolus, or known LV thrombus). *Comment: It is recommended that heparin be withheld for 6 h and that aPTT testing begin at that time. Heparin should be started when aPTT returns to <2 times control (70 s), then infused to keep aPTT 1.5 to 2.0 times control (initial infusion rate 1000 U/h). After 48 h, a change to subcutaneous heparin, warfarin, or aspirin alone should be considered.*

Class IIb

1. Patients treated with nonselective thrombolytic agents, not at high risk, subcutaneous heparin, 7500 U to 12,500 U twice a day until completely ambulatory.

Class III

1. Routine intravenous heparin within 6 h to patients receiving a nonselective fibrinolytic agent (streptokinase, anistreplase, urokinase) who are not at high risk for systemic embolism.

SOURCE: From Ryan et al.[137] With permission.

Secondary Prevention

ORAL ANTICOAGULATION

The role of long-term anticoagulation with warfarin as effective secondary prevention continues to evolve. This therapeutic debate has spanned nearly 50 years, as the first studies were performed in the 1950s and large randomized studies have been published in each of the past few years. This is because randomized trials have produced conflicting results, some showing a clear benefit and some showing no benefit and increased harm. Unlike antiplatelet therapy, oral anticoagulation is inconvenient to use due to difficulty in dosing and the need for careful monitoring to prevent overanticoagulation.

Many of the early trials produced conflicting results and are subject to major criticisms on several points, some of which are crucial. Most trials were open- or single-blind and not properly randomized; they all had small sample sizes, and historical controls were often used. A further criticism is that the intensity of the anticoagulation was not well maintained because of inadequate quality control. Because of these shortcomings, the International Review Group[366] in 1970 reviewed the results of nine prospective trials in 2487 men following MI, and adequate levels of anticoagulation were found in only 50 percent of the trials. Based on these pooled data, mortality was reduced by 20 percent but was restricted to patients with prolonged angina or previous infarction on admission to the trial. Given these equivocal results and the high frequency of bleeding complications, the practice of maintaining patients on long-term anticoagula-

tion was abandoned in many countries in spite of the observed decrease in death rate. Due to these uncertainties regarding the value of long-term anticoagulant therapy, a new series of well-designed clinical studies was started in the mid-1980s in an effort to address this unresolved issue (Table 54-13).

Warfarin versus Placebo The Norwegian Warfarin Re-Infarction Study (WARIS) trial randomized 1214 patients within 30 days of MI to either oral anticoagulation with a goal INR of 2.8 to 4.8 or placebo.[367] During a mean follow-up of 37 months, risk reduction with warfarin by intention-to-treat analysis in total mortality was 24 percent (95 percent CI, 4 to 44 percent, $p < 0.03$), in nonfatal MI, 34 percent (95 percent CI, 19 to 54 percent, $p < 0.001$), and in cerebrovascular accidents 55 percent (95 percent CI, 33 to 77 percent, $p < 0.002$). The incidence of major bleeding was 0.6 percent per year, which represented a twofold increase in major hemorrhage. Quality control revealed that two-thirds of the patients were in the preset INR range of between 2.8 and 4.8.

The Dutch trial of Anticoagulants in the Secondary Prevention of Events in Coronary Thrombosis (ASPECT) recruited 3404 hospital survivors of MI and randomly assigned them to coumarin (INR range between 2.4 and 4.8) or placebo within 8 weeks of hospital admission.[368] After a mean follow-up period of 37 months, all-cause mortality was nonsignificantly reduced by 10 percent (95 percent CI, 11 to 27 percent), but statistically significant reductions were seen in recurrent MI (RR 53 percent, 95 percent CI, 41 to 62 percent) and cere-

TABLE 54-13 Comparison of Secondary Prevention Studies of Oral Anticoagulation

Study	Date	Patients, n	Endpoint	Follow-up	ASA	Warfarin	Combination
WARIS	1990	1214	Mortality	4 years	—	INR 2.8–4.8	—
WARIS-2	2002	3630	Death, MI, stroke	4 years	160 mg	INR 2.8–4.2	75 mg + INR 2.0–2.5
ASPECT	1994	3404	Mortality	4 years	—	INR 2.4–4.8	—
ASPECT-2	2002	999	Death, MI, stroke	1 year	80 mg	INR 3.0–4.0	80 mg + INR 2.0–2.5
APRICOT	1993	300	Patency	3 months	325 mg	INR 2.8–4.0	—
APRICOT-2	2002	308	Patency	3 months	80 mg	—	80 mg + INR 2.0–3.0
CARS	1997	8803	Death, MI, stroke	14 months	160 mg	—	80 mg + 1 or 3 mg
CHAMP	2002	5059	Death, MI, stroke	2.7 years	162 mg	—	81 mg + INR 1.5–2.5
OASIS	2001	3712	Death, MI, stroke	5 months	[a]	INR 2.0–2.5	[a]

[a]Patients were randomized to anticoagulation or standard therapy. The majority of subjects in both groups were receiving aspirin.

brovascular events (RR 40 percent, 95 percent CI, 10 to 60 percent). Quality control demonstrated that two-thirds of all INR values were in the range of 2.4 to 4.8. The combined endpoint (vascular death, MI, or cerebral event) was reduced from 17.5 percent in the control group to 9.5 percent in the anticoagulated group, but at the cost of a 3.87-fold increase in major bleeding with anticoagulation. This translates into the prevention of 3.1 vascular events per 100 patient-years at the cost of one episode of major bleeding.

Warfarin versus Aspirin The Antithrombotics in the Prevention of Reocclusion in Coronary Thrombolysis (APRICOT) trial enrolled 300 subjects following MI successfully treated with thrombolytics as demonstrated at angiography and assigned them to either warfarin, aspirin, or placebo while still hospitalized.[369] At 3 months, 248 subjects had repeat angiography, which found no statistically significant difference in vessel patency rates (30, 25, and 32 percent) or mortality. A statistically significant improvement was seen with aspirin in reinfarction, revascularization, and left ventricular ejection fraction, but not with warfarin.

Warfarin plus Aspirin Considering the importance of both platelets and coagulation in the pathogenesis of acute MI, the combination of both aspirin and oral anticoagulants would seem to be a logical proposition. And, in fact, a metanalysis of the use of anticoagulation in patients with coronary heart disease published in 1999 suggested that both high-dose warfarin alone and moderate-dose warfarin with aspirin were superior to aspirin alone.[370]

The Coumadin Aspirin Reinfarction Study (CARS) trial enrolled 8803 patients following MI and compared aspirin (160 mg) to a combination of either 1 or 3 mg of fixed dose warfarin in combination with aspirin (80 mg).[371] This study showed no significant benefit of combination therapy in reducing the primary endpoint of reinfarction, stroke, or cardiovascular death after a median of 14 months of follow-up, with event rates of 8.6 percent with aspirin alone, 8.4 percent for 3 mg of warfarin plus aspirin, and 8.8 percent with 1 mg of warfarin and aspirin. While the higher-dose warfarin group achieved only a mean INR of 1.3 over the course of the study period, spontaneous major hemorrhage was doubled in this group compared to aspirin alone (1.4 vs. 0.74 percent).

The Organization to Assess Strategies for Ischemic Syndromes (OASIS) trial evaluated anticoagulation therapy in addition to aspirin in patients with unstable angina.[98] Overall, in the 3712 patients randomized to warfarin (goal INR 2.0 to 2.5) or standard therapy, there was a small, nonsignificant trend of reduction in the primary end-

point of cardiovascular death, MI, and stroke (RR 0.90, 95 percent CI 0.72 to 1.14, $p = 0.40$) in the anticoagulation group at 5 months. When subjects were divided into groups based on location in countries with good or bad compliance, there was a significant reduction in the primary outcome in the anticoagulation group in countries with good compliance (6.1 vs. 8.9 percent, RR 0.68, 95 percent CI 0.48 to 0.95). Again, there was an excess of major bleeding (2.7 vs. 1.3 percent) in the warfarin group, which was more dramatic in the good-compliance countries. Over the course of the study, anticoagulated patients had an INR > 2.0 approximately 70 percent of the time.

The Combination Hemotherapy and Mortality Prevention (CHAMP) study also found no significant benefit to combination therapy after randomizing 5059 patients within 2 weeks of MI and following them for a median of 2.7 years.[372] There were no significant differences in endpoints of mortality, MI, and stroke between the aspirin (162 mg) and aspirin (81 mg) plus warfarin (INR goal 1.5 to 2.5) groups. Again, there was almost a doubling of the major bleeding rate in the combination arm compared to the aspirin-only group (1.28 vs. 0.72 events per 100 person-years). The mean INR achieved during the study duration was 1.8, which, along with the data from the other negative trials, supports the concept of a threshold INR needed to show benefit of antithrombotic therapy or combination therapy over traditional antiplatelet therapy.

The Dutch APRICOT 2 trial randomized subjects treated with thrombolytics to 80 mg of aspirin or combination therapy with a goal INR of 2.0 to 3.0.[373] Patients had repeat angiograms at 3 months to reevaluate vessel patency. After achieving a mean INR of 2.6, there was a statistically significant relative risk reduction of 45 percent in ≤ TIMI 2 flow, with 15 percent in the combination group versus 28 percent in the aspirin-only arm ($p < 0.02$). There was also a significant reduction in reinfarction and revascularization, with survival rates free from events of 66 and 86 percent, respectively ($p < 0.01$). In this small study, bleeding complications were infrequent, with TIMI major and minor bleeding occurring in 5 and 3 percent of patients ($p = $ NS).

The ASPECT-2 trial strove to further clarify the issue of a threshold of anticoagulation and the use of combination therapy for secondary prevention of MI.[374] At total of 999 patients were randomized to low-dose aspirin (80 mg), high-dose warfarin (INR 3.0 to 4.0), or combined low-dose aspirin (80 mg) and moderate-dose warfarin (INR 2.0 to 2.5) subsequent to MI and followed for a median length of 12 months. Although the trial was terminated prematurely due to slow patient recruitment, the composite endpoint was reduced with borderline statistical significance in both anticoagulation groups. Reinfarction, stroke, or death saw a 9 percent reduction in aspirin subjects, 5 percent in high-dose warfarin subjects (HR 0.55, 95 percent CI 0.30 to 1.00, $p = 0.0479$), and 5 percent in combination therapy subjects (HR 0.50, 95 percent CI 0.27 to 0.92, $p = 0.03$). All-cause mortality was actually statistically significantly decreased from 4 to 1 percent in the high-dose warfarin group (HR 0.2, 95 percent CI 0.09 to 0.82). There were no significant differences in rates of major bleeding between groups, occurring in 1 percent on aspirin, 1 percent on high-dose warfarin, and 2 percent on combination therapy. The mean INR in the high-dose warfarin group was 3.2, with approximately half of the patients within the range of 3.0 to 4.0, while the mean INR was 2.4 in the combination group, with about 40 percent of subjects in the target range of 2.0 to 2.5.

The WARIS II trial followed up these results in a larger, randomized, open-label multicenter trial of 3630 patients enrolled from 20 Norwegian hospitals.[375] Patients hospitalized for an acute MI were randomized to either 160 mg of aspirin, warfarin adjusted to an INR of 2.8 to 4.2, or 80 mg of aspirin and warfarin adjusted to an INR of 2.0 to 2.5, and were followed for an average of 4 years. In an intention-to-treat analysis of the composite endpoint (death, reinfarction, or ischemic stroke), the study found that there was a statistically significant 29 percent (95 percent CI 17 to 40 percent, $p = 0.001$) reduction in the combination group and a 19 percent (95 percent CI 5 to 31 percent, $p = 0.03$) reduction in the warfarin group compared to aspirin alone. The mean INR achieved in the combination group was 2.2, and 2.8 in patients receiving warfarin alone. The reduction in the composite endpoint was driven by significant reductions in reinfarction (44 and 26 percent) and stroke (48 and 48 percent) in the combination and warfarin-only groups, respectively, in comparison with the aspirin groups. Major bleeding episodes were four times more likely (0.68 percent per year) in patients receiving warfarin and three times as likely (0.57 percent per year) in the combination group compared to aspirin alone (0.17 percent per year), while minor bleeding was increased 3-fold and 2.5-fold in the combination and warfarin arms re-

spectively. Finally, compliance with warfarin therapy proved to be difficult, with 40 percent and 32 percent of patients discontinuing therapy in the combination and warfarin groups compared to only 16 percent in the aspirin arm.

Metanalysis To more reliably determine the role of oral anticoagulation of varying intensity both with and without aspirin therapy, two recent overviews of all of the trials of oral anticoagulation in CAD from 1960 through 2002 were conducted.[370,376] These metanalyses examined over 30 trials involving over 20,000 patients who received oral anticoagulation for at least 3 months and stratified the trials by intensity of anticoagulation and by aspirin use (Table 54-14). The pooled data demonstrated a clear benefit to high-intensity anticoagulation (INR > 2.8) compared to control, with a 10 percent absolute reduction in the occurrence of cardiovascular death, MI, or stroke (OR 0.57, 95 percent CI 0.51 to 0.63, $p < 0.0001$). On the other hand, no significant benefit was seen with low-intensity anticoagulation (INR < 2.0) plus aspirin compared to aspirin (OR 0.91, 95 percent CI 0.79 to 1.06, $p > 0.10$) or with moderate-intensity anticoagulation (INR 2 to 3) compared to control (OR 0.84, 95 percent CI 0.63 to 1.11, $p = 0.20$). Unfortunately, high-intensity anticoagulation was associated with a 4.6 percent incidence of major bleeding, while control patients experienced only 0.7 percent, for an odds increase of 4.5 (95 percent CI 2.5 to 6.0, $p < 0.00001$). There was a 3.6 percent absolute reduction and 12 percent relative reduction in events with moderate- to high-intensity anticoagulation plus aspirin compared to aspirin alone (95 percent CI 3 to 20 percent, $p = 0.01$). This group, however, experienced fewer bleeding complications than the high-intensity group, with major bleeding occurring in 3.0 percent of combination therapy patients compared to 1.7 percent of patients receiving aspirin alone (odds increase 1.7, 95 percent CI 1.39 to 2.17, $p > 0.10$).

The magnitude of the benefit of oral anticoagulation for secondary prevention seen in individual trials and in the metanalyses is likely to be an underestimation of the true benefit of therapy, as it rep-

TABLE 54-14 Summary of Results of Metanalysis of Trials of Oral Anticoagulation for Secondary Prevention[a]

Study Type	Endpoint	OR	95% CI	p Value	Bleeding	OR	95% CI	p Value
High-intensity vs control		−43%	−37 to −49%	<0.0001		+4.5	2.5 to 6.0	<0.00001
OA (INR > 2.8)	20.3%				4.6%			
C	30.3%				0.7%		—	
Moderate-intensity vs control		−16%	−11 to + 37%	0.20		7.67	3.3 to 18	<0.0001
OA (INR 2–3)	31.3%				3.5%		—	
C	33.7%				0%			
Mod- or high-intensity vs ASA		−21%	−6 to −33%	0.008		2.1	1.7 to 2.7	<0.00001
OA	13.5%				5.5%			
ASA	16.3%				2.6%			
Mod- to high-intensity plus ASA vs ASA		−12%	−3 to −20%	0.01		1.74	1.39 to 2.17	0.01
OA plus ASA	15.9%				3.0%			
ASA	17.6%				1.7%			
Mod- to high-intensity plus ASA vs OA		−14%	−6 vs −30%	0.15		0.95	0.60 to 1.51	0.80
OA plus ASA	12.5%				2.2%			
OA	14.3%				2.3%			
Low-intensity plus ASA vs ASA		0.91	0.79 to 1.06%	>0.10		1.2	0.93 to 1.7	NS
OA (INR < 2.0) plus ASA	8.8%				2.3%			
ASA	9.6%				1.8%			

ABBREVIATIONS: OA = oral anticoagulation; C = control; ASA = aspirin.
[a]The composite endpoint examined was a combination of cardiovascular death, MI, or stroke along with the incidence of major bleeding episodes.
SOURCE: From Anand and Yusuf.[376] With permission.

resents conclusions from intention-to-treat analysis that included all patients regardless of their compliance with therapy. The true risk reduction is likely to be higher than these observed reductions when compliance is maximized and the target INR is achieved. For instance, in the OASIS trial—which demonstrated a small, nonsignificant reduction in the primary endpoint of cardiovascular death, MI, and stroke (RR 0.90, 95 percent CI 0.72 to 1.14, $p = 0.40$) with moderate-intensity anticoagulation plus aspirin—only 63.7 percent of patients who had been randomized to anticoagulation plus aspirin were actually receiving their anticoagulation.[377] When patients were analyzed in terms of their compliance (on the basis of residence in a "good compliance" country that had ≥ 70 percent compliance at 35 days vs. a "poor compliance" country that had < 70 percent compliance), a different result emerges. In "good compliance" countries, there was a significant 32 percent reduction in the primary endpoint (RR 0.68, 95 percent CI 0.48 to 0.95, $p = 0.02$), whereas there was no reduction in the primary endpoint for patients residing in "poor compliance" countries.[376] There was, however, along with this benefit, a corresponding increase in major bleeding episodes (2.71 vs. 1.58 percent).

As a whole, these trials demonstrate that long-term anticoagulant treatment after MI results in modest reductions in mortality and substantial reductions in the risk of recurrent MIs and cerebrovascular events. However, this benefit comes at the cost of an increased risk of bleeding (Fig. 54-33), which is probably related to the INR intensity rather than the simultaneous use of antiplatelet agents with oral anticoagulation. Unfortunately, it also appears that a threshold level of anticoagulation is needed in order to demonstrate benefit over aspirin alone, as low-intensity and even moderate-intensity anticoagulation were insufficient to provide a significant advantage. The fear of bleeding complications and the complexity of proper medication adjustment continue to make physicians hesitant to adopt routine anticoagulation as first-line secondary prevention when antiplatelet therapy is available as an effective and safe alternative. Furthermore, recent studies have demonstrated the superiority of dual antiplatelet therapy over aspirin alone for secondary prevention.[160,163] Additional study is needed to determine how the safety and efficacy of dual antiplatelet therapy compares with moderate-intensity oral anticoagulation.

PREVENTION OF VENTRICULAR THROMBUS AND ARTERIAL EMBOLI

The major cause of systemic arterial emboli in patients with acute MI is left ventricular mural thrombosis usually occurring after an acute anterior wall infarction. Among pooled data from several echocardiographic studies, left ventricular thrombi were found in 4 percent of inferior infarctions (range 0 to 15 percent) and in 30 percent of anterior MIs (range 20 to 40 percent).[378] Large anterior infarctions may be associated with mural thrombosis in up to 60 percent of cases.[379] Two-thirds of left ventricular thrombi occur within 2 days after an MI, and systemic emboli, on average, appear 2 weeks later. The incidence of systemic emboli appears to be about 10 percent of the incidence of mural thrombus. One autopsy study found a 50 percent incidence of systemic embolization after MI; but in patients surviving infarction, the incidence of clinically evident systemic emboli resulting from dislodgment of left ventricular thrombi is much lower, ranging from 5 to 26 percent in patients with echocardiographic evidence of mural thrombus.[380–384]

Data from the National Registry of Myocardial Infarction[385] demonstrate that, in the current era of MI therapy, there has been an increase in the prevalence of non-Q-wave infarction (from 45 percent in 1994 to 63 percent in 1999, $p = 0.0001$), with a corresponding decrease in the number of patients presenting with ST-segment elevation or left bundle branch block (LBBB) (from 36.4 percent in 1994 to 27.1 percent in 1999, $p \leq 0.001$). The combination of fewer transmural MIs and the increased used of antithrombotic and antiplatelet agents has caused the occurrence of left ventricular thrombus to be less common. Anticoagulation with immediate warfarin, UFH or LMWH, or treatment with antithrombotic agents (aspirin plus dipyridamole) has been shown to be effective in reducing the formation of left ventricular thrombi,[346,386–390] but aspirin alone does not prevent left ventricular thrombus formation.[391] In patients with left

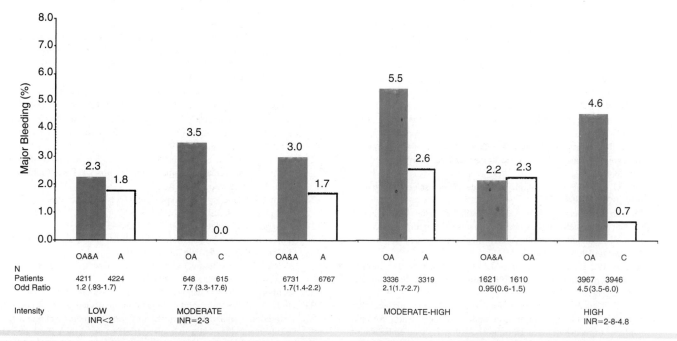

FIGURE 54-33 Major bleeding rates in patients with vascular disease treated with oral anticoagulation for secondary prevention. A = aspirin; C = control; INR = international normalized ratio; N = study population. (From Anand and Yusuf.[376] With permission.)

ventricular thrombus present by echocardiography at hospital dismissal, oral anticoagulation and aspirin were equally effective and better than no treatment in the resolution of left ventricular thrombus and the prevention of arterial thromboemboli.[392] Currently the Consensus Conference on Antithrombotic Therapy of the American College of Chest Physicians (ACCP) recommends the use of warfarin therapy for 1 to 3 months in clinical settings of increased embolic risk following MI such as anterior wall MI, severe left ventricular dysfunction, congestive heart failure, previous emboli, echocardiographic evidence of mural thrombosis, or atrial fibrillation.[142]

Conclusions/Recommendations

In light of the many options for antithrombotic therapy in secondary prevention of MI, it is often the initial management of the infarction that guides subsequent therapy. Patients with large transmural anterior infarctions or those with comorbidities such as atrial fibrillation or prosthetic valves are commonly treated with anticoagulation for secondary prevention, since anticoagulation is indicated for the treatment of the concomitant conditions. The ACCP recommends the use of long-term warfarin therapy in clinical settings of increased embolic risk for a duration of 1 to 3 months following anterior wall MI, MI complicated by severe left ventricular dysfunction, congestive heart failure, previous embolic event, echocardiographic evidence of a mural thrombus, or atrial fibrillation.[142] Recent studies such as WARIS II[375] have shown the benefit of high- or medium-dose anticoagulation plus aspirin over aspirin therapy alone without excessive amounts of bleeding. However, the complexity of managing warfarin therapy and the fear of severe bleeding remain, making this strategy less appealing than the proven effective oral antiplatelet therapy with aspirin alone or aspirin plus clopidogrel. Further study is also needed to determine if oral anticoagulation is superior to combination antiplatelet therapy. Each antithrombotic therapy, then, carries with it risks and benefits whose net balance depends on the type of patient in whom it is used.

References

1. Fuster V, Badimon L, Badimon JJ, et al. The pathogenesis of coronary artery disease and the acute coronary syndromes (1). *N Engl J Med* 1992;326:242–250.
2. Fuster V, Badimon L, Badimon JJ, et al. The pathogenesis of coronary artery disease and the acute coronary syndromes (2). *N Engl J Med* 1992;326:310–318.
3. Ambrose JA, Winters SL, Arora RR, et al. Angiographic evolution of coronary artery morphology in unstable angina. *J Am Coll Cardiol* 1986;7:472–478.
4. Mann JM, Davies MJ. Vulnerable plaque. Relation of characteristics to degree of stenosis in human coronary arteries. *Circulation* 1996;94:928–931.
5. Lee RT, Libby P. The unstable atheroma. *Arterioscler Thromb Vasc Biol* 1997;17:1859–1867.
6. Moreno PR, Bernardi VH, Lopez-Cuellar J, et al. Macrophages, smooth muscle cells, and tissue factor in unstable angina. Implications for cell-mediated thrombogenicity in acute coronary syndromes. *Circulation* 1996;94:3090–3097.
7. Merlini PA, Bauer KA, Oltrona L, et al. Persistent activation of coagulation mechanism in unstable angina and myocardial infarction. *Circulation* 1994;90:61–68.
8. Falk E. Unstable angina with fatal outcome: Dynamic coronary thrombosis leading to infarction and/or sudden death. Autopsy evidence of recurrent mural thrombosis with peripheral embolization culminating in total vascular occlusion. *Circulation* 1985;71:699–708.
9. Davies MJ, Thomas AC. Plaque fissuring—The cause of acute myocardial infarction, sudden ischaemic death, and crescendo angina. *Br Heart J* 1985;53:363–373.
10. Davies MJ. Acute coronary thrombosis—The role of plaque disruption and its initiation and prevention. *Eur Heart J* 1995;16(suppl L):3–7.
11. Falk E, Shah PK, Fuster V. Coronary plaque disruption. *Circulation* 1995;92:657–671.
12. Ambrose JA, Tannenbaum MA, Alexopoulos D, et al. Angiographic progression of coronary artery disease and the development of myocardial infarction. *J Am Coll Cardiol* 1988;12:56–62.
13. Enos WF, Holmes RH, Beyer J. Coronary disease among United States soldiers killed in action in Korea: Preliminary report. *JAMA* 1953;152:1090–1093.
14. Adderley SR, Fitzgerald DJ. Glycoprotein IIb/IIIa antagonists induce apoptosis in rat cardiomyocytes by caspase-3 activation. *J Biol Chem* 2000;275:5760–5766.
15. Kadar A, Glasz T. Development of atherosclerosis and plaque biology. *Cardiovasc Surg* 2001;9:109–121.
16. Stary HC, Blankenhorn DH, Chandler AB, et al. A definition of the intima of human arteries and of its atherosclerosis-prone regions. A report from the Committee on Vascular Lesions of the Council on Arteriosclerosis, American Heart Association. *Circulation* 1992;85:391–405.
17. Stary HC, Chandler AB, Glagov S, et al. A definition of initial, fatty streak, and intermediate lesions of atherosclerosis. A report from the Committee on Vascular Lesions of the Council on Arteriosclerosis, American Heart Association. *Circulation* 1994;89:2462–2478.
18. Stary HC, Chandler AB, Dinsmore RE, et al. A definition of advanced types of atherosclerotic lesions and a histological classification of atherosclerosis. A report from the Committee on Vascular Lesions of the Council on Arteriosclerosis, American Heart Association. *Circulation* 1995;92:1355–1374.
19. Kinlay S, Ganz P. Role of endothelial dysfunction in coronary artery disease and implications for therapy. *Am J Cardiol* 1997;80:11I–16I.
20. Furchgott RF, Zawadzki JV. The obligatory role of endothelial cells in the relaxation of arterial smooth muscle by acetylcholine. *Nature* 1980;288:373–376.
21. Cai H, Harrison DG. Endothelial dysfunction in cardiovascular diseases: The role of oxidant stress. *Circ Res* 2000;87:840–844.
22. Ross R. Atherosclerosis—An inflammatory disease. *N Engl J Med* 1999;340:115–126.
23. Schachinger V, Britten MB, Zeiher AM. Prognostic impact of coronary vasodilator dysfunction on adverse long-term outcome of coronary heart disease. *Circulation* 2000;101:1899–1906.
24. Moncada S, Higgs A. The L-arginine-nitric oxide pathway. *N Engl J Med* 1993;329:2002–2012.
25. Verma S, Anderson TJ. Fundamentals of endothelial function for the clinical cardiologist. *Circulation* 2002;105:546–549.
26. Vita JA, Treasure CB, Nabel EG, et al. Coronary vasomotor response to acetylcholine relates to risk factors for coronary artery disease. *Circulation* 1990;81:491–497.
27. Gimbrone MA Jr, Topper JN, Nagel T, et al. Endothelial dysfunction, hemodynamic forces, and atherogenesis. *Ann N Y Acad Sci* 2000;902:230–239; discussion 239–240.
28. Roth GJ, Calverley DC. Aspirin, platelets, and thrombosis: Theory and practice. *Blood* 1994;83:885–898.
29. George JN. Platelets. *Lancet* 2000;355:1531–1539.
30. Furie B, Furie BC. Molecular and cellular biology of blood coagulation. *N Engl J Med* 1992;326:800–806.
31. Davie EW. Biochemical and molecular aspects of the coagulation cascade. *Thromb Haemost* 1995;74:1–6.
32. Nemerson Y. Tissue factor and hemostasis. *Blood* 1988;71:1–8.
33. Indications for fibrinolytic therapy in suspected acute myocardial infarction: Collaborative overview of early mortality and major morbidity results from all randomised trials of more than 1000 patients. Fibrinolytic Therapy Trialists' (FTT) Collaborative Group. *Lancet* 1994;343:311–322.

34. Jackson KW, Tang J. Complete amino acid sequence of streptokinase and its homology with serine proteases. *Biochemistry* 1982;21: 6620–6625.

35. Reddy KN. Streptokinase—Biochemistry and clinical application. *Enzyme* 1988;40:79–89.

36. Battershill PE, Benfield P, Goa KL. Streptokinase. A review of its pharmacology and therapeutic efficacy in acute myocardial infarction in older patients. *Drugs Aging* 1994;4:63–86.

37. Ryan TJ, Antman EM, Brooks NH, et al. 1999 update: ACC/AHA Guidelines for the Management of Patients With Acute Myocardial Infarction: Executive Summary and Recommendations: A report of the American College of Cardiology/American Heart Association Task Force on Practice Guidelines (Committee on Management of Acute Myocardial Infarction). *Circulation* 1999;100:1016–1030.

38. Effectiveness of intravenous thrombolytic treatment in acute myocardial infarction. Gruppo Italiano per lo Studio della Streptochinasi nell'Infarto Miocardico (GISSI). *Lancet* 1986;1:397–402.

39. Randomised trial of intravenous streptokinase, oral aspirin, both, or neither among 17,187 cases of suspected acute myocardial infarction: ISIS-2. ISIS-2 (Second International Study of Infarct Survival) Collaborative Group. *Lancet* 1988;2:349–360.

40. ISIS-3: A randomised comparison of streptokinase vs tissue plasminogen activator vs anistreplase and of aspirin plus heparin vs aspirin alone among 41,299 cases of suspected acute myocardial infarction. ISIS-3 (Third International Study of Infarct Survival) Collaborative Group. *Lancet* 1992;339:753–770.

41. An international randomized trial comparing four thrombolytic strategies for acute myocardial infarction. The GUSTO investigators. *N Engl J Med* 1993;329:673–682.

42. Smith RA, Dupe RJ, English PD, et al. Fibrinolysis with acyl-enzymes: A new approach to thrombolytic therapy. *Nature* 1981;290:505–508.

43. Monk JP, Heel RC. Anisoylated plasminogen streptokinase activator complex (APSAC). A review of its mechanism of action, clinical pharmacology and therapeutic use in acute myocardial infarction. *Drugs* 1987;34:25–49.

44. Effect of intravenous APSAC on mortality after acute myocardial infarction: Preliminary report of a placebo-controlled clinical trial. AIMS Trial Study Group. *Lancet* 1988;1:545–549.

45. Cannon CP, McCabe CH, Diver DJ, et al. Comparison of front-loaded recombinant tissue-type plasminogen activator, anistreplase and combination thrombolytic therapy for acute myocardial infarction: Results of the Thrombolysis in Myocardial Infarction (TIMI) 4 trial. *J Am Coll Cardiol* 1994;24:1602–1610.

46. Prehospital thrombolytic therapy in patients with suspected acute myocardial infarction. The European Myocardial Infarction Project Group. *N Engl J Med* 1993;329:383–389.

47. Rawles J. Halving of mortality at 1 year by domiciliary thrombolysis in the Grampian Region Early Anistreplase Trial (GREAT). *J Am Coll Cardiol* 1994;23:1–5.

48. Barlow GH. Urinary and kidney cell plasminogen activator (urokinase). *Methods Enzymol* 1976;45:239–244.

49. Nolli ML, Sarubbi E, Corti A, et al. Production and characterization of human recombinant single chain urokinase-type plasminogen activator from mouse cells. *Fibrinolysis* 1989;3:101–106.

50. Declerck PJ, Lijnen HR, Verstreken M, et al. A monoclonal antibody specific for two-chain urokinase-type plasminogen activator. Application to the study of the mechanism of clot lysis with single-chain urokinase-type plasminogen activator in plasma. *Blood* 1990;75: 1794–1800.

51. Scully MF, Ellis V, Watahiki Y, et al. Activation of pro-urokinase by plasmin: Non-Michaelian kinetics indicates a mechanism of negative cooperativity. *Arch Biochem Biophys* 1989;268:438–446.

52. Michels HR, Hoffman JJ, Bar FW. Pharmacokinetics and hemostatic effects of saruplase in patients with acute myocardial infarction: Comparison of infusion, single-bolus, and split-bolus administration. *J Thromb Thrombolysis* 1999;8:213–221.

53. Tebbe U, Windeler J, Boesl I, et al. Thrombolysis with recombinant unglycosylated single-chain urokinase-type plasminogen activator (saruplase) in acute myocardial infarction: Influence of heparin on early patency rate (LIMITS study). Liquemin in Myocardial Infarction During Thrombolysis With Saruplase. *J Am Coll Cardiol* 1995;26:365–373.

54. Pennica D, Holmes WE, Kohr WJ, et al. Cloning and expression of human tissue-type plasminogen activator cDNA in E. coli. *Nature* 1983;301:214–221.

55. Hoylaerts M, Rijken DC, Lijnen HR, et al. Kinetics of the activation of plasminogen by human tissue plasminogen activator. Role of fibrin. *J Biol Chem* 1982;257:2912–2919.

56. Van de Werf F, Bergmann SR, Fox KA, et al. Coronary thrombolysis with intravenously administered human tissue-type plasminogen activator produced by recombinant DNA technology. *Circulation* 1984; 69:605–610.

57. The Thrombolysis in Myocardial Infarction (TIMI) trial. Phase I findings. TIMI Study Group. *N Engl J Med* 1985;312:932–936.

58. Chesebro JH, Knatterud G, Roberts R, et al. Thrombolysis in Myocardial Infarction (TIMI) Trial, Phase I: A comparison between intravenous tissue plasminogen activator and intravenous streptokinase. Clinical findings through hospital discharge. *Circulation* 1987;76: 142–154.

59. Verstraete M, Bernard R, Bory M, et al. Randomised trial of intravenous recombinant tissue-type plasminogen activator versus intravenous streptokinase in acute myocardial infarction. Report from the European Cooperative Study Group for Recombinant Tissue-type Plasminogen Activator. *Lancet* 1985;1:842–847.

60. Granger CB, Califf RM, Topol EJ. Thrombolytic therapy for acute myocardial infarction. A review. *Drugs* 1992;44:293–325.

61. Neuhaus KL, Feuerer W, Jeep-Tebbe S, et al. Improved thrombolysis with a modified dose regimen of recombinant tissue-type plasminogen activator. *J Am Coll Cardiol* 1989;14:1566–1569.

62. Carney RJ, Murphy GA, Brandt TR, et al. Randomized angiographic trial of recombinant tissue-type plasminogen activator (alteplase) in myocardial infarction. RAAMI Study Investigators. *J Am Coll Cardiol* 1992;20:17–23.

63. Neuhaus KL, von Essen R, Tebbe U, et al. Improved thrombolysis in acute myocardial infarction with front-loaded administration of alteplase: Results of the rt-PA-APSAC patency study (TAPS). *J Am Coll Cardiol* 1992;19:885–891.

64. The effects of tissue plasminogen activator, streptokinase, or both on coronary-artery patency, ventricular function, and survival after acute myocardial infarction. The GUSTO Angiographic Investigators. *N Engl J Med* 1993;329:1615–1622.

65. GISSI-2: A factorial randomised trial of alteplase versus streptokinase and heparin versus no heparin among 12,490 patients with acute myocardial infarction. Gruppo Italiano per lo Studio della Sopravvivenza nell'Infarto Miocardico. *Lancet* 1990;336:65–71.

66. In-hospital mortality and clinical course of 20,891 patients with suspected acute myocardial infarction randomised between alteplase and streptokinase with or without heparin. The International Study Group. *Lancet* 1990;336:71–75.

67. Hsia J, Hamilton WP, Kleiman N, et al. A comparison between heparin and low-dose aspirin as adjunctive therapy with tissue plasminogen activator for acute myocardial infarction. Heparin-Aspirin Reperfusion Trial (HART) Investigators. *N Engl J Med* 1990;323:1433–1437.

68. Bleich SD, Nichols TC, Schumacher RR, et al. Effect of heparin on coronary arterial patency after thrombolysis with tissue plasminogen activator in acute myocardial infarction. *Am J Cardiol* 1990;6: 1412–1417.

69. de Bono DP, Simoons ML, Tijssen J, et al. Effect of early intravenous heparin on coronary patency, infarct size, and bleeding complications after alteplase thrombolysis: Results of a randomised double blind European Cooperative Study Group trial. *Br Heart J* 1992;67: 122–128.

70. Purvis JA, McNeill AJ, Siddiqui RA, et al. Efficacy of 100 mg of double-bolus alteplase in achieving complete perfusion in the treatment of acute myocardial infarction. *J Am Coll Cardiol* 1994; 23:6–10.

71. Bleich SD, Adgey AA, McMechan SR, et al. An angiographic assessment of alteplase: Double-bolus and front-loaded infusion regimens in myocardial infarction. DouBLE Study Investigators. Double Bolus Lysis Efficacy. *Am Heart J* 1998;136:741–748.

72. A comparison of continuous infusion of alteplase with double-bolus administration for acute myocardial infarction. The Continuous Infusion versus Double-Bolus Administration of Alteplase (COBALT) Investigators. *N Engl J Med* 1997;337:1124–1130.

73. Torr SR, Nachowiak DA, Fujii S, et al. "Plasminogen steal" and clot lysis. *J Am Coll Cardiol* 1992;19:1085–1090.

74. Fischer S, Kohnert U. Major mechanistic differences explain the higher clot lysis potency of reteplase over alteplase: Lack of fibrin binding is an advantage for bolus application of fibrin-specific thrombolytics. *Fibrinolysis Proteolysis* 1997;11:129–135.

75. Martin U, von Mollendorff E, Akpan W, et al. Dose-ranging study of the novel recombinant plasminogen activator BM 06.022 in healthy volunteers. *Clin Pharmacol Ther* 1991;50:429–436.

76. Seifried E, Muller MM, Martin U, et al. Bolus application of a novel recombinant plasminogen activator in acute myocardial infarction patients: Pharmacokinetics and effects on the hemostatic system. *Ann N Y Acad Sci* 1992;667:417–420.

77. Tebbe U, von Essen R, Smolarz A, et al. Open, noncontrolled dose-finding study with a novel recombinant plasminogen activator (BM 06.022) given as a double bolus in patients with acute myocardial infarction. *Am J Cardiol* 1993;72:518–524.

78. Smalling RW, Bode C, Kalbfleisch J, et al. More rapid, complete, and stable coronary thrombolysis with bolus administration of reteplase compared with alteplase infusion in acute myocardial infarction. RAPID Investigators. *Circulation* 1995;91:2725–2732.

79. Bode C, Smalling RW, Berg G, et al. Randomized comparison of coronary thrombolysis achieved with double-bolus reteplase (recombinant plasminogen activator) and front-loaded, accelerated alteplase (recombinant tissue plasminogen activator) in patients with acute myocardial infarction. The RAPID II Investigators. *Circulation* 1996;94:891–898.

80. Randomised, double-blind comparison of reteplase double-bolus administration with streptokinase in acute myocardial infarction (INJECT): Trial to investigate equivalence. International Joint Efficacy Comparison of Thrombolytics. *Lancet* 1995;346:329–336.

81. A comparison of reteplase with alteplase for acute myocardial infarction. The Global Use of Strategies to Open Occluded Coronary Arteries (GUSTO III) Investigators. *N Engl J Med* 1997;337:1118–1123.

82. Cannon CP, McCabe CH, Gibson CM, et al. TNK-tissue plasminogen activator in acute myocardial infarction. Results of the Thrombolysis in Myocardial Infarction (TIMI) 10: A dose-ranging trial. *Circulation* 1997;95:351–356.

83. Modi NB, Eppler S, Breed J, et al. Pharmacokinetics of a slower clearing tissue plasminogen activator variant, TNK-tPA, in patients with acute myocardial infarction. *Thromb Haemost* 1998;79:134–139.

84. Benedict CR, Refino CJ, Keyt BA, et al. New variant of human tissue plasminogen activator (TPA) with enhanced efficacy and lower incidence of bleeding compared with recombinant human TPA. *Circulation* 1995;92:3032–3040.

85. Cannon CP, Gibson CM, McCabe CH, et al. TNK-tissue plasminogen activator compared with front-loaded alteplase in acute myocardial infarction: Results of the TIMI 10B trial. Thrombolysis in Myocardial Infarction (TIMI) 10B Investigators. *Circulation* 1998;98:2805–2814.

86. Tanswell P, Tebbe U, Neuhaus KL, et al. Pharmacokinetics and fibrin specificity of alteplase during accelerated infusions in acute myocardial infarction. *J Am Coll Cardiol* 1992;19:1071–1075.

87. Gibson CM, Cannon CP, Murphy SA, et al. Weight-adjusted dosing of TNK-tissue plasminogen activator and its relation to angiographic outcomes in the thrombolysis in myocardial infarction 10B trial. TIMI 10B Investigators. *Am J Cardiol* 1999;84:976–980.

88. Van de Werf F, Cannon CP, Luyten A, et al. Safety assessment of single-bolus administration of TNK tissue-plasminogen activator in acute myocardial infarction: The ASSENT-1 trial. The ASSENT-1 Investigators. *Am Heart J* 1999;137:786–791.

89. Giugliano RP, McCabe CH, Antman EM, et al. Lower-dose heparin with fibrinolysis is associated with lower rates of intracranial hemorrhage. *Am Heart J* 2001;141:742–750.

90. Fox NL, Cannon CP, Berioli S, et al. Rates of serious bleeding requiring transfusion in AMI patients treated with TNK. *J Am Coll Cardiol* 1999;33(suppl A):353A.

91. Single-bolus tenecteplase compared with front-loaded alteplase in acute myocardial infarction: The ASSENT-2 double-blind randomised trial. Assessment of the Safety and Efficacy of a New Thrombolytic Investigator. *Lancet* 1999;354:716–722.

92. Ware JH, Antman EM. Equivalence trials. *N Engl J Med* 1997;337:1159–1161.

93. Zeymer U, Tebbe U, Essen R, et al. Influence of time to treatment on early infarct-related artery patency after different thrombolytic regimens. ALKK-Study Group. *Am Heart J* 1999;137:34–38.

94. Barron HV, Fox NL, Berioli S, et al. Comparison of intracranial hemorrhage rates in patients treated with rt-PA and TNK-tPA: Impact of gender, age and low body weight. *Circulation* 1999;100 (suppl I):I-1.

95. Simoons ML, Maggioni AP, Knatterud G, et al. Individual risk assessment for intracranial haemorrhage during thrombolytic therapy. *Lancet* 1993;342:1523–1528.

96. Gurwitz JH, Gore JM, Goldberg RJ, et al. Risk for intracranial hemorrhage after tissue plasminogen activator treatment for acute myocardial infarction. Participants in the National Registry of Myocardial Infarction 2. *Ann Intern Med* 1998;129:597–604.

97. Van de Werf F, Barron HV, Armstrong PW, et al. Incidence and predictors of bleeding events after fibrinolytic therapy with fibrin-specific agents: A comparison of TNK-tPA and rt-PA. *Eur Heart J* 2001;22:2253–2261.

98. Efficacy and safety of tenecteplase in combination with enoxaparin, abciximab, or unfractionated heparin: The ASSENT-3 randomised trial in acute myocardial infarction. *Lancet* 2001;358:605–613.

99. Verstraete M. Third-generation thrombolytic drugs. *Am J Med* 2000;109:52–58.

100. White HD, Van de Werf FJ. Thrombolysis for acute myocardial infarction. *Circulation* 1998;97:1632–1646.

101. den Heijer P, Vermeer F, Ambrosioni E, et al. Evaluation of a weight-adjusted single-bolus plasminogen activator in patients with myocardial infarction: A double-blind, randomized angiographic trial of lanoteplase versus alteplase. *Circulation* 1998;98:2117–2125.

102. Kostis JB, Dockens RC, Thadani U, et al. Comparison of pharmacokinetics of lanoteplase and alteplase during acute myocardial infarction. *Clin Pharmacokinet* 2002;41:445–452.

103. Intravenous NPA for the treatment of infarcting myocardium early; InTIME-II, a double-blind comparison of single-bolus lanoteplase vs accelerated alteplase for the treatment of patients with acute myocardial infarction. *Eur Heart J* 2000;21:2005–2013.

104. Giugliano RP, Antman EM, McCabe CH, et al. Omission of heparin bolus lowers rate of intracranial hemorrhage with lanoteplase. *J Am Coll Cardiol* 2000;35 (suppl A):407A.

105. Kawai C, Hosoda S, Motomiya T, et al. Multicenter trial of a novel modified t-PA, E6010, by bolus injection in patients with acute myocardial infarction. *Circulation* 1994;86(suppl I):I-409.

106. Kawai C, Yui Y, Hosoda S, et al. A prospective, randomized, double-blind multicenter trial of a single bolus injection of the novel modified t-PA E6010 in the treatment of acute myocardial infarction: Comparison with native t-PA. E6010 Study Group. *J Am Coll Cardiol* 1997;29:1447–1453.

107. Kimura K, Tsukahara K, Usui T, et al. Low-dose tissue plasminogen activator followed by planned rescue angioplasty reduces time to reperfusion for acute myocardial infarction treated at community hospitals. *Jpn Circ J* 2001;65:901–906.

108. Inoue T, Yaguchi I, Takayanagi K, et al. A new thrombolytic agent, monteplase, is independent of the plasminogen activator inhibitor in patients with acute myocardial infarction: Initial results of the COmbining Monteplase with Angioplasty (COMA) trial. *Am Heart J* 2002;144:E5.

109. Nagao K, Hayashi N, Kanmatsuse K, et al. An early and complete reperfusion strategy for acute myocardial infarction using fibrinolysis

and subsequent transluminal therapy—The FAST trial. *Circ J* 2002; 66:576–582.

110. Hashimoto K, Oikawa K, Miyamoto I, et al. Phase 1 study of a novel modified t-PA. *Jpn J Med Pharm Sci* 1996;36:623–646.

111. Haze K, Kawai C, Hosoda S, et al. Efficacy and safety of intracoronary administration of YM866 (modified tissue-type plasminogen activator) in patients with acute myocardial infarction. *Jpn Pharmacol Ther* 1996;24:2468–2990.

112. Yui Y, Haze K, Kawai C, et al. Randomized, double-blind multicenter trial of YM866 (modified t-PA) by intravenous bolus injection in patients with acute myocardial infarction in comparison with tisokinase (native t-PA). *J New Remed Clin* 1996;45:2175–2221.

113. Collen D, Lijnen HR. Staphylokinase, a fibrin-specific plasminogen activator with therapeutic potential? *Blood* 1994;84:680–686.

114. Schlott B, Hartmann M, Guhrs KH, et al. Functional properties of recombinant staphylokinase variants obtained by site-specific mutagenesis of methionine-26. *Biochim Biophys Acta* 1994;1204: 235–242.

115. Lijnen HR, Van Hoef B, Vandenbossche L, et al. Biochemical properties of natural and recombinant staphylokinase. *Fibrinolysis* 1992;6: 214–225.

116. Collen D, Van de Werf F. Coronary thrombolysis with recombinant staphylokinase in patients with evolving myocardial infarction. *Circulation* 1993;87:1850–1853.

117. Vanderschueren SM, Stassen JM, Collen D. On the immunogenicity of recombinant staphylokinase in patients and in animal models. *Thromb Haemost* 1994;72:297–301.

118. Vanderschueren S, Collen D, van de Werf F. A pilot study on bolus administration of recombinant staphylokinase for coronary artery thrombolysis. *Thromb Haemost* 1996;76:541–544.

119. Vanderschueren S, Barrios L, Kerdsinchai P, et al. A randomized trial of recombinant staphylokinase versus alteplase for coronary artery patency in acute myocardial infarction. The STAR Trial Group. *Circulation* 1995;92:2044–2049.

120. Vanderschueren S, Dens J, Kerdsinchai P, et al. Randomized coronary patency trial of double-bolus recombinant staphylokinase versus front-loaded alteplase in acute myocardial infarction. *Am Heart J* 1997;134:213–219.

121. Collen D, Bernaerts R, Declerck P, et al. Recombinant staphylokinase variants with altered immunoreactivity. I: Construction and characterization. *Circulation* 1996;94:197–206.

122. Collen D, Sinnaeve P, Demarsin E, et al. Polyethylene glycol-derivatized cysteine-substitution variants of recombinant staphylokinase for single-bolus treatment of acute myocardial infarction. *Circulation* 2000;102:1766–1772.

123. Gardell SJ, Duong LT, Diehl RE, et al. Isolation, characterization, and cDNA cloning of a vampire bat salivary plasminogen activator. *J Biol Chem* 1989;264:17947–17952.

124. Gardell SJ, Hare TR, Bergum PW, et al. Vampire bat salivary plasminogen activator is quiescent in human plasma in the absence of fibrin unlike human tissue plasminogen activator. *Blood* 1990;76: 2560–2564.

125. Witt W, Maass B, Baldus B, et al. Coronary thrombolysis with *Desmodus* salivary plasminogen activator in dogs. Fast and persistent recanalization by intravenous bolus administration. *Circulation* 1994; 90:421–426.

126. Ohman EM, Harrington RA, Cannon CP, et al. Intravenous thrombolysis in acute myocardial infarction. *Chest* 2001;119: 253S–277S.

127. Aversano T, Aversano LT, Passamani E, et al. Thrombolytic therapy vs primary percutaneous coronary intervention for myocardial infarction in patients presenting to hospitals without on-site cardiac surgery: A randomized controlled trial. *JAMA* 2002;287:1943–1951.

128. Awtry EH, Loscalzo J. Aspirin. *Circulation* 2000;101:1206–1218.

129. FitzGerald GA. Mechanisms of platelet activation: Thromboxane A2 as an amplifying signal for other agonists. *Am J Cardiol* 1991;68: 11B–15B.

130. Williams CS, DuBois RN. Prostaglandin endoperoxide synthase: Why two isoforms? *Am J Physiol* 1996;270:G393–G400.

131. Smith WL. Prostanoid biosynthesis and mechanisms of action. *Am J Physiol* 1992;263:F181–F191.

132. Hawkey CJ. COX-2 inhibitors. *Lancet* 1999;353:307–314.

133. Patrono C. Aspirin as an antiplatelet drug. *N Engl J Med* 1994;330: 1287–1294.

134. Final report on the aspirin component of the ongoing Physicians' Health Study. Steering Committee of the Physicians' Health Study Research Group. *N Engl J Med* 1989;321:129–135.

135. Peto R, Gray R, Collins R, et al. Randomised trial of prophylactic daily aspirin in British male doctors. *Br Med J (Clin Res Ed)* 1988;296: 313–316.

136. Hennekens CH, Peto R, Hutchison GB, et al. An overview of the British and American aspirin studies. *N Engl J Med* 1988;318: 923–924.

137. Collaborative overview of randomised trials of antiplatelet therapy—I: Prevention of death, myocardial infarction, and stroke by prolonged antiplatelet therapy in various categories of patients. Antiplatelet Trialists' Collaboration. *Br Med J* 1994;308:81–106.

138. de Gaetano G. Low-dose aspirin and vitamin E in people at cardiovascular risk: A randomised trial in general practice. Collaborative Group of the Primary Prevention Project. *Lancet* 2001;357:89–95.

139. Thrombosis prevention trial: Randomised trial of low-intensity oral anticoagulation with warfarin and low-dose aspirin in the primary prevention of ischaemic heart disease in men at increased risk. The Medical Research Council's General Practice Research Framework. *Lancet* 1998;351:233–241.

139a. Manson JE, Stampfer MJ, Colditz GA, et al. A prospective study of aspirin use and primary prevention of cardiovascular disease on women. *JAMA* 1991;266:521–527.

140. Hansson L, Zanchetti A, Carruthers SG, et al. Effects of intensive blood-pressure lowering and low-dose aspirin in patients with hypertension: Principal results of the Hypertension Optimal Treatment (HOT) randomised trial. HOT Study Group. *Lancet* 1998;351:1755–1762.

141. Pearson TA, Blair SN, Daniels SR, et al. AHA Guidelines for Primary Prevention of Cardiovascular Disease and Stroke: 2002 Update: Consensus Panel Guide to Comprehensive Risk Reduction for Adult Patients Without Coronary or Other Atherosclerotic Vascular Diseases. American Heart Association Science Advisory and Coordinating Committee. *Circulation* 2002;106:388–391.

142. Cairns JA, Theroux P, Lewis HD Jr, et al. Antithrombotic agents in coronary artery disease. *Chest* 2001;119:228S–252S.

143. Aspirin for the primary prevention of cardiovascular events: Recommendation and rationale. *Ann Intern Med* 2002;136:157–160.

144. Lewis HD Jr, Davis JW, Archibald DG, et al. Protective effects of aspirin against acute myocardial infarction and death in men with unstable angina. Results of a Veterans Administration Cooperative Study. *N Engl J Med* 1983;309:396–403.

145. Cairns JA, Gent M, Singer J, et al. Aspirin, sulfinpyrazone, or both in unstable angina. Results of a Canadian multicenter trial. *N Engl J Med* 1985;313:1369–1375.

146. Theroux P, Ouimet H, McCans J, et al. Aspirin, heparin, or both to treat acute unstable angina. *N Engl J Med* 1988;319:1105–1111.

147. Risk of myocardial infarction and death during treatment with low dose aspirin and intravenous heparin in men with unstable coronary artery disease. The RISC Group. *Lancet* 1990;336:827–830.

148. Collaborative meta-analysis of randomised trials of antiplatelet therapy for prevention of death, myocardial infarction, and stroke in high risk patients. *BMJ* 2002;324:71–86.

149. Savi P, Pereillo JM, Uzabiaga MF, et al. Identification and biological activity of the active metabolite of clopidogrel. *Thromb Haemost* 2000;84:891–896.

150. Sharis PJ, Cannon CP, Loscalzo J. The antiplatelet effects of ticlopidine and clopidogrel. *Ann Intern Med* 1998;129:394–405.

151. Quinn MJ, Fitzgerald DJ. Ticlopidine and clopidogrel. *Circulation* 1999;100:1667–1672.

152. Defreyn G, Gachet C, Savi P, et al. Ticlopidine and clopidogrel (SR 25990C) selectively neutralize ADP inhibition of PGE1-activated platelet adenylate cyclase in rats and rabbits. *Thromb Haemost* 1991; 65:186–190.

153. Geiger J, Brich J, Honig-Liedl P. Thienopyridine-based antiplatelet drugs inhibit ADP effects on prostaglandin-stimulated, cAMP/PKA-mediated phosphorylation of the cytoskeletal protein VASP in human platelets (abstr). *Circulation* 1998;98(suppl I):I-595.

154. Gachet C, Savi P, Ohlmann P, et al. ADP receptor induced activation of guanine nucleotide binding proteins in rat platelet membranes—An effect selectively blocked by the thienopyridine clopidogrel. *Thromb Haemost* 1992;68:79–83.

155. Gill S, Majumdar S, Brown NE, et al. Ticlopidine-associated pancytopenia: Implications of an acetylsalicylic acid alternative. *Can J Cardiol* 1997;13:909–913.

156. Bennett CL, Weinberg PD, Rozenberg-Ben-Dror K, et al. Thrombotic thrombocytopenic purpura associated with ticlopidine. A review of 60 cases. *Ann Intern Med* 1998;128:541–544.

157. Bennett CL, Connors JM, Carwile JM, et al. Thrombotic thrombocytopenic purpura associated with clopidogrel. *N Engl J Med* 2000;342:1773–1777.

158. Mehta SR, Yusuf S. The Clopidogrel in Unstable angina to prevent Recurrent Events (CURE) trial programme; Rationale, design and baseline characteristics including a meta-analysis of the effects of thienopyridines in vascular disease. *Eur Heart J* 2000;21:2033–2041.

159. Balsano F, Rizzon P, Violi F, et al. Antiplatelet treatment with ticlopidine in unstable angina. A controlled multicenter clinical trial. The Studio della Ticlopidina nell'Angina Instabile Group. *Circulation* 1990;82:17–26.

160. Yusuf S, Zhao F, Mehta SR, et al. Effects of clopidogrel in addition to aspirin in patients with acute coronary syndromes without ST-segment elevation. *N Engl J Med* 2001;345:494–502.

161. Peters RJG, Zao F, Lewis BS, et al. Aspirin dose and bleeding events in the CURE study. *Eur Heart J* 2002;23:510.

162. Mehta SR, Yusuf S, Peters RJ, et al. Effects of pretreatment with clopidogrel and aspirin followed by long-term therapy in patients undergoing percutaneous coronary intervention: The PCI-CURE study. *Lancet* 2001;358:527–533.

163. Steinhubl SR, Berger PB, Mann JT III, et al. Early and sustained dual oral antiplatelet therapy following percutaneous coronary intervention: A randomized controlled trial. *JAMA* 2002;288:2411–2420.

164. Lefkovits J, Plow EF, Topol EJ. Platelet glycoprotein IIb/IIIa receptors in cardiovascular medicine. *N Engl J Med* 1995;332:1553–1559.

165. Topol EJ, Byzova TV, Plow EF. Platelet GPIIb-IIIa blockers. *Lancet* 1999;353:227–231.

166. Pytela R, Pierschbacher MD, Ginsberg MH, et al. Platelet membrane glycoprotein IIb/IIIa: Member of a family of Arg-Gly-Asp–specific adhesion receptors. *Science* 1986;231:1559–1562.

167. Shattil SJ, Ginsberg MH. Integrin signaling in vascular biology. *J Clin Invest* 1997;100:S91–S95.

168. Cierniewski CS, Byzova T, Papierak M, et al. Peptide ligands can bind to distinct sites in integrin alphaIIbbeta$_3$ and elicit different functional responses. *J Biol Chem* 1999;274:16923–16932.

169. Du XP, Plow EF, Frelinger AL III, et al. Ligands "activate" integrin alpha IIb beta 3 (platelet GPIIb-IIIa). *Cell* 1991;65:409–416.

170. Coller BS, Peerschke EI, Scudder LE, et al. A murine monoclonal antibody that completely blocks the binding of fibrinogen to platelets produces a thrombasthenic-like state in normal platelets and binds to glycoproteins IIb and/or IIIa. *J Clin Invest* 1983;72:325–338.

171. Coller BS. Blockade of platelet GPIIb/IIIa receptors as an antithrombotic strategy. *Circulation* 1995;92:2373–2380.

172. Lincoff AM, Califf RM, Topol EJ. Platelet glycoprotein IIb/IIIa receptor blockade in coronary artery disease. *J Am Coll Cardiol* 2000;35:1103–1115.

173. Reverter JC, Beguin S, Kessels H, et al. Inhibition of platelet-mediated, tissue factor-induced thrombin generation by the mouse/human chimeric 7E3 antibody. Potential implications for the effect of c7E3 Fab treatment on acute thrombosis and "clinical restenosis." *J Clin Invest* 1996;98:863–874.

174. Kleiman NS, Raizner AE, Jordan R, et al. Differential inhibition of platelet aggregation induced by adenosine diphosphate or a thrombin receptor-activating peptide in patients treated with bolus chimeric 7E3 Fab: Implications for inhibition of the internal pool of GPIIb/IIIa receptors. *J Am Coll Cardiol* 1995;26:1665–1671.

175. Crenshaw BS, Harrington R, Tcheng JE. Novel antiplatelet agents: The glycoprotein IIb/IIIa inhibitors. *Exp Opin Invest Drugs* 1995;4:1033–1044.

176. Inhibition of platelet glycoprotein IIb/IIIa with eptifibatide in patients with acute coronary syndromes. The PURSUIT Trial Investigators. Platelet Glycoprotein IIb/IIIa in Unstable Angina: Receptor Suppression Using Integrilin Therapy. *N Engl J Med* 1998;339:436–443.

177. Harrington RA, Lincoff MA, Berdan LG, et al. Maintenance of clinical benefit at six-months in patients treated with the platelet glycoprotein IIb/IIIa inhibitor eptifibatide versus placebo during an acute ischemic coronary event. *Circulation* 1998;98:I-359.

178. A comparison of aspirin plus tirofiban with aspirin plus heparin for unstable angina. Platelet Receptor Inhibition in Ischemic Syndrome Management (PRISM) Study Investigators. *N Engl J Med* 1998;338:1498–1505.

179. Heeschen C, Hamm CW, Goldmann B, et al. Troponin concentrations for stratification of patients with acute coronary syndromes in relation to therapeutic efficacy of tirofiban. PRISM Study Investigators. Platelet Receptor Inhibition in Ischemic Syndrome Management. *Lancet* 1999;354:1757–1762.

180. Inhibition of the platelet glycoprotein IIb/IIIa receptor with tirofiban in unstable angina and non-Q-wave myocardial infarction. Platelet Receptor Inhibition in Ischemic Syndrome Management in Patients Limited by Unstable Signs and Symptoms (PRISM-PLUS) Study Investigators. *N Engl J Med* 1998;338:1488–1497.

181. Mark DB, Cowper PA, Berkowitz SD, et al. Economic assessment of low-molecular-weight heparin (enoxaparin) versus unfractionated heparin in acute coronary syndrome patients: Results from the ESSENCE randomized trial. Efficacy and Safety of Subcutaneous Enoxaparin in Non-Q wave Coronary Events [unstable angina or non-Q-wave myocardial infarction]. *Circulation* 1998;97:1702–1707.

182. Moliterno DJ. Patient-specific dosing of IIb/IIIa antagonists during acute coronary syndromes: Rationale and design of the PARAGON B study. The PARAGON B International Steering Committee. *Am Heart J* 2000;139:563–566.

183. Harrington RA. *PARAGON B*. 49th Annual Scientific Session of the American College of Cardiology. Anaheim, CA: American College of Cardiology; 2000.

184. Newby LK, Ohman EM, Christenson RH, et al. Benefit of glycoprotein IIb/IIIa inhibition in patients with acute coronary syndromes and troponin T–positive status: The PARAGON-B troponin T substudy. *Circulation* 2001;103:2891–2896.

185. Simoons ML. Effect of glycoprotein IIb/IIIa receptor blocker abciximab on outcome in patients with acute coronary syndromes without early coronary revascularisation: The GUSTO IV-ACS randomised trial. *Lancet* 2001;357:1915–1924.

186. Braunwald E, Antman EM, Beasley JW, et al. ACC/AHA guideline update for the management of patients with unstable angina and non-ST-segment elevation myocardial infarction—2002: Summary article: a report of the American College of Cardiology/American Heart Association Task Force on Practice Guidelines (Committee on the Management of Patients With Unstable Angina). *Circulation* 2002;106:1893–1900.

187. Roffi M, Chew DP, Mukherjee D, et al. Platelet glycoprotein IIb/IIIa inhibition in acute coronary syndromes. Gradient of benefit related to the revascularization strategy. *Eur Heart J* 2002;23:1441–1448.

188. Roux S, Christeller S, Ludin E. Effects of aspirin on coronary reocclusion and recurrent ischemia after thrombolysis: A meta-analysis. *J Am Coll Cardiol* 1992;19:671–677.

189. Baigent C, Collins R, Appleby P, et al. ISIS-2: 10 year survival among patients with suspected acute myocardial infarction in randomised comparison of intravenous streptokinase, oral aspirin, both, or neither. The ISIS-2 (Second International Study of Infarct Survival) Collaborative Group. *BMJ* 1998;316:1337–1343.

190. Cannon CP, Braunwald E. GUSTO, TIMI and the case for rapid reperfusion. *Acta Cardiol* 1994;49:1–8.

191. Ito H, Tomooka T, Sakai N, et al. Lack of myocardial perfusion immediately after successful thrombolysis. A predictor of poor recovery of left ventricular function in anterior myocardial infarction. *Circulation* 1992;85:1699–705.

192. Ohman EM, Califf RM, Topol EJ, et al. Consequences of reocclusion after successful reperfusion therapy in acute myocardial infarction. TAMI Study Group. *Circulation* 1990;82:781–791.

193. Cannon CP. Overcoming thrombolytic resistance: Rationale and initial clinical experience combining thrombolytic therapy and glycoprotein IIb/IIIa receptor inhibition for acute myocardial infarction. *J Am Coll Cardiol* 1999;34:1395–1402.

194. Coller BS. Platelets and thrombolytic therapy. *N Engl J Med* 1990; 322:33–42.

195. Weitz JI, Hudoba M, Massel D, et al. Clot-bound thrombin is protected from inhibition by heparin-antithrombin III but is susceptible to inactivation by antithrombin III-independent inhibitors. *J Clin Invest* 1990;86:385–391.

196. Owen J, Friedman KD, Grossman BA, et al. Thrombolytic therapy with tissue plasminogen activator or streptokinase induces transient thrombin activity. *Blood* 1988;72:616–620.

197. Trial of abciximab with and without low-dose reteplase for acute myocardial infarction. Strategies for Patency Enhancement in the Emergency Department (SPEED) Group. *Circulation* 2000;101: 2788–2794.

198. Antman EM, Giugliano RP, Gibson CM, et al. Abciximab facilitates the rate and extent of thrombolysis: Results of the thrombolysis in myocardial infarction (TIMI) 14 trial. The TIMI 14 Investigators. *Circulation* 1999;99:2720–2732.

199. Topol EJ. Reperfusion therapy for acute myocardial infarction with fibrinolytic therapy or combination reduced fibrinolytic therapy and platelet glycoprotein IIb/IIIa inhibition: The GUSTO V randomised trial. *Lancet* 2001;357:1905–1914.

200. Lincoff AM, Califf RM, Van de Werf F, et al. Mortality at 1 year with combination platelet glycoprotein IIb/IIIa inhibition and reduced-dose fibrinolytic therapy vs conventional fibrinolytic therapy for acute myocardial infarction: GUSTO V randomized trial. *JAMA* 2002;288:2130–2135.

201. Ohman EM, Kleiman NS, Gacioch G, et al. Combined accelerated tissue-plasminogen activator and platelet glycoprotein IIb/IIIa integrin receptor blockade with Integrilin in acute myocardial infarction. Results of a randomized, placebo-controlled, dose-ranging trial. IMPACT-AMI Investigators. *Circulation* 1997;95:846–854.

202. Brener SJ, Zeymer U, Adgey AA, et al. Eptifibatide and low-dose tissue plasminogen activator in acute myocardial infarction: The integrilin and low-dose thrombolysis in acute myocardial infarction (INTRO AMI) trial. *J Am Coll Cardiol* 2002;39:377–386.

203. Ronner E, van Kesteren HA, Zijnen P, et al. Safety and efficacy of eptifibatide vs placebo in patients receiving thrombolytic therapy with streptokinase for acute myocardial infarction; A phase II dose escalation, randomized, double-blind study. *Eur Heart J* 2000;21: 1530–1536.

204. Roe MT, Green C, Crater S, et al. Improved speed and stability of reperfusion with reduced-dose tenecteplase and eptifibatide for acute myocardial infarction. *Circulation* 2002;106(suppl):II-629.

205. Zeymer U, Roe MT, Giugliano RP, et al. Effects of facilitated percutaneous coronary intervention on myocardial perfusion and clinical outcome in patients treated with reduced dose tenecteplase and eptifibatide for acute myocardial infarction. *Circulation* 2002;106 (suppl):II-445.

206. Gibson CM, Murphy SA, Marble SJ, et al. Combination therapy with eptifibatide and TNK is associated with an improved rate of dye entry into the myocardium (TIMI myocardial frame count) in ST elevation myocardial infarction (STEMI): An INTEGRITI substudy. *Circulation* 2002;106(suppl):II-363.

207. Giugliano RP, Roe MT, Zeymer U, et al. Restoration of epicardial and myocardial perfusion in acute ST-elevation myocardial infarction with combination eptifibatide + reduced-dose tenecteplase: Dose-finding results from the INTEGRITI trial. *Circulation* 2001;104 (suppl):II-538.

208. Combining thrombolysis with the platelet glycoprotein IIb/IIIa inhibitor lamifiban: Results of the Platelet Aggregation Receptor Antagonist Dose Investigation and Reperfusion Gain in Myocardial Infarction (PARADIGM) trial. *J Am Coll Cardiol* 1998;32:2003–2010.

209. Schwartz L, Bourassa MG, Lesperance J, et al. Aspirin and dipyridamole in the prevention of restenosis after percutaneous transluminal coronary angioplasty. *N Engl J Med* 1988;318:1714–1719.

210. Lembo NJ, Black AJ, Roubin GS, et al. Effect of pretreatment with aspirin versus aspirin plus dipyridamole on frequency and type of acute complications of percutaneous transluminal coronary angioplasty. *Am J Cardiol* 1990;65:422–426.

211. Leon MB, Baim DS, Popma JJ, et al. A clinical trial comparing three antithrombotic-drug regimens after coronary-artery stenting. Stent Anticoagulation Restenosis Study Investigators. *N Engl J Med* 1998; 339:1665–1671.

212. Urban P, Macaya C, Rupprecht HJ, et al. Randomized evaluation of anticoagulation versus antiplatelet therapy after coronary stent implantation in high-risk patients: The multicenter aspirin and ticlopidine trial after intracoronary stenting (MATTIS). *Circulation* 1998;98: 2126–2132.

213. Schomig A, Neumann FJ, Kastrati A, et al. A randomized comparison of antiplatelet and anticoagulant therapy after the placement of coronary-artery stents. *N Engl J Med* 1996;334:1084–1089.

214. Hall P, Nakamura S, Maiello L, et al. A randomized comparison of combined ticlopidine and aspirin therapy versus aspirin therapy alone after successful intravascular ultrasound-guided stent implantation. *Circulation* 1996;93:215–222.

215. Bertrand ME, Legrand V, Boland J, et al. Randomized multicenter comparison of conventional anticoagulation versus antiplatelet therapy in unplanned and elective coronary stenting. The full anticoagulation versus aspirin and ticlopidine (fantastic) study. *Circulation* 1998;98:1597–1603.

216. Moussa I, Oetgen M, Roubin G, et al. Effectiveness of clopidogrel and aspirin versus ticlopidine and aspirin in preventing stent thrombosis after coronary stent implantation. *Circulation* 1999;99: 2364–2366.

217. Berger PB, Bell MR, Rihal CS, et al. Clopidogrel versus ticlopidine after intracoronary stent placement. *J Am Coll Cardiol* 1999;34: 1891–1894.

218. Muller C, Buttner HJ, Petersen J, et al. A randomized comparison of clopidogrel and aspirin versus ticlopidine and aspirin after the placement of coronary-artery stents. *Circulation* 2000;101:590–593.

219. Bertrand ME, Rupprecht HJ, Urban P, et al. Double-blind study of the safety of clopidogrel with and without a loading dose in combination with aspirin compared with ticlopidine in combination with aspirin after coronary stenting: The clopidogrel aspirin stent international cooperative study (CLASSICS). *Circulation* 2000;102:624–629.

220. Mishkel GJ, Aguirre FV, Ligon RW, et al. Clopidogrel as adjunctive antiplatelet therapy during coronary stenting. *J Am Coll Cardiol* 1999;34:1884–1890.

221. Brener SJ, Barr LA, Burchenal JE, et al. Randomized, placebo-controlled trial of platelet glycoprotein IIb/IIIa blockade with primary angioplasty for acute myocardial infarction. ReoPro and Primary PTCA Organization and Randomized Trial (RAPPORT) Investigators. *Circulation* 1998;98:734–741.

222. Neumann FJ, Kastrati A, Schmitt C, et al. Effect of glycoprotein IIb/IIIa receptor blockade with abciximab on clinical and angiographic restenosis rate after the placement of coronary stents following acute myocardial infarction. *J Am Coll Cardiol* 2000;35:915–921.

223. van den Merkhof LF, Zijlstra F, Olsson H, et al. Abciximab in the treatment of acute myocardial infarction eligible for primary percutaneous transluminal coronary angioplasty. Results of the Glycoprotein Receptor Antagonist Patency Evaluation (GRAPE) pilot study. *J Am Coll Cardiol* 1999;33:1528–1532.

224. Neumann FJ, Blasini R, Schmitt C, et al. Effect of glycoprotein IIb/IIIa receptor blockade on recovery of coronary flow and left ventricular function after the placement of coronary-artery stents in acute myocardial infarction. *Circulation* 1998;98:2695–2701.

225. Schomig A, Kastrati A, Dirschinger J, et al. Coronary stenting plus platelet glycoprotein IIb/IIIa blockade compared with tissue plasminogen activator in acute myocardial infarction. Stent versus Thrombolysis for Occluded Coronary Arteries in Patients with Acute Myocardial Infarction Study Investigators. *N Engl J Med* 2000;343: 385–391.

226. Montalescot G, Barragan P, Wittenberg O, et al. Platelet glycoprotein IIb/IIIa inhibition with coronary stenting for acute myocardial infarction. *N Engl J Med* 2001;344:1895–1903.

227. Stone GW, Grines CL, Cox DA, et al. Comparison of angioplasty with stenting, with or without abciximab, in acute myocardial infarction. *N Engl J Med* 2002;346:957–966.

228. Cutlip DE, Cove CJ, Irons D, et al. Emergency room administration of eptifibatide before primary angioplasty for ST elevation acute myocardial infarction and its effect on baseline coronary flow and procedure outcomes. *Am J Cardiol* 2001;88:A6,62–64.

229. L'Allier PL, Brener SJ. Evidence of more complete arterial patency with immediate percutaneous intervention and eptifibatide plus reduced-dose t-PA in acute myocardial infarction. Final results from the INTRO-AMI trial. *Circulation* 2001;104 (suppl):II-465.

230. Smith SC Jr, Dove JT, Jacobs AK, et al. ACC/AHA guidelines for percutaneous coronary intervention (revision of the 1993 PTCA guidelines)—Executive summary: A report of the American College of Cardiology/American Heart Association task force on practice guidelines (Committee to revise the 1993 guidelines for percutaneous transluminal coronary angioplasty) endorsed by the Society for Cardiac Angiography and Interventions. *Circulation* 2001;103: 3019–3041.

231. Popma JJ, Ohman EM, Weitz J, et al. Antithrombotic therapy in patients undergoing percutaneous coronary intervention. *Chest* 2001; 119:321S–336S.

232. Keeley EC, Boura JA, Grines CL. Primary angioplasty versus intravenous thrombolytic therapy for acute myocardial infarction: A quantitative review of 23 randomised trials. *Lancet* 2003;361: 13–20.

233. Morbidity & mortality: *2002 Chart Book on Cardiovascular, Lung, and Blood Diseases*. Bethesda, MD: National Heart, Lung, and Blood Institute; May 2002.

234. Patrono C, Coller B, Dalen JE, et al. Platelet-active drugs: The relationships among dose, effectiveness, and side effects. *Chest* 2001; 119:39S–63S.

235. He J, Whelton PK, Vu B, et al. Aspirin and risk of hemorrhagic stroke: A meta-analysis of randomized controlled trials. *JAMA* 1998;280: 1930–1935.

236. Derry S, Loke YK. Risk of gastrointestinal haemorrhage with long term use of aspirin: Meta-analysis. *BMJ* 2000;321:1183–1187.

237. Roderick PJ, Wilkes HC, Meade TW. The gastrointestinal toxicity of aspirin: An overview of randomised controlled trials. *Br J Clin Pharmacol* 1993;35:219–226.

238. United Kingdom transient ischaemic attack (UK-TIA) aspirin trial: Interim results. UK-TIA Study Group. *BMJ (Clin Res Ed)* 1988; 296:316–320.

239. Weisman SM, Graham DY. Evaluation of the benefits and risks of low-dose aspirin in the secondary prevention of cardiovascular and cerebrovascular events. *Arch Intern Med* 2002;162:2197–2202.

240. Eikelboom JW, Hirsh J, Weitz JI, et al. Aspirin-resistant thromboxane biosynthesis and the risk of myocardial infarction, stroke, or cardiovascular death in patients at high risk for cardiovascular events. *Circulation* 2002;105:1650–1655.

241. Gum PA, Kottke-Marchant K, Poggio ED, et al. Profile and prevalence of aspirin resistance in patients with cardiovascular disease. *Am J Cardiol* 2001;88:230–235.

242. A randomised, blinded, trial of clopidogrel versus aspirin in patients at risk of ischaemic events (CAPRIE). CAPRIE Steering Committee. *Lancet* 1996;348:1329–1339.

243. Cannon CP. Effectiveness of clopidogrel versus aspirin in preventing acute myocardial infarction in patients with symptomatic atherothrombosis (CAPRIE trial). *Am J Cardiol* 2002;90:760–762.

244. Bhatt DL, Chew DP, Hirsch AT, et al. Superiority of clopidogrel versus aspirin in patients with prior cardiac surgery. *Circulation* 2001;103:363–368.

245. The CRUSADE Registry. *European Society of Cardiology Scientific Sessions*. Berlin: European Society of Cardiology; 2002.

246. Kong DF, Califf RM, Miller DP, et al. Clinical outcomes of therapeutic agents that block the platelet glycoprotein IIb/IIIa integrin in ischemic heart disease. *Circulation* 1998;98:2829–2835.

247. Chew DP, Moliterno DJ. A critical appraisal of platelet glycoprotein IIb/IIIa inhibition. *J Am Coll Cardiol* 2000;36:2028–2035.

248. Trip MD, Cats VM, van Capelle FJ, et al. Platelet hyperreactivity and prognosis in survivors of myocardial infarction. *N Engl J Med* 1990; 322:1549–1554.

249. Giugliano RP, McCabe CH, Sequeira RF, et al. First report of an intravenous and oral glycoprotein IIb/IIIa inhibitor (RPR 109891) in patients with recent acute coronary syndromes: Results of the TIMI 15A and 15B trials. *Am Heart J* 2000;140:81–93.

250. Ferguson JJ, Deedwania PD, Kereiakes DJ, et al. Sustained platelet GP IIb/IIIa blockade with oral orofiban: Interim pharmacodynamic results of the SOAR study (abstr). *J Am Coll Cardiol* 1998;31(suppl A):185A.

251. Mousa SA, Kapil R, Mu DX. Intravenous and oral antithrombotic efficacy of the novel platelet GPIIb/IIIa antagonist roxifiban (DMP754) and its free acid form, XV459. *Arterioscler Thromb Vasc Biol* 1999;19:2535–2541.

252. Cannon CP, McCabe CH, Borzak S, et al. Randomized trial of an oral platelet glycoprotein IIb/IIIa antagonist, sibrafiban, in patients after an acute coronary syndrome: Results of the TIMI 12 trial. Thrombolysis in Myocardial Infarction. *Circulation* 1998;97:340–349.

253. Kereiakes DJ, Kleiman NS, Ferguson JJ, et al. Pharmacodynamic efficacy, clinical safety, and outcomes after prolonged platelet glycoprotein IIb/IIIa receptor blockade with oral xemilofiban: Results of a multicenter, placebo-controlled, randomized trial. *Circulation* 1998; 98:1268–1278.

254. Akkerhuis KM, Neuhaus KL, Wilcox RG, et al. Safety and preliminary efficacy of one month glycoprotein IIb/IIIa inhibition with lefradafiban in patients with acute coronary syndromes without ST-elevation: A phase II study. *Eur Heart J* 2000;21:2042–2055.

255. Harrington RA, Armstrong PW, Graffagnino C, et al. Dose-finding, safety, and tolerability study of an oral platelet glycoprotein IIb/IIIa inhibitor, lotrafiban, in patients with coronary or cerebral atherosclerotic disease. *Circulation* 2000;102:728–735.

256. Comparison of sibrafiban with aspirin for prevention of cardiovascular events after acute coronary syndromes: A randomised trial. The SYMPHONY Investigators. Sibrafiban versus Aspirin to Yield Maximum Protection from Ischemic Heart Events Post-acute Coronary Syndromes. *Lancet* 2000;355:337–345.

257. Randomized trial of aspirin, sibrafiban, or both for secondary prevention after acute coronary syndromes. The Second SYMPHONY Investigators. *Circulation* 2001;103:1727–1733.

258. O'Neill WW, Serruys P, Knudtson M, et al. Long-term treatment with a platelet glycoprotein-receptor antagonist after percutaneous coronary revascularization. EXCITE Trial Investigators. Evaluation of oral xemilofiban in controlling thrombotic events. *N Engl J Med* 2000;342:1316–1324.

259. Cannon CP, McCabe CH, Wilcox RG, et al. Oral glycoprotein IIb/IIIa inhibition with orbofiban in patients with unstable coronary syndromes (OPUS-TIMI 16) trial. *Circulation* 2000;102:149–156.

260. Topol EJ, Easton JD, Amarenco P, et al. Design of the blockade of the glycoprotein IIb/IIIa receptor to avoid vascular occlusion (BRAVO) trial. *Am Heart J* 2000;139:927–933.

261. Hughes S. BRAVO trial stopped: Lotrafiban increases mortality: www.theheart.org, December 12, 2000.

262. Mousa SA, Bozarth JM, Lorelli W, et al. Antiplatelet efficacy of XV459, a novel nonpeptide platelet GPIIb/IIIa antagonist: Comparative platelet binding profiles with c7E3. *J Pharmacol Exp Ther* 1998;286:1277–1284.

263. Chew DP, Bhatt DL, Sapp S, et al. Increased mortality with oral platelet glycoprotein IIb/IIIa antagonists: A meta-analysis of phase III multicenter randomized trials. *Circulation* 2001;103:201–206.

264. Newby LK, Califf RM, White HD, et al. The failure of orally administered glycoprotein IIb/IIIa inhibitors to prevent recurrent cardiac events. *Am J Med* 2002;112:647–658.

265. Use of a monoclonal antibody directed against the platelet glycoprotein IIb/IIIa receptor in high-risk coronary angioplasty. The EPIC Investigation. *N Engl J Med* 1994;330:956–961.

266. Platelet glycoprotein IIb/IIIa receptor blockade and low-dose heparin during percutaneous coronary revascularization. The EPILOG Investigators. *N Engl J Med* 1997;336:1689–1696.

267. Peter K, Schwarz M, Ylanne J, et al. Induction of fibrinogen binding and platelet aggregation as a potential intrinsic property of various glycoprotein IIb/IIIa (alphaIIbbeta3) inhibitors. *Blood* 1998;92: 3240–3249.

268. Willerson JT, McNatt JM, Clubb FJ, et al. Xemilofiban, an oral GP IIb/IIIa receptor antagonist is enhanced by aspirin in inhibiting neointimal proliferation following percutaneous coronary angioplasty (abstr). *Circulation* 1997;96(suppl I):I-168.

269. Byrne A, Moran N, Maher M, et al. Continued thromboxane A2 formation despite administration of a platelet glycoprotein IIb/IIIa antagonist in patients undergoing coronary angioplasty. *Arterioscler Thromb Vasc Biol* 1997;17:3224–3229.

270. Cox D, Smith R, Quinn M, et al. Evidence of platelet activation during treatment with a GPIIb/IIIa antagonist in patients presenting with acute coronary syndromes. *J Am Coll Cardiol* 2000;36: 1514–1519.

271. Holmes MB, Sobel BE, Cannon CP, et al. Increased platelet reactivity in patients given orbofiban after an acute coronary syndrome: An OPUS-TIMI 16 substudy. Orbofiban in Patients with Unstable coronary syndromes. Thrombolysis In Myocardial Infarction. *Am J Cardiol* 2000;85:491–493, A10.

272. Ault KA, Cannon CP, Mitchell J, et al. Platelet activation in patients after an acute coronary syndrome: Results from the TIMI-12 trial. Thrombolysis in Myocardial Infarction. *J Am Coll Cardiol* 1999;33: 634–639.

273. Schneider DJ, Taatjes DJ, Sobel BE. Paradoxical inhibition of fibrinogen binding and potentiation of alpha-granule release by specific types of inhibitors of glycoprotein IIb-IIIa. *Cardiovasc Res* 2000;45:437–446.

274. Steinhubl SR, Talley JD, Braden GA, et al. Point-of-care measured platelet inhibition correlates with a reduced risk of an adverse cardiac event after percutaneous coronary intervention: Results of the GOLD (AU-Assessing Ultegra) multicenter study. *Circulation* 2001;103: 2572–2578.

275. Casey M, Fornari C, Bozovich G, et al. Increased expression of platelet P-selectin in patients treated with oral orbofiban in the OPUS TIMI 16 study (abstr). *Circulation* 1999;100(suppl I):I-681.

276. Buckley CD, Pilling D, Henriquez NV, et al. RGD peptides induce apoptosis by direct caspase-3 activation. *Nature* 1999;397:534–539.

277. DiSalveo TG, Webster MWI, Cheseboro JH, et al. Dipyridamole. In: Messerli FH, ed. *Cardiovascular Drug Therapy*. Philadelphia: Saunders; 1996:1498.

278. Gent AE, Brook CG, Foley TH, et al. Dipyridamole: A controlled trial of its effect in acute myocardial infarction. *BMJ* 1968;4:366–368.

279. Persantine and aspirin in coronary heart disease. The Persantine-Aspirin Reinfarction Study Research Group. *Circulation* 1980;62: 449–461.

280. Klimt CR, Knatterud GL, Stamler J, et al. Persantine-Aspirin Reinfarction Study. Part II. Secondary coronary prevention with persantine and aspirin. *J Am Coll Cardiol* 1986;7:251–269.

281. European Stroke Prevention Study. ESPS Group. *Stroke* 1990;21: 1122–1130.

282. Diener HC, Cunha L, Forbes C, et al. European Stroke Prevention Study. 2. Dipyridamole and acetylsalicylic acid in the secondary prevention of stroke. *J Neurol Sci* 1996;143:1–13.

283. Levine GN, Ali MN, Schafer AI. Antithrombotic therapy in patients with acute coronary syndromes. *Arch Intern Med* 2001;161:937–948.

284. Weitz JI, Leslie B, Hudoba M. Thrombin binds to soluble fibrin degradation products where it is protected from inhibition by heparin-antithrombin but susceptible to inactivation by antithrombin-independent inhibitors. *Circulation* 1998;97:544–552.

285. Telford AM, Wilson C. Trial of heparin versus atenolol in prevention of myocardial infarction in intermediate coronary syndrome. *Lancet* 1981;1:1225–1228.

286. Neri Serneri GG, Gensini GF, Poggesi L, et al. Effect of heparin, aspirin, or alteplase in reduction of myocardial ischaemia in refractory unstable angina. *Lancet* 1990;335:615–618.

287. Theroux P, Waters D, Qiu S, et al. Aspirin versus heparin to prevent myocardial infarction during the acute phase of unstable angina. *Circulation* 1993;88:2045–2048.

288. Neri Serneri GG, Modesti PA, Gensini GF, et al. Randomised comparison of subcutaneous heparin, intravenous heparin, and aspirin in unstable angina. Studio Epoorine Sottocutanea nell'Angina Instobile (SESAIR) Refrattorie Group. *Lancet* 1995;345:1201–1204.

289. Cohen M, Adams PC, Hawkins L, et al. Usefulness of antithrombotic therapy in resting angina pectoris or non-Q-wave myocardial infarction in preventing death and myocardial infarction (a pilot study from the Antithrombotic Therapy in Acute Coronary Syndromes Study Group). *Am J Cardiol* 1990;66:1287–1292.

290. Cohen M, Adams PC, Parry G, et al. Combination antithrombotic therapy in unstable rest angina and non-Q-wave infarction in nonprior aspirin users. Primary end points analysis from the ATACS trial. Antithrombotic Therapy in Acute Coronary Syndromes Research Group. *Circulation* 1994;89:81–88.

291. Cohen M, Xiong J, Parry G, et al. Prospective comparison of unstable angina versus non-Q-wave myocardial infarction during antithrombotic therapy. Antithrombotic Therapy in Acute Coronary Syndromes Research Group. *J Am Coll Cardiol* 1993;22:1338–1343.

292. Holdright D, Patel D, Cunningham D, et al. Comparison of the effect of heparin and aspirin versus aspirin alone on transient myocardial ischemia and in-hospital prognosis in patients with unstable angina. *J Am Coll Cardiol* 1994;24:39–45.

293. Gurfinkel EP, Manos EJ, Mejail RI, et al. Low molecular weight heparin versus regular heparin or aspirin in the treatment of unstable angina and silent ischemia. *J Am Coll Cardiol* 1995;26:313–318.

294. Oler A, Whooley MA, Oler J, et al. Adding heparin to aspirin reduces the incidence of myocardial infarction and death in patients with unstable angina. A meta-analysis. *JAMA* 1996;276:811–815.

295. Hirsh J, Warkentin TE, Shaughnessy SG, et al. Heparin and low-molecular-weight heparin: Mechanisms of action, pharmacokinetics, dosing, monitoring, efficacy, and safety. *Chest* 2001;119:64S–94S.

296. Monrad ES. Role of low-molecular-weight heparins in the management of patients with unstable angina pectoris and non-Q-wave acute myocardial infarction. *Am J Cardiol* 2000;85:2C–9C.

297. Waters D, Azar RR. Low-molecular-weight heparins for unstable angina. A better mousetrap? *Circulation* 1997;96:3–5.

298. Prager NA, Abendschein DR, McKenzie CR, et al. Role of thrombin compared with factor Xa in the procoagulant activity of whole blood clots. *Circulation* 1995;92:962–967.

299. Turpie AG, Gallus AS, Hoek JA. A synthetic pentasaccharide for the prevention of deep-vein thrombosis after total hip replacement. *N Engl J Med* 2001;344:619–625.

300. Wong GC, Giugliano RP, Antman EM. Use of low-molecular-weight heparins in the management of acute coronary artery syndromes and percutaneous coronary intervention. *JAMA* 2003; 289:331–342.

301. Cohen M, Demers C, Gurfinkel EP, et al. A comparison of low-molecular-weight heparin with unfractionated heparin for unstable coronary artery disease. Efficacy and Safety of Subcutaneous Enoxaparin in Non-Q-Wave Coronary Events Study Group. *N Engl J Med* 1997;337:447–452.

302. Goodman SG, Cohen M, Bigonzi F, et al. Randomized trial of low molecular weight heparin (enoxaparin) versus unfractionated heparin for unstable coronary artery disease: One-year results of the ESSENCE Study. Efficacy and Safety of Subcutaneous Enoxaparin in Non-Q-Wave Coronary Events. *J Am Coll Cardiol* 2000;36: 693–698.

303. Dose-ranging trial of enoxaparin for unstable angina: Results of TIMI 11A. The Thrombolysis in Myocardial Infarction (TIMI) 11A Trial Investigators. *J Am Coll Cardiol* 1997;29:1474–1482.

304. Antman EM, McCabe CH, Gurfinkel EP, et al. Enoxaparin prevents death and cardiac ischemic events in unstable angina/non-Q-wave myocardial infarction. Results of the thrombolysis in myocardial infarction (TIMI) 11B trial. *Circulation* 1999;100:1593–1601.

305. Antman EM, Cohen M, McCabe C, et al. Enoxaparin is superior to unfractionated heparin for preventing clinical events at 1-year follow-up of TIMI 11B and ESSENCE. *Eur Heart J* 2002;23:308–314.

306. Antman EM, Cohen M, Radley D, et al. Assessment of the treatment effect of enoxaparin for unstable angina/non-Q-wave myocardial infarction. TIMI 11B-ESSENCE meta-analysis. *Circulation* 1999;100:1602–1608.

307. Klein W, Buchwald A, Hillis WS, et al. Fragmin in unstable angina pectoris or in non-Q-wave acute myocardial infarction (the FRIC study). Fragmin in Unstable Coronary Artery Disease. *Am J Cardiol* 1997;80:30E–34E.

308. Swahn E, Wallentin L. Low-molecular-weight heparin (Fragmin) during instability in coronary artery disease (FRISC). FRISC Study Group. *Am J Cardiol* 1997;80:25E–29E.

309. Comparison of two treatment durations (6 days and 14 days) of a low molecular weight heparin with a 6-day treatment of unfractionated heparin in the initial management of unstable angina or non-Q-wave myocardial infarction: FRAXIS (FRAxiparine in Ischaemic Syndrome). *Eur Heart J* 1999;20:1553–1562.

310. Michalis LK, Papamichail N, Katsouras CS, et al. Enoxaparin versus Tinzaparin in the management of unstable coronary artery disease. *J Am Coll Cardiol* 2001;37:365A.

311. Simoons M. *The PENTUA study. Double-Blind Dose-Ranging Study of Fondaparinux (Pentasaccharide) in Unstable Angina.* American Heart Association Scientific Sessions. Anaheim, CA: AHA; 2001.

312. Verstraete M. Direct thrombin inhibitors: Appraisal of the antithrombotic/hemorrhagic balance. *Thromb Haemost* 1997;78:357–363.

313. Eikelboom JW, White H, Yusuf S. The evolving role of direct thrombin inhibitors in acute coronary syndromes. *J Am Coll Cardiol* 2003;41:70S–78S.

314. Markwardt F. Past, present and future of hirudin. *Haemostasis* 1991;21(suppl 1):11–26.

315. Wallis RB. Hirudins: From leeches to man. *Semin Thromb Hemost* 1996;22:185–196.

316. Maraganore JM, Bourdon P, Jablonski J, et al. Design and characterization of hirulogs: A novel class of bivalent peptide inhibitors of thrombin. *Biochemistry* 1990;29:7095–7101.

317. Comparison of the effects of two doses of recombinant hirudin compared with heparin in patients with acute myocardial ischemia without ST elevation: A pilot study. Organization to Assess Strategies for Ischemic Syndromes (OASIS) Investigators. *Circulation* 1997;96:769–777.

318. Frostfeldt G, Ahlberg G, Gustafsson G, et al. Low molecular weight heparin (dalteparin) as adjuvant treatment of thrombolysis in acute myocardial infarction—A pilot study: Biochemical markers in acute coronary syndromes (BIOMACS II). *J Am Coll Cardiol* 1999;33:627–633.

319. A comparison of recombinant hirudin with heparin for the treatment of acute coronary syndromes. The Global Use of Strategies to Open Occluded Coronary Arteries (GUSTO) IIb investigators. *N Engl J Med* 1996;335:775–782.

320. Antman EM, Braunwald E. A second look at bivalirudin. *Am Heart J* 2001;142:929–931.

321. Fuchs J, Cannon CP. Hirulog in the treatment of unstable angina. Results of the Thrombin Inhibition in Myocardial Ischemia (TIMI) 7 trial. *Circulation* 1995;92:727–733.

322. Kong DF, Topol EJ, Bittl JA, et al. Clinical outcomes of bivalirudin for ischemic heart disease. *Circulation* 1999;100:2049–2053.

323. Klootwijk P, Lenderink T, Meij S, et al. Anticoagulant properties, clinical efficacy and safety of efegatran, a direct thrombin inhibitor, in patients with unstable angina. *Eur Heart J* 1999;20:1101–1111.

324. A low molecular weight, selective thrombin inhibitor, inogatran, vs heparin, in unstable coronary artery disease in 1209 patients. A double-blind, randomized, dose-finding study. Thrombin Inhibition in Myocardial Ischaemia (TRIM) study group. *Eur Heart J* 1997;18:1416–1425.

325. Direct thrombin inhibitors in acute coronary syndromes: Principal results of a meta-analysis based on individual patients' data. *Lancet* 2002;359:294–302.

326. Cohen M, Theroux P, Borzak S, et al. Randomized double-blind safety study of enoxaparin versus unfractionated heparin in patients with non-ST-segment elevation acute coronary syndromes treated with tirofiban and aspirin: The ACUTE II study. The Antithrombotic Combination Using Tirofiban and Enoxaparin. *Am Heart J* 2002;144:470–477.

327. Ferguson JJ. The use of enoxaparin and IIb/IIIa antagonists in acute coronary syndromes, including PCI: Final results of the NICE 3 study. *J Am Coll Cardiol* 2001;37(suppl A):365A.

328. James S, Armstrong P, Califf R, et al. Safety and efficacy of abciximab combined with dalteparin in treatment of acute coronary syndromes. *Eur Heart J* 2002;23:1538–1545.

329. Mukherjee D, Mahaffey KW, Moliterno DJ, et al. Promise of combined low-molecular-weight heparin and platelet glycoprotein IIb/IIIa inhibition: Results from Platelet IIb/IIIa Antagonist for the Reduction of Acute coronary syndrome events in a Global Organization Network B (PARAGON B). *Am Heart J* 2002;144:995–1002.

330. Collet JP, Montalescot G, Lison L, et al. Percutaneous coronary intervention after subcutaneous enoxaparin pretreatment in patients with unstable angina pectoris. *Circulation* 2001;103:658–663.

331. Fox KA, Antman EM, Cohen M, et al. Comparison of enoxaparin versus unfractionated heparin in patients with unstable angina pectoris/non-ST-segment elevation acute myocardial infarction having subsequent percutaneous coronary intervention. *Am J Cardiol* 2002;90:477–482.

332. Invasive compared with non-invasive treatment in unstable coronary-artery disease: FRISC II prospective randomised multicentre study. FRagmin and Fast Revascularisation during InStability in Coronary artery disease Investigators. *Lancet* 1999;354:708–715.

333. Goodman SG, Fitchett D, Armstrong PW, et al. Randomized evaluation of the safety and efficacy of enoxaparin versus unfractionated heparin in high-risk patients with non-ST-segment elevation acute coronary syndromes receiving the glycoprotein IIb/IIIa inhibitor eptifibatide. *Circulation* 2003;107:238–244.

334. Lincoff AM, Bittl JA, Harrington RA, et al. Bivalirudin and provisional glycoprotein IIb/IIIa blockade compared with heparin and planned glycoprotein IIb/IIIa blockade during percutaneous coronary intervention. *JAMA* 2003;289:853–863.

335. Collins R, Peto R, Baigent C, et al. Aspirin, heparin, and fibrinolytic therapy in suspected acute myocardial infarction. *N Engl J Med* 1997;336:847–860.

336. Topol EJ, George BS, Kereiakes DJ, et al. A randomized controlled trial of intravenous tissue plasminogen activator and early intravenous heparin in acute myocardial infarction. *Circulation* 1989;79:281–286.

337. O'Connor CM, Meese R, Carney R, et al. A randomized trial of intravenous heparin in conjunction with anistreplase (anisoylated plasminogen streptokinase activator complex) in acute myocardial infarction: The Duke University Clinical Cardiology Study (DUCCS) 1. *J Am Coll Cardiol* 1994;23:11–18.

338. Mahaffey KW, Granger CB, Collins R, et al. Overview of randomized trials of intravenous heparin in patients with acute myocardial infarction treated with thrombolytic therapy. *Am J Cardiol* 1996;77:551–556.

339. Collins R, MacMahon S, Flather M, et al. Clinical effects of anticoagulant therapy in suspected acute myocardial infarction: Systematic overview of randomised trials. *BMJ* 1996;313:652–659.

340. Granger CB, Hirsch J, Califf RM, et al. Activated partial thromboplastin time and outcome after thrombolytic therapy for acute myocardial infarction: Results from the GUSTO-I trial. *Circulation* 1996;93:870–878.

341. Becker RC, Bovill EG, Seghatchian MJ, et al. Pathobiology of thrombin in acute coronary syndromes. *Am Heart J* 1998;136:S19–S31.

342. Ross AM, Molhoek P, Lundergan C, et al. Randomized comparison of enoxaparin, a low-molecular-weight heparin, with unfractionated heparin adjunctive to recombinant tissue plasminogen activator thrombolysis and aspirin: Second trial of Heparin and Aspirin Reperfusion Therapy (HART II). *Circulation* 2001;104:648–652.

343. Simoons M, Krzeminska-Pakula M, Alonso A, et al. Improved reperfusion and clinical outcome with enoxaparin as an adjunct to streptokinase thrombolysis in acute myocardial infarction. The AMI-SK study. *Eur Heart J* 2002;23:1282.

344. Antman EM, Louwerenburg HW, Baars HF, et al. Enoxaparin as adjunctive antithrombin therapy for ST-elevation myocardial infarction: Results of the ENTIRE-Thrombolysis in Myocardial Infarction (TIMI) 23 Trial. *Circulation* 2002;105:1642–1649.

345. Baird SH, Menown IB, McBride SJ, et al. Randomized comparison of enoxaparin with unfractionated heparin following fibrinolytic therapy for acute myocardial infarction. *Eur Heart J* 2002;23:627–632.

346. Kontny F, Dale J, Abildgaard U, et al. Randomized trial of low molecular weight heparin (dalteparin) in prevention of left ventricular thrombus formation and arterial embolism after acute anterior myocardial infarction: The Fragmin in Acute Myocardial Infarction (FRAMI) Study. *J Am Coll Cardiol* 1997;30:962–969.

347. Wallentin L, Dellborg DM, Lindahl B, et al. The low-molecular-weight heparin dalteparin as adjuvant therapy in acute myocardial infarction: The ASSENT PLUS study. *Clin Cardiol* 2001;24:I12–I14.

348. Coussement PK, Bassand JP, Convens C, et al. A synthetic factor-Xa inhibitor (ORG31540/SR9017A) as an adjunct to fibrinolysis in acute myocardial infarction. The PENTALYSE study. *Eur Heart J* 2001;22:1716–1724.

349. Cannon CP, McCabe CH, Henry TD, et al. A pilot trial of recombinant desulfatohirudin compared with heparin in conjunction with tissue-type plasminogen activator and aspirin for acute myocardial infarction: Results of the Thrombolysis in Myocardial Infarction (TIMI) 5 trial. *J Am Coll Cardiol* 1994;23:993–1003.

350. Lee LV. Initial experience with hirudin and streptokinase in acute myocardial infarction: Results of the Thrombolysis in Myocardial Infarction (TIMI) 6 trial. *Am J Cardiol* 1995;75:7–13.

351. Antman EM. Hirudin in acute myocardial infarction. Safety report from the Thrombolysis and Thrombin Inhibition in Myocardial Infarction (TIMI) 9A Trial. *Circulation* 1994;90:1624–1630.

352. Randomized trial of intravenous heparin versus recombinant hirudin for acute coronary syndromes. The Global Use of Strategies to Open Occluded Coronary Arteries (GUSTO) IIa Investigators. *Circulation* 1994;90:1631–1637.

353. Antman EM. Hirudin in acute myocardial infarction. Thrombolysis and Thrombin Inhibition in Myocardial Infarction (TIMI) 9B trial. *Circulation* 1996;94:911–921.

354. Zeymer U, von Essen R, Tebbe U, et al. Recombinant hirudin and front-loaded alteplase in acute myocardial infarction: Final results of a pilot study. HIT-I (hirudin for the improvement of thrombolysis). *Eur Heart J* 1995;16(suppl D):22–27.

355. von Essen R, Zeymer U, Tebbe U, et al. HBW 023 (recombinant hirudin) for the acceleration of thrombolysis and prevention of coronary reocclusion in acute myocardial infarction: Results of a dose-finding study (HIT-II) by the Arbeitsgemeinschaft Leitender Kardiologischer Krankenhausarzte. *Coron Artery Dis* 1998;9:265–272.

356. Neuhaus KL, von Essen R, Tebbe U, et al. Safety observations from the pilot phase of the randomized r-Hirudin for Improvement of Thrombolysis (HIT-III) study. A study of the Arbeitsgemeinschaft Leitender Kardiologischer Krankenhausarzte (ALKK). *Circulation* 1994;90:1638–1642.

357. Neuhaus KL, Molhoek GP, Zeymer U, et al. Recombinant hirudin (lepirudin) for the improvement of thrombolysis with streptokinase in patients with acute myocardial infarction: Results of the HIT-4 trial. *J Am Coll Cardiol* 1999;34:966–973.

358. Theroux P, Perez-Villa F, Waters D, et al. Randomized double-blind comparison of two doses of hirulog with heparin as adjunctive therapy

to streptokinase to promote early patency of the infarct-related artery in acute myocardial infarction. *Circulation* 1995;91:2132–2139.

359. White HD, Aylward PE, Frey MJ, et al. Randomized, double-blind comparison of hirulog versus heparin in patients receiving streptokinase and aspirin for acute myocardial infarction (HERO). Hirulog Early Reperfusion/Occlusion (HERO) Trial Investigators. *Circulation* 1997;96:2155–2161.

360. White H. Thrombin-specific anticoagulation with bivalirudin versus heparin in patients receiving fibrinolytic therapy for acute myocardial infarction: The HERO-2 randomised trial. *Lancet* 2001;358:1855–1863.

361. Vermeer F, Vahanian A, Fels PW, et al. Argatroban and alteplase in patients with acute myocardial infarction: The ARGAMI Study. *J Thromb Thrombolysis* 2000;10:233–240.

362. Serebruany VL, Jang IK, Giugliano RP, et al. A randomized, blinded study of two doses of Novastan (brand of argatroban) versus heparin as adjunctive therapy to recombinant tissue plasminogen activator (accelerated administration) in acute myocardial infarction: Rationale and design of the Myocardial Infarction using Novastan and T-PA (MINT) Study. *J Thromb Thrombolysis* 1998;5:49–52.

363. Jang IK, Brown DF, Giugliano RP, et al. A multicenter, randomized study of argatroban versus heparin as adjunct to tissue plasminogen activator (TPA) in acute myocardial infarction: Myocardial infarction with Novastan and TPA (MINT) study. *J Am Coll Cardiol* 1999;33:1879–1885.

364. Fung AY, Lorch G, Cambier PA, et al. Efegatran sulfate as an adjunct to streptokinase versus heparin as an adjunct to tissue plasminogen activator in patients with acute myocardial infarction. ESCALAT Investigators. *Am Heart J* 1999;138:696–704.

365. Multicenter, dose-ranging study of efegatran sulfate versus heparin with thrombolysis for acute myocardial infarction: The Promotion of Reperfusion in Myocardial Infarction Evolution (PRIME) trial. *Am Heart J* 2002;143:95–105.

366. Collaborative analysis of long-term anticoagulant administration after acute myocardial infarction. An international anticoagulant review group. *Lancet* 1970;1:203–209.

367. Smith P, Arnesen H, Holme I. The effect of warfarin on mortality and reinfarction after myocardial infarction. *N Engl J Med* 1990;323:147–152.

368. Effect of long-term oral anticoagulant treatment on mortality and cardiovascular morbidity after myocardial infarction. Anticoagulants in the Secondary Prevention of Events in Coronary Thrombosis (ASPECT) Research Group. *Lancet* 1994;343:499–503.

369. Meijer A, Verheugt FW, Werter CJ, et al. Aspirin versus Coumadin in the prevention of reocclusion and recurrent ischemia after successful thrombolysis: A prospective placebo-controlled angiographic study. Results of the APRICOT Study. *Circulation* 1993;87:1524–1530.

370. Anand SS, Yusuf S. Oral anticoagulant therapy in patients with coronary artery disease: A meta-analysis. *JAMA* 1999;282:2058–2067.

371. Randomised double-blind trial of fixed low-dose warfarin with aspirin after myocardial infarction. Coumadin Aspirin Reinfarction Study (CARS) Investigators. *Lancet* 1997;350:389–396.

372. Fiore LD, Ezekowitz MD, Brophy MT, et al. Department of Veterans Affairs Cooperative Studies Program Clinical Trial comparing combined warfarin and aspirin with aspirin alone in survivors of acute myocardial infarction: Primary results of the CHAMP study. *Circulation* 2002;105:557–563.

373. Brouwer MA, van den Bergh PJ, Aengevaeren WR, et al. Aspirin plus coumarin versus aspirin alone in the prevention of reocclusion after fibrinolysis for acute myocardial infarction: Results of the Antithrombotics in the Prevention of Reocclusion In Coronary Thrombolysis (APRICOT)-2 Trial. *Circulation* 2002;106:659–665.

374. van Es RF, Jonker JJ, Verheugt FW, et al. Aspirin and coumadin after acute coronary syndromes (the ASPECT-2 study): A randomised controlled trial. *Lancet* 2002;360:109–113.

375. Hurlen M, Abdelnoor M, Smith P, et al. Warfarin, aspirin, or both after myocardial infarction. *N Engl J Med* 2002;347:969–974.

376. Anand SS, Yusuf S. Oral anticoagulants in patients with coronary artery disease. *J Am Coll Cardiol* 2003;41:S62–S69.

377. Effects of long-term, moderate-intensity oral anticoagulation in addition to aspirin in unstable angina. The Organization to Assess Strategies for Ischemic Syndromes (OASIS) Investigators. *J Am Coll Cardiol* 2001;37:475–484.

378. Israel DH, Stein B, Cheseboro JH, et al. Antithrombotic therapy for the prevention of cardiac and arterial thromboembolism. In: Messerli FH, ed. *Cardiovascular Drug Therapy.* Philadelphia: Saunders; 1990.

379. Meltzer RS, Visser CA, Fuster V. Intracardiac thrombi and systemic embolization. *Ann Intern Med* 1986;104:689–698.

380. Haugland JM, Asinger RW, Mikell FL, et al. Embolic potential of left ventricular thrombi detected by two-dimensional echocardiography. *Circulation* 1984;70:588–598.

381. Visser CA, Kan G, Lie KI, et al. Left ventricular thrombus following acute myocardial infarction: A prospective serial echocardiographic study of 96 patients. *Eur Heart J* 1983;4:333–337.

382. Friedman MJ, Carlson K, Marcus FI, et al. Clinical correlations in patients with acute myocardial infarction and left ventricular thrombus detected by two-dimensional echocardiography. *Am J Med* 1982;72:894–898.

383. McEntee CW, Van Reet RE, Winters WL. Incidence and natural history of mural thrombi in acute myocardial infarction by two-dimensional echocardiography. *Circulation* 1981;64:IV-93.

384. Visser CA, Kan G, Meltzer RS, et al. Embolic potential of left ventricular thrombus after myocardial infarction: A two-dimensional echocardiographic study of 119 patients. *J Am Coll Cardiol* 1985;5: 1276–1280.

385. Rogers WJ, Canto JG, Lambrew CT, et al. Temporal trends in the treatment of over 1.5 million patients with myocardial infarction in the US from 1990 through 1999: The National Registry of Myocardial Infarction 1, 2 and 3. *J Am Coll Cardiol* 2000;36:2056–2063.

386. Anticoagulants in acute myocardial infarction: Results of a cooperative clinical trial. *JAMA* 1973;225:724–729.

387. Reeder GS, Lengyel M, Tajik AJ, et al. Mural thrombus in left ventricular aneurysm: Incidence, role of angiography, and relation between anticoagulation and embolization. *Mayo Clin Proc* 1981;56: 77–81.

388. Nordrehaug JE, Johannessen KA, von der Lippe G. Usefulness of high-dose anticoagulants in preventing left ventricular thrombus in acute myocardial infarction. *Am J Cardiol* 1985;55:1491–1493.

389. Johannessen KA, Stratton JR, Taulow E, et al. Usefulness of aspirin plus dipyridamole in reducing left ventricular thrombus formation in anterior wall acute myocardial infarction. *Am J Cardiol* 1989;63: 101–102.

390. Iacono A. Mean-term calcium heparin treatment in acute transmural anterior myocardial infarction: Effects on left ventricular thrombosis and its complications. *Cardiologia* 1997;42:1251–1255.

391. Kupper AJ, Verheugt FW, Peels CH, et al. Effect of low dose acetylsalicylic acid on the frequency and hematologic activity of left ventricular thrombus in anterior wall acute myocardial infarction. *Am J Cardiol* 1989;63:917–920.

392. Kouvaras G, Chronopoulos G, Soufras G, et al. The effects of long-term antithrombotic treatment on left ventricular thrombi in patients after an acute myocardial infarction. *Am Heart J* 1990;119:73–78.

393. Rauch U, Osende JI, Fuster V, et al. Thrombus formation on atherosclerotic plaques: Pathogenesis and clinical consequences. *Ann Intern Med* 2001;134:224–238.

394. Quyyumi AA. Endothelial function in health and disease: New insights into the genesis of cardiovascular disease. *Am J Med* 1998;105: 32S–39S.

395. Corti R, Farkouh ME, Badimon JJ. The vulnerable plaque and acute coronary syndromes. *Am J Med* 2002;113:668–680.

396. Shah PK. Mechanisms of plaque vulnerability and rupture. *J Am Coll Cardiol* 2003;41:S15–S22.

397. Cohen M. The role of low-molecular-weight heparin in the management of acute coronary syndromes. *J Am Coll Cardiol* 2003;41: S55–S61.

398. Llevadot J, Giugliano RP, Antman EM. Bolus fibrinolytic therapy in acute myocardial infarction. *JAMA* 2001;286:442–449.

399. Cannon CP. Multimodality reperfusion therapy for acute myocardial infarction. *Am Heart J* 2000;140:707–716.

400. Bhatt DL, Topol EJ. Current role of platelet glycoprotein IIb/IIIa inhibitors in acute coronary syndromes. *JAMA* 2000;284:1549–1558.

401. Weitz JI, Buller HR. Direct thrombin inhibitors in acute coronary syndromes: Present and future. *Circulation* 2002;105:1004–1011.

402. Effects of recombinant hirudin (lepirudin) compared with heparin on death, myocardial infarction, refractory angina, and revascularisation procedures in patients with acute myocardial ischaemia without ST elevation: A randomised trial. Organisation to Assess Strategies for Ischemic Syndromes (OASIS-2) Investigators. *Lancet* 1999;353: 429–438.

PERCUTANEOUS CORONARY INTERVENTION

John S. Douglas, Jr. / Spencer B. King III

The treatment of patients with coronary heart disease changed dramatically with the advent of surgical coronary artery revascularization techniques in the 1970s and percutaneous coronary intervention in the next decade; accelerated change occurred in the United States with the introduction of drug-eluting stents in 2003. This chapter addresses the development and contemporary use of catheter-based coronary artery intervention, including the selection of patients and devices, procedural issues, results, complications, and long-term outcome.

DEVELOPMENT OF BALLOON ANGIOPLASTY

Percutaneous transluminal coronary angioplasty (PTCA) was conceived and shepherded into worldwide acceptance and application by Andreas R. Gruentzig, but the stage was set by the pioneering work of Dotter and Judkins,[1] who in 1964 mechanically dilated femoral arteries with a coaxial double-catheter system, and of Zeitler,[2] who applied this technique successfully in West Germany and introduced it to Gruentzig. After Gruentzig's development of a polyvinyl chloride balloon catheter with fixed maximal inflated diameters in 1974, modern balloon angioplasty evolved rapidly.[3–5] In September 1977, the first PTCA was performed in Zurich in a 37-year-old insurance salesman with severe angina pectoris and high-grade stenosis of the proximal left anterior descending (LAD) coronary artery.[6–8] Balloon angioplasty was successful in relieving the stenosis; on the 10th and 23d anniversaries of this landmark procedure, coronary arteriography revealed wide patency of the LAD and stress testing remained normal (Fig. 55-1).[9]

Following the report of Gruentzig's first five patients in 1978[10] and 50 patients in 1979,[11] worldwide interest in the technique was assured. Under the auspices of the National Heart, Lung, and Blood Institute (NHLBI), multicenter registries were formed to report experiences with the evolving technique of coronary angioplasty.[12–13] Development of an over-the-wire balloon catheter by Simpson et al.,[14] combined with advances in guidewire and balloon catheter technology, resulted in a steerable balloon catheter system capable of crossing and dilating heretofore unreachable coronary stenoses (Fig. 55-2). By 1986 at Emory University Hospital, catheter-based revascularization techniques were performed more frequently than coronary artery bypass grafting (CABG) for relief from symptoms of ischemic heart disease. The use of percutaneous coronary intervention (PCI) exceeded 130,000 procedures in the United States in 1986, 400,000 in 1995, and 1 million in 1999, about a twofold dominance over the use of surgical revascularization.

Initially, coronary balloon angioplasty was performed for discrete, proximal, noncalcified, subtotal lesions located in one coronary artery. Gruentzig was able to dilate successfully 64 percent of the initial 50 patients and 78 percent of the first 169.[10,15] Most of the patients dilated successfully were improved symptomatically. A 10-year follow-up of Gruentzig's early Zurich series revealed an overall survival rate of 90 percent and 95 percent for those with single-vessel disease.[15,16] Five-year survival in the NHLBI Registry was 93 percent for single-vessel disease and 87 percent for patients with multivessel disease[17]; 70 percent of patients were free of target vessel revascularization at 10 years.[18] Large observational studies comparing medical, surgical, and PTCA therapy suggested that revascularization benefit surpassed medical therapy for most anatomic subsets and that surgery provided a survival benefit over PTCA in severe multivessel disease.[19,20] Observational data from the New York State Cardiac Procedure Registry of 60,000 CABG and PTCA procedures reported better 3-year survival with CABG in patients with three-vessel disease and with two-vessel disease and proximal LAD stenosis while those with one-vessel disease without

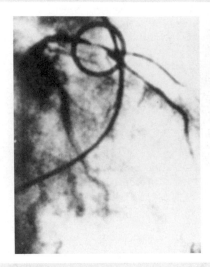 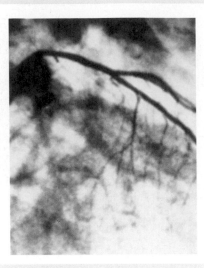

FIGURE 55-1 Right anterior oblique coronary arteriogram of the first patient who underwent transluminal coronary angioplasty on September 16, 1977 (*left*) and on September 16, 1987 (*right*). During this 10-year period, the patient remained completely asymptomatic, and the arteriogram at 10 years showed no narrowing in the coronary arteries. Subsequent angiographic follow-up at 23 years revealed continued patency of this first PTCA site. (From Meier.[9] With permission.)

LAD stenosis had better survival with PTCA. All other patients had similar survival with PTCA and CABG.[21] Subsequently, outcomes for similar anatomic subsets were reported from randomized trials,[22] and these results did not indicate a survival superiority of CABG over PTCA except in diabetics with three-vessel disease (see "Randomized Trials of Balloon Angioplasty," below).

RANDOMIZED TRIALS OF BALLOON ANGIOPLASTY

PTCA versus Medical Therapy

The favorable results of observational studies reporting patients with single and multivessel disease[23,24] led to a series of randomized trials comparing

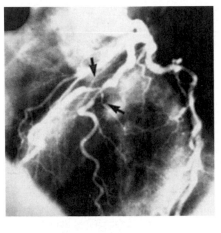 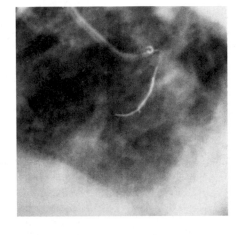 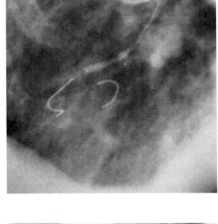

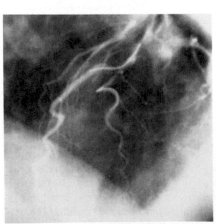 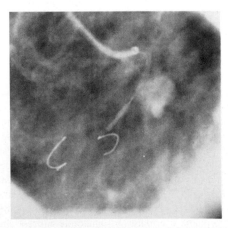 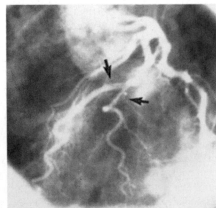

FIGURE 55-2 Angioplasty of high-grade stenoses of the LAD and diagonal bifurcation (*arrows*) using a single guiding catheter through which two dilatation devices were passed. The LAD artery was dilated with a 2.5-mm balloon (note the "waist" of the balloon, produced by the lesion), and the diagonal was dilated with a 2-mm balloon. Treatment of bifurcation lesions continues to present a challenge due to relatively high subsequent cardiac events and restenosis even with the latest stent and/or atherectomy approaches. Stenting of the parent vessel (LAD) and balloon angioplasty of the branch is the most common approach currently.

balloon angioplasty with medical therapy[25–33] and with CABG.[34–40] The Angioplasty Compared to Medical Therapy Evaluation (ACME), involving 212 patients with single-vessel disease and abnormal stress tests, revealed greater freedom from angina in the angioplasty group at 6 months (64 vs. 46 percent) as well as better treadmill performance (2.1- vs. 0.5-min increase). There was no difference in death or MI (MI).[25] The second Randomized Intervention Treatment of Angina (RITA-2) trial randomized 1018 patients with stable angina to PTCA or medical therapy.[28] The majority (60 percent) had single-vessel disease, and 33 percent had two-vessel disease. Angina relief and treadmill performance were significantly better in the PTCA patients, but complications also were more frequent. At 5 years, death or MI occurred in 9.4 percent of PTCA patients compared with 7.6 percent of medically treated patients and the mortality rates were similar, 4.6 versus 4.7 percent.[41] In the Veterans Affairs Non-Q-Wave Infarction Strategies in Hospital (VANQWISH) trial, 920 patients were randomly assigned to either an invasive strategy (routine coronary angiography and myocardial revascularization) or conservative management (medical therapy and noninvasive testing).[26] Although there was no difference in mortality during 12 to 44 months of follow-up, there was a higher incidence of a composite endpoint (death or nonfatal infarction) in the invasive group at 1 month and at 1 year (111 vs. 85 events; $p = 0.05$). Although stents, ticlopidine, and IIb/IIIa inhibitors were not used, there were no deaths at 30 days in the invasive group treated with PTCA but an 11.6 percent 30-day mortality in the group treated with CABG. Whereas the VANQWISH investigators recommended the conservative ischemia-driven approach, the recently reported and larger Fast Revascularization During Instability in Coronary Disease (FRISC II) study, the Treat Angina with Aggrastat and determine Cost of Therapy with Invasive or Conservative Strategy (TACTICS-TIMI 18), and RITA-3 strongly supported an invasive approach.[30–33] (See "Non-ST-Segment Elevation Acute Coronary Syndromes," below).

In 341 mildly symptomatic patients (59 percent asymptomatic or class I, 40 percent class II) in the Atorvastatin versus Revascularization Treatment (AVERT) trial, PTCA was compared with aggressive lipid-lowering therapy (atorvastatin 80 mg).[29] At 18-month follow-up, angina relief was significantly better ($p < 0.009$) in the PTCA group, with 54 percent having improvement, versus 41 percent in the aggressive lipid-lowering group, but quality-of-life scores were similar, and there was a trend toward more events (primarily hospitalization for ischemia) in the PTCA group. In AVERT, stents were used in 30 percent of patients. This study suggests that in low-risk patients with no or mild symptoms, aggressive lipid lowering is as effective as PTCA with limited stenting in reducing subsequent ischemic events and emphasizes the importance of extending aggressive lipid lowering in all patients with obstructive coronary artery disease. The Medicine, Angioplasty or Surgery Study (MASS) randomized 214 patients with stable angina, normal left ventricular function, and severe proximal LAD stenosis to bypass surgery [with left internal mammary artery (LIMA) graft], PTCA (without stent use), or medical therapy.[27] At 3 years, there was no difference in death or MI. Both revascularization strategies yielded better symptom relief, but subsequent procedures were more common in the PTCA group.

PTCA versus CABG

Over 5000 patients were randomized in nine trials comparing balloon angioplasty with CABG surgery. Two of these trials were sponsored by the NHLBI and performed in the United States. The first, the Emory Angioplasty versus Surgery Trial (EAST), was a single-center study,[34] whereas the larger Bypass Angioplasty Revascularization Investigation (BARI)[35,36] involved 18 centers. In-hospital mortality was similar for angioplasty and bypass surgery (approximately 1 percent) in these two studies of patients with multivessel disease, and 5-year survival also was similar (Table 55-1). Repeat revascularization procedures, however, were more common in the angioplasty group. Freedom from angina was better in the CABG group in both EAST and BARI. Metanalyses of eight randomized published trials comparing PTCA and CABG (BARI not included) reported no difference in mortality or MI at 1 year after angioplasty or CABG, but 18 percent of the angioplasty patients had required bypass surgery and 20 percent had an additional angioplasty—a significantly higher rate of repeat revascularization than in the surgery group.[37,38] This increased need for additional revascularization procedures in angioplasty patients, largely due to restenosis, eroded the initial cost advantage of angioplasty; by 3 years in the EAST study, angioplasty had been 95 percent as costly as bypass surgery[39,40]; at 8 years, total costs were $46,548 for CABG and $44,491 for PTCA ($p = 0.37$).[42]

TABLE 55-1 Randomized Comparisons of PTCA and CABG

	EAST		BARI	
	PTCA	CABG	PTCA	CABG
Patient characteristics				
Age (years)	62	61	62	61
Ejection fraction, %	61	62	57	58
Heart failure, %	3	4	9	9
Prior MI, %	41	41	54	44
Diseased vessels, %				
Two	60	60	57	58
Three	40	40	41	41
In-hospital outcome, %				
Myocardial infarction	3	10	2.1	4.6
Death	1	1	1.1	1.3
Repeat revascularization				
PTCA	0	0	3.4	0
CABG	10	0	10.2	0.1
Five-year outcome, %				
Death	12.1	8.8	13.7	10.7
Additional PTCA	48.6	15.5	34.0	7.3
Additional CABG	25.1	0.5	31.3	1.1
Any additional revascularization	61.2	16.1	54.5	8.0

ABBREVIATIONS: EAST = Emory Angioplasty vs. Surgery Trial; BARI = Bypass Angioplasty Revascularization Investigation; PTCA = percutaneous transluminal coronary angioplasty; CABG = coronary artery bypass grafting.

Considerable interest was generated by a subset analysis of treated diabetics in BARI. Among the 353 diabetics treated with insulin or oral hypoglycemic agents, 5-year survival was significantly better in patients who underwent surgery compared to patients who underwent PTCA (80.6 vs. 65.5 percent; $p = 0.003$).[43] Analysis of 7-year survival for all patients in BARI revealed for the first time a significantly better survival with CABG compared with PTCA (84.4 vs. 80.9 percent; $p = 0.0425$) (Fig. 55-3A). This difference was accounted for entirely by the poorer survival of treated diabetics revascularized with PTCA (55.7 vs. 76.4 percent for CABG; $p = 0.0011$)[44] (see Fig. 55-3B). There was no difference in the survival of nondiabetics (see Fig. 55-3C). Further analysis of treated diabetics in BARI revealed that the survival benefit with CABG was conferred only to those patients who received an internal mammary artery (IMA) graft. The 7-year survival of patients treated with an IMA graft was 83.2 percent compared with 54.5 percent for patients receiving a saphenous vein graft only—a figure comparable with that attained with PTCA. EAST, which initially showed no difference between PTCA and CABG in diabetics, at 8 years showed the same trend as BARI.[45] Considering the rather late manifestation of these outcome differences, it is likely that factors other than early restenosis must be operative. Development of new lesions, perhaps unrecognized, probably accounts for those events occurring many years after revascularization. Significantly poorer PTCA outcomes were reported for insulin-requiring diabetics in the Emory database.[46] In the BARI Registry, where revascularization therapy of diabetics was chosen by the physician for patients with two- and three-vessel disease, there was no significant difference in cardiac mortality even after adjusting for baseline differences.[47] In the northern New England observational study, survival was enhanced by CABG in diabetics with three-vessel disease but not in those with two-vessel disease.[48] In these randomized trials and observational reports, balloon angioplasty was the predominant interventional strategy. Use of stents has been shown to reduce restenosis, and their use in trials of stents versus CABG (see "Drug-Eluting Stents: The New Dominant Strategy?") and in diabetic patients is discussed below. Pending clarification by these trials, caution should exercised in the use of PTCA in diabetic patients with multivessel disease[49]; the use of arterial grafts should be emphasized in diabetic patients.[50,51]

Only recently have data become available from BARI analyzing long-term outcomes based on more specific anatomic subsets.[22] At 7 years, there was no difference in survival of PTCA- versus CABG-treated patients without diabetes who had three-vessel disease (85 vs. 87 percent; $p = 0.4$, $n = 592$); three-vessel disease with decreased left ventricular ejection fraction (LVEF) (70 vs. 74 percent; $p = 0.6$, $n = 176$); two-vessel disease

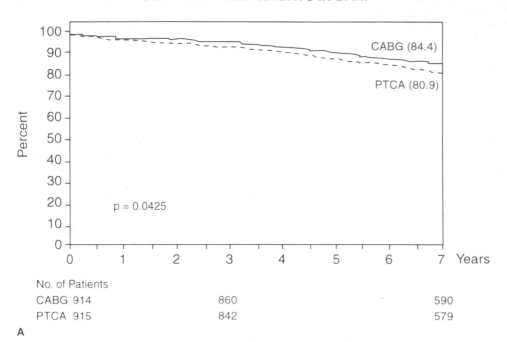

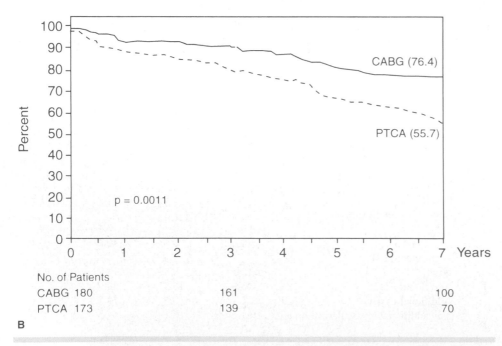

FIGURE 55-3 Survival curves for patients treated with CABG and coronary angioplasty (PTCA) in the Bypass Angioplasty Revascularization Investigation (BARI) (A to C). (From the BARI Investigators.[43,44] With permission.)

with proximal LAD stenosis (87 vs. 84 percent; $p = 0.9$, $n = 352$); and two-vessel disease with proximal LAD stenosis and decreased LVEF (78 vs. 71 percent; $p = 0.7$, $n = 72$). These findings of a prospective, randomized trial tend to support the appropriateness of PTCA in nondiabetics with multivessel disease when the anatomy is permissive and the patient prefers a percutaneous approach.

NEW DEVICES AND STRATEGIES FOR CORONARY INTERVENTION

Atherectomy, Laser, Cutting Balloon, Thrombectomy, and Embolic Protection

The directional atherectomy catheter (Fig. 55-4A) developed by Simpson[52] was, in 1990, the first nonballoon device approved for coronary intervention and the first to undergo randomized comparison with balloon

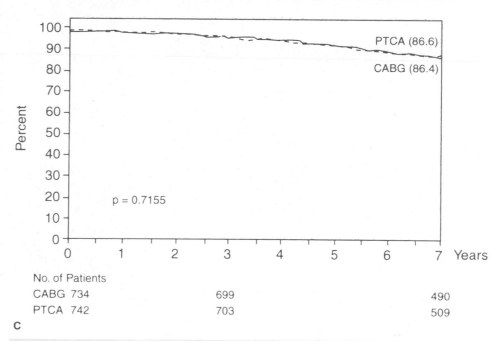

SURVIVAL - PATIENTS WITHOUT TREATED DIABETES IN BARI

PTCA (86.6)
CABG (86.4)

$p = 0.7155$

No. of Patients		
CABG 734	699	490
PTCA 742	703	509

C

FIGURE 55-3 (Continued)

angioplasty. In native coronary artery[53,54] and saphenous vein graft lesions[55] judged suitable for either procedure, however, the more costly directional atherectomy did not show a substantial advantage over balloon angioplasty. Additional trials using techniques to achieve optimal atherectomy (<20 percent residual stenosis) have been reported.[56,57] The randomized Balloon versus Optimal Atherectomy Trial (BOAT) showed no increase in in-hospital death, Q-wave MI, or CABG with directional atherectomy but there *was* a higher rate of non-Q-wave infarction (16 vs. 6 percent; $p < 0.0001$).[56] Restenosis was lower in the atherectomy arm (31 vs. 39.8 percent; $p = 0.016$), but there was no difference in late clinical events. The use of directional atherectomy declined significantly in most but not all centers[58–60] because of its complexity, added cost, and marginal benefit. In some centers, this technique is used to debulk lesions prior to stenting in the hope of reducing restenosis and to treat lesions at bifurcations as well as left main (see below) and ostial lesions of the LAD coronary artery.[60–62] However, in the Atherectomy Before Multi-Link Improves Luminal Gain and Clinical Outcomes (AMIGO) study, in which 753 patients were randomized to directional coronary atherectomy (DCA) plus stent or stent alone, no benefit of debulking prior to stenting was shown.[63] Thirty-day major adverse cardiac events (MACE) (1.6 vs. 1.1 percent) and binary restenosis (24 vs. 20 percent) were not significantly different. Excimer laser angioplasty was approved by the U.S. Food and Drug Administration (FDA) in 1992 for lesions not favorable for balloon angioplasty, but this technology has not been shown to be superior to balloon angioplasty[64] and is used infrequently in most centers—and then primarily for treating in-stent restenosis, where it is safe and initially effective but has no proven superiority.[65] In 1994, an additional atherectomy device, the Rotablator (Scimed/Boston Scientific, Maple Grove, MI) (Fig. 55-4B) was approved for marketing by the FDA. The Rotablator's principal advantage is in the treatment of calcified and undilatable stenoses, but it is also used to treat bifurcation lesions and in-stent restenosis and to debulk prior to stent-

ing.[66–69] In 1999, a rheolytic thrombectomy device known as the Angiojet (POSSIS Medical, Inc., Minneapolis, MN) (Fig. 55-4C) became available for the treatment of intracoronary thrombus; it has proved useful in the setting of acute coronary syndromes associated with large thrombi and in the treatment of stent thrombosis.[70–76] The Export catheter (Medtronic-AVE, Santa Rosa, CA), a much simpler aspiration catheter, has also proved useful in removing intracoronary thrombus. The cutting balloon (Scimed, Boston Scientific, Maple Grove, MI), which consists of longitudinally mounted microsurgical blades on an angioplasty balloon, has been used for bifurcations, small vessels, ostial lesions, in-stent restenosis, and nondilatable lesions with favorable clinical results but without convincing randomized trials indicating incremental benefit.[77] Use of the X-Sizer helical atherectomy device (Endicor Medical, San Clemente, CA) was first reported in 2002, and a multicenter trial was reported in 2003.[78–79] This relatively simple device has promise for use in thrombus-associated lesions, acute infarction, and saphenous vein grafts.

Because of increased awareness of the frequency and clinical significance of PCI-associated microvascular embolization–induced myocardial necrosis, devices to effect "embolic protection" have been developed.[80–88] The first to receive FDA approval was the PercuSurge system (distal occlusion balloon and aspiration) (Medtronic-AVE, Santa Rosa, CA) (Fig. 55-4D). A pivotal randomized study compared saphenous vein grafting (SVG) PCI outcomes with and without PercuSurge (The Safer Trial) in 801 patients; in-hospital MACE was reduced by almost 50 percent (16.5 to 9.6 percent, $p < 0.001$) with distal protection.[81] Q-wave MI was reduced from 2.2 to 1.1 percent and non-Q-wave MI from 14.4 to 7.3 percent. Additional distal protection strategies include use of a variety of filters to catch atherosclerotic and thrombotic debris released during PCI procedures for treatment of SVGs and acute MI, where improved outcomes compared to matched patients were reported.[82–83] A randomized comparison of a filter (the Filter wire, Scimed-Boston

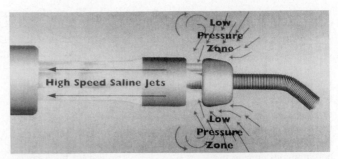

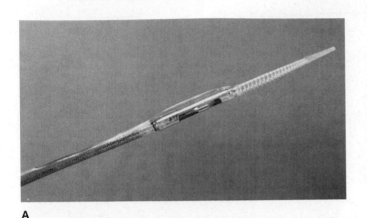

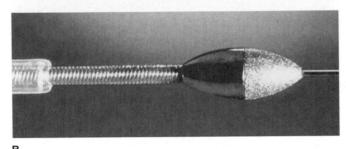

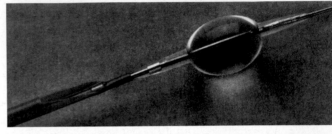

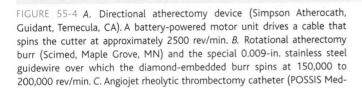

FIGURE 55-4 *A.* Directional atherectomy device (Simpson Atherocath, Guidant, Temecula, CA). A battery-powered motor unit drives a cable that spins the cutter at approximately 2500 rev/min. *B.* Rotational atherectomy burr (Scimed, Maple Grove, MN) and the special 0.009-in. stainless steel guidewire over which the diamond-embedded burr spins at 150,000 to 200,000 rev/min. *C.* Angiojet rheolytic thrombectomy catheter (POSSIS Med-ical, Inc., Minneapolis, MN); high-velocity jets, by virtue of the Bernoulli effect, pull thrombus into the catheter lumen, where it is evacuated. *D.* PercuSurge system (Medtronic AVE, Santa Rosa, CA) using balloon occlusion followed by aspiration of debris to achieve embolic protection. *E.* Filter wire (Scimed-Boston Scientific, Maple Grove, MN) a filter device shown to be comparable to Percu Surge in the FIRE trial. (From Stone et al.[88] With permission.)

Scientific, Maple Grove, MI) with PercuSurge occlusion-aspiration in 650 patients undergoing SVG PCI reported similar rates of periprocedural MI and 30-day MACE (9.9 vs. 11.6 percent), duplicating the MACE rates reported with distal protection in the SAFER Trial.[88] The observations that microembolization occurred in 80 percent of SVG PCI procedures[84,85] and CK-MB elevation was measured in 38 percent of unselected PCI procedures[86] with negative impact on long-term survival[86,87] suggest that protection strategies to protect against embolism will have an increasing role in PCI in the future.

Metallic Stents: After a Decade, the Dominant Strategy

None of the devices described above had the impact on interventional cardiology that was produced by the development of stainless steel intracoronary stents and subsequently by drug-eluting stents. The first coronary stents were implanted in patients in 1986 by Puel in Toulouse and Sigwart in Lausanne for the prevention of restenosis,[89,90] an unproven hypothesis at the time, whereas the initial implantation in a patient in the United States was performed by the authors at Emory University in 1987 in the setting of abrupt closure,[91,92] following encouraging results in a canine model by Roubin et al.[93] The initial European experience was with a self-expanding mesh stent, whereas the experience at Emory was with a balloon-mounted coil stent that subsequently was marketed as the Gianturco-Roubin flex stent (Cook, Inc., Bloomington, IN) following FDA approval for abrupt or threatened closure in 1993. This stent made balloon angioplasty considerably safer by providing effective therapy for coronary dissections and reducing the need for emergency coronary bypass surgery, but the use of this stent, despite intensive anticoagulation with heparin and warfarin, was complicated by stent thrombosis in 5 to 10 percent of patients, and bleeding was a common complication. The device that revolutionized interventional cardiology was the Palmaz-Schatz stent (Fig. 55-5) (Johnson & Johnson Interventional Systems, Warren, NJ). On the basis of two carefully conducted randomized trials that showed reduced restenosis compared with balloon angioplasty,[94,95] this device was granted FDA approval for marketing in 1994 for the elective treatment of de novo lesions in native coronary arteries. Over 100,000 implantations of this stent were performed in the first year of its availability. The interest in stenting was greatly heightened by a pivotal observation that complete stent expansion by high-pressure balloon inflation—confirmed by intravascular ultrasound—when aspirin and ticlopidine were substituted for warfarin yielded a very low stent thrombosis rate and fewer hemorrhagic complications.[96] A randomized trial of stent placement without ultrasound guidance comparing aspirin and ticlopidine with phenprocoumon (a warfarin derivative) (ISAR) revealed a low 30-day incidence of cardiac events and bleeding in the aspirin-ticlopidine patients, supporting this simplified antithrombotic strategy.[97,98] These findings were confirmed by the Stent Anticoagulation

Restenosis Study (STARS) investigation, which showed that aspirin and ticlopidine resulted in a lower rate of stent thrombosis than aspirin alone or a combination of aspirin and warfarin.[99] This conclusion was extended by a multicenter comparison of aspirin and ticlopidine against aspirin and oral anticoagulation in medium- and high-risk patients that showed a better outcome with the simpler approach,[100,101] and by a report suggesting that 14 days of ticlopidine and aspirin would be adequate for prophylaxis against stent thrombosis in most patients.[102] However, rare reports of thrombotic thrombocytopenia purpura related to the use of ticlopidine, accounting for at least 20 deaths,[103,104] led most centers to abandon ticlopidine in favor of clopidogrel, also an antagonist of platelet ADP receptors, with similar pharmacologic activity but with far fewer side effects.[105] Clopidogrel proved equal to ticlopidine in observational reports[106,107]; in a randomized investigation, the Clopidogrel Aspirin Stent Interventional

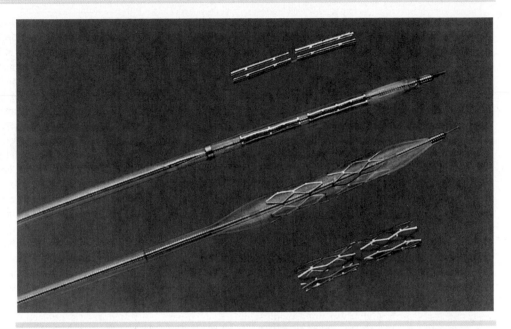

FIGURE 55-5 The Palmaz-Schatz coronary stent (Johnson & Johnson Interventional Systems, Warren, NJ). The free unexpanded stent (*top*) is mounted on a balloon and covered with a sheath. Withdrawal of the sheath and balloon inflation expand the stent (*bottom*). This stent, relatively stiff compared to current stents, revolutionized interventional cardiology.

Cooperative Study (CLASSICS), it was observed that neutropenia, thrombocytopenia, or early discontinuation of the drug were more common in the ticlopidine group (9.1 vs, 2.9 percent) than in the clopidogrel group, which received 300 mg as a loading dose and 75 mg subsequently,[108] and that major cardiac events were similar at 1 month.[109] Currently, most centers use a loading dose of 300 to 600 mg of clopidogrel when prolonged pretreatment is not possible plus aspirin 160 to 325 mg daily and 75 mg clopidogrel plus aspirin for 30 days to 6 months after stent implantation. (See "Adjunctive Strategies," below, for further discussion of clopidogrel therapy).

A number of randomized stent trials have been conducted using dual antiplatelet therapy. The important Belgium Netherlands Stent II (BENESTENT II) study, which randomized the heparin-coated Palmaz-Schatz stent and standard balloon angioplasty, found better event-free survival at 12 months in the stent group (89 vs. 79 percent; $p = 0.004$), lower restenosis (16 vs. 31 percent; $p = 0.0008$), and higher costs in stent patients by $1020 at 1 year.[110] This study raised fundamental questions as to whether a strategy of elective stenting is justified in all patients, and further analysis of long-term follow-up suggested that stent implantation in some subsets was both superior and cost-effective (i.e., unstable angina, proximal LAD stenosis). To investigate these issues, the Optimal Angioplasty versus Primary Stenting (OPUS-1) trial randomized 479 patients to primary stenting or balloon angioplasty followed by provisional stenting only when necessary and reported that after 6 months the combined incidence of death, MI, and target-vessel revascularization was significantly lower in the primary stenting arm (6.1 vs, 14.9 percent; $p = 0.003$); at 6 months, primary stenting was slightly less expensive ($10,206 vs. $10,490).[111] This provocative study, in which 99 percent of patients in the primary stent arm received a stent compared with 37 percent in the provisional stenting arm, supported routine stenting when the anatomy is appropriate as opposed to primary balloon angioplasty with stent backup, a strategy that has been advocated by some investigators[112–114] and that, of course, was the dominant strategy in the

early days of stenting. Routine stent implantation was also supported by the EPISTENT trial, in which patients receiving stents plus abciximab had lower target lesion revascularization (TLR) (8.7 vs. 15 percent, $p < 0.001$) and death (0.5% versus 1.8 percent, $p < 0.02$) than patients undergoing PTCA (with stent backup plus abciximab) (see below) and by a recent metanalysis of 29 trials of routine stenting versus balloon angioplasty (with provisional stenting for inadequate results). This study showed no difference in death, MI, or the need for coronary bypass surgery. Restenosis, as reflected by the need for repeat PCI, was reduced by routine stenting (odds ratio 0.59). Routine stenting resulted in the avoidance of a repeat procedure in approximately 5 patients per 100 treated.[115] Lesion subsets for which there is the most convincing data supporting stent implantation include native coronary arteries 3.0 to 4.0 mm in diameter, stenotic saphenous vein grafts, chronic total occlusions, restenotic lesions following nonstent intervention, and in the setting of acute MI. Less convincing data are available for use of stents in bifurcations, vessel diameters ≤2.5 mm in diameter, long lesions, diffuse disease, ostial lesions, and multivessel disease. The use of coronary stents was reviewed extensively in an American College of Cardiology Expert Consensus Document[116] and in other reports.[117–121] This document and these newer studies provide perspectives on which to base everyday decisions regarding contemporary coronary intervention, but they do not provide data on drug eluting stents.

Metallic Stents versus CABG in Multivessel Disease

The issue of whether to recommend CABG or PCI in patients with multivessel disease should be significantly influenced by the long-term outcome of randomized trials comparing bare metallic stents with bypass surgery and by future trials comparing drug-eluting stents with CABG. Intermediate-term data are available from the Arterial Revascularization Therapy Study (ARTS), which randomized 1205 patients with multivessel disease in 68 clinical centers to bare stent or standard CABG. At 1 year, there was no difference in death or MI; however, repeat interventions were higher in the stent group.[122] One-year survival free of death, MI, and reintervention was seen in 89.4 percent of the surgical group and 75.2 percent of the stent group ($p < 0.04$), but at a higher total 1-year cost (13,645 vs. 10,860 euros). The occurrence of late events in 26 percent of ARTS-stented patients was approximately one-half the incidence seen following balloon angioplasty in multivessel disease in BARI and EAST due to a reduced need for repeat revascularization in stented patients. As in BARI, the mortality rate in ARTS of diabetics treated percutaneously was significantly higher than that of nondiabetics (6.3 vs. 3.1 percent; $p < 0.01$).[123] In the smaller Argentine Randomized Study of Stents versus CABG in Multivessel Disease (ERACI II), 450 patients were randomized; at 14.7 months, survival was better in the stent group (97.4 vs. 92.5 percent; $p < 0.015$) and freedom from MI was higher (97.7 vs. 93.4 percent; $p < 0.017$), but repeat revascularization was needed more often in the stent group and costs were similar.[124] The Stent or Surgery Trial (SOS) conducted in 53 European and Canadian centers randomized 500 patients with multivessel disease to CABG and 488 to bare stent; at 1 year, repeat revascularization was higher with stents (21 vs. 6 percent, $p < 0.0001$).[125] The incidence of death or Q-wave MI was similar in the two groups. At 2 years, 8 CABG patients had died, compared with 22 stented patients, 8 due to cancer. Both PCI and CABG are evolving, and it is important to note that off-pump coronary surgery, IIb/IIIa platelet receptor inhibitors, and, of course, drug-eluting stents were not used in these studies.

A recent metanalysis of 13 trials of percutaneous intervention versus CABG showed a lower 5-year mortality with surgery.[126] There were 1.9 fewer deaths per 100 patients in the surgical group. Trials limited to multivessel disease showed an advantage for surgery that was not apparent at 1 or 3 years but became significant at 5 and 8 years. In aggregate, trials limited to stenting versus surgery showed no difference in survival, but data were available for only 3 years.[126]

Drug-Eluting Stents: The New Dominant Strategy?

Although metallic stents have conferred a significant advantage over balloon angioplasty in reducing both initial complications and late events, in-stent restenosis remains a major obstacle to wider application of percutaneous revascularization, especially in complex lesions and clinical subsets, where restenosis rates can exceed 50 percent. Although a number of systemic drug trials aimed at reducing neointimal hyperplasia are ongoing and brachytherapy may yet play a significant role in the treatment of de novo lesions, the most exciting strategy for the prevention of restenosis is the drug-eluting stent, combining mechanical scaffolding with local pharmacologic action.[127–131] Multiple agents are undergoing testing currently; the most promising have antiproliferative or antineoplastic properties. Sirolimus is an immunosuppressive macrolide antifungal agent that blocks the G1S phase of cellular replication, whereas paclitaxel is an antimicrotubular agent that acts at the Go/G1 and G1/m phases. Both agents decrease smooth muscle migration and proliferation and have been shown to be effective in reducing restenosis in randomized clinical trials where polymers were used to bind the agent to the stent. The largest body of information and longest follow-up is with the sirolimus-eluting stent. Among 45 patients with de novo lesions in vessels 3.0 to 3.5 mm in diameter and lesion length <18 mm, there was no in-stent restenosis or stent thrombosis at 2 years.[129–131] In RAVEL (Randomized Study with the Sirolimus Coated Bx Velocity Balloon-Expandable Stent in the Treatment of Patients with denovo Native Coronary Artery Lesions), 238 patients at 19 international

centers were randomized to either the bare metal or sirolimus-eluting stent, with 6-month angiographic follow-up in 89 percent. The mean lesion length was 9.6 mm, 19 percent had diabetes, and approximately 40 percent had stable angina. No patient in the sirolimus-eluting-stent group had restenosis of 50 percent or more of the luminal diameter, compared to 27 percent in the bare stent group ($p < 0.001$).[132] The restenosis rate for diabetic patients was zero versus 42 percent ($p < 0.02$). There were no stent thromboses and at 1 year the major cardiac event rates were 5.8 percent for the drug-eluting-stent group and 20 percent for those treated with bare stents ($p < 0.001$), a difference entirely attributable to more repeat revascularizations in the bare-stent group. The zero percent restenosis achieved in RAVEL with relatively simple lesions was not achieved in the subsequent U.S. multicenter SIRIUS trial, where 1058 patients with longer lesions (>15 mm to <30 mm by visual estimate; actual length 14.4 mm by core lab) were randomized to receive a sirolimus-coated or bare Bx Velocity stent.[133] In-stent restenosis was reduced from 35 percent with the bare stent to 3.2 percent ($p < 0.001$) with the sirolimus, but when the stent edges (5 mm proximal or distal to the stent) were included, the reduction was less but quite significant (restenosis was reduced from 37 to 9 percent, $p < 0.001$). Target lesion revascularization was reduced from 17 to 4 percent ($p < 0.001$) and major cardiac events from 19 to 7 percent ($p < 0.001$). In addition to longer lesions in SIRIUS compared to RAVEL, there were more diabetics (25 vs. 19 percent) and more patients with other risk factors such as hyperlipidemia and hypertension. Based on these favorable safety and efficacy data, the FDA approved the sirolimus-eluting stent for marketing in the United States in 2003.

Several clinical trials evaluating paclitaxel-coated stents have been reported. In TAXUS I, a safety trial involving 61 patients, there was no restenosis in the paclitaxel group and an 11 percent restenosis rate in the bare-stent group.[134] In TAXUS II, an international efficacy trial, 532 patients were randomized to receive a bare 15-mm metal stent or one of two polymeric formulations of paclitaxel (slow- and moderate-release). Restenosis occurred in 2.3 percent receiving slow-release paclitaxel stents, 4.7 percent in the moderate-release group, and 20 percent ($p < 0.002$ for both) with bare stents.[135] There was no increase in stent thrombosis or aneurysm formation in the paclitaxel groups. TAXUS IV, a pivotal U.S. multicenter trial in which over 1000 patients were randomized to paclitaxel-coated or bare stents with angiographic and clinical follow-up, gave similar results to SIRIUS and led to FDA approval. TAXUS III reported use of a paclitaxel-coated stent in 28 patients with in-stent restenosis, 8 of whom (29 percent) had subsequent adverse cardiac events[136]; 3 of 16 (19 percent) had adverse events following sirolimus-eluting-stent implantation for complex in-stent restenosis (including brachytherapy failure) in a European experience.[137] In 26 patients with more simple in-stent restenosis lesions, placement of a sirolimus-coated stent resulted in only one restenosis (4 percent) at 12 months.[138] Brachytherapy failures and gaps between the drug-eluting stents were associated with late events in these limited experiences. Although drug-eluting stents have great promise, much work is needed to determine how and where they should be applied for optimal benefit.[139] Since the randomized trials have utilized routine angiography prior to determining the clinical endpoints, the difference in events may have been magnified. The clinical difference between drug-eluting stenting and modern bare-metal stenting seems to be significantly less in postmarketing practice. Few or no data are available regarding their use in more complex lesions (bifurcations, total occlusions, lesions >30 mm in length, or in vessels ≤2.5 mm in diameter, saphenous vein grafts, and multivessel disease). It is clear that the substantially higher cost of this technology, which is only partially offset by health insurance reimbursement, limited to a degree its application in multivessel/multilesion disease. The Freedom Trial, a randomized comparison of modern surgery versus sirolimus-eluting stents in diabetics with multivessel disease with a primary endpoint of 5-year mortality, has been proposed and may guide therapy in the future. Similar trials are needed for nondiabetics.

Adjunctive Strategies

ANTIPLATELET THERAPY

Thienopyridines Clopidogrel inhibits platelet aggregation and decreases platelet activation by blocking the adenosine diphosphate (ADP) (P_2Y_{12}) receptor. It has better tolerability and fewer side effects and is at least as effective as ticlopidine; along with aspirin, it is routinely administered prior to stent implantation.[140] Recent evidence supports its use in nonstent PCI as well.[141,142] Although initial clopidogrel doses of 525 to 600 mg are needed to produce potent inhibition of ADP-induced platelet aggregation within 2 h,[143] a 300-mg loading dose is commonly used and has been shown to produce maximal platelet inhibition within 24 h.[144] In the CREDO (Clopidogrel for the Reduction of Events During Observation) trial, patients who received clopidogrel at least 6 h before PCI had a 28-day relative risk reduction of 39 percent ($p = 0.051$) compared to no reduction in those receiving a 300-mg loading dose less than 6 h before intervention.[145] Following PCI, long-term (1 year) clopidogrel was associated with a 27 percent relative reduction in adverse ischemic events ($p = 0.02$). These findings extended and amplified the similar findings in PCI-CURE.[142] Recent reports suggest that inadequate inhibition of platelet aggregation may occur in patients with a higher body mass index[146] and that insensitivity to clopidogrel is more common than previously thought—both factors that may contribute to stent thrombosis. A growing body of evidence supports use of clopidogrel beyond the 2- to 4-week poststent interval that has commonly been recommended for routine PCI procedures; the most convincing evidence for prolonged usage is in patients with delayed healing due to brachytherapy; 3 to 9 months of therapy is recommended following implantation of drug-eluting stents.

IIb/IIIa Platelet Receptor Inhibitors Among the arrows in the quiver of the interventionalist are the potent platelet glycoprotein IIb/IIIa receptor inhibitors.[147–150] The first to be approved by the FDA, the monoclonal antibody abciximab (ReoPro, Centocor, Malvern, PA), was shown to reduce ischemic complications and late clinical events in high-risk angioplasty.[151] The other IIb/IIIa receptor inhibitors approved by the FDA, unlike the antibody abciximab, are competitive inhibitors: eptifibatide (Integrilin, COR Therapeutics, San Francisco, CA) is a peptide and tirofiban (Aggrastat, Merck, White House Station, NJ) is a small nonpeptide molecule. Each of these IIb/IIIa agents has been shown to reduce a composite endpoint of death or nonfatal MI in the setting of coronary intervention and in acute coronary syndromes[98,147,151] (Fig. 55-6). Further, at 3-year following in the EPIC trial, the first major study of abciximab during coronary intervention, a subgroup of 555 patients with acute coronary syndromes treated with bolus abciximab and infusion had a significant reduction in mortality at 3 years.[152] A metanalysis of 19 randomized trials of IIb/IIIa agents (20,137 patients) during PCI reported a significant and sustained decrease (20 to 30 percent) in the risk of death.[153] The relative risk reduction was similar in patients with and without acute MI and with and without stents. In a recent review of the use of the three FDA-approved IIb/IIIa receptor inhibitor

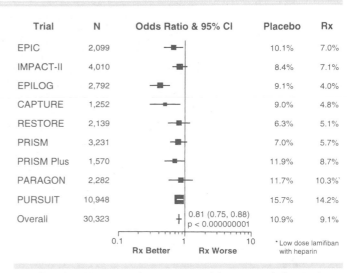

Trial	N	Odds Ratio & 95% CI	Placebo	Rx
EPIC	2,099		10.1%	7.0%
IMPACT-II	4,010		8.4%	7.1%
EPILOG	2,792		9.1%	4.0%
CAPTURE	1,252		9.0%	4.8%
RESTORE	2,139		6.3%	5.1%
PRISM	3,231		7.0%	5.7%
PRISM Plus	1,570		11.9%	8.7%
PARAGON	2,282		11.7%	10.3%*
PURSUIT	10,948		15.7%	14.2%
Overall	30,323	0.81 (0.75, 0.88) $p < 0.000000001$	10.9%	9.1%

0.1   1   10
Rx Better   Rx Worse

* Low dose lamifiban with heparin

FIGURE 55-6 Odds ratios and 95 percent confidence intervals for nine large-scale randomized trials of IIb/IIIa platelet receptor inhibitors for percutaneous coronary interventions or unstable angina/non-Q-wave MI. Overall, in 30,323 patients, a 19 percent reduction in death or MI at 30 days was demonstrated. (From Topol.[98] With permission.)

agents in acute coronary syndromes, it was noted that they were each effective in reducing a composite endpoint of death or MI when administered prior to or at the time of percutaneous coronary intervention[154] (Fig. 55-7). In most centers, the use of these agents, slowed initially by bleeding complications and high costs, has been increasing in high-risk patients. Also contributing to this trend is the favorable outcome of IIb/IIIa receptor inhibitor–treated patients in the Evaluation of Platelet IIb/IIIa Inhibitors of Stenting (EPISTENT) trial, in which abciximab therapy in patients undergoing stent implantation or balloon angioplasty was evaluated.[155,156] At 6 months, the incidence of a composite endpoint of death or MI was 5.6 percent in patients receiving a stent and abciximab compared with 11.4 percent in those receiving a stent and placebo ($p < 0.001$) and 7.8 percent in patients treated with balloon angioplasty and abciximab (Fig. 55-8). There was a further advantage in diabetics, in whom the combination of abciximab and stenting was associated with a lower rate of repeat target vessel revascularization (8.1 percent) than was observed with stenting and placebo (16.6 percent; $p = 0.02$) or angioplasty and abciximab (18.4 percent; $p = 0.008$), and this benefit persisted through 1-year follow-up.[157] The mechanism by which target-vessel revascularization was reduced in the abciximab-treated patients is unclear.[158] Previous reports indicate that abciximab did not prevent neointimal proliferation or reduce instent restenosis.[159] EPISTENT does, however, raise the question of whether all diabetic patients and, further, all patients receiving stents should receive IIb/IIIa platelet inhibitors. A recent metanalysis of diabetics in six large trials indicated that 30-day mortality following PCI was reduced by IIb/IIIa inhibitors from 4.0 to 1.2 percent, $p = 0.0002$.[160] A recently reported head-to-head comparison of tirofiban and abciximab during stenting showed higher adverse events with tirofiban at 30 days but similar outcomes at 6 months.[161,162] The improved outcome with abciximab was related to reduced infarction in patients with acute coronary syndromes.[163] Further trials of these agents in stented patients may shed light on these important questions. Clearly, however, these potent new strategies enhance the ability to provide safe and effective percutaneous revascularization.[153,164] Recently published data from CAPTURE have indicated the presence of a

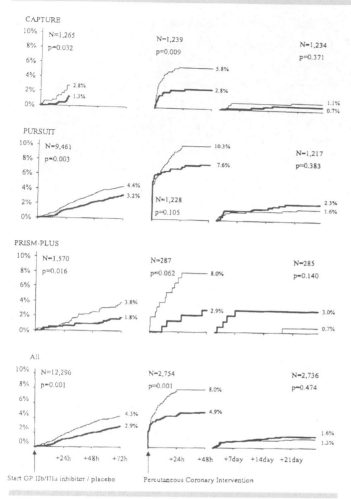

CAPTURE

PURSUIT

PRISM-PLUS

All

Start GP IIb/IIIa inhibitor / placebo   Percutaneous Coronary Intervention

FIGURE 55-7 Kaplan-Meier curves showing cumulative incidence of death or nonfatal myocardial (re)infarction in patients randomly assigned to glycoprotein IIb/IIIa inhibition (*bold lines*) or placebo. Data were derived from CAPTURE, PURSUIT, and PRISM-PLUS.[147–149] (*Left*) Event rates during initial period of pharmacologic treatment until moment of a percutaneous coronary intervention (PCI) or coronary bypass grafting, if any. (*Center*) Event rates among PCI patients during 48-h period after procedure. During and shortly after PCI, all patients were on study medication. (*Right*) Event rates in period starting 48 h after PCI, during which all patients were off study medication. At the beginning of each period, event rates were (re)set at 0 percent. Any patient still alive contributes to event estimates in each period. In PURSUIT, procedure-unrelated MI was defined as any elevation of creatine kinase (CK)-MB above upper limit of normal (ULN). For consistency with CAPTURE and PRISM-PLUS, in present analyses only CK or CK-MB elevations greater than 2 times ULN were considered to be infarctions during medical therapy. In all three trials, procedure-related infarcts were defined by an elevation of CK or CK-MB of greater than 3 times ULN. (From Boersma et al.[154] With permission.)

gradient in the benefit obtained from IIb/IIIa receptor inhibition with abciximab in unstable angina. Death or MI was significantly less frequent in patients with elevated baseline troponin treated with abciximab compared with placebo (9.5 vs. 23.9 percent; $p = 0.002$), but this endpoint was not different in troponin-negative patients (7.5 vs. 9.4 percent; $p = 0.47$).[165] Stated differently, without an elevated troponin level, there was no benefit of treatment with respect to risk of death or MI. While there was no difference in death, MI, or urgent intervention in simple lesions, the situation was otherwise for complex lesions (ACC/AHA classes B2 and C); the incidence of this end-

point was 19.1 percent for placebo versus 11.5 percent for abciximab ($p = 0.03$). Also of interest is the fact that when flow in the culprit artery was less than TIMI grade 3 after angioplasty, the incidence of death and MI at 30 days was 11.5 percent with placebo and 4.1 with abciximab, supporting a role for abciximab in ameliorating the consequences of postprodural slow flow. The observation that IIb/IIIa receptor inhibitors appear to be more effective in patients with refractory unstable angina, complex anatomy, and slow flow[150,151,167] may help to determine the place of these agents (see "Non-ST-Segment Elevation Myocardial Infarction," below).

Thrombin Inhibitors Unfractionated heparin (UFH) has been the thrombin inhibitor utilized for the first two decades of PCI, but the appearance of low-molecular-weight heparin (LMWH) as the antithrombin of choice in the ACC/AHA Unstable Angina Guidelines (a class IIA recommendation) and FDA approval of three direct thrombin inhibitors for use in PCI challenges the interventional cardiologist to provide optimal antithrombotic therapy for a diverse population of complex patients. Clearly UFH has a number of disadvantages, including nonlinear anticoagulant kinetics, the requirement for cofactor antithrombin III, inability to inactivate clot-bound thrombin, platelet activation, stimulation of antibody formation, and a prothrombotic rebound phenomenon. Optimal anticoagulation for balloon angioplasty procedures with UFH requires monitoring of activated clotting time (ACT) to achieve an ACT target of approximately 300 s without IIb/IIIa inhibitors and 200 to 250 s when these agents are used.[168] Several investigators have suggested that ACT targets with stent implantation can safely be reduced to 200 to 250 s to minimize hemorrhagic risks.[169,170]

LMWH (molecular weights of approximately 4000 to 6000 Da) inactivates thrombin less than UFH and binds factor Xa more avidly with anti-IIa:anti-Xa ratios that vary from 1:2 to 1:4, depending on the LWMH agent used. LMWH is more bioavailable than UFH, is less inhibited by platelet factor 4, and causes less thrombocytopenia; moreover, its predictable anticoagulant effect eliminates to a degree the need for laboratory monitoring. The absence of easy monitoring of LMWH activity has been a stumbling block to broad acceptance of LMWH during PCI by interventionalists accustomed to the readily available ACT monitoring of UFH. The National Investigators Collaborating and Enoxaparin (NICE-1) study reported use of LMWH during PCI in a nonrandomized trial in which PCI outcomes following enoxaparin 1 mg/kg intravenously were shown to be similar to the outcomes of the EPISTENT placebo group.[171] The addition of abciximab to a smaller intravenous dose of enoxaparin (0.75 mg/kg) was also shown to be safe and effective in NICE-4.[172] The ideal LMWH regimen for PCI has not been determined, although achieving an anti-Xa level of >0.5 IU/mL has been a suggested target[173,174]; this was achieved in over 97 percent of 242 patients with an intravenous bolus of 0.5mg/kg of enoxaparin, and PCI safety was preserved.[175] A dose of 60 IU/kg of dalteparin plus abciximab was shown to yield favorable results, but a dose of 40 IU/kg resulted in an increased rate of periprocedural thrombosis. The Superior Yield of the New Strategy of Enoxaparin Revascularization and Glycoprotein IIb/IIIa Inhibitors (SYNERGY) study will evaluate the efficacy of LMWH versus UFH plus IIb/IIIa inhibitors in high-risk patients. If PCI is performed within 8 h of LMWH, no further LMWH will be given. If the PCI is between 8 and 12 h, a bolus of 0.3 mg/kg of enoxaparin or 40 IU/kg of dalteparin will be given intravenously. The two LMWH preparations currently available, enoxaparin and dalteparin, are appreciably different with respect to molecular weights, pharmacokinetics, and anti-IIa:Xa ratios. Further studies are clearly needed to guide the use of these agents during PCI in a heterogenous patient population.

The direct thrombin inhibitor (DTI) hirulog (bivalirudin) was approved by the FDA in 2000 for high-risk PCI, whereas hirudin, argatroban, and lipirudin are all FDA-approved for heparin-induced thrombocytopenia. The advantages of DTIs for PCI include the ease of monitoring their action with ACT measurement, their ability to inactivate clot-bound thrombin, and a favorable safety profile. In 4098 patients with unstable angina randomized to UFH or bivalirudin, similar outcomes were reported on initial analysis; but on reanalysis of isoenzyme samples, a 22 percent reduction ($p = 0.039$) in 7-day ischemic endpoints and reduced bleeding was noted with bivalirudin.[176,177] In a more contemporary, stent-based PCI experience, the Randomized Evaluation of Percutaneous Coronary Intervention Linking Angiomax to Reduced Clinical Events (REPLACE-1) trials, bivalirudin (0.75 mg/kg bolus plus 1.75 mg/kg/h infusion during PCI) demonstrated reduced adverse events and major bleeding compared to UFH.[178] In REPLACE-II, bivalirudin was compared to UFH plus abciximab and was found not to be inferior to the more expensive alternative strategy.[179] Taken together, these studies suggest that DTI (primarily bivalirudin) administered during PCI is as effective in avoiding ischemic complications as UFH or UFH plus IIb/IIIa in certain patient subsets with less bleeding risk. It has been suggested that optimal antithrombin therapy for PCI in certain complex patient subgroups—such as those with a high risk of bleeding, renal failure, and/or heparin-induced thrombocytopenia—is perhaps best accomplished with a DTI; whereas those with troponin positivity, diabetes, thrombus-containing lesions, and ST-segment-elevation infarction are probably best managed with an indirect thrombin inhibitor and IIb/IIIa platelet receptor inhibitor.[180] Further studies are needed to determine the safety and efficacy of DTIs combined with IIb/IIIa inhibitors.

Other Peri-PCI Pharmacotherapy At the time of PCI or shortly thereafter, administration of a variety of therapeutic agents not directed at the clotting cascade or platelets has been associated with improved patient outcomes. Preprocedural statin therapy has been associated with a reduction in poststent MI[181] and improvement in survival at 30 days, 6 months, and at 1 year poststenting independent of patient characteristics.[182,183] Similarly, beta-blocker therapy at the time of elective PCI was associated with a 1-year survival benefit (3.9 versus 6.0 percent, $p = 0.0014$) independent of ventricular function, diabetic status, hypertension, or history of MI.[184] A number of orally administered agents—including pioglitazone, sirolimus, cilostazol, chemotherapy for cancer, systemic immunosuppressants, and antioxidants—have, in smaller trials, been associated with reduced restenosis. Some of these agents are undergoing further study. Variable effects on the prevention of contrast nephropathy by the use of the free-radical scavenger *N*-acetylcysteine and by the selective dopamine-1 (DA_1) receptor agonist fenoldopam have been reported.[185-189] (see "Complications," below).

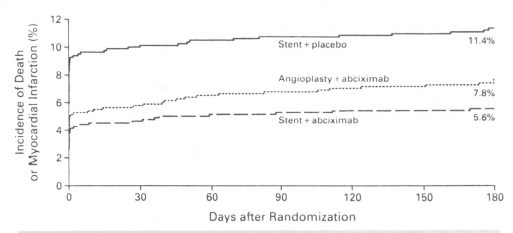

FIGURE 55-8 Kaplan-Meier estimates from EPISTENT of the incidence of the composite endpoint of death or MI within 6 months of randomization according to treatment assignment. For the composite endpoint of death or MI, $p < 0.001$ for the comparison between the stent-plus-abciximab group and the stent-plus-placebo group, $p = 0.01$ for the comparison between angioplasty plus abciximab and stent plus placebo, and $p = 0.07$ for the comparison between stent plus abciximab and angioplasty plus abciximab. (From Lincoff et al.[156] With permission.)

Intravascular Ultrasound Intravascular ultrasound (IVUS) also has been used extensively in some centers to evaluate coronary lesions for device therapy and to assess the results of device and balloon treatment,[96] but the increased cost of this approach is a limiting factor. Although IVUS has had significant impact on the evolution of interventional cardiology, on the understanding of restenosis, and in evaluation of difficult lesions, its routine use in most centers is limited.

Intracoronary Brachytherapy Vascular brachytherapy using beta and gamma emitters, approved by the FDA in 2000, revolutionized the treatment of in-stent restenosis, providing a robust strategy for the management of native coronary artery and saphenous vein graft lesions (see In-Stent Restenosis," below).[190-192] The future role of this strategy for the prevention of restenosis will depend on the effectiveness of drug-eluting stents, the extent of their use, and the potential for the application of brachytherapy beyond in-stent restenosis, perhaps to peripheral vascular application.[192]

INDICATIONS FOR CORONARY INTERVENTION

In general, when one is selecting percutaneous coronary intervention, there should be assurance that the operator can treat, with a high probability of success, the coronary lesion(s) accounting for the symptoms or signs of myocardial ischemia. Further, the associated risk and durability of the revascularization should be acceptable as compared with bypass surgery or medical therapy during both early and long-term follow-up. The latter estimate requires consideration of the likelihood and consequences of abrupt vessel closure, restenosis, and incomplete revascularization. In addition, one cannot disregard the comparative costs of the initial intervention, its complications, and the need for subsequent revascularization procedures. The American College of Cardiology/American Heart Association (ACC/AHA) Guidelines for Percutaneous Transluminal Coronary Angioplasty and Coronary Bypass Surgery provide a detailed analysis of many of these issues.[50,193-195] The ACC/AHA PCI Guideline recommendations for patients with mild or no symptoms and moderate or severe symptoms are summarized in Table 55-2.

TABLE 55-2 Recommendations for PCI from the ACC/AHA Guidelines in Patients with Asymptomatic Ischemia or with Class I Angina Pectoris

Class I (level of evidence: B)	Nondiabetic with one or more significant lesions in one or more coronary arteries suitable for PCI with high likelihood of success and low procedural risk; vessels should subtend a large area of viable myocardium
Class IIa (level of evidence: B)	Same as class I except the myocardial area at risk is of moderate size or the patient has treated diabetes
Class IIb (level of evidence: B)	Three or more coronary arteries suitable for PCI with high likelihood of success and low risk; vessels subtend at least moderate area of viable myocardium; evidence of ischemia
Class III (level of evidence: C)	Small area of myocardium at risk, absence of ischemia, low likelihood of PCI success, absence of symptoms of ischemia, increased PCI risk, left main, <50% stenosis

Selection of Patients

SINGLE-VESSEL DISEASE

Percutaneous revascularization is an attractive option for many symptomatic patients having single-vessel coronary disease who are anatomically suitable. It is important, however, to remember that there are few studies comparing angioplasty with surgery in this group of patients and none that show a statistically significant survival benefit of angioplasty compared with surgery or medical therapy. Data from Emory University indicated that of 692 patients with single-vessel disease who were newly diagnosed in 1988, a total of 46 percent underwent angioplasty, 50 percent were treated medically, and 4 percent underwent coronary bypass surgery. Of 7604 patients with single-vessel disease treated at Emory with angioplasty between 1980 and 1991, angiographic success was 90 percent and complications were infrequent (Q-wave MI, 0.8 percent; emergency CABG, 1.7 percent; and death, 0.2 percent).[196] In these patients with single-vessel disease, 1-, 5-, and 10-year survival was 99, 93, and 86 percent, respectively, whereas 80, 69, and 58 percent were PTCA-free and 92, 87, and 77 percent were CABG-free at 1, 5, and 10 years. In the Duke Data Bank experience, 5-year survival with angioplasty in single-vessel disease compared favorably with bypass surgery (95 vs. 93 percent with CABG).[197]

The ACME study showed that angioplasty in single-vessel disease can lead to improved quality of life compared with medical therapy at 6 months, with reduced angina and improved exercise performance out to 3 years.[25,198,199] Clearly, it is an improvement in symptoms rather than prolongation of life that is achieved by angioplasty in this patient subset. The ACME data suggest, however, that using the angioplasty techniques available at that time resulted in a slightly increased risk of acute complications (2 percent emergency CABG, 1 percent Q-wave MI) and repeat revascularization (23 vs. 9 percent) at 6 months, but no difference in late revascularization at 3 years.[199]

In an observational report from Kansas City of 704 patients with single-vessel LAD artery revascularization, 2-year mortality was 3.9, 2.6, and 1 percent in PTCA, stent, and LIMA-LAD revascularization groups, respectively ($p = 0.33$); repeat procedures occurred in 30, 24, and 5 percent, respectively ($p = 0.001$).[200] In the randomized Medicine, Angioplasty, or Surgery Study (MASS) of isolated LAD disease, there was no difference in MI or mortality at 5 years, but there were fewer late events in the surgery group.[201] In a relatively

small, randomized trial of angioplasty and IMA surgery for isolated disease of the LAD artery, there was no difference in mortality or MI, but angioplasty patients had more repeat revascularizations (25 vs. 3 percent; $p < 0.01$).[202] Clear superiority of stenting over balloon angioplasty for isolated LAD disease was demonstrated in a randomized comparison of these strategies in 120 patients.[203] One-year rates of event-free survival were 87 percent after stenting and 70 percent after angioplasty ($p = 0.04$); restenosis rates were 19 and 40 percent, respectively ($p = 0.02$).

When 220 patients with severe proximal LAD stenosis were randomized to stent implantation or minimally invasive bypass surgery, MACE was significantly higher following stenting (31 vs. 15 percent, $p = 0.02$).[204] The difference was predominately due to repeat revascularizations for restenosis (29 vs. 8 percent, $p = 0.003$). Death or MI occurred in 3 percent of the stent group and 6 percent of surgery patients ($p = 0.50$). A study comparing drug-eluting stents with CABG or medical therapy in single-vessel disease has not been performed, but a low rate of restenosis and reduced need for target-vessel revascularization make PCI a more durable and attractive strategy. In diabetic patients in RAVEL, there was no restenosis in patients receiving the Cypher stent; in SIRIUS, restenosis occurred in 18 percent of diabetics receiving a Cypher stent compared to 50 percent in diabetics receiving a bare stent ($p < 0.001$). Long-term outcome analysis of these trials and ongoing registries will provide important additional information.

Studies from the Cleveland Clinic analyzing the importance of repeat procedures in determining 2-year cardiac cost suggest that coronary intervention is more cost-effective than medical and surgical therapy when the probability of repeat procedures is low.[205] One would infer from this analysis that the presence of multiple or complex lesions, which are likely to recur, may tilt the scale sufficiently to modify adversely the favorable comparative cost-effectiveness of percutaneous intervention in single-vessel disease.

MULTIVESSEL DISEASE

A dramatic increase in the use of percutaneous intervention in multivessel disease, fueled by improved angioplasty technology and new devices, accounts for the growth in these procedures worldwide. *Rational selection of patients, however, requires a careful analysis of multiple issues, including a risk-benefit assessment of each ischemia-producing lesion, a projection of the possible completeness and durability of the physiologic revascularization, and an estimate of resource consumption compared with surgery and medical therapy.*

In general, as stated in "Guidelines for PTCA,"[194,195] patients selected for intervention are symptomatic, have evidence of ischemia, need noncardiac surgery, are recovering from cardiac arrest or malignant arrhythmia, or have compelling anatomy. Patient preferences must be considered, since repeat interventions are a common and integral aspect of percutaneous intervention in multivessel disease (see Table 55-1). Complete revascularization, which has been shown in the surgical experience to produce superior long-term results, has been associated with fewer late interventions after angioplasty,[206] but it is not frequently attained due to the presence of total occlusions, noncritical stenoses, and diffuse disease. In the 1985–1986 NHLBI PTCA Registry, complete revascularization was achieved in 19 percent of multivessel patients.[207]

At Emory University, among 10,783 patients who underwent coronary intervention, complete revascularization was achieved in 84 percent of patients with single-vessel disease and 25 percent with two-vessel disease but in only 5 percent with triple-vessel disease.[196] In the experience of EAST, 71 percent of index segments were revascularized in PTCA patients.[208] Culprit-lesion angioplasty is clearly an accepted strategy, but care must be taken to avoid significant residual ischemia after intervention. This approach was reflected in EAST, where revascularization was attempted in 96 percent of high-priority lesions in PTCA patients and in 99 percent of surgical patients. (*High-priority lesions* were defined as 70 to 100 percent stenoses located proximally or in large vessels $\geq$2.5 mm). This strategy yielded similar 3-year EAST primary endpoints for CABG and PTCA and an identical frequency of patients with all index segments free of severe stenosis of 70 to 100 percent (82 vs. 82 percent).[208] Recently published data from BARI indicated that planned incomplete revascularization was unrelated to 5-year risk of cardiac death or death/MI but *was* related to risk of CABG.[209]

The risks of percutaneous coronary intervention are increased in the presence of unstable angina, advanced age, poor left ventricular function, extensive coronary artery disease, comorbid conditions, and female gender.[210] At Emory, in-hospital mortality for one-, two-, and three-vessel disease was 0.2, 0.4, and 1.2 percent, respectively ($p < 0.0001$), and emergency bypass surgery was needed in 1.7, 3.0, and 3.2 percent, respectively.[196] In general, the risk of intervention is directly related to the probability and consequences of abrupt closure. In multivessel disease, both are frequently higher, and impaired left ventricular function is commonly present. Application of stenting in multivessel percutaneous intervention has improved outcomes significantly.[211–214] In a report from the Washington Hospital Center, in-hospital and long-term outcomes of 398 consecutive patients undergoing multivessel stenting were quite similar to those of patients undergoing single-vessel stenting with respect to mortality (1.4 vs. 0.7 percent; $p = 0.26$), repeat revascularization (20 vs. 21 percent; $p = 0.73$), and Q-wave MI (zero vs. 1.2 percent; $p = 0.02$). Overall event-free survival was similar.[213] Although the major randomized trials of angioplasty versus bypass surgery also showed no overall difference in mortality on long-term follow-up, BARI reported that patients being treated for diabetes had significantly worse 5-year mortality with angioplasty compared with surgery (35 vs. 19 percent).[43] In a smaller cohort of diabetic patients in EAST, however, there were no differences in outcome until almost 8 years following revascularization. The BARI findings question the safety of angioplasty in the diabetic population, who frequently have diffuse multivessel disease, more frequent restenoses, more rapid disease progression, and in many cases a reduced recognition of recurrent ischemia.[49,215] ARTS extended this cautionary theme in diabetics with multivessel disease by observing that stented diabetics had roughly twice the mortality of nondiabetics[123] (see "Randomized Trials of Balloon An-

gioplasty," above). Studies to analyze the outcomes and cost-effectiveness of the much more expensive drug-eluting stents in multivessel disease are needed.

NON-ST-SEGMENT-ELEVATION ACUTE CORONARY SYNDROMES

Patients with unstable angina, who account for a majority of coronary interventions, are at increased risk for periprocedural ischemic complications (see also Chap. 51).[193,194,210] These complications, which are presumed to be related to the presence of thrombus and ruptured complex plaque[216] as demonstrated elegantly by angioscopy,[217,218] have led many operators to pursue a conservative ischemia-driven approach or to defer intervention for a few days while stabilizing the patient on aggressive antianginal therapy, thrombin inhibition, and antiplatelet therapy[219–221] (particularly in the presence of angiographic thrombus).[222] Alternatively, the favorable results achieved with angioplasty in randomized trials of interventional strategies in unstable angina—such as TIMI-IIIB (96 percent angiographic success, 0.4 percent mortality, 2.9 percent MI, 0.7 percent emergency CABG, 2.2 percent abrupt closure)[223]—encouraged many to pursue a more aggressive approach, particularly in patients at highest risk of a coronary event, i.e., those with postinfarction angina[224] and angina refractory to medical therapy.[225] The argument for an early invasive approach in non-ST-segment-elevation acute coronary syndromes was greatly strengthened by three large randomized trials, each including about 2000 patients and utilizing comtemporary strategies of aspirin, UFH or LMWH, IIb/IIIa inhibitors if desired, stents, and thienopyridines.[30–33] In these studies, early angiography and revascularization, if appropriate, was associated with higher survival without recurrence of severe symptoms necessitating urgent procedures or readmission. Death or MI was shown to be reduced by an early invasive strategy in a metanalysis in the RITA 3 study.[33] However, there was a benefit gradient. Benefit was confined to higher-risk patients (age over 65, male, diabetes, previous MI, ST-segment depression, and positive troponin). The ACC/AHA 2002 Guidelines for Unstable Angina and Non-ST-Segment Elevation Myocardial Infarction recommend an early invasive strategy for patients with high-risk indications (see Tables 55-3 and 55-4) and either an early conservative or early invasive strategy in the absence of these findings.[226] The use of platelet glycoprotein IIb/IIIa inhibitors[151] has been shown to be

TABLE 55-3 Recommendations for PCI from the ACC/AHA Guidelines in Patients with Moderate or Severe Symptoms (Angina Class II to IV), Unstable Angina, or Non-ST-Segment-Elevation Myocardial Infarction on Medical Therapy

Class I (level of evidence: B)	Patients with one or more significant lesions in one or more coronary arteries suitable for PCI with high likelihood of success and low procedural risk; vessels should subtend at least a moderate area of viable myocardium
Class IIa (level of evidence: C)	Patients with focal saphenous vein graft lesions or multiple stenoses who are poor candidates for reoperative surgery
Class IIb (level of evidence: B)	Patients with one or more lesions with reduced likelihood of success or less than moderate area of myocardium at risk
	Multivessel-disease patients with significant proximal LAD disease and treated diabetes or abnormal LV function
Class III (level of evidence: C)	Untreated patients without ischemia or only small area of myocardium at risk, low likelihood of success, high procedural risk; patients with <50% stenosis
(level of evidence: B)	Patients with left main stenoses who are candidates for CABG

TABLE 55-4 Early Invasive Strategy Is Recommended in Unstable Angina or Non-ST-Segment Elevation MI

Class I

Any of the high-risk indications

Recurrent angina at rest or minimal activity despite therapy
Elevated troponin
New ST-segment depression
Recurrent angina/ischemia with symptoms or signs of CHF
    or new or worsening mitral regurgitation
Positive stress test
EF <40%
Hemodynamic instability
Sustained ventricular tachycardia
PCI within 6 months or prior CABG

ABBREVIATIONS: CHF = congestive heart failure; EF = ejection fraction; PCI = percutaneous coronary intervention; CABG = coronary artery bypass grafting.
SOURCE: From the 2002 ACC/AHA Unstable Angina Guidelines[226]

effective in reducing complications of intervention in unstable angina, whereas the routine administration of thrombolytic agents has reduced the thrombus burden but with an unfavorable impact on complications (i.e., in-hospital ischemic events: 12.9 vs. 6.3 percent without thrombolytics; $p = 0.02$).[227] Data from CAPTURE in pa-

tients with unstable angina also indicated that the benefit of IIb/IIIa receptor inhibition was confined to troponin-positive patients and those with complex coronary anatomy.[165,166,229]

ST-SEGMENT-ELEVATION MYOCARDIAL INFARCTION (SEE CHAPTER 56)

Selection of Lesions

LESION CHARACTERISTICS

The importance of coronary stenosis angiographic morphology in predicting the outcome of coronary angioplasty was reflected in the early ACC/AHA PTCA Guidelines.[193,194] Lesions were classified as type A for anticipated high success, low risk; type B for anticipated moderate success, moderate risk; and type C for anticipated low success, high risk. The general validity of this classification in predicting the outcome of balloon angioplasty was confirmed in low- and high-risk patients.[230–233] It appears, however, that in many centers the complexity of lesions to be treated has increased (see Fig. 55-9) and that new devices (especially stents) and antithrombotic strategies have, to a certain extent, weakened the prognostic value of this scoring system.[234] In an effort to update this classification based on the results of contemporary coronary intervention using stents and IIb/IIIa platelet receptor inhibitors, Ellis and colleagues analyzed results from 10,907 lesions and proposed a new classification scheme for risk stratification.[235] Over 4000 patients treated in 1995 through 1996 constituted a training set. Nine preintervention variables were independently correlated with adverse outcome. A proposed classifi-

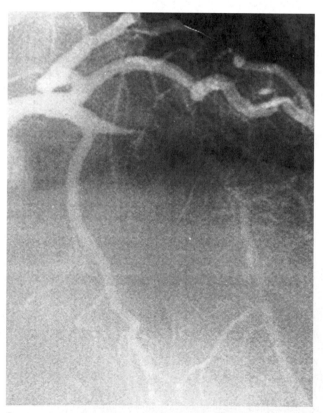

A

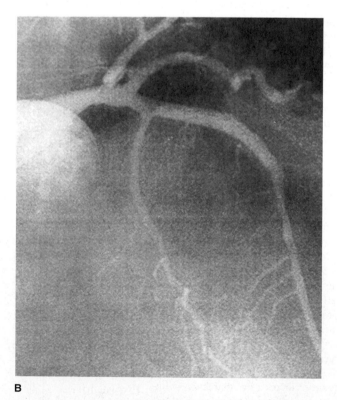

B

FIGURE 55-9 An 82-year-old man with disabling angina and an occluded LAD artery of uncertain duration (A, right anterior oblique view). It was possible to recanalize the long LAD occlusion (B) using a hydrophilic-coated wire and conventional balloon angioplasty followed by placement of two stents. Stents have been shown to be superior to conventional balloon angioplasty in a randomized trial in chronic total occlusions.[278]

cation (Table 55-5) validated against 2146 patients treated in 1997 had greater predictive value than the early ACC/AHA classification, but not by as much as expected. Importantly, lesion characteristics previously thought to be associated with a heightened risk but absent in the new classification include lesion angulation per se, bifurcation location, ostial site, proximal tortuosity, and small thrombus. When the new model was tested against the 1997 validation set, adverse outcomes (death, MI or emergency CABG) occurred in 2.1 percent of low-risk patients, 3.4 percent at moderate risk, 8.2 percent at high risk, and 12.7 at highest risk (compared with 2.5, 3.0, 5.2 and 6.6 percent for ACC/AHA types A, B_1, B_2, and C, respectively). Whether bifurcation location should be included as a predictor of complications is debatable. In our own experience, bifurcation has represented increased risk, and this was confirmed in CAPTURE, where placebo-treated patients with bifurcations had a higher rate of death, MI, or early revascularization than placebo-treated patients without bifurcations (23 vs. 11.7 percent; $p < 0.05$).[166] Importantly, this increased risk of complications with bifurcations was neutralized by treatment with abciximab. It should be recognized, however, that other factors are important in determining risk in the era of stents and IIb/IIIa inhibitors—including patient age, left ventricular ejection fraction, acute MI presentation, and operator experience. These must also be considered.[236–238] In the 2001 ACC/AHA PCI guideline statement, the ABC classification was revised to reflect low, moderate, and high risk (Table 55-6).

LEFT MAIN CORONARY ARTERY LESIONS

Whereas percutaneous intervention in protected left main coronary artery disease has been an accepted strategy for many years,[239] significant narrowing of an unprotected left main coronary artery has been considered a contraindication to this approach since Gruentzig's early recognition of increased mortality.[9,10] With the advent of improved technology in the form of atherectomy devices and stents, percutaneous revascularization has been applied increasingly in patients with unprotected left main coronary artery lesions.[240–243] Although reports of unprotected left main angioplasty/stenting indicated reasonably good results in carefully selected patients and especially when disease is confined to the proximal vessel,[241,243] CABG remains the treatment of choice according to ACC/AHA guidelines.[50,195] Patients considered for percutaneous intervention in an unprotected left main coronary artery lesion in our hospitals include those with significant comorbidity, making CABG impractical, and

patients experiencing abrupt left main coronary artery closure as a complication of coronary angiography or presenting in cardiogenic shock without immediately available surgery.[243,244]

SAPHENOUS VEIN AND LIMA GRAFTS

PCI of distal anastomotic stenoses of SVG and LIMA grafts occurring within a year of CABG is safe and associated with good long-term patency, whereas proximal SVG anastomotic and midgraft lesions have high recurrence rates, especially when long lesions are present. PCI of proximal and mid-LIMA grafts is rarely needed, as this conduit is "immune" to atherosclerosis, but stent implantation has been performed successfully. Atheromatous SVG lesions begin to appear about 3 years post-CABG and PCI is frequently associated with periprocedural MI due to atheroembolization, a complication not prevented by IIb/IIIa platelet receptor inhibitors.[245] Stent implantation was more effective than balloon angioplasty in SVG PCI in a

TABLE 55-5 New Risk Assessment Schema Based on Analysis of 10,907 Lesions Treated in the Stent and IIb/IIIa Era

Strongest correlates	Nonchronic total occlusion
	Degenerated SVG[a]
Moderately strong correlates	Length ≥10 mm
	Lumen irregularity
	Large filling defect
	Calcium + angle ≥45 degrees
	Eccentric
	Severe calcification
	SVG age ≥10 years
Highest risk	Either of strongest correlates
High risk	> moderate correlates and the absence of strong correlates
Moderate risk	1–2 moderate correlates and the absence of strong correlates
Low risk	No risk factors

[a]Saphenous vein graft.
SOURCE: From Ellis et al.[235] With permission.

TABLE 55-6 Lesion Classification From ACC/AHA PCI Guidelines

Low risk	
Discrete (length <10 mm)	Little or no calcification
Concentric	Less than totally occluded
Readily accessible	Not ostial
Nonangulated segment (<45 degrees)	No major side branch
Smooth contour	Absence of thrombus
Moderate risk	
Tubular (length 10–20 mm)	Moderate or heavy calcification
Eccentric	Total occlusion <3 months
Moderate proximal tortuosity	Ostial location
Moderately angulated (>45, <90 degrees)	Bifurcation
Irregular contour	Thrombus present
High risk	
Diffuse (length >20 mm)	Total occlusion >3 months
Excessive proximal tortuosity	Inability to protect side branch
Extreme angulation >90 degrees	Degenerated SVG

SOURCE: From Smith et al.[195] With permission.

randomized trial (6-month MACE 26 vs. 38 percent, $p = 0.05$).[246] Use of embolic protection with the PercuSurge occlusion-aspiration strategy resulted in a 42 percent reduction in 30-day MACE in a randomized trial of 801 patients undergoing SVG stenting,[247] and use of a filter device produced comparable protection when 650 patients were randomized to the filter or PercuSurge during SVG stent procedures.[88] Restenosis following SVG stenting is more frequent than in native vessels and limits the benefit of PCI in spite of relatively favorable results with the subsequent use of brachytherapy to treat in-stent restenoses in SVGs.[248] Whether drug-eluting stents will have an important role in SVG PCI has not been determined.

PREDICTORS OF RESTENOSIS

Characteristics of native coronary artery lesions that were associated with increased restenosis rates following balloon angioplasty alone or after stent implantation include length, total occlusion (Fig. 55-10), vessel size less than 3 mm, ostial location, SVG, and previous angioplasty to the same site.[249–256] The assessment of lesion characteristics by IVUS and angioscopy has also been shown to have prognostic value for determining PCI success and long-term outcome[252–256]; in some centers, these strategies are used to guide therapy. The ability of drug-eluting stents to prevent restenosis in all subsets has not been determined, but data from the SIRIUS trial suggest good efficacy in lesions <2.75 mm in size (TLR 6.3 vs. 18.7 percent in controls, $p < 0.001$) and in lesions >15 to 30 mm in length (TLR 5.2 vs. 17.4 in controls, $p < 0.0001$). Selection of lesions for intervention is strongly based on the operator's assessment of his or her ability to treat the ischemia-producing lesion safely and in a cost-conscious manner and to achieve long-term patency and symptomatic benefit.

IN-STENT RESTENOSIS

One of the most vexing lesions confronting the interventionist is in-stent restenosis, a new "disease" created by the explosion of stent use worldwide. PCI of this lesion, solely the result of neointimal proliferation as opposed to a combination of negative remodeling and intimal proliferation seen in nonstented lesions,[256] was reported by Yokoi et al.[257] to have an overall recurrence rate of 37 percent, but this rate was 85 percent for diffuse in-stent restenosis. Among 288 lesions, recurrent restenosis was highly correlated with the pattern of restenosis (target lesion revascularization in 19 percent of focal lesions less than 10 mm, 35 percent for lesions longer than 10 mm but confined to the stent, 50 percent for lesion longer than 10 mm and extending beyond the stent, and 83 percent for total occlusions; $p < 0.0001$). Additional correlates were the presence of diabetes (odds ratio, 2.8) and previous in-stent restenosis (odds ratio, 2.7).[258] In-stent lesions have been shown by IVUS to have significant reintrusion of tissue shortly after catheter-based intervention not apparent by quantitative angiography.[259] Debulking with atherectomy and laser techniques has been advocated and, although safe and associated with a larger postprocedure minimal lumen diameter (MLD), has not been shown to be superior to balloon angioplasty.[260–263] Although preliminary results from a U.S.-based multicenter randomized comparison of rotational atherectomy and balloon angioplasty were encouraging,[264] results of the ARTIST study indicated that rotablation was inferior to balloon angioplasty (restenosis in 65 percent compared with 51 percent with balloon angioplasty; $p = 0.039$).[265] Yokoi[266] reported results of repeated balloon angioplasty of in-stent restenosis in 310 patients, observing a first recurrence in 51 percent and subsequent recurrences following repetitive procedures in 68, 78, 74, and 92 percent of patients. Although 98 percent of patients were free of death and 90 percent were free of

death/MI/CABG at 3 years, the increasingly high restenosis rate makes this approach impractical. The use of radiation to inhibit neointimal proliferation has produced the most promising strategy for the treatment of this difficult problem. In randomized trials, beta and gamma radiation has reduced restenosis rates by 50 to 60 percent to approximately 20 percent[267,268] with a reduction in 2-year death, MI, or target vessel revascularization (TVR) from 52 to 23 percent ($p = 0.03$).[269] Radiation brachytherapy devices are approved by the FDA for treating in-stent restenosis. Only preliminary reports are available regarding the use of drug-eluting stents for in-stent restenosis, and these have been mixed.[136–138]

MYOCARDIAL BRIDGING

In a small minority of patients with myocardial bridging, clinical symptoms and cardiac events are shown to be attributable to this phenomenon; treatment strategies include stent implantation, which was complicated by restenosis in about 50 percent of patients in small series.[270,271]

CORONARY ARTERY FISTULAS

Coronary artery fistulas (CAFs) are rare anomalies that are usually asymptomatic, requiring no treatment, but can be associated with myocardial ischemia, aneurysmal enlargement, rupture, arrythmias, heart failure, and endocarditis. CAFs drain from either or both coronary arteries to the right heart, pulmonary artery, or coronary sinus. Although surgical ligation is effective, transcatheter closure has been increasingly utilized, employing coils, umbrellas, or vascular occlusive devices.[272,273]

SPASM

When coronary artery spasm occurs in a patient with significant coronary stenosis, it is at the site of organic fixed stenosis in approximately 90 percent of patients; PCI may be required to manage recurrent symptoms and/or associated malignant arrythmias.[274] Results of stenting have been favorable in our small experience.

Selection of Devices

Conventional balloon angioplasty is a simple, relatively low-cost, and reasonably effective method of reducing coronary stenosis, but stents are being used with increasing frequency due to improved initial outcome and reduced restenosis (see Table 55-7). At Emory University Hospital in 1990, balloon angioplasty was the sole technique used in 88 percent of 1863 patients who underwent coronary intervention (directional atherectomy, 3 percent; excimer laser, 3 percent; stents, 2 percent; laser balloon, 1 percent); whereas in 2003, a majority of lesions that were discrete and not involving bifurcations were treated with stent implantation.

The superb results reported in the Benestent II study[110] (overall clinical success 99 percent, stent thrombosis 0.2 percent, restenosis 16 percent, and 1-year mortality 1 percent) coupled with the availability of more flexible, user-friendly, and cheaper metallic stents led to routine stent implantation by most operators by the end of the decade of the 90s. Anatomic subsets of unproven stent benefit include long lesions, small vessels, and bifurcations. Randomized trials confirmed the superiority of stents in total occlusion, SVGs, and restenotic lesions.[275–279] Improvements in stent design included thinner struts, which were associated with lower restenosis, excellent scaffolding, and adequate cell size to access side branches if necessary.[280] The approval of the Cypher drug-eluting stent for marketing in the United States in 2003 provided a powerful tool to the interventionist—one whose benefits appeared clear in "SIRIUS-type" lesions

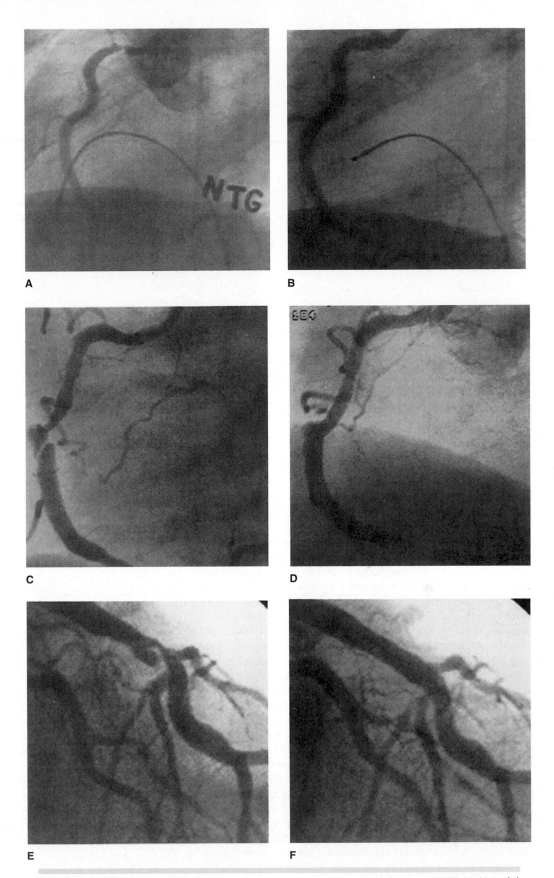

FIGURE 55-10 High-grade de novo stenosis of the ostium of the right coronary artery in a middle-aged man (*A*) was free of calcification. Percutaneous intervention was successful (*B*). This type of lesion is currently treated with stent implantation in most centers, preceded by rotational atherectomy if calcified. A very complex shelf-like de novo stenosis of the right coronary artery (*C*) and the site 2 years after successful percutaneous intervention with directional atherectomy (*D*). Histology showed atheroma and organized thrombus. Flap-like de novo stenosis of the LAD (*E*). This type of lesion responds well to stent implantation or directional coronary atherectomy, (*F*). Sites *A, C,* and *E* are poor lesions for conventional percutaneous balloon angioplasty. Drug-eluting stents have not been tested in these types of lesions.

TABLE 55-7 New Coronary Interventional Strategies

Technique	Indications	Contraindications	Advantages and Limitations
Balloon angioplasty	Focal stenosis	Insignificant narrowing, no ischemia, unimportant artery	Broad applicability, lower cost; poor outcome in thrombotic, ostial, and calcified lesions; significant restenosis
Stents	Focal stenosis	Heavy calcification or thrombus, vessel diameter <2.0 mm	Reduced emergency CABG and restenosis; more expensive, rare stent thrombosis
Directional atherectomy	Focal noncalcified	Diffuse disease, severe tortuosity or bend	Debulks, reduced restenosis; more frequent non-Q-wave MI, more expensive, technically difficult
Rotational atherectomy	Focal calcified stenosis, ostial site	Thrombus, large plaque burden, severe tortuosity or bend	Effective in calcified lesions, reduced elastic recoil; more expensive, similar restenosis, transient left ventricular dysfunction
Laser	Ostial lesion, SVG, in-stent restenosis	Severe calcification, tortuosity or bend	Debulks effectively; increased cost, similar restenosis
Rheolytic thrombectomy	Thrombus	No thrombus	Effective thrombus removal; no plaque removal
Distal protection	SVG, thrombotic lesions	Inadequate anatomy	Reduced embolic complications; anatomic constraints

(see "Drug-Eluting Stents," above) but unclear in the complex anatomy encountered daily (total occlusions, SVGs, bifurcations, vessel <2.5 mm or >3.5 mm, lesions >30 mm long, left main stenosis, ostial lesions, thrombotic lesions, acute MIs).[139]

Currently, DCA is used infrequently in most centers as primary therapy or adjunctively prior to stent implantation due to marginal or no benefit in randomized trials, increased complexity and cost, and an increased rate of non-Q-wave MI. (see "Atherectomy, Laser, Cutting Ballon, Thrombectomy, and Embolic Protection," above).

Rotational atherectomy has proved useful in the presence of calcium, in the treatment of aortoostial and branch ostial lesions, and in nondilatable lesions. Highly angulated or thrombotic lesions or those with impaired distal runoff (recent infarction, fixed thallium defect) and segments with myocardial bridging should be avoided.[281–284] Care is needed in the selection of rotablation in patients with reduced left ventricular function due to the transient regional ventricular dysfunction shown to persist for over 2 h after the procedure.[285]

Although ablative laser angioplasty (XeCl excimer) has been shown to be effective in the treatment of aortoostial sites, undilatable lesions, total occlusions, calcification, long lesions, in-stent restenosis, and saphenous vein grafts,[286–289] its superiority to simpler and less costly balloon and stent strategies has not been demonstrated.[290–292] Lesions that should not be selected for ablative laser angioplasty include those on bend points or in tortuous segments, those associated with severe calcification or thrombus, or lesions with a suspected subintimal wire passage. In general, bifurcation lesions should not be selected for ablative laser therapy unless an eccentrically directed device can be used so as to avoid a perforation at the flow divider of the vessel. The cutting balloon has been used in some centers primarily to treat bifurcation lesions, undilatable le-

sions, and in-stent resenosis (see" In-Stent Restenosis," above), but there are no randomized trial data supporting its use.

When obvious large intracoronary thrombi are present, PCI is associated with increased complications. In the SAFER trial, in which 50 percent of patients undergoing SVG PCI received distal protection, the presence of a thrombus was associated with a 10 percent incidence of no reflow and a 3 percent mortality rate; use of PercuSurge was associated with reduced complications (OR 0.625, $p = 0.02$). Alternatives include dissolving the thrombus (thrombolytic; prolonged treatment with an antithrombin ± IIb/IIIa inhibitor), thrombectomy (guide catheter, Export catheter, Angiojet, Xsizer), embolic protection with a filter, or a combination of thrombectomy and embolic protection. Treatment of a SVG restenotic lesion is one of the few SVG PCI conditions where embolic protection is not required (see "Atherectomy, Laser, Cutting Balloon, Thrombectomy, and Embolic Protection," above). The place of distal protection in native coronary lesions has not been well studied.

PERFORMANCE OF CORONARY INTERVENTION

Operator Proficiency

Current guidelines recommend that cardiologists who wish to become competent in coronary intervention receive special training in diagnostic and therapeutic catheterization during an additional year after the standard fellowship training program and maintain their skills by the performance of 75 procedures per year.[194,195,293–299] Ideally, operators with an annual procedural volume <75 should work only at active centers (>600 procedures per year). An adequate case mix is an important aspect of a physician's training in interventional cardiology that has not yet been addressed by practice guidelines.[301,302] Assurance of quality by the surveillance of procedural outcomes is made difficult by such complex issues as a need to adjust for high-risk patients, low incidence and subjectivity of major adverse events, and low volume of many operators.[163,236–238,302–304] At least five mortality risk models of PCI outcome have been developed; however, validation of these models using a stent and IIb/IIIa platelet receptor inhibitor era multicenter registry revealed that only three models (New York State, Northern New England, and the Cleveland Clinic) predicted mortality rates that were not significantly different from those observed.[305]

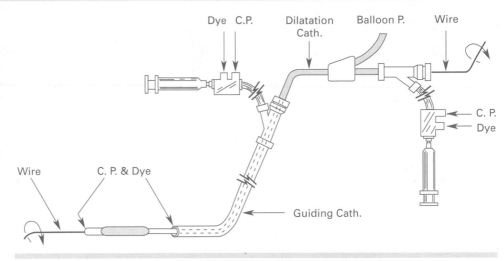

FIGURE 55-11 Diagram of the over-the-wire catheter system used currently for balloon angioplasty and stent deployment. The floppy guidewire is steerable. (From Aueron FM, Gruentzig AR. Percutaneous transluminal coronary angioplasty: Indications and current status. *Prim Cardiol* 1984;10:91. With permission.)

Interventional Laboratory

Optimal conditions for the performance of coronary angioplasty procedures require sophisticated imaging systems; trained personnel; a large inventory of dilation, thrombectomy, atherectomy, and stent hardware and software; and a variety of therapeutic safety nets to protect the patient when intervention fails or is complicated. Most studies suggest that laboratory procedural volume is important and inversely related to adverse procedural outcomes.[236,306–308] The quality of the video image of the coronary arteries is an important determinant of angioplasty success. A freeze-frame storage and display capability is required for use during the procedure, as is a high-quality video replay with slow-motion and stop-frame capability. The ability to solve specific problems such as lesion eccentricity or rigidity, vessel tortuosity, and unusual position or orientation of the coronary ostia often depends on specific device characteristics. Consequently, it is necessary to have available dilating catheters, stents, atherectomy devices, guidewires, and guiding catheters in a variety of shapes and sizes (see Figs. 55-11, 55-12, and 55-13). The 2001 ACC/AHA PCI Guidelines recommend that elective PCI be performed only in centers with cardiac surgery available for emergency situations.[195]

The Coronary Intervention Procedure

Prior to coronary intervention, patients receive an explanation of the procedure, including the operator's estimate of success, possible complications, risks, and benefits. A booklet and videotape describing the procedure and an explanation by the nursing staff help to reduce anxiety and ensure that both patient and family are well informed.

Antiplatelet therapy is used routinely, and patients in whom stenting is planned receive clopidogrel, usually a 300- to 600-mg loading dose unless pretreatment for several days has been performed. A platelet glycoprotein IIb/IIIa receptor antagonist is commonly utilized when there is perceived to be an increased risk of abrupt closure or distal embolization (e.g., suspected or definite thrombus, troponin-positive acute coronary syndrome, complex lesion, diabetes, or multisite intervention). Restenosis trials have failed to show a clear advantage of one antiplatelet regimen over another and have not shown inhibition of restenosis by calcium channel blockers, warfarin

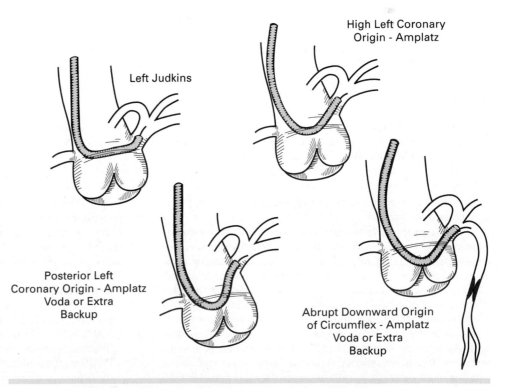

FIGURE 55-12 Guide catheter shapes commonly used for left coronary angioplasty.

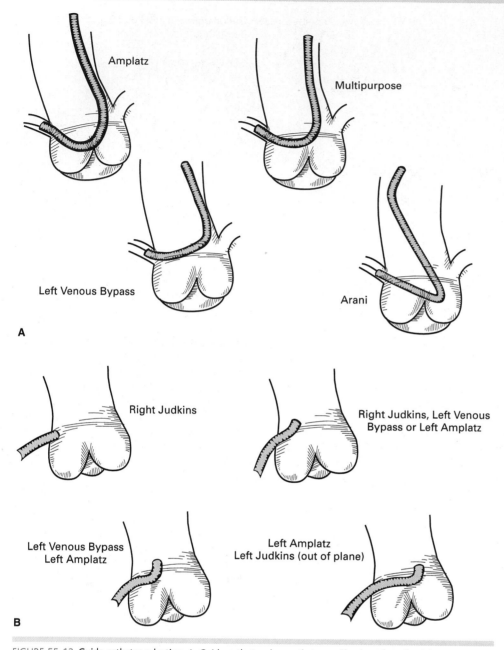

FIGURE 55-13 Guide catheter selection. *A.* Guide catheter shapes that are effective when the right coronary artery has a steep upward initial course, *B.* Guide catheter shapes that are effective when the right coronary artery has an anterior and leftward origin.

preferred by some operators in patients with unstable ischemic syndromes or frank intracoronary thrombus.[310–312] Recently published studies have compared ionic (Ioxaglate) and nonionic (Iomeprol) agents in a randomized format[313]; ionic versus nonionic contrast material in EPIC, EPILOG, and CAPTURE in a metanalysis[314]; and ionic versus nonionic in stenting;[315] however, they have revealed no increase in thrombotic complications, whereas nonionic agents were associated with more bailout stenting in a randomized study.[316] These studies reported outcomes with contrast agents with osmolalities in the range of 600 to 700 mosmol/kg. Recent reports of the use of the isoosmolar nonionic dimer iodixanol in high-risk PTCA were promising,[317] and further evaluation of this agent is warranted.

Intracoronary stenting is conducted most often as a primary strategy but may be utilized for suboptimal outcomes after balloon angioplasty or other interventions. Deployment strategies vary depending on stent designs, since some are balloon-mounted and others are self-expanding. Stent deployment with a properly sized balloon is performed (usually to >12 atm) to expand the stent optimally throughout its length. A recently reported randomized trial of stent implantation showed no advantage of routine inflation to more than 15 atm.[318] Although some operators advocate IVUS guidance, there is no consensus regarding its routine use.[319,320]

If there is concern about the adequacy of the lumen at the treatment site, use of a Doppler flow wire or pressure gradients may be helpful in addition to ultrasound in assessing the result. Studies suggest that a normal coronary hyperemic flow response and a low transluminal gradient are associated with reduced risk of restenosis. *It is clear that optimizing the lumen size is the goal, since final lumen size is an important determinant of the probability of restenosis.* When the operator is confident that the best possible result has been obtained, the patient is returned to his or her room. Puncture-site closure devices are used with increasing frequency. Creatine kinase determinations are performed immediately and every 8 h for three determinations. Because of the dehydrating effect of the osmotic load, most patients receive at least 1 L of intravenous fluids after the procedure. Delayed sheath removal is performed at 2 to 4 h when the ACT is below 150s. If an intimal tear, suboptimal result, or intraluminal thrombus is present, or if multiple stents are implanted, a IIb/IIIa receptor inhibitor is often used.[321] There is evidence that routine heparin administration following uncomplicated angioplasty is not helpful in reducing acute occlusion or restenosis.[322]

anticoagulation, angiotensin-converting enzyme (ACE) inhibitors, steroids, or other agents.

Once the patient is in the catheterization laboratory, electrocardiographic monitoring leads are applied, a peripheral intravenous line is started, and midazolam 1 mg or an equivalent drug is given intravenously. In most laboratories, a femoral approach is employed; use of a radial artery approach, however, is increasing.[309] A thrombin inhibitor is administered (see above). Patients with a history of allergy to contrast material are premedicated with prednisone 40 to 60 mg orally the night before and the day of the procedure and with diphenhydramine (Benadryl) 50 mg intravenously at the time of the procedure. Due to the reported increased thrombotic complications with nonionic agents (attributed to comparatively less thrombin inhibition and enhanced platelet activation), ionic agents have been

RESULTS OF CORONARY INTERVENTION

The results obtained with coronary intervention procedures have been influenced significantly by technologic advances, operator experience, and the difficulty of patients selected. With pioneering equipment, Gruentzig was able to dilate the coronary arteries in 64 percent of his first 50 patients and 78 percent of his first 169 patients.[10,15] Defining primary success as less than 50 percent residual stenosis and freedom from complications, a success rate of 91 percent in over 34,000 patients treated at Emory University was seen between 1980 and 1999 (Table 55-8).[323] Complication rates generally declined despite increasingly difficult cases. Experienced operators should achieve primary success rates in excess of 95 percent in ideal proximal lesions, compared with a reduced success rate of approximately 75 percent in recent (<3 months) total occlusions or in attempting to treat fibrotic, calcified, eccentric stenoses located distally in tortuous coronary arteries. In all techniques, including stenting, lesion characteristics are a major determinant of the outcome of the procedure.[193–195,230–235] Long-term outcome has been reported out to 10 years in patients treated in Zurich, Atlanta, and Rotterdam,[15–17,196,324] and detailed 5- to 8-year follow-up data are available from randomized trials,[25–47,208] (see above and Table 55-1 and Fig. 55-4).

Complications

Patients undergoing coronary intervention are subject to the same complications encountered with the performance of coronary arteriography. In addition, because instrumentation of the atherosclerotic lesion takes place, coronary artery dissection, thrombus formation, and coronary artery spasm may occur, leading to acute occlusion of the coronary artery or of side branches arising from it. Atheroembolism may lead to MI in an otherwise successful procedure. Atheroembolic MI has replaced occlusion of the treated artery as the most common serious complication of coronary intervention; the need for emergency bypass surgery has been reduced from 30 to 50 per thousand in the 1980s to about 1 per thousand in 2003.

Of Gruentzig's first 50 patients, 5 experienced an acute deterioration necessitating emergency bypass surgery and 3 showed electrocardiographic evidence of MI.[10] The results of 3500 patients undergoing elective balloon angioplasty at Emory were analyzed and reported in detail.[325] Angioplasty was attempted in 3933 lesions, with a success rate of 91 percent. No complications occurred in 89 percent of patients, minor complications in 6.9 percent, and major complications (emergency surgery, MI, death) in 4.1 percent. Emergency CABG was performed in 2.7 percent of patients, who had an MI rate of 49 percent and a Q-wave MI rate of 23 percent. In patients sent for emergency surgery, the mortality rate was 2 percent. The overall MI rate was 2.6 percent. There were two nonsurgical deaths, giving a total mortality rate of 0.1 percent (4 of 3500). *Five preprocedural predictors of a major complication were identified: multivessel coronary artery disease, lesion eccentricity, presence of calcium in the lesion, female gender, and lesion length. The strongest predictor of a major complication was the appearance of an intimal dissection during the procedure.* Intimal dissection was evident in 29 percent of patients, and its presence resulted in a sixfold increase in the risk of a major complication. This early series of patients was treated with balloon angioplasty alone.

Although angiographic variables are important predictors of abrupt closure, of equal or greater importance is an estimate of the consequences of abrupt closure. This estimate is determined in large part by the amount of myocardium that is supplied by the artery in jeopardy. An analysis of 294 acute occlusions occurring during 8207 consecutive coronary angioplasty procedures performed in two centers revealed 13 cardiac deaths (4.4 percent of acute occlusions) and an overall cardiac mortality of 0.16 percent.[326] Of 13 patients who died, 12 were women. Multivariate analysis identified three independent predictors of death: collaterals originating from the dilated vessel, female gender, and multivessel disease. In an analysis of 32 deaths associated with 8052 PTCA procedures in three centers, left ventricular failure due to vessel occlusion, the most common cause of death, was independently correlated with female sex, "jeopardy score," and PTCA of a proximal right coronary artery (RCA) site but not ejection fraction or presence of multivessel disease.[327] Right ventricular failure due to occlusion of the proximal RCA and left main coronary dissections accounted for most of the remaining deaths.

The use of stents in the course of a failing angioplasty (Fig. 55-14) and prospectively in patients with unfavorable anatomy has significantly reduced the risk of urgent bypass surgery and Q-wave

TABLE 55-8 Twenty-Year Experience With 34,508 Patients Who Underwent PCI at Emory University

	1980–1983	1984–1987	1988–1991	1992–1995	1996–1999
Age	55 ± 10	58 ± 10	60 ± 11	62 ± 11	62 ± 12
Diabetes	9%	14%	19%	23%	26%
Multivessel disease	17%	34%	48%	56%	58%
Class 3–4 angina	46%	66%	70%	76%	75%
Site length	6.0 ± 4.0	7.9 ± 5.2	6.9 ± 5.2	8.7 ± 6.8	12.8 ± 10.7
Stent	0	0	2.8%	6.1%	47%
Ang. success	89%	86%	90%	94%	95%
Non-Q-wave MI	—	4.3%	3.3%	3.2%	4.0%
Q-wave MI	1.9%	2.0%	1.0%	0.9%	0.3%
CABG	6.7%	5.8%	3.5%	2.7%	1.2%
Death	0.1%	0.6%	0.6%	0.6%	0.6%
Stay (days)	3.0 ± 2.7	3.2 ± 2.8	2.8 ± 3.9	2.7 ± 3.6	1.9 ± 2.8
Hosp. cost (dollars)	—	5233	8549	9552	7856

ABBREVIATIONS: Ang. success = angiographic success; MI = myocardial infarction.
SOURCE: From Douglas et al.[323] With permission.

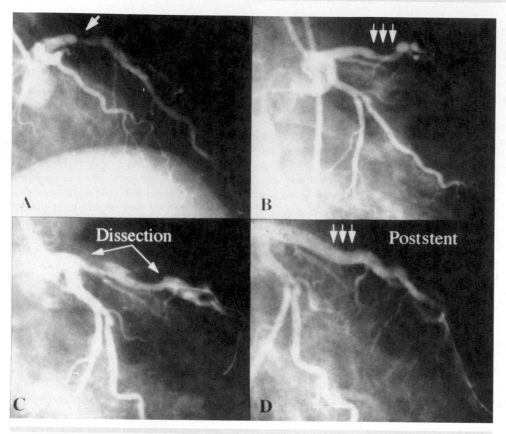

FIGURE 55-14 Complex stenosis of tortuous proximal LAD. *A.* Right anterior oblique, cranial angulation. *B.* Caudal angulation. Following an initial attempt at treatment of the lesion, a long dissection occurred. *C.* Prompt stent implantation stabilized the patient, preventing the need for emergency CABG. *D.*

New complications related in part to the use of nonballoon devices include coronary perforation, distal atheroembolization, arterial access complications, and "domino stenting" (additional stents to treat end-of-stent dissections). Among 8932 patients treated at William Beaumont Hospital, perforation was reported in 0.4 percent (balloon, 0.14 percent; transluminal extraction catheter (TEC), 1.3 percent; DCA, 0.25 percent; excimer laser, 2 percent).[333] This risk of perforation is highest in tortuous and smaller vessels and in laser angioplasty of right coronary lesions. In patients experiencing free perforations, Ellis reported that 75 percent required surgery, 29 percent had a Q-wave MI, and 14 percent died.[334] Perforation was reported in 10 of 432 stent patients (2.3 percent), resulting in cardiac tamponade (50 percent), MI (40 percent), emergency surgery (50 percent), and death (30 percent).[335] The manifestations of perforation were delayed (5 to 24 h) in 20 percent of patients. Angiographic features associated with stent-related perforation were complex lesion morphology, small vessel diameter (2.6 ± 0.2 mm), oversized stents (stent/artery ratio 1.4 ± 0.1), tapering vessel (40 percent), and recrossing dissections (20 percent).[335] These results should engender a cautious approach to stenting in small vessels and when there is uncertainty regarding wire position. One of the new causes of perforation is the hydrophilic coronary guidewire, which easily penetrates the wall of small distal arteries, causing bleeding and cardiac tamponade sometimes many hours post-PCI, especially when IIb/IIIa receptor inhibitors have been used. Prompt application of strategies for the management of vessel perforation can be lifesaving, and angioplasty operators must be facile with them. The availability of a covered stent to treat perforations is a substantial advance.

Fortunately, the risk of vascular access-site complications, a frequent accompaniment of stenting when heparin and warfarin anticoagulation were used adjunctively, has been reduced with less aggressive antithrombotic strategies. In our experience, complications at the femoral artery puncture site were more often related to advanced age, female sex, hypertension, and postprocedure heparin use than to the size of the catheter.[336–338] Prolonged compression of pseudoaneurysms using ultrasound guidance or local thrombin injection obviates surgery in many patients with this complication.[339–341] Closure devices are used actively in some centers but add significantly to the cost of the procedure and have their own complications, including infection.[342,343]

Distal coronary atheroembolization is only occasionally recognized clinically with balloon angioplasty but probably occurs frequently[344] and is a clinically important limitation of debulking strategies such as atherectomy and laser ablation, where its manifestations are slow coronary flow, ischemia, and infarction.[345,346] Reports from directional atherectomy trials indicate that postproce-

MI. We studied outcomes of 34,508 patients who underwent elective or urgent PCI at Emory University from 1980 to 1999.[323] Patients were divided into five 4-year periods (see Table 55-8; all $p < 0.0001$, except non-Q-wave MI and death). Corrected for baseline differences, death fell period to period (odds ratio 0.76, $p = 0.0075$). Other correlates of death were increased urgency, female sex, age, heart failure, multivessel disease, calcium and thrombus. Corrected for baseline differences, CABG fell dramatically (odds ratio 0.63, $p < 0.0001$). Other correlates of CABG were increased urgency, younger age, severe angina, multivessel disease, no prior CABG, lesion calcium, thrombus, and lesion at a branch point. Corrected for baseline differences, the occurrence of Q-wave MI fell significantly from period to period ($p < 0.0001$). Correlates of Q-wave MI were increased urgency, female sex, higher ejection fraction, long lesions, diffuse disease, lesion calcium, thrombus, or lesion ulceration. Length of stay fell from period to period and was significantly correlated with the occurrence of complications. Stent use was less than 10 percent until FDA approval of the Palmaz-Schatz stent in the mid 1990s; it increased to 70 percent in 1999 and to about 90 percent since then. Clearly PCI has changed over the past 20 years, with the treatment of sicker patients being undertaken. However, acute outcome has improved related to multiple technical improvements, including stents and new antithrombotic drugs, heralding a "new era" of percutaneous intervention.[164] Recent reports from multicenter regional registries,[328] multicenter national registries,[329,330] and single-center registries[331,332] have confirmed improved outcomes but differed as to whether female gender was a predictor of adverse outcome.

dural CK elevations were associated with worse long-term outcomes (death, MI, repeat intervention).[346] Although procedural modifications with rotational atherectomy appear to have reduced the immediate impact of microparticulate embolization,[281] the issue remains a source of concern and needs further study. Patients at increased risk include those with bulky, thrombotic, or long native vessel lesions and nonfocal or thrombotic saphenous vein graft lesions, where embolization was noted in about 20 percent; about one-third of patients with this complication in one report died.[347,348] Atheroembolization also complicates stenting, accounting for an increased rate of non-Q-wave MI compared with balloon angioplasty. Particulate embolism to the coronary microcirculation may lead to otherwise silent infarction, reflected by CK elevation, a topic of intense interest due to the finding of adverse late outcome, even with small elevations,[349,350] as well as the recognition that IIb/IIIa platelet receptor inhibitors, filters, and "occlusion-aspiration" systems can protect against this complication. Not all studies, however, have found a correlation between enzyme elevations and adverse late outcome.[351] The use of thrombectomy devices and distal protection strategies plays a major and increasing role in PCI of thrombotic and SVG lesions, similarly aimed at preventing embolic complications (see above).

Acute contrast nephropathy requiring dialysis is a costly complication of coronary intervention, which occurred in 15 of 1828 (0.8 percent) patients and was associated with a high (33.8 percent) in-hospital mortality.[352] Independent predictors of contrast nephropathy included decreased baseline creatinine clearance, diabetes, and contrast dose (no dialysis was required in patients receiving less than 100 mL of contrast agent). Adequate periprocedural hydration and limitation of contrast volume are the most important measures in high-risk patients.[353] The use of the antioxidant acetylcysteine has been associated with a significant reduction in contrast nephropathy in several randomized trials; however, other studies have failed to show benefit,[186–188] and the use of the dopamine antagonist fenoldopam was not protective in a recently reported randomized trial.[189] It had been suggested that an isoosmolar contrast agent may be preferred in patients at high risk for contrast nephropathy.[354–355]

POSTINTERVENTION THERAPY

The most recent ACC/AHA PCI Guideline statement emphasizes the importance of behavior and risk-factor modification and the institution of medical therapy for secondary prevention of atherosclerosis prior to hospital discharge. Recommendations should include dual antiplatelet therapy with aspirin and a thienopyridine in most patients,[141,145] a statin aimed at a target LDL of <100 mg/dL,[183] smoking cessation, weight control, regular exercise, and ACE inhibitor therapy as recommended in the AHA/ACC consensus statement on secondary prevention. Preliminary data suggest that beta blockade after successful elective PCI provides a mortality benefit.[184] The optimal duration of thienopyridine therapy is a topic of considerable interest. Observational studies of patients receiving bare metal stents have indicated that 14 days of treatment was adequate for prophylaxis against stent thrombosis.[102] However, longer treatment has been recommended for the sirolimus-eluting stent (3 months), the paclitaxel-eluting stent (9 months), and following brachytherapy (6 months), and brachytherapy + stent (12 months) due to delayed healing at the PCI site. Recent data from PCI-Cure and CREDO indicate that long-term therapy (1 year) with clopidogrel is associated with a 20 to 30 percent relative reduction in ischemic events following elective PCI in a broad spectrum of patients.

FUTURE DIRECTIONS

The future of coronary intervention with the new availability of drug-eluting stents seems bright indeed. The problem of subacute stent thrombosis, greatly diminished by current deployment and dual antiplatelet strategies, was not exacerbated in the trials by delayed healing induced by drug-eluting stents, thus opening the arena of small-vessel stenting (2- to 2.5-mm vessels) and further expanding intervention for multiple lesions in multiple vessels. Whether any late complications of uncovered stent wires will occur must await long-term follow-up. The major impediment to this strategy is cost. This should be ameliorated somewhat by market competition. Information is being acquired that should guide therapy with drug-eluting stents in complex lesion subsets (total occlusions, bifurcations, SVGs, diffuse disease, left main and calcified lesions). Improved methods of embolic protection are becoming available that will have application in native vessels and in saphenous vein grafts. New methods for opening chronic total occlusions are needed.

References

1. Dotter CT, Judkins MP. Transluminal treatment of arteriosclerotic obstruction: Description of a new technique and a preliminary report of its application. *Circulation* 1964;30:654–670.
2. Zeitler EJ, Schmidtke J, Schoop W. Die Perkutane Behandlung von Arteriellen Durchbluteungasstorungen der Estremiaten mit Katheter. *Vasa* 1973;2:401–404.
3. Gruentzig AR, Turina MI, Schneider JA. Experimental percutaneous dilatation of coronary artery stenosis (abstract). *Circulation* 1976; 54(suppl II):II–81.
4. Gruentzig AR, Kumpe DA. Technique of percutaneous transluminal angioplasty with the Gruentzig balloon catheter. *AJR* 1979;132:547–552.
5. Sheldon WC, Sones FM Jr. Stormy petrel of cardiology. *Clin Cardiol* 1994;17:405–407.
6. Hurst JW. History of cardiac catheterization. In: King SB III, Douglas JS Jr, eds. *Coronary Arteriography and Angioplasty.* New York: McGraw-Hill; 1985:1–9.
7. King SB III. Angioplasty from bench to bedside to bench. *Circulation* 1996;93:1621–1629.
8. King SB III. The development of interventional cardiology. *J Am Coll Cardiol* 1998;31(suppl B):64B–88B.
9. Meier B. The first patient to undergo coronary angioplasty—23-year follow-up. *N Engl J Med* 2001;344:144–145.
10. Gruentzig A. Transluminal dilatation of coronary artery stenosis. *Lancet* 1978;1:263.
11. Gruentzig AR, Senning A, Siegenthaler WE. Nonoperative dilatation of coronary artery stenosis: Percutaneous transluminal coronary angioplasty. *N Engl J Med* 1979;301:61–68.
12. Kent KM, Bentivoglio LG, Block PC. Percutaneous transluminal coronary angioplasty: Report from the Registry of the National Heart, Lung, and Blood Institute. *Am J Cardiol* 1982;49:2011–2020.
13. Detre K, Holubkov R, Kelsey S, et al. Percutaneous transluminal coronary angioplasty in 1985–1986 and 1977–1981: The National Heart, Lung, and Blood Institute Registry. *N Engl J Med* 1988;318:265–270.
14. Simpson JB, Baim DS, Robert EW, et al. A new catheter system for coronary angioplasty. *Am J Cardiol* 1982;49:1216–1222.
15. Gruentzig AR, King SB III, Schlumpf M, et al. Long-term follow-up after percutaneous transluminal coronary angioplasty: The early Zurich experience. *N Engl J Med* 1987;316:1127–1132.
16. King SB, Schlumpf M. Ten year completed follow-up after percutaneous transluminal coronary angioplasty: The early Zurich experience. *J Am Coll Cardiol* 1993;22:353–360.
17. Detre K, Yeh W, Kelsey S, et al. Has improvement in PTCA intervention affected long-term prognosis? The NHLBI PTCA Registry experience. *Circulation* 1995;91:2868–2875.

18. Cannon CR, Yeh W, Kelsey S, et al. Incidence and predictors of target vessel revascularization following percutaneous transluminal coronary angioplasty: A report from the National Heart, Lung, and Blood Institute Percutaneous Transluminal Coronary Angioplasty Registry. Am J Cardiol 1999;84:170–175.

19. Jones RH, Kesler K, Phillips K, et al. Long-term survival benefits of coronary artery bypass grafting and percutaneous transluminal angioplasty in patients with coronary artery disease. J Thorac Cardiovasc Surg 1996;111:1013.

20. Mark DB, Nelson CL, Califf RM, et al. Continuing evolution of therapy for coronary artery disease: Initial results from the era of coronary angioplasty. Circulation 1994;89:2015–2025.

21. Hannan EL, Racz MJ, McCallister BD, et al. A comparison of three-year survival after coronary artery bypass graft surgery and percutaneous transluminal coronary angioplasty. J Am Coll Cardiol 1999;33: 63–72.

22. Velianou JL, Jacobs AK, Feit F, et al. Does angioplasty prolong survival in patients with multivessel disease? Results from the Bypass Angioplasty Revascularization Investigation (BARI). Circulation 1999;100(suppl I):I-84.

23. Cowley MJ, Vetrovec GW, DiSciasio G, et al. Coronary angioplasty of multiple vessels: Short-term outcome and long-term results. Circulation 1985;72:1314–1320.

24. O'Keefe JH Jr, Rutherford BD, McConahay DR, et al. Multivessel coronary angioplasty from 1980–1989: Procedural results and long-term outcome. J Am Coll Cardiol 1990;16:1097–1102.

25. Parisi AF, Folland ED, Hartigan P. A comparison of angioplasty with medical therapy in the treatment of single-vessel coronary artery disease. N Engl J Med 1992;326:10–16.

26. Boden WE, O'Rourke RA, Crawford MH, et al. Outcomes in patients with acute non-Q-wave myocardial infarction randomly assigned to an invasive as compared with a conservative management strategy. N Engl J Med 1998;338:1785–1792.

27. Hueb WA, Bellotti G, deOliveira SA, et al. The Medicine, Angioplasty or Surgery Study (MASS): A prospective, randomized trial of medical therapy, balloon angioplasty or bypass surgery for single proximal left anterior descending artery stenoses. J Am Coll Cardiol 1995;26: 1600–1605.

28. Coronary angioplasty versus medical therapy for angina: The Second Randomized Intervention Treatment of Angina (RITA-2) trial. Lancet 1997;350:461–468.

29. Pitt B, Waters D, Brown WV, et al. Aggressive lipid-lowering therapy compared with angioplasty in stable coronary artery disease. N Engl J Med 1999;341:70–76.

30. Wallentin L. Fast revascularization during instability in coronary artery disease (FRISC II): An early invasive versus early noninvasive strategy in unstable coronary artery disease. J Am Coll Cardiol 1999; 34:1.

31. Fragmin and Fast Revascularization during Instability in Coronary Artery Disease Investigators. Invasive compared with non-invasive treatment in unstable coronary-artery disease: FRISC II prospective randomised multicentre study. Lancet 1999;354:708–715.

32. Cannon CP, Weintraub WS, Dempoulos LA, et al. Comparison of early invasive and conservative strategies in patients with unstable coronary syndromes treated with the glycoprotein IIb/IIIa inhibitor tirofiban. N Engl J Med 2001;344:1879–1887.

33. Fox KAA, Poole-Wilson PA, Henderson RA, et al. Interventional versus conservative treatment for patients with unstable angina or non-ST-elevation myocardial infarction: the British Heart Foundation RITA 3 randomised trial. Lancet 2002;360:743–751.

34. King SB III, Lembo NJ, Weintraub WS, et al. A randomized trial comparing coronary angioplasty with coronary bypass surgery. N Engl J Med 1994;331:1044–1050.

35. The Bypass Angioplasty Revascularization Investigation (BARI) Investigators. Comparison of coronary bypass surgery with angioplasty in patients with multivessel disease. N Engl J Med 1996;335:217–225.

36. Chaitman BR, Schwartz L, Roubin GS, et al. Comparative 5 year incidence of ischemic events for PTCA and CABG in the Bypass Angio-

37. Pocock SJ, Henderson RA, Rickards AF, et al. Metaanalysis of randomized trials comparing coronary angioplasty with bypass surgery. Lancet 1995;346:1184–1189.

38. Sim I, Gupta M, McDonald K, et al. A meta-analysis of randomized trials comparing coronary artery bypass grafting with percutaneous transluminal coronary angioplasty in multivessel coronary artery disease. Am J Cardiol 1995;76:1025–1029.

39. Kosinski AS, Barnharat HX, Weintraub WS, et al. Five year outcome after coronary surgery or coronary angioplasty: Results from the Emory Angioplasty versus Surgery Trial (EAST) (abstr). Circulation 1995;92:I-543.

40. Weintraub WS, Mauldin PD, Becker E, et al. A comparison of the costs and quality of life after coronary angioplasty or coronary surgery for multivessel coronary artery disease: Results from the Emory Angioplasty versus Surgery Trial (EAST). Circulation 1995;92:2831–2840.

41. Henderson RA, Pocock SJ, Clayton TC, et al. Seven-year outcome of RITA-2 Trial: Coronary angioplasty versus medical therapy. J Am Coll Cardiol 2003;42:1161–1170.

42. Weintraub WS, Becker ER, Mauldin PD, et al. Costs of revascularization over eight years in the randomized and eligible patients in the Emory Angioplasty versus Surgery Trial (EAST). Am J Cardiol 2000;747–752.

43. The BARI Investigators. Influence of diabetes on 5-year mortality and morbidity in a randomized trial comparing CABG and PTCA in patients with multivessel disease: The Bypass Angioplasty Revascularization Investigation (BARI). Circulation 1997;96:1761–1769.

44. The BARI Investigators. Seven-year mortality in the Bypass Angioplasty Revascularization Investigation (BARI) by treatment and diabetic status. J Am Coll Cardiol 2000;35:1122–1129.

45. King SB III, Kosinski AS, Guyton RA, et al. Eight-year mortality in the Emory Angioplasty versus Surgery Trial (EAST). J Am Coll Cardiol 2000;35:1116–1121.

46. Weintraub WS, Stein B, Kosinski A, et al. Outcome of coronary bypass surgery versus coronary angioplasty in diabetic patients with multivessel coronary artery disease. J Am Coll Cardiol 1998;31:10–19.

47. Detre KM, Guo P, Holubkov R, et al. Coronary revascularization in diabetic patients: A comparison of the randomized and observational components of the Bypass Angioplasty Revascularization Investigation (BARI). Circulation 1999;99:633–640.

48. Niles NW, McGrath PD, Malenka D, et al. Survival of patients with diabetes and multivessel coronary artery disease after surgical or percutaneous coronary revascularization: results of a large regional prospective study. J Am Coll Cardiol 2001;37:1008–1015.

49. Kuntz RE. Importance of considering atherosclerosis progression when choosing a coronary revascularization strategy: The diabetics-percutaneous transluminal coronary angioplasty dilemma. Circulation 1999;99:847–851.

50. Eagle KA, Guyton RA, Davidoff R, et al. ACC/AHA guidelines for coronary artery bypass graft surgery: Executive summary and recommendations. A report of the American College of Cardiology/American Heart Association Task Force on Practice Guidelines (Committee to Revise the 1991 Guidelines for Coronary Artery Bypass Graft Surgery). Circulation 1999;100:1464–1480.

51. Hirotani T, Kameda T, Kumamoto T, et al. Effects of coronary artery bypass grafting using internal mammary arteries for diabetic patients. J Am Coll Cardiol 1999;34:532–538.

52. Robertson GC, Simpson JB, Selmon MR, et al. Experience of directional coronary atherectomy over four years. J Am Coll Cardiol 1991; 17:384A.

53. Topol EJ, Leya F, Pinkerton CA, et al. A comparison of directional coronary atherectomy with coronary angioplasty in patients with coronary artery disease. N Engl J Med 1993;329:221–227.

54. Adelman AG, Cohen EA, Kimball BP, et al. A comparison of directional atherectomy with balloon angioplasty for lesions of the left anterior descending coronary artery. N Engl J Med 1993;329:228–233.

55. Holmes DR Jr, Topol EJ, Califf RM, et al. A multicenter, randomized trial of coronary angioplasty versus directional atherectomy for pa-

tients with saphenous vein bypass graft lesions. *Circulation* 1995;91:
1966–1974.

56. Baim DS, Cutlip DE, Sharma SK, et al. Final results of the balloon versus optimal atherectomy trial (BOAT). *Circulation* 1998;97:
322–331.

57. Simonton CA, Leon MB, Baim DS, et al. "Optimal" directional coronary atherectomy: Final results of the Optimal Atherectomy Restenosis Study (OARS). *Circulation* 1998;97:332–339.

58. Williams DO, Fahrenbach MC. Directional coronary atherectomy: But wait, there's more. *Circulation* 1998;97:309–311.

59. Tsuchikane E, Kobayashi T, Kirino M, et al. Which is better for STRESS and BENESTENT equivalent lesions, stenting or atherectomy? Results of Stent versus Directional Atherectomy Randomized Trial (START). *Circulation* 1999;100(suppl I):I-727.

60. Moussa I, Moses J, Di Mario C, et al. Stenting after optimal lesion debulking (SOLD) registry: Angiographic and clinical outcomes. *Circulation* 1998;98:1604–1609.

61. Karvouni E, Di Mario C, Nishida T, et al. Directional atherectomy prior to stenting in bifurcation lesions : A matched comparison study with stenting alone. *Catheter Cardiovasc Interv* 2001;53:12–20.

62. Dauerman HL, Higgins PJ, Sparano AM, et al. Mechanical debulking versus balloon angioplasty for the treatment of true bifurcation lesions. *J Am Coll Cardiol* 1998;32:1845–1852.

63. Colombo A. Atherectomy Before MULTI-LINK Improves Luminal Gain and Clinical Outcomes (AMIGO): A comparison of coronary stenting with or without adjunctive directional coronary atherectomy. *J Am Coll Cardiol* 2002;40:4.

64. Reifart N, Vandormael M, Krajcar M, et al. Randomized comparison of angioplasty of complex coronary lesions at a single center: Excimer Laser, Rotational Atherectomy, and Balloon Angioplasty Comparison (ERBAC) study. *Circulation* 1997;96:91–98.

65. Koster R, Hamm CW, Seabra-Comes R, et al. Laser angioplasty of restenosed coronary stents: Results of a multicenter surveillance trial. *Am Coll Cardiol* 1999; 34:25–32.

66. Bersin RM, Cedarholm JC, Kowalchuk GJ, et al. Long-term clinical follow-up of patients treated with the coronary Rotablator: A single-center experience. *Catheter Cardiovasc Interv* 1999; 46:399–405.

67. Kini A, Marmur JD, Duvvuri S, et al. Rotational atherectomy: Improved procedural outcome with evolution of technique and equipment: Single-center results of first 1000 patients. *Catheter Cardiovasc Interv* 1999;46:305–311.

68. Kobayashi Y, De Gregorio J, Kobayashi N, et al. Lower restenosis rate with stenting following aggressive versus less aggressive rotational atherectomy. *Cathet Cardiovasc Intervent* 1999;46:406–414.

69. Sharma SK, Bhalla N, Dangas G, et al. Rotational atherectomy prior to coronary stenting prevents side branch occlusion. *J Am Coll Cardiol* 1997;29(suppl A):498A.

70. Whisenant BK, Baim DS, Kuntz RE, et al. Rheolytic thrombectomy with the Possis AngioJet: Technical considerations and initial clinical experience. *J Invasive Cardiol* 1999;11:421–426.

71. Scott LRP, Silva JA, White C, et al. Rheolytic thrombectomy: A new treatment for stent thrombosis. *Catheter Cardiovasc Interv* 1999;47:
97–101.

72. Nakagawa Y, Matsuo S, Yokoi H, et al. Stenting after thrombectomy with the AngioJet catheter for acute myocardial infarction. *Catheter Cardiovasc Diagn* 1998;43:327–330.

73. Rodes J, Bilodeau L, Bonan R, et al. Angioscopic evaluation of thrombus removal by the Possis AngioJet thrombectomy catheter. *Catheter Cardiovasc Diagn* 1998;43:338–343.

74. Nakaawa Y, Matsuo S, Kimura T, et al. Thrombectomy with Angiojet catheter in native coronary arteries for patients with acute or recent myocardial infarction. *Am J Cardiol* 1999;83:994–999.

75. Silva JA, White CJ, Ramee SR, et al. Treatment of coronary stent thrombosis with rheolytic thrombectomy: Results from a multicenter experience. *Catheter Cardiovasc Interv* 2003;58:11–17.

76. Singh M, Tiede DJ, Mathew V, et al. Rheolytic thrombectomy with angiojet in thrombus-containing lesions. *Catheter Cardiovasc Interv* 2002;56:1–7.

77. Mauri L, Bonan R, Weiner BH, et al. Cutting balloon angioplasty for the prevention of restenosis: Results of the cutting balloon global randomized trial. *Am J Cardiol* 2002;90:1079–1083.

78. Stone GW, Cox DA, Babb JD, et al. A prospective randomized trial of thromboatherectomy during intervention of thrombotic native coronary arteries and saphenous vein graft: the X-TRACT Trial. *J Am Coll Cardiol* 2003;41:43A.

79. Kwok O, Prpic R, Gaspar J, et al. Angiographic outcome after intracoronary X-Sizer Helical atherectomy and thrombectomy: First use in humans. *Catheter Cardiovasc Interv* 2002;55:133–139.

80. Topol EJ, Yadav JS. Recognition of the importance of embolization in atherosclerotic vascular disease. *Circulation* 2000;101:570–580.

81. Baim DS, Wahr D, George B, et al. Randomized trial of a distal embolic protection device during percutaneous intervention of saphenous vein aorto-coronary bypass grafts. *Circulation* 2002;105:1285–1290.

82. Gerckens U, Mueller R, Rowold S, et al. The filter wire: First evaluation of a new protection catheter device for distal embolization in native coronary arteries and SVGs. *J Am Coll Cardiol* 2001;37(suppl A):34A.

83. Limbruno U, Micheli A, Petronio AS, et al. Prevention of no-reflow during primary percutaneous coronary angioplasty with a porous distal embolic protection device. *Circulation* 2002;106:II-446.

84. Gerckens U, Mueller R, Solblik S, et al. Prevention of distal embolization during interventions in CABG and native coronary lesions using a new protection filter device. *J Am Coll Cardiol* 2000;35(suppl A):10A.

85. Popma J, Cox N, Hauptmann K, et al. Initial clinical experience with distal protection using the FilterWire in patients undergoing coronary artery and saphenous vein graft percutaneous intervention. *Catheter Cardiovasc Interv* 2002;57:125–134.

86. Brener S, Lytle B, Schneider J, et al. Association between CK-MB elevation after percutaneous or surgical revascularization and three-year mortality. *J Am Coll Cardiol* 2002;40:1961–1967.

87. Hong MK, Mehran R, Dangas G, et al. Creatine kinase-MB enzyme elevation following successful saphenous vein graft intervention is associated with late mortality. *Circulation* 1999;100:2400–2405.

88. Stone GW, Rogers C, Hermiller J, et al: A prospective randomized multicenter trial comparing distal protection during saphenous vein graft intervention with a filted-based device compared to balloon occlusion and aspiration: The FIRE Trial. *J Am Coll Cardiol* 2003;41:
43A.

89. Sigwart U, Puel J, Mirkovitch V, et al. Intravascular stents to prevent occlusion and restenosis after transluminal angioplasty. *N Engl J Med* 1987;316:701–706.

90. Puel J, Joffrc F, Rousseau H, et al. Endo-protheses coronanennes and auto-expansive dans la preventions des restenoses apres angioplastie transluminale. *Arch Mal Coeur Vaiss* 1987;8:131–132.

91. Roubin GS, King SB III, Douglas JS Jr, et al. Intracoronary stenting during percutaneous transluminal coronary angioplasty. *Circulation* 1990;81(suppl IV):IV-92–IV-100.

92. Hearn JA, King SB III, Douglas JS Jr, et al. Clinical and angiographic outcomes after coronary artery stenting for acute or threatened closure after percutaneous transluminal coronary angioplasty: Initial results with a balloon-expandable, stainless steel design. *Circulation* 1993;88:
2086–2096.

93. Roubin GS, Robinson KA, King SB, et al. Early and late results of intracoronary arterial stenting after coronary angioplasty in dogs. *Circulation* 1987;76:891–897.

94. Fischman DL, Leon MB, Baim DS, et al. A randomized comparison of coronary-stent placement and balloon angioplasty in treatment of coronary artery disease. *N Engl J Med* 1994;331:496–501.

95. Serruys PW, de Jaegere P, Kiemeneij F, et al. A comparison of balloon-expandable-stent implantation with balloon angioplasty in patients with coronary artery disease. *N Engl J Med* 1994;331:489–495.

96. Colombo A, Hall P, Nakamura S, et al. Intracoronary stenting without anticoagulation accomplished with intravascular ultrasound guidance. *Circulation* 1995;91:1676–1688.

97. Schoemig A, Newmann FJ, Kastrati A, et al. A randomized comparison of antiplatelet and anticoagulant therapy after the placement of coronary artery stents. *N Engl J Med* 1996;334:1084–1089.

98. Topol EJ. Toward a new frontier in myocardial reperfusion therapy: Emerging platelet preeminence. *Circulation* 1998;97:211–218.

99. Leon MB, Baim DS, Popma JJ, et al. A clinical trial comparing three antithrombotic-drug regimens after coronary-artery stenting. *N Engl J Med* 1998;339:1665–1671.

100. Urban P, Macaya C, Rupprecht HJ, et al. Randomized evaluation of anticoagulation versus antiplatelet therapy after coronary stent implantation in high-risk patients: The Multicenter Aspirin and Ticlopidine Trial after Intracoronary Stenting (MATTIS). *Circulation* 1998;98: 2126–2132.

101. Bertrand M, Legrand V, Boland J, et al. Randomized multicenter comparison of conventional anticoagulation versus antiplatelet therapy in unplanned and elective coronary stenting: The Full Anticoagulation versus Aspirin and Ticlopidine (FANTASTIC) study. *Circulation* 1998;98:1597–1603.

102. Berger PB, Bell MR, Hasdai D, et al. Safety and efficacy of ticlopidine for only 2 weeks after successful intracoronary stent placement. *Circulation* 1999;99:248–253.

103. Steinhubl SR, Tan WA, Foody JM, et al. Incidence and clinical course of thrombotic thrombocytopenic purpura due to ticlopidine following coronary stenting. *JAMA* 1999;281:806–810.

104. Bennett CL, Davidson CJ, Raisch DW, et al. Thrombotic thrombocytopenic purpura associated with ticlopidine in the setting of coronary artery stents and stroke prevention. *Arch Intern Med* 1999;159: 2524–2528.

105. Quinn MJ, Fitzgerald DJ. Ticlopidine and clopidogrel. *Circulation* 1999;100:1667–1672.

106. Berger PB, Bellot V, Melby S, et al. Clopidogrel versus ticlopidine for coronary stents. *J Am Coll Cardiol* 1999;33:34A.

107. Moussa I, Oetgen M, Roubin G, et al. Effectiveness of clopidogrel and aspirin versus ticlopidine and aspirin in preventing stent thrombosis after coronary stent implantation. *Circulation* 1999;99:2364–2366.

108. Bertrand ME. Clopidogrel aspirin stent international study (CLASSICS) trial. *J Am Coll Cardiol* 1999;34:7.

109. Urban P, Gershlick AH, Rupprecht HJ, et al. Efficacy of ticlopidine and clopidogrel on the rate of cardiac events after stent implantation: Evidence from CLASSICS. *Circulation* 1999;100(suppl I):I-379.

110. Serruys PW, van Hout B, Bonnier H, et al. Randomised comparison of implantation of heparin-coated stents with balloon angioplasty in selected patients with coronary artery disease (Benestent II). *Lancet* 1998;352:673–681.

111. Weaver WD. Late-breaking trials in interventional cardiology: Optimal angioplasty versus primary stenting (OPUS). *J Am Coll Cardiol* 1999;34:1.

112. Narins CR, Holmes DR, Topol EJ. A call for provisional stenting: The balloon is back! *Circulation* 1998;97:1298–1305.

113. Ten Berg JM, Kelder JC, Suttorp M, et al. A plea for plain old balloon angioplasty with a low rate of provisional stenting: An unselected consecutive group of 1058 patients. *Circulation* 1999;100(suppl I):I-455.

114. Rodriquez A. Optimal coronary balloon angioplasty versus stent. *J Am Coll Cardiol* 1998;32:1351–1357.

115. Brophy JM, Belisle P, Lawrence J. Evidence for use of coronary stents. *Ann Intern Med* 2003;138:777–786.

116 Holmes DR, Hirshfeld J, Faxon D, et al. ACC expert consensus document on coronary artery stents: Document of the American College of Cardiology. *J Am Coll Cardiol* 1998;32:1471–1482.

117. Rankin JM, Spinelli JJ, Carere RG, et al. Improved clinical outcome after widespread use of coronary-artery stenting in Canada. *N Engl J Med* 1999;341:1957–1965.

118. Jacobs AK. Coronary stents: Have they fulfilled their promise? *N Engl J Med* 1999;341:2005–2006.

119. Ashby DT, Dangas G, Mehran R, et al. Coronary artery stenting. *Catheter Cardiovasc Interv* 2002;56:83–102.

120. Kandzari DE, Tcheng JE, Zidar JP. Coronary artery stents: Evaluating new designs for contemporary percutaneous intervention. *Catheter Cardiovasc Interv* 2002;56:562–576.

121. Colombo A, Stankovic G, Moses JW. State of the art paper: Selection of coronary stents. *J Am Coll Cardiol* 2002;40:1021–1033.

122. Serruys PW, Unger F, Sousa JE, et al, for the Arterial Revascularization Therapies Study Group: Comparison of coronary artery bypass surgery and stenting for the treatment of multivessel disease. *N Engl J Med* 2001;344:1117–1124.

123. Serruys PW, Costa MA, Betriu A, et al. The influence of diabetes mellitus on clinical outcome following multivessel stenting or CABG in the ARTS Trial. *Circulation* 1999;100(suppl I):I-364.

124. Rodriquez A, Palacios IF, Navia J, et al. Argentine randomized study: Coronary angioplasty with stenting versus coronary artery bypass surgery in patients with multiple vessel disease (ERACI II): 30-day and long-term follow-up results. *Circulation* 1999;100(suppl I):I-234.

125. The SOS Investigators. Coronary artery bypass surgery versus percutaneous intervention with stent implantation in patients with multivessel coronary artery disease (the Stent or Surgery Trial): a randomized controlled trial. *Lancet* 2002;360:965–970.

126. Hoffman SN, TenBrook JA, Wolf M, et al. A meta-analysis of randomized controlled trials comparing coronary artery bypass graft with percutaneous transluminal coronary angioplasty: One to eight year outcomes. *J Am Coll Cardiol* 2003;41:1293–1304.

127. Sousa JE, Serruys PW, Costa MA. New frontiers in cardiology—Drug-eluting stents: Part I. *Circulation* 2003;107:2274–2279.

128. Sousa JE, Serruys PW, Costa MA. New frontiers in cardiology—Drug-eluting stents: Part II. *Circulation* 2003;107:2383–2389.

129. Sousa JE, Costa MA, Abizaid A, et al. Lack of neointimal proliferation after implantation of sirolimus-coated stents in human coronary arteries: A quantitative coronary angiography and three-dimensional intravascular ultrasound study. *Circulation* 2001;103:192–195.

130. Sousa JE, Costa MA, Abizaid AC, et al. Sustained suppression of neointimal proliferation by sirolimus-eluting stents: One-year angiographic and intravascular ultrasound follow-up. *Circulation* 2001;104: 2007–2011.

131. Degertekin M, Serruys PW, Foley DP, et al. Persistent inhibition of neointimal hyperplasia after sirolimus-eluting stent implantation: Long-term (up to 2 years) clinical, angiographic, and intravascular ultrasound follow-up. *Circulation* 2002;106:1610–1613.

132. Morice MC, Serruys PW, Sousa JE, et al. A randomized comparison of a sirolimus-eluting stent with a standard stent for coronary revascularization. The RAVEL trial. *N Engl J Med* 2002;346:1773–1780.

133. Moses JW, Leon MB, Popma JJ, et al. Drug-eluting stent trials: A multicenter randomized clinical study of the sirolimus-eluting stent in native coronary lesions: clinical outcomes. *Circulation* 2002;106:II-392.

134. Grube E, Siber MS, Hauptmann KE, et al. Prospective, randomized, double-blind comparison of NIRx stents coated with paclitaxel in a polymer carrier in de novo coronary lesions compared with uncoated controls. *Circulation* 2001;104(suppl):II-463.

135. Ellis SG. *Transcatheter Cardiovascular Therapeutics* 2002.

136. Tanabe K, Serruys PW, Grube E, et al. TAXUS III Trial. In-stent restenosis treated with stent-based delivery of paclitaxel incorporated in a slow-release polymer forulation. *Circulation* 2002;107:559–564.

137. Degertkin M, Regar E, Tanabe K, et al. Sirolimus-eluting stent for treatment of complex in-stent restenosis. *J Am Coll Cardiol* 2003;41: 184–189.

138. Sousa JE, Gosta MA, Abizaid A, et al. Sirolimus-eluting stent for treatment of in-stent restenosis. A quantitative coronary angiography and three-dimensional intravascular ultrasound study. *Circulation* 2003; 107:24–27.

139. Hodgson J, King SB III, Feldman T, et al. SCAI statement on drug-eluting stents: practice and health care delivery implications. *Catheter Cardiovasc Interv* 2003;58:397–399.

140. Bhatt DL, Bertrand ME, Berger PB, et al. Meta-analysis of randomized and registry comparisons of ticlopidine with clopidogrel after stenting. *J Am Coll Cardiol* 2002;39:9–14.

141. Mehta S, Yusuf S, Peters R, et al. Effects of pretreatment with clopidogrel and aspirin followed by long-term therapy in patients undergoing percutaneous coronary intervention: The PCI-CURE study. *Lancet* 2001;358:527–533.

142. Berger PB, Steinhubl S. Clinical implications of percutaneous coronary intervention-clopidogrel in unstable angina to prevent recurrent

events (PCI-CURE) study—A US perspective. *Circulation* 2002;106: 2284–2287.

143. Pache J, Kastrati A, Mehilli J, et al. Clopidogrel therapy in patients undergoing coronary stenting: Value of a high-loading dose regimen. *Catheter Cardiovasc Interv* 2002;55:436–441.

144. Gurbel PA, Bliden KP, O'Connor CM. The antiplatelet effects of clopidogrel loading for coronary stenting: Pretreatment versus administration in the catheterization laboratory. *Circulation* 2002;106:II-517.

145. Steinhubl SR, Berger PB, Mann JT III, et al. Early and sustained dual oral antiplatelet therapy following percutaneous coronary interventional: A randomized controlled trial. *JAMA* 2002;288:2411–2420.

146. Angiolillo DJ, Fernandez-Ortiz A, Bernardo E, et al. Platelet aggregation varies according to body mass index in patients undergoing coronary stent implantation. Should clopidogrel load-dose be weight adjusted? *Circulation* 2002;106:II-79.

147. The PURSUIT Investigators. Inhibition of platelet glycoprotein IIb/IIIa with eptifibatide in patients with acute coronary syndromes. *N Engl J Med* 1998;339:436–443.

148. PRISM-PLUS Investigators. Inhibition of the platelet glycoprotein IIb/IIIa receptor with tirofiban in unstable anigna and non-Q wave myocardial infarction. *N Engl J Med* 1998;338:1488–1497.

149. The CAPTURE Investigators. Randomized placebo-controlled trial of abciximab before and during coronary intervention in refractory unstable angina: The CAPTURE study. *Lancet* 1997;349:1429–1435.

150. The EPILOG Investigators. Platelet glycoprotein IIb/IIIa receptor blockade and low-dose heparin during percutaneous coronary revascularization. *N Engl J Med* 1997;336:1689–1696.

151. The EPIC Investigators. Use of a monoclonal antibody directed against the platelet glycoprotein IIb/IIIa receptor in high-risk coronary angioplasty. *N Engl J Med* 1994;330:956–961.

152. Topol EJ, Ferguson JJ, Weisman HF, et al. Long term protection from myocardial ischemic events after brief integrin β_3 blockade with percutaneous coronary intervention. *JAMA* 1997;278:479–484.

153. Karvouni E, Katritsis DG, Ioannidis JPA. Intravenous glycoprotein IIb/IIIa receptor antagonists reduce mortality after percutaneous coronary interventions. *J Am Coll Cardiol* 2003;41:26–32.

154. Boersma E, Akkerhuis M, Theroux P, et al. Platelet glycoprotein IIb/IIIa receptor inhibition in non-ST-elevation acute coronary syndromes: Early benefit during medical treatment only, with additional protection during percutaneous coronary intervention. *Circulation* 1999;100:2045–2048.

155. The EPISTENT Investigators. Randomized placebo-controlled and balloon angioplasty-controlled trial to access safety of coronary stenting with use of platelet glycoprotein-IIb/IIIa blockade. *Lancet* 1998; 352:87–92.

156. Lincoff AM, Califf RM, Moliterno DJ, et al. Complementary clinical benefits of coronary artery stenting and blockade of platelet glycoprotein IIb/IIIa receptors. *N Engl J Med* 1999;341:319–327.

157. Marso SP, Bhatt DL, Tanguay JF, et al. Synergy of stenting plus abciximab in diabetic patients: Persistence through 1-year follow-up from EPISTENT. *Circulation* 1999;100(suppl I):365.

158. King SB III, Mahmud E. Will blocking the platelet save the diabetic? *Circulation* 1999;100:2466–2468.

159. The ERASER Investigators. Acute platelet inhibition with abciximab does not reduce in-stent restenosis (ERASER study). *Circulation* 1999;100:799–806.

160. Roffi M, Chew DP, Mukherjee D, et al. Platelett glycoprotein IIb/IIIa inhibitors reduce mortality in diabetic patients with non-ST-segment-elevation acute coronary syndomes. *Circulation* 2001;104: 2767–2771.

161. Topol E, Moliterno D, Hermann H, et al. Comparison of two platelet glycoprotein IIb/IIIa inhibitors, tirofiban and abciximab, for the prevention of ischemic events with percutaneous coronary revascularization. *N Engl J Med* 2001;344:1888–1894.

162. Moliterno DJ, Yakubov SJ, DiBattiste M, et al. Outcomes at 6 months for the direct comparison of tirofiban and abciximab during percutaneous coronary revascularization with stent placement: The TARGET follow-up study. *Lancet* 2002;360:355–360.

163. Stone GW, Moliterno DJ, Bertrand M, et al. Impact of clinical syndrome acuity on the differential response to 2 glycoprotein IIb/IIIa inhibitors in patients undergoing coronary stenting. The TARGET Trial. *Circulation* 2002;105:2347–2354.

164. Ellis SG, Whitlow PL, Guetta V, et al. A highly significant 40 percent reduction in ischemic complications of percutaneous coronary intervention in 1995: Beginning of a new era. *J Am Coll Cardiol* 1996;27 (suppl A):253A.

165. Hamm CW, Heeschen C, Goldman B, et al. Benefit of abciximab in patients with refractory unstable angina in relation to serum troponin T levels. *N Engl J Med* 1999;340:1623–1629.

166. Van den Brand M, Laarman GJ, Steg PG, et al. Assessment of coronary angiograms prior to and after treatment with abciximab, and the outcome of angioplasty in refractory unstable angina patients: Angiographic results from the CAPTURE trial. *Eur Heart J* 1999;20: 1572–1578.

167. Ellis SG, Lincoff AM, Miller D, et al. Reduction in complications of angioplasty with abciximab occurs largely independent of baseline lesion morphology. *J Am Coll Cardiol* 1998;32:1619–1623.

168. Chew DP, Bhatt DL, Lincoff MA, et al. Defining the optimal activated clotting time during percutaneous coronary intervention:aggregate results from 6 randomized, controlled trials. *Circulation* 2001;103:961–966.

169. Tolleson TR, O'Shea JC, Bittl JA, et al. Relationship between heparin anticoagulation and clinical outcomes in coronary stent intervention—Observations from the ESPRIT Trial. *J Am Coll Cardiol* 2003;41: 386–393.

170. Ashby DT, Dangas G, Mehran T, et al. Relationship of the degree of procedural anticoagulation to outcomes after stent implantation. *J Am Coll Cardiol* 2002;39:27A

171. Kereiakes DJ, Kleiman NS, Fry E, et al. Dalteparin in combination with abciximab during percutaneous coronary intervention. *Am Heart J* 2001;141:348–352.

172. Muller I, Seyfarth M, Rudiger S, et al. Effect of a high loading dose of clopidogrel on platelet function in patients undergoing coronary stent placement. *Heart* 2001;85:92–93.

173. Collet JP, Montalescot G, Lison L, et al. Percutaneous coronary intervention after subcutaneous enoxaparin pretreatment in patients with unstable angina pectoris. *Circulation* 2001;103:658–663.

174. Martin JL, Fry ETA, Serano A, et al. Pharmacokinetic study of enoxaparin in patients undergoing coronary intervention after treatment with subcutaneous enoxaparin in acute coronary syndromes. The PEPCI study. *Eur Heart J* 2001;22:143.

175. Choussat R, Montalescot G, Philippe J, et al. A unique, low dose of intravenous enoxaprin in elective percutaneous coronary intervention. *J Am Coll Cardiol* 2002;40:1943–1950.

176. Bittl JA, Strony J, Brinker JA, et al. Treatment with bivalirudin (Hirulog) as compared with heparin during coronary angioplasty for unstable or postinfarction angina. Hirulog Angioplasty Study Investigators. *N Engl J Med* 1995;333:764–769.

177. Bittl J. Chaitman B, Feit F, et al: Bivalirudin versus heparin during coronary angioplasty for unstable or postinfarction angina: Final report reanalysis of the Bivalirudin Angioplasty Study. *Am Heart J* 2001; 142:952–959.

178. Lincoff AM, Bittl JA, Kleiman NS, et al. The REPLACE I Trial: A pilot study of bivalirudin versus heparin during percutaneous coronary intervention. *J Am Coll Cardiol* 2002;39:16a.

179. Lincoff AM, Bittl JA, Harrington RA, et al. Bivalirudin and provisional glycoprotein IIb/IIIa blockade compared with heparin and planned glycoprotein IIb/IIIa blockade during percutaneous coronary intervention. *JAMA* 2003;289:853–863.

180. Antman EM. Should bivalirudin replace heparin during percutaneous coronary interventions? *JAMA* 2003;289:903–905.

181. Herrmann J, Lerman A, Baumgart D, et al. Preprocedural statin medication reduces the extent of periprocedural non-Q wave myocardial infarction. *Circulation* 2002;106:2180–2183.

182. Chan AW, Bhatt DL, Chew DP, et al. Early and sustained survival benefit associated with statin therapy at the time of percutaneous coronary intervention. *Circulation* 2002;105:691–696.

183. Schomig A, Mehilli J, Holle H, et al. Statin treatment following coronary artery stenting and one-year survival. *J Am Coll Cardiol* 2002;40: 854–861.

184. Chan AW, Quinn MJ, Bhatt DL, et al. Mortality benefit of beta-blockade after successful elective percutaneous coronary intervention. *J Am Coll Cardiol* 2002;40:669–675.

185. Kini AS, Mitre CA, Kim M, et al. A protocol for prevention of radiographic contrast nephropathy during percutaneous coronary intervention: Effect of selective dopamine receptor agonist fenoldopam. *Cathet Cardiovasc Intervent* 2002;55:169–173.

186. Kay J, Chow WH, Chan TM, et al. Acetylcysteine for prevention of acute deterioration of renal function following elective coronary angiography and intervention—A randomized controlled trial. *JAMA* 2003;289:553–558.

187. Curhan GC. Prevention of contrast nephropathy. *JAMA* 2003;289: 606–608.

188. Lepor NE. A review of contemporary prevention strategies for radiocontrast nephropathy: A focus on fenoldopam and n-acetylcysteine. *Rev Cardiovasc Med* 2003;4(suppl 1):S15–S20.

189. Stone GW, McCullough P, Tumlin J, et al. A prospective, randomized placebo-controlled multicenter trial evaluating fenoldopam mesylate for the prevention of contrast induced nephropathy: the CONTRAST Trial. *J Am Coll Cardiol* 2003;41:83A.

190. Sheppard R, Eisenberg MJ. Intracoronary radiotherapy for restenosis. *N Engl J Med* 2001;344:295–296.

191. Sapirstein W, Zuckermanbraum DT. FDA approval of coronary artery brachytherapy. *N Engl J Med* 2001;344:297–299.

192. Waksman R. Vascular brachytherapy: applications in the era of drug-eluting stents. *Rev Cardiovasc Med* 2002;3(suppl 5):S23–S30.

193. Ryan TJ, Faxon DP, Gunnar RM, et al. Guidelines for percutaneous transluminal coronary angioplasty: A report of the American College of Cardiology/American Heart Association Task Force on Assessment of Diagnostic and Therapeutic Cardiovascular Procedures (Subcommittee of Percutaneous Transluminal Coronary Angioplasty). *J Am Coll Cardiol* 1988;12:519–540.

194. Ryan TJ, Bauman WB, Kennedy JW, et al. Guidelines for percutaneous transluminal coronary angioplasty: A report of the American Heart Association/American College of Cardiology Task Force on Assessment of Diagnostic and Therapeutic Cardiovascular Procedures (Committee on Percutaneous Transluminal Coronary Angioplasty). *Circulation* 1993;88:2987–3007.

195. Smith SC Jr, Dove JT, Jacobs AK, et al. ACC/AHA Guidelines for Percutaneous Coronary Intervention (Revision of the 1993 Guidelines for Percutaneous Transluminal Coronary Angioplasty). *J Am Coll Cardiol* 2001;37:2239.

196. Weintraub WS, King SB III, Douglas JS Jr, et al. Percutaneous transluminal coronary angioplasty as a first revascularization procedure in single, double, and triple-vessel coronary artery disease. *J Am Coll Cardiol* 1995;26:142–151.

197. Mark DB, Nelson CL, Califf RM, et al. Continuing evaluation and therapy for coronary artery disease: Initial results from the era of coronary angioplasty. *Circulation* 1994;89:2015–2025.

198. Strauss WE, Fortin T, Hartigan P, et al. A comparison of quality of life scores in patients with angina pectoris after angioplasty compared with after medical therapy: Outcomes of a randomized clinical trial. *Circulation* 1995;92:1710–1719.

199. Giacomini JC, Parisi AF, Folland ED, et al. Three year follow-up of patients in the VA ACME trial. *Circulation* 1993;88(suppl I):I-218.

200. O'Keefe JH, Kreamer TR, Jones PG, et al. Isolated left anterior descending coronary artery disease: Percutaneous transluminal coronary angioplasty versus stenting versus left internal mammary artery bypass grafting. *Circulation* 1999;(suppl II):II-114–II-118.

201. Hueb WA, Soares PR, de Oliveiras A, et al. Five-year follow-up of the Medicine, Angioplasty, or Surgery Study (MASS): A prospective, randomized trial of medical therapy, balloon angioplasty, or bypass surgery for single proximal left anterior descending coronary artery stenosis. *Circulation* 1999;100(suppl II):II-107–II-113.

202. Goy JJ, Eickhout E, Burnand B. Coronary angioplasty versus left internal mammary artery grafting for isolated proximal left anterior descending artery stenosis. *Lancet* 1994;343:1449–1454.

203. Versaci F, Gaspardone A, Fabrizio P, et al. A comparison of coronary artery stenting with angioplasty for isolated stenosis of the proximal left anterior descending coronary artery. *N Engl J Med* 1997;336: 817–822.

204. Diegeler A, Thiele H, Falk V, et al. Comparison of stenting with minimally invasive bypass surgery for stenosis of the left anterior descending coronary artery. *N Engl J Med* 2002;347:561–566.

205. Ellis SG, Brown K, Howell G, et al. Two-year cardiac cost after cardiac catheterization: Profound impact of revascularization after first PTCA compared with initial medical or surgical therapy. *J Am Coll Cardiol* 1996;27(suppl A):72A.

206. Cowley MJ, Vandermael M, Topol EJ. Is traditionally defined complete revascularization needed for patients with multivessel disease treated with elective coronary angioplasty? *J Am Coll Cardiol* 1993; 22:1289–1297.

207. Bourassa MG, Holubkov R, Yeh W, et al. Strategy of complete revascularization in patients with multivessel coronary artery disease: A report from the 1985–1986 NHLBI PTCA Registry. *Am J Cardiol* 1992; 70:174–178.

208. Zhao XQ, Brown BG, Stewart DK, et al. Effectiveness of revascularization in the Emory Angioplasty versus Surgery Trial: A randomized comparison of coronary angioplasty with bypass surgery. *Circulation* 1996;93:1954–1962.

209. Kip KE, Bourassa MG, Jacobs AK, et al. Influence of pre-PTCA strategy and initial PTCA result in patients with multivessel disease: The Bypass Angioplasty Revascularization Investigation (BARI). *Circulation* 1999;100:910–917.

210. Ellis SG, Roubin GS, King SB III, et al. Angiographic and clinical predictors of acute closure after native vessel coronary angioplasty. *Circulation* 1988;77:372–379.

211. Laham RJ, Ho KL, Baim DS, et al. Palmaz-Schatz stenting: Early results and one-year outcome. *J Am Coll Cardiol* 1997;30:180–185.

212. Moussa I, Reiners B, Moses J, et al. A long-term angiographic and clinical outcome of patients undergoing multivessel coronary stenting. *Circulation* 1997;96:3873–3979.

213. Kornowski R, Mehran R, Satler LF, et al. Procedural results and late clinical outcomes following multivessel coronary stenting. *J Am Coll Cardiol* 1999;33:420–426.

214. Hernandez-Antolin RA, Alfonso F, Goicolea J, et al. Results (>6 months) of stenting of >1 major coronary artery in multivessel coronary artery disease. *Am J Cardiol* 1999;84:147–151.

215. O'Neill W. Multivessel balloon angioplasty should be abandoned in diabetic patients! *J Am Coll Cardiol* 1998;31:20–22.

216. Fuster V, Badimon L, Badimon JJ, et al. The pathogenesis of coronary artery disease and acute coronary syndromes. *N Engl J Med* 1991;326: 242–250, 320–328.

217. Mizuno K, Satomura K, Miyamoto A, et al. Angioscopic evaluation of coronary artery thrombi in acute coronary syndromes. *N Engl J Med* 1992;326:287–291.

218. Waxman S, Mittleman MA, Manzok, et al. Culprit lesion morphology in subtypes of unstable angina as assessed by angioscopy. *Circulation* 1995;92(suppl I):I-79.

219. Laskey MA, Deutsch E, Hirshfield JWJ, et al. Influence of herapin therapy on percutaneous transluminal coronary angioplasty outcome in patients with coronary arterial thrombus. *Am J Cardiol* 1990;65:179–182.

220. Laskey MA, Deutsch E, Barnathan E, et al. Influence of herapin therapy on percutaneous transluminal coronary angioplasty outcome in unstable angina pectoris. *Am J Cardiol* 1990;65:1425–1429.

221. Rosenman Y, Gilon D, Zelingher J, et al. Importance of delaying balloon angioplasty in patients with unstable angina pectoris. *Clin Cardiol* 1996; 19:111–114.

222. Douglas JS Jr, Lutz JF, Clements SD, et al. Therapy of large intracoronary thrombi in candidates for percutaneous transluminal coronary angioplasty. *J Am Coll Cardiol* 1988;11:238.

223. The TIMI-IIIB Investigators. Effects of tissue plasminogen activator and a comparison of early invasive and conservative strategies in unstable angina and non-Q wave myocardial infarction. *Circulation* 1994;89:1545–1556.

224. Cannon CP, McCabe CH, Stone PH, et al. Prospective validation of the Braunwald classification of unstable angina: Results from the Thrombolysis in Myocardial Ischemia (TIMI) III Registry. *Circulation* 1995; 92(suppl I):I-19.

225. Ghigliotti G, Brunelli C, Corsiglia L, et al. Identification of high-risk patients with unstable angina. *J Am Coll Cardiol* 1996;27(suppl A):332A.

226. Braunwald E, Antman EM, Beasley JW, et al. ACC/AHA 2002 Guidelines for the Management of Patients with Unstable Angina and Non-ST-Segment Elevation Myocardial Infarction. *J Am Coll Cardiol* 2002; 40:1366–1374.

227. Ambrose JA, Almeida OD, Sharma SK, et al. Adjunctive thrombolytic therapy during angioplasty for ischemic rest angina: Results of the TAUSA trial. *Circulation* 1994;90:69–77.

228. Antman EM, McCabe CH, Gurfinkel EP, et al. Enoxaparin prevents death and cardiac ischemic events in unstable angina/non-Q-wave myocardial infarction: Results of the Thrombolysis in Myocardial Infarction (TIMI) IIB Trial. *Circulation* 1999;100:1593–1601.

229. Hamm CW. Unstable angina: The breakthrough. *Eur Heart J* 1999;20: 1517–1519.

230. Ellis SG, Vandormael MG, Cowley MJ, et al. Coronary morphologic and clinical determinants of procedural outcome with angioplasty for multivessel coronary disease. *Circulation* 1990;82:1193–1203.

231. Ellis SG, de Cesare NB, Pinkerton CA, et al. Relation of stenosis morphology and clinical presentation to the procedural results of directional coronary atherectomy. *Circulation* 1991;84:644–653.

232. Tan K, Sulke N, Taub N, et al. Clinical and lesion morphologic determinants of coronary angioplasty success and complications: Current experience. *J Am Coll Cardiol* 1995;25:855–865.

233. Herrman JR, Melkert R, Simon R, et al. ABC-lesion type as a risk factor for the occurrence of early and late clinical events in unstable patients following transluminal coronary angioplasty (PTCA). *J Am Coll Cardiol* 1996;27(suppl A):390A.

234. Fry ET, Hermiller JB, Peters TF, et al. Is ACC/AHA classification predictive of successful coronary intervention in the era of new devices? *J Am Coll Cardiol* 1996;27(suppl A):152A.

235. Ellis SG, Guetta V, Miller D, et al. Relation between lesion characteristics and risk with percutaneous intervention in the stent and glycoprotein IIb/IIIa era: An analysis of results from 10,907 lesions and proposal for new classification scheme. *Circulation* 1999;100: 1971–1976.

236. Hannan EL, Racz M, Rytan TJ, et al. Coronary angioplasty volume-outcome relationships for hospitals and cardiologists. *JAMA* 1997;279: 892–898.

237. Ellis SG, Weintraub W, Holmes D, et al. Relation of operator volume and experience to procedural outcome with percutaneous coronary revascularization at hospitals with high intervention volumes. *Circulation* 1997;95:2479–2484.

238. Kastrati A, Neumann FJ, Schomig A. Operator volume and outcome of patients undergoing coronary stent placement. *J Am Coll Cardiol* 1998;32:970–976.

239. O'Keefe JH, Hartzler GO, Rutherford BD, et al. Left main coronary angioplasty: Early and late results of 127 acute and elective procedures. *Am J Cardiol* 1989;64:144–147.

240. Ellis SG, Tamai H, Nobuyoshi M, et al. Contemporary percutaneous treatment of unprotected left main coronary stenoses: Initial results from a multicenter registry analysis 1994–1996. *Circulation* 1997;96: 3867–3872.

241. Park SJ, Park SW, Hong MK, et al. Stenting of unprotected left main coronary artery stenoses: Immediate and late outcomes. *J Am Coll Cardiol* 1998;31:37–42.

242. Macaya C, Alfonso F, Iniques GJ, et al. Stenting for elastic recoil during coronary angioplasty of the left main coronary artery. *Am J Cardiol* 1992;70:105–107.

243. Keeley EC, Aliabadi D, O'Neill WW, et al. Immediate and long-term results of elective and emergent percutaneous interventions on protected and unprotected severely narrowed left main coronary arteries. *Am J Cardiol* 1999;83:242–246.

244. Marso SP, Gabriel S, Plokker T, et al. Catheter-based reperfusion of unprotected left main stenosis during an acute myocardial infarction (the ULTIMA experience). *Am J Cardiol* 1999;83: 1513–1517.

245. Roffi M, Mukherjee D, Chew DP, et al. Lack of benefit from intravenous platelet glycoprotein IIb/IIIa receptor inhibition as adjunctive treatment for percutaneous interventions of aortocoronary bypass grafts—A pooled analysis of five randomized clinical trials. *Circulation* 2002;106:3063–3067.

246. Savage MP, Douglas JS, Fischman DL, et al. Stent placement compared with balloon angioplasty for obstructed coronary bypass grafts. *N Engl J Med* 1997;337:740–747

247. Baim DS, Wahr D, George B, et al. Randomized trial of distal embolic protection device during percutaneous intervention of saphenous vein aorto-coronary bypass grafts. *Circulation* 2002;105: 1285–1290.

248. de Feyter PJ. Percutaneous treatment of saphenous vein bypass graft obstruction—A continuing obstinate problem. *Circulation* 2003;107: 2284–2286.

249. Kobayashi N, Finci L, Ferraro M, et al. Restenosis after coronary stenting: Clinical and angiographic predictors in 1906 lesions. *J Am Coll Cardiol* 1999;33(suppl A):32A.

250. Kastrati A, Elezi S, Dirschinger J, et al. Influence of lesion length on restenosis after coronary stent placement. *Am J Cardiol* 1999;83: 1617–1622.

251. Topol EJ, Nissen SE. Our preoccupation with coronary luminology: The dissociation between clinical and angiographic findings in ischemic heart disease. *Circulation* 1995;92:2333–2342.

252. Tuzcu EM, Berkalp B, De Franco AC, et al. The dilemma of diagnosing coronary calcification: Angiography versus intravascular ultrasound. *J Am Coll Cardiol* 1996;27:832–838.

253. Mintz GS, Popma JJ, Pichard AD, et al. Intravascular ultrasound predictors of restenosis after percutaneous transcatheter coronary revascularization. *J Am Coll Cardiol* 1996;27:1678–1687.

254. Stone GW, Linnemeier T, St Goar FG, et al. Improved outcome of balloon angioplasty with intracoronary ultrasound guidance: Core lab angiographic and ultrasound results from the Clout study. *J Am Coll Cardiol* 1996;27(suppl A):155A.

255. Bauters C, LaBlanche JM, McFadden E, et al. Angioscopic thrombus is associated with a high risk of angiographic restenosis. *Circulation* 1995;92(suppl I):I-401.

256. Hoffman R, Mintz GS, Dussaillant GR, et al. Patterns and mechanisms of in-stent restenosis: A serial intravascular ultrasound study. *Circulation* 1996;94:1247–1254.

257. Yokoi H, Kimura T, Nakagawa Y, et al. Long-term clinical and quantitative angiographic follow-up after the Palmaz-Schatz stent restenosis. *J Am Coll Cardiol* 1996;27:224.

258. Mehran R, Dangas G, Abizaid AS, et al. Angiographic patterns of in-stent restenosis: Classification and implications for long-term outcome. *Circulation* 1999;100:1872–1878.

259. Shiran A, Mintz GS, Waksman R, et al. Early lumen loss after treatment of in-stent restenosis: An intravascular ultrasound study. *Circulation* 1998;98:200–203.

260. Sharma SK, Duvvuri S, Dangas G, et al. Rotational atherectomy for in-stent restenosis: Acute and long-term results of the first 100 cases. *J Am Coll Cardiol* 1998;32:1358–1365.

261. Radke PW, Klues HG, Haager PK, et al. Mechanisms of acute lumen gain and recurrent restenosis after rotational atherectomy of diffuse in-stent restenosis: A quantitative angiographic and intravascular ultrasound study. *J Am Coll Cardiol* 1999;34:33–39.

262. Mehran R, Mintz GS, Satler LF, et al. Treatment of in-stent restenosis with excimer laser coronary angioplasty: Mechanisms and results compared with PTCA alone. *Circulation* 1997;96:2183–2189.

263. Sakamoto T, Kawarabayashi T, Taguchi H, et al. Intravascular ultrasound-guided balloon angioplasty for treatment of in-stent restenosis. *Catheter Cardiovasc Interv* 1999;47:298–303.

264. Sharma SK, Kini A, Duvvuri S, et al. Randomized trial of rotational atherectomy versus balloon angioplasty for in-stent restenosis (ROSTER): Interim analysis of 100 cases. *Circulation* 1998;98(suppl I): I-717.

265. Vom Dahl j, Dietz U, Haager PK, et al. Rotational atherectomy does not reduce recurrent in-stent restenosis. Results of the Angioplasty Versus Rotational Atherectomy for Treatment of Diffuse In-stent Restenosis Trial (ARTIST). *Circulation* 2001;105–588.

266. Yokoi H, Tamurat, Nakagawa Y, et al. Refractory stent restenosis following balloon angioplasty. *Circulation* 1999;100(suppl I):I-301.

267. Waksman R, White LR, Chan RC, et al. Intracoronary beta radiation therapy for patients with in-stent restenosis: The 6 months clinical and angiographic results. *Circulation* 1999;100(suppl I):I-75.

268. Leon MB, Moses JW, Lansky AJ, et al. Intracoronary gamma radiation for prevention of recurrent in-stent restenosis: Final results from the Gamma-1 Trial. *Circulation* 1999;100(suppl I):I-75.

269. Teirstein PS, Massullo V, Jani S, et al. Two-year follow-up after catheter-based radiotherapy to inhibit coronary restenosis. *Circulation* 1999;99:243–247.

270. Bourassa MG, Butnaru A, Lesperance J, et al. Symptomatic myocardial bridges: overview of ischemic mechanisms and current diagnostic and treatment strategies. *J Am Coll Cardiol* 2003;41: 351–359.

271. Mohlenkamp S, Hort W, Ge J, et al. Update on myocardial bridging. *Circulation* 2002;106:2616–12622.

272. Boccalandro F, Awadalla H, Smalling RW. Percutaneous transcatheter coil embolization of two coronary fistulas originating from the left main ostium and left anterior descending artery. *Catheter Cardiovasc Interv* 2002;57:221–223.

273. Armsby LR, Keane JF, Sherwood MC, et al. Management of coronary artery fistulae—Patient selection and results of transcatheter closure. *J Am Coll Cardiol* 2002;39:1026–1032.

274. Tanabe Y, Itoh E, Suzuki K, et al. Limited role of coronary angioplasty and stenting in coronary spastic angina with organic stenosis. *J Am Coll Cardiol* 2002;39:1120–1126.

275. Sawada Y, Nosaka H, Kimura T, et al. Initial and six month outcome of Palmaz-Schatz stent implantation: Stress/Benestent equivalent versus non-equivalent lesions (abstr). *J Am Coll Cardiol* 1996;27(suppl A): 252A.

276. Pan M, de Lezo JS, Medina A, et al. Simple and complex stent strategies for bifurcated coronary arterial stenosis involving the side branch origin. *Am J Cardiol* 1999;83:1320–1325.

277. Savage MP, Douglas JS Jr, Fischman DL, et al. Stent placement compared with balloon angioplasty for obstructed coronary bypass grafts. *N Engl J Med* 1997;337:740–747.

278. Buller CE, Dzavik V, Carere RG, et al. Primary stenting versus balloon angioplasty in occluded coronary arteries: The Total Occlusion Study of Canada (TOSCA). *Circulation* 1999;100:236–242.

279. Erbel R, Haude M, Hopp HW, et al. Coronary-artery stenting compared with balloon angioplasty for restenosis after initial balloon angioplasty. *N Engl J Med* 1998;339:1672–1678.

280. Kastrati A, Mehilli J, Dirschinger J, et al. Intracoronary stenting and angiographic results: strut thickness effect on restenosis outcome (ISAR-STEREO) trial. *Circulation* 2001;103:2816–2821.

281. Stertzer SH, Pomerantsev EV, Fitzgerald PJ, et al. Effects of technique modification on immediate results of high speed rotational atherectomy in 710 procedures on 656 patients. *Catheter Cardiovasc Diagn* 1995;36:304–310.

282. MacIsaac AI, Bass TA, Buchbinder M, et al. High speed rotational atherectomy: Outcome in calcified and non-calcified coronary artery lesions. *J Am Coll Cardiol* 1995;26:731–736.

283. Ellis SG, Popma JJ, Buchbinder M, et al. Relation of clinical presentation, stenosis morphology, and operator technique to the procedural results of rotational atherectomy and rotational atherectomy-facilitated angioplasty. *Circulation* 1994;89:882–892.

284. Broderick TM, Kereiakes DJ, Whang DD, et al. Myocardial bridging may predispose to coronary perforation during rotational atherectomy. *J Invasive Cardiol* 1996;8:161–163

285. Williams MJA, Dow CJ, Newell JB, et al. Prevalence and timing of regional myocardial dysfunction after rotational coronary atherectomy. *J Am Coll Cardiol* 1996;28:861–869.

286. Douglas JS Jr, Ghazzal ZMG, Ba'albaki HA, et al. Excimer laser coronary angioplasty of ostial lesions: Acute success and complications. *Catheter Cardiovasc Diagn* 1991;23:75.

287. Eigler NL, Douglas JS Jr, Margolis JR, et al. Excimer laser coronary angioplasty of aorto-ostial stenosis: Results of the ELCA Registry. *Circulation* 1993;88:2049–2057.

288. de Marchena EJ, Mallon SM, Knopf WD, et al. Effectiveness of holmium laser-assisted coronary angioplasty. *Am J Cardiol* 1994;73: 117–121.

289. Litvack F, Eigler N, Margolis J, et al. Percutaneous excimer laser coronary angioplasty: Results in the first consecutive 3000 patients. *J Am Coll Cardiol* 1994;23:323–329.

290. Appelman YE, Piek JJ, deFeyter PJ, et al. Excimer laser coronary angioplasty versus balloon angioplasty used in long-term lesions: The long-term results of the AMRO Trial. *J Am Coll Cardiol* 1995; 25(suppl A):329A.

291. Appelman JY, Koolen JJ, deFeyter PJ, et al. Long-term outcome of excimer laser angioplasty versus balloon angioplasty in functional and total coronary occlusions. *J Am Coll Cardiol* 1995;25(suppl A): 330A.

292. Vandormael M, Riefart N, Preusler W. Six month follow-up results following excimer laser angioplasty, rotational atherectomy and balloon angioplasty for complex lesions: ERBAC study. *Circulation* 1994;90 (suppl I):I-213.

293. Pepine CJ, Babb JD, Brinker JA, et al. Task Force 3: Training in cardiac catheterization and interventional cardiology. *J Am Coll Cardiol* 1995;25:14–16.

294. Cowley MJ, Faxon DP, Holmes DR Jr. Guidelines for training, credentialing, and maintenance of competence for the performance of coronary angioplasty: A report from the Interventional Cardiology Committee and the Training Program Standards Committee of the Society for Cardiac Angiography and Interventions. *Catheter Cardiovasc Diagn* 1993;30:1–4.

295. Douglas JS Jr, Pepine CJ, Block PC, et al. Recommendations for development and maintenance of competence in coronary interventional procedures. *J Am Coll Cardiol* 1993;22:629–631.

296. Ryan TJ, Klocke FJ, Reynolds WA, et al. Clinical competence in percutaneous transluminal coronary angioplasty: A statement for physicians from the ACP/ACC/AHA Task Force on Clinical Privileges in Cardiology. *J Am Coll Cardiol* 1990;15:1469–1474.

297. Conti CR. Credentialing cardiologists who perform therapeutic cardiac interventions. *Clin Cardiol* 1995;18:689–691.

298. Hirshfeld JW, Ellis SG, Faxon DP, et al. Recommendations for the assessment and maintenance of proficiency in coronary interventional procedures: Statement of the American College of Cardiology. *J Am Coll Cardiol* 1998;31:722–743.

299. Teirstein PS. Credentialing for coronary interventions: Practice makes perfect. *Circulation* 1997;95:2467–2470.

300. Eisenberg MJ, Rice S, Schiller NB. Guidelines for physician training in advanced cardiac procedures: The importance of case mix. *J Am Coll Cardiol* 1994;23:1723–1725.

301. Eisenberg MJ, St Claire DA, Mak K, et al. Importance of case mix during training in interventional cardiology. *Am J Cardiol* 1996;77: 1010–1013.

302. Ellis SG, Nowamagbe O, Bittl JA, et al. Analysis and comparison of operator-specific outcomes in interventional cardiology. *Circulation* 1996;93:431–439.

303. Califf RM, Jollis JG, Peterson ED. Operator-specific outcomes: A call to professional responsibility. *Circulation* 1996;93:403–406.

304. McGrath PD, Wennberg WE, Malenka DJ, et al. Operator volume and outcomes in 12,988 percutaneous coronary interventions. *J Am Coll Cardiol* 1998;31:570–576.

305. Holmes DR, Selzer F, Johnston JM, et al. Modeling and risk prediction in the current era of interventional cardiology: A report from the National Heart, Lung, and Blood Institute Dynamic Registry. Circulation 2003;107:1871–1876.

306. Ritchie JL, Phillips KA, Luft HS. Coronary angioplasty: Statewide experience in California. Circulation 1993;88:2735–2743.

307. Jollis JG, Peterson ED, DeLong ER, et al. The relation between the volume of coronary angioplasty procedures at hospitals treating Medicare beneficiaries and short-term mortality. N Engl J Med 1995;331:1625–1629.

308. Ryan TJ. The critical question of procedure volume minimums for coronary angioplasty. JAMA 1995;274:1169–1170.

309. Fajadet J, Brunel P, Jordan C, et al. Transradial approach for interventional coronary procedures: Analysis of complications (abstract). J Am Coll Cardiol 1996;27(suppl A):392A.

310. Ritchie JL, Nissen SE, Douglas JS Jr, et al. Use of nonionic or low osmolar contrast agents in cardiovascular procedures. J Am Coll Cardiol 1993;21:269–273.

311. Grines CL, Schreiber TL, Savas V, et al. A randomized trial of low osmolar ionic versus nonionic contrast media in patients with myocardial infarction or unstable angina undergoing percutaneous transluminal coronary angioplasty. J Am Coll Cardiol 1996;27:1381–1386.

312. Lembo NJ, King SB III, Roubin GS, et al. Effects of nonionic contrast media on complications of percutaneous transluminal coronary angioplasty. Am J Cardiol 1991;67:1046–1050.

313. Shrader R, Esch I, Ensslen R, et al. A randomized trial comparing the impact of a nonionic (Iomeprol) versus an ionic (Ioxaglate) low osmolar contrast medium on abrupt vessel closure and ischemic complications after coronary angioplasty. J Am Coll Cardiol 1999;33:395–402.

314. Aguirre FV, Simoons ML, Ferguson JJ, et al. Impact of contrast media on clinical outcomes following percutaneous coronary interventions with platelet glycoprotein IIb/IIIa inhibition: Meta-analysis of clinical trials with abciximab. Circulation 1997;96(suppl I):I-161.

315. Chevalier B, Royer T, Glatt B, et al. Does nonionic contrast medium still modify angioplasty results in the stent era? J Am Coll Cardiol 1999;33(suppl A):85A.

316. Fleisch M, Mulhauser B, Garachemani A, et al. Impact of ionic (Ioxaglate) and nonionic (Loversol) contrast media on PTCA related complications. J Am Coll Cardiol 1999;33(suppl A):85A.

317. Davidson CJ, Laskey WK, Harrison JK, et al. A randomized trial of contrast media utilization in high risk PTCA (the COURT trial). J Am Coll Cardiol 1999;33(suppl A):11A.

318. Dirschinger J, Kastrati A, Neumann F, et al. Influence of balloon pressure during stent placement in native coronary arteries on early and late angiographic and clinical outcome: A randomized evaluation of high-pressure inflation. Circulation 1999;100:918–923.

319. Tobis JM, Colombo A. Do you need IVUS guidance for coronary stent deployment? Catheter Cardiovasc Diagn 1996;37:360–361.

320. Russo RJ, Teirstein PS, for the AVID Investigators. Angiography versus intravascular ultrasound-directed stent placement (abstr). J Am Coll Cardiol 1996;27(suppl A):306A.

321. Kereiakes DJ, Lincoff M, Miller DP, et al. Abciximab therapy and unplanned coronary stent deployment: Favorable effects on stent use, clinical outcomes, and bleeding complications. Circulation 1998;97:857–864.

322. Ellis SG, Roubin GS, Wilentz J, et al. Results of a randomized trial of heparin and aspirin vs aspirin alone for prevention of acute closure and restenosis after angioplasty (abstr). Circulation 1987;76(suppl IV):IV-213.

323. Douglas JS Jr, Ghazzal GMB, Morris DC, et al. Twenty years of angioplasty at Emory University. Circulation 2000;102(suppl II):II-753.

324. Ruygrok PN, De Jaegere PT, Van Domburg RT, et al. Clinical outcome 10 years after attempted percutaneous transluminal coronary angioplasty in 856 patients. J Am Coll Cardiol 1996;27:1669–1677.

325. Bredlau CE, Roubin GS, Leimbruger PP, et al. In-hospital morbidity and mortality in patients undergoing elective coronary angioplasty. Circulation 1985;72:1044–1052.

326. Ellis SG, Roubin GS, King SB III, et al. In-hospital cardiac mortality following acute closure after percutaneous transluminal coronary angioplasty: Analysis of risk factors from 8207 procedures. J Am Coll Cardiol 1988;11:211–216.

327. Ellis SG, Myler RK, King SB III, et al. Causes and correlates of death after unsupported coronary angioplasty: Implications for use of angioplasty and advanced support techniques in high-risk settings. Am J Cardiol 1991;68:1447–1451.

328. Malenka DJ, Wennberg DE, Quinton HA, et al. Gender-related changes in the practice and outcomes of percutaneous coronary interventions in northern New England from 1994 to 1999. J Am Coll Cardiol 2002;40:2092–2101.

329. Anderson HV, Shaw RE, Brindis RG, et al. A contemporary overview of percutaneous coronary interventions. J Am Coll Cardiol 2002;39:1096–1103.

330. Jacobs AK, Johnston JM, Haviland M, et al. Improved outcomes for women undergoing contemporary percutaneous coronary intervention. Circulation 2002;106:2346–2350.

331. Seshadri N, Whitlow PL, Acharya N, et al. Emergency coronary artery bypass surgery in the contemporary percutaneous coronary intervention era. Circulation 202;106:2346–2350.

332. Singh M, Lennon RJ, Holmes DR, et al. Correlates of procedural complications and a simple integer risk score for percutaneous coronary intervention. J Am Coll Cardiol 2002;40:387–393.

333. Ajluni SC, Glazier S, Blankenship L, et al. Perforations after percutaneous coronary interventions: Clinical, angiographic, and therapeutic observations. Cathet Cardiovasc Diagn 1994;32:206–212.

334. Ellis SG, Arnold AZ, Raymond RE, et al. Increased coronary perforation in the new device era: Incidence, classification, management and outcome. Circulation 86(suppl I):I-787.

335. Bensuly KH, Glazier S, Grines CL, et al. Coronary perforation: An unreported complication after intracoronary stent implantation (abstr). J Am Coll Cardiol 1996;27(suppl A):252A.

336. Waksman R, King SB III, Douglas JS Jr, et al. Predictors of groin complications after balloon and new-device coronary intervention. Am J Cardiol 1995;75:886–889.

337. Moscucci M, Mansour KA, Kent C, et al. Peripheral vascular complications of directional coronary atherectomy and stenting: Predictors, management, and outcome. Am J Cardiol 1994;74:448–453.

338. Popma JJ, Satler LF, Pichard AD, et al. Vascular complications after balloon and new device angioplasty. Circulation 1993;88:1569–1578.

339. Rocha-Singh KJ, Schwend RB, Otis SM, et al. Frequency and nonsurgical therapy of femoral artery pseudoaneurysm complicating interventional cardiology procedures. Am J Cardiol 1994;73:1012–1014.

340. Kang SS, Labropoulos N, Mansour MA, et al. Percutaneous ultrasound guided thrombin injection: A new method for treating postcatheterization femoral pseudoaneurysms. J Vasc Surg 1998;27:1032–1038.

341. Liau C, Ho F, Chen M, et al. Treatment of iatrogenic femoral artery pseudoaneurysm with percutaneous thrombin injection. J Vasc Surg 1997;26:18–23.

342. Carey D, Martin JR, Moore CA, et al. Complications of femoral artery disease devices. Catheter Cardiovasc Interv 2001;52:30–37.

343. Assali AR, Sdringola S, Moustapha A, et al. Outcome of access site in patients treated with platelet glycoprotein IIb/IIIa inhibitors in the era of closure devices. Catheter Cardiovasc Interv 2003;58:1–5.

344. Saber RS, Edwards WD, Bailey KR, et al. Coronary embolization after balloon angioplasty or thrombolytic therapy: An autopsy study of 32 cases. J Am Coll Cardiol 1993;22:1283–1288.

345. Waksman R, Scott NA, Douglas JS Jr, et al. Distal embolization is common after directional atherectomy in coronary arteries and vein grafts. Circulation 1993;88(suppl I):I-299.

346. Harrington RA, Lincoff AM, Califf RM, et al. Characteristics and consequences of myocardial infarction after percutaneous coronary intervention: Insights from the Coronary Angioplasty versus Excisional Atherectomy Trial (CAVEAT). J Am Coll Cardiol 1995;25:1693–1699.

347. Moses JW, Teirstein PS, Sketch MR Jr, et al. Angiographic determinants of risk and outcome of coronary embolus and myocardial infarction (MI) with the transluminal extraction catheter (TEC): A report

from the New Approaches to Coronary Intervention (NACI) Registry (abstr). *J Am Coll Cardiol* 1994;23:220A.

348. Safian RD, Grines CL, May MA, et al. Clinical and angiographic results of transluminal extraction coronary atherectomy in saphenous vein bypass grafts. *Circulation* 1994;89:302–312.

349. Abdelmeguid AE, Topol EJ, Whitlow PL, et al. Significance of mild transient release of creatine kinase-MB fraction after percutaneous coronary interventions. *Circulation* 1996;4:1528–1536.

350. Brener SJ, Lytle BW, Schneider JP, et al. Association between CK-MB elevation after percutaneous or surgical revascularization and three-year mortality. *J Am Coll Cardiol* 2002;40:1961–1967.

351. Kini A, Marmur JD, Dangas G, et al. Creatine kinase-MB elevation after coronary intervention correlates with diffuse atherosclerosis, and low-to-medium level elevation has a benign clinical course: Implications for early discharge after coronary intervention. *J Am Coll Cardiol* 1999;34:663–671.

352. McCullough PA, Wolyn R, Rocher LL, et al. Acute contrast nephropathy after coronary intervention: Incidence, risk factors and relationship to mortality. *J Am Coll Cardiol* 1996;17(suppl A):304A.

353. Stevens MA, McCullough PA, Tobin KJ, et al. A prospective randomized trial of prevention measures in patients at high risk for contrast nephropathy. *J Am Coll Cardiol* 1999;33:403–411.

354. Aspelin P, Aubry P, Fransson S, et al. Nephrotoxic effects in high-risk patients undergoing angiography. *N Engl J Med* 2003;348:491–499.

355. Sandler CM. Contrast-agent-induced acute renal dysfunction—Is iodixanol the answer? *N Engl J Med* 2003;348:551–552.

MECHANICAL INTERVENTIONS IN ACUTE MYOCARDIAL INFARCTION

William O'Neill / Bruce R. Brodie

This chapter reviews the historical development of mechanical reperfusion for acute myocardial infarction (AMI), summarizes the results of randomized clinical trials, defines subsets most likely to benefit from this approach, and offers a glimpse into future research directions.

HISTORICAL OVERVIEW

Mechanical reperfusion for AMI had its inception with Fletcher and Tillet's initial treatise describing the use of intravenous thrombolytic therapy in thromboembolic disorders, including myocardial infarction.[1] Shortly after this, Boucek and colleagues published their observations using catheters to deliver fibrinolytic therapy to the aortic root of patients presenting with AMI.[2] Subsequently, Favaloro and associates developed saphenous vein aortocoronary bypass surgery and applied it to patients presenting with acute infarction.[3] Two groups, one in Spokane, Washington, and one in Göttingen, Germany, performed emergency catheterization prior to surgical revascularization for AMI, and for the first time knowledge of the coronary anatomy during AMI became available.[4,5] DeWood and colleagues described the high prevalence of total coronary occlusion in the early hours after acute transmural myocardial infarction and defined the role of the electrocardiographic injury current in identifying a population of patients most likely to have acute total occlusion of the infarct artery and thus most likely to benefit from emergency revascularization.[6,7]

In 1978, Rentrop and colleagues performed emergency guidewire recanalization of a catheter-related acute thrombotic coronary occlusion and subsequently reported on the first 13 patients with AMI treated with mechanical reperfusion.[8,9] These investigators also reported their results with selective catheter infusion of intracoronary streptokinase at the American Heart Association meetings in 1979, and the modern era of reperfusion therapy was born.[10] Once the works of DeWood and Rentrop were disseminated, enormous research interest in reperfusion therapy was generated in both Europe and the United States, and a number of randomized trials quickly followed. Khaja and associates[11] first demonstrated the efficacy of intracoronary streptokinase administration in establishing coronary reperfusion, and the Western Washington investigators[12] documented improved survival in patients with AMI treated with intracoronary streptokinase therapy. Because of the necessity of selective coronary angiography for this treatment, it quickly became apparent that a severe residual stenosis persisted in most patients after successful thrombolysis. The Ann Arbor group demonstrated that balloon angioplasty could more effectively relieve the residual stenosis than thrombolytic therapy, and that this resulted in less recurrent ischemia and better preservation of ventricular function.[13] Lack of trained operators, lack of catheterization facilities, and logistic constraints hindered the development of both intracoronary streptokinase and primary angioplasty as reperfusion strategies in the mid-1980s.

The large GISSI and ISIS-2 trials,[14,15] published in 1984 and 1986, established the efficacy of intravenous streptokinase in improving survival in patients with AMI. Intravenous streptokinase with aspirin gained widespread use and became the standard of care as reperfusion therapy for AMI. Research interest soon focused on the development of new fibrin-specific thrombolytic drugs that could be administered intravenously. Many investigators were still concerned about the severe underlying residual stenosis remaining after thrombolytic therapy, and three major randomized trials, the TAMI, TIMI II-A and European Cooperative trials, were designed to determine the value of routine percutaneous transluminal coronary angioplasty (PTCA) after thrombolytic therapy.[16–18] These studies gave surprising and disappointing results. Not only was routine PTCA unnecessary, it appeared actually to be harmful, and angioplasty was mostly abandoned as an adjunct to thrombolytic therapy in the 1990s.

However, interest still persisted in the use of PTCA without antecedent thrombolytic therapy or primary PTCA. Large credit should be given to the pioneering work of Hartzler and colleagues in Kansas City, Kansas, who demonstrated the feasibility of primary PTCA.[19,20] At the same time, Brodie in Greensboro, North Carolina, and O'Neill and Grines in Royal Oak, Michigan, concluded that primary PTCA had been inadequately tested as a reperfusion

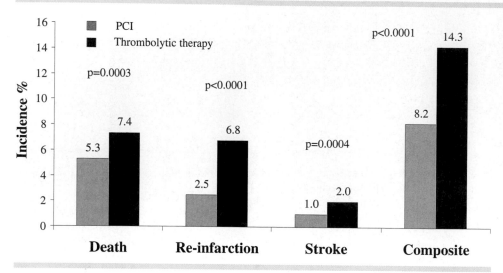

FIGURE 56-1 Metanalysis of 23 randomized trials comparing short-term outcomes with primary percutaneous coronary intervention versus thrombolytic therapy for acute myocardial infarction. (Adapted from Keeley et al. [26] With permission.)

modality.[21,22] These three groups joined forces and organized the original PAMI study group. This group and investigators from the Zwolle group and the Mayo Clinic published the results of the first large randomized trials comparing primary PTCA with thrombolytic therapy in 1993.[23–25] These trials demonstrated the benefit of primary PTCA over thrombolytic therapy and established primary PTCA as a legitimate and competing reperfusion strategy for AMI.

PRIMARY PERCUTANEOUS CORONARY INTERVENTION

Despite the results of the PAMI and Zwolle trials, great controversy persisted in the early 1990s regarding the relative benefit of primary percutaneous coronary intervention (PCI) versus thrombolytic therapy for the treatment of AMI. Primary PCI was recognized as a legitimate reperfusion strategy but was not widely employed because of logistical problems with its use and limited data to support its bene-

fit. This controversy has now been largely settled, based on the results of a number of randomized trials comparing these reperfusion strategies.

Comparison of Outcomes with Thrombolytic Therapy

RANDOMIZED TRIALS

There are now 23 randomized trials incorporating 7739 patients comparing primary PCI with thrombolytic therapy for AMI. These trials have been summarized in a recent metanalysis.[26] Primary PCI was superior to thrombolytic therapy in reducing short-term mortality (5.3 vs. 7.4 percent, $p = 0.0003$), nonfatal reinfarction (2.5 vs. 6.8 percent, $p < 0.0001$), stroke (1.0 vs. 2.0 percent, $p = 0.0004$) and the composite endpoint of death, nonfatal reinfarction, and stroke (8.2 vs. 14.3 percent, $p = 0.0001$) (Fig. 56-1). These results were maintained at long-term follow-up and were independent of the type of thrombolytic agent used (streptokinase vs. fibrin-specific thrombolytics) and whether patients were transferred emergently for primary PCI. The incidence of intracranial hemorrhage was significantly less with primary PCI (0.05 vs. 1.1 percent, $p < 0.0001$), but the overall risk of major bleeding (mostly related to access-site bleeding) was higher with primary PCI (6.8 vs. 5.3 percent, $p = 0.03$) (Fig. 56-2). The risk of access-site bleeding with primary PCI appears to be less in more recent trials with better management of anticoagulation and earlier femoral artery sheath removal.

The survival benefit of primary PCI compared with thrombolytic therapy reported in this metanalysis was substantial (21 lives saved per 1000 patients treated) and is of similar magnitude to the survival benefit of thrombolytic therapy compared with placebo reported by the Fibrinolytic Therapy Trialists' (FTT) Collaborative Group (19 lives saved per 1000 patients treated) (Fig. 56-3).[27] The relative reduction in death and nonfatal reinfarction is similar across all subgroups of patients treated, including elderly patients, women, diabetics, patients with anterior or nonanterior infarction, patients with prior infarction, and patients classified as at low risk or not at low risk.[28] The greatest absolute benefit occurs in patients at highest risk, and several randomized trials have specifically evaluated these high-risk subgroups. The SHOCK trial, which randomized 302 patients with cardiogenic shock to emergency revascularization versus medical stabilization, found a lower 6-month mortality with emergency revascularization (50 versus 63 percent, $p = 0.03$).[29] The survival benefit was especially pronounced in patients treated within 6 h of symptom onset and was seen only in patients under the age of 75 years. Garcia and colleagues randomized 220 patients with anterior infarction to primary PCI ver-

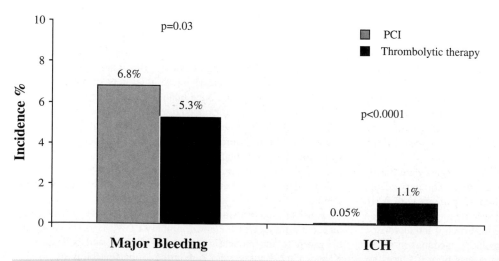

FIGURE 56-2 Metanalysis of 23 randomized trials comparing hemorrhagic complications with primary percutaneous coronary intervention versus thrombolytic therapy for acute myocardial infarction. (Adapted from Keeley et al. [26] With permission.)

sus alteplase and found substantially lower mortality with primary PCI (2.8 vs. 10.8 percent, $p = 0.02$).[30] The Zwolle group randomized 87 elderly patients (>75 years) to primary PCI versus streptokinase and found a lower incidence of the composite endpoint of death, nonfatal reinfarction, or stroke at 30 days with primary PCI (8.7 vs. 29.3 percent, $p = 0.01$).[31]

IMPORTANCE OF TIMI FLOW IN THE INFARCT ARTERY

The importance of achieving timely restoration of normal blood flow in the infarct artery in patients with AMI was convincingly demonstrated in the GUSTO trial.[32] Patients with normal (TIMI-3) antegrade flow in the infarct artery at 90 min after treatment had the best left ventricular function at follow-up catheterization and the lowest 30-day mortality (Table 56-1). Patients with slow (TIMI-2) flow had left ventricular function and 30-day mortality that were significantly worse than those of patients with TIMI-3 flow, and similar to those of patients with no flow (TIMI-0 to -1). A similar relationship between TIMI flow and mortality has been found with primary PCI (Table 56-1).[33] These data indicate that only restoration of TIMI-3 flow is associated with optimal outcomes and that only TIMI-3 flow should be regarded as "true patency." A comparison of the rates of TIMI-3 flow with various thrombolytic strategies[32,34] and with primary PCI[35,36] are shown in Fig. 56-4. The ability of primary PCI to achieve significantly higher TIMI-3 flow rates than thrombolytic therapy probably explains most of the mortality advantage seen with primary

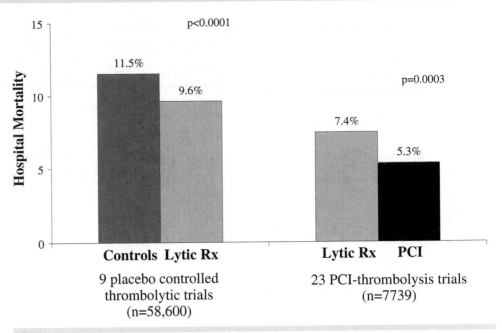

FIGURE 56-3 Comparison of mortality reduction with thrombolytic therapy versus placebo[27] and primary percutaneous coronary intervention versus thrombolytic therapy.[26]

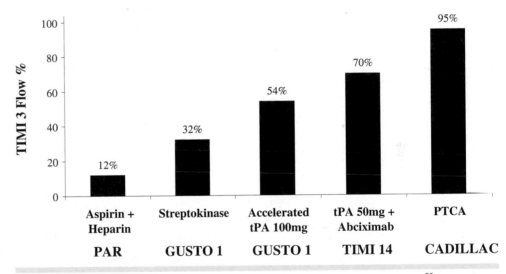

FIGURE 56-4 Frequency of achieving TIMI-3 flow in the infarct artery with aspirin and heparin,[35] several thrombolytic regimens,[32,34] and primary angioplasty (percutaneous transluminal coronary angioplasty).[36]

TABLE 56-1 Relationship between TIMI Flow and 30-Day Mortality after Reperfusion Therapy for Acute Myocardial Infarction

	30-DAY MORTALITY	
TIMI Flow	GUSTO-I[32] (Lytic Therapy)	PAMI-1 and PAMI-2[33] (Primary PTCA[a])
TIMI 0–1	8.9%	17.2%
TIMI 2	7.4%	7.6%
TIMI 3	4.4%	2.1%

[a]Percutaneous transluminal coronary angioplasty.

PCI. Indeed, there appears to be a tight inverse relationship between short-term mortality and the ability to achieve TIMI-3 flow with various thrombolytic regimens and with primary PCI (Fig. 56-5).[23,32,35–41] Newer thrombolytic strategies using combination therapy with low-dose thrombolytics and platelet glycoprotein IIb/IIIa inhibitors have shown improved TIMI-3 flow rates in small pilot trials,[34] but these rates are well below the TIMI-3 flow rates achieved with primary PCI, and they have not shown any mortality advantage in the large GUSTO V and ASSENT-3 trials.[42,43]

While achieving TIMI-3 flow in the *epicardial* coronary artery is important, optimal outcomes with reperfusion therapy also require optimum reperfusion of the microvasculature or optimum *myocardial* reperfusion. This is discussed further in this chapter.

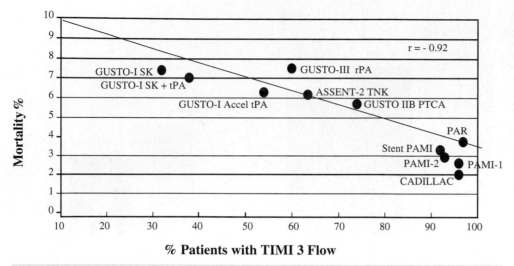

FIGURE 56-5 Relationship between short-term mortality and the frequency of achieving TIMI-3 flow measured acutely in the infarct artery with thrombolytic therapy from the GUSTO-I,[32] GUSTO-III,[37] and ASSENT-2[38] trials and several primary angioplasty (percutaneous transluminal coronary angioplasty) trials. [23,35,36,39–41]

LATE CLINICAL AND ANGIOGRAPHIC OUTCOMES AND MYOCARDIAL SALVAGE

The initial clinical benefit of primary PCI over thrombolytic therapy in reducing death and reinfarction appears to be maintained at late follow-up. The PAMI investigators found that death or reinfarction was lower at 2 years with primary PCI versus thrombolytic therapy (14.9 vs. 23.0 percent, $p = 0.03$) (Fig. 56-6).[44] Similarly, the Zwolle investigators found lower mortality (13.4 vs. 23.9 percent, $p = 0.01$) and less reinfarction (6.2 vs. 21.9 percent, $p < 0.0001$) with primary PCI compared with streptokinase at 5 years.[45] Both studies found a lower frequency of hospital readmissions with primary PCI. Keeley's

recent metanalysis also showed that the initial benefit with primary PCI was maintained at late follow-up at 6 to 18 months.[26]

Late angiographic outcomes following primary PCI have been substantially improved with stenting (Table 56-2).[36,40,46] With stenting, restenosis rates have been reduced to 20 to 22 percent, reocclusion to 5 to 6 percent, and ischemia-driven target vessel revascularization to 7 to 8 percent.[36,40] With thrombolytic therapy, late reocclusion of the infarct artery occurs in 20 to 28 percent of patients when adjunctive PCI is not employed, and this has been reduced to 15 percent with intensive anticoagulant therapy.[47–49] While late angiographic outcomes are better with primary PCI than with thrombolytic therapy, restenosis and reocclusion remain a significant problem and clinical challenge with both reperfusion strategies. The use of drug-eluting stents holds great promise for further improvement of late angiographic outcomes with primary PCI.

Myocardial salvage following primary PCI and thrombolytic therapy have been evaluated in direct comparisons using paired technetium-99m sestamibi scintigraphy.[50,51] Primary stenting plus adjunctive abciximab has resulted in better myocardial salvage (13.5 vs. 8 percent, $p = 0.007$) and greater salvage index (ratio of myocardium salvaged to initial perfusion defect, 0.60 vs. 0.41, $p = 0.001$) compared with thrombolysis using a combination of half dose alteplase plus abciximab.[51] The greater myocardial salvage with primary PCI is probably related to higher patency rates, less reocclusion, and possibly better *myocardial* reperfusion.

Adjunctive Therapy with Stents and Platelet Glycoprotein IIb/IIIa Inhibitors

The Stent PAMI trial documented a clear benefit with stenting vs. balloon angioplasty in reducing restenosis, reocclusion, and the need for target vessel revascularization after primary PCI for AMI.[40] However, using the first-generation Palmaz-Schatz heparin-coated stent, stented patients had lower TIMI-3 flow rates post-PCI and a disturbing trend toward higher mortality at 1 year. Consequently stenting had not been recommended for routine use and was reserved for selected patients, especially patients with coronary dissection and suboptimal PTCA results. More recently, the CADILLAC trial evaluated the role of stenting and platelet glycoprotein IIb/IIIa inhibition with abciximab in

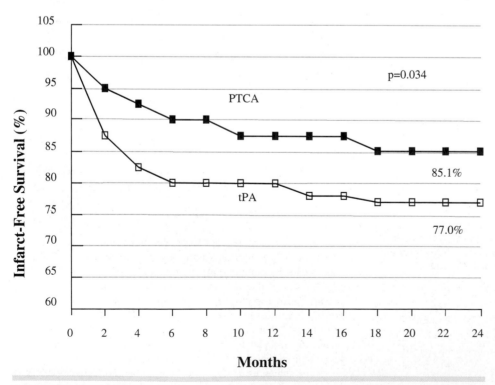

FIGURE 56-6 Actuarial infarction-free survival curves for patients with acute myocardial infarction treated with primary angioplasty (percutaneous transluminal coronary angioplasty) (*solid boxes*) versus tissue plasminogen activator (tPA) (*open boxes*). (From Nunn, et al.[44] With permission.)

2082 patients with AMI treated with primary PCI.[36] Patients were randomized to one of four treatment strategies: PTCA alone, PTCA plus abciximab, stenting alone, and stenting plus abciximab. As in Stent PAMI, stented patients had a clear benefit over balloon angioplasty alone in reducing 6-month restenosis (22.2 vs. 40.8 percent, $p < 0.01$), reocclusion (5.7 vs. 11.3 percent, $p = 0.01$), ischemic target vessel revascularization (6.8 vs. 14.7 percent, $p < 0.001$), and MACE (10.9 vs. 18.3 percent, $p < 0.001$). In contrast to Stent PAMI, using the newer-generation MultiLink stent (Guidant Corporation), there was no degradation of TIMI flow poststenting and no difference in 6-month mortality (3.6 percent with stenting vs. 3.5 percent with PTCA). Based on these data from CADILLAC, stenting can now be recommended for routine use in eligible patients with AMI treated with mechanical intervention.

There are now five randomized trials evaluating abciximab as adjunctive therapy with primary PCI and all five trials have shown a reduction in the composite endpoint of death, reinfarction, or urgent target-vessel revascularization (TVR) at 30 days (Table 56-3).[36,52–55] The greatest benefit was seen in the ADMIRAL trial, in which abciximab was given early, at the time of randomization before primary PCI.[53] In addition to better clinical outcomes, the ADMIRAL trial found improved infarct artery patency prior to PCI and improved left ventricular ejection fraction at 6 months with abciximab. The CADILLAC trial showed improvement in 30-day outcomes with abciximab, but most of the benefit with abciximab vs. placebo in reducing the composite endpoint was seen in patients treated with PTCA alone (4.8 vs. 8.4 percent, $p = 0.02$) without benefit in stented patients (4.5 vs. 5.7 percent, $p = NS$).[36] There was no benefit in left ventricular ejection fraction at 7 months. Abciximab did reduce acute thrombosis in stented patients (0 vs. 1.0 percent, $p = 0.03$) as well as in all patients (0.4 vs. 1.4 percent, $p = 0.01$). Based on the data from these trials, it appears that abciximab is most beneficial when given upstream, before primary PCI, or in the catheterization laboratory in patients treated with PTCA alone who are not eligible for stenting—without much benefit in patients who receive stents. The use of other platelet glycoprotein IIb/IIIa inhibitors with mechanical reperfusion in AMI has not yet been studied.

Primary PCI in Thrombolytic-Ineligible Patients

In most U.S. thrombolytic trials, the majority of patients with AMI screened have been considered ineligible for thrombolytic therapy because of advanced age, late presentation, prior bypass surgery, cardiogenic shock, or bleeding predisposition.[56] These patients constitute a high-risk subset with a significantly increased in-hospital mortality. One of the major advantages of primary PCI compared with thrombolytic therapy is that, where available, primary PCI can be applied to a large majority of patients with AMI. The only contraindications are lack of vascular access, renal insufficiency, and active hemorrhage.

TABLE 56-2 Infarct Artery Restenosis and Reocclusion Rates at 3–12 Months after Reperfusion Therapy for Acute Myocardial Infarction

	Restenosis	Reocclusion Rate
Primary angioplasty		
Primary Angioplasty Registry ($n = 203$)[46]	46%	13%
Stent PAMI Trial (PTCA) ($n = 345$)[40]	34%	9%
CADILLAC trial (PTCA) ($n = 311$)[36]	41%	11%
Primary stenting		
Stent PAMI trial (stent) ($n = 346$)[40]	20%	5%
CADILLAC trial (stent) ($n = 325$)[36]	22%	6%
Thrombolytic therapy		
APRICOT-1 trial ($n = 248$)[47]	83%[a]	28%
White et al ($n = 215$)[48]		25%
APRICOT-2 trial ($n = 308$)[49]		
Aspirin		28%
Warfarin + aspirin		15%

[a]Residual stenosis at 3 months as indicated by angiography after thrombolytic therapy, like primary angioplasty, was defined as >50% luminal diameter narrowing. Angiography was performed at 6–7 months in the primary PCI trials and 3 months in the APRICOT trials.

TABLE 56-3 Randomized Trials Comparing 30-Day Outcomes with Abciximab vs. Placebo with Primary PCI for Acute Myocardial Infarction[a]

	Abciximab (%)	Placebo (%)	p Value
RAPPORT ($n = 483$)[52]			
Death	2.5	2.1	NS
Reinfarction	3.3	4.1	NS
Urgent TVR	1.7	6.6	0.006
Composite	5.8	11.2	0.03
ADMIRAL ($n = 300$)[53]			
Death	3.4	6.6	NS
Reinfarction	1.3	2.6	NS
Urgent TVR	1.3	6.6	0.02
Composite	6.0	14.6	0.01
ISAR-2 ($n = 401$)[54]			
Death	2.5	4.5	NS
Reinfarction	0.5	1.5	NS
Urgent TVR	3.0	5.0	NS
Composite	5.0	10.5	0.04
CADILLAC ($n = 2082$)[36]			
Death	1.9	2.3	NS
Reinfarction	0.8	0.9	NS
Urgent TVR	2.5	4.4	0.02
Stroke	0.1	0.2	NS
Composite	4.6	7.0	0.02
ACE ($n = 400$)[55]			
Death	3.5	4.0	NS
Reinfarction	0.5	4.5	0.01
Urgent TVR	0.5	1.5	NS
Stroke	0.0	0.5	NS
Composite	4.5	10.5	0.02

ABBREVIATIONS: PCI = percutaneous coronary intervention; TVR = target vessel revascularization; TLR = target lesion revascularization.
[a]Patients in the ADMIRAL, ISAR-2, and ACE trials were treated with primary stenting, and half of CADILLAC patients were treated with stents.

Among patients who are usually not considered good candidates for thrombolytic therapy but who may benefit greatly from reperfusion therapy with primary PCI are those with cardiogenic shock, elderly patients, and patients with a predisposition to bleeding. As discussed earlier, patients with cardiogenic shock have a substantial mortality benefit with emergency revascularization compared to medical treatment, including thrombolytic therapy.[29] Elderly patients are frequently excluded from thrombolytic trials, but those who have been enrolled in trials comparing thrombolytic therapy with primary PCI have had a substantial mortality benefit with primary PCI.[31,57,58] Patients with AMI and contraindications to thrombolytic therapy due to bleeding risk have a high mortality; observational data suggest that mortality may be reduced by reperfusion with primary PCI.[59]

There are very few data supporting a benefit of reperfusion therapy in patients who present >12 h after the onset of symptoms. One exception to this is in patients who present late but have persistent ischemic chest pain. These patients frequently have collateral flow to the infarct zone and show substantial recovery of left ventricular function following reperfusion with primary PCI.[60] Patients with AMI who do not have electrocardiographic ST-segment elevation or left bundle branch block have shown no benefit with thrombolytic therapy in randomized trials and appropriately are not considered candidates for thrombolytic therapy.[27] The TACTICS trial documented benefit in these patients with early catheterization (24 to 48 h) and PCI if indicated,[61] but there are no data to support benefit from *emergent* PCI.

Although prior bypass surgery is not a contraindication to thrombolytic therapy, these patients have usually been excluded from thrombolytic trials. Reperfusion rates with thrombolytic therapy in patients with AMI due to saphenous vein graft occlusion are significantly less than with native vessel occlusion (TIMI-2 to -3 flow in the GUSTO I trial: 48 vs. 69 percent, respectively, $p < 0.01$).[62] Reperfusion rates with primary PCI in patients with saphenous vein graft occlusion are better than with thrombolytic therapy but not as good as with primary PCI in native vessel occlusion. The PAMI-2 trial achieved TIMI-3 flow in 70 percent of patients with saphenous vein graft occlusion, compared with 94 percent of patients with native coronary artery occlusion.[63] Patients with prior bypass surgery also had higher in-hospital mortality compared with patients without prior bypass surgery (6.9 vs. 2.6 percent, $p = 0.05$).[63] While primary PCI appears to have an advantage over thrombolytic therapy in treating patients with acute infarction due to saphenous vein graft occlusion, new approaches, such as distal protection, are needed to improve outcomes.

The Role of Cardiac Surgery in the Primary PCI Approach

Not all patients with AMI brought emergently to the cardiac catheterization laboratory undergo PCI.[35] Approximately 10 percent of patients are triaged to either medical treatment or are treated with coronary bypass surgery as the primary reperfusion strategy [primary coronary artery bypass grafting (CABG)]. Patients may be selected for primary CABG when there is severe left main disease or severe three-vessel coronary artery disease with preserved (TIMI-3) flow in the infarct artery, which allows time for transfer to the operating room. The remaining patients not treated with PCI are treated medically. These include patients with no myocardial infarction (mistaken diagnosis), patients with no significant stenosis in the infarct artery (resolution of spasm or thrombus), patients in whom the infarct artery could not be identified, and occasionally patients with unsuitable anatomy or a very small infarct artery.

Bypass surgery may also be performed emergently after failed angioplasty, urgently for reinfarction or recurrent ischemia, and electively for definitive treatment of left main or severe multivessel disease. In experienced centers and with the availability of stents, emergency bypass surgery after failed PCI is rare (about 0.4 percent); the need for urgent bypass surgery for reinfarction or recurrent ischemia that cannot be managed with repeat PCI is also rare (0.1 percent).[40] Elective bypass surgery for treatment of residual coronary artery disease after initial successful primary angioplasty has been used in about 2 to 5 percent of patients.[40,64] Altogether, bypass surgery is performed in about 6 to 10 percent of patients with the primary angioplasty approach.[40,64] Considering the severity of illness of these patients, surgical mortality has been very acceptable (6.4 percent with emergency or urgent bypass surgery and 2.0 percent with elective bypass surgery in the PAMI-2 trial).[64]

Cardiac surgery is also used in patients with mechanical complications of AMI. Those with ventricular septal rupture, acute mitral regurgitation from papillary muscle rupture, and contained myocardial rupture with tamponade usually develop cardiogenic shock and have a very poor outcome without surgical intervention; these patients are candidates for emergent surgery. Patients with cardiogenic shock with severe left main disease (without mechanical complications) may also be candidates for emergent bypass surgery.

Transfer for Primary PCI and Primary PCI at Nonsurgical Centers

The use of primary PCI for AMI has been limited because most hospitals do not have interventional facilities and skilled personnel to perform PCI. Until recently, the transfer of patients presenting at community hospitals with AMI has not been widely recommended because of the potential deleterious effects of treatment delay on clinical outcomes and myocardial salvage. Recent studies suggest that the time delay in transferring patients for primary PCI may not be prohibitive.[65,66]

There are now five randomized trials comparing outcomes in patients with AMI transferred for primary PCI versus those in patients treated at community hospitals with lytic therapy (Table 56-4).[67–71] The largest trial, the DANAMI-2 trial, randomized 1129 patients with AMI presenting at referral hospitals and found less death, reinfarction, and stroke at 30 days in patients transferred for primary PCI compared with patients treated with alteplase at the referring hospitals (8.5 vs. 14.2 percent, $p = 0.002$).[70] The most recent trial, PRAGUE-2, randomized 850 patients with AMI presenting at community hospitals to streptokinase given locally versus transport for primary PCI; lower mortality (6.8 vs.10.0 percent, $p = 0.12$) and a lower composite event rate (death, reinfarction, or stroke) (8.4 vs.15.2 percent, $p = 0.003$) was found in patients transferred for primary PCI.[71] When these cases were analyzed by actual treatment received, mortality was significantly lower with primary PCI (6.0 vs.10.4 percent, $p < 0.05$). These trials have generated great interest and support for the concept of heart attack centers, similar to trauma centers, from which AMI patients would be transported directly to high-volume centers known for excellence with mechanical reperfusion.

Cardiac surgery is an integral part of the primary PCI approach, but it has now been demonstrated that primary PCI can be performed safely and effectively at community hospitals without on-site cardiac surgery when rigorous criteria are established.[72] The C-PORT trial evaluated primary PCI at hospitals with catheterization laboratories but without cardiac surgery or elective PCI.[73] Using skilled operators

TABLE 56-4 Randomized Trials Comparing 30-Day Outcomes in Patients Transferred for Primary PCI[a] vs. Treated Locally with Thrombolytic Therapy

	Death	Reinfarction	Stroke	Composite	p Value[b]	Treatment Delay[c]
Vermeer (n = 150)[67]						
PCI	6.7	1.3	2.7	10.7	0.25	90 min
Alteplase	6.7	9.3	2.7	18.7		
PRAGUE-1 (n = 200)[68]						
PCI	6.9	1.0	0	7.9	0.005	88 min
Streptokinase	14.1	10.1	1.0	23.2		
AIR PAMI (n = 137)[69]						
PCI	8.4	1.4	0	8.5	0.33	104 min
Alteplase	12.1	0	4.5	13.6		
DANAMI-2 (n = 1572)[70]						
PCI	6.6	1.6	1.1	8.0	0.0004	61 min
Alteplase	7.5	6.3	2.0	13.5		
PRAGUE-2 (n = 850)[71]						
PCI	6.8			8.4	0.003	92 min
Streptokinase	10.0			15.2		

[a]Percutaneous coronary intervention.
[b]Compares composite endpoints.
[c]Treatment delay is the difference between symptom onset to balloon inflation with PCI and symptom onset to thrombolytic therapy.

who perform PCI at nearby tertiary centers, the C-PORT investigators documented lower 6-month composite event rates of death, reinfarction, or stroke with primary PCI versus lytic therapy (12.4 vs.19.9 percent, $p = 0.03$). Based on this randomized trial and other observational studies, the American College of Cardiology/American Heart Association (ACC/AHA) Clinical Guidelines now acknowledge that primary PCI can be performed in such institutions when it is done by experienced operators with access to surgical facilities using rigorous protocols and proper case selection.[74] There are no trials testing this approach against transfer to high-volume centers for PCI and surgery if needed.

Technical Aspects of Primary PCI

TREATMENT IN THE EMERGENCY DEPARTMENT
When primary PCI is planned for patients with known or suspected AMI, only a limited history and physical examination should be performed so as to avoid delays in initiating the catheterization procedure. Patients are given 325 mg of soluble chewable aspirin, 5000 U of intravenous heparin, sublingual nitroglycerin, intravenous beta blockers unless contraindicated, and supplemental oxygen and are transported promptly from the emergency department to the catheterization laboratory.

CARDIAC CATHETERIZATION AND ANGIOGRAPHY
Femoral access is usually preferred because this allows for the use of larger devices if necessary and facilitates the use of adjunctive therapy with intraaortic balloon pumping or transvenous pacing when indicated. An activated clotting time (ACT) is measured and additional heparin is given to prolong the ACT to >300 s or 200 to 300 s if platelet glycoprotein IIb/IIIa inhibitors are used. Left ventriculography should be performed prior to intervention, even in patients who are hemodynamically unstable, to assess the severity of ventricular

and valvular dysfunction, help identify the infarct artery (if this is uncertain), and aid in making decisions regarding the necessity for adjunctive therapy, such as intraaortic balloon pumping and pulmonary artery catheter insertion. Occasionally, papillary muscle rupture, ventricular septal defect, or rarely even frank free wall rupture will be demonstrated when not previously suspected, prompting urgent surgery. Alternatively, demonstration of normal left ventricular function may raise early concerns of nonischemic diagnoses such as aortic dissection or pericarditis. A femoral venous sheath may be helpful in patients with occlusion of the right coronary artery to allow access for temporary transvenous pacing if necessary. In patients with hypotension or those are hemodynamically unstable, placement of a pulmonary artery catheter is important to define and monitor hemodynamics. The use of a pulse oximeter to monitor oxygen saturation is also helpful. Following diagnostic coronary and left ventricular angiography, patients are triaged to the most appropriate therapy. About 10 percent of patients undergoing emergency coronary angiography do not undergo primary angioplasty and are triaged to bypass surgery or medical therapy using criteria described earlier.

PRIMARY PCI PROCEDURE
Primary PCI is generally performed with 6- or 7F standard guiding catheters and soft or floppy tipped 0.014-in. steerable guidewires. The soft tip can almost always cross the soft fresh thrombus (in contrast to a chronic total occlusion) and is less traumatic than stiffer wires. The guidewire is advanced well down the infarct artery to ensure that it is in the true lumen and not in a small side branch or under an intimal dissection, since navigation is usually done blindly distal to the occlusion. If the infarct-related artery is initially totally occluded, reperfusion will often be established after the occlusion is crossed with the guidewire. If not, it may be preferable to cross the occlusion with a balloon and then withdraw the balloon without inflating it ("Dottering" the lesion) to establish reperfusion. The more gradual reperfusion provided with the wire or Dottering technique

may result in less reperfusion arrhythmias than rapidly inflating the balloon immediately after crossing. Balloon angioplasty or stenting of the infarct lesion is performed with techniques similar to conventional PCI. No flow (TIMI-0 to -1 flow) or slow flow (TIMI-2 flow) may occur after successful opening of the epicardial infarct artery obstruction. This is generally due to microvascular dysfunction from spasm, distal emboli, or endothelial injury and should be treated with intracoronary verapamil, adenosine, or nitroprusside, which often helps to improve flow. Abciximab may also help with no reflow. With a few exceptions (such as refractory cardiogenic shock), primary PCI should be performed only on the infarct artery. Tandem lesions in the infarct vessel can be dilated, but dilating a noninfarct artery places too much myocardium acutely in jeopardy.

CATHETERIZATION LABORATORY COMPLICATIONS

With increasing operator experience, improved equipment, better patient selection, and the availability of stents, major catheterization laboratory complications with primary PCI have become infrequent. Acute catheterization laboratory complications from the Stent PAMI trial in nonshock patients are shown in Table 56-5.[40] Laboratory deaths and emergency bypass surgery for failed PCI are rare. Ventricular tachycardia or fibrillation, asystole and bradycardia (including second- and third-degree atrioventricular block), and hypotension are the most common complications and usually occur immediately after reperfusion. With increased operator experience and anticipation, these complications can usually be managed effectively and often prevented.

ADJUNCTIVE INTRAAORTIC BALLOON COUNTERPULSATION

Several studies have evaluated the prophylactic use of intraaortic balloon counterpulsation after reperfusion with primary or rescue PCI in high-risk patients.[75,76] Initial studies[75] suggested benefit in terms of less infarct artery reocclusion and less recurrent ischemia, but larger more recent studies, including the large PAMI-2 trial, have shown little or no benefit.[76,77] The results of these trials and the advent of coronary stenting, which has reduced the incidence of reocclusion and recurrent ischemia, have diminished the role of intraaortic balloon counterpulsation after primary PCI in hemodynamically stable patients. Intraaortic balloon counterpulsation is usually indicated prior to primary PCI in hemodynamically unstable patients with congestive heart failure or shock, in patients with mechanical complications of acute infarction, and in those whose anatomy is unsuitable for PCI as a bridge to surgery. There may also be a role for prophylactic intraaortic balloon pumping before primary angioplasty in selected high-risk patients to prevent hemodynamic deterioration.[78]

POST-PCI CARE

Postprocedure care has been standardized in the Stent PAMI and CADILLAC trials.[36,40] Following the interventional procedure, heparin should be held for 2 to 4 h until the ACT is <170 s, at which time the sheath should be removed. Heparin is resumed 2 h after sheath removal without a bolus at 15 U/kg/h and titrated to maintain the aPTT at 60 to 80 s. Full-dose heparin is continued until 48 h postintervention; it is then decreased to one-half dose for 12 h to prevent a rebound hypercoagulable state and then discontinued. In patients who receive abciximab, no postprocedural heparin is given. Low-risk patients can be transferred from the catheterization laboratory directly to the subacute unit (rather than the coronary care unit) and can be targeted for discharge on day 3 (day 0 = day of admission).[79] Aspirin should be given routinely. Clopidogrel 75 mg/day PO should be given to stented patients and continued for 4 weeks. If no contraindications are present, angiotensin-converting enzyme (ACE) inhibitors should be used in patients with congestive heart failure, hypertension, or low ejection fraction (<40 percent). Oral beta blockade should also be routinely administered in the absence of contraindications. Patients who develop symptoms or electrocardiographic changes of recurrent ischemia or reinfarction should undergo emergency repeat catheterization and intervention as indicated.

Cost Issues

Data from several early randomized trials provide direct cost and length-of-stay comparisons between primary PCI and thrombolytic therapy and show an advantage in favor of primary PCI.[79,80] Patients treated with primary PCI have a less complicated hospital course with less reinfarction and less recurrent ischemia, resulting in a shorter length of hospital stay and lower costs. Initial catheterization laboratory costs with primary PCI are more than offset by higher drug charges for alteplase and costs related to high utilization of catheterization and PCI in patients treated with thrombolysis.

A strategy of early discharge with primary PCI may reduce costs further. Primary PCI appears to have two advantages over thrombolytic therapy in allowing a strategy for early discharge. First, the incidence of recurrent ischemic events and reinfarction is substantially less with primary PCI and, unlike the case in thrombolytic therapy, ischemic events are usually confined to the first 2 days. Second, angiographic data obtained at cardiac

TABLE 56-5 Acute Catheterization Laboratory Complications with Primary Angioplasty (PTCA[a]) and Primary Stenting from the Stent PAMI Trial[40]

Complication	Stent (n = 451) (%)	PTCA (n = 448) (%)	Combined (n = 899) (%)
Laboratory death	0.2	0	0.1
Emergency bypass surgery	0.2	0.2	0.2
Cardiac arrest			
Ventricular tachycardia/fibrillation[b]	3.1	4.7	3.9
Cardiopulmonary resusitation[c]	0.9	0.4	0.7
Intubation	0.2	0.7	0.4
Asystole/bradycardia[d]	9.3	8.5	8.9
Sustained hypotension[e]	7.8	8.3	8.0

[a]Percutaneous transluminal coronary angioplasty.
[b]Requiring electric cardioversion.
[c]Requiring chest compression.
[d]Requiring atropine or temporary pacing.
[e]Requiring vasopressors or intraaortic balloon counterpulsation.

TABLE 56-6 ACC/AHA Guidelines for Primary Percutaneous Transluminal Coronary Angioplasty in Acute Myocardial Infarction[83]

Class I
1. As an alternative to thrombolytic therapy in patients with AMI and ST-segment elevation or new or presumed new LBBB who can undergo angioplasty of the infarct-related artery within 12 hours of onset of symptoms or >12 hours if ischemic symptoms persist, if performed in a timely fashion by persons skilled in the procedure and supported by experienced personnel in an appropriate laboratory environment.
2. In patients who are within 36 hours of an acute ST-elevation/Q-wave or new LBBB MI who develop cardiogenic shock, are <75 years of age, and revascularization can be performed within 18 hours of onset of shock.

Class IIa
1. As a reperfusion strategy in candidates for reperfusion who have a contraindication to thrombolytic therapy.

Class IIb
1. In patients with AMI who do not present with ST elevation but who have reduced [less than TIMI (Thrombolysis in Myocardial Infarction) grade 2] flow of the infarct-related artery and when angioplasty can be performed within 12 hours of onset of symptoms.

Class III
This classification applies to patients with AMI who:
1. Undergo elective angioplasty of a non-infarct-related artery at the time of AMI.
2. Are >12 hours after onset of symptoms and have no evidence of myocardial ischemia.
3. Have received fibrinolytic therapy and have no symptoms of myocardial ischemia.
4. Are eligible for thrombolysis and are undergoing primary angioplasty performed by a low volume operator in a laboratory without surgical capability.

ABBREVIATIONS: AMI = acute myocardial infarction; LBBB = left bundle branch block

catheterization with primary PCI provide powerful information for risk stratification. The PAMI-2 trial has documented the safety and cost savings of early discharge in low-risk patients treated with primary PCI.[41] The feasibility of early discharge on day 2 or 3 has also been shown in the Stent PAMI and CADILLAC trials.[36,40]

The impact of adjunctive treatment with coronary stents and platelet inhibitors on costs with primary PCI is evolving. The Stent PAMI Investigators found that the initial increased costs of stenting versus angioplasty alone are partially recovered by decreased posthospital costs in the stented group due to less target-vessel revascularization.[81] The net increased cost of stenting at 1 year, after adjusting for technical improvements and pricing changes, was about $350 per patient. The costs needed to avoid revascularization with stenting in patients with AMI are similar to those in elective stenting. The incremental costs and effectiveness of abciximab and other platelet inhibitors in the setting of primary PCI are currently being evaluated.

ACC/AHA Guidelines for Primary PCI

Based on the results of numerous randomized trials, primary PCI has a class I indication as reperfusion therapy for AMI with ST-segment elevation or left bundle branch block when performed by experienced operators in a timely fashion (Table 56-6).[82] Primary PCI is preferred over thrombolytic therapy for reperfusion in patients with cardiogenic shock and is indicated for patients who have contraindications to thrombolytic therapy. Primary PCI may be performed at certain hospitals without cardiac surgery programs when it is done by experienced operators with access to surgical facilities using rigorous protocols and proper case selection.[74] Such hospitals must have

set up a program of primary PCI conforming to those established standards.

RESCUE PCI

With current fibrinolytic therapy, successful reperfusion (TIMI-3 flow) is achieved in only 55 to 60 percent of patients.[32] Rescue PCI, the mechanical reopening of an occluded infarct artery after failed thrombolysis, has been used as adjunctive therapy in an attempt to improve outcomes in patients with failed thrombolysis. Observational studies have documented that rescue PCI can achieve successful reperfusion in 82 to 92 percent of patients with an occluded infarct artery after failed thrombolysis,[83,84] but reocclusion of the infarct artery has been common[85] and recovery of left ventricular function variable.[83]

Two moderately sized randomized trials have evaluated the efficacy of rescue PCI. The TAMI-5 trial randomized 575 patients with acute infarction treated with alteplase or urokinase to emergency angiography with rescue PCI for failed thrombolysis versus conservative care.[86] Rescue PCI was performed in 30 percent of the emergency catheterization group, with a success rate of 83 percent. At hospital discharge, the emergency catheterization group had a slightly higher infarct artery patency rate (94 vs. 90 percent, $p = 0.07$), better regional wall motion, and less recurrent ischemia but no difference in mortality, reinfarction, or global left ventricular ejection fraction. The Randomized Evaluation of Salvage Angioplasty with Combined Utilization of Endpoints (RESCUE) trial randomized 151 patients with first anterior wall myocardial infarction treated with thrombolytic therapy who had an occluded infarct artery within 8 h of the onset of chest pain to rescue PCI versus conservative care.[87] The rescue PCI group had a lower composite event rate of death or congestive heart failure (6.4 vs. 16.6 percent, $p = 0.05$) and better exercise left ventricular ejection fraction (43 vs. 38 percent, $p = 0.04$). These benefits occurred despite, what the authors felt, was a strong investigator bias not to randomize patients presenting very early in the course of their infarction.

Rescue PCI, especially after alteplase, is associated with lower angiographic success rates and higher reocclusion rates than primary PCI, and this limits its effectiveness. However, recent observational studies using coronary stenting with rescue PCI have reported high procedural success rates and low reocclusion rates.[88–90] The largest of these studies included 167 patients and reported a success rate of 98 percent, a reocclusion rate of only 1.2 percent, and a combined endpoint of death or reinfarction of 1.4 percent at 30 days in non-shock patients.[90] Glycoprotein IIb/IIIa platelet inhibitors may also potentially enhance outcomes with rescue PCI, but this has not been well studied, and the risk of bleeding when aspirin, heparin, ticlopidine or clopidogrel, and glycoprotein IIb/IIIa platelet inhibitors are used in conjunction with thrombolytic therapy may be high.[89]

A major limitation of the rescue PCI approach is the lack of a reliable noninvasive method to detect reperfusion after thrombolytic therapy. The electrocardiogram is very specific in predicting patency of the infarct artery when there is complete (>70 percent) resolution of ST-segment elevation, but this occurs in only a minority of patients.[91] In most patients there is partial or no resolution of ST-segment elevation and the patency status of the infarct artery is uncertain. Consequently, acute angiography is often required to determine infarct artery patency. Based on the available data, acute angiography with rescue PCI should be considered in patients with anterior or large myocardial infarctions who are thought to have failed thrombolysis, as evidenced by persistent chest pain, lack of resolution of ST-segment elevation, or hemodynamic compromise persisting for more than 90 min after treatment.

Rescue PCI should be differentiated from facilitated PCI (described below). Facilitated PCI is the use of pharmacologic therapy followed by planned emergent PCI. With facilitated PCI, the pharmacologic therapy is synergistic with PCI, and PCI is planned. Rescue PCI is generally not planned.

FUTURE DIRECTIONS

Beyond TIMI Flow: Importance of Microvascular Reperfusion

Primary PCI is effective in restoring normal *epicardial* coronary flow (TIMI-3 flow) in more than 90 percent of patients with AMI, but more than half of these patients will have suboptimal flow at the tissue level, as evidenced by poor angiographic blush scores, suboptimal myocardial contrast by echocardiography, or lack of complete electrocardiographic ST-segment resolution.[92–94] While achieving TIMI-3 flow in the *epicardial* coronary artery is important, optimal outcomes with reperfusion therapy also require optimal reperfusion of the micovasculature or optimal *myocardial* reperfusion.

The cause of abnormal myocardial reperfusion after primary PCI is not clear. One potential cause is distal embolization of thrombus and fragments of atherosclerotic plaque at the time of PCI, resulting in obstruction of the distal microcirculation. A number of devices and pharmacologic agents are being tested in clinical trials to reduce distal embolization, in the hope that this will result in improved myocardial reperfusion and better outcomes. The GuardWire embolic protection device (Medtronic PercuSurge, Sunnyvale, California) has been shown to be effective in reducing distal embolization during elective PCI of saphenous vein grafts.[95] The EMERALD (Enhance Myocardial Efficacy and Recovery by Aspiration of Liberalized Debris) trial is evaluating the role of distal protection with the GuardWire device during primary PCI in native coronary arteries, with the hypothesis that this will improve ST-segment resolution and enhance myocardial salvage.

Thrombus plays a major role in the pathogenesis of AMI and can compromise procedural results and cause distal embolization. The AngioJet Rheolytic Thrombectomy Catheter (Possis Medical, Minneapolis, Minnesota) is currently approved for thrombus removal and is commonly used to treat thrombotic lesions during PCI. The AIMI (AngioJet Rheolytic Thrombectomy In Patients Undergoing Primary PCI for AMI) trial is currently under way to evaluate the role of thrombectomy in improving procedural outcomes, preventing distal embolization, and enhancing myocardial salvage. A second thrombectomy catheter, the investigational X-SIZER catheter (ev3, Plymouth, Minnesota) has shown promise as an adjunctive device with primary PCI. A small randomized study has shown improved ST-segment resolution using the X-SIZER thrombectomy catheter prior to stenting, suggesting improved microvascular reperfusion.[96]

There is evidence that deleterious effects to the myocardium, other than from distal embolization, may occur at the time of reperfusion, resulting in suboptimal *myocardial* reperfusion. The pathogenesis of this *reperfusion injury* is poorly understood but may be related to a complement-dependent inflammatory response, to the formation of oxygen free radicals, or several other mechanisms. Adenosine could potentially reduce reperfusion injury by suppressing the formation of free radicals and preventing neutrophil activation. AMISTAD I (Acute Myocardial Infarction Study of Adenosine) found a 33 percent reduction in infarct size in patients with anterior wall infarction treated with adenosine but no benefit in inferior infarction.[97] AMISTAD II, which evaluated adenosine in patients with anterior wall infarction treated with either lytic therapy or primary PCI, found no significant reduction in clinical events or infarct size.[98] However, patients who had successful reperfusion with primary PCI and received adenosine had fewer clinical events (11 vs. 15 percent, $p = 0.043$), and patients treated with high-dose adenosine had smaller infarcts (11 vs. 26 percent, $p = 0.03$). In another reperfusion injury trial, the investigational complement inhibitor pexelizumab (Alexian Pharmaceuticals and Procter & Gamble), showed a surprising mortality benefit in patients with AMI treated with primary PCI.[99] This surprising result occurred despite the lack of reduction in infarct size, and it raised questions regarding the potential mechanisms of this mortality benefit. The results of these two clinical trials may be encouraging enough to warrant further investigation with these and other agents to reduce reperfusion injury.

Systemic Hypothermia

Systemic hypothermia resulting in myocardial cooling has shown promise in reducing infarct size. Myocardial cooling, by decreasing the metabolic activity of the myocardium, may prolong the period of viability in the setting of AMI and may also help to prevent reperfusion injury. A recent pilot study has evaluated the SetPoint Endovascular Temperature Management System (Radiant Medical Incorporated, Redwood City, California), which uses a heat-exchange catheter inserted into the femoral vein and positioned in the inferior vena cava.[100] This system allows the body temperature to be lowered quickly and maintained precisely. Results of a pilot study showed no major adverse effects from the cooling system and indicated a trend toward reduction in infarct size. A randomized trial with the Radiant System is under way, and at least two other cooling systems are being evaluated in clinical trials.

Facilitated PCI

The time delay required to initiate primary PCI has led to a great deal of interest in pharmacologic reperfusion combined with mechanical reperfusion or facilitated PCI. Facilitated PCI is the use of pharmacologic reperfusion to establish TIMI-3 flow as rapidly as possi-

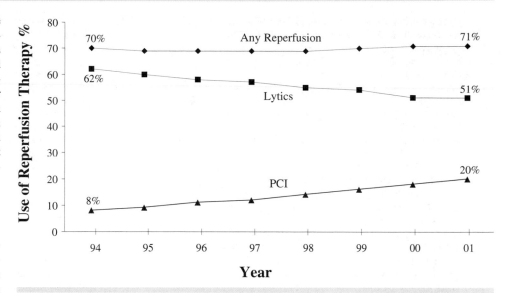

FIGURE 56-7 Temporal trends in the use of reperfusion therapy for patients with ST-segment-elevation acute myocardial infarction of <12 h duration, from the National Registry of Myocardial Infarction.[104]

ble, followed by immediate PCI in those patients without TIMI-3 flow to maximize reperfusion and to stabilize the ruptured plaque. There are several pieces of evidence suggesting that facilitated PCI may prove to be beneficial. Patients undergoing primary PCI for AMI who arrive at the catheterization laboratory with an open versus closed infarct artery have higher procedural success rates, smaller infarcts, better recovery of left ventricular function, and lower early and late mortality.[101,102] The PACT (Plasminogen Activator Angioplasty Compatibility Trial) tested half-dose thrombolysis and then transport for coronary arteriography and PCI in those arteries that remained closed versus PCI without thrombolysis. Initial angiography showed TIMI-2 or -3 flow in 61 percent of the thrombolysis group and 34 percent of the controls. Since both groups had very early treatment with primary or rescue PCI, a significant difference in convalescent left ventricular function could not be shown, but the strategy may prove effective when longer delays are anticipated.[103] The pharmacologic agents recently used in facilitated PCI trials (half-dose lytics plus platelet glycoprotein IIb/IIIa inhibitors) have been shown to be synergistic with PCI. The hypothesis that facilitated PCI may improve outcomes compared with primary PCI alone will be tested in several upcoming trials, including the FINESSE (Facilitated INterventions with Enhanced reperfusion Speed to Stop Events) trial. The FINESSE Trial will evaluate three strategies: half-dose reteplase plus abciximab versus abciximab alone initiated more than 1 h prior to PCI versus abciximab alone given in the catheterization laboratory, all followed by emergent PCI. Whether the benefit of facilitated PCI will be sufficient to outweigh the increased bleeding risks known to occur with combined lytic therapy and platelet glycoprotein IIb/IIIa inhibition[42,43] remains to be determined.

CONCLUSION

Mechanical reperfusion therapy for AMI has become an attractive alternative to thrombolytic therapy. Reperfusion rates are higher, reocclusion rates are lower, myocardial salvage is better; and mortality, nonfatal reinfarction, and stroke are significantly less with primary PCI compared with thrombolytic therapy. Mechanical reperfusion

has become the preferred therapy for patients presenting to institutions equipped to perform PCI, and there is promise that outcomes can become even better with new methods to enhance *myocardial reperfusion* and reduce reperfusion injury. Despite the advantages and despite trends showing increased use of primary PCI, the proportion of patients with ST-segment-elevation AMI treated with primary PCI is relatively small (Fig. 56-7).[104] The major challenge for clinicians in the next decade will be to find new ways to make mechanical reperfusion more available to patients with AMI.

References

1. Fletcher AP, Sherry S, Alkjaersig N, et al. The maintenance of a sustained thrombolytic state in man: II. Clinical observations on patients with myocardial infarction and other thromboembolic disorders. *J Clin Invest* 1959;38:1111.
2. Boucek RJ, Murphy WP Jr. Segmental perfusion of the coronary arteries with fibrinolysin in man following a myocardial infarction. *Am J Cardiol* 1960;6:525–533.
3. Favaloro RG, Effler DB, Cheanvechai C, et al. Acute coronary insufficiency (impending myocardial infarction and myocardial infarction): Surgical treatment by saphenous vein graft technique. *Am J Cardiol* 1971;28:598–607.
4. Berg R, Everhart FJ, Duvoisin G, et al. Operation for acute coronary occlusion. *Am Surg* 1976;42(7):517–521.
5. Rentrop KP. Development and pathophysiological basis of thrombolytic therapy in acute myocardial infarction: Part II: 1977–1980. The pathogenetic role of thrombus is established by the Göttingen pilot studies of mechanical interventions and intracoronary thrombolysis in acute myocardial infarction. *J Intervent Cardiol* 1998;11(4):265–285.
6. DeWood MA, Spores J, Notske R, et al. Prevalence of total coronary occlusion during the early hours of transmural myocardial infarction. *N Engl J Med* 1980;303:897–902.
7. DeWood MA, Stifter WF, Simpson CS, et al. Coronary arteriographic findings soon after non-Q-wave myocardial infarction. *N Engl J Med* 1986;315:417–423.
8. Rentrop P, DeVivie ER, Karsch KR, et al. Acute coronary occlusion with impending infarction as an angiographic complication relieved by guide-wire recanalization. *Clin Cardiol* 1978;1:101–106.
9. Rentrop KP, Blanke H, Karsch KR, et al. Initial experience with transluminal recanalization of the recently occluded infarct-related

coronary artery in acute myocardial infarction—comparison with conventionally treated patients. *Clin Cardiol* 1979;2:92–105.

10. Rentrop KP, Blanke H, Karsch KR, et al. Acute myocardial infarction: Intracoronary application of nitroglycerin and streptokinase. *Clin Cardiol* 1979;2:354–363.

11. Khaja F, Walton JA Jr, Brymer JF, et al. Intracoronary fibrinolytic therapy in acute myocardial infarction: Report of a prospective randomized trial. *N Engl J Med* 1983;308:1305–1311.

12. Kennedy JW, Ritchie JL, Davis KB, et al. Western Washington randomized trial of intracoronary streptokinase in acute myocardial infarction. *N Engl J Med* 1983;390:1477–1482.

13. O'Neill W, Timmis G, Bourdillon P, et al. A prospective randomized clinical trial of intracoronary streptokinase versus coronary angioplasty for acute myocardial infarction. *N Engl J Med* 1986;314:812–818.

14. Gruppo Italiano per lo Studio della Streptochinasi nell'Infarto Miocardico (GISSI): Effectiveness of intravenous thrombolytic treatment in acute myocardial infarction. *Lancet* 1986;1:397–402.

15. ISIS-2 Collaborative Group. Randomized trial of intravenous streptokinase, oral aspirin, both, or neither among 17,187 cases of suspected acute myocardial infarction. *Lancet* 1988;2(8607):349–360.

16. TIMI Research Group. Immediate vs delayed catheterization and angioplasty following thrombolytic therapy for acute myocardial infarction. *JAMA* 1988;260:2849–2858.

17. Topol EJ, Califf RM, George BS, et al. A randomized trial of immediate versus delayed elective angioplasty after intravenous tissue plasminogen activator in acute myocardial infarction. *N Engl J Med* 1987;317:581–588.

18. Simoons ML, Arnold AER, Betriu A, et al. Thrombolysis with tissue plasminogen activator in acute myocardial infarction: No additional benefit from immediate percutaneous coronary angioplasty. *Lancet* 1988;1:197–202.

19. Hartzler GO, Rutherford BD, McConahay DR, et al. Percutaneous transluminal coronary angioplasty with and without thrombolytic therapy for treatment of acute myocardial infarction. *Am Heart J* 1983;106:965–973.

20. O'Keefe JM, Rutherford BD, McConahay DR, et al. Early and late results of coronary angioplasty without antecedent thrombolytic therapy for acute myocardial infarction. *Am J Cardiol* 1989;64:1221–1230.

21. Brodie B, Weintraub R, Stuckey T, et al. Outcomes of direct coronary angioplasty for acute myocardial infarction in candidates and non-candidates for thrombolytic therapy. *Am J Cardiol* 1991;67:7–12.

22. O'Neill WW, Weintraub R, Grines CL, et al. A prospective, placebo-controlled, randomized trial of intravenous streptokinase and angioplasty versus lone angioplasty therapy of acute myocardial infarction. *Circulation* 1992;86:1710–1717.

23. Grines CL, Brown KF, Marco J, et al. A comparison of immediate angioplasty with thrombolytic therapy for acute myocardial infarction. *N Engl J Med* 1993;328:673–679.

24. Zijlstra F, Jan de Boer M, Hoorntje JCA, et al. A comparison of immediate coronary angioplasty with intravenous streptokinase in acute myocardial infarction. *N Engl J Med* 1993;328:680–684.

25. Gibbons RJ, Holmes ZR, Reeder GS, et al. Immediate angioplasty compared with the administration of a thrombolytic agent followed by conservative treatment for myocardial infarction. *N Engl J Med* 1993;328:685–691.

26. Keeley EC, Boura JA, Grines CL. Primary angioplasty vs. intravenous thrombolytic therapy for acute myocardial infarction, a quantitative review of 23 randomized trials. *Lancet* 2003;361:13–20.

27. Fibrinolytic Therapy Trialists' (FTT) Collaborative Group: Indications for fibrinolytic therapy in suspected acute myocardial infarction: Collaborative overview of early mortality and major morbidity results from all randomized trials of more than 1000 patients. *Lancet* 1994;343:311–322.

28. Grines CL, Ellis S, Jones M, et al. Primary coronary angioplasty vs thrombolytic therapy for acute myocardial infarction: Long term follow up of ten randomized trials (abstr). *Circulation* 1999;100(18):I-499.

29. Hochman JS, Sleeper LA, Webb JG, et al. Early revascularization in acute myocardial infarction complicated by cardiogenic shock. *N Engl J Med* 1999;341:625–634.

30. Garcia E, Elizaga J, Perez-Castellano N, et al. Primary angioplasty vs systemic thrombolysis in anterior myocardial infarction. *J Am Coll Cardiol* 1999;33:605–611.

31. de Boer M-J, Ottervanger JP, van't Hof AW, et al. Reperfusion therapy in elderly patients with acute myocardial infarction: A randomized comparison of primary angioplasty and thrombolytic therapy. *J Am Coll Cardiol* 2002;39(11):1729–1732.

32. GUSTO Angiographic Investigators. The effects of tissue plasminogen activator, streptokinase, or both, on coronary artery patency, ventricular function, and survival after acute myocardial infarction. *N Engl J Med* 1993;329:1615–1622.

33. Stone GW, O'Neill WW, Jones B, et al. The central unifying concept of TIMI-3 flow after primary PTCA and thrombolytic therapy in acute myocardial infarction (abstr). *Circulation* 1996;94(8,suppl I):I-515.

34. Antman EM, Giugliano RP, Gibson CM, et al. Abciximab facilitates the rate and extent of thrombolysis: Results of the thrombolysis in myocardial infarctions (TIMI) 14 trial. *Circulation* 1999;99:2720–2732.

35. O'Neill WW, Brodie BR, Ivanhoe R, et al. Primary coronary angioplasty for acute myocardial infarction (The Primary Angioplasty Registry). *Am J Cardiol* 1994;73:627–634.

36. Stone GW, Grines CL, Cox DA, et al. Comparison of angioplasty with stenting, with or without abciximab, in acute myocardial infarction. *N Engl J Med* 2002;346;957–966.

37. GUSTO III Investigators. A comparison of reteplase with alteplase for acute myocardial infarction. The global use of strategies to open occluded coronary arteries. *N Engl J Med* 1997;337:1118–1123.

38. ASSENT-2 Investigators. Single-bolus tenecteplase compared with front-loaded alteplase in acute myocardial infarction: ASSENT-2 double-blind randomized trial. *Lancet* 1999;354:716–722.

39. The Global Use of Strategies to Open Occluded Coronary Arteries in Acute Coronary Syndromes (GUSTO IIb) Angioplasty Substudy Investigators. A clinical trial comparing primary coronary angioplasty with tissue plasminogen activator for acute myocardial infarction. *N Engl J Med* 1997;336:1621–1628.

40. Grines CL, Cox DA, Stone GW, et al. for the stent primary angioplasty in myocardial infarction study group. Coronary angioplasty with or without stent implantation for acute myocardial infarction. *N Engl J Med* 1999;341:1949–1956.

41. Grines CL, Marsalese DL, Brodie BR, et al. Safety and cost-effectiveness of early discharge after primary angioplasty in low risk patients with acute myocardial infarction. *J Am Coll Cardiol* 1998;31:967–972.

42. The GUSTO V Investigators. Reperfusion therapy for acute myocardial infarction with fibrinolytic therapy or combination reduced fibrinolytic therapy and platelet glycoprotein IIb/IIIa inhibition: The GUSTO V randomised trial. *Lancet* 2001;357:1905–1914.

43. The ASSENT-3 Investigators. Efficacy and safety of tenecteplase in combination with enoxaparin, abciximab, or unfractionated heparin: ASSENT-3 randomised trial in acute myocardial infarction. *Lancet* 2001;358:605–613.

44. Nunn CM, O'Neill WW, Rothbaum D, et al. Long-term outcome after primary angioplasty: Report from the Primary Angioplasty in Myocardial Infarction (PAMI-1) Trial. *J Am Coll Cardiol* 1999;33:640–646.

45. Zijlstra F, Hoorntje JCA, de Boer M-J, et al. Long-term benefit of primary angioplasty as compared with thrombolytic therapy for acute myocardial infarction. *N Engl J Med* 1999;341:1413–1419.

46. Brodie BR, Grines CL, Ivanhoe R, et al. Six month clinical and angiographic follow-up after direct angioplasty for acute myocardial infarction: Final results from the primary angioplasty registry. *Circulation* 1994;25:156–162.

47. Veen G, de Boer M-J, Zijlstra F, et al. Improvement in three-month angiographic outcome suggested after primary angioplasty for acute myocardial infarction (Zwolle Trial) compared with successful thrombolysis (APRICOT Trial). *Am J Coll Cardiol* 1999;84: 763–767.

48. White HD, French JK, Hamer AW, et al. Frequent re-occlusion of patent infarct-related arteries between four weeks and one year: Effects of anti-platelet therapy. *J Am Coll Cardiol* 1995;25:218–223.

49. Brouwer MA, van den Bergh PJ, Aengevaeren WR, et al. Aspirin plus coumarin versus aspirin alone in the prevention of reocclusion after fibrinolysis for acute myocardial infarction: Results of the antithrombotics in the prevention of reocclusion in coronary thrombolysis (APRICOT-2) trial. *Circulation* 2002;106:659–665.

50. Schömig A, Kastrati A, Dirschinger J, et al. Coronary stenting plus platelet glycoprotein IIb/IIIa blockade compared with tissue plasminogen activator in acute myocardial infarction. *N Engl J Med* 2000;343: 385–391.

51. Kastrati A, Mehilli J, Dirschinger J, et al. Myocardial salvage after coronary stenting plus abciximab vs fibrinolysis plus abciximab in patients with acute myocardial infarction: A randomized trial. *Lancet* 2002;359:920–925.

52. Brener SJ, Barr LA, Burchenal JEB, et al. Randomized placebo-controlled trial of platelet glycoprotein IIb/IIIa blockade with primary angioplasty for acute myocardial infarction. *Circulation* 1998;98: 734–741.

53. Montalescot G, Barragan P, Wittenberg O, et al. Platelet glycoprotein IIb/IIIa inhibition with coronary stenting for acute myocardial infarction. *N Engl J Med* 2001;344:1895–1903.

54. Neumann FJ, Kastrati A, Schmitt C, et al. Effect of glycoprotein IIb/IIIa receptor blockade with abciximab on clinical and angiographic restenosis rate after the placement of coronary stents following acute myocardial infarction. *J Am Coll Cardiol* 2000;35:915–921.

55. Antoinucci D. The ACE trial. Presented at the Annual Scientific Sessions of the American Heart Association, November 2002, Chicago.

56. Cragg BR, Friedman HC, Bonema JD, et al. Outcome of patients with acute myocardial infarction who are ineligible for thrombolytic therapy. *Ann Intern Med* 1991; 115:173–177.

57. Stone GW, Grines CL, Browne KF, et al. Predictors of in-hospital and six-month outcome after acute myocardial infarction in the reperfusion era: The primary angioplasty and myocardial infarction (PAMI) trial. *J Am Coll Cardiol* 1995;25:370–377.

58. Holmes DR Jr., White HD, Pieper KS, et al. Effect of age on outcome with primary angioplasty versus thrombolysis. *J Am Coll Cardiol* 1999;33:412–419.

59. Zahn R, Schuster S, Schiele R, et al. Comparison of primary angioplasty with conservative therapy in patients with acute myocardial infarction and contraindications for thrombolytic therapy. Maximum individual therapy in acute myocardial infarction (MITRA) study group. *Catheter Cardiovasc Interv* 1999;46:127–133.

60. Brodie BR, Stuckey TD, Hansen C, et al. Benefit of late coronary reperfusion in patients with acute myocardial infarction and persistent ischemic chest pain. *Am J Cardiol* 1994;74:538–543.

61. Cannon C, Weintraub WS, Demopoulos LA, et al. For the TACTICS investigators. Comparison of early invasive and conservative strategies in patients with unstable coronary syndrome treated with glycoprotein IIb/IIIa inhibitor tirosiban. *N Engl J Med* 2001;344:1879–1887.

62. Reiner JS, Lundergan CF, Kopecky SL, et al. Ineffectiveness of thrombolysis for acute myocardial infarction following vein graft occlusion (abstr). *Circulation* 1996;94(8,suppl I):I-570.

63. Stone GW, Brodie BR, Griffin JJ, et al. Clinical and angiographic outcomes in patients with previous coronary artery bypass grafting treated with primary balloon angioplasty for acute myocardial infarction. *J Am Coll Cardiol* 2000;35:605–611.

64. Stone GW, Brodie BR, Griffin JJ, et al. for the PAMI-2 Investigators. The role of cardiac surgery in the hospital phase management of patients treated with primary angioplasty for acute myocardial infarction. *Am J Cardiol* 2000;85:1292–1296.

65. Brodie BR, Stuckey TD, Wall TC, et al. Importance of time to reperfusion for 30-day and late survival and recovery of left ventricular function after primary angioplasty for acute myocardial infarction. *J Am Coll Cardiol* 1998;32:1312–1319.

66. Brodie BR, Stuckey TD, Hansen CJ, et al. Effect of treatment delay on outcomes in patients with acute myocardial infarction transferred from community hospitals for primary percutaneous coronary intervention. *Am J Cardiol* 2002;89:1243–1247.

67. Vermeer F, Oude Ophuis AJ, van der Berg EJ, et al. Prospective randomized comparison between thrombolysis, rescue PTCA, and primary PTCA in patients with extensive myocardial infarction admitted to a hospital without PTCA facilities: A safety and feasibility study. *Heart* 1999;82(4):426–431.

68. Widimsky P, Groch L, Zelizko M, et al. Multi-center randomized trial comparing transport to primary angioplasty vs. immediate thrombolysis vs. combined strategy for patients with acute myocardial infarction presenting to a community hospital without a catheterization laboratory. *Eur Heart J* 2000;21:823–831.

69. Grines CL, Westerhausen DR Jr, Grines LL, et al. A randomized trial of transfer for primary angioplasty vs on-site thrombolysis in patients with high-risk myocardial infarction: The air primary angioplasty in myocardial infarction study. *J Am Coll Cardiol* 2002;39: 1713–1719.

70. Anderson HR. Danish trial in acute myocardial infarction (DANAMI-2). Paper presented at the American College of Cardiology Scientific Session; March 2002; Atlanta.

71. Widimsky P. Primary angioplasty in acute myocardial infarction patients in general community hospitals transported to PTCA units vs. emergency thrombolysis (PRAGUE-2). Presented at the European Society of Cardiology, 2002, Berlin, Germany.

72. Wharton TP Jr, McNamara NS, Febele FA, et al. Primary angioplasty for the treatment of acute myocardial infarction: Experience at two community hospitals without cardiac surgery. *J Am Coll Cardiol* 1999;33:1257–1265.

73. Aversano T, Aversano LT, Passamani E, et al. Thrombolytic therapy vs. primary percutaneous coronary intervention for myocardial infarction in patients presenting to hospitals without on-site cardiac surgery: A randomized control trial. *JAMA* 2002;287:1943–1951.

74. Smith S, Dove J, Jacobs A, et al. ACC/AHA guidelines for percutaneous coronary intervention. *J Am Coll Cardiol* 2001;37(8):2239, i–lxvi

75. Ohman EM, George BS, White CJ, et al. The use of aortic counterpulsation to improve sustained coronary artery patency during acute myocardial infarction: Results of a randomized trial. *Circulation* 1994; 90:792–799.

76. Stone GW, Marsalese D, Brodie BR. A prospective, randomized evaluation of prophylactic intra-aortic balloon counterpulsation in high risk patients with acute myocardial infarction treated with primary angioplasty. *J Am Coll Cardiol* 1997;29:1459–1467.

77. van't Hof AWJ, Liem AM, de Boer MJ, et al. A randomized comparison of intra-aortic balloon pumping after primary coronary angioplasty in high risk patients with acute myocardial infarction. *Eur Heart J* 1999;20:659–665.

78. Brodie BR, Stuckey TD, Hansen C, et al. Intra-aortic balloon counterpulsation before primary percutaneous transluminal coronary angioplasty reduces catheterization laboratory events in high risk patients with acute myocardial infarction. *Am J Cardiol* 1999;84:18–23.

79. Reeder GS, Bailey KR, Gersh BJ, et al. Cost comparison of immediate angioplasty versus thrombolysis followed by conservative therapy for acute myocardial infarction: A randomized prospective trial. *Mayo Clin Proc* 1994;69:5–12.

80. Stone G, Grines C, Rothbaum D, et al. Analysis of the relative cost and effectiveness of primary angioplasty vs tissue type plasminogen activator: The Primary Angioplasty in Myocardial Infarction (PAMI) trial. *J Am Coll Cardiol* 1997;29:901–907.

81. Cohen DJ, Taira DA, Berezin R, et al. Cost-effectiveness of coronary stenting in acute myocardial infarctions: Results from the Stent PAMI trial. *Circulation* 2001;104:3039–3045.

82. Ryan TJ, Antman EM, Brooks NH, et al. 1999 update: ACC/AHA guidelines for the management of patients with acute myocardial infarction: Executive summary and recommendations. *Circulation* 1999;100:1016–1030.

83. Gibson CM, Cannon CP, Grenne RM, et al. Rescue angioplasty in the thrombolysis in myocardial infarction (TIMI-4) trial. *Am J Cardiol* 1997;80:21–26.

84. Flachskampf FA, Ellis FG. Rescue percutaneous transluminal coronary angioplasty. *Curr Opin Cardiol* 1998;13:289–293.

85. Ellis SG, Van de Werf F, Riberiro-daSilva E, et al. Present status of rescue coronary angioplasty: Current polarization of opinion in randomized trials. *J Am Coll Cardiol* 1992;19:681–686.

86. Califf RM, Topol EJ, Stack RS, et al. Evaluation of combination thrombolytic therapy and timing of cardiac catheterization in acute myocardial infarction: Results of thrombolysis and angioplasty in myocardial infarction—Phase 5 randomized trial. *Circulation* 1991; 83:1543–1556.

87. Ellis SG, da Silva ER, Heyndrickx G, et al. Randomized comparison of rescue angioplasty with conservative management of patients with early failure of thrombolysis for acute anterior myocardial infarction. *Circulation* 1994;90:2280–2284.

88. Cafri C, Denktas AE, Crystal E, et al. Contribution of stenting to the results of rescue PTCA. *Catheter Cardiovasc Interv* 1999;47: 411–414.

89. Moreno R, Garcia E, Abeytua M, et al. Coronary stenting during rescue angioplasty after failed thrombolysis. *Catheter Cardiovasc Interv* 1999;47:1–5.

90. Dirschinger J, Pocat J, Kastrati A, et al. Clinical outcome after rescue stenting in patients with acute myocardial infarction (abstr). *J Am Coll Cardiol* 1999;33(2 suppl A):30A.

91. Zeymer U, Schröder R, Molhoek P, et al. Noninvasive detection of early infarct vessel patency by resolution of ST-segment elevation in patients with thrombolysis for acute myocardial infarction: Results of the angiographic substudy of the hirudin for improvement of thrombolysis (HIT)-4 trial. *Eur Heart J* 2001;22:769–775.

92. van 't Hof AWJ, Liem A, Suryapranata H, et al. Angiographic assessment of myocardial reperfusion in patients treated with primary angioplasty for acute myocardial infarction. *Circulation* 1998;97:2302–2306.

93. Ito H, Maruyama A, Iwakura K, et al. Clinical implications of the "no reflow" phenomenon: A predictor of complications and left ventricular remodeling in reperfused anterior wall myocardial infarction. *Circulation* 1996;93:223–228.

94. van 't Hof AWJ, Liem A, de Boer M-J, et al. Clinical value of 12-lead electrocardiogram after successful reperfusion therapy for acute myocardial infarction. *Lancet* 1997;350:615–619.

95. Baim DS, Wahr D, George B, et al. A randomized trial of a distal embolic protection device during percutaneous intervention in saphenous vein aorto-coronary bypass grafts. *Circulation* 2002;105:1285–1290.

96. Beran G, Lang I, Schreiber W, et al. Intracoronary thrombectomy with the X-sizer catheter system improves epicardial flow and accelerates ST-segment resolution in patients with acute coronary syndrome: A prospective, randomized, controlled study. *Circulation* 2002;105: 2355–2360.

97. Mahaffey KW, Puma JA, Barbagelata NA, et al. Adenosine as an adjunct to thrombolytic therapy for acute myocardial infarction: Results of a multi-center randomized, placebo controlled trial: The acute myocardial infarction study of adenosine (AMISTAD) trial. *J Am Coll Cardiol* 1999;34(6):1711–1720.

98. Ross A. Acute myocardial infarction study of adenosine (AMISTAD-II). Paper presented at the American College of Cardiology Scientific Session, March 2002, Atlanta.

99. Granger C. Complement and reduction of infarct size after angioplasty or lytics (CARDINAL) trial. Presented at the Annual Scientific Session of the American Heart Association, November 2002, Chicago.

100. Dixon SR, Whitbourn RJ, Dae MW, et al. Induction of mild systemic hypothermia with endovascular cooling during primary percutaneous coronary intervention for acute myocardial infarction. *J Am Coll Cardiol* 2002;40:1928–1934.

101. Brodie BR, Stuckey TD, Hansen C, et al. Benefit of coronary reperfusion before intervention on outcomes after primary angioplasty for acute myocardial infarction. *Am J Cardiol* 2000;85:13–18.

102. Stone GW, Cox D, Garcia E, et al. Normal flow (TIMI-3) before mechanical reperfusion therapy is an independent determinant of survival in acute myocardial infarction: Analysis from the primary angioplasty in myocardial infarction trials. *Circulation* 2001;104: 636–641.

103. Ross AM, Coyne KS, Reiner JS, et al. A randomized trial comparing primary angioplasty with a strategy of short acting thrombolysis and immediate planned resuce angioplasty in acute myocardial infarction: The PACT Trial. *J Am Coll Cardiol* 1999;34:1954–1962.

104. Rogers WJ, Canto JG, Lambrew CT, et al. Temporal trends in the treatment of over 1.5 million patients with myocardial infarctions in the U.S. from 1990–1999. *J Am Coll Cardiol* 2000;36:2056–2063.

DIAGNOSIS AND MANAGEMENT OF PATIENTS WITH CHRONIC ISCHEMIC HEART DISEASE

Robert A. O'Rourke / Patrick O'Gara / John S. Douglas, Jr.

Ischemic heart disease continues to be a major public health problem.[1] Chronic stable angina is the first indicator of ischemic heart disease in about 50 percent of patients. The reported annual incidence of angina is 213 per 100,000 people over the age of 30. The number of patients with stable angina in the United States approximates 16.5 million, not including individuals who do not seek medical attention for their chest pain or who are shown to have a noncardiac cause of chest discomfort. Angina pectoris is a clinical syndrome that consists of discomfort or pain in the chest, jaw, shoulder, back, or arm. Typically it is precipitated or aggravated by exertion or emotional stress and relieved by nitroglycerin. Angina usually occurs in patients with coronary artery disease (CAD) affecting one or more large epicardial arteries. However, angina is often present in individuals with valvular heart disease, hypertrophic cardiomyopathy, and uncontrolled hypertension. It also occurs in patients with normal coronary arteries and myocardial ischemia due to coronary artery spasm or endothelial dysfunction. The symptom of angina is often observed in patients with noncardiac disorders affecting the esophagus, chest wall, or lungs. An extensive discussion of the differential diagnosis of chest pain is included in Chap. 12.

HISTORICAL PERSPECTIVE

In 1768, William Herberden presented his classic description of angina pectoris in a lecture before the Royal College of Physicians; it was published in 1772.[2] This classic description was published again with minor changes in a chapter entitled "Pectoris Dolor" in his *Commentaries on the History and Cure of Diseases,* which was translated from the Latin and published by his son, also named William Herberden, in 1802.[3] The following quotation is from the original lecture:

> There is a disorder of the breast, marked with strong and peculiar symptoms, considerable for the kind of danger belonging to it, and extremely rare, of which I do not recollect any mention among medical authors. The seat of it, and sense of strangling and anxiety, with which it is attended, may make it not improperly be called angina pectoris. Those who are afflicted with it are seized, while they are walking, and more particularly when they walk soon after eating, with a painful and most disagreeable sensation in the breast, which seems as if it would take their life away, if it were to increase or to continue: the moment they stand still all this uneasiness vanishes.
>
> After it has continued some months, it will not cease so instantaneous upon standing still; and it will come on, not only when the persons are walking, but when they are lying down, and oblige them to rise up from their beds every night for many months together; and in one or two very inveterate cases it has been brought on by the motion of a horse or a carriage, and even by swallowing, coughing, going to stool or speaking, or by any disturbance of mind.
>
> . . . but all the rest, whom I have seen, who are at least twenty, were men, and almost all above 50 years old, and most of them with a short neck, and inclining to be fat. When a fit of this sort comes on by walking, its duration is very short, as it goes off almost immediately upon stopping. If it comes on in the night, it will last an hour or two; and I have met one, in whom it once continued for several days, during all which time the patient seemed to be in imminent danger of death.
>
> But the natural tendency of this illness be to kill the patients suddenly, yet unless it have a power of preserving a person from all other ails, it will easily be believed that some of those, who are afflicted with it, may die in a different manner, since this disorder will last, as I have known it more than once, near twenty years, and most usually attacks only those who are above fifty years of age. I have accordingly observed one, who sunk under a lingering illness of a different nature.
>
> The os sterni is usually pointed to as the seat of this malady, but it seems sometimes as if it was under the lower part of it, and at other times under the middle or upper part, but always inclining more to the left side, and sometimes there is with it a pain about the middle of the left arm.

The syndrome of angina pectoris was described as rare in textbooks of medicine in 1866 (Austin Flint) and 1892 (William Osler). Paul Dudley White wrote: "[angina pectoris] was uncommon in my early professional years. But when the automobile came in the 1920s and the population at large became more prosperous and over nourished, the current epidemic of coronary heart disease, as shown mainly by the symptom angina pectoris, began and incidentally involved younger and younger men."[4] In the United States, the peak mortality rate from coronary heart disease (CHD) occurred about 1962 to 1965; since then, it has been decreasing steadily.[5]

ETIOLOGY AND CLASSIFICATION

Coronary atherosclerosis is the cause of angina pectoris in most patients (Chaps. 44 to 46). Many nonatherosclerotic causes of CAD (Tables 47-1 and 47-2) can also produce angina pectoris or myocardial infarction. Other conditions particularly associated with angina pectoris include congenital coronary artery abnormalities (Chap. 74), aortic stenoses (Chap. 66), mitral stenoses with resulting severe right ventricular hypertension (Chap. 67), hypertrophic cardiomyopathy (Chap. 77), and systemic arterial hypertension[6] (Chap. 61).

Disorders in which angina occurs less frequently include aortic regurgitation (Chap. 61), idiopathic dilated cardiomyopathy (Chap. 76), and luetic heart disease. Mitral valve prolapse (Chap. 68) rarely causes true angina pectoris. Certain conditions may alter the balance between myocardial oxygen supply-demand and precipitate or aggravate angina pectoris, including severe anemia, tachycardia, fever, hyperthyroidism, and Paget's disease of bone.

The Canadian Cardiovascular Society Grading Scale (Table 12-2) is commonly used to classify the severity of angina pectoris, with the most severe symptoms occurring at rest and the least severe only with excessive exercise.

DIAGNOSIS

History and Physical Examination

The first step is to obtain a detailed description of the symptom complex in order to characterize the chest pain or discomfort. Five descriptors typically are considered: (1) location, (2) quality, (3) duration of the discomfort, (4) inciting factors, and (5) factors relieving the pain.[1]

The most commonly used classification scheme for chest pain divides patients into three groups: *typical angina, atypical angina,* or *noncardiac chest pain*[7,8] (Table 57-1).

Angina is further labeled as *stable* when its characteristics are usually unchanged for 60 days (Chaps. 48 and 51). The presence of *unstable angina* predicts a much higher short-term risk of an acute coronary event. *Unstable angina* is defined as angina that presents in one of three major ways: *rest angina, severe new-onset angina,* or *prior angina increasing in severity* (Chap. 51). Recently, the acute coronary syndromes of unstable angina and non-ST-segment elevation myocardial infarction have been linked together by their similar presentation and treatment[9] (Chap 48).

TABLE 57-1 Clinical Classification of Angina

Typical angina (definite)
1. Substernal chest discomfort with a characteristic quality and duration that is
2. provoked by exertion or emotional stress and
3. relieved by rest or nitroglycerin.

Atypical angina (probable)
  Meets two of the above characteristics.

Noncardiac chest pain
  Meets one or none of the typical anginal characteristics.

SOURCE: Modified from Diamond et al.[7]

Usually, the discomfort of chronic stable angina pectoris is precipitated by physical activity, emotions, eating, or cold weather. Certain patients are able to describe accurately the extent and type of exercise at which they reproducibly experience their chest pain (Chap. 12). Many patients will develop angina if they walk up a hill against a cold wind after a large meal. Emotions, particularly anger, excitation, and frustration, often precipitate angina in patients with CAD. Cigarette smoking induces chest discomfort or lowers the exertion threshold for angina in some patients. A history of cocaine use should be sought because it can precipitate myocardial ischemia with or without infarction by coronary vasoconstriction.[10]

When stable angina pectoris develops, it often increases to a plateau over 10 to 30 s and usually disappears within minutes if the exertion is discontinued. Occasionally, the angina will disappear despite continued physical activity ("walk-through angina"), which is attributed to the opening of collaterals. Most patients have discomfort that lasts only several minutes, sometimes up to 10 to 15 min and rarely up to 30 min (Chap. 12).

The discomfort of angina is most often located substernally or just to the left of the sternum. Some patients, in describing the discomfort, clench their fist over their upper sternum (Levine's sign)—a sign of high diagnostic accuracy. Less often, angina is located over the precordium. The discomfort is rarely localized only to the apex of the heart. Nevertheless, angina can be located anywhere from the epigastrium to the neck; rarely, it may be located only in the neck, throat, arm, or back.

The pain often radiates down the arms or to the neck, jaw, teeth, shoulders, or back. Radiation to the left side is more common, but both sides can be involved. The radiation, characteristically down the ulnar aspect of the arm, is often described as numbness. Increased heat or humidity also may lower the exertional threshold at which angina occurs.

Disorders that increase the myocardial oxygen requirement (MVo_2) may exacerbate the occurrence of angina pectoris and sometimes may be associated with angina in the absence of moderate or severe CAD stenosis on coronary arteriography. Patients with stable angina may have many episodes of myocardial ischemia that are asymptomatic or silent. Also, myocardial ischemia may result in symptoms due to either systolic or diastolic left ventricular (LV) dysfunction without the characteristic chest discomfort. *Angina equivalent* symptoms usually are associated with exertion and are relieved by rest and nitroglycerin. *Exertional dyspnea* likely is due to reduced diastolic LV compliance resulting from myocardial ischemia. *Exertional fatigue* or exhaustion probably results from an acute decrease in cardiac output due to diminished systolic LV function and/or associated mitral regurgitation from transient papillary muscle dysfunction.

In general, when myocardial ischemia is produced, an *ischemic cascade* occurs. Regional diastolic and systolic dysfunction precede global diastolic and then systolic dysfunction, which in turn often occurs prior to changes in the electrocardiogram (ECG) and before the symptoms of angina pectoris (Fig. 57-1). Noninva-sive testing is often useful in detecting ischemia (see below). The detection of LV diastolic dysfunction by Doppler mitral valve recording or by diastolic filling curves using radionuclide ventriculography has many limitations (Chaps. 15 and 19). Although diaphoresis and alterations in blood pressure and heart rate may occur, the physical examination is often normal. An examination performed during an episode of pain, however, can be useful. A fourth (most common) or third heart sound, a mitral regurgitant systolic murmur, reversed splitting of the S_2, bibasilar pulmonary rates, or palpable ectopic cardiac impulses that disappear when the pain subsides are all predictive of CAD (Chap. 12). Carotid sinus pressure often terminates anginal chest pain. Evidence of noncoronary atherosclerotic disease such as a carotid bruit, diminished pedal pulse, or abdominal aneurysm increases the likelihood of CAD. An elevated blood pressure, xanthomas, and retinal exudates point to the presence of CAD risk factors[6] (Chap. 12).

Clinical Assessment of the Likelihood of CAD

The clinicopathologic study performed by Diamond and Forrester[11] demonstrated that it is possible to predict the probability of CAD after the history and the physical examination. By combining data from several angiographic studies performed before 1980, they showed that simple clinical observations of pain type, age, and sex were powerful predictors of the probability of CAD.

The utility of this approach was confirmed subsequently in prospective studies at Duke and Stanford.[12–14] In both men and women, the initial clinical characteristics most helpful in predicting CAD were determined. In these studies, age, sex, and pain type were the most powerful predictors (Table 57-2). Smoking, Q waves, or ST-segment–T-wave changes on ECG, hyperlipidemia, and diabetes further strengthened the predictive abilities of these models.[1,14]

Special Tests for Diagnosis

Most special tests in patients with suspected stable angina are performed either to establish the diagnosis and/or to determine the risk for coronary events.[1] Table 57-2 indicates the likelihood for each

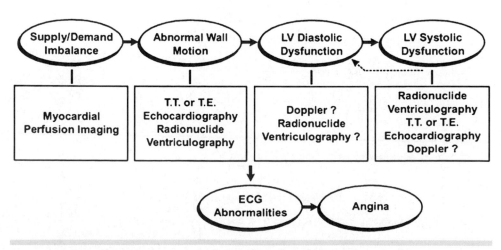

Sequence of Events during Myocardial Ischemia

FIGURE 57-1 Sequence of events in the ischemic cascade plus noninvasive tests for detecting its presence. T.T., transthoracic; T.E., transesophageal.

TABLE 57-2 Pretest Likelihood of CAD in Symptomatic Patients According to Age and Sex[a] (Combined Diamond/Forrester and CASS Data)[7–10]

Age, years	NONANGINAL CHEST PAIN		ATYPICAL ANGINA		TYPICAL ANGINA	
	Men	Women	Men	Women	Men	Women
30–39	4	2	34	12	76	26
40–49	13	3	51	22	87	55
50–59	20	7	65	31	93	73
60–69	27	14	72	51	94	86

[a]Each value represents the percent with significant CAD on catheterization.
SOURCE: Modified from Gibbons et al.[1]

gender by age and characteristics of the chest discomfort. It also indicates why women have more false-positive responses to ECG exercise testing than do men (Chap. 16). Terms useful in the evaluation and selection of diagnostic tests for CAD are listed in Table 57-3. Bayes' theorem states that the pretest prevalence of disease influences the posttest likelihood of significant CAD (Chap. 16). Figure 57-2 illustrates the impact of Bayes' theorem when evaluating several diagnostic tests for CAD. More accurate data on the sensitivity and specificity of noninvasive testing for diagnosis of CAD are provided in Chaps. 14, 15, 17, and 19.

If an exercise ECG test was performed on a 55-year-old woman with atypical chest pain and a pretest likelihood for coronary disease of 0.46, a positive ECG stress test response would indicate her posttest likelihood to be 0.86. However, if she had a positive thallium scan, her likelihood of disease would increase to 0.98. If her thallium scan was negative, the probability of disease would decrease to 0.63.

Diagnostic tests should be performed only when necessary to answer a specific clinical question. Thus a diagnostic test may be of limited additional diagnostic value in patients with either a very high (>0.90) or a very low (<0.10) pretest risk for CAD.[1]

ELECTROCARDIOGRAM AND CHEST ROENTGENOGRAM

A resting 12-lead ECG should be recorded in all patients with symptoms suggestive of angina; however, it will be normal in up to 50 percent of patients with chronic stable angina. ECG evidence of LV hypertrophy or ST-segment–T-wave changes consistent with myocardial ischemia favors the diagnosis of angina pectoris. Evidence of prior Q-wave myocardial infarction (MI) on the ECG makes CAD very likely. Patients with a completely normal resting ECG *rarely have* significant LV systolic dysfunction.

The presence of arrhythmias (e.g., atrial fibrillation or ventricular tachyarrhythmias) on the ECG in patients with chest pain also increases the probability of underlying CAD; however, these arrhythmias frequently are caused by other types of cardiac disease. Various degrees of atrioventricular (AV) block occur in patients with chronic CAD but have a very low specificity for the diagnosis. Left anterior fascicular block, right bundle branch block (RBBB), and left bundle branch block (LBBB) are often present in patients with CAD and frequently indicate multivessel CAD but are not specific.

An ECG obtained during chest pain is abnormal in about 50 percent of patients with angina and a normal resting ECG. Sinus tachycardia is frequent; bradyarrhythmias are less common. ST-segment elevation or depression establishes a high likelihood of angina and indicates ischemia at a low workload, suggesting an unfavorable prognosis. Many high-risk patients with severe episodes of angina need no further noninvasive testing. Coronary arteriography usually defines the severity of CAD and determines the necessity and feasibility of myocardial revascularization. In patients with ST-segment–T-wave depression or inversion on the resting ECG, pseudonormalization of these abnormalities during pain is another indicator that CAD is likely.[15] The occurrence of tachyarrhythmias, AV block, left anterior fascicular block, or bundle branch block during chest pain also increases the probability of CHD and often leads to coronary arteriography.

TABLE 57-3 Glossary of Terms

True positive (TP): Positive result in patient with disease
True negative (TN): Negative result in patient without disease
False positive (FP): Positive result in patient without disease
False negative (FN): Negative result in patient with disease

Sensitivity: $\dfrac{TP}{TP + FN}$

Specificity: $\dfrac{TN}{TN + FP}$

Predictive value of a positive test: $\dfrac{TP}{TP + FP}$

Predictive value of a negative test: $\dfrac{TN}{TN + FN}$

Bayes' theorem:
Probability of disease presence with a positive test =

$$\frac{\text{sensitivity} \times \text{prevalence}}{(\text{sensitivity} \times \text{prevalence}) + [(1 - \text{specificity}) \times (1 - \text{prevalence})]}$$

Probability of disease presence with a negative test =

$$\frac{(1 - \text{sensitivity}) \times \text{prevalence}}{[(1 - \text{sensitivity}) \times \text{prevalence}] + [\text{specificity} \times (1 - \text{prevalence})]}$$

The *chest roentgenogram* often is normal in patients with stable angina pectoris. Its usefulness as a routine test is *not* well established. It is more likely to be abnormal in patients with previous or acute MI, those with a noncoronary artery cause of chest pain, and those with noncardiac chest pain.

Coronary artery calcification increases the likelihood of symptomatic CAD. *Fluoroscopically detectable coronary calcification* is correlated with major vessel occlusion in 94 percent of patients *with* chest pain[16]; however, the sensitivity of the test is less than 40 percent.

Electron beam computed tomography (EBCT) (Chap. 17) is being used with increased frequency for screening asymptomatic individuals. However, the specificity of a positive result may be as low as 49 percent, and the predictive accuracy is less than 70 percent. The role of EBCT in CAD diagnosis and risk stratification continues to be controversial.[17] The most recent report of an American College of Cardiology/American Heart Association (ACC/AHA) expert consensus writing group does not recommend EBCT for *routine screening* of asymptomatic patients for CAD or for its use in most patients with chest pain.[18] It also is of little use in detecting high-risk plaques[19] (see below).

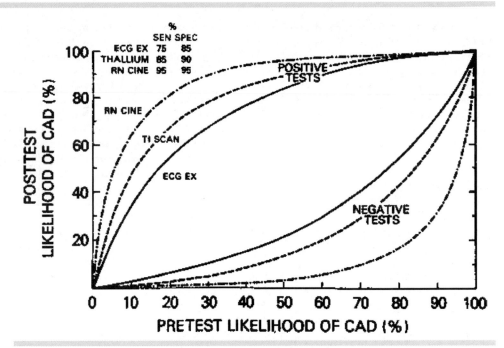

FIGURE 57-2 Probability of CAD. Comparison of ECG exercise testing (ECG Ex), thallium perfusion imaging (TI Scan), and radionuclide cineangiography (RN CINE). Sensitivity (SEN) and specificity (SPEC) values are approximations derived from published series. (From Epstein et al. *Am J Cardiol* 1980;46:491. Reproduced with permission from the publisher and authors.)

EXERCISE ECG STRESS TESTING

Exercise ECG stress testing is a well-established procedure that has been in widespread clinical use for many decades.[20] Although usually a safe procedure, both MI and death occur at a rate of up to 1 per 2500 tests[21] (Chap. 16). Absolute contraindications include acute MI within 2 days, symptomatic cardiac arrhythmias causing hemodynamic compromise, symptomatic and severe aortic stenoses, symptomatic heart failure, acute pulmonary embolus or infarction, acute myocarditis or pericarditis, and acute aortic dissection.

For optimizing the information obtained, the protocol should be tailored to the individual patient, with exercise lasting at least 6 min.[22] Exercise capacity should be reported in estimated metabolic equivalents (METs) of exercise (1 MET is the standard basal oxygen uptake of 3.5 mL/kg/min) as well as in minutes.

The ECG, heart rate, and blood pressure should be monitored carefully and recorded during each stage of exercise, as well as during ST-segment abnormalities and chest pain, as detailed in Chap. 16.

Interpretation of the exercise ECG should include symptomatic response, exercise capacity, hemodynamic response, and ECG changes. The most important ECG abnormalities are ST-segment depression and ST-segment elevation (in leads without diagnostic Q waves) of greater than 1 mm for at least 60 to 80 ms after the end of the QRS complex. Although exercise testing is often terminated when subjects reach a standard percentage (often 85 percent of age-predicted maximum heart rate), there is a *great variability* in maximum heart rate among individuals (Chap. 16). Many stress testing laboratories still utilize approaches that are not up to date.

A metanalysis of 147 published reports describing 24,074 patients who underwent both coronary angiography and exercise testing found wide variation in sensitivity and specificity.[18] The mean sensitivity was 68 percent and the mean specificity 77 percent. In a prospective study of 814 men that minimized workup bias, sensitivity was 45 percent and specificity 85 percent.[23] Therefore the true diagnostic value of the exercise ECG relates to its *relatively high specificity*. The modest sensitivity of the exercise ECG is generally lower than that of imaging procedures.[23a]

To improve the clinical usefulness of exercise ECG testing in the diagnosis of CAD, a treadmill score[22,24] was developed as well as a prognostic score that predicted 5-year survival using the amount of ST-segment depression, the degree of angina during exercise, and the duration of exercise[25] (Chap. 16). Other methods employed include the ST/HR slope, calculated from linear regression of ST-segment depression against heart rate (HR) during peak exercise,[26] and the simple ST/HR index, in which additional ST-segment depression is divided by the overall change in heart rate throughout the exercise period.[27] The cost-effectiveness of these techniques remains unknown.

Diagnostic testing is most valuable when the pretest probability of obstructive CAD is intermediate. In these conditions, the test result has the largest effect on the posttest probability of disease and thus on clinical decisions. Intermediate probability has been defined arbitrarily as between 10 and 90 percent; this definition has been used in several reports, including the ACC/AHA Exercise Test Guidelines.[20]

Special issues in ECG exercise testing include the effect of digoxin on ST–T wave changes, the usefulness of withholding beta-blocking drugs when possible, changes in ST-segment depression in patients with LBBB or RBBB, changes in the exercise ECG in patients with LV hypertrophy on ECG with or without repolarization abnormalities, and the usefulness of ECG testing in patients with resting ST-segment depression; these are discussed in great detail in Chap. 16 and Ref. 20.

Exercise-induced ST-segment depression usually occurs with LBBB and does not necessarily indicate ischemia.[28] However, in RBBB, ST-segment depression in the left chest leads (V_{5-6}) or inferior leads (II and aVF) during exercise has the same significance as when the resting ECG is normal.

The difficulties of using exercise testing for diagnosing obstructive CAD in women have led to speculation that initial stress imaging may be preferable to standard ECG stress testing. However, *women with a completely normal resting ECG* do not have a greater incidence of false-positive tests than men.[1]

REST ECHOCARDIOGRAPHY

Echocardiography can be useful for establishing a diagnosis of CAD and in defining the consequences of CAD in selected patients with chronic stable angina[1] (Chap. 15). However, most patients undergoing a diagnostic evaluation for angina do not need a resting echocardiogram.[1]

Chronic ischemic heart disease, with or without angina, can result in impaired systolic LV function. The extent and severity of regional and global abnormalities are important considerations in choosing appropriate medical or surgical therapy.[27] Echocardiographic findings that may help establish the diagnosis of chronic ischemic heart disease include regional systolic wall motion abnormalities, such as hypokinesis, akinesis, dyskinesis, and diminished segmental wall thickening.[28,29]

Mitral regurgitation demonstrated by Doppler echocardiography may result from global LV systolic dysfunction, regional papillary muscle dysfunction, scarring and shortening of the chordae tendineae, papillary muscle rupture, or other causes.[29]

STRESS IMAGING FOR DIAGNOSIS

Patients who should undergo cardiac stress testing with imaging for the diagnosis of CAD as opposed to exercise ECG alone include those in the following categories: (1) complete LBBB, electronically paced ventricular rhythm, preexcitation syndromes, and other similar ECG conduction abnormalities; (2) patients who have greater than 1 mm of resting ST-segment depression, including those with LV hypertrophy or those taking drugs such as digitalis; (3) patients who are unable to exercise to a level high enough to give meaningful results on routine stress ECG (pharmacologic stress imaging should be considered); and (4) patients with angina who have undergone prior revascularization, in whom localization of ischemia, establishing the functional significance of lesions, and demonstrating myocardial viability are important considerations. In our experience, false-positive ECG tests often occur in patients with hypertension, no evidence of LV hypertrophy on the ECG, but LV hypertrophy by echocardiography. Stress imaging is utilized in most patients with a history of hypertension even when the resting ECG is normal.

Several methods can be used to induce stress, including (1) exercise (treadmill or bicycle) and (2) pharmacologic techniques (dobutamine or vasodilator drugs). When the patient can exercise to an appropriate level of cardiovascular stress for 6 to 12 min, exercise stress testing is generally preferred to pharmacologic stress.[1]

Myocardial Perfusion Imaging In patients with suspected or known chronic stable angina, the largest accumulated experience in myocardial perfusion imaging (MPI) has been with the isotope thallium –201 (^{201}Tl); however, the available evidence suggests that the newer isotopes technetium-99m (^{99m}Tc) sestamibi and ^{99m}Tc tetrofosmin provide similar diagnostic accuracy (Chap. 19). Thus, for the most part, these isotopes can be used interchangeably, with a similar diagnostic accuracy for CAD.[29]

MPI may use either planar or single-photon-emission computed tomography (SPECT), visual analyses, or quantitative techniques (Chap. 19). Quantification using horizontal or circumferential profiles may improve the test's sensitivity, especially in patients with single-vessel disease. For the less commonly used ^{201}Tl planar scintigraphy, average reported values of sensitivity and specificity (uncorrected for posttest referral bias) have been in the range of 83 and 88 percent, respectively, for visual analysis and 90 and 80 percent, respectively, for quantitative analyses.[30] ^{201}Tl SPECT is generally more sensitive than planar imaging for diagnosing CAD, localizing hypoperfused vascular segments, identifying left anterior descending and left circumflex coronary artery stenoses, and accurately predicting multivessel CAD. The average sensitivity and specificity of exercise ^{201}Tl SPECT imaging (uncorrected for referral bias) are in the range of 89 and 76 percent, respectively, for qualitative analyses and 90 and 70 percent, respectively, for quantitative analyses.[30]

Pharmacologic stress uses dipyridamole or adenosine-induced coronary vasodilatation as an adjunct to myocardial perfusion imaging.[31] Dipyridamole planar scintigraphy has a high sensitivity (90 percent average) and acceptable specificity (70 percent average) for the detection of CAD. Dipyridamole SPECT with ^{201}Tl or ^{99m}Tc sestamibi is as accurate as planar imaging, and results of myocardial perfusion imaging during adenosine infusion are similar to those obtained with dipyridamole and exercise imaging[32] (Chap. 19). Evidence of CAD is demonstrated by redistribution defects comparing stress and resting scintigrams (ischemia), fixed defects at rest (scar), and LV dilatation or lung uptake of isotope during stress[30] (Chap. 19).

Stress Echocardiography Stress echocardiography is based on the assessment of myocardial thickening during stress compared with baseline (Chap. 15). Echocardiographic findings suggestive of myocardial ischemia include (1) decrease in wall motion in one or more LV segments with stress, (2) diminution in systolic wall thickening in one or more segments during stress, and (3) compensatory hyperkinesis in complementary (nonischemic) wall segments.[29] The use of digital acquisition and storage as well as side-by-side display of cine loops of LV images acquired at rest and at different levels of stress has improved efficiency and accuracy in interpretation of stress echocardiograms.[29]

In 36 studies including 3210 patients, the reported overall sensitivities (uncorrected for referral bias) ranged from 70 to 97 percent. The average overall sensitivity was 85 percent for exercise echocardiography and 82 percent for dobutamine stress echocardiography.[26] The reported sensitivity of exercise echocardiography for multivessel disease was higher (approximately 90 percent) than the sensitivity for single-vessel disease (approximately 79 percent). In this series of studies, specificity averaged approximately 86 percent for exercise echocardiography and 85 percent for dobutamine echocardiography.[29]

Pharmacologic stress echocardiography is best accomplished using dobutamine because it enhances myocardial contractile performance and wall motion, both of which can be evaluated directly by echocardiography (Chap. 15). In 36 studies, average sensitivity and specificity (uncorrected for referral bias) of dobutamine stress echocardiography in the detection of CAD were 82 and 85 percent, respectively.[29] Additional information concerning the sensitivity of exercise imaging in patients receiving beta blockers, the need for pharmacologic stress imaging in patients with LBBB, and the accuracy of myocardial perfusion and echocardiographic imaging in selected patient subgroups is included in Chaps. 15, 16, and 20.

Echocardiography and MPI have complementary roles, and both add value to routine stress ECG under appropriate circumstances.

TABLE 57-4 Comparative Advantages of Stress Echocardiography and Stress Radionuclide Perfusion Imaging in Diagnosis of CAD

Advantages of stress echocardiography
1. Higher specificity
2. Versatility. More extensive evaluations of cardiac anatomy and function
3. Greater convenience/efficacy/availability
4. Lower cost

Advantages of stress perfusion imaging
1. Higher technical success rate
2. Higher sensitivity, especially for single-vessel coronary disease involving the left circumflex
3. Better accuracy in evaluating possible ischemia when multiple resting LV wall motion abnormalities are present
4. More extensive published data base, especially in evaluation of prognosis

SOURCE: From Gibbons et al.[1]

The choice of which test to perform depends importantly on issues of local expertise, available facilities, and considerations of cost-effectiveness. A summary of the comparative advantages of stress myocardial perfusion imaging and stress echocardiography is provided in Table 57-4.

Coronary Angiography for Diagnosis   Direct referral for diagnostic coronary angiography in patients with chest pain is appropriate when noninvasive tests are contraindicated or likely to be inadequate due to the patient's illness, disability, or physical characteristics.[1] Many patients with obesity, chronic obstructive pulmonary disease, bronchospasm, and heart failure are likely to have suboptimal imaging tests; diagnostic coronary angiography will provide accurate diagnostic information with minimal risk.

Patients with noninvasive tests that are abnormal but not clearly diagnostic often require clarification of an uncertain diagnosis by coronary angiography. In certain cases a second noninvasive test (imaging modality) may be recommended for a patient with a low likelihood of CAD but an intermediate-risk treadmill result. Coronary angiography is likely to be most appropriate for a patient with a high-risk treadmill outcome.[1]

In individuals with symptoms consistent with but not diagnostic of stable angina, coronary angiography may be a necessity when the patient's occupation or activity could constitute a personal risk or a risk to others (e.g., pilots, firefighters, professional athletes).[1] When typical or atypical symptoms suggest stable angina and there is a high clinical probability of severe CAD, direct referral for coronary angiography may be indicated and cost-effective.[33] In diabetic patients, the diagnosis of chronic stable angina can be particularly difficult because of the absence of characteristic symptoms of myocardial ischemia due to the autonomic and sensory neuropathy (Chap. 78). Thus a lower threshold for coronary angiography is appropriate. Special groups for the consideration of coronary angiography include women, who more often have atypical chest discomfort, and the elderly, in whom symptoms are common but noninvasive testing may be difficult and comorbid conditions that mimic angina pectoris are frequent.[1] Coronary angiography is useful in patients in whom coronary artery spasm is suspected, in younger patients with

signs or symptoms of myocardial ischemia possibly due to coronary anomalies, in patients with a history of cocaine use, and in those who have survived sudden cardiac death or ventricular arrhythmias.[1,34] The ACC/AHA recommendations concerning the value of coronary angiography are listed in Table 57-5. Coronary angiographic findings in patients with chronic stable angina are depicted in Fig. 57-3.[34]

TABLE 57-5 Invasive Testing: Coronary Angiography (Recommendations for Coronary Angiography to Establish a Diagnosis in Patients with Suspected Angina, Including Those with Known CAD Who Have a Significant Change in Anginal Symptoms)

Class I
1. Patients with known or possible angina pectoris who have survived sudden cardiac death

Class IIa
1. Patients with an uncertain diagnosis after noninvasive testing in whom the benefit of a more certain diagnosis outweighs the risk and cost of coronary angiography
2. Patients who cannot undergo noninvasive testing due to disability, illness, or morbid obesity
3. Patients with an occupational requirement for a definitive diagnosis
4. Patients who by virtue of young age at onset of symptoms, noninvasive imaging, or other clinical parameters are suspected of having a nonatherosclerotic cause of myocardial ischemia (coronary artery anomaly, Kawasaki disease, primary coronary artery dissection, radiation-induced vasculoplasty)
5. Patients in whom coronary artery spasm is suspected and provocative testing may be necessary
6. Patients with a high pretest probability of left main or three-vessel CAD

Class IIb
1. Patients with recurrent hospitalization for chest pain in whom a definite diagnosis is judged necessary
2. Patients with an overriding desire for a definitive diagnosis and a greater than low probability of CAD

Class III
1. Patients with significant comorbidity in whom the risk of coronary arteriography outweighs the benefits of the procedure
2. Patients with an overriding personal desire for a definitive diagnosis and a low probability of CAD

Class I:	Conditions for which there is evidence and/or general agreement that a given procedure or treatment is useful and effective.
Class II:	Conditions for which there is conflicting evidence and/or a divergence of opinion about the usefulness/efficacy of a procedure or treatment.
IIa:	Weight of evidence/opinion is in favor of usefulness/efficacy.
IIb:	Usefulness/efficacy is less well established by evidence/opinion.
Class III:	Conditions for which there is evidence and/or general agreement that the procedure/treatment is not useful and in some cases may be harmful.

SOURCE: From Gibbons et al.[1]

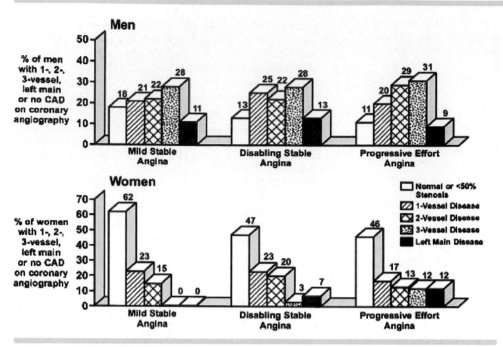

FIGURE 57-3 Prevalence of zero- to three-vessel CAD or coronary angiography in men and women related to severity of angina. (Modified from Douglas JS Jr, Hurst JW. Limitations of symptoms in the recognition of coronary atherosclerotic heart disease. In: Hurst JW, ed. *Update I: The Heart*. New York: McGraw-Hill; 1979:3. Reproduced with permission from the publisher and authors.)

DIFFERENTIAL DIAGNOSIS

Table 12-1 lists the differential diagnoses of angina pectoris. Usually, the distinction is clear if an accurate history is obtained and a complete, accurate physical examination is performed, as discussed in Chap. 12.

PATHOPHYSIOLOGY

In patients with stable angina pectoris due to atherosclerotic CAD, the correlation between the severity or extent of atherosclerosis and the magnitude of anginal symptoms is poor.[35] Also, no definite relation exists between the location of the chest discomfort and the site of the myocardial ischemia. Women have angina as the initial manifestation of CAD more commonly than men, who more often present with acute MI. The pathology of coronary atherosclerosis is discussed in detail in Chap. 44 and the nonatherosclerotic causes of CHD are detailed in Chap. 47.

A disparity between the supply of coronary blood flow (CBF) and the metabolic demands of the myocardium ($M\dot{V}O_2$) is the primary factor in ischemic heart disease. This imbalance may result in clinical manifestations of ischemia when $M\dot{V}O_2$ demand exceeds the capacity of the coronary arteries to deliver an adequate supply of oxygen. In normal hearts there is an excess CBF reserve, so that ischemia does not occur even with very vigorous exercise.[36]

Arteriosclerotic disease in either the epicardial coronary arteries or in the coronary microvasculature may cause an imbalance between supply and demand at even modest levels of exercise. An understanding of the determinants of CBF and myocardial metabolic demand is important in the management of chronic ischemic heart disease.[1]

Myocardial Oxygen Demand

The major relevant determinants of $M\dot{V}O_2$ are heart rate, contractility, and systolic wall stress (Fig. 57-4). A detailed discussion of the major and minor determinants of myocardial oxygen demand is presented in Chaps. 3 and 46. Heart rate is one of the most important determinants of $M\dot{V}O_2$ and can be altered easily by medical therapy in most patients.[37]

Myocardial contractility, partially reflected in the isovolumic rate of change of LV pressure (dP/dt), is a major determinant of $M\dot{V}O_2$ but not usually a primary factor for therapeutic intervention. However, LV systolic wall stress is an important consideration in the medical treatment of angina pectoris.

Systolic wall stress is directly related to the LV systolic pressure (P) and radius (r) and inversely related to wall thickness (h). Thus, reducing systolic pressure afterload (i.e., treating hypertension) can decrease $M\dot{V}O_2$. Decreasing preload by venodilation, and thus reducing LV size and oxygen consumption, is an important mechanism for the efficacy of nitrate therapy in angina pectoris. Positive inotropic agents may actually decrease $M\dot{V}O_2$ in patients with an enlarged left ventricle if the benefits of a diminished LV radius outweigh the negative results of increasing contractility.

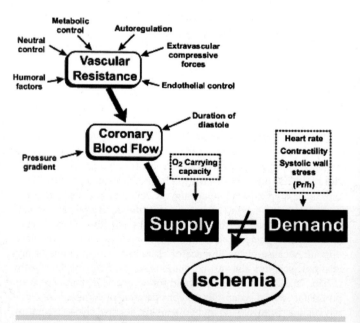

FIGURE 57-4 Factors controlling myocardial oxygen demand. *P*, systolic pressure; *r*, radius; *h*, wall thickness. (Modified from Ardehali A, Ports TA. Myocardial oxygen supply and demand. *Chest* 1990;98:699–705. Reproduced with permission from the publisher and authors.)

Myocardial Oxygen Supply

Oxygen supply to the myocardium depends on the oxygen-carrying capacity of the blood and on CBF (Fig. 57-4). Although a decrease in oxygen-carrying capacity (e.g., anemia) may contribute to the development or exacerbation of myocardial ischemia related to oxygen supply, it usually results from inadequate CBF.

The arteriolar resistance vessels are normally the primary regulators of CBF because the epicardial arteries are low-resistance conduits. Narrowing of the large coronary arteries transiently by vasospasm or permanently by obstructive lesions may increase the coronary resistance sufficiently to reduce CBF.

In the past decade, the pathophysiologic role of the coronary microvasculature has been recognized,[38,39] either concomitantly with atherosclerotic narrowing of the large-conduit arteries or predominantly in anginal syndromes with normal epicardial arteries ("syndrome X").[40,41]

The determinants of CBF are relatively complex and include (1) metabolic control, (2) autoregulation, (3) extravascular compressive forces, (4) duration of diastole, (5) humoral agents composed of both circulating hormones and autocrine and paracrine factors produced within the arterial wall and in particular by the endothelium, (6) neural control, and (7) the difference between aortic diastolic pressure and right atrial pressure[6] (Fig. 57-4).

CBF is relatively constant, being autoregulated during perfusion pressures between 60 and 160 mmHg.[42] Below a perfusion pressure of 60 mmHg, vasodilator reserve disappears and blood flow is directly related to perfusion pressure. Experimentally, loss of vasodilator reserve occurs distal to lesions with an 85 percent decrease in diameter.[43] A decrease in CBF, likely due to vasoconstriction and loss of vasodilator reserve, has been observed despite an increase in blood pressure during cold pressor stimulation in patients with significant CAD.[44]

Extravascular compressive forces—including intrapericardial, intramyocardial, and intraventricular pressures—are important in controlling CBF and account for 30 to 50 percent of the vascular resistance.[6] Since intramyocardial and intraventricular pressures are maximal during systole and are exerted maximally on the subendocardium, LV subendocardial blood flow decreases during systole. Thus, subendocardial blood flow is most vulnerable whenever total blood flow is decreased or $M\dot{V}O_2$ is increased and blood flow is limited. Because of the systolic compressive forces, the subendocardium is also critically dependent on the duration of diastole for its blood flow (Chap. 46).

CBF is regulated by systemic hormones and by neural control mechanisms similar to those of other vascular beds. Angiotensin II is a coronary vasoconstrictor; beta-adrenergic agonists dilate and alpha-adrenergic agonists constrict coronary arteries, although there are some regional differences in distribution of receptors in vessels of different sizes.[6] Importantly, the integrated vasomotor response to the various vasoactive stimuli affecting a coronary artery or arteriole appears greatly influenced by the functional state of the endothelium (Chap. 46).

Endothelial Function and Coronary Vasomotor Control

The phenomenon of endothelium-dependent relaxation[45] and the identification of endothelium-derived relaxing factor as nitric oxide[46] are discussed in detail in Chap. 7. The defect in endothelium-dependent dilatation in atherosclerotic epicardial coronary arteries that vasoconstrict in response to stimuli that normally cause vasodilation—such as acetylcholine, exercise, or cold pressor testing—is discussed in Chap. 46.

The majority view is that endothelium-dependent vasodilator mechanisms are predominant in nondiseased epicardial coronary arteries. Thus interventions such as exercise,[47] mental stress,[48] cold pressor testing,[49] or even pacing-induced tachycardia,[50] that normally induce increases in $M\dot{V}O_2$ and flow, are associated with epicardial coronary artery dilatation that is partially endothelium-dependent. The presence of even nonocclusive, early atherosclerosis appears to attenuate this vasodilator mechanism and results in prevailing constrictor forces.[6]

The local infusion of the alpha-adrenergic agonist phenylephrine does not constrict normal coronary arteries of patients with intact endothelium-dependent dilatation.[51] However, vasoconstriction occurs in even minimally diseased coronary arteries at low concentrations of phenylephrine. Thus, in CAD, there appears to be both loss of endothelium-dependent dilatation and an enhanced vasoconstrictor sensitivity to catecholamines. This disordered vasomotor control is an important contributor to the variability in anginal threshold commonly observed in many patients.[52]

The Microvasculature and Coronary Ischemia

The recognition of the likely importance of the coronary microvascular resistance vessels in the pathogenesis of angina pectoris resulted from studies of patients with angina-like chest pain and angiographically normal epicardial coronary arteries.[53–57]

The coronary etiology of the chest pain is supported by the frequent but not universal evidence of ischemia in these patients during exercise testing[58]; many are found to have abnormal vasodilator reserve.[59] Specifically in patients with angina and angiographically normal coronary arteries, endothelium-dependent vasodilatation of the resistance arteries is often diminished relative to controls.[60]

In contrast, the flow responses to the non-endothelium-dependent dilators, isosorbide dinitrate and papaverine is no different between patients and controls, suggesting that the intrinsic vasodilator capacity of the resistance arteries is not defective. Similar defects in endothelium-dependent coronary vasodilation have been observed in LV hypertrophy associated with hypertension, another condition that may be associated with angina pectoris with normal coronary angiography.[60]

The histopathology of biopsy specimens from patients with normal epicardial coronaries but with anginal syndromes has demonstrated capillary narrowing with swollen endothelium encroaching on the lumen as well as decreased capillary density. Thus, the coronary microvasculature can develop dysfunction of vasomotor control mechanisms and of endothelium-dependent vasodilation that may become clinically significant in the setting of increased $M\dot{V}O_2$. The loss of vasodilator reserve and the actual constriction of resistance arterioles may induce ischemia and chest pain.[61,62]

Spectrum of Pathophysiologic Mechanisms Associated with the Stable Coronary Ischemia Syndromes

Symptomatic myocardial ischemia due primarily to microvascular abnormalities in the control of coronary vascular tone partially explains the characteristics of stable angina syndromes. Angina pectoris or anginal equivalents with a *relatively constant* threshold for inducing ischemic symptoms due to a fixed stenoses of an epicardial coronary artery also in part determine the spectrum of anginal symptoms. Most patients have a somewhat variable threshold for inducing angina from day to day or even at different times of the day.

Interestingly, the same activity that causes chest discomfort in the early morning may not do so in the afternoon or evening. Yet the patient may have a consistent level of exercise for inducing ischemia on protocol exercise testing because of the augmented $M\dot{V}O_2$ that is due to increases in heart rate, contractility, and blood pressure and the associated increment in systolic wall stress. This is explained by the presence of both flow-limiting epicardial coronary stenosis and associated episodic vasoconstriction. Maseri et al.[52] have termed this phenomenon *mixed angina.* Myocardial ischemia is induced by both an increase in $M\dot{V}O_2$ and a decrease in CBF. The site(s) of vasoconstriction may be at an epicardial stenosis, in the microvasculature, or at both locations.[63] The concept of a *variable flow reserve* that interacts with differing metabolic demands to produce intermittent ischemia is depicted in Fig. 57-5A and *B.*

In the stable anginal syndromes, the predominant vasoconstrictors are likely neural and hormonal, whereas in the unstable (acute) coronary syndromes, platelet and coagulation products, as well as inflammatory mediators are important contributors (Chap. 51). Patients with predominantly vasoconstrictor pathophysiology in an epicardial vessel have been classified as having *vasospastic angina* or *Prinzmetal's variant angina* (Chap. 51).

Cellular Basis for the Clinical Manifestations of Ischemia

The cellular effects of myocardial ischemia are discussed in detail in Chaps. 45 and 46. The rapid decreases in systolic function and diastolic compliance that are associated with creatine phosphate deple-

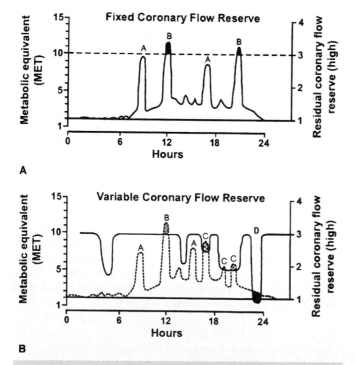

A

B

FIGURE 57-5 Concept of variable coronary flow reserve in the presence of variable atherosclerotic obstruction. *A.* Episodes not associated with ischemia. *B.* Ischemic episode occurring at levels of exercise exceeding threshold of residual coronary flow reserve. *C.* Ischemic episodes occurring at lower levels of exercise when residual coronary flow is reduced. *D.* Ischemic episodes occurring at rest in the presence of maximal reduction in residual coronary flow reserve. ——, residual coronary flow reserve; ---, variable atherosclerotic obstruction as measured by MED. (Modified from Cohn PF. Mechanisms of myocardial ischemia. *Am J Cardiol* 1992;70:14G–18G; and Maseri A. Role of coronary artery spasm in symptomatic and silent myocardial ischemia. *J Am Coll Cardiol* 1987;9:249–262. Reproduced with permission from the authors and publishers.)

tion and ionic shifts will increase LV end-diastolic pressure. Elevated pulmonary vascular pressures often stimulate mechanoreceptors and mediate the dyspnea response. Dyspnea may be associated with angina or may be present as an anginal equivalent in patients who do not develop chest discomfort.

The metabolic abnormalities due to ischemia cause cellular depolarization and the flow of electric currents between normal and ischemic areas that are reflected on the ECG.[6] ST-segment depression reflecting subendocardial underperfusion is the most common ECG manifestation of ischemia in chronic stable angina during ambulatory recordings or exercise testing.[64] The ST-segment depression observed during exercise testing or ambulatory ECG recordings usually is not associated with complex or life-threatening ventricular arrhythmias; exercise-induced ventricular ectopic activity is not a reliable predictor of cardiac events in asymptomatic persons.[65]

The Coronary Ischemia Cascade

Studies in which hemodynamic and ECG recordings have been performed during spontaneous episodes of ischemia, either in unstable patients or during balloon inflation at angioplasty, have provided insights into the sequential responses evoked at the onset of ischemia and are consistent with those described in animals undergoing acute coronary artery ligation[66] (Fig. 57-1).

After balloon inflation, impaired LV compliance occurs within a few seconds and is followed rapidly by systolic contractile dysfunction causing a decrease in LV ejection fraction of up to 30 percent within 10 s.[66] ECG changes occur at about 20 s, and angina, if it occurs, appears at between 25 and 30 s.

Considering this "ischemic cascade," there are likely to be episodes that do not progress to angina. Since many patients do not perceive coronary ischemic pain or have high pain thresholds, the common occurrence of asymptomatic (silent) ischemia in individuals with CAD is not surprising.

Hemodynamic measurements and ECG recording in patients with spontaneous or exercise-induced ischemia provide physiologic explanations for many of the classic clinical observations about angina.

As noted earlier, an anginal episode may be associated with new physical findings, particularly the development of an S_4 and of mitral regurgitation due to papillary muscle dysfunction.

Circadian Rhythm of Coronary Ischemia

The prevalence of MI, unstable angina, variant angina, and silent ischemia is greatest in the morning, during the first few hours after awakening, and the threshold for precipitating anginal attacks in patients with stable angina also appears to be lowest in the morning.[67,69] Patients often develop ST-segment depression and angina at lower thresholds during exercise testing in the morning than later in the day. Studies with ambulatory ECG recordings have confirmed that the incidence of both painful and painless episodes of ST-segment depression is highest in the morning[68] and, in particular, in the first few hours after awakening (Fig. 57-6).

The diurnal variation in ischemic threshold is attributed to the endogenous rhythms of catecholamine secretion and to the sensitivity to coronary vasoconstrictors, both of which appear to peak in the morning. The increase in sympathetic nervous system activity is associated with increases in heart rate, blood pressure, contractility, and $M\dot{V}O_2$. The lowered morning anginal threshold and the higher morning systolic blood pressure have *important therapeutic implications.* A decrease in the frequency of ischemia can be achieved by blunting the morning surge of beta-adrenergic stimulation by the administration of beta blockers. The control of hypertension by the *early morning use of antihypertensive drugs* is also important. In pa-

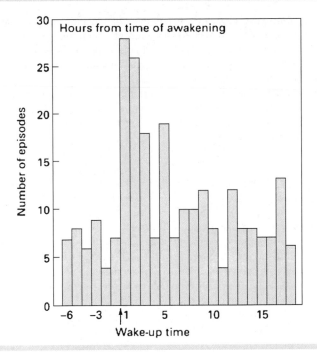

FIGURE 57-6 When the frequency of episodes is displayed hourly from the time of awakening, the peak activity occurs in the first and second hour after arising. (From Rocco et al.[68] Reproduced with permission from the authors and publishers.)

tients with recurrent morning angina, the use of nitroglycerin (NTG) soon after awakening may prevent angina in many instances.

Mechanisms of Anginal Pain

Anginal pain is a useful warning, but it is often too insensitive. Its mechanism is discussed in detail in Chap. 12. Pain stimuli arise within the myocardium and most likely stimulate free nerve endings in or near small coronary vessels. Impulses travel in afferent unmyelinated or small myelinated cardiac sympathetic nerves through the upper five thoracic sympathetic ganglia to dorsal horn cells and through the spinothalamic tract of the thalamus and then to the cortex.[69]

Integration and modification of these impulses occur at several levels, including the cerebral cortex. This modulation may also contribute importantly to the variability in anginal threshold. At the cortical level, psychosocial and cultural factors may alter the perception of pain. The radiation patterns of angina are determined by the levels of the thoracic spinal cord that share the sensory inputs from the heart and from somatic structures.

The nature of the stimuli causing angina has been poorly delineated. The causes are probably chemical, and several molecules—including kinins, serotonin, hydrogen ions, and inflammatory mediators—have been proposed. By contrast, adenosine, which is increased during ischemia, has been shown to cause anginal-type pain during intravenous infusion in normal volunteers.[70]

ASYMPTOMATIC (SILENT) ISCHEMIA IN STABLE CAD

The presence of unrecognized myocardial infarction due to the absence of pain was mentioned by Herrick in 1912.[71] The frequent presence of extensive CAD and MI at autopsies of apparently asymptomatic persons was recognized later.[72] Direct evidence of asympto-

matic (silent) ischemia during ECG exercise testing and ambulatory ECG recording stimulated interest in this clinical entity.[73]

Prevalence of Silent Ischemia

Asymptomatic ischemic episodes may be present in patients with any of the ischemic coronary syndromes and may be observed in patients who are totally asymptomatic or who have chest discomfort with some episodes of ischemia but not others.[74] The prevalence of silent ischemic episodes approximates 40 percent in patients with chronic stable angina and in those with a history of instability.[75] The incidence of asymptomatic ischemia occurring in individuals with extensive CAD has been estimated at 5 percent.[76] ST-segment depression of 60 s or more on ambulatory recordings is uncommon in patients with no evidence of CAD.[77,78]

A prospective study of 68-year-old men with a 9.9 and a 6.6 percent prevalence of a history of angina pectoris or MI, respectively, demonstrated ST-segment depression on ambulatory ECG recordings. In 25 percent,[79] 92 percent of the "ischemic" episodes were asymptomatic, but ST-segment depression was associated with an increased risk of coronary events.

The true prevalence of silent ischemia is difficult to determine and obviously will depend on age and the presence and extent of CAD. In the presence of CAD, however, it is apparent that episodes of asymptomatic ischemia are often more common than are painful episodes.[80]

Screening for Silent Ischemia

In the absence of symptoms, ambulatory ECG monitoring can reveal transient ST-segment depression suggestive of CAD. However, as indicated in the "ACC/AHA Guidelines for Ambulatory Electrocardiography,"[81] there is presently no evidence that ambulatory ECG monitoring provides reliable information concerning ischemia in asymptomatic subjects without known CAD.

In the absence of symptoms, EBCT is sometimes used as a means of screening for CAD. However, as indicated in the "ACC/AHA Expert Consensus Document" on this topic, available data is insufficient to support recommending EBCT for this purpose to asymptomatic members of the general public.

Physicians are often confronted with concerned asymptomatic patients with abnormal findings on ambulatory ECG and EBCT. Although the published data on this situation are scant, in the absence of symptoms, such patients have a low pretest probability of significant CAD. A negative exercise test result only confirms the low probability of disease, and a positive test result may not increase the probability of disease enough to make a clinical difference. The presence of severe coronary calcification on EBCT is common in older individuals. Because the evidence supporting the value of additional testing after EBCT is scant, the ACC/AHA Committee on Chronic Stable Angina suggests that further testing be reserved for individuals with severe calcification, defined as a calcium score greater than the 75th percentile for age and gender-matched populations.[82] Asymptomatic patients with abnormal findings on ambulatory ECG or EBCT who are able to exercise can be evaluated with exercise ECG testing, although the efficacy of exercise ECG testing in asymptomatic patients is not well established. Stress imaging procedures (i.e., either stress myocardial perfusion imaging or stress echocardiography) are generally not indicated as the initial stress test in most such patients. However, in patients with resting ECG abnormalities that preclude adequate interpretation of the exercise ECG, stress imaging procedures are preferable to the exercise ECG for the evaluation of severe coronary calcification on EBCT. If the baseline ECG shows preexcitation or greater than 1 mm of ST-segment depression, exercise stress imaging procedures are preferred. In patients who are unable to exercise, pharmacologic stress imaging is preferable to exercise ECG testing.

Pathophysiology of Silent Ischemia

An obvious possible explanation for painful as opposed to asymptomatic ischemia is that the ischemia, and thus the noxious stimulus, is more severe in the former. The correlation between the duration and severity of an ischemic episode and the development of anginal pain in chronic stable angina, however, is only fair.[82] Symptomatic episodes last slightly longer and have a slightly higher frequency of severe ST-segment depression than do painless ones, but there is considerable overlap.[83]

An alternative reason for lack of pain with myocardial ischemia is neurologic.[84] Neuropathy with defective sensory efferent nerves definitely occurs in some patients and is particularly prevalent in diabetics (Chap. 86). Modification of pain stimuli in the central nervous system (CNS) may contribute importantly to the variable expression of ischemic pain. This modulation may occur in spinal centers because transcutaneous nerve,[84] esophageal,[85] and dorsal column stimulation[86] can increase anginal threshold. Modulation of pain-mediating efferent messages also may occur at supraspinal centers. Psychological or cultural factors also may affect pain perception. Subsets of patients with predominantly painless ischemic episodes tend to have a higher threshold and tolerance for painful stimuli than those who experience pain.[87-89] Thus processing of pain signals in the CNS likely contributes to the variability of anginal threshold or to the absence of pain.

Diabetic patients have a relatively high incidence of painless MI and definite silent ischemic episodes as documented by exercise testing and ambulatory ECG recordings (Chap. 86).[90-93]

Causes and Functional Consequences of Asymptomatic Ischemia

Ischemia caused by the increased $M\dot{V}O_2$ associated with exercise testing is often silent.[94] Ambulatory ECG recordings have provided insights into potential mechanisms of many episodes of painless or painful ischemia during daily living. The heart rate at the onset of ischemia is generally lower with ambulatory ECG recordings than with exercise testing.[95] These observations suggest that coronary vasoconstriction likely contributes to many episodes of silent ischemia.

Clinical Implications of Silent Ischemia

Asymptomatic silent ischemia is a common component of both acute and chronic coronary artery syndromes. Thus it may have the same clinical importance as symptomatic ischemia.[96] The important indicators of risk are the extent and severity of ischemia, regardless of how it is detected or manifest, and whether the disease is in a stable or unstable phase. Whether ECG monitoring for silent ischemia and changing therapy to decrease or eliminate it diminish morbidity and mortality in a cost-effective manner is unproven.[78]

Therapeutically, it is appropriate to treat high-risk ischemia whether or not it is associated with pain. Persistent, severe ischemia despite medical therapy should lead to consideration of myocardial revascularization.

Treatment of Silent Ischemia

Most medical or interventional strategies that reduce symptomatic ischemia will also reduce asymptomatic ischemia.[97-99] The available data from early clinical trials of the treatment of asymptomatic (silent) ischemia in stable CAD have recently been summarized.[97-99] NTG is highly effective, and beta blockers appear to be somewhat more effective than calcium antagonists. Calcium antagonists may be most effective in preventing ischemia occurring at lower heart rates, because coronary artery vasoconstriction may be a predominant factor in this situation. In patients with ischemic CAD, the total ischemic burden and not just symptoms may be the appropriate therapeutic target.

RISK STRATIFICATION OF PATIENTS WITH CHRONIC ISCHEMIC HEART DISEASE

The prognosis for the patient with chronic CHD is usually related to four patient factors.[1] *LV performance* is the strongest predictor of long-term survival in patients with CHD, and the ejection fraction (EF) is the most often used measure of the presence and the degree of LV dysfunction. The second predictive factor is the *anatomic extent and severity* of atherosclerotic involvement of the coronary arteries. The number of stenosed coronary arteries is the most common measure of this factor. The third patient factor affecting prognosis is evidence of a *recent coronary plaque rupture,* indicating a much higher short-term risk for cardiac death or nonfatal MI. Worsening clinical symptoms with unstable features are an important clinical marker of a complicated plaque. The fourth prognostic factor is *general health and noncoronary comorbidity.*

History and Physical Examination for Prognosis

Useful information relative to *risk stratification* can be obtained from the history. This includes demographics such as age and gender as well as a medical history focusing on hypertension, diabetes, hypercholesterolemia, smoking, peripheral vascular disease, and previous MI.

The physical examination can be useful in risk stratification by defining the presence or absence of signs that may alter the probability of *severe* CAD.[1] Useful physical findings include those suggesting vascular disease (abnormal fundi, decreased peripheral pulses, bruits), long-standing hypertension (high blood pressure, abnormal fundi), aortic valve stenoses or hypertrophic obstructive cardiomyopathy (systolic murmur, abnormal carotid arterial pulse, abnormal LV impulse), left-sided heart failure (third heart sounds, displaced LV impulse, bibasilar rales), and right-sided heart failure (elevated jugular venous pressure, hepatomegaly, ascites, peripheral edema).[1] Hubbard et al.[100] identified five clinical markers that independently predicted severe three-vessel and left main CAD—including age, typical angina, diabetes, male gender, and prior MI—which were used to develop a five-point cardiac risk score.

ECG and Chest Roentgenogram for Prognosis

Patients with chronic stable angina who have abnormalities on resting ECG are at greater risk than those with normal ECGs.[101] Evidence of one or more prior MIs on ECG indicates a greater risk for cardiac events. The presence of Q waves in multiple ECG leads, often accompanied by an R wave in lead V_1 (posterior infarction), is commonly associated with a markedly reduced left ventricular ejection fraction (LVEF)—an important factor in the natural history of patients with CAD.[102] Persistent ST-segment–T-wave inversions, particularly in V_1 to V_3, are associated with an increased prevalence of future coronary events and a poor prognosis.[103]

On the chest roentgenogram, the presence of cardiomegaly, a LV aneurysm, or pulmonary venous congestion is associated with a poorer long-term prognosis than would apply to patients with a normal chest x-ray.

The presence of calcium in the coronary arteries on chest x-ray or fluoroscopy in patients with symptomatic CAD suggests an increased risk of cardiac events. Although the presence and amount of coronary artery calcification by EBCT correlate *to some extent* with the severity of CAD, there is considerable patient variation.[17]

Noninvasive Testing for Prognosis

ASSESSMENT OF LV FUNCTION

LV global systolic function and volumes are important predictors of prognosis in patients with cardiac disease.[1] In patients with chronic CHD, LVEF measured at rest by either echocardiography (usually qualitative and less reliable) or radionuclide ventriculography (RVG) is predictive of long-term prognosis. As LVEF decreases, subsequent mortality increases; a resting ejection fraction of greater than 35 percent is associated with an annual mortality rate of more than 3 percent.[1]

Radionuclide LVEF may be measured at rest using a gamma camera, a ^{99m}Tc tracer, and first-pass or gated equilibrium blood pool angiography (RVG) or by gated SPECT perfusion imaging using a technetium-based isotope[29] (Chap. 19). LV diastolic function can also be estimated from RVG diastolic filling curves. LV systolic function can be measured by quantitative two-dimensional echocardiography (Chap. 15), and LV diastolic function can be assessed by transmitral valve Doppler recording.[102]

In patients with chronic stable angina and a history of previous MI, segmental wall motion abnormalities are apparent not only in the zone(s) of prior infarction but also in areas with ischemic "stunning" or "hibernation" of myocardium that are nonfunctional but still viable.[103] In patients with CHD, the presence, severity, and mechanism of mitral regurgitation can be detected reliably using transthoracic and transesophageal two-dimensional imaging and Doppler echocardiographic techniques (Chap. 15).

Echocardiography is the definitive test for detecting intracardiac thrombi.[29] LV thrombi are most common in patients with stable angina pectoris who have significant LV wall motion abnormalities. In patients with anterior and apical infarctions, the presence of LV thrombi denotes an increased risk of both embolism and death (Chap. 52).

ECG EXERCISE TESTING

Unless cardiac catheterization is clearly indicated, symptomatic patients with suspected or known CAD who have no confounding features on their resting ECG and are able to exercise should usually undergo exercise testing to assess the risk of future cardiac events[1] (Chap. 16). Also, demonstration of exercise-induced ischemia is desirable for most patients who are being considered for revascularization.[104]

Several studies have shown that risk assessment in patients with a normal ECG who are not taking digoxin and who are physically capable should *usually* start with the exercise test[1,105] (Chap. 16). In contrast, a stress-imaging technique should be used for patients with ECG evidence of LV hypertrophy, widespread resting ST-segment depression (>1 mm), complete LBBB, ventricular paced rhythm, or preexcitation.[19] The primary evidence that ECG exercise testing can be used to estimate prognosis and assist in management decisions consists of seven observational studies.[1,20] One of the strongest and most consistent prognostic markers is the *maximum exercise capacity.*[106,107]

A second group of *prognostic markers* relates to exercise-induced ischemia (Chap. 16). ST-segment depression and ST-segment elevation (in leads without pathologic Q waves) best summarize the prognostic

TABLE 57-6 Survival According to Risk Groups Based on Duke Treadmill Scores

Risk Group (score)	Percentage of Total	Four-Year Survival	Annual Mortality (percent)
Low (≥ +5)	62	0.99	0.25
Moderate (−10 to +4)	34	0.95	1.25
High (< −10)	4	0.79	5.0

SOURCE: From Gibbons et al.[1]

information related to ischemia. Other variables are less powerful, including angina, the number of leads with ST-segment depression, the configuration of the ST-segment depression, and the duration of ST-segment deviation into the recovery phase.

The *Duke treadmill score* combines this information and provides a way to calculate risk.[108,109] This score equals the exercise time in minutes minus five times the peak ST-segment deviation during or after exercise (in millimeters) minus four times the angina index (which has a value of 0 if there is no angina, 1 if angina occurs, and 2 if angina is the reason for stopping the test). Among outpatients with suspected CAD, two-thirds of those with scores indicating low risk had a 4-year survival of 99 percent (average annual mortality of 0.25 percent); the 4 percent who had scores indicating high risk had a 4-year survival of 79 percent (average annual mortality rate of 5 percent) (Table 57-6). Recent studies indicate that this approach is equally applicable in men and women.[110]

STRESS IMAGING FOR PROGNOSIS

Stress-imaging studies using radionuclide MPI techniques or two-dimensional (2D) echocardiography at rest and during stress are useful for risk stratification and determining the most effective treatment strategy for patients with chronic stable angina.[1] Whenever feasible, treadmill or bicycle exercise should be used as the most desirable forms of stress because exercise provides the most information concerning a patient's symptoms, cardiovascular function, and hemodynamic response during usual activity (Chap. 19). The inability to perform a bicycle or exercise treadmill test has been shown to be a serious and negative prognostic factor for patients with chronic CAD.[1]

In patients unable to exercise adequately, various types of pharmacologic stress are commonly used for *risk stratification*. The type of pharmacologic stress selected will depend on specific patient factors, including the patient's heart rate and blood pressure, evidence of bronchospastic disease, the presence of LBBB or a pacemaker, and the likelihood of ventricular arrhythmias. Pharmacologic agents are often used to increase workload or cause an increase in overall CBF.[111,112]

Myocardial perfusion imaging (MPI) is an important technique in the risk stratification of patients with CAD.[29] Either planar (uncommonly) or SPECT imaging using ^{201}Tl or ^{99m}Tc perfusion tracers with images obtained during stress and at rest provides important information concerning the severity and location of functionally significant CAD (Chap. 19).

Stress echocardiography is also used frequently for detecting the presence and amount of ischemia in patients with chronic stable angina. However, the amount of prognostic data obtained with this approach is less well documented. Nevertheless, the presence or absence of inducible myocardial wall motion abnormalities has useful predictive value in patients undergoing exercise or pharmacologic stress echocardiography.[29,110–115] A negative stress echocardiographic study denotes a low cardiovascular event rate during follow-up.

MYOCARDIAL PERFUSION IMAGING FOR PROGNOSIS

Normal poststress thallium scan results are highly predictive of a benign prognosis even in patients with known CAD.[1] An analysis of 16 studies involving 3594 patients followed for an average of 29 months indicated a rate per year of cardiac death and MI of 0.9 percent, differing little from that of the general population.[116,117] In an often quoted prospective study of 5183 consecutive patients undergoing myocardial perfusion imaging during stress and later at rest, patients with normal scans were at low risk (<0.5 percent per year) for the composite endpoint of cardiac death and MI during 642 ± 226 days of mean follow-up[118] (Chap. 19).

The number, extent, and sites of abnormalities on stress MPI reflect the location and severity of functionally significant coronary artery stenoses (Chap. 19). Lung uptake of ^{201}Tl on postexercise or pharmacologic stress images is an indicator of stress-induced global LV dysfunction and is associated with pulmonary venous hypertension in the presence of multivessel CAD.[119] Transient poststress ischemic LV dilatation also correlates with severe two- or three-vessel CAD (Chap. 19). SPECT may be more accurate than planar imaging for determining the size of defects, detecting particularly left circumflex CAD, and localizing abnormalities in the distribution of individual coronary arteries. More false-positive results are likely to result from photon attenuation during SPECT imaging, however.

The assessment of both myocardial perfusion and LV function at rest may help determine the extent and severity of CAD.[1] This combined information can be obtained by performing two separate exercise tests [e.g., stress MPI and stress radionuclide ventriculography (RVG)] or by combining the studies after a single exercise test (first-pass RVG) with ^{99m}Tc-based agents followed by MPI or by perfusion imaging using ECG gating. The use of ECG-gated ^{99m}Tc sestamibi SPECT imaging at rest and with exercise or pharmacologic stress provides important prognostic information concerning LVEF and the extent of reversible ischemia (Chap. 19).

Pharmacologic stress perfusion imaging for risk stratification is preferable to *exercise perfusion* imaging in patients with LBBB.[1] Recently, 245 patients with LBBB underwent SPECT imaging with ^{201}Tl or ^{99m}Tc sestamibi during dipyridamole or adenosine stress.[1,119] The 3-year survival was 57 percent in the high-risk group compared with 87 percent in the low-risk group ($p = 0.001$).

STRESS ECHOCARDIOGRAPHY FOR PROGNOSIS

Stress echocardiography is both sensitive and specific for detecting inducible myocardial ischemia in patients with chronic stable angina.[29] Compared with standard exercise ECG treadmill testing, stress echocardiography provides additional clinical value for detecting and localizing myocardial ischemia. Several studies indicate that patients can be risk-stratified by the presence or absence of inducible wall motion abnormalities on stress echocardiography.[110–115] The presence of ischemia on the exercise echocardiogram is independent and additive to clinical and exercise data in predicting cardiac events in both men and women.[120,121]

Coronary Angiography for Prognosis

The availability of powerful but expensive therapeutic strategies to reduce the long-term morbidity and mortality of CAD dictates that the patients most likely to benefit because of increased risk be defined. The assessment of cardiac risk and the need for further testing usually

begins with simple, repeatable, and inexpensive use of the history and physical examination, which often leads to noninvasive or invasive testing, depending on outcome. Clinical risk factors are generally additive, and a crude estimate of 1-year mortality can be obtained from these variables. Methods for the accurate identification of vulnerable or high-risk plaques are lacking. However, magnetic resonance imaging (MRI) offers significant promise in this regard.[1]

Risk stratification of patients with chronic stable angina by stress testing with exercise or pharmacologic agents has been shown to permit the identification of groups of patients with low, intermediate, or high risk for subsequent cardiac events.[1,29,30]

The randomized trials of coronary artery bypass grafting (CABG) demonstrated that patients randomized to initial CABG had a lower mortality than those assigned to medical therapy only if they were at substantial risk (annual mortality > 3 percent).[122,123] Coronary angiography is appropriate for patients whose mortality risk is in this range. Noninvasive test findings that identify high-risk patients are listed in Table 57-7 Patients identified as at high risk are generally referred for coronary arteriography independent of their symptomatic status. The ACC/AHA guidelines for risk stratification using

TABLE 57-7 Noninvasive Risk Stratification

High risk (greater than 3% annual mortality rate)
1. Severe resting left ventricular dysfunction (LVEF < 35%)
2. High-risk treadmill score (score ≤ −11)
3. Severe exercise left ventricular dysfunction (exercise LVEF < 35%)
4. Stress-induced large perfusion defect (particularly if anterior)
5. Stress-induced multiple perfusion defects of moderate size
6. Large, fixed perfusion defect with LV dilatation or increased lung uptake (thallium 201)
7. Stress-induced moderate perfusion defect with LV dilatation or increased lung uptake (thallium 201)
8. Echocardiographic wall motion abnormality (involving greater than two segments) developing at low dose of dobutamine (≤10 mg/kg/min) or at a low heart rate (<120 beats/per minute)
9. Stress echocardiographic evidence of extensive ischemia

Intermediate risk (1% < 3% annual mortality rate)
1. Mild/moderate resting left ventricular dysfunction (LVEF = 35% − 49%)
2. Intermediate-risk treadmill score[a] (− 11 < score < 5)
3. Stress-induced moderate perfusion defect without LV dilatation or increased lung intake (thallium 201)
4. Limited stress echocardiographic ischemia with a wall motion abnormality only at higher doses of dobutamine involving less than or equal to two segments

Low risk (less than 1% annual mortality rate)
1. Low-risk treadmill score (score ≥ 5)
2. Normal or small myocardial perfusion defect at rest or with stress
3. Normal stress echocardiographic wall motion or no change of limited resting wall motion abnormalities during stress

[a]Duke treadmill score; see text.
SOURCE: From Gibbons et al.[1]

coronary angiography in patients with stable angina are listed in Table 57-8.

TREATMENT OF ASYMPTOMATIC PATIENTS WITH KNOWN CAD AND CHRONIC STABLE ANGINA

Even in asymptomatic patients, aspirin and beta blockers are recommended in those with prior MI. The data in support of these recommendations are detailed in the "ACC/AHA Guideline for the Management of Patients with Acute Myocardial Infarction."[124]

In the absence of prior MI, patients with documented CAD on the basis of noninvasive testing or coronary angiography probably also benefit from aspirin, although the data on this specific subset of patients are limited.

Several studies have investigated the potential role of beta blockers in patients with asymptomatic ischemia demonstrated on exercise testing and/or ambulatory monitoring.[20,81] The data generally demonstrate a benefit from beta-blocker therapy, but not all trials have been positive.

Lipid-lowering therapy in asymptomatic patients with documented CAD was demonstrated to decrease the rate of adverse ischemic events in the Scandinavian Simvastatin Survival Study (4S) trial as well as in the CARE study and the Long-term Intervention with Pravastatin in Ischaemic Disease (LIPID) trial, as previously mentioned.

ACE inhibitors are indicated in patients with CAD who have diabetes and/or systemic dysfunction (Chap. 43).

TABLE 57-8 Coronary Angiography for Risk Stratification in Patients with Chronic Stable Angina

Class I
1. Patients with disabling [Canadian Cardiovascular Society (CCS) classes III and IV] chronic stable angina despite medical therapy.
2. Patients with high-risk criteria on noninvasive testing regardless of anginal severity.
3. Patients with angina who have survived sudden cardiac death or serious ventricular arrhythmia.
4. Patients with angina and symptoms and signs of CHF.
5. Patients with clinical characteristics that indicate a high likelihood of severe CAD.

Class IIa
1. Patients with significant LV dysfunction (ejection fraction less than 45 percent), CCS class I or II angina, and demonstrable ischemia but less than high-risk criteria on noninvasive testing.
2. Patients with inadequate prognostic information after noninvasive testing.

Class IIb
1. Patients with CCS class I or II angina, preserved LV function (ejection fraction greater than 45 percent), and less than high-risk criteria on noninvasive testing.
2. Patients with CCS class III or IV angina, which with medical therapy improves to class I or II.
3. Patients with CCS class I or II angina but intolerance (unacceptable side effects) to adequate medical therapy.

Class III
1. Patients with CCS class I or II angina who respond to medical therapy and who have no evidence of ischemia on noninvasive testing.
2. Patients who prefer to avoid revascularization.

TREATMENT OF CHRONIC STABLE ANGINA

There are two major purposes in the treatment of stable angina. The first is to prevent MI and death and *thereby increase the quantity of life.* The second is to reduce symptoms of angina and the frequency and severity of ischemia, which should *improve the quality of life.* Therapy directed toward preventing death has the highest priority. The choice of therapy often depends on the clinical response to initial medical therapy, although some patients (and many physicians) prefer coronary revascularization in situations where either may be successful. It must be stressed that the pharmacologic treatment of chronic CAD has greatly improved and may even be superior to revascularization therapy for many patients.[125] Patient education, cost-effectiveness, and patient preference are important components in this decision-making process.

Pharmacotherapy to Prevent MI

ANTIPLATELET AGENTS
Aspirin exerts an antithrombotic effect by inhibiting cyclooxygenase and synthesis of platelet thromboxane A_2. In the Physicians' Health Study, aspirin given on alternative days to asymptomatic individuals was associated with a decreased incidence of MI.[126] In the Swedish Angina Pectoris Aspirin Trial (SAPAT) in patients with stable angina, the addition of 75 mg of aspirin to sotalol resulted in a 34 percent reduction in primary outcome events of MI and sudden death and a 32 percent decrease in secondary vascular events.[127] A recent metanalysis of 200,000 patients showed similar benefits of aspirin doses from 75 to 325 mg.[128]

Ticlopidine is a thienopyridine derivative that inhibits platelet aggregation induced by adenosine diphosphate and low concentrations of thrombin, collagen, thromboxane A_2, and platelet-activating factor.[129] It has *not* been shown to decrease adverse cardiovascular events and may induce neutropenia and often thrombotic thrombocytopenic purpura (TTP).

Clopidogrel, also a thienopyridine derivative, is chemically related to ticlopidine, but it appears to possess a greater antithrombotic effect than ticlopidine. In a randomized trial that compared clopidogrel with aspirin in patients with previous MIs, stroke, or peripheral vascular disease, clopidogrel was slightly more effective than aspirin in decreasing the combined risk of MI, vascular death, and ischemic stroke.[130]

The greater reduction in event rates with clopidogrel in the CURE, PCI CURE, and CREDO studies cannot yet be applied to patients not undergoing revascularization.[131,132]

Aspirin, 75 to 325 mg per day, should be used routinely in all patients with acute and chronic ischemic heart disease and with and without clinical symptoms in the absence of contraindications. In those unable to take aspirin, clopidogrel may be used instead. Warfarin is the third choice.[133]

ANTITHROMBOTIC THERAPY
Disturbed fibrinolytic function after exercise appears to be associated with an increased risk of subsequent cardiovascular death in patients

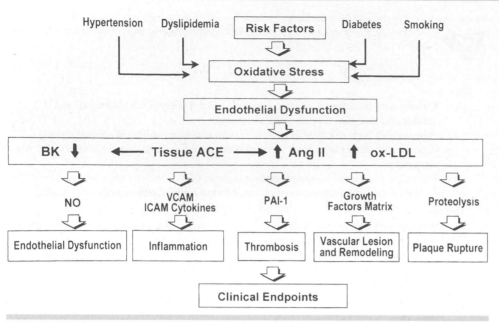

FIGURE 57-7 Interaction among the renin angiotensin system, diabetes. BK = bradykinin; ACE = angiotensin converting enzyme; VCAM = vascular cell adhesion molecule; ICAM = intercellular adhesion molecule; PAI-1 = plasminogen activator inhibitor.

with chronic stable angina, providing the rationale for long-term antithrombotic therapy. In small placebo-controlled trials among patients with chronic stable angina, daily subcutaneous administration of low-molecular-weight heparin deceased the fibrinogen level and improved the exercise time to ST-segment depression.[134] The clinical experience of such therapy, however, is extremely limited. The efficacy of newer antiplatelet and antithrombotic agents such as glycoprotein IIIb/IIa inhibitors and recombinant hirudin in the management of patients with chronic stable angina has not been established. Low-intensity oral anticoagulation with warfarin decreased the risk of ischemic events in a randomized trial of patients with risk factors for atherosclerosis but without symptoms of angina.[135]

LIPID-LOWERING AGENTS

Recent clinical studies have convincingly demonstrated that low-density lipoprotein (LDL)–lowering agents can decrease the risk of adverse ischemic events in patients with established CAD (Chap. 43). In the 4S trial,[136,137] treatment with an HMG-CoA reductase inhibitor in patients with documented CAD (including stable angina) and a baseline total cholesterol concentration between 212 and 308 mg/dL was associated with a 30 to 35 percent reduction in both mortality rate and major coronary events. In the Cholesterol And Recurrent Events (CARE) study,[138] in men and women with previous MI and total cholesterol levels of less than 240 mg/dL and LDL-cholesterol levels of 115 to 174 mg/dL, treatment with an HMG-CoA reductase inhibitor (statin) was associated with a 24 percent reduction in risk for nonfatal MI. Thus lipid-lowering therapy should be recommended even in the presence of mild to moderate elevations of LDL cholesterol in patients with chronic stable angina. Recent studies and ongoing clinical trials (including the Heart Protection Trial)[139,140] suggest that a reduction of LDL-cholesterol below 100 mg/dL will further reduce cardiac events (Chap. 43).

Angiotensin-Converting Enzyme Inhibitors

The potential cardiovascular protective effects of ACE inhibitors have been suspected for some time. As early as 1990, several randomized clinical trials showed that ACE inhibitors reduced the incidence of recurrent MI and that this effect could not be attributed to the effect on blood pressure alone.

The results of the Heart Outcomes Prevention Evaluation (HOPE) trial now confirm that use of the ACE inhibitor ramipril (10 mg per day)[141] reduces the rate of cardiovascular death, MI, and stroke in patients who are at high risk or have vascular disease in the absence of heart failure.

Greater than 90 percent of ACE is tissue-bound, whereas only 10 percent of ACE is present in soluble form in the plasma. In nonatherosclerotic arteries, the majority of tissue ACE is bound to the cell membranes of endothelial cells on the luminal surface of the vessel walls, and there is a large concentration of ACE within the adventitial vasa vasorum endothelium. It is now well appreciated that atherosclerosis represents different stages of a process that is in large part mediated by the endothelial cell (Figure 57-7). Thus, in the early stage, ACE, with its predominant location for the endothelial cells, would be an important mediator of local angiotensin II and bradykinin levels that could have an important impact on endothelial function.

ACE inhibition shifts the balance of ongoing vascular mechanisms in favor of those promoting vasodilatory, antiaggregatory, antiproliferative, and antithrombotic effects (Fig. 57-7).

The HOPE study was unique in that of the 9541 patients in this study, 3577 (37.5 percent) had diabetes. There was a significant reduction in diabetic complications, a composite for the development of diabetic nephropathy, need for renal dialysis, and laser therapy for diabetic retinopathy in those patients receiving ramipril. The Microalbuminuria, Cardiovascular, and Renal Outcomes (MICRO)-HOPE, a substudy of the HOPE study,[142] provided new clinical data on the cardiorenal therapeutic benefits of ACE inhibitor intervention in a broad range of middle-aged patients with diabetes mellitus who are at high risk for cardiovascular events.

ACE inhibitors should be used as routine secondary prevention for patients with known CAD, particularly in diabetics without severe renal disease.

In the ongoing Bypass And Revascularization Investigation (BARI) 2 Diabetes (2-D) and Clinical Outcomes Utilizing Aggressive Drug Evaluation (COURAGE) trials; ACE inhibitors are prescribed for all diabetics with documented ischemic heart disease unless contraindicated. The ACE inhibitor used in the BARI-2D trial is quinapril (an agent with high lipophilicity and enzyme-binding capabilities—a tissue ACE).

Antianginal and Anti-ischemic Therapy

Antianginal and anti-ischemic drug therapy consists of beta-adrenoreceptor blocking agents (beta blockers), calcium antagonists, and nitrates. Drug interactions are described in Chap. 90. There is a tendency for physicians to give *lower doses* of antianginal medications than those proven to be effective in clinical trials; higher doses and combined therapy are often not utilized in patients who could be "angina-free" if treated more appropriately; this is particularly true with beta-blocker therapy. For example, the usual dose for angina is 50 to 200 mg of metoprolol twice daily.

BETA BLOCKERS

The decrease in heart rate, contractility, arterial pressure, and usually LV wall stress with beta blockers is associated with decreased $M\dot{V}O_2$. A reduction in heart rate also increases diastolic coronary artery perfusion time, which may enhance LV perfusion. Although beta blockers have the potential to increase coronary vascular resistance by the formation of cyclic AMP, the clinical relevance of this pharmacodynamic effect remains to be demonstrated.

All beta blockers without intrinsic sympathetic activity appear to be equally effective in angina pectoris. In patients with chronic stable exertional angina, these agents decrease the heart rate–blood pressure product during exercise, and the onset of angina or the ischemic threshold during exercise is delayed or avoided.[1] In treating stable angina, it is essential that the dose of beta blockers be adjusted to lower the resting heart rate to 60 beats or less per minute. In patients with severe angina, the heart rate can be reduced to less than 50 beats per minute if there are no symptoms associated with bradycardia and AV block does not develop (Chap. 90). In patients with exertional angina, beta blockers attenuate the increase in heart rate during exercise, which ideally should not exceed 75 percent of the heart rate response associated with the onset of ischemia. It is often useful for the patient to perform exercise (sit-ups, running in place) before and after the institution of beta-blocker therapy. If the heart rate increase with exercise is not significantly reduced by therapy, the dose of the beta blocker is inadequate. Beta blockers are definitely effective in reducing exercise-induced angina. Three controlled studies comparing beta blockers with calcium antagonists[143–145] report equal efficacy in the treatment of chronic stable angina.

In the International Multicenter Angina Exercise (IMAGE) study,[146] both metoprolol and nifedipine were effective as monotherapy in increasing exercise time, although metoprolol was more effective than nifedipine. The combination therapy also significantly increased the exercise time to ischemia compared with either drug alone. The absolute contraindications to the use of beta blockers are severe bradycardia, preexisting high-degree AV block, sick sinus syndrome, and severe, unstable LV failure (Chap. 90). Asthma and bronchospastic disease, severe depression, and peripheral vascular disease are relative contraindications (Chap. 90). Fatigue, inability to perform exercise, lethargy, insomnia, nightmares, worsening claudication, and impotence are frequently experienced side effects. Most patients with chronic CAD and diabetes can be treated with beta blockers (Chap. 86).

In patients with postinfarction stable angina and those who require antianginal therapy after revascularization, treatment with beta blockers appears to be effective in controlling symptomatic and asymptomatic ischemic episodes. Beta blockers are still the antiischemic drugs of choice in elderly patients with stable angina.[1]

Beta blockers are frequently combined with nitrates for treating chronic stable angina. This combination of therapy appeared to be more effective in several studies than nitrates or beta blockers alone.[147–149] Beta blockers may also be combined with calcium antagonists. For combination therapy, slow-release dihydropyridine derivatives or new-generation long-acting dihydropyridine derivatives are the calcium antagonists of choice.[1]

CALCIUM ANTAGONISTS

These agents, also considered in Chap. 90, reduce the transmembrane flux of calcium by the calcium channels. There are three types of voltage-dependent calcium channels: L type, T type, and N type.

All calcium antagonists exert a negative inotropic effect, depending on dosage. In smooth muscle, calcium ions also regulate the contractile mechanism, and calcium antagonists reduce smooth muscle tension in the peripheral vascular bed, thus causing vasodilation. All the calcium antagonists cause dilatation of the epicardial conduit vessels and the arterial resistance vessels, the former being the primary mechanism for the beneficial effect of calcium antagonists for relieving vasospastic angina. Calcium antagonists also decrease $M\dot{V}O_2$ demand, primarily by reducing the systemic vascular resistance and arterial pressure. The negative inotropic effect of calcium antagonists also decreases the $M\dot{V}O_2$.

Randomized clinical trials comparing calcium antagonists and beta blockers have demonstrated that calcium antagonists are *equally effective* as beta blockers in relieving angina and improving exercise time to onset of angina or ischemia.[1] The calcium antagonists are effective in reducing the incidence of angina in patients with vasospastic angina.[150,151]

In a *retrospective case-controlled study* reported in patients with hypertension, treatment with immediate-acting nifedipine, diltiazem, and verapamil was associated with an increased risk of MI of 31 to 61 percent.[152] Although a subsequent metanalysis of immediate-release and short-acting nifedipine in patients with MI and unstable angina reported a dose-related influence on excess mortality,[153] further analysis of the published reports failed to confirm an increased risk of adverse cardiac events with calcium antagonists.[154,155] Importantly, long-acting calcium antagonists, including slow-release and long-acting dihydropyridine and nondihydropyridine derivatives, are effective in relieving symptoms in patients with chronic stable angina. They should be used in combination with beta blockers when initial treatment with beta blockers is not successful or as a substitute for beta blockers when initial treatment leads to unacceptable side effects. The use of calcium blockers may decrease the incidence of coronary artery spasms, which beta blockers do not. Many patients with two- or three-vessel CAD are asymptomatic on combined beta blocker and calcium antagonist therapy. Some have further improvement on triple therapy (combined beta blocker, calcium antagonist, and long-acting nitrates). Further information concerning the potential side effects of the calcium antagonists is given elsewhere (Chap. 90).

NITROGLYCERIN AND NITRATES

Nitrates are endothelium-independent vasodilators that produce beneficial effects by both reducing the $M\dot{V}O_2$ and improving CBF perfusion. The decreased $M\dot{V}O_2$ results from the reduction of LV volume and arterial pressure primarily due to reduced preload. Nitroglycerin also exerts antithrombotic and antiplatelet effects in patients with stable angina.[1]

Nitrates dilate large epicardial arteries and collateral vessels. The vasodilating effect on epicardial coronary arteries with or without atherosclerotic CAD is beneficial in relieving coronary vasospasm in patients with vasospastic angina.

In patients with exertional stable angina, nitrates improve exercise tolerance, time to onset of angina, and time to ST-segment depression during treadmill exercise testing. In combination with beta blockers or calcium antagonists, nitrates produce greater antianginal and anti-ischemic effects in patients with stable angina.[156–159]

The interaction between nitrates and sildenafil (Viagra) is discussed in detail elsewhere.[160] The coadministration of nitrates and sildenafil greatly increases the risk of potentially life-threatening hypotension.

The major problem with long-term use of nitroglycerin and long-acting nitrates is development of nitrate tolerance.[161] Tolerance develops not only to antianginal and hemodynamic effects but also to platelet antiaggregatory effects.[162] The mechanism for development of nitrate tolerance remains unclear. For practical purposes, the administration of nitrates with an adequate nitrate-free interval (8 to 12 h) appears to be the most effective method of preventing nitrate tolerance. Unfortunately, this means that patients with unpredictable episodes of myocardial ischemia should not be treated with nitrate therapy alone because they will be "unprotected" for part of each 24-h day.

The primary consideration in the choice of pharmacologic agents for treatment of angina should be to *improve prognosis*. Aspirin and lipid-lowering therapies have been shown to reduce the risk of death and nonfatal myocardial infarction in both primary and secondary prevention trials. Beta blockers also reduce cardiac events when used as secondary prevention in postinfarction patients and reduce mortal-

ity and morbidity among patients with hypertension. Nitrates have not been shown to reduce mortality with acute infarction or in patients with chronic CAD.

Recommended drug therapy using calcium antagonists versus beta blockers in patients with angina-associated conditions are listed in Table 57-9.

Treatment of Risk Factors

The recommendations of the AHA for the treatment of risk factors are detailed in Chap. 43. *Interventions that have been shown to reduce the incidence of CAD events include those that lead to declines in* (1) cigarette smoking, (2) low-density lipoprotein (LDL) choles-

TABLE 57-9 Recommended Drug Therapy (Calcium Antagonist versus Beta Blocker) in Patients with Angina and Associated Conditions

Condition	Recommended Treatment and Alternative	Avoid
Medical conditions		
Systemic hypertension	Beta blockers (calcium antagonists)	
Migraine or vascular headaches	Beta blockers (verapamil or diltiazem)	
Asthma or chronic obstructive pulmonary disease with bronchospasm	Verapamil or diltiazem	Beta blockers
Hyperthyroidism	Beta blockers	
Raynaud's syndrome	Long-acting slow-release calcium antagonists	Beta blockers
Insulin-dependent diabetes mellitus	Beta blockers (particularly if prior myocardial infarction) or long-acting slow-release calcium antagonists	
Non-insulin-dependent diabetes mellitus	Beta blockers or long-acting slow-release calcium antagonists	
Depression	Long-acting slow-release calcium antagonists	Beta blockers
Mild peripheral vascular disease	Beta blockers or calcium antagonists	
Severe peripheral vascular disease with rest ischemia	Calcium antagonists	Beta blockers
Cardiac arrhythmias and conduction abnormalities		
Sinus bradycardia	Long-acting slow-release calcium antagonists that do not decrease heart rate	Beta blockers, diltiazem, verapamil
Sinus tachycardia (not due to heart failure)	Beta blockers	
Supraventricular tachycardia	Verapamil, diltiazem, or beta blockers	
Atrioventricular block	Long-acting slow-release calcium antagonists that do not slow AV conduction	Beta blockers, verapamil, diltiazem
Rapid artrial fibrillation (with digitalis)	Verapamil, diltiazem, or beta blockers	
Ventricular arrhythmias	Beta blockers	
Left ventricular dysfunction		
Congestive heart failure		
Mild (LVEF ≥ 40%)	Beta blockers	
Moderate to Severe (LVEF < 40%)	Amlodipine or felodipine (nitrates)	Verapamil, diltiazem
Left-sided valvular heart disease		
Mild aortic stenosis	Beta blockers	
Aortic insufficiency	Long-acting slow-release dihydropyridines	
Mitral regurgitation	Long-acting slow-release dihydropyridines	
Mitral stenosis	Beta blockers	
Hypertrophic cardiomyopathy	Beta blockers, nondihydropyridine calcium antagonist	Nitrates, dihydropyridine, calcium antagonists

SOURCE: From Gibbons et al.[1]

terol, (3) systemic hypertension, (4) LV hypertrophy, and (5) thrombogenic factors (Chap. 43).

The causal role of *LDL cholesterol* in the pathogenesis of atherosclerotic CAD has been affirmed by recent randomized, controlled clinical trials of lipid-lowering therapy. Several primary and secondary prevention trials have shown that the lowering of LDL cholesterol is associated with a reduced risk of CAD (Chap. 43). Angiographic trials provide firm evidence linking cholesterol reduction to favorable trends in coronary anatomy.

Data from numerous observational studies indicate a continuous and graded relation between blood pressure and cardiovascular disease risk.[163] Hypertension predisposes patients to coronary events both as a result of the direct vascular injury caused by increases in blood pressure and by its effects on the myocardium, including increased wall stress and $M\dot{V}O_2$.

CAD, diabetes, LV hypertrophy, heart failure, retinopathy, and nephropathy are indicators of increased cardiovascular disease risk in hypertensive patients. The target of therapy is a reduction in blood pressure to less than 130 mmHg systolic and less than 85 mmHg diastolic in patients with CAD and coexisting diabetes, heart failure, or renal failure.[164] In diabetics, an even lower blood pressure (<120) appears to be of greater benefit.

Treatment of *hypertension* begins with nonpharmacologic means. When lifestyle modifications and dietary alterations adequately reduce blood pressure, pharmacologic intervention may be unnecessary (Chaps. 43 and 61).

When pharmacologic treatment is necessary (as is usually the case), beta blockers or calcium antagonists may be especially useful in patients with hypertension and angina pectoris; however, short-acting calcium antagonists should not be used.[165]

Epidemiologic studies have implicated *LV hypertrophy* as a risk factor for the development of MI, congestive heart failure, and sudden death.[166] LV hypertrophy has also been shown to predict a poorer prognosis in patients with definite CAD.[167] In the Framingham Heart Study,[168] the subjects who demonstrated ECG evidence of LV hypertrophy regression on follow-up were at a substantially reduced risk for cardiovascular events.

Coronary artery thrombosis is a trigger of acute MI. Aspirin has been documented to reduce the risk for CHD in both primary and secondary prevention settings.[1] Elevated plasma fibrinogen levels predict CAD risk in prospective observational studies[169] (Chap. 43).

Interventions that are likely to reduce the incidence of CAD events include those that lead to declines in diabetes mellitus, LDL cholesterol, obesity, physical inactivity, and postmenopausal status (Chap. 43).

Diabetes mellitus, which is defined as a fasting blood sugar level of more than 126 mg/dL,[170] is present in a significant minority of adult Americans. Data supporting an important role of diabetes mellitus as a risk factor for cardiovascular disease come from a number of observational settings. This is true for both type I and type II diabetes. Atherosclerosis accounts for 80 percent of all diabetic mortality[171,172] (Chaps. 43 and 78). The goal is to maintain a blood glucose HbA$_1$c level of less than 7% and a blood glucose level of less than 140 mg/dL. In diabetic patients with hypertension, microalbuminuria, or decreased LV systolic function, ACE inhibitors appear indicated. This may apply to most diabetics with CAD.[1,173] Observational studies and clinical trials have demonstrated a strong inverse association between *HDL cholesterol* and CAD risk (Chap. 43). This inverse relation is observed in both men and women and among asymptomatic persons as well as patients with established CAD.[1] The National Cholesterol Adult Treatment Panel III has defined a low HDL-cholesterol level as less than 40 mg/dL.[173]

Obesity is a common condition associated with increased risk for CHD and mortality (Chap. 43). New AHA guidelines for weight control have recently been published.[174]

Multiple randomized, controlled trials comparing exercise training with a "no exercise" control group have demonstrated a statistically significant improvement in exercise tolerance for the exercise group versus the control group.[1] The threshold for ischemia is likely to increase with exercise training because training reduces the heart rate–blood pressure product at a given submaximal exercise workload[1] (Chap. 38).

POSTMENOPAUSAL HORMONAL REPLACEMENT THERAPY

Both estrogenic and androgenic hormones produced by the ovary have appeared to be protective against the development of atherosclerotic cardiovascular disease. When hormonal production decreases in the perimenopausal period over several years, the risk of CAD rises in postmenopausal women. By age 75 years, the risk of atherosclerotic cardiovascular disease among men and women is equal. Women have an accelerated risk of developing CAD if they experience an early menopause or abrupt onset of menopause through surgical removal or chemotherapeutic ablation of the ovaries. Loss of estrogen and onset of menopause result in an increase in LDL cholesterol, a small decrease in HDL cholesterol, and therefore an increased ratio of total cholesterol to HDL cholesterol. Numerous epidemiologic studies have suggested a favorable influence of estrogen replacement therapy on the primary prevention of CAD in postmenopausal women.

Based on the above, postmenopausal estrogen replacement has previously been advocated for both primary and secondary prevention of CAD in women. However, the first published randomized trial of estrogen plus progestin therapy in postmenopausal women with known CAD did not show any reduction in cardiovascular events over 4 years of follow-up[175] despite an 11 percent lower LDL cholesterol level and a 10 percent higher HDL-cholesterol level in those women receiving hormone replacement therapy.

The Women's Health Initiative, a randomized controlled primary prevention trial of estrogen plus progestin, found that the overall health risks of this therapy exceeded its benefits.[175a] Thus, current information suggests that hormone replacement therapy in postmenopausal women does not reduce risk for major vascular events or coronary deaths in secondary prevention. Women who are taking hormone replacement therapy and who have vascular disease can continue this therapy if it is being prescribed for other well-established indications (e.g., osteoporosis) and no better alternative therapies are appropriate. There is, however, at the present time no basis for adding or continuing estrogens in postmenopausal women with clinically evident CAD or cerebrovascular disease in an effort to prevent or retard progression of their underlying disease.

Other randomized trials of hormone replacement therapy in primary and secondary prevention of CAD in postmenopausal women are being conducted.[175b] As their results become available over the next several years, this recommendation may require modification.

Interventions that may reduce the incidence of CAD events include those that lead to declines in psychosocial factors, triglycerides, lipoprotein(a), homocysteine, oxidative stress, and consumption of alcohol (Chap. 43).

Triglyceride levels are predictive of CHD in a variety of observational studies and clinical settings.[176] However, much of the association of triglycerides with CHD risk is related to other factors, including diabetes, obesity, hypertension, high LDL cholesterol, and low HDL cholesterol[177] (Chap. 43).

Lipoprotein(a) is a lipoprotein particle that has been linked to CHD risk in observational studies. Elevated levels of lipoprotein(a) are largely genetically determined and found in 15 to 20 percent of patients with premature CHD.[178,179] Increased *homocysteine* levels are associated with increased risk of CAD, peripheral arterial disease, and carotid disease.[180,181] Elevated homocysteine levels can occur as a result of inborn errors of metabolism such as homocysteinuria, and they also can be increased by deficiencies of vitamin B_6, vitamin B_{12}, and folate, which are commonly seen in older patients[182] (Chap. 43).

Extensive laboratory data indicate that oxidation of LDL cholesterol promotes and accelerates the atherosclerosis process. Observational studies have documented an association between dietary intake of antioxidant vitamins (vitamin C, vitamin E, and β-carotene) and reduced risk for CHD.[183] Observational studies have repeatedly shown an inverse relation of *moderate alcohol intake* to the risk of CHD events.[184] However, excessive alcohol intake can promote many other medical problems that outweigh its beneficial effects on CHD risk.

Risk factors associated with increased risk but that cannot be modified or when modified are unlikely to change the incidence of CHD events include age, male gender, and a positive family history of premature CHD. The latter is defined as definite MI or sudden death before age 55 in a father or other male first-degree relative or before age 65 in a mother or other female first-degree relative[1] (Chap. 43).

MYOCARDIAL REVASCULARIZATION

There are currently two well-established revascularization approaches to treatment of chronic stable angina caused by coronary atherosclerosis. One is CABG surgery, in which segments of autologous arteries or veins are used to reroute blood around relatively stenotic segments of the proximal coronary artery. The other is percutaneous coronary intervention (PCI) using catheter-borne or laser techniques to open usually short areas of stenosis from within the coronary artery. These techniques are described in greater detail in Chaps. 55 and 58. Revascularization is also potentially feasible with transthoracic (laser) myocardial revascularization in patients in whom neither CABG nor PCI is feasible (Chap. 48). The recommendations of the American College of Cardiology/American Heart Association, American College of Physicians–American Society of Internal Medicine (ACC/AHA/ACP–ASIM) for revascularization with PCIs or CABG in patients with stable angina are listed in Table 57-10.

Patients with stable angina pectoris may be appropriate candidates for revascularization either by CABG surgery or PCI. In general, this is an individual decision to be made by the patient with knowledge of the advantages and disadvantages either of medical therapy alone or revascularization with either CABG or PCI.

There are two general indications for revascularization procedures: the presence of symptoms that are not acceptable to the patient either because of (1) restriction of physical activity and lifestyle as a result of limitations or side effects from medications or (2) the presence of findings that indicate clearly that the patient would have a better prognosis with revascularization than with medical therapy. Considerations regarding revascularization are based on an assessment of the grade or class of angina experienced by the patient, the presence and severity of myocardial ischemia on noninvasive testing, the degree of LV function, and the distribution and severity of coronary artery stenoses.

A recent metanalysis of three major large, multicenter, randomized trials of initial surgery versus medical management (performed in the 1970s) as well as other smaller trials has confirmed the surgical benefits achieved by surgery at 10 postoperative years for patients with three-vessel disease, two-vessel disease, or even one-vessel disease that included a severe stenosis of the proximal left anterior descending coronary artery (Chap. 58).

The advantages of PCI for the treatment of CAD include a low level of procedure-related morbidity, a low procedure-related mortality rate in properly selected patients, a short hospital stay, early return to activity, and the feasibility of multiple procedures. However, PCI is not feasible in all patients; it remains accompanied by a significant incidence of restenosis, and there is an occasional need for emergency CABG surgery (Chap. 45).

Three randomized studies have compared PCI with medical management alone for the treatment of chronic stable angina.[185–187] All these randomized studies of PCI versus medical management have involved patients at a low risk of mortality even with medical management and did not assess patients with moderate to severe CAD (Chap. 55). Multiple trials have compared the strategy of an initial PCI with initial CABG surgery for treatment of multivessel CAD (Chaps. 55 and 58). The results of all these trials have shown that early and late survival rates have been equivalent for the PCI and CABG surgery groups. In the Bypass Angioplasty Revascularization Investigation (BARI) trial, the subgroups of patients with treated diabetes had a significantly better survival rate with CABG surgery.[188] This was true, however, on post hoc analysis of the clinical variables, including diabetes, which was not a prerandomization blocking variable.

The randomized studies of invasive therapy for chronic angina have all excluded patients who developed recurrent angina after previous CABG surgery. Few existing data define outcomes for risk-stratified groups of patients who develop recurrent angina after bypass surgery. Those that do indicate that patients with ischemia produced by late atherosclerotic stenoses in vein grafts are at a higher risk with medical management alone than those with ischemia produced by native-vessel disease.

OTHER THERAPIES IN PATIENTS WITH REFRACTORY ANGINA

Recent evidence has emerged regarding the relative efficacy, or lack thereof, of a number of techniques for the management of refractory chronic angina pectoris. These techniques should only be used in patients who cannot be managed adequately by medical therapy and who are not candidates for revascularization (interventional and/or surgical). Data are reviewed regarding three techniques: spinal cord stimulation, enhanced external counterpulsation, and laser transmyocardial revascularization.[1]

Spinal Cord Stimulation

The efficacy of SCS depends on the accurate placement of the stimulating electrode in the dorsal epidural space, usually at the C7-T1 level. A review of the literature has revealed two small randomized clinical trials involving implanted spinal cord stimulators, one of which directly tested its efficacy. The authors concluded that SCS was effective in the treatment of chronic intractable angina pectoris and that its effect was exerted through an anti-ischemic action.[1]

Enhanced External Counterpulsation

This technique uses a series of cuffs that are wrapped around both of the patient's legs. Using compressed air, pressure is applied via the cuffs to the patient's lower extremities in a sequence synchronized with

TABLE 57-10 Revascularization for Chronic Stable Angina (Recommendations for Revascularization with PTCA or Other Catheter-Based Techniques and CABG in Patients with Stable Angina)

Class I
1. CABG for patients with significant left main coronary disease.
2. CABG for patients with three-vessel disease. The survival benefit is greater in patients with abnormal LV function (ejection fraction < 50%).
3. CABG for patients with two-vessel disease with significant proximal left anterior descending CAD and either abnormal LV function (ejection fraction < 50%) or demonstrable ischemia on noninvasive testing.
4. PCI for patients with two- or three-vessel disease with significant proximal left anterior descending CAD, who have anatomy suitable for catheter-based therapy, normal LV function and who do not have treated diabetes.
5. PCI or CABG for patients with one- or two-vessel disease CAD without significant proximal left anterior descending CAD, but with a large area of viable myocardium and high risk criteria on noninvasive testing.
6. CABG for patients with one- or two-vessel disease CAD without significant proximal left anterior descending CAD who have survived sudden cardiac death or sustained ventricular tachycardia.
7. In patients with prior PCI, CABG, or PCI for recurrent stenosis associated with a large area of viable myocardium or high-risk criteria on noninvasive testing.
8. PTCA or CABG for patients who have not been treated successfully by medical therapy and can undergo revascularization with acceptable risk.

Class IIa
1. Repeat CABG for patients with multiple saphenous vein graft stenoses, especially when there is significant stenosis of a graft supplying the LAD. It may be appropriate to use PTCA for focal saphenous vein graft lesions or multiple stenoses in poor candidates for reoperative surgery.
2. Use of PCI or CABG for patients with one- or two-vessel disease CAD without significant proximal LAD disease but with a moderate area of viable myocardium and demonstrable ischemia on noninvasive testing.
3. Use of PCI or CABG for patients with one-vessel disease with significant proximal LAD disease.

Class IIb
1. Compared with CABG, PCI for patients with two- or three-vessel disease with significant proximal left anterior descending CAD, who have anatomy suitable for catheter-based therapy, and who have treated diabetes or abnormal LV function.
2. Use of PCI for patients with significant left main coronary disease who are not candidates for CABG.
3. PCI for patients with one- or two-vessel disease CAD without significant proximal left anterior descending CAD, who have survived sudden cardiac death or sustained ventricular tachycardia.

Class III
1. Use of PCI or CABG for patients with one- or two-vessel CAD without significant proximal left anterior descending CAD, who have mild symptoms that are unlikely due to myocardial ischemia or who have not received an adequate trial of medical therapy and
   a. Have only a small area of viable myocardium or
   b. Have no demonstrable ischemia on noninvasive testing
2. Use of PCI or CABG for patients with borderline coronary stenoses (50% to 60% diameter in locations other than the left main coronary artery) and no demonstrable ischemia on noninvasive testing.
3. Use of PCI or CABG for patients with insignificant coronary stenosis (<50% diameter).
4. Use of PCI in patients with significant left main coronary disease who are candidates for CABG.

NOTE: PTCA is used in these recommendations to indicate PTCA or other catheter-based techniques, such as stents, atherectomy, and laser therapy. See classes I to III as described at the bottom of Table 57-5.

the cardiac cycle. Specifically, in early diastole, pressure is applied sequentially from the lower legs to the lower and upper thighs, to propel blood back to the heart. The procedure results in an increase in arterial blood pressure and retrograde aortic blood flow during diastole (diastolic augmentation). Treatment was relatively well tolerated and free of limiting side effects in most patients. However, the sample size in this study was relatively small.[1] (Two multicenter registry studies found the treatment to be generally well tolerated and efficacious; anginal symptoms were improved in approximately 75 to 80 percent of patients. However, additional clinical trial data are necessary before this technology can be recommended definitively.)

Laser Transmyocardial Revascularization

Another emerging technique for the treatment of more severe chronic stable angina refractory to medical or other therapies is laser transmyocardial revascularization (TMR). This technique has either been performed in the operating room (using a carbon dioxide or holmium: YAG laser) or by a percutaneous approach with a specialized (holmium: YAG laser) catheter. Eight prospective randomized clinical trials have been performed, two using the percutaneous technique and the other six using an epicardial surgical technique.[1]

PERCUTANEOUS TMR

The two randomized percutaneous TMR trials assessed parameters such as angina class, freedom from angina, exercise tolerance, and quality of life score. In general, these studies have shown improvements in severity of angina class, exercise tolerance, and quality of life, as well as increased freedom from angina.[1] However, percutaneous TMR technology has not been approved by the Food and Drug Administration; therefore, percutaneous TMR should still be considered an experimental therapy.

SURGICAL TMR

The surgical TMR technique has also generally been associated with improvement in symptoms in patients with chronic stable angina. The mechanism for improvement in angina symptoms is still controversial.[1] Three studies also assessed myocardial perfusion using thallium scans. Only one of these studies demonstrated an improvement in myocardial perfusion in patients who underwent TMR versus those continuing to receive only medical therapy. Despite the apparent benefit in decreasing angina symptoms, no definite benefit has been demonstrated in terms of increasing myocardial perfusion.[1]

A NEW CLASS OF ANTIANGINA DRUGS, pFOX INHIBITORS

The potential clinical usefulness of newer antianginal drugs currently being studied include the pFOX inhibitor class of drugs, which partially inhibit fatty acid oxidation and improve cardiac efficiency. Clearly, the development of drugs that modulate myocardial metabolism, have the potential to reduce extent of myocardial ischemia and angina symptoms, yet have no clinically significant effects on heart rate, blood pressure, or coronary blood flow, are of considerable interest. Ranolazine is currently pending FDA approval and is not approved for patient use as of this writing. The biochemical rationale, and progress in development of pFOX inhibitors is the result of approximately two decades of research.

The pFOX inhibitor drugs partially relieve the inhibition of pyruvate dehydrogenase through an inhibition of the enzyme sequence necessary for beta-oxidation of FFA in mitochondria (when there is sufficient residual oxygen supply to the myocardium to allow pyruvate oxidation). The reader is referred to several excellent reviews for a more detailed discussion of these concepts. The sustained release formulation of ranolazine was tested for chronic angina in both the MARISA (Monotherapy Assessment of Ranolazine and Stable Angina) and CARISA (Combination Assessment of Ranolazine and Stable Angina) trials.[188a,b]

The MARISA and CARISA studies indicate that ranolazine is a potentially effective drug to alleviate chronic angina in patients with moderately severe symptoms. The increase in exercise time with monotherapy or when combined with other antianginal drugs averaged about of 30 s with more marked improvements in individual patients. The average increase of 30 s over placebo approximates the magnitude of increase seen with beta blockers or calcium channel antagonists when time-dependent placebo controls were used.

FOLLOW-UP OF PATIENTS WITH CHRONIC STABLE ANGINA

Published evidence of the efficacy of specific strategies for the follow-up of patients with chronic stable angina on patient outcome is nonexistent. The ACC/AHA/ACP-ASIM guidelines[1] for the monitoring of symptoms and antianginal therapy during patient follow-up are as follows:

For the patient with successfully treated chronic stable angina, a follow-up evaluation every 4 to 12 months is appropriate. During the first year of therapy, evaluations every 4 to 6 months are recommended. After the first year of therapy, annual evaluations are recommended if the patient is stable and reliable enough to return for evaluation when anginal symptoms become worse or other symptoms occur.[1] At the time of follow-up, a general assessment of the patient's functional and health status and quality of life may reveal additional issues that affect angina. Symptoms that have worsened should follow reevaluation as outlined above. A detailed history of the patient's daily activity is critical because anginal symptoms may remain stable only because stressful activities have been eliminated.

A careful history of the characteristics of the patient's angina, including provoking and alleviating factors, must be repeated at each visit. Detailed questions should be asked about common drug side effects. The patient's adherence to the treatment program must be assessed.

The physical examination should be focused by the patient's history. Every patient should have his or her weight, blood pressure, and pulse noted. The jugular venous pressure, carotid pulse magnitude and upstroke, and presence or absence of carotid bruits should be noted. Pulmonary examination with special attention to rales, rhonchi, wheezing, and decreased breath sounds is required. A cardiac examination should note the presence of fourth and third heart sounds, a new or changed systolic murmur, the location of the LV impulse, and any change from previous examinations. Clearly, the vascular examination should identify any change in peripheral pulses and new bruits; the abdominal examination should identify hepatomegaly and the presence of any pulsatile mass suggesting an abdominal aortic aneurysm. The presence of new or worsening peripheral edema should be noted.

The American Diabetes Association recommends that patients not known to have diabetes should have a *fasting blood glucose* measured every 3 years and an annual measurement of glycosylated hemoglobin for individuals with established diabetes. Fasting blood work, 6 to 8 weeks after initiating lipid-lowering drug therapy, should include liver function testing and assessment of the cholesterol profile. This should be repeated every 8 to 12 weeks during the first year of therapy and at 4- to 6-month intervals thereafter.

An ECG should be repeated when medications affecting cardiac conduction are initiated or changed. A repeat ECG is indicated for a change in the anginal pattern, symptoms or finding suggestive of an arrhythmia or conduction abnormality, and near or frank syncope. There is no clear evidence showing that routine, periodic ECGs are useful in the absence of a change in history or physical examination.

In the absence of a change in clinical status, low-risk patients with an estimated annual mortality rate of less than 1 percent over each year of the interval do not require repeat stress testing for 3 years after the initial evaluation.[1] *Annual follow-up for noninvasive testing in the absence of a change in symptoms* has not been studied adequately; it may be useful in high-risk patients with an estimated annual mortality rate of greater than 5 percent. Follow-up testing should be performed in a stable high-risk patient only if the initial decision not to proceed with revascularization may change if the patient's estimated risk worsens. Patients with an immediate-risk (>1 and <3 percent) annual mortality rate are more problematic because of limited data. They may need testing at an interval of 1 to 3 years depending on the individual circumstances. The ACC/AHA, ACP–ASIM recommendations for echocardiography, treadmill exercise testing, stress imaging studies and coronary angiography during patient follow-up are also listed in Table 57-11.

TABLE 57-11 Recommendations for Echocardiography, Treadmill Exercise Testing, Stress Imaging Studies, and Coronary Angiography during Patient Follow-up

Class I

1. Chest x-ray for patients with evidence of new or worsening congestive heart failure.
2. Assessment of LV ejection fraction and segmental wall motion in patients with new or worsening congestive heart failure or evidence of intervening MI by history or ECG.
3. Echocardiography for evidence of new or worsening valvular heart disease.
4. Treadmill exercise test for patients without prior revascularization who have a significant change in clinical status, are able to exercise, and do not have any of the ECG abnormalities listed below in number 5.
5. Stress imaging procedures for patients without prior revascularization who have a significant change in clinical status and are unable to exercise or have one of the following ECG abnormalities:
    a. Preexcitation (Wolff-Parkinson-White) syndrome.
    b. Electronically paced ventricular rhythm.
    c. More than 1 mm of rest ST-segment depression.
    d. Complete left bundle branch block.
6. Stress imaging procedures for patients who have a significant change in clinical status and required a stress imaging procedure on their initial evaluation because of equivocal or intermediate-risk treadmill results.
7. Stress imaging procedures for patients with prior revascularization who have a significant change in clinical status.
8. Coronary angiography in patients with marked limitation of ordinary activity. (CCS class III despite maximal medical therapy).

Class IIb

Annual treadmill exercise testing in patients who have no change to clinical status, can exercise, have none of the ECG abnormalities listed in number 5 above, and have an estimated annual mortality of >1%.

Class III

1. Echocardiography or radionuclide imaging for assessment of LV ejection fraction and segmental wall motion in patients with a normal ECG, no history of MI, and no evidence of congestive heart failure.
2. Repeat treadmill exercise testing in <3 years in patients who have no change in clinical status and an estimated annual mortality ≥1% on their initial evaluation as demonstrated by one of the following:
    a. Low-risk Duke treadmill score (without imaging).
    b. Low-risk Duke treadmill score with negative imaging.
    c. Normal LV function and a normal coronary angiogram.
    d. Normal LV function and insignificant CAD.
3. Stress imaging procedures for patients who have no change in clinical status and a normal rest ECG, are not taking digoxin, are able to exercise, and did not require a stress imaging procedure on their initial evaluation because of equivocal or intermediate-risk treadmill results.
4. Repeat coronary angiography in patients with no change in clinical status, no change on repeat exercise testing or stress imaging, and insignificant CAD on initial evaluation.

NOTE: See classes I–III as described at the bottom of Table 57-5.

MANAGEMENT OF SPECIAL CATEGORIES

Systemic Arterial Hypertension

Patients with systemic arterial hypertension (SAH) often have angina pectoris. In most patients, significant coronary atherosclerosis of the epicardial blood vessels is present, but some patients with SAH may have angina pectoris or even fatal MI without significant obstruction of the large epicardial vessels. A major mistake is to send a patient for noninvasive testing when his or her hypertension has not been treated. In many patients, treatment of the hypertension with a beta blocker, calcium antagonist, or ACE inhibitor also will decrease $M\dot{V}O_2$ and prevent the development of angina pectoris. In general, efforts should be made to control the blood pressure both at rest and during exercise. It is now known that many patients with an elevated systolic and/or diastolic blood pressure above the normal variation during exercise will develop severe fixed SAH. Efforts should be made to control the blood pressure both at rest and during exertion.

Chronic Obstructive Pulmonary Disease/Asthma

Beta blockers should be avoided in the subset of patients who have true bronchospastic lung disease; in them, the use of nitrates and calcium antagonists is preferred. Since many of these patients receive medications for their pulmonary disease that may increase their heart rate or even produce supraventricular tachycardia, it is preferable to use a heart rate–slowing calcium antagonist such as diltiazem or verapamil.

Elderly Patients

In general, elderly patients tolerate calcium antagonists better than beta blockers. The presence of sinus tachycardia or atrial fibrillation is a relative contraindication to the selection of dihydropyridines such as nifedipine or amlodipine. In such patients, diltiazem or verapamil or even a beta blocker is preferable. On the other hand, beta blockers, verapamil, and diltiazem can exacerbate AV block, and verapamil produces constipation in many elderly patients. Also, some elderly patients develop postural hypotension from short-acting nitrates.

Peripheral Vascular Disease

Patients with peripheral vascular disease may have a worsening of their symptoms when they are treated with a nonselective beta blocker, permitting unopposed alpha-induced vasoconstriction. Alternatively, the worsening symptoms may be due to a decrease in arterial perfusion pressure. In general, it is preferable to treat patients with chronic stable angina who have peripheral vascular disease with nitrates and a calcium antagonist.

Diabetes Mellitus

Patients with chronic stable angina who have diabetes mellitus and insulin-induced hypoglycemic episodes should probably be treated with nitrates and calcium antagonists (Chap. 78). If it is necessary to use a beta blocker, a cardioselective agent should be chosen, since it is less likely to impair the recognition of and recovery from insulin-induced hypoglycemia. In most diabetics, cardioselective beta blockers are well tolerated. The BARI-2D randomized clinical trial is evaluating the efficacy of *early* myocardial revascularization in diabetes with CAD.

Chronic Renal Disease

While beta blockers and calcium antagonists can normally be used effectively in patients with chronic angina and chronic renal insufficiency, careful monitoring may be necessary, because many beta blockers and calcium antagonists (Chap. 84) are excreted primarily by the kidneys.

LONG-TERM MANIFESTATIONS OF CHRONIC ISCHEMIC HEART DISEASE

Heart Failure

Patients with severe CAD that produces a loss of 20 percent or more of the myocardium or that results in a ventricular septal defect or severe mitral regurgitation may develop important LV failure. While there may be significant hypertrophy of the remaining myocytes and interstitium (Chap. 20), the ventricle is unable to compensate completely and heart failure often results, with a decreased stroke volume and elevated diastolic filling pressures. Such a syndrome of heart failure may be clinically predominant and often more incapacitating than any symptom of angina pectoris (Chap. 66).

Patients with severe LV dysfunction due to CAD have a poor prognosis. Usually it reflects permanent, irreversible loss of myocytes. In some patients, severe chronic CAD is associated with persistently impaired LV function at rest due to reduced CBF that can be partially or completely restored to normal either by improving blood flow (more common) or by reducing oxygen demand. This concept of "hibernating" myocardium is important because there can be significant improvement following good LV revascularization. While this does not occur routinely, it must be considered before concluding that the LVEF of an individual patient is too low to consider revascularization surgery or that the etiology of the heart failure is not CHD. Myocardial perfusion imaging techniques, magnetic resonance imaging (MRI), dobutamine echocardiography, and positron-emission tomography (PET) are useful in detecting myocardial viability (Chap. 19).

The treatment of patients with heart failure due to CHD is the same as for most patients with combined systolic and diastolic LV failure and includes diuretics, an ACE inhibitor, digitalis, beta blockers, and spironolactone.

Cardiac transplantation is also frequently performed for severe heart failure due to CAD (Chap. 26). A patient with heart failure who has a large LV aneurysm may benefit from aneurysmectomy if there is sufficient remaining functioning LV tissue. Similarly, heart failure due to severe mitral regurgitation sometimes can be improved significantly by corrective mitral valve surgery, which is often combined with myocardial revascularization. Mitral valve repair in patients with severe functional mitral regurgitation (MR), with a reduced annular size, can improve symptoms considerably.

Cardiac Arrhythmias, Conduction Disturbances

Chronic ischemic heart disease causes many cardiac arrhythmias. The basic management is discussed in Chap. 27. In general, beta blockers should be employed whenever there is no strong contraindication, and type IC antiarrhythmic agents should be avoided unless the patient is symptomatic. In patients with atrial fibrillation, the ventricular response rate should be controlled with digoxin.

Patients with chronic atrial fibrillation also should be maintained on warfarin (INR = 2 to 3) unless there is a contraindication, in which case aspirin (80 to 325 mg/day) should be used. Patients in heart failure who have atrial fibrillation may benefit from an effective atrial contraction restored by electrical cardioversion. Unfortunately, large percentages revert to atrial fibrillation in the next few months.

Embolic Disease

Patients with ischemic disease are likely to have systemic emboli, particularly patients with a history of systemic embolus, chronic atrial fibrillation, ventricular aneurysm, a large dyskinetic or hypokinetic area of myocardium, or a severely depressed LVEF. Such patients should be considered for chronic, long-term, low-dose warfarin therapy (INR = 2 to 3).

CHEST PAIN WITH NORMAL CORONARY ARTERIES

The combination of chest pain with many of the features of angina pectoris—although frequently atypical—and normal epicardial coronary arteries at cardiac catheterization was first described in the 1960s.[189] The early studies identified many of the features of what was subsequently characterized as a syndrome: female predominance, frequent ischemic ST-segment changes on the exercise ECG, inconsistent relationship between ECG changes and metabolic or hemodynamic evidence of ischemia, and pain that may be very severe, prolonged, variable in location, precipitated by unusual events, and unresponsive to usual anti-ischemic therapy.

The term *syndrome X* was applied to this diagnostic combination in 1973;[190] it is usually used to describe patients with the common features of angina-like pain and normal epicardial coronaries, but the term is also used to categorize groups that undoubtedly are heterogeneous.[191] The continued use of this term is unfortunate and has been discouraged,[192] especially since there is also a *metabolic syndrome X*—characterized by insulin resistance, hyperinsulinemia, and diabetes—that is associated with abnormal lipids, hypertension, and abdominal obesity (Chap. 78). A more specific term such as *angina with normal coronary arteriography* is preferable.

References

1. Gibbons RJ, Chatterjee K, Daley J, et al., American College of Cardiology/American Heart Association, American College of Physicians–American Soceity of Internal Medicine (ACC/AHA/ACP–ASIM) guidelines for the management of patients with chronic stable angina: A report of the ACC/AHA Task Force on Practice Guidelines (Committee on the Management of Patients with Chronic Stable Angina). *J Am Coll Cardiol* 2002;41:160–168.

2. Herberden W. Some account of disorder of the breast. *Med Trans R Coll Phys (Lond)* 1772;2:59–67.

3. Herberden W. *Commentaries on the History and Care of Disease.* London: T Payne; 1802.

4. White PD. Angina pectoris: Historical background. In: Paul O, ed. *Angina Pectoris.* New York: Medcom Press; 1974:1.

5. Fuster V. Epidemic of cardiovascular disease and stroke: The three main challenges. In: *American Heart Association 71st Scientific Sessions.* Dallas: American Heart Association; 1999.

6. Schlant RC, Alexander RW. Diagnosis and management of patients with chronic ischemic disease. In: Alexander RW, Schlant RC, Fuster V, et al, eds. *Hurst's The Heart,* 9th ed. New York: McGraw-Hill; 1998:1275.

7. Diamond GA, Staniloff HM, Forrester JS, et al. Computer-assisted diagnosis in the noninvasive evaluation of patients with suspected coronary disease. *J Am Coll Cardiol* 1983;1:444–455.

8. Chaitman BR, Bourassa MG, Davis K, et al. Angiographic prevalence of high-risk coronary artery disease in patient subsets (CASS). *Circulation* 1981;64:360–367.

9. O'Rourke RA, Hochman JS, Cohen MC, et al. New approaches to diagnosis and management of unstable angina and non-ST-segment elevation myocardial infarction. *Arch Inter Med* 2001;161:674–682.

10. Lange RA, Cigarroa RG, Yancy CWJ, et al. Cocaine-induced coronary-artery vasoconstriction. *N Engl J Med* 1989;321:1557–1562.

11. Diamond GA, Forrester JS. Analysis of probability as an aid in the clinical diagnosis of coronary-artery disease. *N Engl J Med* 1979;300:1350–1358.

12. Pryor DB, Harrell FE, Lee KL, et al. Estimating the likelihood of significant coronary artery disease. *Am J Med* 1983;75:771–790.

13. Sox HC, Hickam DH, Marton KL, et al. Using the patient's history to estimate the probability of coronary artery disease. *N Engl J Med* 1979;300:1350S.

14. Pryor DB, Shaw L, McCants CB, et al. Value of the history and physical in identifying patients at increased risk for coronary artery disease. *Ann Intern Med* 1993;18:81–90.

15. Castellanos A, Kessler KM, Myerburg RJ. The resting electrocardiogram. In: Alexander RW, Schlant RC, Fuster V, et al, eds. *Hurst's The Heart,* 9th ed. New York: McGraw-Hill; 1998:351.

16. Margolis JR, Chen JT, Kong Y, et al. The diagnostic and prognostic significance of coronary artery calcification: A report of 800 cases. *Radiology* 1980;137:609–616.

17. Wexler L, Brundage B, Crouse J, et al. Coronary artery calcification, pathophysiology, epidemiology, imaging methods and clinical implications. *Circulation* 1996;94:1175–1192.

18. O'Rourke R, Brundage B, Froelicher V, et al. American College of Cardiology/American Heart Association consensus document on electron beam computed tomography for the diagnosis of coronary artery disease (Committee on Electron Beam Computer Tomography). *Circulation* 2000;20:126–140.

19. DeTrano RC, Duherty TM, Davies MJ, et al. Predicting coronary events with coronary calcium: Pathophysiologic and clinical problems. *Curr Probl Cardiol* 2000;25:369–404.

20. Gibbons RJ, Balady GJ, Bricker JT, et al. ACC/AHA 2002 guideline update for exercise testing: A report of the American College of Cardiology/American Heart Association Task Force on Practice guidelines (Commiteee on Exercise Testing). *J Am Coll Cardiol* 2002;41:160–168. American College of Cardiology website: http://www.acc.org/clinical/guidelines/exercise/exercise_clean.pdf. Accessed October 17, 2002.

21. Stuart RJ, Ellestad MH. National survey of exercise stress testing facilities. *Chest* 1980;77:94–97.

22. Myers J, Froelicher VF. Optimizing the exercise test for pharmacological investigations. *Circulation* 1990;82:1839–1846.

23. Froelicher VF, Lehmann KG, Thomas R, et al. The electrocardiographic exercise test in a population with reduced workup bias: Diagnostic performance, computerized interpretation, and multivariable prediction. Veterans Affairs Cooperative Study in Health Services 016 (QUEXTA) Study Group, Quantitative Exercise Testing and Angiography. *Ann Intern Med* 1998;128:965–974.

23a. Froelicher V, Shetler K, Ashley E. Better decisions through science: Exercise testing scores. *Curr Probl Cardiol* 2003;28:595–620.

24. Veragari J, Hakki AH, Heo J, Iskandrian AS. Merits and limitations of quantitative treadmill exercise score. *Am Heart J* 1987;114:819–826.

25. Mark DB, Shaw L, Harrell FE, et al. Prognostic value of a treadmill exercise score in outpatients with suspected coronary artery disease. *N Engl J Med* 1991;325:849–853.

26. Kligfield P, Ameisen O, Okin PM. Heart rate adjustment of ST segment depression for improved detection of coronary artery disease. *Circulation* 1989;79:245–255.

27. Lachterman B, Lehmann KG, Detrano R, et al. Comparison of the ST/heart rate index to standard ST criteria for analysis of the exercise electrocardiogram. *Circulation* 1990;82:44–50.

28. Whinnery JE, Froelicher VF, Stuart AJ. The electrocardiographic response to maximal treadmill exercise in asymptomatic men with left bundle branch block. *Am Heart J* 1977;94:316–324.

29. Cheitlin MD, Armstrong WF, Aurigemma GP, et al. ACC/AHA/ASE 2003 guideline update for the clinical application of echocardiography. *J Am Coll Cardiol* 2003;42:954–970.

30. Klocke FJ, Baird MG, Lorell BH, et al. ACC/AHA/ASNC revision of the 1995 guidelines for the clinical use of cardiac radionuclide imaging. *J Am Coll Cardiol* 2003;42:1318–1333.

31. Verani MS. Pharmacologic stress myocardial perfusion imaging. *Curr Probl Cardiol* 1993;18:481–525.

32. Nishimura S, Mahmarian JJ, Boyce TM, Verani MS. Equivalence between adenosine and exercise thallium-201 myocardial tomography: A mulitcenter, prospective, crossover trial. *J Am Coll Cardiol* 1992;20:265–275.

33. Patterson RE, Eisner RL, Horowitz SF. Comparison of cost effectiveness and utility of exercise ECG, single photon emission tomography and coronary angiography for diagnosis of coronary artery disease. *Circulation* 1995;91:54–65.

34. Spaulding CM, Joly LM, Rosenberg A, et al. Immediate coronary angiography in survivors of out-of-hospital cardiac arrest. *N Engl J Med* 1997;336:1629–1633.

35. Douglas JS Jr, Hurst JW. Limitations of symptoms in the recognition of coronary atherosclerotic heart disease. In: Hurst JW, ed. *Update I: The Heart.* New York: McGraw-Hill; 1979:3.

36. Barnard RJ, Duncan HW, Livesay JJ, Buckberg GD. Coronary vasodilator reserve and flow distribution during near-maximal exercise in dogs. *J Appl Physiol Respir Environ Exerc Physiol* 1977;43:988–992.

37. Boerth RC, Covell JW, Pool PE, Ross J Jr. Increased myocardial oxygen consumption and contractile state associated with increase in heart rate in dogs. *Circ Res* 1969;24:725–734.

38. Pupita G, Maseri A, Kaski JC, et al. Myocardial ischemia caused by distal coronary artery constriction in stable angina pectoris. *N Engl J Med* 1990;323:514–520.

39. McGorisk GM, Treasure CB. Endothelial dysfunction in coronary heart disease. *Curr Opin Cardiol* 1996;11:341–350.

40. Egashira K, Inou T, Hirooka Y, et al. Evidence of impaired endothelium-dependent coronary vasodilatation in patients with angina pectoris and normal coronary angiograms. *N Engl J Med* 1993;328:1659–1664.

41. Cannon RO III, Camici PG, Epstein SE. Pathophysiological dilemma of syndrome X. *Circulation* 1992;85:883–892.

42. Dole WP. Autoregulation of the coronary circulation. *Prog Cardiovasc Dis* 1987;29:369–387.

43. Gould KL, Lipscomb K, Calvert C. Compensatory changes of the distal coronary vascular bed during progressive coronary constriction. *Circulation* 1975;51:1085–1094.

44. Mudge GH Jr, Grossman W, Mills RM Jr, et al. Reflex increase in coronary vascular resistance in patients with ischemic heart disease. *N Engl J Med* 1976;295:1333–1337.

45. Furchgott RF, Zawadzski JV. The obligatory role of endothelial cells in the relaxation of arterial smooth muscle by acetylcholine. *Nature* 1980;288:373–376.

46. Palmer RMJ, Ferrige AG, Moncada S. Nitric oxide release accounts for the biological activity of endothelium-derived relaxing factor. *Nature* 1987;327:524–526.

47. Bortone AS, Hess OM, Eberli FR. Abnormal coronary vasomotion during exercise in patients with normal coronary arteries and reduced coronary flow reserve. *Circulation* 1991;83:26–37.

48. Yeung AC, Vekshtein VI, Krantz DS, et al. The effect of atherosclerosis on the vasomotor response of coronary arteries to mental stress. *N Engl J Med* 1991;325:1551–1556.

49. Nabel EG, Ganz P, Gordon JB, et al. Dilation of normal and constriction of atherosclerotic coronary arteries caused by the cold pressor testing. *Circulation* 1988;77:43–52.

50. Nabel EG, Ganz P, Gordon JB, et al. Paradoxical narrowing of atherosclerotic coronary arteries induced by increases in heart rate. *Circulation* 1990;81:850–859.

51. Vita JA, Treasure CB, Yeung AC, et al. Patients with evidence of coronary endothelial dysfunction as assessed by acetylcholine infusion demonstrate marked increase in sensitivity to constrictor effects of catecholamines. *Circulation* 1992;85:1390–1397.

52. Maseri A, Chierchia S, Kaski JC. Mixed angina pectoris. *Am J Cardiol* 1985;56:30E–33E.

53. Maseri A, Crea F, Kaski JC. Mechanisms of angina pectoris in syndrome X. *J Am Coll Cardiol* 1991;17:499–506.

54. Cannon RO III, Camici PG, Epstein SE. Pathophysiological dilemma of syndrome X. *Circulation* 1992;85:883–892.

55. Fuh MM-T, Jeng C-Y, Young MM, et al. Insulin resistance, glucose intolerance, and hyperinsulinemia in patients with microvascular angina. *Metabolism* 1993;42:1090–1092.

56. Quyyumi AA, Cannon RO III, Panza JA, et al. Endothelial dysfunction in patients with chest pain and normal coronary arteries. *Circulation* 1992;86:1864–1871.

57. Opherk D, Schuler G, Wetterauer K, et al. Four-year follow-up study in patients with angina pectoris and normal coronary arteriograms ("syndromes X"). *Circulation* 1989;80:1610–1616.

58. Legrand V, Hodgson JM, Bates ER, et al. Abnormal coronary flow reserve and abnormal radionuclide exercise test results in patients with normal coronary angiograms. *J Am Coll Cardiol* 1985;6:1245–1253.

59. Cannon RO III, Watson RM, Rosing DR, Epstein SE. Angina caused by reduced vasodilator reserve of the small coronary arteries. *J Am Coll Cardiol* 1983;1:1359–1373.

60. Egashira K, Inou T, Hirooka Y, et al. Evidence of impaired endothelium-dependent coronary vasodilatation in patients with angina pectoris and normal coronary angiograms. *N Engl J Med* 1993;328:1659–1664.

61. Treasure CB, Klein JL, Vita JA, et al. Hypertension and left ventricular hypertrophy are associated with impaired endothelium-mediated relaxation in human coronary resistance vessels. *Circulation* 1993;87:86–93.

62. Mosseri M, Schaper J, Admon D, et al. Coronary capillaries in patients with congestive cardiomyopathy or angina pectoris with patent main coronary arteries: Ultrastructural morphometry of endomyocardial biopsy samples. *Circulation* 1991;48:203–210.

63. Maseri A, Crea F, Kaski JC, Davies G. Mechanisms and significance of cardiac ischemic pain. *Prog Cardiovasc Dis* 1992;35:1–18.

64. Deanfield JE. Characteristics of silent and symptomatic ischemia in chronic stable angina: Comparison with unstable and vasospastic angina. In: Singh BM, ed. *Silent Myocardial Ischemia and Angina: Prevalence, Prognostic and Therapeutic Significance.* New York: Pergamon Press; 1988:104–111.

65. Nair CK, Aronow MH, Sketch R, et al. Diagnostic and prognostic significance of exercise-induced premature ventricular complexes in men and women: A four-year follow-up. *J Am Coll Cardiol* 1983;1:1201–1206.

66. Sigwart U, Grbic M, Payot J, et al. Ischemic events during coronary artery balloon occlusion. In: Rutishauser W, Roskamm H, eds. *Silent Myocardial Ischemia.* Berlin: Springer-Verlag; 1984:29.

67. Muller JE, Stone PH, Turi ZG, et al. Circadian variation in the frequency of onset of acute myocardial infarction. *N Engl J Med* 1985; 313:1315–1322.

68. Rocco MB, Barry J, Campbell S, et al. Circadian variation of transient myocardial ischemia in patients with coronary artery disease. *Circulation* 1987;75:395–400.

69. Rosen SD, Paulesu E, Frith CD, et al. Central nervous pathways mediating angina pectoris. *Lancet* 1994;344:147–150.

70. Sylven C, Beerman B, Jonzon B. Angina pectoris-like pain provoked by intravenous adenosine in healthy volunteers. *BMJ* 1986;293:227–230.

71. Herrick JB. Clinical features of sudden obstruction of the coronary arteries. *JAMA* 1912;59:2015–2020.

72. Roseman MD. Painless myocardial infarction: A review of the literature and analysis of 220 cases. *Ann Intern Med* 1954;41:1–8.

73. Froelicher VF, Yanowitz FG, Thompson AJ. The correlation of coronary angiography and the electrocardiographic response to maximal treadmill testing in 76 asymptomatic men. *Circulation* 1973;48:597–604.

74. Cohn PF. Asymptomatic coronary artery disease: Pathophysiology, diagnosis, management. *Mod Concepts Cardiovasc Dis* 1981;50:55–60.

75. Serneri GGN, Doddi M, Arata L, et al. Silent ischemia in unstable angina is related to an altered cardiac norepinephrine handling. *Circulation* 1993;87:1928–1937.

76. Cohn PF. Prevalence of silent myocardial ischemia. In: Cohn PF, ed. *Silent Myocardial Ischemia and Infarction.* New York: Marcel Dekker; 1986:71–80.

77. Deanfield JE, Ribiero P, Oakley K, et al. Analysis of ST-segment changes in normal subjects: Implications for ambulatory monitoring in angina pectoris. *Am J Cardiol* 1984;54:1321–1325.

78. Crawford NH, Bernstein SJ, DiMarco J, et al. ACC/AHA guidelines for ambulatory electrocardiography. *Circulation* 1999;34:912–948.

79. Hedblad B, Juul-Moller S, Svensson K, et al. Increased mortality in men with ST segment depression during 24 h ambulatory long-term ECG recording: Results from prospective population study "Men born in 1914," from Malmo, Sweden. *Eur Heart J* 1989;10:149–158.

80. Pepine CJ, Coy K, Lambert C. Silent myocardial ischemia during daily activities in asymptomatic patients with positive treadmill tests. In: Singh B, ed. *Silent Myocardial Ischemia and Angina.* New York: Pergamon Press; 1988:93–103.

81. Crawford MH, Bernstein SJ, Deedwania PC, et al. ACC/AHA guidelines for ambulatory electrocardiography: A report of the American College of Cardiology/American Heart Association Task Force on Practice Guidelines (Committee to Revise the Guidelines for Ambulatory Electrocardiography): Developed in collaboration with the North American Society for Pacing and Electrophysiology. *J Am Coll Cardiol* 1999;34:912–948.

82. Deanfield JE, Maseri A, Selwyn AP, et al. Myocardial ischaemia during daily life in patients with stable angina: Its relation to symptoms and heart rate changes. *Lancet* 1983;3:753–758.

83. Cannon RO III, Watson RM, Rosing DR, Epstein SE. Angina caused by reduced vasodilator reserve of the small coronary arteries. *J Am Coll Cardiol* 1983;1:1359–1373.

84. Mannheimer C, Carlsson CA, Vedin A, Wilhelmsson C. Transcutaneous electrical nerve stimulation (TENS) in angina pectoris. *Pain* 1986;26:291–300.

85. Davies HA, Page Z, Rush EM, et al. Esophageal stimulation lowers exertional angina threshold. *Lancet* 1985;1:1011–1014.

86. Pepine CJ, Coy K, Lambert C. Silent myocardial ischemia during daily activities in asymptomatic patients with positive treadmill tests. In: Singh B, ed. *Silent Myocardial Ischemia and Angina.* New York: Pergamon Press; 1988:93.

87. Droste C, Roskamm H. Experimental pain measurements in patients with asymptomatic myocardial ischemia. *J Am Coll Cardiol* 1983;1:940–945.

88. Glazier JJ, Chierchia S, Brown MJ, Maseri A. Importance of generalized defective perception of painful stimuli as a cause of silent myocardial ischemia in chronic stable angina pectoris. *Am J Cardiol* 1986;58:667–672.

89. Falcone C, Sconocchia R, Guasti L, et al. Dental pain threshold and angina pectoris in patients with coronary artery disease. *J Am Coll Cardiol* 1988;12:348–352.

90. Bradley RF, Partamian JO. Coronary heart disease in the diabetic patient. *Med Clin North Am* 1993;78:1093–1104.

91. Fearman I, Faccio E, Melei J. Autonomic neuropathy and painless myocardial infarction in diabetic patients: Histology evidence of their relationships. *Diabetes* 1977;26:1147–1158.

92. Nesto RW, Phillips RT, Kett KG. Angina and exertional myocardial ischemia in diabetic and nondiabetic patients: Assessment by exercise thallium scintigraphy. *Ann Intern Med* 1988;108:170–175.

93. Chiariello M, Indolfi C, Cotecchia MR. Asymptomatic transient ST changes during ambulatory ECG monitoring in diabetic patients. *Am Heart J* 1985;110:529–534.

94. Coy KM, Imperi GA, Lambert CR, Pepine CJ. Silent myocardial ischemia during daily activities in asymptomatic men with positive exercise test responses. *Am J Cardiol* 1987;59:45–49.

95. Deanfield JE, Kensett M, Wilson RA, et al. Silent myocardial ischaemia due to mental stress. *Lancet* 1984;2:1001–1005.

96. Bertolet BD, Hill JA, Pepine CJ. Treatment strategies for daily life silent myocardial ischemia: A correlation with potential pathogenic mechanisms. *Prog Cardiovasc Dis* 1992;35:97–118.

97. Rogers WJ, Bourassa MG, Andrews TC, et al. Asymptomatic Cardiac Ischemia Pilot (ACIP) Study: Outcome at 1 year for patients with asymptomatic cardiac ischemia randomized to medical therapy or revascularization. *J Am Coll Cardiol* 1995;26:594–605.

98. Pepine CJ, Sharaf B, Andrews TC, et al. Relation between clinical, angiographic and ischemic findings at baseline and ischemia-related adverse outcomes at 1 year in Asymptomatic Cardiac Ischemia Pilot Study. *J Am Coll Cardiol* 1997;29:1483–1489.

99. Davies RF, Goldberg AD, Forman S, et al. Asymptomatic Cardiac Ischemia Pilot (ACIP) study two-year follow-up: Outcomes of patients randomized to initial strategies of medical therapy versus revascularization. *Circulation* 1997;95:2037–2043.

100. Hubbard BL, Gibbons RJ, Lapeyre AC, et al. Identification of severe coronary artery disease using simple clinical parameters. *Arch Intern Med* 1992;152(2):309–312.

101. Hammermeister KE, DeRouen TA, Dodge HT. Variables predictive of survival in patients with coronary disease: Selection by univariate and multivariate analyses from the clinical, electrocardiographic, exercise, arteriographic, and quantitative angiographic evaluations. *Circulation* 1979;59(3):421–430.

102. Oh JK, Gibbons RJ, Christian TF, et al. Correlation of regional wall motion abnormalities determined by technetium-99m sestamibi imaging in patients treated with reperfusion therapy during acute myocardial infarction. *Am Heart J* 1996;131:32–37.

103. Califf RM, Mark DB, Harrell FE, et al. Importance of clinical measures of ischemia in the prognosis of patients with documented coronary artery disease. *Circulation* 1988;11(1):20–26.

104. Guidelines for percutaneous transluminal coronary angioplasty: A report of the American College of Cardiology/American Heart Association Task Force on Assessment of Diagnostic and Therapeutic Cardiovascular Procedures (Committee on Percutaneous Transluminal Coronary Angioplasty). *J Am Coll Cardiol* 1993;22(7):2033–2054.

105. Christian TF, Miller TD, Bailey KR, Gibbons RJ. Exercise tomographic thallium-201 imaging in patients with severe coronary artery disease and normal electrocardiograms. *Ann Intern Med* 1994;121(11):825–832.

106. Mark DB, Hlatky MA, Harrell FE, et al. Exercise treadmill score for predicting prognosis in coronary artery disease. *Ann Intern Med* 1987;106(6):793–800.

107. Morrow K, Morris CK, Froelicher VF, et al. Prediction of cardiovascular death in men undergoing noninvasive evaluation for coronary artery disease. *Ann Intern Med* 1993;118(9):689–695.

108. Mark DB, Shaw L, Harrell FE, et al. Prognostic value of a treadmill exercise score in outpatients with suspected coronary artery disease. *N Engl J Med* 1991;325:849–853.

109. Alexander KP, Shaw LJ, Shaw LK, et al. Value of exercise treadmill testing in women. *J Am Coll Cardiol* 1998;32(6):1657–1664.

110. Beleslin BD, Ostojic M, Stepanovic J, et al. Stress echocardiography in the detection of myocardial ischemia: Head-to-head comparison of exercise, dobutamine, and dipyridamole tests. *Circulation* 1994;90:1168–1176.

111. Dagianti A, Penco M, Agati L, et al. Stress echocardiography: Comparison of exercise, dipyridamole and dobutamine in detecting and predicting the extent of coronary artery disease [published erratum appears in *J Am Coll Cardiol* 1995;26:114]. *J Am Coll Cardiol* 1995;26(1):18–25.

112. Williams MJ, Odabashian J, Lauer MS, et al. Prognostic value of dobutamine echocardiography in patients with left ventricular dysfunction. *J Am Coll Cardiol* 1996;27:132–139.

113. Afridi I, Quinones MA, Zoghbi WA, Cheirif J. Dobutamine stress echocardiography: Sensitivity, specificity, and predictive value for future cardiac events. *Am Heart J* 1994;127:1510–1515.

114. Kamaran M, Teague SM, Finkelhor RS, et al. Prognostic value of dobutamine stress echocardiography in patients referred because of suspected coronary artery disease. *Am J Cardiol* 1995;76:887–891.

115. Marcovitz PA, Shayna V, Horn RA, et al. Value of dobutamine stress echocardiography in determining the prognosis of patients with known or suspected coronary artery disease. *Am J Cardiol* 1996;78:404–408.

116. Brown KA. Prognostic value of thallium-201 myocardial perfusion imaging: A diagnostic tool comes of age. *Circulation* 1991;83:363–381.

117. National Center for Health Statistics. *Vital Statistics of the United States, 1979,* Vol II: Mortality, Part A (U.S. Department of Health and Human Services publication PHS84–1101). Washington, DC: US Government Printing Office; 1984.

118. Hachamovitch R, Berman DS, Shaw LJ, et al. Incremental prognostic value of myocardial perfusion single photon emission computed tomography for the prediction of cardiac death: Differential stratification for risk of cardiac death and myocardial infarction [published erratum appears in *Circulation* 1999;98(2):190]. *Circulation* 1998;97(6):533–543.

119. Wagdy HM, Hodge D, Christian TF, et al. Prognostic value of vasodilator myocardial perfusion imaging in patients with left bundle-branch-block. *Circulation* 1998;97(16):1563–1570.

120. Marwick T, D'Hondt AM, Baudhuin T, et al. Optimal use of dobutamine stress for the detection and evaluation of coronary artery disease: Combination with echocardiography or scintigraphy, or both? *J Am Coll Cardiol* 1993;22(1):159–167.

121. Marwick TH. Use of exercise echocardiography for the prognostic assessment of patients with stable chronic coronary artery disease. *Eur Heart J* 1997;18(suppl D):D97–D101.

122. Yusuf S, Zucker D, Peduzzi P, et al. Effect of coronary artery bypass graft surgery on survival: Overview of 10-year results from randomized trials by the Coronary Artery Bypass Graft Surgery Trialists Collaboration [published erratum appears in *Lancet* 1994;344(8934):1446]. *Lancet* 1994;344(8922):563–570.

123. Emond M, Mock MB, Davis KB, et al. Long-term survival of medically treated patients in the Coronary Artery Surgery Study (CASS) registry. *Circulation* 1994;90(6):2645–2657.

124. Ryan TJ, Antman EM, Brooks NH, et al. ACC/AHA guidelines for the management of patients with acute myocardial infarction: 1999 update: A report of the American College of Cardiology/American Heart Association Task force on Practice Guidelines (Committee on Management of Acute Myocardial Infacttion). 1999. American College of Cardiology Web site. Available at http://www.acc.org/clinical/guidelines/nov96/1999/index.htm. Accessed October 17, 2002.

125. O'Rourke R, Boden W, Weintraub W, et al. Medical therapy versus percutaneous coronary intervention: Implications of the Avert Study and the Courage Trial. *Curr Pract Med* 1999;2(11):225–227.

126. Final report on the aspirin component of the ongoing Physicians' Health Study. Steering Committee of the Physicians' Health Study Research Group. *N Engl J Med* 1989;321:129–135.

127. Juul-Moller S, Edvardsson N, Jahnmatz B, et al. Double-blind trial of aspirin in primary prevention of myocardial infarction in patients with stable chronic angina pectoris: The Swedish Angina Pectoris Aspirin Trial (SAPAT) group. *Lancet* 1992;340:1421–1425.

128. O'Rourke RA. Hurst's Online—Meta-Analysis of 200,000 patients with low/high doses. (See website for references.)

129. McTavish D, Faulds D, Goa KL. Ticlopidine: An updated review of its pharmacology and therapeutic use in platelet-dependent disorders. *Drugs* 1990;40(2):238–259.

130. Yusuf S, Zhao F, Mehta SR, et al: Effects of clopidogrel in addition to aspirin in patients with acute coronary syndromes without ST-segment-elevation. *N Engl J Med* 2001;345(7):494–502.

131. O'Rourke RA, Hurst's Online Editorial. Are the One Year Results of the CREDO Trial Compelling? http://www.cardiology.accessmedicine.com

132. Khot UN, Nissen SE: Is CURE a cure for acute coronary syndromes? Statistical versus clinical significance. *J Am Coll Cardiol* 2002;40:218–219.

133. CAPRIE Steering Committee. A randomized, blinded trial of clopidogrel versus aspirin in patients at risk of ischemic events (CAPRIE). *Lancet* 1996;348(9038):1329–1339.

134. Melandri G, Semprini F, Cervi V, et al. Benefit of adding low molecular weight heparin to the conventional treatment of stable angina pectoris: A double-blind, randomized, placebo-controlled trial. *Circulation* 1993;88(6):2517–2523.

135. Thrombosis prevention trial: Randomised trial of low-intensity oral anticoagulation with warfarin and low-dose aspirin in the primary prevention of ischaemic heart disease in men at increased risk. The Medical Research Council's General Practice Research Framework. *Lancet* 1998;351:233–241.

136. Randomized trial of cholesterol lowering in 4444 patients with coronary heart disease: The Scandinavian Simvastatin Survival Study (4S). *Lancet* 1994;344:1383–1389.

137. Pedersen T, Olsson A, Faergeman O, et al. Lipoprotein changes and reduction in the incidence of major coronary heart disease events in the Scandinavian Simvastatin Survival Study (4S). *Circulation* 1998;97:1453–1460.

138. Sacks FM, Pfeffer MA, Moye LA, et al. The effect of pravastatin on coronary events after myocardial infarction in patients with average cholesterol levels: Cholesterol and Recurrent Events Trial investigators. *N Engl J Med* 1996;335(14):1001–1009.

139. Gould A, Rossouw J, Santanello N, et al. Cholesterol reduction yields clinical benefit impact of Statin Trials. *Circulation* 1998;86:946–952.

140. MRC/BHF Heart Protection Study of cholesterol lowering with simvastatin in 20,536 high-risk individuals: A randomized placebo-controlled trial. *Lancet* 2002;360:7–22.

141. Yusef S, Sleight P, Pogue J, et al. Effects of an angiotensin-converting-enzyme inhibitor, ramipril, on cardiovascular events in high-risk patients. The Heart Outcomes Prevention Evaluation Study Investigators. *N Engl J Med* 2000;342:145–153.

142. Heart Outcomes Prevention Evaluation Study Investigators. Effects of ramipril on cardiovascular outcomes in people with diabetes mellitus: Results of the HOPE study and MICRO-HOPE sub-study. *Lancet* 2000;355:253–259.

143. Wallace WA, Wellington KL, Chess MA, Liang CS. Comparison of nifedipine gastrointestinal therapeutic system and atenolol on antianginal efficacies and exercise hemodynamic responses in stable angina pectoris. *Am J Cardiol* 1994;73(1):23–28.

144. de Vries RJ, van den Heuvel AF, Lok DJ, et al. Nifedipine gastrointestinal therapeutic system versus atenolol in stable angina pectoris: The Netherlands Working Group on Cardiovascular Research (WCN). *Int J Cardiol* 1996;57:143–150.

145. Fox KM, Mulcahy D, Findlay I, et al. The Total Ischaemic Burden European Trial (TIBET): Effects of atenolol, nifedipine SR and their combination on the exercise test and the total ischaemic burden in 608 patients with stable angina. The TIBET Study Group. *Eur Heart J* 1996;17(1):96–103.

146. Savonitto S, Ardissiono D, Egstrup K, et al. Combination therapy with metoprolol and nifedipine versus monotherapy in patients with stable angina pectoris: Results of the International Multicenter Angina Exercise (IMAGE) study. *J Am Coll Cardiol* 1996;27(2):311–316.

147. van de Ven LL, Vermeulen A, Tana JG, et al. Which drug to choose for stable angina pectoris: A comparative study between bisoprolol and nitrates. *Int J Cardiol* 1995;47(3):217–223.

148. Waysbort J, Meshulam N, Brunner D. Isosorbide-5-mononitrate and atenolol in the treatment of stable exertional angina. *Cardiology* 1991;79(suppl 2):19–26.

149. Krepp HP. Evaluation of the antianginal and anti-ischemic efficacy of slow release isosorbide-5-mononitrate capsules, bupranolol and their combination, in patients with chronic stable angina pectoris. *Cardiology* 1991;79(suppl 2):14–18.

150. Pepine CJ, Feldman RL, Whittle J, et al. Effect of diltiazem in patients with variant angina: A randomized double-blind trial. *Am Heart J* 1981;101(6):719–725.

151. Antman E, Muller J, Goldberg S, et al. Nifedipine therapy for coronary-artery spasm: Experience in 127 patients. *N Engl J Med* 1980;302(23):1269–1273.

152. Psaty BM, Heckbert SR, Koepsell TD, et al. The risk of myocardial infarction associated with antihypertensive drug therapies. *JAMA* 1995;274(8):620–625.

153. Furberg CD, Psaty BM, Meyer JV. Nifedipine: Dose-related increase in mortality in patients with coronary heart disease. *Circulation* 1995;92(5):1326–1331.

154. Opie LH, Messerli FH. Nifedipine and mortality: Grave defects in the dossier. *Circulation* 1995;92(5):1068–1073.

155. Ad Hoc Subcommittee of the Liaison Committee of the World Health Organization and the International Society of Hypertension. Effects of calcium antagonists on the risks of coronary heart disease, cancer and bleeding. *J Hypertens* 1997;15:105–115.

156. Schneider W, Maul FD, Bussmann WD, et al. Comparison of the antianginal efficacy of isosorbide dinitrate (ISDN) 40 mg and verapamil 120 mg three times daily in the acute trial and following two-week treatment. *Eur Heart J* 1998;9:149–158.

157. Ankier SI, Fay L, Warrington SJ, Woodings DF. A multicentre open comparison of isosorbide-5-mononitrate and nifedipine given prophylactically to general practice patients with chronic stable angina pectoris. *J Int Med Res* 1989;17(2):172–178.

158. Emanuelsson H, Ake H, Kristi M, Arina R. Effects of diltiazem and isosorbide-5-mononitrate, alone and in combination, on patients with stable angina pectoris. *Eur J Clin Pharmacol* 1989;36:561–566.

159. Akhras F, Jackson G. Efficacy of nifedipine and isosorbide mononitrate in combination with atenolol in stable angina. *Lancet* 1991;338(8774):1036–1039.

160. Cheitlin MD, Hutter AM Jr, Brindis RG, et al. ACC/AHA expert consensus documents: Use of sildenafil (Viagra) in patients with cardiovascular disease. *J Am Coll Cardiol* 1999;33:273–282.

161. Fung HL, Bauer JA. Mechanisms of nitrate tolerance. *Cardiovasc Drugs Ther* 1994;8(3):489–499.

162. Chirkov YY, Chirkova LP, Horowitz JD. Nitroglycerin tolerance at the platelet level in patients with angina pectoris. *Am J Cardiol* 1997;80(2):128–131.

163. Stamler J, Neaton J, Wentworth DN. Blood pressure (systolic and diastolic) and risk of fatal coronary heart disease. *Hypertension* 1989;13(suppl 5):I2–I12.

164. The sixth report of the Joint National Committee on prevention, detection, evaluation, and treatment of high blood pressure. *Arch Intern Med* 1997;157(21):2413–2446.

165. Alderman MH, Cohen H, Roque R, Madhavan S. Effect of long-acting and short-acting calcium antagonist on cardiovascular outcomes in hypertensive patients. *Lancet* 1997;349(9052):594–598.

166. Kannel WB, Gordon T, Castelli WP, Margolis JR. Electrocardiographic left ventricular hypertrophy and risk of coronary heart disease: The Framingham Study. *Ann Intern Med* 1970;72(6):813–822.

167. Ghali JK, Liao Y, Simmons B, et al. The prognostic role of left ventricular hypertrophy in patients with or without coronary artery disease. *Ann Intern Med* 1992;117(10):831–836.

168. Levy D, Salomon M, D'Agostino RB, et al. Prognostic implications of baseline electrocardiographic features and their serial changes in subjects with left ventricular hypertrophy. *Circulation* 1994;90(4):1786–1793.

169. Ernst E, Resch KL. Fibrinogen as a cardiovascular risk factor: A meta-analysis and review of the literature. *Ann Intern Med* 1993;118(12):956–963.

170. American Diabetes Association. Clinical practice recommendations 1998: Screening for type 2 diabetes. *Diabetes Care* 1998;21(suppl 1):1–98.

171. The effect of intensive treatment of diabetes on the development and progression of long-term complications in insulin-dependent diabetes mellitus: The Diabetes Control and Complications Trial Research Group. *N Engl J Med* 1993;329:977–986.

172. Getz GS. Report on the workshop on diabetes and mechanisms of atherogenesis, September 17 and 18, 1992, Bethesda, Maryland. *Arterioscler Thromb* 1993;13:459–464.

173. National Cholesterol Education Program. Third report of the expert panel on detection, evaluation, and treatment of high blood cholesterol in adults (adult treatment panel III). *Circulation* 2002;106:3143–3421.

174. Eckel RH. Obesity and heart disease: A statement for healthcare professionals from the Nutrition Committee, American Heart Association. *Circulation* 1997;96(9):3248–3250.

175. Hulley S, Grady D, Bush T, et al. Randomized trial of estrogen plus progestin for secondary prevention of coronary heart disease in postmenopausal women: Heart and Estrogen/Progestin Replacement Study (HERS) research group. *JAMA* 1998;280(7):605–613.

175a. Curb JD, McTiernan A, Heckbert SR, et al. Outcomes ascertainment and adjudication methods in the women's health initiative. *Ann Epidemiol* 2003;95:S122–S128.

175b. Barrett-Connor E, Ensrud KE, Harper K, et al. Post hoc analysis of data from the Multiple Outcomes of Raloxifene Evaluation (MORE) trial on the effects of three years of raloxifene treatment on glycemic control and cardiovascular disease risk factors in women with and without type 2 diabetes. *Clin Ther* 2003;25(3):919–930.

176. Jeppesen J, Hein HO, Suadicani P, Gyntelberg F. Triglyceride concentration and ischemic heart disease: An eight-year follow-up in the Copenhagen male study [published erratum appears in *Circulation* 1999;98(2);190]. *Circulation* 1998;97(11):1029–1036.

177. Reaven GM. Insulin resistance and compensatory hyperinsulinemia: Role in hypertension, dyslipidemia, and coronary heart disease. *Am Heart J* 1991;121(4 pt 2):1283–1288.

178. Coronary Heart Disease. Triglyceride, high-density lipoprotein, and coronary heart disease. *JAMA* 1993;269:505–510.

179. Genest JJ, Jenner JL, McNamara JR, et al. Prevalence of lipoprotein (a) [Lp(a)] excess in coronary artery disease. *Am J Cardiol* 1991;67(13):1039–1045.

180. Clarke R, Daly L, Robinson K, et al. Hyperhomocysteinemia: An independent risk factor for vascular disease. *N Engl J Med* 1991;324(17):1149–1155.

181. Stampfer MJ, Malinow MR, Willett WC, et al. A prospective study of plasma homocysteine and risk of myocardial infarction in US physicians. *JAMA* 1992;268(7):877–881.

182. Berliner JA, Navab M, Fogelman AM, et al. Atherosclerosis: Basic mechanisms. Oxidation, inflammation, and genetics. *Circulation* 1995; 91(9):2488–2496.

183. Nyyssonen K, Parviainen MT, Salonen R, et al. Vitamin C deficiency and risk of myocardial infarction: Prospective population study of men from eastern Finland. *BMJ* 1997;314(7081):634–638.

184. Gaziano JM, Buring JE, Breslow JL, et al. Moderate alcohol intake, increased levels of high-density lipoprotein and its subfractions, and decreased risk of myocardial infarction. *N Engl J Med* 1993;329(25):1829–1834.

185. Parisi AF, Folland ED, Hartigan P. A comparison of angioplasty with medical therapy in the treatment of single-vessel coronary artery disease: Veterans Affairs ACME Investigators. *N Engl J Med* 1992;326(1):10–16.

186. Coronary angioplasty versus medical therapy for angina: The second Randomised Intervention Treatment of Angina (RITA-2) trial. RITA-2 trial participants. *Lancet* 1997;350(9076):461–468.

187. Pitt B, Waters D, Brown WV, et al. Aggressive lipid-lowering therapy compared with angioplasty in stable coronary artery disease: Atorvastatin versus Revascularization Treatment Investigators. *N Engl J Med* 1999;341(2):70–76.

188. Comparison of coronary bypass surgery with angioplasty in patients with multivessel disease: The Bypass Angioplasty Revascularization Investigation (BARI) investigators [published erratum appears in *N Engl J Med* 1997;336(2):147]. *N Engl J Med* 1996;335(4):217–225.

188a. Pepine CJ, Wolff AA. A controlled trial with a novel anti-ischemic agent, ranolazine, in chronic stable angina pectoris that is responsive to conventional antianginal agents. *Am J Cardiol* 1999;84:46–50.

188b. Chaitman BR, Skettino S, DeQuattro V. Improved exercise performance on ranolazine in patients with chronic angina and a history of heart failure: The MARISA Trial. *J Am Coll Cardiol* 2001;37(suppl A):149A.

189. Kemp HG, Elliott WC, Gorlin R. The anginal syndrome with normal coronary arteriography. *Trans Assoc Am Physicians* 1967;80:59–70.

190. Kemp HG. Left ventricular function in patients with the anginal syndrome and normal coronary arteriograms. *Am J Cardiol* 1973;32(3):375–376.

191. Cannon RO III, Canici PG, Epstein SE. Pathophysiological dilemma of syndrome X. *Circulation* 1992;85:883–892.

192. Kaplan MN. Syndromes X: Two too many. *J Am Coll Cardiol* 1992;69:1643–1644.

CORONARY BYPASS SURGERY

Bruce W. Lytle

Coronary bypass surgery—as a planned, consistent approach for the treatment of patients with angiographically documented coronary atherosclerosis—was begun by Sones and colleagues in 1967. The concept behind the concerted effort undertaken by cardiologists and cardiac surgeons at the Cleveland Clinic Foundation in 1967 was that the symptoms and clinical events associated with coronary artery disease (CAD) were related to stenotic coronary artery lesions that could be specifically identified by coronary angiography, and if those lesions could be treated with bypass grafting, unfavorable symptoms and events would be less common. Experience has shown that concept to be correct, but it also has shown that atherosclerosis is a progressive disease.

Effective bypass surgery obviously relieves symptoms of angina, and early randomized trials have also shown that it prolong the life expectancy of some subsets of patients with severe CAD. The arrival of an anatomic treatment for CAD, the most common cause of premature death in western countries, initiated a rapid growth in the personnel and medical infrastructure dedicated to bypass surgery. Along with the growth of bypass surgery came the investigation of strategies for endoluminal anatomic treatment for CAD, which have resulted in increasingly effective percutaneous therapy (PCT) for CAD. Also, pharmacologic treatments for CAD have progressed rapidly, particularly in the last decade. The roles of these complementary therapies for the treatment of CAD continue to evolve, and identifying the optimal application of these therapies continues to be a challenge.

Bypass Grafts and Outcomes

Early coronary bypass operations were based almost entirely on aorta-to-coronary reversed saphenous vein grafts (SVG) (Fig. 58-1A). Patency rates of SVGs within the first postoperative year were 80 to 90 percent and were influenced by surgical technique, gender (men > women), coronary artery size (bigger > smaller), and the coronary artery grafted [left anterior descending (LAD)] greater than circumflex or right coronary artery, but they were not influenced by coronary risk factors.[1–3] However, serial angiographic studies of SVGs demonstrated a significant late attrition rate of initially successful grafts that ranged from 2 to 5 percent per year 6 to 11 years after operation.[2,3] Serial Cleveland Clinic Foundation studies of SVGs found that of grafts patent within 5 years of operation, only 55 percent remained angiographically perfect 6 to 12 years after surgery (Fig. 58-2A).[1] Furthermore, the late graft attrition rate was not related to the vessel grafted but was increased for patients with risk factors such as diabetes and hyperlipidemia.[1,3]

Much of the late attrition of SVGs appears to be related to intrinsic pathologic changes in those grafts: intimal fibroplasia and vein graft atherosclerosis.[3,4] Almost all SVGs examined within a few months after operation exhibit intimal fibroplasia, a hypercellular proliferative hyperplasia that involves the intima, is usually concentric, and is distributed throughout the length of the graft. With time it becomes less cellular and more fibrotic. Intimal fibroplasia may cause stenoses and occlusions, but it usually does not.

Vein graft atherosclerosis (VGA) is characterized by lipid infiltration of areas of intimal fibroplasia and is different in distribution and character than native coronary atherosclerosis.

Native coronary artery atherosclerosis is a proximal, eccentric, and intermittent lesion that is usually covered by a fibrous cap. VGA is distributed throughout the length of vein grafts; it is circumferential, not encapsulated, and extremely friable. With time the early circumferential lesion will often progress to eccentric

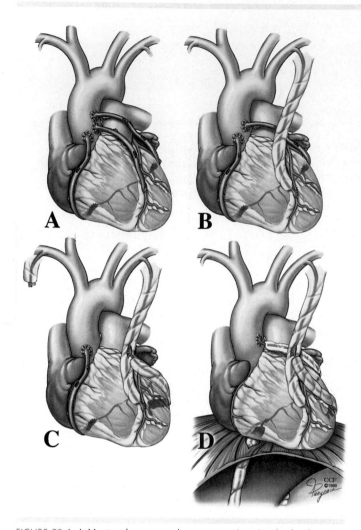

FIGURE 58-1 *A.* Most early coronary bypass operations involved only aorta-to-coronary saphenous vein grafts. *B.* The use of a LITA-to-LAD graft combined with vein grafts has become the standard bypass operation. *C.* Bilateral ITA grafting may be accomplished with a composite ITA graft. Here the RITA is anastomosed to the LITA-LAD graft and used as a graft to the circumflex coronary artery with an SVG used to graft the RCA. *D.* Total arterial revascularization is accomplished here with an aorta-to-coronary RITA-to-circumflex graft. The radial artery is used as a composite graft from the LITA to the diagonal coronary artery, the LITA is used as a graft to the LAD, and an in situ gastroepiploic graft to the RCA.

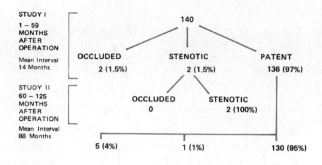

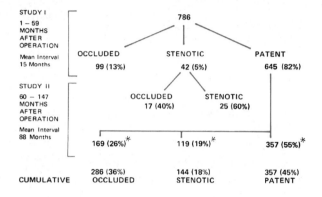

Percentages Refer to Grafts Originally Patent.

FIGURE 58-2 *A.* Data from serial postoperative angiography of ITA-to-coronary grafts (*top*). Percentages not marked with an asterisk refer to the total number of grafts (140). Any graft narrowing was considered a stenosis. [From Lytle BW, Loop FD, Cosgrove DM, et al. Long-term (5 to 12 years) serial studies of internal mammary artery and saphenous vein coronary bypass grafts. *J Thorac Cardiovasc Surg* 1985;89:250. With permission.] *B.* Data from serial postoperative angiography of saphenous vein–to-coronary grafts (*bottom*). Any graft narrowing was considered a stenosis. Percentages not marked with an asterisk refer to the total number of grafts (786). Percentages marked with an asterisk refer to grafts originally patent. [From Lytle BW, Loop FD, Cosgrove DM, et al. Long-term (5 to 12 years) serial studies of internal mammary artery and saphenous vein coronary bypass grafts. *J Thorac Cardiovasc Surg* 1985;89:250. With permission.]

lesions causing severe stenoses (Fig. 58-3). VGA is a dangerous lesion. Because of the friability and nonencapsulated nature of this lesion, embolization of atherosclerotic debris is a major risk during percutaneous interventions on vein grafts and during reoperations, and it is probable that spontaneous embolization may occur. VGA is usually not recognized before 2 to 3 years after operation and does not appear to cause much graft attrition before 5 postoperative years. However, the increased rate of graft attrition seen more than 5 years after operation appears to be in large part due to VGA, and the presence of late stenoses in vein grafts predicts adverse clinical events.

Since the early SVG studies, substantial progress has been made in extending the effectiveness of SVGs. First, perioperative treatment with platelet inhibitors has decreased the occlusion rate of SVGs at 1 year after operation,[5,6] such that approximately 90 percent of SVGs

are functioning at 1 postoperative year. Second, lipid-lowering regimens, including the use of 3-hydroxy-3-methylglutaryl-coenzyme A (HMG-CoA) reductase inhibitors, or statins, have been shown to decrease the rate of vein graft atherosclerosis 5 to 15 years after operation and have decreased the risk of death and nonfatal myocardial infarction (MI) during a 5-year follow-up after bypass surgery.[7,8] It is also important not to lose sight of the fact that despite the imperfections of vein grafts, many SVGs provide substantial long-term benefit, and studies of patients more than 15 years after operation have shown approximately 50 percent of SVGs still to be functioning at that time.[9]

Internal Thoracic Artery Grafts

Grafts from the internal thoracic artery (ITA) to the coronary artery were used in a few centers from the beginning of bypass surgery, usually as grafts to the LAD artery. Early patency rates of ITA grafts are better than those for vein grafts, but more importantly, the late

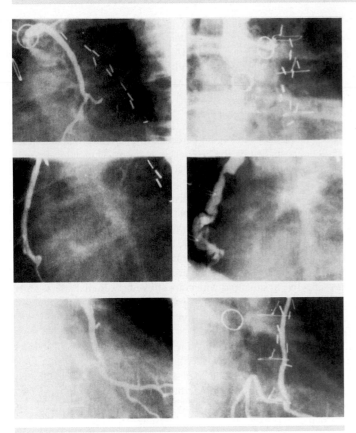

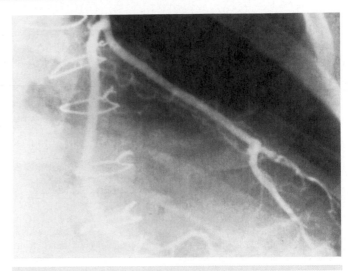

FIGURE 58-4 Early patency studies of composite ITA grafts have been favorable. Here the LITA supplies the diagonal and LAD vessels and the RITA the circumflex.

FIGURE 58-3 Angiographic anatomy 1 year after operation (*left*) showing patent vein grafts to the LAD and RCA and an ITA graft to the circumflex artery. Seven years later (*right*), the LAD vein graft is occluded, the RCA graft exhibits diffuse irregular stenoses characteristic of vein graft atherosclerosis, and the ITA graft is unchanged. [From Lytle BW, Loop FD, Cosgrove DM, et al. Long-term (5 to 12 years) serial studies of internal mammary artery and saphenous vein coronary bypass grafts. *J Thorac Cardiovasc Surg* 1985;89:250. With permission.]

attrition of ITA grafts is extremely low (Fig. 58-2B).[1,2,10,11] Early occlusion of ITA grafts is usually technically related and today is uncommon. Prospective angiographic studies from the multicenter Bypass Angioplasty Revascularization Investigation (BARI) trial noted a 98 percent 1-year patency (<50 percent stenosis) rate for ITA grafts.[10] It is possible for atherosclerosis to involve the ITA, particularly at its subclavian origin, but it is not common, and the late development of a new atherosclerotic lesion in a patent ITA graft is very rare. Thus, the 20-year patency rate of LITA-to-LAD grafts is still approximately 90 percent.[12] The most common cause of late ITA graft failure appears to be competition in blood flow through a native coronary artery that is only moderately stenotic.[13] That may produce a diffuse ITA narrowing or "string sign." It is known that atretic ITA grafts may increase in size if the stenosis of the nonsignificant native coronary artery becomes more severe with time, but this is not a predictable phenomenon.

The success of the left ITA (LITA) to LAD graft has led to the use of the right ITA (RITA) as a bypass graft, usually simultaneously with the LITA (bilateral ITA grafting). The RITA has been used as an in situ graft and as a "free" graft, with the proximal anastomosis constructed either to the LITA (Fig. 58-1C) or the aorta (Fig. 58-1D). Although patency rates of ITA grafts have been highest when the LAD-diagonal system is grafted, Dion et al. restudied 135 pedicled

ITA-to-circumflex artery grafts 13 months after operation and noted a 95 percent patency rate.[14] Longer-term studies of ITA-to-circumflex grafts have also shown favorable outcomes. ITA grafts to the right coronary artery (RCA) have been less frequent and prospective postoperative studies are rare, but long-term patency of ITA grafts to the right coronary system is possible. Studies of aorta-to-coronary ITA grafts have tended to show patency rates not quite as good as those of pedicled grafts. However, these types of grafts can exhibit 20-year patency, and once they are patent they appear to remain free from graft atherosclerosis.

A strategy that greatly expands the capacity to achieve extensive revascularization with ITA grafts is composite arterial grafting, where the RITA is anastomosed to the LITA (Fig. 58-4).[15] This strategy makes use of the free ITA graft more effective, and although long-term data are not available, early studies show patency rates of 91 to 95 percent within a year of operation for this strategy. With experience, the composite ITA grafting strategy may be used to graft the circumflex and right coronary systems as well as the LAD and achieve total revascularization with two ITA grafts.

Clinical Impact of ITA Grafts

The high and stable patency rate of the LITA to LAD graft is important in producing improved clinical outcomes. A large observational study by Loop et al. showed that patients who received a LITA-LAD graft (with or without SVGs to the Cx and RCA systems) had better survival rates, underwent fewer reoperations, and experienced fewer adverse cardiac events over a 10-year follow-up when compared with patients who received only vein grafts. These observations were true regardless of whether patients had single-, double-, or triple-vessel disease.[11] Subsequent to the publication of this study in 1986, the LITA-LAD strategy became a fundamental part of operations for coronary revascularization (Fig. 58-1B). Data from the Coronary Artery Surgery Study (CASS) indicate that the benefits of ITA grafting extend into the second decade after bypass surgery,[16] and 20-year follow-up of patients from the Cleveland Clinic Foundation registry have shown that the benefits of ITA

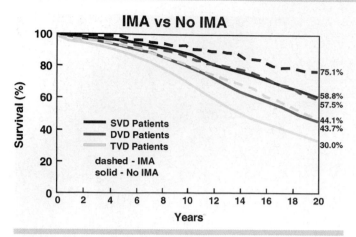

FIGURE 58-5 The 20-year follow-up of Cleveland Clinic Foundation patients from the years 1971–1974 shows superior survival rates for patients receiving left internal mammary artery (IMA) grafts compared with those receiving only vein grafts. These differences widen during the second postoperative decade.

grafts continue to extend out to 20 years after operation (Fig. 58-5). The LITA-LAD graft is the most effective and longest-lasting anatomic treatment of CAD known.

If one ITA graft is good, might two ITA grafts produce even better outcomes (Fig. 58-6)? The strategy of bilateral ITA grafting has not become widespread because it makes the bypass operation technically more difficult, diabetic patients appear to be at increased risk of wound complications, and outcomes for patients receiving LITA-LAD grafts along with vein grafts are so good during the first postoperative decade that improvement is difficult to show. However, there are now series containing enough patients with long enough follow-up that the benefit of two ITA grafts seems apparent, particularly during the second postoperative decade.[17,18] We have retrospectively reviewed a large nonrandomized, but propensity-matched series of patients and noted improved 12-year survival rates and a decreased risk of reoperation. (Fig. 58-6).[17]

Alternative Arterial Bypass Grafts

The gastroepiploic artery (GEA) has been successfully used as an in situ graft, usually to graft the right coronary artery (Fig. 58-1D).

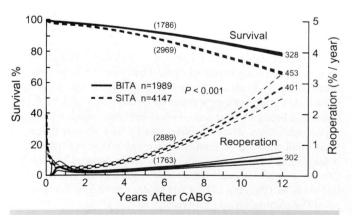

FIGURE 58-6 Comparison of survival and reoperation hazrd function curves in propensity-matched patients receiving bilateral ITA (BITA) grafts and single ITA (SITA) grafts with or without additional vein grafts. (From Lytle BW, Blackstone EH, LOOP FD, et al. Two internal thoracic artery grafts are better than one. J Thoracic Cardiovasc Surg 1999;117:855–872. With permission.)

Suma reported 644 of 685 GEA grafts (94 percent) patent within 1 year and 43 of 52 previously patent grafts with persistent patency 5 to 10 years after operation.[19] GEA grafts are adversely effective by competitive flow through minimally stenotic native coronary vessels and prone to spasm, intraluminal vasodilators being used intraoperatively by most proponents. The GEA has not become a widely used graft because it is difficult to use.

The inferior epigastric artery (IEA) has been used as a bypass graft with patency rates of 90 percent within a year of operation; 25 of 29 grafts studied by Buche et al. were patent 25 months after operation.[20] The IEA is useful as a composite arterial graft but is relatively short.

The most widely used alternative arterial graft is the radial artery. The radial artery is a long graft that is somewhat larger than the ITA; it is easily procured and has favorable size and handling characteristics. Five-year patency rates of 80 to 85 percent have been reported for radial artery grafts, and anecdotal patency beyond that time frame has been noted.[21,22] As with other arterial grafts, the radial artery is less effective in situations with competitive flow. Radial artery grafts are not as reliable as left ITA grafts but may be superior to vein grafts over the long term if they prove to be resistant to late graft atherosclerosis.

Total arterial revascularization is an appealing concept, but its clinical importance is not yet certain. Total arterial revascularization can be achieved in selected patients solely with the use of ITA grafts; for many patients, however, alternative arterial grafts are needed to complement the ITA grafts (Fig. 58-1D). Bergsma et al. reported on a group of 256 selected patients with triple-vessel disease who were revascularized with two ITA grafts and a GEA graft. These relatively good-risk patients had both a good survival rate and a very low incidence of angina (86 percent with no angina over 51 months).[23] If the radial artery proves to be a reliable graft that is resistant to atherosclerosis, total arterial revascularization will be more easily achievable.

EVOLUTION OF THE BYPASS SURGERY PATIENT POPULATION

In the early years of bypass surgery, surgical candidates were usually relatively young; they had limited CAD, good LV function, and few comorbid conditions. Today the surgical population had evolved into an older group of patients with more extensive coronary stenoses and more left main stenoses; there are also increased numbers of diabetics. Table 58-1 shows the changes in preoperative descriptors for patients undergoing primary coronary surgery at the Cleveland Clinic Foundation for selected years from 1967 through 2002, and Table 58-2 shows data concerning patient characteristics for the years 1980, 1990, and 2001 in the countrywide Society of Thoracic Surgeons (STS) National Database.[24–25] The bypass surgery population has changed for multiple reasons. Improved technology and experience have made it possible to operate on more complex and sicker patients with reasonable risk. Also, the randomized trials demonstrated that the patients who have the most to gain from surgery are patients with left main or multivessel disease and abnormal left ventricular (LV) function. Furthermore, the U.S. population has been aging, and older patients have high expectations for their activity level. Finally, in the early 1980s, the advent of percutaneous anatomic treatments (percutaneous transluminal coronary angioplasty, or PTCA) for coronary stenoses provided an alternative treatment for patients with limited coronary lesions, removing many of those patients from the surgical population.

TABLE 58-1 Preoperative Clinical Characteristics for the First 1000 Patients per Year Undergoing Elective Primary Isolated Coronary Bypass Grafting (Cleveland Clinic Foundation)

Clinical Variable	1967–1970	1976	1982	1988	1994	1999	2002
Age (years, median)	50	55	59	64	64	66	67
Men (%)	85	89	84	78	75	73	71
Diabetes (%)	7	6	9	19	24	32	33
Age ≥ 70 years (%)	0.2	3	10	26	28	36	39
Single-vessel disease[a] (%)	56	15	8	3	9	10	10
Double-vessel disease[a] (%)	31	28	25	19	29	27	20
Triple-vessel disease[a] (%)	13	57	67	78	60	62	68
Left main coronary stenosis (≥50%) (%)	9	12	13	16	19	23	24
Left ventricular asynergy (%)	41	45	55	57	48	45	47

[a]The terms *single*, *double-*, and *triple-vessel disease* refer to the number of the three main coronary vessels (left anterior descending, circumflex, and right coronary arteries) that have stenoses ≥50%.

CURRENT OPERATIVE STRATEGIES AND RISKS

Standard Operative Strategies

Most operations for bypass surgery are performed using a median sternotomy incision and cardiopulmonary bypass (CPB). Aortic occlusion and cold potassium-based cardioplegia (delivered through the aortic root or retrograde through a catheter in the coronary sinus) are usually used to achieve a combination of an immobile surgical field and myocardial protection. The development of effective cardioplegic arrest allowed major advances in the complexity of surgical revascularization to be carried out with a low risk of significant perioperative myocardial damage. Today, standard revascularization techniques most commonly involve the use of a single ITA graft (82 percent of year 2001 patients in the STS database),[25] with vein grafts employed to graft other vessels (Fig. 68-1B). More extensive use of ITA grafts, common in some centers, has not become widespread, as only 3.7 percent of STS reported patients received bilateral ITA grafts in 2001.

Differently Invasive Bypass Surgery

The strategies described above have provided effective revascularization operations and are widespread. However, changes in operative techniques have been evolving that are designed to decrease the perioperative morbidity and possibly the mortality of bypass surgery. These new concepts include surgery through small incisions (minimally invasive bypass surgery) and operations performed without the use CPB (beating-heart or off-pump surgery). Small incisions have the advantage of patient preference, a decrease in the risk of major wound complications, and an early return to full activity. Off-pump surgery offers the possibility of decreasing CPB-related

complications. An operation that combines both concepts involves preparation of a LITA graft through a small left thoracotomy, then an off-pump anastomosis to the LAD coronary artery under direct vision—the MIDCAB operation (Fig. 58-7). The evolution of this procedure has included thoracoscopic ITA preparation, allowing for an incrementally smaller anterior thoracotomy and, in a few cases, true port access surgery using robotics technology and involving only small port access incisions. The limited-incision off-pump combination has become a consistently utilized strategy to achieve limited revascularization, the LITA-LAD graft constituting the vast majority of cases performed this way.[26,27] However, grafts from the GEA to the LAD or RCA or SVG or radial artery grafts from the descending aorta to the circumflex system are also possible. To achieve more extensive revascularization, some institutions have used the minimally invasive LITA-LAD graft in combination with percutaneous stenting of other vessels, a "hybrid" procedure. The outcomes of such alternative procedures have been reported as favorable by some authors, although others have noted imperfect early angiographic and clinical outcomes.[27]

TABLE 58-2 Comparison of Patient Characteristics 1980, 1990, 2001—The Society of Thoracic Surgery Database

Characteristic	1980	1990	2001	P Value
Age (years)	58.5 ± 9.11	64.1 ± 10.2	65	<0.001
EF	0.62 ± 0.15	0.51 ± 0.14	51	<0.001
Female	17.04	26.98	29	<0.005
Diabetes mellitus	11.73	22.8	34	<0.005
MI <21 days before CABG	0.34	12.47	25.7	<0.005
Cardiogenic shock	0.51	1.61	1.7	<0.010
Unstable angina	28.51	47.84	50.9	<0.005
Left main disease	6.93	11.7	24	<0.005
Reoperation	1.88	7.01	9.9	<0.005
Nonelective operation	4.11	18.22	45.0	<0.005

KEY: CABG = coronary artery bypass grafting; EF = ejection fraction; IABP = intraaortic balloon pump; MI = myocardial infarction.
[a]Values are shown as percentages except for age and EF, which are shown as mean ± standard deviation.
SOURCES: Edwards et al.[24] and *STS Annual Report.*[25] With permission.

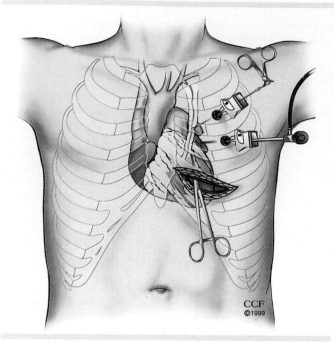

FIGURE 58-7 A small left anterior thoracotomy may be used to construct limited anastomosis without the use of CPB; with the use of percutaneous CPB, more vessels are accessible through this small incision. Endoscopic preparation of the LITA graft may be employed.

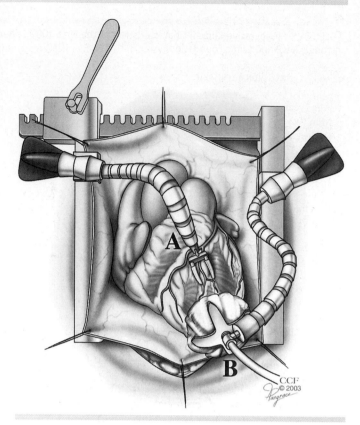

FIGURE 58-8 Myocardial stabilizers allow multivessel revascularization to be accomplished without cardiopulmonary bypass.

The most common alternative strategy is the use of a full median sternotomy incision without the use of CPB.[28–32] Termed "off-pump," "beating-heart," or OPCAB surgery, this strategy was used for approximately 19 percent of STS-reported cases in 2001.[25] The avoidance of CPB has many possible advantages, including decreasing the inflammatory response, avoiding activation of the coagulation system, maintaining pulsatile flow, decreasing myocardial ischemia, and decreasing the risk of micro- or macroembolization that might contribute to end-organ failure.

Most surgeons would now agree that OPCAB offers real advantages in decreasing the risk of noncardiac complications for some subgroups of high-risk patients, including those with known atherosclerosis of the ascending aorta, previous neurologic events, and disorders of the coagulation system. For standard-risk patients, the advantages of OPCAB are less clear. Studies comparing OPCAB surgery with standard strategies have shown consistent advantage for OPCAB in blood utilization and intensive care unit (ICU) stay. Other advantages have been noted in individual studies, but all studies are not consistent and the differences in outcomes, when noted, have not been large.

The possible major disadvantage of the OPCAB approach, and of all alternative revascularization strategies, is that the extent and effectiveness of revascularization might be compromised relative to that achieved with the median sternotomy, CPB, cardioplegic arrest (CPBCAB) approach. Early in the OPCAB, learning-curve the revascularization disadvantages were real and consistent, but surgeons and OPCAB technologies have steadily improved, such that the gap between OPCAB and CPBCAB revascularization has narrowed. Improvements in immobilization technology (Fig. 58-8) have allowed more consistent graft-to-coronary anastomoses, and early angiographic studies have shown favorable patency rates following OPCAB surgery.[29,30] Today, OPCAB revascularization is still difficult in settings of calcified or intramyocardial coronary arteries, diffuse small vessel disease requiring multiple grafts, reoper-ations for patients with atherosclerotic vein grafts, severe cardiac hypertrophy, and a desire to achieve complex ITA and complete revascularization.

The ultimate fruition of differently invasive bypass surgery would be port-access, off-pump, multivessel revascularization with ITA grafts. Strategies similar to this have been attempted in small numbers of highly selected cases using robotics technology. The technological horizon includes mechanical suture devices and graft to coronary and aortic connectors—parallel technologies that may make robotic surgery more accurate and efficient.

HOSPITAL MORTALITY

Overall hospital mortality rates for primary bypass surgery usually vary between 1 and 4 percent. Mortality rates in the voluntary country-wide STS database ranged from 2.69 to 2.37 percent in the 1999–2001 time frame[25] and the New York State Registry (a compulsory registry with subsequent public disclosure) noted an in-hospital mortality rate from 1998 to 2000 of 2.15 to 2.32 percent (Hannan EL, personal communication, 2003). Single-institution reviews have noted overall mortality rates of 1 percent or less for elective surgery.[28] Overall risks are associated in part with patient-related characteristics. Review of large datasets from the early and mid-1990s identified seven variables that were predictive of in-hospital death in all datasets: acuteness of operation, age, prior cardiac surgery, gender, LV ejection fraction, percent of left main coronary artery stenosis, and number of coronary systems with >70 percent stenosis.[33] Acuteness of operation, age, and previous surgery had the greatest predictive value. Also identified were 13 variables that added some predictive value to the core variables: PTCA during the same admission, MI less than 1 week prior to operation, angina, ventricular arrhythmia, congestive heart failure (CHF), mitral regurgitation, diabetes, cerebrovascular disease, peripheral vascular disease, chronic obstructive pulmonary disease (COPD), and elevated serum creatinine.

In the spectrum of clinical settings including stable angina, unstable angina with electrocardiographic (ECG) changes, recent subendocardial infarction, recent Q-wave MI, and cardiogenic shock, there has been an increased operative risk associated with increasing degrees of ischemia and decreasing degrees of LV dysfunction. Modern methods of myocardial protection have diminished the impact of unstable angina, but operations for postinfarction ischemia and shock still generate substantial risk, and the mortality rate of bypass surgery after MI decreases with increasing post-MI interval.[34] Thus, the usual strategy for patients post-MI is to control acute ischemia with medical treatment and undertake operation more electively.

The use of historical data to elucidate the association of patient-, surgeon-, and institution-related variables with outcomes and to then predict outcomes for future patients has become common. This *risk stratification* process has value for both physicians and patients in selecting treatment and in the clarification of likely outcomes and complications. However, the risk-stratification process is not perfect, particularly when data from multiple institutions are combined. First, variables are measured differently in different institutions. Second, only variables that can be measured and recorded are analyzed. Some variables, such as the diffuse nature of distal CAD, are difficult to define and quantify. Third, some variables are not measured in all patients. For example, echocardiography is not routinely employed in all institutions; therefore ascending aortic atherosclerosis is inconsistently identified. Fourth, for a variable to be predictive of risk, it must occur with some frequency. Examples of uncommon variables that have a strong impact on operative mortality include hepatic cirrhosis, congenital clotting disorders, severe protamine allergies, and previous mediastinal radiation therapy.

The setting in which bypass surgery is performed appears to have some impact on outcomes.[35] There is evidence from Medicare data that the risks of coronary artery bypass grafting (CABG) are less in high-volume centers and that those decreased risks are not based on patient selection. Other studies suggest that states with a certificate of need for cardiac surgery and/or public reporting of outcomes have lower procedure-related risks for CABG.[36] Whether these statewide outcomes are based on improved treatment or patient selection is not known. Patient selection, with the exclusion of high-risk patients, will dramatically influence overall outcomes, and evidence does exist that high-risk patients are sometimes denied surgical treatment in areas of intense scrutiny of outcomes. Certainly not all institutions should perform all operations, and it probably is of benefit for high-risk patients to undergo surgery in selected institutions. However, in a milieu of medical economics where patient mobility may be limited, care must be taken that high-risk patients are not denied potentially lifesaving operations.

One advantage of identifying characteristics that predict high risk is that patients who are at extremely low risk may also be identified. For example, during the years 1995–1998, the STS database recorded 25,776 patients who underwent a primary elective bypass operation, had a LV ejection fraction of >50 percent, and did not have peripheral vascular disease, carotid disease, renal failure, a prior myocardial infarction, or an intraaortic balloon pump. For those good-risk patients, 98 deaths occurred, for a 0.38 percent mortality rate (Edwards FH for the STS database, personal communication, 1999).

HOSPITAL MORBIDITY

Perioperative Myocardial Infarction

The introduction of cardioplegic arrest increased the effectiveness of myocardial protection. Cardioplegic solutions usually have a high concentration of potassium and are injected into the aortic root after aortic cross-clamping to arrest the heart and decrease energy consumption. Modifications of this basic strategy have included addition of blood, addition of metabolic substrates, warming of some or all of the cardioplegic solution, and the delivery of cardioplegia retrograde through the coronary sinus into the cardiac venous system. The low risk of perioperative MI has made it difficult to show a clinical advantage for one strategy over another. For example, in a trial of warm blood cardioplegia versus cold crystalloid cardioplegia in primary elective bypass operations, rates of MI (1.4 versus 0.8 percent), IABP use (1.4 versus 2.0 percent), and death (1.0 versus 1.6 percent) were equivalent.[37] For patients undergoing operation in the face of acute ischemia based either on failed PTCA or unstable angina, blood cardioplegia does appear to provide incremental benefit.[38] Retrograde delivery through the coronary sinus and coronary venous system provides more effective delivery during reoperations, in the setting of acute coronary ischemia, or if the aortic valve is insufficient.[39]

The metabolic environment created by these cardioplegic strategies appears to be sufficient for protection. When significant perioperative MI occurs, it is often based on anatomic causes, acute coronary occlusion, graft failure, incomplete revascularization, or embolization of atherosclerotic debris. Some comparative studies of OPCAB and CPBCAB have shown cardiac enzyme release to be decreased after OPCAB. However, the significance of these differences is not known, and studies of focal MI have often not shown differences.

Neurologic Complications

Neurologic complications of bypass surgery include focal stroke (type I) and diffuse encephalopathy (type II). In a multicenter trial examining patients undergoing CPBCAB type bypass surgery, Roach et al. found that the total number of adverse outcomes was 6.1 percent divided between type I (3.1 percent) and type II (3.0 percent). Focal strokes appear to have multiple causes, including carotid or intracranial vascular disease, embolic phenomena based on intraventricular or atrial thrombus or postoperative atrial fibrillation, and atheroembolization from the aorta, probably the most common cause.[40–42] Multiple techniques are available to diminish the risk of stroke when aortic atherosclerosis is present, including alternative arterial cannulation sites, single aortic cross-clamping, circulatory arrest and aortic replacement, and OPCAB surgery. Two nonrandomized studies have cited a lower stroke risk with OPCAB compared with CPBCAB surgery, although a randomized trial of good-risk patients showed no differences in neurologic complications.[31,43,45] To be fully effective in avoiding neurologic complications, OPCAB strategies must avoid manipulation of an atherosclerotic aorta. This can be accomplished by using composite grafts from the ITAs and may be aided by graft to aortic connectors.

An issue that is currently unresolved is the degree of cognitive dysfunction associated with OPCAB and CPBCAB surgery. Cognitive dysfunction, particularly late out-of-hospital cognitive dysfunction, has been noted after bypass surgery but seems to improve over time. A randomized trial comparing OPCAB and CPBCAB showed no cognitive differences 1 year after surgery. Microemboli of gas and debris can be caused by CPB, but their frequency and extent with modern oxygenators and filters is unclear. This continues to be an area of intense investigation.

The presence of carotid stenoses, symptomatic or asymptomatic, in a patient undergoing bypass surgery creates a short- and a long-term risk of stroke. Multiple management strategies have been employed. Staged procedures with carotid endarterectomy or carotid stenting performed first are safe but can be applied only in very select patients with stable CAD. Staged operations with patients undergoing bypass surgery first is associated with a risk of stroke for patients with severe uncorrected carotid stenoses, patients with bilateral stenoses being at greatly increased risk.[46] Combined carotid endarterectomy and coronary surgery has been employed for many patients, but overall risks have been increased relative to those for patients undergoing isolated bypass surgery.

Wound Complications

Deep sternal wound complications represent a serious adverse outcome and occur in 0.5 to 4 percent of cases, depending on patient selection. Obesity and diabetes have been associated with increased risk, but aggressive treatment of blood glucose levels with intravenous insulin may mitigate this. No studies have shown that the use of a single ITA graft increases the risk of sternal wound complications, but some authors have implicated bilateral ITA grafting, particularly for diabetic patients.[47] Dissection of the ITA as a skeletonized artery rather than a pedicle may leave collateral circulation to the sternum intact and diminish the impact of ITA use.[48]

Long-Term Outcomes after Bypass Surgery

Late survival after bypass surgery is related to the patient's cardiac status at the time of operation, the bypass operation, progression of atherosclerosis, noncardiac comorbidity, and fate. Recent follow-up of 8221 surgical patients from the CASS registry documented overall survival of 96, 90, 74, 56, and 45 percent at 1, 5, 10, 15, and 18 postoperative years, respectively.[49] These figures are inferior to those for the age-sex-matched U.S. population and inferior to series of patients receiving ITA grafts at operation (Fig. 58-6).

Patient-related variables have a strong impact on the overall survival rate, and the longer the follow-up interval, the more important those variables become. Age is a major determinant of survival. However, elderly patients, while having a diminished survival as compared with younger patients, actually have survival rates better than those of age-matched controls, an effect that begins to be observed around age 60.

LV function (LVF), left main stenosis, a proximal LAD stenosis, and the number of significantly stenotic coronary arteries are cardiac variables that have been noted to decrease the long-term survival of cardiac patients regardless of the form of treatment used. While the late survival of patients treated medically is dramatically influenced by these cardiac variables, surgery partially or totally negates their impact. In our study analyzing the impact of arterial revascularization, a proximal LAD stenosis had no effect on late survival and left main disease, and the number of systems diseased had minor influence.[17] In no long-term study has bypass surgery completely obliterated the impact of abnormal LV function on late survival.

Studies from the past have noted that risk factors for atherosclerosis—particularly cigarette smoking, hypercholesterolemia, hypertension, and diabetes—have been associated with a decreased survival rate. Stopping smoking after surgery appears to return the patient to a nonsmoker's prognosis.[50] There is now evidence that

postoperative treatment with statins decreases the angiographic progression of atherosclerosis in grafts and native coronary arteries and decreases the risk of late postoperative cardiac events, even for patients without hyperlipidemia.[7,8] Diabetes severe enough to require treatment is associated with a decreased late survival rate.

Operation-related variables also affect late outcome. As discussed previously, the surgical strategies of the LITA-LAD graft and bilateral ITA grafting incrementally improve late survival.[11,17] The impact of incomplete revascularization on long-term outcome is of increasing importance with the emergence of PTCA and minimally invasive bypass operations, strategies that may involve less complete revascularization than can be achieved with standard bypass surgical techniques. Definitions of "incomplete revascularization" have varied, and it is difficult to separate incomplete revascularization as a surgical strategy from incomplete revascularization as a marker of bad coronary and noncoronary atherosclerosis. Retrospective multivariate analyses of the Cleveland Clinic Foundation data identified incomplete revascularization as a risk factor for late death, an effect also noted by Weintraub et al.[51,52] A CASS registry study by Bell et al. noted a strong negative effect of incomplete revascularization on the survival of patients with abnormal LVF who underwent bypass surgery even within a 5-year follow-up.[53]

REOPERATION

Atherosclerosis is a progressive disease, and some surgical patients will eventually undergo reoperation because of graft failure, progression of atherosclerosis in native coronary arteries, or both. A study of patients undergoing bypass surgery in the 1970s noted a cumulative incidence of reoperation of 2.7, 11.4, and 17.3 percent at 5, 10, and 12 postbypass years, respectively.[54] Young age, normal left ventricular function, single- or double-vessel disease, severe symptoms, incomplete revascularization, and not having an ITA graft were all factors that increased the likelihood of a reoperation. In the early 1980s it was feared that reoperation would overwhelm the surgical world. That has not happened for multiple reasons, including the use of ITA grafts, better risk-factor control, an aging population of patients undergoing primary operation, and the availability of PCT as an alternative treatment. However, recurrent ischemic syndromes will develop and some patients will need reoperation, presenting coronary surgeons with their greatest challenges.

Patients who are candidates for reoperation are different from those having primary surgery. Today typical candidates for reoperation underwent primary surgery more than 10 years ago and had triple-vessel disease at that time. Their atherosclerosis is advanced and they have a higher prevalence of aortic atherosclerosis, left main stenosis, severe distal CAD, abnormal LVF, and noncardiac atherosclerosis than patients undergoing primary surgery. They usually have the unique characteristics of having their myocardial blood supply dependent on ITA grafts (at risk for injury) or atherosclerotic vein grafts that create the possibility of coronary atheroembolism.

Few data are available that help to define the indications for reoperation, particularly for patients that are not severely symptomatic. Because the myocardium of reoperative candidates is usually jeopardized by vascular pathology that differs from that in native coronary artery atherosclerosis, generalizations from the randomized studies of patients without previous surgery is unwise. We examined outcomes for patients with prior surgery who developed recurrent ischemic syndromes in two retrospective nonrandomized studies. These studies showed that late (5 years) stenoses in vein grafts, caused by vein graft atherosclerosis, are more dangerous lesions than native coronary lesions.[55] For example, patients 5 years after operation with a 50 percent stenosis in LAD vein graft had survival of 70 and 50 percent 2 and 5 years after angiography, compared with survival rates of 97 and 70 percent for patients whose LAD coronary artery was jeopardized by a 50 percent native vessel stenosis. When we compared outcomes for patients with stenotic vein grafts who underwent repeat surgery with those who were treated without initial reoperation, we found that patients with late (5 years) stenoses in vein grafts had better survival rates with surgery and that the patients who particularly benefited were those with an atherosclerotic vein graft to the LAD coronary artery (Fig. 58-9).[56] The patients with a 50 percent LAD graft stenosis had immediate and obvious benefit, but even those with a 20 to 50 percent stenosis had an improved survival rate with surgery when followed for 5 years. Patients with late stenoses in non-LAD grafts also appeared to have improved late survival unless they had a patent ITA-to-LAD graft. Patients with early vein graft stenoses did not have an improved late survival rate with surgery, although those who underwent reoperation had fewer symptoms at late follow-up.

All studies that have examined large numbers of patients undergoing reoperation have noted an increased in-hospital risk as compared with patients undergoing primary surgery. The STS National Database noted an overall risk of 7.14 percent for reoperations from 1980 to 1990 and 7.2 to 4.7 percent for the years 1998–2001. The Cleveland Clinic Foundation studies have documented a risk of 3 to 4 percent for a first reoperation from 1967 through 1991[57] and 2 percent from that time to the present.

The increased risk of reoperation is related in large part to an increased risk of perioperative MI. Graft injury, atherosclerotic embolization from vein grafts or the aorta, incomplete revascularization due to diffuse disease or lack of bypass conduit, and technical difficulty with severely atherosclerotic coronary vessels are anatomic causes of perioperative MI that are either unique to reoperation or more common in that setting. The use of retrograde cardioplegia has been of major benefit in the management of atherosclerotic vein grafts and patent ITA grafts, but avoiding perioperative MI during reoperation still represents a challenge.

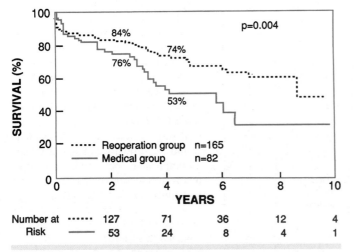

FIGURE 58-9 Patients with late (≥ 5 years after operation) stenoses in venous grafts to the LAD coronary artery have better survival with reoperation than with medical treatment. (From Lytle BW, Loop FD, Taylor PC, et al. The effect of coronary reoperation on the survival of patients with stenoses in saphenous vein bypass grafts to coronary arteries. *J Thorac Cardiovasc Surg* 1993:105:605–614. With permission.)

In the reoperative setting, emergency operation produces a large increase in risk. Definitions of "emergency" vary among studies, but the lesson is the same. For example, in the STS database for 1997, mortality rates were 5.2 percent for elective, 7.4 percent for urgent, 13.5 percent for emergency, and 40.7 percent for "salvage" reoperations.[25] Left main stenosis, advanced age, CHF, female gender, and number of stenotic vein grafts have been other factors associated with increased risk.

In general, the long-term outcomes after reoperation are slightly inferior to those after primary surgery. Loop et al. noted a 69 percent 10-year survival for 2429 hospital survivors of a first reoperation.[58] LVF was the variable having the strongest impact on survival. Reoperations tend to achieve less perfect revascularization than primary procedures, and by 5 to 6 postoperative years, about 50 percent of reoperative patients have some angina, although it is severe in only a few.[59]

COMPARATIVE TRIALS INVOLVING BYPASS SURGERY

For an invasive treatment of any disease to be widely applied, it must provide outcomes superior outcomes to those of less invasive therapies. Since its inception, bypass surgery has been carefully scrutinized, and its status relative to alternative treatments such as medical therapy and PCT has been tested with randomized trials and nonrandomized comparisons. Randomized trials of widely differing treatments—such as surgery versus medical treatment or surgery versus PCT—are difficult to carry out. They are expensive, recruitment is difficult, and vast allowances must be made for changes in physician opinions and patient outcomes. The strength of randomized trials is that they eliminate bias in the selection of the initial treatment once the patient has been entered into the trial. However, they do not eliminate physician and patient bias at the point of entry into the trial, and in the randomized trials involving bypass surgery, only subsets of patients with CAD were eligible, and the majority of patients eligible to be randomized were not randomized. Also, randomized trials do not eliminate bias in the selection of further therapy once the initial therapy has been carried out. If the alternative therapy is selected once the initial therapy has been carried out, that is called "crossover," and rarely is crossover a random event. Nonrandomized trials have the disadvantage of bias in the selection of treatment but the advantage of inclusiveness. Therefore both randomized and nonrandomized trials provide information that is useful in the selection of therapies for patients with CAD.

Trials of Surgery versus Medical Treatment

During the 1970s, multicenter randomized trials of patients with chronic angina were initiated to test the effectiveness of bypass grafting versus medical management. The most influential of these trials were the Veterans Administration Study of patients with Chronic Stable Angina. (VA Study),[60] the European Coronary Surgery Study (ECSS),[61] and the Coronary Artery Surgery Study (CASS).[62, 63] These trials randomized patients either to initial medical management or to initial treatment with bypass surgery, and their primary emphasis was survival. In the two largest trials (ECSS and CASS), severely symptomatic patients were excluded from randomization. These trials showed that prompt surgery improved the life expectancy of some patients, and those who benefited the most from surgery were patients at the highest risk of death without operation. Individual trials noted improved survival rates for patients with significant left main stenosis, three-vessel

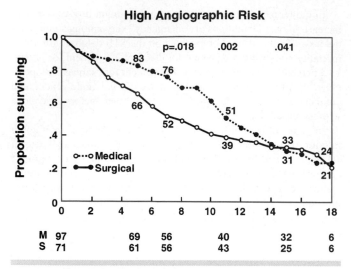

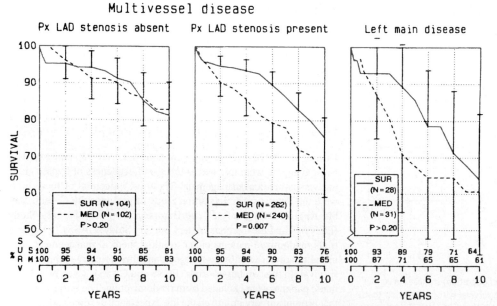

FIGURE 58-10 In the initial trial of bypass surgery versus medical management, the VA study, patients with abnormal LV function and three-vessel disease had a better survival rate with surgery. (From The VA Coronary Artery Bypass Surgery Cooperative Study Group. Eighteen-year follow-up in the
Veterans Affairs Cooperative Study of Coronary Artery Bypass Surgery for Stable Angina. Circulation 1992;86:121–130. With permission.)

disease with abnormal LVF (Fig. 58-10), and two- or three-vessel disease with a >75 percent stenosis in the proximal LAD coronary artery
(Fig. 58-11). The clinical descriptors of an abnormal baseline ECG or
a strongly positive exercise test helped to define patient subsets who
experienced improved survival rates with surgery. A metanalysis of
randomized trials confirmed the observations of the individual trials
but also showed a significant survival benefit for patients with triple-,
double-, or even single-vessel disease that included a proximal LAD
stenosis regardless of whether they had normal or abnormal LVF.[64] For
patients without a proximal LAD stenosis, surgery improved the sur-

vival rate only for those with left main stenosis or triple-vessel disease.
It was also noted that the surgically treated patients had fewer symptoms at 5 years after surgery and took fewer antianginal medications.

The degree of benefit achieved with initial bypass surgery diminished with time both in terms of survival and in regard to symptom
status. There were multiple reasons for this. First, the status of the
surgically treated patients deteriorated based on late vein graft failure
and the progression of native vessel atherosclerosis. Few patients in
these early trials received ITA grafts or were treated with platelet inhibitors or lipid lowering agents, strategies that we now know significantly extend the benefits of surgery. Second, the status of the "medically treated" patients improved slightly because a large proportion
of those patients "crossed over" and underwent bypass surgery, although they were still analyzed as part of the medically treated
group. In the three major studies, 40 to 44 percent of the total medically treated patient population had undergone bypass surgery by 10
postoperative years, including 65 percent of patients with left main
disease and 48 percent of those with three-vessel disease.[65] Finally,
when all-cause mortality is the endpoint, any two survival curves will
eventually meet at zero.

In all these trials a minority of patients presenting for evaluation
met the criteria for entry into the trial, and of those that met the criteria for entry, a minority were actually randomized. In the case of the
CASS study, however, patients who were not randomized were
prospectively followed in a nonrandomized registry that has provided
useful information. Among the important conclusions from the
CASS registry are that asymptomatic patients with 50 percent left
main stenosis and those with left main equivalent (70 percent stenosis of proximal LAD and circumflex vessels) have improved survival
with surgery.[66,67] For severely symptomatic patients, bypass surgery
improved the survival rates of those with three-vessel disease regardless of whether they had normal or abnormal LVF, even if they did
not have severe proximal coronary artery stenoses.[68]

Outcomes for patients with unstable angina were tested in another
VA trial. Patients with rest angina and abnormal LVF had greatly improved survival with initial surgery. Pa-
tients with progressive angina did not
appear to have a worse survival rate if
they were initially treated with medical
therapy, but 19 percent of this group
crossed over to surgery within 30 days
of randomization; by 96 months, 45
percent had crossed over to surgery.[69]

Are the conclusions from these
older trials still valid today, when both
medical and surgical therapies have improved? To repeat the trials of randomized surgery versus medical treatment
would be difficult and has not been
accomplished, but there are some
relatively modern comparative studies
that appear to show a persistent advantage for revascularization over even
modern medical therapy. First, the randomized three-armed MASS trial (surgery versus PCT versus medicine) for
the treatment of isolated LAD stenosis
showed that the surgically treated patients experienced fewer symptoms and
cardiac events during a 5-year follow-
up, although the low incidence of cardiac death was not different in the three

FIGURE 58-11 In the European Coronary Surgery Study, patients with multivessel disease and a proximal LAD lesion (center) experienced an improved survival rate with surgery, whereas those without an LAD lesion (left) did
not. (From Varnauskas E and the European Coronary Surgery Study Group. Twelve-year follow-up of survival in the
randomized European Coronary Surgery Study. N Engl J Med 1988;319:332–337. With permission.)

groups.[70] Second, the Asymptomatic Cardiac Ischemia Pilot (ACIP) trial showed that good-risk patients with asymptomatic ischemia experienced a better survival rate with initial revascularization (PCT or surgery) than with medical treatment alone.[71] Third, analysis of the Studies of Left Ventricular Dysfunction (SOLVD) trial involving high-risk patients (ejection fraction <35 percent) showed that patients with bypass surgery had a 26 percent lower mortality rate than those without revascularization.[72] Finally, fourth, a study of nonrandomized data from the Alberta (APPROACH) registry showed better-risk survival rates for surgically treated patients compared with those treated medically, the largest difference being noted in patients >70 years of age.[73]

Bypass Surgery versus PCT

Multiple studies have compared surgery and PCT. Balloon angioplasty (BA), the first PCT generation, was compared with bypass surgery and medical management for the treatment of isolated LAD disease in the MASS trial.[70] This trial randomized 214 patients and found that, at a 5-year follow-up, the adverse events of MI, severe angina, and death occurred for 6 surgery patients, 29 BA patients, and 17 medically treated patients. The percentage of patients free from angina at follow-up were surgery, 72.7 percent, BA, 64.7 percent, and medical treatment, 25.8 percent, respectively. There was not a significant difference in survival rate.

Multiple trials of patients with multivessel disease randomized favorable-risk patients with lesions suitable for PCT and, in general, showed that BA produced less effective revascularization than surgery. In the largest of these trials, the BARI, 54 percent of BA patients required reintervention compared with 8 percent of those receiving surgery. Despite the large number of reinterventions, the BA group experienced more symptoms, took more medications, and were less completely revascularized.[10,74,75] In addition, patients who had treated diabetes had significantly worse survival (Fig. 58-12) over a 7-year follow-up if they were treated with PCT.[75,76] Smaller trials showed trends toward an increased risk for diabetic patients, and large risk-adjusted observational studies have also shown excess mortality for diabetic patients treated with PCT over a 5- to 7-year follow up interval.[77–79] The advantage of

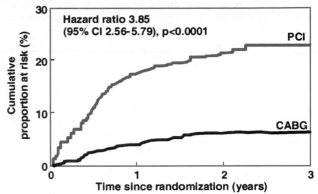

Cumulative Risk of Repeat Revascularization

Hazard ratio 3.85
(95% CI 2.56–5.79), p<0.0001

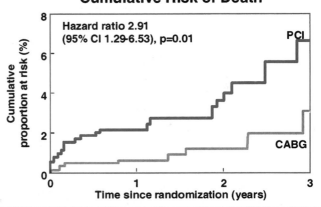

Cumulative Risk of Death

Hazard ratio 2.91
(95% CI 1.29–6.53), p=0.01

FIGURE 58-13 In the SOS (surgery versus stent) trial, patients with percutaneous intervention experienced an increased risk of repeat revascularization (*top*) and a higher death rate (*bottom*). [From the SOS Investigators. Coronary artery bypass surgery versus percutaneous coronary intervention with stent implantation in patients with multivessel coronary artery disease (the Stent or Surgery trial): A randomised controlled study. *Lancet* 2002:360:965–970. With permission.]

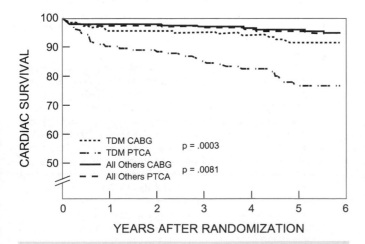

FIGURE 58-12 BARI trial patients with treated diabetes had worse survival following PTCA than following CABG (*p* = 0.003). Patients without diabetes had equivalent survival. (From BARI Investigators. Influence of diabetes on 5-year mortality and morbidity in a randomized trial comparing CABG and PTCA in patients with mutivessel disease. *Circulation* 1997;96:1761–1769.)

surgery appears most pronounced for patients with three-vessel disease and, in BARI, was present only for patients receiving at least one ITA graft.

Since completion of those "first generation" trials, the use of coronary stents has lowered the procedure-related risks, and the restenosis rate associated with PCT, off-pump, and minimally invasive surgery. These procedures have therefore become more common in the surgical domain. Two randomized trials of stenting (second-generation PCT) versus surgery for patients with isolated LAD disease showed stenting to be less effective than surgery, as the PCT patients experienced more symptoms, took more medications, and had a higher incidence of adverse cardiac events.[26,27] Again, there were no significant survival differences.

Two randomized trials of surgery versus stenting for patients with multivessel disease (the ARTS and SOS trials) show many similar findings. Again, patients with PCT experienced more angina, took more antianginal medications, and underwent many more repeat revascularization procedures than did those who had surgery.[80,81] However, when compared with BA, stenting decreased the first-year reintervention rate to 17 percent in ARTS and 21 percent in SOS, approximately half of that seen with BA. In ARTS, there was no overall survival difference between PCT and surgery, but in SOS there was a significant excess mortality associated with PCT at a 3-year follow-up (Fig. 58-13). SOS did not examine diabetics as a separate subset, but in ARTS the 1-year event-free survival rate of diabetics treated with PCT was 63.4 percent, compared with 84.4 percent for surgical patients ($p < 0.001$).[82]

Third-generation PCT and drug-coated stents promise to decrease the restenosis rate of PCT. Detailed information is not yet available, but early reported data show a 1-year restenosis rate of 10 percent or less for vessels 2.5 mm in diameter. It appears that patients with diabetes have an increased restenosis rate even with coated stents, but the precise levels are not yet known. Saphenous vein graft disease and complex small vessel disease have not been tested with coated stents. The clinical impact of a decrease in the risk of in-stent restenosis will certainly be favorable, but these very early outcomes for selected patients receiving coated stents do not justify ignoring the lessons of previous trials. For example, the excess mortality of diabetic patients who undergo PCT may not be entirely related to restenosis. Surgery bypasses large areas of native vessel disease and is thus more protective against native vessel progression. Also, the benefits of coated stents are known to extend for small numbers of months, whereas the effectiveness of ITA grafts extends for more than 20 years.

INDICATIONS FOR BYPASS SURGERY

For Prognosis

Patients who experience an improved survival rate with bypass surgery even in the absence of severe symptoms include those with a left main coronary stenosis of 50 percent or multivessel disease with a proximal LAD lesion and abnormal LVF. In addition, patients with previous bypass surgery who have large amounts of myocardium in jeopardy should undergo reoperation even in the absence of severe symptoms. These situations are anatomic indications for surgery.[83] The worse the patient's symptoms and the worse the LVF, the stronger the survival benefit of surgery. Modern imaging allows the identification of patients with abnormal LVF and viable myocardium, a subset that appears to experience great benefit from surgery.[84]

For nondiabetic patients with multivessel disease, a proximal LAD lesion, and normal LVF, revascularization should be recommended even without severe symptoms. For patients in this subgroup, midterm follow-up of good candidates for PCT appears to show equivalent survival as compared with surgery; the advantages and disadvantages of both revascularization strategies should be discussed with the patient. For diabetic patients with multivessel disease, data from multiple sources indicate an excess mortality associated with PCT; therefore surgery should be the first choice of revacularization for these patients.[85]

For Symptom Relief

Patients without life-threatening CAD who are, however, symptomatic with angina, usually enjoy significant and persistent symptom relief after surgery. Before suggesting operation for symptom relief, ischemia in areas supplied by graftable vessels should be demonstrated. The choice of revascularization strategies is usually based on coronary vascular anatomy, the likelihood of complete revascularization with PCT, diabetic status, and patient preference.

TRANSMYOCARDIAL LASER REVASCULARIZATION

The concept of achieving myocardial revascularization by the creation of channels in the myocardium has been investigated since the 1950s, and the increasing population of patients with severe distal native vessel atherosclerosis (usually occurring years after previous bypass surgery) who may not be well treated with either bypass surgery alone or PCT has provided impetus to the search for such alternative revascularization strategies. Laser energy has been used to create such channels, and randomized clinical trials of transmyocardial laser revascularization (TMLR) versus medical management have been conducted involving patients with angina and severe CAD judged untreatable by conventional invasive means. Both CO_2 and holmium lasers have been tested; in both studies, over 70 percent of TMLR patients noted improvement in angina at 1 year after surgery compared with 13 to 32 percent improvement in the medically treated group (p 0.001).[86] Five-year follow-up has shown persistence of the benefit in the CO_2 study.[87] Survival data on the TMLR- and medically treated patients were the same in both studies. Although there is some apparent benefit from TMLR, the mechanism of improvement is not clear (see also Chap. 57). Autopsy studies have noted granulation tissue occluding the myocardial channels within a few days of operation, and anginal relief may not be immediate. Denervation and microcollateral stimulation have been suggested as possible mechanisms of angina relief. TMLR appears to have a role in revascularization but currently does not appear to produce the degree or the consistency of improved myocardial perfusion that can be achieved when bypass surgery or PTCA is possible. The indications for TMLR are still in evolution.

References

1. Lytle BW, Loop FD, Cosgrove DM, et al. Long-term (5 to 12 years) serial studies of internal mammary artery and saphenous vein coronary by-pass grafts. *J Thorac Cardiovasc Surg* 1985;89:248–258.
2. Fitzgibbon GM, Kafka HP, Leach AJ, et al. Coronary bypass graft fate and patient outcome: Angiographic follow-up of 5065 grafts related to survival and reoperation in 1388 patients during 25 years. *J Am Coll Cardiol* 1996;28:616–626.
3. Bourassa MG, Campeau L, Lesperance J. Changes in grafts and coronary arteries after coronary bypass surgery. *Cardiovasc Clin* 1991;21:83–100.
4. Neitzel GF, Barboriak JJ, Pintar K, et al. Atherosclerosis in aortocoronary bypass grafts. Morphologic study and risk factor analysis 6 to 12 years after surgery. *Arteriosclerosis* 1986;6:594–600.
5. Gavaghan TP, Gebski V, Baron DW. Immediate postoperative aspirin improves vein graft patency early and late after coronary artery bypass graft surgery. A placebo-controlled, randomized study. *Circulation* 1991;83:1526–1533.
6. Goldman S, Copeland J, Moritz T, et al. Starting aspirin therapy after operation. Effects on early graft patency. *Circulation* 1991;84:520–526.
7. The Post Coronary Artery Bypass Graft Trial Investigators. The effect of aggressive lowering of low-density lipoprotein cholesterol levels and low-dose anticoagulation on obstructive changes in saphenous-vein coronary-artery bypass grafts. *N Engl J Med* 1997;336:153–162.
8. Flaker GC, Warnica JW, Sacks FM, et al. Pravastatin prevents clinical events in revascularized patients with average cholesterol concentrations. Cholesterol and Recurrent Events CARE Investigators. *J Am Coll Cardiol* 1999;34:106–112.
9. Lawrie GM, Morris GC Jr, Earle N. Long-term results of coronary by-pass surgery. Analysis of 1698 patients followed 15 to 20 years. *Ann Surg* 1991;213:377–385.
10. Whitlow PL, Dimas AP, Bashore TM, et al. Relationship of extent of revascularization with angina at one year in the Bypass Angioplasty

Revascularization Investigation (BARI). *J Am Coll Cardiol* 1999;34: 1750–1759.

11. Loop FD, Lytle BW, Cosgrove DM, et al. Influence of the internal-mammary artery graft on 10-year survival and other cardiac events. *N Engl J Med* 1986;314:1–6.

12. Lytle BW, Cosgrove DM. Coronary artery bypass surgery. In: Wells SA, ed. *Current Problems in Surgery*. St. Louis:Mosby–Year Book, 1992; 29:733–807.

13. Sabik JF, Lytle BW, Blackstone EH, et al. Does Competitive flow reduce internal thoracic artery graft patency? *J Thorac Cardiovasc Surg.* In press.

14. Dion R, Etienne PY, Verhelst R, et al. Bilateral mammary grafting. Clinical, functional, and angiographic assessment in 400 consecutive cases. *Eur J Cardiothorac Surg* 1993;7:287–294.

15. Tector AJ, Amundsen S, Schmahl TM, et al. Total revascularization with T grafts. *Ann Thorac Surg* 1994;57:33–39.

16. Cameron A, Davis KB, Green G, et al. Coronary bypass surgery with internal-thoracic-artery grafts—Effects on survival over a 15-year period. *N Engl J Med* 1996;334:216–219.

17. Lytle BW, Blackstone EH, Loop FD, et al. Two internal thoracic artery grafts are better than one. *J Thorac Cardiovasc Surg* 1999;117:855–872.

18. Buxton BF, Komeda M, Fuller JA, Gordon I. Bilateral internal thoracic artery grafting may improve outcome of coronary artery surgery. Risk-adjusted survival. *Circulation* 1998;98:III-1–III-6.

19. Suma H, Isomura T, Horii T, et al. Late angiographic result of using the right gastroepiploic artery vein graft. *J Thorac Cardiovasc Surg* 2000; 120:496–498.

20. Buche M, Schroeder E, Gurne O, et al. Coronary artery bypass grafting with the inferior epigastric artery. Midterm clinical and angiographic results. *J Thorac Cardiovasc Surg* 1995;109:553–560.

21. Acar C, Ramsheyi A, Pagny JY, et al. The radial artery for coronary artery bypass grafting: clinical and angiographic results at five years. *J Thorac Cardiovasc Surg* 1998;116:981–989.

22. Possati G, Gaudino M, Alessandrini F, et al. Mid-term clinical and angiographic results of radial artery grafts used for myocardial revascularization. *J Thorac Cardiovasc Surg* 1998;116:1015–1021.

23. Bergsma TM, Grandjean JG, Voors AA, et al. Low recurrence of angina pectoris after coronary artery bypass graft surgery with bilateral internal thoracic and right gastroepiploic arteries. *Circulation* 1998;97:2402–2405.

24. Edwards FH, Grover FL, Shroyer AL, et al. The Society of Thoracic Surgeons National Cardiac Surgery Database: Current risk assessment. *Ann Thorac Surg* 1977;63:903–908.

25. STS Annual Report: 2001.

26. Drenth DJ, Veeger NJ, Winter JB, et al. A prospective randomized trial comparing stenting with off-pump coronary surgery for high-grade stenosis in the proximal left anterior descending coronary artery: three-year follow-up. *J Am Coll Cardiol* 2002;40:1955–1960.

27. Diegeler A, Thiele H, Falk UF, et al. Comparison of stenting with minimally invasive bypass surgery for stenosis of the left anterior descending coronary artery. *N Eng J Med* 2002;347:561–566.

28. Sabik JF, Gillinov AM, Blackstone EH, et al. Does off-pump coronary surgery reduce morbidity and mortality? *J Thorac Cardiovasc Surg* 2002;124:698–707.

29. Calafiore AM, Teodori G, Giammarco G, et al. Multiple arterial conduits without cardiopulmonary bypass: Early angiographic results. *Ann Thorac Surg* 1999;67:450–456.

30. Puskas JD, Thourani VH, Marshall JJ, et al. Clinical outcomes, angiographic patency and resource utilization in 200 consecutive off-pump coronary bypass patients. *Ann Thorac Surg* 2001;71:1477–1484.

31. Nathoe HM, van Dijk D, Jansen EW, et al. A comparison of on-pump and off-pump coronary bypass surgery in low-risk patients. *N Engl J Med* 2003;348:394–402.

32. Angelini GD, Taylor FC, Reeves BC, et al. Early and midterm outcome after off-pump and on-pump surgery in Beating Heart Against Cardioplegic Arrest Studies (BHACAS 1 and 2): A pooled analysis of two randomised controlled trials. *Lancet* 2002;359:1194–1199.

33. Jones RH, Hannan EL, Hammermeister KE, et al. Identification of preoperative variables needed for risk adjustment of short-term mortality after coronary bypass graft surgery: The Working Group Panel on the Cooperative CABG Database Project. *J Am Coll Cardiol* 1996;28: 1478–1487.

34. Lee DC, Oz MC, Weinberg AD, et al. Appropriate timing of surgical intervention after transmural acute myocardial infarction. *J Thorac Cardiovasc Surg* 2003;125:115–120.

35. Birkmeyer JD, Siewers AE, Finlayson EV, et al. Hospital volume and surgical mortality in the United States. *N Engl J Med* 2002;346: 1128–1137.

36. Vaughan-Sarrazin MS, Hannan EL, Gormley CJ, et al. Mortality in medicare beneficiaries following coronary artery bypass graft surgery in states with and without certificate of need regulation. *JAMA* 2002;288: 1859–1866.

37. Martin TD, Craver JM, Gott JP, et al. Prospective, randomized trial of retrograde warm blood cardioplegia: myocardial benefit and neurologic threat. *Ann Thorac Surg* 1994;57:298–302.

38. Christakis GT, Fremes SE, Weisel RD, et al. Reducing the risk of urgent revascularization for unstable angina: A randomized clinical trial. *J Vasc Surg* 1986;3:764–772.

39. Buckberg GD. Strategies and logic of cardioplegic delivery to prevent, avoid and reverse ischemic and reperfusion damage. *J Thorac Cardiovasc Surg* 1987;93:127–139.

40. Roach GW, Kanchuger M, Mangano CM, et al. Adverse cerebral outcomes after coronary bypass surgery. Multicenter study of Perioperative Ischemia Research Group and the Ischemia Research and Education Foundation Investigators. *N Engl J Med* 1996;335:1857–1863.

41. Hartman GS, Yao FS, Bruefach M III. Severity of aortic atheromatous disease diagnosed by transesophageal echocardiography predicts stroke and other outcomes associated with coronary artery surgery: A prospective study. *Anesth Analg* 1996;83:701–708.

42. Blauth CI, Cosgrove DM, Webb BW, et al. Atheroembolism from the ascending aorta. An emerging problem in cardiac surgery. *J Thorac Cardiovasc Surg* 1992;103:1104–1112.

43. Iaco AL, Contini M, Teodori G, et al. Off or on bypass: What is the safety threshold? *Ann Thorac Surg* 1999;68:1486–1489.

44. Cleveland JC Jr, Shroyer AL, Chen AY, et al. Off-pump coronary artery bypass grafting decreases risk-adjusted mortality and morbidity. *Ann Thorac Surg* 2001;72:1282–1289.

45. Van Dijk D, Jansen EW, Hijman R, et al. Cognitive outcome after off-pump and on-pump coronary artery bypass graft surgery: A randomized trial. *JAMA* 2002;287:1405–1412.

46. Hertzer NR, Loop FD, Beven EG, et al. Surgical strategy for simultaneous coronary and carotid disease: A study including prospective randomization. *J Vasc Surg* 1989;9:455–463.

47. Loop FD, Lytle BW, Cosgrove DM, et al. Sternal wound complications after isolated coronary bypass grafting: Early and late mortality, morbidity and cost of care. *Ann Thorac Surg* 1990;49:179–187.

48. Matsa M, Paz Y, Gurevitch J, et al. Bilateral skeletonized internal thoracic artery grafts in patients with diabetes mellitus. *J Thorac Cardiovasc Surg* 2001;121:668–674.

49. Myers WO, Blackstone EH, Davis K, et al. CASS Registry long term surgical survival. *J Am Coll Cardiol* 1999;33:488–498.

50. Cavender JB, Rogers WJ, Fisher LD, et al. Effects of smoking on survival and morbidity in patients randomized to medical or surgical therapy in the Coronary Artery Surgery Study (CASS): 10 year follow-up. *J Am Coll Cardiol* 1992;20:287–294.

51. Cosgrove DM, Loop FD, Lytle BW, et al. Determinants of 10-year survival after primary myocardial revascularization. *Ann Surg* 1985;202:480–490.

52. Jones EL, Weintraub WS. The importance of completeness of revascularization during long-term follow-up after coronary artery operations. *J Thorac Cardiovasc Surg* 1996;112:227–237.

53. Bell MR, Gersh BJ, Schaff HV, et al. Effect of completeness of revascularization on long-term outcome of patients undergoing coronary artery bypass surgery: A report from the Coronary Artery Surgery Study (CASS) Registry. *Circulation* 1992;86:446–457.

54. Cosgrove DM, Loop FD, Lytle BW, et al. Predictors of reoperation after myocardial revascularization. *J Thorac Cardiovasc Surg* 1986;92: 811–821.

55. Lytle BW, Loop FD, Taylor PC, et al. Vein graft disease: The clinical impact of stenoses in saphenous vein grafts to coronary arteries. *J Thorac Cardiovasc Surg* 1992;103:831–840.

56. Lytle BW, Loop FD, Taylor PC, et al. The effect of coronary reoperation on the survival of patients with stenoses in saphenous vein to coronary bypass grafts. *J Thorac Cardiovasc Surg* 1993;105:605–614.

57. Lytle BW, McElroy D, McCarthy PM, et al. Influence of arterial coronary bypass grafts on the mortality in coronary reoperations. *J Thorac Cardiovasc Surg* 1994;107:675–683.

58. Loop FD, Lytle BW, Cosgrove DM, et al. Reoperation for coronary atherosclerosis: Changing practice in 2509 consecutive patients. Ann Surg 1990;212:378–386.

59. Lytle BW, Loop FD, Cosgrove DM, et al. Fifteen hundred coronary reoperations: Results and determinants of early and late survival. *J Thorac Cardiovasc Surg* 1987;93:847–859.

60. Peduzzi P. Eighteen-year follow-up in the Veterans Affairs Cooperative Study of coronary artery bypass surgery for stable angina. The VA Coronary Artery Bypass Surgery Cooperative Study Group. *Circulation* 1992;86:121–130.

61. Varnauskas E and The European Coronary Surgery Study Group. Twelve-year follow-up of survival in the randomized European Coronary Surgery Study. *N Engl J Med* 1988;319:332–337.

62. Passamani E, Davis KB, Gillespie MJ, et al. A randomized trial of coronary artery bypass surgery. Survival of patients with a low ejection fraction. *N Engl J Med* 1985;312:1665–1671.

63. Alderman EL, Bourassi MG, Cohen LS, et al. Ten year follow-up of survival and myocardial infarction in the randomized Coronary Artery Surgery Study. *Circulation* 1990;82:1629–1646.

64. Yusuf S, Zucker D, Peduzzi P, et al. Effect of coronary artery bypass graft surgery on survival: Overview of 10-year results from randomised trials by the Coronary Artery Bypass Graft Surgery Trialists Collaboration. *Lancet* 1994;344:563–570.

65. Rogers WJ, Coggin CJ, Gersh BJ, et al. Ten-year follow-up of quality of life in patients randomized to receive medical therapy or coronary artery bypass graft surgery. The Coronary Artery Surgery Study (CASS). *Circulation* 1990;82:1647–1658.

66. Taylor HA, Deumite NJ, Chaitman BR, et al. Asymptomatic left main coronary artery disease in the Coronary Artery Surgery Study (CASS) registry. *Circulation* 1989;79:1171–1179.

67. Caracciolo EA, Davis KB, Sopko G, et al. Comparison of surgical and medical group survival in patients with left main equivalent coronary artery disease. Long-term CASS experience. *Circulation* 1995;91:2335–2344.

68. Myers WO, Schaff HV, Gersh BJ, et al. Improved survival of surgically treated patients with triple vessel coronary artery disease and severe angina pectoris. A report from the Coronary Artery Surgery Study (CASS) registry. *J Thorac Cardiovasc Surg* 1989;97:487–495.

69. Sharma GV, Deupree RH, Khuri SF, Parisi AF, et al. Coronary bypass surgery improves survival in high-risk unstable angina. Results of a Veterans Administration Cooperative study with an 8-year follow-up. Veterans Administration Unstable Angina Cooperative Study Group. *Circulation* 1991;84[suppl III]:III260–III267.

70. Hueb WA, Soares, PR, Almeida DeOliveira S, et al. Five-year follow-up of the Medicine, Angioplasty, or Surgery Study (MASS). A prospective randomized trial of medical therapy, balloon angioplasty, or bypass surgery for single proximal left anterior descending coronary artery stenosis. *Circulation* 1999;100(supp II):II-107–II-113.

71. Davies RF, Goldberg AD, Forman S, et al. Asymptomatic Cardiac Ischemia Pilot (ACIP) study two-year follow-up. Outcomes of patients randomized to initial strategies of medical therapy versus revascularization. *Circulation* 1997;95:2037–2043.

72. Veenhuyzen GD, Singh SN, McAreavey D, et al. Prior coronary artery bypass surgery and risk of death among patients with ischemic left ventricular dysfunction. *Circulation* 2001;104:1489–1493.

73. Graham MM, Ghali WA, Faris PD, et al. Survival after coronary revascularization in the elderly. *Circulation* 2002;105:2378–2384.

74. Bypass Angioplasty Revascularization Investigation (BARI). Comparison of coronary bypass surgery with angioplasty in patients with multivessel disease. *N Engl J Med* 1996;335:217–225.

75. BARI Investigators. Influence of diabetes on 5-year mortality and morbidity in a randomized trial comparing CABG and PTCA in patients with multivessel disease. *Circulation* 1997;96:1761–1769.

76. BARI Investigators. Seven-year outcome in the Bypass Angioplasty Revascularization Investigation by treatment and diabetic studies. *J Am Coll Cardiol* 2000;35:1122–1129.

77. King SB III, Lembo NJ, Weintraub WS, et al. A randomized trial comparing coronary angioplasty with coronary bypass surgery: Emory Angioplasty vs. Surgery Trial (EAST). *N Engl J Med* 1994;331:1044–1050.

78. Detre KM, Guo P, Holubkov R, et al. Coronary revascularization in diabetic patients: a comparison of the randomized and observational components of the Bypass Angioplasty Revascularization Investigators (BARI). *Circulation* 1999;99:632–640.

79. Niles NW, McGrath PD, Malenka, D, et al. Survival of patients with diabetes and multivessel coronary artery disease after surgical or percutaneous coronary revascularization: Results of a large regional prospective study. Northern New England Cardiovascular Disease Study Group. *J Am Coll Cardiol* 2001;37:1008–1015.

80. Serruys PW, Unger F, Sousa JE, et al. Comparison of coronary artery bypass surgery and stenting for the treatment of multivessel disease. *N Engl J Med* 2001;344:1117–1124.

81. The SOS Investigators. Coronary artery bypass surgery versus percutaneous coronary intervention with stent implantation in patients with multivessel coronary artery disease (the Stent or Surgery trial): A randomised controlled trial. *Lancet* 2002;360:965–970.

82. Abizaid A, Costa MA, Centemero M, et al. Clinical and economic impact of diabetes mellitus on percutaneous and surgical treatment of multivessel coronary disease patients: Insights from the Arterial Revascularization Therapy Study (ARTS) Trial. *Circulation* 2001;104:533–538.

83. Eagle KA, Guyton RA, Davidoff R, et al. ACC/AHA guidelines for coronary arterybypass graft surgery: Executive summary and recommendations: a report of the American College of Cardiology/American Heart Association Task Force on Practice Guidelines (Committee to Revise the 1991 Guidelines for Coronary Artery Bypass Graft Surgery). *J Am Coll Cardiol* 1999;34:1262–1346.

84. Allman KC, Shaw LJ, Hachamovitch R, et al. Myocardial viability testing and impact of revascularization on prognosis in patients with coronary artery disease and left ventricular dysfunction: A meta-analysis. *J Am Coll Cardiol* 2002;39:151–158.

85. Kip KE, Alderman EL, Bourassa MG, et al. Differential influence of diabetes mellitus on increased jeopardized myocardium after initial angioplasty or bypass surgery: Bypass Angioplasty Revascularization Investigation. *Circulation* 2002;105:1914–1920.

86. Allen KB, Dowling RD, Fudge TL, et al. Comparison of transmyocardial revascularization with medical therapy in patients with refractory angina. *N Engl J Med* 1999;341:1029–1036.

87. Horvath KA, Aranki SF, Cohn LH, et al. Sustained angina relief 5 years after transmyocardial laser revascularization with a CO_2 laser. *Circulation* 2001;104:I-81–I-84.

MANAGEMENT OF THE PATIENT AFTER CARDIAC SURGERY

Douglas C. Morris / Stephen D. Clements, Jr. / James M. Bailey

The initial management of most patients following cardiac surgery occurs in specialized intensive care units (ICUs). The unique pathophysiologic alterations associated with hypothermia and cardiopulmonary bypass (CPB) mandated that a specialized environment, including sophisticated electrophysiologic and hemodynamic monitoring and intensive attention and supervision by specially trained critical care nurses, be available. While CPB is no longer universally applied in cardiac surgery, the multiple management problems posed by cardiac patients continue to demand specialized treatment.

ROLE OF VASCULAR CANNULAS, LIFE SUPPORT, AND MONITORING IN THE IMMEDIATE POSTOPERATIVE PERIOD

The patient typically arrives in the ICU or postcardiac surgery recovery area from the operating room with the necessary apparatus for monitoring the following parameters: heart rate and rhythm; arterial, central venous, pulmonary artery, and pulmonary artery occlusion pressures (PAOPs); cardiac output; urinary output; mediastinal drainage; body temperature; arterial oxygen saturation (SpO_2), and end-tidal carbon dioxide ($ETCO_2$) tension.

Most of the apparatus attached to the patient upon arrival in the ICU serves a dual purpose. A pulmonary artery catheter not only allows monitoring of pulmonary artery pressures but can also be used to estimate the filling pressure of the left ventricle, cardiac output, and body core temperature. The peripheral arterial cannula provides a continuous pulse-wave tracing of systemic blood pressure and ready access to arterial blood sampling for laboratory analysis. Regular periodic assessments of arterial blood gases, especially after a major change in ventilator settings, are essential unless continuous

$ETCO_2$ and SpO_2 by pulse oximetry are being monitored. $ETCO_2$ and SpO_2 are reliable in guiding the weaning of mechanical ventilation and tracheal extubation. Monitoring of these parameters has been used very effectively in "fast-track" protocols. Assessment of volume loss is based on chest and mediastinal tube drainage plus urine output. The endotracheal tube secured in the correct position with an appropriately inflated cuff is essential for positive-pressure ventilation of the lungs. Confirmation of bilateral breath sounds and absence of tracheal air leak versus cuff inflation should be made upon arrival in the ICU. The endotracheal tube's position should be ascertained on the initial chest x-ray. The endotracheal tube also allows for suctioning of bronchial secretions and reduces (but does not eliminate) the risk of oropharyngeal and gastric reflux secretions entering the trachea and bronchi. The endotracheal tube can often be removed the evening of surgery if the patient is conscious, is able to protect the airway, has good ventilatory mechanics and muscle strength, and is able to take on the work of breathing. Most patients can have the pulmonary artery catheter removed within 12 to 24 h if cardiovascular drug therapy is at minimum levels. The peripheral arterial cannula can be removed once cardiovascular function is satisfactory and the need for blood sampling is at a routine daily level. The urinary catheter is usually removed when the patient is ambulatory unless there is a vigorous diuresis or an increased risk of urinary retention. Chest tubes are generally removed when the total drainage is less than 100 mL per tube over 8 h.

The primary factor that differentiates cardiac surgery from other forms of surgery is CPB. With such improvements in extracorporeal technology as membrane oxygenation, arterial blood filtration, and blood sparing techniques, the noncardiac complications have been significantly reduced. Major improvements in myocardial protection coupled with changes in anesthetic and CPB techniques now frequently allow extubation within several hours of surgery.

The patient can often be safely and comfortably transferred from the ICU within the first 6 to 24 h, a process that has been termed *fast tracking*.[1] Individuals undergoing "off pump" procedures also have the potential for rapid recovery and early extubation and removal of catheters and chest tubes; they can be sitting up in the chair the next morning ready for transfer.

Fast tracking requires that the patient's status be characterized as follows: awake or easily aroused, neurologically intact, cooperative, and comfortable; stable, satisfactory hemodynamics; normothermia; satisfactory spontaneous ventilation; normal coagulation with minimal chest tube drainage; satisfactory urine output, electrolyte, and acid-base balance.[2]

EARLY POSTOPERATIVE MANAGEMENT

Pathophysiologic Consequences of Cardiopulmonary Bypass

The basic pathophysiology during the early postoperative period revolves around the following variables: transient left ventricular dysfunction, capillary leak, warming from hypothermia, mediastinal bleeding, and emergence from anesthesia.

While improvements in surgical techniques, cardioplegia delivery, and other myocardial protection features achieved in the past decade were expected to lessen the likelihood of developing transient left ventricular systolic dysfunction following CPB, the reported prevalence of this complication (90 percent) did not change between 1979 and 1990.[3] This transient myocardial depression has been attributed by some authors to inadequate myocardial protection or the effects of cold cardioplegia,[4,5] but the bulk of the evidence incriminates the inflammatory state induced by CPB as the primary causative factor.[6]

The inflammatory state induced by CPB involves platelet–endothelial cell interactions and vasospastic responses that result in low-flow states in the coronary circulation.[7] The inflammatory reaction causes vascular endothelial adhesion molecules to attract inflammatory cells that subsequently adhere to the vascular endothelium. These inflammatory cells mediate much of the subsequent injury by the release of oxygen-free radicals or proteolytic enzymes.[8] This release of oxygen-free radicals in response to reperfusion injury is now generally accepted as the explanation for the transient postoperative ventricular dysfunction.[9,10] Depressed myocardial function seems to be unrelated to CPB time, number of coronary artery grafts, preoperative medications, or postoperative core temperature. Ventricular function is generally depressed by 2 h and is at its worst at 4 to 5 h after CPB. Significant recovery of function usually occurs by 8 to 10 h, and full recovery is reached by 24 to 48 h.[11] Systemic vascular resistance, while not rising immediately after surgery, increases as ventricular function worsens. This rise in systemic vascular resistance is likely secondary to reduced ventricular function and the need to maintain systemic blood pressure and is not per se a major causative factor of depressed cardiac contractility. The confounding effect of vasopressor drugs used in an attempt to increase systemic blood pressure must be recognized.

The inflammation-mediated production of oxygen-free radicals and release of proteolytic enzymes by neutrophils also damages the endothelial cells. The "gatekeeper" function of the endothelium is disturbed and capillary permeability increases, resulting in edema.[8] The capillary leak syndrome may last from a few hours up to 1 to 2 days, depending to a large degree on the duration of CPB. When the capillary leak ceases and interstitial edema fluid is mobilized, intravascular volume overload is a threat.

Hypothermia predisposes the patient to cardiac dysrhythmias, increases systemic vascular resistance, precipitates shivering (which increases O_2 consumption and CO_2 production), and impairs coagulation.[11] Hypothermia with the patient's core temperature below 35°C frequently recurs after rewarming to 37°C (98.6°F) at the end of CPB. This fall in core temperature reflects the loss of heat from the surgical field after CPB, exposure of the patient to ambient temperature, and incomplete rewarming of peripheral tissues, especially fat and muscle. If the patient is hypothermic upon arrival in the ICU, monitoring the temperature of noncore body sites such as a finger or toe can assure complete assessment of rewarming. Hypothermia causes peripheral vasoconstriction and contributes to the hypertension frequently seen after cardiac surgery. Furthermore, hypothermia causes a decrease in cardiac output by producing bradycardia along with the increase in vascular resistance. Most believe that the patient should be passively rewarmed by warm air (e.g., Bear Hugger) and that shivering should be eliminated by the administration of meperidine (25 to 50 mg) and muscle relaxants.[12] As body temperature increases, the vasoconstriction and hypertension associated with hypothermia are replaced by vasodilatation, tachycardia, and hypotension. Volume loading during the rewarming process helps reduce the rapid swings in blood pressure. Vasopressors (e.g., norepinephrine) may be required to maintain an adequate systemic blood pressure. As the patient is rewarmed, large increases in O_2 consumption and CO_2 production can occur, with a consequent increase in demand on cardiovascular and pulmonary functions.[13]

Hypercarbia will cause catecholamine release, tachycardia, and pulmonary hypertension. If the patient cannot increase the cardiac output and O_2 delivery, venous hemoglobin desaturation and metabolic acidosis will result.

The commonly reported prevalence of severe postoperative bleeding (more than 10 U of blood transfused) following cardiac surgery is between 3 and 5 percent. While approximately half of the patients who undergo reoperation for excessive bleeding exhibit incomplete surgical hemostasis, the remainder bleed because of various acquired hemostatic defects, most often related to platelet dysfunction.[14] The factors that predispose to bleeding following CPB are residual heparin effect, platelet dysfunction (which may be intensified by preoperative drug therapy—e.g., aspirin, clopidogrel, and GPIIb/IIIa inhibitors), clotting-factor depletion, inadequate surgical hemostasis, hypothermia, and postoperative hypertension. CPB decreases both platelet count and function. Hemodilution causes platelet counts to fall rapidly to about 50 percent of preoperative values. Within minutes after instituting CPB, the bleeding time is prolonged and platelet aggregation impaired. The bleeding time usually normalizes by 2 to 4 h after CPB. The platelet count usually requires several days to return to normal levels. While the exact mechanism responsible for the transient platelet dysfunction remains undefined, it appears to be related to contact of platelets with the synthetic surfaces of the extracorporeal oxygenator and to hypothermia. Reductions in the plasma concentrations of coagulation factors II, V, VII, IX, X, and XIII due to hemodilution occur during CPB, but these coagulation factors remain well above levels considered adequate for hemostasis and generally normalize within the first 12 h after surgery. Moreover, while bleeding after CPB is often attributed to excessive fibrinolysis, the decrease in both plasminogen and fibrinogen levels during CPB is due to hemodilution and not consumption.[14] Exploration for postoperative bleeding commonly identifies no localized site of bleeding but only diffuse oozing. Less frequently, a specific site such as an internal mammary pedicle will be identified.

MANAGEMENT OF COMMON POSTOPERATIVE SYNDROMES

Vasoconstriction with Hypertension and Borderline Cardiac Output

Increased arteriolar resistance as a consequence of hypothermia and increased levels of circulating catecholamines, plasma renin, or angiotensin II is present in most postoperative cardiac patients. The usual criterion for pharmacologic lowering of blood pressure in postoperative patients is a mean arterial blood pressure 10 percent above the upper level of normal (>90 mmHg). Patients with a friable aorta or friable suture lines might be subjected to a lower mean arterial pressure to prevent dehiscence. The mean arterial blood pressure is monitored because it is most reflective of systemic vascular resistance. As the hypothermic patient is rewarmed, a short-acting vasodilator (nitroprusside, nitroglycerin, or nicardipine) can be infused intravenously to maintain mean arterial pressure at 80 to 90 mmHg. Intravascular volume should be maintained at a relatively high level (PAOP of 14 to 16 mmHg) in anticipation of vasodilation upon rewarming and to enhance cardiac output and peripheral perfusion. If the cardiac index is marginal (2.0 to 2.2 L/min/m^2), an inotropic drug should be administered in addition to the vasodilator.

Vasodilatation and Hypotension

This condition, which generally appears during rewarming, is most effectively prevented and best treated by fluid administration. There is a paucity of data indicating that any specific volume expander is better than another, although colloids remain in the intravascular space longer than crystalloid solutions. Fluid should be administered until cardiac output no longer increases or appropriate left ventricular filling pressures have been restored (PAOP approximately 14 to 16 mmHg for a normal ventricle or 18 to 22 mmHg for a noncompliant ventricle).[15]

If the blood pressure is marginal despite fluid administration and the cardiac index is over 2.5 L/min/m^2, norepinephrine is the preferable agent. More recently, the use of low dose vasopressin (≤ 0.1 U/min) has been recommended for systemic hypotension with a high cardiac output, since endogenous vasopressin levels are depressed after CPB. It is important to emphasize that this therapy is recommended only for a high cardiac output state. If the cardiac index is marginal (less than 2.0 L/min/m^2), an inotropic agent should be administered.

Normal Ventricular Systolic Function and Low Cardiac Output

This set of circumstances is often noted in small women with systemic hypertension and in patients undergoing aortic valve replacement for aortic stenosis. The likely explanation is diastolic dysfunction. The problem should be managed by volume expansion with the intent to elevate PAOP to levels as high as 20 to 25 mmHg if necessary as long as right ventricular function is adequate to fill the left ventricle. Sinus rhythm and atrioventricular synchrony are essential and, if not present, should be restored. In the absence of other reasons for diastolic dysfunction, the possibility of cardiac compression from clots in the mediastinum and pericardial space should be considered. If volume expansion does not lead to hemodynamic improvement, transesophageal echocardiography (TEE) should be used to establish or exclude the presence of clots or other causes of low output.

APPROACH TO POSTOPERATIVE CARDIOVASCULAR PROBLEMS

Low-Cardiac-Output Syndrome

Satisfactory cardiac performance following cardiac surgery is usually indicated by a cardiac index greater than 2.2, L/min/m^2 with a heart rate below 100 beats per minute. Marginal cardiac function is present with a cardiac index between 2.0 and 2.2 L/min/m^2. A cardiac index below 2.0 L/min/m^2 is unacceptably low, and therapeutic intervention is indicated. Clinical signs of the adequacy or inadequacy of organ perfusion must be incorporated into any assessment of cardiac performance. It is also useful to measure the mixed-venous oxygen saturation, as a subset of patients who are hypothermic may have a low cardiac index but an acceptable mixed venous oxygen tension.

ASSESSMENT

The most common causes of low cardiac output postoperatively are related to a decreased left ventricular preload. The decreased preload, in turn, can likely be attributed to hypovolemia (due to bleeding or to vasodilatation as a consequence of warming or of drugs), cardiac tamponade, or right ventricular dysfunction. Alternative explanations for low cardiac output include decreased contractility due to a preexisting low ejection fraction or to intra- or postoperative ischemia or infarction. Tachy- or bradyarrhythmias decrease cardiac output by reducing ventricular preload (e.g., decreased diastolic filling time, loss of atrial contraction or atrioventricular synchrony) or by reducing the number of effective ventricular contractions per minute. Substantial increases in systemic vascular resistance (i.e., vasoconstriction) impede ventricular ejection and lower cardiac output. Vasodilatation from sepsis or anaphylaxis resulting in systemic hypotension can lead to reduced coronary blood flow and myocardial ischemia. Sepsis (an unlikely occurrence in the immediate postoperative period) is also associated with the production of myocardial depressant factors. Anemia may result in reduced blood viscosity (a major determinant of total peripheral resistance) leading to hypotension and decreased oxygen delivery to the heart. The hypotension in anemia, however, is most often due to changes in effective blood volume rather than to the changes in viscosity.

ETIOLOGY AND MANAGEMENT

The multiple variables constantly monitored usually provide sufficient clues as to the cause of low cardiac output. If there is no obvious noncardiac cause then the first step is to optimize the heart rate by either cardiac pacing or antiarrhythmic drugs. Postoperative myocardial performance is usually best at a rate of 90 to 100 beats per minute. The next step is to increase preload until cardiac output is no longer increasing (PAOP of 15 to 18 mmHg). If these measures prove unsuccessful, pharmacologic intervention with inotropic agents, vasodilators, vasopressors, or a combination of these drugs must be considered. The selection of drugs should be based upon the balance of their effects on heart rate, contractility, ventricular preload, and systemic vasculature resistance (Table 59-1). Many clinicians find that a combination of a phosphodiesterase inhibitor and inotrope/vasopressor is the optimal pharmacological therapy for low cardiac output syndrome secondary to impaired ventricular function. Phosphodiesterase inhibitors, such as amrinone and milrinone, may offer advantages for patients who were in heart failure preoperatively since beta receptors may be downregulated and catecholamines may be less effective. The presence of elevated left- and right-sided filling

TABLE 59-1 Medications Used in Low-Cardiac-Output Syndrome

Medication	Hemodynamic Properties	Dosage Range
Dopamine	Low dose—dopaminergic effect Moderate dose—inotropic effect High dose—vasopressor effect	2–20 μg/kg/min
Dobutamine	Positive inotropic agent	2–20 μg/kg/min
Epinephrine	Positive inotropic agent	1–4 μg/min
Amrinone	Positive inotropic agent	10–15 μg/kg/min
Isoproterenol	Potent inotropic agent Pronounced chronotropic effect	0.5–10 μg/min
Norepinephrine	Potent vasopressor effect; inotropic effect	1–100 μg/min
Phenylephrine	Potent vasopressor agent	10–500 μg/min

pressures, a recent cessation of mediastinal drainage, and progressively increasing dosage requirements for inotropic drugs suggests tamponade, which should be relieved emergently.

Hypertension

MANAGEMENT

A variety of medications are available for control of hypertension; the drug selected should depend on the hemodynamic status of the patient, the cardiovascular effects of the drug, and the patient's other medical problems. Systemic hypertension in the presence of a high left ventricular filling pressure and marginal cardiac output is most appropriately treated by an arterial vasodilator. Nitroprusside relaxes vascular smooth muscle in arterial resistance vessels (both systemic and pulmonary) and in venous capacitance vessels. The advantages of the drug are its very rapid onset and the rapid dissipation of its effects. The risks with this agent are rapid and excessive hypotension, production of a coronary steal syndrome by dilatation of the coronary resistance vessels, and the potential for either acute cyanide toxicity or thiocyanate toxicity with prolonged use.

Nitroglycerin is primarily a venous dilator, although it produces varying degrees of arterial vasodilatation, especially at high doses. Its major role in treating systemic hypertension is in the patient with high filling pressures and active myocardial ischemia. Nicardipine is a potent systemic and coronary vasodilator without the risk of coronary steal, and it has no significant effect on the venous system. While its onset of action is rapid (1 to 2 min), its elimination half-life is about 40 min. Unlike some calcium-channel blockers, this agent lacks a negative inotropic effect and has no effect on atrioventricular conduction.

When the hypertension is associated with a normal cardiac output and a relatively rapid sinus heart rate or a propensity toward dysrhythmias, a drug with negative inotropic and chronotropic properties is desirable. Esmolol is a cardioselective, ultra-short-acting beta blocker, which also produces a rapid and titratable control of the blood pressure accompanied by a decrease in heart rate. The drug is usually tolerated satisfactorily by patients with a history of bronchospasm because of its relatively high selectivity for beta$_1$-type adrenergic receptors. It is not ideal for patients with impaired cardiac contractility, particularly in the presence of elevated filling pressures. Diltiazem is an arterial vasodilator that has a mild negative inotropic effect and a more potent negative chronotropic effect. Labetalol has both alpha- and beta-blocking properties as well as a direct vasodilatory effect. Its predominant effect is as a beta blocker, especially in the intravenous form. The angiotensin converting enzyme inhibitor enalaprilat can be administered intermittently by the intravenous route. This agent is usually reserved for the patient who is hemodynamically stable with either a normal or reduced cardiac output but with hypertension expected to persist (Table 59-2).

Arrhythmias

GENERAL CONSIDERATIONS AND SINUS TACHYCARDIA

The most common rhythm disturbance immediately after cardiac surgery is sinus tachycardia. This condition is appropriately treated by searching for and correcting the underlying cause (pain, anxiety, low cardiac output, anemia, fever, or beta-blocker withdrawal). The second most common arrhythmia is ventricular ectopy. Again, an underlying cause such as myocardial ischemia, hypokalemia, hypomagnesemia, hypoxia, or administration of sympathomimetic drugs must be sought and corrected if possible. Occasionally repositioning of a ventricular pacemaker lead or a pulmonary artery catheter that slipped back into the right ventricle will stop the ectopy. It is also important to review the patient's preoperative record to determine if the patient had preexisting ectopy. Patients with chronic ventricular ectopy frequently have their ectopy exaggerated postoperatively. In the presence of active myocardial ischemia, pharmacologic suppression is advisable for complex

TABLE 59-2 Intravenous Antihypertensive Agents

Drug	Peak Effect	Duration	Dosage
Nitroprusside	Immediate	2–5 min	0.3–1.0 μg/kg/min
Nitroglycerine	Immediate	2–5 min	5–100 μg/min infusion
Nicardipine	5–60 min	20–40 min	2.5 mg over 5 min; may repeat times 4 at 10-min intervals; infusion 2–15 mg/h
Esmolol	2–5 min	8–10 min	1-min loading infusion of 0.25–0.5 mg/kg; sustained infusion of 50–200 μg/kg/min
Enalaprilat	15–30 min	6 h or more	0.625–1.25 mg slowly over 5 min every 6 h
Hydralazine	15–20 min	3–4 h	5- to 10-mg bolus may be repeated every 15 min; up to total of 40 mg
Diltiazem	3–30 min	3 h	20- to 25-mg bolus may repeat; infusion of 10–20 mg/h
Verapamil	2–3 min	20–40 min	5- to 10-mg bolus; may repeat in 10 min; infusion of 3–25 mg/h
Labetalol	5–15 min	2–6 h	20-mg bolus over 2 min; then 40- to 80-mg boluses every 15 min until effect achieved (to total dose of 300 mg)

ventricular ectopy. If suppression of ventricular ectopy seems necessary, the most effective agent is intravenous amiodarone. The drug should be administered through a three-phase infusion over the first 24 h: 150 mg over 10 min, 300 mg over the next 6 h, and a 0.5- to1.0-mg/min infusion.

VENTRICULAR TACHYCARDIA AND FIBRILLATION

After cardiac surgery, a few patients develop sustained ventricular tachycardia (either monomorphic or polymorphic) or ventricular fibrillation. These profound rhythm disturbances may develop in the absence of evidence of acute myocardial ischemia or infarction or electrolyte imbalance. In most cases the patients have had previous myocardial infarction and have undergone "complete" revascularization, including regions likely to be nonviable. Reperfusion of these areas that probably include viable as well as nonviable myofibrils embedded in the healed infarct may lead to altered dispersion of repolarization. These changes support development of reentry arrhythmias.[16] The ventricular tachycardia in these patients uncommonly responds to lidocaine and usually requires amiodarone. In some instances, a combination of amiodarone and a beta blocker is required. In a rare circumstance, aortic counterpulsation has seemed to be of benefit.

Every encounter with a wide complex tachycardia requires careful consideration as to the possibility of supraventricular tachycardia with aberrant conduction. In the presence of atrial fibrillation with a rapid ventricular response, right bundle branch aberrant conduction often mimics ventricular tachycardia. Care must be given to avoid lidocaine in these situations, because it may result in an even more rapid ventricular rate. Wide complex tachyarrhythmias in the range of 250 to 300 beats per minute should suggest the presence of an anomalous conduction pathway. The mechanism of this arrhythmia usually involves atrial flutter, with one-to-one conduction or atrial fibrillation with a very fast ventricular response involving an anomalous pathway. Once this is recognized, procainamide becomes the drug of choice, since it does have favorable therapeutic effects on the bypass track tissue. Lidocaine and verapamil should be avoided if the presence of an anomalous pathway is suspected (see also Chap. 24).

SUPRAVENTRICULAR ARRHYTHMIAS

The most common supraventricular dysrhythmias with the exception of sinus tachycardia are atrial fibrillation and atrial flutter. These rhythm disturbances occur in 10 to 30 percent of patients following cardiac surgery. The predominant predisposing factor in the development of atrial fibrillation is the patient's age. The prevalence of atrial fibrillation in postoperative cardiac patients <40 years of age is as low as 3.7 percent, while the prevalence is at least 28 percent in patients >70 years. Atrial fibrillation is most likely to appear on the second postoperative day. Within 1 to 3 days, 80 percent of these patients will return to sinus rhythm with only digoxin or beta-blocker therapy.[17,18] The prophylactic use of beta blockers has a protective effect against the development of atrial fibrillation or flutter. This beneficial effect has been demonstrated with any one of several beta blockers, administered in low or high doses and started preoperatively or postoperatively. Neither digoxin nor verapamil has demonstrated effective prophylaxis against atrial fibrillation or flutter.[19]

Preoperative oral administration of amiodarone also reduces the prevalence of postoperative atrial fibrillation.[20] The major limitation to the widespread application of this prophylactic approach is the apparent need for a 7-day preoperative treatment period. An accelerated loading regimen over 1 to 2 days may be effective but is unproved.[20] Intravenous infusions of either esmolol or diltiazem can be used to control the ventricular rate with atrial fibrillation or flutter. Esmolol is given as a 1-min loading infusion of 0.25 to 0.5 mg/kg, followed

by a sustained infusion of 50 to 200 μg/kg/min. Diltiazem is administered as a bolus of 20 to 25 mg (which may be repeated), followed by an infusion of 10 to 15 mg/h. Diltiazem is preferred in patients with impaired ventricular function. Atrial epicardial pacing wires provide the means of atrial pacing to convert some cases of atrial flutter to sinus rhythm. Short bursts (15 to 30 s) of atrial pacing at rates of 300 to 600 per minute may be effective in converting atrial flutter. Approximately 10 percent of patients with atrial fibrillation require electrical cardioversion to restore sinus rhythm. If hemodynamic compromise is present and aggravated by a supraventricular tachyarrhythmia, cardioversion should be used immediately rather than later.

Intravenous ibutilide (1 mg infused over 10 min to be repeated once if necessary) is the most effective pharmacologic means of converting recent-onset atrial flutter. The drug is much less effective (in the range of 30 to 50 percent) for conversion of recent-onset atrial fibrillation. The disadvantage of ibutilide is the propensity for causing torsades de pointes in 2 to 4 percent of patients.

CONDUCTION DEFECTS

The prevalence of intraventricular conduction abnormalities after coronary bypass surgery is reported to be from 1 to 45 percent, with approximately 10 percent being the most commonly reported frequency. The most common conduction defect is right bundle branch block, which may be due to selective sensitivity of the right bundle to the effects of hypothermia and the extracorporeal circulation process. Only about 5 percent of the patients are left with a permanent conduction abnormality, and the prognosis for these patients is no worse than it is for comparable patients with no conduction defect.[21,22] The development of high-degree (second- or third-degree) atrioventricular block is an indication for temporary pacing via epicardial pacing wires. Atrioventricular block is not as common as either bundle branch block or fascicular block, but it does occur, especially after aortic valve surgery.

Respiratory Management

EXPECTED RESPIRATORY CHANGES
AFTER CARDIAC SURGERY

Pulmonary problems are the most significant cause of morbidity following cardiac surgery. Splinting due to chest pain, phrenic nerve damage, cephalad displacement of the diaphragm by abdominal contents, and alveolar edema due to elevated left heart filling pressures may all contribute to pulmonary dysfunction.

Atelectasis is the most common pulmonary complication, occurring in about 70 percent of patients following cardiac surgery with CPB.[23] During CPB, the lungs are not perfused and are usually allowed to collapse. Once the lungs are reexpanded, a variable amount of atelectasis remains. The preponderance of atelectasis occurs in the left lower lobe because of its compression during cardiac surgery, the tendency to suction more thoroughly the right mainstem bronchus during blind nasoorotracheal suctioning, and the frequent surgical practice of opening the left pleural space to facilitate dissection of the left internal mammary artery.

After thoracotomy, both lung and chest wall compliance decrease significantly. The maximum decrease occurs at approximately 3 days, but the decrease persists to a lesser degree 6 or more days after sternotomy. Alterations in chest wall mechanics lead to a decrease in the forced expiratory volume in one second (FEV_1) and the functional residual capacity (FRC). The changes in the FEV_1 may persist for 6 weeks. In addition to these changes in flows and volumes, reduced inspiratory strength and uncoordinated rib cage expansion occur. These changes result in an increase in respiratory rate and a decrease in tidal volume, a decrease in respiratory efficiency, and an increase in oxygen cost of breathing. The atelectasis and decrease in lung volume result in ventilation: perfusion mismatch and shunting. The clinical manifestation is a decrease in arterial PO_2 and hemoglobin saturation.[23]

BASIC CONCEPTS OF OXYGENATION AND ALVEOLAR VENTILATION

The goals of mechanical ventilation are the maintenance of satisfactory arterial oxygenation and CO_2 removal. An $SpO_2 > 90$ percent is considered to be acceptable, but it may be associated with a marginal PaO_2. A PaO_2 below 65 mmHg will result in a precipitous fall in the oxygen saturation of hemoglobin. The FIO_2 should be gradually decreased to 0.4 as tolerated, to minimize adsorption atelectasis and pulmonary O_2 toxicity. Mechanical ventilation is also used to maintain alveolar ventilation, which regulates the arterial blood CO_2 tension ($PaCO_2$). Alveolar ventilation is regulated by controlling the tidal volume and the respiratory rate. Generally, the ventilator should maintain an exhaled minute ventilation of 6 to 8 L/min. Decreasing the tidal volume below 8 to 10 mL/kg may result in alveolar hypoventilation and atelectasis. Mild hypocarbia ($PaCO_2$ of 30 to 35 mmHg) is satisfactory immediately after surgery, but more profound respiratory alkalosis should be avoided because it leads to hypokalemia and a leftward shift of the oxygen-hemoglobin dissociation curve (decreased oxygen release to the tissues). Hypercarbia in the immediate postoperative period usually indicates that minute ventilation is inadequate. The problem can be rectified primarily by increasing the ventilator rate; in some cases it is appropriate to increase the tidal volume as well. Later, as the patient is weaned from the ventilator, hypercarbia may reflect opioid analgesia (a necessary side effect of satisfactory analgesia) or compensatory hypoventilation in response to a metabolic alkalosis, most likely due to excessive diuresis. Severe hypercarbia should raise a concern about mechanical problems such as ventilator malfunction, endotracheal tube malposition, or a pneumothorax. Occasionally, hypoxemia and even hypotension may develop in the mechanically ventilated patient due to a tension pneumothorax or hemothorax.

VENTILATORY WEANING AND EXTUBATION

Ventilatory support should be reduced as tolerated when the cardiovascular system has become stable and the arterial oxygen tension is satisfactory [a PaO_2/FIO_2 ratio > 300 mmHg with PEEP (peak end-expiratory pressure) of 5 cmH$_2$O]. The patient should also be alert, normothermic, and have no active bleeding. Monitoring of SpO_2 and $ETCO_2$ is helpful and allows the weaning process to be done safely and expeditiously. Weaning should be discontinued if any of the following signs appear: $SpO_2 < 90$; $PaO_2 < 60$ mmHg; $ETCO_2 > 50$ mmHg; $PaCO_2 > 55$ mmHg; pH < 7.30; 10-mmHg rise in pulmonary artery pressure; respiratory rate > 30; 20-mmHg rise in systemic blood pressure; or 20-beat rise in heart rate.[3]

Most patients require low to moderate doses of morphine or another opioid in order to tolerate the endotracheal tube. As long as the spontaneous ventilatory rate remains greater than 15 breaths per minute, the patient will almost certainly be able to maintain adequate ventilation after the endotracheal tube is removed.

BRONCHOSPASM

Severe bronchospasm during CPB is an unusual event, but it can occur. The most likely cause of this fulminant bronchospasm is activation of human C5a anaphylatoxin by the extracorporeal circulation. Other likely causes of bronchospasm in the postoperative period are cardiogenic pulmonary edema; simple exacerbation of preexisting bronchospastic disease triggered by instrumentation, secretions, or cold anesthetic gas; beta-adrenergic blockers in susceptible individuals; and allergic reaction to protamine. The initial therapy of bronchospasm in the postoperative patient, once a diagnosis of heart failure is excluded, should be inhaled beta$_2$-agonists (terbutaline, metaproterenol, albuterol) and/or inhaled cholinergic agents (ipratropium bromide or glycopyrrolate). In the inhaled form, these rather potent bronchodilators have minimal cardiovascular effects. In addition to their bronchodilator effect, these agents may augment mucociliary transport and aid in clearing secretions. A combination of beta$_2$-agonists and cholinergic agents should be tried in the patient refractory to a single agent. Even more refractory bronchospasm requires either a short course of systemic steroids or intravenous aminophylline.

Postoperative Oliguria and Renal Insufficiency

ETIOLOGY

The use of radiocontrast agents in the days immediately preceding cardiac surgery may embarrass renal function, as manifest by a rise in blood urea nitrogen and serum creatinine values. Following CPB, there is a substantial incidence of postoperative renal dysfunction (up to 30 percent) but a relatively low incidence of severe renal impairment requiring dialysis (1 to 5 percent). Renal blood flow and glomerular filtration rate are reduced by 25 to 75 percent during bypass, with partial but not complete recovery in the first day after CPB. This reduction in renal function is attributed to renal artery vasoconstriction, hypothermia, and loss of pulsatile perfusion during CPB. Angiotensin II levels are higher with nonpulsatile flow as compared to pulsatile flow. While renal dysfunction cannot be consistently related to the systemic blood pressure and pump flow rate during nonpulsatile bypass, there is a definite relation between the incidence of postbypass renal dysfunction and the duration of CPB. In addition to the duration of CPB, the risk of developing postbypass renal failure seems to be a function of the patient's underlying renal function (also affected by age) and the perioperative circulatory status. The histologic changes that accompany renal impairment after cardiopulmonary bypass are characteristic of tubular necrosis. The tubular cells seem to be the most susceptible to acute reductions in renal perfusion.

MANAGEMENT

There are three agents (so-called renoprotective drugs) that might be used during CPB to prevent an ischemic insult to the kidneys. Mannitol used in the CPB priming fluid may moderate ischemic insult, probably by volume expansion and hemodilution. It also initiates an osmotic diuresis, which prevents tubular obstruction and may serve as a free radical scavenger. Furosemide appears to improve renal blood flow when given during bypass. So-called renal-dose dopamine (1 to 2.5 μg/kg/min based on ideal body weight) may maintain renal blood flow and urine output. Once renal failure has developed, none of these drugs is likely to offer any beneficial effect. A megadose of furosemide (200 to 300 mg) may be tried, but if there is no diuretic response, it should not be repeated. Similarly, a single dose of mannitol (12.5 to 25 mg) either with or without furosemide could be tried, but it should not be repeated if there is no effect.

Postoperative Gastrointestinal Dysfunction

GASTROINTESTINAL CONSEQUENCES OF CARDIOPULMONARY BYPASS

The gastrointestinal consequences of CPB appear to be minimal. Reviews of the subject report a 1 percent prevalence.[24,25] Most patients eat within 24 to 48 h after an uncomplicated elective procedure. The limited investigations of the gastrointestinal tract after cardiac surgery have found a slight decrease in hepatic and pancreatic blood flow during cooling and rewarming on bypass and a decrease in gastric pH.[26] Transient elevations in liver function tests and hyperamylasemia may occur after cardiac surgery; the risk factors include long CPB time, multiple transfusions, and multiple valve replacements. Appearance of jaundice portends a poor prognosis.[27] Severe gastrointestinal complications are usually ischemic in nature and are often associated with a low-output syndrome.[32] The use of opioids as part of general anesthesia and postoperative pain management contributes to gastrointestinal dysfunction (cramping, ileus, and constipation) and to postoperative nausea and vomiting. The nausea and vomiting can be minimized by use of a naso- or orogastric tube to maintain gastric decompression intraoperatively and early in the postoperative period, with the additional benefit of improving thoracoabdominal compliance to positive-pressure ventilation.

Postoperative Metabolic Disorders

POTASSIUM IMBALANCE

There are multiple factors that can produce large and rapid shifts in the serum potassium levels during and after CPB. The principal detrimental effects of these potassium shifts involve the electrical activity of the heart. The electrocardiographic signs of hyperkalemia and hypokalemia are described in Chap. 13. The electrocardiographic changes of hyperkalemia do not necessarily appear in the classic progressive manner; they are more related to the rate of rise in serum potassium rather than to the absolute serum concentration. The therapy of severe hyperkalemia should include counteracting the toxic cardiac effects of the elevated potassium with intravenous calcium gluconate or calcium chloride and lowering the serum level of potassium with sodium bicarbonate and/or administration of regular insulin and glucose. Hypokalemia is treated with the intravenous administration of KCl at a rate of no more than 10 to 15 meq/h. The serum potassium rises approximately 0.1 meq/L for each 2 meq of KCl administered. Large doses of KCl should be administered by a central venous catheter because of the caustic effect of potassium on peripheral veins.

HYPOMAGNESEMIA

Hypomagnesemia is common following cardiac surgery using CPB. Magnesium mimics potassium in its effects on the electrical activity of the heart. The cause of the hypomagnesemia is unknown, but it is probably multifactorial. Many patients will be hypomagnesemic preoperatively due to the use of loop diuretics, thiazides, digoxin, or alcohol and to the effects of type I diabetes mellitus. Magnesium is usually lost in the urine during CPB. Patients with postoperative hypomagnesemia develop atrial and ventricular dysrhythmias more frequently and require more prolonged mechanical ventilatory support than do patients with normal magnesium levels.[28] Magnesium administration also seems to improve stroke volume and cardiac index in the early postoperative period.[29] Magnesium can be administered as magnesium sulfate (2 g in 100-mL solution) to raise serum levels to 2 meq/L.

HYPERGLYCEMIA

During CPB there is a rise in blood glucose levels. The elevation is modest during hypothermia and becomes more marked during rewarming. This rise in glucose is due in part to increased glucose mobilization related to dramatic increases in cortisol, catecholamine, and growth hormone levels during CPB. Also, there is an apparent failure of insulin secretion, particularly during hypothermia, probably related to inhibition of the insulin secretory response by the elevated catecholamines. This blunting of the insulin response persists for the first 24 h after surgery. These changes are exaggerated in the diabetic patient.[30] Insulin requirements are likely to be seven times greater than the preoperative requirements during the first 4 h postoperatively. Furthermore, such insulin resistance is exacerbated by catecholamines, diuretics, and blood transfusions.[31] These multiple factors make the diabetic patient susceptible to hyperosmolar hyperglycemia and nonketotic diabetic coma.[32]

Postoperative Fever

Fever is a common occurrence in the postoperative patient. It is generally a consequence of pleuropericarditis, atelectasis, or phlebitis. A reasonable assumption in a patient with a core temperature <38°C (100.4°F) and no evidence of phlebitis or presence of a pericardial or pleural rub is that the source of the fever is atelectasis. The appropriate therapeutic approach is to encourage intensified efforts at incentive spirometry and coughing. Any fever >38.5°C (101.3°F) warrants blood, sputum, and urine cultures. A white blood cell count (total and differential) and a chest x-ray should also be obtained. Sternal wound infections occur in 0.4 to 5 percent of patients after sternotomy.[33–35] Multiple factors have been identified as increasing the risk of developing sternal wound infection. These include pneumonia, prolonged mechanical ventilation (especially with tracheostomy), emergency operations, postoperative hemorrhage with mediastinal hematoma, early reexploration, obesity, diabetes mellitus, and use of bilateral internal mammary grafts. The greatest risk for sternal infection seems to be in diabetic patients who receive bilateral internal mammary grafts.[35] Debate continues as to whether the most appropriate initial treatment is debridement and closure or open packing and subsequent plastic surgical closure with a muscle flap.

Approximately 1 percent of patients who have had coronary artery bypass surgery experience leg wound infections that necessitate extra care. Leg infections seem to occur more frequently in obese women, especially if the thigh veins are harvested.[36]

Neurologic and Neurophysiologic Dysfunction

MECHANISM

The mechanisms thought to account for most cerebral injury during cardiac surgery are macroembolization of air, debris from aortic atheroma or left ventricular thrombus; microembolization of aggregates of granulocytes, platelets, and fibrin; and cerebral hypoperfusion. Death or disabling stroke occurs in about 2 percent of patients, with another 3 percent experiencing transient or minor functional disability secondary to cerebral infarction.[37] Focal neurologic deficits resulting from intraoperative events are usually noted within the first 24 to 48 h after surgery.

ENCEPHALOPATHY AND DELIRIUM

Alteration of mental status (encephalopathy and delirium) will be seen in approximately 30 percent of patients after cardiopulmonary bypass.[37] While the appearance of these encephalopathic symptoms likely reflects cerebral injury, other causes must be excluded, including drugs, sepsis, fever, hypoxemia, ethanol withdrawal, renal failure, and hyperosmolar state. Postoperative encephalopathic changes, varying from mild confusion and disorientation to protracted somnolence or agitation and hallucinations, may appear at any time during the hospital stay.[38] Studies of this condition have not identified any consistent risk factors, but advancing age, duration of CPB, and sleep deprivation have frequently been associated. The prevalence of this condition has remained rather constant since the early days of cardiac surgery involving CPB, but there has been a shift in the clinical presentation. Currently, the condition seems to present with disorientation rather than with hallucinations, paranoid ideation, and the agitation that had been noted earlier.[38] Recognition of this entity is important because the family can be assured that the patient's mental status is likely to recover. Agitation and acute psychosis in these patients usually respond to intravenous haloperidol, 2 to 10 mg, repeated as needed to produce adequate sedation.

BRACHIAL PLEXOPATHY AND ULNAR NERVE DYSFUNCTION

Another serious neurologic complication of cardiac surgery is brachial plexopathy. This neurologic dysfunction, involving C8 and T1, usually results from mechanical trauma secondary to sternal retraction, but it may be due to penetration by a posterior fractured segment of the first rib or injury during internal jugular cannulation. There is no specific therapy for this condition, and recovery can take as long as 6 months, with a few cases being permanent.[39] Ulnar nerve dysfunction may result from malpositioning of the upper extremities during surgery, which results in pressure being exerted on the ulnar nerve at the elbow.

References

1. Aps C. Fast-tracking in cardiac surgery. *Br J Hosp Med* 1995;54:139–142.
2. Jindosi A, Aps C, Neville E, et al. Postoperative cardiac surgical care: An alternative approach. *Br Heart J* 1993;69:59–64.
3. Bojar RM. *Manual of Perioperative Care in Cardiac and Thoracic Surgery*, 2d ed. Boston: Blackwell Scientific; 1994.
4. Levy JH, Salemenpera MT, Bailey JM, Ramsey JG. Postoperative circulatory control. In: Kaplan JA, ed. *Cardiac Anesthesia*, 3d ed. Philadelphia: Saunders; 1993:1168–1193.
5. Swanson DK, Myerowitz PD. Effect of reperfusion temperature and pressure on the functional and metabolic recovery of preserved hearts. *J Thorac Cardiovasc Surg* 1983;86:242–251.
6. Cameron D. Initiation of white cell activation during cardiopulmonary bypass: Cytokines and receptors. *J Cardiovasc Pharmacol* 1996; 27(suppl 1):S1–S5.
7. Gold JP, Roberts AJ, Hoover EL, et al. Effects of prolonged aortic cross clamping with potassium cardioplegia on myocardial contractility in man. *Surg Forum* 1979;30:252–254.
8. Spiess BD. Ischemia as a coagulation problem? *J Cardiovasc Pharmacol* 1996;27(suppl 1):S38–S41.
9. Bolli R. Oxygen derived free radicals and postischemic myocardial dysfunction. *J Am Coll Cardiol* 1988;12:239–249.
10. Przyklenk K, Kloner RA. "Reperfusion injury" by oxygen derived free radicals? *Circ Res* 1989;64:86–96.
11. Breisblatt WM, Stein KI, Wolfe CJ, et al. Acute myocardial dysfunction and recovery: A common occurrence after coronary bypass surgery. *J Am Coll Cardiol* 1990;15:1261–1269.
12. Ralley FE, Wynando JE, Rams JG, et al. The effects of shivering on oxygen consumption and carbon dioxide production in patients rewarming from hypothermic cardiopulmonary bypass. *Can J Anaesth* 1988;35:332–337.
13. Donati F, Maille JG, Blain R, et al. End-tidal carbon dioxide tension and temperature changes after coronary artery bypass surgery. *Can Anaesth Soc J* 1985;32:272–277.
14. Harker L, Malpass TW, Branson HE, et al. Mechanism of abnormal bleeding in patients undergoing cardiopulmonary bypass: Acquired transient platelet dysfunction associated with selective alpha-granule release. *Blood* 1980;56:824–834.
15. Ellis RJ, Mangano DT, Van Dyke DC. Relationship of wedge pressure to end diastolic volume in patients undergoing myocardial revascularization. *J Thorac Cardiovasc Surg* 1979;78:605–613.
16. Topol EJ, Lerman BB, Baughman KL, et al. De novo refractory ventricular tachyarrhythmias after coronary revascularization. *Am J Cardiol* 1986;57:57–59.
17. Leith JW, Thomson D, Baird DK, Harris PJ. The importance of age as a predictor of atrial fibrillation and flutter after coronary artery bypass grafting. *J Thorac Cardiovasc Surg* 1990;100:338–342.
18. Hashimoto K, Ilstrup DM, Schaff HV. Influence of clinical and hemodynamic variables on risk of supraventricular tachycardia after coronary artery bypass. *J Thorac Cardiovasc Surg* 1991;101:56–65.
19. Andrews TC, Reimold SC, Berlin JA, Antman EM. Prevention of supraventricular arrhythmias after coronary artery bypass surgery. A meta-analysis of randomized controlled trials. *Circulation* 1991; 84(suppl III):III-236–III-244.
20. Daoud EG, Strickberger SA, Man KC, et al. Peroperative amiodarone as prophylaxis against artrial fibrillation after heart surgery. *N Engl J Med* 1997;337:1785–1791.
21. Baerman JM, Kirsch MM, de Buitleir M, et al. Natural history and determinates of conduction defects following coronary artery bypass surgery. *Ann Thorac Surg* 1987;44:150–153.
22. Tuzcu EM, Emre A, Goormastic M, Loop FD. Incidence and prognostic significance of intraventricular conduction abnormalities after coronary bypass surgery. *J Am Coll Cardiol* 1990;16:607–610.
23. Sladden RN, Berkowitz DE. Cardiopulmonary bypass and the lung. In: Gravlee GP, Davis RF, Utley IR, eds. *Cardiopulmonary Bypass*. Baltimore: Williams & Wilkins; 1993:468–487.
24. Hanks JB, Curtis SE, Hanks BB, et al. Gastrointestinal complications after cardiopulmonary bypass. *Surgery* 1982;92:394–400.
25. Welling RE, Rath R, Albers JE, Glaser RS. Gastrointestinal complications after cardiac surgery. *Arch Surg* 1986;121:1178–1180.
26. Mori A, Watanabe K, Onoe M, et al. Regional blood flow in the liver, pancreas, and kidney during pulsatile and nonpulsatile perfusion under profound hypothermia. *Jpn Circ J* 1988;52:219–227.
27. Collins JD, Bassendine MF, Ferner R, et al. Incidence and prognostic importance of jaundice after cardiopulmonary bypass surgery. *Lancet* 1983;1:1119–1123.
28. Aglio LS, Stanford GG, Maddi R, et al. Hypomagnesemia is common following cardiac surgery. *J Cardiothorac Anesth* 1991;5:201–208.
29. England MR, Gordon G, Salem M, Chernow B. Magnesium administration and dysrhythmias after cardiac surgery: A placebo-controlled, double-blind, randomized trial. *JAMA* 1993;269:2369–2370.
30. Frater RW, Oka Y, Kadish A, et al. Diabetes and coronary artery surgery. *Mt Sinai J Med* 1982;49:237–240.
31. Elliott MJ, Gill GV, Home PD, et al. A comparison of two regimens for the management of diabetes during open-heart surgery. *Anesthesiology* 1984;60:364–368.
32. Seki S. Clinical features of hyperglycemia, nonketotic diabetic coma associated with cardiac operations. *J Thorac Cardiovasc Surg* 1986;91: 8678–8687.
33. Ulicny KS, Hiradzka SF. The risk factors of median sternotomy infection: A current review. *J Cardiac Surg* 1991;6:338–351.
34. Hazelrigg SR, Wellons HA, Schneider JA, Kolm P. Wound complications after median sternotomy: Relationship to internal mammary grafting. *J Thorac Cardiovasc Surg* 1989;98:1096–1099.
35. Grossi EA, Esposito R, Harris LJ, et al. Sternal wound infections and use of internal mammary artery grafts. *J Thorac Cardiovasc Surg* 1991;102: 342–347.
36. De Laria GA, Hunter JA, Goldin MD, et al. Leg wound complications associated with coronary revascularization. *J Thorac Cardiovasc Surg* 1981;81:403–407.
37. Breuer AC, Furlan AJ, Hanson MR, et al. Central nervous system complications of coronary artery bypass graft surgery: Prospective analysis of 421 patients. *Stroke* 1983;14:82–87.
38. Smith LW, Dimsdale JE. Postcardiotomy delirium: Conclusions after 25 years? *Am J Psychiatry* 1989;146:452–458.
39. Shaw PJ, Bates D, Cartlidge NE, et al. Early neurological complications of coronary artery bypass surgery. *BMJ* 1985;91:1384–1387.

REHABILITATION OF THE PATIENT WITH CORONARY HEART DISEASE

Nanette K. Wenger

Cardiac rehabilitation, an essential component of long-term comprehensive management for coronary patients, includes individualized prescriptive exercise training and health education and counseling appropriate for each patient's needs, specific cardiac problem, and risk status.[1,2] *Cardiac rehabilitation* is described by the U.S. Public Health Service as "comprehensive, long-term programs involving medical evaluation, prescribed exercise, cardiac risk factor modification, education, and counseling." Initially, these services were recommended following myocardial infarction (MI); subsequently, they were applied after coronary artery bypass graft (CABG) surgery, for patients with chronic stable angina pectoris, for heart transplant patients, and for patients following percutaneous coronary intervention (PCI).[3] The Clinical Practice Guideline *Cardiac Rehabilitation*[4] documented the benefits of rehabilitative services for patients with heart failure and left ventricular (LV) systolic dysfunction and recommended their application.

The goal of cardiac rehabilitation is the restoration and maintenance of optimal physiologic, psychological, social, and vocational status compatible with the underlying disease.[4]

The current short hospital stay for uncomplicated MI necessitates early ambulation and an accelerated educational regimen, with deferral of most teaching and counseling to the outpatient setting. Early discharge is characteristic for patients after successful reperfusion by coronary thrombolysis or acute primary PCI. Patients recovering from CABG surgery typically undergo rapid ambulation, have a short hospital stay, and constitute an increasing percentage of patients referred for cardiac rehabilitation. Such patients without prior MI characteristically have good ventricular function and favorable survival and are at low risk for proximate coronary events. Many require protracted guidance in coronary risk reduction for secondary prevention; early counseling aids in averting physiologic and psychological disability. Most patients following successful PCI have brief hospital stays, good functional status, and early resumption of employment and other activities. Patients with stable angina without recent MI constitute almost one-fourth of the total coronary population but are undeserved in rehabilitative care. They are frequently not referred for formal rehabilitation, often due to lack of insurance reimbursement. They often have substantial loss of productivity and reduction in quality of life; they require comprehensive medical management, with needs that may exceed those of patients after uncomplicated MI. With the aging of the U.S. population, coronary rehabilitation is now provided to many elderly patients[5,6] as well as to many with severe, complicated coronary illness. There is contemporary emphasis on education and counseling as cornerstones of rehabilitation,[2] using the behavioral approach to assist patients in coronary risk reduction, prevention of progression of atherosclerosis, and reduction in the risk of subsequent cardiovascular events.[7–9] Psychosocial assessment and interventions (see Chap. 107) as well as occupational assessment and vocational counseling are also stressed.

Each year almost 1 million U.S. survivors of MI are candidates for cardiac rehabilitation, in addition to more than 7 million patients with stable angina pectoris and patients following CABG surgery (367,000 in 1996, 44 percent under age 65) or PCI (482,000 in 1996, 51 percent younger than age 65). Rehabilitation services are underutilized, with only 11 to 20 percent of patients currently participating in formal programs.[4,10] Among MI patients in the Global Utilization of Streptokinase and tissue plasminogen activator (tPA) for Occluded Coronary Arteries (GUSTO) trial, 38 percent of U.S. and 32 percent of Canadian patients attended cardiac rehabilitation programs.[11] A U.S. national survey of 500 cardiac rehabilitation programs highlighted the underrepresentation of women, nonwhites, and those older than age 65.[12] Heart failure is the most common discharge diagnosis for hospitalized U.S. Medicare patients and the fourth most common discharge diagnosis for all hospitalized patients. Coronary heart disease is a substantial contributor to heart failure. Rehabilitation for patients with heart failure (and after cardiac transplantation) has increased as its benefits and safety have been documented.[13] An estimated 4.7 million patients with heart failure are candidates for cardiac rehabilitation.[4]

Rehabilitation remains underutilized despite its efficacy and cost-effectiveness (see Chap. 104).[14,15] Contributors include lack of physician referral, lack of insurance coverage or other reimbursement, lack of patient motivation, lack of perceived benefits of cardiac rehabilitation, poor self-esteem, and lack of accessibility of formal programs.[16–18] Home-based rehabilitation may increase access at more modest cost. A 72 percent participation rate at 6 months and 41 percent at 4 years is described with medically directed home exercise, comparable to supervised exercise regimens.[19]

EXERCISE TRAINING

Although no single randomized trial of exercise training demonstrated reduced mortality and morbidity following MI—in part owing to inadequate sample size and/or duration of follow-up, high dropout rates, etc.—favorable trends were seen in several. Metanalysis[14,20] of over 30 large prospective, randomized exercise trials suggests a survival advantage as high as 25 percent for exercising patients at 3 years following MI. Similar data derive from a systematic review.[21] Exercise training significantly decreased the risk of sudden cardiac death in the first year following initial MI. This benefit cannot be attributed independently to exercise, since many studies also included coronary risk reduction. The reduction in mortality approaches that of pharmacologic management following MI with beta-blocking drugs and of heart failure patients with angiotensin-converting enzyme (ACE) inhibitor therapy. Reduction in cardiovascular mortality was 26 percent in multifactorial trials of cardiac rehabilitation, compared with 15 percent in trials solely of exercise training. Exercise training does not change rates of nonfatal reinfarction.[4,8,21] A British observational study showed that regular light-to-moderate physical activity versus inactivity in men with coronary heart disease was associated with significantly decreased 5-year cardiovascular and all-cause mortality.[22]

Limitations of extrapolation of these data include that patients were predominantly middle-aged men, only postinfarction patients were studied, and most studies (1960–1984) antedated contemporary medical and revascularization therapies. Nonetheless, a recent observational study of MI patients showed association of regular physical activity with reduced fatal and nonfatal reinfarction and all-cause mortality.[23]

The Clinical Practice Guideline *Cardiac Rehabilitation,* from the U.S. Department of Health and Human Services,[4] highlights the beneficial effect of cardiac rehabilitation exercise training on exercise tolerance as one of the most clearly established favorable outcomes for patients with angina, MI, CABG surgery, PCI, and patients with compensated heart failure or a decreased LV ejection fraction. Exercise training particularly benefits the least physically fit patients with decreased exercise tolerance (see Chap. 95).[24] Improvement in functional capacity and exercise tolerance occurred for both women and men and for elderly patients. The most consistent benefit resulted from exercise training at least three times weekly for 12 or more weeks. The duration of exercise varied from 20 to 40 min at an intensity 70 to 85 percent of the baseline exercise test heart rate. Improvement in exercise tolerance occurred with lower-intensity exercise as well.[25] Maintenance of exercise training is required to sustain improved exercise tolerance.

No increased cardiovascular complications or other serious adverse outcomes occurred in any randomized, controlled trial of exercise training in coronary patients. Trials involved 3932 patients following MI, 745 with catheterization-documented coronary disease, 215 following CABG surgery, and 139 following PCI. No deterioration in exercise tolerance was reported in any patients, nor did any controlled study document greater improvement in exercise tolerance in control compared with exercising patients. Improvement in functional capacity with exercise training, averaging 20 percent after recovery from MI, is associated with an increase in cardiorespiratory reserve and a reduction in activity-related symptoms: angina, dyspnea, fatigue, and at times claudication. Exercise training (1) improves oxygen transport, evident as increased maximal cardiac output and oxygen consumption; (2) reduces heart rate, systolic blood pressure, and thereby myocardial oxygen requirement at rest and submaximal work levels; and (3) and returns exercise heart rate to normal more rapidly.

Endurance exercise is associated with a number of antiatherosclerotic, anti-ischemic, antithrombotic, and antiarrhythmic physiologic adaptations with potential clinical benefits.[2] However, there is no evidence that exercise as a sole intervention alters the angiographic characteristics of coronary lesions, increases coronary blood flow or myocardial oxygen supply, or stimulates formation of coronary collaterals in humans. Nonetheless, short-term endurance exercise training improved endothelium-dependent vasodilation in a small randomized trial of coronary patients.[26,27] Comprehensive coronary risk reduction also improves endothelial function, but clinical trial outcomes of lessened cardiovascular events are needed. No consistent improvement in cardiac hemodynamic measurements or ventricular systolic function has resulted from exercise training,[28] although exercise may improve skeletal muscle function in patients with heart failure.[29] Exercise training decreases myocardial ischemia, as measured by exercise electrocardiogram (ECG) testing, ambulatory ECG recording, and radionuclide perfusion imaging.[30,31] In several randomized clinical trials, apparent spontaneous improvement in resting ejection fraction after MI in both exercising and control populations renders suspect improvements in ejection fraction described in observational studies. No consistent changes in ventricular arrhythmia are related to exercise rehabilitation.

Clinical benefits of exercise training include a decrease in angina in patients with coronary disease[30] and symptoms of heart failure in patients with LV systolic dysfunction.[32,33] Improvement in electrocardiographic and nuclear cardiology measures of myocardial ischemia provides objective support for the symptomatic improvement. Exercise training of patients with LV systolic dysfunction provided added symptomatic improvement to that achieved by medication.[33] Exercise training aids in weight management, control of dyslipidemia, reduction in elevated blood pressure, and improvement of insulin sensitivity.[34–39] Improvement in blood rheology is also described.[40]

Decrease in symptoms and improvement in functional status can enable return to remunerative employment and leisure and recreational activities.[41] For more impaired coronary patients, including many elderly ones, modest increases in functional capacity can help maintain independent living.[5,6,42–44]

Guidelines for Prescriptive Exercise Training

Individualized medically prescribed physical activity is the hallmark of rehabilitative exercise training.[2,45–50] The prescriptive components of exercise training include its "dosage" (intensity, frequency, and duration of exercise); types of exercise; and rate of progression of exercise intensity. Coronary patients should exercise only at a level documented to produce an appropriate cardiovascular response during testing. The prediscarge (or early posthospitalization) exercise test, performed for risk stratification, can guide initial exercise recommendations. It is inappropriate to use age-predicted target heart rates for coronary patients; disease, therapies, and prior training or fitness may influence the heart rate response to exercise.

Prescription of target heart rate range is based on exercise testing. Although in prior years patients exercised to a target heart rate range between 70 and 85 percent of the highest level safely achieved at exercise testing,[51] exercise intensities in the 50 to 70 percent heart rate range produce comparable improvement in functional capacity and endurance and provide greater safety with unsupervised exercise.[1,25,52] This documented efficacy of lower-intensity exercise training to improve aerobic capacity has increased its applicability.[1,25] Particularly for unfit patients or those with lower exercise capacities, the greater comfort of lower-intensity exercise may encourage adherence, although increased duration of training may be required. Comparably favorable effects on quality of life occurred with low- and high-intensity exercise.[53]

The design of an exercise session involves an initial 5 to 10 min of warmup exercise—i.e., stretching and range-of-motion activities that enable musculoskeletal and circulatory readiness for exercise. A 20- to 40-min endurance component initially involves walk-run sequences or exercise on a stationary bicycle or treadmill; for these activities, skill is a minimal component of the intensity of work demand.

When space for exercise is limited, "station" training may be preferable, with participants serially using bicycle ergometry, arm ergometry, rowing machines, and treadmills. When more space is available, gymnasium-type programs can accommodate larger numbers of patients for walk-jog and floor exercises; some facilities have indoor or outdoor tracks. A final 5- to 10-min cool-down period of gradually decreased intensity allows the heart rate to slow and averts postexercise hypotension. Three exercise sessions weekly appear adequate; greater frequency does not significantly improve aerobic capacity. Aerobic recreational games add variety and improve adherence; they also provide upper body exercise. Because the oxygen cost of these activities varies with skill and competitiveness, they should be limited early in exercise training.

As the level of training increases, recreational activities in which skill often influences work intensity add variety to the regimen. Enjoyable endurance activities include rope skipping, bicycling, skating, swimming, rowing, and aerobic dancing; both rope-skipping and swimming (for unskilled swimmers) impose higher workloads and should be undertaken carefully.

Characteristics of Aerobic (Dynamic) and Strength (Isometric) Exercise Training

The physiologic response to aerobic (dynamic) exercise—rhythmic repetitive movements of large muscle groups—increases heart rate, parallel to the activity intensity, and increases stroke volume in young and middle-aged patients. In most elderly patients, the increase in heart rate predominates. Systolic blood pressure increases progressively with exercise intensity, with maintenance of or slight decrease in diastolic blood pressure and widening of the pulse pressure.

With strength (isometric) training, the increase in heart rate is modest and the increase in cardiac output slight. There is substantial increase in systolic blood pressure with high-intensity isometric activity, particularly in unfit individuals; this may provoke angina, ven-

tricular dysfunction, and/or arrhythmias and is the basis for limiting isometric activity in coronary patients with low exercise capacity. Once reasonable aerobic capacity is achieved, combined aerobic and strength training exercises in clinically stable patients may improve muscle strength, with improvement in endurance and the ability to return to weight-bearing activities of daily living and active occupational and recreational lifestyles.[54] Studies document the effectiveness of mild to moderate resistive exercise training in selected coronary patients.[55-58] The absence of myocardial ischemia, abnormal hemodynamic changes, and cardiovascular complications suggests that resistance exercise training is safe for coronary patients following aerobic exercise training. Most reported studies involved small numbers of low-risk male patients 70 years of age or younger with minimal functional aerobic impairment and normal or near-normal LV function. Whether the safety and effectiveness of this resistance training can be extrapolated to other populations of coronary patients (e.g., women, older patients of both sexes with low aerobic fitness, or patients at moderate to high cardiovascular risk) is not known.[4]

Arm versus Leg Exercise Training

Because exercise training is predominantly muscle-specific, both arm and leg exercises should be included in exercise rehabilitation.[59] The heart rate and blood pressure responses to leg work decrease following leg training, with only modest improvement in the response to arm work and vice versa. In one study, improvement in exercise response of the untrained limb was only 50 to 75 percent of the trained limb, suggesting that half the improved trained-limb performance is due to a generalized training effect; the remainder reflects predominantly improved oxygen extraction by trained skeletal muscle. Arms and legs respond comparably to aerobic training.

Since walk-run sequences or stationary bicycle or treadmill exercise train primarily leg muscles, supplementary arm exercise training is accomplished by selected repetitive calisthenics, shoulder wheels, rowing machines, and arm ergometers. When data from leg exercise testing are used to prescribe arm exercise, a reduction of about 10 beats per minute in target heart rate range is appropriate. The workload for arm training is about half that for leg training.[59] Since most occupational and recreational activities entail both arm and leg work, arm training should be included in rehabilitative exercise.

The Effect of Cardiovascular Drugs on Exercise Training

Exercise training can occur in patients receiving antianginal drugs, which may lessen symptoms and improve the ability to exercise. Although beta-blocking drugs decrease heart rate and blood pressure response to exercise training, they do not attenuate improvement in physical work capacity. Exercise testing for exercise prescription should be performed with patients receiving medications planned for their training.

The Role of Exercise Testing in Coronary Rehabilitation

Graded exercise testing, using either a treadmill or bicycle protocol, is safely performed in the initial weeks following MI. Most centers currently test patients to a sign- or symptom-limited endpoint because heart rate limits are often inaccurate as a result of antianginal therapy effects on heart rate. Treadmill testing typically entails serial 3-min stages of walking at increasing speed and elevations; comparable test protocols are available for a bicycle ergometer (see Chap. 16). Arm testing may be undertaken in patients with claudication or musculoskeletal problems that make leg testing not feasible.[60]

The results of predischarge exercise tests, with or without radionuclide studies, contribute independent prognostic information for risk stratification.[61] High-risk patients are characterized by a low exercise capacity [peak workload below 4 to 6 metabolic equivalents (METs)]; occurrence of angina, ischemic ST-segment abnormalities, and/or exercise-induced hypotension at low levels of exercise; and development of ventricular arrhythmias at low levels of exercise. Radionuclide evidence of myocardial ischemia or LV dysfunction with exercise indicates an adverse prognosis. Predischarge exercise testing also identifies low-risk patients who do not require additional diagnostic testing, are well suited for accelerated rehabilitation, and for whom early discharge home and prompt resumption of preinfarction activities, including return to work, can be recommended.[61,62] The exercise test can help define safe activity levels and guide the surveillance necessary during exercise rehabilitation. This permits simple, accelerated, and less costly rehabilitation for low-risk patients, reserving financial and personnel resources for high-risk patients who may derive substantial benefit from supervised training. Satisfactory performance of an exercise test, coupled with explanation of its relationship to activities at home, may lessen the fear of MI patients that physical activity may result in reinfarction or death. Such counseling has been associated with early return to work.[41]

Safety of Rehabilitative Exercise Training

The Clinical Practice Guideline *Cardiac Rehabilitation*[4] documents the safety of cardiac rehabilitation exercise training; randomized, controlled trials involving over 4500 coronary patients showed no increase in morbidity or mortality. A survey of 142 U.S. cardiac rehabilitation programs (1980 and 1984) reported a low rate of nonfatal MI of 1 per 294,000 patient-hours and a cardiac mortality rate of 1 per 784,000 patient-hours.[63] Twenty-one episodes of cardiac arrest occurred, with successful resuscitation of 17 patients. A 1978 report[51] also described a low rate of fatal cardiac events with exercise training: 1 per 116,400 patient-hours. Adverse events predominated in patients with ischemic ECG changes at exercise testing, above average functional capacity, and those who exceeded prescribed training heart rates. Definitive information is lacking regarding the effect of levels of supervision and ECG monitoring of exercise training on safety.

IMPLEMENTATION OF CARDIAC REHABILITATIVE CARE

Inpatient, or Hospital, Phase

Rehabilitative care for patients hospitalized for a coronary event includes progressive resumption of physical activity (early ambulation) and education and counseling of patient and family (see also Chap. 52).

EARLY AMBULATION
Early ambulation limits the detrimental effects of deconditioning: reduced physical work capacity and maximal oxygen uptake; orthostatic intolerance, characterized by orthostatic hypotension and tachycardia (due both to hypovolemia and to a lessened cardiovascular reflex response); increase in blood viscosity owing to decreased plasma volume disproportionate to decreased red blood cell mass; and decrease in pulmonary ventilation. Decreased muscle mass and muscular contractile strength renders muscular contraction inefficient, with more oxygen required for comparable work.

Guidelines[64] for physical activity in the coronary or surgical intensive care unit are for initial low-intensity exercise (1 to 2 METs), with gradual progression in work demand; supervision of progressive ambulation permits detection of inappropriate responses. Patients feed themselves, perform personal care, use a bedside commode, and sit in a bedside chair. Cardiac work is less in the seated than the supine position. Sitting in a chair two or three times daily limits the hypovolemia of immobilization and resulting orthostatic hypotension. Exposure to gravitational stress, rather than physical activity intensity, appears the determinant in limiting hypovolemia, cardiac underfilling, and deterioration of oxygen transport capacity with effort intolerance. Patients perform arm and leg exercises to maintain muscle tone and increase flexibility and joint mobility. Incentive spirometry is important for postoperative patients.

Disproportionate responses[64] to low-level activity include chest discomfort, dyspnea, or palpitations; a heart rate in excess of 100 beats per minute or lower than 50 beats per minute; ST-segment displacement on the electrocardiographic monitor; appearance of arrhythmias; or a decrease of more than 10 to 15 mmHg in systolic blood pressure. Although the latter usually indicates ischemic ventricular dysfunction, the vasodilator effect of nitrate, calcium channel blocking drugs, or ACE inhibitors must also be considered. A systolic blood pressure response during low-level activity of more than 180 mmHg or a diastolic pressure of more than 110 mmHg is an indication for antihypertensive therapy. Appropriate responses to ambulation indicate that the patient can progress to higher-intensity activity; disproportionate responses require activity restriction and clinical reassessment for unrecognized myocardial ischemia or LV dysfunction.

The major prescriptive hospital activity is walking, with stepwise increases in pace and distance. Most household tasks require a work intensity of 2 to 3 METs.

Electrocardiographic telemetry monitoring during ambulation is indicated for patients with serious ventricular arrhythmias or asymptomatic myocardial ischemia. A protocol for early ambulation and concomitant educational activities for patients with MI is applicable, with minor modifications, to postoperative coronary patients (Table 60-1).

Benefits of early ambulation include prevention of deconditioning, decrease in pulmonary atelectasis and thromboembolic complications, lessened anxiety and depression, and an enhanced sense of well-being related to improved functional status.[64]

EDUCATION AND COUNSELING OF HOSPITALIZED PATIENTS AND THEIR FAMILIES
The current abbreviated hospital stay limits the ability to address the informational and learning needs of the patient, spouse, and family; to assist them through recovery; and to prepare them for convalescence.[65] Answering questions or concerns of patients in a coronary or surgical intensive care unit (or during the preprocedure phase for elective PCI or CABG surgery) can provide reassurance. Education includes explanation of the medical or surgical problem(s), tests planned, and familiarization with procedures and equipment; this helps patients adjust to a situation perceived as life-threatening. The temporary nature of most restrictions should be emphasized, citing that recovery lessens the intensity of surveillance and care.

Increased knowledge can anxiety and improve adherence to recommendations. Patients should be instructed about medications—the purpose, dosage, desired effects, and potential adverse responses of each. Patients and family members should be taught the appropriate response to new or recurrent symptoms and how to gain access to emergency medical care.

TABLE 60-1 Inpatient Rehabilitation: Five-Step Myocardial Infarction Program (Revised 1996: Grady Memorial Hospital/Emory University School of Medicine)

Step	Date	M.D. Initials	Nurse/Exer Specialist Notes	Supervised Exercise	CCU/Step Down Unit Activity	Educational Activity
				CCU		
1	—			Active and passive ROM all extremities in bed Teach patient ankle plantar and dorsiflexion—repeat hourly when awake	Partial self-care Feed self Dangle legs on side of bed Use bedside commode Sit in chair 15 min, 1–2 times/day	Orientation to CCU Personal emergencies, social service aid as needed Bedside teaching (CCU staff)
2	—			Active ROM all extremities, sitting on side of bed or bedside chair	Sit in chair 15–30 min, 2–3 times/day Complete self-care	Orientation to rehabilitation team, program Smoking cessation Educational literature if requested Planning transfer from CCU
				Step Down Unit		
3	—			Warm-up exercises, 2–2.5 METs: Stretching ROM Calisthenics Walk in hall 50–75 ft and back at slow pace	Sit in chair ad lib Walk in room Walk to class with supervision Out of bed as tolerated	Normal cardiac anatomy and function Development of atherosclerosis What happens when myocardial infarction occurs Coronary risk factors and their control Diet
4	—			Teach pulse counting, Borg Scale ROM and calisthenics, 3 METs Practice walking few stairsteps Walk 300–500 ft bid Instruct on home exercise	Tepid shower or tub bath, with supervision Walk in corridor prn	Heart attack management: Medications Exercise Surgery Response to symptoms Family, community adjustments on return home Work simplification techniques (as needed)
5	—			Continue above activities Check pulse counting Walk up flight of steps Walk 500 ft bid Continue home exercise instruction; present information regarding outpatient exercise program	Continue all previous activities Predischarge exercise test (as appropriate)	Discharge planning Medications, diet, activity Return appointments Schedules tests Return to work Community resources Educational literature Medication cards

ABBREVIATIONS: bid = twice a day; MET = maximal exercise test; multistage exercise test; prn = as required; ROM = range of motion.
NOTE: 1 foot = 0.30 meter.
SOURCE: Reprinted with permission of Grady Memorial Hospital/Emory University School of Medicine.

Outpatient, or Ambulatory, Phase

About 70 percent of survivors of MI younger than age 70[7] and many patients following myocardial revascularization are at low risk for proximate coronary events. Exercise rehabilitation for these patients begins shortly after discharge from the hospital; these patients usually progress rapidly in increasing their intensity and duration of exercise, often without supervision. Coronary patients who are elderly; have significant comorbidity, myocardial ischemia, heart failure, or serious arrhythmias; have complications of MI or CABG surgery; or those with severe angina may require exercise surveillance of variable duration.[46,61] Outpatient exercise rehabilitation is best described by the characteristics of the exercise training and the requirements and complexity of surveillance, based on each patient's clinical and risk factor status, rather than by traditional phases of earlier years that typically had fixed durations and composition. This responds to an individual patient's needs for exercise training rather than requiring a patient to conform to program phases or requirements.

THERAPEUTIC EXERCISE TRAINING

Therapeutic exercise training typically lasts 8 to 12 weeks. In the early years of outpatient exercise rehabilitation, ECG telemetry was not widely available. In subsequent years, complication rates were described as lower in exercise programs with continuous ECG monitoring.[51] It remains unknown whether ECG monitoring, closer medical supervision, and/or differences in exercise intensity were the safety determinants. More recently, continuous ECG monitoring has not been shown to provide added safety for low-risk patients during supervised exercise[63]; ECG monitoring is currently recommended only for high-risk patients and selected patients with problems in exercising,[1,4] although some recommend more extensive ECG monitoring. Often, ECG monitoring is undertaken solely as a requirement for insurance reimbursement rather than based on medical need. Many patients in supervised exercise programs without continuous ECG monitoring or patients exercising independently can be taught to check their heart rate response intermittently or to estimate exercise intensity by the rating of perceived exertion, as described by Borg.[66] In supervised settings, heart rate response can be documented by intermittent use of defibrillator paddles as ECG leads. A technique of value in unsupervised settings is the "talk test," wherein patients exercise only to the level that permits continued conversation with an exercising companion, a level generally below the anaerobic threshold at which respiratory rate accelerates.

High-risk coronary patients—those with a markedly reduced exercise capacity, severely depressed LV function, complex ventricular arrhythmias, exercise-induced angina, ischemia, or hypotension at low exercise intensities, and/or the inability to self-monitor exercise heart rate—may require supervised and often ECG-monitored exercise. The need and duration of ECG surveillance of exercise for these high-risk patients remain uncertain. The uniform success of resuscitation with supervised exercise, despite the rarity of its application, suggests that exercise supervision may be beneficial for such patients.[63]

Initial home exercise may involve progressive walking and walk-jog sequences or serial increases in the intensity and duration stationary bicycle exercise. Videotapes may help guide and pace home exercise and are available for varying intensities of exercise training. Home-based exercise rehabilitation optimally includes planned communication and management by rehabilitation nurses and other specially trained personnel.[7,8] Although recent studies document the efficacy of home-based exercise training and risk reduction guided by a specialized cardiac nurse manager, data are not available as to the efficacy of long-term risk reduction or long-term compliance with unsupervised exercise in the absence of such strategies. All training regimens appear to increase functional capacity more rapidly than occurs spontaneously.[8,32,33] No differences in outcomes were observed between a standard cardiac rehabilitation program, a physician-supervised nurse case-managed cardiovascular risk reduction program, or a community-based cardiovascular risk reduction program by exercise physiologists.[67] Supervision of exercise may not entail an "all or nothing" approach; intermittent supervision may be feasible in a community facility, there may be periodic telephone

transmission of the exercise ECG of patients who exercise at home, patients may use inexpensive heart rate monitors during home exercise, or a combination of these techniques may be used. It is not known whether any of these approaches improves exercise adherence or safety; several studies of independent exercise showed a lack of coronary risk reduction.

The Clinical Practice Guideline *Cardiac Rehabilitation*[4] highlights these alternative approaches to cardiac rehabilitation as effective and safe for selected clinically stable patients.[68] Transtelephonic and other means of monitoring and surveillance of patients can extend cardiac rehabilitation beyond the setting of supervised, structured, group-based rehabilitation. The feasibility, safety, and efficacy of these strategies for exercise rehabilitation must be assessed in more diverse populations of patients with stable coronary heart disease, particularly elderly patients, those with LV dysfunction, and other patients of higher risk status.

MAINTENANCE EXERCISE TRAINING

Maintenance training can be undertaken or continued in community recreational facilities or at home. Because lifetime physical activity is necessary to maintain fitness, patients must achieve reasonable independence in exercising and remain involved in an exercise regimen that is social, enjoyable, convenient, and appropriate. Most coronary patients with prior exercise restrictions who attain a 7- to 8-MET level can safely progress to unsupervised exercise. Patients leaving supervised programs may require counseling regarding long-term exercise in the community or at home.

EDUCATION AND COUNSELING OF AMBULATORY CORONARY PATIENTS

The behavioral approach to coronary risk reduction enables coronary patients to manage their illness, maintain healthy lifestyles, and improve adherence to medications and other recommended regimens.[65,69] Metanalysis of 28 controlled trials of patient education showed that "education programs have demonstrated a measurable impact on blood pressure, mortality, exercise, [and] diet" and that other parameters are positively affected, although less consistently.[70] A combination of education, counseling, and behavioral intervention strategies seems most effective.[4,7] Whether the same interventions are equally effective for men and women and across the life span remains unanswered because few studies have enrolled patients over age 70 or included women. Patients with coronary disease are at the highest risk for disability and death and constitute patients for whom untreated risk factors are most damaging.[71] Cardiac rehabilitation provides an integrating structure for identification and management of cardiovascular risk-reduction, targeting national intervention goals.[2]

There is no evidence that CABG surgery per se encourages favorable modification of coronary risk status postoperatively.[72] Postoperative recurrence of coronary symptoms or deterioration of function following saphenous vein CABG surgery relates predominantly to progression of atherosclerosis in the graft vessels and native circulation. Core components of secondary prevention include control of hypertension, diabetes, hyperlipidemia, and obesity and cessation of cigarette smoking,[73] with adoption of a physically active lifestyle; even at advanced age, these may slow progression or induce regression of atherosclerosis. Clinical trial evidence documents significant reduction in cardiovascular morbidity and mortality based on such comprehensive interventions.

Community resources that may be helpful in rehabilitation include counseling and guidance services, home-care agencies, vocational rehabilitation services for job training and placement, services for financial aid, outpatient coronary rehabilitation programs, and postcoronary groups or clubs. Participation in community heart clubs or educational groups may facilitate rehabilitation; coronary risk reduction and other skills learned and practiced in these settings may encourage health-related behaviors and aid in reinforcing maintenance of these changes.

CORONARY POPULATIONS WITH SPECIAL REHABILITATION NEEDS

Women

Women have less favorable outcomes than their male peers following MI and myocardial revascularization, in part related to older age and greater comorbidities but also reflecting lesser application of proved beneficial therapies (see Chap. 97).[74] Women are less likely to be referred to and to participate in cardiac rehabilitation,[14] despite documentation of comparable or greater improvement than men in functional capacity with exercise training.[75] Underrepresentation of elderly patients in cardiac rehabilitation doubly jeopardizes women, who are more likely to be elderly.

Elderly Coronary Patients

Elderly patients constitute a high percentage of those with MI, CABG surgery, and transcatheter revascularization (see Chap. 96). More than half of patients currently eligible for cardiac rehabilitation are older than age 65.[76] Complications of MI and myocardial revascularization are more frequent in the elderly, with prolongation of hospitalization predisposing to deconditioning; early ambulation can limit functional deterioration and decrease depression. Teaching energy-conserving techniques for self-care and performance of houschold tasks helps maintain independent living, an outcome valued by elderly patients. Modification of conventional coronary risk factors is feasible and warranted, given the greater prevalence and severity of coronary disease in the elderly.[4]

Elderly patients are at high risk of disability following a coronary event. They are less fit after a coronary event, in part because of decreased fitness prior to the event. Although few studies and no randomized trials have addressed the efficacy and safety of exercise training and multifactorial rehabilitation at elderly age, available studies document that elderly patients benefit from exercise training and secondary prevention; functional independence and self-esteem are improved.[4,76]

Elderly coronary patients have trainability comparable with that of younger patients,[44,77] with elderly women and men showing comparable improvement. Increases in functional capacity of 10 to 60 percent are described with 12 weeeks of posthospital exercise training. Exercise testing before hospital discharge was feasible in about half of MI patients aged 70 years or older, enabling accurate risk stratification and exercise prescription. No complications or adverse outcomes of exercise training in elderly patients were described in any cardiac rehabilitation study. Nonetheless, rates of physician referral to and patient participation in exercise rehabilitation were substantially lower among elderly than younger patients,[6,76] and older women were even less likely to be referred than older men.[43] Adherence to exercise training was high (90 percent) in the reported studies,[44] and significant reduction in coronary risk factors occurred in elderly patients with multifactorial cardiac rehabilitation.[6] Psychologic benefits include lesser social isolation and decrease in depression.

The importance of warmup and cool-down activities warrants emphasis because of the delayed return of the exercise heart rate to normal in the elderly. Walking provides an adequate training stimulus for many elderly patients because it constitutes a significant percentage of the decreased aerobic capacity of aging.[78] Running, jumping, and other high-impact activities should be limited to avoid musculoskeletal complications. Walking, bicycle ergometry, and/or walking in a pool in shallow water can favorably modify the decreased joint mobility of aging; enhance neuromuscular coordination, balance, and stability and lessen propensity for falls; and improve endurance.

Coronary Patients with Heart Failure

Impairment of exercise capacity with heart failure appears in part due to inadequate nutritive blood flow to skeletal muscle; important factors other than lack of increase in cardiac output with exercise include the ability to decrease peripheral vascular resistance and possibly adequacy of right ventricular function (see also Chap. 24). Patients with heart failure and normal cardiac output responses to exercise frequently improve their functional capacity with exercise training, whereas those with severe hemodynamic dysfunction with exercise often do not.[79] A combination of LV systolic dysfunction and residual myocardial ischemia may limit trainability. The LV ejection fraction predicts poorly both exercise capacity and the potential for improvement with training; some patients with substantial LV dysfunction have a normal exercise capacity and no symptoms or impairment of lifestyle.

Most studies of exercise training of patients with heart failure and moderate to severe LV systolic dysfunction do not demonstrate deterioration in LV volume, wall thickness, or function.[80,81] A review of exercise training clinical trials in patients with moderate-to-severe heart failure showed a 17 to 37 percent increased peak VO_2 with training, associated decreased symptoms and improvement in quality-of-life scores. Adverse effects were absent.[82] Randomized, controlled clinical trial data of exercise training in postinfarction patients with an ejection fraction less than 40 percent showed that long-term home-based exercise may attenuate the unfavorable remodeling response and even improve ventricular function.[80] Peripheral (skeletal muscle) adaptations appear to mediate the improvement in exercise tolerance; exercise training substantially corrects the impaired oxidative capacity of skeletal muscle in chronic heart failure.[83] Exercise training also may improve peripheral artery endothelial function[84] and augment both the symptomatic and functional benefits of ACE inhibitor therapy.[33] Even small improvements in symptomatic status and functional capacity can exert a favorable impact on quality of life. Improved clinical outcomes are also described,[85] although no large trials have studied survival. Importantly, most studies antedate current increased use of beta-blocking drugs. In both supervised and at-home settings, low- to moderate-intensity exercise regimens provide benefit, although adverse events may occur in this high-risk patient group.[4] Overall, exercise training appears safe and beneficial in improving exercise capacity and quality of life.[13]

Although initial exercise training of patients with LV systolic dysfunction was predominantly supervised, typically with continuous ECG monitoring, other studies have described moderate-intensity, unsupervised exercise as safe and effective.[13] The optimal duration of exercise supervision and the duration and need for ECG monitoring remain uncertain but should be guided by clinical evidence of exercise-related ischemia and/or arrhythmia.[32] In 105 ambulatory cardiac transplant candidates, nonsupervised prescribed walking at a target heart rate range close to baseline exercise test-determined anaerobic threshold produced significant improvement in peak maximal oxygen consumption and peak exercise tolerance in 38 of 68 clinically stable patients without adverse effects. After an average of 6 months, 31 of 38 patients improved sufficiently to be removed from the transplant list, with improvement persisting to 2 years.[86]

Additional components of rehabilitative care for these patients include teaching work simplification, particularly the pacing of daily living activities; working in a seated rather than a standing position; and taking rest periods between activities.

Patients with Implanted Pacemakers and Defibrillators

Exercise prescription is determined by the characteristics of the pacemaker (Chaps. 31 and 32). Because most patients likely to exercise currently receive rate-responsive pacemakers, exercise testing can ascertain the appropriateness of the sensor response to exercise intensity,[87] and reprogramming can be undertaken as needed.

The exercise target heart rate range for patients with implanted defibrillators should be set at 20 to 30 beats per minute below the threshold rate of the device to fire. This also enables appropriate work-related activities.[88] Coparticipants in the exercise setting must be reassured that they cannot be harmed by physical contact with a patient whose defibrillator discharges.

PSYCHOLOGICAL ASPECTS OF CORONARY REHABILITATION

Psychosocial variables are important in the prognosis of coronary disease[45] (see Chap. 10). Although type A behavior pattern previously received emphasis, currently the hostility component of type A behavior is regarded as its most adverse feature. High levels of anger and hostility appear associated with increased cardiac morbidity and mortality.[89]

Other major psychological problems in coronary patients involve anxiety, depression, denial, and dependence. Denial of presenting symptoms may limit or delay access to care. "Appropriate" denial, characterized by confidence in a favorable outcome, often an effective coping strategy of coronary patients, is associated with a favorable prognosis. Anxiety, often the initial psychological manifestation at hospitalization, is related to a fear of dying and may progress to depression as patients contemplate their potential inability to resume former family, occupational, and community roles. Anxiety and depression contribute to failure to make satisfactory life adjustments, return to work, to return to sexual function, and engage in social activities following MI. Depression may precede MI in 30 to 50 percent of patients. Depression is associated with increased morbidity and mortality following MI and CABG surgery[90]; patients with depression were five times more likely to die during the initial 6 months following MI than nondepressed patients.[91] Depression may be associated with social isolation, an independent risk factor. The 6-month mortality of patients living alone was double that of patients living with others (16 vs. 8 percent), and follow-up of patients with coronary disease showed a 50 percent 5-year mortality rate among those most socially isolated, compared with 17 percent without these characteristics. The impact of social isolation on prognosis appeared independent of LV ejection fraction and other physiologic prognostic factors. Interventions against depression and social isolation follow-

ing MI have failed to show reinfarction or survival benefit in a randomized clinical trial.[92]

Many patients with successful physical recovery following MI or myocardial revascularization often have residual psychological impairment. Two major strategies that appear to limit this complication are education and counseling and initiation of physical activity. Many patients remain psychologically disabled because, inappropriately, they perceive an excessive severity of MI and vulnerability to sudden death; resumption of physical activity provides reassurance and restores self-confidence. In randomized exercise trials, exercising patients returned to sexual activity, work, and a near-normal lifestyle more rapidly and had greater improvements in work capacity, income, and job responsibility.[93] Both physical and psychosocial benefits occurred even with low-intensity exercise, particularly among older and sicker coronary patients. Despite the paucity of controlled studies, consistent moderate psychosocial benefit appears to result from combinations of structured exercise, education, and counseling.[94] Although the contribution of peer support in a group program has not been ascertained, it may be helpful given the predictive power of social isolation for coronary mortality.[95]

VOCATIONAL ASPECTS OF CORONARY REHABILITATION

A major goal of rehabilitation for nonelderly patients recovered from MI or myocardial revascularization is resumption of gainful employment, change in occupation if needed, and the resulting economic and psychological benefits.[45,96] In the 1980s, about 80 percent of patients below 65 years of age and employed at the time of MI who recovered from uncomplicated MI returned to work within 2 to 3 months, typically resuming their former jobs.[97] Despite this, subsequent cessation of employment was high, up to 20 percent between 6 months and 1 year. Comparable data are not available for patients with complications of MI or residual functional impairment, although their return to work is estimated at 25 to 33 percent.

These data contrast markedly with work resumption following CABG surgery. Despite a substantial decrease in symptoms, improvement in functional capacity, and reported enhancement of life quality and participation in leisure activities, return to work following CABG surgery is less favorable than anticipated.[98,99] No difference in 10-year employment status was described between patients randomized to medical and surgical treatment in the Coronary Artery Surgery Study (CASS).[100] Return to work following PCI is comparable to that following CABG surgery, although PCI patients return to work more promptly.[99] Some reports describe lack of confidence in the ability to return to work following PCI, even when patients were physically able to do so.[101]

Most studies of return to work involved predominantly or exclusively men; recent examination of working women with coronary disease showed them to have a longer convalescence and lesser return to work; whether this is a gender issue or reflects older age or greater occurrence of depression among women warrants study.[102]

For patients younger than age 65 following MI or myocardial revascularization, the indirect health care costs of disability, including lessened productivity, loss of income, welfare payments, and unemployment insurance costs, must be considered when the cost-effectiveness of rehabilitation is determined.[62,103–105] Coronary disease is the leading problem for which adults receive premature disability benefits under the U.S. Social Security system; almost one-fourth of men and women receiving disability have permanent disability due to coronary disease. Symptomatic and functional improvement correlate poorly with return to work and resumption of preillness lifestyle, with psychosocial status appearing as a more important determinant.[98] Since only about 15 percent of the U.S. labor force currently performs manual labor, the severity of angina or heart failure in coronary patients rarely precludes return to work. Many nonmedical factors negatively influence resumption of employment: older age, adequate nonwork income, anxiety or depression, activity-induced symptoms, lower social class and less education, jobs involving high-level physical activity (more common among blue-collar workers), and perception of the coronary illness as job-related. Patients who fail to resume employment within 6 months after a coronary event are unlikely ever to do so.

Exercise testing performed for risk stratification can be used for work evaluation; it permits a relatively precise assessment of function that may help allay the apprehensions of the patient, family,[106] physician, and employer about the capability and safety of return to work.[107] A randomized, controlled trial of occupational work assessment early following MI, identifying low-risk patients and counseling them about the appropriateness of prompt return to work, effected a 32 percent reduction in the duration of convalescence.[41] Patients without or arrhythmia during a symptom-limited exercise test typically are free of these problems when occupational static and dynamic work are combined. Arm ergometry may be preferable for occupational assessment of patients who perform predominantly arm work.[59]

Furthermore, since most occupational work is intermittent, occupational myocardial work demand is lower than for the same level of steady-state exercise; cardiac output, blood pressure, and oxygen uptake do not approach steady state until about 2 min after the onset of work, explaining the tolerance of patients with modest cardiac impairment for significant workloads of short duration, when adequate rest periods are interspersed. Recommendations for full-time work should approximate 30 percent of measured physical work capacity. Guidelines are available to assist physicians in assessing and establishing the employment of patients with coronary heart disease.[108]

Other nonmedical considerations also influence postinfarction or postrevascularization employment, particularly the financial, social, disability, and compensation benefits of not returning to work. In several studies, the patient's preoperative perception about ability to return to work appeared the most important determinant.

Benefits to employers of cardiac rehabilitative care for their employees include earlier return to work, less disability, less absenteeism, reduced financial expenditures for sickness and disability payments, reduced training costs for replacement of personnel, and greater productivity.[1] Employers thus should encourage coronary rehabilitative care as a component of their managed care plans.

References

1. Report of the WHO Expert Committee, Wenger NK, Expert Committee Chairman. *Rehabilitation after Cardiovascular Diseases, with Special Emphasis on Developing Countries.* WHO Tech. Rep. Series No. 831, Geneva: World Health Organization; 1993.

2. Leon AS, Franklin BA, Costa F, et al. Cardiac Rehabilitation and Secondary Prevention of Coronary Heart Disease. An American Heart Association Scientific Statement from the Council on Clinical Cardiology, Committee on Exercise, Rehabilitation and Prevention, *Circulation*. In press.

3. Agency for Health Care Policy and Research. *Cardiac Rehabilitation Programs.* Health Technology Assessment Report No. 3, DHHS Publication No. AHCPR 92-0015. Rockville, MD: U.S. Department of Health and Human Services, Public Health Service, Agency for Health Care Policy and Research; December 1991.

4. Wenger NK, Froelicher ES, Smith LK, et al. *Cardiac Rehabilitation.* Clinical Practice Guideline No. 17, AHCPR Publication No. 96-0672. Rockville, MD: U.S. Department of Health and Human Services, Public Health Service, Agency for Health Care Policy and Research and the National Heart, Lung, and Blood Institute; October 1995.

5. Ades PA, Waldmann ML, Gillespie C. A controlled trial of exercise training in older patients. *J Gerontol* 1995;50A:M7–M11. In press.

6. Lavie CJ, Milani RV, Littman AB. Benefits of cardiac rehabilitation and exercise training in secondary coronary prevention in the elderly. *J Am Coll Cardiol* 1993;22:678–683.

7. DeBusk RF, Houston Miller N, Superko HR, et al. A case-management system for coronary risk factor modification after acute myocardial infarction. *Ann Intern Med* 1994;120:721–729.

8. Haskell WL, Alderman EL, Fair JM, et al. Effects of intensive multiple risk factor reduction on coronary atherosclerosis and clinical cardiac events in men and women with coronary artery disease. The Stanford Coronary Risk Intervention Project (SCRIP). *Circulation* 1994;89: 975–990.

9. Schuler G, Hambrecht R, Schlierf G, et al. Regular physical exercise and low-fat diet: Effects on progression of coronary artery disease. *Circulation* 1992;86:1–11.

10. Leon AS, Certo C, Comoss P, et al. Scientific evidence of the value of cardiac rehabilitation services with emphasis on patients following myocardial infarction: I. Exercise conditioning component (position paper). *J Cardiopulm Rehabil* 1990;10:79–87.

11. Mark DB, Naylor CD, Hlatky MA, et al. Use of medical resources and quality of life after acute myocardial infarction in Canada and the United States. *N Engl J Med* 1994;331:1130–1135.

12. Thomas RJ, Houston Miller N, Lamendola C, et al. National survey on gender differences in cardiac rehabilitation programs: Patient characteristics and enrollment patterns. *J Cardiopulm Rehabil* 1996;16: 402–412.

13. Piña IL, Apstein CS, Balady GJ, et al. Exercise and Heart Failure. A Statement from the American Heart Association Committee on Exercise, Rehabilitation, and Prevention. *Circulation* 2003;107:1210–1225.

14. O'Connor GT, Buring JE, Yusuf S, et al. An overview of randomized trials of rehabilitation with exercise after myocardial infarction. *Circulation* 1989;80:234–244.

15. Oldridge N, Furlong W, Feeny D, et al. Economic evaluation of cardiac rehabilitation soon after acute myocardial infarction. *Am J Cardiol* 1993;72:154–161.

16. Livingston MD, Dennis C. Economic issues: The value and effectiveness of cardiac rehabilitation. In: Wenger NK, Smith LK, Froelicher ES, et al, eds. *Cardiac Rehabilitation. A Guide to Practice in the 21st Century.* New York: Marcel Dekker; 1999:447–466.

17. Ades PA. Cardiac rehabilitation and secondary prevention of coronary heart disease. *N Engl J Med* 2001;345:892–902.

18. Daly J, Sindone AP, Thompson DR, et al. Barriers to participation in a adherence to cardiac rehabilitation programs: A critical literature review. *Prog Cardiovasc Nurs* 2002;17:8–17.

19. Burke LE. Adherence to a heart-healthy lifestyle—what makes the difference? In: Wenger NK, Smith LK, Froelicher ES, et al, eds. *Cardiac Rehabilitation. A Guide to Practice in the 21st Century.* New York: Marcel Dekker, 1999:385–393.

20. Oldridge NB, Guyatt GH, Fischer ME, et al. Cardiac rehabilitation after myocardial infarction: Combined experience of randomized clinical trials. *JAMA* 1988;260:945–950.

21. Jolliffe JA, Rees K, Taylor RS, et al. Exercise-based rehabilitation for coronary heart disease. *Cochrane Database of Syst Rev* 2001; (1):CD001800.

22. Wannamethee SG, Shaper AG, Walker M. Physical activity and mortality in older men with diagnosed coronary heart disease. *Circulation* 2000;102:1358–1363.

23. Steffen-Batey L, Nichaman MZ, Goff DC Jr, et al. Change in level of physical activity and risk of all-cause mortality or reinfarction. The Corpus Christi Heart Project. *Circulation* 2000;102:2204–2209.

24. Balady GJ, Jette D, Scheer J, et al and the Massachusetts Association of Cardiovascular and Pulmonary Rehabilitation Database Co-Investigators.

Changes in exercise capacity following cardiac rehabilitation in patients stratified according to age and gender: Results of the Massachusetts Association of Cardiovascular and Pulmonary Rehabilitation Multicenter Database. *J Cardiopulm Rehabil* 1996;16:38–46.

25. Goble AJ, Hare DL, Macdonald PS, et al. Effect of early programmes of high and low intensity exercise on physical performance after transmural acute myocardial infarction. *Br Heart J* 1991;65:126–131.

26. Ehsani AA, Biello DR, Schultz J, et al. Improvement of left ventricular contractile function by exercise training in patients with coronary artery disease. *Circulation* 1986;74:350–358.

27. Hambrecht R, Wolf A, Gielen S, et al. Effect of exercise on coronary endothelial function in patients with coronary artery disease. *N Engl J Med* 2000;342:454–460.

28. Hung J, Gordon EP, Houston N, et al. Changes in rest and exercise myocardial perfusion and left ventricular function 3 to 26 weeks after clinically uncomplicated acute myocardial infarction: Effects of exercise training. *Am J Cardiol* 1984;54:943–950.

29. Sullivan MJ, Higginbotham MB, Cobb FR. Exercise training in patients with severe left ventricular dysfunction: Hemodynamic and metabolic effects. *Circulation* 1988;78:506–515.

30. Todd IC, Ballantyne D. Effect of exercise training on the total ischaemic burden: An assessment by 24-hour ambulatory electrocardiographic monitoring. *Br Heart J* 1992;68:560–566.

31. Sebrechts CP, Klein JL, Ahnve S, et al. Myocardial perfusion changes following 1 year of exercise training assessed by thallium-201 circumferential count profiles. *Am Heart J* 1986;112:1217–1226.

32. Coats AJS, Adamopoulos S, Meyer TE, et al. Effects of physical training in chronic heart failure. *Lancet* 1990;335:63–66.

33. Meyer TE, Casadei B, Coats AJS, et al. Angiotensin-converting enzyme inhibition and physical training in heart failure. *J Intern Med* 1991;230:407–413.

34. Ross R, Janssen I. Physical activity, total and regional obesity: Dose response considerations. *Med Sci Sports Exerc* 2001;33(suppl): S521–S527.

35. Jakicic JM, Clark K, Coleman E, et al. American College of Sport Medicine. Appropriate intervention strategies for weight loss and prevention of weight regain for adults. *Med Sci Sports Exerc* 2001;33: 2145–2156.

36. Leon AS, Rice T, Mandel S, et al. Blood lipid response to 20 weeks of supervised exercise in a large biracial population: The HERITAGE family study. *Metabolism* 2000;49:513–520.

37. Leon AS, Sanchez OA. Response of blood lipids to exercise training alone or combined with dietary intervention. *Med Sci Sports Exerc* 2001;33(suppl):S502–S515.

38. Fagard RH. Exercise characteristics and the blood pressure response to dynamic physical training. *Med Sci Sports Exerc* 2001;33(suppl): S484–S492.

39. Kelley DE, Goodpaster BH. Effects of exercise on glucose homeostasis in type 2 diabetes mellitus. *Med Sci Sports Exerc* 2001;33(suppl): S495–S501.

40. Church TS, Lavie CJ, Milani RV, et al. Improvement in blood rheology after cardiac rehabilitation and exercise training in patients with coronary heart disease. *Am Heart J* 2002;143:349–355.

41. Dennis C, Houston-Miller N, Schwartz RG, et al. Early return to work after uncomplicated myocardial infarction: Results of a randomized trial. *JAMA* 1988;260:214–220.

42. Ades PA, Grunvald MH. Cardiopulmonary exercise testing before and after conditioning in older coronary patients. *Am Heart J* 1990;120: 585–589.

43. Ades PA, Waldman ML, Polk DM, et al. Referral patterns and exercise response in the rehabilitation of female coronary patients aged ≥62 years. *Am J Cardiol* 1992;69:1422–1425.

44. Williams MA, Maresh CM, Esterbrooks DJ, et al. Early exercise training in patients older than age 65 years compared with that in younger patients after acute myocardial infarction or coronary artery bypass grafting. *Am J Cardiol* 1985;55:263–266.

45. Wenger NK, Smith LK, Froelicher ES, et al, eds. *Cardiac Rehabilitation: A Guide to Practice in the 21st Century.* New York: Marcel Dekker; 1999.

46. Fletcher GF, Balady G, Amsterdam EA, et al. Exercise Standards for Testing and Training. A Statement for Healthcare Professionals from the American Heart Association. *Circulation* 2001;104:1694–1740.

47. American College of Sports Medicine Position Stand. Exercise for patients with coronary artery disease. *Med Sci Sports Exerc* 1994;26:i–v.

48. American College of Sports Medicine. *ACSM's Guidelines for Exercise Testing and Prescription,* 6th ed. Philadelphia: Lippincott, Williams & Wilkins; 2000.

49. American Association of Cardiovascular and Pulmonary Rehabilitation. *Guidelines for Cardiac Rehabilitation and Secondary Prevention Programs,* 3rd ed. Champaign, IL: Human Kinetics; 1999.

50. NIH Consensus Development Panel on Physical Activity and Cardiovascular Health. Physical activity and cardiovascular health. *JAMA* 1996;276:241–246.

51. Haskell WL. Cardiovascular complications during exercise training of cardiac patients. *Circulation* 1978;57:920–924.

52. DeBusk RF, Haskell WL, Miller NH, et al. Medically directed at-home rehabilitation soon after uncomplicated acute myocardial infarction: A new model for patient care. *Am J Cardiol* 1985;55:251–257.

53. Worcester MC, Hare DL, Oliver RG, et al. Early programmes of high and low intensity exercise and quality of life after acute myocardial infarction. *BMJ* 1993;307:1244–1247.

54. Franklin BA, Bonzheim K, Gordon S, et al. Resistance training in cardiac rehabilitation. *J Cardiopulm Rehabil* 1991;11:99–107.

55. Kelemen MH. Resistive training safety and assessment guidelines for cardiac and coronary prone patients. *Med Sci Sports Exerc* 1989;21: 675–677.

56. Sparling PB, Cantwell JD, Dolan CM, et al. Strength training in a cardiac rehabilitation program: A six-month follow-up. *Arch Phys Med Rehabil* 1990;71:148–152.

57. Pollock ML, Franklin BA, Balady GJ, et al. Resistance exercise in individuals with or without cardiovascular disease. Benefits, rationale, safety, and description. An advisory from the Committee on Exercise, Rehabilitation, and Prevention, Council on Clinical Cardiology, American Heart Association. *Circulation* 2000;101:828–833.

58. Wilke NA, Sheldahl LM, Levandoski SG, et al. Transfer effect of upper extremity training to weight carrying in men with ischemic heart disease. *J Cardiopulm Rehabil* 1991;11:365–372.

59. Franklin BA. Exercise testing, training and arm ergometry. *Sports Med* 1985;2:100–119.

60. Balady GJ, Weiner DA, Rose L, et al. Physiologic responses to arm ergometry exercise relative to age and gender. *J Am Coll Cardiol* 1990;16:130–135.

61. Ryan TJ, Antman EM, Brooks NH, et al. 1999 Update: ACC/AHA Guidelines for the Management of Patients with Acute Myocardial Infarction: A report of the American College of Cardiology/American Heart Association Task Force on Practice Guidelines (Committee on Management of Acute Myocardial Infarction). *J Am Coll Cardiol* 1999;34:890–911, and (Executive Summary and Recommendations) *Circulation* 1999;100:1016–1030.

62. Picard MH, Dennis C, Schwartz RG, et al. Cost-benefit analysis of early return to work after uncomplicated acute myocardial infarction. *Am J Cardiol* 1989;63:1308–1314.

63. Van Camp SP, Peterson RA. Cardiovascular complications of outpatient cardiac rehabilitation programs. *JAMA* 1986;256:1160–1163.

64. Wenger NK. In-hospital exercise rehabilitation after myocardial infarction and myocardial revascularization: Physiologic basis, methodology, and results. In: Wenger NK, Hellerstein H, eds. *Rehabilitation of the Coronary Patient,* 3d ed. New York: Churchill-Livingstone; 1992:351–365.

65. Comoss PM. Education of the coronary patient and family: Principles and Practice. In: Wenger NK, Hellerstein HK, eds. *Rehabilitation of the Coronary Patient,* 3d ed. New York: Churchill-Livingstone; 1992:439–460.

66. Borg GA. Psychophysical bases of perceived exertion. *Med Sci Sports Exerc* 1982;14:377–381.

67. Gordon NF, English CD, Contractor AS, et al. Effectiveness of three models for comprehensive cardiovascular disease risk reduction. *Am J Cardiol* 2002;89:1263–1268.

68. Berra KA, Haskell WL. Program models for cardiac rehabilitation. Part C. Home-based. In: Pashkow FJ, Dafoe WA, eds. *Clinical Cardiac Rehabilitation. A Cardiologist's Guide,* 2d ed. Baltimore: Williams & Wilkins, 1999:1–25.

69. Ornish D, Brown SE, Scherwitz LW, et al. Can lifestyle changes reverse coronary heart disease? The Lifestyle Heart Trial. *Lancet* 1990; 336:129–133.

70. Mullen PD, Mains DA, Velez R. A meta-analysis of controlled trials of cardiac patient education. *Patient Educ Couns* 1992;19:143–162.

71. Fuster V, Pearson TA. 27th Bethesda Conference: Matching the intensity of risk factor management with the hazard for coronary disease events. *J Am Coll Cardiol* 1996;27:957–1047.

72. CASS Principal Investigators and Their Associates. Coronary Artery Surgery Study (CASS): A randomized trial of coronary artery bypass surgery. Quality of life in patients randomly assigned to treatment groups. *Circulation* 1993;68:951–960.

73. Fiore MC, Smith SS, Jorenby DE, et al. The effectiveness of the nicotine patch for smoking cessation: A meta-analysis. *JAMA* 1994;271: 1940–1947.

74. Wenger NK. Coronary heart disease: The female heart is vulnerable. *Prog Cardiovasc Dis.* 46(3). In press.

75. Cannistra LB, Balady GJ. Exercise training in special populations: Women. In: Wenger NK, Smith LK, Froelicher ES, et al, eds. *Cardiac Rehabilitation. A Guide to Practice in the 21st Century.* New York: Marcel Dekker; 1999:117–125.

76. Williams MA, Fleg JL, Ades PA, et al. Secondary prevention of coronary heart disease in the elderly (with emphasis on patients ≥75 years of age). An American Heart Association Scientific Statement from the Council on Clinical Cardiology Subcommittee on Exercise, Cardiac Rehabilitation, and Prevention. *Circulation* 2002;105:1735–1743.

77. Shephard RJ. The scientific basis of exercise prescribing for the very old. *J Am Geriatr Soc* 1990;38:62–70.

78. Bruce RA, Larson EB, Stratton J. Physical fitness, functional aerobic capacity, aging, and responses to physical training or bypass surgery in coronary patients. *J Cardiopulm Rehabil* 1989;9:24–34.

79. Wilson JR, Groves J, Rayos G. Circulatory status and response to cardiac rehabilitation in patients with heart failure. *Circulation* 1996;94: 1567–1572.

80. Giannuzzi P, Temporelli PL, Corrà U, et al for the ELVD Study Group. Attenuation of unfavorable remodeling by exercise training in postinfarction patients with left ventricular dysfunction: Results of the Exercise in Left Ventricular Dysfunction (ELVD) Trial. *Circulation* 1997;96:1790–1797.

81. Dubach P, Myers J, Dziekan G, et al. Effect of exercise training on myocardial remodeling in patients with reduced left ventricular function after myocardial infarction: Application of magnetic resonance imaging. *Circulation* 1997;95:2060–2067.

82. Piña IL. Exercise training in special population: Heart failure and posttransplantation patients. In: Wenger JK, Smith LK, Froelicher ES, et al, eds. *Cardiac Rehabilitation. A Guide to Practice in the 21st Century.* New York: Marcel Dekker; 1999:127–140.

83. Adamopoulos S, Coats AJS, Brunotte F, et al. Physical training improves skeletal muscle metabolism in patients with chronic heart failure. *J Am Coll Cardiol* 1993;21:1101–1106.

84. Hornig B, Maier V, Drexler H. Physical training improves endothelial function in patients with chronic heart failure. *Circulation* 1996;93: 210–214.

85. Belardinelli R, Georgiou D, Cianci G, et al. Randomized, controlled trail of long-term moderate exercise training in chronic heart failure: Effects on functional capacity, quality of life, and clinical outcome. *Circulation* 1999;99:1173–1182.

86. Stevenson LW, Steimle E, Fonarow G, et al. Improvement in exercise capacity of candidates awaiting heart transplantation. *J Am Coll Cardiol* 1995;25:163–170.

87. Tamarisk NK. Enhancing activity levels of patients with permanent cardiac pacemakers. *Heart Lung* 1988;17:698–707.

88. Kalbfleisch KR, Lehmann MH, Steinman RT, et al. Reemployment following implantation of the automatic cardioverter defibrillator. *Am J Cardiol* 1989;64:199–202.

89. Helmers KF, Krantz DS, Howell RH, et al. Hostility and myocardial ischemia in coronary artery disease patients: Evaluation by gender and ischemic index. *Psychosom Med* 1993;55:29–36.

90. Frasure-Smith N, Lesperance F, Talajic M. Depression and 18-month prognosis after myocardial infarction. *Circulation* 1995;91:999–1005.

91. Frasure-Smith N, Lesperance F, Talajic M. Depression following myocardial infarction: Impact on 6-month survival. *JAMA* 1993;270: 1819–1825.

92. Louis AA, Manousos IR, Coletta AP, et al. Clinical trials update: The Heart Protection Study, IONA, CARISA, ENRICHD, ACUTE, ALIVE, MADIT II AND REMATCH. *Eur J Heart Fail* 2002;4: 111–116.

93. Stern MJ, Cleary P. National Exercise and Heart Disease Project: Psychosocial changes observed during a low-level exercise program. *Arch Intern Med* 1981;141:1463–1467.

94. Maeland JG, Havlik OE. Psychological predictors for return to work after a myocardial infarction. *J Psychosom Res* 1987;31:471–481.

95. Orth-Gomer K, Unden A-L, Edwards M-E. Social isolation and mortality in ischemic heart disease: A 10-year follow-up study of 150 middle-aged men. *Acta Med Scand* 1988;224:205–215.

96. Pravikoff DS. Return to work: Factors and issues of vocational counseling. In: Wenger NK, Smith LK, Froelicher ES, et al, eds. *Cardiac Rehabilitation. A Guide to Practice in the 21st Century.* New York: Marcel Dekker; 1999:295–302.

97. Wenger NK, Hellerstein HK, Blackburn H, et al. Physician practice in the management of patients with uncomplicated myocardial infarction: Changes in the past decade. *Circulation* 1982;65:421–427.

98. Walter PJ, ed. *Return to Work after Coronary Artery Bypass Surgery: Psychosocial and Economic Aspects.* Berlin: Springer-Verlag; 1985.

99. Russell RO Jr, Abi-Mansour P, Wenger NK. Return to work after coronary bypass surgery and percutaneous transluminal angioplasty: Issues and potential solutions. *Cardiology* 1986;73:306–322.

100. Rogers WJ, Coggin CJ, Gersh BJ, et al, for the CASS Investigators. Ten-year follow-up of quality of life in patients randomized to receive medical therapy or coronary artery bypass graft surgery. The Coronary Artery Surgery Study (CASS). *Circulation* 1990;82:1647–1658.

101. Fitzgerald ST, Becker DM, Celentano DD, et al. Return to work after percutaneous transluminal coronary angioplasty. *Am J Cardiol* 1989; 64:1108–1112.

102. Walling A, Tremblay GJ, Jobin J, et al. Evaluating the rehabilitation potential of a large population of post-myocardial infarction patients: Adverse prognosis for women. *J Cardiopulm Rehabil* 1988;8:99–106.

103. Ades PA, Huang D, Weaver SO. Cardiac rehabilitation participation predicts lower rehospitalization costs. *Am Heart J* 1992;123:916–927.

104. Levin LA, Perk J, Hedback B. Cardiac rehabilitation: A cost analysis. *J Intern Med* 1991;230:427–434.

105. Oldridge N, Furlong W, Feeny D, et al. Economic evaluation of cardiac rehabilitation soon after acute myocardial infarction. *Am J Cardiol* 1993;72:154–161.

106. Taylor CB, Bandura A, Ewart CK, et al. Exercise testing to enhance wives' confidence in their husbands' cardiac capability soon after clinically uncomplicated acute myocardial infarction. *Am J Cardiol* 1995;55:635–638.

107. Hellerstein HK. Vocational aspects of rehabilitation: Work evaluation. In: Wenger NK, Hellerstein HK, eds. *Rehabilitation of the Coronary Patient,* 3d ed. New York: Churchill-Livingstone; 1992:523–542.

108. 20th Bethesda Conference. Insurability and employability of the patient with ischemic heart disease, October 3–4, 1988. *J Am Coll Cardiol* 1989;14:1003–1044.

SYSTEMIC ARTERIAL HYPERTENSION

HYPERTENSION: EPIDEMIOLOGY, PATHOPHYSIOLOGY, DIAGNOSIS, AND TREATMENT

William J. Elliott / George L. Bakris / Henry R. Black

Hypertension is the most common disease-specific reason for which Americans visit a physician. It is one of the leading causes of morbidity and mortality in the world and will increase in worldwide importance as a public health problem by 2020.[1] In addition to the morbidity and mortality directly attributable to hypertension, high blood pressure (BP) is a powerful risk factor (a condition or characteristic of an individual or a population) that increases the likelihood of developing a wide variety of cardiovascular (CV) diseases (Table 61-1).[2,3]

All health care providers routinely encounter patients who are likely to benefit from lowered BP. These include not only patients with definite hypertension but also those with prehypertension (systolic BP 120 to 139 mmHg or diastolic BP 80 to 89 mmHg),[4] who have a higher risk of cardiovascular events than individuals with "optimal" or "normal" BP.[5] In the next decade, more patients will likely become candidates for antihypertensive therapy, as clinical trials demonstrate the benefits of treatment and pharmacologic approaches become safer and more effective. Furthermore, many people, perhaps the majority of those over 40 years of age, who do not yet meet the criteria for drug treatment for hypertension will benefit from lifestyle modifications, a presumably safe and cost-effective public health approach to reducing BP.[6] Many of the therapeutic lifestyle changes that lower BP or slow the rate of rise of BP should be incorporated into everyone's lifestyle very early.[6]

This chapter reviews the risks imparted by an elevated BP, discusses the pathophysiology of hypertension, and analyzes currently available and recommended tools to measure BP and evaluate patients with hypertension. Treatment both with and without drugs is discussed in light of the explosion of information furnished by clinical trials and newer approaches to lowering BP created by an enhanced understanding of the mechanisms responsible for raising it. The techniques of molecular biology and the contribution of genetics to hypertension have dramatically increased physicians' appreciation of the complexity of the problem.

Hypertension is a disorder of circulatory regulation. The now classic mosaic theory of the etiology of hypertension, which was first proposed in 1949 by Irvine Page, can be endorsed even more enthusiastically in light of current knowledge. One can no longer expect a simple explanation of why BP is elevated in an individual patient or that a single approach to therapy will be successful in the majority of those who are treated.

Despite progress in identifying the risks associated with elevated BP and development of many ways to lower BP—and demonstration that these methods reduce death and other "hard endpoints"—BP control remains suboptimal.[7,8] In preliminary data from the most recent national survey, only 34 percent of hypertensive Americans ages 18 to 74 had a BP of <140/90 mmHg, the current goal.[4] The prevalence of uncontrolled hypertension is even higher for those ≥75 years of age, and the threshold for "control" should be lower in some hypertensives, particularly those with diabetes mellitus (DM) and/or renal disease with proteinuria. Although the United States generally does better in controlling hypertension than other countries,[9]

TABLE 61-1 Risks Associated with Hypertension

Cerebrovascular disease
Coronary artery disease
Heart failure
Renal insufficiency
Peripheral vascular disease
Premature mortality

improvement is needed, both here and elsewhere. Otherwise, the 1.2 billion hypertensives predicted to be living by the year 2010 will continue to suffer higher morbidity and premature mortality rates, much of which could have been prevented.

DEFINITION

BP is a continuous variable, and whatever number is used to define hypertension will be arbitrary.[3] In the past several decades, the lower limit for the definition of definite hypertension has changed from 160/95 mmHg to 140/90 mmHg. Although there is still some disagreement, most authorities now agree on several important principles:

- Hypertension should be diagnosed if either the systolic or the diastolic BP level is elevated.
- Simply defining and consequently categorizing individuals as hypertensive or not, only on the basis of their BP levels, neglects the value of using the presence or absence of other risk factors, comorbidities, and target organ damage (TOD) to assess prognosis and ultimately to guide therapy. Thus, all current guidelines use a more comprehensive system to stratify risk. The diagnosis of hypertension is based on properly measured office BP readings, although home and ambulatory measurements have similar but lower threshold values (Table 61-2). Although home or ambulatory measurements are sometimes useful, it is not appropriate to routinely use these techniques to diagnose most individuals. Office readings remain the standard. In certain situations, especially when an individual claims to have multiple "normal" readings outside the physician's office (see below), it may be reasonable to rely more on out-of-office measurements.
- The approach to treatment for individuals with elevated BP should not focus simply on the BP level, which assesses the relative risk that is imparted by that BP, but also on the remainder of the CV risk profile. This approach combines the BP with other risk factors to estimate the absolute risk of adverse events that an individual faces. In the scheme for classification and stratification of hypertension in the Seventh Report of the Joint National Committee on Prevention, Detection, Evaluation, and Treatment of High Blood Pressure (JNC 7), for example (Table 61-3), the stages (normal to prehypertension through stages 1 or 2) represent increasing relative risk as BP rises.[4]

It is not of major significance whether hypertensives are classified as being in a stage as recommended by JNC 7 or a class per the World Health Organization/International Society of Hypertension (WHO/ISH).[4,10] What is important is to base the evaluation and care of hypertensive patients on more than the BP number. In several quantitative risk estimators, pretreatment BP does not affect overall risk; it matters only whether the treated BP is <140/90 mmHg.[11,12]

EPIDEMIOLOGY AND RISK

Physicians are seldom concerned about reducing elevated BP solely because of the specific symptoms or conditions associated with it. Instead, hypertension is treated because of the increased risk of morbidity and mortality that results from having an elevated BP (Table 61-1).

These risks have been well documented in numerous epidemiologic studies, beginning with the Framingham Heart Study and extending to the present.[2,13,14] Metanalyses of pooled data have confirmed the robust, continuous relationship between BP level and cerebrovascular disease and coronary artery disease (CAD) in both western and eastern populations.[3,15,16] In addition, BP is directly related to left ventricular hypertrophy (LVH), heart failure (HF), peripheral vascular disease (PVD), carotid atherosclerosis, renal disease, and "subclinical CV disease."[2] Cardiovascular risk factors tend to cluster; thus, hypertensives are more likely than normotensive people to have type 2 diabetes mellitus (DM) or dyslipidemia, especially elevated triglycerides and low high-density lipoprotein cholesterol (HDL-C).[17] The common denominator may be insulin resistance, perhaps as a result of the frequent coexistence of hypertension and obesity.[18]

Since 1993 in the United States, systolic BP has been given equal weight to diastolic BP in the diagnostic scheme for hypertension. Elevated systolic BPs have been identified as a major public health problem, for several reasons.[19] The lifetime risk in Framingham for 55- or 65-year-old men or women to develop hypertension is 90 percent[20]; among those 65 to 89 years old, systolic elevations were found in 87 percent of the hypertensive men and 93 percent of the hypertensive women. Systolic BP is less likely to be controlled than diastolic.[8] Most importantly, for people over age 50 or 60 years, systolic BP is a much better predictor of TOD and future CV and renal events than diastolic BP.[19,21] Overall, each 20 mmHg increase in systolic BP doubles cardiovascular risk.[3]

Some have argued that one should not measure diastolic BP other than perhaps to calculate pulse pressure (PP).[22] Pulse pressure, the difference between systolic and diastolic BP, was not a better predictor of risk than systolic BP in the most recent metanalysis of 61 epidemiologic studies of more than 1 million people.[3] A wide PP, unless it is a result of aortic insufficiency or an arteriovenous malformation, is a simple clinical indicator of less

TABLE 61-2 Threshold Values for "Normal" versus "Abnormal" BP (in mmHg)

Source	Office Readings	Home Readings	Ambulatory BP Monitor Readings
JNC 7[4]	140/90		
Tsuji et al.[89]	140/90	137/84	
de Guademaris et al.[269]	140/90	127/83	
Pickering[270]	140/90	135/85	135/85
Staessen et al.[271]	140/90		133/82

SOURCES: Adapted from Refs. 4, 89, and 269–271.

TABLE 61-3 Stratification of Cardiovascular Risk and Links to Initial Treatment Strategy

| | | | CONSIDERATIONS FOR INITIAL DRUG THERAPY | |
BP Category	Blood Pressure Range[a] (systolic; diastolic, mmHg)	Role of Lifestyle Modifications	No Compelling Indication	Compelling Indication (see Table 61-22)
Normal	<120 **and** <80	Encouraged	Not indicated	As indicated for other condition
Prehypertension	120–139 **or** 80–89	Recommended	Not indicated	As indicated for other condition
Stage 1	140–159 **or** 90–99	Recommended	Thiazide-type diuretic for most patients; other drug(s)[b] as needed	Use drug(s) for the compelling indications, thiazide-type diuretics and other drug(s)[b] as needed
Stage 2	≥160 **or** ≥100	Recommended	Two-drug combinations for most patients (usually thiazide-type diuretic + other drug[b])	

[a]Categorization of blood pressure is determined by higher blood pressure (systolic or diastolic).
[b]Other initial antihypertensive drugs most commonly recommended include: angiotensin converting-enzyme inhibitors (ACE-Is), angiotensin-receptor blockers (ARBs), beta blockers (BB); calcium channel blockers (CCBs).
SOURCE: Adapted from JNC 7.[4]

compliant ("stiffer") large central arteries and significant arterial damage. For all levels of systolic BP (even as low as 110 to 130 mmHg), risk varies little with increasing diastolic BPs in people under 60 years of age. One should not ignore elevated diastolic BPs if the systolic readings are >140 mmHg, especially in younger individuals. So far, no classification system for hypertension includes PP, either in defining hypertension, stratifying risk, or recommending treatment. This seems reasonable until more data and support are marshaled for the use of PP as a prognostic indicator.[19]

With the exception of hypertensive encephalopathy, few (if any) clinical symptoms have traditionally been attributed to elevated BPs themselves. This may have to be reevaluated, however, as newer and very well tolerated drugs are developed and as improved methods of assessing subtle symptoms are perfected. Hypertensive subjects given angiotensin receptor blockers (ARBs), for example, consistently have fewer adverse reactions (especially headache) than do subjects given placebo.[23,24] Furthermore, in the Treatment of Mild Hypertension Study (TOMHS) and the Hypertension Optimal Treatment (HOT) trial, the groups with the lowest BPs had the fewest complaints.[25,26] These trials utilized a wide variety of drugs to reduce BP and clearly showed not only that lowering BP is safe but that hypertensives treated to lower levels feel better. Hypertension may not be the asymptomatic condition it has long been thought to be.

ECONOMICS

Cost considerations are increasingly important in the pharmacologic management of hypertension in the United States, and they have always been a major consideration in the rest of the world. No regimen, no matter how carefully and appropriately selected, will be effective if the patient cannot afford it. Moreover, if an antihypertensive agent does not appear on the national formulary or the formulary of the insurance company from which a patient receives medication, the cost will not be covered and the patient may not be willing or able to purchase it. Generic preparations tend to be the least expensive options for initial therapy and are available for every class of antihyper-

tensive agent except ARBs. In general, branded calcium antagonists (CAs) are the most expensive, with ARBs and angiotensin-converting enzyme (ACE) inhibitors the next most expensive drugs. For many of the fixed-dose combinations now available, the cost is less than what would be paid for the individual components if they were purchased separately. It is also customary for fixed-dose combinations that include a thiazide diuretic to cost no more than does the nondiuretic component alone.

A careful analysis of the economics of hypertension treatment must include more than what is spent on drugs, patient visits, or laboratory tests.[27,28] For many affected (and especially high-risk) patients, the extremely expensive complications of under- and/or untreated hypertension far outweigh the inconvenience and costs associated with effective treatment.[27] In the United States in the year 2003, hypertension costs approximately $50.3 billion for cardiovascular disease and probably another $28 billion for renal disease.[29] Approximately 36 percent of the expenditures for hypertension pays for antihypertensive drugs; this proportion and the total could be reduced if hypertension treatment were more effective in controlling BP and reducing the risk of myocardial infarction (MI), HF, stroke, and end-stage renal disease (ESRD).[27]

PATHOPHYSIOLOGY

Hypertension, a disorder of BP regulation, can result from a multitude of causes.[30] Control of BP involves complex interactions among the kidneys, the central nervous system (CNS) and peripheral nervous system (PNS), and the vascular endothelium throughout the body as well as a variety of the other organs, such as the adrenal and pituitary glands. While a smaller number of nephrons may predispose to hypertension (either because of low birth weight[31] or anatomy[32]), the heart is the organ that responds to many of the changes mediated by these systems. It also secretes hormones locally and systemically that help regulate BP. In people genetically predisposed to develop hypertension, an imbalance occurs among the various systems that modulate BP. The sympathetic nervous system (SNS), the reninangiotensin-aldosterone (RAA) system, vasopressin (VP), nitric oxide (NO), and a host of vasoactive peptides, including endothelin, adrenomedullin, and others produced by the heart and many different cells (endothelial and vascular smooth cells, for example), modulate the responses of these systems and help maintain BP over a range commensurate with optimum physical and mental activity. Additionally, these systems affect the ability of the kidney to handle sodium (Na^+) and volume, which some feel is the primary controller of BP.[33]

Sympathetic Nervous System and Renal Sodium Handling

While the SNS and the RAA system control BP in the short term, ultimately it is the kidney that is responsible for long-term blood volume and BP control.[33] High-pressure baroreceptors in the carotid sinus and aortic arch respond to acute elevations in systemic BP by causing a reflex vagal bradycardia that is mediated through the parasympathetic system and inhibition of sympathetic output from the CNS. Low-pressure cardiopulmonary receptors in the atria and ventricles likewise respond to increases in atrial filling by increasing heart rate (HR) through inhibition of the cardiac SNS, increasing atrial natriuretic peptide (ANP) release, and inhibiting VP release.[34–36] These reflexes are largely controlled centrally, particularly in the nucleus tractus solitarius of the dorsal medulla. This vasomotor center also receives input from the limbic system and hypothalamus in response to emotional or psychological stress.

The consequences of SNS stimulation are peripheral vasoconstriction, an increase in HR, release of norepinephrine from the adrenals, and a resultant rise in systemic BP. The increase in SNS activity also plays a role in mediating local vascular hypertrophy and stiffness. Renal efferent sympathetics are also activated and cause internal vasoconstriction, with a fall in renal blood flow and an increase in renal vascular resistance.[37] The renal SNS also directly stimulates Na^+ reabsorption and renin release from the juxtaglomerular apparatus.[37] Thus, the SNS and CNS have effects on renal handling of Na^+.

Hyperactivity of the SNS has been described in patients with essential hypertension, particularly in the young and those with prehypertension (120 to 139/80 to 89 mmHg).[38] Elevated plasma norepinephrine levels with increased HR and cardiac indices have been described in people with newly diagnosed hypertension.[38] These individuals frequently show exaggerated BP responses to emotional (e.g., mental arithmetic) and physical stressors (e.g., ice-water immersion). Additionally, a subset of these patients exhibits elevated plasma renin levels that may reflect beta-adrenergic stimulation of renin secretion.

A defect in baroreceptor sensitivity has been postulated to be responsible for abnormal responsiveness of the SNS and thus may contribute to the increase in BP and HR variability noted in some hypertensive patients.[39] SNS activity also is increased in certain high-risk groups with hypertension, including African Americans, those who are obese or insulin-resistant, and those who ingest or inhale agents such as nicotine, alcohol, cyclosporine, and cocaine.[40–42] A very small subset of patients may have hypertension caused by compression of the lateral medulla by cranial nerves and/or vessels.[37] This results in increased SNS activity. Selective decompression of these nerves may ameliorate the hypertension in rare instances. Activation of the CNS/SNS may also result from renal afferent sympathetics from the kidney in hypertensive patients. In experimental models of hypertension, renal sympathectomy lowers BP.[37,38]

The influence of the SNS on Na^+ handling in the kidney also has been examined in detail.[43] Several classic studies have linked SNS hyperactivity with supranormal increases in BP in response to a given Na^+ load. Patients with essential hypertension and associated renal failure have sometimes been cured of the underlying hypertension by renal transplantation from a normotensive donor.[33]

Most authorities believe that the mechanism by which the kidney causes hypertension is impairment in the excretion of Na^+.[33,44] This impairment may be related to genetic changes in various Na^+ exchangers in the proximal and distal tubules that result in altered responses to stimulation by the SNS and the RAA system. Epidemiologic studies have linked the relative Na^+ content in the diet with the prevalence of hypertension in various populations, although the value of dietary Na^+ restriction in reducing BP remains controversial (see below).[6] Interventional studies with Na^+ restriction and/or loading have revealed that the BP responses in many hypertensive patients are "salt-sensitive": their BP rises after a salt load.[45] In addition, salt loading of patients with essential hypertension results in a net total body Na^+ accumulation. Three genetic diseases associated with hypertension in childhood (Liddle's syndrome, the syndrome of apparent mineralocorticoid excess, and glucocorticoid-remediable aldosteronism) all are associated with increased reabsorption of Na^+ by the kidney.[46]

Genetically mediated defects in the ability of the kidney to excrete Na^+ do not readily explain several observations:

- Young hypertensive subjects appear to excrete Na^+ normally or supranormally.
- Individuals with high-normal BP may have a low blood volume.
- As many as 40 percent of people with hypertension do not show a change in BP with Na^+ loading ("salt resistance").
- With aging, salt sensitivity increases both in frequency and in degree, such that by age 70, the majority of hypertensive patients are salt-sensitive.

In fact, several metanalyses suggest that salt restriction is not important, especially in normotensives or hypertensives under age 40.[47–49] All these findings are consistent with the idea that the defect in Na^+ excretion in hypertensive patients may be acquired rather than genetically determined. However, abnormal Na^+ handling is a mechanism that contributes to elevating BP in many but probably not all patients with hypertension.

The Renin-Angiotensin-Aldosterone System

The RAA system is one of the most important physiologic mediators that regulate blood volume and BP. Plasma angiotensinogen, released primarily from the liver, is catabolized by renin from the kidney to generate angiotensin I, which is further degraded by angiotensin-converting enzyme to angiotensin II (A II). In addition to the systemic RAA system, there is now evidence that a local RAA system is present in blood vessels, heart, kidney, and other tissues, where it may mediate local effects (such as tissue remodeling) independent of circulating renin or angiotensinogen levels.

Most of the actions of A II are mediated by the AT_1 receptor. Activation of this constantly expressed receptor results in vasoconstriction, vascular smooth muscle proliferation, deposition of connective tissue and LDL-cholesterol transport into arterial media, inhibition of endothelial function, increased cardiac contractility, CNS stimulation, NO production, aldosterone and VP release, renal tubular absorption of Na^+, and thirst.[50] Within the kidney, stimulation of the AT_1 receptor by A II also causes renal vasoconstriction (especially of the efferent arteriole and vasa rectae), a fall in renal blood flow, and an increase in renal vascular resistance. Angiotensin II also increases Na^+ reabsorption, both by increasing aldosterone release and through direct effects on the proximal tubule. Additionally, A II increases the sensitivity of the tubuloglomerular (TG) feedback response.

Angiotensin subtype 2 (AT_2) receptors also are stimulated by angiotensin II. Activation of these receptors, which are clearly active during fetal development, produces virtually opposite actions (to stimulation of AT_1 receptors) in some experimental systems. The role of the activated AT_2 receptors in healthy adults and even in adults with cardiac or vascular disease is being intensely investigated.

The role of the RAA system in essential hypertension is complex. Plasma renin activity (PRA) is elevated in about 20 percent of hypertensive patients; it is either normal (50 percent) or low (30 percent) in the majority. However, in many patients with normal plasma renin levels, PRA may be inappropriately high in relation to total body Na^+. Sodium depletion accentuates and Na^+ infusion blunts changes in PRA levels in patients with hypertension. Additionally, BP in these patients is frequently reduced after the use of ACE inhibitors or ARBs.[51]

One reason for widely varying PRA levels across populations and Na^+ intakes may be nephron heterogeneity within individual kidneys. According to this hypothesis, some ischemic nephrons make excess renin, while other hyperfiltering nephrons generate less renin.[52] The ischemic nephrons secrete renin, which enters the circulation and then leads to A II generation, which causes inappropriate vasoconstriction and Na^+ reabsorption in the other hyperfiltering nephrons. This, then, results in Na^+ retention and the development of hypertension.

Unfortunately, this is only part of the explanation, since PRA is relatively low in African Americans and the elderly, two populations with a high prevalence of hypertension and a high rate of hypertension-associated complications. Low PRA, however, does not necessarily mean that the RAA is not active, since tissue effects and local actions are not necessarily evident from the measurement of plasma renin activity alone.

Vasopressin

While VP has been clearly shown *not* to play a role in the genesis of essential hypertension, it does play an important role in the maintenance of established hypertension, especially in African Americans.[53] In African Americans, selective inhibition of V_1A receptors reduces systolic BP by an additional 8 to 12 mmHg in the presence of a high-salt diet (suppression of the RAA system) and clonidine (suppression of SNS).[54] This was not observed in Caucasians.[55] In light of the interaction between arginine vasopressin (AVP), A II, and endothelin on cellular growth and vascular responsiveness, it appears that AVP may have a potentiating effect on one of these other hormones.

Endothelin

Endothelin is the most potent endogenous vasoconstrictor in humans. Comparative studies with A II have demonstrated not only that the endothelin family of hormones has cellular actions similar to those of A II but also that the two hormones work in concert to potentiate each other's vascular and cellular effects.[56] Given this, however, the specific role of endothelin in the etiology of essential hypertension is minimal.[57] It plays a far more important role in pulmonary hypertension, cyclosporine-induced hypertension, and decreased renal function as well as in maintaining BP in people with HF.[58,59]

Endothelin is the major mechanism by which cyclosporine constricts the afferent arteriole of the kidney and reduces renal function. Calcium antagonists and endothelin receptor blockade prevent this reduction. Additionally, endothelin A receptors have been shown to play a major role in contributing to the maintenance of elevated renal perfusion pressure in patients with HF.[60]

Nitric Oxide

Nitric oxide is a major intrinsic vasodilator produced by the endothelium in response to vasoconstrictor hormones (including A II); it plays a vital role in the maintenance of normal BP.[61,62] Defects in NO release or synthesis that are induced by atherosclerosis or that are genetically programmed predispose individuals to the development of atherosclerosis and hypertension.[63] NO serves as a major counterbalancing factor that maintains BP within the range necessary to maintain organ perfusion, but avoid injury. It counterbalances vasoconstrictive hormones and cytokines, such as A II, platelet-derived growth factor (PDGF), tumor necrosis factor alpha, and other hormones that stimulate its release. Transgenic animal models that do not have the ability to synthesize NO have very high BP and typically die of CV causes earlier than do animals that can produce NO.

Additionally, NO plays a major role in the genesis of hypertension in people who are insulin-resistant. The underlying mechanisms and the factors that contribute to the interaction between insulin and NO have been studied extensively in healthy people and insulin-resistant subjects. A genetic and/or acquired defect of NO synthesis could represent a central defect that triggers many of the metabolic, vascular, and sympathetic abnormalities characteristic of insulin-resistant states, all of which may predispose to cardiovascular disease (CVD).[64]

Ion Transport Abnormalities

A number of dietary factors affect the SNS, the CNS, and the RAA system in people and animals genetically predisposed to develop hypertension. High Na^+ and low potassium (K^+) intake, low Ca^{2+}, and/or low magnesium (Mg^{2+}) intake, can increase BP. Substantial evidence from animal models of hypertension as well as diabetic and nondiabetic hypertensive individuals supports an association between the development or worsening of hypertension and changes in intracellular pH, which is related to changes in electrolyte composition.[6,65] These observations have led to several hypotheses regarding the importance of one ion relative to others.

Numerous investigators have documented increases in cytosolic free Na^+ concentrations in cells of hypertensive or diabetic patients compared with age- and sex-matched normotensive or nondiabetic controls. These result from altered activity of the Na^+/H^+ antiporter and the Na^+/Li^+ countertransporter and are correlated with diastolic BP.

The relationship between intracellular Mg^{2+} and BP is less clearly defined.[6] Data from animals and humans demonstrate an inverse relation between intracellular Mg^{2+} concentration and BP elevation. The primary mechanism responsible for this relative reduction in intracellular Mg^{2+} relates to Na^+-dependent Mg^{2+} efflux through the plasma membrane.

Increases in the intracellular Ca^{2+} concentration are seen commonly in obese and essential hypertensive subjects. Like Na^+, these changes reflect altered membrane ion transport activity. Early clinical studies in small numbers of patients demonstrated that oral Ca^{2+} ingestion reduced BP, but larger clinical trials did not confirm these results.[6,65,66]

Increased K^+ intake is well known to have effects on BP control through multiple mechanisms, including opening K^+ channels in the vasculature, altering sympathetic neuronal output, and increasing vasodilatory prostaglandins.[67] In hypertensive patients, hypokalemia will blunt reductions in BP by antihypertensive medication, perhaps because it results in the closure of K^+ channels.

Potassium also modulates vascular responsiveness in salt-sensitive individuals. After dietary potassium supplementation, a nocturnal fall in BP was seen in all "nondipper" subjects, whether salt-sensitive or salt-resistant.[68] These results suggest that a inverse relationship between dietary K^+ intake and high BP can exist, even when daytime BP is unchanged by a high-K^+ diet.[68]

Taken together, these data suggest that both univalent and divalent cations can affect vascular responses to stimuli such as those mediated by the RAA and the SNS. Changes in vascular response are linked to altered function of membrane ion transporters (Na^+/H^+ antiporter, Na^+/K^+/ATPase, Mg^{2+}/Na^+ exchanger, Ca^{2+}/H^+ exchanger, Ca^{2+} ATPase, and others). Both the Na^+/K^+/ATPase and the Ca^{2+}/ATPase pumps are important in maintaining the Ca^{2+} homeostasis of the cell.

Extracellular Volume Homeostasis

Although an acute infusion of saline administered to animals with experimentally induced hypertension will initially raise blood volume and cardiac output, the increase in cardiac output is transient and is replaced soon thereafter by a rise in systemic vascular resistance (SVR). There are several potential mechanisms for this observation. First, the normal response to a salt load is inhibition of the SNS. However, in salt-sensitive patients, the SNS is not inhibited and even may be activated with a salt load.[69] A possible explanation is that in the setting of renal dysfunction or intrarenal ischemia, salt loading triggers an intense tuboglomerular feedback signal that activates the renal afferent SNS. This renal response subsequently triggers a CNS response. Renal afferent nerves can activate CNS sympathetic activity in both experimental hypertension and chronic renal disease.

Second, parabiotic experiments have suggested there may be circulating factors in salt-loaded animals with hypertension that are responsible for some of the increase in SVR. One candidate is a circulating Na^+/K^+/ATPase inhibitor, which has been documented in some patients with essential hypertension. These substances, one of which is ouabain, are digitalis-like and adrenally derived.[70] They are presumably secreted in an attempt to facilitate Na^+ excretion, may have the adverse consequence of increasing intracellular Na^+ and thus facilitating Na^+-Ca^{2+} exchange in vascular smooth muscle cells. This would lead to a rise in intracellular Ca^{2+} and stimulate vascular smooth muscle contraction, vasoconstriction, and a rise in SVR.

A third mechanism is the loss of a vasodepressor substance, probably adrenomedullin, which is expressed in some of the interstitial cells in the renal medulla and the juxtamedullary region.[71] Release of adrenomedullin into the circulation depends on medullary blood flow and can be inhibited if activation of renal SNS or inhibition of NO reduces blood flow.[37] Thus, either tubulointerstitial (TI) injury and/or intrarenal ischemia would lower circulating levels of adrenomedullin.

Fourth, the increase in pressure associated with a saline load could cause increased tension in the peripheral vasculature, leading to microvascular rarefaction (which has been observed in the forearms and nail beds of patients with essential hypertension), which could raise the SVR. An increased pressure load on the vessels also could result in compensatory vascular hypertrophy mediated by local growth factors and the local RAA system. Indeed, there is evidence that A II, PDGF, and basic fibroblast growth factor are involved in these processes.

Mechanisms of Na^+ Retention in Essential Hypertension

A rise in systemic BP normally is associated with brisk natriuresis. This is probably due to a transient rise in pressure in the peritubular capillaries in the juxtamedullary region, with a subsequent increase in interstitial pressure and a backflow of Na^+ through the paracellular space of the proximal tubule. Most patients with essential hypertension have an abnormality in the pressure-natriuresis curve, in which higher systemic pressures are required to excrete a Na^+ load.

A second mechanism for decreased Na^+ excretion is an enhancement of tubuloglomerular (TG) feedback. TG feedback is a reflex vasoconstriction that occurs with chloride delivery to the macula densa, and the vasoconstrictive response will reduce both glomerular filtration and Na^+ excretion. TG feedback can be enhanced in the setting of increased local vasoconstrictors such as A II and adenosine or by a reduction in local vasodilators such as NO. TG feedback appears to be enhanced in models of experimental hypertension.[72]

Finally, alterations in intrarenal vasoactive mediators may be involved in the impairment of Na^+ excretion in patients with hypertension. In both experimental and human hypertension, there may be low concentrations of renal vasodilators—such as prostaglandins, dopamine, and NO—as well as elevated concentrations of renal vasoconstrictors such as A II and adenosine and increased activity of the renal SNS. In addition to their effects of enhancing TG feedback, alterations in the levels of these agents could contribute to net Na^+ reabsorption because of their direct effects on tubular Na^+ transport.

Some studies have shown that TI injury can be induced in rats with either catecholamine (phenylephrine) or A II infusion and that subsequently these animals will develop hypertension when placed on a high-salt diet.[72] Evaluation of biopsied kidneys from these rats demonstrated focal areas of peritubular capillary rarefaction. This also has been observed in renal biopsies of patients with essential hypertension. The loss of peritubular capillaries could help explain the impairment of pressure-natriuresis. The ischemia related to the vasoconstriction and capillary loss could lead to alterations in the various vasoactive mediators. Indeed, there is some evidence that NO levels fall and adenosine levels rise with TI injury and ischemia, and this could contribute to the enhanced TG feedback that has been observed.[73,74]

While this pathway links a hyperactive SNS or RAA system with TI injury and salt-dependent hypertension, it is likely that TI injury induced in other ways could result in salt-sensitive hypertension. TI disease is associated with reflux nephropathy, chronic pyelonephritis, DM, cyclosporine, radiation, lead and analgesic nephropathy, hypercalcemia/nephrocalcinosis, and gout, all of which are strongly associated with hypertension. In addition, many high-risk groups associated with salt-dependent essential hypertension, such as older persons, obese persons, and African Americans, have a high prevalence of TI disease.

Insulin Resistance

Insulin resistance is a metabolic disorder that is manifest by a reduction in peripheral skeletal muscle utilization of glucose.[18] To fully understand the contribution of insulin resistance to the genesis of hypertension, one has to evaluate the effects of insulin resistance and hyperinsulinemia on factors that contribute to BP elevation. High circulating levels of insulin cause sodium retention and other vascular effects, such as cellular proliferation and matrix expansion.[75] In the presence of hyperinsulinemia, neurohumoral factors such as A II, endothelin, and VP also potentiate proliferation of endothelial and vascular smooth muscle cells. Last, the effect of insulin on various growth factors contributes to the development of vascular injury through its potentiation of the atherosclerotic process. In a person genetically predisposed to hypertension and/or nephropathy, these factors can potentiate injury to the vasculature and end organs.

Not all subjects with insulin resistance have each of the associated components of insulin resistance syndrome (or syndrome X): dyslipidemia, hyperuricemia, type 2 DM/glucose intolerance, hypertension, microalbuminuria, left ventricular hypertrophy, salt sensitivity, and obesity, among others. Both normotensive offspring of hypertensive nondiabetic parents and nondiabetic first-degree relatives of patients with type 2 DM have several of the hallmarks of insulin resistance.[76] Thus, a genetic predisposition may be needed to develop this syndrome.

Genetic Factors

Commonly accepted candidate genes associated with essential hypertension are summarized in Table 61-4. Aside from single-gene mutations that manifest as rare or unusual hypertensive phenotypes (e.g., those discussed below), most genetic investigations have resulted in contradictory findings. For example, specific variants in the angiotensinogen gene were first associated with a higher risk of hypertension, but this has not been seen in all laboratories or across all populations. Because hypertension probably results from a multitude of different genes, it will likely take another 5 to 10 years to identify those associated with a higher risk of hypertension. A number of federally funded studies to identify these genes from sibling pairs and families are under way. Until these genetic profiles are delineated, it will still be necessary to rely on data gathered from epidemiologic studies to identify subjects at risk for the development of hypertension and CV events.

These are several clear examples of genetically mediated syndromes in hypertension.[46,77]

GLUCOCORTICOID-REMEDIABLE ALDOSTERONISM

This is an inherited autosomal dominant disorder that mimics an aldosterone-producing adenoma.[78] An important clinical clue to diagnosing this disease is the age at onset of hypertension. Patients with glucocorticoid-remediable aldosteronism (GRA) typically manifest high BP as children, whereas patients with other mineralocorticoid excess states, such as aldosterone-producing adenomas (APA) and idiopathic adrenal hyperplasia, are usually diagnosed in the third through sixth decades of life. A strong family history of hypertension is the rule, often associated with early death of affected family members from cerebrovascular accidents, which is characteristic of some GRA families.

In GRA, the RAA system is suppressed and aldosterone secretion is regulated solely by adrenocorticotropic hormone (ACTH). As a result, plasma aldosterone levels usually decline during the course of an upright posture study, similar to what is seen in patients with APA. The administration of exogenous ACTH to patients with GRA is associated with aldosterone hyperresponsiveness, compared with normal subjects. Moreover, in contrast to normal subjects, in whom continuous ACTH administration is associated with a rise and a subsequent fall in aldosterone to basal levels over days, patients with GRA exhibit an exuberant aldosterone response that is sustained as long as ACTH is infused.

In 1992, Lifton and colleagues[78a,b] showed that GRA is caused by a genetic mutation that results in a hybrid or chimeric gene product resulting from unequal crossing between nucleotide sequences of the 11-hydroxylase and aldosterone synthase genes. These two genes are located in close proximity on human chromosome 8, are 95 percent homologous in nucleotide sequence, and have an identical intron-exon structure. The structure of the duplicated gene contains the 5′ regulatory sequences that confer the ACTH responsiveness of 11-hydroxylase fused to more distal coding sequences of the aldosterone synthase gene. Therefore this hybrid gene is regulated by ACTH and has aldosterone synthase activity, allowing ectopic expression of aldosterone synthase activity in the ACTH-regulated zona fasciculata, which normally produces cortisol. This abnormal gene duplication can be readily detected by Southern blot analysis, allowing for direct genetic screening for this disorder with a small sample of white blood cells.

GLUCOCORTICOID RESISTANCE

The structure, growth, and secretory activity of the adrenal cortical zona fasciculata are regulated largely by ACTH, release of which is inhibited by cortisol. Normally, an increase in ACTH release raises the levels of cortisol, which then inhibits the release of ACTH. This continuous inhibitory feedback of cortisol on ACTH release is interrupted in patients with glucocorticoid resistance. In this disorder, although cortisol levels are exceedingly high, ACTH release is not inhibited, leading to uninhibited ACTH secretion, which in turn stimulates the adrenal cortex to produce 11-deoxycorticosterone (DOC). If sufficient DOC is secreted, salt and water retention ensue, precipitating hypertension and hypokalemia. Animal studies indicate that the mechanism for this may be related to changes in hippocampal steroid receptor building and downregulation of endothelial cell nitric oxide synthase.[79,80]

LIDDLE'S SYNDROME

Liddle's syndrome is an autosomal dominant disorder that mimics the signs and symptoms of mineralocorticoid excess. The fault appears to lie with continuously avid Na^+ channels in the distal nephron, resulting in severe hypertension and excessive salt absorption with K^+ wasting despite negligible aldosterone production.[81] A prominent feature is premature death from stroke or HF. The clinical manifestations can be corrected by triamterene or amiloride (which block the Na^+ channel), but not by spironolactone (which binds the aldosterone receptor).

The cellular defect associated with this syndrome is located on the apical membrane of the tubule, where the epithelial Na^+ channel (ENaC) plays a critical role in Na^+ absorption. Liddle's syndrome has been traced to a defect in the ENaC gene, which regulates cyclic adenosine monophosphate (cAMP)-mediated translocation of EnaC to the cell surface.[82,83]

TABLE 61-4 Candidate Genes Associated with Hypertension and Cardiovascular Risk

Monogenic forms
  Glucocorticoid-remediable aldosteronism
  Liddle's syndrome
Polygenic forms that affect the following:
  Angiotensinogen gene
  Na^+-Li^+ countertransport
  Epithelial amiloride-sensitive sodium channel
  Nitric oxide generation
  Alpha-adducin
  G beta$_3$ subunit (intracellular signal transduction)
  Insertion/deletion of ACE gene

DIAGNOSIS OF HYPERTENSION

The pressure generated by the heart during its normal contractile cycle has been estimated for more than 100 years. Since the early 1930s, insurance companies have recognized the value of BP readings for predicting mortality. Prior to Riva-Rocci's sphygmomanometer,[84] palpation of the pulse and appreciation of the contour and pressure within a peripheral artery were skills learned only through extensive experience. Objective measurements were made easier by the instruments of Janeway and Korotkoff, who characterized the sounds heard when using a stethoscope placed over the compressed artery in 1905. The terminology introduced by Korotkoff is still used today: systolic BP is recognized when clear and repetitive tapping sounds are heard; diastolic BP is recorded when the sounds disappear. An exception is recognized among patients who have audible sounds even down to zero millimeters of mercury; the "muffling" of the sounds (Korotkoff phase IV) is then recorded before the zero.[85]

Techniques of Measuring Blood Pressure

The proper technique for accurate BP measurement is typically taught very early during medical training but then seldom followed. Many expert panels have made recommendations regarding the methodology of BP measurement; these frequently do not agree in all details, but several general principles can be extracted[85]:

- There are six sizes of commonly available BP cuffs: newborn, infant, child, normal adult, large adult, and thigh. Using a smaller-than-recommended cuff on a larger arm typically results in an overestimation of casual BP. In obese or muscular persons, the large adult-size cuff is required for all those with an arm circumference at the midhumerus of more than 38 cm. In very large individuals, the thigh cuff is often necessary.
- To accurately measure BP, the deflation rate of the column of mercury should be 2 to 3 mmHg/s. The lower rate of deflation should be used for persons with HRs less than 72 beats per minute (bpm); the more rapid deflation is appropriate only for those with resting tachycardia. If the precision of measurement is to be at least 2 mmHg, the observer should have the opportunity to hear at least one Korotkoff sound at each 2-mmHg gradation of the mercury column. Thus, the proper deflation rate depends on the HR of the subject and is unlikely to be more than 3 mmHg/s if a precise BP measurement is desired.
- It is unusual for a single BP measurement to be an accurate indicator of future CV risk; multiple measurements made on different occasions are more likely to be helpful in deciding whether a particular person ought to have his or her BP lowered. Although it is traditional to average the second and third of a series of BP measurements in a single position (e.g., supine, seated, or standing) and to record this as the "average BP" at a given visit, recent "quality care guidelines" mandate instead the recording of individual BP measurements, with the lowest on a given date being the one of greatest interest to auditors. For these reasons, it is quickly becoming "standard practice" to record individual readings and is especially important to measure BP in several positions (including standing), since the auditors record only the lowest BP reading (in any position) as the "BP taken at that visit."[86] The BP readings of many physicians participating in managed care audits are being judged as a "quality of care" indicator, and by recording a large number of BP measurements in several positions, one has the best chance that at least one will be deemed "acceptable."[86]

- Most long-term data on hypertension and its treatment have been derived from "casual" measurements made with a mercury sphygmomanometer and stethoscope in a health care provider's office. Physicians and patients are often more interested and impressed by BP readings taken in other settings (e.g., with home monitors or ambulatory BP monitoring devices, both of which are discussed further below). However, nearly all data linking BP measurements to adverse clinical sequelae (including MI, stroke, and death) were gathered a medical office. For now, office readings taken by a trained professional should be the BPs used for diagnosing and treating hypertensives in all but a few special situations.

BP is subject to a large degree of intrinsic variability. Several steps can be taken to minimize this variability, including the following:

- Taking multiple measurements, especially when the pulse is irregular (e.g., atrial fibrillation). This is necessary because ventricular filling pressures vary considerably as a result of variability of diastolic filling time. BP variability is especially pronounced in older persons with primarily or exclusively systolic BP evaluations.
- Centering the bladder of the cuff over the brachial artery with its lower edge within 2.5 cm of the antecubital fossa. This leaves enough space so that the stethoscope head can be applied inferiorly without touching the cuff (and generating background noise).
- Having the subject rest silently and comfortably (with back support if seated) for at least 5 min before the measurement.
- Abstaining from drinking caffeine or alcohol-containing beverages or tobacco use within 30 min before a BP measurement.
- Questioning the subject regarding the most recent meal or evacuation of bowels or bladder. Distended abdominal viscera can not only be painful but also routinely cause BP to be elevated, presumably because of anxiety or pain. Older persons typically have a lower BP postprandially; thus it is often necessary to inquire about and record when the last meal was eaten.
- Assuring that the arm is supported at the level of the heart. Both muscular work (of tensed muscles around the elbow) and hydrostatic pressure caused by a "dangling arm" increase the pressure necessary to obliterate the pulse and lead to overestimation of systolic BP.
- Listening over the brachial artery by using the bell of the stethoscope with minimal pressure exerted on the skin. At the conclusion of the BP measurement, there should be no lasting indentations in the area where the head of the stethoscope was placed. Otherwise the systolic BP is likely to be overestimated and the diastolic BP to be underestimated because too great a pressure was exerted directly over the artery.
- The "peak inflation level" of the mercury column should be determined by using palpation of the radial artery *before* the stethoscope is applied. For all subsequent BP measurements, the cuff typically should be inflated 20 mmHg higher than the pressure at which the palpable pulse at the radial artery disappears. Important prognostic information may be missed if the "auscultatory gap" is not detected; this risk is minimized by determining the peak inflation level by palpation before the stethoscope is applied.[87]
- Although mercury columns traditionally have been used in the measurement of BP, environmental concerns associated with elemental mercury are increasing. In Sweden and many other countries, elemental mercury is forbidden in the workplace. Nonetheless, sphygmomanometers used in the measurement of BP should be calibrated frequently and routinely against such standards (typically every 6 months) to assure accuracy.
- Attempting to avoid "terminal digit preference." Traditionally, BP measurements have been made to the nearest 2 mmHg (the typi-

cal markings on a mercury sphygmomanometer). Theoretically, in a large collection of systolic and diastolic BP measurements, there should be an equal number of readings ending in 0, 2, 4, 6, or 8 mmHg. It is often instructive to compare the actual distribution of terminal digits with the 20 percent expected for each one. This typically reveals a preference for 0 in inpatient medical services, where BP readings are typically precise to ± 10 mmHg.

- Measurements of BP in both arms typically are obtained at the initial visit, and the arm with the higher BP is used thereafter if the difference is greater than 10/5 mmHg. In such situations, there is often concern about coarctation of the aorta or Takayasu's arteritis or moyamoya disease, but seldom is this seen on ultrasonography or other confirmatory testing. BP measurement in a leg should be commonplace in all young hypertensives at the first visit and may be useful in older people as a peripheral indicator of aortic insufficiency ("Hill's sign").

- Assuring that the equipment used to measure BP is in good working order. Many sphygmomanometers (even in hospitals) are in poor repair and should be cleaned, calibrated, and fitted with non-leaking tubing and properly sized cuffs. The interest in BP measurements recently demonstrated by agencies that certify health systems for quality has improved the chance that any given patient will be hospitalized in a bed with properly maintained BP measuring equipment.

Home Blood Pressure Measurements

The technology for obtaining accurate and reproducible BP measurements outside the traditional medical environment has improved greatly in the last 25 years. Many available devices are convenient, inexpensive, and relatively accurate. Even persons with hearing difficulties, problems with hand-eye coordination, and other disabilities can operate semiautomatic (usually oscillometric) devices with digital readouts and printers to record BPs. Some authorities believe that such devices should be provided to every person with elevated BP. Others are concerned about overinterpretation of the data, as these methods have not been used in decision making in clinical trials and therefore should not be used routinely in practice to make diagnostic or therapeutic decisions.[88]

Home BP readings are typically lower (by an average of about 12/7 mmHg) than measurements taken in the traditional medical environment, even in normotensive subjects.[89] Home readings tend to be better correlated with both the extent of TOD and the risk of future mortality than are readings taken in the physician's office.[90] Home readings can be helpful in evaluating symptoms suggestive of hypotension, especially if the symptoms are intermittent or infrequent. During treatment, reliable home readings can lower costs by substituting for multiple visits to health care providers.[91] Persons who routinely measure BP at home probably have a better prognosis than do those who do not, because of both selection bias (they tend to be more interested in their BP than are those who refuse to purchase and use a home BP machine) and social support (when a friend or spouse becomes involved in measurement and overseeing pill-taking and appointment-keeping behaviors).

Home BP readings should be interpreted cautiously, carefully, and conservatively.[92-94] There are no long-term clinical trials that based all treatment decisions solely on home readings, but several reports show benefit from supplementing office BP measurements with home readings.[95-99] Unlike ambulatory BP monitoring, home BP readings have not yet become widely accepted for demonstrating the efficacy of antihypertensive drugs.[100,101] Several studies have shown that prognosis is better predicted by home readings than by one or two "casual" BP measurements.[90,102] Many of the factors that contribute to BP variability are more difficult to control in the home environment, including intrinsic circadian variation, food and alcohol ingestion, exercise, and stress. The possibility that home BP measurements will become an obsession is also a disadvantage. If home readings are to be taken, the instrument should be calibrated against a mercury sphygmomanometer by using a Y-tube and the technique of the measurer checked. Home readings can be a useful adjunct to information obtained in the physician's office, especially when the two are widely disparate. One long-term study showed that people with much lower home BP readings (compared with those in the physician's office) suffer fewer major CV events than do people who have elevated readings both in the office and at home.[102] Patients who are interested in and capable of measuring their BP at home should do it at a fixed time of the day and record all the readings obtained. The physician can then review them during the office visit and strive to educate the patients about the difficulties of interpretation of the readings.[88,93]

Ambulatory Blood Pressure Monitoring

Extensive research has led to a better definition of the role of automatic recorders that measure BP frequently over a 24-h period during a person's usual daily activities (including sleep).[103] The use of these devices by practitioners in the United States was very limited until April 1, 2002, when the Center for Medicare and Medicaid Services authorized reimbursement (of approximately $40 to 55 per session) for ambulatory BP monitoring only for the evaluation of "white coat hypertension."[104] Despite the low reimbursement, this decision may remove one of the barriers to more widespread use of this important diagnostic modality. As a research tool, the advantages and disadvantages of ambulatory BP monitoring (ABPM) have been well documented (Table 61-5), normal values have been defined (Table 61-2),[105,106] and publications correlating abnormal results of ABPM with adverse outcomes have appeared.[107-109] Several expert panels have defined the special situations in which ABPM is particularly useful (Table 61-6).[7,110]

TABLE 61-5 Advantages and Disadvantages of Ambulatory Blood Pressure Monitoring

Advantages
Many BP and pulse measurements during 24-h period
Measures diurnal variation (including during sleep)
Measures BP and pulse during daily activities
Can identify "white coat" hypertension
No "alerting response"
No placebo effect
Better correlation with target-organ damage than other methods of BP measurement

Disadvantages
Cost
Limited availability of equipment
Disruption of daily activities due to noise/discomfort (e.g., sleep quality, flaccid arm during measurement)
Limited "normative" data
Limited guidelines (or consensus) for interpretation of data in individuals
Few long-term prospective studies demonstrating utility compared to traditional (and much less expensive) BP measurements

SOURCE: From Elliott and Black.[272] With permission.

TABLE 61-6 Situations in which Ambulatory Blood Pressure Monitoring Is Useful

Diagnosing office or "white-coat" hypertension in patients with office hypertension but no target-organ damage[a]
Diagnosis of "high normal" blood pressure without target-organ damage
Assessing refractory or resistant hypertension[a]
Evaluating episodic hypertension (at least once a day)
Evaluating symptoms consistent with hypotension[a]
Deciding if drug treatment is warranted in older patients
Assuring efficacy of antihypertensive drug therapy over 24 h
Evaluating hypertension with autonomic dysfunction
Identifying nocturnal hypertension[a]
Managing hypertension during pregnancy
Evaluation of efficacy of antihypertensive drugs in clinical research

[a]Denotes situations for which a repeat ambulatory blood pressure monitoring session may be considered; some would include "after major changes in drug therapy" to this list.
SOURCE: Adapted from O'Brien et al.[110] With permission.

Several varieties of ABPM devices are currently available. In the United States, those that measure BP indirectly (i.e., without arterial cannulation) use either an auscultatory or an oscillometric technique. The former type uses a microphone placed over the artery to detect Korotkoff sounds in the traditional fashion. The latter measures biophysical oscillations of the brachial artery, which are compared (using a standardized algorithm) with those observed with a mercury sphygmomanometer: systolic BP is determined directly from the threshold oscillation, mean arterial pressure is estimated, and diastolic BP is calculated. Both types of monitors are small (<450 g), simple to apply and use, accurate, relatively quiet and tolerable, and powered by two to four small batteries. Data from 80 to 120 measurements of BP and pulse are typically stored in a small microprocessor and then downloaded into a desktop computer, which then edits the readings and prints the report.

None of the currently available ABPM devices is completely without problems. Devices that rely on direct measurements require 24 h of arterial cannulation, which is potentially dangerous, and are rarely used even for research. Indirect measurements of BP using auscultatory techniques can be confused by ambient noise levels, even if R-wave gating is used (this requires the electrocardiographic leads to be attached to the chest). Oscillometric techniques require that the subject keep the arm straight and flaccid during the measurement and can be completely confused if the subject has a tremor. The interpretation of ABPM readings may be enhanced by a diary of the subject's activities, but such diaries are not always completed.

ABPM makes it possible to measure BP routinely during sleep and has reawakened interest in the circadian variation of HR and BP. Most normotensives and perhaps 80 percent of hypertensives have at least a 10 percent drop in BP during sleep compared with the daytime average. Although there may be some important demographic confounders (blacks and the elderly have less prominent "dips"[111]), several prospective studies have shown an increased risk of CV events (and proteinuria in type 1 diabetics[112]) among those with a nocturnal "nondipping" BP or pulse pattern.[107,113–115] However, there is concern, based on several Japanese studies, that elderly persons with more than a 20 percent difference between nighttime and daytime av-

erage BPs ("excessive dippers") may suffer unrecognized ischemia in "watershed areas" (of the brain and other organs) during sleep if their BP declines below the autoregulatory threshold.[108,116,117]

During the last 20 years, research has demonstrated an important correlation between ABPM readings and the prevalence and extent of TOD in hypertensives. Compared with "casual" BP measurements (obtained in the health care provider's office), ABPM measurements clearly are a better predictor of LVH, cardiac function, and overall scores summing optic, carotid, cardiac, renal, and peripheral vascular damage resulting from elevated BP. Ambulatory BP monitoring may also be useful in identifying "white coat normotensives." This term describes a small minority of patients [61 of 234 (26 percent) in the original series from New York City] who have normal BP readings in the physician's office but elevated ABPM readings with LVH and carotid wall thickening similar to that usually seen in sustained hypertensives.[118]

Perhaps the most important data demonstrating the value of ABPM have come from recent studies that included CV events (death, MI, stroke). In the first published study of outcomes in central Italy, ABPM was the best predictor of future CV events; "nondipper hypertensives" had approximately three times the risk of hypertensives whose BP was ≥10 percent lower at night compared to daytime ("dippers"). Continued follow-up and refinements in these analyses come to the same conclusions.[114,115] A population-based study involving 1572 men and women of ABPM versus casual and home BPs has been ongoing since 1987 in Ohasama, Japan. After an average of approximately 5 years of follow-up, there was no significant relationship between one casual BP measurement and future CV mortality. However, there was a highly significantly increased risk of CV death in the quintile with the highest ABPM, and the lowest risk was found in those in the lowest quintile of ABPM.[119] The value of ABPM in refractory hypertension was demonstrated in another study of 86 hypertensive people taking on average three antihypertensive medications daily.[120] Follow-up data were collected approximately 4 years after an ABPM was performed; the patients having ABPM results in the lowest tertile had significantly lower rates of CV complications: 2.2 versus 9.5 versus 13.5 events per 100 patient-years. These data suggest that ABPM may be helpful in sorting out which patients with elevated office BP measurements who already are taking multiple antihypertensive medications ought to have intensified treatment and which ones can be spared the additional expense and risk. Perhaps most impressive were the results of a substudy of the Systolic Hypertension in Europe (Syst-EUR) trial, which involved 808 patients who had ABPM in addition to the usual clinic BP measurements before randomization to placebo or active treatment.[107] In the group randomized to placebo, ABPM was clearly a better predictor of future CV events than was the office BP measurement. Active treatment reduced the difference in prognosis among ambulatory and office measurements. Furthermore, the risk of a CV event was much higher in patients who did not display a nocturnal decline in BP. These data suggest (but do not prove) that the poor prognosis seen with nondipping hypertension can be mitigated by active antihypertensive treatment.

White Coat Hypertension

Approximately 10 to 20 percent of American hypertensives have substantially lower BP measurements outside the health care provider's office than in it[121]; in Italy, the prevalence is 30 percent in pregnancy.[122] The name *white coat hypertension* has been given to the situation in which BP measurements outside the health care setting are considerably lower than those in it, even though the "white coat" itself is unlikely to be the only factor that increases BP. Careful studies originally done in Italy and later corroborated in other countries show that BP rises in response to an approaching physician who is not previously known to the subject. This apparently does not happen if the subject is approached by a nurse even if she or he is wearing a white coat. The pathophysiologic and psychological "reasons" for this exaggerated BP response are obscure.[123]

The clinical consequences and prognostic significance of white coat hypertension continue to be hotly debated in the medical literature. One school of thought suggests that if a person has an acute rise in BP caused by stress related to an approaching physician, similar elevations in BP are likely whenever a stressful stimulus is encountered. Thus, some of the literature supports the concept that the white coat response is merely a precursor to "more substantial and more sustained hypertension." This point of view is buttressed by several clinical and population-based studies in which people with "white coat hypertension" have a greater prevalence of subclinical risk factors for cardiovascular disease (CVD), including LVH, a family history of hypertension and heart disease, hypertriglyceridemia, elevated fasting insulin levels, and lower levels of HDL cholesterol.[124–128]

A second school of thought, based on careful and more conservative definitions of the white coat effect, proposes that some individuals consistently show a similar and marked elevation in BP in response to the health care environment. Using somewhat more stringent criteria than the studies cited above, several long-term studies have shown a greatly reduced risk of either TOD or major CV sequelae among people with lower BPs measured either at home or by 24-h BP monitoring compared with measurements taken in the same person in the physician's office.[102,129] Whether the future risk of such individuals for CV events is similar (or even identical) to that of completely normotensive people is open to question. Another intermediate possibility is that white coat hypertension simply represents regression to the mean in those with considerable BP variability.

The best approach to the treatment of white coat hypertension is unresolved. Clearly, such individuals should benefit from lifestyle modifications, which presumably would reduce the probability of progression to sustained hypertension. Giving no antihypertensive medication to "white coat hypertensives" appears unwise.[130] Even in the largest and longest experience, the risk of future CV events did not differ between white coat and sustained hypertensives when both were treated with antihypertensive medications.[131] Whether intensive treatment with continuous antihypertensive medication is warranted for only temporary increases in BP is debatable. Clearly, the treatment and repeated ABPM sessions required to monitor therapy would not be very cost-effective, compared to the initial session, which has the possibility to limit therapy in 20 percent of those monitored. One ABPM session annually is usually the upper limit.[110] Several authoritative groups have recommended that ABPM be used sparingly in the general hypertensive population but may be more widely used in managed care, veterans' hospitals, and other situations where minimal incremental direct costs are involved.[110]

EVALUATION OF THE HYPERTENSIVE PATIENT

Six key issues must be addressed during the initial office evaluation of a person with elevated BP readings:

- Documenting an accurate diagnosis of hypertension (see above)
- Defining the presence or absence of TOD related to hypertension
- Screening for other CV risk factors that often accompany hypertension
- Stratifying risk for CVD

- Assessing whether the person is likely to have an identifiable cause of hypertension (secondary hypertension) and should have further diagnostic testing to confirm or exclude the diagnosis
- Obtaining data that may be helpful in the initial choice and subsequent choice of therapy

There are many diagnostic possibilities for explaining a single set of elevated BP readings (Tables 61-7 and 61-8). Aside from those who take one of several types of drugs known to elevate BP, many persons with only one elevated BP reading will have their BP decline and return to the normal range. This is the reason for recommending multiple encounters (at least two or three) before a diagnosis of hypertension is firmly established.

Routine Evaluation in All Hypertensive Patients

The recommendations of JNC 7 and other national and international expert panels limit the number of initial tests and the expense related to them for the routine evaluation of a hypertensive patient[4,10,132] (Table 61-9). Those that are used in assessing the presence or absence of TOD include physical examination, blood urea nitrogen (BUN)/creatinine, electrolytes, urinalysis, and an electrocardiogram (ECG). Assessing the number of CV risk factors can be accomplished with the medical history, chemistry panel (glucose, lipid profile), and urinalysis. Although JNC 7 no longer includes a formal risk-stratification system (see Table 61-3), other expert panels have very elaborate systems for linking the assessment of CV risk and the intensity of antihypertensive treatment.[11,132,133]

Several elements of the evaluation of a hypertensive patient warrant further comment. The physical examination should be "directed" toward looking for clues to an identifiable secondary cause of hypertension, such as an abdominal or flank bruit, which would be a sign of renal artery disease, or an abdominal or flank mass, which might be a pheochromocytoma or a polycystic kidney.

Proper examination of the optic fundus is often neglected even though it is a valuable tool for evaluating hypertensive patients. Before effective antihypertensive drug therapy became available, the most important predictor of future CV events was not the BP level but the appearance of the optic fundi. Although the prognosis of hypertensive patients has improved greatly since that time, the appreciation of hypertension-related changes in the optic fundus is still important in the assessment of both the severity and the duration of elevated BP. The optic fundus is the only site in the entire body where blood vessels can be examined directly. Very few patients with a recent onset of hypertension have Keith-Wagener-Barker (KWB) grade III or IV fundi (Table 61-10).

Arteriosclerosis can be directly recognized and the severity and duration of previous hypertension can be estimated through the appreciation of abnormalities of the retinal arteries. The normal yellowish-white color of the retinal arteries gradually changes to a reddish-brown tone ("copper wire"), and the ratio of artery/vein diameters is reduced from the normal 2:3 to less than 1:3. Over time, the column of blood within the artery gradually diminishes and the artery is reduced to a whitish thread ("silver wire") despite a persistent (albeit reduced) flow of blood. "AV nicking" is perhaps the most easily recognized ocular abnormality in hypertension. When the thickened artery containing blood at elevated pressure compresses a low-pressure, thin-walled vein within the shared adventitial sheath, the vein disappears from view. Hypertension is therefore both epidemiologically and pathophysiologically a risk factor for the rare condition retinal vein occlusion.[134] When arterial blood flow is reduced sufficiently to cause infarction of underlying retinal tissue,

TABLE 61-7 Causes of Hypertension

I. Systolic and diastolic hypertension
  A. Primary, essential or idiopathic
  B. Secondary
    1. Renal
      a. Renal parenchymal disease
        (1) Acute glomerulonephritis
        (2) Chronic nephritis
        (3) Polycystic disease
        (4) Diabetic nephropathy
        (5) Hydronephrosis
      b. Renovascular
        (1) Renal artery stenosis
        (2) Intrarenal vasculitis
      c. Renin-producing tumors
      d. Renoprival
      e. Primary sodium retention (Liddle's syndrome, Gordon's syndrome)
    2. Endocrine
      a. Acromegaly
      b. Hypothyroidism
      c. Hyperthyroidism
      d. Hypercalcemia (hyperparathyroidism)
      e. Adrenal
        (1) Cortical
          (a) Cushing's syndrome
          (b) Primary aldosteronism
          (c) Congenital adrenal hyperplasia
          (d) Apparent mineralocorticoid excess (licorice)
        (2) Medullary: pheochromocytoma
      f. Extraadrenal chromaffin tumors
      g. Carcinoid
      h. Exogenous hormones
        (1) Estrogen
        (2) Glucocorticoids
        (3) Mineralocorticoids
        (4) Sympathomimetics
        (5) Tyramine-containing foods and monoamine oxidase inhibitors
    3. Coarctation of the aorta
    4. Pregnancy-induced hypertension
    5. Sleep apnea
    6. Neurologic disorders
      a. Increased intracranial pressure
        (1) Brain tumor
        (2) Encephalitis
        (3) Respiratory acidosis
      b. Quadriplegia
      c. Acute porphyria
      d. Familial dysautonomia
      e. Lead poisoning
      f. Guillain-Barré syndrome
    7. Acute stress, including surgery
      a. Psychogenic hyperventilation
      b. Hypoglycemia
      c. Burns
      d. Pancreatitis
      e. Alcohol withdrawal
      f. Sickle cell crisis
      g. Postresuscitation
      h. Postoperative
    8. Increased intravascular volume
    9. Alcohol and drug use
II. Systolic hypertension
  A. Increased cardiac output
    1. Aortic valvular regurgitation
    2. Atrioventricular fistula, patent ductus arteriosus
    3. Thyrotoxicosis
    4. Paget's disease of bone
    5. Beriberi
    6. Hyperkinetic circulation
  B. Rigidity of aorta
III. Iatrogenic hypertension (see Table 61–8)

SOURCE: Adapted from Kaplan NM: Systemic hypertension: Mechanisms and diagnosis. In: Braunwald E, ed. *Heart Disease,* 5th ed. Philadelphia: Saunders; 1997:807–839.

TABLE 61-8 Partial List of Drugs Known to Elevate Blood Pressure

Nonsteroidal anti-inflammatory drugs
Sympathomimetic amines (e.g., phenylpropanolamines)
Estrogen and estrogen analogues (e.g., oral contraceptive pills and hormone replacement therapy)
Corticosteroids
Methylxanthines (e.g., theophylline, caffeine, theobromine)
Cyclosporine
Erythropoietin
Cocaine
Nicotine
Phencyclidine ("angel dust")
"Herbal ecstasy" (and other ephedra-containing substances)
Withdrawal from certain drugs (e.g., beta blockers, alpha agonists, opioids, ethanol, calcium antagonists)

TABLE 61-9 Tests Recommended by JNC 7 for the Initial Evaluation of a Hypertensive Patient

Serum chemistry (glucose, potassium, creatinine)
Urinalysis
Electrocardiogram
Fasting lipid profile (including HDL cholesterol, triglycerides, and calculated LDL cholesterol)

Optional tests:
  Estimate of urinary albumin excretion (24-h urine or urinary albumin/creatinine ratio)
Serum calcium

SOURCE: Adapted from JNC 7.[4]

TABLE 61-10 Keith-Wagener-Barker Classification of Optic Fundi

Grade	Characteristic Finding
I	Arterial tortuosity, localized arterial spasm or narrowing (relative to neighboring vein), "silver wiring"
II	Extensive or generalized arteriolar narrowing, resulting in arteriovenous crossing changes ("arterial nicking")
III	Hemorrhages or exudates
IV	Papilledema

round to oval white patches with fluffy borders are formed ("cytoid bodies" or "cotton-wool spots"). After breakdown in the blood-retinal barrier (caused by a ruptured aneurysm, neovascularization—typically in diabetics—or "blowout" hemorrhages resulting from hypertension), intraretinal "flame shaped" hemorrhages can be recognized by direct ophthalmoscopy. The leakage of plasma into the macular space often causes an acute reduction in vision and leaves behind the "macular star figure" for years thereafter. Grade IV retinopathy (papilledema), which is the hallmark of either retinal vein occlusion or a hypertensive emergency, is usually caused by ischemia in the optic nerve circulation resulting from increased intraocular or intracranial pressure and diminished axoplasmic flow in the optic nerve fibers. In some cases, particularly when BP is not exceedingly high and there is no other evidence of acute TOD from a hypertensive emergency, another cause should be sought. Papilledema without other evidence of hypertensive retinopathy is generally due to another etiology.

The impact of controlling hypertension on ophthalmic endpoints (e.g., vision loss, retinal hemorrhages, and laser photocoagulation procedures) has not received much attention in the recent medical literature. There are nonetheless several reports of reduced risk of these endpoints in several clinical trials that assessed their incidence prospectively, particularly among diabetic hypertensives.[135]

Cardiac Evaluation

One of the most important elements of the physical examination of hypertensive patients is the cardiac examination. An atrial (S_4) gallop is an extremely common finding and may be a vital clue to the presence of hypertensive heart disease.

A key part of the laboratory evaluation is directed at determining whether LVH is present. The ECG is currently recommended as part of the initial evaluation of all persons with hypertension. Not only is the ECG useful in documenting previously undetected MI, myocardial ischemia, and/or cardiac rhythm disturbances but it is also the least expensive and possibly the most cost-effective way to diagnose and/or exclude LVH. Compared with echocardiography, computed tomography (CT), or magnetic resonance imaging (MRI) of the heart, the ECG is perhaps only 10 to 50 percent sensitive (depending on which criteria are used) and at best 80 percent specific. Nonetheless, the greater expense of these more accurate methods of screening for LVH limits their use. A "limited echocardiogram" that accurately calculates left ventricular (LV) size at a very affordable price and also provides information about ventricular geometry has been recommended but has not been commonly endorsed by third-party or other payers.

The prognostic significance of LVH among hypertensive patients is well established. LVH is often considered the "hemoglobin A_{1c} of BP," since it is an objective measure of both the severity and the duration of elevations in BP. In the Framingham Heart Study, ECG evidence of LVH was associated with an approximately threefold increase in the incidence of CV events. Echocardiographically detected LVH appears to predict an even greater incremental increase in the risk of future CV events, although the geometry of the ventricle may also play a role. Hypertension is typically associated with concentric hypertrophy of the ventricle, perhaps as a result of concentric remodeling, which in one series carried a fourfold increased risk of cardiac morbidity and mortality (compared with nonhypertrophied hearts). Eccentric hypertrophy, typically seen in response to exercise in athletes, imparted only a twofold increased risk of events in the same series. In several reports from various locales, in both univariate and multivariate models, LVH was the most powerful of any of the traditional CV risk factors in predicting not only death or MI but also stroke, HF, and other CV endpoints.[136] Although research studies including thousands of people have demonstrated the importance of echocardiographically determined measurements of LV mass, there is concern that the intrinsic variability of a single echocardiogram is sufficiently high (perhaps 10 to 15 percent) that serial determinations in a usual hypertensive individual are unlikely to be cost-effective. An exception may be a person with stage 1 hypertension, in whom the presence of this form of LVH would indicate the need for antihypertensive drug therapy earlier than it might have been given if the clinician had thought the patient was free of TOD.

LVH is associated both epidemiologically and pathophysiologically with intimal hyperplasia of the epicardial coronary arteries, increased coronary vascular resistance, increased severity and frequency of ventricular dysrhythmias, decreased flow reserve, and reduced diastolic relaxation. At the extreme, diastolic dysfunction and restrictive cardiomyopathy result clinically in "flash pulmonary edema" despite a normal ejection fraction and carry a poor prognosis, even when carefully defined.[137,138] Although this phenomenon is not well understood, some feel that hypertension plays the major role in the pathogenesis of this syndrome, which has been identified in up to 40 percent of patients presenting to the hospital with HF. Because of its status as a powerful risk factor for cardiovascular events, LVH (by the new Cornell voltage-duration method) was the major inclusion criterion for the recent LIFE (Losartan Intervention For Endpoint reduction) Study. In this important clinical trial, the ARB ± diuretic was more effective at reducing cardiovascular risk than a beta blocker ± diuretic; nearly all of the benefit was in the reduction of stroke.[139]

The most difficult aspect of LVH is the importance of its reversal and how to achieve it. The results of short-term clinical studies evaluating changes in LVH have come to different conclusions about which class of antihypertensive drug regresses LVH better or quicker. The LIFE Study is, so far, the only outcome study to show, as a primary or secondary endpoint, a correlation between reduction in LVH and an improvement in prognosis. Most studies agree that LVH is unlikely to regress without reducing BP; most authorities therefore recommend spending resources on achieving BP control rather than on serial echocardiograms to see if the LV mass index is returning toward normal.

Renal Evaluation

Current recommendations for the evaluation of renal function include only serum BUN and creatinine, and a dipstick for proteinuria. An additional test for microalbuminuria (MA) (albumin in the urine between 30 and 300 mg/day, below the detectable range of the conventional dipstick) is recommended by the National Kidney Foundation.[140] MA is a powerful independent risk factor for CV events, in both diabetics and nondiabetics.[140–143]

The prevalence of MA in type 2 diabetics is about 20 percent (range, 12 to 36 percent), and is more common (about 30 percent) in those older than 55.[140,141] The prevalence of MA ranges from 5 to 40 percent in nondiabetic hypertensives.[141] Lipid abnormalities (especially elevated LDL cholesterol), duration of hypertension, and BP control all contribute to this variability in MA prevalence in essential hypertensives. MA may be a marker for BP control, since BP control using all agents except dihydropyridine CA and central or peripheral sympathetic blockers reduces albuminuria.[144] The degree of MA is proportional to the severity of systolic, diastolic, and mean BP elevation as measured by either clinic or 24-h ambulatory BP monitoring.[145–147] Last, circadian abnormalities of BP observed in nondippers (see above), who are known to be at higher risk for CVD, are also associated with a higher prevalence of MA.

The pathophysiology of how MA contributes to or accelerates the atherosclerotic process is uncertain. MA may be due to increased vascular permeability and, hence, altered barrier function of the endothelium.[145,146] People with MA have an elevated transcapillary escape rate of albumin, regardless of whether they have preexisting DM. Moreover, when albumin leaks into the interstitial space, cellular injury occurs secondary to free radicals and cytokine production enhanced by the presence of albumin. MA may be another manifestation of the metabolic components of syndrome X[75] (see above).

By simply using a conventional dipstick, which can detect only higher levels of urinary protein (>300 mg/24 h), the clinician may miss an opportunity to characterize a patient's prognosis more precisely at the initial visit. Dipsticks that detect MA are available and inexpensive. Some recommend that all hypertensives with "trace" proteinuria by conventional dipstick (generally 300 to 500 mg/day) should have a spot urine measurement of the albumin/creatinine ratio.[140] Routine assessment of MA for diabetic patients is well advised, but in hypertensives without DM, its value is still debatable. In part this is due to the relatively low prevalence of MA and the uncertainty of the significance of its modification in the nondiabetic population.

Subjects with MA and type 2 DM have an annual total and CV mortality about four times higher than that of diabetics without MA.[140] In several series, the CV event and mortality rates in nondiabetic hypertensives with MA were two- to fourfold higher than in those without MA.[143,148] MA is also associated with other types of hypertension-related TOD, including LVH. These associations are not as commonly seen in younger individuals or those with stage 1 hypertension, suggesting that the association of MA and LVH may be related to a higher BP load.

Evaluation of the Vasculature

One of the hallmarks of the hypertensive circulation is decreased vascular compliance. Acutely elevated BP affects the elastic behavior of both large and small arteries, such that the muscular layers of the arterial wall are unable to relax as quickly and transmit pressure waves as easily and reproducibly as they can when BP is lower. This is a passive and reversible phenomenon that typically lasts minutes to hours. Over a prolonged period, however, there is a gradual infiltration of the internal elastic lamina of blood vessels with thinned, split, and frayed elastic fibers and a laying down of new intercellular matrix; in extreme cases, medial necrosis is found within the arterial wall. This process—which is attributed to aging, hypertension, or a

combination of the two—is often described as "arteriosclerosis," since it leads to chronic and generally irreversible stiffening of the arterial tree.

There are several methods of assessing arterial compliance, but most are invasive, expensive, or not widely used in clinical medicine.[149] Several new methods for calculating total arterial compliance are based on pulse contour analysis[150] but are only now being used in large clinical studies.[151–153] Whether arterial compliance measurements should be used routinely to evaluate hypertensives remains to be seen.[154]

Pseudohypertension is the name given to the rare circumstance in which BP measurements by the usual indirect sphygmomanometry are much higher than direct intraarterial measurements; these differences are usually attributed to very "stiff" and calcified arteries that are nearly impossible to compress with the bladder in the usual BP cuff. The "Osler maneuver" (palpating the walls of the brachial artery when blood flow has been interrupted by inflating the cuff higher than systolic pressure) has been recommended as a simple measure to diagnose this condition. This technique is less accurate than initially reported, and the authors do not recommend it. Because the diagnosis requires an expensive and potentially dangerous intraarterial measurement (and perhaps an infusion of an intravenous antihypertensive agent to "calibrate" the difference between indirect and direct BP measurements), few clinicians routinely check for and diagnose pseudohypertension.

The benefits of lowering BP in older patients with "stiff" arteries, however, are well established.[155] Three clinical trials specifically involving isolated systolic hypertension [systolic BP (SBP) ≥160 mmHg with diastolic BP (DBP) <90 or <95 mmHg] each showed that older individuals with BP elevations only in systolic BP (a typical finding in patients with reduced vascular compliance) have a reduced risk of CV events with pharmacologic treatment.[155–157] Whether arterial compliance should be measured as a predictor of CV risk and measured serially over time is controversial; perhaps it would not be as cost-effective as serial BP determinations during treatment.

Other Evaluation

Other blood tests such as PRA and serum insulin have been abandoned for routine or even specialized evaluation for all hypertensive patients. Some newly appreciated markers of CV risk, such as C-reactive protein and homocysteine, have not yet been shown to be sensitive or specific enough to warrant routine testing, but interest in these markers is growing.[158,159]

Evaluation for Identifiable Causes of Hypertension

There are many identifiable causes of hypertension (secondary hypertension). In patients with some of these causes, the elevation of BP can be eliminated with specific treatment such as angioplasty or surgical therapy or by removing the agent that caused the hypertension. By far the most common identifiable cause is chronic renal failure. Although chronic renal disease can almost never be cured, the hypertension associated with it can often be controlled with adequate diuresis or dialysis and the use of other drugs. Renal artery stenosis, pheochromocytoma, and primary aldosteronism, however, are potentially curable. These conditions are encountered commonly enough that the clinician seeing a hypertensive patient must have a high index of suspicion in the appropriate clinical setting and should order the specialized tests necessary to screen for and confirm the diagnosis. Other etiologies—such as specific enzyme deficiencies, coarctation of the aorta, and Ask-Upmark kidney—are distinctly rare. This section covers only the most common of all the etiologies listed in Table 61-7. If a secondary cause of hypertension is suspected, a referral to a hypertension specialist may be appropriate.[7,132]

RENOVASCULAR HYPERTENSION

Patients with this form of secondary hypertension often have stage 2 hypertension and considerable TOD and are at risk of losing renal function. At least 90 percent of cases of renovascular hypertension now are due to renal artery atherosclerosis, with only 10 percent being due to fibromuscular dysplasia or unusual causes.[160] Atherosclerotic renal artery stenosis is a disease of older individuals. Characteristically, these patients develop hypertension after age 50 or have a history of hypertension that had been relatively easy to control and became refractory. A large proportion of these patients have evidence of vascular disease elsewhere (carotids, coronaries, and peripheral circulation in particular), and the majority are or were cigarette smokers, often heavy smokers. Although it is more common in whites, blacks also can develop atherosclerotic renovascular hypertension. Fibromuscular dysplasia tends to affect young white women, in whom BP tends to rise abruptly to stage 2 during the third decade of life. Abdominal or frank bruits are heard commonly, and renal function is usually normal when the diagnosis is entertained.

Laboratory Testing   The objective of laboratory testing in patients suspected of having renovascular hypertension is not only to verify that arterial lesions are present but also to determine that the lesion that is discovered is in fact the cause of the patient's hypertension.[160] The clinical situations in which renovascular disease should be suspected are listed in Table 61-11. The tests used to screen for renovascular hypertension are biochemical or depend on a variety of imaging techniques (Table 61-12).

Biochemical   Measurement of serum K^+ (which, if low, may indicate hyperaldosteronism) or PRA (which, if high, may confirm activation of the RAA system) plays no role in case finding for renovascular hypertension because the sensitivity and specificity are too low. Even measuring the PRA after captopril (the so-called captopril test) has a sensitivity of only 60 to 70 percent, although better results have been obtained in some series. Measuring the concentration and activity of renin simultaneously from each renal vein and computing the renal vein renin ratio was once a very popular approach, but the sensitivity and specificity for detection of renovascular hypertension with this test are both approximately 75 percent, unacceptably low for an invasive procedure that requires special expertise and sophisticated measurements. This ratio may still be useful to help prove that an anatomic lesion is also the cause of a patient's hypertension, but it should not be used as a screening tool.[161]

Imaging   Rapid-sequence intravenous pyelography and standard renal scanning were the earliest noninvasive imaging studies used for diagnosing renovascular hypertension. Even though in expert hands each has reasonable sensitivity (65 to 70 percent for scanning and 75 percent for pyelography), neither has a place in the diagnostic approach any longer. Renal duplex ultrasound has the advantage of being noninvasive and widely available. In some laboratories, the sensitivity of this test approaches 90 to 95 percent.[162] However, abdominal gas or fat may make it difficult to visualize the renal arteries, and the test is very operator-dependent. In specialized centers with special expertise and in selected patients, it is a useful test. In many settings, however, little is gained by using this technique. Gadolinium-enhanced MRI and CT angiography are new and more

expensive approaches to visualization of the renal arteries; they are becoming more widely available and are noninvasive.[163] However, until the image quality improves and the cost decreases, these techniques are not likely to replace angiography when visualization of the renal arteries is required.

TABLE 61-11 Testing for Renovascular Hypertension: Clinical Index of Suspicion as a Guide to Selecting Patients for Workup

Low (should not be tested)
Stage 1 or 2 hypertension in the absence of clinical clues

Moderate (noninvasive screening test recommended)
Stage 3 hypertension (JNC VI: $\geq 180/\geq 110$ mmHg)
Hypertension refractory to standard therapy
Abrupt onset of sustained stages 2–3 hypertension at age <20 years
Hypertension with a suggestive abdominal bruit (long, high-pitched, and localized to the region of the renal artery)
Stages 2–3 hypertension (diastolic BP exceeding 105 mmHg) in a smoker, in a patient with evidence of occlusive vascular disease (cerebrovascular, coronary, peripheral vascular), or in a patient with unexplained but stable elevation of serum creatinine

High (may consider proceeding directly to arteriography)
Stage 3 hypertension with either progressive renal insufficiency or refractoriness to aggressive treatment, particularly in a patient who has been a smoker or has other evidence of occlusive arterial disease
Accelerated or malignant hypertension (grade III or IV retinopathy)
Hypertension with recent elevation of serum creatinine, either unexplained or reversibly induced by an angiotensin-converting enzyme inhibitor or angiotensin II receptor blocker
Moderate to severe hypertension with incidentally detected asymmetry of renal size

SOURCE: Adapted from Mann SL, Pickering TG. Detection of renovascular hypertension: State of the art: 1992. *Ann Intern Med* 1992;117:845.

TABLE 61-12 Detection of Renovascular Hypertension

Biochemical
Serum K^+
PRA (peripheral renin assay, or originally "activity")[a]
Renal vein renin activity[a]
Split renal function tests[a]

Imaging
Rapid-sequence intravenous pyelography[a]
Renography[a]
Captopril (or enalaprilat) renography
Intraarterial digital subtraction angiography
Standard angiography
Duplex renal ultrasound
Magnetic resonance angiography

[a]Designates tests that are seldom used today.

Isotopic renography with labeled diethylenetriamine pentaacetic acid (DTPA, a measure of glomerular filtration) or MAG-3 (a measure of renal blood flow) with captopril is a minimally invasive test that detects a discrepancy between perfusion and function of the kidneys. The overall sensitivity and specificity are 90 percent when done carefully, especially in patients whose prior probability of having renovascular hypertension is high.[164] Only ACE inhibitors and ARBs need to be stopped before the test is performed, and adverse reactions from the single dose of captopril are rare. Isotopic renography with captopril also provides functional information. If the time to peak activity is initially normal and becomes abnormal after captopril ("captopril-induced changes"), the likelihood of cure or improvement after revascularization is high.

Intraarterial digital subtraction angiography is most frequently performed to define the renal artery anatomy and determine whether an arterial narrowing is present. In addition, the type of lesion (ostial, nonostial, or branch) can be determined. The disadvantages of this technique are the intraarterial puncture, high cost, and risk of contrast-induced renal impairment. In many centers, percutaneous renal angioplasty is done at the same time if indicated.

A recent clinical trial and a large series have shown little benefit to routine revascularization of renal arteries as compared to medical treatment.[165,166] The authors are generally not in favor of revascularization unless hypertension is resistant, renal function declines, or evidence has been obtained (a positive captopril renogram with captopril-induced changes or a renal vein renin ratio >1.5) that the lesion is functionally significant. The presence of anatomic renal artery stenosis does not mean that the lesion is responsible for the elevation in BP (functional renal artery stenosis).

In considering whether to proceed with screening for renovascular disease, the clinician must consider how the data will be used. In many hypertensive patients with renovascular hypertension, BP can be controlled adequately with medical therapy.[165] If the risk of surgery or angioplasty is viewed as unacceptably high or if the patient will not consent to having a revascularization procedure if a remediable lesion is discovered, any specific further evaluation may not be appropriate.

PHEOCHROMOCYTOMA

Patients with pheochromocytoma are almost always symptomatic on presentation, usually with a characteristic cluster of complaints that occurs in paroxysms or "spells."[167] The description of the spell tends to be typical and is usually the same in each patient. The spells may occur many times a day or may be separated by weeks or months. Often there is a characteristic trigger (change in position, certain foods, trauma, pain, or drugs) that should increase the clinician's index of suspicion for pheochromocytoma. Hypertension is not usually paroxysmal, as has often been stated, with some BPs elevated and some normal. Most measurements are in fact in the hypertensive range, although wide variability is the rule. The three most common symptoms of pheochromocytoma are headache, diaphoresis, and palpitations (Table 61-13). Many other symptoms—particularly anxiety, weakness, and tremulousness—are also quite common. The pattern of symptoms can provide guidance about the predominant hormone secreted by the tumor. When norepinephrine is the primary hormone produced, pallor is usually the symptom. Flushing is more likely if substantial amounts of epinephrine are produced.

Laboratory Testing for Pheochromocytoma Whereas it is possible and sometimes desirable to manage hypertensive patients with renovascular hypertension or states of mineralocorticoid excess using medical therapy, it is almost always imperative to remove a

TABLE 61-13 Symptoms and Signs of Pheochromocytoma

Symptoms[a]	Frequency, %
Headaches	40–96
Diaphoresis	40–74
Palpitations	45–70
Pallor	40–45
Nervousness and/or anxiety	22–43
Tremulousness	29–31
Signs[b]	**Frequency, %**
Hypertension	>90
Sustained	50–60
Intermittent	2–50
Paroxysms	50
Weight loss (hypermetabolic state)	80
Funduscopic changes	50–70
Orthostatic hypotension	40–70

[a]Infrequent symptoms: flushing, Raynaud's phenomenon, nausea, seizures, dizziness, dyspnea, and abdominal, chest, or arm pain.
[b]Infrequent signs: acrocyanosis, bradycardia, fever, and glucose intolerance.

pheochromocytoma. As with renovascular hypertension, once the clinical presentation suggests that a pheochromocytoma may be the cause of a patient's hypertension, a variety of tests are available to confirm the diagnosis (Table 61-14). If a pheochromocytoma is suspected, biochemical confirmation of an increase in catecholamine production should be sought. Despite recent enthusiasm for plasma metanephrines in some centers,[168,169] measurement of 24-h urinary excretion of total catecholamines (norepinephrine, epinephrine, and dopamine) or their metabolites (vanillylmandelic acid or metanephrines) costs much less and is only a little less sensitive and specific.[170] Whether urine or plasma is assayed, attention must be paid to the conditions under which the sample is collected; creatinine should be measured in the same urine sample to verify that there was a full 24-h collection. To reduce the number of false-positive results, the patient should be in a nonstressful situation when the sample is obtained.

When urinary values are nondiagnostic, the measurement of plasma catecholamines and/or metanephrines can be very useful.[168,169]

TABLE 61-14 Diagnostic Tests for Pheochromocytoma

Biochemical
  Urinary free catecholamines
  Urinary vanillylmandelic acid
  Urinary metanephrines
  Plasma catecholamines (or metanephrines)
  Clonidine suppression test
  Glucagon stimulation test
Imaging studies
  Computed axial tomography
  Magnetic resonance imaging (especially T_2-weighted images)
  ^{123}I–meta-iodobenzylguanidine
  Abdominal ultrasound
  Adrenal vein or vena caval drainage
  Angiography

If plasma catecholamines (norepinephrine plus epinephrine) levels exceed 2000 pg/mL in the basal state, the presence of a pheochromocytoma is highly likely. If the levels are less than 1000 pg/mL, the diagnosis is very unlikely; whereas in patients with plasma catecholamine levels between 1000 and 2000 pg/mL, the clonidine suppression test may be useful.[167] If plasma catecholamine levels do not suppress after the administration of 0.3 mg of oral clonidine in an appropriately prepared and monitored patient, a further aggressive search for a pheochromocytoma is warranted.

The choice of which initial imaging procedure to obtain is also somewhat controversial.[171] CT scanning is a highly sensitive imaging modality that will locate nearly all pheochromocytomas, especially those in the adrenal gland or the abdomen. MRI has the advantage of not requiring contrast material (which is sometimes necessary with CT scanning) and is also helpful in localizing nonadrenal or nonabdominal pheochromocytomas. Enhancement of the T2-weighted images happens virtually only with pheochromocytomas and adrenal carcinomas, helping distinguish adrenal masses that are not biochemically active (so-called incidentalomas) from metabolically active or malignant tumors.

The use of iodine-123 metaiodobenzylguanidine (^{123}I MIBG) scanning has been particularly helpful when a pheochromocytoma is suspected but is not clearly located with CT or MRI. This radiopharmaceutical is a guanethidine analogue that is concentrated in pheochromocytomas and other neural crest tumors.[172] Using total-body scanning helps localize the tumor if the initial CT or MRI scans are negative or equivocal. The sensitivity of this test exceeds 90 percent, but it is not widely available.

PRIMARY ALDOSTERONISM

In an untreated hypertensive patient with significant hypokalemia (serum K^+ ≤3.2 meq/L), renal K^+ wasting (24-h urinary K^+ >30 meq), PRA below 1 ng/mL per hour, and elevated plasma or urinary aldosterone values, the diagnosis is unequivocal. Often, however, the diagnosis is not so obvious because the values are not as definitive; in such cases, multiple measurements are needed during salt loading.

The single best test in people with normal renal function for identifying patients with primary aldosteronism is the measurement of 24-h urinary aldosterone excretion during salt loading[173,174] (Table 61-15). An excretion rate of >14 μg of aldosterone in 24 h after 3 days of salt loading (greater than 200 meq/day) distinguishes most patients with primary aldosteronism from those with essential hypertension. Only 7 percent of patients with primary aldosteronism have values that fall within the range for essential hypertension. In contrast, about 39 percent of patients with primary aldosteronism have plasma aldosterone values that fall within the range for essential hypertension.[173] The findings of hypokalemia and suppressed PRA provide corroborative evidence, but the absence of either or both does not preclude the diagnosis.

A substantial number of patients with primary aldosteronism, however, do not present with hypokalemia; serum K^+ concentration is normal in 7 to 38 percent of reported cases. In addition, 10 to 12 percent of patients with proven tumors may not have hypokalemia during short-term salt loading. Plasma renin activity <1 ng/mL per hour or one that fails to rise above 2 ng/mL per hour after salt and water depletion and upright posture has been used as an additional test to exclude primary aldosteronism. However, about 35 percent of patients with the disease have values that rise >2 ng/mL per hour when appropriately stimulated. In addition, about 40 percent of subjects with essential hypertension have suppressed PRA, and 15 to 20 percent of these patients have values <2 ng/mL per hour under conditions of stimulation.[175]

The plasma aldosterone/renin ratio has been used to define the appropriateness of PRA for the circulating concentrations of aldosterone and probably has low specificity as a screening test.[175] It is assumed that the volume expansion associated with excessive aldosterone production inhibits the synthesis of renin without affecting the autonomous production of aldosterone. Both tests are subject to the same limitations: first, there is inherent variability of plasma levels of aldosterone even in the presence of a tumor, and this translates into variability in the absolute value of the ratio; second, the use of drugs that result in marked and prolonged stimulation of renin long after their discontinuation may alter the ratio.

The most common cause of primary aldosteronism is an aldosterone-producing adenoma (70 to 80 percent of all proven cases). Approximately 20 to 30 percent of cases are caused by hyperplasia of the zona glomerulosa layer of the adrenal cortex (bilateral adrenal hyperplasia). Some reports suggest the occurrence of a syndrome intermediate between adenoma and hyperplasia. The distinction between these two processes is important, because surgical intervention is likely to be curative in the majority of adenomas and fails to reduce BP in patients with bilateral adrenal hyperplasia.[176]

An adenoma is likely in the presence of spontaneous hypokalemia <3.0 meq/L, plasma 18-hydroxycorticosterone values >100 ng/dL, and an anomalous postural decrease in plasma aldosterone concentration. In addition, adenomas are largely unresponsive to changes in sodium balance and appear to be exquisitely sensitive to ACTH, unlike hyperplasias, which are more sensitive to angiotensin II infusions. Plasma 18-hydroxycorticosterone values <100 ng/dL, a postural increase in aldosterone, or both are findings usually associated with hyperplasia, but they do not completely rule out the presence of an adenoma.

An adrenal CT scan should be the initial step in tumor localization. It is noninvasive, and all adenomas ≥1.5 cm in diameter can be located accurately. Only 60 percent of nodules measuring between 1 and 1.4 cm in diameter are detected by CT scanning. Nodules <1 cm in diameter are very difficult if not impossible to demonstrate. The overall sensitivity of localizing adenomas by high-resolution CT scanning exceeds 90 percent. Adrenal venous aldosterone levels should be measured when the biochemical findings are highly suggestive of an adenoma, but the adrenal CT scan is ambiguous.

Medical therapy is indicated in patients with adrenal hyperplasia, patients with an adenoma who are poor surgical risks, and those with

---

TABLE 61-15 Diagnostic Studies for Mineralocorticoid Excess States

Biochemical
Serum potassium
Plasma renin activity
Plasma aldosterone
Plasma aldosterone/renin ratio
24-h urinary aldosterone excretion
Plasma 18-hydroxycorticosterone
Plasma 18-oxocortisol
Plasma 18-hydroxycortisol
Adrenal vein sampling for aldosterone

Imaging studies
Abdominal ultrasound
Computed axial tomography
Iodocholesterol scanning
Adrenal venography

bilateral adrenal adenomas that may require bilateral adrenalectomy. Total bilateral adrenalectomy has no place in the management of primary aldosteronism. The long-standing experience has been that the hypertension associated with primary aldosteronism is salt- and water-dependent and is best treated with sustained salt and water depletion.[177,178] The usual doses of diuretic agents are hydrochlorothiazide 25 to 50 mg/day or furosemide 80 to 160 mg/day in combination with either spironolactone 100 to 200 mg/day or amiloride 10 to 20 mg/day. These combinations usually result in prompt correction of hypokalemia and normalization of BP within 2 to 4 weeks.

In the majority of patients with an aldosterone-producing adenoma, surgical excision leads to normotension as well as reversal of the biochemical defects.[176] One year postoperatively, about 70 percent of patients are normotensive, but 5 years postoperatively, only 53 percent remain normotensive. The restoration of normal K^+ homeostasis is permanent. Patients undergoing surgery should receive drug treatment for a least 8 to 10 weeks both to decrease BP and to correct metabolic abnormalities. These patients have a significant K^+ deficiency that must be corrected preoperatively because hypokalemia increases the risk of cardiac arrhythmias during anesthesia.

After the removal of an aldosterone-producing adenoma, selective hypoaldosteronism usually occurs, even in patients whose PRA had been stimulated with chronic diuretic therapy. Potassium supplementation should be given cautiously and serum K^+ values monitored closely. Sufficient residual mineralocorticoid activity is often left to prevent excessive renal retention of K^+ provided that Na^+ intake is adequate. Abnormalities in aldosterone production can persist for as long as 3 months after tumor removal.

OTHER FORMS OF IDENTIFIABLE SECONDARY HYPERTENSION

In addition to these three most common and potentially curable forms of identifiable secondary hypertension, there are a vast number of rare conditions in which the genetic defect leading to hypertension is unknown. These include enzyme deficiencies such as 11-α-hydroxylase deficiency and 17-β-hydroxylase deficiency, other congenital disorders such as the Ask-Upmark kidney, trauma such as the Page kidney, urologic causes such as hydronephrosis, endocrine abnormalities such as Cushing's syndrome and Cushing's disease, and even infectious etiologies such as renal tuberculosis. The elevated BP may be the first clue to these diagnoses. Two causes of identifiable hypertension are not rare, and all clinicians will see patients with iatrogenic hypertension (Table 61-8) and with sleep apnea. Any of the drugs or other substances listed in the table should be stopped before one concludes that a patient has hypertension. The relation of sleep apnea to hypertension and obesity has long been recognized.[179] The typical clinical presentation of sleep apnea (daytime drowsiness, snoring) in an obese hypertensive should alert the clinician to this disorder.

TREATMENT OF HYPERTENSION

Patients with JNC 7 stage 2 hypertension (SBP $\geq$160 mmHg or DBP $\geq$100 mmHg) should receive drug therapy, usually with two agents, once their hypertension has been diagnosed and confirmed (Table 61-3).[4] Patients with stage 1 hypertension should receive lifestyle modifications (Table 61-16) and pharmacologic therapy (typically beginning with a thiazide-type diuretic; Table 61-17) unless goal BP is achieved without drugs.[4] Individuals with prehypertension should receive lifestyle modifications unless they have diabetes or renal impairment. Whenever these conditions are present, the BP should be

TABLE 61-16 Lifestyle Modifications for Prevention and Treatment of Hypertension

Primary lifestyle modifications that lower blood pressure

Attain and maintain normal body weight for adults (body mass index, 18.5–24.9 kg/m^2)

Reduce dietary sodium intake to no more than 100 mmol/day (approximately 6 g of sodium chloride or 2.4 g of sodium per day)

Engage in regular aerobic physical activity, such as brisk walking (at least 30 min per day, most days of the week)

Limit alcohol consumption to no more than 1 oz (30 mL) of ethanol [e.g., 24 oz (720 mL) of beer, 10 oz (300 mL) of wine, or 2 oz (60 mL) of 100-proof spirits] per day in most men; no more than 0.5 oz (15 mL) of ethanol per day in women and lighter-weight persons

Maintain adequate intake of dietary potassium [>90 mmol (3500 mg) per day]

Consume a diet that is rich in fruits and vegetables and in low-fat dairy products, with a reduced content of saturated and total fat [e.g., the Dietary Approaches to Stop Hypertension (DASH) diet]

Routinely recommended lifestyle modifications

Avoid tobacco (lowers cardiovascular risk independently of any effect on blood pressure)

Consume fish (improves lipid profile and reduces cardiovascular risk more than blood pressure–lowering effect could)

Increase dietary fiber (improves lipid profile and reduces cancer risk independently of any effect on blood pressure)

Lifestyle modifications not routinely recommended

Biofeedback
Dietary calcium supplementation
Dietary magnesium supplementation
Micronutrient supplementation

SOURCE: Adapted from Whelton et al.[6] With permission.

less than 130/80 mmHg, and drug therapy plus lifestyle modifications are recommended. In all situations, if there is a "compelling indication" for the use of a specific type of antihypertensive drug (see Table 6-18), that drug should be given, because it improves the prognosis in that condition, according to clinical trial data.[4]

Lifestyle Modifications

The JNC 7 report builds on a recent Advisory from the National High Blood Pressure Education Program to recommended weight loss for obese hypertensive patients, modification of dietary Na^+ intake to $\leq$100 mmol/day, and modification of alcohol intake to no more than two drinks per day.[4,6] Both also recommended an increase in physical activity for all patients with hypertension who have no specific condition that would make such a recommendation not applicable or safe. For many patients these suggestions are not practicable or are already being implemented; therefore drug therapy may be indicated even sooner in these situations.

There is little doubt that lifestyle factors such as diet, exercise, and stress can affect BP.[6] There is a strong positive correlation between the level of body weight and body mass index (weight/height^2)

TABLE 61-17 Commonly Used Oral Antihypertensive Drugs by Pharmacologic Class

Drug	Dose, mg/day	Doses per Day	Mechanism of Action	Special Considerations
Diuretics				
Thiazides and related drugs			Decrease body sodium and extracellular fluid volume	More effective antihypertensive agents than loop diuretics unless serum creatinine is > 2 mg/dL, or creatinine clearance is ≤50 mL/min
Chlorthalidone	12.5–25	1		
Hydrochlorothiazide	12.5–25	1		
Loop diuretics			Inhibit $2Cl^-Na^+$ pump in ascending loop of Henle	Effective even in patients with advanced renal failure or heart failure
Furosemide	20–320	2		
Torsemide	5–100	1		
Potassium-sparing diuretics			Increase K^+ reabsorption	Weak diuretics if used alone; may cause hyperkalemia in patients with serum creatinine > 2.5 mg/dL, particularly if combined with ACE-I, ARBs, K^+ supplements, or NSAIDs
Amiloride	5–20	1		
Triamterene	37.5–75	1		
Spironolactone	12.5–50	2–3	Aldosterone antagonist	
Eplerenone	25–100	1	Selective aldosterone antagonist	
Adrenergic inhibitors				
Beta blockers				
Cardioselective			Inhibit beta$_1$ receptors, decrease CO, decrease heart rate, increase SVR	In higher doses, inhibit beta$_2$ receptors
Atenolol	25–100	1		
Metoprolol	50–200	1–2		
Noncardioselective			Inhibit both beta$_1$ and beta$_2$ receptors	Asthma more likely
Nadolol	20–240	1		
Propranolol	40–360	1–3		
Timolol	20–40	2		
With intrinsic sympathomimetic activity (ISA)			Have partial agonist activity	Less bradycardia and hypertriglyceridemia than those without ISA
Acebutolol	200–1200	2		
Pindolol	10–60	2		
Antiadrenergic agents				
Centrally acting			Stimulate alpha$_2$-adrenergic receptors in the brain, resulting in inhibition of efferent sympathetic activity; decrease SVR	Sudden withdrawal may result in hypertensive crisis
α-Methyldopa	250–1500	2		
Clonidine	0.1–0.6	2		
Clonidine TTS (patch)	0.1–0.3	Once **weekly**		
Selective α_1-blockers			Inhibit α_1-adrenergic receptors; decrease SVR, CO may increase slightly	First dose hypotension; cause orthostatic hypotension
Doxazosin	1–16	1		
Terasozin	1–20	1		
α,β Blockers			Block both α and β adrenergic receptors	
Labetalol	200–800	2–3		
Carvedilol	6.25–50	2		
Calcium Antagonists			Block entry of calcium into vascular smooth muscle cells; decrease SVR	
Nondihydropyridine			Reduce heart rate	
Verapamil	120–480	1–2		May cause heart block, especially if used with beta blocker
Diltiazem	120–540	1–3		

(continued)

TABLE 61-17 Commonly Used Oral Antihypertensive Drugs by Pharmacologic Class (*Continued*)

Drug	Dose, mg/day	Doses per Day	Mechanism of Action	Special Considerations
Dihydropyridine			Little inhibitory effect on SA, AV nodes	More potent vasodilators than those above; side-effects: pedal edema, dizziness, tachycardia, headache
Nifedipine	30–150	1–3		
Felodipine ER	2.5–10	1		
Amlodipine	2.5–10	1		
ACE inhibitors			Block conversion of Angiotensin I to Angiotensin II; decrease aldosterone; increase bradykinin and vasodilatory prostaglandins; decrease SVR, no change in CO	May cause hyperkalemia, especially with renal impairment, K^+-sparing diuretics, potassium supplements, or NSAIDs; can cause renal failure with renovascular hypertension (see text) may cause cough
Captopril	25–300	2–3		
Enalapril	2.5–40	1–2		
Lisinopril	2.5–40	1		
Benazepril	10–40	1		
Ramipril	2.5–10	1		
Quinapril	10–40	1		
Trandolapril	1–4	1		
Perindopril	1–8	1		
Angiotensin receptor blockers			Block AT_1 receptor	Less cough, angioedema than with ACE-I
Losartan	25–100	1–2		
Valsartan	40–320	1		
Irbesartan	75–300	1		
Candesartan	4–32	1		
Telmisartan	20–40	1		
Eprosartan	400–800	1		
Olmesartan	20–40	1		
Direct Vasodilators			Directly relax vascular smooth muscle by opening K^+ channels	Fluid retention and reflex tachycardia make these poor choices for monotherapy; used with diuretic and beta blocker usually
Hydralazine	20–300	1–2		
Minoxidil	2.5–30	1–2		

ABBREVIATIONS: SVR = systemic vascular resistance; ACE-I = angiotensin-converting enzyme inhibitor; ARBs = angiotensin II receptor blockers; NSAIDs = nonsteroidal anti-inflammatory drugs; TTS = transdermal therapeutic system; ISA = intrinsic sympathomimetic activity.

and the level of BP.[180] The relationship of dietary Na^+ and BP is equally clear, especially at low and modest intakes of Na^+ and in those deemed to be salt-sensitive.[181] Other nutrients, such as K^+, the omega-3 fatty acids present in fish oil, and possibly Ca^{2+} and Mg^{2+}, are inversely related to BP level. Sedentary individuals who do little if any aerobic exercise usually have higher BPs than do appropriately matched controls even when one controls for other confounding variables. The relationship of stress to BP is somewhat less clear. Physical or mental stress will raise BP temporarily, but the relationship of chronic anxiety and stress has been more difficult to demonstrate.

The appreciation of these relationships has naturally led to numerous attempts to lower BP by modifying lifestyles (Table 61-16). A systematic review (18 trials, 2611 patients) of dietary advice to reduce weight indicates that a reduction in weight of 3–9 percent correlated with about 3 mm Hg reduction in systolic and diastolic BP.[182] In all comparative clinical trials (including the Trial of Hypertension Prevention-1 and Trial of Nutrition in the Elderly) weight loss has been the most effective lifestyle modification to lower BP.[49] A systematic review (58 trials, 2161 patients) indicated that salt restriction (by 118 mmol/24 hrs) lowers BP by 3.9/1.9 mm Hg (both $p < 0.001$).[47] Most randomized clinical trials involving other nonpharmacological modalities, including potassium, magnesium, omega-3 fatty acids (from fish oils), or garlic supplementation, have shown much less impressive changes in BP.[6,183,184]

Three recent studies have combined the two most successful lifestyle modifications (weight loss and Na^+ restriction) in prospective, randomized, and well-controlled trials. The shortest of these was the PREMIER Clinical Trial that randomized 810 adults with BPs between 120–159/80–95 mmHg to 1 of 3 intervention groups. After 6 months, those who received a behavioral intervention with both exercise, weight loss, and sodium restriction reduced BP by 3.7/1.7 mmHg ($p < .001/.002$), compared to an "advice only" group. The individuals who received advice about the DASH diet in addition to their behavioral intervention had an even greater fall in BP (4.3/2.6 mmHg, $p < .001/.001$).[185] Even more impressive results were obtained when the data were analyzed according to cut points for BP used in JNC VI. Longer follow-up will be required before comparisons with other studies are possible.

In an earlier, but longer-term trial, the Trials of Hypertension Prevention-2 (TOHP-2) studied the value of weight loss and Na^+ restriction in a 2×2 factorial design against usual care.[186] At 6 months, the group assigned to both Na^+ reduction and weight loss did the best (BP fell 4.0/2.8 mmHg, with usual care subtracted), while those receiving a single modality did not experience as much of a BP reduction (3.7/2.7 mmHg for the weight loss only group, 2.9/1.6 mmHg for the Na^+ reduction only group, also usual care subtracted). At 3 years of follow-up, however, BP reductions were greatly attenuated: the combined treatment had a BP reduction of only 1.1/0.6 mmHg. This finding highlights another difficulty with lifestyle modifications: the high recidivism rate seen in virtually all long-term studies. While adherence to a drug regimen is notoriously poor, adherence to lifestyle modifications is, if anything, even worse. As in TOHP-1, the regimen was delivered by highly trained nutritionists in group and individual sessions and is consequently not an inexpensive way to reduce BP.

A second long-term, randomized, well-controlled study directly assessing the value of lifestyle modifications was the Trial of Nonpharmacologic Interventions in the Elderly (TONE).[187] This study also evaluated the efficacy of weight loss and Na^+ reduction, but in a different population and with a somewhat different objective. Only hypertensives 60 to 80 years of age were enrolled, and all were already receiving single-drug pharmacologic treatment. The objective of TONE was to see whether the imposition of a formal lifestyle approach, again taught by highly trained professionals, would allow hypertensives to stay healthy and go off their medications. The results were equally disappointing. After 30 months, when the study ended, 44 percent of the actively treated subjects were able to stay well without antihypertensive drugs, compared with 38 percent of those not receiving active lifestyle modifications. While this was statistically significant ($p <0.001$), it means that 56 percent of successfully treated hypertensives needed to resume drug therapy even when given the best possible lifestyle regimen administered by experts.

The value of alcohol reduction has also been addressed by a randomized clinical trial (PATHS).[188] This study enrolled 641 patients at seven Department of Veterans Affairs clinics who were actively employed and completely functional but reported consuming at least six alcoholic drinks per day. The subjects reduced their alcohol intake by nearly 20 percent once they entered into the study and before randomization to intensive counseling or usual care. Those in the intensive counseling group were seen frequently and were able to reduce their average reported alcohol consumption to 2.0 drinks per day, which was significantly better than the usual care group (3.3 drinks per day). In spite of this, BP and events were not different at the end of this 2-year trial. A recent metanalysis of trials of alcohol reduction on BP concluded that the effect is less than that due to weight reduction, dietary sodium restriction, and physical activity but is statistically significant at about 2.5 to 4.0/0.9 to 1.2 mmHg.[189]

TABLE 61-18 "Compelling" Conditions for which Specific Antihypertensive Drug Therapy Reduced Morbidity and Mortality in Clinical Trials

"Compelling Condition"	1997	2003
Heart failure (systolic type)	ACE-I (CONSENSUS, SAVE, etc.)	β Blockers (MERIT-HF, etc.); spironolactone (RALES); ARB (Val-HeFT)
Diabetes mellitus, type 1	ACE-I (CCSG)	
Diabetes type 2 (CV events)		ACE-I (MICRO-HOPE)
Diabetic nephropathy		ARBs (IDNT, RENAAL); ARB + ACE-I (COOPERATE)
Diabetes type 2: progression of microalbuminuria		ACE-I (MICRO-HOPE); ARB (IRMA-2)
Known CV disease		ACE-I (HOPE)
Older persons	Diuretic (SHEP) DHP-CA (Syst-Eur)	ACE-I or DHP-CA (STOP-2) DHP-CA (Syst-China) ARB (SCOPE, second-line)
Nondiabetic renal impairment		ACE-I (REIN, AASK)
Poststroke/TIA		ACE-I (PROGRESS)
LVH (strict criteria)		ARB I (LIFE)

ABBREVIATIONS: ACE-I = angiotensin-converting enzyme inhibitor, ARB = angiotensin receptor blocker, DHP-CA = dihydropyridine calcium antagonist; CV = cardiovascular; LVH = left ventricular hypertrophy; TIA = transient ischemic attack.
SOURCES: CONSENSUS = COoperative North Scandinavian ENalapril SUrvival Study (*N Engl J Med* 1987; 316:1429–1435).
SAVE = Survival And Ventricular Enlargement study (*N Engl J Med* 1992;327:669–677).
CCSG = Captopril Cooperative Study Group (*N Engl J Med* 1993;323:1456–1462).
SHEP = Systolic Hypertension in the Elderly Program (*JAMA,* 1991;265:3255–3264).
Syst-Eur = Systolic Hypertension in Europe trial.[156]
MERIT-HF = MEtoprolol Randomized Intervention Trial in congestive Heart Failure (*JAMA* 2000;283:1295–1320).
RALES = Randomized Aldactone Evaluation Study.[232]
Val-HeFT = Valsartan Heart Failure Trial.[235]
MICRO-HOPE = MIcroalbuminuria, Cardiovascular and Renal Outcomes substudy of the Heart Outcomes Prevention Evaluation.[211]
IDNT = Irbesartan Diabetic Nephrophathy Trial.[200]
RENAAL = Reduction of Endpoints in Non-insulin dependent diabetes mellitus with the Angiotensin II Antagonist Losartan.[201]
COOPERATE = Combination treatment of angiotensin-II receptor blocker and angiotensin-converting enzyme inhibitor in nondiabetic renal disease.[213]
IRMA-2 = Irbesartan Microalbuminuria study 2.[237]
STOP-2 = Swedish Trial in Old Patients with hypertension 2 (*Lancet* 1999;354:1751–1756).
Syst-China = Systolic Hypertension in China trial.[157]
SCOPE = Study on COgnition and Prognosis in the Elderly.[208]
REIN = Ramipril Evaluation In Nephropathy trial (*Lancet* 1998;352:1252–1256).
AASK = African American Study of Kidney disease and hypertension.[219]
PROGRESS = Perindopril pROtection aGainst REcurrent Stroke Study.[199]
LIFE = Losartan Intervention For Endpoint reduction.[139]

Appel and associates showed in the Dietary Approaches to Stop Hypertension (DASH) trial that a diet rich in fruit and vegetables lowered BP by 2.8/1.1 mmHg more than did the control diet.[190] The fruit and vegetable diet was designed to contain K^+ and Mg^{2+} at the 75th percentile of the usual American diet, while the control diet was at the 25th percentile. A "combination" diet that also contained foods rich in Ca^{2+} was lower in total and saturated fat; it lowered BP by 5.5/3.0 mmHg more than did the control diet. In the hypertensive subjects in DASH ($n = 133$ of 459), the BP reduction was impressive (11.4/5.5 mmHg). Although this study was short (only 8 weeks) and may not be generalizable to the population since it was carried out in four centers with special expertise, this approach offers great promise for using nutritional management to prevent hypertension in individuals with high-normal BP. The DASH diet provides high amounts of K^+, Mg^{2+}, and Ca^{2+} in the food eaten, not as supplements, and also limits the intake of dietary and saturated fat. Even more impressive results were obtained in the DASH-Sodium Study.[191] Those who received the low-salt control diet had a very significant 6.7/2.5 mmHg lower BP than those randomized to the high-salt control diet; for the DASH diet, the difference was smaller, 3.0/1.6 mmHg. Further studies done over longer periods in a less highly selected cohort will be needed to verify these results and determine whether the DASH and/or DASH-Sodium diets will be valuable therapeutic tools for the general population.

All recommendations for lifestyle modifications include smoking cessation and tobacco avoidance.[6,7,10,132] The reason for the inclusion of this recommendation was to improve CV health rather than because of a proven direct relationship between smoking and hypertension. A direct relationship between smoking and BP, in fact, has not been demonstrated in epidemiologic studies, and often the opposite (BP lower in smokers) was observed.[192] It is now clear, however, that cigarette smoking increases BP and HR transiently (for about 15 min) and that the rise in both is gone by 30 min. The mechanism is the increase in catecholamine secretion induced by smoking. Since the authors recommend that office readings be taken no sooner than 30 min after smoking or caffeine ingestion (another substance that transiently raises BP), one may well miss the elevation of BP caused by smoking if it is measured when the patient has not smoked. Indeed, ABPM studies have shown that smokers have significantly higher BP on days when they smoke compared with days when they do not.[193] The recommendation not to smoke is clearly appropriate, and it is worthwhile not only because of enhanced CV health but also because smoking induces a rise in BP.

Perhaps the most important long-term clinical trial that included lifestyle modifications as a randomized choice was the Treatment of Mild Hypertension Study (TOMHS).[194] This study compared five classes of antihypertensives (diuretics, CAs, ACE inhibitors, alpha blockers, and beta blockers) to placebo in middle-aged subjects with only minimal elevations of BP (average BP of 140/91 mmHg when the study started) and superimposed these pharmacologic treatments on a comprehensive lifestyle regimen that included weight loss, Na^+ restriction, alcohol reduction, and exercise. One arm of the study received lifestyle modifications and a placebo (i.e., no drug therapy). In TOMHS, the nutritional advice and exercise program were monitored by certified nutritionists and trained exercise physiologists. The subjects were seen frequently in group and individual sessions. The group given placebo reduced BP from 140/91 to 132/82 mmHg (a reduction of 9.1/8.6 mmHg) and sustained that level for the 4.4 years of study follow-up, even though the reduction in Na^+ intake, amount of weight loss, and increase in exercise were diminished over time. Perhaps the most important finding in TOMHS was the statistically significantly fewer number of CV events ($p < 0.03$) in the group given pharmacologic treatment plus lifestyle modifications compared to those who received no active drug. Those who received drug therapy, in aggregate, achieved an average BP of 125/79 mmHg, a reduction of 16/12 mmHg. Even though the lifestyle modifications were successful in reducing BP, the group given drugs had significantly fewer CV events, probably because their BP was lower.

The inevitable conclusion from this trial is that even successful lifestyle modifications that bring BP to goal do not reduce morbidity and probably mortality as well as the combination of drugs and therapeutic lifestyle changes that lower BP even further. The fact that the value of BP reduction in preventing CV complications with pharmacologic agents could be demonstrated in a group at such low risk calls into question the current emphasis on delaying drug treatment,

even in low-risk individuals. Furthermore, in TOMHS, the patients' quality of life, as assessed by a very extensive questionnaire delivered on multiple occasions, showed that subjects felt best when their BP was lowest.[25] This result was seen whether they were on combined treatment or on lifestyle modifications alone. Physicians should strive to get the maximum safe BP reduction by combining drug treatments and lifestyle modifications and not to neglect either approach in treating hypertensive patients.

The lack of proof for lifestyle modifications to reduce CV events does not mean that physicians should abandon nondrug treatments. In general patients should be encouraged to lose weight; restrict Na^+ intake; eat generous amounts of K^+, Mg^{2+}, Ca^{2+}, and fish; exercise regularly; moderate alcohol consumption (if they drink); stop smoking; and reduce stress. The most important thing is to lower BP, perhaps to the lowest tolerable level, and to do so safely and without excessive personal or societal cost. The tension between advocates of lifestyle modifications and those who consider it at best no more than an adjunct is not useful. The recommendations for therapeutic lifestyle changes are still very appropriate for the general population. If adopted, they may well prevent or delay the virtually inevitable rise in BP that occurs with age, and many hypertensives will be able to reduce BP further than might be achieved with drugs alone. Lifestyle modifications are the primary public health approach to trying to reduce the prevalence of hypertension and the average BP in the society.[4,6] If successful, such modification is likely to save more lives and prevent more MIs, strokes, and episodes of HF than can be prevented by using drugs in those who are already hypertensive.

PHARMACOLOGIC THERAPY

The ultimate goal of hypertension treatment is to reduce cardiovascular and renal morbidity and mortality; the short-term goal is to achieve the recommended goal BP by using the least intrusive means possible.[4] *Intrusive* has several interpretations: economic, office visits, adverse effects, and convenience. The choice of the drug with which to begin therapy is probably the most important decision the clinician must make when treating hypertensive patients. Approximately one-third of patients will respond to the first choice and can tolerate most rational options. If the clinician chooses wisely, the first choice may be successful in getting BP to goal, and that will be the drug on which the patient stays indefinitely. Since the remainder will need additional treatment, the choice of the first drug must be done with an eye toward what can be added to achieve that goal. Fortunately, the "preferred" first-line antihypertensive agent for most patients has now been defined by data from clinical trials.[195]

Classification of Antihypertensive Agents

Antihypertensive agents can be classified in a number of ways. Some drugs are effective parentally and are indicated only for a hypertensive crisis, while the overwhelming majority are used orally as chronic therapy. Antihypertensive agents are further classified by pharmacologic class and alleged primary mechanism of action (Table 61-17). There are more than 100 effective antihypertensive drugs and 50 fixed-dose combinations from which to choose.[196]

Surrogate versus Clinical Endpoints

Physicians should no longer be willing simply to look at the degree of BP reduction in making a choice of antihypertensive therapy. Clinical endpoints are the events that physicians are ultimately trying to prevent in treating hypertension. So-called surrogate (or intermediate) endpoints are factors that may contribute to clinical endpoints and can be affected favorably or unfavorably by treatment. Some surrogate endpoints do not correlate well with mortality/morbidity endpoints, such as reduction of ventricular extrasystoles in the Cardiac Arrhythmia Suppression Trial, changes in serum lipid values in the Women's Health Initiative (WHI), or glucose or cholesterol changes in the Antihypertensive and Lipid Lowering prevention of Heart Attack Trial (ALLHAT, see below).[197,198] BP reduction is a surrogate or intermediate endpoint, since the real reason for treating hypertension is to reduce the morbidity and mortality associated with elevated BP, and not simply to lower BP. Physicians now expect and demand proof that the selection made will prevent hypertension-related clinical endpoints. Data from large, prospective clinical trials that are designed to evaluate the ability of a drug to reduce hypertension-related CV events as well as or better than an otherwise reasonable alternative drug are the most reliable means to use in choosing from among the otherwise bewildering number of options.

Initial Drug Therapy

Many considerations can enter the clinician's decision-making process when lifestyle modifications are insufficient to bring a patient's BP to goal. While many feel that a simple and uniform recommendation should be provided for all hypertensive individuals, principles of "evidence-based medicine" can be marshaled for exceptional cases.

COMPELLING CONDITIONS

Both JNC VI and JNC 7 recognized that hypertensive patients often present with concomitant illnesses or conditions that benefit from therapy with specific antihypertensive drugs. In 1997, there were only a few situations in which antihypertensive drugs reduced morbidity and mortality; the list (Table 61-18) is much longer today. For example, a hypertensive person who fulfills the new Cornell voltage-duration criteria for LVH should be treated with an ARB, rather than a beta blocker, based on the results of LIFE.[139] In the current treatment algorithm (Fig. 61-1), this is the first consideration in developing an antihypertensive regimen and it is independent of the level of BP.

SYMPTOMATIC IMPROVEMENT

Both JNC VI and JNC 7 recognized that patients sometimes have other conditions that may improve symptomatically (rather than by reduced morbidity or mortality) when a specific type of antihypertensive drug is given.

Despite the lack of long-term data about CV risk reduction, treatment of these conditions may be useful in improving a patient's adherence to therapy and might tend to override the general guidelines for beginning treatment with a specific type of medication. For example, a person with chronic diarrhea due to "dumping syndrome" after a partial gastrectomy might enjoy a better quality of life if verapamil were prescribed as the initial drug for hypertension.

COMPARATIVE EFFICACY VERSUS PLACEBO IN PREVENTING EVENTS

Before 1997, only initial diuretics and beta blockers had been shown to reduce morbidity and mortality in clinical trials against placebo in hypertension. Dihydropyridine (DHP) CAs were added to this list after the Syst-EUR and Syst-China trials were completed.[156,157] These trials used the DHP CA nitrendipine, followed by enalapril (or

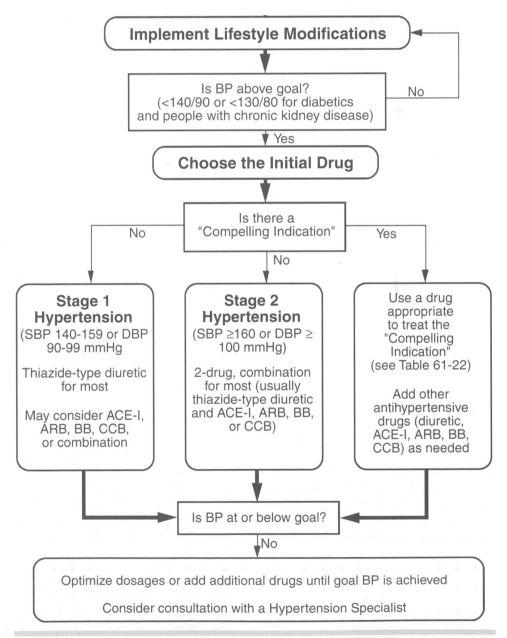

FIGURE 61-1 The authors' suggested algorithm for the treatment of hypertension based on outcomes data from large clinical trials and modified from JNC 7.[4] BP = blood pressure; SBP = systolic blood pressure; DBP = diastolic blood pressure; ACE-1 = angiotensin-converting enzyme inhibitor; ARB = angiotensin receptor blocker; BB = beta blocker; CCB = calcium channel blocker.

captopril) and then hydrochlorothiazide (if needed) to get BP to goal. An initial ACE inhibitor ($\pm$ diuretic) was more effective than an initial placebo (or two) for reducing CV events in the Perindopril pROtection aGainst REcurrent Stroke Study (PROGRESS) study.[199] An initial ARB was more effective in preventing a composite renal endpoint than an initial placebo in both the Irbesartan Diabetic Nephropathy Trial (IDNT) and Reduction of Endpoints in Non-Insulin Dependent Diabetes Mellitus with the Angiotensin II Antagonist Losartan (RENAAL) studies.[200,201] A summary of the relative efficacy of different initial drug therapies against placebo or no treatment in preventing stroke, coronary heart disease (CHD) events, and CV death is shown in Fig. 61-2. An initial beta blocker was significantly more effective than placebo/no treatment in preventing only stroke; this conclusion was also reached in a earlier and smaller metanalysis of trials involving only older patients.[202]

COMPARATIVE EFFICACY OF INITIAL DRUGS IN PREVENTING EVENTS

Only a very important few of the recent clinical trials of different initial antihypertensive treatments that involved ACE inhibitors or CAs showed significant differences between initial drug strategies regarding prevention of major adverse CV events. To summarize these data, many metanalyses have been published.[203,204] A recent paper suggested a slight benefit with CAs on stroke, but at the risk of more MIs and HF.[16] Perhaps most importantly, this paper contains the results of a meta–regression analysis across 27 trials involving 136,124 patients, suggesting that the differences across drug classes could easily be explained by achieved differences in systolic BP.[16]

The major problem with the interpretation of large clinical trials involving comparisons across drug classes involves attribution of the observed difference(s) in endpoints. When there are differences in achieved BPs across randomized groups, most authors attribute the difference to an inferiority of the drug, rather than its BP-lowering ability, as the "cause" of the poor results. Fairer comparisons that are easier to interpret are obtained when BP-lowering is equivalent across randomized treatments. Public health officials, however, remind us that intent-to-treat analyses of clinical trials provide us with comparisons of treatment strategies, not comparisons of drugs themselves. When a particular strategy starting with a specific drug is

found to be inferior (in either BP-lowering efficacy or CV endpoints) to another, we can more easily adopt *the strategy* with better results.

Four very recent clinical trials are of special interest. Compared to an initial diuretic, an initial ACE inhibitor was not significantly better in preventing a first cardiovascular event or death in the Second Australian National Blood Pressure Trial (ANBPT-2).[205] An initial ARB ($\pm$ diuretic) was superior to an initial beta blocker ($\pm$ diuretic) in patients with LVH for reducing major cardiovascular events in LIFE; although the group given losartan had both lower systolic BP as well as a major reduction in stroke, they had no reduction in CHD events or death.[139] The Controlled ONset Verapamil INvestigation of Cardiovascular Endpoints (CONVINCE) trial was stopped early and failed to demonstrate "equivalence" of a regimen beginning with a novel formulation of verapamil and a traditional regimen beginning with the physician's choice of either a diuretic or a beta blocker.[206]

Perhaps most importantly, the recent ALLHAT study directly compared the thiazide-like diuretic, chlorthalidone, with three newer antihypertensive drugs: amlodipine (a CA), doxazosin (an alpha blocker), and lisinopril (an ACE inhibitor). The doxazosin arm was stopped early, and showed a significant increase (compared to the diuretic) in CVD, an endpoint that included CHD, heart failure, and peripheral arterial disease.[207] Although there were no significant differences between the diuretic and either of the two remaining newer drugs in the primary endpoint (CHD death or nonfatal MI), the diuretic was significantly better at preventing heart failure than both other drugs, and also better in reducing BP, stroke, and CV events than lisinopril. Because of its superiority in preventing one or more CV complications of hypertension and its lower cost, a thiazide diuretic was recommended as the only "preferred" initial antihypertensive drug therapy by the ALLHAT Research Group.[195,198]

Although there are many possible confounders and interpretations of the ALLHAT data, it is difficult to overlook the many strengths of this large, randomized, double-blind, well-done study. It is likely that, for individuals over 55 years of age without any specific medical reason to use another antihypertensive drug, a thiazide-type diuretic should be the first choice. Whether the benefits of the diuretic used in ALLHAT (chlorthalidone) are also applicable to others, such as hydrochlorothiazide, cannot be answered definitively, but it is likely.

Some feel that the conclusions of a single clinical trial, no matter how well done, must be interpreted in context with the results of all other studies. With the possible exception of ACE inhibitors in the ANBPT-2,[205] no other agent has ever been superior to a thiazide in preventing CV events. The next set of metanalyses from the World Health Organization/International Society of Hypertension's Blood Pressure Lowering Treatment Trialists' Collaboration is likely to show very few significant differences across most CV endpoints for either a CA or an ACE inhibitor versus a diuretic/beta blocker as initial therapy (Fig. 61-3). Under these circumstances, the lower acquisition cost of the diuretic makes it the most attractive option, since no other drug class is superior to it in either BP lowering or in CV event reduction or is better in any specific subgroup of hypertensive patients.

SEQUENCE OF ADDITIONAL DRUGS

There have so far been no clinical trials comparing well-tolerated active drugs as "second-line" treatment options, and this remains an area of potential future research. Most people would consider an ACE inhibitor, ARB, beta blocker, or CA to be a reasonable second choice if a diuretic is the initial therapy. Beta blockers have been the conventional second-line treatment in many previous clinical trials

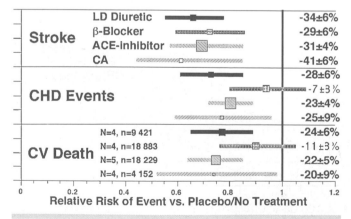

FIGURE 61-2 A summary of the relative efficacy of different initial drug therapies against placebo or no treatment in preventing stroke, coronary heart disease (CHD) events, and cardiovascular (CV) death. LD = low dose. (Adapted from Elliott WJ. Cardiovascular events during long-term antihypertensive drug treatment: Meta-analysis of four major drug classes vs placebo or no treatment (abstr). *Am J Hypertens* 2003;16:113A. With permission.)

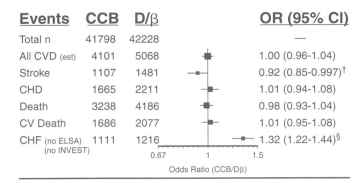

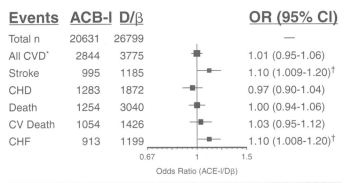

FIGURE 61-3 Results of metanalyses of 10 clinical trials comparing an initial calcium antagonist with an initial diuretic or beta blocker (*top panel*) and 8 clinical trials comparing an initial ACE inhibitor with an initial diuretic or beta blocker (*bottom panel*). CCB = calcium channel blocker; D = diuretic; β = beta blocker; *n* = number of patients; CVD = cardiovascular disease events, estimated for ALLHAT (Ref.198); CHD = coronary heart disease events (primarily myocardial infarction); CHF = congestive heart failure, which was not reported for ELSA or INVEST; †p = 0.04; §p < 0.0001. (Updated from Elliott WJ. Cardiovascular events during initial antihypertensive therapy with either a calcium antagonist or a diuretic/beta blocker: Meta-analysis of 7 clinical trials (abstr). *Am J Hypertens* 2003;16:9A-10A. With permission.)

that used a diuretic first. An ARB (candesartan) was more effective than placebo and/or other treatments (not including an ACE inhibitor) following the initial diuretic in the recently completed Study on COgnition and Prognosis in the Elderly (SCOPE) trial, which showed a significant reduction in stroke.[208] The most successful trial of ACE-inhibitor therapy in CV event protection was the Heart Outcomes Prevention Evaluation (HOPE), in which ramipril or placebo was given in addition to whatever other antihypertensive therapy was required (i.e., as "add-on" treatment). Although the overall BP reduction with ramipril was said to be only 3/2 mm Hg compared to placebo, some patients were not hypertensive at enrollment, and this (and the possible addition of other antihypertensive drugs to the placebo arm) may have diluted the BP changes. A recent report of major BP differences across randomized groups in a small subset of patients who underwent ambulatory BP monitoring suggests a much larger BP difference between the groups, especially at night.[209] Nonetheless, the major significant reductions in the composite CV endpoint (stroke, MI, or CV death), as well as in each of its individual components in both diabetics and nondiabetics prove that an ACE inhibitor is certainly better than placebo as "add-on" therapy.[210,211] Because several beta blockers, ACE inhibitors, and ARBs are available in fixed-dose combination with low-dose thiazide diuretics, some would argue that one of these should be the second-line treatment when a diuretic is insufficient—for cost, convenience, and probably adherence reasons. There is no outcome-based clinical trial information to support the use of a CA as second-line therapy. Only one successful factorial design study of the BP-lowering efficacy of the combination of a CA and diuretic has been published, as opposed to many studies of diuretic + ACE inhibitor or + ARB combinations.[212] Although promising, the addition of an ARB to an ACE inhibitor requires more clinical trial data before it can be routinely recommended to lower BP; the few outcomes data that exist with this combination are controversial.[213]

Blood Pressure Goal during Treatment

In all hypertensive patients, the goal should be a SBP below 140 mmHg and a DBP below 90 mmHg; for some, it should be lower (Table 61-19).[4,10,132] The primary clinical trial evidence for the recommendation for 140/90 mmHg comes from the Hypertension Optimal Treatment (HOT) Study, which randomized 18,790 hypertensives to three different diastolic BP targets; the optimal achieved BP to reduce major CV events was 138.5/82.6 mmHg. There was no significant CV benefit to reducing BP more, and the number and cost of extra pills was greater.[214]

For diabetic patients, the recommended goal is lower (SBP <130 mmHg and DBP <80 mmHg).[4,215,216] The recommendation for a lower-than-usual BP is based on the United Kingdom Prospective Diabetes Study (UKPDS), which randomized 1148 type 2 diabetics to a BP of either <180/105 or <150/85 mmHg. After 8.4 years of average follow-up, those treated to the lower BP goal had an average BP that was 10/5 mmHg lower than those randomized to the higher goal as well as a significant 24 percent reduction in diabetes-related endpoints along with other major CV benefits.[135] Despite a larger number of pills and more frequent office visits, overall the lower BP goal saved money because of the significantly reduced risk of stroke and other diabetes-related complications.[217] A similar cost-effectiveness analysis of American epidemiologic and clinical trial data concluded that, for diabetics over age 60, achieving a BP goal of <130/85 saved

TABLE 61-19 Goal Blood Pressures

Population of Hypertensives	Goal Blood Pressure	Recommended by
"Uncomplicated" (i.e., no diabetes, cardiovascular or renal complications)	<140/90 mmHg	JNC 7, HOT study
Renal disease (elevated serum creatinine or proteinuria)	<130/80 mmHg	Compromise between National Kidney Foundation, JNC 7 and AASK study results
Diabetics	<130/80 mmHg	UKPDS 38, HOT study, American Diabetes Association
Cardiovascular complications	<130/85 mmHg	JNC 7

ABBREVIATIONS: JNC 7 = Seventh report of the Joint National Committee on Prevention, Detection, Evaluation, and Treatment of High Blood Pressure[4]; HOT = Hypertension Optimal Treatment study[214]; AASK = African American Study of Kidney disease and hypertension[219]; UKPDS 38 = United Kingdom Prospective Diabetes Study 38[135]; American Diabetes Association 2003 guidelines.[216]

money overall as long as the annual cost to lower BP from 140/90 mm Hg was less than $414. Again this was due to a reduction in high-cost complications of hypertension, including MI, stroke, ESRD, and HF.[218] The recommendation to achieve a diastolic BP <80 mmHg in diabetics is supported by the HOT study, in which the best reduction in major CV events was seen in those randomized to the diastolic BP target of <80 mmHg.[214]

For patients with renal disease, JNC 7 also recommends the BP target of <130/80 mmHg.[4] Although this is not yet completely evidence-based, the results of the African-American Study of Kidney disease (AASK) and hypertension study did not support the lower goal (<125/75 mmHg) recommended by JNC VI.[219]

One of the perceived limitations to achieving these lower levels of BP was the fear that lowering BP too far might be harmful—the concept of the "J" curve. Several investigators had pointed out that subjects treated to diastolic BP level below 85 mmHg had higher rates of MI than did those whose on-treatment diastolic BP was between 85 and 90 mmHg. However, an increased risk for those with low diastolic BP is also evident in large untreated populations and placebo groups of several trials. Furthermore, the Systolic Hypertension in the Elderly Program (SHEP) treated individuals down to an average diastolic BP of 67 mmHg and prevented MIs compared to placebo-treatment (average of 71 mmHg). Similarly, an analysis of SHEP provided no evidence for an increase in risk of stroke with decreasing levels of on-treatment systolic BPs.[220] The HOT and UKPDS 38 studies provided proof that intensive BP lowering was not harmful.[135,214]

Factors to Consider in Building an Antihypertensive Drug Regimen

There are 10 factors that should always be considered when antihypertensive drug therapy is chosen: efficacy, comorbidities, safety, patient demographics, special situations (e.g., pregnancy), dosing schedule, drug interactions, adherence, mechanism(s) of action, and cost. These considerations are important not only in choice of initial therapy but also for subsequent antihypertensive agents. In recent clinical trials, most patients required two or more drugs to achieve goal BPs; a recent meta–regression analysis suggested that there is only a 2.5 percent chance of achieving goal BP with monotherapy when the initial DBP is >10 mmHg higher than goal.

EFFICACY

JNC VI made the distinction between surrogate and clinical endpoints when it provided guidelines for selecting treatments that were based on efficacy, defined as the reduction of morbidity and mortality. Now five classes of drugs (thiazide diuretics, beta blockers, long-acting CAs, ACE inhibitors, and ARBs) have been shown to reduce CV or renal endpoints when used as initial therapy for hypertension in appropriately designed and implemented clinical trials. Other agents, such as peripheral sympatholytics (reserpine and guanethidine), centrally acting alpha agonists (alpha-methyldopa), and vasodilators (hydralazine), have also been used in clinical trials as the second, third, or even fourth agent added to achieve BP control. None is an option for initial therapy because they are relatively poorly tolerated or need to be taken together with other drugs to lower BP effectively in the long term. Alpha/beta blockers are effective as monotherapy and are well tolerated but have not yet been shown to reduce clinical endpoints in hypertensive patients. Alpha blockers are valuable as adjunctive therapy, not as initial therapy according to ALLHAT.[207]

COMORBIDITIES AND OTHER RISK FACTORS

JNC VI or JNC 7 recognized two other factors that may alter the choice of initial treatment in an individual hypertensive patient:

- Data from events trials that were conducted in subjects with other conditions but in which many subjects with hypertension were enrolled. These trials were the basis for "compelling" indications for specific antihypertensive drugs in both JNC VI and JNC 7 (see Table 61-18).

- JNC VI recognized that individual patients may have certain comorbid conditions for which a specific agent may be appropriate even though no clinical trial data exist to prove it. Good examples are osteoporosis and thiazide diuretics and angina pectoris and beta blockers (Table 61-20). These "specific" indications try to codify clinical judgment,

TABLE 61-20 Effects of Antihypertensive Drug Classes on Other Conditions

May have favorable effects on comorbid conditions	
Angina	β blocker, Ca^{2+} antagonist
Atrial tachycardia and fibrillation	β blocker, non-DHP CA
Cyclosporine-induced hypertension	Ca^{2+} antagonist (caution with the dose of cyclosporine)
Liver disease	β blocker
Peripheral vascular disease	α blocker, CA
Dyslipidemia	α blocker
Essential tremor	β blocker
Hyperthyroidism	β blocker
Migraine	β blocker (non-cardioselective), non-DHP CA
Post-MI	β blocker (cardioselective)
Osteoporosis	Thiazide diuretic
Preoperative hypertension	β blocker
Prostatism (benign prostatic hyperplasia)	α blocker
May have unfavorable effects on comorbid conditions	
Bronchospastic disease	β blocker
Depression	β blocker, central α-agonist, reserpine
DM (types 1 and 2)	β blocker, high-dose diuretic
Dyslipidemia	β blocker (non-ISA), diuretic (high-dose)
Gout	Diuretic
Second- or third-degree heart block	β blocker, non-DHP CA
Renal insufficiency/renovascular disease	ACE-I, ARB

ABBREVIATIONS: MI = myocardial infarction; DM = diabetes mellitus; DHP CA = dihydropyridine calcium antagonist; ISA = intrinsic sympathomimetic activity; ACE-I = angiotensin-converting enzyme inhibitor; ARB = angiotensin receptor blocker.

which any reasonable clinician would use to care for all the health needs of his or her patients. For the most part, these recommendations do not add classes of drugs to the list of those that are favored because of a reduction in clinical endpoints but instead alter the choice of which class should be selected for initial therapy.

Thus, other risk factors and active clinical problems can sometimes influence the choice of specific drugs for individual patients. This approach, using somewhat different language, was also adopted by the British Hypertension Society in their guidelines.[132]

Dyslipidemias Hypertensive patients who have lipid abnormalities (which may be present in as many as 50 percent of treated hypertensives) may wish to avoid drugs that worsen their particular dyslipidemia. Although it has not been proved that the changes in serum lipids caused by certain classes of antihypertensive agents are harmful, it is certainly reasonable to choose a drug that is lipid-neutral or one that may improve the lipid profile, all else being equal. In large doses (>25 mg/day), thiazide diuretics and related compounds such as chlorthalidone raise TC and LDL cholesterol 5 to 10 percent and may lower HDL cholesterol 2 to 4 percent. Serum triglycerides may increase 15 to 30 percent. With currently recommended doses (up to 25 mg of chlorthalidone or equivalent), the long-term changes are less troublesome.[198] Beta blockers that do not have intrinsic sympathomimetic activity lower HDL cholesterol even more (10 percent) and also raise triglycerides (approximately 20 percent) without affecting TC or LDL. Beta blockers that do have intrinsic sympathomimetic activity and alpha/beta blockers are lipid-neutral. Alpha blockers reduce TC and LDL cholesterol approximately 8 to 10 percent, triglycerides 15 percent, and HDL cholesterol 10 to 15 percent. Putatively beneficial changes in serum lipids correlated *inversely* with CV events in recent trials with estrogens (Heart and Estrogen/progestin Replacement Study[221] and WHI[197]) and alpha blockers (ALLHAT[207]). ACE inhibitors generally do not affect serum lipids in nondiabetics. ARBs and CAs are lipid-neutral. Other sympatholytics do not affect the lipid profile, and direct vasodilators (e.g., hydralazine) raise HDL cholesterol and lower triglycerides and TG, even when combined with thiazide diuretics. (see also Chap. 43).

Glucose, Insulin and New Diabetes Mellitus Some antihypertensive drugs may affect glucose metabolism and worsen or improve insulin sensitivity.[207] The magnitude and direction of the drug-induced changes seen in glucose and insulin are very similar to what occurs with lipids. Peripheral alpha blockers and some ACE inhibitors (captopril, enalapril, trandolapril, and perindopril) improve insulin sensitivity.[222] Every ACE inhibitor and ARB so far studied reduces urinary protein excretion, which may contribute to the renal benefit seen in patients with DM treated with these drugs. Both moderate- and high-dose thiazides and beta blockers worsen insulin sensitivity and can precipitate glucose intolerance and frank diabetes.[139,198,223] In HOPE, the Captopril Primary Prevention Project (CAPPP), LIFE, and ALLHAT, incident diabetes was less common when an ACE inhibitor or ARB was the randomized choice.[139,198,210] Patients at high risk of becoming diabetic (the obese and those with glucose intolerance or other components of syndrome X) thus may reduce their risk of new diabetes during treatment with an ACE inhibitor or ARB.

Hypertensives with Diabetes Mellitus As discussed above, the combination of hypertension and DM confers a much higher risk for CV events and renal failure than does either one alone. According to JNC VI, type 1 diabetics with renal impairment and proteinuria should re-

ceive an ACE inhibitor, which has been shown to reduce ESRD by 50 percent. Little other information is available about optimal treatment of hypertension in type 1 diabetics.

The American Diabetes Association has recently published guidelines for treatment of hypertension in type 2 diabetics, which include a lower-than-usual goal for BP during treatment (<130/80 mmHg, discussed above), and a recommendation for an ARB to be a component of the antihypertensive drug regimen (i.e., initial drug therapy).[216] An ARB has been beneficial in two studies with renal endpoints (IDNT, RENAAL) and for CV event prevention in the diabetic subset of LIFE.[200,201,224] An ACE inhibitor provided impressive CV event reduction in MICRO-HOPE, although the number of subjects reaching ESRD was only 18, insufficient to see a significant difference between the ACE inhibitor and placebo-treated groups.[211] In UKPDS 38, there was no significant difference between captopril or atenolol as initial therapy, whereas the group achieving the lower BP did much better.[135] An initial ACE inhibitor was less effective than chlorthalidone in reducing BP, stroke, combined CVD, and HF in ALLHAT; these results may also have been confounded by the difference in achieved systolic BP.[198] Some argue that BP control, rather than how it is accomplished, is the key factor in reducing CV and renal events in type 2 diabetic patients.

The role of CAs in treatment of hypertension in diabetics is controversial. Although an initial DHP-CA was successful in reducing CV events (compared to placebo) in Syst-Eur,[225] a different DHP-CA was significantly less effective than an ARB in reducing renal events (but not CV events) in IDNT.[200] The National Kidney Foundation recommends that a CA be used as third-line therapy after a diuretic and either an ACE inhibitor or ARB.[215] It also favors nondihydropyridine (non-DHP) CAs over DHP CAs because they reduce proteinuria and slow the progression of diabetic nephropathy.[144,226]

In diabetics, reducing BP to goal may be a more important factor in reducing mortality and preserving renal function than the initial drug chosen to do so, as it usually takes several drugs to achieve a BP <130/80 mmHg (Table 61-19).

Left Ventricular Hypertrophy Left ventricular hypertrophy (LVH) results from chronic elevations in arterial pressure that cause cardiac myocyte hypertrophy and remodeling of the coronary resistance vessels. This leads to perivascular fibrosis of the intramyocardial arteries and arterioles. Over time, these changes in the myocardium contribute to the development of ventricular wall stiffness and diastolic dysfunction.

LVH is a robust independent risk factor for CV and premature mortality, probably because it reflects the degree of BP control over the long term. LVH is especially common in the elderly, particularly in elderly women, and is often associated with diastolic dysfunction. All antihypertensive agents except direct vasodilators reduce LV mass. In metanalyses, agents that block the RAA system reduce LV mass better or more quickly than do other antihypertensive agents. However, TOMHS and the Veterans Administration (VA) study of monotherapy found no differences among antihypertensive agents in their ability to regress LVH.[227] Moreover, in TOMHS, measures to improve nutritional hygiene—such as weight loss, reduced Na^+ and alcohol intake—as well as exercise were effective by themselves in regressing LV mass. Perhaps the most important factor responsible for LV mass regression is the prolonged reduction of systolic BP.

So far, the only completed clinical trial to enroll only patients with LVH was the LIFE study.[139] The group randomized to losartan (± diuretic) had a significant reduction in LVH and composite CV events (mostly due to stroke) compared to the group receiving atenolol (± diuretic), despite a BP difference between groups of only

1.3/0.4 mmHg. Significant differences in cardiac events between randomized groups were seen best in diabetics.[224] These are the first randomized, prospective data to suggest that reducing LVH prevents CV events.

Heart Failure Hypertension is a major risk factor for the subsequent development of HF, typically many years later.[228] For many untreated or undertreated hypertensives, LVH is an important intermediate step, resulting in "hypertensive heart disease" with impaired LV filling and increased ventricular stiffness. This type of HF (which has been seen in up to 40 percent of hospitalized patients with an antecedent history of hypertension) is commonly called *diastolic dysfunction.*[137] The more common type of "systolic dysfunction" associated with a reduced LV ejection fraction is most often due to previous MI (for which hypertension is also an important risk factor). In a metanalysis of placebo-controlled clinical trials in hypertension, there was a 42 percent reduction in the incidence of HF among hypertensives randomized to either a low-dose diuretic or a beta blocker.[229]

Distinguishing between the two subtypes of HF is most easily done by estimation of the LV ejection fraction; the results dictate therapy.[230] Patients with low ejection fractions ("systolic HF") improve both their BP and long-term prognosis with ACE inhibitors and diuretics, to which can be added beta blockers, spironolactone, and/or other drugs as needed.[231,232] Two trials directly comparing an ARB with an ACE inhibitor showed significant differences mainly in better tolerability of the ARB.[233,234] In the valsartan in heart failure (Val-HeFT) trial, an ARB or placebo was given to HF patients taking "conventional therapy" (which included an ACE inhibitor in 93 percent but a beta blocker in only 13 percent). Although there were no differences between randomized groups in mortality, the group receiving valsartan had a significant 13 percent reduction in HF-related morbidity or mortality, mostly due to a 27 percent reduction in hospitalization for HF.[235] Valsartan has received approval from the U.S. Food and Drug Administration (FDA) for HF because of the very significant reduction in morbidity and mortality in the 366 patients who did not take an ACE inhibitor in Val-HeFT. In those who took a beta blocker in addition to the ACE inhibitor, valsartan was associated with a significantly higher morbidity or mortality rate. This limits enthusiasm for valsartan as a third-line HF drug; other studies will determine whether other ARBs share this drawback. The role of DHP CAs and other direct-acting vasodilators (e.g., hydralazine in combination with isosorbide dinitrate) remains controversial. Most authorities recommend these drugs as adjunctive therapy (after diuretics, maximum doses of ACE inhibitors and/or ARBs, a beta blocker, and sometimes spironolactone) if BP is still elevated.

Treatment of hypertension in patients with diastolic dysfunction and HF has not been as well studied, but most authorities recommend using drugs that reduce HR, increase diastolic filling time, and allow the heart muscle to relax more fully: beta blockers or nondihydropyridine CAs. Although these suggestions make physiologic sense, there are no clinical trial data to support them.

Valvular Disease The coexistence of hypertension and valvular heart disease is, for most affected patients, simply an occurrence of two common conditions in the same person. There are few syndromes or scenarios in which the two are pathophysiologically connected, but there are some circumstances in which their coexistence has clinical importance, especially in regard to choosing antihypertensive drug therapy.

A murmur of aortic sclerosis is found in approximately 21 to 26 percent of adults over 65 years of age. In the CV Health Study, 29 percent of the 5621 subjects age 65 and over had this valvular abnormality detected on echocardiography; it was found much more commonly among hypertensives and those with LVH.[236] Perhaps most important, its presence was associated with a 50 percent increased risk of CV events over an average of 5 years of follow-up. After adjustment for risk factor differences at baseline (e.g., hypertension), only one of four studied endpoints retained statistical significance. Calcific aortic stenosis is about 10 times less common but must often be evaluated more extensively, usually with an echocardiogram. Aortic insufficiency in hypertensives is found almost exclusively in patients with isolated systolic hypertension and is most easily recognized by the characteristic murmur and peripheral signs. Unloading the left ventricle with arteriolar vasodilators (e.g., nifedipine) prolongs the time until valve replacement surgery.

Mitral valve disease is less common than it was in past decades, primarily because of efforts to treat streptococcal pharyngitis. Mitral stenosis is still seen occasionally in citizens of developing countries but is not commonly associated with systemic hypertension. Since digoxin is typically used to control the ventricular rate in atrial fibrillation, antihypertensive drugs that interfere with the excretion of digoxin should be used cautiously. Mitral insufficiency is also less common than it was in the past, but there are few problems specific to this disease that affect hypertension and its therapy.

The right-sided cardiac valves seldom need be considered in the treatment of patients with systemic hypertension. In patients with primary (or secondary) pulmonary hypertension (which can be treated with the usual antihypertensive drugs, although with less success), the status of the right-sided heart valves takes on increased significance. Occasionally, insufficiency of the tricuspid valve is the major diagnostic clue to carcinoid heart disease.

Microalbuminuria and Proteinuria MA is a predictor of CV and renal death in patients with DM (see above). ACE inhibitors are associated with the most data showing reductions in MA and delaying its progression to proteinuria,[211] but ARBs are also more effective than placebo, especially at higher doses.[237] These agents reduce albuminuria by reducing intraglomerular pressure as well as decreasing glomerular size selectivity and partially restoring membrane charge. Both ACE inhibitors and nondihydropyridine CAs reduce albuminuria and together have additive antialbuminuric effects, in part independently of further reductions in BP.[238] The effects of different classes of antihypertensive agents on MA and proteinuria are summarized in Table 61-21.

TABLE 61-21 Effects of Different Classes of Antihypertensive Agents on Microalbuminuria/Proteinuria

Decrease levels
   ACE inhibitors
   Angiotensin receptor blockers
   α-β blockers
   Nondihydropyridine CA
   β blockers
   Diuretics

Increase levels
   Short-acting dihydropyridine CA
   Minoxidil

No effect
   Dihydropyridine CA
   α blockers
   Central alpha agonist (clonidine, methyldopa)

CA = Calcium antagonist.

The ACE inhibitors and ARBs are the antihypertensive agents that most consistently reduce proteinuria. Even in the absence of hypertension, these agents can prevent the increase of MA to proteinuria or normalize protein excretion in patients with MA.[211,237,239] Nondihydropyridine CAs (diltiazem and verapamil) also have some utility in reducing urinary protein excretion in hypertensive patients with kidney disease.[238] A high Na^+ intake blunts the antiproteinuric and antihypertensive effects of ACE inhibitors and diltiazem; therefore the restriction of dietary Na^+ is recommended for patients with MA or proteinuria.

Renal Dysfunction   Lowering of the BP will slow the progression of nephropathy, but the recommended target BP is controversial. The recent African American Study of Kidney disease and hypertension showed no benefit to lowering BP to <125/75 mmHg, as compared to <140/90 mmHg,[219] but there are concerns about whether this finding can be generalized to all hypertensives with renal impairment. ARBs and ACE inhibitors will slow the progression of diabetic and nondiabetic nephropathy assuming that they are given with sufficient other drugs to reduce BP <140/90 mmHg.[240]

In spite of the evidence from many long-term clinical trials, there is a general hesitancy among some clinicians to prescribe ACE inhibitors (or ARBs) for patients with serum creatinine >1.4 mg/dL because it often rises, by up to 25 percent, after the drug is given. An analysis of long-term clinical trials has confirmed that this reduction in renal function plateaus within a month.[241] If the serum creatinine increases by >30 percent or continues to rise after 1 month of therapy, overdiuresis, renal artery stenosis, or unsuspected LV dysfunction should be considered.[241] There are also concerns about hyperkalemia associated with an ACE inhibitor or ARB; this should be worrisome only if the serum K^+ rises ≥0.5 meq/L.

Thus, while any class of antihypertensive agent may be used to achieve this new recommended lower level of BP to preserve renal function, certain principles should be kept in mind:

- BP will seldom if ever be controlled adequately in patients with significant renal impairment (serum creatinine >1.8 mg/dL) without the use of a loop diuretic.
- A long-acting loop diuretic (such as torsemide) is preferred; furosemide or bumetanide should given twice daily.
- Combinations of antihypertensive medications will be needed to achieve goal BP. One of these drugs should be an ACE inhibitor or ARB. Some authors recommend both an ACE inhibitor and an ARB simultaneously, but this requires more study.[213,242]

Coronary Artery Disease   Since hypertension is a major risk factor for CAD, it is not surprising that a large number of patients have both conditions. It is unlikely on ethical grounds that a placebo-controlled trial will be done with any single antihypertensive drug in such patients. The presence of CAD in a patient with hypertension is likely to influence both the choice of drugs used to treat the patient and the BP goal to be achieved. Because both beta blockers and CAs are effective antihypertensive agents with major antianginal efficacy, they are often the preferred agents for initial treatment, especially in the common setting of unstable angina pectoris.[243] A recent metanalysis suggested that the former are more effective, although the latter are more commonly used.[244] The recent HOPE trial showed a large survival benefit for high-risk hypertensives (most of whom had known CAD) treated with ramipril.[210] None of the volunteers in HOPE had known HF at enrollment, for which this degree of benefit would have been expected. This has been interpreted by some as evidence in favor of this class of medication or even for this specific agent for all hypertensive patients with CAD.

The issue of how low to reduce BP in the setting of CAD is controversial. Since coronary artery filling occurs during diastole, reducing perfusion pressure at this time might increase coronary ischemia. It is unlikely that a study similar to the HOT study will be done in patients with CAD, but some still recommend caution in lowering BP below 85 mmHg in patients with angina and/or known CAD. JNC VI indicated that "BP should be lowered to the usual target range (<140/90 mmHg), and even lower BP is desirable if angina persists."[7] A post hoc analysis comparing levels of achieved BP control among 270,000 hypertensives with or without CAD enrolled in recent clinical trials is planned by the World Health Organization/International Society of Hypertension's Collaborative Trialists' Group.[245] Even after such data become available, it probably will be advisable to use beta blockers, CAs, and perhaps nitrates for hypertensive patients with CAD, in order to achieve a slightly lower than usual BP target, and to recommend aspirin and intensive treatment of dyslipidemias. Sildenafil citrate (Viagra) appears to have no major interactions with any antihypertensive drugs, but all nitrate-containing preparations are contraindicated.

After Stroke   Although hypertension is the risk factor for stroke with the highest population-attributable risk, and "clinically evident cerebrovascular disease is an indication for antihypertensive treatment," optimal BP management depends on the nature, cause, and chronology of the neurologic symptoms. In the immediate setting of acute stroke, most neurologists avoid antihypertensive drugs unless BP is very high (e.g., BP >185/110 mmHg). If treatment is necessary, an intravenously administered, short-acting drug is preferred because it can be discontinued quickly if a patient's neurologic condition deteriorates acutely.

The PROGRESS Study proved that lowering BP in people who had suffered a prior stroke or TIA was beneficial, not only in preventing recurrent stroke but also in reducing CV events.[199] Although a significant benefit was seen only in the group receiving both the ACE inhibitor perindopril, and the diuretic indapamide (and not in those whose physicians chose to give them only perindopril), there was benefit for every group, regardless of baseline BP. *There should no longer be fear in lowering BP in patients who survive a stroke or TIA, once the acute phase has passed.*

SAFETY (ADVERSE REACTIONS AND SIDE EFFECTS)

The two primary types of adverse reactions and side effects that occur with antihypertensive therapy are clinical and biochemical (Table 61-17). Clinical side effects are directly evident to the patient and are perceived by the patient or the clinician to be related to the drug. The appearance of these adverse reactions requires that the drug be stopped or the dose be reduced, or the patient must be willing to remain on therapy until he or she becomes able to tolerate the side effect or it disappears. The drugs recommended for first- and second-line therapy (in Fig. 61-2) and ARBs generally cause fewer clinical side effects than do other drugs at doses that lower BP.

Biochemical side effects may lead to clinically evident adverse reactions (e.g., hypokalemia from thiazide diuretics causing muscle weakness, palpitations, nocturia, or polyuria), but usually the biochemical problems that occur with antihypertensive agents are more troublesome to the clinician than they are to the patient. The importance of biochemical side effects is usually not that they result in clinically evident problems but that these drug-related changes in lipids, glucose, or insulin may aggravate other risk factors and accelerate the clinical impact of dyslipidemias, glucose intolerance, or insulin resistance. It is unlikely that the relatively minor changes in glucose, triglycerides, HDL cholesterol, or TG that result from therapy with thiazides or beta blockers are responsible for an increase in

TABLE 61-22 Combination Products Currently Approved for Hypertension in the United States—Listed within subtype in Chronological Order of FDA Approval

Diuretic/diuretic combinations[a]	
Triamterene/hydrochlorothiazide (37.5/25, 50/25, 75/50)	Dyazide,[b] Maxzide[b]
Spironolactone/hydrochlorothiazide (25/25, 50/50)	Aldactone[b]
Amiloride/hydrochlorothiazide (5/50)	Moduretic[b]
Beta blocker/diuretic combinations	
Propranolol/hydrochlorothiazide (40/25, 80/25)	Inderide
Metoprolol/hydrochlorothiazide (50/25, 100/25)	Lopressor/HCT
Atenolol/chlorthalidone (50/25, 100/25)	Tenoretic
Nadolol/bendroflumethiazide (40/5, 80/5)	Corzide
Timolol/hydrochlorothiazide (10/25)	Timolide
Propranolol LA (long-acting)/hydrochlorothiazide (80/50, 120/50, 160/50)	Inderide LA
Bisoprolol/hydrochlorothiazide (2.5/6.25, 5/6.25, 10/6.25)	Ziac[c]
Centrally acting drug/diuretic combinations	
Guanethidine/hydrochlorothiazide (10/25)	Esimil
Methyldopa/hydrochlorothiazide (250/15, 250/25, 500/30, 500/50)	Aldoril
Methyldopa/chlorothiazide (250/150, 250/250)	Aldochlor
Reserpine/chlorothiazide (0.125/250, 0.25/500)	Diupres
Reserpine/chlorthalidone (0.125/25, 0.25/50)	Demi-Regroton
Reserpine/hydrochlorothiazide (0.125/25, 0.125/50)	Hydropres
Clonidine/chlorthalidone (0.1/15, 0.2/15, 0.3/15)	Combipres
ACE inhibitor/diuretic combinations	
Captopril/hydrochlorothiazide (25/15, 25/25, 50/15, 50/25)	Capozide[c]
Enalapril/hydrochlorothiazide (5/12.5, 10/25)	Vaseretic
Lisinopril/hydrochlorothiazide (10/12.5, 20/12.5, 20/25)	Prinzide, Zestoretic
Fosinopril/hydrochlorothiazide (10/12.5, 20/12.5)	Monopril/HCT
Quinapril/hydrochlorothiazide (10/12.5, 20/12.5, 20/25)	Accuretic
Benazepril/hydrochlorothiazide (5/6.25, 10/12.5, 20/12.5, 20/25)	Lotensin/HCT
Moexipril/hydrochlorothiazide (7.5/12.5, 15/25)	Uniretic
Angiotensin II receptor antagonist/diuretic combinations	
Losartan/hydrochlorothiazide (50/12.5, 100/25)	Hyzaar
Valsartan/hydrochlorothiazide (80/12.5, 160/12.5)	Diovan/HCT
Irbesatan/hydrochlorothiazide (75/12.5, 150/12.5, 300/12.5)	Avalide
Candesartan/hydrochlorothiazide (16/12.5, 32/12.5)	Atacand/HCT
Telmisartan/hydrochlorothiazide (40/12.5, 80/12.5)	Micardis/HCT
Eprosartan/hydrochlorothiazide (400/12.5, 600/12.5)	Teveten/HCT
Olmesartan/hydrochlorothiazide (20/12.5, 40/12.5, 40/25)	Benicor/HCT
Calcium antagonist/ACE inhibitor combinations	
Amlodipine/benazepril (2.5/10, 5/10, 5/20, 10/20)	Lotrel
Diltiazem/enalapril (180/5)	Teczem
Verapamil (extended release)/trandolapril (180/2, 240/1, 240/2, 240/4)	Tarka
Felodipine (extended release)/enalapril (5/5)	Lexxel
Vasodilator/diuretic combinations	
Hydralazine/hydrochlorothiazide (25/25, 50/25, 100/25)	Apresazide
Prazosin/polythiazide (1/0.5, 2/0.5, 5/0.5)	Minizide
Triple combination	
Reserpine/hydralazine/hydrochlorothiazide (0.10/25/15)	Ser-Ap-Es

[a]Numbers in parentheses indicate the dose (in milligrams) of each drug in a particular combination product.
[b]Indicated for initial therapy only for individuals in whom the development of hypokalemia cannot be risked.
[c]Approved by the U.S. Food and Drug Administration for initial therapy.

ischemic heart disease; the exact opposite has been seen in secondary MI prevention studies with several beta blockers. In ALLHAT, the biochemical profile of the group receiving the alpha blocker seemed favorable (lower cholesterol, TG, and glucose and higher K^+) compared with the group on chlorthalidone, yet the diuretic prevented CV events more successfully.[207] Similarly, chlorthalidone prevented at least one or more serious forms of CVD compared to either amlodipine or lisinopril, despite a significantly lower serum potassium and higher glucose and cholesterol at 4 years.[198]

At the doses that are now recommended, these changes and the electrolyte disturbances noted with thiazides are quite modest, although it is still possible that thiazides at high doses could reduce serum K^+ sufficiently to cause sudden cardiac death. Whether the increases in insulin resistance seen with thiazide diuretics and beta blockers and the hypokalemia seen with thiazide diuretics have precipitated DM sooner or in patients who would not otherwise have become diabetic is uncertain. It may be prudent to select another option for patients with DM or dyslipidemia as long as BP is reduced to goal. Certain types of dual therapy also may ameliorate biochemical adverse reactions. Thiazides and either ACE inhibitors or ARBs, when given together, produce few if any of the metabolic abnormalities associated with thiazides alone. Several fixed-dose combinations of these classes of drugs are available and may be appropriate as initial therapy[7] (Table 61-22).

The incidence of clinical side effects tends to rise with increasing doses with all classes of drugs with the exception of ACE inhibitors and ARBs. Patients who develop an adverse reaction on a high dose of a drug or on a dose they previously tolerated do not necessarily need to have that drug discontinued. Instead, the dose can be lowered and another antihypertensive can be added to reduce BP to goal. The primary problems with ACE inhibitors are cough and angioedema, both of which tend to be idiosyncratic and occur with all representatives of that class of agents. Reducing the dose or changing to a different ACE inhibitor is rarely helpful. ACE inhibitors should be increased to the maximum recommended dose before therapy is abandoned or another agent is added unless a low-dose combination is felt to be more appropriate. Angiotensin II receptor blockers are the best tolerated of all currently available antihypertensive agents, and patients persist in taking them at higher rates than other drugs.[246]

DEMOGRAPHIC CONSIDERATIONS

Blacks and Other Ethnic Minorities Some classes of antihypertensive agents reduce BP more or less effectively in certain ethnic groups. Thiazide diuretics, for example, are more effective in blacks than in whites, whereas ACE inhibitors, ARBs, and beta blockers are more effective, at lower doses, in whites than in blacks.[247] Peripheral alpha blockers, alpha/beta blockers, and CAs are equally effective in all ethnic groups. In general, the response rates to antihypertensive agents in Hispanics is intermediate between that seen in whites and that in blacks, while east Asians but not necessarily south Asians (patients from the Indian subcontinent) often need lower doses than do whites.

African Americans bear a larger population burden of hypertension and have a higher risk for hypertensive complications than whites. Because data on the benefits of treatment were limited, a larger sample than was present in the U.S. population was recruited for ALLHAT. The significantly poorer stroke, HF, and combined CVD rates in blacks treated with lisinopril (compared to chlorthalidone) may be due to the relative ineffectiveness of the ACE inhibitor in reducing BP when a diuretic cannot be added to the regimen.[198] However, the importance of ACE-inhibitor therapy in blacks was shown in AASK, in which diuretics were used in nearly all patients. In this study, patients randomized to ramipril did much better both in loss of glomerular filtration rate (GFR) and clinical events than those given either amlodipine or metoprolol.[219,248] Despite the slightly higher risk of angioedema and cough, there is no reason to avoid ACE inhibitors in black hypertensive patients but perhaps more reason to consider concomitant therapy with a diuretic.

The Elderly All classes of antihypertensive agents lower BP effectively in older persons, although the doses needed to reach goal are often lower than those necessary in young and middle-aged hypertensive patients. Certain drugs and certain classes of drugs, however, should be used with caution in older hypertensives. These include agents, such as peripheral alpha blockers, which can exacerbate the postural fall in BP seen more frequently in older individuals with baroreceptor dysfunction; nondihydropyridine CAs and beta blockers, which may aggravate subtle or subclinical conduction defects or precipitate systolic dysfunction and HF; and verapamil, which may not be well tolerated in some older persons already bothered by constipation. Cough from an ACE inhibitor is more common in older women. Although, compared to placebo, both diuretics and DHP CAs reduce morbidity and mortality in older persons with stage 2 isolated systolic hypertension,[155] chlorthalidone was more effective than amlodipine in preventing HF in ALLHAT and is much less expensive.[198] The benefits of effective treatment are more evident in older hypertensives, who are at higher absolute risk of CV events than are younger hypertensives. Even hypertensive patients above 80 years of age benefit significantly from treatment, especially in stroke prevention.[249] Therapy should not be withheld from the elderly for fear of toxicity or lack of efficacy.

Children The diagnosis and treatment of hypertension in children are different from those in adults, primarily because of the limited experience with antihypertensive drug therapy in children and the low risk of CV events in younger individuals.[250,251] Most pediatricians are very comfortable measuring and monitoring BP in their patients, but few nonnephrologists commit the expected 1 percent of their patients to drug therapy. Because of a higher incidence of secondary hypertension than there is in adults, most hypertensive children have at least an evaluation of the kidneys and urinary tract before beginning treatment.[251]

The diagnosis of hypertension in pediatric patients is truly population-based, since the 5 percent of children with the highest BP are diagnosed with "significant hypertension" and the highest 1 percent are deemed eligible for pharmacologic treatment.[251] The diagnostic cutoffs for hypertension in youth are age- and weight-dependent, and "growth charts" for plotting the progress of a child's BP against age are often completed by pediatricians for height, weight, and, more recently, BP. More frequent measurements and attention to BP are warranted when a child's BP exceeds the 90th percentile. Treatment of hypertension in children begins with lifestyle modifications, since they are likely to be beneficial as a child grows into adolescence and adulthood. There are limited data on the benefits of specific drugs in hypertensive children, although data about BP lowering with drugs in children are now being gathered. Although the recommended treatment algorithm is based on time-tested drug use in adults, there is a growing awareness of the possibility of long-term adverse effects with diuretics and especially beta blockers (which make exercise more difficult and may lead to weight gain) and a growing use of both ACE inhibitors and CAs. Doses of antihypertensive drugs in children are typically based on the body weight of the child.[251]

SPECIAL SITUATIONS

Pregnancy Hypertension is found in about 10 percent of pregnancies and is the major cause of perinatal morbidity and mortality in most developed countries. Because of the unique patient population, hypertension in pregnancy has a special definition, four specific types, and a treatment algorithm that recognizes the need to assess outcomes in both mother and baby. Since most pregnancies are managed by obstetricians, most of the authoritative pronouncements about this condition have been advanced by expert panels drawn from that discipline.[252,253] In the United States, hypertension in pregnancy is defined as either BP >140/90 mmHg on two measurements at least 4 h apart or a diastolic BP >110 mmHg at any time during pregnancy or up to 6 weeks postpartum.[253]

The classification of hypertension in pregnancy typically requires some knowledge of BP status before conception.[253] If there was preexisting hypertension, the patient is said to have "chronic hypertension," which can be diagnosed before 20 weeks' gestation and persists at least 42 days postpartum. Preeclampsia is hypertension appearing after 20 weeks' gestation, associated with proteinuria (at least 300 mg per 24-h collection or 1+ on a random dipstick without urinary tract infection), which typically resolves within 42 days after delivery. Other criteria help to make the diagnosis more likely.[253] Preeclampsia with superimposed chronic hypertension is a combination of the two. Gestational hypertension is diagnosed when and if the BP returns to normal within 42 days after delivery.

A large number of demographic, genetic, and laboratory parameters as well as other factors have been associated with a higher risk of preeclampsia, but none has been accepted as the underlying "cause" (Table 61-23). Despite many smaller studies claiming that low-dose aspirin or Ca^{2+} supplementation prevented preeclampsia in high-risk women, the large NIH-sponsored megatrials have been unsuccessful in showing benefit from these inexpensive preventive measures.[254,255]

TABLE 61-23 Factors Associated with Altered Risk for the Development of Preeclampsia

> Genetic markers
>> Angiotensinogen gene polymorphism
>> Tumor necrosis factor alpha (TNF-α) gene polymorphism
>> Mitochondrial transfer RNA gene mutation
> Congenital thrombophelias
>> Resistance to activated protein C (factor V Leiden, perhaps the most common form of hereditary thrombocytosis)
>> Mutation in gene for prothrombin factor II
>> Hyperhomocysteinemia (mutation C677T)
>> Protein S deficiency
>> Antiphospholipid antibody syndrome
>> Protein C and antithrombin deficiencies

SOURCE: Adapted from the 2000 Report of the National High Blood Pressure Education Program Working Group on High Blood Pressure in Pregnancy.[253]

These may be two situations in which the large, NIH-sponsored, well-done clinical trial ranks higher in medical evidence than a met-analysis.[256] Since aspirin tends to delay parturition and increase the likelihood of bleeding, few obstetricians routinely recommend it.

Treatment of elevated BP during pregnancy traditionally begins with bed rest, followed by methyldopa as the primary drug, based on its long history of efficacy and lack of adverse effects on babies. For severe hypertension (BP >160/109 mmHg) in outpatients that is not controlled with these measures to a diastolic BP between 90 and 100 mmHg, hydralazine, labetalol, and nifedipine are routinely added in succession.[253] ACE inhibitors and ARBs are contraindicated because of the risk of renal and other abnormalities in the fetus, and diuretics are typically avoided because of the risk of oligohydramnios. For intrapartum management, until delivery can be achieved, intravenous magnesium sulfate has been a mainstay for the prevention of progression of preeclampsia to seizures and other more serious complications.

Hypertension during pregnancy also carries prognostic significance for future health problems as the woman ages. Sixty percent of women with early-onset preeclampsia have abnormalities on renal biopsy and a higher risk of persistent hypertension after delivery. Women who develop hypertension during pregnancy are not only at higher risk for hypertension later in life but also have a roughly twofold increase in the risk of death from CAD.

Hypertensive Emergencies and Urgencies   Although rare, hypertensive crises still are seen in physicians' offices and emergency rooms.[257] Fortunately, there now are excellent medications available for both acute, in-hospital treatment and outpatient management; these improvements have led to a decrease in the 1-year mortality rate after a hypertensive emergency from 80 percent (1928) to 50 percent (1955) to less than 10 percent (Fig. 61-4).

The primary pathophysiologic abnormality in patients who experience hypertensive crises is the alteration of autoregulation in certain vascular beds (especially cerebral and renal), which often is followed by frank arteritis and ischemia in vital organs.[258] Autoregulation is the ability of blood vessels to dilate or constrict to maintain normal organ perfusion. Normal arteries from normotensive individuals can maintain flow over a wide range of mean arterial pressures, usually 60 to 150 mmHg. Chronic elevations of BP cause compensatory functional and structural changes in the arterial circulation and shift the autoregulatory curve to the right; this allows hypertensive patients to maintain normal perfusion and avoid excessive blood flow at higher BP levels. When BP increases above the autoregulatory range, tissue damage occurs. An understanding of autoregulation is also important for therapy, since the sudden lowering of BP into a range that would otherwise be considered normal may reduce BP below the autoregulatory capacity of the hypertensive circulation and lead to inadequate tissue perfusion (Fig. 61-5). In the later stages of a hypertensive crisis, pathologists can demonstrate cerebral edema and both acute and chronic inflammation of the medium and small arteries and arterioles, often associated with necrosis.

Hypertensive crises occur in a variety of clinical settings.[258] The most common is a chronic and often untreated patient with JNC VI–defined stage 3 essential hypertension (i.e., usual BP ≥180/110) whose BP rises above the autoregulatory range, triggering the pathophysiologic sequence outlined above. Identical crises can occur, however, any time there is an acute or rapid rise in BP in a normotensive or minimally hypertensive individual, such as a child or a woman during pregnancy. Hypertensive crises can most easily be recognized by the association of an extremely elevated BP with physical examination or laboratory findings that indicate acute TOD. The actual levels of BP are of little import.

The initial evaluation of a severely hypertensive patient includes a thorough inspection of the optic fundi (looking for acute hemorrhages, exudates, or papilledema); a mental status assessment; a careful cardiac, pulmonary, and neurologic examination; a quick search for clues that might indicate secondary hypertension (e.g., abdominal bruit, striae, radial-femoral delay); and laboratory studies to assess

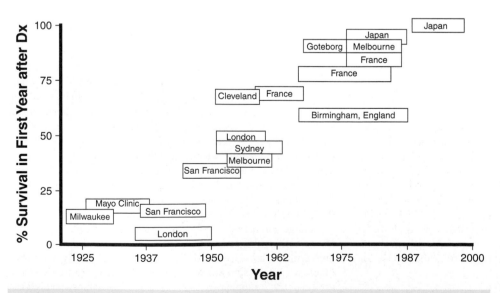

FIGURE 61-4 Improvement in 1-year survival from 1925 to 1999 among patients presenting with a hypertensive emergency. Dx = diagnosis. (From Elliott.[258] With permission.)

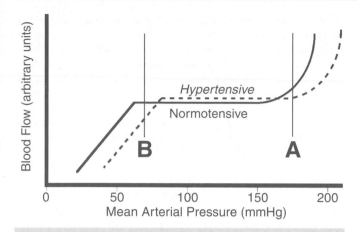

FIGURE 61-5 Blood pressure versus flow relationships in normotensive (dark curve) and hypertensive (dotted curve) persons, based on cerebral blood flow data. Chronically hypertensive persons can autoregulate their blood flow within the normal range despite higher blood pressures (e.g., vertical line A). Lowering BP in the setting of a hypertensive emergency to what might be considered "normal" (in a normotensive person, e.g., vertical line B) probably will put BP below the autoregulatory threshold and may compromise local circulation. (Adapted from Johansson B, Strandgaard S, Lassen NA. The hypertensive "breakthrough" of autoregulation of cerebral blood flow with forced vasodilation, flow increase, and blood-brain barrier damage. *Circ Res* 1974:34–35 (suppl I):I-167.)

renal function (dipstick and microscopic urinalysis, serum creatinine).[258]

There are several different types of common clinical presentations of hypertensive emergencies; the neurologic crises are the most difficult to distinguish from one another (Table 61-24). Hypertensive encephalopathy is typically a diagnosis of exclusion; hemorrhagic and thrombotic strokes usually are diagnosed after focal neurologic deficits are corroborated by CT. Subarachnoid hemorrhage is diagnosed by the typical findings on lumbar puncture. The management of each of these conditions is somewhat different in that nimodipine may be the drug of choice for subarachnoid hemorrhage because of its antihypertensive and anti-ischemic effects. Many physicians still prefer nitroprusside or another intravenous vasodilator because it can be discontinued rapidly if BP goes too low.[258] Goal BP also depends on the presenting diagnosis and is usually lower for encephalopathy than it is for acute stroke in evolution (Table 61-24). For hemorrhagic stroke and subarachnoid hemorrhage, BP lowering is usually not recommended unless the BP is "very high" (>180/105 mmHg).

Patients who present with hypertensive crises involving cardiac ischemia/infarction or pulmonary edema can be managed with either nitroglycerin or nitroprusside, although typically a combination of drugs (including an ACE inhibitor when there is HF) is used in these settings. Efforts to preserve myocardium and open the obstructed coronary artery (by thrombolysis, angioplasty, or surgery) also are indicated.

TABLE 61-24 Types of Hypertensive Crises with Suggested Drug Therapy and BP Targets

Type of Crisis	Drug of Choice	BP Target
Neurologic		
Hypertensive encephalopathy	Nitroprusside[a]	25% reduction in mean arterial pressure over 2–3 h
Intracranial hemorrhage or acute stroke in evolution	Nitroprusside[a] (controversial)	0–25% reduction in mean arterial pressure over 6–12 h (controversial)
Acute head injury/trauma	Nitroprusside[a]	0–25% reduction in mean arterial pressure over 2–3 h (controversial)
Subarachnoid hemorrhage	Nimodipine	Up to 25% reduction in mean arterial pressure in previously hypertensive patients, 130–160 systolic in normotensive patients
Cardiac		
Ischemia/infarction	Nitroglycerin or nicardipine	Reduction in ischemia
Heart failure	Nitroprusside[a] or nitroglycerin	Improvement in failure (typically 10–15% decrease in BP)
Aortic dissection	Beta blocker + nitroprusside[a]	120 mmHg systolic in 30 min (if possible)
Renal		
Hematuria or acute renal impairment	Fenoldopam	0–25% reduction in mean arterial pressure over 1–12 h
Catecholamine-excess states		
Pheochromocytoma	Phentolamine	To control paroxysms
Drug withdrawal	Drug withdrawn	Typically only one dose necessary
Pregnancy-related		
Eclampsia	MgSO$_4$, methyldopa, hydralazine	Typically <90 mmHg diastolic, but often lower

[a]Some physicians prefer an intravenous infusion of either fenoldopam or nicardipine, neither of which has potentially toxic metabolites, over nitroprusside. Recent studies have also shown improvements in renal function during therapy with the former as compared to nitroprusside.
SOURCE: Adapted from Elliott.[258] With permission.

Patients with aortic dissection are managed in a somewhat different fashion.[259] A beta blocker is added to the intravenous vasodilator and the goal BP is much lower: Typically 120 mmHg systolic is recommended, but 100 mmHg systolic may be even better. Pharmacologic therapy is only a temporary adjunct to definitive surgical therapy, which should be planned with dispatch, although long-term medical therapy may be more appropriate in some patients.[260]

Hypertensive crises involving the kidney commonly are followed by a further deterioration in renal function even when BP is lowered properly.[257] Some physicians prefer fenoldopam to nicardipine or nitroprusside in this setting because of its lack of toxic metabolites and specific renal vasodilating effects.[261] BP should be reduced about 10 percent during the first hour and a further 10 to 15 percent during the next 1 to 3 h. The need for acute dialysis often is precipitated by BP reduction, but many patients are able to avoid dialysis in the long term if BP is carefully and well controlled during follow-up.

Hypertensive crises resulting from catecholamine excess states [pheochromocytoma, monoamine oxidase (MAO) inhibitor crisis, cocaine intoxication, etc.] are best managed with an intravenous alpha blocker (phentolamine), with a beta blocker added later if needed. Many patients with severe hypertension caused by sudden withdrawal of antihypertensive agents (e.g., clonidine) are easily managed by reinstituting the previous therapy.

Hypertensive crises during pregnancy must be managed in a more careful and conservative manner because of the presence of the fetus. Magnesium sulfate, methyldopa, and hydralazine are the drugs of choice, with oral labetalol and nifedipine being drugs of second choice in the United States. Delivery of the infant often assists in the management of hypertension in pregnancy and often is hastened by the obstetrician under these conditions.

Hypertensive urgencies are situations in which acute TOD is not present; they require somewhat less aggressive management and nearly always can be handled with oral antihypertensive agents without admission to the hospital. Nifedipine, clonidine, captopril, labetalol, and several other short-acting antihypertensive drugs have been used for this problem. Nifedipine has been reported to cause precipitous hypotension, stroke, MI, and death and, according to the FDA, "should be used with great caution, if at all."[262] Otherwise, none of these drugs seems to have a major advantage over all the others, and all are effective in most patients.[263] *The most important aspect of managing a hypertensive urgency is to assure adherence to antihypertensive therapy during long-term follow-up.*

Patients presenting with a hypertensive emergency should be diagnosed quickly and started promptly on effective parenteral therapy (often nitroprusside 0.5 μg/kg per minute) in an intensive care unit. BP should be reduced about 25 percent gradually over 2 to 3 h. Oral antihypertensive therapy should be instituted after 6 to 12 h of parenteral therapy; evaluation for secondary causes of hypertension may be considered after transfer from the intensive care unit. Because of advances in antihypertensive therapy and management, "malignant hypertension" should be malignant no longer.

DOSE SCHEDULE (DOSAGE AND CHRONOTHERAPY)

It is clear that BP needs to be controlled for 24 h. Drug preparations that are given once a day are easier for patients to remember to take, but adherence to treatment is usually only slightly worse if twice-a-day preparations are used. In fact, patients may be better protected if they forget to take one dose of a twice-a-day medication and thus are uncovered for 12 h than if they skip a once-a-day pill and are unprotected for a considerably longer period.

In addition to controlling BP over 24 h, long-acting and some newer agents may blunt the early-morning increase in BP and HR. Many of the major sequelae of hypertension have a strong circadian

variation, with a peak incidence in the early morning. Recent met-analyses have estimated the excess risk of heart attack during the period from 6 A.M. to noon at 40 percent, sudden cardiac death at 29 percent, and stroke at 49 percent compared with what would be expected if these events happened evenly or randomly throughout the day.[264,265] Since most patients take antihypertensive agents in the morning, most authorities recommend long-acting drugs that should cover the early-morning period, when BP, pulse, and cardiovascular risk are highest. Although many of the currently used medications have short intrinsic elimination half-lives, pharmaceutical technology has made available several methods of making sustained-release compounds from short-acting drugs.[266,267]

Three preparations of CAs have been formulated to be taken in the evening and release either verapamil or diltiazem mostly in the early morning hours. No drug is released during the sleeping hours, which might cause excessive lowering of BP during the middle of the night. The same matching of drug delivery to the circadian pattern of BP is not achieved by giving other preparations of the same drugs at night. Although these newer preparations lower the early morning rise in BP and HR, the CONVINCE study was stopped by its sponsor before sufficient events were observed to allow evaluation of the first of these "chronotherapeutic" preparations in preventing major CV events. Although statistical power was low and the results were confounded by non-adherence to therapy, there was no evidence that the Controlled-Onset, Extended Release (COER)-verapamil preparation prevented morning CV events more than the traditional morning dose of either a diuretic or beta blocker.[206]

DRUG INTERACTIONS

The selection of the initial agent to treat hypertension must be done with the understanding that many hypertensive patients may not reach goal BP on that agent alone and will therefore need additional antihypertensive therapy. Furthermore, many hypertensive patients need to take chronic medications for other conditions, and so drug-drug interactions are of concern.

Certain combinations of antihypertensive agents are particularly effective, such as thiazide diuretics with beta blockers, ACE inhibitors, or ARBs. Combinations of ACE inhibitors with CAs (both DHP and non-DHP) are also effective. Moreover, combinations of the two subtypes of CAs are synergistic with regard to BP reduction. DHP CAs and beta blockers are also very effective combinations. Non-DHP CAs and beta blockers should not be used together because of the risk of excessive bradycardia and conduction defects. Thiazide diuretics are also effective with all other antihypertensive drugs, including CAs and should always be included in a triple-drug regimen. Little is known about the efficacy of combining alpha blockers with central and peripheral sympatholytics or with ACE inhibitors or ARBs.

Recently a series of low-dose combinations have been introduced that have fewer clinical side effects than occur when the components are used as monotherapy (Table 61-22). The best example is the combination of a DHP CA with an ACE inhibitor. These fixed-dose combinations are associated with a significantly lower incidence of edema than that seen when a DHP CA is given alone. The incidence of cough, however, is not lessened when these drugs are combined. The appeal of a low-dose fixed-dose combination is that BP can be reduced more quickly and effectively, with fewer adverse reactions using two drugs at lower doses than might occur when one or the other component is pushed to the maximum dose. The added advantage is that the patient needs to take fewer pills to get BP to goal; thus adherence to the regimen tends to improve (see below).

Most commonly used antihypertensives do not have any serious drug-drug interactions with anticoagulants, platelet inhibitors, or antibiotics. Non-DHP CAs, beta blockers, and telmisartan (an ARB) must be used with care in patients who are taking digoxin. Nonsteroidal anti-inflammatory agents may raise BP and interfere with the activity of all antihypertensive agents; it is still controversial whether the specific inhibitors of cyclooxygenase-2 interfere as much or as widely as the older cyclooxygenase-1 inhibitors.

ADHERENCE

Overall, fewer than 50 percent of patients continue taking the initially prescribed antihypertensive drug therapy for 4 years.[246] The proportion who adhere to therapy properly improves only modestly when the drugs and medical care are provided free of charge.[198] About 10 percent of the overall expenditures on hypertension in the United States are wasted because of nonadherence to medical advice and antihypertensive drug therapy. Patients who do not follow the advice of their physicians and do not take their medications correctly have an *infinite* cost/benefit ratio because they incur all the cost associated with the therapy but derive *none* of the benefits of treatment.

To assess adherence with antihypertensive medications precisely is generally difficult, but several simple measures often are recommended.[7] Some medications induce physical signs that are absent in those who have not recently taken them—e.g., bradycardia with beta blockers, orthostatic BP change with alpha blockers, and an increase in serum urate with diuretics. A telephone call to the patient's pharmacy generally will reveal how many times the patient's prescriptions have been refilled during the preceding year. Several interventions have been advocated to improve adherence with medications (Table 61-25).

MECHANISM OF ACTION OF THE DRUG AND PATHOPHYSIOLOGY OF THE PATIENT'S HYPERTENSION

Some have felt that physicians could be much more successful in treating hypertensive patients if they could match their choice of drug therapy with the reason why the patient is hypertensive (the pathophysiologic abnormality responsible for the patient's hypertension). If physicians truly could know precisely why an individual was hypertensive and easily and safely obtain such information, treating hypertension would be not be complicated. If it really were known

exactly how drugs work, those decisions would be much simpler. This approach, while intellectually appealing, has problems.

The first difficulty is that attempts to profile patients either biochemically using PRA, for example, or hemodynamically by measuring cardiac output and peripheral vascular resistance are expensive. In addition, these methods are not precise enough to provide the kind of necessarily definitive information needed to predict the response to therapy in a particular patient. Furthermore, trying to base therapy on the presumed pathophysiology in an individual would be expected to have is also imprecise, even when it might work well in large populations. This approach runs the risk of denying certain patients the potential benefits of certain classes of drugs. Although it is true that blacks and older persons tend on the average to have low or suppressed PRA, many do not. Also, many patients with a low PRA will respond to drugs such as ACE inhibitors or ARBs that are less effective on the average in hypertensives with this renin profile. When sequential monotherapy was rotated among five drugs, only 18 percent of the 34 young subjects had BP that was >10 mmHg lower than on any other therapy.[268] In the VA trial of monotherapy, the selection of initial treatment on the basis of PRA was less effective than simply using age and ethnicity (thiazide diuretics and CAs for older patients and blacks and ACE inhibitors and beta blockers for whites and in those less than 60 years of age).[247] However, neither method correctly predicted a good response in more than 63 percent of the patients.[247]

The second issue that complicates this approach is that many drugs have complex mechanisms of action and may work well in patient subgroups in which they were supposed to be ineffective. For example, thiazide diuretics not only reduce plasma volume but also act as vasodilators after 4 weeks of therapy. These agents are effective and very well tolerated in older persons even though many have a modestly decreased plasma volume compared with younger hypertensives. Although ACE inhibitors usually suppress the endocrine renin-angiotensin-aldosterone (RAA) system, the antihypertensive effect is still evident even when plasma A II concentration returns to pretreatment levels. This is good evidence for a tissue site of action for these drugs or for the possibility that other mechanisms, perhaps the stimulation of bradykinin or nitric oxide, participate in the way ACE inhibitors lower BP; that is, there is the suggestion that the initial formulation of their mechanism of action was incomplete. This also explains why some patients with low PRA (a measure of the activity of the *endocrine* RAA system) respond well to these agents or to ARBs, which suppress the RAA system at the angiotensin AT_1 receptor in tissues throughout the body. Calcium antagonists were presumed to work best in older hypertensives and in those with suppressed PRA, but these agents are equally effective in all subgroups of hypertensives.

Perhaps the major flaw in the reasoning that drugs can be used to "probe" the pathophysiologic abnormality causing a patient's hypertension is the concept that there is a single overriding abnormality responsible for that patient's elevated BP. In all likelihood, more than one or perhaps many of the systems that control BP (see above) are dysfunctional simultaneously, and single drugs or combinations of pharmacologic agents that reduce BP do so by correcting more than one abnormality.

COST

The economics of hypertension and its therapy are complex, but the simple fact is that if a person cannot afford to pay for the drug chosen by the health care provider, the written prescription will do little good in the long term.[28] Many pharmacists and businesspeople associated with health care believe that the agent with the lowest purchase price is the best, but this oversimplification omits the costs of extra visits to health care providers, laboratory testing, and adverse

---

TABLE 61-25 Interventions That Promote Adherence to Medications

Educate the patient regarding the proper use of medications
Improve patient's social support network (e.g., spouse or caretaker)
Increase patient's autonomy and involvement in decision making when appropriate
Remove barriers to compliance with pill taking
Integrate into activities of daily living (e.g., brushing teeth)
Avoid large ("horse") pills
Avoid bad-tasting formulations (e.g., lactulose, quinine)
Simplify the therapeutic regimen
Minimize the number of pills
Minimize the frequency of pill taking
Minimize the inconvenience of pill taking
Provide a positive attitude and positive reinforcement about achieving therapeutic goals
Maintain continuity of care with the same practitioner
Use well-tolerated antihypertensive drug therapy, individualized for each patient

drug experiences that result in emergency room visits or hospitalization. Such global evaluations of the economics of hypertension and its therapy are rare. It is possible for a more expensive but better-tolerated drug (e.g., an ARB) to actually be less expensive in the long term than another agent that produces many side effects or other conditions, some of which must be evaluated by laboratory testing, physician visits, and even hospitalization.

Generically available drugs are usually less expensive to purchase than their branded counterparts and are strongly favored in most managed care pharmacy plans by both mandates to physicians and lower copayments by patients.[196] Generic formulations are available for at least one agent from each of the major drug classes except ARBs, which have produced the least data in outcomes trials. ALLHAT was the most recent demonstration of the value of inexpensive, generically available drugs; its conclusion recommended the thiazide not only because of efficacy in preventing one or more forms of CVD but also because of its low cost.[198]

Many authorities are concerned that achieving the new, lower target BPs for diabetic and renally impaired hypertensives will cost more, as it will require more visits to health care providers and more antihypertensive medications. These increases in short-term expenditures are likely, however, to be offset by a lower future incidence of expensive outcomes, including heart attack, stroke, ESRD, and HF, at least for diabetic patients over age 60 in the United States.[218]

Many proposals for reducing the high cost of antihypertensive therapy have been advanced. In stage 2 hypertension, initial combination drug tablets have been recommended by JNC 7, as these tablets typically cost much less than two separate prescriptions for the same doses of individual agents.[4] Some formularies and pharmacy benefits managers prefer agents that have all doses priced identically, in the belief that a pill splitter can then be used to divide one tablet into treatment for 2 days or more.

Until a universal pharmacy benefits program is instituted, there are likely to be wide variations in the pricing and cost of antihypertensive agents. Although it is difficult for physicians to stay abreast of fluctuations in these costs, it is important that all health care providers attempt to provide tolerable antihypertensive medications at the lowest possible cost for the benefit of the patient, the health plan, and the national budget.

SUMMARY AND RECOMMENDATIONS

Although there are numerous options and many sources of error, the successful pharmacologic treatment of a hypertensive patient need not be complicated. Once the diagnosis has been established and the routine evaluation and other necessary tests have been completed, lifestyle modifications should begin. Lifestyle modifications should be given time to work unless the patient is in a group for which drug therapy should be added. Drug therapy is indicated in all hypertensive patients if goal BP is not reached with lifestyle modifications alone.

The following steps are recommended for choosing a regimen and then altering it until the goal is reached:

- Deal first with cost. If the patient is unable to afford any but the least expensive drugs or cannot pay for the one that is selected, price becomes the primary issue.
- Ascertain whether other risk factors or comorbidity are present. Avoid drugs that may worsen these factors or conditions and choose the ones that may improve them.
- Find out what clinical adverse reactions the patient would or did find most troublesome and avoid agents that are likely to cause or

exacerbate these problems. Some patients are not concerned by certain side effects that are very troublesome to others.
- Consider demographic issues and select the class of drug with a higher probability of success if options are available. A thiazide-like diuretic (preferably chlorthalidone) is recommended if there is a free choice of drug treatment for a patient over 55 years of age.
- Start with the lowest effective dose and plan to see the patient within 4 weeks unless the severity of the patient's hypertension or another problem warrants an earlier visit. Carry out appropriate biochemical monitoring when necessary. Start with a fixed-dose combination when appropriate (e.g., stage 2 hypertension).
- Increase the dose if goal BP has not been reached or if there has been only a suboptimal response. Do not increase the first dose or any dose prematurely. Give each dose enough time to be fully effective. If intolerable side effects occur and are likely to be drug-related or if there has been no response, only then switch to another appropriate agent as monotherapy.
- Continue the process of dose titration and monitoring until the maximum recommended dose has been reached. Stopping before the full dose has been reached leads to a situation in which the patient is treated with multiple agents at subtherapeutic doses when only one or two drugs may be necessary.
- If the maximum-tolerated dose of the first drug fails to reduce BP to goal, add a second agent that has a different mechanism of action and is known to have additive antihypertensive effects to the first-choice agent. A fixed-dose combination that combines two drugs in the desired doses also could be used at this time.
- Titrate the second drug to the full dose, as was done for the first drug, and continue appropriate monitoring. If the two-drug combination fails, consider a specific cause for the patient's refractory hypertension, and if none is evident, add a third drug, being sure that a diuretic is part of the regimen. Consider a referral to a hypertension specialist.
- Plan to see a patient who is at goal at least once every 3 months to be sure that BP control is sustained.
- Reinforce the need for adherence to the regimen (including lifestyle modifications) and inquire about adverse reactions. Although some patients will not reach goal with this approach even with the many available treatment options, most will come under control or close to it. Patients who do this can anticipate substantial long-term benefit with an extended life expectancy and a much reduced risk of stroke, ischemic heart disease, HF, and probably renal failure and quite possibly, dementia.

CONCLUSION

Although treating high BP can be costly and at times may seem unrewarding, the benefits to individual patients and to society make the effort worthwhile. Physicians must be careful not to become apathetic about hypertension. This important public health problem has not been solved and will not be solved until all hypertensive patients are able to avail themselves of what has been among the most successful examples of preventive medicine.

References

1. Murray CJ, Lopez AD. Alternative projections of mortality and disability by cause 1990–2020: Global Burden of Disease Study. *Lancet* 1997;349:1498–1504.
2. Kannel WB. Blood pressure as a cardiovascular risk factor: Prevention and treatment. *JAMA* 1996;275:1571–1576.

3. Age-specific relevance of usual blood pressure to vascular mortality: A meta-analysis of individual data for one million adults in 61 prospective studies. Prospective Studies Collaborative. *Lancet* 2002;360:1903–1913.

4. Chobanian AV, Bakris GL, Black HR, et al. The seventh report of the Joint National Committee on Prevention, Detection, Evaluation, and Treatment of High Blood Pressure: The JNC 7 Report. *JAMA* 2003; 289:2560–2572.

5. Vasan RS, Larson MG, Leip EP, et al. Impact of high-normal blood pressure on the risk of cardiovascular disease. *N Engl J Med* 2001;345: 1291–1297.

6. Whelton PK, He J, Appel LJ, et al. Primary prevention of hypertension: Clinical and public health advisory from the National High Blood Pressure Education Program. *JAMA* 2002;288:1882–1888.

7. The sixth report of the Joint National Committee on Prevention, Detection, Evaluation, and Treatment of High Blood Pressure (JNC VI). *Arch Intern Med* 1997;157:2413–2446.

8. Hyman DJ, Pavlik VN. Characteristics of patients with uncontrolled hypertension in the United States. *N Engl J Med* 2001;345:479–486.

9. Erdine S. How well is hypertension controlled in Europe? *J Hypertens* 2000;18:1348–1349.

10. 1999 World Health Organization–International Society of Hypertension Guidelines for the Management of Hypertension: Guidelines Subcommittee. *J Hypertens* 1999;17:151–183.

11. Wallis EJ, Ramsay LE, Haq IU, et al. Coronary and cardiovascular risk estimation for primary prevention: Validation of a new Sheffield table in the 1995 Scottish health survey population. *Br Med J* 2000;320: 671–676.

12. Executive Summary of the Third Report of the National Cholesterol Education Program (NCEP) Expert Panel on Detection, Evaluation, and Treatment of High Blood Cholesterol in Adults (Adult Treatment Panel III). *JAMA* 2001;285:2486–2497.

13. Lee ML, Rosner BA, Weiss ST. Relationship of blood pressure to cardiovascular death: The effects of pulse pressure in the elderly. *Ann Epidemiol* 1999;9:101–107.

14. van den Hoogen PCW, Feskens EJM, Nagelkerke NJD, et al. The relation between blood pressure and mortality due to coronary heart disease among men in different parts of the world. *N Engl J Med* 2000; 342:1–8.

15. Blood pressure, cholesterol, and stroke in eastern Asia: Eastern Stroke and Coronary Heart Disease Collaborative Research Group. *Lancet* 1998;352:1801–1807.

16. Staessen JA, Wang JG, Thijs L. Cardiovascular protection and blood pressure reduction: A meta-analysis. *Lancet* 2001;358:1305 1315.

17. Kannel WB. Risk stratification in hypertension: New insights from the Framingham Study. *Am J Hypertens* 2000;13(suppl 2):3S–10S.

18. Ferrannini E, Natali A, Capaldo B, et al. Insulin resistance, hyperinsulinemia, and blood pressure. *Hypertension* 1997;30:1144–1149.

19. Izzo JL Jr, Levy D, Black HR. Clinical advisory statement: Importance of systolic blood pressure in older Americans. *Hypertension* 2000; 35:1021–1024.

20. Vasan RS, Beiser A, Seshadri S, et al. Residual lifetime risk for developing hypertension in middle-aged women and men: The Framingham Heart Study. *JAMA* 2002;287:1003–1010.

21. Black HR, Kuller LH, O'Rourke MF, et al. The first report of the Systolic and Pulse Pressure (SYPP) Working Group on systolic and pulse pressure. *J Hypertens.* 1999;17(suppl 5):S3–S14.

22. Dart AM, Kingwell BA. Pulse pressure—A review of mechanisms and clinical relevance. *J Am Coll Cardiol* 2001;37:975–984.

23. Grossman E, Messerli FH, Neutel JM. Angiotensin II receptor blockers: Equal or preferred substitutes for ACE inhibitors? *Arch Intern Med* 2000;160:1905–1911.

24. Hansson L, Smith DH, Reeves R, Lapuerta P. Headache in mild-to-moderate hypertension and its reduction by irbesartan therapy. *Arch Intern Med* 2000;160:1654–1658.

25. Grimm RH, Grandits GA, Cutler JA, et al. Relationships of quality of life measures to long-term lifestyle and drug treatment in the Treatment of Mild Hypertension Study (TOMHS). TOMHS Research Group. *Arch Intern Med* 1997;157:638–648.

26. Wiklund I, Halling K, Ryden-Bergsten T, Fletcher A. Does lowering the blood pressure improve the mood? Quality-of-life results from the Hypertension Optimal Treatment (HOT) study. *Blood Pressure* 1997; 6:357–364.

27. Elliott WJ. Improving the cost-effectiveness of treating hypertension. In: Epstein M, ed. *Calcium Antagonists in Clinical Medicine,* 3d ed. Philadelphia: Hanley & Belfus; 2002:733–748.

28. Elliott WJ. Economic considerations in the management of hypertension. In: Izzo J, Black HR, eds. *Hypertension Primer,* 3d ed. Baltimore: Lippincott, Williams & Wilkins; 2003:317–319.

29. *American Heart Association's Heart & Stroke Facts, Statistical Supplement.* Dallas: American Heart Association; 2003:40.

30. Beevers G, Lip GY, O'Brien E. ABC of hypertension: The pathophysiology of hypertension. *Br Med J* 2001;322:912–916.

31. David RJ, Collins JW Jr. Differing birth weight among infants of U.S.-born blacks, African-born blacks, and U.S.-born whites. *N Engl J Med* 1997;337:1209–1214.

32. Keller G, Zimmer G, Mall G, et al. Nephron number in patients with primary hypertension. *N Engl J Med.* 2003;348:101–108.

33. Cowley AW Jr, Roman RJ. The role of the kidney in hypertension. *JAMA* 1996;275:1581–1589.

34. Morimoto S, Sasaki S, Itoh H, et al. Sympathetic activation and contribution of genetic factors in hypertension with neurovascular compression of the rostral ventrolateral medulla. *J Hypertens* 1999;17: 1577–1582.

35. Laitinen T, Hartikainen J, Niskanen L, et al. Sympathovagal balance is major determinant of short-term blood pressure variability in healthy subjects. *Am J Physiol* 1999;276(4 Part 2):H1245–H1252.

36. Adamopoulos S, Rosano GM, Ponikowski P, et al. Impaired baroreflex sensitivity and sympathovagal balance in syndrome X. *Am J Cardiol* 1998;82:862–868.

37. DiBona GF, Kopp UC. Neural control of renal function. *Physiol Rev* 1997;77:76–97.

38. Julius S, Valentini M. Continuing on J. P. Henry's path: Studies of physiology and pathophysiology of cardiopulmonary receptors in humans. *Acta Physiol Scand Suppl* 1997;640:122–124.

39. Narkiewicz K, Pesek CA, Kato M, et al. Baroreflex control of sympathetic nerve activity and heart rate in obstructive sleep apnea. *Hypertension* 1998;32:1039–1043.

40. Ryuzaki M, Stahl LK, Lyson T, et al. Sympathoexcitatory response to cyclosporin A and baroreflex resetting. *Hypertension* 1997;29: 576–582.

41. Ligtenberg G, Blankestijn PJ, Oey PL, et al. Reduction of sympathetic hyperactivity by enalapril in patients with chronic renal failure. *N Engl J Med* 1999;340:1321–1328.

42. Watanabe K, Sekiya M, Tsuruoka T, et al. Relationship between insulin resistance and cardiac sympathetic nervous function in essential hypertension. *J Hypertens* 1999;17:1161–1168.

43. Yuasa S, Li X, Hitomi H, et al. Sodium sensitivity and sympathetic nervous system in hypertension induced by long-term nitric oxide blockade in rats. *Clin Exp Pharmacol Physiol* 2000;27:18–24.

44. Weir MR. Impact of salt intake on blood pressure and proteinuria in diabetes: Importance of the renin-angiotensin system. *Miner Electrolyte Metab* 1998;24:438–445.

45. Cappuccio FP, Markandu ND, Carney C, et al. Double-blind randomized trial of modest salt restriction in older people. *Lancet* 1997;350: 850–854.

46. Lifton RP, Gharavi AG, Geller DS. Molecular mechanisms of human hypertension. *Cell* 2001;104:545–556.

47. Graudal NA, Galloe AM, Garred P. Effects of sodium restriction on blood pressure, renin, aldosterone, catecholamines, and triglycerides: A meta-analysis. *JAMA* 1998;279:1383–1391.

48. Alam S, Johnson AG. A meta-analysis of randomized controlled trials (RCT) among healthy normotensive and essential hypertensive elderly patients to determine the effect of high salt (NaCl) diet of blood pressure. *J Hum Hypertens* 1999;13:367–374.

49. He J, Whelton PK, Appel LJ, et al. Long-term effects of weight loss and dietary sodium reduction on incidence of hypertension. *Hypertension* 2000;35:544–549.

50. Timmermans PB. Angiotensin II receptor antagonists: An emerging new class of cardiovascular therapeutics. *Hypertens Res* 1999;22: 147–153.

51. Weber MA. Angiotensin II receptor antagonists in the treatment of hypertension. *Cardiol Rev* 1997;5:72–80.

52. Laragh JH. Abstract, closing summary, and table of contents for Laragh's 25 lessons in pathophysiology and 12 clinical pearls for treating hypertension. *Am J Hypertens* 2001;14:1173–1177.

53. Thibonnier M, Kilani A, Rahman M, et al. Effects of the nonpeptide V(1) vasopressin receptor antagonist SR49059 in hypertensive patients. *Hypertension* 1999;34:1293–1300.

54. Bakris GL, Kusmirek SL, Smith AC, et al. Calcium antagonism abolishes the antipressor action of vasopressin (V1) receptor antagonism. *Am J Hypertens* 1997;10:1153–1158.

55. Bakris G, Bursztyn M, Gavras I, et al. Role of vasopressin in essential hypertension: Racial differences. *J Hypertens* 1997;15:545–550.

56. Gardener SM, March JE, Kemp PA, Bennett T. Cardiovascular responses to angiotensins I and II in normotensive and hypertensive rats: Effects of NO synthase inhibition or ET receptor antagonism. *Br J Pharmacol* 1999;128:1795–1803.

57. Krum H, Viskoper RJ, Lacourciere Y, et al. The effect of an endothelin-receptor antagonist, bosentan, on blood pressure in patients with essential hypertension: Bosentan Hypertension Investigators. *N Engl J Med* 1998;338:784–790.

58. Kim NH, Rubin IJ. Endothelin in health and disease: Endothelin receptor antagonists in the management of pulmonary artery hypertension. *J Cardiovasc Pharmacol Ther* 2002;7:9–19.

59. Taler SJ, Textor SC, Canzanello VJ, Schwartz GL. Cyclosporin-induced hypertension: Incidence, pathogenesis and management. *Drug Saf* 1999;20:437–449.

60. Moe GW, Albermaz A, Naik GO, et al. Beneficial effects of long-term selective endothelin type A receptor blockade in canine experimental heart failure. *Cardiovasc Res* 1998;39:571–579.

61. Higashi Y, Oshima T, Ozono R, et al. Effect of L-arginine infusion on systemic and renal hemodynamics in hypertensive patients. *Am J Hypertens* 1999;12:8–15.

62. Cardillo C, Panza JA. Impaired endothelial regulation of vascular tone in patients with systemic arterial hypertension. *Vasc Med* 1998;3: 138–144.

63. Vogel RA. Cholesterol lowering and endothelial function. *Am J Med* 1999;107:479–487.

64. Sartori C, Scherrer U. Insulin, nitric oxide and the sympathetic nervous system: At the crossroads of metabolic and cardiovascular regulation. *J Hypertens* 1999;17:1517–1525.

65. Kotchen TA, McCarron DA. Dietary electrolytes and blood pressure: A statement for healthcare professionals from the American Heart Association Nutrition Committee. *Circulation* 1998;98:613–617.

66. McCarron DA, Reusser ME. Finding consensus in the dietary calcium-blood pressure debate. *J Am Coll Nutr* 1999;18(suppl 5): 398S–405S.

67. Tobian L. Dietary sodium chloride and potassium have effects on the pathophysiology of hypertension in humans and animals. *Am J Clin Nutr* 1997;65(suppl 2):606S–611S.

68. Wilson DK, Sica DA, Miller SB. Effects of potassium on blood pressure in salt-sensitive and salt-resistant black adolescents. *Hypertension* 1999;34:181–186.

69. Campese VM. Salt-sensitive hypertension: Renal and cardiovascular implications. *Nutr Metab Cardiovasc Dis* 1999;9:143–156.

70. Takahashi H. Endogenous digitalislike factor: An update. *Hypertens Res Clin Exp* 2000;23 (suppl):S1–S5.

71. Charles CJ, Lainchbury JG, Lewis LK, et al. The role of adrenomedullin. *Am J Hypertension* 1999;12:166–173.

72. Johnson RJ, Schreiner GF. Hypothesis: The role of acquired tubulointerstitial disease in the pathogenesis of salt-dependent hypertension. *Kidney Int* 1997;52:1169–1179.

73. Zou AP, Nithipatikom K, Li PL, Cowley AW Jr. Role of renal medullary adenosine in the control of blood flow and sodium excretion. *Am J Physiol* 1999;276(3 Part 2):R790–R798.

74. Szentivanyi M Jr, Zou AP, Maeda CY, et al. Increase in renal medullary nitric oxide synthase activity protects from norepinephrine-induced hypertension. *Hypertension* 2000;35:418–423.

75. Stehouwer CDA, Lambert J, Donker AJM, van Hinsbergh VWM. Endothelial dysfunction and pathogenesis of diabetic angiopathy. *Cardiovasc Res* 1997;34:55–68.

76. Andersen UB, Dige-Petersen H, Frandsen EK, et al. Basal insulin-level oscillations in normotensive individuals with genetic predisposition to essential hypertension exhibit an irregular pattern. *J Hypertens* 1997;15:1167–1173.

77. Luft FC. Molecular genetics of human hypertension. *J Hypertens* 1998;16:1871–1878.

78. Takeda Y. Genetic alterations in patients with primary hyperaldosteronism. *Hypertens Res Clin Exp* 2001;24:469–474.

78a. Lifton R. Molecular genetics of human blood pressure measurement. *Science* 1996;272:676–680.

78b. Lifton RP, Dluhy RG, Powers M, et al. A chimaeric 11-hydroxylase/aldosterone synthase gene causes glucocorticoid-remediable aldosteronism and human hypertension. *Nature* 1992;355:262–265.

79. Hastings NB, Orchinik M, Aubourg MV, McEven BS. Pharmacological characterization of central and peripheral type I and type II adrenal steroid receptors in the prairie vole, a glucocorticoid-resistant rodent. *Endocrinology* 1999;140:4459–4469.

80. Wallerath T, Witte K, Schafer SC, et al. Down-regulation of the expression of endothelial NO synthase is likely to continue to glucocorticoid-mediated hypertension. *Proc Natl Acad Sci USA* 1999;96:13,357–13,362.

81. Warnock DG. Liddle syndrome: Genetics and mechanisms of Na$^+$ channel defects. *Am J Med Sci* 2001;322:302–307.

82. Kellenberger S, Gautschi I, Rossier BC, Schild L. Mutations causing Liddle syndrome reduce sodium-dependent downregulation of the epithelial sodium channel in the Xenopus oocyte expression system. *J Clin Invest* 1998;101:2741–2750.

83. Gao PJ, Zhang KX, Zhu DL, et al. Diagnosis of Liddle syndrome by genetic analysis of beta and gamma subunits of epithelial sodium channel— A report of five affected family members. *J Hypertens* 2001;19:885–889.

84. Mancia G. Scipione Riva-Rocci. *Clin Cardiol* 1997;20:503–504.

85. Perloff D, Grim C, Flack J, et al. Special Report: Human blood pressure determination by sphygomanometry [AHA Medical/Scientific Statement]. *Circulation* 1993;88:2460–2470.

86. National Committee for Quality Assurance (NCQA). HEDIS 3.0, Vol. 1. Washington, DC: NCQA; 1997.

87. Cavallini MC, Roman MJ, Blank SG, et al. Association of the auscultatory gap with vascular disease in hypertensive patients. *Ann Intern Med* 1996;124:877–883.

88. Yarows SA, Julius S, Pickering TG. Home blood pressure monitoring. *Arch Intern Med* 2000;160:1251–1257.

89. Tsuji I, Imai Y, Nagai K, et al. Proposal of reference values for home blood pressure measurement: Prognostic criteria based on a prospective observation of the general population in Ohasama, Japan. *Am J Hypertens* 1997;10:409–418.

90. Ohkubo T, Imai Y, Tsuji I, et al. Home blood pressure measurement has a stronger predictive power for mortality than does screening blood pressure measurement: A population-based observation in Ohasama, Japan. *J Hypertens* 1998;16:971–975.

91. Pickering T, Gerin W, Holland JK. Home blood pressure teletransmission for better diagnosis and treatment. *Curr Hyperten Rep* 1999;1:489–494.

92. Aylett M, Marples G, Jones K. Home blood pressure monitoring: Its effect on the management of hypertension in general practice. *Br J Gen Pract* 1999;49:725–728.

93. Johnson KA, Partsch DJ, Rippole LL, McVey DM. Reliability of self-reported blood pressure measurements. *Arch Intern Med* 1999;159: 2689–2693.

94. Herpin D, Pickering T, Stergiou G, et al. Consensus conference on self-blood pressure measurement. Clinical applications and diagnosis. *Blood Press Monit* 2000;5:131–135.

95. Zarnke KB, Feagan BG, Mahon JL, Feldman RD. A randomized study comparing a patient-directed hypertension management strategy with usual office-based care. *Am J Hypertens* 1997;10:58–67.

96. Broege PA, James GD, Pickering TG. Management of hypertension in the elderly using home blood pressures. *Blood Press Monit* 2001;6: 139–144.

97. Campo C, Fernandez G, Gonzalez-Estaban J, et al for the ESPADA Study Group. Comparative study of home and office blood pressure in hypertensive patients treated with enalapril/HCTZ 20/6 mg: The ESPADA study. *Blood Press* 2000;9:355–362.

98. Leeman MJ, Lins RL, Sternon JE, et al. Effect of antihypertensive treatment on office and self-measured blood pressure: The Autodil study. *J Hum Hypertens* 2000;14:525–529.

99. Kjeldsen SE, Hedner J, Jamerson K, et al. Hypertension optimal treatment (HOT) study: Home blood pressure in treated hypertensive subjects. *Hypertension* 1998;31:1014–1020.

100. Stergiou GS, Baibas NM, Gantzarou AP, et al. Reproducibility of home, ambulatory, and clinic blood pressure: Implications for design of trials for the assessment of antihypertensive drug efficacy. *Am J Hypertens* 2002;15:101–104.

101. Imai Y, Ohkubo T, Hozawa A, et al. Usefulness of home blood pressure measurements in assessing the effect of treatment in a single-blind placebo-controlled open trial. *J Hypertens* 2001;19:179–185.

102. Perloff D, Sokolow M, Cowan RM, Juster RP. Prognostic value of ambulatory blood pressure measurements: Further analyses. *J Hypertens* 1989;7(suppl 3):S3–S10.

103. O'Brien E, Beevers G, Lip GYH. ABC of hypertension: Blood pressure measurement: Part III—Automated sphygmomanometry: Ambulatory blood pressure measurement. *Br Med J* 2001;322:1110–1114.

104. Tunis S, Kendall P, Londner M, Whyte J. Medicare Coverage Policy—Decisions: Ambulatory Blood Pressure Monitoring (#CAG-00067N): Decision Memorandum. Washington, DC: Health Care Financing Administration, October 17, 2001. Found on the Internet at: www.hcfa.gov/coverage/8b3-ff2.htm; accessed 01 APR 02 at 18:32 CST.

105. Staessen JA, Bieniaszewski L, O'Brien ET, Fagard R. What is normal blood pressure in ambulatory monitoring? *Nephrol Dial Transplant* 1996;11:241–245.

106. Rasmussen SL, Torp-Pedersen C, Borch-Johnsen K, Ibsen H. Normal values for ambulatory blood pressure and differences between casual blood pressure and ambulatory blood pressure: Results from a Danish population survey. *J Hypertens* 1998;16:1415–1424.

107. Staessen JA, Thijs L, Fagard R, et al. Predicting cardiovascular risk using conventional vs. ambulatory blood pressure in older patients with systolic hypertension. *JAMA* 1999;282:589–596.

108. Kario K, Pickering TG, Matsuo T, et al. Stroke prognosis and abnormal nocturnal blood pressure falls in older hypertensives. *Hypertension* 2001;38:852–857.

109. Bur A, Herkner H, Vlcek M, et al. Classification of blood pressure levels by ambulatory blood pressure in hypertension. *Hypertension* 2002; 40:817–822.

110. O'Brien E, Coats A, Owens P, et al. Use and interpretation of ambulatory blood pressure monitoring: Recommendations of the British Hypertension Society. *Br Med J* 2000;320:1128–1134.

111. Staessen JA, Bieniaszewski L, O'Brien E, et al. Nocturnal blood pressure fall on ambulatory monitoring in a large international database. *Hypertension* 1997;29:30–39.

112. Lurbe E, Redon J, Kesani A, et al. Increase in nocturnal blood pressure and progression to microalbuminuria in type 1 diabetes. *N Engl J Med* 2002;347:797–805.

113. Verdecchia P, Schillaci G, Borgioni C, et al. Adverse prognostic value of a blunted circadian rhythm of heart rate in essential hypertension. *J Hypertens* 1998;16:1335–1343.

114. Verdeccia P, Schillaci G, Reboldi G, et al. Different prognostic impact of 24-hour mean blood pressure and pulse pressure on stroke and coronary artery disease in essential hypertension. *Circulation* 2001;103: 2579–2584.

115. Verdecchia P, Reboldi G, Porcellati C, et al. Risk of cardiovascular disease in relation to achieved office and ambulatory blood pressure control in treated hypertensive subjects. *J Am Coll Cardiol* 2002;39: 878–885.

116. Elliott WJ. Circadian variation in blood pressure: Implications for elderly patients. *Am J Hypertens* 1999;12:43S–49S.

117. Kario K, Eguchi K, Hoshide S, et al. U-curve relationship between orthostatic blood pressure change and silent cerebrovascular disease in elderly hypertensives: Orthostatic hypertension as a new cardiovascular risk factor. *J Am Coll Cardiol* 2002;40:133–141.

118. Liu JE, Roman MJ, Pini R, et al. Cardiac and arterial target organ damage in adults with elevated ambulatory and normal office blood pressure. *Ann Intern Med* 1999;131:564–572.

119. Ohkubo T, Imai Y, Tsuji I, et al. Prediction of mortality by ambulatory blood pressure monitoring versus screening blood pressure measurements: A pilot study in Ohasama. *J Hypertens.* 1997;15:357–364.

120. Redon J, Campos C, Narciso ML, et al. Prognostic value of ambulatory blood pressure monitoring in refractory hypertension: A prospective study. *Hypertension* 1998;31:712–718.

121. Verdeccia P, Staessen JA, White WB, et al. Properly defining white coat hypertension. *Eur Heart J* 2002;23:106–109.

122. Bellomo G, Narducci PL, Rondoni F, et al. Prognostic value of 24-hour blood pressure in pregnancy. *JAMA* 1999;282:1447–1452.

123. Pierdomenico SD, Bucci A, Constantini F, et al. Twenty-four hour autonomic nervous function in sustained and "white coat" hypertension. *Am Heart J* 2000;140:672–677.

124. Muscholl MW, Hense HW, Brockel U, et al. Changes in left ventricular structure and function in patients with white coat hypertension: Cross sectional survey. *Br Med J* 1998;317:565–570.

125. Owens PE, Lyons SP, Rodriguez SA, O'Brien ET. Is elevation of clinic blood pressure in patients with white coat hypertension who have normal ambulatory blood pressure associated with target organ changes? *J Hum Hypertens* 1998;12:743–748.

126. Palatini P, Mormini P, Santonastaso M, et al for the HARVEST Study Investigators. Target organ damage in stage 1 hypertensive subjects with white coat and sustained hypertension: Results from the HARVEST Study. *Hypertension* 1998;31:57–63.

127. Grandi AM, Broggi R, Colombo S, et al. Left ventricular changes in isolated office hypertension: A blood pressure-matched comparison with normotension and sustained hypertension. *Arch Intern Med* 2001; 161:2677–2681.

128. Sega R, Trocino G, Lanzarotti A, et al. Alterations of cardiac structure in patients with isolated office, ambulatory, or home hypertension: Data from the general population (Pressione Arteriose Monitorate E Loro Associazioni [PAMELA] Study). *Circulation* 2001;104: 1385–1392.

129. Verdeccia P, Schillaci G, Borgioni C, et al. White-coat hypertension: Not guilty when correctly defined. *Blood Press Monit* 1998;3: 147–152.

130. Moser M. White-coat hypertension: To treat or not to treat: A clinical dilemma (editorial). *Arch Intern Med* 2001;161:2655 2656.

131. Verdecchia P, Schillaci G, Borgioni C, et al. Prognostic significance of the white coat effect. *Hypertension* 1997;29:1218–1224.

132. Ramsay LE, Williams B, Johnston GD, et al. British Hypertension Society guidelines for hypertension management 1999: Summary. *Br Med J* 1999;319:630–635.

133. Wallis EJ, Ramsay LE, Jackson PR. Cardiovascular and coronary risk estimation in hypertension management. *Heart* 2002;88:306–312.

134. The Eye Disease Case–Control Study Group. Risk factors for central retinal vein occlusion. *Arch Ophthalmol* 1996;114:545–554.

135. Tight blood pressure control and risk of macrovascular and microvascular complications in type 2 diabetes: UKPDS 38: UK Prospective Diabetes Study Group. *Br Med M* 1998;317:703–713.

136. Verdecchia P, Schillaci G, Borgioni C, et al. Prognostic significance of serial changes in left ventricular mass in essential hypertension. *Circulation* 1998;97:48–54.

137. Kitzman DW, Little WC, Brubaker PH, et al. Pathophysiological characterization of isolated diastolic heart failure in comparison to systolic heart failure. *JAMA* 2002;288:2144–2150.

138. Redfield MA, Jacobsen SJ, Burnett JC Jr, et al. Burden of systolic and diastolic ventricular dysfunction in the community: Appreciating the scope of the heart failure epidemic. *JAMA* 2003;289:194–202.

139. Dahlöf B, Devereux RB, Kjeldsen SE, et al for the LIFE study group. Cardiovascular morbidity and mortality in the Losartan Intervention For Endpoint reduction in hypertension study (LIFE): A randomised trial against atenolol. *Lancet* 2002;359:995–1003.

140. Keane WF, Eknoyan G. Proteinuria, albuminuria, risk, assessment, detection, elimination (PARADE): A position paper of the National Kidney Foundation. *Am J Kidney Dis* 1999;33:1004–1010.

141. Dinneen SF, Gerstein HC. The association of microalbuminuria and mortality in non-insulin-dependent diabetes mellitus: A systemic overview of the literature. *Arch Intern Med* 1997;157:1413–1418.

142. Borch-Johnsen K, Feldt-Rasmussen B, Strandgaard S, et al. Urinary albumin excretion: An independent predictor of ischemic heart disease. *Arterioscler Thromb Vasc Biol* 1999;19:1992–1997.

143. Gerstein GC, Mann JEF, Yi Q, et al. Albuminuria and risk of cardiovascular events, death, and heart failure in diabetic and nondiabetic individuals. *JAMA* 2001;286:421–426.

144. Tarif N, Bakris GL. Preservation of renal function: The spectrum of effects by calcium channel blockers. *Nephrol Dial Transplant* 1997;12:2244–2250.

145. Pontremoli R, Sofia A, Ravera M, et al. Prevalence and clinical correlates of microalbuminuria in essential hypertension: The MAGIC study. *Hypertension* 1997;30:1135–1143.

146. Cirillo M, Senigalliese L, Laurenzi M, et al. Microalbuminuria in nondiabetic adults: Relation of blood pressure, body mass index, plasma cholesterol levels, and smoking: The Gubbio Population Study. *Arch Intern Med* 1998;158:1933–1939.

147. Pedrinelli R, Dell'Omo G, Penno G, et al. Microalbuminuria and pulse pressure in hypertensive and atherosclerotic men. *Hypertension* 2000;35:48–54.

148. Agewall S, Wikstrand J, Ljungman S, Fagerberg B. Usefulness of microalbuminuria in predicting cardiovascular mortality in treated hypertensive men with and without diabetes mellitus. *Am J Cardiol* 1997;80:164–169.

149. Glasser SP, Arnett DK, McVeigh GE, et al. Vascular compliance and cardiovascular disease: A risk factor or marker? *Am J Hypertens* 1997;10:1175–1189.

150. Simon A, Megnien JL, Levenson J. Detection of preclinical atherosclerosis may optimize the management of hypertension. *Am J Hypertens* 1997;10:813–824.

151. Asmar RG, London GM, O'Rourke ME, Safar ME, for the REASON Project coordinators and investigators. Improvement in blood pressure, arterial stiffness, and wave reflections with a very-low-dose perindopril/indapamide combination in hypertensive patients: A comparison with atenolol. *Hypertension* 2001;38:922–926.

152. Asmar R, Topouchain J, Pannier B, et al. Pulse wave velocity as endpoint in large-scale intervention trial. The Complior Study. Scientific, Quality Control, Coordination, and Investigation Committees of the Complior Study. *J Hypertens* 2001;19:813–818.

153. Williams B, O'Rourke M. The Conduit Artery Functional Endpoint (CAFE) study in ASCOT. *J Hum Hypertens* 2001;15(suppl 1):S69–S74.

154. Blacher J, Asmar R, Djane S, London GM. Aortic pulse wave velocity as a marker of cardiovascular risk in hypertensive patients. *Hypertension* 1999;33:1111–1117.

155. Staessen JA, Gasowski J, Wang JG, et al. Risks of untreated and treated isolated systolic hypertension in the elderly: Meta-analysis of outcome trials. *Lancet* 2000;355:865–872.

156. Staessen JA, Fagard R, Thijs L, et al for the Systolic Hypertension in Europe (Syst-EUR) Trial Investigators. Morbidity and mortality in the placebo-controlled European Trial on Isolated Systolic Hypertension in the Elderly. *Lancet* 1997;360:757–764.

157. Liu L, Wang J, Gong L, et al for the Systolic Hypertension in China (Syst-China) Collaborative Group. Comparison of active treatment and placebo in older Chinese patients with isolated systolic hypertension. *J Hypertens* 1998;16:1823–1829.

158. Homocyteine and risk of ischemic heart disease and stroke: A meta-analysis. Homocysteine Studies Collaboration. *JAMA* 2002;288:2015–2022.

159. Ridker PM, Rifai N, Rose L, et al. Comparison of C-reactive protein and low-density lipoprotein cholesterol levels in the prediction of first cardiovascular events. *N Engl J Med* 2002;347:1557–1565.

160. Safian RD, Textor SC. Medical progress: Renal-artery stenosis. *N Engl J Med* 2001;344:431–442.

161. Alcazar JM, Rodicio JL. European Society of Hypertension: How to handle renovascular hypertension. *J Hypertens* 2001;19:2109–2111.

162. Helenon O, Melki P, Correas JM, et al. Renovascular disease: Doppler ultrasound. *Semin Ultrasound CT MR* 1997;18:136–146.

163. Vasbinder GB, Nelemans PJ, Kessels AG, et al. Diagnostic tests for renal artery stenosis in patients suspected of having renovascular hypertension: A meta-analysis. *Ann Intern Med* 2001;135:401–411.

164. van Jaarsveld BC, Krijnen P, Derkx FH, et al. The place of renal scintigraphy in the diagnosis of renal artery stenosis. Fifteen years of clinical experience. *Arch Intern Med* 1997;157:1226–1234.

165. Chàbovà V, Schirger A, Stanson AW, et al. Outcomes of atherosclerotic renal artery stenosis managed without revascularization. *Mayo Clin Proc* 2000;75:437–444.

166. van Jaarsveld BC, Krijnen P, Pieterman H, et al. The effect of balloon angioplasty on hypertension in atherosclerotic renal-artery stenosis. Dutch Renal Artery Stenosis Intervention Cooperative Study Group. *N Engl J Med* 2000;342:1007–1014.

167. Bravo EL. Pheochromocytoma. *Cardiol Rev* 2002;10:44–50.

168. Raber W, Raffesberg W, Bischof M, et al. Diagnostic efficacy of unconjugated plasma metanephrines for the detection of pheochromocytoma. *Arch Intern Med* 2000;160:2957–2963.

169. Lenders JW, Pack K, Walther MM, et al. Biochemical diagnosis of pheochromocytoma: Which test is best? *JAMA* 2002;287:1427–1434.

170. Witteles RM, Kaplan EL, Roizen MF. Sensitivity of diagnostic and localization tests for pheochromocytoma in clinical practice. *Arch Intern Med* 2000;160:2521–2524.

171. Pacak K, Linehan WM, Eisenhofer G, et al. Recent advances in genetics, diagnosis, localization, and treatment of pheochromocytoma. *Ann Intern Med* 2001;134:315–329.

172. Jalil N, Pattou FN, Combemale F, et al. Effectiveness and limits of preoperative imaging studies for the localization of pheochromocytomas and paragangliomas: A review of 282 cases: French Association of Surgery (AFC), The French Association of Endocrine Surgeons (AFCE). *Eur J Surg* 1998;164:23–28.

173. Ganguly A. Primary aldosteronism. *N Engl J Med* 1998;339:1828–1834.

174. Stewart PM. Mineralocorticoid hypertension. *Lancet* 1999;353:1341–1347.

175. Kaplan NM. Cautions over the current epidemic of primary hyperaldosteronism. *Lancet* 2001;357:953–954.

176. Sawka AM, Young WF, Thompson GB, et al. Primary hyperaldosteronism: Factors associated with normalization of blood pressure after surgery. *Ann Intern Med* 2001;135:258–261.

177. Bravo EL. Medical management of primary hyperaldosteronism. *Curr Hypertens Rep* 2001;3:406–409.

178. Lim PO, Young WF, MacDonald TM. A review of the medical treatment of primary hyperaldosteronism. *J Hypertens* 2001;19:353–361.

179. Nieto FJ, Young TB, Lind BK, et al. Association of sleep-disordered breathing, sleep apnea, and hypertension in a large community-based study. *JAMA* 2000;283:1829–1836.

180. Ledoux M, Lambert J, Reeder BA, Depres JP. Correlation between cardiovascular disease risk factors and simple anthropometic measures: Canadian Heart Health Surveys Research Group. *Can Med Assoc J* 1997;157(suppl 1):S46–S53.

181. Chobanian AV, Hill M. National Heart, Lung, and Blood Institute Workshop on Sodium and Blood Pressure: A critical review of current scientific evidence. *Hypertension* 2000;35:858–863.

182. Mulrow CD, Chiquette E, Angel L, et al. *Dieting to Reduce Body Weight for Controlling Hypertension in Adults* (Cochrane Review). Oxford, UK: Update Software; 2001.

183. Whelton PK, He J, Cutler JA, et al. Effects of oral potassium on blood pressure: Meta-analysis of randomized controlled clinical trials. *JAMA* 1997;277:1624–1632.

184. Issacsohn JL, Moser M, Stein EA, et al. Garlic powder and plasma lipids and lipoproteins: A multicenter, randomized, placebo-controlled trial. *Arch Intern Med* 1998;158:1189–1194.

185. Writing Group of the PREMIER Collaborative Research Group. Effects of comprehensive lifestyle modification on blood pressure con-

trol: Main results of the PREMIER clinical trial. *JAMA* 2003;289: 2083–2093.

186. The Trials of Hypertension Prevention Collaborative Research Group. Effects of weight loss and sodium reduction intervention on blood pressure and hypertension incidence in overweight people with high-normal blood pressure: The Trials of Hypertension Prevention, phase II. *Arch Intern Med* 1997;157:657–667.

187. Whelton PK, Appel LJ, Espeland MA, et al. Sodium reduction and weight loss in the treatment of hypertension in older persons: A randomized controlled trial of nonpharmacologic interventions in the elderly (TONE). TONE Collaborative Research Group. *JAMA* 1998;279: 839–846.

188. Cushman WC, Cutler JA, Hanna E, et al for the PATHS Group. The Prevention and Treatment of Hypertension Study (PATHS): Effects of an alcohol treatment program on blood pressure. *Arch Intern Med* 1998;152:1197–1207.

189. Xin X, He J, Frontini MG, et al. Effects of alcohol reduction on blood pressure: A meta-analysis of randomized controlled trials. *Hypertension* 2001;38:1112–1117.

190. Appel LJ, Moore TJ, Obarzanek E, et al. A clinical trial of the effects of dietary patterns on blood pressure. *N Engl J Med* 1997;336:1117–1124.

191. Sacks FM, Svetkey LP, Vollmer WM, et al. Effects on blood pressure of reduced dietary sodium and the Dietary Approaches to Stop Hypertension (DASH) diet. *N Engl J Med* 2001;344:3–9.

192. Minami J, Ishimitus T, Matsouka H. Effects of smoking cessation on blood pressure and heart and heart rate variability in habitual smokers. *Hypertension* 1999;33:586–590.

193. Bolinder G, de Faire U. Ambulatory 24 hour blood pressure monitoring in healthy, middle-aged smokeless tobacco users, smokers, and nontobacco users. *Am J Hypertens* 1998;11:1153–1163.

194. Neaton JD, Grimm RH, Prineas RJ, et al. Treatment of mild hypertension study: Final results. *JAMA* 1993;270:713–724.

195. Appel LJ. The verdict from ALLHAT: Thiazide diuretics are the preferred initial therapy for hypertension (editorial). *JAMA* 2002;288: 3039–3042.

196. Drugs for hypertension. Treatment guidelines from the medical letter. *Med Lett* 2003;1:31–42.

197. Risks and benefits of estrogen plus progestin in healthy postmenopausal women: Principal results from the Women's Health Initiative Randomized Clinical Trial. *JAMA* 2002;288:321–333.

198. Major outcomes in high-risk hypertensive patients randomized to angiotensin-converting enzyme inhibitor or calcium channel blocker vs. diuretic: The Antihypertensive and Lipid Lowering Treatment to Prevent Heart Attack Trial (ALLHAT). The ALLHAT Officers and Coordinators for the ALLHAT Collaborative Research Group. *JAMA* 2002; 288:2981–2997.

199. Randomised trial of a perindopril-based blood-pressure-lowering regimen among 6105 individuals with previous stroke or transient ischaemic attack. PROGRESS Collaborative Group. *Lancet* 2001;358: 1033–1041.

200. Lewis EJ, Hunsicker LG, Clarke WR, et al. Renoprotective effect of the angiotensin-receptor antagonist irbesartan in patients with nephropathy due to Type 2 diabetes. Collaborative Study Group. *N Engl J Med* 2001;345:841–860.

201. Brenner BM, Cooper ME, de Zeeuw D, et al. Effects of losartan on renal and cardiovascular outcomes in patients with Type 2 diabetes and nephropathy. Reduction of Endpoints in Non-Insulin Dependent Diabetes Mellitus with the Angiotensin II Antagonist Losartan (RENAAL) Study Group. *N Engl J Med* 2001;345:861–869.

202. Messerli FH, Grossman E, Goldboourt U. Are beta-blockers efficacious as first-line therapy for hypertension in the elderly: A systematic review. *JAMA* 1998;279:1903–1907.

203. Pahor M, Psaty BM, Alderman MH, et al. Health outcomes associated with calcium antagonists compared with other first-line antihypertensive therapies: A meta-analysis of randomised controlled trials. *Lancet* 2000;356:1949–1951.

204. Blood Pressure Lowering Treatment Trialists' Collaborative. Effects of ACE-inhibitors, calcium antagonists, and other blood-pressure-lowering drugs: Results of prospectively designed overviews of randomised trials. *Lancet* 2000;356:1955–1964.

205. Wing LMH, Reid CM, Ryan P, et al. A comparison of outcomes with angiotensin-converting-enzyme inhibitors and diuretics for hypertension in the elderly. Second Australian National Blood Pressure Study Group. *N Engl J Med* 2003;348:583–592.

206. Black HR, Elliott WJ, Grandits G, et al for the CONVINCE Research Group. Principal results of the Controlled ONset Verapamil INvestigation of Cardiovascular Endpoints (CONVINCE) Trial. *JAMA* 2003; 289:2073–2082.

207. The ALLHAT Collaborative Research Group. Major cardiovascular events in hypertensive patients randomized to doxazosin vs. chlorthalidone: The Antihypertensive and Lipid-Lowering Treatment to Prevent Heart Attack Trial (ALLHAT). *JAMA* 2000;283:1967–1975.

208. Lithell L, Hansson L, Skoog I, et al. The Study on Cognition and Prognosis in the Elderly (SCOPE): Principal results of a randomized double-blind intervention trial. *J Hypertens* 2003;21:875–886.

209. Svensson P, de Faire U, Sleight P, et al. Comparative effects of ramipril on ambulatory and office blood pressures: A HOPE Substudy. *Hypertension* 2001;38:E28–E32.

210. Effects of an angiotensin-converting-enzyme inhibitor, ramipril, on death from cardiovascular causes, myocardial infarction, and stroke in high-risk patients. The Heart Outcomes Prevention Evaluation (HOPE) Study Investigators. *N Engl J Med* 2000;342:145–153.

211. Heart Outcomes Prevention Evaluation (HOPE) Study Investigators. Effects of ramipril on cardiovascular and microvascular outcomes in people with diabetes mellitus: The HOPE study and MICRO-HOPE substudy. *Lancet* 2000;355:253–259.

212. Burris J, Weir M, Oparil S, et al. An assessment of diltiazem and hydrochlorothiazide in hypertension. *JAMA* 1990;263:1507–1512.

213. Nakao N, Yoshimura A, Morita H, et al. Combination treatment of angiotensin-II receptor blocker and angiotensin-converting-enzyme inhibitor in non-diabetic renal disease (COOPERATE): A randomised controlled trial. *Lancet* 2003;361:117–124.

214. Hansson L, Zandretti A, Carruthers SG, et al. Effects of intensive blood pressure lowering and low-dose aspirin in patients with hypertension: Principal results of the Hypertension Optimal Treatment (HOT) randomised trial: The HOT Study Group. *Lancet* 1998;351: 1755–1762.

215. Bakris GL, Williams M, Dworkin L, et al for the National Kidney Foundation Hypertension and Diabetes Executive Committee Working Group. Preserving renal function in adults with hypertension and diabetes: A consensus approach. *Am J Kidney Dis* 2000;35:646–661.

216. American Diabetes Association. Treatment of hypertension in adults with diabetes. *Diabetes Care* 2003;26(suppl 1):S80–S83.

217. Raikou M, Gray A, Briggs A, et al. Cost-effectiveness analysis of improved blood pressure control in hypertensive patients with type 2 diabetes: UKPDS 40. UK Prospective Diabetes Study Group. *Br Med J* 1998;317:720–726.

218. Elliott WJ, Weir DR, Black HR. Cost-effectiveness of lowering treatment goal of JNC VI for diabetic hypertensives. *Arch Intern Med* 2000; 160:1277–1283.

219. Wright JT Jr., Bakris GL, Greene T, et al. Effect of blood pressure lowering and antihypertensive drug class on progression of hypertensive kidney disease: Results from the AASK Trial. *JAMA* 2002;288:2421–2431.

220. Perry HM Jr, Davis BR, Price TR, et al. Effect of treating isolated systolic hypertension on the risk of developing various types and subtypes of stroke. The Systolic Hypertension in the Elderly Program (SHEP). *JAMA* 2000;284:465–471.

221. Hulley S, Grady D, Bush T, et al. Randomized trial of estrogen plus progestin for secondary prevention of coronary heart disease in postmenopausal women. Heart and Estrogen/progestin Replacement Study (HERS) Research Group. *JAMA* 1998;280:605–613.

222. Elisaf MS, Theodorou J, Pappas H, et al. Effectiveness and metabolic effects of perindopril and diuretics combination in primary hypertension. *J Hum Hypertens* 1999;13:787–791.

223. Gress TW, Nieto FJ, Shahar E, et al for the Atherosclerosis Risk in Communities Study. Hypertension and antihypertensive therapy and

the risk factors for the type 2 diabetes mellitus. *N Engl J Med* 2000; 342:905–912.

224. Lindholm L, Ibsen H, Dahlöf B, et al for the LIFE study group. Cardiovascular morbidity and mortality in patients with diabetes in the Losartan Intervention For Endpoint reduction in hypertension study (LIFE): A randomised trial against atenolol. *Lancet* 2002;359:1004–1010.

225. Tuomilehto J, Rastenye D, Birkenhager WH, et al. Effects of calcium-channel blockade in older patients with diabetes and systolic hypertension: Systolic Hypertension in Europe Trial Investigators (Syst-Eur). *N Engl J Med* 1999;340:677–684.

226. Bakris GL, Weir MR, DeQuattro V, McMahon FG. Effects of an ACE inhibitor/calcium antagonist combination on proteinuria in diabetic nephropathy. *Kidney Int* 1998;54:1283–1289.

227. Gottdiener JS, Reda DJ, Massie BM, et al. Effect of single-drug therapy on reduction of left ventricular mass in mild to moderate hypertension: Comparison of six antihypertensive agents; The Department of Veterans Affairs Cooperative Study Group on Antihypertensive Agents. *Circulation* 1997;95:2007–2014.

228. Levy D, Larson MG, Vasan RS, et al. The progression from hypertension to congestive heart failure. *JAMA* 1996;275:1557–1562.

229. Psaty BM, Smith NL, Siscovick DS, et al. Health outcomes associated with antihypertensive therapies used as first-line agents: A systematic review and meta-analysis. *JAMA* 1997;277:739–745.

230. Gomberg-Maitland M, Baran DA, Fuster V. Treatment of congestive heart failure: Guidelines for the primary care physician and the heart failure specialist. *Arch Intern Med* 2001;161:342–352.

231. Bonet S, Agusti A, Arnau JM, et al. Beta-adrenergic blocking agents in heart failure: Benefits of vasodilating and non-vasodilating agents according to patients' characteristics. A meta-analysis of clinical trials. *Arch Intern Med* 2000;160:621–627.

232. Pitt B, Zannad F, Remme WJ, et al for the Randomized Aldactone Evaluation Study (RALES) Investigators. The effect of spironolactone on morbidity and mortality in patients with severe heart failure. *N Engl J Med* 1999;341:709–717.

233. Pitt B, Segal R, Martinez FA, et al for the ELITE Investigators. Results of the Evaluation of Losartan In The Elderly (ELITE) Trial. *Lancet* 1997;349:757–762.

234. Pitt B, Poole-Wilson PA, Segal R, et al. Effect of losartan compared with captopril on mortality in patients with symptomatic heart failure: randomised trial. The Losartan Heart Failure Survival Study ELITE II. *Lancet* 2000;355:1582–1587.

235. Cohn JN, Tognoni G for the Val-HeFT Investigators. A randomized trial of the angiotensin-receptor blocker valsartan in chronic heart failure. *N Engl J Med* 2001;345:1667–1675.

236. Otto CM, Lind BK, Kitzman DW, et al. Association of aortic-valve sclerosis with cardiovascular mortality and morbidity in the elderly. *N Engl J Med*. 1999;341:142–147.

237. Parving H-H, Lehnert H, Brochner-Mortensen J, et al. The effect of irbesartan on the development of diabetic nephropathy in patients with type 2 diabetes. The Irbesartan in Patients with Type 2 Diabetes and Microalbuminuria Study Group. *N Engl J Med* 2001;345:870–878.

238. Kloke HJ, Branten AJ, Huysmans FT, Wetzels JF. Antihypertensive treatment of patients with proteinuric renal diseases: Risks or benefits of calcium channel blockers? *Kidney Int* 1998;53:1559–1573.

239. Ravid M, Brosh D, Levi Z, et al. Use of enalapril to attenuate decline in renal function in normotensive, normoalbuminuric patients with type 2 diabetes mellitus: A randomized, controlled trial. *Ann Intern Med* 1998;128:982–988.

240. Jafar TH, Schmid CH, Landa M, et al. Angiotensin-converting enzyme inhibitors and progression of nondiabetic renal disease: A meta-analysis of patient-level data. *Ann Intern Med* 2001;135:73–87.

241. Bakris GL, Weir MR. ACE inhibitor associated elevations in serum creatinine: Is this a cause for concern? *Arch Intern Med* 2000;160:685–693.

242. Mogensen CE, Neldam S, Tikkanen I, et al. Randomised controlled trial of dual blockade of renin-angiotensin system in patients with hypertension, microalbuminuria, and non-insulin dependent diabetes: The candesartan and lisinopril microalbuminuria (CALM) study. *Br Med J* 2000;321:1440–1444.

243. Yeghiazarians Y, Braunstein JB, Askari A, Stone PH. Medical progress: Unstable angina pectoris. *N Engl J Med* 2000;342:101–114.

244. Heidenreich PA, McDonald KM, Hastie T, et al. Meta-analysis of trials comparing beta-blockers, calcium antagonists, and nitrates for stable angina. *JAMA* 1999;281:1927–1936.

245. Protocol for prospective collaborative overviews of major randomized trials of blood-pressure-lowering treatments. World Health Organization/International Society of Hypertension Blood Pressure Lowering Treatment Trialists' Collaboration. *J Hypertens* 1998;16:127–137.

246. Conlin PR, Gerth WC, Fox J, et al. Four-year persistence patterns among patients initiating therapy with the angiotensin II receptor antagonist losartan versus other antihypertensive drug classes. *Clin Ther* 2001;23:1999–2010.

247. Preston RA, Materson BJ, Reda DJ, et al for the Department of Veterans Affairs Cooperative Study Group on Antihypertensive Agents. Age-race subgroup compared to renin profile as predictors of blood pressure response to antihypertensive therapy in 1031 patients: Results of the VA cooperative study. *JAMA* 1998;280:1168–1172.

248. Agodoa LY, Appel L, Bakris GL, et al. Effect of ramipril vs amlodipine on renal outcomes in hypertensive nephrosclerosis: A randomized controlled trial. African American Study of Kidney Disease and Hypertension (AASK) Study Group. *JAMA* 2001;285:2719–2728.

249. Gueyffier F, Bulpitt C, Boissel J-P, et al for the INDANA Group. Antihypertensive drugs in very old people: A subgroup meta-analysis of randomised controlled trials. *Lancet* 1999;353:793–796.

250. Update on the Task Force Report (1987) on High Blood Pressure in Children and Adolescents: A Working Group Report from the National High Blood Pressure Education Program. National High Blood Pressure Education Program Working Group on Hypertension Control in Children and Adolescents. *Pediatrics* 1996;98:649–658.

251. Sinaiko AR. Current concepts: Hypertension in children. *N Engl J Med* 1996;335:1968–1973.

252. Helewa ME, Burrows RF, Smith J, et al. Report of the Canadian Hypertension Society Consensus Conference: Definition, evaluation, and classification of hypertensive disorders in pregnancy. *Can Med Soc J* 1997;157:715–725.

253. Report of the National High Blood Pressure Education Program Working Group on High Blood Pressure in Pregnancy. *Am J Obstet Gynecol* 2000;183:S1–S22.

254. Caritis S, Sibai B, Hauth J, et al. Low-dose aspirin to prevent preeclampsia in women at high risk. *N Engl J Med* 1998;338:701–705.

255. Levine RJ, Hauth JC, Curet LB, et al. Trial of calcium to prevent preeclampsia. *N Engl J Med* 1997;337:69–76.

256. DerSimonian R, Levine RJ. Resolving discrepancies between a meta-analysis and a subsequent large controlled trial. *JAMA* 1999;282:664–670.

257. Kitiyakara C, Guzman NJ. Malignant hypertension and hypertensive emergencies. *J Am Soc Nephrol* 1998;9:133–142.

258. Elliott WJ. Hypertensive emergencies. *Crit Care Clin* 2001;17:435–451.

259. Dmowski AT, Carey MJ. Aortic dissection. *Am J Emerg Med* 1999;17:372–375.

260. Chen K, Varon J, Wenker OC, et al. Acute thoracic aortic dissection: The basics. *J Emerg Med* 1997;15:859–867.

261. Murphy MB, Murray C, Shorten GD. Fenoldopam: A selective peripheral dopamine-receptor agonist for the treatment of severe hypertension. *N Engl J Med* 2001;345:1548–1557.

262. Stason WB, Schmid CH, Niedzwiecki D, et al. Safety of nifedipine in patients with hypertension: A meta-analysis. *Hypertension* 1997;30:7–14.

263. Grossman E, Ironi AN, Messerli FH. Comparative tolerability profile of hypertensive crises treatments. *Drug Saf* 1998;19:99–122.

264. Cohen MC, Rohtla KM, Lavery CE, et al. Meta-analysis of the morning excess of acute myocardial infarction and sudden cardiac death. *Circulation* 1997;79:1512–1515.

265. Elliott WJ. Circadian variation in the timing of stroke onset: A meta-analysis. *Stroke* 1998;29:992–996.

266. Elliott WJ, Prisant LM. Drug delivery systems for antihypertensive agents. *Blood Pressure Monit.* 1997; 2:53–60.

267. Smolensky MH, Portaluppi F. Chronopharmacology and chronotherapy of cardiovascular medications: Relevance to prevention and treatment of coronary heart disease. *Am Heart J* 1999;137:S14–S24.

268. Deary AJ, Schumann AL, Murfet H, et al. Double-blind, placebo-controlled crossover comparison of five classes of antihypertensive drugs. *J Hypertens* 2002;20:771–777.

269. de Gaudemaris R, Chau NP, Maillion JM. Home blood pressure variability, comparison with office readings and proposal for reference values. Groupe de la Mesure, French Society of Hypertension. *J Hypertens* 1994;12:831–838.

270. Pickering T. Recommendations for the use of home (self) and ambulatory blood pressure monitoring. American Society of Hypertension Ad Hoc Panel. *Am J Hypertens* 1996;9:1–11.

271. Staessen JA, Bieniaszewski L, O'Brien ET, Fagard R. What is normal blood pressure in ambulatory monitoring? *Nephrol Dial Transplant* 1996;11:241–245.

272. Elliott WJ, Black HR. Special situations in the management of hypertension. In: Hollenberg NK, ed. *Atlas of Hypertension,* 4th ed. Philadelphia: Current Medicine; 2003:257–281.

PART EIGHT

CARDIOPULMONARY DISEASE

PULMONARY HYPERTENSION

Lewis J. Rubin

Pulmonary hypertension is a hemodynamic abnormality common to a variety of conditions that is characterized by increased right ventricular (RV) afterload and work. The clinical manifestations, natural history, and reversibility of pulmonary hypertension depend heavily on the nature of the pulmonary vascular lesions and the etiology and severity of the hemodynamic disorder. For example, subacute or chronic hypoxia predominantly causes increased muscularization of the small muscular pulmonary arteries and arterioles with the intima relatively intact. Relief of the hypoxia improves or occasionally reverses the process with little or no pathologic residue.[1,2] In contrast, the lesions of systemic sclerosis (scleroderma), mostly confined to the intima of the small pulmonary arteries and arterioles, are usually progressive and irreversible. Unlike these two examples, which spare the pulmonary capillary bed, the pulmonary capillaries are the primary site of involvement in pulmonary capillary hemangiomatosis.[3] Because of its large capacity, its great distensibility, its low resistance to blood flow, and the modest amounts of smooth muscle in the small arteries and arterioles, the *pulmonary circulation is not predisposed to become hypertensive*. When total cross-sectional area is decreased by destruction or obliteration of lung tissue or occlusive lesions in the resistance vessels, pulmonary arterial pressures increase. The degree of pulmonary hypertension that develops is a function of the amount of the pulmonary vascular tree that has been eliminated. Pulmonary hypertension is usually secondary to cardiac or pulmonary disease. Although primary pulmonary hypertension (PPH) is uncommon, it is well recognized as a distinctive clinical entity in which intrinsic pulmonary vascular disease is free of the complicating features of secondary pulmonary hypertension contributed by diseases of the heart and/or lungs. Mild pulmonary hypertension can exist for a lifetime without becoming evident clinically. For example, native residents at high altitude, in whom mild to moderate pulmonary hypertension is a natural result of sustained exposure to hypoxia, can adapt and function normally. When pulmonary hypertension does become manifest clinically, the symptoms tend to be nonspecific (Table 62-1).

DEFINITIONS

Pulmonary *arterial* hypertension (PAH) can be either acute or chronic. The acute form is usually a result of either pulmonary embolism (Chap. 63) or the adult respiratory distress syndrome. This chapter deals with *chronic* pulmonary arterial hypertension.

Pulmonary *venous* hypertension usually is encountered clinically as a consequence of left ventricular (LV) failure or mitral valvular disease. Occasionally, it may occur in the course of fibrosing mediastinitis. Only rarely is the entity known as pulmonary venoocclusive disease (PVOD) encountered. Even though pulmonary hypertension may be confined, at the outset, to the pulmonary veins (e.g., acute mitral regurgitation), sooner or later pulmonary arterial hypertension supervenes. The hallmarks of pulmonary venous hypertension are pulmonary congestion and edema. For practical purposes, pulmonary venous hypertension exists when pulmonary venous (or LA) pressure rises above approximately 15 mmHg.

Cor pulmonale signifies the presence of pulmonary hypertension in the setting of chronic respiratory disease.[4] Pulmonary hypertension in patients with chronic lung disease tends to be less severe than in connective tissue diseases, chronic thromboembolic disease, or primary pulmonary hypertension. Pulmonary hypertension may be severe, however, in some patients with interstitial lung disease.

NORMAL PULMONARY CIRCULATION

Structure

Immediately before birth, pulmonary and systemic arterial blood pressures are near equal and about 70/40 mmHg, with a mean of 50 mmHg. Immediately after birth, with closure of the ductus arteriosus and initiation of ventilation, pulmonary arterial pressure falls rapidly to about one-half of systemic levels. Thereafter, pulmonary

TABLE 62-1 Symptoms of Primary Pulmonary Hypertension

Dyspnea	Palpitations
Fatigue	Orthopnea
Dizziness	Cough
Syncope	Hoarseness
Chest pain	

TABLE 62-2 Values for Normal Pulmonary Circulation at Sea Level and High Altitude

	Sea Level	Altitude (~15,000 ft)
Pulmonary arterial pressure (P_{PA}), mmHg	20/12, 15	38/14, 25
Cardiac output (Q), L/min	6.0	6.0
Left atrial pressure (P_{LA}), mmHg	5.0	5.0
Pulmonary vascular resistance (PVR),[a] (mmHg/L)/min (R units)	1.7	3.3

$$^{a}PVR = \frac{P_{PA} - P_{LA}}{Q} = \frac{15 - 5}{6} = 1.67 \text{ R units.}$$ To convert R units to CGS units (dynes $\cdot$ s/cm^5), multiply R units by 80.

arterial pressures gradually decrease over several weeks to reach adult levels.[5]

In some neonates, the normal pulmonary hypertension of the fetus fails to recede normally, generally due to either a developmental anomaly or a relentless increase in pulmonary vascular tone. In such infants, the persistent pulmonary hypertension and right ventricular (RV) failure may become life-threatening. Surgical intervention or temporizing measures, such as the use of inhaled nitric oxide (NO) or extracorporeal membrane oxygenation (ECMO), may be useful in reversing the pulmonary vascular abnormalities.[6]

In the normal adult at sea level, the small muscular arteries and arterioles in the lungs are thin-walled and contain very little smooth muscle. In contrast, in the fetus or the adult who has lived under hypoxic conditions (e.g., native residents at high altitude), the media of the arterioles are thickened, and the muscle extends distally into precapillary vessels that are ordinarily devoid of muscle; i.e., the precapillary vessels undergo "remodeling."[7]

Endothelium and Endothelium–Smooth Muscle Interactions

In addition to its role as a semipermeable barrier between blood and interstitium, the endothelium provides many biologically important functions, the net effect of which is the processing of blood flowing through the lungs. Among these functions are the synthesis, uptake, storage, release, and metabolism of vasoactive substances; transduction of blood-borne signals; modulation of coagulation and thrombolysis; regulation of cell proliferation; engagement in the local inflammatory and proliferative reactions to injury; involvement in immune reactions; and angiogenesis (Chap. 4). Some of the enzymes involved in these processes, such as the angiotensin-converting enzyme, are found on the surface of endothelial cells; others, such as 5'-nucleotidase, are found within the cell.[8] Hence it is appropriate to regard endothelium as an organ with diverse metabolic and endocrine functions, one that is unique because of its strategic location as a continuous, monolayered lining of blood vessels throughout the body. Importantly, the lungs contain the largest expanse of endothelium in the body.

The cells that make up the monolayered endothelial lining communicate not only with each other by anatomic junctions and bridges but also with the underlying smooth muscle by way of biologically active substances.[9] This interaction participates in regulating normal vasomotor tone as well responding to the administration of vasoactive substances. Thus, damage to the lining cells, proliferation of the intima, or hypertrophy of the smooth muscle will each upset the normal interplay.

Hemodynamics

For the adult pulmonary circulation, the definition of *normal* depends on the altitude. The normal pulmonary hemodynamics of adults residing at sea level and above sea level are compared in Table 62-2. At

sea level, a cardiac output of 5 to 6 L/min is associated with a pulmonary arterial pressure of about 20/12 mmHg, with a mean of about 15 mmHg. At an altitude of 15,000 ft, the same level of blood flow is associated with somewhat higher pressures (Table 62-2). Pulmonary arterial pressures also tend to increase somewhat with age.

A pressure drop of only 5 to 10 mmHg between the pulmonary artery and left atrium accompanies the cardiac output of 5 to 6 L/min (Table 62-2). Determination of pulmonary vascular resistance (PVR), calculated as the ratio of the difference in mean pressure at the two ends of the pulmonary vascular bed (pulmonary arterial pressure minus LA pressure divided by the cardiac output) (Table 62-2), is a practical clinical tool for assessing the hemodynamic state of the pulmonary circulation and for distinguishing between active and passive changes in the pulmonary resistance vessels (e.g., the effect of administering a vasodilator agent to a patient with pulmonary hypertension). In practice, since the left atrium (LA) may not be readily accessible, pulmonary artery wedge pressure is generally substituted for LA pressure.

Another approach to defining certain characteristics of the pulmonary arterial tree and its behavior—i.e., elastic properties and geometry—is the calculation of pulmonary arterial input impedance. This approach has more physiologic than clinical value. It takes into account the pulsatile nature of pulmonary arterial pressures and flow. Like vascular resistance, it is defined as a ratio. But instead of a ratio involving *mean* pressures and blood flow, the ratio uses the amplitudes of pulsatile pressure to oscillatory flow near the beginning of the pulmonary artery at a particular frequency. Values for the ratio are obtained by resolving mathematically the pulsatile pressure and flow curves into their sinusoidal components.

Although calculated PVR has proved useful in assessing the state of the normal and abnormal pulmonary circulation and even though a change in calculated resistance can often aid in deciding whether pulmonary vasoconstriction or vasodilatation has occurred, translation of a calculated ratio into vasomotor activity must be done with caution.[4] For example, changes in calculated PVR are not readily interpretable when a vasodilator agent evokes multiple hemodynamic changes simultaneously (e.g., simultaneous changes in pulmonary vascular pressures and blood flow). Also, a clinical shortcut, such as the substitution in the numerator of the pulmonary arterial pressure for the pressure *drop* between the pulmonary artery and left atrium, may be useful empirically but deprives the calculation of any physiologic meaning. Finally, the clinical significance of a value calculated for PVR depends heavily on the implications of the hemodynamic changes on the work of the right ventricle (RV). For example, the same decrease in calculated PVR brought about by two different pulmonary vasodilators may affect the work of the RV differently: Should one agent elicit a *decrease* in pulmonary arterial pressure along with an *increase* in cardiac output (an ideal response), it is more apt to be of long-term benefit than another agent that, while increasing the cardiac output, fails to decrease the pulmonary arterial pressure.

In the normal lung, a considerable increase in cardiac output, i.e., two to three times that at rest, generally increases pulmonary arterial pressure by only a few millimeters of mercury. On the other hand, in pulmonary hypertensive states, in which the distensibility and extent of the pulmonary vascular bed have been restricted by disease, pulmonary arterial pressure increases along with even small increments in pulmonary blood flow. Changes in pulmonary blood volume are much more subtle than changes in blood pressure or flow in their hemodynamic effects; they are also much more difficult to quantify. Clinical clues can be helpful in recognizing that the pulmonary blood volume has increased. Often a fullness of the pulmonary vascular pattern on the chest radiograph along with evidences of interstitial edema suggest that pulmonary blood volume has increased acutely. In chronic mitral stenosis or LV failure, the pulmonary blood volume is not only increased but is also redistributed toward the apices of the lungs, i.e., "cephalization" (Chap. 14).

Autonomic innervation of the pulmonary vascular tree plays a lesser role in modulating vasomotor tone than do local stimuli, particularly hypoxia. Indeed, hypoxia can exert its pulmonary pressor effect in the isolated lung—i.e., one that is devoid of external innervation. The mechanism by which hypoxia exerts its local pressor effect is not fully characterized but appears to involve altered smooth muscle cell membrane ion channel activity.[2] Acidosis potentiates the hypoxic pressor effect. Hypercapnia also exerts a pulmonary pressor effect, presumably by way of the local acidosis that it generates, but it is less powerful than hypoxia as a pulmonary vasoconstrictor agent.

PULMONARY HYPERTENSION: GENERAL FEATURES

Clinical Manifestations

Pulmonary hypertension is a final common hemodynamic consequence of multiple etiologies and diverse mechanisms. As noted earlier, most cases of pulmonary hypertension are secondary (Table 62-3). Among the underlying causes of pulmonary hypertension are mechanical compression and distortion of the resistance vessels of the lungs (e.g., by diffuse pulmonary fibrosis), hypoxic vasoconstriction (e.g., in severe obstructive airways or diffuse parenchymal diseases), intravascular obstruction (e.g., thromboemboli or tumor emboli), and combinations of mechanical and vasoconstrictive influences. The significance of pulmonary hypertension, however, is that if it is uncontrolled, it leads to RV failure. Once pulmonary arterial pressures reach systemic levels, RV failure becomes inevitable.

Special Studies

The "gold standard" for the diagnosis of pulmonary hypertension is right-sided heart catheterization. This technique enables the direct determination of right atrial and ventricular pressures, pulmonary arterial pressure, pulmonary artery wedge pressure (as an approxi-

TABLE 62-3 Nomenclature and Classification of Pulmonary Hypertension

DIAGNOSTIC CLASSIFICATION

1. Pulmonary arterial hypertension
   1.1 Primary pulmonary hypertension
      (a) Sporadic
      (b) Familial
   1.2 Related to
      (a) Collagen-vascular disease
      (b) Congenital systemic to pulmonary shunts
      (c) Portal hypertension
      (d) HIV infection
      (e) Drugs/toxins
         (1) Anorexigens
         (2) Other
      (f) Persistent pulmonary hypertension of the newborn
      (g) Other
2. Pulmonary venous hypertension
   2.1 Left-side atrial or ventricular heart disease
   2.2 Left-side valvular heart disease
   2.3 Extrinsic compression of central pulmonary veins
      (a) Fibrosing mediastinitis
      (b) Adenopathy/tumors
   2.4 Pulmonary venoocclusive disease
   2.5 Other
3. Pulmonary hypertension associated with disorders of the respiratory system and/or hypoxemia
   3.1 Chronic obstructive pulmonary disease
   3.2 Interstitial lung disease
   3.3 Sleep-disordered breathing
   3.4 Alveolar hypoventilatory disorders
   3.5 Chronic exposure to high altitude
   3.6 Neonatal lung disease
   3.7 Alveolar-capillary dysplasia
   3.8 Other
4. Pulmonary hypertension due to chronic thrombotic and/or embolic disease
   4.1 Thromboembolic obstruction of proximal pulmonary arteries
   4.2 Obstruction of distal pulmonary arteries
      (a) Pulmonary embolism (thrombus, tumor, ova and/or parasites, foreign material)
      (b) In-situ thrombosis
      (c) Sickle cell disease
5. Pulmonary hypertension due to disorders directly affecting the pulmonary vasculature
   5.1 Inflammatory
      (a) Schistosomiasis
      (b) Sarcoidosis
      (c) Other
   5.2 Pulmonary capillary hemangiomatosis

mation of pulmonary venous pressure), pulmonary blood flow (cardiac output), and the responses of these parameters to interventions (vasodilators, oxygen, exercise). However, the skilled clinician can often suspect pulmonary hypertension on the basis of the assessment of an elevated jugular venous pressure pulsation and a loud P_2

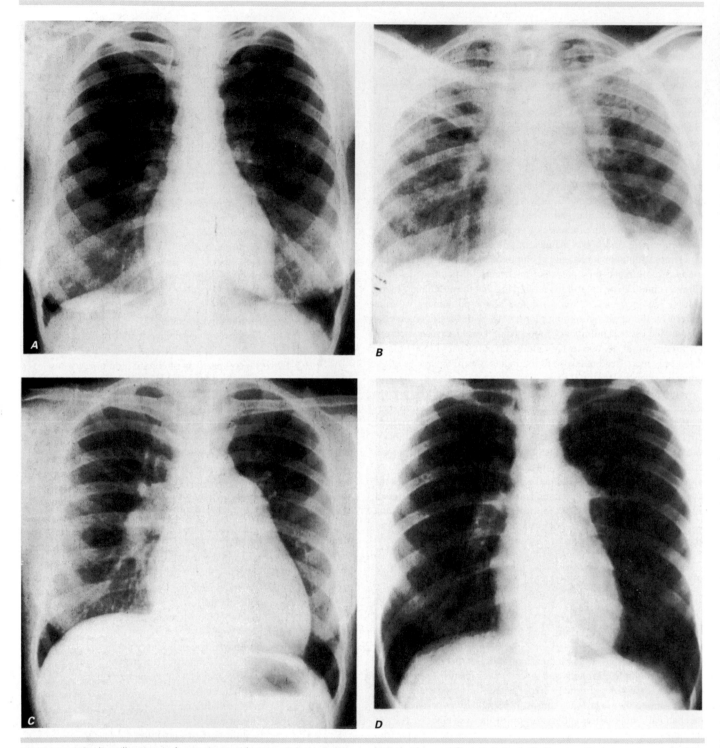

FIGURE 62-1 Cardiac silhouette in four patients with severe pulmonary hypertension on admission to the hospital: *A,B.* Primary pulmonary hypertension showing different stages in the evolution of right-sided heart failure. *C.* Wide-spread pulmonary fibrosis. *D.* Systemic lupus erythematosus proven by lung biopsy. This radiograph is indistinguishable from that of primary pulmonary hypertension.

(Chap. 12). PVR can be calculated from the measurements and samples obtained during cardiac catheterization, (Table 62-2). As a rule, noninvasive methods are less reliable and less informative.

CHEST RADIOGRAPHY

The findings on the chest radiograph depend on the duration of the pulmonary hypertension and its etiology (Chap.14). The characteris-

tic findings of pulmonary hypertension are enlargement of the pulmonary trunk and hilar vessels in association with attenuation (pruning) of the peripheral pulmonary arterial tree (Fig. 62-1). Right-sided heart enlargement can best be detected radiographically on the lateral view as fullness in the retrosternal airspace. In secondary pulmonary hypertension, changes in the lungs (e.g., hyperinflation, fibrosis) and in the position of the heart and diaphragm often mask the radiologic changes of pulmonary hypertension. Contrast angiography has a role in the workup for pulmonary hypertension when chronic thromboembolic disease, which may be treated surgically, is suspected.[8]

THE ELECTROCARDIOGRAM

The electrocardiogram (ECG) can disclose hypertrophy of the RV and is more reliable in respiratory disorders that do not involve the parenchyma of the lungs (e.g., alveolar hypoventilation and sleep apnea) than in obstructive airways disease or parenchymal lung disease (Chap 13).

ECHOCARDIOGRAPHY

The amount of reliable information obtained by Doppler and two-dimensional echocardiography depends greatly on the commitment of individual clinics to standardizing and perfecting these noninvasive techniques (Chap. 15). In general, echocardiographic techniques have proved useful in providing a measure of RV thickness as an index of RV hypertension. In some clinics, reliable estimates of the level of pulmonary hypertension have been obtained by determining regurgitant flows across the tricuspid and pulmonic valves using continuous-wave Doppler echocardiography.[9] In patients in whom the pulmonic valve has been visualized, its behavior during the cardiac cycle has also been used to estimate the level of pulmonary arterial pressure. Echocardiography is an attractive alternative to repeated cardiac catheterization in following the course of the disease and assessing the effects of therapeutic interventions in some patients (Chap. 15).

LUNG SCANS

Ventilation/perfusion scans are of most value in the diagnosis and exclusion of pulmonary thromboembolic disease (see below).

RADIONUCLIDE STUDIES

The response of the RV ejection fraction to exercise is assessed in some clinics using radionuclide angiography. Scintigraphy using thallium 201 also has been useful in detecting hypertrophy of the RV due to pulmonary hypertension (Chap. 19).

LUNG BIOPSY

The sampling of lung tissue by open thoracotomy or thoracoscopy occasionally is helpful in identifying the etiology of the pulmonary hypertension—e.g., in the setting of suspected pulmonary vasculitis. However, the procedure carries substantial risk in these hemodynamically compromised individuals. Attempts to predict responsiveness to vasodilators on the basis of lung biopsy have had limited success.[10]

SECONDARY PULMONARY HYPERTENSION

Cardiac and/or respiratory diseases are the most common causes of secondary pulmonary hypertension. Cardiac disease leads to pulmonary hypertension by increasing pulmonary blood flow (e.g., large left-to-right shunts) or by increasing pulmonary venous pressure (e.g., LV failure). Almost invariably, secondary influences such as intimal proliferation in the pulmonary resistance vessels add a component of obstructive pulmonary vascular disease.[11] In respiratory disease, the predominant mechanism for the pulmonary hypertension is an increase in resistance to pulmonary blood flow arising from perivascular parenchymal changes coupled with pulmonary vasoconstriction due to hypoxia. In pulmonary thromboembolic disease, clots in various stages of organization and affecting pulmonary vessels of different size increase resistance to blood flow.[11]

Cardiac Disease

The mechanisms of pulmonary hypertension usually are quite different in acquired disorders of the left side of the heart than in those of congenital heart disease.

ACQUIRED DISORDERS OF THE LEFT SIDE OF THE HEART

LV failure is the most common cause of pulmonary hypertension. Among the various etiologies, myocardial disorders and lesions of the mitral and aortic valves predominate. Both categories of lesions lead to an increase in pulmonary venous pressure that, in turn, evokes an increase in pulmonary arterial pressure. Presumably, the increase in pulmonary arterial pressure is reflex in origin. In time, three types of morphologic changes supervene: (1) occlusive intimal and medial changes not only in pulmonary venules and veins but also in the precapillary vessels, (2) perivascular interstitial edema and fibrosis that, under the influence of gravity, cause vascular and perivascular changes to be most marked in the dependent portions of the lungs, and (3) occlusion of small pulmonary vessels by emboli or thrombi when the RV fails and cardiac output decreases. The medical management of myocardial failure is discussed in Chap. 25. The treatment of congenital heart disease and of mitral valvular disease is usually mechanical (e.g., surgical or balloon mitral valvuloplasty). The prospect for relief of the pulmonary venous hypertension, as by mitral valve commissurotomy or replacement, depends on the reversibility of the pulmonary vascular and perivascular lesions (Chap. 67).

Although LV failure is the most common cause of RV failure, the level of pulmonary hypertension that accompanies LV failure rarely is sufficient to account for the RV failure. RV failure, secondary to LV failure, is usually attributed in part to failure of the muscle in the shared ventricular septum.

CONGENITAL HEART DISEASE

Pulmonary hypertension is part of the natural history of many types of congenital heart disease and is often a major determinant of the clinical course, the feasibility of surgical intervention, and the outcome (Chaps. 73 and 74). Congenital defects of the heart associated with large left-to-right shunts (e.g., atrial septal defect) or abnormal communications between the great vessels (e.g., patent ductus arteriosus) are commonly associated with pulmonary arterial hypertension. Pulmonary hypertension occurs in both "pretricuspid" congenital defects (e.g., secundum atrial septal defect) and "posttricuspid" congenital defects (e.g., ventricular septal defect). Important differences exist in the natural history of these two categories. Their differences are considered elsewhere in this book (Chap. 73). The major cause of pulmonary hypertension in congenital heart disease is an increase in blood flow, an increase in resistance to blood flow, or, most often, a combination of the two. In congenital heart disease with right-to-left shunting (systemic hypoxemia), pulmonary vasoconstriction adds to the resistance to blood flow. Erythrocytosis, acting by way of increased viscosity and propensity to thrombosis, also contributes to the increase in resistance. Although the increase in pulmonary vascular tone elicited by hypoxia contributes to the increase in PVR, the predominant resistance is offered by anatomic changes in the walls of the small muscular arteries and arterioles. Patients with congenital heart disease and pulmonary hypertension who become pregnant are at increased risk of sudden death both in the course of delivery and in the immediate postpartum period.

Depending on the nature of the congenital cardiac defect, vasodilators are sometimes helpful in diminishing heightened pulmonary vasomotor tone. Caution is required in administering such agents to such patients because of the potential to increase right-to-left shunting by reducing systemic vascular resistance to a greater degree than its pulmonary counterpart. Phlebotomy, with replacement of fluid (e.g., plasma or albumin) is helpful in congenital cyanotic heart disease in which severe hypoxemia has evoked a large increase in red cell mass. Once again, caution is required to avoid depletion of iron stores and a reduction in the circulating blood volume.

THROMBOEMBOLIC DISEASE

Thromboembolic disease is a form of occlusive pulmonary vascular disease that may be acute or chronic. In the United States and Europe, clots originating in peripheral veins represent a common cause of chronic occlusive pulmonary vascular disease. Elsewhere in the world, other intravascular particulates may cause pulmonary vascular occlusive disease. For example, in Egypt, where schistosomiasis is endemic, pulmonary vascular disease stemming from ova lodged in pulmonary vessels and hypersensitivity reactions to the organism (usually situated outside the lungs) is common. In some parts of Asia, filariasis is reputed to be an important cause of pulmonary hypertension. Tumor emboli to the lungs from extrapulmonary sites (e.g., the breast) can cause pulmonary hypertension by invading the adjacent minute vessels of the lungs. Intravenous drug use may be associated with talc or cotton fiber embolism to the lungs, which can result in a granulomatous pulmonary arteritis.

The *syndromes of thromboembolic pulmonary hypertension* can be categorized according to the segments of the pulmonary arterial tree that are primarily affected: (1) small (muscular pulmonary arteries and arterioles), (2) intermediate arteries, and (3) large central arteries. Some overlap is inevitable because clots lodged in large vessels are fragmented by the churning motion of the heart, and both the parent clot and its derivatives tend to move peripherally for final lodging.

Occlusion of Small Muscular Arteries and Arterioles by Organized Thrombi   At autopsy, small thrombi, predominantly recent in origin, are commonplace in the small pulmonary vessels of patients with pulmonary hypertension who have developed heart failure preterminally. In contrast is the syndrome of widespread pulmonary vascular occlusion by organized thrombi in the small pulmonary arteries and arterioles. Once attributed to multiple pulmonary emboli, these lesions are now regarded as organized, in situ thrombi.[12] The syndrome is rare and indistinguishable during life from primary pulmonary hypertension except by lung biopsy. However, histologic identification of these lesions serves little purpose in management. After a ventilation/perfusion scan has excluded chronic proximal thromboembolism (see below), treatment consists of long-term anticoagulation to prevent further clotting using warfarin or related agents, antiplatelet agents, or both.

Occlusion of Intermediate Pulmonary Arteries by Emboli   This syndrome is by far the most common of the three.[12] It is thought to be caused by multiple emboli released from vessels in the upper legs and thighs that progressively amputate the pulmonary arterial tree. Ventilation/perfusion scans and selective angiography demonstrate the pulmonary vascular occlusion, although both studies tend to underestimate the degree of obstruction compared with direct inspection of the vascular tree at surgery or postmortem (Chap. 63). The major therapeutic concern in these patients is to exclude chronic proximal pulmonary thromboembolism (see below) and to prevent recurrent thromboemboli. Treatment involves the use of anticoagulants of the warfarin type and antiplatelet agents.

Chronic Proximal Pulmonary Thromboembolism   In some patients who have survived large to massive pulmonary emboli, resolution fails to occur, and the clots become organized and incorporated into the walls of the major pulmonary arteries, leading to pulmonary hypertension (Fig. 62-2). Overwhelming the capacity of the local fibrinolytic mechanisms also allows the clot to propagate, to obstruct large segments of the pulmonary vascular bed, and to decrease the compliance of the central pulmonary vessels. By the time the diagnosis is made, the obstructing lesions in the central pulmonary arteries have become an integral part of the vascular wall through the processes of endothelialization and recanalization.[12]

The importance of recognizing *proximal* pulmonary thromboembolism as a cause of pulmonary hypertension is the possibility of relieving the pulmonary hypertension by surgical intervention, i.e., by pulmonary thromboendarterectomy. Ventilation/perfusion lung scanning is the critical diagnostic test. As a rule, patients with proximal pulmonary thromboembolism show two or more segmental perfusion defects. If the perfusion defects are segmental or larger, selective pulmonary angiography is called for to define the location, extent, and number of pulmonary vascular occlusions.[13,14] Cardiac catheterization for selective pulmonary angiography also enables hemodynamic assessment. Fiberoptic angioscopy, helical computed tomographic scanning, and magnetic resonance imaging may be helpful in defining the lesions of proximal thromboembolic pulmonary hypertension[15] (Chap. 63).

Surgery is advocated for patients with pulmonary hypertension who have persistent clots in lobar or more proximal pulmonary arteries after at least 6 months of anticoagulation. Thromboendarterectomy is done using a median sternotomy and deep hypothermic cardiopulmonary bypass with intermittent periods of circulatory arrest. Postoperatively, hemodynamic improvement is usually quite dramatic.[8,14] Reperfusion pulmonary edema can be a severe complication immediately after the obstruction has been relieved. In experienced hands, mortality is about 5 percent. After the operation, patients are placed on lifelong anticoagulants. A filter is usually placed in the inferior vena cava to further prevent recurrence.

Respiratory Diseases and Disorders

In addition to intrinsic pulmonary diseases, disturbances in respiratory muscle function or in the control of breathing also can cause pulmonary hypertension. Among the intrinsic lung diseases are those affecting the airways (e.g., chronic bronchitis) as well as those affecting the parenchyma (i.e., emphysema, pulmonary fibrosis). Among the ventilatory disorders are the syndromes of alveolar hypoventilation due to respiratory muscle weakness and sleep-disordered breathing.

INTRINSIC DISEASES OF THE LUNGS AND/OR AIRWAYS

Diseases that affect the parenchyma of the lungs or the tracheobronchial tree can elicit pulmonary hypertension in different ways depending on the underlying disease (Fig. 62-3). In obstructive airways disease, ventilation/perfusion abnormalities cause vasoconstriction due to arterial hypoxemia. In diffuse fibrosis, several mechanisms act in concert: Loss of vascular surface area due to lung destruction, loss of vascular compliance due to hyperinflation-induced vascular compression, and vascular remodeling due to hypoxic vasoconstriction all promote an increased PVR.

INTERSTITIAL FIBROSIS

Pulmonary sarcoidosis, asbestosis, and idiopathic and radiation-induced fibrosis commonly cause widespread pulmonary fibrosis that results in cor pulmonale. Dyspnea and tachypnea dominate the clini-

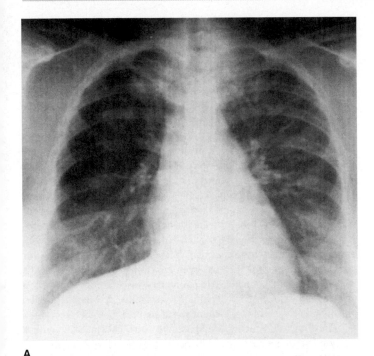

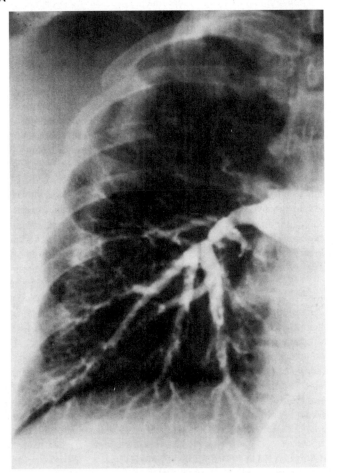

A

B

FIGURE 62-2 Pulmonary hypertension due to organized clot in central pulmonary arteries. Dramatic relief after pulmonary thromboendarterectomy. *A.* Chest radiograph. The right upper lobe is strikingly hypoperfused, and the vasculature on the left is quite prominent, reflecting redirection of the pulmonary blood flow to open vessels. *B.* Angiogram. The flow to the right upper lung is interrupted by the large central clot.

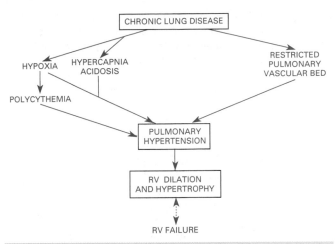

FIGURE 62-3 The evolution of RV failure in chronic obstructive airways disease (chronic bronchitis and emphysema; COPD). The factors on the left arise primarily from the bronchitis; those on the right from emphysema.

cal picture of interstitial fibrosis; cough is rarely prominent. Usually, severe pulmonary hypertension occurs toward the end of the illness, when hypoxemia and hypercapnia are present at rest (Fig. 62-1). RV failure is a common sequel.

Systemically administered vasodilators have no proven place in treating the pulmonary hypertension associated with interstitial fibrosis and may worsen intrapulmonary gas exchange. Recent experience with inhaled vasodilators, such as the prostacyclin analogue iloprost, is encouraging and suggests the possibility of producing selective pulmonary vasodilator and/or antiproliferative effects in this population.[16] Oxygen therapy, particularly during daily activity or sleep, can be important in attenuating the hypoxic pulmonary pressor response. Glucocorticoids and other potent immunosuppressive agents are the mainstay of therapy and often effect some symptomatic relief. The advent of lung transplantation has widened greatly the therapeutic horizons for dealing with widespread interstitial fibrosis.

CHRONIC OBSTRUCTIVE AIRWAYS DISEASE

Chronic bronchitis and emphysema [chronic obstructive pulmonary disease (COPD)] are the most common causes of cor pulmonale in patients with intrinsic pulmonary disease.[17,18] Cystic fibrosis is an example of a mixed airways and parenchymal lung disease in which pulmonary hypertension plays a significant role in outcome.

Cor pulmonale is encountered in two different settings: *acutely* in the setting of decompensation, which is often due to an acute respiratory infection, and *chronically* when progressive lung disease and worsening gas exchange lead to unremitting vascular remodeling.

The gold standard for diagnosing pulmonary hypertension in patients with COPD is right heart catheterization. Noninvasive studies, such as echocardiography, have proved useful in some centers.[19,20] RV enlargement, the cardinal sign of pulmonary hypertension, can be difficult to discern in obstructive airways disease because of hyperinflation and cardiac rotation.[21] Once suspicion is raised that the clinical picture of RV failure stems from gas exchange abnormalities, an arterial blood sample will confirm that the Po_2 is low ($Po_2 < 50$ mmHg) and the Pco_2 is high ($Pco_2 > 50$ mmHg). Derangement in gas exchange to this degree is rare in LV failure unless overt pulmonary edema is present.

ECG evidence of RV hypertrophy is also often equivocal in patients with chronic obstructive airways disease (chronic bronchitis and emphysema, COPD) because of rotation and displacement of the heart, widened distances between electrodes and the cardiac surface, and the predominance of right-sided heart dilatation over hypertrophy. Because of these limitations, standard ECG criteria for RV enlargement apply in about only one-third of patients with COPD who have cor pulmonale at autopsy. Consecutive changes in the ECG are often more useful than a single ECG in detecting RV overload. As the arterial P_{O_2} drops to abnormal levels (e.g., <60 to 70 mmHg while awake), T waves tend to become inverted, biphasic, or flat in the right, precordial leads (V_1 to V_3); the mean electrical axis of the QRS shifts 30 degrees or more to the right of the patient's usual axis; ST segments become depressed in leads II, III, and aVF; and right bundle branch block (incomplete or complete) often appears. These changes tend to reverse as arterial oxygenation improves (Chap. 13).

In the patient with COPD with acute cor pulmonale precipitated by a bout of bronchitis or pneumonia, the goal of therapy is to maintain tolerable levels of arterial oxygenation while waiting for the upper respiratory infection to subside. Supplemental oxygen, such as 28% oxygen delivered by a Venturi mask, generally suffices to relieve arterial hypoxemia and to restore pulmonary arterial pressures to normal. Considerable improvement also may be accomplished even in the individual who has chronic pulmonary hypertension by sustained (>18 h/day) breathing of oxygen-enriched air. Once the RV has failed, inotropic agents should be used cautiously because of the threat of arrhythmias posed by arterial hypoxemia and respiratory acidosis. Moreover, after adequate oxygenation has been achieved, the need for digitalis and diuretics often decreases because the hemodynamic burden on the RV decreases. Even though acute cor pulmonale is largely reversible, each bout appears to leave behind a slightly higher level of pulmonary hypertension after recovery.[17]

Arterial blood gas composition is the therapeutic compass to the control of pulmonary hypertension in COPD. The degree of hypoxia may be underestimated by blood sampling while the patient is awake and at rest, since hypoxemia is more marked during sleep and with physical activity. Determinations of the oxygen saturation during sleep or with ambulation using pulse oximetry are helpful in optimally prescribing supplemental oxygen.

Ensuring the return of arterial oxygenation toward normal is much more vital than the administration of inotropic agents.[22] When respiratory infection has triggered the episode of pulmonary hypertension, a vital strategy for improving arterial oxygenation is the administration of an appropriate antibiotic. While awaiting the salutary effects of antibiotic therapy, attention is paid to hydration, to postural drainage, and to adequate alveolar ventilation.

Phlebotomy has fallen into disuse. Polycythemia is rarely severe enough to be a serious problem in cor pulmonale associated with bronchitis and emphysema; when it is present, it is usually indicative of suboptimal use of supplemental oxygen. Vasodilators recently have been tried in various types of secondary pulmonary hypertension, including that due to COPD.[23] The agents tried are the same as those outlined for *primary* pulmonary hypertension. They may aggravate arterial hypoxemia by exaggerating ventilation/perfusion abnormalities. Unfortunately, the efficacy of vasodilator agents in secondary pulmonary hypertension has proved to be far less impressive or predictable than in primary pulmonary hypertension. To date, the safest and most effective approach to pulmonary vasodilatation in obstructive lung disease with arterial hypoxemia is the use of supplemental oxygen.[23]

CONNECTIVE TISSUE DISEASES

Pulmonary vascular disease is an important component of certain connective tissue diseases, most commonly systemic lupus erythematosus (SLE), the scleroderma spectrum of diseases, and dermatomyositis (Chap. 84).[24] The lesions may take the form of interstitial inflammation and fibrosis, obliterative disease, or vasculitis, either singly or in combination. Although pulmonary hypertension can complicate many connective tissue diseases, it has been documented most often in SLE and progressive systemic sclerosis (scleroderma) and its variant syndromes. The possibility has been raised that primary pulmonary hypertension is an inflammatory, or autoimmune, disease. This prospect has gained support from the occasional instances in which the lesions are confined to the pulmonary arterial tree without interstitial involvement and similarities in the histologic appearance of the vascular lesions. The high frequency of both collagen-vascular disease and primary pulmonary hypertension in women and the occurrence of Raynaud's phenomenon in up to 20 percent of patients with primary pulmonary hypertension has been used as additional evidence.[25] Finally, there is a high incidence of positive serologic tests for antibodies (ANA, anti-Ku), particularly in women with primary pulmonary hypertension. With respect to the pathogenesis of the two disorders, the idea has been raised that both the Raynaud's phenomenon and an increase in pulmonary vascular tone represent a widespread vasoconstrictive pulmonary-systemic disorder. However, this hypothesis has not gained universal support.

The lungs and pleura are frequently involved in SLE, with a reported frequency of up to 70 percent. Patients with pulmonary hypertension and SLE are predominantly women; most of these patients also exhibit Raynaud's phenomenon.

The histopathologic lesions in these patients resemble those of primary pulmonary hypertension. Pulmonary hypertension in these patients may originate in microthrombi secondary to the hypercoagulable state caused by lupus anticoagulant or anticardiolipin antibodies in the blood. Unfortunately, treatment of pulmonary hypertension associated with SLE using either anticoagulants or pulmonary vasodilators has had only modest success. This poor outcome contrasts with the results obtained in patients with active pulmonary vasculitis, who may either improve or stabilize their vascular disease with immunosuppressive agents.

In progressive systemic sclerosis (scleroderma) and its variants, such as the CREST syndrome (*c*alcinosis, *R*aynaud's syndrome, *e*sophageal involvement, *s*clerodactyly, and *t*elangiectasia), and in overlap syndromes (e.g., mixed connective tissue disease), the incidence of pulmonary vascular disease is high. In these patients, pulmonary hypertension is the cause of considerable morbidity and mortality. In a prospective study involving cardiac catheterization of patients with progressive systemic sclerosis or the CREST syndrome variant, pulmonary hypertension, either as an isolated finding or in association with pulmonary parenchymal or cardiac disease, was found in up to one-third of patients with progressive systemic sclerosis and in up to one-half of patients with the CREST syndrome.[26] The pulmonary vascular disease may be independent of pulmonary or other visceral disease. As in the case of SLE, the pathology of these lesions is often indistinguishable from that of primary pulmonary hypertension. Vasodilator therapy has not proved to be highly effective; however, continuous intravenous epoprostenol recently has been shown to improve hemodynamics and exercise tolerance.[27]

ALVEOLAR HYPOVENTILATION IN PATIENTS WITH NORMAL LUNGS

In patients who hypoventilate despite normal lungs (alveolar hypoventilation), the primary pathogenetic mechanism is alveolar hypoxia potentiated by respiratory acidosis.[28] These abnormal alveolar and arterial blood gases play the same role in eliciting pulmonary hypertension in patients with alveolar hypoventilation as in those in whom the abnormal alveolar and blood gases are the result of ventilation/perfusion abnormalities. In individuals with normal lungs, the alveolar hypoventilation generally originates from an inadequate ventilatory drive (e.g., after encephalitis), covert obstruction of the upper airways (e.g., in the sleep apnea syndromes), an ineffective chest bellows (e.g., after poliomyelitis or polymyositis), or lungs entrapped by neoplasm or fibrosis (e.g., in trapped lung caused by asbestosis).

Regardless of etiology, whether pulmonary hypertension will occur in patients with alveolar hypoventilation and normal lungs depends on the whether there is sufficient alveolar and arterial hypoxia to raise pulmonary arterial pressures considerably. In the sleep apnea syndromes, severe arterial hypoxemia and pulmonary hypertension that develop initially only during sleep may become self-perpetuating and carry over into wakefulness, although this only occurs in those with severe disturbances in respiration during sleep.[29]

For the patient with alveolar hypoventilation with combined respiratory and cardiac (RV) failure, the highest therapeutic priority is to improve oxygenation. Assisted ventilation, particularly during sleep, may be particularly helpful in improving oxygenation and reducing hypercapnia (e.g., continuous positive airway pressure) breathing. Pharmacologic therapy is rarely needed for patients with alveolar hypoventilation because of the efficiency of assisted ventilation coupled with oxygen therapy in promoting pulmonary vasodilatation.

PRIMARY (UNEXPLAINED) PULMONARY HYPERTENSION

Definition

Primary pulmonary hypertension (PPH) is a disorder intrinsic to the pulmonary vascular bed that is characterized by sustained elevations in pulmonary artery pressure and vascular resistance that generally lead to RV failure and death.[25] The diagnosis of PPH requires the exclusion on clinical grounds of other conditions that can result in pulmonary artery hypertension[30] (Table 62-3). PPH is a rare disease, with an incidence of 1 to 2 per million.[31] Its prevalence is about 0.1 to 0.2 percent of all patients who come to autopsy.

The clinical diagnosis of PPH rests on three different types of evidence: (1) clinical, radiographic, and ECG manifestations of pulmonary hypertension; (2) hemodynamic features consisting of abnormally high pulmonary arterial pressures and PVR in association with normal left-sided filling pressures and a normal or low cardiac output; and (3) exclusion of the causes of secondary pulmonary hypertension.

SPECIAL TYPES
Certain associations of PPH have attracted interest because of their prospects for shedding light on some etiologies. These include anorexigen-induced pulmonary hypertension, familial pulmonary hypertension, human immunodeficiency virus (HIV) infection–associated pulmonary hypertension, and portal-pulmonary hypertension.[30–33] In each of these, the clinical findings and the histologic appearance of the lungs at autopsy are identical to those characterizing the sporadic form of PPH. This diversity in associations underscores the likelihood that so-called PPH is the final common expression of heterogeneous etiologies.

General Features

After puberty, females predominate, those between 10 and 40 years of age being most often affected. Before puberty, no sex difference is discernible. The textbook picture of a patient with PPH is that of a young woman in the prime of life who develops one or more of the symptoms in Table 62-1 without discernible cause. Gender and age are sometimes useful in distinguishing clinically between the likelihood of PPH and pulmonary thromboembolic disease. The latter generally favors men, particularly in their later years.[25]

As a rule, median survival of patients can be predicted on the basis of the New York Heart Association functional classification: 6 months for class IV, 2 to 2.5 years for class III, and 6 years for classes I and II. Unless interrupted by sudden death, which occurs in approximately 15 percent of patients, the usual downhill course terminates in intractable RV failure.[34]

Etiology

The common denominator in the pathogenesis of PPH appears to be injury to the layers of the vascular wall of the small muscular pulmonary arteries and arterioles.[35] In response to injury, the intima of these vessels proliferates, so that the endothelium changes from a single flat layer to a piled-up projection that narrows the caliber of the vascular lumen. Also, the media of the affected vessels hypertrophy.[36]

The primary site of injury in PPH remains uncertain. Recently, an intrinsic defect in ion channel function and calcium homeostasis in vascular smooth muscle has been implicated.[37] Other studies have shown that endothelial function is disturbed, leading to altered production or handling of a variety of endothelium-derived vasoactive substances.[35] These abnormalities, coupled with altered platelet-endothelial interactions that predispose to intravascular thrombosis, lead to an inexorable course of enhanced vascular reactivity, proliferation and remodeling, and progressive obliterative vasculopathy. Diverse etiologies seem to be capable of eliciting PPH[38] (Table 62-4). For example, ingestion of the anorexigens fenfluramine and its isomer dexfenfluramine has been demonstrated to markedly increase the risk of PPH,[31] ingestion of toxic oil elicited an outbreak of pulmonary hypertension in Spain,[39] and HIV infection also has been implicated.[32]

An epidemic of PPH in Europe between 1967 and 1970 that was linked to the use of aminorex, an anorectic agent, raised the prospect

TABLE 62-4 Suggested Mechanisms for Primary Pulmonary Hypertension

Proposed Mechanism	Evidence
Early/sustained vasoconstriction kinetics	Altered smooth muscle cell calcium Endothelial dysfunction
Genetic predisposition identified	Familial disease with gene locus ?Susceptibility with exposures, e.g., anorexigens, HIV, portal hypertension
Pulmonary thrombosis/embolism arteries/arterioles	Widespread occlusion of ?Altered endothelial-platelet interaction
Autoimmune disease	Raynaud's phenomenon and antinuclear antibodies common, female gender predilection

of hereditary predisposition, since only 1 in 1000 who took the drug developed pulmonary hypertension. More recently, the fenfluramines have been associated with both severe pulmonary hypertension and valvular heart disease.[31,40] The toxic oil epidemic in Spain has reinforced the concept of individual susceptibility to pulmonary vasotoxic agents.[39]

In recent years, an increasing number of patients have been identified in whom PPH is genetically linked.[41] In these individuals, the hereditary pattern is that of autosomal dominance with incomplete penetrance. The gene responsible for familial disease recently has been identified as the *BMPR2* (bone morphogenic protein receptor 2) gene, a member of the transforming growth factor beta (TGF-β) family.[42] One major insight provided by the families with PPH is the diversity of pulmonary vascular lesions in members of the same family.[41]

Pathology

The evolution of PPH depends on progressive attenuation of the pulmonary arterial tree, which gradually increases PVR to the point of eliciting RV strain and failure. The seat of the disease is in the small pulmonary arteries (between 40 and 100 μm in diameter) and arterioles. The obliterative lesions can affect one or more layers of these vessels. In some instances, medial hypertrophy predominates; in others, it is the intima that proliferates. In addition, evidence of inflammation may be present[36] (Fig. 62-4).

Histologic examination of the lung identifies a constellation of pulmonary precapillary lesions that are consistent with the clinical diagnosis of PPH—i.e., plexiform lesions, angiomatoid lesions, concentric intimal fibrosis, and necrotizing arteritis. The pathologist is often hard pressed to distinguish between organized clots in small vessels that initiate the pulmonary hypertension and those that result from the obliterative pulmonary vascular disease. Recent clots in small pulmonary arteries and arterioles are common at autopsy in patients with PPH, particularly when the RV has failed and cardiac output falls. Although similar clots may not have initiated the pulmonary hypertension process in PPH, it seems reasonable that more often they are complicating features that aggravate and exaggerate pulmonary vascular obstruction.

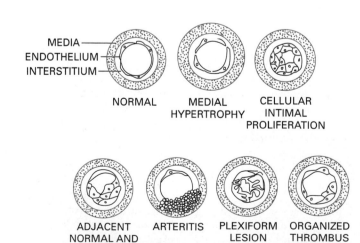

FIGURE 62-4 Vascular lesions in primary pulmonary hypertension. The plexiform lesion, once believed to be the histologic hallmark of primary pulmonary hypertension, has emerged as only one feature of a constellation of lesions.

Pathophysiology

The hemodynamic hallmarks of PPH in the resting patient were indicated earlier: a combination of a high pulmonary arterial pressure, a normal or low cardiac output, and a normal LA or pulmonary artery wedge pressure. Calculated PVR is high, generally leading to the logical conclusion that the resistance vessels, i.e., the small muscular arteries and arterioles, are the predominant sites of vascular obstruction. During exercise, as cardiac output increases, pulmonary arterial pressures increase further; the increments in pressure in the pulmonary hypertensive circuit are much more striking than in the normotensive pulmonary circulation owing to the inability of the existing vasculature to dilate or recruit unused vessels to accommodate the rise in pulmonary blood flow.

Pulmonary vasodilators are currently administered acutely for testing the responsiveness of the pulmonary circulation.[30] Among these, inhaled nitric oxide (NO) and intravenous prostacyclin or adenosine have become the gold standards. Several clinical and hemodynamic changes are sought as desirable endpoints: (1) improvement in exercise tolerance and in the quality of life, as the increase in physical capacity, attributable to an increase in cardiac output, in turn improves oxygen delivery to peripheral organs and tissues; (2) a decrease in the level of pulmonary arterial hypertension, with evidence of regression of RV hypertrophy or dilatation, or both; (3) a decrease in calculated PVR; optimally, this decrease should entail an increase in cardiac output (with minimal increase in heart rate) accompanied by a decrease in pulmonary arterial pressure; and (4) since pulmonary vasodilators are also systemic vasodilators, pulmonary vasodilatation must be effected without evoking undue systemic hypotension and tachycardia.

The combination of right heart catheterization and vasodilator testing is particularly useful not only for defining the hemodynamic state of the patient but also in providing a hemodynamic baseline for future invasive and noninvasive studies, such as serial echocardiograms.

Clinical Picture

In its early stages, the disease is difficult to recognize. In the sporadic case, the first clue is often an abnormal chest radiograph (Fig. 62-1) or ECG indicative of RV hypertrophy (Fig. 62-5). Both are late manifestations. The existence of RV enlargement is generally confirmed by echocardiography. By the time these changes appear, however, pulmonary hypertension is moderate to severe. Initial complaints—particularly easy fatigability and dyspnea—tend to be discounted, i.e., attributed to being "out of shape" except when the index of suspicion is high, as with a history of ingestion of anorectic agents or of familial pulmonary hypertension (Table 62-1).

When the disease is advanced, increasing nonspecific discomfort progressively reduces the activities of daily life. Dyspnea, particularly during physical activity, becomes incapacitating. Some patients develop an anginal type of chest pain along with breathlessness. Other common symptoms are weakness, fatigue, and exertional or postexertional syncope (Table 62-1). Infrequently, an enlarged pulmonary artery causes hoarseness because of compression of the left recurrent laryngeal nerve. In time, right heart failure develops.

Patients with severe pulmonary hypertension seem vulnerable to sudden death. Death has occurred unexpectedly during normal activities, cardiac catheterization, and surgical procedures and after the administration of barbiturates or anesthetic agents. The mechanisms of sudden death are not clear and may include arrhythmias or acute pulmonary thromboembolism. It was noted earlier that as far as clinical manifestations and physical examination are concerned, PPH has an advantage over secondary pulmonary hypertension in that signs and symptoms of underlying cardiac or respiratory disease do not obscure its manifestations. On physical examination, the jugular venous pulse usually shows a prominent *a* wave. RV hypertrophy causes a heave along the left sternal border, and a distinct systolic impulse is palpable over the region of the main pulmonary artery (Chap. 12). The pulmonic component of the second sound is markedly accentuated, the second heart sound is narrowly split, and an ejection sound is heard in the pulmonic area. Often a fourth heart sound emanating from the hypertrophied RV is heard at the lower left sternal border. The murmur of tricuspid regurgitation is best heard along the sternal border with the patient in the supine position and can be accentuated with inspiration (Chap. 12). In some patients, a midsystolic murmur is audible at the pulmonic area; as pulmonary arterial pressures approximate systemic arterial levels, the murmur of pulmonary valvular regurgitation often appears (Chap. 12).

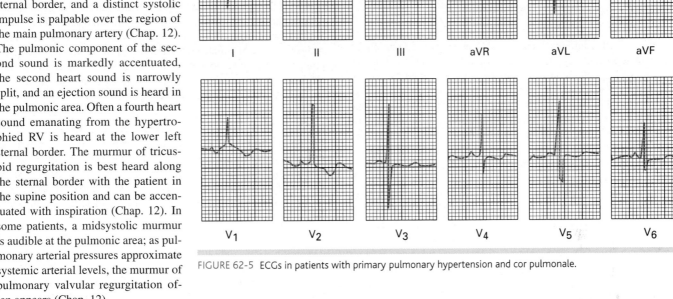

MD, 56 F

FIGURE 62-5 ECGs in patients with primary pulmonary hypertension and cor pulmonale.

The onset of RV failure is accompanied by jugular venous distention and a gallop (S_3); inspiration intensifies the gallop. The liver becomes enlarged and tender, and abdominojugular reflux can be elicited. Hydrothorax and ascites are seen as RV failure progresses.

Special Studies

Direct determination of pulmonary circulatory pressures by right heart catheterization is the only way to definitively establish the diagnosis of pulmonary hypertension; however, other studies that are less direct can strongly suggest that it is present. Since the diagnosis of "primary" is one of exclusion, a number of tests are undertaken, usually in the hope of identifying a more treatable disease than PPH.[38]

CHEST RADIOGRAPHY AND ELECTROCARDIOGRAPHY
In the early stages, the chest radiograph is generally normal. Later it shows cardiac enlargement in association with enlargement of the pulmonary trunk, while the peripheral pulmonary arterial branches are attenuated; the lung fields appear oligemic (Fig. 62-1). Although fullness of the central pulmonary arterial trunks and peripheral "pruning" are distinctive, appearances vary somewhat from patient to patient in accord with the level and pace of the pulmonary hypertension and the age of the patient. Radiographic evidence of RV enlargement usually becomes overt only late in the course of the pulmonary hypertension (Chap. 14). The ECG usually shows right axis deviation, RV hypertrophy, and, usually, right atrial enlargement (Chap. 13).

THE ECHOCARDIOGRAM
Two-dimensional echocardiography (TDE) confirms the enlargement and hypertrophy of the right atrium and RV, tricuspid regurgitation, and pulmonic valvular regurgitation. At the same time, LV

structure and function are normal. The magnitude of the velocity of the tricuspid regurgitant jet using Doppler techniques can provide a noninvasive estimate of RV peak systolic pressure. The determination of RV ejection fraction using radionuclide techniques can be helpful in evaluating the extent to which the excessive RV afterload has compromised the RV (Chap 19).

LUNG SCANS
Lung scans are particularly helpful in suggesting the possibility of large, long-standing organized clots in the major pulmonary arteries that may be amenable to surgical removal (thromboendarterectomy). The lung scan in PPH fails to disclose major perfusion defects. Angiography is done to exclude pulmonary emboli in cases where the scan is equivocal. Scanning over the brain or kidneys may disclose the presence of an intracardiac or intrapulmonary right-to-left shunt.

RIGHT-SIDED HEART CATHETERIZATION
Cardiac catheterization is invaluable in quantifying the hemodynamic abnormalities, in excluding cardiac causes of pulmonary arterial hypertension, and in assessing the hemodynamic responses of the heart and pulmonary circulation to vasodilator agents.[4]

Diagnosis

The diagnosis of PPH rests on two pillars: (1) the detection of pulmonary hypertension and (2) the exclusion of known causes of high pulmonary arterial pressure. The history is of utmost importance. Before categorizing pulmonary hypertension as "primary" or "unexplained," due regard must be paid to the exclusion of known etiologies (Table 62-3), particularly thromboembolic disease and connective tissue disorders. Account also should be taken of the likelihood of familial disease. Pulmonary function tests are useful in excluding diffuse pulmonary disorders, particularly interstitial fibrosis and granuloma. Serologic testing can point the way to covert connective tissue disorders. Abnormal liver function tests can signal the coexistence of portal and pulmonary hypertension. The value of cardiac catheterization in eliminating acquired or congenital heart disease was indicated earlier. Unfortunately, by the time pulmonary hypertension complicating heart disease is recognized, the anatomic lesions are often too far advanced for the obliterative pulmonary vascular disease to be reversible.

Treatment

Treatment of PPH initially focused on the use of vasodilators in the hope that an increase in pulmonary vascular tone contributed importantly to the high pulmonary arterial pressures. Although the bulk of the pulmonary vascular obstruction was clearly anatomic, vasodilators offered the prospect not only of decreasing pulmonary arterial pressures somewhat, and therefore the hemodynamic burden on the RV, but also of prompting reversibility of the anatomic lesions. Unfortunately, the use of vasodilators, which could affect the systemic as well as the pulmonary circulation, led to progressive disenchantment with one agent after another.

The situation has changed considerably during the past decade. The introduction of acute vasodilator testing for responsiveness helped to confirm the idea that in only about one-quarter of patients, heightened pulmonary vasomotor tone helped to sustain the pulmonary hypertension. An optimal "responder" to acute testing manifested an increase in cardiac output along with a decrease in pulmonary arterial pressure and in PVR with no undue effect on systemic arterial pressure. Improvement in exercise tolerance accompanied the increase in cardiac output. Calcium channel blocking agents that could be taken orally could maintain those patients who were highly responsive during acute testing at lower pulmonary arterial pressures. A landmark development for patients who failed to satisfy the criteria for a good hemodynamic response to acute vasodilator testing was the demonstration that such patients respond to continuous infusion of epoprostenol. Indeed, a substantial number of such patients have been treated in this way for years or have used continuous intravenous epoprostenol as a transition to transplantation. During this evolution, heart-lung and then lung transplantation became increasingly feasible and available, although the donor supply is still a limiting factor. More recently, the development of oral medications that block the receptors for endothelin have been shown to be effective therapy and may obviate the need for prostanoid therapy in many severely afflicted patients.

As a result of these advances, a patient with PAH has several therapeutic options, ranging from oral calcium channel blocking agents to oral endothelin receptor antagonists to continuous infusion of prostacyclin to lung transplantation. However, none of these modalities is free of complications. The oral calcium channel blocking agents must generally be administered in large doses that are often accompanied by undesirable side effects.[43] Endothelin receptor antagonists can cause hepatic injury. The continuous infusion of prostacyclin runs the risks of a permanently placed intravenous catheter.[44,45] Transplantation offers the substitution of immunosuppression and its attendant risk of infection as a better option than chronic cor pulmonale and RV failure.[46] Despite the limitations of each of these therapeutic modalities, together they provide a graduated therapeutic approach that has provided, at each stage, a better quality of life for many individuals with PPH. Moreover, they have prompted the search for agents that can be used in place of prostacyclin, which, until now, has required intravenous infusion; prostacyclin analogues that are delivered subcutaneously and by aerosol are

currently available in many parts of the world or are under investigation. Other novel approaches include chronic ambulatory NO, which can be administered by inhalation.

VASODILATOR AGENTS

Various agents have been tried over the years as pulmonary vasodilators. These include α-adrenergic antagonists, β-adrenergic agonists, diazoxide, hydralazine, nitrates, and angiotensin-converting enzyme inhibitors. In general, these have not withstood the test of time. Experience has taught that untoward reactions can occur with any pulmonary vasodilator, even when low doses are used. Four categories of agents, some of which have antiproliferative as well as vasodilator properties, continue to hold promise, however: calcium channel blocking agents, prostacyclin and its analogues, endothelin receptor antagonists, and NO or NO-enhancing agents.

DRUGS THAT BLOCK CALCIUM TRANSPORT

The designation *calcium channel blocker* refers to a heterogeneous group of agents of different structural, pharmacologic, and electrophysiologic properties. The agents in this category currently receiving the most clinical attention as potential pulmonary vasodilators are nifedipine, diltiazem, and amlodipine. Of these, nifedipine is the most popular.

Nifedipine   Note that this use is not listed in the manufacturer's directive. Nifedipine is a synthetic agent that is unrelated to other vasoactive or cardiotonic drugs. Although it has significant direct negative inotropic effects, these are usually not prominent clinically because of the reflex sympathetic stimulation of the heart; it does not possess antiarrhythmic properties. It is widely used for therapy of patients who manifest acute vasoreactivity when tested with short-acting agents under hemodynamic monitoring. Sustained-release preparations are used, with the dosage generally titrated to the maximal tolerable level based on avoiding untoward systemic effects, i.e., hypotension, headache, dizziness, and flushing. Considerable caution is necessary in administering the higher dosages, however, because side effects can occur precipitously and be life-threatening. In one study, 64 patients with PPH were treated acutely with high doses of calcium channel blockers. Seventeen patients responded to treatment with nifedipine (13 patients) or diltiazem (4 patients) and were alive after 5 years.[43]

In experienced centers, the trial of calcium channel blockers orally is preceded by use of testing of acute vasoreactivity using one or more of three agents: (1) inhaled NO, in concentrations of 10 to 40 ppm for 5 to 10 min; (2) prostacyclin (PGI$_2$, epoprostenol, Flolan), administered intravenously in increasing doses (starting dose of 1–2 ng/kg/min followed by successive increments every 15 min of 2 ng/kg/min until a maximal dose of 12 ng/kg/min is reached or until side effects preclude further increases), and (3) adenosine (50–200 ng/kg/min). Only patients who manifest substantial reductions in PVR (usually to values below 5–6 mmHg/L/min), resulting from a fall in pulmonary artery pressure without systemic hypotension and accompanied by an unchanged or increased cardiac output, are considered candidates for chronic therapy with oral calcium channel antagonists.

Prostacyclin and Its Analogues   Epoprostenol (Flolan, prostacyclin, PGI$_2$), a metabolite of arachidonic acid, and its analogues continue to be a major focus of attention as treatments for a variety of forms of pulmonary hypertension. The pulmonary endothelium elaborates prostacyclin into the bloodstream, where it has a short biological half-life (2 to 3 min). In principle, it is attractive for the treatment of pulmonary hypertension on several accounts: (1) it is a pulmonary vasodilator, (2) it inhibits platelet aggregation, and (3) it inhibits proliferation of vascular smooth muscle. Unfortunately, it suffers the disadvantage of requiring continuous intravenous infusion, which is accomplished using portable pumps.[44,45] Success in short-term randomized trials and in long-term management has recently been reported using aerosolized iloprost, a stable prostacyclin analogue.[16,47]

Endothelin Receptor Antagonists Endothelin (ET) is a potent mitogen and vasoconstrictor that is produced in excess by the hypertensive pulmonary endothelium. Circulating levels of endothelin are increased in patients with PAH, and the magnitude of elevation correlates with survival. Bosentan (Tracleer), an orally active dual ET-A and -B receptor antagonist, has been demonstrated to improve hemodynamics and exercise tolerance and delay the time to clinical worsening in PAH.[48] Although the drug is generally well tolerated, liver function must be monitored monthly since it can produce significant hepatic dysfunction in approximately 5 percent of patients.

Nitric Oxide NO is synthesized in endothelial cells from one of the guanidine nitrogens of L-arginine by the enzyme NO synthase. It has proved to be the endothelium-derived relaxing factor that contributes to the low initial tone of the pulmonary circulation. It has the advantage of other vasodilators of selectively relaxing pulmonary vessels without affecting systemic arterial pressure. It is currently being used as a test of vasoreactivity in a wide variety of pulmonary hypertensive states including PPH and also has been used to control pulmonary hypertension in the syndrome of persistent pulmonary hypertension in the newborn.[49–51]

Agents that enhance nitric oxide activity by inhibiting its catabolism, such as the phosphodiesterase-5 (PDE5) inhibitor sildenafil, may pose a novel approach to therapy and are undergoing investigation.

Anticoagulants Since 1984, when Fuster et al.,[52] in a retrospective study, showed that long-term survival was improved in patients with PPH by anticoagulant therapy (warfarin in low doses), the use of anticoagulants has been incorporated into the therapeutic regimens of patients with PPH. This practice is supported by the high incidence of antemortem clots found at autopsy in the small pulmonary arteries and arterioles of patients with PPH. Moreover, in a nonrandomized trial that separated "responders" from "nonresponders" to calcium channel blockers, survival was significantly better in those given warfarin than in those who were not anticoagulated.[43] The usual goal of anticoagulation is to achieve and maintain an international normalized ratio (INR) of 2 to 2.5.[53]

ATRIAL SEPTOSTOMY

Blade-balloon atrial septostomy has been performed in patients with severe RV pressure and volume overload refractory to maximal medical therapy.[54] The goal of this approach is to decompress the overloaded right heart and improve systemic output of the underfilled left ventricle. Improvements in exercise function and signs of severe right heart dysfunction such as syncope and ascites have been observed. Since the creation of an interatrial communication will result in an increased venous admixture, worsening hypoxemia is an expected outcome. The size of the septostomy that is created should be monitored carefully to achieve the ideal balance of optimizing systemic oxygen transport and reducing right heart filling pressures without overfilling a noncompliant left ventricle or producing extreme degrees of venous admixture.

LUNG TRANSPLANTATION

Only one-quarter of patients with PPH and even fewer with other forms of PAH are responsive to long-term oral vasodilator therapy. Of the remainder, approximately 65 to 75 percent maintain sustained clinical improvement with long-term continuous intravenous therapy using prostacyclin. When pulmonary hypertensive disease has progressed, or threatens to progress, to the stage of RV failure, the physician and patient are left with few therapeutic options other than lung transplantation. Lung transplantation is currently being done at specialized centers and is almost invariably handicapped by a shortage of donor lungs, which can lead to long delays. Single- or double-lung transplantation has largely replaced heart-lung transplantation. Often, hemodynamic improvement is dramatic,[55] but transplantation for PPH poses not only a considerable surgical risk but also the prospect of opportunistic infections that accompany lifelong immunosuppression.[56] Rejection phenomena, notably bronchiolitis obliterans, are the major limiting factor to prolonged survival. The median survival after lung transplantation is approximately 3 years.[46]

Prognosis

The diagnosis of PPH carries with it a poor prognosis unless medical or surgical therapy succeeds in decreasing PVR. Although death usually occurs within a few years after the onset of symptoms, instances of long-term survival do occur. Although sudden death accounts for 10 to 15 percent of all PPH-related deaths, the prognosis is largely determined by the severity of pulmonary hypertension and right heart dysfunction.[34]

PULMONARY VENOOCCLUSIVE DISEASE AND PULMONARY CAPILLARY HEMANGIOMATOSIS

These are the least common of all types of unexplained pulmonary hypertension.[57] Not infrequently, the patient is thought to have primary pulmonary hypertension until manifestations inconsistent with pulmonary precapillary disease, such as pulmonary congestion and edema or severe hypoxemia, redirect attention to the vascular bed distal to the arterioles. The pathogenetic mechanism of pulmonary venoocclusive disease (POVD) is unknown, but the disease may begin as an inflammatory-thrombotic process in the small pulmonary veins and venules and end in fibrous obliteration of the venous and venular lumens. Presumably as a secondary phenomenon, the distal pulmonary arterial tree also develops obstructive lesions that are generally proliferative ("reactive") rather than inflammatory in nature; the intervening capillary bed is generally normal. The pulmonary venoocclusive lesions have been attributed to an inflammatory response to vascular injury, followed by thrombosis and scarring. Among the postulated etiologies are viral illness, chemotherapy, toxins, autoimmune disease, and mediastinal fibrosis.[36]

Both POVD and capillary hemangiomatosis can be familial. When the pulmonary hypertension is suspected of originating distal to the pulmonary capillary bed, mitral valve disease, myocardial dysfunction, or even LA myxoma has a greater likelihood of being the cause than does POVD.

Clinical Picture

Predominantly children and young adults are affected, but the age has ranged from infancy to 48 years. Clinical suspicion of this disorder generally arises when a patient with congested and edematous lungs proves to have a normal mitral valve and left ventricle.

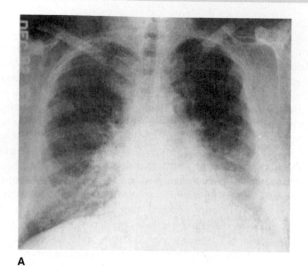

A

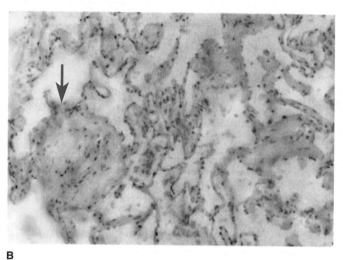

B

FIGURE 62-6 Pulmonary venoocclusive disease (POVD) proven by open lung biopsy. *A.* Chest radiography. Pulmonary interstitial edema is marked at both bases. *B.* Lung biopsy. In addition to obliterative pulmonary venular disease, the pulmonary arterioles (*arrow*) showed intimal proliferation and medical hypertrophy. (Courtesy of Dr. G. G. Pietra.)

The cardinal signs are dyspnea and fatigue on exertion in conjunction with evidence of pulmonary hypertension; the pulmonary venous rather than pulmonary arterial etiology is suggested by radiologic evidence of postcapillary pulmonary hypertension without evidence of involvement of the left side of the heart (Fig. 62-6*A*). Pleural effusions are common. Cyanosis, syncope, hemoptysis, and finger clubbing have been inconsistent findings. Moderate to severe hypoxemia, due to intrapulmonary shunting through the abnormal capillary network, is a hallmark of capillary hemangiomatosis. Rarely, systemic embolization may occur.

Hemodynamics

Cardiac catheterization discloses a high pulmonary arterial pressure with a normal pulmonary wedge (and LV end-diastolic) pressure. The low wedge pressure has been attributed to discontinuities and channels of high resistance between the pulmonary capillaries and the pulmonary and bronchial venous channels so that wedging interrupts all sources of flow distal to the area blocked by the catheter.[30] When epoprostenol is administered to a patient with POVD, an acute pulmonary edema pattern may ensue, resulting from increasing pulmonary blood flow in the face of downstream vascular obstruction.[45,58] This response, when present, is virtually diagnostic of POVD. Patients with capillary hemangiomatosis may experience worsening hypoxemia with epoprostenol, attributable to increased shunting through the low-resistance capillary meshwork.

Pathology

At autopsy, both lungs are involved. The lungs are the seat of congestion, edema, and focal fibrosis, which may become extensive. The venous lesions may be more marked in one region than in another. Although the small pulmonary arteries as well as the small pulmonary veins are affected, the lesions are different (Fig. 62-6*B*). Most striking are the morphologic changes in the pulmonary veins and venules, which are narrowed or occluded by intimal proliferation and fibrosis; up to 95 percent of the veins and venules may be affected in this way, but complete occlusion is uncommon. Bronchial veins and bronchopulmonary anastomoses share in the occlusive process. Hypertrophy in the walls of the pulmonary arteries may be quite striking. POVD, to varying degrees, may also coexist with capillary hemangiomatosis. Thrombi in the pulmonary arteries are common.[36]

Treatment

Medical management has been disappointing, since the lesions generally are irreversible. An occasional patient has been reported to do well with medical therapy, although most experienced clinicians consider both POVD and capillary hemangiomatosis to be contraindications to the use of oral vasodilators or intravenous epoprostenol. The usual duration of life after recognition ranges from a few weeks in infants to several years in adults, with 7 years being the maximum. The treatment of choice is probably lung transplantation.

References

1. Fishman AP. Pulmonary circulation. In: Fishman AP, Fisher A, eds. *The Handbook of Physiology*, Sec 3: *The Respiratory System*, Vol I: *Circulation and Nonrespiratory Functions*. Bethesda, MD: American Physiological Society; 1985:93–165.

2. Fishman AP. The enigma of hypoxic pulmonary vasoconstriction. In: Fishman AP, ed. *The Pulmonary Circulation: Normal and Abnormal*. Philadelphia: University of Pennsylvania Press; 1990:109–130.

3. Eltorky MA, Headley AS, Winer-Muram H, et al. Pulmonary capillary hemangiomatosis: A clinicopathologic review. *Ann Thorac Surg* 1994; 57:772–776.

4. Fishman AP, ed. *The Pulmonary Circulation: Normal and Abnormal*. Philadelphia: University of Pennsylvania Press; 1990:1–551.

5. Harris P, Heath D. The structure of the normal pulmonary blood vessels after infancy. In: Harris P, Heath D, eds. *The Human Circulation: Its Form and Function in Health and Disease*. Edinburgh: Churchill-Livingstone; 1986:30–47.

6. Kinsella JP, Abman SH. Recent developments in the pathophysiology and treatment of persistent pulmonary hypertension of the newborn. *J Pediatr* 1995;126:853–864.

7. Reid LM. Vascular remodeling. In: Fishman AP, ed. *The Pulmonary Circulation: Normal and Abnormal*. Philadelphia: University of Pennsylvania Press; 1990:259–282.

8. Fedullo PF, Auger WR, Kerr KM, Rubin LJ. Chronic thromboembolic pulmonary hypertension. *N Eng J Med* 2001;345:1465–1472.

9. Beard JT II, Bryd BF III. Saline contrast enhancement of trivial Doppler tricuspid regurgitation signals for estimating pulmonary arterial pressure. *Am J Cardiol* 1988;62:486–488.

10. Palevsky HI, Schloo BL, Pietra GG, et al. Primary pulmonary hypertension: Vascular structure, morphometry, and responsiveness to vasodilator agents. *Circulation* 1989; 80:1207–1221.

11. Edwards WD. The pathology of secondary pulmonary hypertension. In: Fishman AP, ed. *The Pulmonary Circulation: Normal and Abnormal.* Philadelphia: University of Pennsylvania Press; 1990:329–342.

12. Williamson TL, Kim NH, Rubin LJ. Chronic thromboembolic pulmonary hypertension. *Prog Cardiovasc Dis* 2002;45:203–212.

13. Ryan KL, Fedullo PF, Davis GB, et al. Perfusion scans underestimate the severity of angiographic and hemodynamic compromise in chronic thromboembolic pulmonary hypertension. *Chest* 1988;93: 1180–1185.

14. Jamieson SW, Auger WR, Fedullo PF, et al. Experience and results with 150 pulmonary thromboendarterectomy operations over a 29-month period. *J Thorac Cardiovasc Surg* 1993;106:116–127.

15. Ricou F, Nicod PH, Moser KM, Peterson KL. Catheter-based intravascular ultrasound imaging of chronic thromboembolic pulmonary disease. *Am J Cardiol* 1991;67:749–752.

16. Olschewski H, Ardeschir H, Walmrath D, et al. Inhaled prostacyclin and iloprost in severe pulmonary hypertension secondary to lung fibrosis. *Am J Respir Crit Care Med* 1999;160:600–603.

17. Weitzenblum E, Oswald M, Mirhom R, et al. Evolution of pulmonary haemodynamics in COPD patients under long-term oxygen therapy. *Eur Respir J* 1989;2(suppl 7):669S–673S.

18. Fishman AP. A century of primary pulmonary hypertension. In: Rubin LJ, Rich S, eds. *Primary Pulmonary Hypertension*. New York: Marcel Dekker; 1997:1–18.

19. Matthay RA, Shub C. Imaging techniques for assessing pulmonary artery hypertension and right ventricular performance with special reference to COPD. *J Thorac Imaging* 1990;5:47–67.

20. Tramarin R, Torbicki A, Marchandise B, et al. Doppler echocardiographic evaluation of pulmonary artery pressure in chronic obstructive pulmonary disease: A European multicentre study. *Eur Heart J* 1991; 12:103–111.

21. Maeda S, Katsura H, Chida K, et al. Lack of correlation between P pulmonale and right atrial overload in chronic obstructive airways disease. *Br Heart J* 1991;65:132–136.

22. Weitzenblum E, Sautegeau A, Ehrhart M, et al. Long-term oxygen therapy can reverse the progression of pulmonary hypertension in patients with chronic obstructive pulmonary disease. *Am Rev Respir Dis* 1985;131:493–498.

23. Brown G. Pharmacologic treatment of primary and secondary pulmonary hypertension. *Pharmacotherapy* 1991;11:137–156.

24. Yousem SA. The pulmonary pathologic manifestations of the CREST syndrome. *Hum Pathol* 1990;21:467–474.

25. Rich S, Dantzker DR, Ayres SM, et al. Primary pulmonary hypertension: A national prospective study. *Ann Intern Med* 1987;107: 216–223.

26. Shuck JW, Oetgen WJ, Tesar JT. Pulmonary vascular response during Raynaud's phenomenon in progressive systemic sclerosis. *Am J Med* 1985;78:221–227.

27. Badesch D, Brundage B, Tapson V, et al. Continuous intravenous epoprostenol for pulmonary hypertension due to scleroderma: Spectrum of disease. *Ann Intern Med* 2000;132:425–434.

28. Fishman AP. Pulmonary hypertension and cor pulmonale. In: Fishman AP, ed. *Pulmonary Diseases and Disorders*, 2d ed. New York: McGraw-Hill; 1988:999–1048.

29. Chaouat AE, Weitzenblum E, Krieger J, et al. Pulmonary hemodynamics in the obstructive sleep apnea syndrome: Results in 220 consecutive patients. *Chest* 1996;109:380–386.

30. Rubin LJ. Primary pulmonary hypertension. *N Eng J Med* 1997;336: 111–117.

31. Abenhaim L, Moride Y, Brenot F, et al. Appetite-suppressant drugs and the risk of primary pulmonary hypertension. *N Engl J Med* 1996;335: 609–616.

32. Speich R, Jenni R, Opravil M, et al. Primary pulmonary hypertension in HIV infection. *Chest* 1991;100:1268–1271.

33. Kuo PC, Plotkin JS, Rubin LJ. Distinctive clinical features of portopulmonary hypertension. *Chest* 1997;112:980–986.

34. D'Alonzo GE, Barst RJ, Ayres SM, et al. Survival in patients with primary pulmonary hypertension. *Ann Intern Med* 1991;115:343–349.

35. Voelkel NF, Tuder RM, Weir EK. Pathophysiology of primary pulmonary hypertension: In Rubin LJ, Rich S, eds. *Primary Pulmonary Hypertension*. New York: Marcel Dekker; 1997:83–133.

36. Pietra G. Pathology of primary pulmonary hypertension. In: Rubin LJ, Rich S, eds. *Primary Pulmonary Hypertension*. New York: Marcel Dekker, 1997:19–62.

37. Yuan JXJ, Aldinger AM, Juhaszova M, et al. Dysfunctional voltage-gated K^+ channels in pulmonary artery smooth muscle cells of patients with primary pulmonary hypertension. *Circulation* 1998;98: 1400–1406.

38. Gaine SP, Rubin LJ. Primary pulmonary hypertension. *Lancet* 1998; 353:719–725.

39. Lopez-Sendon J, Sanchez MAG, De Juan MJM, Coma-Canella I. Pulmonary hypertension in the toxic oil syndrome. In: Fishman AP, ed. *The Pulmonary Circulation: Normal and Abnormal*. Philadelphia: University of Pennsylvania Press; 1990:385–396.

40. Connolly HD, Crary JL, McGoon MD, et al. Valvular heart disease associated with fenfluramine-phentermine. *N Engl J Med* 1997;337: 581–588.

41. Loyd J, Newman J. Familial primary pulmonary hypertension: Clinical patterns. *Am Rev Respir Dis* 1984;129:194–197.

42. The International PPH Consortium, Lane KB, Machado RD, Pauciulo MW, et al. Heterozygous germline mutations in BMPR2, encoding a TGF-beta receptor, cause familial primary pulmonary hypertension. *Nat Genet* 2000;26:81–84.

43. Rich S, Kaufmann E, Levy PS. The effect of high doses of calcium-channel blockers on survival in primary pulmonary hypertension. *N Engl J Med* 1992;327:76–81.

44. Barst RJ, Rubin LJ, McGoon MD, et al. Survival in primary pulmonary hypertension with long-term continuous intravenous prostacyclin. *Ann Intern Med* 1994;121:409–415.

45. Barst RJ, Rubin LJ, Long WA, et al. A comparison of continuous intravenous epoprostenol (prostacyclin) with conventional therapy for primary pulmonary hypertension. *N Engl J Med* 1996;334: 296–302.

46. Arcasoy SM, Kotloff RM. Lung transplantation. *N Engl J Med* 1999; 340:1081–1091.

47. Olschewski H, Simonneau G, Galie N, et al. Inhaled iloprost for severe pulmonary hypertension. *N Engl J Med* 2002;347:322–329.

48. Rubin LJ, Badesch DB, Barst RJ, et al. Bosentan therapy for pulmonary arterial hypertension. *N Engl J Med* 2002;346:896–903.

49. Sitbon O, Brenot F, Denjean A, et al. Inhaled nitric oxide as a screening vasodilator agent in primary pulmonary hypertension: A dose-response study and comparison with prostacyclin. *Am J Respir Crit Care Med* 1995;151:384–389.

50. Krasuski RA, Warner JJ, Wang A, et al. Inhaled nitric oxide selectively dilates pulmonary vasculature in adult patients with pulmonary hypertension, irrespective of etiology. *J Amer Coll Cardiol* 2000;36: 2204–2211.

51. Pepke-Zaba J, Higenbottam T, Dinh-Xuan AT, et al. Inhaled nitric oxide as a cause of selective pulmonary vasodilation in pulmonary hypertension. *Lancet* 1991;338:1173–1174.

52. Fuster V, Steele PM, Edwards WD, et al. Primary pulmonary hypertension: Natural history and the importance of thrombosis. *Circulation* 1984;70:580–585.

53. Hoeper M, Galie N, Simonneau G, Rubin LJ. Pulmonary perspective: New treatments for pulmonary arterial hypertension. *Am J Resp Crit Care Med* 2002;165:1209–1216.

54. Sandoval J, Gaspar J, Pulido T, et al. Graded balloon dilation atrial septostomy in severe primary pulmonary hypertension. A therapeutic alternative for patients nonresponsive to vasodilator treatment. *J Am Coll Cardiol* 1998;32(2):297–304.

55. Pasque MK, Kaiser LR, Dresler CM, et al. Single lung transplantation for pulmonary hypertension. *J Thorac Cardiovasc Surg* 1992;103: 475–481.

56. Katayama Y, Cremona G, Wallwork J, Higenbottam T. Transplantation for primary pulmonary hypertension. In: Rubin LJ, Rich S, eds. *Primary Pulmonary Hypertension*. New York: Marcel Dekker; 1996:287–304.

57. Mandel JME, Hales CA. Pulmonary veno-occlusive disease. *Am J Respir Crit Care Med* 2000;162(5):1964–1973.

58. Davis LL, deBoisblanc BP, Glynn CE, et al. Effect of prostacyclin on microvascular pressures in a patient with pulmonary veno-occlusive disease. *Chest* 1995;108:1754–1756.

PULMONARY EMBOLISM

Nils Kucher / Victor F. Tapson

Approximately 100,000 patients in the United States die each year directly due to acute pulmonary embolism (PE), with another 100,000 deaths occurring in patients with concomitant disease in whom PE contributes significantly to their demise.[1,2] Three-month mortality in unselected patients with acute PE is as high as 15 percent.[3] A substantial number of patients die from PE prior to being diagnosed. Autopsy studies have repeatedly documented the high frequency with which PE has gone unsuspected and undetected.[4] Despite advances in diagnostic imaging tests and therapeutic interventions, PE remains underdiagnosed and prophylaxis continues to be dramatically underutilized.

Deep venous thrombosis (DVT) and PE have a high recurrence rate. The most important breakthrough in therapy is among patients with idiopathic venous thromboembolism (VTE), who benefit from long-term, low-intensity anticoagulation with warfarin to prevent recurrent events. A second breakthrough in therapy is among hemodynamically stable PE patients with evidence of right ventricular dysfunction, in whom thrombolysis should be considered in the absence of a high bleeding risk. Accurate risk assessment in patients with PE is paramount in selecting the appropriate management strategy. In addition to findings from the past medical history and physical examination, modern risk stratification of acute PE includes echocardiography and the cardiac biomarkers troponin and brain natriuretic peptide.

Anticoagulation with heparin as a "bridge" to warfarin is still considered the standard treatment of PE. The spectrum of anticoagulant drugs has been recently expanded. Low-molecular-weight heparins (LMWH) have been shown to be effective and safe not only for treatment but also for the prevention of VTE, particularly in hospitalized medical patients. Fondaparinux, a new pentasaccharide, is very effective in a fixed low dose in preventing VTE after orthopedic surgery. Ximelagatran, an oral direct thrombin inhibitor, does not re-quire dose adjustment and serial blood testing and may be at least as effective and safe as warfarin.

RISK FACTORS AND PATHOGENESIS OF VENOUS THROMBOEMBOLISM

In 1856, Virchow proposed his triad of factors leading to intravascular coagulation, including stasis, vessel wall injury, and hypercoagulability. Risk factors for DVT are based on these processes (Table 63-1). Extensive investigation has been undertaken of the veins of the lower extremities, since most significant PEs originate from this location. Although thrombi may form at any point along the vein wall, most originate in valve pockets. The veins of the calf are the most common site of origin, with subsequent extension of the clot prior to embolization.[5] Eventually, the thrombus may expand to fill the vessel entirely, with both retrograde and further proximal extension. If embolization does not occur, the thrombosis can partially or completely resolve via three mechanisms: recanalization, organization, and lysis. Chronic thrombophlebitis with recurrent pain and swelling can be incapacitating. Frequently, more than one risk factor for venous thrombosis is present; knowledge of these risk factors provides the rationale for both prophylaxis and clinical suspicion.

Acquired Risk Factors

Comorbidities enhance the risk of VTE. In the DVT FREE prospective registry of 5451 patients with ultrasound-confirmed DVT, the most common comorbidities were arterial hypertension (50 percent), surgery within 3 months (38 percent), immobility within 30 days (34 percent), cancer (32 percent), and obesity (27 percent).[6]

TABLE 63-1 Risk Factors for Venous Thromboembolism

Acquired factors
Age greater than 40
Prior history of venous thromboembolism
Prior major surgical procedure
Trauma
Hip fracture
Immobilization/paralysis
Venous stasis
Varicose veins
Congestive heart failure
Myocardial infarction
Obesity
Pregnancy/postpartum period
Oral contraceptive therapy
Cerebrovascular accident
Malignancy
Severe thrombocythemia
Paroxysmal nocturnal hemoglobinuria
Antiphospholipid antibody syndrome (including lupus anticoagulant)
Inherited factors
Antithrombin III deficiency
Factor V Leiden (activated protein C resistance)
Prothrombin gene (G20210A) defect
Protein C deficiency
Protein S deficiency
Dysfibrinogenemia
Disorders of plasminogen
Hyperhomocysteinemia

Acute paraplegia significantly increases the risk of DVT (particularly in the paralyzed limb), and the period of highest risk appears to be the first 2 weeks after the onset of the paralysis.[7] Long automobile or airplane trips are risk factors for VTE. The proportion of subjects who develop acute PE during or after airplane travel correlates with the flight distance. The risk of PE significantly increases with a flight distance >5000 km.[8]

Obesity merits further investigation, because recent studies have implicated obesity as a risk factor for VTE, particularly in the United States, where obesity represents a major health issue.[9,10] The Nurses' Health Study explored risk factors for PE in women and found that a body mass index ≥ 29 kg/m^2 was an independent risk factor.[11] The Framingham Study has confirmed that obesity is a risk factor for PE, particularly in women.[12] In addition to increased venous stasis, obesity may also increase the risk for VTE as a consequence of elevated plasma levels of certain clotting factors—such as fibrinogen, factor VII, and plasminogen activator inhibitor-1[13–15]—and as a result of platelet activation due to enhanced lipid peroxidation.[16]

Age appears to increase mortality due to PE,[17] and PE is suspected less commonly prior to death in the elderly patient.[18]

Prior VTE forecasts increase the risk of recurrence. Surgical patients with a previous history of VTE who do not receive prophylaxis develop postoperative DVT in more than 50 percent of cases.[19] Surgery itself significantly enhances the risk. Surgery patients without additional risk factors develop DVT in nearly 20 percent of cases if neither pharmacologic nor mechanical prophylaxis is applied.[20] Prophylactic anticoagulation is initiated either prior to surgery or shortly thereafter to prevent the development of intraoperative and early postoperative thrombosis. Total hip and total knee replacement

patients not receiving prophylaxis develop DVT in more than 50 percent of cases.[21] These orthopedic settings have been comprehensively investigated, prompted by the increasing use of LMWH. Spinal surgery, pelvic surgery, and neurosurgery place patients at a particularly high risk for VTE.

Trauma, particularly of the lower extremities and pelvis, heightens the risk of DVT. PE has been identified at autopsy in as many as 60 percent of patients with lower extremity fractures,[22] and mortality has been attributed to PE in as many as 50 percent of patients dying after hip fracture.[23] The incidence of VTE increases with time after the traumatic event. Autopsy-confirmed PE in patients surviving for less than 24 h after trauma has been demonstrated in 3.3 percent, increasing to 5.5 percent in those surviving up to 7 days. Pulmonary emboli occurred in 18.6 percent of those surviving for a longer period.[24]

Upper extremity DVT has become more important because of an increasing use of pacemakers, implantable defibrillators, and long-term indwelling central venous catheters. Venous catheters traumatize veins as well as serving as potential nidi for thrombosis. Symptomatic PE can originate from upper extremity thrombi, although this appears much less common than embolization from lower extremity DVT. An upper extremity DVT is at increased risk for superior vena cava syndrome and loss of vascular access.[25] Upper extremity (axillary-subclavian) thrombosis may also occur due to the effort-induced syndrome described by Paget-Schroetter.[26]

Epidemiologic analyses as well as autopsy data suggest that patients with cardiac disease are predisposed to VTE.[17] Although myocardial infarction without anticoagulation has been associated with a significant incidence of DVT, more recent therapeutic strategies have had a beneficial impact.[27] Large, placebo-controlled acute myocardial infarction trials have indicated that the use of thrombolytic therapy has reduced the incidence of VTE.[28,29]

Cancer clearly augments the risk of VTE, although the precise pathogenesis of thromboembolism in cancer is not well understood. Numerous mechanisms, including intrinsic tumor procoagulant activity and extrinsic factors such as chemotherapeutic agents and indwelling access catheters contribute to this process. The thrombophilic tendency associated with cancer is often amplified by weakness and reduced ambulation with venous stasis. An analysis based on data from PIOPED found that of 399 patients with PE, 73 (18.3 percent) had cancer.[17] Pancreatic, lung, gastric, genitourinary tract, and breast malignancies are associated with a particularly high risk of DVT and PE. About half of all cancer patients and about 90 percent of those with metastases exhibit abnormalities of one or more coagulation parameters. The most common abnormalities include elevation of clotting factor levels (fibrinogen and factors V, VIII, IX, and XI), fibrinogen and fibrin degradation products, and thrombocytosis. Most tumor cells produce both tissue factor and cancer procoagulant.[30] Tissue factor appears to be the primary coagulant factor implicated in promoting fibrin deposition and is expressed in situ as well as in isolated cells of numerous cancers.[31] Tumor cell expression of tissue factor also promotes metastatic dissemination.[31] One cancer procoagulant is a cysteine protease that activates factor X. Mucin, a glycoprotein produced by certain tumors, possesses a sialic acid moiety that may cleave factor X to Xa. Plasminogen activator inhibitor type 1 (PAI-1) is secreted by numerous tumor cells and inhibits plasmin generation, augmenting the thrombophilic state as well as possibly also promoting tumor metastasis dissemination.[31] Other procoagulant properties of tumor cells include expression of cytokines such as IL-1β and tumor necrosis factor alpha (TNF-α), which, in turn, regulate expression of procoagulants and mediate interactions between tumor cells, platelets, leukocytes, and endothelial cells. Thrombin, certain cytokines, and growth factors such as vascular endothelial growth factor (VEGF) can stimulate endothelial cells to synthesize tissue factor, further potentiating a procoagulant surface and leading to fibrin deposition on vessel walls. Activated protein C inhibitor may contribute to a prothrombotic state, as it can inhibit both fibrinolysis and the protein C anticoagulant pathway.[31]

Chemotherapy, with resulting neutropenia and sepsis, often necessitates hospitalization and bed rest, which contributes further to the risk of VTE. Following the administration of various chemotherapeutic agents, changes in the levels of coagulation factors, suppression of anticoagulant and fibrinolytic activity, and direct endothelial damage have been documented clinically and experimentally.[32] Hormonal therapy, particularly tamoxifen in breast cancer adjuvant therapy, is also associated with an increased risk of thromboembolism, particularly when combined with chemotherapy. There is no convincing evidence that an aggressive search for cancer is warranted in patients presenting with apparently idiopathic DVT.[32,33]

Pregnancy and the postpartum period are the most common settings in which women under age 40 acquire thromboembolic disease. Venous thrombosis develops in these settings five times more often than in age-matched women not on oral contraceptives.[34] Although DVT appears to be more common in the third trimester and postpartum than prior to delivery, the risk is clearly considerable throughout pregnancy.[34] Cesarean section further augments the risk. Oral contraceptives are associated with the development of VTE.[35] Third-generation agents (agents containing desogestrel or gestodene as the progestogen component) appear to cause acquired resistance to activated protein C and double the risk of VTE.[36,37] Results from a clinical trial evaluating hormonal replacement therapy indicated that such therapy increased the incidence of VTE in women 45 to 64 years of age. A yearly total of 16.5 cases of VTE per 100,000 women may be attributed to hormonal replacement therapy.[38] The risk of VTE also appears to be highest during the first year of exposure to hormonal replacement.[39] It has not been clearly established that previous use increases the risk.[40] Although such therapy is associated with obvious benefits, physicians must consider other potential risk factors for VTE before prescribing hormonal replacement therapy.

Inherited Risk Factors

Inherited thrombophilias result in variable degrees of VTE risk. The factor V Leiden mutation, a single base mutation (sustitution of A for G at position 506), is a common genetic polymorphism associated with activated protein C resistance. It is present in approximately 4 to 6 percent of the general population.[41] The relative risk of a first idiopathic DVT among men heterozygous for the mutation has been shown to be three- to sevenfold higher than that of those not affected.[41] This genetic mutation is also a risk factor for recurrent pregnancy loss, probably due to placental thrombosis.[42] Oral contraceptives in patients with factors V Leiden is associated with a tenfold higher risk of VTE.[43]

Another, less frequent thrombophilic mutation has been identified in the 3′ untranslated region of the prothrombin gene (substitution of A for G at position 20210). This mutant allele is present in 2 to 4 percent of the general population and causes increased levels of prothrombin.[44] This prothrombin gene defect increases the risk of DVT by a factor of 2.7 to 3.8.[44,45] It appears that carriers of both factor V Leiden and the prothrombin G20210A defect have an increased risk of recurrent DVT after a first episode and are candidates for lifelong anticoagulation.[46]

Homocysteine has potentially thrombogenic effects, including injury to vascular endothelium and antagonism of the synthesis and function of nitric oxide.[47] Coexisting hyperhomocysteinemia has been shown to increase the risk for thrombosis in patients with factor V Leiden.[48] However, the thermolabile methylenetetrahydrofolate reductase gene variant is not independently associated with thrombosis, emphasizing that the precise role of homocysteine in venous thrombosis is unclear. Thus, interactions between the genetic factors (defects in enzymes) that control homocysteine metabolism and nutritional factors (folate, vitamin B_6, and vitamin B_{12} deficiencies) that affect homocysteine metabolism warrant additional investigation with regard to VTE.

PATHOPHYSIOLOGY OF ACUTE PULMONARY EMBOLISM

Gas-Exchange Abnormalities

The effect of PE on oxygenation and hemodynamics depends on the extent of obstruction of the pulmonary vascular bed and the severity of underlying cardiopulmonary disease. Hypoxemia develops in the preponderance of patients with PE and has been attributed to various mechanisms. When no previous cardiopulmonary disease is present, lung regions with low ventilation/perfusion ratios and shunting due to perfusion of atelectatic areas appear to be the predominant mechanisms of hypoxemia. Hypoxemia leads to an increase in sympathetic tone, with systemic vasoconstriction, and may actually increase venous return with augmentation of stroke volume, at least initially, if there is no significant underlying cardiac or pulmonary pathology already present.

Hemodynamic Alterations

PE leads to an increase in pulmonary vascular resistance depending on clot burden and the dynamics of embolic events. An increase in pulmonary artery pressure increases right ventricular shear stress. The extent of pulmonary artery obstruction and the presence of underlying cardiac disease determine whether right ventricular dysfunction develops. When the extent of embolic occlusion approaches 75 percent, the right ventricle must generate a systolic pressure in excess of 50 mmHg and a mean pulmonary artery pressure (PAP) of greater than 40 mmHg to preserve cardiac output.[49] Although a hypertrophied right ventricle (in an otherwise normal patient) may theoretically be capable of achieving pressures this high, a normal right ventricle is unable to and will fail.[49] Right ventricular dilatation and dysfunction evolve rapidly, and a reduced right heart cardiac output causes diminished left ventricular filling. Left ventricular distensibility is further compromised by ventricular interdependence due to a shift of the interventricular septum toward the left ventricle. As a consequence, systemic cardiac output and pressure decrease. Myocardial ischemia and microinfarction are probably caused by two mechanisms: (1) increased oxygen demand of the failing right ventricle and (2) reduced coronary perfusion as a consequence of a decreased systemic cardiac output. Flow in the right coronary artery may be further compromised due to increased right ventricular wall tension. As cardiogenic shock worsens, pulseless electric activity is occasionally seen prior to cardiac arrest.

Right ventricular failure develops more frequently in the setting of PE when the patient has underlying coronary artery disease.[50]

DIAGNOSIS OF DEEP VENOUS THROMBOSIS AND PULMONARY EMBOLISM

VTE represents the spectrum of one disease. Most clinically significant PEs arise from the prior development of DVT in the lower extremities, with subsequent embolization to the lungs. Patients may present with symptoms of either DVT, PE, or both. At the present time, the diagnostic strategy involves assessment of clinical pretest probability, D-dimer testing, chest computed tomography, venous ultrasound, and pulmonary angiography. Ventilation/perfusion scanning has been the diagnostic cornerstone for patients with suspected PE for decades. Lower extremity ultrasound is the most common leg study utilized, and contrast-enhanced computed tomography (CT) of the chest has increasingly replaced ventilation/perfusion scanning in most institutions.

History and Physical Examination

The clinical diagnosis of both DVT and PE, based upon the history and physical examination, is insensitive and nonspecific. Patients with lower extremity DVT may be asymptomatic or may have erythema, warmth, pain, swelling, and/or tenderness. These findings are not specific for DVT but suggest the need for further evaluation.

PE must always be considered when unexplained dyspnea is present. Pleuritic chest pain and hemoptysis are also common in PE. Coughing may be present, and while sometimes caused by PE, it more commonly occurs with bronchitis or pneumonia. Anxiety and light-headedness are symptoms that may be caused by PE but may also be due to a number of other entities that result in hypoxemia or hypotension. Severe dyspnea and syncope are the principal symptoms that may suggest massive, life-threatening PE.

Tachypnea and tachycardia are the most common signs of PE, but they are also nonspecific. A pleural rub or accentuated pulmonic component of the second heart sound may suggest PE but can also be explained by other disorders. In some patients, a tricuspid regurgitation systolic murmur may be heard. A low systolic arterial pressure combined with distended neck veins are signs of right ventricular dysfunction.

Assessment of the clinical pretest probability may be helpful to improve the diagnostic accuracy in patients with suspected PE. Wells and coworkers have prospectively tested a rapid seven-item bedside assessment to estimate the clinical pretest probability for PE.[51] The following clinical variables are required to calculate the score: signs or symptoms of DVT (3 points), an alternative diagnosis is less likely than PE (3 points), a heart rate > 100 beats per minute (1.5 points), immobilization or surgery within 4 weeks (1.5 points), a history of DVT or PE (1.5 points), hemoptysis (1.0 points), and active cancer (1.0 points). A score ≤ 4.0 makes PE unlikely. Half of the patients with suspected PE and a Wells score ≤ 4.0 can be correctly classified as "PE-negative."

Differential Diagnosis

PE may mimic a large spectrum of diseases. The most common differential diagnoses are chronic lung disease, asthma, congestive heart failure, pneumonia, acute myocardial infarction, aortic dissection, primary pulmonary hypertension, chronic thromboembolic hypertension, pericarditis, cancer, pneumothorax, costochondritis, musculoskeletal pain, and anxiety states.

Nonimaging Studies for Pulmonary Embolism

D DIMER

The plasma D dimer is a specific derivative of cross-linked fibrin. Measurement of circulating plasma D dimer has been comprehensively evaluated as a diagnostic test for acute VTE. A normal enzyme-linked immunosorbent assay (ELISA) is highly sensitive in excluding PE and DVT. When the D-dimer level is below 500 μg/L, the sensitivity

and negative predictive value for VTE are ≥98 percent, respectively.[52] In another prospective analysis, 96 percent of 79 patients with high-probability ventilation perfusion scans had elevated D-dimer levels.[53] Thus, increased levels of cross-linked fibrin degradation products are an indirect but suggestive marker of intravascular thrombosis indicating endogenous fibrinolysis. However, an increased D-dimer level is nonspecific for PE and may be seen in patients with various diseases, including infections, cancer, myocardial infarction, the postoperative state, and second- and third-trimester pregnancies.

When clinical studies comparing D dimer with the results of other diagnostic tests for VTE are reviewed, there appear to be appreciable differences in assay performance, heterogeneity among the patient population, and inconsistent use of definitive diagnostic criteria for VTE.[54,55] The number of available D-dimer assays, including rapid bedside assays, is increasing. The results of clinical studies utilizing one manufacturer's D-dimer assay cannot be extrapolated to another study using another manufacturer's assay. No single assay has been established as superior to all the others. The ELISA assays are sensitive but cannot be performed rapidly. The latex tests, while rapid, have not proven to be sufficiently sensitive. A rapid, quantitative, immunoturbidimetric technique has been evaluated that recognizes the D-dimer epitope by using antibody-coated latex particles.[56]

Recently, it has been shown that the specificity of the ELISA D-dimer (μg/L) may be increased when the D-dimer/fibrinogen (D/F) ratio is used to predict PE.[57] Functional fibrinogen, measured by the Clauss method (g/L), is increased in most conditions that mimic PE symptoms and signs. However, in PE, the fibrinogen level decreases with increasing pulmonary occlusion rate. In the mentioned study, a D/F ratio >1000 was highly specific for the presence of PE.[57]

ARTERIAL BLOOD GAS ANALYSIS

Hypoxemia is common in acute PE. Some patients, particularly young individuals without underlying cardiopulmonary disease, may have a normal Pa_{O_2}. In a retrospective study of hospitalized patients with PE, the Pa_{O_2} was greater than 80 mmHg in 29 percent of patients less than 40 years old, compared with 3 percent in the older group.[58] However, the alveolar-arterial (A-a) difference was elevated in all patients. Thus, as age increases, it becomes even less likely that a patient with PE will have a normal room-air Pa_{O_2}. In PIOPED, a subset of patients with suspected PE without a history or evidence of underlying cardiac or pulmonary disease was evaluated, and the Pa_{O_2} and A-a gradient were compared.[59] Patients with and without PE could not be distinguished based on either of these values. However, the A-a gradient was elevated by more than 20 mmHg in 76 of 88 (86 percent) patients with PE. The diagnosis of acute PE cannot be excluded based on a normal Pa_{O_2}, and although the A-a gradient is usually elevated, it may be normal in patients without preexisting cardiopulmonary disease. An important tenet should be that unexplained hypoxemia, particularly in the setting of risk factors for DVT, should suggest the possibility of PE.

ELECTROCARDIOGRAPHY

Approximately 20 percent of patients with PE have no electrocardiographic (ECG) changes. The ECG cannot be relied upon to rule in or rule out PE, though ECG proof of a clear alternative diagnosis, such as myocardial infarction, is useful when PE is among the possible diagnoses. The potential coexistence of PE together with another process must, however, be a consideration. ECG findings in acute PE are generally nonspecific and include T-wave changes, ST-segment abnormalities, incomplete or complete right bundle branch block, right axis deviation in the extremity leads, and clockwise rotation of the QRS vector in the precordial leads. The changes that do occur are likely caused by right heart dilatation. The "classic" S1 Q3 T3 pattern described by McGinn and White[60] in 1935 in seven patients with acute cor pulmonale secondary to PE was subsequently demonstrated to be present in about 10 percent of PE cases.[61] In patients without underlying cardiac or pulmonary disease from the Urokinase Pulmonary Embolism Trial (UPET), ECG abnormalities were documented in 87 percent of patients with proven PE.[62] These findings were not specific for PE, however. In this clinical trial, 26 percent of patients with massive or submassive PE and 32 percent of those with massive PE had manifestations of acute cor pulmonale, such as the S1 Q3 T3 pattern, right bundle branch block, a P-wave pulmonale, or right axis deviation. The low frequency of specific ECG changes associated with PE was confirmed in the PIOPED study.[59]

Despite its lack in diagnostic accuracy, ECG may be helpful in predicting adverse clinical outcomes in patients with PE. It has recently been suggested that a T-wave inversion in V_2 or V_3 is the most frequent ECG sign of massive PE.[63] In another PE study, both the pseudoinfarction pattern (Qr in V_1) (Fig. 63-1) and T-wave inversion in V_2 were closely related to the presence of right ventricular dysfunction and were independent predictors of adverse clinical outcome.[64]

Imaging Studies for Pulmonary Embolism

CHEST RADIOGRAPHY

The chest radiograph is abnormal in the majority of patients with PE, but the findings are nonspecific. Atelectasis, pulmonary infiltrates, pleural effusion, and mild elevation of a hemidiaphragm may be present.[59] Classic radiographic evidence of pulmonary infarction (Hampton's hump) or decreased vascularity (Westermark's sign) are suggestive but uncommon. A normal chest radiograph in the presence of significant dyspnea and hypoxemia without evidence of bronchospasm or anatomic cardiac shunt is strongly suggestive of PE. In most situations, however, the chest radiograph cannot be used to definitively diagnose or exclude PE. Although exclusion of other processes such as pneumonia, congestive heart failure, pneumothorax, or rib fracture (which may cause symptoms similar to acute PE) is important, PE often coexists with other underlying lung diseases.

COMPUTED TOMOGRAPHY OF THE CHEST

Contrast-enhanced computed tomography (CT) of the chest has become the most useful imaging test in patients with clinically suspected acute PE.

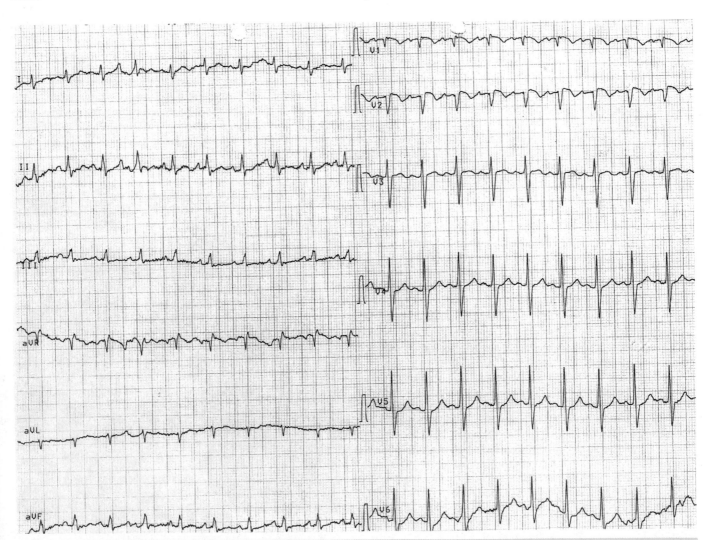

FIGURE 63-1 Twelve-lead ECG from a 54-year-old man with massive pulmonary embolism (PE) and cardiogenic shock. Several signs of right ventricular strain are present: sinus tachycardia with a heart rate of 100 beats per minute; right axis deviation; SI SII SIII; clockwise rotation of QRS vector in the precordial leads; Qr in V_1; and T-wave inversion in V_2.

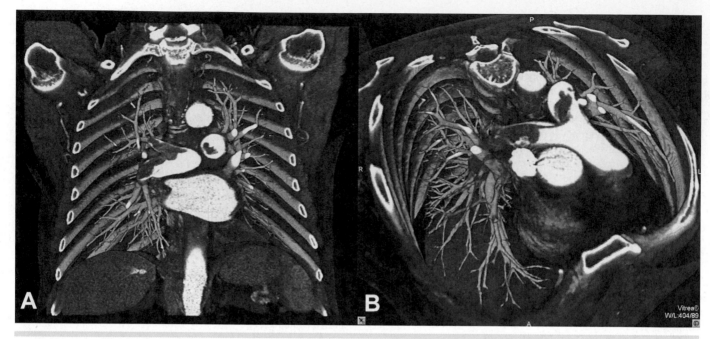

FIGURE 63-2 Contrast-enhanced 16-slice computed tomography in a 72-year-old man with extensive, acute central pulmonary embolism showing a "saddle embolus" (*arrows*) extending into both central pulmonary arteries. Colored volume rendering technique seen from an anterocranial (1*A*) and anterior (1*B*) perspective allows intuitive visualization of location and extent of embolism.

First-generation scanners have poor resolution in the segmental pulmonary arteries and a limited sensitivity for subsegmental clots. However, they appear to predict a benign clinical course over the ensuing 3 months.[65]

Second-generation scanners involve continuous movement of the patient through the scanner with concurrent scanning by a constantly rotating gantry and detector system.[66–72] A helix of projecting data is obtained. Continuous volume acquisitions can be obtained during a single breath. Rapid scans can be obtained, facilitating imaging in critically ill patients.

The latest generation of multidetector CT scanners (Figs. 63-2 and 63-3) permits image acquisition of the entire chest with 1-mm or submillimeter resolution with a breathhold of less than 10 s.[73]

Limitations of chest CT in early clinical studies included poor visualization of horizontally oriented vessels in the right middle lobe and lingula because of volume averaging.[67] The peripheral areas of the upper and lower lobes may be inadequately scanned, and the presence of intersegmental lymph nodes may result in false-positive studies. Multiplanar reconstructions in coronal, sagittal, or oblique planes aid in distinguishing lymph nodes from emboli. CT may reveal emboli in the main, lobar, or segmental pulmonary arteries with >90 percent sensitivity and specificity.[67–70] Accurate results have been reported for large PEs.[70,71] However, for subsegmental emboli, the sensitivity and specificity are lower. The incidence of isolated subsegmental emboli with first- and second-generation scanners appears to be approximately 6 to 30 percent.[55,72] When CT is being used for PE diagnosis, it should be incorporated into a diagnostic strategy, including pretest probability, D-dimer testing, ventilation/perfusion scanning, and ultrasound of the deep veins.[73] An additional advantage is evaluating a patient for the entire spectrum of VTE in one imaging session by scanning the legs and pelvis as well as the lungs.

Another important advantage of chest CT is the concomitant ability to define nonvascular and vascular structures such as airway, parenchymal, and pleural abnormalities; lymphadenopathy; and cardiac and pericardial disease. This is very important for rapid detection of alternative diagnoses (aortic dissection, pneumonia, pericardial tamponade, etc.) in patients with acute "chest syndromes" in the emergency setting. The intravenous contrast agent may precipitate renal failure in patients with renal insufficiency. Those patients with a history of allergy to contrast agents should receive preprocedure treatment with steroids.

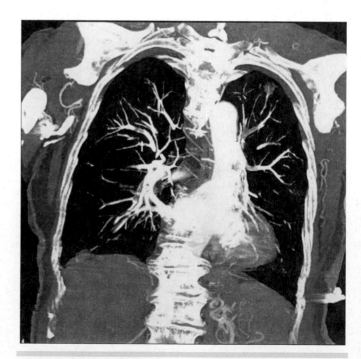

FIGURE 63-3 Contrast-enhanced 16-slice computed tomography (coronal reconstruction) in a 63-year-old man with multiple segmental pulmonary emboli (*arrows*). As an incidental finding, the examination also revealed a focal lung lesion in the left upper lobe which was later confirmed to be stage I small cell lung cancer.

VENTILATION/PERFUSION SCANNING

Ventilation/perfusion or lung scanning has been the pivotal diagnostic test for suspected PE for many years. Chest CT has virtually replaced lung scanning. An increasing number of hospitals use lung scanning to rule out PE only in patients with proven allergy to radiographic contrast agents, severe renal insufficiency, or pregnancy.

Ventilation/perfusion scanning is nondiagnostic in up to 70 percent of consecutive patients with suspected PE. Normal and high-probability scans are considered diagnostic. A normal perfusion scan excludes the diagnosis of PE with enough certainty that further diagnostic testing is unnecessary. Matching areas of decreased ventilation and perfusion in the presence of a normal chest radiograph suggests a process other than PE.

In the PIOPED study, the utility of lung scanning combined with clinical assessment of patients with suspected PE was prospectively evaluated.[74] Patients with PE had scans that were of high, intermediate, or low probability, but so did most individuals without PE. Although the specificity of high-probability scans was 97 percent, the sensitivity was only 41 percent. Of interest, 33 percent of patients with intermediate-probability scans and 12 percent of those with low-probability scans were diagnosed definitively with PE by pulmonary arteriography. Forty percent of low-probability scans in the presence of high clinical suspicion were followed by documentation of PE at angiography. When the clinical suspicion of PE was considered very high, the positive predictive value of high-probability scans for PE was 96 percent. In patients with nondiagnostic lung scans, further diagnostic testing for PE should be undertaken.

PULMONARY ANGIOGRAPHY

Standard contrast pulmonary arteriography is the established "gold standard" imaging test for the diagnosis of PE. The risk of subsequent VTE in patients with a negative test and without anticoagulation is less than 2 percent. Pulmonary angiography is highly sensitive and specific for PE. Nowadays, pulmonary angiography is rarely performed because multiplanar chest CT scanning seems to be equally accurate and is less invasive.

For smaller (subsegmental) emboli, pulmonary angiography appears less accurate. Two referee readers from the PIOPED study agreed on the presence or absence of subsegmental emboli in only 66 percent of cases.[75] In another study, using selective pulmonary arteriography, there was excellent agreement on main, lobar, and segmental emboli but only 13 percent agreement on subsegmental emboli.[76] The significance of such emboli is unclear, however, and may depend upon the presence of underlying cardiopulmonary disease, the extent of concurrent DVT, and the continued presence or absence of risk factors for DVT. Arteriography is safe in most instances. Complications related to this technique among 1111 patients suspected of PE in the PIOPED study included death in 0.5 percent and major nonfatal complications in 1 percent.[75]

Technique Prior to injecting contrast agents into the pulmonary artery, optimal recording of right heart pressure tracings is important. If pressure curves "wedge" in the main pulmonary arteries, massive PE should be suspected. If systolic pulmonary artery pressure exceeds 50 mmHg, chronic thromboembolic pulmonary hypertension is included in the differential diagnosis. A reduced amount of contrast agent is recommended in patients with right heart failure and extremely high pulmonary artery pressures.

A pigtail catheter is preferred because it permits a high contrast injection rate with optimal images and side holes for contrast that maximize safety. At least two views of each lung should be obtained. The standard procedure includes the ipsilateral posterior oblique and the anteroposterior or ipsilateral anterior oblique view.

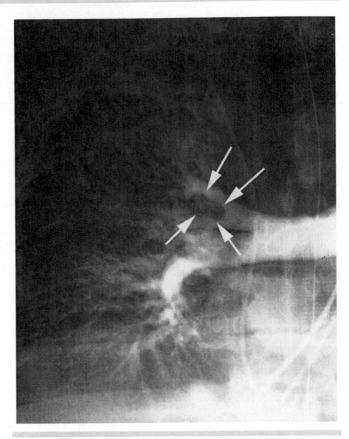

FIGURE 63-4 Selective conventional angiography of the right pulmonary artery in a 67-year-old woman with acute onset of dyspnea and chest pain, an elevated D-dimer ELISA level, and an inconclusive ventilation/perfusion scan. The right-upper-lobe artery is obstructed with visualization of the tail of the embolus in the proximal right-upper-lobe artery.

The primary sign for PE is an intraluminal filling defect in an arterial branch or cutoff of a branch with the visualized tail of the embolus (Fig. 63-4). Secondary signs of PE are decreased abrupt occlusion of a vessel, oligemia or avascularity of a segment, a prolonged arterial phase with slow filling and emptying of veins, and tortuous peripheral vessels.

In chronic pulmonary hypertension, the pulmonary arteries are pouched and contain organized thrombi with usually concave edges. Bands and webs within the arteries may be present. Lobar and segmental vessels may show abrupt narrowing or occlusion.

MAGNETIC RESONANCE IMAGING

Gadolinium-enhanced magnetic resonance (MR) angiography is also being utilized to evaluate clinically suspected PE.[77,78] In a clinical trial comparing MR with chest CT, the average sensitivity of chest CT for five observers was 75 percent and of MR 46 percent.[79] The average specificity of chest CT was 89 percent, compared with 90 percent for MR. A more recent study showed that when MR is performed under optimal conditions, it appears to be highly sensitive and specific even for segmental PE in comparison to pulmonary angiography.[80] MR has several attractive advantages over chest CT, including excellent sensitivity and specificity for the diagnosis of DVT and no requirement of ionizing radiation or iodinated contrast agents. Furthermore, MR technology also allows assessment of left and right ventricular size and function—potentially important for the risk stratification of PE patients.

ECHOCARDIOGRAPHY

Transthoracic echocardiography has emerged as the most important tool for risk assessment and treatment guidance in patients with acute PE. The presence of right ventricular dysfunction on the baseline echocardiogram is an independent predictor of early death.[3,81–84] In the Management and Prognosis in Acute Pulmonary Embolism Thrombolysis (MAPPET-3) trial,[85] most PE patients underwent echocardiography for risk stratification prior to enrollment.

Echocardiography is not useful to routinely diagnose PE because it is normal in about half of consecutive patients with suspected PE. However, emergency bedside echocardiography is highly useful to diagnose PE in hemodynamically unstable patients with a clinical suspicion of PE. This is very important because potentially life-saving therapy, including thrombolysis, catheter fragmentation, or surgical embolectomy can be rapidly initiated based on the presence of severe right ventricular dysfunction in the echocardiogram without obtaining time-consuming PE imaging tests.[86]

Transesophageal echocardiography has been shown to be useful to visualize centrally located clots and is an alternative to transthoracic echocardiography for patients with poor image quality of the right ventricle.[87]

Intravascular ultrasound imaging has been utilized as an investigational technique to image large emboli.[88–90]

Technique Right ventricular systolic dysfunction in routine clinical practice is semiquantitatively assessed by examination of the right ventricular free wall motion using a four-point scale: normal/near-normal right ventricular function and mild, moderate, or severe right ventricular dysfunction. Patients with severe right ventricular dysfunction may show regional wall motion abnormalities of the right ventricle known as the "McConnell sign": evidence of severe hypokinesis of the right ventricular free wall combined with preserved systolic contraction of the right ventricular apex.[91]

Right ventricular dilatation is an indirect sign of right ventricular pressure overload in the setting of acute PE. The ratio of right ventricular to left ventricular size should be measured using M-mode echocardiography in the parasternal long-axis view at the level between the mitral valve and the papillary muscle. An alternative is to measure the size ratio of both ventricles in the apical four-chamber view at the level of the atrioventricular valves (Fig. 63-5*B*). A ratio of right ventricular to left ventricular size of ≥ 1 in the apical four-chamber view and ≥ 0.5 in the parasternal long-axis view indicates

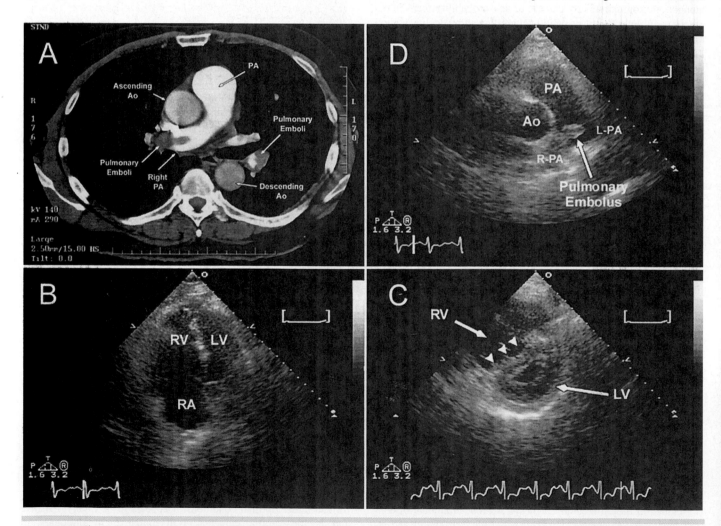

FIGURE 63-5 Chest computed tomography and echocardiographic findings in a 55-year-old man with submassive PE. *A.* Chest computed tomogram demonstrating multiple segmental emboli, including a central embolus in main pulmonary artery and extending into right pulmonary artery. *B.* Transthoracic apical four-chamber view with severe right ventricular dilatation. *C.* Transthoracic parasternal short-axis view showing flattening of interventricular septum ("D-shaped" left ventricle, *arrowheads*). *D.* Transthoracic short-axis view demonstrating the central clot in the main and right pulmonary arteries. Ao = aorta; PA = pulmonary artery; R-PA = right pulmonary artery; L-PA = left pulmonary artery; RA = right atrium; LV = left ventricle. (From Clark RK, Bednarz J, Spencer KT, Lang RM. Acute pulmonary embolism. *Circulation* 2000;102:2441. With permission.)

right ventricular dilation. In patients with severe right ventricular pressure overload, a constant shift of the interventricular septum toward the left ventricle or a paradoxical (systolic) septal movement toward the left ventricle may be observed. In the parasternal short-axis view, a constant shift of the septum to the left side often causes a "D-shaped" left ventricle (Fig. 63-5C). Further indirect signs of right ventricular dysfunction are systolic pulmonary artery hypertension manifest by an increased tricuspid regurgitant velocity > 2.6 m/s and reduced inspiratory collapse of a dilated inferior vena cava due to elevated central venous pressure.

Echocardiography is also useful to diagnose a patent foramen ovale in patients with suspected paradoxical embolism,[92] directly visualizing thrombi in the main pulmonary artery (Fig. 63-5D), right heart chambers, or vena cava.

Imaging Studies for Deep Venous Thrombosis

A number of diagnostic techniques can be utilized to evaluate the patient with suspected DVT. Compression ultrasound is the most common technique used in the United States and in many other areas of the world. Impedance plethysmography is used at some centers, and a number of important clinical trials have been performed utilizing this now outdated technique. Magnetic resonance imaging (MRI) appears to have some important advantages, but it has not generally been used as a first-line test. Venography remains the gold standard, but it has been necessary less often at many centers in view of the accuracy of ultrasound. Each diagnostic technique has advantages and limitations. Although diagnostic algorithms may be suggested for suspected DVT, these are institution-specific, depending on resources and available expertise with certain techniques.

ULTRASONOGRAPHY

Compression ultrasound with venous imaging is a portable, accurate, and widely available diagnostic technique for DVT. The primary criterion to diagnose DVT by ultrasound is the noncompressibility of the vein. Combined with a Doppler reading, this technique is referred to as *duplex ultrasonography*. Ultrasound technology has been further improved by the development of color duplex instrumentation that displays Doppler frequency shifts as color superimposed on the gray-scale image. The color duplex images display both mean blood-flow *velocity,* expressed as a change in hue or saturation, and *direction* of blood flow, displayed as red or blue. Ultrasound imaging techniques can also identify or suggest the presence of pathology other than DVT—for example, Baker's cysts, hematomas, lymphadenopathy, arterial aneurysms, superficial thrombophlebitis, or abscesses.[93] The sensitivity and specificity of ultrasound for symptomatic proximal DVT has been well above 90 percent in most recent clinical trials.[94,95] There are limitations, including insensitivity for asymptomatic DVT (less than 50 percent), operator dependence, the inability to accurately distinguish acute from chronic DVT in symptomatic patients, and insensitivity for calf vein thrombosis.[96–98] Compared with other technology, ultrasound is relatively inexpensive and is the preferred diagnostic modality for symptomatic suspected proximal DVT.

Ultrasound is considered diagnostic for PE if it confirms DVT in patients with PE symptoms. The majority of patients with PE have no imaging evidence of DVT, however.[99] Thus, PE cannot safely be ruled out in patients with suspected PE without evidence of DVT.

CONTRAST VENOGRAPHY

Contrast venography is a costly and invasive procedure that may result in superficial phlebitis or hypersensitivity reactions, but it is generally safe and accurate. Although contrast venography is the gold standard for DVT diagnosis,[100] it is now rarely performed. DVT is usually diagnosed with compression or Doppler ultrasonography, which is widely available, noninvasive, and accurate. Alternative diagnostic approaches are contrast CT and MRI.

Venography is performed whenever noninvasive testing is nondiagnostic or impossible to perform or during interventional procedures such as catheter-directed thrombolysis, catheter embolectomy, percutaneous angioplasty, or insertion of an inferior vena caval filter.

IMPEDANCE PLETHYSMOGRAPHY

Impedance plethysmography (IPG) has been used in patients presenting with suspected acute DVT but is rarely obtained in the era of ultrasound. It has proven reliable for the detection of completely obstructive proximal DVT but can fail to detect massive, nonobstructive DVT as well as most calf DVT.[101,102] The specificity of IPG is adversely affected by disorders that obstruct venous outflow, such as tumor or hematoma.[103,104]

MAGNETIC RESONANCE IMAGING

MRI has clear advantages as a diagnostic test for suspected DVT and appears to be an accurate, noninvasive alternative to venography.[105] A major feature of this technique is excellent resolution of the inferior vena cava and pelvic veins.[106,107] Preliminary experience with MRI suggests that it is at least as accurate as contrast venography or ultrasound imaging and more sensitive than ultrasound for pelvic vein thrombosis.[105–107] Simultaneous bilateral lower extremity imaging can be accomplished, and MRI appears to accurately distinguish acute from chronic DVT. This technique is also useful in differentiating other entities such as cellulitis or a Baker's cyst from acute DVT. As with many other diagnostic techniques, its utility depends to a certain degree on the experience of the reader.

DIAGNOSTIC STRATEGY

The overall diagnostic approach depends on the hemodynamic presentation of the patient. While rapid diagnosis and therapeutic intervention is required in patients with shock and suspected massive PE, there is sufficient time to obtain imaging tests in hemodynamically stable patients with suspected PE.

Patients with Suspected Pulmonary Embolism and Shock

In patients with cardiogenic shock and suspected massive PE, rapid initiation of reperfusion therapy, including thrombolysis or surgical embolectomy, is potentially lifesaving. Time-consuming imaging tests can be avoided when emergency bedside echocardiography is available. In patients with suspected massive PE and evidence of severe right ventricular dysfunction on the echocardiogram, thrombolysis or embolectomy may be rapidly initiated.[86]

Patients with Suspected Pulmonary Embolism without Shock

The initial assessment includes the history, physical examination, ECG, and a chest radiograph. We recommend calculating the Wells bedside score to assess the clinical pretest probability for PE. A plasma D-dimer ELISA should be obtained in all emergency department or other outpatients. If the pretest probability is not exceedingly

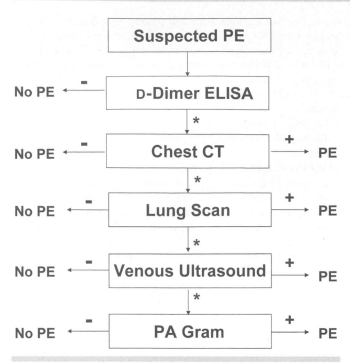

FIGURE 63-6 Diagnostic strategy for patients with suspected pulmonary embolism (PE) without shock. In this strategy, chest computed tomography is used as the principal imaging test. * Further testing should be considered if the test is inconclusive or negative, with a persistent suspicion of PE.

high and the D dimer below the assay-specific cutoff level, PE is safely excluded. In patients with elevated D-dimer levels, spiral chest CT should be obtained (Fig. 63-6). In patients with significant impairment of renal function, pregnancy, or allergy to contrast agents, ventilation/perfusion scanning may be preferred as the primary imaging test. A ventilation/perfusion scan can also be performed in patients with a nondiagnostic or negative chest CT when the clinical suspicion of PE persists. A venous ultrasound study is the next step in the cascade to diagnose or exclude PE. If a high clinical suspicion for PE persists despite a negative ultrasound study, pulmonary angiography can be performed. This strategy is safe and requires pulmonary angiography in less than 10 percent of patients.[108]

PREVENTION OF VENOUS THROMBOEMBOLISM

Background

Prophylaxis for DVT is effective.[109] A substantial reduction in the incidence of DVT can be accomplished when individuals at risk receive appropriate preventive care; however, such measures appear to be grossly underutilized. A review of the use of prophylaxis for DVT in 16 Massachusetts hospitals revealed that prophylaxis was administered to only 44 percent of high-risk patients in teaching hospitals and only 19 percent in nonteaching hospitals.[110] The frequency of prophylaxis ranged from 9 to 56 percent among hospitals. Another retrospective analysis revealed that only 97 of 250 patients (39 percent) at *very high risk* for DVT received any form of prophylaxis and that, of these 97, only 64 (66 percent) received appropriate regimens.[111]

Prophylaxis can be pharmacologic or nonpharmacologic. Pharmacologic prophylaxis options include unfractionated heparin,[112,113] LMWH,[114] fondaparinux,[115] and warfarin.[116] Aspirin has a slight

benefit[117] but not enough to be used as a standard therapy to prevent VTE. LMWHs have been increasingly utilized in clinical practice for both prevention and treatment of established VTE. The LMWH preparations are advantageous in that they produce a more predictable dose response and are administered subcutaneously only once or twice daily (without monitoring), depending on the preparation.[118] Early ambulation whenever possible is always recommended in postoperative patients.

General Medical Patients

Prophylactic measures to prevent VTE are not widely implemented among patients with medical illness. In the DVT FREE Registry of 5451 DVT patients, 59 percent who did not receive prophylaxis were medical patients.[6]

Patients should be stratified according to DVT risk, and certain prophylactic measures are more appropriate for some patients than for others. Generally, low-dose anticoagulation with standard, unfractionated heparin or LMWH is indicated in medical or surgical patients deemed at risk for DVT. When standard heparin is used for prophylaxis in general medical patients, 5000 U given subcutaneously every 8 to 12 h is generally adequate. LMWHs have also been studied in general medical patients. In a large double-blind, randomized clinical study comparing two different doses of subcutaneous LMWH (enoxaparin) delivered once daily to acutely ill medical patients, the higher dose (40 mg) proved effective and the lower dose (20 mg) was no better than placebo.[119] The incidence of DVT was 5.5 percent in the former group and 14.9 percent in the latter.

When prophylactic anticoagulation is contraindicated, mechanical devices, such as gradual vascular compression stockings or intermittent pneumatic compression boots, are utilized. Anticoagulation together with pneumatic compression is appropriate in patients deemed at exceptionally high risk or with multiple risk factors for DVT.

General Surgical Patients

In general surgical patients, a number of prophylactic strategies have been employed. An overview of the results of randomized trials in surgical patients demonstrated the substantial benefit of DVT prophylaxis.[109] In this review of more than 70 randomized trials involving 16,000 patients, it was found that perioperative use of subcutaneous heparin could prevent about half of all PEs and about two-thirds of all DVTs. In a large metanalysis, the value of prophylaxis to reduce the incidence of DVT was confirmed; it was also suggested that intermittent pneumatic compression plus the use of gradient compression stockings may result in the lowest incidence of postoperative DVT.[120] Other combined treatments were associated with lower rates than heparin alone and appear appropriate in patients at exceptionally high risk. For those patients undergoing minor operations who are less than 40 years old and have no additional risk factors for DVT, no prophylaxis other than early ambulation is recommended. Older patients undergoing major operations without additional risk factors should receive either standard unfractionated heparin, LMWH, or intermittent pneumatic compression. When additional risk factors are present in the latter group, standard heparin every 8 h or LMWH should be administered. Enoxaparin has been approved by the U.S. Food and Drug Administration (FDA) for prophylaxis in patients undergoing elective abdominal surgery (40 mg subcutaneously once daily). A second preparation, dalteparin, has also been approved in the United States for once-daily use as prophylaxis for elective abdominal surgery.

Other High-Risk Patients

Certain orthopedic populations at particularly high risk for acute DVT have been carefully studied with well-designed randomized clinical trials, which led to the approval of enoxaparin by the FDA for prophylaxis against DVT in patients undergoing elective total hip or knee replacement. The approved dosing regimens are 30 mg subcutaneously twice daily initiated within 12 to 24 h after surgery (rarely used) and 40 mg once daily initiated preoperatively (commonly used). The duration of prophylaxis depends upon whether the patient is ambulatory and upon additional risk factors. A large randomized, placebo-controlled clinical trial suggested a lower incidence of DVT with more prolonged (1 month) outpatient prophylaxis in this patient population.[121] LMWHs have also been evaluated in trauma patients at risk for DVT and have proven efficacious in this patient population.[122] Intermittent pneumatic compression should be utilized if anticoagulation prophylaxis is contraindicated. For prophylaxis after total hip or knee replacement, the oral direct thrombin inhibitor ximelagatran appears promising when compared with warfarin[123] or enoxaparin.[124]

MANAGEMENT

Risk Stratification

PE encompasses a wide range of acuity, with varying prognoses and treatment modalities. Therefore risk assessment is paramount in selecting the appropriate management strategy. With therapeutic levels of anticoagulation, most patients will likely have a benign clinical course. Unfortunately, some PE patients suffer rapid clinical deterioration, including death from right ventricular failure or the need for cardiopulmonary resuscitation, mechanical ventilation, administration of pressors for systolic arterial hypotension, rescue thrombolysis, or surgical embolectomy.

Severe dyspnea, cyanosis, and syncope usually indicate life-threatening PE. The clinical examination may show signs of acute right ventricular dysfunction, including tachycardia, a low arterial blood pressure, distended neck veins, an accentuated pulmonic component of the second heart sound, or a tricuspid regurgitation murmur. On the ECG, T-wave inversion and a pseudoinfarction pattern (Qr) in the anterior precordial leads indicate severe right ventricular dilation and dysfunction. Chest CT or MRI may not only confirm PE but also shows significant right ventricular dilatation in some patients.

Modern risk stratification in PE includes (1) the clinical evaluation, (2) ECG, (3) echocardiography, and (4) cardiac biomarkers, including troponins and natriuretic peptides.

CLINICAL EVALUATION

The Geneva Prognostic Index is a predictive model of clinical outcome in PE.[125] This index was used to identify low-risk patients who were managed successfully on a completely outpatient basis. Risk stratification was performed using a clinical score with a maximum of 8 points. The score had to be less than or equal to 2 to qualify the patient for outpatient treatment. The scoring system was as follows: history of cancer (+2), congestive heart failure (+1), DVT (+1), hypoxemia (+1), systolic blood pressure <100 mm Hg (+1), or evidence of DVT by ultrasound (+1). During 3-month follow-up, none of the 43 patients died, and there was no major bleeding. One of the 43 outpatients had an objectively confirmed DVT during follow-up. In conclusion, this study showed that carefully selected PE patients at low risk for right heart failure and recurrent VTE can be treated safely on an entirely outpatient basis.

ECHOCARDIOGRAPHY

Transthoracic echocardiography is the most important tool for risk stratification in PE because right ventricular dysfunction on the echocardiogram is a powerful and independent predictor of mortality.[3] From a prognostic point of view, echocardiography helps to classify PE into three groups: (1) low-risk PE (no right ventricular dysfunction) with a hospital mortality of <4 percent, (2) submassive PE (right ventricular dysfunction and a preserved arterial pressure) with a hospital mortality of 5 to 10 percent, and (3) massive PE (right ventricular dysfunction and cardiogenic shock) with a hospital mortality of approximately 30 percent.[126] A limitation of echocardiography is its limited availability on a 24-h basis 365 days per year as well as its cost. Another problem is occasional poor imaging quality of the right ventricle, particularly in obese patients or those with chronic lung disease.

CARDIAC BIOMARKERS

Cardiac troponins I and T as well as N-terminal pro-brain natriuretic peptide (NT-proBNP) and brain natriuretic peptide (BNP) have emerged as promising tools for risk assessment of patients with acute PE.

Cardiac troponins are the most sensitive and specific markers of myocardial cell damage.[127] Elevations of troponin levels in PE patients are mild and of short duration compared to those in patients with acute coronary syndromes.[129] In acute PE, troponin levels correlate well with the presence of right ventricular dysfunction.[129–131] Some PE patients have initially negative troponin test results but may show a "troponin leak" 6 to 12 h later.[129–131] Myocardial ischemia due to alterations in oxygen supply and demand of the failing right ventricle probably plays a major role in the pathogenesis of troponin release (Fig. 63-7). This is supported by the observation of a troponin

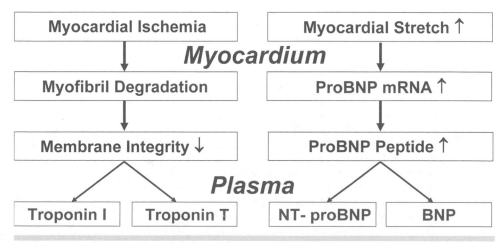

FIGURE 63-7 Mechanism of cardiac biomarker release in patients with acute pulmonary embolism. Right ventricular pressure overload with increased myocardial shear stress are responsible for myocardial synthesis and secretion of natriuretic peptides. Troponin release is due to myocardial ischemia and microinfarction (see also discussion under "Pathophysiology of Acute Pulmonary Embolism, Hemodynamic Alterations").

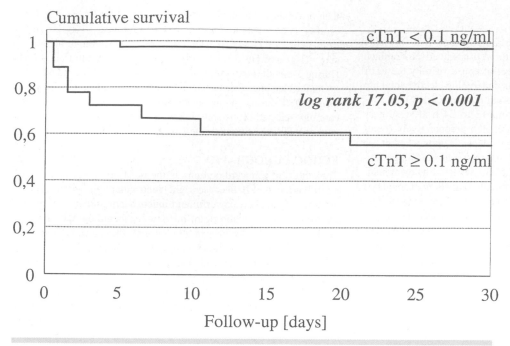

FIGURE 63-8 Cumulative survival rate at 30 days in patients with acute pulmonary embolism according to the level of troponin T. A level > 0.1 ng/mL identifies patients at high risk for adverse clinical outcome. (From Giannitsis et al.[131] With permission.)

leak in patients with severe PE in the absence of angiographic coronary artery disease.[131]

The natriuretic peptides are useful diagnostic and prognostic markers for patients with congestive heart failure. The stimulus for BNP synthesis and secretion is cardiomyocyte stretch (Fig. 63-7). The intact 108–amino acid prohormone (proBNP), the biologically active BNP (32 amino acids, plasma half-life 20 min), and the amino-terminal part of the prohormone NT-proBNP (76 amino acids, plasma half-life 60 to 120 min) can be measured with commercially available assays. Prohormone in normal ventricular myocytes is not stored in a significant amount. Thus it takes a few hours for the levels of plasma natriuretic peptides to increase significantly after the onset of acute cardiomyocyte stretch.[132] This includes synthesis of myocardial BNP messenger ribonucleic acid (mRNA), synthesis of prohormone, and release into the circulation. Elevations in BNP and NT-proBNP are associated with the presence of right ventricular dysfunction in acute PE.[133–135]

Levels of natriuretic peptide are also increased in patients with primary pulmonary hypertension, chronic thromboembolic pulmonary hypertension, and chronic lung disease.[136–139]

Troponins and natriuretic peptides are similarly accurate in identifying low-risk PE patients (Figs. 63-8 and 63-9). The negative predictive value (NPV) for in-hospital death is high for the biomarker assays (Table 63-2). The cutoff levels for troponins are the lower detection limits for myocardial ischemia reported by the manufacturer. The cutoff level for the BNP triage assay to predict a benign clinical outcome in PE patients is lower (<50 pg/mL) than the "congestive heart failure" cutoff level of 90 pg/mL.

At this time, none of the biomarkers have been shown to be superior over others. Keeping in mind that BNP synthesis and release into the circulation is an active process that takes several hours, an initially negative BNP test result in a symptomatic PE patient with a symptom duration <6 h should be interpreted with caution.[134]

At present, elevated cardiac biomarkers alone cannot be recommended to guide treatment decisions. In hemodynamically stable PE patients with increased troponin and/or BNP levels, further risk stratification with echocardiography should be undertaken due to the low specificity of the assays for PE-related right ventricular dysfunction. In patients with biomarker levels below the assay-specific cutoff, echocardiography will not add prognostic information. The prognostic implications of abnormal echocardiography combined with elevated biomarkers require further investigation.

Anticoagulation

When DVT or PE is diagnosed or strongly suspected, anticoagulation therapy should be initiated immediately unless contraindications exist. The diagnosis should be confirmed if anticoagulation is to be continued.

STANDARD UNFRACTIONATED HEPARIN

Standard heparin has been the time-honored parenteral anticoagulant based upon its prompt antithrombotic effect in preventing thrombus growth. The major anticoagulant effect of heparin is accounted for by a unique pentasaccharide with a high-affinity binding sequence to antithrombin III, which is present on only one-third of heparin molecules.[142] The interaction of heparin with antithrombin III markedly accelerates its ability to inactivate thrombin, factor Xa, and factor

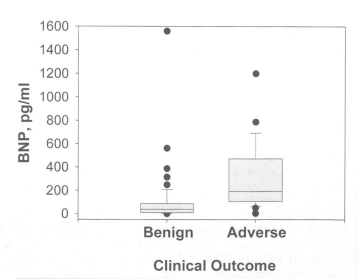

FIGURE 63-9 Brain natriuretic peptide (BNP) levels (median, confidence interval, and outliers) in patients with acute pulmonary embolism according to clinical outcome. Although BNP levels between patients with benign and adverse outcome overlap, the negative predictive value for the absence of adverse outcomes for BNP triage levels < 50 pg/mL was 97 percent. (From Kucher et al.[134] With permission.)

TABLE 63-2 Cardiac Biomarkers and In-Hospital Death in Patients with Pulmonary Embolism

Embolism Biomarker	Assay	Cutoff Level	Test + %	NPV %	PPV %
cTnI	Centaur, Bayer[129]	0.07 ng/mL	41	98	14
cTnT	Elecsys, Roche[129]	0.04 ng/mL	37	97	12
cTnT	TropT, Roche[131]	0.10 ng/mL	32	97	44
cTnT	Elecsys, Roche[140]	0.09 ng/mL	11	99	34
cTnT	Elecsys, Roche[130]	0.01 ng/mL	50	100	25
BNP	Shionoria, CIS[141]	21.7 pmol/L	33	99	17
BNP	Triage, Biosite[134]	50 pg/mL	58	100	12
NT-proBNP	Elecsys, Roche[135]	500 pg/mL	58	100	12

ABBREVIATIONS: NPV = negative predictive value; PPV = positive predictive value; cTnI = cardiac troponin I; cTnT = cardiac troponin T; BNP = brain natriuretic peptide; NT-proBNP = N-terminal pro-brain natriuretic peptide.

IXa. Heparin also catalyzes the inactivation of thrombin by a second plasma cofactor, heparin cofactor II. Heparin does not directly dissolve thrombus, but it allows the fibrinolytic system to act unopposed and more readily reduces the size of the thromboembolic burden.[142] Although thrombus growth can be prevented, early recurrence can develop even during therapeutic anticoagulation. The efficacy of heparin is limited because clot-bound thrombin is protected from heparin-antithrombin III inhibition. Furthermore, heparin resistance can occur because unfractionated heparin binds to plasma proteins.[143] The dose response to intravenous heparin is highly variable. Even when a therapeutic activated partial thromboplastin time (aPTT) between 55 and 85 s is achieved, subsequent consecutive measurements are often not within the desired therapeutic range.[144]

When intravenous standard, unfractionated heparin is instituted, the aPTT should be aggressively followed at 6-h intervals until it is consistently in the therapeutic range of 1.5 to 2.0 times control values.[145] This range corresponds to a heparin level of 0.2 to 0.4 U/mL as measured by protamine sulfate titration. Heparin can be administered by several protocols, but a weight-based approach has been shown to substantially enhance the chances of attaining the therapeutic range quickly. Heparin can be administered as an intravenous bolus of 5000 U followed by a maintenance dose of at least 30,000 U every 24 h by continuous infusion.[146] This aggressive approach decreases the risk of subtherapeutic anticoagulation and, although excessive levels are sometimes achieved initially, bleeding complications do not appear to be increased.[146] An alternative regimen consisting of a bolus of 80 U/kg followed by 18 U/kg/h has been recommended.[147,148] Subsequent adjusting of the heparin dose should also be weight-based (Table 63-3). This approach was recommended by the recent American College of Chest Physicians (ACCP) Consensus Conference on Antithrombotic Therapy.[148] Warfarin therapy may be initiated as soon as the aPTT is therapeutic, and heparin should be maintained until a therapeutic international normalized ratio (INR) of 2.0 to 3.0 has overlapped with a therapeutic aPTT for 2 consecutive days. This initial anticoagulation approach applies to both acute DVT and PE. Although proximal lower extremity thrombus is more likely to result in PE, calf thrombi should still be treated aggressively with anticoagulation or followed with noninvasive testing over 10 to 14 days for extension into the popliteal vein.[149,150]

The spectrum of upper extremity venous thrombosis is variable and includes patients with peripherally and centrally placed intravenous catheters as well as those with underlying malignancy. Symptomatic patients with documented upper extremity DVT should be anticoagulated.[151] Prophylactic anticoagulation in patients with long-term indwelling catheters should also be instituted.[152]

LOW-MOLECULAR-WEIGHT HEPARIN

Mechanisms of Action and Pharmacology Low-molecular-weight heparin (LMWH) is being utilized increasingly for acute VTE. These agents differ in a number of respects from standard, unfractionated heparin (Tables 63-4 and 63-5). A major advantage of these preparations over unfractionated heparin is substantially enhanced bioavailability. Standard heparin consists of lengthy glycosaminoglycan polymers that are heterogenous in size, with a mean molecular mass of approximately 15,000 Da. LMWHs, also glycosaminoglycans, are prepared by chemical or enzymatic depolymerization and are approximately one-third of the size of unfractionated heparin. These

TABLE 63-3 Nomogram for Heparin Therapy in Acute Venous Thromboembolism

The initial heparin dose is 80-U/kg bolus, then 18 U/kg/h.
Subsequent dose modifications, based on aPTT as follows:

aPTT		Heparin Dose Adjustment
Seconds	Times Control	
<35	<1.2	80-U/kg bolus, then increase by 4 U/kg/h
35 to 45	1.2 to 1.5	40-U/kg bolus, then increase by 2 U/kg/h
46 to 70	1.5 to 2.3	No change
71 to 90	2.3 to 3	Decrease infusion rate by 2 U/kg/h
>90	>3	Hold infusion 1 h, then decrease rate by 3 U/kg/h

ABBREVIATION: aPTT = activated partial thromboplastin time.
SOURCE: American College of Chest Physicians Guidelines[148] and Raschke et al.[147]

TABLE 63-4 A Comparison of Low-Molecular-Weight Heparin with Unfractionated Heparin

Characteristic	UFH[a]	LMWH[b]
Mean molecular weight	12,000–15,000	4000–6000
Protein binding	Substantial	Minimal
Anti-Xa activity	Substantial	Substantial
Anti-IIa activity	Substantial	Minimal
Platelet inhibition	Substantial	Minimal
Vascular permeability	Moderate	None
Microvascular permeability	Substantial	Minimal
Elimination (predominant)	Hepatic/macrophages	Renal

[a]Unfractionated heparin.
[b]Low-molecular-weight heparin.

LMWH fractions are also diverse, with a mean molecular mass of 4000 to 5000 Da. The difference in size between unfractionated heparin and LMWH results in an altered anticoagulant profile.[153] Only one-third of the LMWH molecules contain the pentasaccharide required for antithrombin III binding. Maximal inhibition of thrombin requires the binding of heparin to both antithrombin III and the activated enzyme. In contrast, the accelerated inactivation of factor Xa by the heparin/antithrombin III combination requires only the binding of unfractionated heparin to antithrombin III and does not require the formation of the ternary complex. Heparin molecules smaller than 18 saccharide units are unable to bind thrombin and antithrombin III simultaneously, precluding maximal acceleration of the inactivation of thrombin by antithrombin III. These smaller LMWH molecules do, however, retain their ability to catalyze the inhibition of factor Xa by antithrombin III. For this reason, LMWH fractions appear to have relatively more anti-Xa than antithrombin activity and significantly less effect upon the aPTT. While the ratio of anti-Xa to antithrombin of unfractionated heparin is 1:1, the LMWH preparations have significantly higher ratios. In addition, other anticoagulant properties such as stimulation of tissue factor pathway–inhibitor release appear to be responsible for the effect of these agents, suggesting more reason for variability among them.[153]

While the different preparation methods result in products with similar molecular profiles, structural variations remain, which impart significant differences in their biological actions. Chemical modifications of various portions of the molecules, charge density, and the

TABLE 63-5 Potential Advantages of Low-Molecular-Weight Heparins over Unfractionated Heparin

Efficacy: Comparable or superior[a]
Safety: Comparable or superior[b]
Bioavailability: Superior
Subcutaneous administration
Once- or twice-daily dosing
No laboratory monitoring[c]
Less phlebotomy
Earlier ambulation
Home therapy in certain patient subsets

[a]Based upon objectively documented recurrence rates in clinical trials.
[b]Based upon rates of major and minor bleeding in clinical trials.
[c]In certain patient populations (significant obesity, renal insufficiency), monitoring has been suggested.

degree of desulfation all affect the characteristics of the final product. Because of these differences, antithrombin III activity, the effects on tissue-factor-pathway inhibitor, platelet factor 4, and heparin cofactor II would be expected to differ for the various LMWH preparations. There may be other potential differences with respect to stimulation of the release of tissue plasminogen activator and prostacyclin.

Clinical Trials and Indications Numerous clinical trials have demonstrated the efficacy and safety of LMWH for treatment of acute proximal DVT, using recurrent symptomatic VTE as the primary outcome measure.[154–160] Treatment with LMWH is more convenient for the patient and the nursing staff for several reasons. A continuous intravenous line is not required, as these agents can be administered once or twice per day subcutaneously at fixed therapeutic doses, usually without laboratory monitoring.

In certain settings, therapy can be monitored by measuring anti-Xa levels. A therapeutic anticoagulant level is achieved in the range of approximately 0.5 to 1.0 units/mL for the HEPRN pack (Dupont) assay. This is a chromogenic assay based on the inhibition of factor Xa by heparin-activated antithrombin III. The peak level is reached 3 to 6 h after subcutaneous injection. Prophylactic doses of LMWH usually result in anti-Xa levels of 0.1 to 0.3 U/mL. The peak anti-Xa level is useful in monitoring (1) heparin therapy with baseline elevated aPTTs due to a antiphospholipid antibodies, (2) LMWH dosing in obese patients, (3) LMWH dosing in patients with renal dysfunction, (4) pregnancy, and (5) for the etiology of an unexpected bleeding or clotting event while the patient is on heparin or LMWH.

In two large, randomized (Canadian and European) trials, therapy with LMWH was compared with that using standard weight-based unfractionated heparin.[154,155] The LMWH patients were treated entirely as outpatients or continued at home after a brief hospitalization. The outpatient LMWH regimens proved safe and effective. Three metanalyses examined the use of LMWH compared with unfractionated heparin in the initial treatment of acute proximal DVT.[161–163] Although there was overlap among the clinical trials included in the analyses, they have helped to confirm the efficacy and safety of LMWH for the treatment of established DVT. At the present time, only one LMWH (enoxaparin) is FDA-approved for use in the United States for treatment of established DVT in the outpatient setting or for DVT (with or without PE) in the inpatient setting. Unlike the regimen for prophylaxis, in which a fixed dose of enoxaparin is utilized, a weight-based dosing regimen is employed for treatment of established VTE. For outpatient and inpatient therapy, the FDA has approved a dosing regimen of 1 mg/kg subcutaneously every 12 h. For inpatient treatment, the FDA has also approved use of 1.5 mg/kg of enoxaparin once every 24 h. In addition to being more convenient, the LMWH preparations appear to be cost-effective, particularly when outpatient therapy is utilized.[120] Some of the different LMWH products and their prophylaxis and treatment regimens are listed in Table 63-6.

In patients with symptomatic PE, LMWH appears at least as effective as intravenous unfractionated heparin as a "bridge" to warfarin.[165] Extended 3-month treatment with enoxaparin as monotherapy without warfarin for symptomatic acute PE is feasible and shortens the duration of hospitalization compared with that of patients receiving standard treatment.[166]

COMPLICATIONS OF HEPARIN

Heparin-Induced Thrombocytopenia
Heparin-induced thrombocytopenia (HIT) typically develops 5 or more days after the initiation of heparin therapy and occurs in 5 to 10 percent of patients.[167–169] If a patient is placed on heparin for VTE and the platelet count progressively decreases either by 50 percent or to 100,000/mm^3 or less, heparin therapy should be discontinued. Although the risk of HIT appears to be lower with LMWH, it is important for clinicians to realize that HIT can occur with the use of either form of heparin.[170]

Over the past decade, there have been many important advances in the pathogenesis, diagnosis, and treatment of HIT, which represents one of the most common immune-mediated adverse drug reactions.[171] This entity is caused by heparin-dependent IgG antibodies that recognize complexes of heparin and platelet factor 4, leading to activation of platelets via platelet Fc gamma IIa receptors. Formation of procoagulant, platelet-derived microparticles, and possibly activation of endothelium generate thrombin in vivo. The generation of thrombin helps to account for the strong association between HIT and thrombosis, including the syndrome of warfarin-induced venous limb gangrene. This syndrome develops during warfarin treatment of HIT and DVT when acquired protein C deficiency leads to the inability to regulate thrombin generation in the microvasculature.

Both argatroban and lepirudin are FDA approved for management of heparin-induced thrombocytopenia. Argatroban, metabolized by the liver, is optimal for patients with renal dysfunction. Lepirudin, metabolized by the kidneys, is preferred in patients with hepatic dysfunction. However, these direct thrombin inhibitors can cause major bleeding and there is no antidote. Alternative therapies that can be considered for off-label use are the direct thrombin inhibitor bivalirudin[172] and the pentasaccharide fondaparinux.[173]

OTHER ADVERSE EFFECTS OF HEPARIN Prolonged administration of unfractionated heparin may cause asymptomatic osteopenia, osteoporosis, and rarely pathologic bone fractures. After discontinuation of heparin, bone metabolism by densitometry usually improves within a year. LMWHs should not be given for at least 12 h prior to placement of an epidural catheter due to the risk of epidural or spinal hematoma, which can cause permanent paraplegia.

WARFARIN
The vitamin K antagonist warfarin sodium inhibits gamma carboxylation activation of coagulation factors II, VII, IX, and X as well as proteins C and S. The full anticoagulant effect of warfarin may take up to several days even if the INR is in the intended therapeutic range. Elevation in the prothrombin time may initially reflect depletion of coagulation factor VII, which has a half-life of about 6 h, whereas factor II has a half-life of about 5 days.

Warfarin is a difficult drug to dose and monitor, and it has multiple drug-drug and drug-food interactions. Quinolone antibiotics and

TABLE 63-6 Doses of Low-Molecular-Weight Heparin for Prevention and Treatment of Venous Thromboembolism

LMWH	Prevention	Treatment
Enoxaparin	30 mg q12h or 40 mg qd	1 mg/kg bid, 1.5 mg/kg qd^a
Dalteparin	2500 to 5000 Xa U qd	200 Xa U/kg qd
Tinzaparin	75 Xa U/kg qd	175 Xa U/kg qd
Nadroparin	41 to 62 U/kg qd	<50 kg 4100 Xa U q12h
		50 to 75 kg 6150 Xa U q12h
		>70 kg 9200 Xa U q12h
Reviparin	4200 Xa U qd	35 to 45 kg 3500 Xa U q12h
		46 to 60 kg 4200 Xa U q12h
		>60 kg 6300 Xa U q12h
Ardeparin	50 Xa U/kg q12h	Not evaluated

^{a}Enoxaparin is the only LMWH approved for use in the United States for established DVT. It is indicated in patients who present with DVT (with or without concomitant PE). A dose of either 1.5 mg/kg or 1 mg/kg q12h has proven effective for inpatients with DVT +/− PE. Outpatient studies have been with 1 mg/kg q12h. It would appear highly likely that the once-daily dose would be adequate for outpatients, particularly since these patients tend to be stable and *may* have smaller thrombotic burdens.

amiodarone, often concomitantly used with warfarin, may cause a marked increase in the INR. High doses of acetaminophen also increase the INR.[174] Vitamin K–containing green vegetables lower the INR.

Warfarin therapy should be initiated with concomitant unfractionated heparin or LMWH. Otherwise the first few days of warfarin administration may lead to a paradoxical prothrombotic state due to rapid depletion of proteins C and S. The procoagulant effect of warfarin can be inhibited by overlapping heparin with warfarin for at least 5 days.

The initial dose should ordinarily be approximately 5 mg, and it should be lowered for debilitated and elderly patients.[175,176] A few patients have extremely low daily warfarin dose requirements of 1 to 2 mg, with an increased bleeding risk due to CYP2C9 variant alleles.[177]

In carefully selected patients, self-management of warfarin therapy using INR measurement with "point of care" devices may be effective and safe.[178]

Adverse Effects of Warfarin
Warfarin has a narrow therapeutic window, and the risk of bleeding increases with increasing INR. A large retrospective survey of more than 42,000 patients taking vitamin K antagonists suggested that an INR of 2.2 to 2.3 has the highest benefit-risk ratio.[179] In this study, a twofold increase in the hazard of mortality per unit INR elevation greater than 2.5 was observed. Risk factors for warfarin-related bleeding include hepatic disease, renal dysfunction, alcoholism, drug interactions, trauma, cancer, and history of gastrointestinal bleeding. The risk of bleeding is greatest in the first month after initiation of anticoagulation.[180]

Major bleeding can routinely be treated with vitamin K, cryoprecipitate, or fresh-frozen plasma. In patients with excessive INR values without bleeding, withholding one or two doses of warfarin with administration of oral vitamin K 2.5 mg is an effective strategy.

Rare complications of warfarin are skin necrosis and cholesterol microembolization, causing the "purple toes" syndrome by enhancing crystal release from ulcerated plaques.[181]

Reliable contraception is mandatory in women of childbearing potential because warfarin is teratogenic, particularly during weeks 6 to 12 of gestation.[182]

OPTIMAL DURATION AND INTENSITY OF ANTICOAGULATION

VTE should be treated for at least 3 months with oral warfarin, keeping the INR at 2.0 to 3.0. Individuals unable to take warfarin can be treated with 3-month LMWH monotherapy.

Several trials have established that patients with idiopathic VTE benefit from extended anticoagulation.[183–186] The optimal intensity and duration were controversial until the results of the PREVENT trial were published.[187] This double-blind, randomized, controlled study showed that indefinite-duration anticoagulation can be administered safely and effectively with a low-intensity target INR of 1.5 to 2.0 after completion of 6-month full-intensity anticoagulation. The incidence of PE and DVT was reduced by two-thirds, and patients required INR testing only once every 8 weeks.[187] In PREVENT, the strategy of long-term, low-intensity warfarin was highly effective in preventing recurrence in all subgroups, even in patients with factor V Leiden or the prothrombin gene mutation. In conclusion, we recommend 6 months of full-intensity anticoagulation followed by indefinite-duration, low-intensity anticoagulation for patients with idiopathic VTE—i.e., in the absence of surgery/trauma within 90 days, metastatic cancer, gastrointestinal bleeding, hemorrhagic stroke, or antiphospholipid antibodies.

Ximelagatran, an oral fixed-dose direct thrombin inhibitor, appears to be promising for long-term anticoagulation in patients with idiopathic VTE. In the THRIVE-3 study,[188] 1233 patients with idiopathic VTE were randomized after completing 6 months of full-intensity warfarin anticoagulation to treatment with ximelagatran (24 mg twice daily) or placebo. Ximelagatran group patients had 85 percent fewer VTE recurrent events without increase in major bleeding. The principal advantage of ximelagatran is that there is no monitoring of coagulation parameters required. However, in a large-scale trial of anticoagulation in patients with chronic atrial fibrillation, ximelagatran caused asymptomatic increases in liver function tests in about 6 percent of patients.

Vena Cava Interruption

In patients with established VTE in whom heparin therapy cannot be continued, inferior vena cava (IVC) filter placement can be undertaken to prevent lower extremity thrombi from embolizing to the lungs. The essential indications for filter placement include contraindications to anticoagulation, recurrent embolism while on adequate therapy, and significant bleeding complications during anticoagulation.[189] Filters are sometimes placed in the setting of massive PE when it is believed that any further emboli might be lethal.[189]

Patients with filters after a VTE event are more than twice as likely as non-filter patients to require rehospitalization for DVT.[190] Thus, anticoagulation is generally continued when a filter is placed unless it is contraindicated. A number of filter devices exist, but the Greenfield filter design has been most widely used. These devices can be inserted via the jugular or femoral vein and are effective. Possible mechanisms of IVC filter failure include filter migration; improper filter positioning; allowing thrombi to bypass the filter; and formation of thrombosis proximal to the filter or on the proximal tip of the filter with subsequent embolization. Rare complications include clinically significant perforation of the IVC, migration to the heart, and displacement of the filter during insertion. Rarely, these devices may erode into the wall of the IVC. Occasionally, IVC obstruction due to thrombosis at the filter site may occur. Deaths due to filter placement are extraordinarily uncommon. Temporary filters have been placed in individuals deemed at extremely high risk for DVT yet unable to receive anticoagulant prophylaxis, such as certain trauma patients.[191] Retrievable filters can be removed within 2 weeks after placement or can remain permanently if necessary because of a trapped large thrombus or a persistent contraindication to anticoagulation.[192]

Thrombolytic Therapy

SYSTEMIC THROMBOLYSIS

Thrombolysis is standard therapy in patients with massive PE and cardiogenic shock. In the largest thrombolysis study (MAPPET-3),[85] it was shown that thrombolysis with alteplase is also effective in patients with submassive PE—i.e., in the presence of preserved arterial pressure and evidence of right ventricular dysfunction. Compared to therapy with heparin alone, thrombolysis significantly reduced adverse clinical outcomes, including the need for cardiopulmonary resuscitation, mechanical ventilation, administration of pressors, secondary "rescue" thrombolysis, or surgical embolectomy. There was no significant increase of major bleeding with alteplase in these carefully selected PE patients. Nevertheless, the use of thrombolysis in any patient with preserved systemic arterial pressure is somewhat controversial in the United States.

Thrombolysis may prevent the development of right ventricular failure by dissolution of pulmonary arterial thrombi and the continued release of neurohumoral factors that might otherwise lead to chronic pulmonary hypertension. Thrombolysis may also dissolve much of the source of the residual thrombus in the deep veins, thereby minimizing the likelihood of recurrent PE. In patients with acute PE, thrombolysis is effective up to 2 weeks after the onset of symptoms.[193]

There are only 10 randomized PE trials of thrombolysis versus heparin to date, with a total of 717 patients with varying severity of PE.[62,74,85,194–200] In an overview, there is a trend toward mortality reduction with thrombolysis (Table 63-7).

TABLE 63-7 Relative Risk of In-Hospital Death for Thrombolysis versus Heparin Alone in the Pulmonary Embolism Trials

Study	HEPARIN/THROMBOLYSIS		
	n/n	Mortality (n/n)	Relative Risk (95% CI)
UPET, 1973[62]	78/82	7/6	0.82 (0.29–2.32)
Tibbutt, 1974[199]	17/13	1/0	0.43 (0.02–9.74)
Ly, 1978[200]	11/14	2/1	0.39 (0.04–3.79)
Marini, 1988[194]	10/20	0/0	—
PIOPED, 1990[74]	4/9	0/1	1.50 (0.07–30.59)
Levine, 1990[195]	25/33	0/1	2.29 (0.10–54.05)
PAIMS 2, 1992[197]	16/20	1/2	1.60 (0.16–16.10)
Goldhaber, 1993[198]	55/46	2/0	0.24 (0.01–4.84)
Jerjes-Sanchez, 1995[196]	4/4	4/0	0.11 (0.01–1.57)
MAPPET-3, 2002[85]	138/118	3/4t	1.56 (0.36–6.83)
Metanalysis	358/359	20/15	0.75 (0.39–1.44)

TABLE 63-8 Regimens for Systemic Thrombolytic Therapy in Pulmonary Embolism

Lytic Agent	Dose regimen
Streptokinase	Loading dose: 250,000 U IV Continuous infusion: 100,000 U/h for 24 h
Urokinase	Loading dose: 2000 U/lb IV over 10 min Continuous infusion: 2000 U/lb/h for 12–24 h
Alteplase (t-PA)	Loading dose: none Continuous infusion: 100 mg over 2 h
Reteplase	1. Bolus: 10 U IV 2. Bolus: 10 U IV after 30 min

None of the thrombolytic agents have been shown to be superior to others. The only contemporary FDA-approved thrombolytic regimen is a continuous intravenous infusion of 100 mg alteplase over 2 h. Other available thrombolytic regimens for the treatment of PE are presented in Table 63-8.

The major complication resulting from thrombolytic therapy is bleeding. The potential benefit of PE thrombolysis must be weighed against the increased risk of major hemorrhage. In an overview, there is a twofold increase in the hazard of major hemorrhage with thrombolysis in comparison to treatment with heparin alone (Table 63-9). There is a 1 to 2 percent risk of intracranial hemorrhage.[201] Therefore, low-risk PE patients with a normal arterial pressure without right ventricular dysfunction should not be treated with thrombolysis because the risk of bleeding exceeds the expected benefits from pulmonary artery reperfusion. Absolute and relative contraindications to thrombolysis are listed in The Task Force on Pulmonary Embolism Guidelines from the European Society of Cardiology.[126]

Heparin should be withheld until the thrombolytic infusion is completed. The aPTT is then determined and heparin is initiated without a loading dose if this value is less than twice the upper limit of normal. If the aPTT exceeds this value, the test is repeated every 4 h until it is safe to proceed with heparin.

The use of thrombolytic therapy for DVT without PE is even more controversial than its use in patients with symptomatic PE. Thrombolysis may be associated with a reduction in post-phlebitic syndrome when used for acute DVT, but at the cost of an increased risk of bleeding.[202] It is reasonable to consider systemic thrombolytic therapy in patients with proximal occlusive DVT associated with significant swelling and symptoms when there are no contraindications.

LOCAL THROMBOLYSIS

For acute PE, the peripheral intravenous route is the primary method of drug delivery. A number of investigators have employed standard or low-dose intrapulmonary arterial thrombolytic infusions in order to deliver a high concentration of drug in close proximity to the clot.[203–205]

Intraembolic thrombolytic infusions may offer advantages over merely infusing the agents into the pulmonary artery. Such techniques have been applied in both animal models of PE and in patients, with enhanced thrombolysis.[206,207] Lower than conventional doses of t-PA or urokinase are delivered via a catheter imbedded directly within massive emboli over 10 to 20 min.[206,207] Combining thrombolytic therapy via direct delivery (at low doses) with the possible mechanical benefits of direct intraembolic infusion could prove advantageous over the intravenous route, particularly in the setting of contraindications to thrombolytic therapy.

Catheter Fragmentation And Embolectomy

Interventional thrombus fragmentation with or without embolectomy is an alternative to systemic thrombolysis or surgical embolectomy. If the bleeding risk it not exceedingly high, catheter fragmentation may be combined with local or systemic thrombolysis.

An ideal catheter for PE has not yet been developed.[208] Several fragmentation and embolectomy devices have been tested in patients with massive PE (Table 63-10).[209–212] Most of the devices appear to be effective, safe, and potentially life-saving in the presence of large "fresh" clots. However, none of the devices has been investigated in a large controlled trial, and all commercially available devices have important limitations.

Catheter-directed techniques have been successfully employed in the setting of acute iliofemoral DVT utilizing doses of urokinase ranging from 1.4 to 16 million U delivered over an average of 30 h.[213,214] Results from a national registry of patients with iliofemoral thrombosis treated with local, catheter-directed therapy indicates that this approach is frequently successful.[214]

Surgical Embolectomy

Emergency pulmonary embolectomy with cardiopulmonary bypass is an effective method in patients with acute massive PE in the presence of (1) a high bleeding risk, (2) right heart thrombi, and (3) an atrial septal defect or patent foramen ovale with the risk of systemic (paradoxical) embolism.

TABLE 63-9 Relative Risk of Major Bleeding for Thrombolysis versus Heparin alone in the Pulmonary Embolism Trials

Study	HEPARIN/THROMBOLYSIS		
	n/n	Major Bleeding (n/n)	Relative Risk (95% CI)
UPET, 1973[62]	78/82	11/22	1.90 (0.99–3.66)
Tibbutt, 1974[199]	17/13	1/1	1.31 (0.09–19.0)
Ly, 1978[200]	11/14	2/4	1.57 (0.35–7.06)
Marini, 1988[194]	10/20	0/0	—
PIOPED, 1990[74]	4/9	0/1	1.50 (0.07–30.59)
Levine, 1990[195]	25/33	0/0	—
PAIMS 2, 1992[197]	16/20	2/3	1.20 (0.23–6.34)
Goldhaber, 1993[198]	55/46	1/2	2.39 (0.22–25.54)
Jerjes-Sanchez, 1995[196]	4/4	0/0	—
MAPPET-3, 2002[85]	138/118	1/5	5.85 (0.69–49.35)
Metanalysis	358/359	18/38	2.11 (1.23–3.62)

TABLE 63-10 Catheter Fragmentation and Embolectomy Devices for Pulmonary Embolism

Device	Mechanism	Risk / Disadvantage
Greenfield catheter[209]	Suction embolectomy	Ineffective for older clots
Pigtail catheter[210]	Fragmentation via pigtail catheter rotation	Distal macroembolization
Amplatz device[211] ("clot buster")	Clot maceration via high-speed impeller rotation	Distal microembolization, hemolysis
Angioget[212]	Embolectomy via high-pressure saline injection (Venturi effect)	Ineffective for older clots
Hydrolyzer[213]	Embolectomy via rheolytic effect	Ineffective for older clots

In one case series of 71 embolectomies performed for acute PE using cardiopulmonary bypass, hospital mortality was 29 percent.[215] However, the mortality in those patients who had not sustained a cardiac arrest preoperatively was only 11 percent. In another cohort study of 29 patients with massive PE undergoing emergency embolectomy without aortic cross-clamping on a warm beating heart, total mortality was 11 percent (Fig. 63-10).[216]

Supportive Measures

When massive PE associated with hypotension and/or severe hypoxemia is suspected, supportive treatment is immediately initiated. Intravenous saline can be rapidly infused, but caution is recommended because right ventricular function is often markedly compromised. Dopamine or norepinephrine appear to be the favored choices of vasoactive therapy in massive PE and should be administered if the blood pressure is not rapidly restored.[217] Death from massive PE results from right ventricular failure, and dobutamine has been recommended by some as a means by which to augment right ventricular output.[218,219] A vasopressor such as norepinephrine combined with dobutamine might offer optimal results. Intubation and mechanical ventilation are instituted to manage respiratory failure.

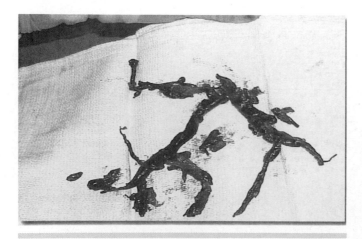

FIGURE 63-10 Extensive clot was removed from a 58-year-old patient with massive pulmonary embolism and shock who had a benign clinical course following emergency embolectomy on cardiopulmonary bypass.

CHRONIC THROMBOEMBOLIC PULMONARY HYPERTENSION

In a few patients with acute PE, the residual thromboembolic burden becomes extensive and causes thromboembolic pulmonary hypertension.[220,221] At least 50 percent of patients who develop chronic thromboembolic pulmonary hypertension have no documented history of DVT or PE, and this feature greatly impedes the diagnosis. Most patients have no identifiable coagulopathy. Dyspnea with exertion and fatigue are the most common complaints. The nonspecific nature of these findings may substantially delay the correct diagnosis. The physical examination generally reveals a right ventricular heave, a loud P_2, a right ventricular S_3, and tricuspid regurgitation consistent with pulmonary hypertension. In 20 percent of patients, one or more murmurs may be auscultated over the lung fields.

The chest radiograph usually reveals right ventricular enlargement and enlarged main pulmonary arteries. ECG changes are consistent with pulmonary hypertension. Arterial blood gases generally reveal hypoxemia with a widened A-a gradient, although some patients may demonstrate only exercise-induced hypoxemia. Echocardiography documents pulmonary hypertension as well as right ventricular dilation and dysfunction. Chest CT will usually demonstrate chronic thrombi and may reveal other rare causes of pulmonary hypertension, such as mediastinal fibrosis. With chronic thromboembolic pulmonary hypertension, the ventilation/perfusion scan nearly always indicates a high probability of PE, but occasionally it is less impressive. Right heart catheterization and pulmonary arteriography are performed both to establish the diagnosis with certainty and to determine operability. Although anticoagulation should be instituted and IVC filters are recommended in patients with chronic thromboembolic pulmonary hypertension, the only means by which to alleviate symptoms and improve survival is with surgery. The University of California at San Diego has been the leading center for the evaluation and surgical therapy of chronic thromboembolic hypertension in more than 2000 patients.[222] Optimal candidates for surgery are patients with New York Heart Association class II and III symptoms.

Pulmonary thromboendarterectomy is performed via median sternotomy on cardiopulmonary bypass in deep hypothermia with circulatory arrest periods, and the overall mortality, which has continued to improve, is now less than 5 percent. Repeated balloon angioplasty of the pulmonary arteries (Fig. 63-11) may be considered in patients who are not candidates for surgery.[223] Lung transplantation is rarely performed but can be considered in patients in whom thrombi are too distal to extract.

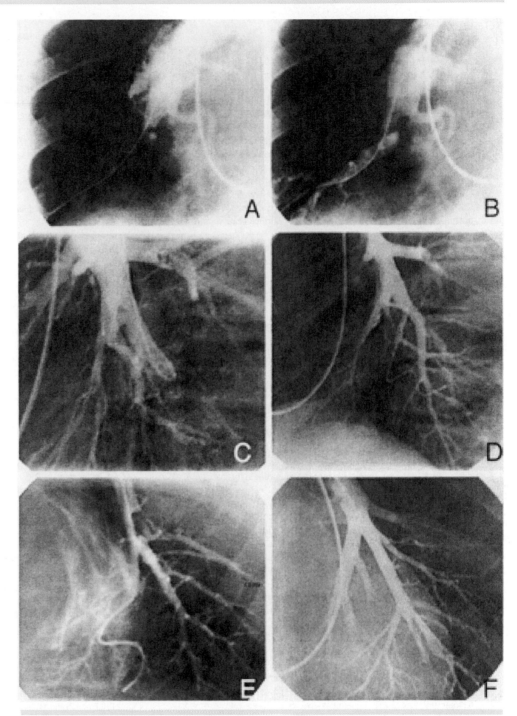

FIGURE 63-11 Percutaneous balloon pulmonary angioplasty (BPA) as an alternative to surgical embolectomy for patients with chronic thromboembolic pulmonary hypertension. Angiographic appearance of occluded (*A, C*) and stenotic (*E*) lower lobe pulmonary artery segmental branches. They are horizontally paired with angiograms performed immediately after successful BPA (*B, D,* and *F*). (From Feinstein et al.[223] With permission.)

References

1. Anderson FA, Wheeler HB. Venous thromboembolism: Risk factors and prophylaxis. *Clin Chest Med* 1995;16:235–251.

2. Dalen JE, Alpert JS. Natural history of pulmonary embolism. *Prog Cardiovasc Dis* 1975;17:257–270.

3. Goldhaber SZ, Visani L, De Rosa M. Acute pulmonary embolism: Clinical outcomes in the International Cooperative Pulmonary Embolism Registry (ICOPER). *Lancet* 1999;353:1386–1389.

4. Lindblad B, Eriksson A, Bergquist D. Autopsy-verified pulmonary embolism in a surgical department: Analysis of the period from 1951 to 1988. *Br J Surg* 1991;78:849–852.

5. Cotton LT, Clark C. Anatomical localization of venous thrombosis. *Ann R Coll Surg Engl* 1965;36:214–224.

6. Goldhaber SZ, Tapson VF, for the DVT FREE Steering Committee. A prospective registry of 5451 patients with confirmed deep vein thrombosis. *Am J Cardiol* 2004. In press.

7. Lamb GC, Tomski MH, Kaufman J, et al. Is chronic spinal cord injury associated with increased risk of venous thromboembolism? *J Am Paraplegia Soc* 1993;16:153–156.

8. Lapostolle F, Surget V, Borron SW, et al. Severe pulmonary embolism associated with air travel. *N Engl J Med* 2001;345:779–783.

9. Flegal KM, Carroll MD, Ogden CL, et al. Prevalence and trends in obesity among US adults, 1999–2000. *JAMA* 2002;288:1723–1727.

10. Freedman DS, Khan LK, Serdula MK, et al. Trends and correlates of class 3 obesity in the United States from 1990 through 2000. *JAMA* 2002;288:1758–1761.

11. Goldhaber SZ, Grodstein F, Stampfer MJ, et al. A prospective study of risk factors for pulmonary embolism in women. *JAMA* 1997;277:642–645.

12. Goldhaber SZ, Savage DD, Garrison RJ, et al. Risk factors for pulmonary embolism. The Framingham Study. *Am J Med* 1983;74:1023–1028.

13. Primrose JN, Davies JA, Prentice CR, et al. Reduction in factor VII, fibrinogen and plasminogen activator inhibitor-1 activity after surgical treatment of morbid obesity. *Thromb Haemost* 1992;68:396–399.

14. Sundell IB, Nilsson TK, Ranby M, et al. Fibrinolytic variables are related to age, sex, blood pressure, and body build measurements: a cross-sectional study in Norsjo, Sweden. *J Clin Epidemiol* 1989;42:719–723.

15. Landin K, Stigendal L, Eriksson E, et al. Abdominal obesity is associated with an impaired fibrinolytic activity and elevated plasminogen activator inhibitor-1. *Metabolism* 1990;39:1044–1048.

16. Davi G, Guagnano MT, Ciabattoni G, et al. Platelet activation in obese women: role of inflammation and oxidant stress. *JAMA* 2002;288:2008–2014.

17. Carson JL, Kelley MA, Duffy A, et al. The clinical course of pulmonary embolism. *N Engl J Med* 1992;326:1240–1245.

18. Goldhaber SZ, Hennekens CH, Evans DA, et al. Factors associated with correct antemortem diagnosis of major pulmonary embolism. *Am J Med* 1982;73:822–826.

19. Kakkar VV, Howe CT, Nicolaides AN, et al. Deep vein thrombosis of the legs: Is there a "high risk" group? *Am J Surg* 1970;120:527–530.

20. Clagett GP, Reisch JS. Prevention of venous thromboembolism in general surgical patients: Results of a meta-analysis. *Ann Surg* 1988;208:227–240.

21. Clagett GP, Anderson FA Jr, Geerts W, et al. Prevention of venous thromboembolism. *Chest* 1998;114:531S–560S.

22. Fisher M, Michele A, McCann W. Thrombophlebitis and pulmonary infarction associated with fractured hip. *Clin Res* 1963;11:407.

23. Fitts WT Jr, Lehr HB, Bitner RL, et al. An analysis of 950 fatal injuries. *Surgery* 1964;56:663–668.

24. Coon WW. Risk factors in pulmonary embolism. *Surg Gynecol Obstet* 1976;143:385–390.

25. Joffe HV, Goldhaber SZ. Upper-extremity deep vein thrombosis. *Circulation* 2002;106:1874–1880.

26. Haire WD. Arm vein thrombosis. *Clin Chest Med* 1995;16:341.

27. Handley AJ, Emerson PA, Fleming PR. Heparin in the prevention of deep vein thrombosis after myocardial infarction. *Br Med J* 1972;2:436–438.

28. Gruppo Italiano per lo Studio della Streptochinasi nell'Infarto Miocardico (GISSI). Effectiveness of intravenous thrombolytic treatment in acute myocardial infarction. *Lancet* 1986;1:397–402.

29. ISIS-2 Collaborative Group. Randomized trial of IV streptokinase, oral aspirin, both or neither among 17,187 cases of suspected acute myocardial infarction. *Lancet* 1988;2:349–360.

30. Rickles FR, Levine MN, Edwards RL. Hemostatic alterations in cancer patients. *Cancer Met Rev* 1992;11:291–311.

31. Carroll VA, Binder BR. The role of the plasminogen activation system in cancer. *Semin Thromb Hemostas* 1999;25:183–198.

32. Lee AYY, Levine MN. The thrombophilic state induced by therapeutic agents in the cancer patient. *Semin Thromb Hemost* 1999;25:137–146.

33. Sorensen HT, Mellemkjaer L, Steffensen FH, et al. The risk of a diagnosis of cancer after primary deep venous thrombosis or pulmonary embolism. *N Engl J Med* 1993;38:1169–1173.

34. Toglia MR, Weg JG. Current concepts: Venous thromboembolism during pregnancy. *N Engl J Med* 1996;335:108–114.

35. Stadel BV. Oral contraceptives and cardiovascular disease. *N Engl J Med* 1981;305:672–677.

36. Weiss N. Third-generation oral contraceptives: How risky? *Lancet* 1995;346:1570.

37. World Health Organization Collaborative Study of Cardiovascular Disease and Steroid Hormone Contraception. Venous thromboembolic disease and combined oral contraceptives: Results of international multicentre case-control study. *Lancet* 1995;346:1575–1582.

38. Daly E, Vessey MP, Hawkins MM, et al. Risk of venous thromboembolism in users of hormone replacement therapy. *Lancet* 1996;348:977–980.

39. Jick H, Derby LE, Wald Myers M, et al. Risk of hospital admission for idiopathic venous thromboembolism among users of postmenopausal estrogens. *Lancet* 1996;348:981–983.

40. Grodstein F, Stampfer MJ, Goldhaber SZ, et al. Prospective study of exogenous hormones and risk of pulmonary embolism in women. *Lancet* 1996;348:983–987.

41. Ridker PM, Hennekens CH, Lindpainter K, et al. Mutation in the gene coding for coagulation factor V and the risk of myocardial infarction, stroke, and venous thrombosis in apparently healthy men. *N Engl J Med* 1995;332:912.

42. Ridker PM, Miletich JP, Buring JE, et al: Factor V Leiden as a risk factor for recurrent pregnancy loss. *Ann Intern Med* 1998;128:1000.

43. Vandenbroucke JP, Rosing J, Bloemenkamp KW, et al. Oral contraceptives and the risk of venous thrombosis. *N Engl J Med* 2001;344:1527–1535.

44. Poort SR, Rosendaal FR, Reitsma PH, et al. A common genetic variation in the 3'-untranslated region of the prothrombin gene is associated with elevated plasma prothrombin levels and an increase in venous thrombosis. *Blood* 1996;88:3698–3703.

45. Hillarp A, Zoller B, Svensson PJ, Dahlback B. The 20210A of the prothrombin gene is a common risk factor among Swedish outpatients with verified deep venous thrombosis. *Thromb Haemost* 1997;78:990–992.

46. DeStefano V, Martinelli I, Mannucci PM, et al. The risk of recurrent deep venous thrombosis among heterozygous carriers of both factor V Leiden and the G20210A prothrombin mutation. *N Engl J Med* 1999;341:801–806.

47. D'Angelo A, Selhub J. Homocysteine and thrombotic disease. *Blood* 1997;90:1–11.

48. Ridker PM, Hennekens CH, Selhub J, et al. Interrelation of hyperhomocysteinemia, factor V Leiden, and risk of future venous thromboembolism. *Circulation* 1997;95:1777–1782.

49. Benotti JR, Dalen JE. The natural history of pulmonary embolism. *Clin Chest Med* 1984;5:403.

50. McIntyre KM, Sasahara AA. The ratio of pulmonary artery pressure to pulmonary vascular obstruction. *Chest* 1997;71:692.

51. Wells PS, Anderson DR, Rodger M, et al. Derivation of a simple clinical model to categorize patients' probability of pulmonary embolism: Increasing the models utility with the SimpliRED D-dimer. *Thromb Haemost* 2000;83:416–420.

52. Bounameaux H, Cirafici P, DeMoerloose P, et al. Measurement of D-dimer in plasma as diagnostic aid in suspected pulmonary embolism. *Lancet* 1991;337:196.

53. Rowbotham BJ, Egerton-Vernon J, Whitaker AN, et al. Plasma cross-linked fibrin degradation products in pulmonary embolism. *Thorax* 1990;45:684–687.

54. Becker DM, Philbrick JT, Bachhuber TL, Humphries JE. D-Dimer testing and acute venous thromboembolism: A shortcut to accurate diagnosis? *Arch Intern Med* 1996;156:939–946.

55. Moser KM. Diagnosing pulmonary embolism: D-dimer needs rigorous evaluation. *Br Med J* 1994;309:1525–1526.

56. Knecht MF, Heinrich F. Clinical evaluation of an immunoturbidimetric D-dimer assay in the diagnostic procedure of deep vein thrombosis and pulmonary embolism. *Thromb Res* 1997;88:413–417.

57. Kucher N, Doernhoefer T, Wallmann D, et al. Accuracy of D-dimer/fibrinogen ratio to predict pulmonary embolism: a prospective diagnostic study. *J Thromb Haemost* 2003;1:708–713.

58. Green RM, Meyer TJ, Dunn M, Glassroth J. Pulmonary embolism in younger adults. *Chest* 1992;101:1507–1511.

59. Stein PD, Terrin ML, Hales CA, et al. Clinical, laboratory, roentgenographic, and electrocardiographic findings in patients with acute pulmonary embolism and no pre-existing cardiac or pulmonary disease. *Chest* 1991;100:598–603.

60. McGinn S, White PD. Acute cor pulmonale resulting from pulmonary embolism. *JAMA* 1935;104:1473–1480.

61. Sokolow M, Katz LN, Muscovitz AN. The electrocardiogram in acute pulmonary embolism. *Am Heart J* 1940;19:166–184.

62. The Urokinase Pulmonary Embolism Trial. A national cooperative study. *Circulation* 1973;47(suppl II):1–108.

63. Ferrari E, Imbert A, Chevalier T, et al. The ECG in pulmonary embolism. Predictive value of negative T waves in precordial leads: 80 case reports. *Chest* 1997;111:537–543.

64. Kucher N, Walpoth N, Wustmann K, et al. QR in V_1—An ECG sign associated with right ventricular dysfunction and adverse clinical outcome in pulmonary embolism. *Eur Heart J* 2003;24:1113–1119.

65. van Strijen MJ, de Monye W, Schiereck J, et al. Single-detector helical CT as the primary diagnostic test in suspected pulmonary embolism: A multicenter clinical management study of 510 patients. *Ann Intern Med* 2003;138:307–314.

66. Remy-Jardin M, Remy J. Spiral CT angiography of the pulmonary circulation. *Radiology* 1999;212:615–636.

67. Remy-Jardin M, Remy J, Wattinne L, Giraud F. Central pulmonary thromboembolism: Diagnosis with spiral volumetric CT with the single-breath-hold technique: Comparison with pulmonary angiography. *Radiology* 1992;185:381–387.

68. Remy-Jardin M, Remy J, Deschildre F, et al. Diagnosis of pulmonary embolism with spiral CT: Comparison with pulmonary angiography and scintigraphy. *Radiology* 1996;200:699–706.

69. Goodman LR, Curtin JJ, Mewissen MW, et al. Detection of pulmonary embolism in patients with unresolved clinical and scintigraphic diagnosis: Helical CT versus angiography. *AJR* 1995;164:1369–1374.

70. Teigen CL, Maus TP, Sheedy PF, et al. Pulmonary embolism: Diagnosis with contrast-enhanced electron-beam CT and comparison with pulmonary angiography. *Radiology* 1995;194:313–319.

71. van Rossum AB, Pattynama PM, Treurniat FE, et al. Spiral CT angiography for detection of pulmonary embolism: Validation in 124 patients. *Radiology* 1995;197(P):303.

72. van Rossum AB, Treurniat FE, Kieft GJ, et al. Role of spiral volumetric computed tomographic scanning in the assessment of patients with clinical suspicion of pulmonary embolism and an abnormal ventilation perfusion scan. *Thorax* 1996;51:23–28.

73. Schoepf UJ, Holzknecht N, Helmberger TK, et al. Subsegmental pulmonary emboli: Improved detection with thin-collimation multidetector row spiral CT. *Radiology* 2002;222:483–490.

74. The PIOPED Investigators. Value of the ventilation/perfusion scan in acute pulmonary embolism: Results of the prospective investigation of pulmonary embolism diagnosis. *JAMA* 1990;263:2753–2759.

75. Stein PD, Athanasoulis C, Alavi A, et al. Complications and validity of pulmonary angiography in acute pulmonary embolism. *Circulation* 1992;85:462–468.

76. Quinn MF, Lundell CJ, Klotz TA, et al. Reliability of selective pulmonary arteriography in the diagnosis of acute pulmonary embolism. *AJR* 1987;149:469–471.

77. Meaney JFM, Weg JG, Chenevert TL, et al. Diagnosis of pulmonary embolism with magnetic resonance angiography. *N Engl J Med* 1997;336:1422–1427.

78. Tapson VF. Pulmonary embolism—New diagnostic approaches. *N Engl J Med* 1997;336:1449–1451.

79. Sostman HD, Layish DT, Tapson VF, et al. Prospective comparison of helical CT and MR imaging in clinically suspected acute pulmonary embolism. *JMRI* 1996;6:275.

80. Oudkerk M, van Beek EJ, Wielopolski P, et al. Comparison of contrast-enhanced magnetic resonance angiography and conventional pulmonary angiography for the diagnosis of pulmonary embolism: A prospective study. *Lancet* 2002;359:1643–1647.

81. Goldhaber SZ. Echocardiography in the management of pulmonary embolism. *Ann Intern Med* 2002;136:691–700.

82. Miniati M, Monti S, Pratali L, et al. Value of transthoracic echocardiography in the diagnosis of pulmonary embolism: Results of a prospective study in unselected patients. *Am J Med* 2001;110:528–535.

83. Grifoni S, Olivotto I, Cecchini P, et al. Short-term clinical outcome of patients with acute pulmonary embolism, normal blood pressure, and echocardiographic right ventricular dysfunction. *Circulation* 2000;101:2817–2822.

84. Ribeiro A, Lindmarker P, Johnsson H, et al. Pulmonary embolism: One-year follow-up with echocardiography Doppler and five-year survival analysis. *Circulation* 1999;99:1325–1330.

85. Konstantinides S, Geibel A, Heusel G, et al. Heparin plus alteplase compared with heparin alone in patients with submassive pulmonary embolism. *N Engl J Med* 2002;347:1143–1150.

86. Kucher N, Windecker S, Meier B, Hess OM. Novel management strategy for patients with suspected pulmonary embolism. *Eur Heart J* 2003;24:366–376.

87. Pruszczyk P, Torbicki A, Kuch-Wocial A, et al. Diagnostic value of transoesophageal echocardiography in suspected haemodynamically significant pulmonary embolism. *Heart* 2001;85:628–634.

88. Tapson VF, Davidson CJ, Gurbel PA, et al. Rapid and accurate diagnosis of pulmonary emboli in a canine model using intravascular ultrasound imaging. *Chest* 1991;100:1410–1413.

89. Tapson VF, Davidson CJ, Kisslo KB, et al. Rapid visualization of massive pulmonary emboli utilizing intravascular ultrasound. *Chest* 1994;105:888–890.

90. Ricou F, Nicod PH, Moser KM, Peterson KL. Catheter-based intravascular ultrasound imaging of chronic thromboembolic pulmonary disease. *Am J Cardiol* 1991;67:749–752.

91. McConnell MV, Rayan ME, Solomon SD, et al. Echocardiographic diagnosis of acute pulmonary embolism: A distinct pattern of abnormal right ventricular wall motion. *Am J Cardiol* 1996;78:469.

92. Konstantinides S, Geibel A, Kasper W, et al. Patent foramen ovale is an important predictor of adverse outcome in patients with major pulmonary embolism. *Circulation* 1998;97:1946.

93. Borgstede JP, Clagett GE. Types, frequency, and significance of alternative diagnoses found during duplex Doppler venous examinations of the lower extremities. *J Ultrasound Med* 1992;11:85–89.

94. Lensing AW, Levi MM, Buller HR, et al. Diagnosis of deep-vein thrombosis using an objective Doppler method. *Ann Intern Med* 1990;113:9–13.

95. White R, McGahan JP, Daschbach MM, Hartling MM. Diagnosis of deep-vein thrombosis using duplex ultrasound. *Ann Intern Med* 1989;111:297–304.

96. Cronan JJ, Leen V. Recurrent deep venous thrombosis: Limitations of ultrasound. *Radiology* 1989;170:739–742.

97. Killewich LA, Bedford GR, Beach KW, Strandness DE. Diagnosis of deep venous thrombosis: A prospective study comparing duplex scanning to contrast venography. *Circulation* 1989;79:810–814.

98. Davidson BL, Elliott CG, Lensing AWA. Low accuracy of color Doppler ultrasound in the detection of proximal leg vein thrombosis in asymptomatic high-risk patients. *Ann Intern Med* 1992;117:735–738.

99. Mac Gillavry MR, Sanson BJ, Buller HR, Brandjes DP. Compression ultrasonography of the leg veins in patients with clinically suspected pulmonary embolism: Is a more extensive assessment of compressibility useful? *Thromb Haemost* 2000;84:973–976.

100. Rabinov K, Paulin S. Roentgen diagnosis of venous thrombosis in the leg. *Arch Surg* 1972;104:134.

101. Hull R, Hirsh J, Powers P. Impedance plethysmography: The relationship between venous filling and sensitivity and specificity for proximal vein thrombosis. *Circulation* 1978;58:898–902.

102. Hull R, van Aken WG, Hirsh J, et al. Impedance plethysmography using the occlusive cuff technique in the diagnosis of venous thrombosis. *Circulation* 1976;53:696–700.

103. Anderson DR, Lensing AWA, Wells PS, et al. Limitations of impedance plethysmography in the diagnosis of clinically suspected deep-vein thrombosis. *Ann Intern Med* 1993;118:25–30.

104. Tapson VF, Carroll BA, Davidson BL, et al. The diagnostic approach to acute venous thromboembolism. American Thoracic Society Consensus Statement and Clinical Practice Guidelines. *Am J Resp Crit Care Med* 1999;160:1043–1066.

105. Evans AJ, Tapson VF, Sostman HD, et al. The diagnosis of deep venous thrombosis: A prospective comparison of venography and magnetic resonance imaging. *Chest* 1992;102:120S.

106. Witty LA, Tapson VF, Evans AJ, et al. MRI versus ultrasound: A radiologic and clinical evaluation of DVT. *Am Rev Respir Dis* 1993;147:A998.

107. Burke B, Sostman HD, Carroll BA, Witty LA. The diagnostic approach to deep venous thrombosis: Which technique? *Clin Chest Med* 1995;16:253–268.

108. Musset D, Parent F, Meyer G, et al. Diagnostic strategy for patients with suspected pulmonary embolism: A prospective multicentre outcome study. *Lancet* 2002;360:1914–1920.

109. Collins R, Scrimgeour A, Yusuf S, Peto R. Reduction in fatal pulmonary embolism and venous thrombosis by perioperative administration of subcutaneous heparin. *N Engl J Med* 1988;318:1162–1173.

110. Anderson FA Jr, Brownell W, Goldberg RJ, et al. Physician practices in the prevention of venous thromboembolism. *Ann Intern Med* 1991;115:591–595.

111. Bratzler DW, Raskob GE, Murray CK, et al. Underuse of venous thromboembolism prophylaxis for general surgery patients: Physician practices in the community hospital setting. *Arch Intern Med* 1998;158:1909–1912.

112. Prevention of fatal postoperative pulmonary embolism by low doses of heparin. An international multicentre trial. *Lancet* 1975;2:45–51.

113. Collins R, Scrimgeour A, Yusuf S, Peto R. Reduction in fatal pulmonary embolism and venous thrombosis by perioperative administration of subcutaneous heparin: Overview of results of randomized trials in general, orthopedic, and urologic surgery. *N Engl J Med* 1988;318:1162.

114. Lassen MR, Bauer KA, Eriksson BI, Turpie AG. Postoperative fondaparinux versus preoperative enoxaparin for prevention of venous thromboembolism in elective hip-replacement surgery: A randomised double-blind comparison. *Lancet* 2002;359:1715–1720.

115. Bounameaux H, Perneger T. Fondaparinux: A new synthetic pentasaccharide for thrombosis prevention. *Lancet* 2002;359:1710–1711.

116. Colwell CW, Collis DK, Paulson R, et al. Comparison of enoxaparin and warfarin for the prevention of venous thromboembolic disease after total hip arthroplasty. Evaluation during hospitalization and three months after discharge. *J Bone Joint Surg* 1999;81-A:932.

117. Antithrombotic Trialists' Collaboration. Collaborative meta-analysis of randomised trials of antiplatelet therapy for prevention of death, myocardial infarction, and stroke in high-risk patients. *Br Med J* 2002;324:71–86.

118. Tapson VF, Hull R. Management of venous thromboembolic disease: The impact of low-molecular-weight heparin. *Clin Chest Med* 1994;16:281–294.

119. Samama MM, Cohen AT, Darmon JY, et al. A comparison of enoxaparin with placebo for the prevention of venous thromboembolism in acutely ill medical patients. *N Engl J Med* 1999;341:793–800.

120. Colditz GA, Tuden RL, Oster G. Rates of venous thrombosis after general surgery: Combined results of randomised clinical trials. *Lancet* 1986;2:143.

121. Bergqvist D, Benoni G, Bjorgello XX, et al. Low-molecular-weight heparin (enoxaparin) as prophylaxis against venous thromboembolism after total hip replacement. *N Engl J Med* 1996;335:696–700.

122. Geerts WH, Jay RM, Code KI, et al. A comparison of low-dose heparin with low-molecular-weight heparin as prophylaxis against venous thromboembolism after major trauma. *N Engl J Med* 1996;335:701–707.

123. Francis, CW, Davidson BL, Berkowitz SD, et al. Ximelagatran versus warfarin for the prevention of venous thromboembolism after total knee arthroplasty. A randomized, double- blind trial. *Ann Intern Med* 2002;137:648–655.

124. Eriksson BI, Agnelli G, Cohen AT, et al. Direct thrombin inhibitor melagatran followed by oral ximelagatran in comparison with enoxaparin for prevention of venous thromboembolism after total hip or knee replacement. *Thromb Haemost* 2003;89:288–296.

125. Wicki J, Perrier A, Perneger TV, et al. Predicting adverse outcome in patients with acute pulmonary embolism: A risk score. *Thromb Haemost* 2000;84:548–552.

126. Guidelines on diagnosis and management of acute pulmonary embolism. Task Force on Pulmonary Embolism, European Society of Cardiology. *Eur Heart J* 2000;21:1301–1336.

127. Alpert JS, Thygesen K, Antman E, et al. Myocardial infarction redefined—A consensus document of The Joint European Society of Cardiology/American College of Cardiology Committee for the redefinition of myocardial infarction. *J Am Coll Cardiol* 36:959–969.

128. Muller-Bardorff M, Weidtmann B, Giannitsis E, et al. Release kinetics of cardiac troponin T in survivors of confirmed severe pulmonary embolism. *Clin Chem* 2002;48:673–675.

129. Konstantinides S, Geibel A, Olschewski M, et al. Importance of cardiac troponins I and T in risk stratification of patients with acute pulmonary embolism. *Circulation* 2002;106:1263–1268.

130. Pruszczyk P, Bochowicz A, Torbicki A, et al. Cardiac troponin T monitoring identifies high-risk group of normotensive patients with acute pulmonary embolism. *Chest* 2003;123:1947–1952.

131. Giannitsis E, Muller-Bardorff M, Kurowski V, et al. Independent prognostic value of cardiac troponin T in patients with confirmed pulmonary embolism. *Circulation* 2000;102:211–217.

132. Hama N, Itoh H, Shirakami G, et al. Rapid ventricular induction of brain natriuretic peptide gene expression in experimental acute myocardial infarction. *Circulation* 1995;92:1558–1564.

133. Tulevski II, Hirsch A, Sanson BJ, et al. Increased brain natriuretic peptide as a marker for right ventricular dysfunction in acute pulmonary embolism. *Thromb Haemost* 2001;86:1193–1196.

134. Kucher N, Printzen G, Goldhaber SZ. Prognostic role of brain natriuretic peptide in acute pulmonary embolism. *Circulation* 2003;107:2545–2547.

135. Kucher N, Printzen G, Doernhoefer T, et al. Low pro-brain natriuretic peptide levels predict benign clinical outcome in acute pulmonary embolism. *Circulation* 2003;107:1576–1578.

136. Nagaya N, Nishikimi T, Okano Y, et al. Plasma brain natriuretic peptide levels increase in proportion to the extent of right ventricular dysfunction in pulmonary hypertension. *J Am Coll Cardiol* 1998;31:202–208.

137. Nagaya N, Nishikimi T, Uematsu M, et al. Plasma brain natriuretic peptide as a prognostic indicator in patients with primary pulmonary hypertension. *Circulation* 2000;102:865–870.

138. Bando M, Ishii Y, Sugiyama Y, et al. Elevated plasma brain natriuretic peptide levels in chronic respiratory failure with cor pulmonale. *Respir Med* 1999;93:507–514.

139. Tulevski II, Groenink M, van Der Wall EE, et al. Increased brain and atrial natriuretic peptides in patients with chronic right ventricular pressure overload: correlation between plasma neurohormones and right ventricular dysfunction. *Heart* 2001;86:27–30.

140. Janata K, Holzer M, Laggner AN, et al. Cardiac troponin T in the severity assessment of patients with pulmonary embolism: cohort study. *Br Med J* 2003;326:312–313.

141. ten Wolde M, Tulevski II, Mulder JW, et al. Brain natriuretic peptide as a predictor of adverse outcome in patients with pulmonary embolism. *Circulation* 2003;107:2082–2084.

142. Hirsh J, Warkentin TE, Raschke R, et al. Heparin and low-molecular-weight heparin. Mechanisms of action, pharmacokinetics, dosing considerations, monitoring, efficacy, and safety. *Chest* 1998;114:489S–510S.

143. Hirsh J, Anand SS, Halperin JL, Fuster V. Guide to anticoagulant therapy. Heparin: A statement for healthcare professionals from the American Heart Association. *Circulation* 2001;103:2994–3018.

144. Hylek EM, Regan S, Henault LE, et al. Challenges to the effective use of unfractionated heparin in the hospitalized management of acute thrombosis. *Arch Intern Med* 2003;163:621–627.

145. Hull RD, Raskob GE, Hirsh J, et al. Continuous intravenous heparin compared with intermittent subcutaneous heparin in the initial treatment of proximal vein thrombosis. *N Engl J Med* 1986;315:1109–1114.

146. Hull R, Raskob G, Rosenbloom D, et al. Optimal therapeutic level of heparin therapy in patients with venous thrombosis. *Arch Intern Med* 1992;152:1589–1595.

147. Raschke RA, Reilly BM, Guidry JR, et al. The weight-based heparin dosing nomogram compared with a "standard care" nomogram. *Ann Intern Med* 1993;119:874.

148. Hyers TM, Agnelli G, Hull RD, et al. Antithrombotic therapy for venous thromboembolic disease. *Chest* 1998;114:561S–578S.

149. Lagerstedt CI, Olsson C-G, Fagher BO, Oqvist BW. Need for long-term anticoagulant treatment in symptomatic calf-vein thrombosis. *Lancet* 1985;2:515–518.

150. Moser KM, Le Moine JR. Is embolic risk conditioned by location of deep venous thrombosis? *Ann Intern Med* 1981;94:439–444.

151. Prandoni P, Polistena P, Bernardi E, et al. Upper extremity deep vein thrombosis. *Arch Intern Med* 1997;157:57–62.

152. Randolph AG, Cook DJ, Gonzalez CA, et al. Benefit of heparin in central venous and pulmonary artery catheters: A meta-analysis of randomized controlled trials. *Chest* 1998;113:165–171.

153. Nader HB, Walenga JM, Berkowitz SD, et al. Preclinical differentiation of low molecular weight heparins. *Semin Thromb Hemost* 1999;25(suppl 3):63–72.

154. Levine M, Gent M, Hirsh J, et al. A comparison of low-molecular-weight heparin administered primarily at home with unfractionated heparin administered in the hospital for proximal deep vein thrombosis. *N Engl J Med* 1996;334:677–681.

155. Koopman MM, Prandoni P, Piovella F, et al. Low-molecular-weight heparin versus heparin for proximal deep vein thrombosis. *N Engl J Med* 1996;334:682–687.

156. A Collaborative European Multicentre Study. A randomized trial of subcutaneous low-molecular-weight heparin (CY216) compared with intravenous unfractionated heparin in the treatment of deep vein thrombosis. *Thromb Haemost* 1991;65:251–256.

157. Hull RD, Raskob GE, Pineo GF, et al. Subcutaneous low-molecular-weight heparin compared with continuous intravenous heparin in the treatment of proximal-vein thrombosis. *N Engl J Med* 1992;326:975–983.

158. Prandoni P, Lensing AWA, Buller HR, et al. Comparison of subcutaneous low-molecular-weight heparin with intravenous standard heparin in proximal deep vein thrombosis. *Lancet* 1992;339:441–445.

159. Simonneau G, Charbonnier B, Decousus H, et al. Subcutaneous low-molecular-weight heparin compared with continuous intravenous unfractionated heparin in the treatment of proximal deep vein thrombosis. *Arch Intern Med* 1993;153:1541–1546.

160. Lindmarker P, Holmstrom M, Granqvist S, et al. Fragmin once daily subcutaneously in a fixed dose compared with continuous intravenous unfractionated heparin in the treatment of deep venous thrombosis. *Thromb Haemost* 1993;69:648.

161. Siragusa S, Cosmi B, Piovella F, et al. Low-molecular-weight heparins and unfractionated heparin in the treatment of patients with acute venous thromboembolism: Results of a meta-analysis. *Am J Med* 1996;100:269–270.

162. Lensing AWA, Prins MH, Davidson BL, Hirsh J. Treatment of deep venous thrombosis with low-molecular-weight heparins: A meta-analysis. *Arch Intern Med* 1995;155:601–607.

163. Leizorovicz A, Simonneau G, Decousus H, Boissel JP. Comparison of efficacy and safety of low molecular weight heparins and unfractionated heparin in initial treatment of deep venous thrombosis. *Br Med J* 1994;309:299–304.

164. O'Brien B, Levine M, Willan A, et al. Economic evaluation of outpatient treatment with low-molecular-weight heparin for proximal vein thrombosis. *Arch Intern Med* 1999;159:2298–2304.

165. Simonneau G, Sors H, Charbonnier B, et al. A comparison of low-molecular-weight heparin with unfractionated heparin for acute pulmonary embolism. *N Engl J Med* 1997;337:663.

166. Beckman JA, Dunn K, Sasahara AA, Goldhaber SZ. Enoxaparin monotherapy without oral anticoagulation to treat acute symptomatic pulmonary embolism. *Thromb Haemost* 2003;89:953–958.

167. Kelton JG, Sheridan D, Santos A, et al. Heparin-associated thrombocytopenia: Laboratory studies. *Blood* 1998;79:925–930.

168. Amiral J, Bridey F, Dreyfus M, et al. Platelet factor 4 complexed to heparin is the target for antibodies generated in heparin-induced thrombocytopenia. *Thromb Haemost* 1992;68:95–96.

169. Visentin GP, Ford SE, Scott JP, Aster RH. Antibodies from patients with heparin-induced thrombocytopenia/thrombosis are specific for platelet factor 4 complexed with heparin or bound to endothelial cells. *J Clin Invest* 1994;93:81–88.

170. Warkentin TE, Levine MN, Hirsh J, et al. Heparin-induced thrombocytopenia in patients treated with low-molecular-weight heparin or unfractionated heparin. *N Engl J Med* 1995;332:1330–1335.

171. Warkentin TE. Heparin-induced thrombocytopenia: A ten-year retrospective. *Annu Rev Med* 1999;50:129–147.

172. Bittl JA, Strony J, Brinker JA, et al. Treatment with bivalirudin (Hirulog) as compared with heparin during coronary angioplasty for unstable or postinfarction angina. Hirulog Angioplasty Study Investigators. *N Engl J Med* 1995;333:764–769.

173. Gallus AS, Coghlan DW. Heparin pentasaccharide. *Curr Opin Hematol* 2002;9:422–429.

174. Hylek EM, Heiman H, Skates SJ, et al. Acetaminophen and other risk factors for excessive warfarin anticoagulation. *JAMA* 1998;279:657.

175. Harrison L, Johnston M, Massicotte MP, et al. Comparison of 5-mg and 10-mg loading doses in initiation of warfarin therapy. *Ann Intern Med* 1997;126:133.

176. Joffe HV, Goldhaber SZ. Effectiveness and safety of long-term anticoagulation of patients ≥90 years of age with atrial fibrillation. *Am J Cardiol* 2002;90:1397–1398.

177. Higashi MK, Veenstra DL, Kondo LM, et al. Association between CYP2C9 genetic variants and anticoagulation-related outcomes during warfarin therapy. *JAMA* 2002;287:1690–1698.

178. Sawicki PT. A structured teaching and self-management program for patients receiving oral anticoagulation. *JAMA* 1999;281:145.

179. Oden A, Fahlen M. Oral anticoagulation and risk of death: A medical record linkage study. *Br Med J* 2002;325:1073–1075.

180. White RH, Beyth RJ, Zhou H, Romano PS. Major bleeding after hospitalization for deep-venous thrombosis. *Am J Med* 1999;107:414–424.

181. The Global Use of Strategies to Open Occluded Coronary Arteries (GUSTO) IIB Investigators. A comparison of recombinant hirudin with heparin for the treatment of acute coronary syndromes. *N Engl J Med* 1996;335:775–782.

182. Toglia M, Weg JG. Venous thromboembolism during pregnancy. *N Engl J Med* 1996;335:108.

183. Schulman S, Rhedin A-S, Lindmarker P, et al. A comparison of 6 weeks with 6 months of oral anticoagulant therapy after a first episode of venous thromboembolism. *N Engl J Med* 1995;332:1661.

184. Kearon C, Gent M, Hirsh J, et al. A comparison of three months of anticoagulation with extended anticoagulation for a first episode of idiopathic venous thromboembolism. *N Engl J Med* 1999;340:901.

185. Agnelli G, Prandoni P, Santamaria MG, et al. Three months versus one year of oral anticoagulant therapy for idiopathic deep venous thrombosis. Warfarin Optimal Duration Italian Trial Investigators. *N Engl J Med* 2001;345:165–169.

186. Kearon C, Ginsberg JS, Kovacs M et al. Low-intensity (INR 1.5–1.9) versus conventional-intensity (INR 2.0–3.0) anticoagulation for extended treatment of unprovoked VT: A randomized double blind trial (abstr). *Blood* 2002;100:150a.

187. Ridker PM, Goldhaber SZ, Danielson E, et al. Long-term, low-intensity warfarin therapy for the prevention of recurrent venous thromboembolism. *N Engl J Med* 2003;348:1425–1434.

188. Schulman S, Wahlander K, Lundstrom T, et al. Secondary prevention of venous thromboembolism with the oral direct thrombin inhibitor ximelagatran. *N Engl J Med* 2003;349:1713–1721.

189. Greenfield LJ. Vena caval interruption and pulmonary embolectomy. *Clin Chest Med* 1984;5:495–505.

190. White RH, Zhou H, Kim J, Romano PS. A population-based study of the effectiveness of inferior vena cava filter use among patients with venous thromboembolism. *Arch Intern Med* 2000;160:2033–2041.

191. Hughes GC, Smith TP, Eachempati SR, et al. The use of a temporary vena caval interruption device in high-risk trauma patients unable to receive standard venous thromboembolism prophylaxis. *J Trauma* 1999;46:246–249.

192. Millward SF, Oliva VL, Bell SD, et al. Gunther Tulip Retrievable Vena Cava Filter: Results from the Registry of the Canadian Interventional Radiology Association. *J Vasc Intervent Radiol* 2001;12:1053–1058.

193. Daniels LB, Parker JA, Patel SR, et al. Relation of duration of symptoms with response to thrombolytic therapy in pulmonary embolism. *Am J Cardiol* 1997;80:184.

194. Marini C, Di Ricco G, Rossi G, et al. Fibrinolytic effects of urokinase and heparin in acute pulmonary embolism: A randomized clinical trial. *Respiration* 1988;54:162–173.

195. Levine M, Hirsh J, Weitz J, et al. A randomized trial of a single bolus dosage regimen of recombinant tissue plasminogen activator in patients with acute pulmonary embolism. *Chest* 1990;98:1473–1479.

196. Jerjes-Sanchez C, Ramirez-Rivera A, de Lourdes Garcia M, et al. Streptokinase and heparin versus heparin alone in massive pulmonary embolism: A randomized controlled trial. *J Thromb Thrombolysis* 1995;2:227–229.

197. Dalla-Volta S, Palla A, Santolicandro A, et al. PAIMS 2: Alteplase combined with heparin versus heparin in the treatment of acute pulmonary embolism. Plasminogen activator Italian multicenter study 2. *J Am Coll Cardiol* 1992;20:520–526.

198. Goldhaber SZ, Haire WD, Feldstein ML, et al. Alteplase versus heparin in acute pulmonary embolism: Randomised trial assessing right-ventricular function and pulmonary perfusion. *Lancet* 1993;341:507–511.

199. Tibbutt DA, Davies JA, Anderson JA, et al. Comparison by controlled clinical trial of streptokinase and heparin in treatment of life-threatening pulmonary embolism. *Br Med J* 1974;1:343–347.

200. Ly B, Arnesen H, Eie H, et al. A controlled clinical trial of streptokinase and heparin in the treatment of major pulmonary embolism. *Acta Med Scand* 1978;203:465–470.

201. Kanter DS, Mikkola KM, Patel SR, et al. Thrombolytic therapy for pulmonary embolism. Frequency of intracranial hemorrhage and associated risk factors. *Chest* 1997;111:1241.

202. Rogers LQ, Lutcher CL. Streptokinase therapy for deep vein thrombosis: A comprehensive review of the literature. *Am J Med* 1990;88:389–395.

203. Leeper KV Jr, Popovich J Jr, Lesser BA, et al. Treatment of massive acute pulmonary embolism. The use of low doses of intrapulmonary arterial streptokinase combined with full doses of systemic heparin. *Chest* 1988;93:234–240.

204. The UKEP study. Multicentre clinical trial on two local regimens of urokinase in massive pulmonary embolism. *Eur Heart J* 1987;8:2–10.

205. Verstraete M, Miller GAH, Bounameaux H, et al. Intravenous and intrapulmonary recombinant tissue-type plasminogen activator in the treatment of acute massive pulmonary embolism. *Circulation* 1988;77:353–360.

206. Tapson VF, Gurbel PA, Royster R, et al. Pharmacomechanical thrombolysis of experimental pulmonary emboli: Rapid low-dose intraembolic therapy. *Chest* 1994;106:1558–1562.

207. Tapson VF, Davidson CJ, Bauman R, et al. Rapid thrombolysis of massive pulmonary emboli without systemic fibrinogenolysis: Intraembolic infusion of thrombolytic therapy. *Am Rev Respir Dis* 1992;145:A719.

208. Goldhaber SZ. Integration of catheter thrombectomy into our armamentarium to treat acute pulmonary embolism. *Chest* 1998;114(5):1237–1238.

209. Greenfield LJ, Proctor MC, Williams DM, et al. Long-term experience with transvenous catheter pulmonary embolectomy. *J Vasc Surg* 1993;18:450–458.

210. Schmitz-Rode T, Janssens U, Duda SH, et al. Massive pulmonary embolism: Percutaneous emergency treatment by pigtail rotation catheter. *J Am Coll Cardiol* 2000;36:375–380.

211. Uflacker R, Strange C, Vujic I. Massive pulmonary embolism: Preliminary results in treatment with the Amplatz thrombectomy device. *J Vasc Intervent Radiol* 1996;7:519–528.

212. Koning R, Cribier A, Gerber L, et al. A new treatment for pulmonary embolism: Percutaneous rheolytic thrombectomy. *Circulation* 1997;96:2498–2500.

213. Semba CP, Dake MD. Iliofemoral deep venous thrombosis: Aggressive therapy with catheter-directed thrombolysis. *Radiology* 1994;191:487–494.

214. Mewissen MW, Seabrook GR, Meissner MH, et al. Catheter-directed thrombolysis for lower extremity deep venous thrombosis: Report of a national multicenter registry. *Radiology* 1999;211:39–49.

215. Gray HH, Morgan JM, Paneth M, Miller GAH. Pulmonary embolectomy: Indications and results. *Br Heart J* 1987;57:572.

216. Aklog L, Williams CS, Byrne JG, Goldhaber SZ. Acute pulmonary embolectomy: a contemporary approach. *Circulation* 2002;105:1416–1419.

217. Tapson VF, Witty LA. Massive pulmonary embolism: Diagnostic and therapeutic strategies. *Clin Chest Med* 1996;16:329.

218. Jardin F, Genevray B, Brunney D, Margairaz A. Dobutamine: A hemodynamic evaluation in pulmonary embolism shock. *Crit Care Med* 1985;13:1009–1012.

219. Manier G, Castaing Y. Influence of cardiac output on oxygen exchange in acute pulmonary embolism. *Am Rev Respir Dis* 1992;145:130–136.

220. Shure D. Chronic thromboembolic pulmonary hypertension: Diagnosis and treatment. *Semin Respir Crit Care Med* 1996;17:7.

221. Fedullo PF, Auger WR, Channick RN, et al. Chronic thromboembolic pulmonary hypertension. *Clin Chest Med* 1995;16:353–374.

222. Fedullo PF, Auger WR, Kerr KM, Rubin LJ. Chronic thromboembolic pulmonary hypertension. *N Engl J Med* 2001;345:1465–1472.

223. Feinstein JA, Goldhaber SZ, Lock JE, et al. Balloon pulmonary angioplasty for treatment of chronic thromboembolic pulmonary hypertension. *Circulation* 2001;103:10–13.

CHRONIC COR PULMONALE

E. Clinton Lawrence / Kenneth L. Brigham

HISTORY

In the first edition of his seminal textbook *Heart Disease,* published in 1931, Paul Dudley White devotes a chapter to "Pulmonary Heart Disease—Cor Pulmonale."[1] Expanding on the concept of "the emphysema heart," he defined *cor pulmonale* as right ventricular disease resulting from primary disorders of the lungs, in contradistinction to that resulting from mitral valvular or left ventricular disease. Thus, the sine qua non of cor pulmonale was pulmonary hypertension (PH) resulting from "increased resistance in the pulmonary circulation."[1] White separated the causes for this process into either: (1) damage to small pulmonary vessels (arterioles and capillaries) resulting from diseases of the lungs and associated structures; or (2) the rare condition of *endarteritis obliterans* of the larger pulmonary arteries, usually of unknown cause but occasionally resulting from syphilis.[2,3] In subsequent editions he expanded the chapter to include *acute cor pulmonale,* but in the first edition published more than 70 years ago he presented the etiology, pathology, and clinical features of *chronic cor pulmonale* with such precision and insight as to still be relevant today.

Although the term *cor pulmonale* was popularized by White, the concept that conditions of the lungs could affect right ventricular (RV) function was more long-standing. Sir William Osler, for example, recognized that "…obliteration of any number of blood vessels within the lungs, such as occurs in emphysema or cirrhosis, is followed by hypertrophy of the right ventricle," due to increased resistance in the pulmonary circulation.[4]

DEFINITION

The term *pulmonary heart disease* (i.e., cor pulmonale) refers to cardiac dysfunction resulting from altered structure or function of the lungs. Since the lungs are interposed in the cardiovascular circuit between the RV and left side of the heart, alterations in lung structure or function will selectively affect the right side of the heart.

Cor pulmonale has been variably defined. Some definitions provide a useful classification of disease for clinicians while others are based more on alterations in organ structure and function. The best general definition of the term *cor pulmonale* remains the one articulated in 1963 by an expert committee appointed by the director general of the World Health Organization (WHO). They defined *chronic cor pulmonale* as "hypertrophy of the RV resulting from diseases affecting the function and/or structure of the lung, except when these pulmonary alterations are the result of diseases that primarily affect the left side of the heart or congenital heart disease." [5]

Acute dilatation of the RV of the heart, that is, acute cor pulmonale is a disorder in which the RV is dilated and the muscular wall is stretched thin. This is most often the result of massive pulmonary embolism as described in Chap. 63. The chronic form of the disorder, the principal subject of this chapter, is characterized by RV hypertrophy with eventual dilatation and right side of the heart failure.

The RV is ill suited to excessive mechanical demands, being adapted to pump blood through the normally low-resistance, high-capacitance lung circulatory bed. RTH Laennec, in his *Treatise on Diseases of the Chest* published early in the nineteenth century, gives an elegant description of the gross anatomy of cardiac dilatation and hypertrophy, including findings limited to the RV (in fact, his tour de force elegantly describes the gross pathology of virtually every lung disease).[6]

The final common pathophysiologic event that causes chronic cor pulmonale is pulmonary hypertension (PH), that is, chronically increased resistance to blood flow through the pulmonary circulation. Unlike systemic hypertension, PH is difficult to diagnose clinically so that pulmonary vascular pressures may be elevated for prolonged periods before the disorder is recognized. In fact, dysfunction of the RV (i.e., cor pulmonale) is often recognized as the initial clinical diagnosis in patients with either primary or secondary PH. Newer noninvasive techniques can provide more information about pulmonary circulatory function than in the past. However, suspecting PH early in its course still depends largely on the skill of the experienced clinician.

Although lung disorders that cause chronic cor pulmonale can be classified in many ways, this chapter will use a classification based on the mechanism by which the disorder increases pulmonary vascular resistance.

INCIDENCE

Estimates of the incidence of chronic cor pulmonale, as well as estimates of morbidity and even mortality directly attributable to right heart dysfunction secondary to lung disease, are difficult to obtain. It is difficult to separate epidemiologic data relevant to cor pulmonale from the lung disease that is its primary cause. In addition, a definitive diagnosis most often requires invasive diagnostic procedures often at a time when treating the lung disease is the most paramount clinical issue. However, the magnitude of the clinical problem can be appreciated from data on chronic obstructive pulmonary disease (COPD), undoubtedly the most common cause of cor pulmonale.

The estimated total prevalence of COPD in the world is currently 400 million individuals. In 1999, there were 713,000 hospital discharges with a diagnosis of COPD in the United States, a discharge rate of 25.9 per 10,000 population. In the United States, there were 123,550 deaths due to COPD in the year 2000.[7] According to a WHO report, COPD accounted for 4.8 percent of all deaths in the United States in 1998. Worldwide, the problem is even more dramatic. WHO estimates that COPD accounted for 4.73 percent of all deaths in member nations (Table 64-1). Thus, for every 100,000 people in the world, 43 died of COPD in 2001.[7]

It has been estimated that up to 14 percent of patients with COPD suffer from secondary PH.[7] The fraction of patients with right side of the heart dysfunction resulting from secondary PH is unknown. A study from the United Kingdom estimates that 0.3 percent of the population had both an arterial oxygen tension less than 55 mmHg and clear evidence of airways obstruction by pulmonary function testing.[8] These data would predict 60,000 subjects in England and Wales at serious risk for secondary PH.[8] Again, the number of these subjects who had cor pulmonale cannot be determined.

It is clear from the available epidemiologic data that diseases predisposing to cor pulmonale are an enormous health problem throughout the world. Undoubtedly cor pulmonale is a major contributor to the morbidity and mortality in these diseases.

ETIOLOGIES

Diseases that affect lung structure and function can increase pulmonary vascular resistance either directly or indirectly through effects on the lungs' gas exchange function. Any cause of persistent PH of sufficient magnitude and duration can cause cor pulmonale.

PH is discussed in detail in Chap. 62. However, an understanding of where the causes of PH fit in a pathophysiologic schema that relates lung dysfunction to dysfunction of the RV is essential for understanding cor pulmonale. Table 64-2 presents a pathophysiologic classification of potential causes of chronic cor pulmonale.

A classification of this sort is somewhat arbitrary. In fact, there is enormous overlap in mechanisms in virtually all of the diseases listed in Table 64-2. It is probably more accurate to perceive relations among the various basic mechanisms as interacting with the eventual outcome of a remodeling of the pulmonary vascular bed resulting in a largely irreversible increase in pulmonary vascular resistance. The Venn diagram in Fig. 64-1 illustrates this concept.

PATHOPHYSIOLOGY OF INCREASED PULMONARY VASCULAR RESISTANCE

Persistent Pulmonary Vasoconstriction

The lung has the daunting task of constantly removing carbon dioxide from and reoxygenating all of the blood destined for the systemic circulation with each heartbeat. For the lung to perform its principal function of gas exchange efficiently, it must not only maintain the integrity of the vast gas exchange surface that brings blood into intimate contact with air, but must match the amount of blood perfusing with the amount of air ventilating each gas exchange unit. This matching of ventilation and perfusion is accomplished primarily by the unique property of pulmonary vessels to constrict when exposed to a hypoxic environment (systemic vessels dilate in response to hypoxia). Since laminar flow of blood through tubes is governed by Poiseuille's law, (i.e., resistance to flow is a function of vessel radius to the fourth power), this is a very sensitive mechanism. Small changes in resistance vessel diameter can have major effects on perfusion.

Viewed teleologically, hypoxic pulmonary vasoconstriction must be a local phenomenon. To optimize gas exchange, blood flow needs to be selectively reduced to areas of lung that are poorly ventilated (and thus hypoxic). Since the normal pulmonary vascular bed has a very large capacitance and a reserve of capacity to exchange carbon dioxide and oxygen, blood shunted away from poorly ventilated areas will be shunted to well-ventilated areas and thus contribute ar-

TABLE 64-1 Worldwide Mortality Attributable to COPD

WHO region	Total Population (000's)	Total Deaths	COPD Deaths	COPD % of Total Deaths	Deaths per 100,000
Africa	655,476,000	10,680,871	116,045	1.09	17.7
The Americas	837,967,000	5,910,811	221,682	3.75	26.5
Eastern Mediterranean	493,091,000	4,156,667	88,318	2.12	17.9
Europe	874,178,000	9,702,763	284,581	2.93	32.6
Southeast Asia	1,559,810,000	14,466,690	614,555	4.25	39.4
Western Pacific	1,701,689,000	11,636,373	1,347,093	11.58	79.2
Total	**6,122,211,000**	**56,554,175**	**2,672,274**	**4.73**	**43.6**

World Health Organization. *Consultation on the Development of a Comprehensive Approach for the Prevention and Control of Chronic Respiratory Diseases.* WHO, 2001: 6.

terialized blood to the systemic blood supply with essentially no increase in overall pulmonary vascular resistance in the normal lung. The diagram in Fig. 64-2 illustrates this phenomenon.[9]

But what if all (or a very large fraction) of the lung is hypoxic? In that case, there will be global constriction of the resistance vessels in the lung circulation with an obligatory increase in pulmonary vascular resistance and PH. The purest clinical example of this is the persistent PH (and cor pulmonale) that develops in people living at high enough altitude so that ambient air is deficient in oxygen because of the low barometric pressure.[10] Alveolar hypoventilation resulting either from decreased central ventilatory drive or from physical distortions of the lung relative to the ventilatory apparatus due to deformities of the chest can also result in hypoxia. If hypoxia is sufficiently extensive, the normal hypoxic vasoconstrictive response will result in PH. That chronic hypoventilation can result in cor pulmonale is graphically illustrated in drawings of the "fat boy" in Dicken's *Pickwick Papers,* who is generally said to have suffered from obesity-hypoventilation (thus Pickwickian) syndrome. The peripheral edema characteristic of right side of the heart failure is evident in both Dickens' elegant description and in the classic illustration.[11]

Loss of Cross-Sectional Area of the Pulmonary Vascular Bed

Resistance to blood flow through the pulmonary vasculature depends on the radius of individual resistance vessels and on the total cross-sectional area of the vascular bed. If the area of the vascular bed is sufficiently decreased, then PH will develop.

TABLE 64-2 Pathophysiologic Classification of Diseases of the Lungs that can cause Cor Pulmonale

Principal Pathophysiologic Mechanism	Disease Entity
Persistent vasoconstriction	• High altitude dwellers • Hypoventilation syndromes • Chest deformities • ? Primary pulmonary hypertension
Loss of cross-sectional area of the vascular bed	• Thromboembolic disease • Emphysema • Lung resection • Fibrotic lung diseases • Cystic fibrosis
Obstruction of large vessels	• Extrinsic compression of pulmonary veins • Fibrosing mediastinitis • Adenopathy/tumors • Pulmonary veno-occlusive disease
Chronically increased blood flow Vascular remodeling	• Eisenmenger's syndrome • Primary pulmonary hypertension • Secondary pulmonary hypertension • Collagen vascular diseases • Cystic fibrosis

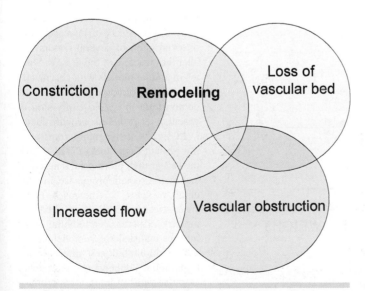

FIGURE 64-1 Venn diagram illustrating interactions among pathophysiologic mechanisms of pulmonary hypertension.

It is intuitively obvious that resistance to flow should increase if the total amount of vascular bed is decreased. However, the relation for the lungs is not linear, at least in situations where the remaining lung vessels are intrinsically normal. The large capacitance of the normal lung vascular bed allows large reductions in the amount of the bed that is perfused without an increase in resistance. The clearest example of the direct effects of reducing the size of the vascular bed is with lung resection. Figure 64-3 is from a group of studies in animals in which careful measurements of pulmonary hemodynamics were made with the lungs intact and following resection of different amounts of lung tissue.[12] The total lung mass could be decreased in half before there was any increase in pulmonary artery pressure. That observation is consistent with clinical experience with lung resection in humans. If the unresected lung is essentially normal, a total pneumonectomy does not result in PH at rest. Once the capacitance of the pulmonary vascular bed is exceeded, there is a steep relation between pulmonary artery pressure and the amount of vascular bed. In the experiments from which the data in Fig. 64-3 are derived, this was done by resecting more lung tissue. Following pneumonectomy in humans, PH on exercise may occur because of increased pulmonary blood flow in a vascular bed with little remaining capacitance.[13]

In the most common clinical settings in which there is loss of lung vessels, the remaining perfused vessels are either functionally or structurally abnormal. For example, destruction of lung parenchyma with COPD reduces the area of the vascular bed, but there may be vasoconstriction in the perfused bed as a result of an abnormal ventilatory pattern. Pulmonary emboli directly obstruct lung vessels, but even patent vessels may be constricted due to release of humoral mediators. In addition, chronic pulmonary embolic disease can result in structural remodeling of the pulmonary vascular bed with irreversible PH and cor pulmonale.[14]

Pulmonary artery pressure in patients with COPD increases with exercise even though resting pulmonary artery pressure may be normal. Figure 64-4 shows data from studies in patients with COPD and a range of resting pulmonary artery pressures.[15] Pressure during

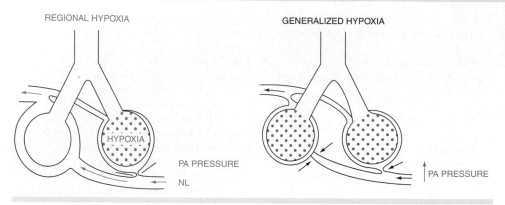

FIGURE 64-2 Illustration of the pulmonary hemodynamic consequences of alveolar hypoxia. Local hypoxia causes local vasoconstriction, matching perfusion to alveolar ventilation. Generalized hypoxia causes global vasoconstriction resulting in pulmonary hypertension. PA, posteroanterior, NL, normal lung. (Reprinted here with permission.[9])

In addition, the rare but devastating disorder, fibrosing mediastinitis, can enmesh large pulmonary arteries or veins (or bronchi) in an inexorably advancing mass of connective tissue with progressive occlusion.[16] Occlusion of the main pulmonary artery imposes a direct resistance against which the RV must pump, analogous physiologically to stenosis of the pulmonary valve or hypertrophic stenosis of the pulmonary outflow tract of the RV. If progression of the obstruction is sufficiently slow, chronic cor pulmonale can be a principal clinical picture in the presence of normal lungs. Obstruction of pulmonary veins will also elevate overall pulmonary vascular resistance, but in this case the lung microvasculature will bear the brunt of the pressure increase. The consequences for the pulmonary circulation and the right side of the heart are analogous to those of either left side of the heart failure or mitral valve stenosis. Depending on the chronicity and pace of the obstruction, cor pulmonale may result.

exercise was a steep function of resting pressure, although exercise increased pressure even in subjects with normal resting pressures indicating loss of pulmonary vascular capacitance. In the compromised vascular bed, hemodynamic reserve is lost so that physiologic changes such as local hypoxic vasoconstriction or increased pulmonary blood flow, which are easily accommodated in the normal lung circulation, result in increased afterload to the RV, the proximate cause of cor pulmonale.

Obstruction of Large Pulmonary Vessels

The most common cause of acute cor pulmonale is occlusion of the large proximal pulmonary artery by a massive embolus. However, large pulmonary vessels may also be compromised more insidiously by disorders of the mediastinum.

Direct compression of either pulmonary arteries or veins can result from enlarging mediastinal lymph nodes or mediastinal tumors.

Chronically Increased Pulmonary Blood Flow

Although the definition of cor pulmonale given earlier excludes congenital heart disease, chronically increased flow through the pulmonary circulation results in functional and structural alterations in the pulmonary vascular bed, and these changes in the lung come to dominate the pathophysiology. This clinical situation develops most often as a result of an abnormal shunting of blood from the left side of the circulation back to the right side, bypassing the systemic circulation (e.g., septal defects). In order to maintain blood supply to systemic organs, the right side of the heart must pump a larger volume of blood per unit time (the shunted blood in addition to the systemic venous return).

Increased flow through pulmonary vessels causes remodeling of the lung circulation and progressive PH. The remodeling process involves apparently direct effects of increased flow on expression of several factors that alter the structure of the vessels. Studies in animal models with chronically increased pulmonary blood flow demonstrate increased expression of vascular endothelial growth factor (VEGF) and its receptors, transforming growth factor beta (TGF-β) and the cell growth promoters, tenascin-C and matrix metalloproteinase, in muscular vessels.[17–19] Increased linear shear stress imposed on cultured pulmonary vascular endothelial cells induces cytoskeleton remodeling and other endothelial cell alterations.[20] Endothelial dependent pulmonary vascular relaxation is also compromised in experimentally induced increased pulmonary blood flow,[21] so

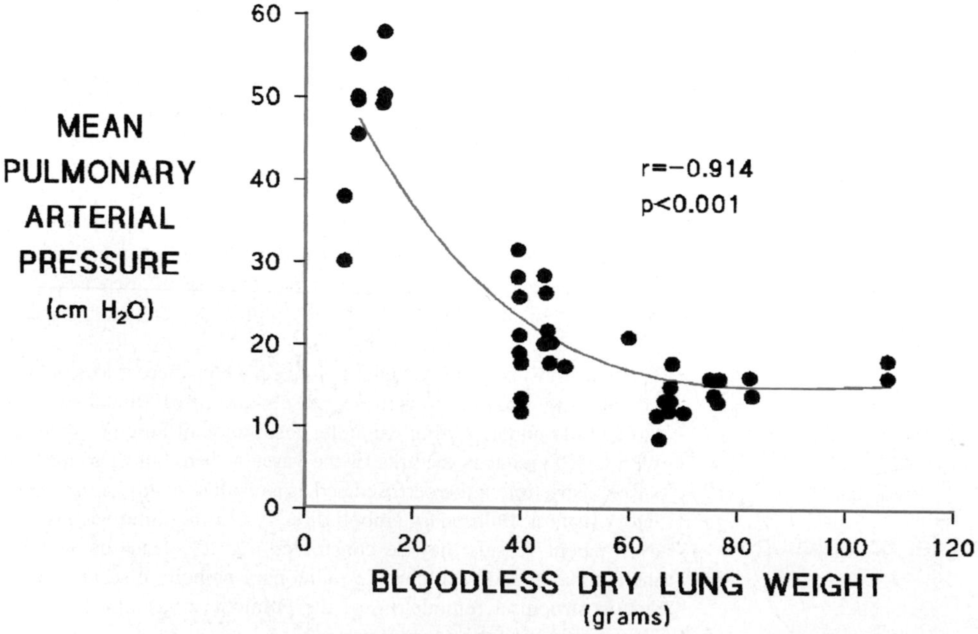

FIGURE 64-3 Effects of resecting progressively more lung tissue on pulmonary artery pressure in anesthetized sheep. About half of the lung tissue can be removed before pulmonary artery pressure rises at rest. When sufficient tissue has been removed to cause pressure to increase, pulmonary artery pressure becomes a steep function of the amount of lung tissue perfused. (Reprinted here with permission.[12])

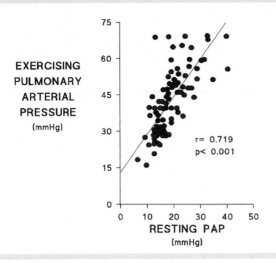

FIGURE 64-4 Pulmonary artery pressures at rest and exercise in a group of patients with chronic obstructive pulmonary disease and a wide range of resting pressures. In this group of subjects, pulmonary artery pressure during exercise was a steep function of resting pressure. (Reprinted here with permission.[15])

that loss of normal homeostatic mechanisms for maintaining low pulmonary vascular resistance may contribute to the development of persistent PH in this circumstance.

The ultimate result of persistent increased pulmonary blood flow and the worsening PH is reversal of flow through the shunt. As pulmonary vascular resistance increases, right side of the heart pressures rise, finally reaching levels approaching systemic pressures, reversing the pressure gradient and forcing blood to flow through the shunt from the right side of the circulation to the left. Clinically, this condition is termed *Eisenmenger's complex*[22] (see Chaps. 73 and 74). Although patients with this syndrome appear to tolerate high right-sided pressures better than do those with other causes of PH, eventually right side of the heart failure, cor pulmonale, occurs.

Pulmonary Vascular Remodeling

A low baseline resistance to blood flow, a large vascular capacitance, and the ability to create flow heterogeneities in order to match perfusion to ventilation are all essential to normal function of the lung circulation. Structural remodeling of the pulmonary arterial circulation that occurs in several lung diseases resulting in PH compromises each of these essential characteristics.

The clearest example of vascular remodeling in the lungs is the unusual disorder, primary PH, which occurs as both a familial, inherited, and a sporadic disorder (see Chap. 74). The etiology of this progressive fatal disease remains unknown, although an inherited abnormality in the gene encoding bone morphogenic protein receptor-2 (a member of the TGF-β receptor superfamily) is apparently responsible for the disease in at least some families[23,24] (see Chap. 9). Exactly how this genetic predisposition fits into the pathogenesis of PH is not yet clear. Remodeling also occurs in secondary PH with functional consequences such as those in the primary form of the disease. For example, pulmonary complications of collagen vascular diseases include remodeling of the lung vasculature[25] (see Chap. 84).

Much has been learned about how remodeling of the pulmonary arterial circulation occurs from studies in animals in which pulmonary vascular resistance is elevated chronically by various experimental interventions. Remodeling is a complex process that, anatomically, includes hypertrophy of smooth muscle in arterial resistance vessels, extension of vascular smooth muscle peripherally to previously nonmuscular arteries, and loss of microvascular bed resulting from intimal proliferation.[26] These structural changes act in concert to increase resistance to blood flow through the lung circulation. In addition, in some forms of persistent PH, there is a tonic vasoconstrictive component that compounds the problem.[27]

RESPONSE OF THE RIGHT CARDIAC VENTRICLE TO INCREASED PULMONARY VASCULAR RESISTANCE

Normal Right Ventricular Structure and Function

Mechanical demands on the RV under normal conditions are minimal compared to demands on the left ventricle (LV) because the work required to pump blood through the low resistance, low impedance lung circulation is a fraction of that required to perfuse the high pressure systemic circulation. The structure of the RV compared to the left reflects the difference in their physiologic requirements. A cross-section through a normal heart is shown in Fig. 64-5.[28] The LV is symmetrical with a thick muscular wall. In contrast, the RV wall is much thinner and the cavity is crescent shaped, because the convexity of the septum bulges toward the right. Both the geometry of the two ventricles and the mass of their muscular walls reflect their different functions. The symmetrical, thick-walled left ventricle is suited to generating high outflow pressures, while the thin-walled asymmetric RV is not.

Figure 64-6 compares the responses of the normal right and left ventricles to increased afterload in an experimental preparation.[29] When aortic pressure is increased (i.e., increased afterload to the LV), there is a marked increase in stroke work, but stroke volume is maintained. However, RV stroke volume decreases as a steep function of increasing pulmonary artery pressure (i.e., increased afterload to the RV) with only a modest increase in stroke work. Note that the

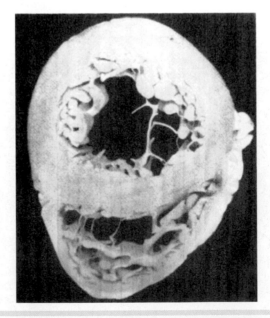

FIGURE 64-5 A cross-section of a gross specimen of a normal heart illustrating a thick-walled spherical left ventricle contrasted to a thin-walled-crescent-shaped right ventricle. (Printed here with permission.[28])

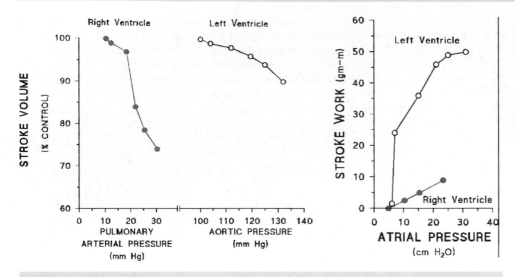

FIGURE 64-6 Responses of the right and left ventricles to experimental increases in afterload to each ventricle contrasting responses of the two ventricles. (Reprinted here with permission.[29])

massively enlarged trabeculae carnae are exactly as described by Laennec.[6] In this advanced case, it is not difficult to imagine that the RV could sustain pulmonary artery pressures as high as systemic arterial pressures.

However, the robust appearance of the hypertrophied ventricle is misleading; the complex process of hypertrophy is not entirely homeostatic. As the RV hypertrophies in response to a chronic pressure load, several alterations occur that result in less efficient function. Such changes include loss of cardiac myocytes[30] and myocardial edema followed by fibrosis.[31] In addition, the hypertrophied ventricle becomes stiff resulting in an increase in end-diastolic RV pressure that compromises endocardial perfusion and creates a mismatch of myocardial oxygen demand and supply.

In addition to these pathologic changes at the organ level, hypertrophy is accompanied by changes in the architecture and mechanical function of individual cardiac myocytes. Alterations such as subcellular relocation of critical cell proteins,[32] alterations in microtubules,[33] changes in calcium handling,[34] and depressed sarcomere contraction[35] occur in experimental RV hypertrophy and are likely important parts of the pathogenesis of cor pulmonale in humans.

degree of elevation of pulmonary artery pressure in the studies depicted in Fig. 64-6 were modest, well below those in both primary and secondary PH in humans.

Remodeling of the Right Ventricle: Structure and Function

The RV dilates enough with even modest acute increases in afterload that its effectiveness as a pump is compromised; this results in right side of the heart failure—acute cor pulmonale. However, with prolonged increases in pulmonary artery pressure that are not high enough initially to precipitate RV failure, the RV, like the LV, undergoes hypertrophy. Figure 64-7, a cross-section of a gross specimen of a heart from a patient who died of PH,[28] should be compared to the normal heart in Fig. 64-5. The grossly thickened myocardium and

As RV hypertrophy progresses, failure of its pump function with either persistence of increased pulmonary artery pressure or acute increases resulting from altered status of the underlying lung disease is increasingly likely. The sequence of events is initial dilatation of the hypertrophied ventricle, an elevation in RV end-diastolic pressure resulting in increased systemic venous pressure and clinically apparent peripheral edema. In patients with COPD, bouts of increasing respiratory failure, and hypoxemia may result in acute worsening of RV function and peripheral edema that is a transient function of the severity of the respiratory failure, resolving if treatment of the lung disease is effective. Figure 64-8 shows data from a study of 9 patients with COPD who had right side of the heart catheterizations while they were edema free and during an episode of exacerbation of their lung disease and cor pulmonale.[36] During an acute episode of respiratory decompensation, decreased arterial oxygenation was accompanied by marked increases in pulmonary artery pressure and in RV end-diastolic pressure, reflecting worsening RV failure. Interestingly, acute edematous episodes in patients with COPD are not invariably accompanied by increased RV end-diastolic pressure, so that factors other than RV failure may be responsible for peripheral edema in those cases.[36]

There may also be primary abnormalities in the RV that account for the unique clinical features of Eisenmenger's syndrome. One study reported extensive evaluations of ventricular morphology in patients with Eisenmenger's complex (i.e., PH with right to left shunts), a group with "pre-Eisenmenger's" syndrome (i.e., ventricular septal defect with left to right shunting), and fetuses with healthy hearts.[37] They found the same ventricular morphology in all groups—a flat ventricular septum and equal thickness of the right and left ventricular free walls, concluding that the usual regression of RV wall thickness subsequent to birth does not occur in the presence of large shunts so that the right ventricle retains function even with

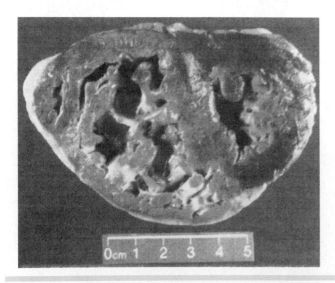

FIGURE 64-7 Cross-section of a gross specimen of a heart from a patient who died of pulmonary hypertension illustrating selective marked hypertrophy of the right ventricle. (Reproduced with permission.[28])

increased mechanical demand. In adults with severe PH due to Eisenmenger's syndrome, the RV may be functionally devoid of sympathetic innervation, contributing to eventual ventricular failure.[38]

In addition to the structural and functional alterations in the RV that occur with hypertrophy, other systemic factors can adversely affect function either by directly affecting cardiac muscle or by exaggerating RV afterload. Obviously generalized hypoxia, regardless of the cause, will exaggerate PH imposing increased mechanical demand on the RV. Increased blood viscosity secondary to polycythemia that develops as a response to chronic hypoxemia will exaggerate the increased afterload resulting from PH. Hypercapnea and the resulting acidemia appear to affect the myocardium directly, compromising the ability of the ventricle to increase work in response to increased afterload.[29] Thus, either hypoventilation syndromes with chronic hypercapnea and acidosis or acute elevations in carbon dioxide that occur with acute exacerbations in patients with COPD will challenge the reserve of the right side of the heart while increasing the mechanical demand.

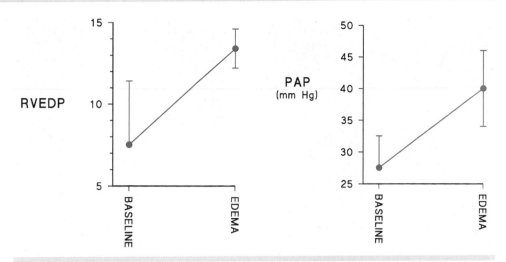

FIGURE 64-8 Right ventricular end-diastolic pressure and pulmonary artery pressure (PAP) in a group of patients with chronic obstructive pulmonary disease measured at a time when they were free of peripheral edema and repeated during an episode of worsening pulmonary symptoms associated with peripheral edema. Elevated right-sided pressures are evidence of cor pulmonale. (Graph constructed from data in Table 64-4.[36])

CLINICAL MANIFESTATIONS

Symptoms

Although cor pulmonale may result from many different pulmonary diseases, the cardinal symptom is shortness of breath, especially with exertion, with progression over months to years.[39] However, shortness of breath is virtually universal with all disorders of the cardiopulmonary system and thus does not serve to differentiate primary pulmonary disorders from secondary RV dysfunction (i.e., *cor pulmonale*). Other nonspecific symptoms of cor pulmonale include fatigue, palpitations, atypical chest pain, swelling of the lower extremities, dizziness, and even syncope. In essence, the symptoms of cor pulmonale are those of PH (see Chap. 62). However, complaints consistent with Raynaud's phenomena suggest either an underlying connective tissue disorder or primary PH; a history of liver disease suggests the possibility of portal-PH; and a history of previous pulmonary emboli and/or deep venous thrombosis may indicate chronic thromboembolic PH (see Chap. 101).

PHYSICAL EXAMINATION

The physical findings in cor pulmonale are a combination of those of the underlying pulmonary disease and those of PH (see Chap. 12). Thus, pursed lip breathing, hyperresonant chest, and diminished breath sounds with prolonged expiratory phase are characteristic of emphysema, whereas coarse "Velcro" rales with small lung volumes, dullness to percussion, egophony, and clubbing are seen in many interstitial lung diseases. Telangiectasias of the skin may be present with either cirrhosis of the liver or CREST syndrome; patients with

the latter disorder may exhibit tightening of the skin circumorally and of the fingers (sclerodactyly), often with digital ulcerations and even loss of distal portions of digits (see Chap. 14). Arthritic changes may be seen with connective tissue diseases but are most pronounced with rheumatoid arthritis.

The physical findings of PH may not be present until the disease process is far advanced (see Chap. 12). However, an increased pulmonic component of the second heart sound (P_2) as demonstrated by splitting of S_2 over the cardiac apex with expiration is a reliable sign of PH and cor pulmonale.[40] With progression of the disease process, one may appreciate a left parasternal (RV) lift, murmurs of tricuspid regurgitation, pulmonic flow and regurgitation (Graham Steele) murmurs, and prominent "A" waves in jugular venous pulsations. With decompensated cor pulmonale (RV failure), distension of jugular neck veins, a tender liver with hepatojugular reflux, peripheral edema, and ascites often ensue, usually accompanied by right-sided S_3 and often by S_4 gallops (see Chap. 12).

Electrocardiogram

Electrocardiographic abnormalities, when present, are helpful in establishing a diagnosis of cor pulmonale, whereas the absence of such findings does not exclude the diagnosis.[41] Characteristic findings in advanced cor pulmonale include tall, peaked P waves anteriorly (i.e., "p pulmonale"), and rightward axis and prominent R waves in early V leads producing an R/S ratio greater than 1 in lead V_1 and R/S ratio less than 1 in V_{5-6} (i.e., "RVH"). However, the triad of "S_1, Q_3, T_3" indicative of RV strain are more commonly found (see Chap. 13).

Chest Radiograph

Characteristic findings on chest radiograph are those of PH (see Chap. 14) and include cardiomegaly on the posteroanterior (PA) view with the lateral view showing the normally clear retrosternal airspace obscured by the enlarged RV. Additional findings include a right main pulmonary artery greater than 16 mm in diameter and left main pulmonary artery prominence below the aortic knob, with "pruning" of the peripheral vasculature (Fig. 64-9).[42] However, some of these

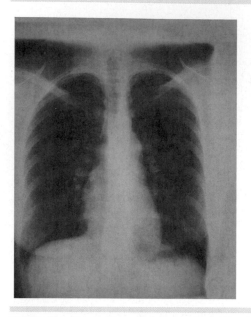

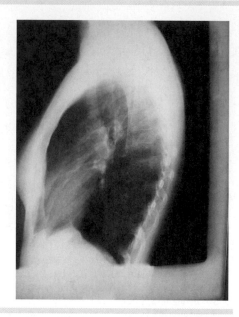

FIGURE 64-9 Chest radiographs from a patient with primary pulmonary hypertension. The posteroanterior view shows prominent central pulmonary arteries with relative oligemia (pruning) of peripheral vessels, while the lateral view demonstrates the enlarged right ventricle filling the retrosternal airspace.

dysfunction not readily apparent on resting studies.[45]

While right side of the heart catheterization may eventually be required for confirmation and more complete assessment of pulmonary hemodynamics, the immediate question to be addressed is the cause of the RV dysfunction. As shown in Fig. 64-11, the possibility of acute and/or chronic pulmonary thromboembolic disease must be addressed by either rapid sequence spiral contrast computed tomography (CT) of chest (i.e., "pulmonary embolism protocol"), radionuclide ventilation/perfusion lung scanning, or pulmonary arteriography. Supplemental studies may include bilateral lower extremity Doppler ultrasound examination and measurements of blood D-dimer levels. Whenever there is concern for acute thromboembolism, immediate anticoagulation

changes can be masked or minimized with the severe hyperinflation that accompanies end-stage emphysema or the smaller lung volumes and severe fibrotic changes seen in certain interstitial lung diseases.

Echocardiogram

Transthoracic echocardiography (TTE) is helpful both in detecting the presence of RV dysfunction and in excluding causation from LV disease processes, mitral valve disease, congenital heart defects, or global disorders of the myocardium (see Chap. 15). The findings of cor pulmonale with two-dimensional echocardiography include RV dilatation and/or hypertrophy, and diminished function.[43] Whenever tricuspid regurgitation is present, Doppler studies can estimate RV and therefore pulmonary artery systolic pressure (PAPs) in millimeters of mercury from the velocity (v) of the regurgitant jet by the formula: $PAPs = (v^2 \times 4) + CVP$, where CVP is central venous pressure.[44] Occasionally, pulmonic regurgitation is present permitting estimation of pulmonary artery diastolic pressure.

DIAGNOSTIC EVALUATION

Strategy

The diagnostic approach ultimately leading to the finding of chronic cor pulmonale is shown in Fig. 64-10. The initial and most basic evaluation should include the history, physical examination, electrocardiogram (ECG), and chest x-ray (PA and lateral). When the initial evaluation suggests some disorder of the cardiopulmonary system, a TTE with two-dimensional and color Doppler modes is indicated. These echocardiographic studies allow assessment of the global myocardium, the LV, and the heart valves, and with the intravenous infusion of agitated saline "bubbles" or color Doppler may detect intracardiac shunts as well (see Chap. 15). Echocardiographic evidence of RV dysfunction and/or PH in the absence of the aforementioned abnormalities is often sufficient to make a diagnosis of cor pulmonale. In some cases, TTE immediately after exercise will reveal RV

Initial Evaluation
- History
- Physical Examination
- Electrocardiogram
- Chest X-Ray

↓

CARDIOPULMONARY DISEASE SUSPECTED

↓

ECHOCARDIOGRAM

↓

RV – Dysfunction Present
LV – Normal
MV – Normal

↓

COR PULMONALE CONFIRMED

FIGURE 64-10 Diagnostic evaluation. Algorithm of process leading to a diagnosis of chronic cor pulmonale. RV, right ventricle; LV, left ventricle; MV, mitral valve.

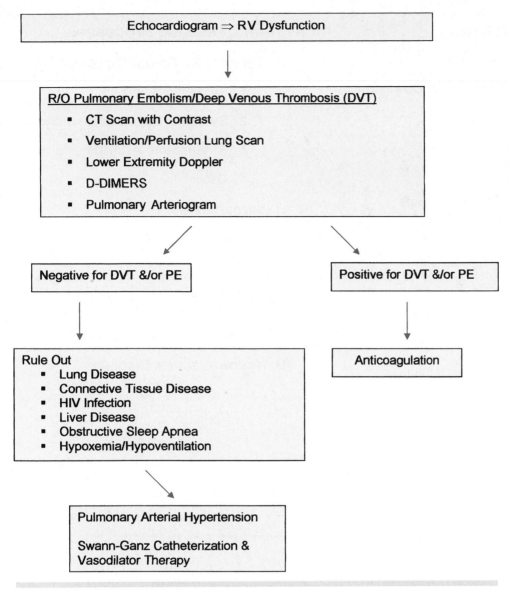

FIGURE 64-11 Evaluation of cor pulmonale. Algorithm of clinical approach to patients with chronic cor pulmonale.

If all of the preceding studies are nonrevealing, by exclusion the diagnosis is primary PH, which is discussed in Chaps. 62 and 73.

Differential Diagnosis

The differential diagnosis of chronic cor pulmonale is the same as that for PH, except that by definition left-sided myocardial or valvular diseases have been excluded. WHO issued a reclassification of PH following a consensus conference in Evian, France, in1998,[46] which is discussed in Chap. 62. Although the diagnostic possibilities are extensive, they may be considered for clinical purposes as due to disorders of (1) lung parenchyma; (2) lung vasculature; (3) systemic disorders; or (4) hypoxic vasoconstriction (Fig. 64-12). The diagnostic strategies outlined in Figs. 64-10 and 64-11 will narrow the diagnostic possibilities to the most likely etiology.

Special Diagnostic Studies

Transesophageal Echocardiogram (TEE) In clinical situations where TTE cannot adequately evaluate either the mitral valve or atrial septum, TEE views may provide valuable information (see Chap. 15). The finding of severe mitral stenosis or regurgitation or an atrial septal defect may lead to surgical correction of these processes with resolution or improvement in PH and cor pulmonale.

Right Heart Catheterization In experienced hands, TTE with or without a TEE study, in concert with available clinical information, is sufficient to make a diagnosis of cor pulmonale (see Chap. 15). Formal catheterization of the right side of the heart with oxygen saturation determinations at various levels is sometimes necessary to determine whether congenital heart defects, such as ventricular or atrial septal defects of patent ductus arteriosus are present and to exclude stenosis of the pulmonic valve or pulmonary arteries.

More commonly, bedside right heart catheterization with a balloon-tipped flow-directed pulmonary artery "Swann-Ganz" catheter is performed to measure pulmonary artery pressures directly. Essential data obtained include right atrial, RV, pulmonary artery, and pulmonary capillary wedge pressures; pulmonary and systemic vascular resistance; and thermodilution cardiac output and cardiac index. In addition to the diagnostic and prognostic information thus obtained, the hemodynamic effects of selective pulmonary vasodilators can be assessed.

Cardiac Magnetic Resonance Imaging (MRI) While echocardiography is excellent for assessing RV function, cardiac MRI may be even more sensitive.[47] Cardiac MRI studies provide such exquisite detail of the heart chambers and valves that serial cardiac catheterizations may be avoided in many instances (see Chap. 22).

with intravenous heparin is indicated while diagnostic studies are being obtained.

When life-threatening pulmonary emboli have been excluded, attention is turned to evaluation of pulmonary or systemic causes for the RV dysfunction. Pulmonary function studies should include spirometry with flow-volume loops, lung volumes by plethysmography, diffusion capacity for carbon monoxide (DLCO), and arterial blood gases. High-resolution CT scanning of the chest may be helpful in evaluation of interstitial lung disorders and may obviate the need for open lung biopsy. Should the history suggest the possibility of sleep-disordered breathing (severe snoring with periods of apnea, daytime somnolence, etc.), a formal sleep study should be ordered. Hypoxia related to underlying lung pathology, altered respiratory drive, or sleep-disordered breathing can be readily assessed by pulse oximetry at rest and with exercise, while overnight monitoring of oxygen saturation may be performed at home. Serologic studies should include screening for connective tissue diseases with ANA and rheumatoid factor levels; antibodies to the HIV virus should be measured in at-risk individuals. Whenever liver disease is expected, antibodies to hepatitis A, B, and C should be measured in addition to standard liver function studies.

I. Parenchymal Lung Disease

A. Obstructive Lung Disease

1. Chronic Obstructive Lung Disease

2. Cystic Fibrosis

3. Bronchiectasis

B. Interstitial Lung Diseases

1. Idiopathic Pulmonary Fibrosis

2. Sarcoidosis

3. Connective Tissue Diseases

4. Miscellaneous

II. Vascular Lung Disease

A. Microvascular

1. Pulmonary Arterial Hypertension

2. Sickle Cell Disease

3. Schistosomiasis

B. Macrovascular

1. Chronic Thromboembolic Pulmonary Hypertension

2. Pulmonary Artery Stenoses

3. Extrinsic Compression

III. Systemic Disease Processes

A. Connective Tissue Diseases

1. Systemic Sclerosis

2. Systemic Lupus Erythematous

3. Rheumatoid Arthritis

4. Other

B. Sarcoidosis

IV. Hypoxemia

A. Altitude

B. Alveolar Hypoventilation

C. Sleep Disordered Breathing

D. Neuromuscular Disorders

FIGURE 64-12 Differential diagnosis of cor pulmonale. Clinical classification of causes of chronic cor pulmonale.

TREATMENT

Supplemental Oxygen Therapy

Regardless of the underlying disease leading to cor pulmonale, alveolar hypoxia will aggravate and compound the pathologic process through compensatory regional pulmonary vasoconstriction. In recognition of this fact, Medicare criteria for supplemental oxygen are less stringent for patients with cor pulmonale, requiring a $Pa_{O_2} < 59$ mmHg or $Sa_{O_2} < 89$ percent for patients with cor pulmonale versus a $Pa_{O_2} < 55$ or $Sa_{O_2} < 88$ percent for other patients. It is imperative that every patient with cor pulmonale be assessed as to his or her need for supplemental oxygen therapy. The need for supplemental oxygen should be assessed at least by measuring oxygen saturation at rest and with ambulation; monitoring for nocturnal oxygen desaturation is appropriate in those patients who remain normoxic with ambulation and those whose history suggest sleep-disordered breathing.

Supplemental oxygen may be supplied in various ways but most easily via nasal cannula in liters per minute sufficient to maintain $Sa_{O_2} < 90$ percent and/or $Pa_{O_2} < 60$ mmHg. It is important that

portable oxygen be prescribed so that patients can remain as mobile and active as their conditions permit. Humidification of the home oxygen delivery helps alleviate the drying effect of oxygen delivered via nasal cannula. The maximal rate of delivery of home oxygen systems is about 6 L/min; selected patients with greater oxygen requirements may maintain higher levels of Sa_{O_2} when oxygen is delivered via a transtracheal catheter.

General Measures

Useful adjuncts in the treatment of cor pulmonale include diuretics, systemic anticoagulation, supplemental oxygen, and perhaps digitalis.[48] Patients often respond well to a combination of a loop diuretic, such as furosemide, and the potassium-sparing diuretic aldactone. Anticoagulation with warfarin (Coumadin) has proven beneficial in patients with primary PH[49] and is often used in patients with cor pulmonale resulting from COPD. Although similar data are not available for other causes of PH and cor pulmonale, Warfarin therapy is generally recommended unless a relative contraindication exists (e.g., history of bleeding varices, liver dysfunction, or hemoptysis). In contrast to full anticoagulation that is proper for treating known thromboembolic disease or other cardiac disorders, the recommended international normalized ratio range is 1.5 to 2.5 for PH and cor pulmonale as prophylaxis. The value of digitalis in the treatment of cor pulmonale is controversial, but in the circumstance of decompensated RV failure it may have some value. Digitalis, calcium channel blockers, and warfarin have comprised the "conventional" treatment arm in studies comparing conventional versus specific pulmonary vasodilators in addition to conventional treatment for primary PH.[50]

Disease-Specific Therapy

Since cor pulmonale by definition results from some pulmonary process, it follows that treatment of the underlying disease, if successful, should improve the function of the RV. Unfortunately, medical treatment for most established diseases of the lungs, such as COPD, idiopathic pulmonary fibrosis, and cystic fibrosis, may at best slow progression of the disease process and in most instances is merely symptomatic. *Smoking cessation* and avoidance of exposure to secondary smoke is critically important for all patients; indeed, patients with COPD who are able to stop smoking have improved survival as compared to those COPD patients who continue. Immunosuppressive therapy is usually administered to patients with connective tissue diseases and those with interstitial lung disorders, although only a minority of patients in the latter category responds. Idiopathic pulmonary fibrosis is a particularly difficult disorder to treat. Although reports of improvements in pulmonary function and oxygenation in patients receiving gamma-interferon injections thrice weekly[51] have engendered hope in both patients and physicians, some patients receiving gamma interferon have fared less well.[52] Supplemental oxygen therapy is specific therapy when hypoxemia without parenchymal lung disease is the cause of cor pulmonale. Hypoxemia resulting from sleep-disordered breathing may be alleviated by use of positive pressure [continuous positive airway pressure (CPAP) or bilevel positive airway pressure] masks along with supplemental oxygen for obstructive sleep apnea, by central nervous system stimulants for central sleep apnea, and by weight reduction for the obesity-hypoventilation syndrome. Hypoxemia with resultant cor pulmonale as a consequence of neuromuscular disorders may respond to supplemental oxygen along with nocturnal ventilation using positive pressure masks, negative pressure body suits, or mechanical ventilation delivered through a tracheostomy tube. Chronic thromboembolic PH with cor pulmonale is treated with lifelong anticoagulation using warfarin; placement of an inferior vena cava filter is recommended. Patients with clots in more central pulmonary vessels may benefit from thromboendarterectomy (see Chap. 101). However, none of the aforementioned "specific treatments" is curative and cor pulmonale usually progresses over time.

Pulmonary Vasodilator Therapy

A variety of pulmonary vasodilator agents is available for the treatment of cor pulmonale caused by pulmonary arterial hypertension. PH and cor pulmonale resulting from other processes such as left-sided heart or valve disease, disorders of respiration and/or hypoxemia, or chronic thromboembolic disease would not be expected to respond to pulmonary vasodilator therapy and such therapy is generally not approved and often contraindicated. In some instances, however, a pulmonary vasoconstrictor component coexists such that a trial of specific pulmonary vasodilator therapy may be warranted. Some patients with sarcoidosis present with PH and cor pulmonale disproportionate to the degree of parenchymal disease and may respond to pulmonary vasodilators.[53] Patients with chronic thromboembolic PH and cor pulmonale may partially respond to pulmonary vasodilator therapy indicating a component of vasoconstriction in the smaller pulmonary vessels.[54]

A variety of pulmonary vasodilator agents have been used in the treatment of PH and cor pulmonale (see also Chap. 62). There was initial enthusiasm for calcium channel blockers in the 1990s when Rich et al. demonstrated that those patients with primary PH who responded acutely to high doses of diltiazem or verapamil, as demonstrated by >20 percent reduction in mean PAP and pulmonary vascular resistance ("responders"), had an excellent prognosis over 5 years compared to the group of "nonresponders."[49] However, these data applied only to patients with primary PH and the percentage of "responders" now appears closer to 10 percent of patients referred to centers specializing in the treatment of PH. Thus, calcium channel blockers have only a minor role in the treatment of patients with most forms of cor pulmonale.

The medical treatment of primary PH and other forms of PH has been transformed by continuous intravenous infusion of *prostacyclin and its analogues (epoprostenol, PGI₂, Flolan).*[50] Prostacyclin has relatively specific vasodilatory effects on the pulmonary microvasculature along with antiplatelet effects; over time it may also promote vascular remodeling.[55] Prostacyclin is the "gold standard" in the medical treatment of primary pulmonary arterial hypertension, but is ineffective in the larger group of patients with severe COPD or interstitial pulmonary fibrosis or when hypoxemia is the cause for PH. Prostacyclin may also be administered subcutaneously,[56] orally[57] or by inhalation,[58] albeit with less effect than the intravenous route (see also Chap. 62).

Endothelin receptor blockers (ERBs) are the most recent class of drugs for the treatment of PH. The ERBs prevent the binding of the potent vasoconstrictor endothelin-1 (ET-1) to its receptors on pulmonary vascular smooth muscle cells, thereby producing vasodilatation of the pulmonary vascular bed. There is one currently commercially available ERB, bosentan (Tracleer), which blocks the binding of endothelin to its A and B receptors (ET_A, ET_B).[59] Bosentan has proven effective in improving the pulmonary hemodynamics and functional class of patients with PH and has received Food and Drug Administration approval for these indications. There are additional ERBs in clinical trials that selectively block ET_A. The receptor ET_A regulates vasoconstriction, whereas ET_B regulates the inflammatory and fibroproliferative actions of ET-1. Oral Sildenafil may play a role in the treatment of PH.[60]

Lung Transplantation

Lung transplantation has become an accepted form of treatment for a variety of end-stage lung and pulmonary vascular diseases. Indeed, the first successful lung transplant was actually a combined heart–lung transplant performed for PH and cor pulmonale in 1981 at Stanford. As the discipline of lung transplantation has evolved over the past two decades, heart–lung transplantation has been supplanted by single or bilateral lung transplantation,[61] with bilateral lung transplantation becoming the transplantation procedure of choice for primary PH.[62] In fact, unless the PH is totally reversed with medical therapy, an unlikely scenario, bilateral lung transplantation offers the *only* definitive treatment for cor pulmonale. One argument in favor of combined heart–lung transplantation for PH was concern that the extremely dilated and hypocontractile RV of advanced cor pulmonale was irreversibly damaged. However, studies have shown that the RV almost immediately begins to diminish in size with improved contractility following lung transplantation with restoration of more normal pulmonary vascular resistance.[63] The recuperative abilities of the RV are described in Fig. 64-13, which shows a patient with

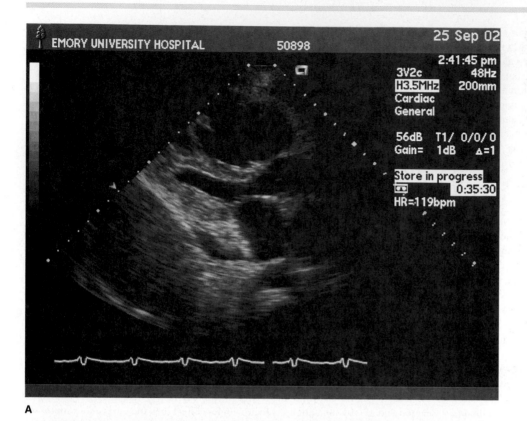

A

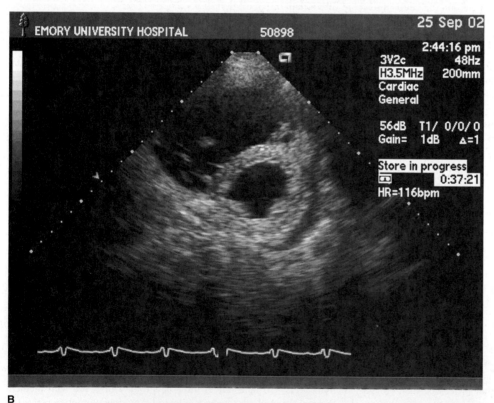

B

FIGURE 64-13 Resolution of chronic cor pulmonale by lung transplantation. Panels A-C represent echocardiographic findings 2 months prior to bilateral lung transplantation in a patient with primary pulmonary hypertension. Panels D-F represent echocardiographic findings 2 months following transplant. Panels A & D depict the horizontal long axis; Panels B & E show the short axis; Panels C & F represent the apical 4-chamber view. Note the diminution in right ventricle (RV) size, resolution of RV impingement on the left ventricle (LV) with normalization of LV size following transplant.

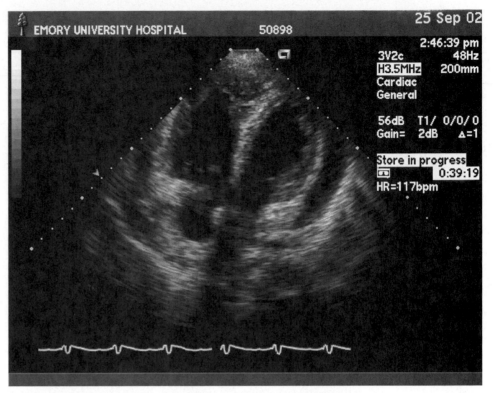

C

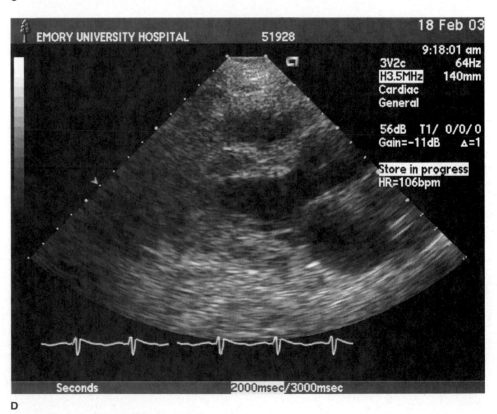

D

FIGURE 64-13 *(Continued)*

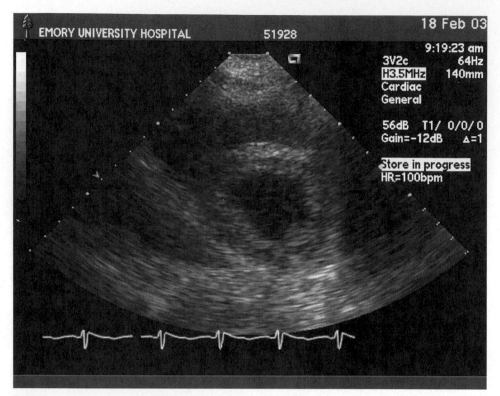

E

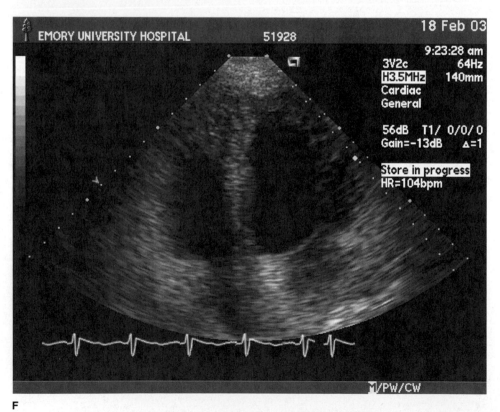

F

FIGURE 64-13 (*Continued*)

primary PH and New York Heart Association (NYHA) class IV right-sided heart failure who received a bilateral lung transplant at Emory University Hospital. The transthoracic echocardiogram demonstrated severe RV dilatation and hypocontractility 2 months prior to the transplant procedure, which was markedly improved at 2 months posttransplant.

PROGNOSIS

The prognosis for patients with chronic cor pulmonale may be most quantitatively assessed by review of the natural history of primary PH before there was effective treatment, as documented in the National Institutes of Healths Registry begun in the 1970s.[64] The median survival was 2.8 years, with 1-, 3-, and 5-year survival of 65, 50, and 33 percent, respectively. However, the initial hemodynamic data from right side of the heart catheterization identified subgroups with greater likelihood of death. Subjects at greatest risk were those with systemic levels of mean pulmonary artery pressure (>85 mmHg), cardiac index < 2.0 L/min/m^2, and/or mean right atrial pressure > 20 mmHg. Moreover, clinical assessment by NYHA functional class was highly predictive of outcome with median survival for patients in class I and II at 58.6 months, class III at 31.5 months, and class IV at 6 months. Treatment of primary PH with continuous intravenous infusion of prostacyclin (Flolan), which is indicated for treatment of NYHA class III and IV patients, has roughly doubled survival.[65] Patients with cor pulmonale resulting from COPD have a greater likelihood of dying than similar patients with COPD alone.[66] While information is not readily available for other disease processes resulting in cor pulmonale, clinical experience strongly supports the notion that cor pulmonale, regardless of etiology, is an independent risk factor for earlier demise.

References

1. White PD. Pulmonary heart disease-cor pulmonale (pulmonary hypertension): The emphysema heart. In: White PD, ed. *Heart Disease.* New York: Macmillan; 1931:404–409.

2. White PD. Pulmonary heart disease-acute and chronic cor pulmonale (pulmonary hypertension). In: White PD, ed. *Heart Disease,* 2d ed. New York: Macmillan; 1937:332–343.

3. White PD. pulmonary heart disease-acute and chronic cor pulmonale (pulmonary hypertension). In: White PD, ed. *Heart Disease,* 3d ed. New York: MacMillan; 1944:458–473.

4. Osler W. Hypertrophy and dilatation. In: Fye WB, ed. *William Osler's Collected Papers on the Cardiovascular System,* 2d ed. Birmingham: The Classics of Cardiology Library;1985:628–640.

5. World Health Organization. Chronic cor pulmonale. A report of the expert committee. *Circulation* 1963;27:594–598.

6. Laennec RTH. *A Treatise on Diseases of the Chest.* London: T. and G. Underwood; 1821.

7. World Health Organization. *Consultation on the Development of a Comprehensive Approach for the Prevention and Control of Chronic Respiratory Diseases.* WHO, 2001:6.

8. Williams BT, Nicholl JP. Prevalence of hypoxaemic chronic obstructive lung disease with reference to long-term oxygen therapy. *Lancet* 1985; I:369–372.

9. Brigham KL, Newman JH. The pulmonary circulation. In: Basics of Respiratory Disease, *Am Thorac Soc* 1979;5:15–19.

10. Reeves JT, Weil JV. Chronic mountain sickness: A view from the crow's nest. *Adv Exp Med Biol* 2001;502:419–437.

11. Dickens C. *The Works of Charles Dickens: The Pickwick Papers.* Boston: Houghton, Osgood and Co.; 1879.

12. Snapper JR, Harris, TR, Brigham, KL. Effect of changing lung mass on lung water and permeability-surface area in sheep. *J Appl Physiol: Respirat Environ Exercise Physiol* 1982;52:1591–1597.

13. Van Miegham W, Demedts M: Cardiopulmonary function after lobectomy or pneumonectomy for pulmonary neoplasm. *Respir Med* 1989; 83:199.

14. Fedillo PF, Auger WR, Channick RN, et al. Chronic thromboembolic pulmonary hypertension. *Clin Chest Med* 1995;16:353–374.

15. Weitzenblum E. Chronic cor pulmonale. *BMJ Heart* 2003;89:225–230.

16. Loyd JE, Tillman BF, Atkinson, JB, et al. Mediastinal fibrosis complicating histoplasmosis. *Medicine* 1988;67:295–310.

17. Mata-Greenwood E, Meyrick B, Soifer SJ, et al. Expression of VEGF and its receptors FLT-1 and FLK-1/KDR are altered in lambs with increased pulmonary blood flow and pulmonary hypertension. *Am J Physiol Lung Cell Mol Physiol* 2003;285:L209–L221.

18. Mata-Greenwood E, Meyrick B, Fineman JR, et al. Alterations in TGF-β_1 expression in lambs with increased pulmonary blood flow and pulmonary hypertension. *Am J Physiol Lung Cell Mol Physiol* 2003; 285(1):L209–L221.

19. Jones PL, Chapados R, Baldwin HS, et al. Altered hemodynamics controls matrix metalloproteinase activity and tenascin-C expression in neonatal pig lung. *Am J Physiol Lung Cell Mol Physiol* 2002;282: L26–35.

20. Birukov KG, Birukova AA, Dudek SM, et al. Shear stress-mediated cytoskeletal remodeling and cortactin translocation in pulmonary endothelial cells. *Am J Respir Cell Mol Biol* 2002;26:453–464.

21. Vitvvitsky EV, Griffin JP, Collins MH, et al. Increased pulmonary blood flow produces endothelial cell dysfunction in neonatal swine. *Ann Thorac Surg* 1998;66:1372–1377.

22. Berman EB, Barst RJ. Eisenmenger's syndrome: Current management. *Prog Cardiovasc Dis* 2002;45:129–138.

23. Lane KB, Machado RD, Pauciulo MW, et al. Heterozygous germline mutations in BMPR2, encoding a TGF-beta receptor, cause familial primary pulmonary hypertension. The International PPH Consortium. *Nat Genet* 2000;26:81–84.

24. Thomas AQ, Gaddipati R, Newman JH, et al. Genetics of primary pulmonary hypertension. *Clin Chest Med* 2001;22:477–491.

25. Fagan KA, Badesch DB. Pulmonary hypertension associated with connective tissue disease. *Prog Cardiovasc Dis* 2002;45:225–234.

26. Meyrick B, Reid L. Pulmonary hypertension. Anatomic and physiologic correlates. *Clin Chest Med* 1983;4:199–217.

27. Perkett EA, Brigham KL, Meyrick B. Continuous air embolization into sheep causes sustained pulmonary hypertension and increased pulmonary vasoreactivity. *Am J Pathol* 1988;132:444–454.

28. Rappaport E. Cor pulmonale. In: Murray J., Nadel J. eds. *Textbook of Respiratory Medicine,* 3rd ed. New York: Saunders; 2000:1635.

29. Macnee W. Pathophysiology of cor pulmonale in chronic obstructive pulmonary disease. *Am J Respir Crit Care Med* 1994;150:833–852.

30. Yamamoto S, Sawada K, Shimomura H, et al. On the nature of cell death during remodeling of the hypertrophied human myocardium. *J Mol Cell Cardiol* 2000;32:161–175.

31. Davis KL, Laine GA, Geissler HJ, et al. Effects of myocardial edema on the development of myocardial interstitial fibrosis. *Microcirculation* 2000;7:269–280.

32. Ecarnot-Laubriet A, De Luca K, Vandroux D, et al. Downregulation and nuclear relocation of MLP during the progression of right ventricular hypertrophy induced by chronic pressure overload. *J Mol Cell Cardiol* 2000;32:2385–2395.

33. Sato H, Nagai T, Kuppuswamy D, et al. Microtubule stabilization in pressure overload cardiac hypertrophy. *J Cell Biol* 1997;139: 963–973.

34. Kuramochi T, Honda M, Tanaka K, et al. Calcium transients in singly myocytes and membraneous ultrastructures during the development of cardiac hypertrophy and heart failure in rats. *Clin Exp Pharmacol Physiol* 1994;21:1009–1018.

35. Hamrell BB, Dey SK. Sarcomere shortening velocity in pressure overload hypertrophied rabbit right ventricular myocardium at physiological sarcomere lengths. *J Mol Cell Cardiol* 1993;25:1483–1500.

36. Weitzenblum E, Apprill M, Oswald M, et al. Pulmonary hemodynamics in patients with chronic obstructive pulmonary disease before and during an episode of peripheral edema. *Chest* 1994;105:1377–1382.

37. Hopkins WE, Waggoner AD. Severe pulmonary hypertension without right ventricular failure: The unique hearts of patients with Eisenmenger syndrome. *Am J Cardiol* 2002;89:34–38.

38. Hirose Y, Ishida Y, Hayashida K, et al. Viable but denervated right ventricular myocardium: A case of Eisenmenger reaction. *Cardiology* 1997;88:609–612.

39. Rich S, Dantzker D, Ayres S, et al. Primary pulmonary hypertension: A national prospective study. *Ann Intern Med* 1987;107:216–223.

40. Rappaport E. Cor pulmonale. In: Murray F, Nadel J, eds. *Textbook of Respiratory Medicine,* 3rd ed. Philadelphia: Saunders; 2000:1631–1648.

41. Ahearn GS, Tapson VF, Rebeiz A, et al. Electrocardiography to define clinical status in primary pulmonary hypertension and pulmonary arterial hypertension secondary to collagen vascular disease. *Chest* 2002; 122(2):524–527.

42. Fraser RG, Paré JAP, Paré PD, et al, eds. Pulmonary hypertension and edema. In Fraser WD. *Diagnosis of Diseases of the Chest,* 3rd ed, Philadelphia: Saunders, 1990:1823–1968.

43. Jardin F, Dubourg O, Bourdarias JP. Echocardiographic pattern of acute cor pulmonale. *Chest* 1997;111(1):209–217.

44. Berger M, Haimowitz A, Van Tosh A, et al. Quantitative assessment of pulmonary hypertension in patients with tricuspid regurgitation using continuous wave Doppler ultrasound. *J Am Coll Cardiol* 1985;(2): 359–365.

45. Bossone E, Avelar E, Bach DS, et al. Diagnostic value of resting tricuspid regurgitation velocity and right ventricular ejection flow parameters for the detection of exercise induced pulmonary arterial hypertension. *Int J Cardiovasc Imaging* 2000;(6):429–436.

46. Rich S, ed. *Primary Pulmonary Hypertension—Executive Summary from the World Symposium—Primary Pulmonary Hypertension.* WHO 1998:1–27.

47. Saba TS, Foster J, Cockburn M, et al. Ventricular mass index using magnetic resonance imaging accurately estimates pulmonary artery pressure. *Eur Respir J* 2002;6:1519–1524.

48. Rubin L. Primary pulmonary hypertension. *Curr Concept Mass Med Soc* 1997;336(2):111–117.

49. Rich S, Kaufmann E, Levy PS. The effect of high doses of calcium-channel blockers on survival in primary pulmonary hypertension. *N Engl J Med* 1992;327(2):76–81.

50. Barst R, Rubin L, Long W, et al. A comparison of continuous intravenous epoprostenol (prostacyclin) with conventional therapy for primary pulmonary hypertension. *N Engl J Med* 1996;334(5):296–301.

51. Ziesche R, Hofbauer E, Wittmann K, et al. A preliminary study of long-term treatment with interferon gamma-1b and low-dose prednisolone in patients with idiopathic pulmonary fibrosis. *N Engl J Med* 1999; 341(17):1264–1269.

52. Honoré I, Nunes H, Groussard O, et al. Acute respiratory failure after interferon-γ therapy of end-stage pulmonary fibrosis. *Am J Respir Crit Care Med* 2003;167:953–957.

53. Preston IR, Klinger JR, Landzberg MJ, et al. Vasoresponsiveness of sarcoidosis-associated pulmonary hypertension. *Chest* 2001;120(3): 866–872.

54. Dantzker DR, Bower JS. Partial reversibility of chronic pulmonary hypertension caused by pulmonary thromboembolic disease. *Am Rev Respir Dis* 1981;124(2):129–131.

55. Archer S, Rich S. Primary pulmonary hypertension: A vascular biology and translational research "work in progress." *Circulation* 2000;28: 2781–2791.

56. Simonneau G, Barst RJ, Galie N, et al. Continuous subcutaneous infusion of trepostinil, a prostacyclin analogue, in patients with pulmonary arterial hypertension. *Am J Respir Crit Care Med* 2002;165:800–804.

57. Galie N, Humbert M, Vachiery JL, et al. Effects of beraprost sodium, an oral prostacyclin analogue, in patients with pulmonary arterial hypertension: A randomized, double-blind, placebo-controlled trial. *J Am Coll Cardiol* 2002;39(9):1496–1502.

58. Olschewski H, Simonneau G, Galie N, et al. Inhaled iloprost for severe pulmonary hypertension. *N Engl J Med* 2002;347(5):322–329.

59. Channick R, Simonneau G, Sitbon O, et al. Effects of the dual endothelin-receptor antagonist bosentan in patients with pulmonary hypertension: A randomized placebo-controlled study. *Lancet* 2001;358(9288): 1119–1123.

60. Ghofrani HA, Wiedemann R, Rose F, et al. Combination therapy with oral sildenafil and inhaled iloprost for severe pulmonary hypertension. *Ann Intern Med* 2002;136(7):515–522.

61. Mendeloff EN, Meyers BF, Sundt TM, et al. Lung transplantation for pulmonary vascular disease. *Ann Thorac Surg* 2002;73(1):209–217.

62. Conte JV, Borja MJ, Patel CB, et al. Lung transplantation for primary and secondary pulmonary hypertension. *Ann Thorac Surg* 2001;72(5): 1673–1679.

63. Katz WE, Gasior TA, Quinlan JJ, et al. Immediate effects of lung transplantation on right ventricular morphology and function of patients with variable degrees of pulmonary hypertension. *J Am Coll Cardiol* 1996; 27(2):384–391.

64. D'Alonzo GE, Barst RJ, Ayres SM, et al. Survival in patients with primary pulmonary hypertension. *Ann Intern Med* 1991;115(5):343–349.

65. Barst RJ, Rubin LJ, McGoon MD, et al. Survival in primary pulmonary hypertension with long-term continuous intravenous prostacyclin. *Ann Intern Med* 1994;121(6):409–415.

66. Incalzi RA, Fuzo L, De Rosa M, et al. Electrocardiographic signs in chronic cor pulmonale: A negative prognostic finding in chronic obstructive pulmonary disease. *Circulation* 1999;99(12):1600–1605.

VALVULAR HEART DISEASE

ACUTE RHEUMATIC FEVER

Simon Chakko / Alan L. Bisno

DEFINITION

Rheumatic fever is an inflammatory disease that appears as a delayed nonsuppurative sequel to group A streptococcal infection of the pharynx. It affects the heart, joints, central nervous system, skin, and subcutaneous tissues with varying frequency. Its clinical manifestations include migratory polyarthritis, fever, carditis, and less frequently, Sydenham's chorea, subcutaneous nodules, and erythema marginatum. Rheumatic fever is a clinical syndrome for which no specific diagnostic test exists. No symptom, sign, or laboratory test result is pathognomonic, although several combinations of them are diagnostic.[1] Its importance relates to involvement of the heart, which, though rarely fatal during the acute stage, may lead to rheumatic valvular disease, a chronic and progressive condition that causes cardiac disability or death many years after the initial event.

ETIOLOGY

Antecedent infection of the upper respiratory tract with group A streptococcus is necessary for the development of rheumatic fever. This etiologic relation has been clearly established by clinical, immunologic, and epidemiologic studies.[1,2] Cutaneous streptococcal infection may lead to acute glomerulonephritis but has never been demonstrated to cause acute rheumatic fever (ARF).

At least one third of patients deny previous sore throat, and cultures of the pharynx are often negative for group A streptococci at the onset of ARF. However, an antibody response to streptococcal extracellular products can be demonstrated in almost all cases, and the attack rate of ARF is strongly correlated with the magnitude of the antibody response.

A clear sequential relation between outbreaks of streptococcal pharyngitis or scarlet fever and ARF has been demonstrated in epidemiologic studies of military recruit camps; such outbreaks can be eradicated when streptococcal infection is controlled by chemotherapy.[3] Prompt and effective penicillin therapy of streptococcal pharyngitis prevents the initial attack of ARF (so-called primary prevention),[4] and continuous chemoprophylaxis against streptococcal infection (secondary prophylaxis) prevents its recurrences.[5]

EPIDEMIOLOGY

ARF is a major health problem in the developing countries of Asia, Africa, Middle East, and Latin America. A World Health Organization survey conducted between 1986 and 1990 estimated the prevalence of ARF and chronic rheumatic heart disease per 1000 schoolchildren to be 12.6 in Zambia, 10.2 in Sudan, and 7.9 in Bolivia.[6] Hospital statistics from many developing countries reveal that 10 to 35 percent of all cardiac admissions are for ARF and rheumatic heart disease.[6,7] Exceedingly high attack rates have been reported among aboriginal populations in New Zealand and Australia.[8]

ARF is most common among children in the 5 to 15 year age group. There is no clear-cut sex predilection, although there is a female preponderance in rheumatic mitral stenosis and in Sydenham's chorea occurring after puberty. The attack rate of ARF following untreated exudative tonsillitis varies, depending upon the epidemiologic circumstances and the rheumatogenic potential of prevalent streptococcal strains. This rate has been reported to approximate 3 percent during epidemics in military recruit camps[9] but only 0.4 percent after endemically occurring infections in untreated children in civilian populations in the United States. One third or more[10] of the cases occur after asymptomatic streptococcal infections. A striking feature of the epidemiology of ARF is the propensity of patients who have suffered an initial attack to experience recurrences of the disease following group A streptococcal infections.

Strains of group A streptococci vary in their propensity to elicit ARF. Although the precise factor or factors that confer this property are unknown, highly rheumatogenic strains share certain biologic characteristics. Only a limited number of the more than 90 streptococcal M-protein types have been strongly and repetitively associated with ARF.[11] These strains are often heavily encapsulated, a feature manifested by the formation of mucoid colonies on blood-agar plates. Their M-protein molecules share a particular surface-exposed antigenic domain against which ARF patients mount a strong immunoglobulin G response.[12] These characteristics were established, however, by study of ARF cases and outbreaks in the United States and Great Britain; they remain to be validated for cases occurring in third world countries or among aboriginal populations.

The twentieth century witnessed a dramatic decline in the incidence of ARF and rheumatic heart disease in industrialized nations.[13]

The reasons for this decline are unclear, but they most likely relate to improved living standards (including decreases in household crowding), efficacy of antimicrobials in treatment of acute streptococcal pharyngitis and prevention of recurrent rheumatic attacks, and changes in the rheumatogenicity of prevalent streptococcal strains. The incidence of ARF and the prevalence of rheumatic heart disease are now very low in North America and Western Europe. The disease is very rare in affluent suburban populations[14] but persists among disadvantaged families dwelling in the crowded urban inner cities.[15] The higher incidence rates reported in blacks as compared to whites appear to be due to socioeconomic rather than genetic factors.

There is no evidence of a decline in the frequency of streptococcal pharyngitis concomitant with the dramatic decline in ARF incidence. This strongly suggests that there have been changes in the rheumatogenicity of streptococcal strains currently prevalent in civilian populations of North America and Western Europe.

In the mid-1980s, after decades of decline, outbreaks of ARF occurred in numerous cities and in two military recruit camps in the United States.[13] The largest epidemic occurred in Salt Lake City, Utah, and the surrounding intermountain area[16] where over 500 cases were diagnosed between 1985 and 2000.

PATHOGENESIS

The exact mechanism by which group A streptococcus causes ARF remains unexplained. Possibilities include (1) toxic effects of streptococcal products, particularly streptolysins S or O, which are capable of inducing tissue injury; (2) a serum sickness–like reaction; and (3) autoimmune phenomena induced by similarity or identity of certain streptococcal antigens to a wide variety of human tissue antigens. Although no mechanism has been unequivocally proven, autoimmunity, or, more precisely, molecular mimicry, appears to be most likely. There are shared epitopes between cardiac myosin and streptococcal M protein that lead to cross-reactive humoral and T-cell immunity against group A streptococci and the heart.[17] Epitopes of streptococcal M protein also share antigenic determinants with heart valves, sarcolemmal membrane proteins, synovium, and articular cartilage.[18] Circulating antibodies that react with neurons of the caudate and subthalamic nuclei and with group A streptococcal cell membranes have been found in many children with Sydenham's chorea.[19,20] These cross-reactive and toxic phenomena could explain many of the clinical manifestations of ARF, but in the absence of a credible animal model of the disease, there is no direct proof that they do so.

Even in severe epidemics of exudative pharyngitis, ARF affects only a small proportion of infected persons. This fact, coupled with the known familial aggregation of ARF cases, has long suggested the possibility of a genetic predisposition to rheumatic attacks. Studies of the distribution of class 1 HLA antigens in patients with rheumatic fever versus healthy patients have been inconclusive. An intriguing potential link between the genetic constitution of the human host and susceptibility to ARF is the identification of certain alloantigens that are expressed in a higher proportion of circulating B lymphocytes of patients with rheumatic fever and their family members than in those of patients with poststreptococcal glomerulonephritis or normal controls.[21]

PATHOLOGY

ARF is characterized by exudative and proliferative inflammatory lesions of the connective tissue, most notably of the heart, joints, and subcutaneous tissue. When carditis ensues, all layers of the heart are involved. Pericarditis is common, and fibrinous pericarditis is occasionally present. The pericardial inflammation usually resolves over time with no clinically significant sequelae. In the myocardium initially there is fragmentation of collagen fibers, lymphocytic infiltration, and fibrinoid degeneration. This is followed by the appearance of myocardial Aschoff nodules that are considered pathognomonic of ARF. The Aschoff nodule consists of an area of central necrosis surrounded by lymphocytes, plasma cells, and large mononuclear and giant multinucleate cells. Many of these cells have an elongated nucleus with a clear area just within the nuclear membrane ("owl-eyed" nucleus). These cells are called Anitschkow myocytes, although histochemical studies suggest that they are of macrophage-histiocyte origin. Aschoff nodules may also be found in endomyocardial biopsy specimens obtained from patients with acute rheumatic carditis.[22]

Endocardial involvement is responsible for chronic rheumatic valvulitis.[23] Small fibrinous, verrucous vegetations, 1 to 2 mm in diameter, are seen on the atrial surface at sites of valve coaptation and on the chordae tendineae. Even when no vegetations are present, there is edema and inflammation of the valve leaflets. A thickened and fibrotic patch (MacCallum's patch) may be found in the posterior left atrial wall. It is believed to be the effect of the mitral regurgitant jet impinging on the left atrial wall.[23] Healing of the valvulitis leads to granulation and fibrosis of the leaflets and fusion of the chordae. Valvular stenosis or incompetence may result. The mitral valve is involved most frequently, followed by the aortic valve. Tricuspid and pulmonic valves are usually spared.

CLINICAL MANIFESTATIONS

ARF may involve different organ systems such as heart, joints, skin, and central nervous system. The clinical picture depends upon the systems involved, and the manifestations may appear singly or in various combinations (Table 65-1). Five clinical features (carditis, polyarthritis, chorea, subcutaneous nodules, and erythema marginatum) are so characteristic of the disease that they are classified as major manifestations according to the Jones criteria (Table 65-2).[24] Additional findings such as fever, arthralgia, heart block, and acute phase reactants in the blood (i.e., elevation of erythrocyte sedimentation rate and serum concentration of C-reactive protein) are com-

TABLE 65-1 Clinical Manifestations of Acute Rheumatic Fever

General
  High fever, lassitude, prostration, tachycardia
Cardiac
  Cardiomegaly, congestive heart failure
  Acute pericarditis, pericardial effusion
  Apical pansystolic murmur (mitral regurgitation)
  Apical mid-diastolic murmur (Carey Coombs)
  Basal diastolic (aortic regurgitation)
Dermatologic
  Subcutaneous nodules
  Erythema marginatum
Rheumatologic
  Arthralgia
  Migratory polyarthritis
Neurologic
  Sydenham's chorea

monly present in ARF but are nonspecific in nature and are therefore classified as minor manifestations.

The latent period from the onset of streptococcal sore throat to the onset of initial and recurrent attacks of ARF varies between 1 and 5 weeks with a median of 19 days. The mode of onset is quite variable. An abrupt onset with fever and toxicity is common in patients in whom acute polyarthritis is the presenting complaint. The onset may be insidious or even subclinical when mild carditis is the initial manifestation. Most attacks begin with polyarthritis, and occasionally this may be preceded by abdominal pain and fleeting signs of peritoneal inflammation, which may be misdiagnosed as acute appendicitis. Overall, arthritis occurs in approximately 75 percent of first attacks, carditis in 40 to 50 percent, chorea in 15 percent, and subcutaneous nodules and erythema marginatum in less than 10 percent.[25] These figures may vary widely, however.

TABLE 65-2 Guidelines for the Diagnosis of the Initial Attack of Rheumatic Fever (Jones Criteria, Updated in 1992)*

Major Manifestations	Minor Manifestations	Supporting Evidence for Antecedent Group A Streptococcal Infection
Carditis	Clinical findings	Positive throat culture
Polyarthritis	Arthralgia	or rapid streptococcal
Chorea	Fever	antigen test
Erythema marginatum	Laboratory findings	Elevated or rising strep-
Subcutaneous nodules	Elevated acute phase	tococcal antibody titer
	reactants	
	Erythrocyte sedimentation	
	rate	
	C-reactive protein	
	Prolonged P-R interval	

*If supported by evidence of preceding group A streptococcal infection, the presence of two major manifestations or one major and two minor manifestations indicates a high probability of acute rheumatic fever.
SOURCE: From Dajani AS, Ayoub E, Bierman FZ, et al. Guidelines for the diagnosis of rheumatic fever: Jones criterion, updated 1992. Reproduced by permission of *JAMA* 1992;268:2069–2073, copyrighted 1992, American Medical Association.

Carditis

Carditis is the only manifestation of ARF that has the potential to cause long-term disability and death. Severe valvular regurgitation may precipitate intractable heart failure and may be fatal during the acute phase of the disease. Fortunately, this complication is quite rare. Carditis, if present, usually appears within the first 3 weeks of the illness. The cardiac involvement is frequently mild or even asymptomatic, but occasionally the course can be fulminant. In most patients with acute rheumatic fever, cardiac enzymes, such as troponin I, are normal or only minimally elevated.[26–28] The diagnosis of carditis requires the presence of one of the following four manifestations: (1) organic cardiac murmurs not previously present, (2) cardiomegaly, (3) pericarditis, and (4) congestive heart failure.

Valvulitis is characterized by characteristic murmurs that are almost always present unless they are obscured by a loud pericardial friction rub, a large pericardial effusion, or low cardiac output. Mitral regurgitation (MR) leads to a blowing holosystolic murmur best heard at the apex and radiating to the axilla and occasionally to the base of the heart or the back (see Chap. 12). Hemodynamic and surgical pathologic studies indicate that mitral annular dilatation is usually the initial abnormality and predisposes to lengthening or rupture of the chordae tendineae and prolapse of the anterior leaflet.[29] Increased flow across the mitral valve in the presence of valvulitis may produce a mid-diastolic murmur (Carey Coombs murmur) that follows an S_3 gallop. This murmur is not diagnostic of ARF because other conditions that lead to increased flow across the mitral valve can cause a similar murmur, and in children an S_3 gallop can be physiologic (see Chap. 12). The Carey Coombs murmur can be differentiated from the diastolic rumble of mitral stenosis by the absence of an opening snap, presystolic accentuation, and loud first sound. A high-pitched decrescendo basal diastolic murmur of aortic regurgitation (AR) may also be heard. It is best heard along the left sternal border over the aortic area in expiration with the patient leaning forward (see Chap. 12).

Myocarditis in the absence of valvulitis is not likely to be rheumatic in origin. Tachycardia is common. S_3, S_4, or summation gallops may be audible. Cardiomegaly may be noted on the chest roentgenogram or echocardiogram. In acute congestive heart failure, rapid distention of the hepatic capsule may lead to right upper quadrant discomfort and tenderness. Congestive heart failure is usually caused by left ventricular volume overload associated with severe MR or AR.

In the presence of pericarditis, a pericardial friction rub or muffled heart sounds due to a large effusion may be noted. The presence of effusion should be confirmed by echocardiography. Large effusions leading to tamponade are rare. Pericarditis in the absence of valvular involvement is rarely due to ARF, and other causes should be sought.[24]

Polyarthritis

Arthritis is the most frequent major manifestation of ARF. Any joint may be affected, but involvement of larger joints such as knees, ankles, elbows, and wrists is more common. Several joints are involved in quick succession, and each for a brief period, resulting in the typical picture of migratory polyarthritis accompanied by signs and symptoms of an acute febrile illness. A striking feature of rheumatic arthritis is its dramatic response to salicylate therapy. Thus, the typical migratory polyarthritis pattern may not be present if effective anti-inflammatory therapy is administered early in the course of the disease. Moreover, the classic migratory pattern is not invariable. In some cases the pattern may be initially additive, persisting in several joints simultaneously,[30] or even, rarely, monoarthritic.[31]

The synovial fluid contains numerous white blood cells with a marked preponderance of polymorphonuclear leukocytes. Bacterial cultures are sterile. Inflammation of any one joint subsides spontaneously within a week, and the entire bout of polyarthritis rarely lasts more than 4 weeks. Resolution is complete with no residual joint damage. A possible exception is the so-called Jaccoud deformity of the metacarpophalangeal joints. This is a periarticular fibrosis and not a true synovitis, and its relation to ARF is unclear.[32]

A much-debated issue is the nature and significance of an entity known as *poststreptococcal reactive arthritis* (PSRA). This designation is applied to a group of patients with a nonmigratory arthritis that is poorly responsive to salicylates or nonsteroidal anti-inflammatory agents and that may persist for several months.[33] Some observers believe it is a distinct entity. Of practical importance is whether such patients are at risk of developing carditis. In view of reports suggesting that some PSRA patients have developed rheumatic valvulitis, the authors' believe they should be maintained on antistreptococcal prophylaxis according to the recommended American Heart Association guidelines (see later).

Subcutaneous Nodules

These nodules are seen in only 1 to 21 percent of patients with ARF.[34] They are most often associated with carditis and rarely appear as an isolated manifestation of ARF. They are round, firm, painless, freely movable subcutaneous lesions varying in size from 0.5 to 2.0 cm. They occur in crops and are usually found over bony surfaces and over tendons such as elbows, knees, wrists, the occiput, and vertebrae. They last for a week or two and disappear spontaneously. Similar nodules also occur in rheumatoid arthritis and systemic lupus erythematosus.

Erythema Marginatum

This rash is usually found on the trunk and proximal parts of the extremities, with the face being spared. It begins as an erythematous macule or papule that extends outward while skin in the center returns to normal. Lesions may merge and form serpiginous patterns. They blanch on pressure, are never pruritic or indurated, and are not influenced by anti-inflammatory therapy. The rash is evanescent, migrating from place to place and leaving no residual scarring. Individual lesions may appear and disappear in minutes to hours. Erythema marginatum has also been reported in sepsis, drug reactions, and glomerulonephritis.

Sydenham's Chorea (St. Vitus' Dance)

This neurologic disorder often occurs in isolation, either unaccompanied by other major manifestations of ARF or after a latent period of several months, at a time when all other manifestations of ARF have subsided. It is characterized by rapid, purposeless, involuntary movements, most noticeable in the extremities and face. The arms and legs flail about in erratic, jerky, uncoordinated movements. The speech is usually slurred and jerky. The involuntary movements disappear during sleep and may be suppressed by sedation. The patient is unable to sustain a tetanic muscular contraction. Emotional lability is characteristic of Sydenham's chorea and may often precede other neurologic manifestations.

The duration of the chorea is variable, and its severity may wax and wane. Most patients recover in 6 months. Long-term sequelae such as convulsions, learning disabilities, and behavior problems are rare but have been reported in a small number of patients.

Rarely, chorea may be due to other conditions that affect the basal ganglia, including collagen vascular, endocrine, neoplastic, genetic, metabolic, and infectious disorders. Perhaps the most frequent differential diagnostic consideration is systemic lupus erythematosus. The relation of chorea occurring during pregnancy (chorea gravidarum) to ARF remains unclear.

Interest has focused on the possibility that certain other neurologic conditions, including tics, obsessive-compulsive disorder, and Tourette's syndrome may be poststreptococcal sequelae.[35,36] Studies of this putative entity, known as *poststreptococcal autoimmune neuropsychiatric disorders associated with streptococci* (PANDAS), are continuing.[36]

Minor Manifestations

Minor manifestations of ARF include fever, arthralgia, and laboratory evidences of inflammation (see Table 65-2). Fever usually ranges from 38.4° to 40°C (101.12°F to 104°F) and rarely lasts for more than 3 to 4 weeks. Arthralgia is pain in one or more joints without objective evidence for inflammation. When diagnosing ARF using the Jones criteria, arthralgia should not be considered a minor manifestation when arthritis is present.

Other Clinical Features

Abdominal pain in ARF is the result of peritoneal inflammation and may be confused with acute appendicitis or sickle cell crisis. Because it occurs at the onset of the illness, other manifestations of ARF may not yet be present. Epistaxis has been reported as a manifestation of ARF, but it is not clear to what extent it may be attributable to the large doses of aspirin administered for treatment of the disease. Tachycardia may be out of proportion to fever and persists during sleep.

LABORATORY FINDINGS

A mild-to-moderate normochromic normocytic anemia and leukocytosis with an increased proportion of polymorphonuclear leukocytes are common. Elevated serum levels of C-reactive protein and an increased erythrocyte sedimentation rate are almost always present, indicating the presence of acute inflammation. An exception is "pure" chorea that may appear after these markers of inflammation have returned to normal.

Throat cultures are usually negative for group A streptococci by the time ARF appears. Streptococcal antibody tests provide evidence for antecedent streptococcal infection and include antistreptolysin O (ASO), anti-DNAse B, and antihyaluronidase. These antibodies reach peak titer at about the time of onset of ARF. The ASO is elevated in 80 percent or more of patients with ARF. A battery of these three tests will establish the presence of immunologically significant infection with group A streptococcus in 95 percent of patients. The normal ranges for these titers vary depending upon the test used, patient's age, and geographic locale. ASO titers greater than 200 Todd U/mL in adults and 320 Todd U in children are generally considered elevated. In patients seen early during the course of ARF, rising antibody titers may be seen. An elevated streptococcal antibody titer is not diagnostic of ARF, but the diagnosis is very unlikely if all three tests (ASO, anti-DNAse B, and antihyaluronidase) are negative.

Electrocardiogram

Persistent sinus tachycardia that does not resolve during sleep is common in the presence of carditis.[37] Sinus bradycardia and sinus arrhythmia may be present in some patients and can be abolished by the administration of atropine. Prolongation of the PR interval is a common abnormality. In various studies, the incidence varied from 10 to 84 percent.[37] A study of the resurgence of ARF[16] described the ECG findings in 232 patients. Alterations in atrioventricular conduction were noted in 74 patients (32 percent). Of these, 66 patients had a prolonged PR interval, 4 had transient episodes of AV block, and 4 had transient episodes of AV dissociation.

Some investigators have suggested that the AV conduction delay is a manifestation of carditis. However, the response to atropine and the lack of correlation with clinical carditis suggests that this is a nonspecific finding.[24] Transient complete heart block that causes Stokes-Adams attacks has been described. Bundle branch blocks are rare. Atrial flutter and fibrillation have been described in the presence of carditis. Low QRS voltage may be noted if a large pericardial effusion is present.

Echocardiogram

Few studies have used transthoracic echocardiography (TTE) to evaluate and follow-up patients with rheumatic carditis.[38] During the resurgence of ARF in Salt Lake City, TTE was performed in children with ARF.[16] During the acute phase of rheumatic carditis there is valvular thickening, and nodular lesions are visible on the body and tips of the mitral leaflets.[39] These are most likely TTE equivalents of rheumatic verrucae. The key features of rheumatic mitral valvulitis were annular dilation and elongation of the chordae to the anterior leaflet resulting in MR with a posterolaterally directed jet.[16] In a TTE study of 73 patients with active rheumatic carditis and MR, it was noted that 90 percent of patients had elongated mitral valve chordae, 94 percent had failure of leaflet edge coaptation, and 96 percent had annular dilation.[40] The failure of mitral leaflet coaptation results in the systolic displacement or prolapse of the free edge of the anterior leaflet toward the left atrium.

Rheumatic carditis can be differentiated from the common mitral valve prolapse syndrome because only the coapting portion of the anterior mitral leaflet prolapses, and there is no billowing of the medial portion of the leaflet.[40] The resulting mitral regurgitant jet is directed toward the posterolateral wall of the left atrium. The site where this jet strikes the posterior left atrial wall corresponds to the site of endocardial thickening described at autopsy as McCallum's patch.

In the past congestive heart failure seen in ARF was attributed to myocarditis. TTE studies have shown that patients with ARF and congestive heart failure have preserved left ventricular systolic function and severe MR.[39,41] Thus the etiology of heart failure appears to be acute MR and not myocarditis (see prior discussion of troponin levels).[38,42]

TTE evaluation has revealed that some patients with ARF have Doppler evidence for MR or AR in the absence of an audible murmur, which has been described a subclinical or silent carditis. The incidence of such subclinical carditis reported from various countries ranges from 16 to 47 percent.[16,43–45] The regurgitation detected by Doppler was mild when there was no audible murmur. Silent MR was more common than aortic. Doppler evaluation of normal subjects has demonstrated that mild MR may be detected in 19 to 45 percent and AR in 0 to 3 percent of children and young adults in the absence of any valvular abnormality.[46,47] Thus it is important not to misinterpret physiologic MR as pathologic. Doppler regurgitant flows that are holosystolic, visible in two planes, and have a mosaic pattern are considered to be pathologic. However, quality and gain settings of the instrument, and the patients' body habitus and hemodynamics during a febrile illness affect such mild regurgitant flows. The natural history and clinical significance of silent carditis is not clear since the number of patients studied is small and the follow-up is limited.[43,44] These studies suggest that the Doppler regurgitation persists in a significant number of patients, but development of a clinically detectable lesion during follow-up is rare. TTE has some incremental diagnostic value when added to the clinical findings in the diagnosis of carditis, but management is not altered and prognosis appears to be very good in silent carditis.[45,47,48] The cost of TTE is a major concern since ARF is common in areas where medical resources are limited.[47,48]

Endomyocardial Biopsy

ARF is basically a clinical syndrome for which no specific diagnostic test exists. However, the presence of Aschoff nodules on histologic specimens obtained at surgery and autopsy can be considered diagnostic of ARF. Percutaneous transvenous myocardial biopsy is now feasible. Aschoff nodules and interstitial mononuclear infiltrates with or without myocyte necrosis have been described in the myocardial biopsy specimens of a few patients with ARF. In a prospective study of patients with suspected or definite rheumatic carditis,[22] however, myocardial specimens were diagnostic in only a minority of cases. Thus, the role of myocardial biopsy in the diagnosis of rheumatic carditis is limited.

DIAGNOSIS

The diagnostic criteria for ARF were originally proposed by T. Duckett Jones in 1944 and have been later modified and updated by the American Heart Association (Table 65-2).[24] Based on their diagnostic importance, clinical and laboratory findings are divided into major and minor manifestations. If supported by evidence of a preceding group A streptococcal infection, the presence of two major manifestations, or of one major and two minor manifestations, indicates a high probability of ARF. Supporting evidence of a previous group A streptococcal infection is a prerequisite for fulfilling the criteria. There are some circumstances in which the diagnosis of ARF can be made without strictly adhering to the Jones criteria. Chorea may not occur until several months after the antecedent streptococcal pharyngeal infection. Isolated carditis that does not provoke congestive failure may not be recognized during the acute phase of illness yet may persist for months. In these situations, markers of inflammation may no longer be present and antistreptococcal antibody titers may have returned to normal by the time the illness comes to light. Moreover, in patients with previous ARF or established rheumatic heart disease, recurrences are common and a presumptive diagnosis of a recurrence may be made in the presence of a single major or several minor manifestations.[24]

Overdiagnosis must be avoided. Following well-documented group A streptococcal pharyngitis, vague signs and symptoms and nonspecific laboratory abnormalities may occur. Discomfort in the extremities, borderline temperature elevation, increased intensity of functional murmurs, tachycardia, elevated erythrocyte sedimentation rate, and prolonged PR interval may occur in the absence of major manifestations. These patients do not develop rheumatic heart disease on follow-up.[24] Thus the diagnosis of ARF should not be made in the absence of major manifestations. There is no evidence that temporarily withholding salicylates or corticosteroids has any adverse effect on the long-term prognosis.

Because ARF can have such diverse manifestations (acute polyarthritis, congestive heart failure, chorea, or combinations of these) and because there is no specific diagnostic test for the disease, the differential diagnostic possibilities in an individual case may be quite broad. Among the diseases that need most frequently to be differentiated are rheumatoid arthritis, juvenile rheumatoid arthritis, systemic lupus erythematosus, serum sickness, sickle cell crisis or cardiopathy, rubella arthritis, septic arthritis (especially gonococcal arthritis in adolescent patients), Lyme disease, infective endocarditis, viral myocarditis, and early stages of Henoch-Schönlein purpura.[49] Choreiform movements have been described in patients with systemic lupus erythematosus, neoplasms involving the basal ganglia, legionnaires' disease, hypoparathyroidism, antiphospholipid syndrome, Wilson's disease, and Huntington's disease. Chorea is also seen occasionally in women taking oral contraceptives and during pregnancy ("chorea gravidarum").

In areas of low ARF incidence, the Jones criteria are perhaps most useful in excluding the diagnosis. The specificity of the criteria is most problematic when the diagnosis is based upon acute polyarthritis as a single major manifestation plus laboratory findings indicative of acute inflammation. In such cases, there must be clear-cut supporting laboratory evidence of recent streptococcal infection and alternative diagnoses must be carefully ruled out.

TREATMENT

Antibiotics neither modify the course of the disease nor prevent the development of rheumatic carditis. Nevertheless, a course of antibiotics to eradicate group A streptococci remaining in the pharynx and tonsils is usually given.[50] Penicillin G benzathine (1.2 million U intramuscularly as a single injection) is the treatment of choice for patients who are not allergic to penicillin. Erythromycin is prescribed for the penicillin-allergic patient. An oral cephalosporin is an acceptable alternative if the penicillin allergy is not of the immediate type. Following this, continuous prophylactic therapy is given to prevent streptococcal pharyngitis (see later).

Anti-inflammatory drugs provide dramatic clinical improvement but are not curative and do not prevent development of rheumatic heart disease.[51] Aspirin is very effective in reducing fever, toxicity, and inflammation of the joints. It is given as tolerated in a dosage of 90 to 100 mg/kg per day in children and 6 to 8 g/day in adults in divided doses, every 4 h. A serum salicylate level of 20 to 25 mg/dL is adequate. Adverse effects include salicylism and gastrointestinal bleeding. The precise dose of aspirin is determined by the severity of symptoms, clinical response, salicylate levels, and tolerance to the drug. After 2 weeks of therapy, a reduced dose of aspirin may be used for another 6 weeks.

Corticosteroids are used in patients with carditis manifested by heart failure and in patients who do not tolerate aspirin or whose symptoms do not respond well to this drug. Prednisone 40 to 60 mg/day in divided doses is given for 2 to 3 weeks, and the dosage is gradually reduced over the following 3 weeks. In some patients symptoms of ARF may reappear when the anti-inflammatory therapy, especially steroids, is stopped. Continuing aspirin therapy for 1 month after steroids are discontinued can prevent this. Although the use of nonsteroidal anti-inflammatory drugs is a reasonable alternative to salicylates in patients who cannot tolerate salicylates and who do not require corticosteroids, there is a paucity of data on the use of these agents in ARF. Thus, specific regimens remain to be defined.

Congestive heart failure is managed in the conventional manner. Digoxin should be used cautiously in the presence of myocarditis. After the acute attack subsides, the level of physical activity is determined by the cardiac status. Patients without residual cardiac disease do not require restriction of physical activity.

PROGNOSIS

Manifestations of chronic rheumatic heart disease include MR and aortic regurgitation or stenosis, congestive heart failure, and atrial fibrillation. The ultimate cardiac prognosis of an individual ARF episode is rather directly related to the severity of cardiac involvement during the acute phase, provided that the patient is protected from recurrent attacks (see later). In the United Kingdom–United States Collaborative Study,[52] only 6 percent of the patients with no carditis or only questionable carditis during their attack of ARF were found to have heart murmurs when reexamined 10 years later. Heart disease was present at follow-up in 30 percent of the patients initially found to have only apical systolic murmurs, in 40 percent of those with basal diastolic murmurs during the acute phase, and in 68 percent of those who initially suffered from congestive heart failure, pericarditis, or both. Some patients with "pure" chorea may later develop rheumatic heart disease, even though carditis was not recognized during the initial attack. It may be in such cases, however, that the initial findings of carditis were no longer prominent by the time that chorea (which often occurs after a long latent period) manifested itself.

Prevention

The risk of developing ARF following a symptomatic or asymptomatic streptococcal infection is much higher in patients who have experienced a previous attack than it is in those who are nonrheumatic. In some studies, the recurrence rate following immunologically confirmed streptococcal upper respiratory infection has been as high as 16 percent.[53] In patients with rheumatic heart disease, recurrent attacks lead to progressive damage. Although patients who did not suffer carditis initially are less prone to develop it in the event of a recurrence, exceptions do occur. It is therefore crucial that ARF patients be protected optimally from streptococcal infections. This is accomplished by continuous antimicrobial prophylaxis.[54]

The recommended prophylactic regimens are shown in Table 65-3. The optimal duration of antibiotic prophylaxis remains contro-

TABLE 65-3 Secondary Prevention of Rheumatic Fever (Prevention of Recurrent Attacks)

Agent	Dose	Mode
Benzathine penicillin G	1,200,000 U every 4 weeks* or	Intramuscular
Penicillin V	250 mg twice daily or	Oral
Sulfadiazine	0.5 g once daily for ≤27 kg (60 lb) 1.0 g once daily for patients >27 kg (60 lb)	Oral
For individuals allergic to penicillin and sulfadiazine		
Erythromycin	250 mg twice daily	Oral

*In high-risk situations, administration every 3 weeks is justified and recommended.

SOURCE: Dajani A, Taubert K, Ferrieri P, et al. Treatment of acute streptococcal pharyngitis and prevention of rheumatic fever: A statement for health professionals. Committee on Rheumatic Fever, Endocarditis, and Kawasaki Disease of the Council on Cardiovascular Disease in the Young, the American Heart Association. Reproduced by permission of *Pediatrics* 1995;96:758–764.

versial. The risk of ARF declines with age and the number of years since previous attack. The recommendations of the American Heart Association for the duration of secondary prophylaxis are given in Table 65-4. The decision to discontinue ARF prophylaxis must be individualized on the basis of risk for recurrence and the probable consequence of a recurrence. It should be noted that health care workers, individuals who have contact with schoolchildren, military recruits, and residents of areas with a high incidence of ARF are at increased risk for streptococcal infection.

TABLE 65-4 Duration of Secondary Rheumatic Fever Prophylaxis

Category	Duration
Rheumatic fever with carditis and residual heart disease (persistent valvular disease*)	At least 10 years since last episode and at least until age 40 years, sometimes lifelong prophylaxis
Rheumatic fever with carditis but no residual heart disease (no valvular disease*)	10 years or well into adulthood, whichever is longer
Rheumatic fever without carditis	5 years or until age 21 years, whichever is longer

*Clinical or echocardiographic evidence.
SOURCE: From Dajani A, Taubert K, Ferrieri P, et al. Treatment of acute streptococcal pharyngitis and prevention of rheumatic fever: A statement for health professionals. Committee on Rheumatic Fever, Endocarditis, and Kawasaki Disease of the Council on Cardiovascular Disease in the Young, the American Heart Association. Reproduced by permission of *Pediatrics* 1995;96:758–764.

Reference

1. Jones TD. Diagnosis of rheumatic fever. *JAMA* 1944;26:481–484.
2. Kurahara D, Tokuda A, Grandinetti A, et al. Ethnic differences in risk for pediatric rheumatic illness in a culturally diverse population. *J Rheumatol* 2002;29(2):379–383.
3. Frank PF, Stollerman GH, Miller LF. Protection of a military population from rheumatic fever. *JAMA* 1965;193:755–783.
4. Wannamaker LW, Rammelkamp CH Jr, Denny FW, et al. Prophylaxis of acute rheumatic fever by treatment of preceeding streptococcal infection with various amounts of depot penicillin. *Am J Med* 1951;10: 673–695.
5. Wood HF, Feinstein AR, Taranta A, et al. Rheumatic fever in children and adolescents. A long-term epidemiologic study of subsequent prophylaxis, streptococcal infections, and clinical sequelae. III. Comparative effectiveness of three prophylaxis regimens in preventing streptococcal infections and rheumatic recurrences. *Ann Intern Med* 1964; 60(suppl 5):31–46.
6. WHO programme for the prevention of rheumatic fever/rheumatic heart disease in 16 developing countries: Report from Phase I (1986–90). *Bull World Health Organ* 1992;70:213–218.
7. Vijaykumar M, Narula J, Reddy KS, et al. Incidence of rheumatic fever and prevalence of rheumatic fever disease in India. *Int J Cardiol* 1994; 43(3):221–228.
8. Carapetis JR, Wolff DR, Currie BJ. Acute rheumatic fever and rheumatic heart disease in the top end of Australia's Northern Territory. *Med J Aust* 1996;164(3):146–149.
9. Rammelkamp CH, Denny FW, Wannamaker LW. Studies on the epidemiology of rheumatic fever in the armed services. In: Thomas L, ed. *Rheumatic Fever*. Minneapolis: University of Minnesota Press; 1952: 72–89.
10. Siegel AC, Johnson EE, Stollerman GH. Controlled studies of streptococcal pharyngitis in a pediatric population: I. Factors related to the attack rate of rheumatic fever. *N Engl J Med* 1961;265:559–566.
11. Bisno AL. The concept of rheumatogenic and non-rheumatogenic group A streptococci. In: Read SE, Zabriskie JB, eds. *Streptococcal Diseases and the Immune Response*. New York: Academic Press; 1980:789–803.
12. Bessen DE, Veasy LG, Hill HR, et al. Serologic evidence for a class I group A streptococcal infection among rheumatic fever patients. *J Infect Dis* 1995;172:1608–1611.
13. Bisno AL. Group A streptococcal infections and acute rheumatic fever. *N Engl J Med* 1991;325:783–793.
14. Land MA, Bisno AL. Acute rheumatic fever: a vanishing disease in suburbia. *JAMA* 1983;249:895–898.
15. Ferguson GW, Shultz JM, Bisno AL. Epidemiology of acute rheumatic fever in a multi-ethnic, multi-racial U.S. urban community: The Miami-Dade experience. *J Infect Dis* 1991;164:720–725.
16. Veasy LG, Tani LY, Hill HR. Persistence of acute rheumatic fever in the intermountain area of the United States. *J Pediatr* 1994;124:9–16.
17. Cunningham M. Molecular mimicry between group A streptococci and myosin in the pathogenesis of acute rheumatic fever. In: Narula J, Virmani R, Reddy KS, Tandon R (eds). *Rheumatic Fever*. Washington, DC: Armed Forces Institute of Pathology; 1999:135–165.
18. Baird RW, Bronze MS, Kraus W, et al. Epitopes of group A streptococcal M protein shared with antigens of articular cartilage and synovium. *J Immunol* 1991;146:3132–3137.
19. Husby G, van de Rijn I, Zabriskie JB, et al. Antibodies reacting with cytoplasm of subthalamic and caudate nuclei neurons in chorea and rheumatic fever. *J Exp Med* 1976;144:1094–1110.
20. Church AJ, Cardoso F, Dale RC, et al. Anti–basal ganglia antibodies in acute and persistent Sydenham's chorea. *Neurology* 2002;59(2):227–231.
21. Khanna AK, Buskirk DR, Williams RC Jr, et al. Presence of a non–HLA B cell antigen in rheumatic fever patients and their families as defined by a monoclonal antibody. *J Clin Invest* 1989;83:1710–1716.
22. Narula J, Chopra P, Talwar KK, et al. Does endomyocardial biopsy aid in the diagnosis of active rheumatic carditis? *Circulation* 1993;88(part 1):2198–2205.
23. Virmani R, Farb A, Burke AP, et al. Pathology of acute rheumatic carditis. In: Narula J, Virmani R, Reddy KS, Tandon R (ed). *Rheumatic Fever*. Washington, DC: Armed Forces Institute of Pathology; 1999:217–234.
24. Dajani AS, Ayoub E, Bierman FZ, et al. Guidelines for the diagnosis of rheumatic fever: Jones criteria, updated 1992. *JAMA* 1992;268: 2069–2073.
25. Sanyal SK, Thapar MK, Ahmed SH, et al. The initial attack of acute rheumatic fever during childhood in North India: A prospective study of the clinical profile. *Circulation* 1974;49:7–12.
26. Gupta M, Lent RW, Kaplan EL, et al. Serum cardiac troponin I in acute rheumatic fever. *Am J Cardiol* 2002;89(6):779–782.
27. Kamblock J. Serum cardiac troponin I in acute rheumatic fever. *Am J Cardiol* 2002;90(11):1277–1278.
28. Kamblock J, Payot L, Jung B, et al. Does rheumatic myocarditis really exist? Systematic study with echocardiography and cardiac troponin I blood levels. *Eur Heart J* 2003;24(9):855–862.
29. Marcus RH, Sareli P, Pocock WA, et al. The spectrum of severe rheumatic mitral valve disease in a developing country: Correlations among clinical presentation, surgical pathologic findings, and hemodynamic sequelae. *Ann Intern Med* 1994;120:177–183.
30. Stollerman GH. Current issues in the prevention of rheumatic fever. *Minerva Med* 2002;93(5):371–387.
31. Carapetis JR, Currie BJ. Rheumatic fever in a high incidence population: The importance of monoarthritis and low grade fever. *Arch Dis Child* 2001;85(3):223–227.

32. Stollerman GH. *Rheumatic Fever and Streptococcal Infection.* New York: Grune & Stratton; 1975.

33. Shulman ST, Ayoub EM. Poststreptococcal reactive arthritis. *Curr Opin Rheumatol* 2002;14(5):562–565.

34. Bisno AL. Noncardiac manifestations of rheumatic fever. In: Narula J, Virmani R, Reddy KS, Tandon R (eds). *Rheumatic Fever.* Washington, DC: Armed Forces Institute of Pathology; 1999:245–256.

35. Swedo SE, Leonard HL, Garvey M, et al. Pediatric autoimmune neuropsychiatric disorders associated with streptococcal infections: Clinical description of the first 50 cases. *Am J Psychiatry* 1998;155(2):264–271.

36. Murphy ML, Pichichero ME. Prospective identification and treatment of children with pediatric autoimmune neuropsychiatric disorder associated with group A streptococcal infection (PANDAS). *Arch Pediatr Adolesc Med* 2002;156(4):356–361.

37. Krishnan SC, Kushwaha SS, Josephson ME. Electrocardiographic abnormalities and arrhythmias in patients with acute rheumatic fever. In: Narula J, Virmani R, Reddy KS, Tandon R (eds). *Rheumatic Fever.* Washington, DC: Armed Forces Institute of Pathology, 1999:287–298.

38. Minich LL, Tani LY, Veasy LG. Role of echocardiography in the diagnosis and follow-up evaluation of rheumatic fever. In: Narula N, Virmani R, Reddy KS, Tandon R (eds). Rheumatic fever. Washington, DC: Armed Forces Institute of Pathology; 1999:307–318.

39. Vasan RS, Shrivastava S, Vijayakumar M, et al. Echocardiographic evaluation of patients with acute rheumatic fever and rheumatic carditis. *Circulation* 1996;94(1):73–82.

40. Marcus RH, Sareli P, Pocock WA, et al. Functional anatomy of severe mitral regurgitation in active rheumatic carditis. *Am J Cardiol* 1989;63:577–584.

41. Essop MR, Wisenbaugh T, Sareli P. Evidence against a myocardial factor as the cause of left ventricular dilation inactive rheumatic carditis. *J Am Coll Cardiol* 1993;22(3):826–829.

42. Veasy LG. Lessons learned from the resurgence of rheumatic fever in the United States. In: Narula J, Virmani R, Reddy KS, Tandon R (eds). *Rheumatic Fever.* Washington, DC: Armed Forces Institute of Pathology; 1999:69–78.

43. Figueroa FE, Fernandez MS, Valdes P, et al. Prospective comparison of clinical and echocardiographic diagnosis of rheumatic carditis: Long-term follow-up of patients with subclinical disease. *Heart* 2001;85(4):407–410.

44. Ozkutlu S, Ayabakan C, Saraclar M. Can subclinical valvitis detected by echocardiography be accepted as evidence of carditis in the diagnosis of acute rheumatic fever? *Cardiol Young* 2001;11(3):255–260.

45. Narula J, Chandrashekher Y, Rahimtoola S. Diagnosis of active carditis. The echos of change. *Circulation* 1999;100:1576–1581.

46. Yoshida K, Yoshikawa J, Shakudo M, et al. Color Doppler evaluation of valvular regurgitation in normal subjects. *Circulation* 1988;78:840–847.

47. Choong CY, Abascal VM, Weyman J, et al. Prevalence of valvular regurgitation by Doppler echocardiography in patients with structurally normal hearts by two-dimensional echocardiography. *Am Heart J* 1989;117(3):636–642.

48. Stollerman GH. Rheumatic fever in the 21st century. *Clin Infect Dis* 2001;33(6):806–814.

49. Robson WL, Leung AK. Acute rheumatic fever and Henoch-Schönlein purpura. *Acta Paediatr* 2003;92(4):513.

50. Bisno AL. Rheumatic fever. In: Goldman L, Bennett JC, eds. *Cecil's Textbook of Medicine,* 21st ed Philadelphia: Saunders; 2000:1624–1630.

51. Thatai D, Turi ZG. Current guidelines for the treatment of patients with rheumatic fever. *Drugs* 1999;57(4):545–555.

52. United Kingdom and United States Joint Report on Rheumatic Heart Disease. The natural history of rheumatic fever and rheumatic heart disease: Ten-year report of a cooperative clinical trial of ACTH, cortisone and aspirin. *Circulation* 1965;194:1284.

53. Taranta A, Wood HF, Feinstein AR, et al. Rheumatic fever in children and adolescents. A long-term epidemiologic study of subsequent prophylaxis, streptococcal infections, and clinical sequelae. IV. Relation of the rheumatic fever recurrence rate per streptococcal infection to the titers of streptococcal antibodies. *Ann Intern Med* 1964;60(suppl 5):47–57.

54. Dajani A, Taubert K, Ferrieri P, et al. Treatment of acute streptococcal pharyngitis and prevention of rheumatic fever: A statement for health professionals. Committee on Rheumatic Fever, Endocarditis, and Kawasaki Disease of the Council on Cardiovascular Disease in the Young, the American Heart Association. *Pediatrics* 1995;96(4 pt 1):758–764.

AORTIC VALVE DISEASE

Shahbudin H. Rahimtoola

Rheumatic heart disease is not the most important cause of valve disease in the developed countries. Mitral valve prolapse and congenital aortic valve disease are the most common valvular lesions. Most patients with severe valve disease are considered candidates for surgery. Echocardiography/Doppler ultrasound has a very important role in the diagnosis and follow-up of these patients. Cardiac catheterization/angiography remains an extremely important diagnostic procedure that is needed in almost all patients considered for interventional therapy.

AORTIC VALVE STENOSIS

Aortic stenosis (AS) is obstruction to outflow of blood from the left ventricle (LV), which may be at the valve, above the valve (supravalvular), or below the valve (subvalvular).[1] Supravalvular AS is a congenital lesion. Subvalvular AS results either from a congenital discrete fibromuscular obstruction or from a muscular obstruction (hypertrophic cardiomyopathy).

Etiology

The most common causes of AS are congenital, rheumatic, and calcific (degenerative).[1] Calcific AS is seen in patients 35 years of age or older and is the result of calcification of a congenital or rheumatic valve or of a normal valve. Degenerative or calcific AS is related to atherosclerosis[2] and may represent an immune reaction to antigens present in the valve.[3] Other causes of AS[1] are rare (Table 66-1). At the present time, calcific AS in the older patient is the most common valve lesion requiring aortic valve replacement (AVR).[1,4] Among patients under the age of 70, congenital bicuspid valve accounted for one-half of the surgical cases; "degenerative" changes were the cause in 18 percent.[4] In those aged 70 or older, degenerative changes accounted for almost one-half of the surgical cases and a congenital bicuspid valve accounted for approximately one-quarter of the cases (Fig. 66-1).

Pathology

In congenital AS, the valve may be unicuspid, bicuspid, or tricuspid, depending on the patient's age.[1] In patients under the age of 15 years, over 80 percent of stenotic valves are either unicuspid or bicuspid and 15 to 20 percent are tricuspid.[5] In patients aged 15 to 65 years, 60 percent are bicuspid, 10 percent are unicuspid, and 25 to 30 percent are tricuspid.[5] In patients 65 years of age or over, 90 percent of the valves are tricuspid and 10 percent are bicuspid.[5] Unicuspid valves produce severe obstruction in infancy. Congenital bicuspid valves can produce severe obstruction to LV outflow after the first few years of life.[1] The valvular abnormality produces turbulent flow, which traumatizes the leaflets and eventually leads to fibrosis, rigidity, and calcification of the valve. In a congenitally abnormal tricuspid aortic valve, the cusps are of unequal size and have some degree of commissural fusion; the third cusp may be diminutive. Eventually, the abnormal structure leads to changes similar to those seen in a bicuspid valve, and significant LV outflow obstruction often results. In calcific AS early changes show chronic inflammatory cell infiltrate (macrophages and T lymphocytes), lipids in lesions and in adjacent fibrosa, and thickening of fibrosa with collagen and elastin.[2] These patients also have a higher incidence of risk factors for coronary atherosclerosis.[6]

Rheumatic AS results from adhesions and fusion of the commissures and cusps. The leaflets and the valve ring become vascularized, which leads to retraction and stiffening of the cusps. Calcification occurs, and the aortic valve orifice is reduced to a small triangular or round opening, which is frequently regurgitant as well as stenotic. Importantly, the heart exhibits other evidence of rheumatic heart disease, namely, involvement of the mitral valve and presence of Aschoff's nodules in the myocardium.

The LV is concentrically hypertrophied.[7] The hypertrophied cardiac muscle cells are increased in size, with their transverse diameters ranging from 15 to 70 μm (normal, 10 to 15 μm). There is an increase of connective tissue[8,9] and a variable amount of fibrous tissue (collagen fibrils) in the interstitial tissue. Usually, the cardiac muscle cells do not degenerate in patients with AS. Myocardial ultrastructural changes[1] may account for the LV systolic dysfunction that occurs late in the disease; such changes include unusually large nuclei, loss of myofibrils, accumulation of mitochondria, large cytoplasmic areas devoid of contractile material, and proliferation of fibroblasts and collagen fibers in the interstitial space. Subclinical calcific emboli are commonly found in calcific AS if diligently sought at autopsy.

TABLE 66-1 Etiology of Aortic Valve Stenosis

I. Congenital
II. Acquired
   A. Rheumatic
   B. Calcific (degenerative/autoimmune)
   C. Rare causes
      1. Obstructive infective vegetations
      2. Homozygous type II hyperlipoproteinemia
      3. Paget's disease of bone
      4. Systemic lupus erythematosus
      5. Rheumatoid involvement
      6. Ochronosis (alkaptonuria)
      7. Irradiation

Pathophysiology

With reduction in the *aortic valve area* (AVA), energy is dissipated during the transport of blood from the LV to the aorta. The AVA has to be reduced by about 50 percent of normal before a measurable gradient can be demonstrated in humans.[10] When a pressure gradient develops between the LV and the ascending aorta, LV pressure rises; aortic pressure remains within the normal range until end-stage heart failure occurs. The relationship of AVA to cardiac output and pressure gradient is discussed in Chap. 20. As LV pressure rises, ventricular wall stress increases, which leads to impaired LV function. Hypertrophy develops in proportion to increased intraventricular pressure, and myocardial stress remains normal.[11] *Thus, the major compensatory mechanism by which the heart copes with LV outflow obstruction is left ventricular hypertrophy (LVH).* LV mass in patients with severe AS undergoing AVR averages 229 g/m^2 (normal, 105 g/m^2)[11]; LV volume is within the normal range,[12] and so there is a considerable thickening of the LV wall.

The diastolic properties of the LV are affected in AS.[12,13] This diastolic abnormality results from a combination of impaired myocardial relaxation with altered chamber compliance, because the LVH per se offers increased resistance to filling, and from increased myocardial stiffness because of structural alterations.[13] As a result, LV

end-diastolic pressure is elevated. Powerful left atrial (LA) contraction produces the required LV filling and results in an elevated LV end-diastolic pressure (atrial booster pump function).[14] The necessary LV filling and fiber length to achieve an adequate stroke volume are achieved by LA systole, which occupies only a small part of the cardiac cycle. Therefore, there is a transient increase in LA pressure due to the large *a* wave, but mean LA pressure remains in the normal range or is only minimally increased (Fig. 66-2). LA contraction is therefore of considerable benefit to these patients. Loss of effective atrial contraction, either because of atrial fibrillation or because of an inappropriately timed atrial contraction [e.g., that associated with first-degree heart block or with atrioventricular (AV) dissociation], results in elevations of mean LA pressure, reduction of cardiac output, or both and may precipitate clinical heart failure with pulmonary congestion.

Patients with severe LVH may exhibit LV diastolic dysfunction, which may produce the syndrome of clinical heart failure (paroxysmal nocturnal dyspnea, orthopnea, and even pulmonary edema) even if LV systolic pump function is normal. In patients 60 years of age or older, a higher percentage of women (41 percent) than men (14 percent) have "excessive" LVH, that is, greater amounts of LVH in spite of similar degrees of severity of AS.[15] They have "supernormal" LV systolic pump function (high LV ejection fraction) and a small, thick-walled chamber with lower end-systolic wall stress.

LV systolic pump function is determined by myocardial (muscle) function and by a combination of LV afterload and preload. Thus, impaired LV systolic pump function (as measured by ejection fraction) may be the result of afterload preload mismatch,[16] impaired myocardial function, or both. LV systolic pump function is normal in most patients with severe AS. When LVH alone is not adequate to overcome the outflow obstruction, the LV uses the Frank-Starling mechanism (preload reserve) to maintain systolic pump function. When the preload reserve is no longer adequate, a reduction of LV systolic pump function occurs (see Fig. 66-2). In AS, major use of the preload reserve is not a good compensatory mechanism. Even small increases in LV volume may result in major increases in LV end-diastolic pressure because the LV is on the very steep portion of its diastolic pressure-volume curve, and the corresponding increase in mean LA pressure produces pulmonary edema. Thus, clinical heart failure may be a result of either LV diastolic dysfunction in the presence of normal LV systolic function or impaired myocardial function producing LV systolic dysfunction, with or without associated LV diastolic dysfunction. Eventually, pulmonary artery, right ventricular, and right atrial pressures are elevated. Peripheral edema results from increases in systemic venous pressure and salt and water retention.

In most patients with AS, cardiac output is in the normal range and initially increases normally with exercise. Later, as the severity of AS increases progressively, the cardiac output remains within the normal range at rest, but, on exercise, it no longer increases in proportion to the amount of exercise undertaken or does not increase at all (fixed cardiac output). With the development of heart

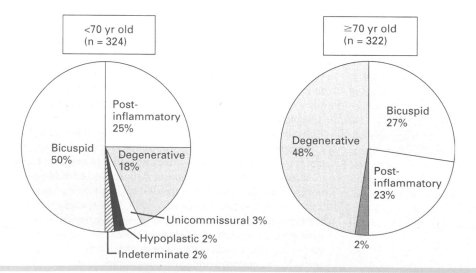

FIGURE 66-1 Etiology of aortic stenosis in patients under the age of 70 years (*left panel*); congenital bicuspid valve accounted for one-half of the surgical cases. In those aged 70 or older (*right panel*), "degenerative" changes accounted for almost one-half of the surgical cases. (From Passik et al.,[4] with permission.)

failure, there is a reduction in the resting cardiac output and a tachycardia. As a result, stroke volume may be so lowered that it results in a small gradient across the LV outflow tract in spite of severe AS. As the patient's age increases, there is a progressive decrease of cardiac output with exercise and a progressive increase of LV end-diastolic pressure at equal levels of AVA. This may be related only to LV diastolic dysfunction and is most marked in the older patient.[17]

In severe AS, myocardial oxygen needs are increased (Fig. 66-3). Total coronary blood flow is increased because of the severe LVH; however, coronary blood flow per 100 g of LV mass is reduced.[18] As a result, blood flow to the subendocardium[19] is inadequate at rest; and because coronary vasodilator reserve is reduced,[20] myocardial blood flow is also reduced further, relative to need, on exercise. Coronary blood flow is diminished because of a reduced coronary perfusion pressure (the elevated LV end-diastolic pressure lowers the diastolic aortic–LV pressure gradient) and also because the hypertrophied myocardium compresses the coronary arteries as they traverse the myocardium to supply blood to the subendocardium (systolic "milking" of intramural arteries). As a result, patients may have classic angina pectoris even in the absence of *coronary artery disease* (CAD). Associated obstructive CAD further increases the imbalance between myocardial oxygen needs and supply (see Fig. 66-3).

Clinical Findings

HISTORY

Patients with congenital valve stenosis may give a history of a murmur since childhood or infancy; those with rheumatic stenosis may have a history of rheumatic fever. Most patients with valvular AS, including some with severe valve stenosis, are asymptomatic. The symptoms of AS are angina pectoris, syncope, exertional presyncope, dyspnea (on exertion, orthopnea, paroxysmal nocturnal dyspnea, pulmonary edema), and the symptoms of heart failure. Once symptoms occur in a patient with severe AS, the life span of the patient is very short without surgical treatment. Sudden cardiac death is stated to occur in 5 percent of patients with AS. It occurs only in those with severe valve stenosis, most of whom have had some cardiac symptoms before the fatal episode. Typical angina pectoris occurs with or without associated CAD (see Fig. 66-3).

Syncope is the result of reduced cerebral perfusion. Syncope occurring on effort is caused by either systemic vasodilatation in the presence of a fixed or inadequate cardiac output, an arrhythmia, or both.[21–23] Syncope at rest is usually due to a transient ventricular

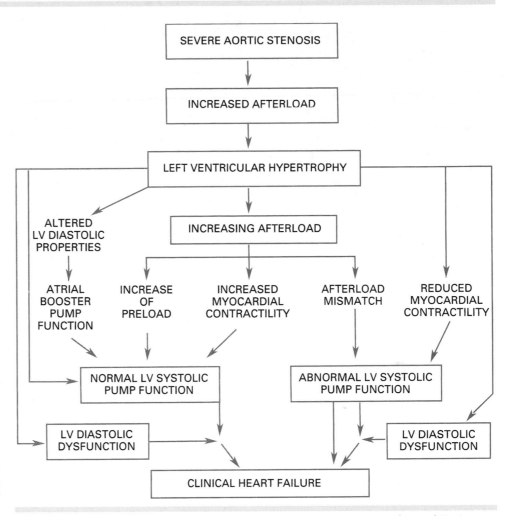

FIGURE 66-2 Illustration of some aspects of the pathophysiology in severe aortic stenosis (see text). The heart responds to aortic stenosis by hypertrophy, and left ventricular (LV) systolic pump function remains normal. LV hypertrophy may alter the LV diastolic properties. As a result, LV end-diastolic pressure is elevated, but powerful atrial contraction produces the required LV filling and fiber length (atrial booster pump function).

As LV afterload continues to increase, the LV uses two additional compensatory mechanisms, namely, increase of preload and increase of myocardial contractility. Both of these help maintain normal LV systolic pump function. When the limit of the preload reserve has been reached (afterload mismatch) or myocardial contractility is reduced, LV systolic pump function becomes abnormal.

Clinical heart failure is usually a result of abnormal LV systolic pump function; diastolic dysfunction may also be present in some patients. Clinical heart failure in those with normal LV systolic pump function is a result of LV diastolic dysfunction. (Copyright by SH Rahimtoola.[64])

tachyarrhythmia, from which the patient recovers spontaneously. Other possible causes of syncope include transient atrial fibrillation or transient AV block, during which the ventricle is deprived of the powerful atrial booster pump function and/or the ventricular rate is slow.

Dyspnea on exertion, orthopnea, paroxysmal nocturnal dyspnea, and pulmonary edema result from varying degrees of pulmonary venous hypertension. Systemic venous congestion with enlargement of the liver and peripheral edema result from increased systemic venous pressure and salt and water retention. There is an increased incidence of gastrointestinal arteriovenous malformations.[1] As a result, these patients are susceptible to gastrointestinal hemorrhage and anemia. Bleeding is often caused by an acquired defect in the structure of von Willebrand's factor.[23a] Calcific systemic embolism may occur.[1]

PHYSICAL FINDINGS

There is a spectrum of physical findings in patients with AS, depending on the severity of the stenosis, stroke volume, LV function, and

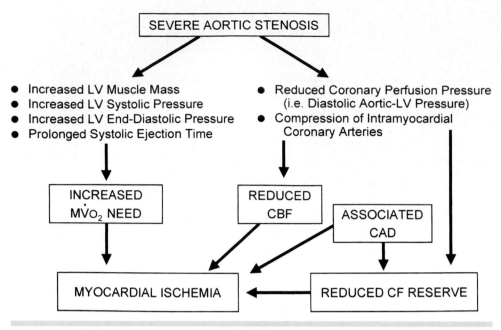

FIGURE 66-3 In severe aortic stenosis (AS), myocardial oxygen needs are increased because of increased muscle mass (hypertrophy), increases in LV pressures, and prolongation of the systolic ejection time. Total coronary blood flow is increased; however, coronary blood flow per 100 g of LV mass is reduced because of a reduction in diastolic aortic-LV pressure gradient and "systolic milking" of the coronary arteries in the hypertrophied LV as they traverse the myocardium from the epicardium to the endocardium to supply the subendocardial myocardial region. Thus, these patients may have myocardial ischemia, particularly in the subendocardial region. Coronary vasodilator reserve (i.e., the ability of the coronary blood flow to increase with vasodilatation) is also significantly reduced, and thus the myocardial ischemia can be markedly exacerbated on effort. Associated obstructive coronary artery disease can be expected to further exacerbate the myocardial ischemia. (Copyright by SH Rahimtoola.[64])

the rigidity and calcification of the valve (Table 66-2). The arterial pulse rises slowly, taking a longer time than normal to reach peak pressure, and the peak is reduced (*parvus et tardus*);[24] the pulse pressure may be narrowed. The anacrotic notch on the upstroke is best appreciated in the carotid arteries. The more severe the valve stenosis, the lower the anacrotic notch on the arterial pulse. A systolic thrill may be felt in the carotid arteries. The jugular venous pulse is normal unless the patient is in heart failure. In the absence of heart failure, the heart size is normal. The cardiac impulse is heaving and sustained in character, and there may be a palpable fourth heart sound (S_4). An aortic systolic thrill is often present at the base of the heart. In 80 to 90 percent of adult patients with severe AS, there is an S_4 gallop sound, a midsystolic ejection murmur that peaks late in systole, and a single second heart sound (S_2) because A_2 and P_2 are superimposed or A_2 is absent or soft. There is often a faint early diastolic murmur of minimal aortic regurgitation (AR). In the young patient with valvular AS, a systolic ejection sound (systolic ejection click) initiates the systolic murmur but later tends to disappear as AS becomes severe. The S_2 may be paradoxically split due to late A_2, and there may be no early diastolic murmur. In many patients, particularly the elderly, the systolic ejection murmur is atypical, may be soft, is described as a seagull sound (or musical, or cooing), and may be heard only at the apex of the heart (Gallavardin phenomenon). In the presence of heart failure, the jugular venous pressure is often increased, the LV is dilated, a third heart sound is present, and the systolic murmur may be very soft or absent. Thus, the clinical features on physical examination may resemble those of heart failure from a variety of causes, such as dilated cardiomyopathy, rather than AS (see Chap. 14).

Severe valvular AS is common in patients 60 years of age or older.[25] The clinical features in many of these patients tend to be

TABLE 66-2 Physical Examination of Patients with Varying Severity of Aortic Valve Stenosis

	Mild	Moderate	Severe + Normal LV Function	Severe + LV Dysfunction	Severe + Heart Failure[a]
Arterial pulse	Normal	Slowly rising	*Parvus et tardus*	*Parvus et tardus*	Small volume
Jugular venous pulse	Normal	Normal	Normal	Normal	±
Carotid thrill	±	±	±	±	±
Cardiac impulse	Normal	Heaving	Heaving, sustained palpable *a* wave	Heaving	Heaving or reduced
Precordial thrill	±	±	Usually ++	±	–
Auscultation					
S_4	–	±	++	+	–
S_3	–	–	–	±	+
ESS	+	±	–	–	–
Peak of ESM	Early systole	Mid-systole	Late systole	Late to mid-systole, soft	Mid-systole, soft or absent
S_2	Normal	Normal or single	Single or paradoxical	Single	Single

[a]There may be signs of mitral and tricuspid regurgitation and of pulmonary hypertension.

ABBREVIATIONS: S_4 = fourth heart sounds (presystolic gallop); S_3 = third heart sound (diastolic gallop); ESS = ejection systolic sound; ESM = ejection systolic murmur; S_2 = second heart sound.

somewhat different.[25] Systemic hypertension is present in about 20 percent of the patients, half of whom have moderate or severe systolic and diastolic hypertension. A fifth of the patients first present in heart failure. The male:female ratio is 2:1. Because of thickening of the arterial wall and its associated lack of dispensability, the arterial pulse rises normally or even rapidly, and the pulse pressure is wide. The S_2 is either absent or single. As noted earlier, the murmur may be high pitched and musical and may radiate from the base to the apex or may be heard best at the apex, mimicking mitral regurgitation.

CHEST X-RAY

The characteristic finding is a normal-sized heart with a dilated proximal ascending aorta (poststenotic dilation). Calcium in the aortic valve can often be seen on the lateral film. In the current era, calcification is most easily recognized on two-dimensional echocardiography. Calcium in the aortic valve is the hallmark of AS in adults 40 to 45 years of age.[1] In patients aged ≥45 years, the diagnosis of severe AS is doubtful if there is no calcium in the aortic valve. The presence of calcium, however, does not necessarily mean that the valve is stenotic or that the AS is severe. In patients with heart failure, the cardiac size is increased because of dilatation of the LV and LA; the lung fields show pulmonary edema and pulmonary venous congestion with redistribution of blood flow. In the presence of heart failure, the right ventricle and the right atrium may be dilated.

ELECTROCARDIOGRAM

The *electrocardiogram* (ECG) in severe AS shows LVH with or without secondary ST-T-wave changes. It is important to recognize, however, that in about 10 to 15 percent of patients with severe AS, LVH cannot be appreciated on the ECG. In fact, the ECG may be entirely normal in some of these patients. The P-wave abnormality ($P \geq 0.12$ s) of LA enlargement and/or hypertrophy and/or conduction delay is present in over 80 percent.[1] The ECG may show left bundle branch block, right bundle branch block with left or right axis deviation, or, occasionally, isolated right bundle branch block.[26] In some patients, the conduction abnormality results from aortic valve calcification extending into the specialized conducting tissue, which may even produce heart block. The patients are usually in sinus rhythm. The presence of atrial fibrillation indicates the presence of associated mitral valve disease, CAD, or heart failure secondary to aortic valve disease. Atrial fibrillation is relatively common in the elderly with calcific AS, probably because of the increased presence of associated diseases.

Laboratory Investigations

ECHOCARDIOGRAPHY/DOPPLER ULTRASOUND

Echocardiography/Doppler (echo/Doppler) ultrasound (Chap. 17) is an extremely important and useful noninvasive test. On the echocardiogram, the aortic valve leaflets normally are barely visible in systole. In the presence of a bicuspid aortic valve, eccentric valve leaflets may be seen. The aortic valve leaflets may appear to be thickened as a result of calcification and/or fibrosis; however, the older patient without valve stenosis may also have thickened cusps. The aortic valve may have a reduced opening, but this also occurs in other conditions in which the cardiac output is reduced. The LVH often results in thickening of both the interventricular septum and the posterior LV wall. The LV cavity size is normal. All these abnormalities are better appreciated on two-dimensional echocardiography. When LV systolic function is impaired, the LV and LA are dilated and the percentage of dimensional shortening is reduced.

M-mode, or two-dimensional echocardiography, is not a reliable technique for assessing the severity of AS. The presence of normal movement of thin aortic leaflets on the echocardiogram, however, is strong evidence against severe AS in adults. Echo/Doppler, when properly applied, is extremely useful for estimating the valve gradient and AVA noninvasively.[27,28] When compared with results obtained at cardiac catheterization, the standard error of the estimate of mean gradient in the best laboratories is 10 mmHg.[29] Thus, the mean gradient by Doppler can be expected to be within ±20 mmHg (95 percent confidence level) of that obtained at catheterization.[29] Similarly, the AVA will be within ±0.3 cm² of that obtained at cardiac catheterization.[29] A study of 156 patients compared AVA obtained by cardiac catheterization with that obtained by Doppler ultrasound.[30] Of 125 patients with AVA ≤ 0.8 cm² at cardiac catheterization, 36 patients (29 percent) had a Doppler-estimated AVA ≥ 0.9 cm². In all 7 patients with AVA >1.0 cm² by cardiac catheterization, Doppler-estimated AVA was 1.0 cm²; the findings in these 7 patients must be interpreted cautiously because they were likely to be a highly selected subgroup. Guidelines for assessing severity of AS based on Doppler-obtained gradients are shown in Table 66-3. In a study of 636 patients studied by cardiac catheterization, no single aortic valve gradient was found to be both sensitive and specific for severe AS.[31] A mean gradient of ≥50 mmHg or a peak gradient ≥60 mmHg were "specific" with a 90 percent or more positive predictive value. It was not possible to find a lower limit with 90 percent negative predictive value.[31] Thus, a mean gradient of <50 mmHg is compatible with mild, moderate, or severe AS.

Transesophageal echo/Doppler ultrasound is very useful in defining an aortic valve abnormality and in assessing its severity when an adequate examination cannot be obtained with the transthoracic technique.

CARDIAC CATHETERIZATION AND ANGIOGRAPHY

Cardiac catheterization remains the standard technique to assess the severity of AS "accurately." This is done by measuring simultaneous LV and ascending aortic pressures and measuring cardiac output by either the Fick principle or the indicator dilution technique. It is important to calculate the AVA (see Chap. 20).[31] AS can be considered

TABLE 66-3 Suggested Conservative Guidelines for Relating Severity of Aortic Stenosis to Doppler Gradients in Adults

Peak Gradient, mmHg	Mean Gradient, mmHg	Severe AS
≥80	≥70	Highly likely
60–79	50–69	Probable
<60	<50	Uncertain

A SUGGESTED GRADING OF THE DEGREE OF AORTIC STENOSIS

Aortic Stenosis	AVA, cm²	AVA Index, cm²/m²
Mild	>1.5	>0.9
Moderate	>1.0–1.5	>0.6–0.9
Severe[a]	≤0.8–1.0	≤0.4–0.6

[a]Patients with AVAs that are at borderline values between the moderate and severe grades (0.9–1.1 cm²; 0.55–0.65 cm²/m²) should be considered individually.
ABBREVIATIONS: AVA = aortic valve area.
SOURCE: From Rahimtoola,[29] with permission.

TABLE 66-4 Aortic Valve Disease: Indications for Coronary Arteriography

Patients ≥35 years
Patients <35 years:
    Left ventricular dysfunction
    Symptoms or signs suggesting CAD
    Two or more risk factors for premature CAD
      (excluding gender)

ABBREVIATIONS: CAD = coronary artery disease.
SOURCE: From Rahimtoola,[29] with permission.

to be severe when the AVA is 1.0 cm^2 or less or the AVA index is 0.6 cm^2/m^2 or less (see Table 66-3).[29] The state of LV systolic pump function can be quantitated by measuring LV end-diastolic and end-systolic volumes and ejection fraction. *It must be recognized that the ejection fraction may underestimate myocardial function in the presence of the increased afterload of severe AS.*

The presence of CAD and its site and severity can be estimated only by selective coronary angiography (Table 66-4). The incidence of associated CAD will vary considerably depending on the prevalence of CAD in the population.[29] It was reported to be 50 percent in patients with AS and 20 percent in patients with AR.[29] In general, in persons 50 years of age or older, it is about 50 percent (Table 66-5).[32–34]

GATED BLOOD POOL RADIONUCLIDE SCANS

Gated blood pool radionuclide scans provide information on ventricular function similar to that provided by two-dimensional echocardiography and LV cineangiography. These studies are of value in the patient in whom LV cineangiography is unsuccessful and echocardiographic studies are suboptimal.

EXERCISE TESTS

It is usually recommended that exercise tests of any kind not be undertaken in patients with severe AS unless there is a specific reason

TABLE 66-5 Isolated Aortic Valve Replacement: Incidence of Associated Coronary Artery Disease

	VA Co-op Study*	Mayo Clinic†	MGH‡ (80–89 years)
Total number of patients	643	618	64
Patients with coronary artery disease	312	321	37
%	49%	52%	58%
1 VD	17%	22%	27%
2 VD	17%	14%	19%
3 VD	15%	17%	13%
Additional LMCAD	—	5%	3%

*Sethi GK, et al.[32]
†Mullany CJ, et al.[33]
‡Levinson JR, et al.[34]
ABBREVIATIONS: LMCAD = left main coronary artery disease; MGH = Massachusetts General Hospital; VA = Veterans Administration; VD = vessel disease.

for such studies. Exercise tests in these patients may precipitate ventricular tachyarrhythmias and ventricular fibrillation,[22] particularly if they have significant associated CAD. If there is doubt about the severity of AS and concern that the patient's symptoms may not be caused by AS, it is usually wise to document the absence of severe AS and of associated CAD before performing an exercise test. Occasionally, in a patient with severe AS who denies all symptoms, a closely monitored exercise test by experienced and skilled physicians may be needed to assess exercise capacity but should usually *only* be undertaken after exclusion of associated significantly obstructive CAD.

AMBULATORY ELECTROCARDIOGRAM RECORDING

Ambulatory ECG recordings may be needed occasionally in a patient suspected of having an arrhythmia or painless ischemia (see Chap. 41).

PROVOCATIVE DIAGNOSTIC TEST

Occasionally, the severity of the AS may be in doubt in a patient because of a small mean aortic valve gradient. The AS may be severe or mild to moderate, and the calculated AVA may be very small because of severe stenosis or because the small stroke volume only opens the valve to a limited extent; thus, the AVA will be determined to be small even on echo/Doppler ultrasound. Infusion of an inotropic agent such as dobutamine, which results in increases of cardiac output (and of stroke volume) and heart rate (and of shortening of systolic ejection time), usually helps one to make a correct diagnosis. In these circumstances, it is important to measure cardiac output and LV and aortic pressures simultaneously and meticulously, both before and during dobutamine infusion.[35] Whether the AS is mild or severe, the gradient increases with dobutamine infusion; however, in mild AS the AVA increases significantly; but in severe AS the AVA does not increase or increases minimally (approximately 10 percent).

Clinical Decision Making

There are a number of steps involved in clinical decision making in patients with valvular heart disease (Table 66-6).[29] The first is a complete clinical evaluation, which includes history, physical examination, ECG, and chest x-ray. Next, disease of all cardiac valves, ventricular function, and hemodynamic effects, as well as CAD, other cardiovascular disease, and disease of other organs should be diagnosed and the severity assessed. Before proceeding to additional testing, it is important to list the questions to be answered and to be reasonably certain that these questions need to be answered. The tests that are most likely to provide these answers *in the clinician's own institution* should then be performed, with the following criteria kept in mind: reliability, accuracy, lowest risk to patient, and reasonable (lowest) cost. The results of the tests should be reviewed as they become available, and an overall evaluation/assessment of the patient and, finally, recommendations regarding management should be made.

In a prospective, blinded study of consecutive patients with valvular heart disease, the sensitivity and specificity of diagnosis of AS and the accuracy of assessment of severity of AS were determined (Table 66-7).[36] This study revealed the following important points: (1) Clinical evaluation was sensitive, highly specific, and reasonably accurate in diagnosing AS and was very accurate in assessing its severity when AS was moderate or severe. This emphasizes the importance of a thorough clinical evaluation of the patient. (2) Echo/Doppler ultrasound improved the accuracy of this assessment to a certain extent. (3) The reason clinical evaluation and echo/

TABLE 66-6 Steps in Clinical Decision Making in Patients with Valvular Heart Disease

1. Perform a complete clinical evaluation
   History
   Physical examination
   Electrocardiogram
   Chest x-ray film
2. Diagnose and assess severity of disease
   All valves
   Ventricular function
   Hemodynamic effects
   Coronary artery disease
   Other cardiovascular disease
   Effects on other body organs
   Other organ diseases
3. List questions that need answering
4. Be reasonably certain these questions need to be answered
5. Perform test(s) most likely to provide these answers in one's own institution with the following criteria:
   Reliability
   Accuracy
   Lowest risk to patients
   Reasonable (or lowest) cost
6. Review results of test(s)
7. Make an overall assessment of patient
8. Make recommendations regarding management

SOURCE: From Rahimtoola,[29] with permission.

Doppler do not have a 100 percent specificity is the inability in a patient occasionally to distinguish mild AS from turbulence across a normal or slightly diseased aortic valve. (4) Both clinical evaluation and echo/Doppler ultrasound are excellent in diagnosing the AS as being at least moderate or severe. (5) An important difficulty in diagnosis by clinical evaluation and by echo/Doppler is in not being able to separate accurately all patients with moderate AS from those with severe AS.

Natural History and Prognosis

Valvular AS is frequently a progressive disease, its severity increasing over time.[1,35,37] The factors that control this progression and the

TABLE 66-7 Clinical Decision Making Utilizing Clinical Evaluation and Echo/Doppler in Patients with Aortic Stenosis

	After Clinical Evaluation, %	After Echo/Doppler, %
Diagnosis of AS		
Sensitivity	78	100
Specificity	92	92
Accuracy of diagnosis		
All levels of severity	48	65
Moderate or severe AS	100	100

SOURCE: From Kotlewski et al.,[36] with permission.

TABLE 66-8 Natural History of Mild[a] Aortic Stenosis ($n = 142$)

	10 Years	20 Years	25 Years
Mild	88%	63%	38%
Moderate	4%	15%	25%
Severe	8%	22%	38%

[a]Mild stenosis is defined here as an aortic valve area >1.5 cm^2.
SOURCE: From Horstkotte and Loogen,[38] with permission.

time it takes for severe outflow obstruction to develop are unknown; however, it is possible that in the older patient, AS may progress at a faster rate than it does in the younger patient. In a study of 142 patients with "mild" stenosis (catheterization-proven AVA >1.5 cm^2),[38] the rate of progression to severe stenosis was 8 percent in 10 years, 22 percent in 20 years, and 38 percent in 25 years. At 25 years, 38 percent still had mild AS (Table 66-8). The duration of the asymptomatic period after the development of severe AS is also unknown; some data suggest that it may be less than 2 years. The outcome of the asymptomatic patient with severe AS is not known. In the study of 123 asymptomatic patients aged 63 ± 16 years,[39] the actuarial probability of an event (death or aortic valve surgery) was 7 ± 5 percent at 1 year, 38 ± 8 percent at 3 years, and 74 ± 10 percent at 5 years. The event rate at 2 years for peak aortic jet velocity by Doppler ultrasound of >4 m/s was 79 ± 18 percent, of 3 to 4 m/s was 66 ± 13 percent, and of <3 m/s was 16 ± 16 percent.[39] However, the limitations of gradients and of aortic peak velocity obtained by Doppler ultrasound should be kept in mind.[37] The overwhelming majority of adults with severe AS who are seen by cardiologists have symptoms.

Severe disease in adults is lethal, particularly if the patient is symptomatic, with a prognosis that is worse than for many forms of neoplastic disease.[29] The 3-year mortality is approximately 36 to 52 percent; the 5-year mortality is about 52 to 80 percent; and the 10-year mortality is 80 to 90 percent.[29,35] A study of elderly patients (average age 77 years) showed 1-year and 3-year mortalities were 44 and 75 percent, respectively.[35] With the onset of severe symptoms (angina, syncope, or heart failure), the average life expectancy is 2 to 3 years (Table 66-9).[38,40] Almost all patients with heart failure are dead in 1 to 2 years.[38,40] A combination of symptoms is much more ominous, a sign of a greatly reduced survival. Sudden death, like syncope, occurs in the presence of severe AS. Its exact incidence is difficult to determine but may be about 5 percent.[40] Most but not all of these patients have had some cardiac symptoms before the fatal

TABLE 66-9 Average Survival of Symptomatic Patients with Severe Aortic Stenosis

	Autopsy Data,* Years	Post Cardiac Catheterization,† Months
Overall	3	23
Angina	5	45
Syncope	3	27
Heart failure	<2	11

*From Ross and Braunwald.[40]
†From Horstkotte and Loogen.[38]

episode; at times, the only symptom has been exertional presyncope. Patients with aortic valve "sclerosis" have an approximately 50 percent increase in cardiovascular mortality and myocardial infarction.[41] This incidence is lower than it is in patients with AS, and aortic sclerosis appears to be a marker for vascular atherosclerosis.

Management

All patients with AS need antibiotic prophylaxis against infective endocarditis (see Chap. 90). Those in whom the valve lesion is of rheumatic origin need additional prophylaxis against recurrence of rheumatic fever. Patients with mild or moderate stenosis rarely have symptoms or complications and do not need any specific medical therapy (Table 66-10). In mild stenosis, the patient should be encouraged to lead a normal life. Those with moderate AS should avoid moderate to severe physical exertion and competitive sports. Atrial fibrillation in patients with mild or moderate AS should be reverted rapidly to sinus rhythm. In severe AS, reversion to sinus rhythm often becomes a matter of some urgency.

SURGERY

Operation should be advised for the symptomatic patient who has severe AS. In young patients, if the valve is pliable and mobile, simple commissurotomy or valve repair may be feasible; the operative mortality is <1 percent.[42] It will relieve outflow obstruction to a major degree. In such patients, catheter balloon valvuloplasty (CBV) is the procedure of choice in experienced and skilled centers. Both of these are palliative procedures that postpone AVR for many years. Older patients and even young patients with calcified, rigid valves need AVR. The natural history of symptomatic patients with severe AS is dismal (i.e., a 10-year mortality of 80 to 90 percent), but there is good outcome after AVR, particularly in patients without any comorbid cardiac and noncardiac conditions. Given the unknown natural history of the asymptomatic patient with severe AS, which may not be benign,[29] it is reasonable to recommend AVR even to the asymptomatic patient. There is, however, no consensus about AVR in all asymptomatic patients; it is clearly indicated in those undergoing

TABLE 66-10 Medical Treatment of Patients with Aortic Valve Stenosis

I. Antibiotic prophylaxis
   A. Infective endocarditis (Chap. 92)
   B. Recurrent rheumatic carditis (Chap. 72)
II. Restriction of activities
   A. Severe exercise
   B. Competitive sports
III. Arrhythmias
   A. Prevent and/or control
   B. Restore sinus rhythm, if possible
IV. Cardiac medications (only if essential)
   A. Avoid negative inotropic and proarrhythmic agents if possible
   B. Diuretics—use cautiously
   C. Arteriolar and venodilators—use cautiously
V. Follow-up of asymptomatic patients
   A. Mild AS: Every 2–5 years
   B. Moderate AS: Every 6–12 months
   C. Develop symptoms: Immediate

SOURCE: Copyright SH Rahimtoola.[64]

TABLE 66-11 Severe Aortic Valve Stenosis: Indications for Surgery

I. All symptomatic patients
   A. LV function normal: as soon as possible
   B. LV dysfunction: urgent
   C. Heart failure: emergent
II. Asymptomatic patients
   A. Patients undergoing surgery for CAD, aorta, other valves
   B. Associated significantly obstructed CAD
   C. LV dysfunction
   D. Progressive decline of LVEF
   E. Marked or excessive LVH:
     1. $\geq$11–12 mm in smaller people, e.g., women
     2. $\geq$13–14 mm in larger people, e.g., men
   F. Patients aged $\geq$60–65 years
   G. "Very" severe AS $\leq$0.7 cm^2; 0.4 cm^2/m^2
   H. Others:
     1. Abnormal response to exercise
       a. Hypotension/no or minimal increase of BP
       b. Ischemia
       c. LV dysfunction
       d. Arrhythmias
     2. Arrhythmias
       a. Ventricular/Atrial tachyarrhythmias
       b. A-V block >1° AVB

ABBREVIATIONS: LV = left ventricular; EF = ejection fraction; LVH = left ventricular hypertrophy; AS = aortic stenosis; BP = blood pressure; AVB = atrioventricular block; CAD = coronary artery disease.
SOURCE: Copyright © by Shahbudin H. Rahimtoola.[64]

surgery for CAD, aorta or other valve disease, in those with LV dysfunction, and/or with associated CAD (Table 66-11).

The operative mortality of AVR is about 4 percent.[43] In patients without associated CAD, heart failure, or other comorbid factors, it may be 1 to 2 percent in centers with experienced and skilled staff.[33] In those in New York Heart Association (NYHA) functional classes I, II, III and IV, it was 1.25 percent, 1.81 percent, 3.69 percent and 7.05 percent, respectively.[44] Patients with associated CAD should have coronary bypass surgery at the same time as AVR because it results in a lower operative and late mortality (Table 66-12).[33] The operative mortality for AVR and coronary bypass surgery is 6.8 percent.[43] The operative mortality in octogenarians or in those who are older is much higher: 6 percent for isolated AVR and 10 percent for those undergoing AVR and associated coronary bypass surgery.[45]

In severe AS, AVR results in an improvement of survival (Fig. 66-4),[38,46] even in those with normal preoperative LV function. LV function remains normal postoperatively if perioperative myocardial damage has not occurred.[11,29,47,48] LVH regresses toward normal;[11,29,47,48] after 2 years, the regression continues at a slower rate for up to 8 to 10 years after AVR.[48] In those with excessive LVH preoperatively,[15] the LVH may regress slowly or not at all. These patients may have persistent severe LV diastolic dysfunction, which may be a difficult clinical problem both in the early postoperative period and after hospital discharge. Their clinical picture subsequently resembles that of patients with hypertrophic cardiomyopathy without outflow obstruction, and they may have to be treated as such. Surviving patients are functionally improved.

After AVR, the 10-year survival is 50 percent or better and the 15-year survival is 33 percent or better.[49] Approximately 40 percent of

TABLE 66-12 Aortic Valve Replacement (AVR) Operative Mortality and Late Survival: Effect of Coronary Bypass Surgery (CBS)

	1982–1983	1967–1976					
	Operative Mortality, %	Operative Mortality, %	All Patients, %	1 VD, %	2 VD, %	3 VD, %	LMCAD, %
AVR + no CAD	1.4	4.5	63	—	—	—	—
AVR + CAD + CBS	4.0	6.3	49	38	28	34	11
AVR + CAD + no CBS	9.4	10.3	36	65	22	13	1

ABBREVIATIONS: CAD = coronary artery disease, VD = vessel disease, LMCAD = left main coronary artery disease.
SOURCE: From Mullany et al.,[33] with permission.

the late deaths are not related to the prosthesis but to associated cardiac abnormalities and other comorbid conditions.[49] Thus, the late survival will vary in different subgroups of patients. The older patients (≥65 years) have a relative 10-year survival (actual survival compared to an age- and gender-matched person in the population) after AVR that is significantly better than that of those who are younger (<65 years): 94 versus 81 percent (Fig. 66-5).[50]

HEART FAILURE

Patients who present with heart failure should be hospitalized and treated with digitalis and diuretics and should undergo surgery as soon as possible. *Angiotensin-converting enzyme* (ACE) inhibitors should be used cautiously if at all. The patient must be monitored and hypotension avoided; a "significant" fall in blood pressure is an indication to discontinue or reduce the dose of ACE inhibitor. If heart failure does not respond satisfactorily and rapidly to medical therapy, surgery becomes a matter of considerable urgency. CBV can be an important bridge procedure in selected critically ill patients.[51] It usually improves the patients' hemodynamics and makes them better candidates for valve replacement. AVR in patients with AS and heart failure can be performed at an operative mortality of 10 percent or less.[35,52] Although this is higher than it is in patients not in heart failure, the risk is justified because late survival in those who survive the operation is excellent and is far superior to that which can be expected with medical therapy; the 7-year survival of patients who survive operation is 84 percent.[53] The survival is lower in those with associated CAD.[52] The impaired LV function improves in all such patients provided that there has been no perioperative myocardial damage; it becomes normal in two-thirds of the patients (Fig. 66-6).[54] In some patients the improvement is less marked.[52]

This is more likely in those with longer duration of preoperative LV dysfunction and in those with associated CAD. In addition, the operative survivors are functionally much improved. LV hypertrophy and dilatation (if present preoperatively) regress toward normal. Despite the excellent results of AVR in patients with severe AS who are in heart failure, it is important to recognize that surgery should *not* be delayed until heart failure develops. Patients with severe AS, mean gradient ≥30 mmHg, and LV ejection fraction ≤0.35 have a higher operative mortality; however, the survivors have an improvement in LV function and functional class.[55,56] For patients who have severe AS, heart failure and "severe" pulmonary hypertension have a high

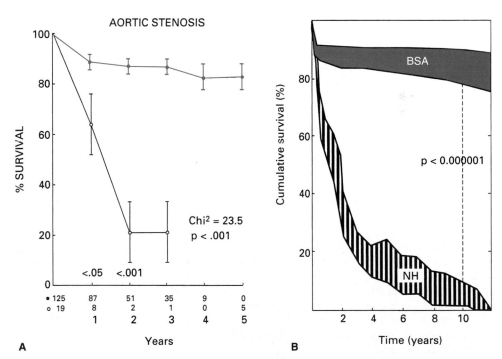

FIGURE 66-4 There are no prospective randomized trials of aortic valve replacement (AVR) in severe aortic stenosis, and there are unlikely to be any in the near future. Two studies have compared the results of AVR with medical treatment during the same time period in symptomatic patients with normal left ventricular (LV) systolic pump function. *Panel A.* Patients who had AVR (*closed circles*) had a much better survival than did those treated medically (*open circles*). (From Schwarz et al.,[46] with permission.) *Panel B.* Patients who were treated with AVR (body surface area, BSA) had a better survival than did those treated medically (natriuretic hormone, NH). (From Horstkotte and Loogen,[38] with permission.)

These differences in survival between those treated medically and surgically are so large that there is a great deal of confidence that AVR significantly improves the survival of those with severe AS.

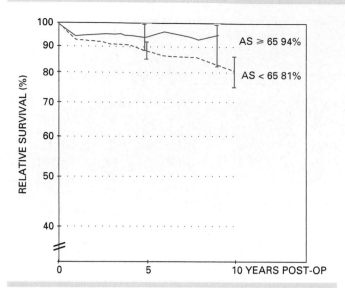

FIGURE 66-5 Data from the Karolinska Institute in Sweden provided an interesting perspective on the long-term survival of patients aged ≥65 years after aortic valve replacement (AVR). They examined the relative survival (i.e., compared the survival of the patient who had undergone AVR with another age- and sex-matched person in the same population). Patients <65 years of age had a relative survival of 81 percent, significantly lower than 100 percent. In contrast, patients aged ≥65 years who underwent AVR had a relative survival of 94 percent at the end of 10 years—not significantly different from 100 percent. These data indicate that (1) survival following AVR for aortic stenosis (AS) in patients aged ≥65 years is identical to an age- and sex-matched individual in the population who does not have AS and (2) the late relative survival of patients ≥65 years is much better than that of patients ≤65. (From Lindblom et al.,[50] with permission.)

operative mortality and poor late survival; however, this is still better than it is for those who have only medical treatment.[57]

Up to 6 percent of the older patients present in cardiogenic shock.[58] The hospital mortality in such patients is very high, almost 50 percent. After hospital discharge, the subsequent mortality is also very high if the patients have not had their stenosis relieved.[51] Thus, these patients need to be treated aggressively with medical therapy using hemodynamic monitoring, and they need emergent surgery with or without CBV as a "bridge" procedure[51] (Table 66-13).

CATHETER BALLOON VALVULOPLASTY

In calcific AS, the average increase in AVA after CBV is 0.3 cm^2 and the final AVA usually averages 0.8 cm^2; thus, many patients continue to have severe AS.[29,51,58] The 30-day, 1-year, and 3-year mortalities average 14, 35, and 71 percent, respectively, in the older patient (average age 78 ± 9 years) with calcific AS[58]—a mortality rate that is similar to the natural history of this lesion. This technique is indicated[51] as a bridge procedure in those who need emergent noncardiac surgery, and in other selected subgroups (Table 66-14) CBV is the procedure of choice in young patients who have pliable, noncalcified valves with commissural fusion.

The recommendations of the American College of Cardiology/American Heart Association (ACC/AHA) Practice Guidelines are shown in Tables 66-13 and 66-15.[59] Guidelines *are not* and *should not* be the law. Application of these guidelines to clinical practice should be based on the following principles: (1) classes I and III apply to all patients in these classes unless there is a specific clinical circumstance not to do so; (2) class II applies to patients in this class, depending on the clinical conditions of the patients and the skill and experience at the individual medical center.

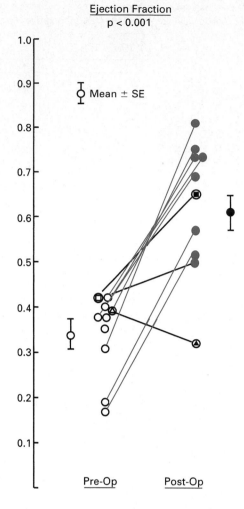

● Peri-Op MI and late CHB

● Post-Op Perivalvular Aortic Imcompetence

FIGURE 66-6 Examination of changes in LV ejection fraction in each individual patient. In those who had aortic stenosis with left ventricular (LV) systolic dysfunction and clinical heart failure, the LV ejection fraction after aortic valve replacement (AVR) increased from 0.34 to 0.63. All but 1 patient showed an improvement in LV ejection fraction. The only patient who showed a deterioration in ejection fraction suffered a perioperative myocardial infarction and had complete heart block. The only patient who showed only a small increase in ejection fraction had had a myocardial infarct prior to AVR. Note that ejection fraction normalized in two-thirds of the patients, and in the two patients with the lowest ejection fraction (0.18 and 0.19), the ejection fraction normalized in both.

These data indicate that there is probably no lower limit of ejection fraction at which time these patients become inoperable. This also indicates that the lower the ejection fraction, the more urgent the need for AVR. (From Smith et al.,[54] with permission.)

ACUTE AORTIC REGURGITATION

Etiology

The two most common causes of acute AR are infective endocarditis and prosthetic valve dysfunction.[60] Other causes include dissection of the aorta, systemic hypertension, and trauma.[61] AR associated with dissection of the aorta indicates that the dissection involves the

TABLE 66-13 Recommendations for Aortic Balloon Valvotomy in Adults with Aortic Stenosis*

Indication	Class
1. A "bridge" to surgery in hemodynamically unstable patients who are at high risk for AVR	IIa
2. Palliation in patients with serious comorbid conditions	IIb
3. Patients who require urgent noncardiac surgery	IIb
4. An alternative to AVR	III

*Recommendations for aortic balloon valvotomy in adolescents and young adults with AS are provided in section VI.A. of the ACC/AHA Guidelines.
ABBREVIATION: AVR = aortic valve replacement.
SOURCE: ACC/AHA Guidelines,[59] with permission.

ascending aorta down to the aortic valve annulus and root. AR associated with systemic hypertension is usually mild and transient; it is associated with severe elevation of aortic pressure, and, when the systemic hypertension is controlled, the AR usually disappears unless permanent changes have occurred in the aortic valve annulus and root or valve leaflets.

Pathophysiology

The LV diastolic pressure–volume relationship plays a very important role in the pathophysiology of acute AR (Fig. 66-7).[62,63] Two features should be considered:[60] (1) The ability of the LV to dilate acutely is limited; as a result, the volume overload of acute AR produces a rapid increase of LV diastolic pressure (curve B in Fig. 66-7). (2) The LV diastolic pressure–volume relationship before the onset

TABLE 66-14 Suggested Indications for Catheter Balloon Valvuloplasty in Patients with Severe Calcific Aortic Valve Stenosis*

  I. "Bridge" procedure to eventual AVR
   A. Cardiogenic shock
   B. Moderate to severe heart failure
   C. Emergent/urgent need for noncardiac therapeutic procedures (e.g., operation)
 II. Patient with limited life span
   A. Noncardiac reasons (e.g., carcinoma)
   B. Cardiac reason(s) other than aortic stenosis
III. Others
   A. Patient at extremely high risk for AVR
   B. AVR not desirable for noncardiac reasons or cardiac causes other than aortic stenosis
   C. Patient refuses surgery
 IV. Rare
   A. "Therapeutic test": patients with small stroke volume and small valve gradient, with valve stenosis suspected to be severe but severity in doubt even after provocative diagnostic tests

*Caution should be exercised in recommending this procedure in asymptomatic patients.
ABBREVIATIONS: AVR = aortic valve replacement.
SOURCE: Adapted from Rahimtoola,[51] with permission.

TABLE 66-15 Recommendations for Aortic Valve Replacement in Aortic Stenosis

Indication	Class
1. Symptomatic patients with severe AS	I
2. Patients with severe AS undergoing coronary artery bypass surgery	I
3. Patients with severe AS undergoing surgery on the aorta or other heart valves	I
4. Patients with moderate AS undergoing coronary artery bypass surgery or surgery on the aorta or other heart valves (see sections III.F.6., III.F.7., and VIII.D. of the ACC/AHA Guidelines)	IIa
5. Asymptomatic patients with severe AS and	
• LV systolic dysfunction	IIa
• Abnormal response to exercise (e.g., hypotension)	IIa
• Ventricular tachycardia	IIb
• Marked or excessive LV hypertrophy (≥15 mm)	IIb
• Valve area <0.6 cm^2	IIb
6. Prevention of sudden death in asymptomatic patients with none of the findings listed under indication 5	III

ABBREVIATIONS: AS = aortic stenosis; ACC/AHA = American College of Cardiology/American Heart Association; LV = left ventricular.
SOURCE: ACC/AHA Guidelines,[59] with permission.

of acute AR. If the LV is already stiff or less compliant than normal from an associated lesion (e.g., AS or systemic hypertension), the LV diastolic pressure will rise more precipitously as a result of the volume overload of acute AR (curve A) than if the LV were normal (curve B). In comparison, if the LV is somewhat dilated from a previous lesion—for example, mild AR (curve C)—initially the LV pressure will rise more gradually with acute AR but may subsequently rise to the same high levels as that seen with a normal or stiff LV.

Acute AR that is mild produces little or no hemodynamic abnormality, for example, when associated with systemic hypertension. Increasing severity of AR produces greater degrees of hemodynamic abnormalities, and severe AR often produces the clinical picture of "heart failure."

Acute AR that is severe results in a large volume of regurgitant blood; therefore, the volume of blood in the LV in diastole is increased. In an acute situation, the LV end-diastolic volume can only increase mildly (no more than 20 to 30 percent) and the LV diastolic pressure–volume relationships are particularly important. The LV systolic pump function is initially normal (Fig. 66-8). The increased LV diastolic pressure results in increases in mean LA and pulmonary venous pressures and produces varying degrees of pulmonary edema.[64] The normal LV systolic pump function in the presence of LV dilatation results in an increase of LV stroke volume. A large percentage of the LV stroke volume is returned to the LV in diastole; however, as a result, the forward stroke volume is reduced. The LV uses two mechanisms: an increase of myocardial contractility and, importantly, a compensatory tachycardia to maintain an adequate forward cardiac output. As a result, the forward cardiac output may be appropriate initially. If the compensatory mechanisms are

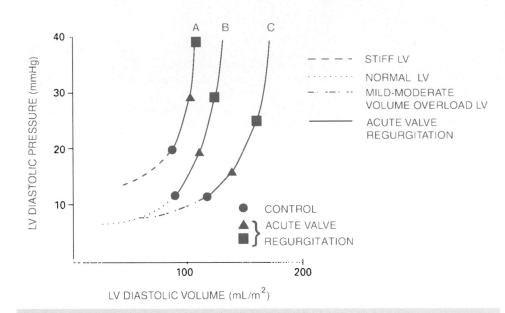

FIGURE 66-7 The left ventricular (LV) diastolic pressure–volume (P–V) relationship in acute valve regurgitation. The volume overload of acute aortic regurgitation (AR) produces a rapid increase of LV diastolic pressure in a patient with normal LV diastolic P–V prior to the acute AR (*curve B*). The LV diastolic pressure will rise more or less precipitously as a result of the volume overload of acute AR, depending on whether the LV is already stiff (*curve A*) or is somewhat dilated from a previous volume overload (*curve C*). (From Rahimtoola,[65] with permission.)

inadequate, forward cardiac output is reduced. Pulmonary edema, with or without an adequate cardiac output, produces the picture of clinical heart failure.[64] Subsequently, LV systolic pump function may become abnormal; when that occurs, the pulmonary edema is further increased and the forward cardiac output is further reduced, leading to more severe manifestations of heart failure.

Clinical Findings

HISTORY AND PHYSICAL FINDINGS

The clinical presentations are those relating to preexisting disorders that have caused the acute AR. For example, patients may have peripheral signs of infective endocarditis, a history of trauma, or severe chest pain of aortic dissection. The other clinical presentations are those related to the AR itself. If the AR is mild, the patient is usually asymptomatic. In the symptomatic patient, the symptoms are those of heart failure.

On physical examination, the symptomatic patient with acute severe AR usually has a tachycardia. The arterial pulse shows an increased rate of rise of pressure. Systolic pressure is usually normal unless there is very severe heart failure; however, the diastolic pressure is in the normal range or may be decreased. The pulse pressure is usually normal. Thus, although the classic peripheral signs of chronic, severe AR are often absent, an important diagnostic clue is the rapid rate of rise of arterial pressure. The usual clinical signs of heart failure may be present. On examination of the precordium, the LV impulse is normal or slightly displaced to the left; it is usually hyperkinetic unless LV systolic dysfunction is present. The first heart sound is soft, and the second heart sound is often single and is soft. If pulmonary hypertension is present, P_2 is loud and there is a loud S_3 gallop sound, an S_4 gallop sound is absent. The clinical sine qua non of

AR is the AR murmur, an early or immediate, blowing, decrescendo diastolic murmur beginning after A_2 that is best heard with the diaphragm of the stethoscope. Having the patient sit up and lean forward with the breath held in expiration facilitates the audibility of the murmur in difficult cases. The murmur may be short and soft if the ascending aortic pressure equalizes with LV pressure in early or mid-diastole. An Austin Flint murmur, if present, occurs in presystole or mid-diastole (see Chap. 14).

An important clinical picture in intravenous drug abusers[60] includes: (1) a peripheral arterial pulse that has a rapid rate of rise and fall, even though the pulse pressure is small; (2) the telltale signs of intravenous drug abuse; (3) sinus tachycardia; and (4) "normal" heart size with pulmonary edema on chest x-ray.

CHEST X-RAY

The chest x-ray shows a "normal" heart size with pulmonary edema; however, some enlargement of all cardiac chambers and the main pulmonary artery may be present. The aorta is not dilated unless aortic annular/root disease or dissection of the aorta is the cause of the acute AR. The aorta may also be dilated in the older patient and/or in those with an associated disease such as systemic hypertension. The lungs may show the signs of infected pulmonary emboli if there is associated tricuspid valve endocarditis.

ELECTROCARDIOGRAM

The ECG often shows nonspecific ST-T-wave changes and a sinus tachycardia; however, it may be normal. The ECG may show signs that are usually found in the associated causative disorder (e.g., LVH with ST-T-wave changes in patients with severe hypertension). The ECG may show a variety of conduction abnormalities (atrioventricular and bundle branch block), including heart block, which, in the presence of infective endocarditis, is a sign of paravalvular or myocardial abscess.

Natural History and Prognosis

The natural history of this condition is variable. If the AR is mild to moderate in severity, these patients are likely to do well with medical therapy. Eventually, the changes of chronic AR will be seen. In patients with severe AR, the natural history depends on whether or not they have heart failure.[65] If heart failure is present, which is common, the prognosis is very poor without AVR unless the heart failure can be very easily controlled with medical therapy.

Management

DIAGNOSIS OF AORTIC REGURGITATION

In most instances, the diagnosis can be made by clinical evaluation. The diagnosis by physical examination in an acutely ill patient who is in extremis may be difficult.

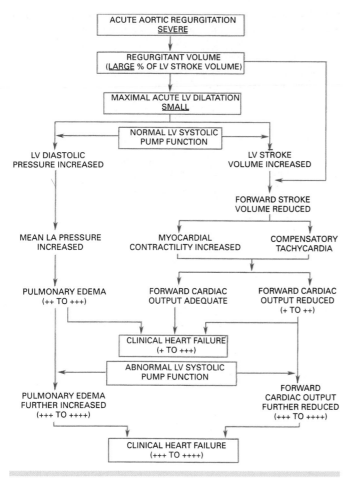

FIGURE 66-8 Pathophysiology of acute severe aortic regurgitation (AR). Acute AR that is severe results in a large volume of regurgitant blood; therefore, the volume of blood in the LV in diastole is increased. In an acute situation, the LV end-diastolic volume can only increase mildly (no more than 20 to 30 percent) and the LV diastolic pressure–volume relationships are particularly important (see Fig. 66-1). The subsequent findings are dependent on LV systolic pump function, LV diastolic pressure–volume relationship, myocardial contractile state, and compensatory tachycardia (see text for details). (Copyright by SH Rahimtoola.[64])

Transthoracic echo/Doppler ultrasound is an important and valuable noninvasive procedure that should be used in every instance. It will demonstrate the AR and its severity and will provide useful information about the size and function of the LV and other valvular and cardiac abnormalities. If the transthoracic method is not adequate, the transesophageal method should be used, which is usually essential in those with infective endocarditis (see Chap. 90).

Echocardiography shows the diastolic flutter of the anterior leaflet of the mitral valve. In addition, the echocardiogram may show vegetations on the aortic valve, prolapse of an aortic valve leaflet into the LV in diastole, and premature mitral valve closure. The mitral valve may be seen to open for only a short time because the stroke volume is limited. Occasionally, the aortic valve leaflets have been totally destroyed, and none are seen on the echocardiogram. Doppler ultrasound demonstrates the AR and an estimate of its severity.

Cardiac catheterization and angiography, including coronary arteriography, show the abnormal physiology described, and aortography shows gross AR. These modalities may be needed to make the diagnosis and are usually indicated before surgical intervention. Coronary arteriography is indicated in the appropriate patient (see

earlier). In the extremely ill patient, there is often a need for clinical judgment regarding which tests are essential.

Other tests may be needed in very special circumstances.

DIAGNOSIS OF THE ETIOLOGY OF ACUTE AORTIC REGURGITATION

The diagnosis of the etiology is usually made during the clinical evaluation. Additional laboratory tests will be needed to confirm the diagnosis; for example, blood cultures in those with suspected infective endocarditis. Echo/Doppler ultrasound examination is also extremely valuable in diagnosing the underlying lesion. Its widespread availability and comparative ease of use, especially in the very acutely ill patient, make it the noninvasive procedure of choice. The availability of biplane and omniplane transesophageal probes should further enhance its value as a diagnostic tool.

Magnetic resonance imaging (MRI) has a very high specificity for the diagnosis of dissection of the aorta[66] and, if available, should be used in all hemodynamically stable patients if the diagnosis has not already been made. The availability of biplane or omniplane transesophageal echocardiography improves the specificity and diagnostic accuracy of transesophageal echocardiography. Angiography is also an effective and time-honored method of diagnosing dissection of the aorta.

In summary, clinical evaluation is available in all institutions; echo/Doppler ultrasound is available in almost all institutions. The use of the other tests depends on the availability of equipment and the skill and experience of personnel using the equipment for this purpose at each institution.

BEDSIDE HEMODYNAMIC MONITORING

In acute disorders affecting the LV, there may be a phase lag between the rise in pulmonary venous pressure and the appearance of pulmonary edema on the chest x-ray film. As a result, the reliability of the chest x-ray in demonstrating the presence and severity of elevated LA pressure initially is less than satisfactory in the acutely ill patient.[67] If the assessment of LA pressure is made by physical examination and chest x-ray, a significant number of errors may be made in these patients with an acute cardiac problem. Therapeutic decisions based on incorrect assessments may result in significant problems. The optimization of filling pressures and cardiac output may not be made accurately in acute heart failure without measuring their actual values. Thus, use of a balloon flotation catheter for bedside hemodynamic monitoring is required in most, if not all, acutely ill patients with acute AR.

TREATMENT

Treatment of heart failure is directed toward reducing pulmonary venous pressure and increasing cardiac output. In all patients, treatment is also directed toward correcting or controlling the etiologic disease/disorder and/or the altered pathophysiologic state (Table 66-16).[60,65]

Intravenous nitroprusside for an acute, severe condition is useful and important in the management of these patients.[68] Combined arteriolar and venous dilators will produce a reduction of LA v-wave and mean LA pressure. They produce a reduction in LV end-diastolic and end-systolic volumes and an increase in LV ejection fraction. The regurgitant fraction and regurgitant volume are reduced; as a result, the forward stroke volume and cardiac output are increased.[68] Digitalis therapy is of significant benefit in the management of heart failure. The combination of various agents (vasodilators, diuretics, and digitalis) tends to produce the maximum benefit in an individual

TABLE 66-16 Treatment of Heart Failure in Acute Valve Regurgitation

I. Correct or control altered pathophysiologic state
  A. Reduce pulmonary venous pressure
    1. Diuresis
    2. Vasodilation
    3. Control heart rate and maintain sinus rhythm (digitalis, cardioversion, antiarrhythmics)
  B. Increase cardiac output
    1. Reduction of valve regurgitation (vasodilators)
    2. Inotropic stimulation (digitalis, dobutamine)
  C. Improve left ventricular systolic dysfunction
    1. Reduce pulmonary venous pressure
    2. Increase cardiac output
    3. Angiotensin-converting enzyme inhibitors
II. Correct or control underlying disease or disorder
  A. Antibiotics for infective endocarditis
  B. Pharmacologic therapy for systemic hypertension
  C. Surgery for valve regurgitation in infective endocarditis, prosthetic valve dysfunction, dissection of the aorta, trauma

SOURCE: From Rahimtoola,[60] with permission.

TABLE 66-17 Indications for Surgery in Infective Endocarditis

Congestive heart failure
Infection
  Uncontrolled by antibiotic therapy
  Fungal
  Usually with staphylococcal infection of aortic or mitral valves
  Serratia
  Usually with gram-negative bacillary infection
Recurrent septic systemic emboli despite adequate antibiotic therapy
Perivalvular and myocardial abscesses
Structural damage to valve in association with other catastrophes (e.g., ruptured sinus of Valsalva)
Very large mobile vegetation

SOURCE: From Rahimtoola,[47] with permission.

patient; intravenous nitroprusside is often necessary in the acutely ill patient.

Surgical therapy (valve replacement/valve repair or appropriate surgery for dissection of the aorta) is the cornerstone of the most definitive therapy currently available for heart failure in these patients. The management of the patient with heart failure or suspected heart failure is outlined in Fig. 66-9.[65] If the AR is due to *dissection of the aorta,* the need for cardiac surgery is an emergency, even if the regurgitation is mild or moderate, because AR indicates involvement of the ascending aorta down to the region of the aortic valve annulus and root. The outcome of the patient with heart failure due to infective endocarditis is very poor with medical therapy but is improved with AVR.[69] The indications for surgery in *infective endocarditis* are listed in Table 66-17.[47] Infective endocarditis due to special organisms (e.g., fungi) can only rarely be controlled by pharmacologic therapy alone, and surgery is almost always needed. In these and some other conditions, valve surgery may be needed even if the AR is only mild or moderate. It must be recognized, however, that in 90 to 95 percent of patients needing surgery for endocarditis, the indication for valve surgery is heart failure. When the heart failure is a result of *prosthetic valve dysfunction* or *trauma,* the need for surgery can be an emergency, an urgent situation, or an elective procedure. Prosthetic valves are inherently stenotic. When regurgitation is superimposed, it produces a pressure plus volume overload on the LV that the ventricle may not handle very well acutely. Furthermore, AR may be a sign of bioprosthetic valve degeneration or prosthetic endocarditis; in both conditions, prosthetic AVR is usually needed even if the AR is mild to moderate.

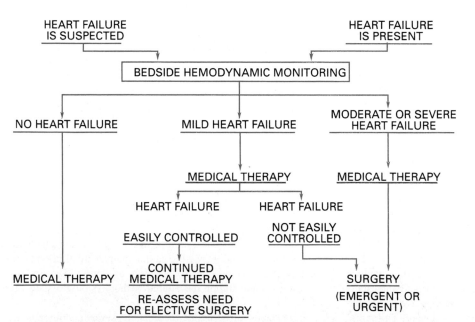

ACUTE SEVERE VALVE REGURGITATION

FIGURE 66-9 Role of bedside hemodynamic monitoring in acute aortic regurgitation (AR). All patients with acute AR probably should have this procedure. If the AR is mild and there are no significant hemodynamic abnormalities, then the balloon flotation catheter can be withdrawn. In comparison, if the AR is moderate to severe and there are significant hemodynamic abnormalities, then the balloon flotation catheter is left in place to guide therapy in the management of these acutely ill patients. If the hemodynamic abnormalities are mild, the patient is treated medically. If these abnormalities are easily controlled, medical therapy is continued and periodic reassessments are made to assess the need for elective surgery. If the hemodynamic abnormalities are not easily corrected or the hemodynamic abnormalities initially are moderate to severe, then surgery is undertaken either emergently or urgently. (From Rahimtoola,[65] with permission.)

Trauma may result in AR from damage to valve leaflets or aortic annulus and root or from dissection of the aorta. If trauma produces dissection of the aorta and AR, the need for surgery may be an emergent one.

In some instances, heart failure can be controlled completely with pharmacologic therapy, and the LV and LA are able to dilate and adapt to the volume overload; in such instances, surgical therapy may be delayed, perhaps for a considerable period.

CHRONIC AORTIC REGURGITATION

Etiology

In North America, the most common cause of chronic, isolated severe AR is aortic root and annular dilatation that is presumably the result of medial disease. Other common causes include a congenital (bicuspid) valve, previous infective endocarditis, and rheumatic disease.[1,61] Chronic AR also occurs in association with a variety of other diseases (Table 66-18). Between 40 and 60 percent of the surgically removed valves from patients with isolated severe AR are classified as idiopathic. Half of these (or 20 to 30 percent of all the valves removed) show histologic criteria of myxomatous degeneration.[70]

Pathology

During systole the aortic root and annulus expands by an increase of 14 to 16 percent of the diameter (twice the radius).[71] This causes the commissural attachments to spread apart, initiating the opening of the valves. These movements are continued during LV systole, which produces the forward motion of the blood. The length of the free edge of the cusps equals the diameter of the aortic root and annulus, or roughly one-third of the perimeter. Therefore, dilatation of the aortic root and annulus, if it is not accompanied by an enlargement of the cusps, results in AR.[71]

Depending on the cause, the valve cusps may show thickening, shortening, commissural lesions, or calcification.[1] Regardless of the cause, the LV is dilated and hypertrophied; some of the largest ventricles have been described in association with chronic severe AR. Little pockets may be seen in the LV outflow tract. These are pouches out of the endocardial lining formed by the regurgitant jets striking the LV.

TABLE 66-18 Etiology of Chronic Aortic Valve Regurgitation

Aortic root dilatation
Congenital bicuspid valve
Previous infective endocarditis
Rheumatic
In association with other diseases
    Congenital lesions, e.g., supravalvular or discrete
       subvalvular aortic stenosis, ventricular septal defect,
       and aneurysm of the sinus of Valsalva
    Connective tissue disease, e.g., Marfan's syndrome,
       osteogenesis imperfecta, and Ehlers-Danlos syndrome
    Autoimmune diseases, e.g., ankylosing spondylitis,
       rheumatoid arthritis, and systemic lupus erythematosus
    Various forms of aortitis and arteritis, e.g., giant-cell
       arteritis and Takayasu's disease
Syphilis

The myocardium is hypertrophied, with replication of sarcomeres in series, elongation of fibers, and wall thickening. The wall is not as thickened as it is in patients with AS.

Ultrastructural changes in the myocardial cells are similar to those seen in AS; an important difference, however, is the frequent presence of degenerated cardiac muscle cells in patients with severe AR.[1] Cardiac muscle cells with mild degeneration show focal myofibrillar lysis, with preferential loss of thick myofilament and focal proliferation of tubules of the sarcoplasmic reticulum. Moderately degenerated muscle cells show a marked decrease in the number of myofibrils and T tubules and proliferation of sarcoplasmic reticulum, mitochondria, or both. Severely degenerated muscle cells usually are present in areas of marked fibrosis; they are often atrophic, have thickened basement membranes, and have lost their intercellular connections. These degenerated cardiac muscle cells may represent the ultrastructural basis for impaired LV function, which is seen more commonly in severe AR than it is in severe AS.

In patients with rheumatoid arthritis and ankylosing spondylitis, nodules on the outer surface of the anterior leaflet of the mitral valve have been described (see Chap. 94).

Pathophysiology

In chronic as opposed to acute AR, the AR becomes severe over time; therefore, the LV diastolic pressure–volume relationships are different from those seen in acute AR (see Fig. 66-7). If the AR is mild to moderate, the LV end-diastolic volume is increased moderately, the LV diastolic pressure–volume curve is moved to the right (curve B) of normal (curve A), and the LV diastolic pressure is usually normal (Fig. 66-10). In severe AR, the LV diastolic pressure–volume curves are moved further to the right (curves C and D). If the LV systolic pump function is normal, the LV end-diastolic volume can be quite large without significant elevation of LV end-diastolic pressure (curve C). If the LV diastolic volume increases further, however, the LV diastolic pressures will be increased. If LV systolic pump

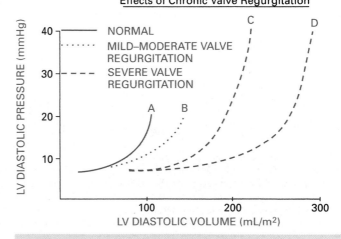

FIGURE 66-10 In chronic aortic regurgitation (AR) as opposed to acute AR, the AR becomes severe over time; therefore, the left ventricular (LV) diastolic pressure–volume (P–V) relationships are different from those seen in acute AR (see Fig. 66-7). If the AR is mild to moderate, the LV diastolic P–V curve is moved to the right (curve B). In severe AR, the LV diastolic P–V curves are moved further to the right, depending on whether the LV systolic pump function is normal (curve C) or abnormal (curve D). (From Rahimtoola,[65] with permission.)

dysfunction supervenes, the LV diastolic pressure–volume curve (curve D) relationships are moved even further to the right, with quite marked LV dilatation and increases in LV diastolic pressure.

The increase of LV end-diastolic volume[72] is a result of the regurgitant volume (and is proportional to the amount of regurgitation) and LV systolic dysfunction. As LV systolic dysfunction supervenes and increases in severity, for any severity of regurgitant volume the LV end-diastolic volume increases further in an attempt to maintain LV stroke volume.

Severe chronic AR results in a large regurgitant volume (a large percentage of LV stroke volume). The LV responds by dilating (average LV end-diastolic volume in patients undergoing surgery was 205 mL/m²)[11]; the dilatation is proportional to the amount of the regurgitant volume. The subsequent large LV stroke volume produces LV systolic hypertension. Both of these increase LV wall stress (afterload), which can result in an impairment of LV function. The heart responds by becoming hypertrophied (average LV mass in patients undergoing valve surgery was 222 g/m²,[11] and LV systolic pump function remains normal. There is also an alteration of the LV diastolic pressure–volume relationship (see Fig. 66-10). As a result, some

patients with normal LV systolic pump function become symptomatic[73] because of the abnormal LV diastolic function (Fig. 66-11).

In AR, the LV is ejecting against systemic resistance, and the myocardial tension that is developed to open the aortic valve and eject the huge stroke volume is great. This contrasts with another volume-overload lesion, mitral regurgitation, in which there is a low-resistance chamber into which the LV is also emptying (the LA). Thus, for the same degree of regurgitant volume, afterload is higher in AR.

As LV afterload (a combination of LV dilatation, LVH, and systolic hypertension) continues to increase, the LV utilizes two additional compensatory mechanisms, namely, increase of preload and an increase of myocardial contractility. Both of these help maintain normal LV systolic pump function.

When the limit of preload reserve has been reached (afterload mismatch)[16] and/or myocardial contractility is reduced, LV systolic pump function becomes abnormal. At this stage, correction of AR will result in normalization or marked improvement of LV systolic function. The additional LV dilatation also results in further alteration of the LV diastolic pressure-volume relationship (see Fig. 66-10). Clinical heart failure is usually a result of the abnormal LV systolic pump function. In patients with normal LV systolic pump function, clinical heart failure is a result of LV diastolic dysfunction.

Because of the leak of blood from the ascending aorta to the LV in diastole, the aortic diastolic pressure is reduced. The large LV stroke volume (a combination of forward stroke volume and regurgitant volume) results in elevation of the aortic systolic pressure, and thus the pulse pressure is considerably increased. Reduction or normalization of aortic systolic pressure is suggestive of LV systolic dysfunction in these patients.

LV stroke volume in AR consists of the forward stroke volume (blood delivered to the body tissues and the heart), which, multiplied by heart rate, makes up the forward cardiac output and the regurgitant volume (the volume of blood that regurgitates back to the LV). In the early stages, even in severe AR, the forward cardiac output and LV ejection fraction are normal at rest. During exercise, as in normal individuals, the systemic vascular resistance is decreased[74] and the heart rate is increased, which reduces the length of diastole. Both these factors reduce the regurgitant volume, and forward stroke volume and cardiac output are increased during exercise.[74] Thus, the ejection fraction on exercise is related to both the myocardial contractile state[75] and the fall in systemic vascular resistance.[74] Accordingly, a decline in ejection fraction on exercise cannot be used as a specific marker of LV

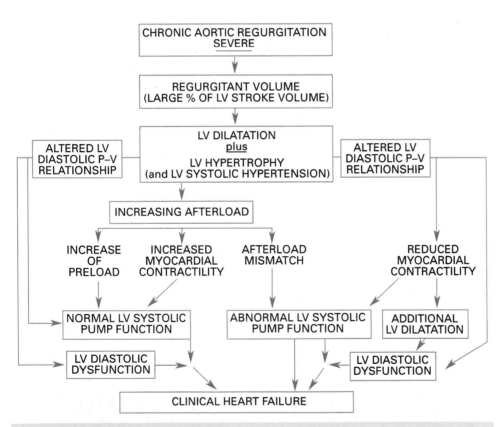

FIGURE 66-11 Severe chronic aortic regurgitation results in a large regurgitant volume [a large percentage of left ventricular (LV) stroke volume]. The LV responds by dilating; the subsequent large LV stroke volume results in the production of LV systolic hypertension. There is an alteration of the LV diastolic pressure–volume (P–V) relationship. However, some patients with normal LV systolic pump function become symptomatic because of the abnormal LV diastolic function. As LV afterload (a result of LV dilatation, hypertrophy, and systolic hypertension) continues to increase, the LV utilizes two additional compensatory mechanisms (i.e., increase of preload and an increase of myocardial contractility). Both of these help maintain normal LV systolic pump function.

When the limit of preload reserve has been reached (afterload mismatch) and/or myocardial contractility is reduced, LV systolic pump function becomes abnormal. The additional LV dilatation also results in further alteration of the LV diastolic P–V relationship.

Clinical heart failure is usually a result of the abnormal LV systolic pump function; diastolic dysfunction may also be present in some patients. Clinical heart failure in those with normal LV systolic pump function is a result of LV diastolic dysfunction. (Copyright by SH Rahimtoola.[64])

function in these patients unless the change in systemic vascular resistance has also been measured. A fall of normal resting ejection fraction to less than 0.50 on exercise, however, has been shown to correlate with reduced total body oxygen consumption and increased LA pressure during exercise.[74,76]

Further impairment of LV function produces demonstrable abnormalities at rest; there is a further increase in LV end-diastolic volume, which helps to maintain forward stroke volume. The resting LV ejection fraction is reduced, and mean LA pressure begins to increase. Even at this stage, the forward cardiac output may be maintained in the normal range. The increases in LA pressure may produce various grades of pulmonary edema. Finally, in the state of severe heart failure, the ejection fraction may be low, LV end-diastolic volume is large, and LV end-diastolic pressure is greatly increased and is associated with increases in LA, pulmonary, right ventricular, and right atrial pressures. Forward cardiac output is no longer normal. An increase in systemic venous pressure in association with salt and water retention produces engorgement of systemic organs (e.g., the liver), as well as peripheral edema.

In severe AR, myocardial oxygen needs are increased because of increases in LV diastolic and systolic volumes, LV muscle mass (hypertrophy), and LV pressures, as well as by prolongation of systolic ejection time. Total coronary blood flow is increased. Coronary reserve, the ability of the coronary blood flow to increase with vasodilatation, however, is significantly reduced,[77–79] probably because of a reduced diastolic aortic–LV pressure gradient and compression of intramyocardial coronary arteries (systolic "milking" of intramural arteries). Therefore, myocardial ischemia is often present on stress in these patients.[77–79] Some patients with severe AR may complain of angina pectoris on effort even in the absence of epicardial CAD. Associated obstructive CAD can be expected to exacerbate further the myocardial ischemia (Fig. 66-12).

PHYSICAL EXAMINATION

A variety of interesting but not very useful clinical signs may be present in patients with chronic severe AR. These include *de Musset's sign* (bobbing of the head with each heartbeat), *Traube's sign* (pistol-shot sound heard over the femoral artery), *Duroziez's sign* (systolic murmur over the femoral artery when it is compressed proximally and diastolic murmur when it is compressed distally), and *Quincke's pulse* (capillary pulsations that can be detected by pressing a glass slide on the patient's lip or transmitting a light through the patient's fingertips).

The arterial pulse is characteristic and consists of an abrupt distention with a rapid rise and a quick collapse *(Corrigan's pulse)*. The arterial pulse may be bisferious, a double impulse during systole. The systolic arterial pressure is increased (in severe AR it averages 145 to 160 mmHg), the diastolic pressure is reduced (in severe AR it averages 45 to 60 mmHg), and the Korotkoff's sounds persist down to 0 mmHg. Even in such instances, however, the recorded intraarterial pressure rarely falls below 30 mmHg. The vasoconstriction that occurs in the presence of heart failure may result in some elevation of the arterial diastolic pressure and should not be interpreted as an improvement in severity of AR. Similarly, LV systolic dysfunction can produce a fall of systolic blood pressure that should not be considered to be an improvement of the AR. The fall of systolic pressure along with elevation of diastolic pressures tends to normalize the pulse pressure. The jugular venous pressure is normal except in heart failure and in those rare instances in which the greatly dilated ascending aorta obstructs the superior vena cava.

On inspection, the chest may rock and the cardiac impulse may be visible. The cardiac impulse is hyperdynamic (Table 66-19). There may be a systolic thrill at the base of the heart, over the carotids, and in the suprasternal notch. This results from a large LV stroke volume

Clinical Features

HISTORY

Patients with mild to moderate AR usually do not have symptoms that can be attributed to the heart. Even patients with severe AR may be asymptomatic. They may complain of pounding of the head or palpitations, which result from their awareness of the beating of a dilated LV that undergoes a large volume change in systole, during either sinus beats or postectopic beats. The main symptoms of severe AR result from elevated pulmonary venous pressures and include dyspnea on exertion, orthopnea, and paroxysmal nocturnal dyspnea. When heart failure occurs, patients complain of fatigue and weakness. Angina pectoris occurs in 20 percent of such patients and may be present even if the coronary arteries are normal. Angina associated with syphilitic AR may be due to associated ostial stenosis of the coronary arteries. In such patients, angina often occurs at rest and is difficult to control.

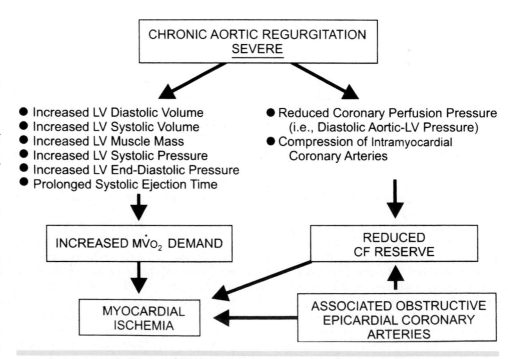

FIGURE 66-12 In severe aortic regurgitation, myocardial oxygen needs are increased. Total coronary blood flow is increased, but coronary reserve (i.e., the ability of the coronary blood flow to increase with vasodilatation) is significantly reduced, probably because of a reduced diastolic aortic–LV pressure gradient and compression (systolic milking) of intramyocardial coronary arteries. Therefore, myocardial ischemia is often present on stress in these patients. Associated obstructive coronary artery disease can be expected to further exacerbate the myocardial ischemia. (Copyright by SH Rahimtoola.[64])

TABLE 66-19 Physical Examination of Patients with Varying Severity of Chronic Aortic Valve Regurgitation

	Mild	Moderate	Severe	Severe + LV Systolic Dysfunction	Severe + Heart Failure + LV Systolic Dysfunction
Arterial pulse	Normal	Corrigan's + to + +	Corrigan's + + +	Corrigan's + +	Corrigan's +
Arterial pressure					
Systolic	Normal	Increased + to + +	Increased + + +	Increased + +	Normal/+
Diastolic	Normal	Decreased + to + +	Decreased + + + to + + + +	Decreased + + to + + +	Decreased +
Pulse pressure	Often normal	Increased + to + +	Increased + + + to + + + +	Increased + + to + + +	Increased +
Cardiac impulse	Often normal	Hyperdynamic	Very hyperdynamic visible ± chest may rock	Hyperdynamic	May be hypodynamic
Precordial thrill:					
Systolic	−	±	±	±	−
Diastolic	−	−	±	±	−
Auscultation:					
S_4	−	−	−	−	−
S_1	Normal	Often soft	Soft	Soft	Soft
S_2	Normal	Normal or single	Often single	Often single	Often single
S_3	−	+	+ + to + + +	+ + +	+ + +
ESM	±	+	+ to + +	+ to + +	+
AoDM	+	+ +	+ + + to + + + +	+ + to + + +	+ to + +
Austin Flint murmur	−	−	±	−	−

ABBREVIATIONS: S_1 and S_2 = first and second heart sounds; S_3 = third heart sound (diastolic gallop); S_4 = fourth heart sound (presystolic gallop); ESM = ejection systolic murmur; AoDM = aortic diastolic murmur; −absent; + + + + most prominent; ± present or absent.

across a diseased aortic valve. A diastolic thrill signifies severe AR. S_1 is usually soft because the mitral valve leaflets are close to each other at the onset of systole, or there may be premature valve closure. This is exaggerated if the PR interval is prolonged. The S_2 is usually single because the aortic valve does not close properly or because the LV ejection time is prolonged and the P_2 may not be heard. Often, a systolic ejection murmur, which is sometimes very loud, is present. The clinical sine qua non of AR is an early or immediate, blowing, decrescendo diastolic murmur beginning after A_2. It is best heard with the diaphragm of the stethoscope at the left sternal border or, in difficult instances, by having the patient sit up and lean forward and by auscultating with the respiration held at the end of a deep expiration. In severe AR, the murmur may be holodiastolic. When it is soft, its intensity can be increased by having the patient perform isometric exercise, for example, a handgrip, which increases aortic diastolic pressure. At times, this murmur is better heard along the right sternal border, which should draw attention to the possibility that the cause of the AR is aortic root and annular disease (see Chap. 14). Classically, rupture of the sinus of Valsalva into the right side of the heart chambers produces a continuous murmur.

In many patients with severe AR, an Austin Flint murmur[80] (see Chap. 12) is present in presystole and/or mid-diastole. Two inferences can be drawn from the presence of an Austin Flint murmur: (1) it signifies that the AR is severe; and (2) it requires that associated mitral stenosis be excluded. The most helpful sign at the bedside is the response of the murmur to the inhalation of amyl nitrite. The vasodilatation produced by amyl nitrite increases forward flow, reduces the regurgitant volume, and results in the Austin Flint murmur becoming much softer or disappearing. In comparison, the increased cardiac output and tachycardia accentuate or increase the murmur of mitral stenosis. Alternatively, echocardiography can easily demonstrate the presence of organic mitral stenosis.

With severe LV dilatation and/or LV systolic dysfunction, secondary mitral regurgitation may be present with the characteristic holosystolic murmur. Heart failure may be associated with pulmonary congestion or edema, pulmonary hypertension, right ventricular enlargement, tricuspid regurgitation, elevated jugular venous pressure, hepatomegaly, and peripheral edema (see Chap. 14).

CHEST X-RAY

The LV is increased in size, resulting in an increase in the cardiothoracic ratio. Since the upper limit of normal of the cardiothoracic ratio is 0.49, many patients with increased LV size have an enlarged LV volume and may still have a cardiothoracic ratio within the normal range. A better noninvasive quantification of LV size can be obtained by echocardiography. The ascending aorta is dilated throughout, and there may be calcium in the aortic valve. With increased filling pressures in the later stages, there might be evidence of an enlarged LA and an increased LA and pulmonary venous pressure, which are manifested in the pulmonary vascular shadows by a redistribution of blood flow, pulmonary congestion, and pulmonary edema. In the presence of heart failure, enlargement of the right atrium and superior vena cava may be appreciated. Calcification that is limited to the ascending aorta is strongly suggestive of luetic aortitis.

ELECTROCARDIOGRAM

The ECG shows LVH with or without associated secondary ST-T-wave changes. In a small percent of patients, ECG evidence of LVH is absent in spite of severe AR. Conduction abnormalities, such as atrioventricular block or left or right bundle branch block with or without axis deviation, may be present. The PR interval may be prolonged, particularly in patients with ankylosing spondylitis. The rhythm is usually sinus. The presence of atrial fibrillation should make one suspect the presence of associated mitral valve disease or heart failure.

ECHOCARDIOGRAPHY

The sign of AR on echocardiography is diastolic fluttering of the anterior leaflet of the mitral valve. Echocardiography can easily exclude the presence of associated mitral stenosis. LV dimensions are increased, and if LV function is normal, the percent of dimensional shortening is normal. The increase in LV dimensions caused by volume overload, results in separation between the open anterior leaflet of the mitral valve and the endocardial surface of the interventricular septum (septal-E point separation). In AR, as in other volume-overload lesions, the response in mild volume overload is an elongation of the heart. Since M-mode echocardiography takes a pencil look at the short axis of the heart, LV dimensions by M-mode echocardiography may appear to be normal. In such patients, two-dimensional echocardiography is much superior to the M-mode technique for assessing LV volumes and systolic function. A dilated ascending aorta can be detected on echocardiography, as can an enlarged LA. Aortic valve vegetations suggest infective endocarditis. Some other conditions can easily be detected by echocardiography: for example, prolapse of the aortic leaflet into the LV in diastole.

Doppler ultrasound is useful for diagnosing and assessing the severity of AR. When using Doppler, there is a high incidence of "false-positive" (physiologic) trivial regurgitation.[81] There is also an overlap between the various grades of severity of assessment of AR by Doppler when compared with angiography (see Chap.15).

Transesophageal echocardiography is a useful technique when transthoracic echocardiogram is unsatisfactory and, in certain instances, when identifying the anatomy of the valve leaflets and aortic root and annulus. It is essential to evaluate if the valve is suitable for repair, especially in patients suspected of having infective endocarditis. Echo/Doppler ultrasound is also very useful for assessing disease of other valves.

CARDIAC CATHETERIZATION AND ANGIOGRAPHY

Cardiac catheterization allows the measurement of intracardiac and intravascular pressures and cardiac output, both at rest and during exercise, and can demonstrate the changes described in the section, "Pathophysiology," earlier. In addition, other valvular disease—for example, mitral stenosis, aortic stenosis, and mitral regurgitation—can be excluded. LV angiography demonstrates enlarged LV volumes and allows the calculation of LV volumes and LV ejection fraction. Angiography performed with injection of contrast medium in the ascending aorta demonstrates AR and allows a semiquantitative assessment of the degree of AR. In addition, the angiogram demonstrates the dimensions of the aortic root and the state of the ascending aorta. The indications for selective coronary angiography are the same as for aortic stenosis (see Table 66-6).

GATED BLOOD POOL RADIONUCLIDE SCANS

Gated blood pool radionuclide scans also allow the measurement of LV volumes and ejection fraction. The scans also allow measurement of LV ejection fraction on exercise and on serial studies. It is also possible to quantify the amount of AR.

TREADMILL EXERCISE TEST

A treadmill exercise test provides an objective assessment of the degree of functional impairment and documentation of arrhythmias related to exertion. In some patients, however, the exercise test may remain normal despite deterioration of LV function.

AMBULATORY ELECTROCARDIOGRAM RECORDING

Ambulatory ECG recording may be needed occasionally in a patient suspected of having an arrhythmia (see Chap. 41).

MAGNETIC RESONANCE IMAGING

MRI can demonstrate AR but is rarely needed clinically (see Chap. 25).

Clinical Decision Making

Please see the equivalent section, "Aortic Valve Stenosis," earlier. The sensitivity, specificity, and accuracy of diagnosis of chronic AR are shown in (Table 66-20).[36] The following should be noted: (1) The sensitivity, specificity, and accuracy of diagnosing AR after clinical evaluation are good but not quite as good as in AS; (2) echo/Doppler ultrasound improves these criteria to a greater extent than it does in AS; (3) the difficulties lie in accurately distinguishing patients with mild[81] AR from healthy individuals and those with moderate AR and in distinguishing between moderate AR and severe AR; and (4) both clinical evaluation and echo/Doppler ultrasound are excellent in diagnosing AR as moderate or severe.

Natural History and Prognosis

Patients with mild AR that does not progress should have a normal life expectancy. Their major risk is the development of infective endocarditis and further valve destruction. Patients with moderate AR, if their disease does not progress, would be expected to have a life expectancy that is reasonably close to the normal range. The disease does progress, however, and mortality at the end of 10 years appears to be about 15 percent.

Patients with severe AR are known to have a long asymptomatic period before the condition is discovered. In asymptomatic patients with normal LV function at rest, symptoms and/or LV dysfunction (and/or sudden death) develop at the rate of about 3 to 6 percent per year.[59] The predictor of development of symptoms is LV systolic dysfunction at rest.[59,82] In patients with normal LV systolic function at rest (Table 66-21), the predictors of development of LV systolic

TABLE 66-20 Clinical Decision Making Utilizing Clinical Evaluation versus Echo/Doppler in Patients with Aortic Regurgitation

	After Clinical Evaluation, %	After Echo/Doppler, %
Diagnosis of AR		
Sensitivity	66	79
Specificity	76	74
Accuracy of diagnosis		
All levels of severity	43	57
Moderate or severe AR	91	100

SOURCE: From Kotlewski et al.,[36] with permission.

TABLE 66-21 Chronic Severe Aortic Regurgitation: Asymptomatic + Normal LV Function at Rest

		Likelihood of Symptoms or LV Dysfunction or Death, % per Year
LV end-diastolic dimension	≥70 mm	10
	<70 mm	2
LV end-systolic dimension	≥50 mm	19
	40–49 mm	6
	<40 mm	0

SOURCE: From Bonow et al.,[82] with permission.

dysfunction and/or symptoms are an increased LV size (LV dimension at end-diastole of ≥70 mm and at end-systole of ≥50 mm,[59–82] and LV end-diastolic volume index of ≥150 mL/m^2)[83] and abnormal LV ejection fraction on exercise of ≥0.50.[76] In small people, for example, in women,[84] these values are too large and have to be corrected for body size. The corrected dimensions for end-diastole and end-systole are 35 mm/m^2 and 25 mm/m^2, respectively. Sudden death in asymptomatic patients appears to occur only in those with a massively dilated LV (LV end-diastolic dimension of ≥80 mm).[82] It is likely that LV dysfunction first appears on exercise and later also at rest; eventually, heart failure ensues. Severe symptoms, however, may occur even when LV systolic pump function is normal at rest. The 5-year mortality of symptomatic patients with severe AR is about 25 percent, and the 10-year mortality averages 50 percent.[85] Once symptoms occur in patients with AR, it is likely that the rate of deterioration will be rapid. Most patients with angina are dead within 4 years.[86] The 2- to 3-year mortality of those with heart failure is 50 to 70 percent. In a study of older patients, the mortality was 4.7 percent per year; in the symptomatic patient it was 9.4 percent per year[87]; and in the asymptomatic patient 2.8 percent, which was not significantly different from age- and gender-matched individuals in the population. In the symptomatic patient, those in the New York Heart Association (NYHA) classes III and IV had an annual mortality of 24.6 percent per year, while in the class II patient it was 6.3 percent per year. In asymptomatic patients, those with LV ejection fraction <0.55, the annual mortality was 5.8 percent per year, and in those with LV end-systolic dimension >25 mm/m^2, it was 7.8 percent per year.[87]

Management

All patients with AR need antibiotic prophylaxis to prevent infective endocarditis. Patients with AR of a rheumatic origin need antibiotic prophylaxis to prevent recurrences of rheumatic carditis. Patients with syphilitic AR need a course of antibiotics to treat syphilis.

Patients with mild AR need no specific therapy (Table 66-22). They do not need to restrict their activities and can lead a normal life. Patients with moderate AR also usually need no specific therapy. These patients, however, should avoid heavy physical exertion, competitive sports, and isometric exercise.

In asymptomatic patients with severe AR,[88,89] a calcium channel blocking agent, long-acting nifedipine, produced significant reductions in blood pressure and LV end-diastolic volume and mass and major increases in LV ejection fraction at the end of 1 year. Almost all patients completed the trial. A prospective randomized trial in *asymptomatic* patients with *normal LV systolic* function[90] showed

TABLE 66-22 Medical Treatment of Patients with Aortic Regurgitation

I. Antibiotic prophylaxis
   A. Infective endocarditis
   B. Recurrent rheumatic carditis
II. Restriction of activities (moderate/severe AR)
   A. Severe exercise
   B. Competitive sports
III. Arrhythmias
   A. Prevent and/or control
   B. Restore sinus rhythm, if possible
IV. Cardiac medications
   A. Asymptomatic, normal LV function
     1. Mild AR: None
     2. Moderate AR: ? Nifedipine long-acting
     3. Severe AR: Nifedipine long-acting
   B. Severe AR symptomatic (while waiting for surgery)
     1. Normal LV function: Nifedipine long-acting
     2. LV dysfunction: Digitalis
                       ACE inhibitors
                       Hydralazine ± nitrates, if needed
                       Diuretics, if needed
                       Dobutamine, if needed
   C. Severe AR + heart failure:
     Digitalis, diuretics, ACE inhibitors
     Hydralazine + nitrates
     IV nitroprusside, if IV therapy needed
     Dobutamine, if needed
V. Follow-up of asymptomatic patient
   A. Mild AR: Every 2–5 years
   B. Moderate AR: Every 1–2 years
   C. Severe AR: Every 6–12 months
   D. Develop symptoms: Early or immediate

SOURCE: Copyright by SH Rahimtoola.[64]

that at the end of 6 years, 34 ± 6 percent of patients treated with digoxin developed LV systolic dysfunction and/or symptoms and thus needed AVR, compared with 15 ± 3 percent of patients treated with long-acting nifedipine ($p < .001$; Fig. 66-13); 89 percent (23 of 26) of those who needed AVR had developed LV systolic dysfunction with or without symptoms; only 3 had become symptomatic without developing LV systolic dysfunction. Accordingly, all asymptomatic patients with severe AR and normal LV systolic function should be treated with a vasodilator (the calcium antagonist long-acting nifedipine) unless there is a contraindication to its use.

The role of nifedipine in patients with moderate AR has not been studied. In view of its beneficial effects in severe AR, long-acting nifedipine could be used in selected patients with moderate AR if there are no contraindications to its use. The value of an ACE inhibitor is not well documented. Moreover, there are no published data to show that ACE inhibitor therapy reduces the need for valve surgery. In brief, ACE inhibitors are not of proven benefit in asymptomatic patients with AR and normal LV systolic function.

Symptomatic patients with severe AR need medical and surgical treatment. Medical treatment (see Table 66-22) consists of the administration of digitalis, diuretics, and vasodilators. Digitalis is clearly indicated in patients with symptoms. The need for and benefits of this therapy in asymptomatic patients have not been well doc-

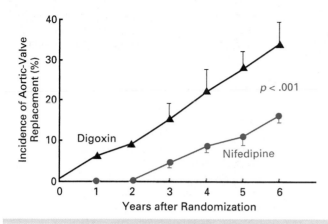

FIGURE 66–13 The role of long-term nifedipine therapy in asymptomatic patients with severe aortic regurgitation (AR) and normal left ventricular (LV) systolic pump function was evaluated in 143 asymptomatic patients in a prospective randomized trial. By actuarial analysis, at 6 years, 34 ± 6 percent of patients in the digoxin group underwent aortic valve replacement (AVR), versus 15 ± 3 percent of those in the nifedipine group, $p < .001$. This randomized trial demonstrates that long-term vasodilator therapy with nifedipine reduces and/or delays the need for AVR in asymptomatic patients with severe AR and normal LV systolic pump function. (From Scognamiglio et al.,[88] with permission.)

umented. Diuretics are of value when the LA pressure is elevated and in the presence of heart failure.

Long-term hydralazine therapy in symptomatic patients results in significant benefit in only 20 to 35 percent of patients.[29] Those who are likely to benefit cannot be predicted. Vasodilators are indicated in patients who refuse surgery or who are not operative candidates for any reason.

Vasodilators are also indicated for short-term therapy in patients awaiting AVR to optimize their hemodynamics (reduce filling pressures and increase cardiac output) and thus reduce their operative risks. If LV systolic function is normal, they can be given long-acting nifedipine. If they have abnormal LV systolic function, they should be treated with digitalis and ACE inhibitors; diuretics and hydralazine, with or without nitrates, can be used if needed. Small doses of hydralazine (50 mg) are without therapeutic effect in AR, and larger doses (≥ 100 mg) need to be given only twice daily;[91] the twice-daily regimen reduces the incidence of side effects. Hydralazine should be started in small doses and gradually increased, depending on patient tolerance of the drug.

Vasodilators are of considerable short-term benefit in patients in functional classes III and IV or heart failure. All such patients need digitalis, diuretics, and ACE inhibitors. In patients in functional class IV with heart failure, vasodilators should ideally be started after the institution of bedside hemodynamic monitoring, that is, measurement of pulmonary artery wedge pressure and cardiac output with the use of balloon flotation catheters. Hemodynamic monitoring accurately identifies patients who need the therapy, since clinical judgments can be wrong. It establishes whether arterial dilators alone will suffice or whether additional venodilators are needed. Finally, it provides information on the optimum dosage of vasodilator therapy. After the initial hemodynamic measurements are made, arterial dilators are given in progressively increasing dosage until an optimum effect on cardiac output has been obtained. If cardiac output does not show any further increase but LA pressure is still very high, additional venodilator therapy should be given. If the patient is very ill or the hemodynamic abnormalities are marked, intravenous therapy (e.g., sodium nitroprusside) is the vasodilator of first choice. In this sit-

uation, intravenous vasodilator therapy should be used only with bedside hemodynamic monitoring. Inotropic agents, such as dobutamine, may be needed to improve LV function and increase cardiac output. Low-dose dopamine may be of value to increase urinary output.

Patients with severe chronic AR need valve surgery. The correct timing of surgical therapy is now better defined but is not fully clarified. AVR should be performed before irreversible LV dysfunction occurs. The major problem, however, is identifying the precise point at which LV dysfunction will occur. Here, two major difficulties are encountered: (1) patients may already have impaired LV systolic pump function at rest when they first present or at the time of the first symptom, and (2) patients with severe symptoms may have normal LV systolic pump function. Patients may be in NYHA functional class III (symptoms with less than ordinary activity), with a normal LV ejection fraction,[70] or they may be in functional class I (asymptomatic), with a reduced LV ejection fraction.[70,70a] A reduced LV ejection fraction demonstrated by two-dimensional echocardiography and/or radionuclide ventriculography is the best noninvasive indicator of depressed LV systolic function.

Decisions about AVR should be based on the clinical functional class and on the LV ejection fraction at rest (Table 66-23).[92] Patients with chronic severe AR who are symptomatic (NYHA functional classes II to IV) need valve replacement. The benefit from AVR has been demonstrated even when the LV ejection fraction is 0.25 or less.[93] As opposed to AS, in which there is no lower level of ejection

TABLE 66-23 Chronic Severe Aortic Regurgitation: Indications for Surgery*

I. Symptomatic patients
   A. LV function normal: As soon as possible
   B. LV dysfunction: Urgent
   C. Heart failure: Emergent
   D. Individualize if:
     1. Very severe LV dysfunction (LVEF ≤ 0.20)
     2. Severe LV dilatation (LVEDD ≥ 80 mm with severe LV dysfunction; LVEDVI ≥ 300 mL/m^2)
     3. Small RgV (RgV/EDV ≤ 0.14)
II. Asymptomatic patients
   A. LV systolic dysfunction (LVEF ≤ 0.50–0.54)
   B. Normal LV systolic function
     1. Associated cardiovascular diseases requiring surgery
       a. CAD
       b. Other valve disease
       c. Ascending aortic aneurysm
     2. Large LV
       LVEDD ≥ 70–75 mm; 35–38 mm/m^2
       LVESD ≥ 50–55 mm; 25–27 mm/m^2
       LVEDVI ≥ 150 mL/m^2
       PLUS PA wedge on exercise ≥ 20–22 mmHg
     3. Progressive changes in LV size and function
       Increase of LVEDD and/or LVESD
       Decrease of LVEF

*Valve replacement/valve repair.
ABBREVIATIONS: CAD = coronary artery disease; EF = ejection fraction; EDD = end-diastolic dimension; EDVI = end-diastolic volume index; RgV = regurgitant volume; EDV = end-diastolic volume; LV = left ventricular; PAW = pulmonary artery wedge.
SOURCE: Copyright by SH Rahimtoola.[64]

fraction that indicates inoperability, it is likely that some patients with AR and a very low ejection fraction become inoperable. This level has not been precisely defined but may be about 0.15 or less. There is a need to individualize the need for AVR in those with very severe LV systolic dysfunction at rest (LV ejection fraction <0.20), in those with very severe LV dilatation (LV end-diastolic volume index ≥300 mL/m^2),[94] and in those with a small regurgitant volume, with a ratio of regurgitant volume to end-diastolic volume of 0.14.[95] Data indicate that patients with severe AR, LV end-diastolic dimension on echocardiography of ≥80 mm, and mild to moderate reduction of LV ejection fraction (mean 0.43) can obtain benefit from AVR.[96] Postoperatively, they are symptomatically improved, LV ejection fraction increases, and LV size is reduced; the 5- and 10-year survivals are 87 and 71 percent, respectively.

Patients who are in NYHA functional class I (asymptomatic) and have a reduced ejection fraction at rest should be offered AVR. If the ejection fraction is normal at rest, one should consider AVR in NYHA functional class I patients if they have severe obstructive CAD and/or need surgery for other valve disease (see Table 66-23). It is suggested that patients undergo an exercise test during right side of the heart catheterization if the LV is large [LV end-diastolic volume ≥150 mL/m^2 and LV internal dimension on M-mode echocardiography of ≥70 mm (≥25 mm/m^2) at end-diastole and ≥50 mm (≥25mm/m^2) at end-systole] and/or the LV ejection fraction shows a new, persistent reduction to 0.54 to 0.60; if the patients have reduced exercise capacity on treadmill testing; or if ambulatory ECG monitoring demonstrates ventricular tachyarrhythmias. AVR is recommended if the pulmonary artery wedge pressure during exercise 15 ≥ 20 to 24 mmHg. Patients with associated significant CAD should have coronary bypass surgery performed at the time of valvular surgery (see "Aortic Valve Stenosis," earlier, and Table 66-12).

AVR, with or without associated coronary bypass surgery for obstructive CAD, can be performed at many surgical centers with an operative mortality of 5 percent or less. If AVR is successful and uncomplicated, LV volume and LVH regress but do not return to normal; the beneficial effects on LV size, volume, and mass continue to be seen up to 5 years after surgery.[48,97,98] Impaired LV systolic pump function improves postoperatively in 50 percent or more of patients;[93] this improvement is more likely to occur if LV dysfunction has been present preoperatively for 12 months or less, and in this subgroup LV ejection fraction usually normalizes.[98] Even if LV systolic pump function does not improve, there is a reduction in end-diastolic volume and LVH;[93] from a cardiac point of view, this is advantageous to the patient. The 5-year survival of patients undergoing AVR in severe AR is 85 percent (this figure includes operative and late cardiac deaths).[92] The 5-year survival of patients with LV ejection fraction ≥0.45 is 87 percent, versus 54 percent in patients with an ejection fraction <0.45.[92] Late survival after valve replacement for chronic severe AR is best predicted by variables indicative of LV systolic pump function. Both the operative mortality and late survival are dependent on cardiac and LV function and associated noncardiac comorbid factors.

Indeed, in general, the major factors influencing outcome in patients with *valvular heart disease* are LV dysfunction and its magnitude, duration of LV dysfunction, degree of LV dilatation, greater NYHA functional class, older age, associated CAD, and comorbid conditions. In the future, it is possible that selected patients may eventually need to have valve repair rather than AVR for AR.

The recommendations of the ACC/AHA Practice Guidelines are shown in Table 66-24.[59] Guidelines are *not* and should *not* be the *law*. Application of such guidelines to clinical practice should be based on the following principles: (1) classes I and III apply to all

TABLE 66-24 Recommendations for Aortic Valve Replacement in Chronic Severe Aortic Regurgitation

Indication	Class
1. Patients with NYHA functional class III or IV symptoms and preserved LV systolic function, defined as normal ejection fraction at rest (ejection fraction ≥0.50)	I
2. Patients with NYHA functional class II symptoms and preserved LV systolic function (ejection fraction ≥0.50 at rest) but with progressive LV dilatation or declining ejection fraction at rest on serial studies or declining effort tolerance on exercise testing	I
3. Patients with Canadian Heart Association functional class II or greater angina with or without CAD	I
4. Asymptomatic or symptomatic patients with mild to moderate LV dysfunction at rest (ejection fraction 0.25 to 0.49)	I
5. Patients undergoing coronary artery bypass surgery or surgery on the aorta or other heart valves	I
6. Patients with NYHA functional class II symptoms and preserved LV systolic function (ejection fraction ≥0.50 at rest) with stable LV size and systolic function on serial studies and stable exercise tolerance	IIa
7. Asymptomatic patients with normal LV systolic function (ejection fraction >0.50) but with severe LV dilatation (end-diastolic dimension >75 mm or end-systolic dimension >55 mm)^a	IIa
8. Patients with severe LV dysfunction (ejection fraction <0.25)	IIb
9. Asymptomatic patients with normal systolic function at rest (ejection fraction >0.50) and progressive LV dilatation when the degree of dilatation is moderately severe (end-diastolic dimension 70 to 75 mm, end-systolic dimension 50 to 55 mm)	IIb
10. Asymptomatic patients with normal systolic function at rest (ejection fraction >0.50) but with decline in ejection fraction during	
• Exercise radionuclide angiography	IIb
• Stress echocardiography	III
11. Asymptomatic patients with normal systolic function at rest (ejection fraction >0.50) and LV dilatation when degree of dilatation is not severe (end-diastolic dimension <70 mm, end-systolic dimension <50 mm)	III

^{a}Consider lower threshold values for patients of small stature of either gender. Clinical judgment is required.

ABBREVIATIONS: NYHA = New York Heart Association; LV = left ventricular; CAD = coronary artery disease.

SOURCE: ACC/AHA Guidelines,[59] with permission.

patients in these classes unless there is a specific clinical circumstance not to do so; (2) class II applies to patients in this class depending on the clinical conditions of the patients and the skill and experience at the individual medical center.

References

1. Rahimtoola SH. Aortic valve disease. In: Fuster V, Alexander RW, O'Rourke RA, eds. *Hurst's The Heart,* 10th ed. New York, McGraw Hill; 1998:1667–1695.

2. Otto CM, Knusisto J, Reichenbach D, et al. Characterization of the early lesion of "degenerative" valvular aortic stenosis: Historical and immunohistochemical studies. *Circulation* 1994;90:844–853.

3. Olsson N, Dalsgaaro C-J, Haegerstrand A, et al. Accumulation of T lymphocytes and expression of interleukin-2 receptors in nonrheumatic stenotic aortic valves. *J Am Coll Cardiol* 1994;23:1162–1170.

4. Passik CS, Ackerman DM, Pluth JR, et al. Temporal changes in the causes of aortic stenosis: A surgical pathological study of 646 cases. *Mayo Clin Proc* 1987;62:119–123.

5. Roberts WC. The structural basis of abnormal cardiac function: A look at coronary, hypertensive, valvular, idiopathic myocardial, and pericardial heart disease. In: Levine JJ, ed. *Clinical Cardiovascular Physiology.* New York: Grune & Stratton; 1976.

6. Stewart BF, Siscovick P, Lind B, et al. Clinical factors associated with calcific aortic valve disease. *J Am Coll Cardiol* 1997;29:630–634.

7. Kennedy JW, Twiss RD, Blackmon JR, et al. Quantitative angiography: III. Relationships of left ventricular pressure, volume, and mass in aortic valve disease. *Circulation* 1968;38:838–845.

8. Bonow RO. Left ventricular structure and function in aortic valve disease. *Circulation* 1989;79:966–969.

9. Krayenbuehl HP, Hess OM, Monrad ES, et al. Left ventricular myocardial structure in aortic valve disease before, intermediate, and later after AVR. *Circulation* 1989;79:744–755.

10. Tobin JR Jr, Rahimtoola SH, Blundell PE, et al. Percentage of left ventricular stroke work loss: A simple hemodynamic concept for estimation of severity in valvular aortic stenosis. *Circulation* 1967;35:868–879.

11. Pantely G, Morton MJ, Rahimtoola SH. Effects of successful, uncomplicated AVR on ventricular hypertrophy, volume, and performance in aortic stenosis and aortic incompetence. *J Thorac Cardiovasc Surg* 1978;75:383–391.

12. Hess OM, Ritter M, Schneider J, et al. Diastolic stiffness and myocardial structure in aortic valve disease before and after replacement. *Circulation* 1984;69:855–865.

13. Hess OM, Villari B, Krayenbuehl HP. Diastolic dysfunction in aortic stenosis. *Circulation* 1993;87(suppl IV):73–76.

14. Stott DK, Marpole DGF, Bristow JD, et al. The role of LA transport in aortic and mitral stenosis. *Circulation* 1970;41:1031–1041.

15. Carroll JD, Carroll EP, Feldman T, et al. Sex-associated differences in left ventricular function in aortic stenosis of the elderly. *Circulation* 1992;86:1099–1107.

16. Ross J Jr. Afterload mismatch and preload reserve: A conceptual framework for the analysis of ventricular function. *Prog Cardiovasc Dis* 1976;18:255–264.

17. Bache RJ, Wang Y, Jorgensen CR. Hemodynamic effects of exercise in isolated valvular aortic stenosis. *Circulation* 1971;44:1003.

18. Johnson LL, Sciacca RR, Ellis K, et al. Reduced left ventricular myocardial blood flow per unit mass in aortic stenosis. *Circulation* 1978; 57:582–590.

19. Vinten-Johansen J, Weiss HR. Oxygen consumption in subepicardial and subendocardial regions of the canine LV: The effect of experimental acute valvular aortic stenosis. *Circ Res* 1980;46:139–145.

20. Marcus ML, Doty DB, Horatzka LF, et al. Decreased coronary reserve: A mechanism for angina pectoris in patients with aortic stenosis and normal coronary arteries. *N Engl J Med* 1982;307:1362–1366.

21. Grech ED, Ramsdale DR. Exertional syncope in aortic stenosis: Evidence to support inappropriate left ventricular baroreceptor response. *Am Heart J* 1991;121:603–606.

22. Schwartz LS, Goldfischer J, Sprague GJ, et al. Syncope and sudden death in aortic stenosis. *Am J Cardiol* 1969;23:647–658.

23. Kulbertus HE. Ventricular arrhythmias, syncope and sudden death in aortic stenosis. *Eur Heart J* 1988;9(suppl E):51–52.

23a. Sadler JE. Aortic stenosis, von Willebrand factor, and bleeding. *N Engl J Med* 2003;349:323–325.

24. Wood P. Aortic stenosis. *Am J Cardiol* 1958;1:553–571.

25. Murphy ES, Lawson RM, Starr A, et al. Severe aortic stenosis in the elderly: State of left ventricular function and result of AVR on ten-year survival. *Circulation* 1981;64(suppl II):184–188.

26. Thompson R, Mitchell A, Ahmed M, et al. Conduction defects in aortic valve disease. *Am Heart J* 1979;98:3–10.

27. Skjaerpe T, Hegrenaes L, Hatle L. Noninvasive estimation of valve area in patients with aortic stenosis by Doppler ultrasound and two-dimensional echocardiography. *Circulation* 1985;72:810–815.

28. Currie PJ, Seward JB, Reeder GS, et al. Continuous-wave Doppler echocardiographic assessment of severity of calcific aortic stenosis: A simultaneous Doppler-catheter correlative study in 100 adult patients. *Circulation* 1985;71:1162–1169.

29. Rahimtoola SH. Perspective on valvular heart disease: Update II. In: Knoebel S, ed. *An Era in Cardiovascular Medicine.* New York: Elsevier; 1991:45–70.

30. Roger VL, Tajik AJ, Reeder GS, et al. Effect of Doppler echocardiography on utilization of hemodynamic cardiac catheterization in the preoperative evaluation of aortic stenosis. *Mayo Clin Proc* 1996;71: 141–149.

31. Griffith MJ, Carey C, Coltart DJ, et al. Inaccuracies of using aortic valve gradients alone to grade severity of aortic stenosis. *Br Heart J* 1989;62:372–378.

32. Sethi GK, Miller DC, Sonchek J, et al. Clinical, hemodynamic and angiographic predictors of operative mortality in patients undergoing single AVR. *J Thorac Cardiovasc Surg* 1987;93:884–887.

33. Mullany CJ, Elveback ER, Frye RL, et al. Coronary artery disease and its management: Influence on survival in patients undergoing AVR. *J Am Coll Cardiol* 1987;10:66–72.

34. Levinson JR, Akins CW, Buckley MJ, et al. Octogenarians with aortic stenosis: Outcome after aortic valve replacement. *Circulation* 1989; 80(suppl.1):49–56.

35. Connolly HM, Rahimtoola SH: Indications for surgery in aortic valve disease. In: Yusuf S, Cairus JA, Canu AJ, et al. eds. *Evidence-Based Cardiology.* London: BMJ Books 2003;767–781.

36. Kotlewski A, Kawanishi DT, McKay CR, et al. The relative value of clinical examination, echocardiography with Doppler and cardiac catheterization with angiography in the evaluation of aortic valve disease. In: Bodnar E, ed. *Surgery for Heart Valve Disease.* London: ICR;1990:66–72.

37. Rahimtoola SH. Prophylactic AVR for mild aortic valve disease at time of surgery for other cardiovascular disease? ... NO. *J Am Coll Cardiol* 1999;33:2009–2015.

38. Horstkotte D, Loogen F. The natural history of aortic valve stenosis. *Eur Heart J* 1988;9(suppl E):57–64.

39. Otto CM, Burwash JG, Legget ME, et al. Prospective study of asymptomatic valvular aortic stenosis: Clinical, echocardiographic, and exercise predictors of outcome. *Circulation* 1997;95:2262–2270.

40. Ross J Jr, Braunwald E. Aortic stenosis. *Circulation* 1968;36(suppl IV):61–67.

41. Otto CM, Lind BK, Kitzman DW, et al. Association of aortic valve sclerosis with cardiovascular mortality and morbidity in the elderly. *N Engl J Med* 1999;341:142–147.

42. Kirklin JW, Barratt-Boyes BG. Congenital valvular aortic stenosis. In: *Cardiac Surgery.* New York: Wiley; 1986:972–988.

43. Edwards FH, Peterson Ed, Coombs LP, et al. Prediction of operative mortality after valve replacement surgery. *J Am Coll Cardiol* 2001; 37:885–892.

44. Society of Thoracic Surgery Database 1997:Internet.

45. Alexander KP, Anstrom KJ, Muhlbaier LH, et al. Outcomes of cardiac surgery in patients age ≥80 years; Results from the National Cardiovascular Network. *J Am Coll Cardiol* 2000;35:731–738.

46. Schwarz F, Banmann P, Manthey J, et al. The effect of aortic valve replacement on survival. *Circulation* 1982;66:1105–1110.

47. Rahimtoola SH. Valvular heart disease: A perspective. *J Am Coll Cardiol* 1983;1:199–215.

48. Monrad ES, Hess OM, Murakami T, et al. Time course of regression of left ventricular hypertrophy after aortic valve replacement. *Circulation* 1988;77:1345–1355.

49. Hammermeister KL, Sethi GK, Henderson WG, et al. Outcomes 15 years after valve replacement with a mechanical valve or bioprosthetic valve: Report of the Veterans Affairs Randomized Trial. *J Am Coll* 2000;36:1152–1158.

50. Lindblom D, Lindblom U, Qvist J, et al. Long-term relative survival rates after heart AVR. *J Am Coll Cardiol* 1990;15:566–573.

51. Rahimtoola SH. Catheter balloon valvuloplasty for severe calcific aortic stenosis: A limited role. *J Am Coll Cardiol* 1994;23:1076–1078.

52. Connolly HM, Oh JK, Orszulak TA, et al. AVR for aortic stenosis with severe left ventricular dysfunction: Prognostic indicators. *Circulation* 1997;95:2395–2400.

53. Rahimtoola SH, Starr A. Valvular surgery. In: Braunwald E, Mock M, Watson J, eds. *Congestive heart failure: Current Research and Clinical Applications.* Orlando, FL: Grune & Stratton; 1982:89–93.

54. Smith N, McAnulty JH, Rahimtoola SH. Severe aortic stenosis with impaired left ventricular function and clinical heart failure: Results of AVR. *Circulation* 1978;58:255–264.

55. Connolly HM, Oh JK, Schaff HV, et al. Severe aortic stenosis with low transvalvular gradient and severe left ventricular dysfunction. Result of aortic valve replacement in 52 patients. *Circulation* 2000; 101:1940–1946.

56. Rahimtoola SH. Severe aortic stenosis with low systolic gradient. The good and bad news. *Circulation* 2000;101:1892–1894.

57. Malouf JF, Enriquez-Serrano M, Pellikka PA, et al. Severe pulmonary hypertension in patients with severe aortic stenosis: Clinical profile and prognostic implications. *J Am Coll Cardiol* 2002;40:789–795.

58. Otto CM, Mickel MC, Kennedy JW, et al. Three-year outcome after balloon aortic valvuloplasty: Insights into prognosis of valvular aortic stenosis. *Circulation* 1994;89:642–650.

59. Bonow RO, Carabello B, de Leon AC Jr, et al. ACC/AHA guidelines for the management of patients with valvular heart disease: A report of the American College of Cardiology/American Heart Association Task Force on Practice Guidelines (Committee on Management of Patients with Valvular Heart Disease). *J Am Coll Cardiol* 1998;32:1486–1588.

60. Rahimtoola SH. Recognition and management of acute aortic regurgitation. *Heart Dis Stroke* 1993;2:217–221.

61. Rahimtoola SH. Valvular heart disease. In: Stein J, ed. *Internal Medicine,* 4th ed. St. Louis: Mosby–Year Book; 1994:202–234.

62. Belenkie I, Rademaker A. Acute and chronic changes after aortic valve damage in the intact dog. *Am J Physiol* 1981;241:H95–H103.

63. Welch GH Jr, Braunwald E, Sarnoff SJ. Hemodynamic effects of quantitatively varied experimental aortic regurgitation. *Circ Res* 1957;5: 546–551.

64. Rahimtoola SH. Aortic regurgitation. In: Rahimtoola SH, ed. *Atlas of Heart Diseases: Valvular Heart Disease,* Vol 11. Philadelphia: Current Medicine; 1997:7.1–7.26.

65. Rahimtoola SH. Management of heart failure in valve regurgitation. *Clin Cardiol* 1992;15(suppl I):22–27.

66. Cigarroa JE, Isselbacher EM, De Sanctis RW, et al. Diagnostic imaging in the evaluation of suspected aortic dissection: Old standards and new directions. *N Engl J Med* 1993;328:35–43.

67. Kostuk W, Barr JW, Simon AL, Ross J Jr. Correlations between the chest film and hemodynamics in acute myocardial infarction. *Circulation* 1973;48:624–632.

68. Chatterjee K, Parmley WW, Swan HJC, et al. Beneficial effects of vasodilator agents in severe mitral regurgitation due to dysfunction of subvalvular apparatus. *Circulation* 1973;48:684–690.

69. Richardson JV, Karp RB, Kirklin JW, et al. Treatment of infective endocarditis: A 10-year comparative analysis. *Circulation* 1978;58:589–597.

70. Tonnemacher D, Reid CL, Kawanishi DT, et al. Frequency of myxomatous degeneration of the aortic valve as a cause of isolated aortic regurgitation severe enough to warrant AVR. *Am J Cardiol* 1987;60: 1194–1196.

70a. Borer JS, Bonow RO. Contemporary approach to aortic and mitral regurgitation. *Circulation* 2003;108:2432–2438.

71. Antunes M. Repair for acquired valvular heart disease. In: Rahimtoola SH, ed. *Atlas of Heart Diseases: Valvular Heart Disease.* Vol 11. Philadelphia: Current Medicine; 1997:12.1–12.23.

72. Miller GAH, Kirklin JW, Swan HJC. Myocardial function and left ventricular volumes in acquired valvular insufficiency. *Circulation* 1965; 31:374–384.

73. Karaian CH, Greenberg BH, Rahimtoola SH. The relationship between functional class and cardiac performance in patients with chronic aortic insufficiency. *Chest* 1985;88:553–557.

74. Kawanishi DT, McKay CR, Chandrarratna PAN, et al. Cardiovascular response to dynamic exercise in patients with chronic symptomatic mild-to-moderate and severe aortic regurgitation. *Circulation* 1986;73: 62–72.

75. Shen WF, Roubin GS, Choong CY-P, et al. Evaluation of relationship between myocardial contractile state and left ventricular function in patients with aortic regurgitation. *Circulation* 1985;71:31–38.

76. Boucher CA, Wilson RA, Kanarek DJ, et al. Exercise testing in asymptomatic or minimally symptomatic aortic regurgitation: Relationship of left ventricular ejection fraction to left ventricular filling pressure during exercise. *Circulation* 1983;67:1091–1100.

77. Falsetti HL, Carroll RJ, Cramer JA. Total and regional myocardial blood flow in aortic regurgitation. *Am Heart J* 1979;97:485–493.

78. Uhl GS, Boucher CA, Oliveros RA, et al. Exercise-induced myocardial oxygen supply-demand imbalance in asymptomatic or mildly symptomatic aortic regurgitation. *Chest* 1981;80:686–691.

79. Nittenburg A, Foult JM, Antony I, et al. Coronary flow and resistance reserve in patients with chronic aortic regurgitation, angina pectoris, and normal coronary arteries. *J Am Coll Cardiol* 1988;11: 478–486.

80. Schaefer RA, McAnulty JH, Starr A et al. Diastolic murmurs in the presence of Starr-Edwards mitral prosthesis: With emphasis on the genesis of the Austin Flint murmur. *Circulation* 1975;51:402–409.

81. Rahimtoola SH. Drug induced valvular heart disease: Here we go again. Will we do better this time? *Mayo Clinic Proc* 2002;77:1275–1277.

82. Bonow RO, Lakatos E, Maron BJ, et al. Serial long-term assessment of the natural history of asymptomatic patients with chronic aortic regurgitation and normal left ventricular systolic function. *Circulation* 1991;84:1625–1635.

83. Siemienczuk D, Greenberg B, Morris C, et al. Chronic aortic insufficiency: Factors associated with progression to AVR. *Ann Intern Med* 1989;110:587–592.

84. Klodas E, Enrique-Sarano M, Tajik AJ, et al. Surgery for aortic regurgitation in women: Contrasting indications and outcomes compared with men. *Circulation* 1996;94:2472–2478.

85. Rapaport E. Natural history of aortic and mitral valve disease. *Am J Cardiol* 1975;35:221–227.

86. McKay CR, Rahimtoola SH. Natural history of aortic regurgitation. In: Gaasch WH, Levine HJ, eds. *Chronic Aortic Regurgitation.* Boston: Kluwer Academic; 1980:1–17.

87. Dujardin KS, Enriquez-Sarano M, Schaff HV, et al. Mortality and morbidity of aortic regurgitation in clinical practice: A long-term follow-up study. *Circulation* 1999;99:1851–1857.

88. Scognamiglio R, Rasoli G, Ponchia A, et al. Long-term nifedipine unloading therapy in asymptomatic patients with chronic severe aortic regurgitation. *J Am Coll Cardiol* 1990;16:424–429.

89. Rahimtoola SH. Vasolidator therapy in chronic severe aortic regurgitation. *J Am Coll Cardiol* 1990;16:430–432.

90. Scognamiglio R, Rahimtoola SH, Fasoli G, et al. Nifedipine in asymptomatic patients with severe aortic regurgitation and normal left ventricular function. *N Engl J Med* 1994;331:689–695.

91. McKay CR, Nanna M, Kawanishi DT, et al. Importance of internal controls, statistical methods, and side effects in acute vasodilator trials: A study of hydralazine kinetics in patients with aortic regurgitation. *Circulation* 1985;72:865–872.

92. Greves J, Rahimtoola SH, McAnulty JH, et al. Preoperative criteria predictive of late survival following AVR for severe aortic regurgitation. *Am Heart J* 1981;101:300–308.

93. Clark DG, McAnulty JH, Rahimtoola SH. Valve replacement in aortic insufficiency with left ventricular dysfunction. *Circulation* 1980;61: 411–421.

94. Taniguchi K, Nakano S, Hirose H, et al. Preoperative left ventricular function: Minimal requirement for successful late results of AVR for aortic regurgitation. *J Am Coll Cardiol* 1987;10:510–518.

95. Levine HJ, Gaasch WH. Ratio of regurgitant volume to end-diastolic volume: A major determinant of ventricular response to surgical correction of chronic volume overload. *Am J Cardiol* 1983;52:406–410.

96. Klodas E, Enriquez-Sarano M, Tajik AJ, et al. Aortic regurgitation complicated by extreme left ventricular dilation: Long-term outcome after surgical correction. *J Am Coll Cardiol* 1996;27:670–677.

97. Gaasch WH, Carroll JD, Levine HJ, et al. Chronic aortic regurgitation: Prognostic value of left ventricular end-systolic dimension and end-diastolic radius/thickness ratio. *J Am Coll Cardiol* 1983;1:775–782.

98. Bonow RO, Dodd JT, Maron BJ, et al. Long-term serial changes in left ventricular function and reversal of ventricular dilatation after AVR for chronic aortic regurgitation. *Circulation* 1988;78:1108–1120.

MITRAL VALVE DISEASE

Shahbudin H. Rahimtoola / Louis J. Dell'Italia

MITRAL STENOSIS*

Etiology

Mitral stenosis (MS), an obstruction to blood flow between the left atrium (LA) and the left ventricle (LV), is caused by abnormal mitral valve function. In virtually all adult patients, the cause of MS is previous rheumatic carditis.[1] About 60 percent of patients with rheumatic mitral valve disease do not give a history of rheumatic fever or chorea, and about 50 percent of patients with acute rheumatic carditis do not eventually have clinical valvular heart disease. Other causes of MS are all uncommon or rare.[2] Congenital MS is uncommon. MS, usually rheumatic, in association with atrial septal defect is called *Lutembacher's syndrome*. A rare cause of MS is massive mitral valve annular calcification. This process occurs most frequently in elderly patients and produces MS by limiting leaflet motion. When stenosis is present, it is usually mild in degree. Other causes of obstruction to LA outflow include a LA myxoma, massive LA ball thrombus, and cor triatriatum, in which a congenital membrane is present in the LA.

Pathology

Acute rheumatic carditis is a pancarditis involving the pericardium, myocardium, and endocardium. In temperate climates and developed countries, there is usually a long interval (averaging 10 to 20 years) between an episode of rheumatic carditis and the clinical presentation of symptomatic MS. In tropical and subtropical climates and in less developed countries, the latent period is often shorter, and MS may occur during childhood or adolescence (see Chap. 65).

The pathologic hallmark of rheumatic carditis is an Aschoff's nodule. The most common lesion of acute rheumatic endocarditis is mitral valvulitis. In this condition the mitral valve has vegetations along the line of closure and the chordae tendineae. Mitral regurgitation (MR) may be present during an acute episode of rheumatic carditis.

MS is usually the result of repeated episodes of carditis alternating with healing and is characterized by the deposition of fibrous tissue. MS may result from fusion of the commissures, cusps, or chordae, or a combination of these.[2] Ultimately, the deformed valve is subject to nonspecific fibrosis and calcification. Lesions along the line of closure result in fusion of the commissures and contracture and thickening of the valve leaflets. The chordal lesions are manifest as shortening and fusion of these structures. The combination of commissural fusion, valve leaflet contracture, and fusion of the chordae tendineae results in a narrow, funnel-shaped orifice, which restricts the flow of blood from the LA to the LV. The rapidity with which patients become symptomatic may depend on the number and severity of repeated bouts of rheumatic valvulitis. Frequently, the rheumatic episodes are not clinically apparent.

In pure MS, the LV is usually normal, but there may be evidence of previous carditis with deposition of fibrous tissue. The LA is enlarged and hypertrophied as a consequence of LA hypertension. Mural thrombi are often found in the LA, particularly if atrial fibrillation has been present. Calcification of the mitral valve frequently also involves the mitral annulus.

Pathophysiology

The pathophysiologic features of MS all result from obstruction of the flow of blood between the LA and the LV. With reduction in the valve area, energy is lost to friction during the transport of blood from the LA to the LV. Accordingly, a pressure gradient is present across the stenotic valve. The relation between valve areas, cardiac output, flow period, and average diastolic gradient between the LA and the LV is defined by the formula of Gorlin and Gorlin (Chap. 17).

---

*Mitral stenosis section written by SH Rahimtoola. Mitral regurgitation section written by LJ Dell'Italia.

It is readily apparent that maintaining cardiac output when the valve area is small requires a large gradient and thus an elevated LA pressure. Similarly, an increased demand for cardiac output (CO), such as occurs during exercise or pregnancy, results in an increase in gradient and high LA pressures. More subtle is the effect of the length of the diastolic flow period on the relation between CO and gradient. The time available for systole is that part of the cardiac cycle occupied by isovolumic contraction and relaxation or by ejection. As the heart rate increases, the total amount of time spent during systole increases despite a reduction in the systolic time per beat.[3] *Thus, time available for diastole decreases as the heart rate increases.* Because blood can flow through the mitral valve only during diastole, the flow rate is inversely proportional to the duration of the flow period at a constant stroke volume. Of course, a higher flow rate results in a greater loss of energy to friction and requires a larger gradient and higher LA pressures. It is important to remember that the gradient from LA to LV is a function per beat, not per minute. Thus, the gradient is dependent on the stroke volume and the diastolic filling time, as well as the LV diastolic pressure.

The pressure gradient between the LA and the LV, which increases markedly with increased heart rate or CO, is responsible for LA hypertension. The LA gradually enlarges and hypertrophies. Pulmonary venous pressure rises with LA pressure increase and is passively associated with an increase in pulmonary arterial (PA) pressure (Fig. 67-1). In up to 20 percent of patients, the pulmonary vascular resistance is also elevated,[4] which further increases PA pressure. PA hypertension results in *right ventricular* (RV) hypertrophy and RV enlargement. The changes in RV function eventually result in *right atrial* (RA) hypertension and enlargement and systemic venous congestion; frequently, tricuspid regurgitation also occurs. In a small percentage of patients, there may be regional or global LV systolic dysfunction, the cause or causes of which are not fully understood.[5–7]

Pulmonary venous hypertension alters lung function in several ways. Distribution of blood flow in the lung is altered, with a relative increase in flow to the upper lobes and therefore in physiologic dead space. Pulmonary compliance generally decreases with increasing pulmonary capillary pressure, increasing the work of breathing, particularly during exercise. Chronic changes in the pulmonary capillaries and pulmonary arteries include fibrosis and thickening. These changes protect the lungs from the transudation of fluid into the alveoli (alveolar pulmonary edema). Indeed, it is not uncommon to find patients with severe MS whose resting PA wedge pressure (indirect LA pressure) exceeds 25 to 30 mmHg. Capillary and alveolar thickening, which help protect against pulmonary edema, further add to the abnormalities of ventilation and perfusion. Pulmonary vascular changes cause an elevated pulmonary vascular resistance.

In some patients with high pulmonary vascular resistance and RV dysfunction, CO may be low. The body maintains oxygen consumption by extracting more oxygen from the arterial blood, and the mixed venous oxygen content falls. The hemoglobin-O_2 dissociation curve is shifted to the right, facilitating the unloading of oxygen from hemoglobin to the tissues. The reduced CO may result in a *surprisingly small gradient* across the mitral valve despite severe stenosis. Although pulmonary congestion may be less striking in these patients, the CO does not increase normally with exercise, and, typically, the patients are severely limited by fatigue.

Long-standing MS with severe PA hypertension and resultant RV dysfunction may be accompanied by chronic systemic venous hypertension. Tricuspid regurgitation is frequently present, even in the absence of intrinsic disease of this valve. Functional pulmonic regurgitation may also be present. Dependent edema formation and visceral congestion directly reflect elevated systemic venous pressure

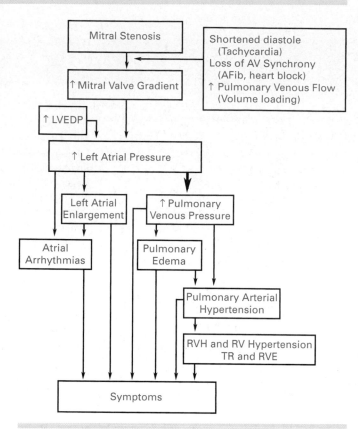

FIGURE 67-1 Pathophysiology of mitral stenosis. Mitral stenosis results in a diastolic pressure gradient from the left atrium (LA) to the left ventricle (LV). The actual gradient is dependent on the mitral valve area and the mitral valve *flow per diastolic second.* As a result, there is an elevation of LA pressure and therefore also of pulmonary venous pressure. Physiologic and pathologic changes μ such as tachycardia and atrial fibrillation (which shorten diastole and may also result in loss of effective atrial contraction) or pregnancy, volume loading, and left-to-right shunts (at ventricular and aortopulmonary levels), which increase pulmonary venous flow μ will increase the mitral valve gradient as well as LA and pulmonary venous pressures. An increased LV diastolic pressure will also result in further increase of LA pressure. An elevated LA pressure has several important effects; these include enlargement of the left atrium, atrial arrhythmias, and an increase of pulmonary venous pressure. Pulmonary venous hypertension may result in pulmonary edema and pulmonary arterial (PA) hypertension. PA hypertension and right ventricular (RV) hypertension results in RV hypertrophy (RVH) and may result in tricuspid regurgitation (TR) and RV enlargement (RVE). All of these changes contribute to producing symptoms. In addition, a fixed or even reduced cardiac output will also contribute to the symptomatic state of the patient. (Copyright by S. H. Rahimtoola.[2])

and salt and water retention. Chronic passive congestion in the liver leads to central lobular necrosis and eventually to cardiac cirrhosis.

Clinical Findings

HISTORY

An asymptomatic interval is usually present between the initiating event of acute rheumatic fever and the presentation of symptomatic MS (averaging 10 to 20 years).[4,8] During this interval, the patient feels well (Table 67-1). Initially, there is little or no gradient at rest, but with increased cardiac output, LA pressure rises and exertional dyspnea develops. As mitral valve obstruction increases, dyspnea occurs at lower work levels. The progression of disability is so subtle

TABLE 67-1 Symptoms Associated with Mitral Stenosis

On exertion
　Dyspnea, wheezing, cough
　Fatigue
　Diminished activity/or pace of activity
　Palpitations
　Feeling faint, presyncope, syncope
At rest
　Cough, wheezing
　Paroxysmal nocturnal dyspnea
　Orthopnea
　Hemoptysis
　Hoarseness (Ortner's syndrome)
From complications of MS (see Table 67-2)

SOURCE: Copyright SH Rahimtoola.[10]

and so protracted that patients may adapt by circumscribing their lifestyles.

As obstruction progresses, the patients note orthopnea and paroxysmal nocturnal dyspnea that apparently results from redistribution of blood to the thorax on assuming the supine position. With severe MS and elevated pulmonary vascular resistance, fatigue rather than dyspnea may be the predominant symptom. Dependent edema, nausea, anorexia, and right-upper-quadrant pain reflect systemic venous congestion resulting from elevated systemic venous pressure and salt and water retention.

Palpitations are a frequent complaint in patients with MS and may represent frequent premature atrial contractions or paroxysmal atrial fibrillation and flutter. Of patients with severe symptomatic MS, 50 percent or more have chronic atrial fibrillation. Paroxysmal atrial fibrillation may produce pulmonary edema in some patients with MS. The acute increase in LA pressure that produces pulmonary edema results both from a decrease in the diastolic flow period caused by increased heart rate and from a loss of atrial transport function.

Systemic embolism, a frequent complication of MS, may result in stroke, occlusion of extremity arterial supply, occlusion of the aortic bifurcation, and visceral or myocardial infarction. Atrial fibrillation, increasing age of the patient, increasing LA size, and a previous history of embolism are associated with an increased incidence of systemic embolism[4] (Table 67-2).

TABLE 67-2 Complications of Mitral Stenosis

Arrhythmias
　Atrial flutter/fibrillation
Embolism
　Systemic-cerebral, coronary, abnormal, peripheral,
　　pulmonary
Acute pulmonary edema
Pulmonary arterial hypertension
Right ventricular hypertrophy/dilatation
Tricuspid regurgitation
Clinical heart failure
Left ventricular dysfunction
Chest pain/angina
Infective endocarditis

SOURCE: Copyright by SH Rahimtoola.[10]

Hemoptysis may result from a variety of causes. It is usually due to increased pulmonary venous pressure. Sputum may be blood-stained with paroxysmal nocturnal dyspnea, pink frothy sputum may result from rupture of alveolar capillaries associated with acute pulmonary edema or from pulmonary infarction due to pulmonary embolism, or hemoptysis may be severe and profuse (pulmonary apoplexy). The latter results from rupture of thin-walled, dilated bronchial veins, and although usually not fatal, it may be life-threatening because of aspiration pneumonia or massive hemorrhage. The edematous bronchial mucosa is more likely to be associated with chronic bronchitis, especially in cold and wet climates; it can also result in blood-stained sputum. Exertional chest pain, typical of angina pectoris, may be present in some patients with severe MS even if the coronary arteries are normal. Severe PA hypertension has been postulated as a cause. Infective endocarditis is an uncommon complication of pure MS.

Progression of symptoms in MS is generally slow but relentless. Thus, a sudden change in symptoms rarely reflects a change in valve obstruction. Rather, there is usually a noncardiac precipitating event or paroxysmal atrial fibrillation. Fever, pregnancy, hyperthyroidism, and noncardiac surgery, all of which increase CO, can precipitate decompensation in patients with moderate to severe MS.

PHYSICAL FINDINGS

During the latent, presymptomatic interval, incidental physical findings may be normal or may provide evidence of mild MS. Frequently, the only characteristic finding noted at rest will be a loud S_1 and a presystolic murmur. A short diastolic decrescendo rumble may be heard only with exercise. In patients with symptomatic stenosis, the findings are more obvious, and careful physical examination usually leads to the correct diagnosis (see Chap. 12).

The general appearance of the patient in MS is usually normal. The MS facies, characterized by malar flush (pinkish-purple patches on the cheeks),[4] is uncommon and is caused by peripheral cyanosis, which is usually associated with a low CO, systemic vasoconstriction, and severe PA hypertension. Tachypnea may be present if LA pressure is high. The arterial pulse is normal except for irregularity in atrial fibrillation and is of low volume when CO is reduced. All peripheral pulses should be carefully examined because of the frequency of systemic embolism. The jugular venous pressure may be normal or may show evidence of elevated RA pressure. A prominent a wave is a result of RV hypertension and hypertrophy or of associated tricuspid stenosis. A prominent v wave is caused by tricuspid regurgitation. Atrial fibrillation produces an irregular venous pulse with absent a waves. The chest findings may be normal or may reveal signs of pulmonary congestion with rales or pleural fluid (dullness and absent breath sounds). Marked LA enlargement may produce egophony at the tip of the left scapula.

The precordium is usually unremarkable on inspection. On palpation, the apical impulse should feel normal or is tapping (palpable mitral valve closure or RV forming the cardiac apex). An abnormal LV impulse suggests disease other than isolated MS. A diastolic thrill is usually appreciated only when the patient is examined in the left lateral position. When PA hypertension is present, a sustained RV lift along the left sternal border and pulmonic valve closure may be palpable.

On auscultation in the supine position, the only abnormality appreciated may be the accentuated S_1, which is caused by flexible valve leaflets and the wide closing excursion of the valve leaflets[9] (see Chap. 12). Failure to examine the patient in the left lateral position accounts for most of the missed diagnoses of symptomatic MS. The diastolic rumble is heard best with the bell of the stethoscope applied at the apical impulse. Nevertheless, the murmur may be localized, and the region around the apical impulse also should be auscultated. The *opening snap* (OS) occurs when the movement of the domed mitral valve into the LV is suddenly stopped.[9] It is heard best with the diaphragm and is often most easily appreciated midway between the apex and the left sternal border. In this intermediate region, the S_1, the pulmonary component of the second heart sound (P_2), and the OS can be identified. The auscultatory signs of MS in sinus rhythm and in atrial fibrillation are illustrated in Figs. 67-2 and 67-3.

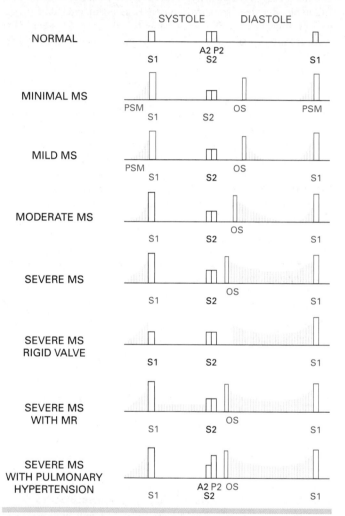

FIGURE 67-2 Auscultatory signs of mitral stenosis (MS) in patients with sinus rhythm are illustrated. These include a presystolic murmur, loud first heart sound (S_1), an opening snap (OS), and a middiastolic murmur (low-pitched, decrescendo diastolic rumble, and rumbling murmur). These signs may be accentuated or at times may be heard only by placing the patient in the left lateral decubitus position. Importantly, these signs are helpful in assessing the severity of the MS; as the MS becomes more severe, the S_2–OS interval is shortened and the length of the middiastolic rumble is increased. In mild MS, the S_2–OS interval is long and the diastolic murmur is short. In moderate MS, the S_2–OS interval is shorter, and although the diastolic murmur is longer at rest, there is usually a gap between the end of the murmur and the onset of the presystolic murmur. In severe MS, the S_2–OS interval is short (usually 0.04 to 0.06 s) and the diastolic murmur is a full-length murmur. With PA hypertension, P_2 is increased in intensity. In the presence of a rigid mitral valve (with or without calcification), S_2 is soft and the OS is usually not heard. A holosystolic murmur of mitral regurgitation may be present. (Adapted and modified from Kawanishi DT, Rahimtoola SH. Mitral stenosis. In: Rahimtoola SH, ed. *Valvular Heart Disease II.* St. Louis: Mosby; 1996:8.1–8.24. Copyright by S. H. Rahimtoola.)

The OS occurs after the LV pressure falls below LA pressure in early diastole. When LA pressure is high, as in severe MS, the snap occurs earlier in diastole (see Fig. 67-2). The converse is true with mild MS. The interval between A_2 and the OS varies from 40 to 120 ms. Although the OS is present in most cases of MS, it is absent in patients with stiff, fibrotic, or calcified leaflets. Thus, absence of the OS in severe MS suggests that mitral valve replacement rather than commissurotomy may be necessary.

The low-pitched diastolic rumble follows the OS and is best heard with the bell of the stethoscope. In some patients with low cardiac output or mild MS, brief exercise, such as situps or walking, is adequate to increase flow and bring out the murmur. The murmur is low-pitched, rumbling, and decrescendo. In general, the more severe the MS, the longer the murmur (see Fig. 67-2). Presystolic accentuation of the murmur occurs in sinus rhythm and has been reported even in atrial fibrillation. In the latter situation, a brief "presystolic" accentuation is due to narrowing of the mitral orifice produced by ventricular systole before the final, complete closure of the mitral valve and the mitral component of S_1. A diastolic rumble is not diagnostic of MS and may be heard with increased flow across a normal mitral valve—for example, in ventricular septal defect with a large left-to-right shunt.

The two most important auscultatory signs of severe MS are a short A_2-OS interval (usually 40 to 60 ms) and a full-length diastolic rumble. The A_2-OS interval may be longer if there is associated moderate to severe aortic regurgitation (AR), and the OS may be absent when the mitral valve is rigid. The diastolic murmur may not be full-length in severe MS if the stroke volume is low and there is no tachycardia.

Systolic murmurs also may be heard in association with the murmur of MS. A blowing, holosystolic murmur at the apex suggests associated MR; whereas a systolic blowing murmur heard best at the lower left sternal border that increases with inspiration usually signifies tricuspid regurgitation. The Graham Steell murmur is a high-pitched diastolic decrescendo murmur of pulmonic regurgitation caused by severe PA hypertension. In most patients with MS, such a murmur usually indicates AR instead. In general, a left-sided S_3 is not compatible with severe MS, with the possible exception of concomitant severe AR and/or significant LV systolic dysfunction. If an S_3 and a rumble are present, MR is usually the predominant lesion (see Chap. 12).

ROENTGENOGRAM

The posteroanterior and lateral chest films are often so typical that experienced clinicians can make the tentative diagnosis from them. The thoracic cage is normal. The lung fields show evidence of elevated pulmonary venous pressure. Blood flow is more evenly redistributed to the upper lobes, resulting in apparent prominence of upper-lobe vascularity. Increased pulmonary venous pressure results in transudation of fluid into the interstitium. Accumulation of fluid in the interlobular septa produces linear streaks in the bases, which extend to the pleura (Kerley B lines).[10] Interstitial fluid may also be seen as perivascular or peribronchial cuffing (Kerley A lines). With transudation of fluid into the alveolar spaces, alveolar pulmonary edema is seen. These changes are not specific for MS but represent long-standing elevated LA pressure. Chronic hemosiderin deposition can result in an interstitial radiodensity that does not resolve after the relief of stenosis. PA hypertension results in enlargement of the main PA and right and left main pulmonary arteries.

The cardiac silhouette usually does not show generalized cardiomegaly, but the LA is invariably enlarged. This is manifest in the posteroanterior chest film by a density behind the RA border (double atrial shadow), prominence of the LA appendage on the left side of the heart border between the main PA and LV apex, and elevation of the left main bronchus. The lateral film shows the LA bulging posteriorly. The LV silhouette is normal. The RV may be enlarged if PA hypertension has been present. RV enlargement is usually noted by filling of the retrosternal space, but this is an unreliable sign in adults. The combination of a normal-sized LV, enlarged LA, and pulmonary venous congestion should immediately raise the possibility of MS. Mitral valve calcification is occasionally seen on the plain chest film (see Chap. 14).

ELECTROCARDIOGRAM

The *electrocardiogram* (ECG) is not usually as helpful as the chest x-ray. Patients in sinus rhythm may have a widened P wave caused by interatrial conduction delay and/or prolonged LA depolarization. Classically, the P wave is broad and notched in lead II and biphasic in lead V_1; it measures 0.12 s or more. Atrial fibrillation is common. LV hypertrophy is almost never present unless there are associated lesions. RV hypertrophy may be present if PA hypertension is marked (see Chap. 62).

CLINICAL INDICATIONS OF SEVERE MITRAL STENOSIS

Some clinical features make it virtually certain that MS is severe. These include (1) moderate to severe PA hypertension as indicated by clinical and ECG evidence of RV hypertrophy or PA hypertension or both, and/or (2) moderate to severe elevation of LA pressure as indicated by orthopnea, a short P_2-OS interval, a diastolic rumble that occupies the whole length of a long diastolic interval in patients with atrial fibrillation, and pulmonary edema on the chest x-ray. In both these clinical circumstances, one must be certain that there is no other cause for elevated LA pressure and that LA hypertension is not caused mainly by a correctable transient elevation of LV diastolic pressure.

Laboratory Tests

ECHOCARDIOGRAPHY/DOPPLER ULTRASOUND

Echocardiography/Doppler ultrasound has proved to be both sensitive and specific for MS when adequate studies are done (see Chap. 15).[11,12] False-positive and false-negative results are uncommon. Doppler studies provide an estimate of mitral valve area (MVA) that is within ± 0.4 cm^2 (prior to interventional therapy) of that obtained by cardiac catheterization.[13] The echographic findings of MS reflect the loss of normal valve function (see Chap. 15).

Echocardiography is of great value in patients with equivocal signs and in patients with gross PA hypertension to differentiate MS from an Austin Flint murmur of aortic regurgitation (AR), and in the rare patient with "silent" MS. When transthoracic echocardiography

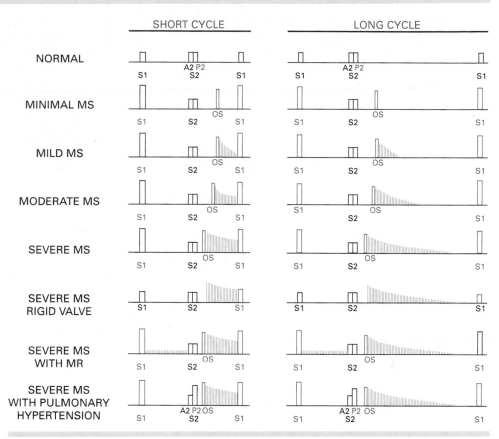

FIGURE 67-3 Auscultatory signs of mitral stenosis (MS) in atrial fibrillation are illustrated. The presystolic murmur is absent. The loud S$_1$ and the OS are still heard. In the short cycles, the duration of diastole is short and the middiastolic rumble occupies the whole of diastole (*left panel*). In the long cycles (*right panel*), the length of middiastolic murmur is related to the severity of MS. As the MS becomes more severe, the length of this murmur is increased. In atrial fibrillation, with a slow ventricular response and very long R-R intervals, the middiastolic rumble may not occupy the whole diastolic period and the presystolic murmur is usually absent. Thus, one may get the impression that the MS is moderate rather than severe. Increasing the heart rate μ, for example, with brief physical exertion μ may produce more characteristic auscultatory findings. Alternatively, when the ventricular rate in atrial fibrillation is rapid or in short cycles, the auscultatory findings may suggest a more severe degree of MS than is really the case (*left panel*). (Adapted and modified from Kawanishi DT, Rahimtoola SH. Mitral stenosis. In: Rahimtoola SH, ed. *Valvular Heart Disease. II.* St. Louis: Mosby; 1996:8.1–8.24. Copyright 1996 by S. H. Rahimtoola.)

is unsatisfactory, transesophageal echocardiography is a useful technique to assess LA thrombus, the anatomy of the mitral valve and subvalvular apparatus, and to assess the suitability of the patient for catheter balloon commissurotomy (CBC) or surgical valve repair.

Echocardiography/Doppler ultrasound is a most useful test in MS and should be performed in all patients. It is essential to determine suitability of the valve for commissurotomy and/or repair and to determine the likely result. The essential information that should be obtained is listed in Table 67-3.[14]

CARDIAC CATHETERIZATION/ANGIOGRAPHY

In most patients with disabling symptoms from presumed MS, right and left side of the heart catheterization should be performed as part of a preoperative assessment. Simultaneous measurement of cardiac output and the gradient between the LA and the LV and calculation of valve area remain the "gold standard" for assessing the severity of MS (see Chap. 17). LV angiography assesses the competence of the mitral valve, an important determinant of operability for mitral commissurotomy. Quantification of LV function provides a useful prognostic indicator of operative and late survival and of the expected functional result. Aortic valve function should be evaluated in all

TABLE 67-3 Assessment of Patient with Mitral Stenosis

Clinical
History
Physical Examination:
    Loud S_1
    A_2 – OS interval, length of MDM
    Loud P_2, RVH
Chest x-ray:
    Pulmonary edema (congestive, interstitial, alveolar)
    Enlargement of LA and other cardiac chambers
ECG:
    Rhythm
    LA enlargement
    RV and LV "hypertrophy"
Echocardiogram/Doppler (BP at time of study must be recorded)
M-mode
    LV and LA dimensions absolute and corrected for BSA
2 Dimensional/Doppler
    MVA (Doppler half time, planimetry)
    Mitral valve morphology
        Score
        Ca^{++} in one or both commissures
    LA Thrombus
    MR Severity
    PA Pressure
    Mean MVG
    LV volumes, measured LV ejection fraction
    Other valve lesions
Transesophageal echocardiography, if necessary
Treadmill Test
    Assessment of exercise capacity, if necessary
Cardiac Catheterization/Angiography
    MVA
    Mean PA wedge/LA pressure
    PA pressures: Systolic, diastolic, mean
    Mean MVG
    Cardiac output/cardiac index
    Pulmonary and systemic vascular resistances
    MR severity
    LV volumes and EF
    Right heart pressures
    Other valve lesions
Coronary Arteriography
    Patients aged ≥35 years
    Patients aged <35 years:
        LV dysfunction
        Symptoms or signs suggestive of CAD
        One or more risk factors for premature CAD
            (excluding gender)

The important tests are highlighted.
ABBREVIATIONS: OS = opening snap; MDM = middiastolic murmer; RVH = right ventricular hypertrophy; LA = left atrial; LV = left ventricular; BP = blood pressure; BSA = body surface area; MVA = mitral valve area; MR = mitral regurgitation; PA = pulmonary artrial; MVG = mitral valve gradient; CAD = coronary artery disease.
SOURCE: From Rahimtoola SH, Durairaj A, Mehra A, Nuno I.[14]

patients. Selective supraventricular aortography should be performed in all patients unless there is a contraindication. Tricuspid valve function can be assessed when there is a question of coexisting lesions. In certain circumstances, for example, in a patient with suspected severe MS who has a small gradient and mildly elevated LA pressure, dynamic exercise in the catheterization laboratory with measurement of mitral valve gradient (MVG), CO, LA, and PA pressures can be extremely useful. Another example is a patient with significant symptoms in whom the findings at rest suggest moderate (or even mild) MS. Selective coronary arteriography establishes the site, severity, and extent of coronary artery disease and should be performed in patients with angina, in those with LV dysfunction, in those with risk factors for coronary artery disease, and in those 35 years of age or older who are being considered for interventional therapy. The essential information that should be obtained is listed in Table 67-3.[14]

OTHER INVESTIGATIONS

In most clinical situations, other investigations are not needed. Occasionally, a treadmill exercise test to evaluate functional capacity may be very useful clinically, for example, when a patient denies symptoms in spite of severe hemodynamic abnormalities.

Clinical Decision Making

The reader is referred to the section on aortic stenosis in Chap. 66. In a prospective blinded study of consecutive patients with valvular heart disease, the sensitivity and specificity of diagnosis of MS by clinical evaluation was 86 and 87 percent, respectively. The accuracy of diagnosis of MS for moderate to severe stenosis was 92 percent by clinical evaluation and 97 percent by echocardiography/Doppler ultrasound.[15] This emphasizes the importance of a thorough clinical evaluation. The principal difficulty with both clinical evaluation and echocardiography/Doppler ultrasound is being able to accurately separate in all instances mild from moderate MS and moderate from severe MS.

Natural History and Prognosis

The population presenting with MS is changing because of the sharp decline in the incidence of acute rheumatic fever in the past 40 years (see Chap. 65). Native-born American citizens with symptomatic MS are presenting at an older age. Young adults in the third and fourth decades with symptomatic MS are more likely to come from low socioeconomic backgrounds and from the inner city or to be immigrants, particularly from the Middle East, Latin America, Africa, or Asia. Therefore, the latent period between acute rheumatic fever and symptomatic MS is variable and appears to be related to the presence of repeated streptococcal infection. Women with MS outnumber men by almost two to one. The most important feature of the asymptomatic interval is the susceptibility to repeated bouts of both rheumatic valvulitis and streptococcal infection. The mechanism for the progression from no symptoms to mild to severe symptoms is progressive stenosis of the mitral valve.

With the onset of exertional dyspnea and fatigue, the valve area is usually reduced to one-half to one-third its normal size. Further small reductions in valve area markedly obstruct flow and result in symptoms with minimal exertion. The interval from initial mild symptoms to disabling symptoms may be 10 years. During this time, the patient is at some risk of death (see later). Permanent injury may result from atrial fibrillation with rapid ventricular rate, resulting in pulmonary edema, and from systemic embolus. Unfortunately, it is not possible to predict who is at risk of embolism. When late functional class (FC) II or FC III symptoms are present, the valve area is usually 1.0 cm² or less (in an occasional patient the valve area is 1.2 or 1.3 cm²), and both rest and exercise hemodynamics are deranged. Further small reductions in valve area result in symptoms at rest.

The 10-year survival of patients with MS who are asymptomatic is approximately 84 percent and that of those who are mildly symptomatic is 34 to 42 percent.[16–18] The 10-year survival of patients who are moderately or severely symptomatic and who do not have therapy is 40 percent or less, and the survival at 20 years is less than 10 percent.[16–18] Patients in the New York Heart Association (NYHA) FC IV have a very poor survival without treatment[16]: 42 percent at 1 year and 10 percent or less at 5 years. All are dead by 10 years.

Management

MS can be prevented through two approaches primary and secondary (see Table 67-4; Chap. 65). Although the incidence of infective endocarditis is low in isolated MS, all patients exposed to bacteremia should receive appropriate prophylaxis against infective endocarditis

TABLE 67-4 Medical Treatment of Mitral Stenosis

Antibiotic prophylaxis:
Recurrent rheumatic fever
Infective endocarditis

Restrict activities (moderate/severe ms):
Severe exercise
Competitive sports

Arrhythmias:
Prevent or control
Atrial fibrillation/flutter:
<Control ventricular rate
<Anticoagulation: Start with IV heparin and warfarin when INR is 2 to 3 discontinue heparin
<Restore sinus rhythm

Cardiac medications:
Warfarin anticoagulation: INR at 2 to 3
<Atrial fibrillation/supraventricular arrhythmias
<Systemic emboli
<LA thrombus
<Pulmonary emboli
<LV Systolic dysfunction
Elevated pulmonary venous pressure: diuretics*
"Heart failure"
<Pulmonary congestion: diuretics*
<Pulmonary edema: diuretics,* venodilators if necessary*
<LV systolic dysfunction: digitalis, ACE-inhibitors
<Elevated systemic venous pressure and fluid retention: digitalis, diuretics, ACE-inhibitors; beta-blockers (second generation) after patients are stabilized and there is LV systolic dysfunction.
Follow-up (see Algorithms 67-1–67-5)[14]

*Use judiciously; Patients with severe MS need an elevated LA pressure to maintain adequate LV filling and CO.
ABBREVIATIONS: MS = mitral stenosis; INR = international normalized ratio; LA = left atrial; ACE = angiotensin-converting enzyme; LV = left ventricular.
SOURCE: From Rahimtoola SH, Durairaj A, Mehra A, Nuno I.[14]

(see Chap. 81). Family and vocational planning should be considered. Women with this disease should consider bearing children before symptoms occur, since pregnancy is usually well tolerated with mild MS. Occupations that require strenuous exertion in middle age and later should probably be avoided if possible. In patients with moderate or severe MS, activities such as strenuous exercise and competitive sports should be restricted.[9]

When patients reach the symptomatic threshold, medical treatment may be of some benefit (see Table 67-4). Medical therapy is directed to (1) prevention or control of arrhythmia, the most common of which is atrial fibrillation; (2) anticoagulation; and (3) treatment of elevated pulmonary venous pressure, LV systolic dysfunction, and heart failure. Follow-up times are shown in Algorithms 67-1 to 67-5.[14]

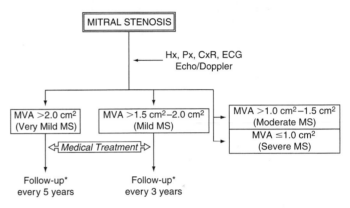

Algorithm 67-1

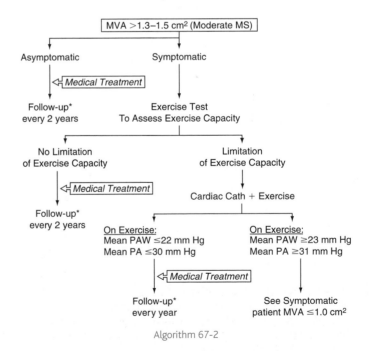

Algorithm 67-2

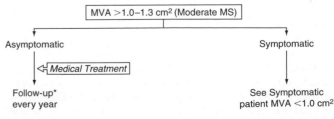

Algorithm 67-3

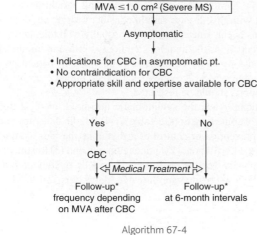

Algorithm 67-4

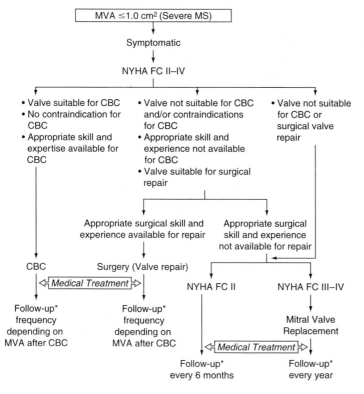

Algorithm 67-5

INTERVENTIONAL THERAPY

Interventional therapy is usually performed in patients with severe MS (MVA $\leq$ 1.0 cm^2) and occasionally in symptomatic patients with moderate MS (MVA > 1.0 to 1.3 cm^2). Patients with moderate MS (MVA > 1.3 to 1.5 cm^2) usually do not need interventional therapy. MVA >1.5 to 2.0 cm^2 is considered mild MS, and MVA >2.0 cm^2 is very mild MS.

Detailed management strategies are shown in algorithms 1 to 5.

Follow-up times in the algorithms relate to when patients are seen by a cardiologist. Patients should be seen sooner by a cardiologist if there is any change in their condition. When seen by a cardiologist, patients should have a history, physical examination, ECG, chest x-ray, and echocardiogram/Doppler. Patients should be seen at more frequent intervals by the primary care physician, family practitioner, internist, or cardiologist at which times only a history, physical examination, ECG, and chest x-ray are performed.

CATHETER BALLOON COMMISSUROTOMY

CBC is the procedure of choice if indicated (see algorithms) and if there are no contraindications (Table 67-5). In the United States, CBC is most commonly performed using the Inoue balloon. CBC is the procedure of choice because of the following:

1. Hospital mortality in the last 10 years is close to 0.[19,20]
2. The success rate is < 95 percent.[19]
3. The MVA increases to an average of 1.9 to 2.0 cm^2.[19,20,21]
4. There are reductions of MVG, LA (PA wedge) and PA pressures, and increase of CO.
5. Sixty percent of patients improve to NYHA FC I and 30 percent to FC II.[19,20]

The improvement has been objectively documented by exercise tests,[20] good immediate results are obtained in about 89 percent of patients,[19] closed mitral commissurotomy in a nonrandomized study in the 1950 to 1960s had shown an improved survival in symptomatic patients (NYHA FC II and III-IV) when compared to medical therapy[17] (Fig. 67-4), and in randomized trials the results of CBC versus closed surgical commissurotomy or surgical "repair" by open procedures are similar.[21] Follow-up to 10 years after CBC shows very good event-free survival (Fig. 67-5). There were no deaths up to 7 years of follow-up, and the event rate (MVR or repeat CBC) was 10 percent[20] in patients who after CBC had MVA > 1.5 cm^2 and mean PA wedge pressure of 18 mmHg (see Fig. 67-5). The 10-year results are also very good, event-free survival (freedom from cardiovascular

TABLE 67-5 Contraindications (Absolute/Relative to Catheter Balloon Commissurotomy for Mitral Stenosis)

Related to valve
• Mitral regurgitation that is truly 3+ to 4+
• Thrombus in left atrium
• Unfavorable valve morphology
    <High score (MGH 9-16; USC 3-4)
    <Commissural calcium
• Mild mitral stenosis
Related to medical center
• Lack of appropriate procedural skill and experience
Need for open heart surgery
• Coronary artery bypass surgery
• Other valve surgery
• Ascending aorta surgery for
    <Aneurysm
    <Dilatation ($\geq$5.5cm)
    <Annular ectasia
Procedural difficulties related to transseptal puncture
• Severe tricuspid regurgitation
• Huge right atrium
• Distorted/displaced atrial septum
• Venous problems
    <Femoral-Iliac veins obstructed or thrombosed
    <Inferior vena cava: Obstructed or thrombosed
      Drainage into azygos vein

Severe kyphoscoliosis (thoracic/abdominal)
SOURCE: From Rahimtoola SH, Durairaj A, Mehra A, Nuno I.[14]

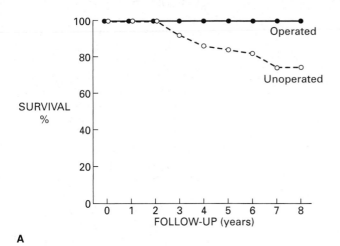

COMPARISON OF 33 OPERATED &
66 UNOPERATED PATIENTS WITH MITRAL STENOSIS
(MILD GROUP : Class II)

A

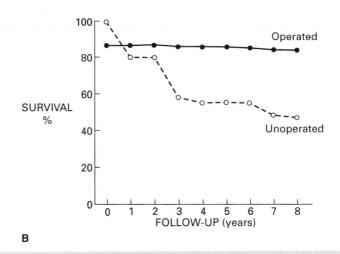

COMPARISON OF 67 OPERATED &
34 UNOPERATED PATIENTS WITH MITRAL STENOSIS
(SEVERE GROUP : Class III & IV)

B

FIGURE 67-4 Comparison of survival of patients with New York Heart Association class II symptoms (*left panel*) and class III and IV symptoms due to mitral stenosis (*right panel*).[29] Survival of patients treated medically (unoperated) is indicated by the broken line and those with surgical closed mitral commissurotomy (operated) by the solid line. In patients treated by surgical commissurotomy, there were no operative or late deaths in those with mild symptoms and no late deaths in those with class III and IV symptoms. There is a clear improvement in survival in operated patients. The 5-year mortality with medical treatment alone in those with class III and IV symptoms approaches 50 percent; with surgery, there is no appreciable mortality following recovery from the procedure. (From Roy SB, Gopinath N. Mitral stenosis. *Circulation* 1968;38(suppl v):68–76.)

deaths, MVR, repeat CBC, and NYHA FC I or II) is 56 ± 4 percent and those with good immediate result is 61 ± 5 percent[19] (Fig. 67-6).

MITRAL VALVE REPAIR

If the valve is suitable for CBC but there are contraindications for CBC, surgical valve repair is the procedure of choice if appropriate skill and experience is available.

MITRAL VALVE REPLACEMENT

MVAs after MVR and CBC are similar. There is a reduction of mean PA wedge and mean PA systolic pressures and of MVG as well as an increase of MVA (Table 67-6); operative mortality is 2 to 7 per-cent,[21–23] prosthesis-related mortality averages 2.5 percent per year (range 2 to 3 percent per year), and prosthesis-related complications average 5 percent per year (range 2 to 6 percent per year).[21,22] Use of a mechanical valve necessitates use of anticoagulant therapy with its resultant problems and complications. The insertion of a bioprosthesis to avoid anticoagulation-related problems and complications is associated with structural valve deterioration. In young people (16 to 40 years of age), structural valve deterioration begins at 2 to 3 years and is >60 percent at 10 years. Even in people aged 41 to 60 years bioprostheses is associated with high structural valve deterioration up to 50 percent and 50 percent of the late mortality is a consequence of structural valve deterioration.

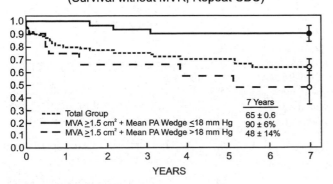

Event Free Survival
(Survival without MVR, Repeat CBC)

Orrange SE et al. Circulation 1997;95:382-389

FIGURE 67-5 Good event-free survival up to 7 years after catheter balloon commissurotomy. (From Orrange SE, Kawanish DT, Lopez BM, et al. Actuarial outcome after catheter balloon commissurotomy in patients with mitral stenosis. *Circulation* 1997;95:382–389.

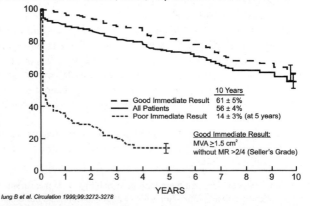

"Good Functional Results"
(Freedom from CV deaths, MVR, Repeat dilatation, & NYHA FC I or II)

Iung B et al. Circulation 1999;99:3272-3278

FIGURE 67-6 Good functional results up to 10 years after catheter balloon commissurotomy. (From Iung B, et al.[19] *Circulation* 1999;99:3272–3278.

TABLE 67-6 Mitral Stenosis: Results of Mitral Valve Replacement in 33 Patients

	Mitral Stenosis	
	Pre-MVR*	Post-MVR
LV end-diastolic pressure, mmHg	11 ± 5	12 ± 6
Mean PA wedge pressure, mmHg	36 ± 15	28 ± 14†
Mean systolic PA pressure, mmHg	54 ± 24	42 ± 22‡
Cardiac index, L/min/m²	2.1 ± 1.5	2.3 ± 0.6
LV EDVI, mL/m²	79 ± 18	72 ± 24
LV ESVI, mL/m²	41 ± 13	39 ± 21
LV ejection fraction	0.48 ± 0.10	0.47 ± 0.14
Mitral regurgitant volume, mL	—	—
Regurgitant volume/end-diastolic volume	—	—
Mitral valve gradient, mmHg	15 ± 7	8 ± 3†
Mitral valve area, cm²	12 ± 0.4	1.8 ± 0.6†

*MVR = mitral valve replacement.
†$p < .001$.
‡$p < .01$ comparing before and after mitral valve replacement artery.
SOURCE: Crawford MH et al.[114]

MITRAL VALVE REGURGITATION VERSUS CATHETER BALLOON COMMISSUROTOMY

MVR is usually recommended in patients who are in NYHA FC III and IV (see algorithm) because of the previously listed increased mortality and morbidity associated with MVR. MVR should also be considered in patients who are in NYHA FC II who have moderate or severe pulmonary hypertension and in those who are in NYHA FC I (asymptomatic) if they have a moderate or severe increase of pulmonary vascular resistance.

It is important to recognize that if the conditions exist for CBC and/or surgical valve repair, then performing MVR is inappropriate because MVR is associated with a higher hospitalization rate and late mortality and a higher complication rate related to the prosthesis.

INDICATIONS FOR CATHETER BALLOON COMMISSUROTOMY IN ASYMPTOMATIC PATIENTS WITH MITRAL STENOSIS

The MVA should be ≤ 1.0 cm² or > 1.0 to 1.5 cm² in selected patients, the valve should be suitable for CBC, there should be no contraindications for CBC, and appropriate skill and experience for CBC should be available. The indications are PA hypertension, episodic acute pulmonary edema, atrial fibrillation or flutter (paroxysmal/permanent), embolism (systemic/pulmonary), no thrombus in the LA or inferior vena cava, and patient should not be contemplating pregnancy and occupations that pose high risk to the patient or public.

TABLE 67-7 Recommendations for Percutaneous Mitral Balloon Valvotomy

Indication	Class
1. Symptomatic patients (NYHA functional class II, III, or IV), moderate or severe MS (mitral valve area ≤1.5 cm²),* and valve morphology favorable for percutaneous balloon valvotomy in the absence of left atrial thrombus or moderate to severe MR	I
2. Asymptomatic patients with moderate or severe MS (mitral valve area ≤1.5 cm²)* and valve morphology favorable for percutaneous balloon valvotomy who have pulmonary hypertension (pulmonary artery systolic pressure >50 mmHg at rest or 60 mmHg with exercise) in the absence of left atrial thrombus or moderate to severe MR	IIa
3. Patients with NYHA functional class III–IV symptoms, moderate or severe MS (mitral valve area ≤1.5 cm²),* and a nonpliable calcified valve who are at high risk for surgery in the absence of left atrial thrombus or moderate to severe MR	IIa
4. Asymptomatic patients, moderate or severe MS (mitral valve area ≤1.5 cm²) and valve morphology favorable for percutaneous balloon valvotomy who have new onset of atrial fibrillation in the absence of left atrial thrombus or moderate to severe MR	IIb
5. Patients in NYHA functional class III–IV, moderate or severe MS (MVA ≤1.5 cm²),* and a nonpliable calcified valve who are low-risk candidates for surgery	IIb
6. Patients with mild MS	III

*The committee recognizes that there may be variability in the measurement of mitral valve area and that the mean transmitral gradient, pulmonary artery wedge pressure, and pulmonary artery pressure at rest or during exercise should also be taken into consideration.
ABBREVIATIONS: NYHA = New York Heart Association; MS = mitral stenosis; MR = mitral regurgitation; MVA = mitral valve area.
SOURCE: ACC/AHA Guidelines,[21] with permission.

Guidelines The recommendations of the American College of Cardiology and the American Heart Association Practice Guidelines are shown in Tables 67-7, 67-8, and 67-9.[21] Guidelines are *not* and should *not* be the law. Application of guidelines to clinical practice should be based on the following principles: (1) classes I and III apply to all patients in these classes unless there is a specific clinical circumstance contradicting this, and (2) class II applies to patients in this class depending on the clinical condition of the patient and the skill and experience at the individual medical center.

MITRAL REGURGITATION

Normal Mitral Structure and Function

The mitral valve is a complex structure formed by four elements.[25,26]

1. The annulus is asymmetrical, with a fixed portion (corresponding to the anterior leaflet) shared with the aortic annulus and a dynamic portion (corresponding to the posterior leaflet) that represents most of the circumference of the annulus.

2. The two leaflets are asymmetrical; the anterior has the greater length of tissue but occupies a smaller portion of the circumference of the annulus than does the posterior portion.

3. The chordae join each papillary muscle to the corresponding commissure and the adjoining halves of both leaflets and maintain the two leaflets in a position allowing coaptation.

The two papillary muscles and the adjacent wall attach the mitral apparatus to the LV. Mitral competence during systole is normally ensured, first by a large area of coaptation between leaflets allowing high-friction resistance to abnormal valve movement and, second by the systolic position to the anterior leaflet parallel to the direction of blood flow.

Mitral Regurgitation

In Western society, the most common causes of chronic mitral regurgitation (MR) are ischemic heart disease and myxomatous degeneration of the valve, resulting in prolapse, ruptured chordae, or partial flail leaflet.[27] Patients with chronic severe degenerative MR and symptoms of heart failure and/or LV dysfunction are clearly candidates for mitral valve repair or replacement. However, the indications for such surgery in asymptomatic patients, especially those with normal LV function, remains controversial, especially in light of data demonstrating structural and biochemical abnormalities in the valve itself

TABLE 67-8 Recommendations for Mitral Valve Repair for Mitral Stenosis

Indication	Class
1. Patients with NYHA functional class III–IV symptoms, moderate or severe MS (mitral valve area ≤1.5 cm^2),* and valve morphology favorable for repair if percutaneous mitral balloon valvotomy is not available	I
2. Patients with NYHA functional class III–IV symptoms, moderate or severe MS (mitral valve area ≤1.5 cm^2),* and valve morphology favorable for repair if a left atrial thrombus is present despite anticoagulation	I
3. Patients with NYHA functional class III–IV symptoms, moderate or severe MS (mitral valve area ≤1.5 cm^2),* and a nonpliable or calcified valve with the decision to proceed with either repair or replacement made at the time of the operation.	I
4. Patients in NYHA functional class I, moderate or severe MS (mitral valve area ≤1.5 cm^2),* and valve morphology favorable for repair who have had recurrent episodes or embolic events on adequate anticoagulation	IIb
5. Patients with NYHA functional class I–IV symptoms and mild MS	III

*The committee recognizes that there may be a variability in the measurement of mitral valve area and that the mean transmitral gradient, pulmonary artery wedge pressure, and pulmonary artery pressure at rest or during exercise should also be considered.
ABBREVIATIONS: NYHA = New York Heart Association; MS = mitral stenosis.
SOURCE: ACC/AHA Guidelines,[21] with permission.

that raise questions regarding the durability and longevity of the repaired valve. In addition, there is a persistent uncertainty about the ability of vasodilator therapy to obviate or delay the need for surgery in asymptomatic patients with chronic MR. These controversial issues are compounded by the difficulty in determining the transition to an irreversible LV dysfunction and, thus, the timing for optimal surgical intervention.

Etiology and Mechanism

MR is often referred to as *organic,* if there is an intrinsic valve disease, or *functional,* if the valve is structurally normal but leaks due to an extravalvular abnormality, such as an alteration in LV chamber geometry and/or dilatation of the mitral annulus that affects normal coaptation of the mitral valve leaflets during systole (Table 67-10). Ischemic MR may be organic (ruptured or ischemic papillary muscle) and/or functional due to LV chamber dilatation. Nonischemic MR may be organic (e.g., rheumatic) or functional (e.g., dilated cardiomyopathy).

Rheumatic Disease

Rheumatic MR is rarely pure and, in most cases, is associated with stenosis and fusion of the commissures (Fig. 67-7, Plate 89). Severe rheumatic MR requiring surgical correction is still frequent in developing countries but is now rare in developed countries.[27] The underlying lesion is retractile fibrosis of leaflets and chordae, causing loss of coaptation. The secondary dilatation of the mitral annulus tends to further decrease the contract between leaflets. Elongated or ruptured chordae are infrequent.

Degenerative Mitral Regurgitation

Mitral annular calcification is a common autopsy finding, especially in the elderly population, and calcification is accelerated by the

TABLE 67-9 Recommendations for Mitral Valve Replacement for Mitral Stenosis

Indication	Class
1. Patients with moderate or severe MS (mitral valve area ≤1.5 cm^2)* and NYHA functional class III–IV symptoms who are not considered candidates for percutaneous balloon valvotomy or mitral valve repair	I
2. Patients with severe MS (mitral valve area ≤1 cm^2)* and severe pulmonary hypertension (pulmonary artery systolic pressure >60 to 80 mmHg) with NYHA functional class I–II symptoms who are not considered candidates for percutaneous balloon valvotomy or mitral valve repair	IIa

*The committee recognizes that there may be a variability in the measurement of mitral valve area and that the mean transmitral gradient, pulmonary artery wedge pressure, and pulmonary artery pressure should also be considered.
ABBREVIATIONS: MS = mitral stenosis; NYHA = New York Heart Association.
SOURCE: ACC/AHA Guidelines,[21] with permission.

TABLE 67-10 Mitral Regurgitation: Mechanisms

Etiology	Mechanism	Echocardiographic Appearance
Rheumatic	Retraction	Thickened chordae/ leaflets
Lupus erythematosus	Thickening	Normal or restricted motion
Anticardiolipin syndrome		
Carcinoid		
Ergot lesions		
Postradiation		
Degenerative	Prolapsed leaflets	Prolapsing/flail leaflets
Marfan's syndrome	Ruptured chords	Redundant tissue
Ehlers-Danlos syndrome		Ruptured chords
Traumatic MR		
Traumatic MR		
Ischemic (infarction)	Ruptured papillary muscle	Flail leaflet
Myocardial disease	Dilatation of annulus	Normal leaflets
Ischemic (chronic)	Traction anterior leaflet	Reduced motion of leaflets
Cardiomyopathies		
Infiltrative disease	Thickened leaflet	Thickened leaflets
Hypereosinophilic syndrome	Loss of coaptation	Reduced motion
Endomyocardial fibrosis		
Hurler's disease		
Endocarditis	Destructive lesions	Perforations
		Flail leaflets
Congenital	Cleft leaflet	Cleft leaflet
	Transposed valve	Tricuspid valve

association with hypertension, aortic stenosis, and diabetes and is also associated with connective tissue diseases such as Marfan's and Hurler's syndromes. (Fig. 67-8, Plate 90). It is usually of little functional consequence; however, it can be a cause of severe MR and in some severe cases cause inflow obstruction that may require surgical management.[28]

Degenerative MR is often associated with valve prolapse, an abnormal movement of the leaflets into the LA during systole due to inadequate chordal support (elongation or rupture) and excessive valvular tissue. In Western countries, mitral prolapse represents the most frequent causes leading to surgery for severe MR.[27] Myxomatous degeneration is the pathological substrate of mitral valve prolapse, characterized by redundant, floppy leaflets and associated with progressive MR.[29,30] Heart valves have a complex, layered architecture and highly specialized, functionally adapted cells and extracellular matrix (ECM). As in other tissues, turnover of the valvular ECM depends on a dynamic balance between synthesis and degradation. In most tissues, degradation of the ECM occurs through the action of matrix metalloproteinases (MMPs) and other proteases, especially those housed within inflammatory cells. Myxomatous valves have significant thickening and highly abnormal layered architecture and ECM components.[29,30] In particular, interstitial cells in myxomatous leaflets exhibited features of activated myofibroblasts, expressed elevated levels of MMPs and other proteolytic enzymes and cytokines, and were significantly increased in number in the spongiosa.[31] It remains to be determined whether high proteolytic activity and cell activation in the mitral leaflets are causal or whether regur-

gitation and abnormal mechanical stress induce matrix remodeling as a reactive mechanism. Nevertheless, this explains why patients with severe MR due to mitral valve prolapse, who are asymptomatic or minimally symptomatic with normal ventricular performance, can be expected to progress to surgical indications at an annual rate of 10.3 percent.[32]

Mechanical properties of myxomatous leaflets and chordae taken from patients demonstrate that myxomatous leaflets were more extensible and half as strong as normal valve tissue, which suggested that the abnormal stresses engendered by progressive stretching of enlarged leaflets and inherent weakness are synergistic in valve degeneration, possibly following as well as preceding valve repair.[32] Most notably, myxoid chordae failed at loads one-half of those of normal chordae.[33] This may explain why chordal rupture is the main indication for repair of myxoid mitral valves. These findings also suggest that chordal preservation should be carried out with caution, as myxoid chordae are clearly abnormal with compromised mechanical strength. Nevertheless, 7 years after repair, the incidence of significant regurgitation remains low (29 percent), with good clinical outcome and low reoperation rates after repair (93 percent to 96 percent freedom at 10 years).[34–36] However, a published study in 242 patients receiving mitral valve repair for degenerative valve regurgitation reported that freedom from nontrivial MR ($> 1/4$) was 94.3 ± 1.6 percent at 1 month, 58.6 ± 4.9 percent at 5 years, and 27.2 ± 8.6 percent at 7 years. Freedom from severe MR ($> 2/4$) was 98.3 ± 0.9 percent at 1 month, 82.8 ± 3.8 percent at 5 years, and 71.1 ± 7.4 percent at 7 years.[37] This is not surprising because genetic evidence suggests that myxoid changes are not entirely acquired and that genetic determinants are at least responsible for permanent cellular alterations in these valves.[38] Therefore, data suggest that the durability of a successful mitral reconstruction for degenerative mitral valve disease is not constant, and this should be taken into account when asymptomatic patients are offered early mitral valve repair.

Infective Endocarditis

Infective endocarditis accounts for about 5 percent of cases of severe MR. Vegetations may produce mild MR by interposition between leaflets. Severe endocarditic MR is usually related to ruptured chordae and less frequently to destruction of mitral tissue involving either the leaflet's edges or a perforation (Fig. 67-9, Plate 91).

Ischemic and Functional Mitral Regurgitation

Ischemic and functional MR, due to LV wall dysfunction secondary to ischemia, scarring, aneurysm, cardiomyopathy, or myocarditis

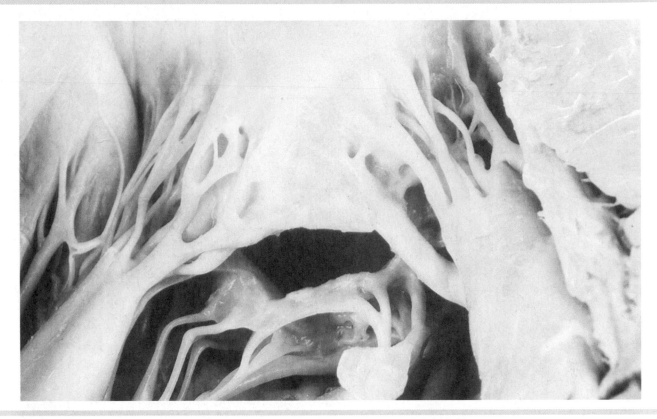

FIGURE 67-7 (Plate 89) Anatomic example of rheumatic mitral regurgitation. Note the thickening of the leaflet and chordae and the retraction of the mitral tissue. (Courtesy of WD Edwards.)

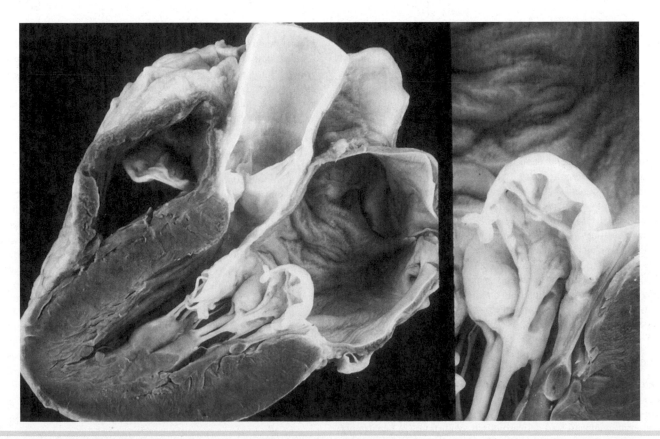

FIGURE 67-8 (Plate 90) Anatomic example of a flail posterior leaflet with ruptured chord. On the right of the picture, close-up view of the ruptured chord. Otherwise the left atrium is enlarged and the valvular tissue normal. (Courtesy of W. D. Edwards.)

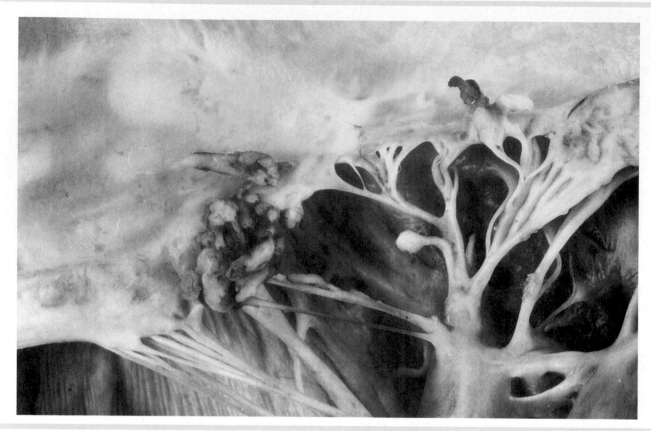

FIGURE 67-9 (Plate 91) Anatomic example of mitral regurgitation due to endocarditis. Note the vegetations of the anterior leaflet and the ruptured chords. (Courtesy of WD Edwards.)

have in common the same mechanism: the coaptation of intrinsically normal leaflets is incomplete. However, MR may be determined more by localized LV deformation than by the systolic function. Studies utilizing real-time three dimensional echocardiography in humans with MR demonstrated that the pattern of MV deformation from the medial to the lateral side was asymmetrical in ischemic MR, whereas it was symmetrical in nonischemic MR of cardiomyopathy.[39] This study supports the hypothesis that the geometry of the MV related to unilateral papillary displacement (regional LV dysfunction) is different from that related to bilateral displacement (global LV dysfunction), since each papillary muscle distributes the chordae only to the ipsilateral half of both leaflets. These types of MR are usually responsive to vasodilators or improvement of ischemia. Rupture of papillary muscle produces MR because of the flail leaflet and involves in 80 percent of cases the posteromedial papillary muscle and is most often associated with infarction of the adjacent ventricular wall.[40] It is the rarest form of heart rupture and of ischemic MR. Complete rupture is rapidly fatal without surgery, and partial- or single-head rupture of the papillary muscle more often allows emergency surgery[40] (Fig. 67-10, Plate 92).

Other Causes of Mitral Regurgitation

Clinically significant MR may be found in (1) *connective tissue disorder,* Marfan's syndrome, Ehlers-Danlos' syndrome, pseudoxanthum elasticum, osteogenesis imperfecta, Hurler's disease, systemic lupus erythematosus, and anticardiolipin syndrome; (2) penetrating or nonpenetrating *cardiac trauma;* (3) *myocardial disease*—hypertrophic cardiomyopathy, amyloidosis, or sarcoidosis; (4) *endocardial*

lesions due to hypereosinophilic syndrome, endocardial fibroelastosis, carcinoid tumors, ergot toxicity, radiation toxicity, diet or drug toxicity[41]; (5) *congenital* lesions such as cleft mitral valve isolated or associated with persistent atrioventricular canal, corrected transposition with or without Ebstein's abnormality of the left atrioventricular valve; and (6) *cardiac tumors.*

Hemodynamics of Mitral Regurgitation

The abnormal coaptation of the mitral leaflets creates a *regurgitant orifice* during systole. The systolic pressure gradient between the LV and LA is the driving force of the regurgitant flow, which results in a *regurgitant volume.* This regurgitant volume represents a percentage of the total ejection of the LV and may be expressed as the *regurgitant fraction.* The regurgitant volume creates a volume overload by entering the LA in systole and the LV in diastole, thereby creating a unique hemodynamic stress by inducing a low pressure form of volume overload due to ejection into the LA. Moderate MR is said to be present when the regurgitant fraction is in the range of 30 to 50 percent; severe MR is defined as a regurgitant fraction >50 percent.

The determinants of mitral regurgitant volume are best understood in the context of the orifice equation. This equation, based on the Torricelli principle, states that flow through an orifice varies by the square root of the pressure gradient across that orifice.

$$MRV = MROA \cdot C \cdot T_s \cdot \sqrt{LVP - LAP}$$

where MRV = mitral regurgiant volume, MROA = mitral regurgitant orifice area, C = constant, T_s = time or duration of systole,

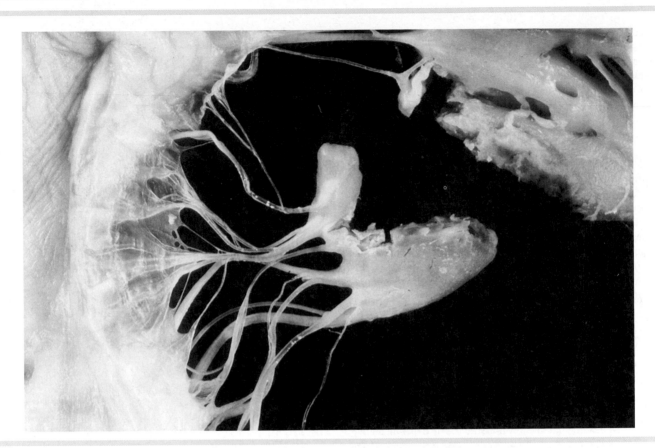

FIGURE 67-10 (Plate 92) Anatomic example of a ruptured posterior papillary muscle. Note the normal valvular tissue otherwise. (Courtesy of WD Edwards.)

LVP = LV mean systolic pressure, and LAP = left atrial mean systolic pressure. In many if not most patients with MR the regurgitant orifice area is dynamic with variations that are dependent on LV geometry. The systolic pressure gradient across the valve can also vary dramatically. These two determinants of regurgitant volume are the primary therapeutic targets in patients with MR.

The pressure gradient between the LV and atrium begins with mitral closure (simultaneous to S_1) and persists after closure of the aortic valve (S_2) until the mitral valve opens.[42] Thus, timing of regurgitant flow is determined by that of the regurgitant orifice and is most often holosystolic. Regurgitant flow and orifice area have been shown to vary throughout systole in distinct patterns characteristic of the underlying mechanism of mitral incompetence.[43] In functional regurgitation in dilated cardiomyopathy, there was a constant decrease in OA throughout systole.[44] In mitral valve prolapse, OA was small in early systole, increasing substantially in midsystole, and decreasing mildly during left ventricular relaxation.[45] In rheumatic MR, there was a roughly constant regurgitant OA during most of systole.

The dynamic changes in OA during systole that differ across various MR etiologies may help explain the response to therapy in chronic MR. Therapy with vasodilators in chronic MR has been shown to reduce LV wall stress and thereby delay or obviate the need for valve replacement in AR.[46] However, no such data are available in patients with chronic MR using standard vasodilators or agents that block renin angiotensin system components,[47–50] but may vary depending on the underlying etiology of MR.[50] The observed efficacy of Angiotensin-converting enzyme (ACE) inhibitor in papillary muscle dysfunction or dilated cardiomyopathy produces a decrease in LV size and thereby regurgitant OA as a result of afterload reduction. In contrast, ACE inhibitor were ineffective in reducing LV volumes in patients with structural valve disease due to rheumatic heart disease or mitral annular calcification, which was attributed to an inability of these agents to decrease the relatively "fixed" mitral regurgitant OA that characterizes these conditions. ACE inhibitors were similarly ineffective in mitral valve prolapse, a condition in which preload or afterload reduction may actually increase the degree of prolapse and subsequently the severity of MR.

Degree and Consequences of Regurgitation

The degree of volume overload depends on three factors, the area of the regurgitant orifice, the regurgitant gradient, and the regurgitant duration. The volume overload is usually less severe in mitral than in AR, despite a usually larger regurgitant gradient and orifice that is in part related to a shorter duration of MR during the cardiac cycle in mitral than in AR. However, another important consideration is related to the unique loading conditions of MR, where the LV is intrinsically unloaded in both early and late systole by ejection into the low pressure LA; whereas in AR, the excess volume is ejected into the high pressure aorta. It is of interest that there was increased myosin heavy chain synthesis after 6 h of pressure overload but no change after 6 h of MR in the dog.[51] Taken together, the inherent differences in the hemodynamics of the volume overload reflect the lower LV mass and mass-to-volume ratio in patients with MR as compared to AR.[51,52]

The height of the LA V wave and, more generally, left atrial pressure is mainly determined by left atrial compliance.[53] In acute MR, the LA is less compliant than it is in chronic MR and the MR produces a marked increase in LA pressure. The atrial V wave, in turn, decreases the ventriculoatrial gradient and, thus, for any effective regurgitant orifice, tends to limit the regurgitant volume. When MR becomes chronic, the LA dilates, the V wave is less prominent and does not limit the regurgitant volume; the LA pressure may be normal even with severe MR at rest.[54] However, a study of patients with ischemic and nonischemic heart failure (LV ejection fraction < 25 percent) and mild-to-moderate MR, there was an increase in exercise-induced changes in MR severity that correlated with $V_{O_{2max}}$ and increases in pulmonary capillary wedge pressure, end-diastolic and end-systolic sphericity indexes and with mitral valvular coaptation distance.[55] There are numerous studies demonstrating the importance of resting RV ejection fraction in determining exercise capacity and morbidity and mortality after mitral valve repair or replacement in patients with chronic MR.[56–58] Taken together, the effect on resting RV function reflects chronic passive pulmonary congestion of MR that may not be impressive at rest but may increase in severity during mild-to-moderate exercise.

Left Ventricular Function

EFFECTS ON MYOCARDIAL OXYGEN CONSUMPTION
The volume overload of chronic MR produces an eccentric pattern of hypertrophy manifested by a decrease in the LV mass to volume ratio in response to the increase in diastolic load, as systolic load is facilitated by ejection into the low pressure LA. In experimentally induced MR in the dog, the volume overload has little initial effect on myocardial oxygen consumption due to the mechanical facilitation of shortening due to ejection into the low pressure LA.[59] However, the marked increase in LV end-diastolic volume, that over time outstrips the increase in LV mass, produces an increase in stress-volume area that is equivalent to dogs with pure pressure overload, suggesting a similar myocardial oxygen consumption.[60] Indeed, chronic MR in the dog produced decreased LV creatine phosphate to adenosine triphosphate (ATP) ratios,[61] while expression of the fetal isoform of creatine kinase was significantly higher[62] when compared to healthy specimens. In patients, the severity of MR, determined by LV volumes, related to the decreased LV creatine phosphate to ATP ratios,[63] suggests that bioenergetic abnormalities occur in the dilated LV in spite of "normal" LV ejection fraction.

EFFECTS ON DIASTOLIC FUNCTION
One of the difficult problems in caring for patients with MR is that they may remain compensated, without symptoms of congestive heart failure, for many years. After experimentally induced MR in the dog, filling fraction during the first 40 percent of diastolic time was increased significantly at 4 days by 67 percent and at 2 and 4 weeks by 76 percent.[64,65] The eccentricity index, which relates the relative sizes of the long and short axes, demonstrated progressive LV sphericity over time that was greatest during the early rapid filling phase and a near four-fold increase in the transmitral pressure gradient. In patients, chronic MR caused the pressure-dimension and volume curve to shift to the right as myocardial stiffness was unchanged (Fig. 67-11).[66] However, as the LV fails in patients with chronic MR, the chamber stiffness and pressure volume curve is shifted toward a less compliant ventricle.[66]

Much has been studied regarding the role of the profibrotic response in the course of pressure overload. In contrast, hearts with volume overload undergo a continual state of remodeling of the ECM

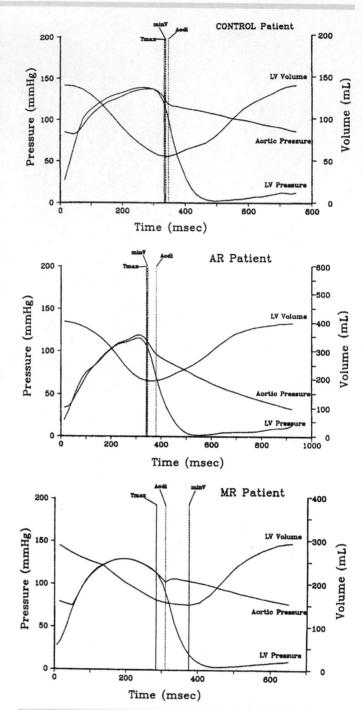

FIGURE 67-11 Shows the LV pressure–volume relationships in a control patient, a patient with aortic regurgitation, and a patient with mitral regurgitation.

that opposes excess collagen deposition, in spite of increased cardiac renin–angiotensin system (RAS) expression.[67] Indeed, in human hearts, there is a greater increase in steady-state mRNA for collagen I and collagen III in the pressure overload of aortic valvular stenosis as compared to the volume overload of AR.[67,68] In addition, in the dog model of MR, there is upregulation of the intracardiac RAS, decreased LV wall thickness to diameter ratio, increased MMP activity, and dissolution of the collagen weave within 2 weeks and lasting for 5 months after induction of MR.[69–71] Taken together, these findings are consistent with the contention that less ECM allows for the necessary LV chamber enlargement and compliance characteristics in volume overload.

EFFECTS ON SYSTOLIC FUNCTION

It is difficult to measure contractility of the LV particularly in the case of MR, because the definition of end-systole and end-ejection has been used interchangeably to assess LV performance based on the assumption that timing of these events is nearly coincident. However, studies in animals,[72] and in humans[73–75] have clearly demonstrated that end-ejection, defined as minimum ventricular volume, dissociates from end-systole in MR because of the shortened time to LV end-systole in association with preserved time to end-ejection (minimum volume) due to the low impedance ejection presented by the LA (Fig. 67-12). Thus, the load-dependent ejection or shortening phase indices of function, such as LV ejection fraction (EF) and velocity of circumferential shortening, can be normal and mask significant myocardial dysfunction in the setting of MR.[75] For this reason it is not surprising that an LV ejection fraction value of 60 percent is considered the lower limit for timing for mitral valve surgery in MR.[76]

Ejection fraction is dependent upon preload and afterload. Plotting ejection fraction against afterload provides a better index of contractile function than ejection fraction alone. As an alternative to ejection fraction, end-systolic volume or dimension is relatively independent of preload and varies linearly with afterload. The slope of this relation describes the end-systolic pressure-stress and volume-dimension relation or systolic elastance. Three months of experimentally produced MR in the dog resulted in decreased LV systolic elastance and decreased shortening of isolated myocytes, but augmented LV ejection fraction.[77] An analysis of LV chamber elastance in patients with chronic MR supported the concepts that contractile function is impaired in some patients with long-term MR and a normal LV ejection fraction.[75] However, use of this methodology in patients is potentially hazardous because it requires invasive hemodynamic monitoring and manipulation of blood pressure to alter loading conditions.

Afterload has been approximated by measuring either end-systolic pressure or end-systolic wall stress; however, wall stress is a better index of afterload because it accounts for ventricular geometry, which is especially important in the case of the spherically dilated heart with MR. A relatively high end-systolic volume for a given end-systolic wall stress indicates relatively less ventricular shortening for a given afterload, therefore depressed myocardial contractility.[78] In patients having surgery for severe MR, the end-systolic stress to end-systolic volume ratio separated patients with a good prognosis for valve replacement.[78] Four of the 5 patients died and 1 patient was unimproved after surgery. There are well-appreciated limitations of the single point ratio in the assessment of contractile function.[79] However, the incorporation of a wall-stress determination adds complementary physiologic and prognostic data to LV end-systolic dimension and volume and LV ejection fraction in the assessment of MR.[76]

Neurohormonal Activation

The adrenergic nervous system provides inotropic support for the overloaded heart and may represent an important mechanism of compensation in the course of MR since Starling (preload) reserve is called upon as an early compensatory mechanism. Indeed, there was a positive relation between norepinephrine release rates (an index of sympathetic activity) with increasing end-systolic dimension and decrease in LV performance in patients with chronic MR.[80] Other studies demonstrated also a decrease in LV myocardial beta-adrenergic receptor density that was related to the severity of symptoms and LV dysfunction.[81] As has been seen throughout this chapter, the canine model of experimentally induced MR demonstrates many similarities to the human condition. This model has been shown to be dependent upon adrenergic support to compensate for innate contractile depression identified both at the LV chamber and isolated cardiomyocyte.[82] However, the cost of incessant increase in local catecholamines has been shown to actually reduce protein synthesis and viability of isolated adult cardiomyocytes.[83] It is of great interest that beta-adrenergic blockade treatment of MR dogs improved LV chamber remodeling and ECM preservation,[84] as well as improved isolated cardiomyocyte contractile function and an increase in the number of contractile elements within cardiomyocytes.[85]

Tumor necrosis factor-α (TNF-α) is a proinflammatory cytokine that has been shown to activate MMPs and to be increased in the myocardium in response to stretch.[86] TNF-α is found to be elevated in the plasma of patients with congestive heart failure[87] and in the plasma of patients with aortic stenosis and MR.[88] Furthermore, in patients with chronic MR, increased TNF-α expression in the myocardium and plasma was related to the extent of LV dilatation.[84] Moreover, correction of the LV volume overload state with MV repair led to reversal of TNF-α expression and reverse LV remodeling. Taken together, these findings suggest that TNF-α may play a key role in inflammatory-mediated changes in the ECM that results in progressive LV dilatation in patients with chronic MR.

Clinical Presentation

Primary MR often is initially diagnosed based on a finding of a systolic murmur in an asymptomatic patient. However, the nature and severity of symptoms with MR are related to its severity that in turn is related to the presence of pulmonary hypertension, coronary artery disease, atrial fibrillation, and associated valvular disease. Fatigue

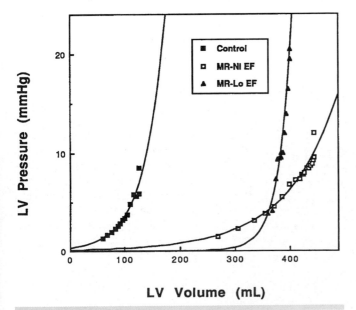

FIGURE 67-12 Shows the LV diastolic pressure–volume relationships in a control patient, two patients with MR one of whom had normal left ventricular ejection fraction (LVEF), and another patient who had reduced LV ejection fraction.

and mild dyspnea on exertion are the most usual symptoms and are rapidly improved by rest. The administration of diuretics and progressive self-limitation of physical activity may prevent the occurrence of more severe symptoms. Severe dyspnea on exertion or, more rarely, paroxysmal nocturnal dyspnea, frank pulmonary edema, or even hemoptysis may be observed later in the course of the disease. Such severe symptoms may be triggered by a new onset of atrial fibrillation, or increase in degree of MR, the occurrence of endocarditis or ruptured chordae, or a change in LV compliance or function.

With severe MR of *acute onset,* symptoms are usually more dramatic with pulmonary edema or congestive heart failure, but will progressively subside with administration of a diuretic, afterload reduction, and increased LA compliance with time. A syndrome of sudden onset of atypical chest pain and dyspnea may occur with abrupt chordal rupture.[89] Sudden death as the initial presentation of MR due to flail leaflet is 1 to 2.5 percent over 6 years and is related to LV systolic dysfunction, leaflet redundancy, severe MR, and associated comorbid conditions.[90] Rupture of papillary muscle in the setting of acute myocardial infarction usually has a dramatic presentation, with cardiogenic shock or a severe pulmonary edema. Pulmonary edema may also be observed in transient severe papillary muscle dysfunction.

Physical Examination

Blood pressure is usually normal. Carotid upstroke is brisk. Cardiac palpation may show laterally displaced, diffuse, and brief apical impulse with enlarged LV. An apical thrill is characteristic of severe MR. The left sternal border lift is observed with RV dilatation and may be difficult to distinguish from the left atrial lift due to the dilated, expansive LA, which is more substernal and lower. S_1 is included in the murmur and is usually normal but may be increased in rheumatic disease. S_2 is usually normal but may be paradoxically split if the LV ejection time is markedly shortened. The presence of a third heart sound (S_3) is directly related to the volume of the regurgitation in patients with organic MR.[91] It is often associated with an early diastolic rumble due to the increased mitral flow in diastole even without MS. The S_3 and diastolic rumble are low-pitched sounds and may be difficult to detect without careful auscultation in the left lateral decubitus position. The S_3 increases with expiration. In ischemic-functional MR, S_3 corresponds more often to restrictive LV filling. An atrial gallop (S_4) is heard mainly in MR of recent onset and in ischemic or functional MR in sinus rhythm. Midsystolic clicks are markers of valve prolapse (see Chaps. 12 and 13).

The hallmark of MR is the systolic murmur, most often holosystolic, including first and second heart sounds.[92] If an opening snap or S_3 is mistakenly interpreted as S_2, the murmur may appear midsystolic. Only a careful examination beginning at the base of the heart to identify the second heart sound and progressing toward the apex will allow clear recognition of the nature of the murmur. The murmur is of the blowing type but may be harsh, especially in valve prolapse. The maximum intensity is usually at the apex, and it may radiate to the axilla in rheumatic or anterior leaflet prolapse, affecting primarily the anterior leaflet. In posterior leaflet prolapse, the jet is usually superiorly and medially directed and the murmur radiates toward the base of the heart. The murmur may be heard in the back, in the neck, and sometimes on the skull. In the cases where the murmur radiates to the base, it may be difficult to distinguish from the murmur of aortic stenosis or obstructive cardiomyopathy, and pharmacologic maneuvers showing that the murmur decreases with amyl nitrite and increases with methoxamine strongly suggest MR. Murmur intensity does not increase with postextrasystolic beats and usually parallels the degree of MR, but in myocardial infarction severe MR may be totally silent. Murmurs of shorter duration usually correspond to mild MR; they may be mid or late systolic in mitral valve prolapse or early systolic in functional MR.

Electrocardiogram

The most frequent feature of MR is atrial fibrillation, which was found in approximately 50 to 60 percent of earlier series and is now present in approximately 50 percent of surgically corrected MR.[93] Patients in sinus rhythm may present with signs of left atrial enlargement (Fig. 67-13). LV hypertrophy is more rarely seen and may be associated with secondary ST-T abnormalities. RV hypertrophy is uncommon. The ECG, especially in acute MR, may be entirely normal, while ischemic MR may manifest Q waves or ST-T wave changes.

Chest Roentgenogram

Cardiomegaly may be present in chronic MR or in ischemic or functional MR (Fig. 67-14). LA body and appendage dilatation is frequent but giant LA is rare and is usually seen in severe mixed valve disease. Although valvular calcifications are rare, annular calcification seen as a C-shaped density below the posterior leaflet is frequent. Because LA pressure is frequently normal even with severe MR, signs of pulmonary hypertension or pulmonary edema are rarely observed.

Doppler Echocardiography

Doppler echocardiography (see Chap. 15) in MR characteristically reveals a high-velocity jet in the LA during sys-

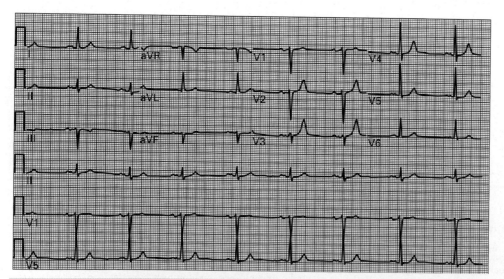

FIGURE 67-13 Electrocardiogram of a patient with severe mitral regurgitation. Note left atrial enlargement, as indicated by notched P waves (lead I and rhythm strip lead II).

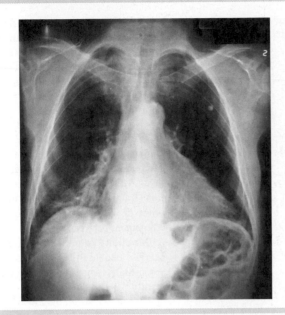

FIGURE 67-14 Chest roentgenogram of a patient with severe mitral regurgitation. Note the cardiomegaly and enlargement of the left atrial body and appendage.

tole, and the severity of the regurgitation is a function of the distance from the valve that the jet can be detected. Most centers grade regurgitation as mild, moderate, or severe using a combination of color-flow, continuous, and pulsed-wave Doppler imaging.[94–95] Area of the mitral jet > 8 cm^2 has also been shown to indicate severe MR. However, jet area is significantly affected by the cause of the MR, which, in some cases, can produce an eccentric jet that limits the accuracy of this approach. Another mean of determining MR severity utilizes the vena contracta defined as the narrowest cross-sectional area of the regurgitant jet by color-flow Doppler. Although Doppler echocardiography provides several methods of quantifying regurgitation, none have been shown to predict clinical outcome.

Echocardiography

The most important aspect of echocardiography is the quantification of LV end-diastolic and end-systolic dimensions, wall thickness, and ejection fraction and fractional shortening. M-mode diameter or volume can assess the LA size by two-dimensional echocardiography. However, the LV ejection fraction may be normal in the setting of myocardial dysfunction resulting in postoperative LV dysfunction, even in the absence of clinical symptoms prior to surgery. For this reason, clinical management requires periodic imaging studies to detect changes, especially in the end-systolic dimension. Surgery should be considered when LV ejection fraction is $<$ 60 percent and LV end-systolic dimension is $>$ 45 mm.[96] One study

demonstrated that the preoperative exercise echocardiographic LV ejection fraction and LV end-systolic volume were the best predictors of postoperative LV dysfunction in patients with minimal symptoms prior to surgery.[97] Such an evaluation can detect latent LV dysfunction that is indicated by a limited contractile reserve by exercise.

Evaluation of the valvular leaflets is an important part of the echocardigraphic exam. *Rheumatic MR* is characterized by thickening of the leaflets and chordae. The posterior leaflet has reduced mobility, whereas the anterior leaflet may be doming if commissural fusion is associated. In *degenerative MR,* prolapse is observed with the passage of valvular tissue beyond the annulus plane in the long-axis view (Fig. 67-15). The valve leaflets are diffusely thickened leaflets and excessive valvular tissue and increased echogenicity of the annulus is consistent with mitral annular calcification. Flail segments can appear as complete eversion of the segment with or without the small floating echo of ruptured chordae (Fig. 67-16).

In ischemic or functional MR, the finding of a dilated annulus is nonspecific and annular descent is reduced. The features of ischemic heart disease may be observed as regional wall motion abnormalities. The leaflet tissue is normal. The mitral tenting due to the abnormal traction by the principal chordae on the anterior leaflet reduces the area of coaptation of the two leaflets and therefore allows for a central jet of MR. With papillary muscle rupture, MR is due to the flail leaflet. The diagnosis is based on visualization of a small mass of muscle, which is attached to chordae and floats freely during the cardiac cycle.

Transesphogeal echocardiography provides superior imaging quality to transthoracic echocardiography. However, its incremental value is notable only when the transthoracic information is suboptimal or incomplete and when questions arise regarding the feasibility of valve repair the presence of endocarditis or other associated complications. It is also utilized on a large scale intraoperatively to monitor the results of valve repair with loading conditions matched to a baseline study performed at the beginning of the surgical procedure.

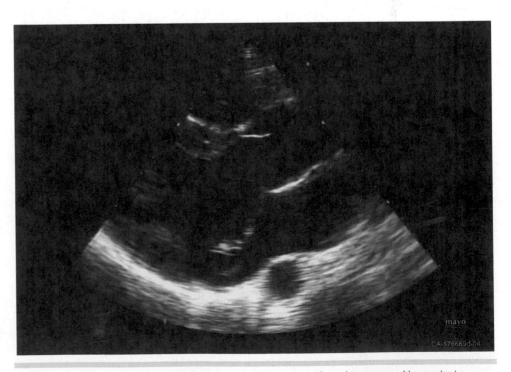

FIGURE 67-15 Echocardiogram of a bileaflet mitral valve prolapse seen from the parasternal long-axis view.

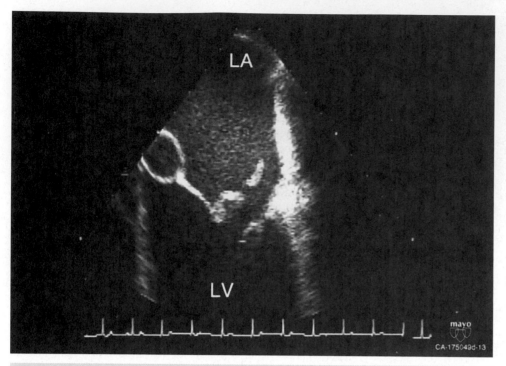

FIGURE 67-16 Transesophageal echocardiography (*horizontal plane*) of a flail anterior leaflet. The ruptured chord is seen at the tip of the anterior leaflet.

Radionuclide Studies

Radionuclide angiography can be used to estimate the LV end-diastolic and end-systolic volume as well as the RV and LV ejection fraction. The detection of exercise-induced LV dysfunction can be helpful in the asymptomatic patient.[96] A comparison of the stroke counts measured over the RV and LV allows the calculation of a regurgitant fraction in the absence of tricuspid and pulmonary regurgitation.

Cardiac Catheterization

Cardiac catheterization is utilized to assess hemodynamic status, the severity of MR, LV function, and coronary anatomy. The large V wave of the pulmonary wedge pressure is more frequent in acute MR than it is in chronic MR but can be observed in other diseases such as ventricular septal defect or heart failure with reduced left atrial compliance without MR (Fig. 67-17). Selective LV cineangiography provides a clinically useful assessment of MR severity, qualitatively grading the degree of opacification of the LA and pulmonary veins. Quantitation of MR regurgitant volume and regurgitant fraction can be obtained by comparing the angiographic stroke volume to the forward stroke volume, calculated by the Fick method. The assessment of LV function can be performed using quantitative angiography, while the use of high-fidelity pressure recording has provided important information on LV elastance[73–75] and LV chamber stiffness[66] in patients with MR. Obstructive coronary atherosclerosis continues to be frequent even in the absence of angina,[98] and coronary angiography is ordinarily performed in patients older than 40 to 50 years of age.

Natural History

In patients with primary MR, there may be a period of several years without sysmptoms. In a prospective study of 300 patients with MR, rate of symptom onset was 2 to 4 percent per year.[99] In patients with unoperated clinically significant MR, the late survival has been found as high as 60 percent at 10 years[100] or as low as 30 percent at 5 years.[101] In patients with flail mitral leaflets, at 10 years survival was 57 percent,[89] and sudden death in patients with MR due to flail leaflets occurs at a rate of 1.8 percent per year.[102] The rates are higher in patients with symptoms or reduced ejection fraction, but even in the absence of these risk factors the rate is 0.8 percent per year.[102]

Morbidity in patients with severe MR is also high. Of patients who are initially asymptomatic, approximately 10 percent per year develop symptoms,[103] which may be hastened by atrial fibrillation. In patients with flail leaflets 10 years after diagnosis, heart failure occurred in 63 percent, and permanent atrial fibrillation in 30 percent of those initially in sinus rhythm[89] (Fig. 67-18). Also at 10 years, 90 percent of the patients had either died or undergone surgery,[89] confirming that in these patients surgery is almost unavoidable (Fig. 67-19).

Management

MEDICAL TREATMENT

Prevention of infective endocarditis using the appropriate prophylaxis is necessary in patients with MR. Young patients with rheumatic MR should receive rheumatic fever prophylaxis. In patients with atrial fibrillation, rate control is achieved using digoxin and/or beta blockers. Long-term maintenance of sinus rhythm after cardioversion in patients with severe MR or enlarged LA is usually not possible in patients who are treated medically. However, return to sinus rhythm after surgery is possible in patients with atrial fibrillation of short duration. Oral anticoagulation should be used in patients with atrial fibrillation.

Although vasodilators are successfully used to increase forward output and decrease LV filling pressure in patients with acute MR[104] and dilated cardiomyopathy, the hemodynamic effects are less clear in patients with primary mitral valve disease.[47–50] Studies to date have reported conflicting results regarding the benefits of chronic ACE inhibitor therapy in patients with MR of heterogeneous etiologies.[104–108] In concordance with these clinical studies, reports from two independent laboratories have demonstrated that blockade of the RAS fails to improve LV function and remodeling in a canine model of MR.[109–111] The canine model of MR is characterized by an absence of fibrosis, activation of MMPs, and by dissolution of the fine collagen weave.[111] As RAS blockade is antifibrotic, it may have accentuated this process resulting in loss of the fine collagen weave that destroys the structural support of the ECM that is necessary for maintenance of normal LV chamber geometry and for the translation of forces from individual cardiomyocytes to the LV chamber. Beta$_1$-adrenergic blockade treatment of MR dogs improved LV chamber remodeling and ECM preservation,[84] as well as improved isolated

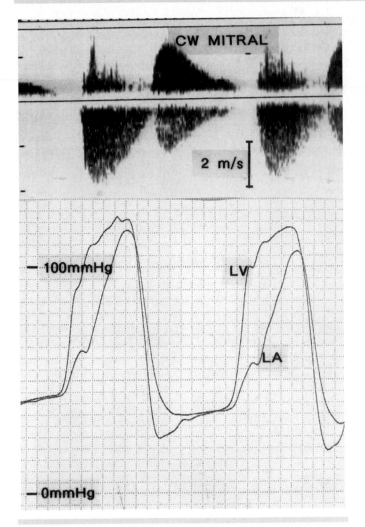

FIGURE 67-17 Simultaneous recording of left ventricular and left atrial pressures and continuous-wave (CW) Doppler in a patient with severe mitral regurgitation. Note the large V wave on the left atrial pressure recording, with a triangular shape of the mitral regurgitant jet obtained by CW Doppler. (Courtesy of Rick Nishimura, Mayo Clinic.)

cardiomyocyte contractile function and an increase in the number of contractile elements within cardiomyocytes.[85] Insights from the canine model of MR, coupled with a lack of conclusive clinical data on treatment, provide a strong rationale for a well-designed clinical trial of Beta-RB in patients with MR that incorporates information on LV size and function, and especially clinical outcome.

SURGICAL TREATMENT

In most patients requiring surgery, the most relevant question is the timing of the surgical indication, which is influenced by the natural history of MR and by the outcome after surgical correction of MR. The determinants of outcome are listed in Table 67-11. The current American College of Cardiology and American Heart Association guidelines for timing of surgery suggest that surgery should be considered in patients with chronic asymptomatic severe MR when LV end systolic dimension is ≥ 45 mm (normal < 40 mm) and LV ejection fraction is ≤ 60 percent (normal 65 percent; Table 67-12). A markedly reduced preoperative ejection fraction (< 50 percent) is associated with a high late mortality.[112–114] In patients with severe MR and an ejection fraction < 30 percent or an end-systolic dimension > 55 mm, very high-risk surgery

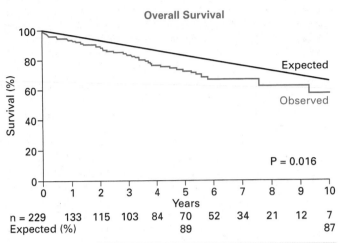

FIGURE 67-18 Survival with medical treatment of patients diagnosed with mitral regurgitation due to flail leaflets. Note the excess mortality in comparison to the expected survival. (Reprinted by permission of the *New England Journal of Medicine* from Ling H, Enriquez-Sarano M, Seward J, et al. Clinical outcome of mitral regurgitation due to flail leaflets. *N Engl J Med*. 1996;335: 1417–1423. Copyright 1996, Massachusetts Medical Society.)

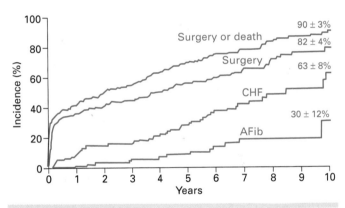

FIGURE 67-19 Cardiac morbidity with medical treatment in patients diagnosed with mitral regurgitation due to flail leaflets. CHF, congestive heart failure, Afib, atrial fibrillation. (Reprinted by permission of the *New England Journal of Medicine* from Ling H, Enriquez-Sarano M, Seward J, et al. Clinical outcome of mitral regurgitation due to flail leaflets. *N Engl J Med*. 1996;335: 1417–1423. Copyright 1996, Massachusetts Medical Society.)

TABLE 67-11 Determinants of Outcome

Unoperated Patients	Operated Patients
Symptoms	Age
Pulmonary hypertension	Preoperative symptoms
LV end-diastolic volume	Coronary disease
AV-O$_2$ difference	End-systolic dimensions
Ejection fraction	Ejection fraction
	LA size?
	Valve repair

ABBREVIATIONS: LV = left ventricular; LA = left atrial.

TABLE 67-12 American College of Cardiology/American Heart Association Guidelines for Surgery for Nonischemic Severe Mitral Regurgitation

Class I (evidence and/or general agreement that surgery is useful and effective)
- Symptoms caused by MR (acute or chronic)
- Asymptomatic patients with severe MR and mild-moderate LV dysfunction defined as an:
  –ejection fraction 30–60% **and**
  –end systolic dimension 45–55 mm

Class IIa (conflicting evidence and/or divergence of opinion but the weight of evidence/opinion favours surgical intervention)
- Asymptomatic patients with normal LV function and
  –atrial fibrillation **or**
  –pulmonary hypertension (>50 mmHg at rest or >60 mmHg with exercise)
- Asymptomatic patients with
  –ejection fraction 50–60% **or**
  –end systolic dimension 45–55 mm
- Severe left ventricular systolic dysfunction (ejection fraction <30% and/or end systolic dimension >55 mm) if chordal preservation is highly likely

ABBREVIATIONS: MR = mitral regurgitation; LV = left ventricular.

should be undertaken if it is highly likely that a valve repair can be performed. Valve repair is highly controversial in dilated cardiomyopathy. In the patient with ischemic heart disease and MR, revascularization can improve MR and valve repair and/or annuloplasty should be considered on a case by case basis.

POSTOPERATIVE OUTCOME

Mitral valve repair offers several advantages including avoidance of long-term anticoagulation and, most importantly, preservation of the continuity between the mitral annulus and papillary muscles. This annular–papillary muscle continuity helps maintain normal left LV geometry and systolic function.[115] When annular–papillary continuity is preserved, ejection fraction typically remains stable or improves after mitral surgery in contrast to a decline by an average of 10 ejection fraction units when this continuity is disrupted.[116–118] The average operative mortality for mitral valve repair is 1 to 2 percent compared to 5 to 10 percent with valve replacement. Age and the existence of coronary artery disease are important predictors of survival. Mitral valve repair has a low rate of reoperation for recurrent MR with an event-free survival ranging from 80 to 90 percent at 5 to 10 years in published series.[119] However, considering the inherent structural abnormalities of the valve of degenerative MR[31] and the data in patients with valve repair,[37] the durability of a successful mitral reconstruction for degenerative mitral valve disease is not constant. This should be taken into account when asymptomatic patients are offered early mitral valve repair, especially when LV functional dimensions are within accepted guidelines for observational treatment.

Atrial fibrillation when present preoperatively usually persists postoperatively—unless it is of brief duration—but the excess risk due this arrhythmia appears modest, although it requires anticoagulation. In the patient with MR and atrial fibrillation, some centers now advocate a concurrent atrial procedure to restore sinus rhythm and prevent recurrent atrial fibrillation.[120] Late risk of thromboembolism after mitral replacement for MR is not different from it as in other mitral valve diseases. Differences in thromboembolic risk after valve repair and valve replacement have been variably estimated but

appear to favor valve repair. In addition, anticoagulation is recommended permanently following valve repair only if atrial fibrillation persists; the occurrence of bleeding is less common than it is when following prosthetic replacement.

References

1. Rahimtoola SH. Valvular heart disease. In: Stein J, ed. *Internal Medicine,* 4th ed. St. Louis: Mosby-Year Book;1994:202–234.
2. Kawanishi DT, Rahimtoola SH. Mitral stenosis. In: Rahimtoola SH, ed. *Valvular Heart Disease II.* St. Louis: Mosby;1996:8.1–8.24.
3. Selzer A. Effects of atrial fibrillation upon the circulation in patients with mitral stenosis. *Am Heart J* 1960;59:518–526.
4. Wood P. An appreciation of mitral stenosis: Part 1. Clinical features. *BMJ* 1954;1:1051–1063. An appreciation of mitral stenosis: Part 2. Investigations and results. *BMJ* 1954;1:1113–1124.
5. Gash AK, Carabello BA, Cepin D, Spann JE. Left ventricular ejection performance and systolic muscle function in patients with mitral stenosis. *Circulation* 1983;67:148–154.
6. Gaasch WH, Folland ED. Left ventricular function in rheumatic mitral stenosis. *Eur Heart J* 1991;12(suppl B):66–69.
7. Mohan JC, Khalilullah M, Arora R. Left ventricular intrinsic contractility in pure rheumatic mitral stenosis. *Am J Cardiol* 1989;64:240–242.
8. Bowe JC, Bland EF, Sprague HB, White PD. The course of mitral stenosis without surgery: 10 and 20 year perspective. *Ann Intern Med* 1960;52:741–749.
9. Barrington WW, Bashore T, Wooley CE. Mitral stenosis: Mitral dome excursion at M_1 and the mitral opening snap μ the concept of reciprocal heart sounds. *Am Heart J* 1988;115:1280–1290.
10. Melhem RE, Dunbar JD, Booth RW. The "B" lines of Kerley and left atrial size in mitral valve disease: Their correlation with mean atrial pressure as measured by left atrial puncture. *Radiology* 1991;76:65–69.
11. Khandheria BK, Tajik AJ, Reeder GS, et al. Doppler color flow imaging: A new technique for visualization and characterization of the blood flow jet in mitral stenosis. *Mayo Clin Proc* 1986;61:623–630.
12. Reid CL, Chandraratna PAN, Kawanishi DT, et al. Influence of mitral valve morphology on double-balloon catheter balloon valvuloplasty in patients with mitral stenosis: An analysis of factors predicting immediate and 3-month results. *Circulation* 1989;80:515–524.

13. Rahimtoola SH. Perspective on valvular heart disease: An update. *J Am Coll Cardiol* 1989;14:1–23.

14. Rahimtoola SH, Durairaj A, Mehra A, Nuno I. Current evaluation and management of patients with mitral stenosis. *Circulation* 2002;106: 1183–1188.

15. Kawanishi DT, Kotlewski A, McKay CR, et al. The relative value of clinical examination, echocardiography with Doppler and cardiac catheterization with angiography in the evaluation of mitral valve disease. In: Bodnar E, ed. *Surgery for Heart Valve Disease.* London: ICR Publishers; 1990:73–78.

16. Olesen KH. The natural history of 271 patients with mitral stenosis under medical treatment. *Br Heart J* 1962;24:349–357.

17. Roy SB, Gopinath N. Mitral stenosis. *Circulation* 1968;38(suppl V): 68–76.

18. Rowe JC, Bland EF, Sprague HB, White P. The course of mitral stenosis without surgery: Ten- and twenty-year perspectives. *Ann Intern Med* 1960;52:741–749.

19. Iung B, Garbanz E, Michand P, et al. Late results of percutaneous mitral commissurotomy in a series of 1024 patients: Analysis of late clinical deterioration: Frequency, anatomic findings, and predictive factors. *Circulation* 1999;99:3272–3278.

20. Orrange SE, Kawanishi DT, Lopez BM, et al. Actuarial outcome after catheter balloon commissurotomy in patients with mitral stenosis. *Circulation* 1997;95:382–389.

21. Bonow RO, Carabello B, de Leon AC Jr, et al. ACC/AHA guidelines for the management of patients with valvular heart disease. *J Am Coll Cardiol* 1998;32:1486–1588.

22. Fuster V, Ryden LE, Asinger RW, et al. ACC/AHA guidelines for the management of patients with valvular heart disease. *J Am Coll Cardiol* 2001;38:1231–1265.

23. Hammermeister K, Sethi GK, Henderson WG, et al. Outcomes 15 years after valve replacement with a mechanical vs. bioprosthetic valve: final report of the VA randomized trial. *J Am Coll Cardiol* 2000;36: 1152–1158.

24. Kirklin JW, Barratt-Boyes BG. Mitral valve disease: with or without tricuspid valve disease. In: Rahimtoola SH, ed. *Cardiac Surgery,* 2nd ed. New York, NY: Churchill Livingstone; 1999:425–489.

25. Lam J, Ranganathan N, Wigle E, Silver M. Morphology of the human mitral valve: I. Chordae tendineae: A new classification. *Circulation* 1970;41:449–458.

26. Ranganathan N, Lam J, Wigle E, Silver M. Morphology of the human mitral valve: II. The valve leaflets. *Circulation* 1970;41:459–467.

27. Olson L, Subramanian R, Ackermann D, et al. Surgical pathology of the mitral valve: A study of 712 cases spanning 21 years. *Mayo Clin Proc* 1987;62:22–34.

28. Carpentier AF, Pellerin M, Fuzellier J-F, Relland JYM. Extensive calcification of the mitral annulus: pathology and surgical management. *J Thorac Cardiovasc Surg* 111:718–730, 1996.

29. Davies MJ, Moore BP, Braimbridge MV. The floppy mitral valve: study of incidence, pathology, and complications in surgical, necropsy, and forensic material. *Br Heart J* 1978;40:468–481.

30. Tamura K, Fukuda Y, Ishizaki M, et al. Abnormalities in elastic fibers and other connective-tissue components of floppy mitral valve. *Am Heart J.* 1995;129:1149–1158.

31. Rabkin E, Aikawa M, Stone JR, et al. Activated interstitial myofibroblasts express catabolic enzymes and mediate matrix remodeling in myxomatous heart valves. *Circulation* 2001;104:2525.

32. Avierinos JF, Gersh BJ, Melton LJ, et al. Natural history of asymptomatic mitral valve prolapse in the community. *Circulation* 2002; 106:1355.

33. Barber JE, Kasper FK, Ratliff NB, et al. Mechanical properties of myxomatous mitral valves. *J Thorac Cardiovasc Surg* 2001;122:955–962.

34. Barber JE, Ratliff NB, Cosgrove DM, et al. Myxomatous mitral valve chordae. I: Mechanical properties. *J Heart Valve Dis* 2001;10: 320–324.

35. Gillinov AM, Cosgrove DM, Blackstone EH, et al. Durability of mitral valve repair for degenerative disease. *J Thorac Cardiovasc Surg.* 1998; 116:734–743.

36. David TE, Omran A, Armstrong S, et al. Long-term results of mitral valve repair for myxomatous disease with and without chordal replacement with expanded polytetrafluoroethylene sutures. *J Thorac Cardiovasc Surg.* 1998;115:1279–1286.

37. Flameng W, Herijgers P, Bogaerts K. Recurrence of mitral valve regurgitation after mitral valve repair in degenerative valve disease. *Circulation* 2003;107:1609.

38. Glesby MJ, Pyeritz RE. Association of mitral valve prolapse and systemic abnormalities of connective tissue: a phenotypic continuum. *J Am Med Assoc* 1989;262:523–528.

39. Kwan J, Shiota T, Agler DA, et al. Geometric differences of the mitral apparatus between ischemic and dilated cardiomyopathy with significant mitral regurgitation. Real-time three-dimensional echocardiography study. *Circulation* 2003;107:1135.

40. McQuillan BM, Weyman AE, Kishon Y, et al. Mitral valve operation in postinfarction rupture of a papillary muscle: Immediate results and long-term follow-up of 22 patients. *Mayo Clin Proc* 1992;67:1023–1030.

41. Connolly H, Crary J, McGoon M, et al. Valvular heart disease associated with fenfluramine-phentermine. *N Engl J Med* 1997;337:581–588.

42. Yellin E, Yoran C, Sonnenblick E, et al. Dynamic changes in the canine mitral regurgitant orifice area during ventricular ejection. *Circ Res* 1979;45:677–683.

43. Schwammenthal E, Chen C, Benning F, et al. Dynamics of mitral regurgitant flow and orifice area. Physiologic application of the proximal flow convergence method: Clinical data and experimental testing. *Circulation* 1994;90:307–322.

44. Yiu SF, Enriquez-Sarano M, Tribouilloy C, et al. Determinants of the degree of functional mitral regurgitation in patients with systolic left ventricular dysfunction. *Circulation* 2000;102:1400.

45. Enriquez-Sarano M, Sinak L, Tajik A, et al. Changes in effective regurgitant orifice throughout systole in patients with mitral valve prolapse: A clinical study using the proximal isovelocity surface area method. *Circulation* 1995;92:2951–2958.

46. Scoglamiglio R, Rahimtoola SH, Fasoli G, et al. Nifedipine in asymptomatic patients with severe aortic regurgitation and normal left ventricular function. *N Eng J Med* 1994;331:689–694.

47. Carabello BA, Crawford FA Jr. Valvular heart disease. *N Eng J Med* 1997;337:32–41.

48. Dell'Italia LJ. The renin-angiotensin system in mitral regurgitation: A typical example of tissue activation. *Curr Cardiol Rep* 2002;4(2): 97–105.

49. Gaasch WH, Aurigemma G. Inhibition of the renin-angiotension system and left ventricular adaptation to mitral regurgitation (editorial). *J Am Coll Cardiol* 2002;39:1380–1381.

50. Levine HJ, Gaasch WH. Vasoactive drugs in chronic regurgitant lesions of the mitral and aortic valves. *J Am Coll Cardiol* 1996;28:1083–1091.

51. Imamura T, McDermott PJ, Kent RL, et al. Acute changes in myosin heavy chain synthesis rate in pressure versus volume overload. *Circ Res* 1994;75:418–425.

52. Wisenbaugh T, Spann J, Carabello B. Differences in myocardial performance and load between patients with similar amounts of chronic aortic versus chronic mitral regurgitation. *J Am Coll Cardiol* 1984;3: 916–923.

53. Grose R, Strain J, Cohen M. Pulmonary arterial V waves in mitral regurgitation: Clinical and experimental observations. *Circulation* 1984; 69:214–222.

54. Braunwald E, Awe W. The syndrome of severe mitral regurgitation with normal left atrial pressure. *Circulation* 1963;27:29–35.

55. Lapu-Bula R, Robert A, Van Craeynest D, et al. Contribution of exercise-induced mitral regurgitation to exercise stroke volume and exercise capacity in patients with left ventricular systolic dysfunction. *Circulation* 2002;106:1342.

56. Hochreiter C, Niles N, Devereux RB, et al. Mitral regurgitation: Relationship of noninvasive descriptors of right and left ventricular performance to clinical and hemodynamic findings and to prognosis in medically and surgically treated patients. *Circulation* 1986;73:900–912.

57. Rosen SE, Borer JS, Hochreiter C, et al. Natural history of the asymptomatic/minimally symptomatic patient with severe mitral regurgitation

secondary to mitral valve prolapse and normal right and left ventricular performance. *Am J Cardiol* 1994;74:374–380.

58. Wencker D, Borer JS, Hochreiter C, et al. Preoperative predictors of late postoperative outcome among patients with nonischemic mitral regurgitation with 'high risk' descriptors and comparison with unoperated patients. *Cardiology* 2000;93:37–42.

59. Urschel CW, Covell JW, Graham TP, et al. Effects of acute valvular regurgitation on the oxygen consumption of the canine heart. *Circ Res* 1968;23:33–43.

60. Carabello BA, Nakano K, Corin W, et al. Left ventricular function in experimental volume overload hypertrophy. *Am J Physiol* 1989;256:H974–H81.

61. Zhang J, Tohler C, Erhard M, et al. Relationships between myocardial bioenergetic and left ventricular function in hearts with volume-overload hypertrophy. *Circulation* 1997;96:334–343.

62. Schultz D, Su X, Bishop SP, et al. Angiotensin-converting inhibitor therapy does not reverse the selective upregulation of B creatine kinase gene in volume overload hypertrophy in the dog. *J Mol Cell Cardiol* 1997;29:2665–2673.

63. Conway MA, Bottomley PA, Ouwerkerk R, et al. Mitral regurgitation. Impaired systolic function, eccentric hypertrophy, and increased severity are linked to lower phosphocreatine/ATP ratios in humans. *Circulation* 1998;97:1716–1723.

64. Katayama K, Tajimi T, Guth BD, et al. Early diastolic filling dynamics during experimental mitral regurgitation in the conscious dog. *Circulation* 1988;78:390–400.

65. Zile MR, Tomita M, Nakano K, et al. Effects of left ventricular volume overload produced by mitral regurgitation on diastolic function. *Am J Physiol* 1991;261:H1471–H1480.

66. Corin WJ, Murakami T, Monrad ES, et al. Left ventricular passive chamber properties in chronic mitral regurgitation. *Circulation* 1991;83:797–807.

67. Fielitz J, Hein S, Mitrovic V, et al. Activation of the cardiac renin-angiotensin system and increase myocardial collagen expression in human aortic valve disease. *J Am Coll Cardiol* 2001;37:14443–14449.

68. Goldfine SM, Pena M, Magid NM, et al. Myocardial collagen in cardiac hypertrophy from chronic aortic regurgitation. *Am J Ther* 1998;5(3):139–146.

69. Dell'Italia LJ, Meng QC, Balcells E, et al. Increased angiotensin converting enzyme and chymase-like activity in cardiac tissue of dogs with chronic mitral regurgitation. *Am J Physiol* 1995;269:H2065–H2073.

70. Dell'Italia LJ, Balcells E, Meng QC, et al. Volume overload cardiac hypertrophy is unaffected by ACE inhibitor treatment in the dog *Am J Physiol* 1997;273:H961–H970.

71. Stewart JA, Wei C-C, Brower GL, et al. Cardiac mast cell and chymase mediated matrix metalloproteinase activity and left ventricular remodeling in mitral regurgitation in the dog. *J Mol Cell Cardiol* 2003;35:311–319.

72. Berko B, Gaasch WH, Tangiawa N, et al. Disparity between ejection and end-systolic indexes of left ventricular contractility in mitral regurgitation. *Circulation* 1987;75(6):1310–1319.

73. Wisenbaugh T. Does normal pump function belie muscle dysfunction in patients with chronic severe mitral regurgitation? *Circulation* 1988;77(3):515–525.

74. Bricker ME, Starling MR. Dissociation of end systole from end ejection in patients withlong-term mitral regurgitataion. *Circulation* 1990;81:1277–1286.

75. Starling M, Kirsch M, Montgomery D, Gross M. Impaired left ventricular contractile function in patients with long-term mitral regurgitation and normal ejection fraction. *J Am Coll Cardiol* 1993;22:239–250.

76. Meier DJ, Landolfo CL, Starling MR. The role of echocardiography in the timing of surgical intervention fro chronic aortic and mitral regurgitation. In: Otto CM, ed. *The Practice of Clinical Echocardiography* 2nd ed. Philadelphia: Saunders, 2002.

77. Urabe Y, Mann DL, Kent RL, et al. Cellular and ventricular contractile dysfunction in experimental canine mitral regurgitation. *Circ Res* 1992;70:131–147.

78. Carabello BA, Nolan SP, McGuire LB. Assessment of preoperative left ventricular function in patients with mitral regurgitation: Value of the end-systolic wall stress-end-systolic volume ratio. *Circulation* 1981;64:1212–1217.

79. Carabello BA, Spann JF. The uses and limitations of end-systolic indices of left ventricular function. *Circulation* 1984;69:1058–1064.

80. Mehta RH, Supiano MA, Oral H, et al. Relation of systemic sympathetic nervous system activation to echocardiographic left ventricular size and performance and its implication in patients with mitral regurgitation. *Am J Cardiol* 2000;86:1193–1197.

81. Sakagoshi N, Nakano S, Taniguchi K, et al. Relation between myocardial beta-adrenergic receptor and left ventricular function in patients with left ventricular volume overload due to chronic mitral regurgitation with and without aortic regurgitation. *Am J Cardiol* 1991;68:81–84.

82. Nagatsu M, Zile MR, Tsutsui H, et al. Native β-adrenergic support for left ventricular dysfunction in experimental mitral regurgitation normalizes indexes of pump and contractile function. *Circulation* 1994;89:818–826.

83. Mann DL, Kent RL, Parsons B, Cooper G. Adrenergic effects on the biology of the adult mammalian cardiocyte. *Circulation* 1992;85:790–804.

84. Tallaj J, Wei CC, Hankes GH, et al. β_1-adrenergic receptor blockade attenuates angiotensin II-mediated catecholamine release into the cardiac interstitium in mitral regurgitation. *Circulation* 2003;108:225–230.

85. Tsutsui H, Spinale FG, Nagatsu M, et al. Effects of chronic β-adrenergic blockade on the left ventricular and cardiocyte abnormalities of chronic canine mitral regurgitation. *J Clin Invest* 1994;93:2639–2648.

86. Mann DL. Inflammatory mediators and the failing heart: past, present, and the foreseeable future. *Circ Res* 2002;91(11):988–998.

87. Kapadia SR, Yakoob K, Nader S, et al. Elevated circulating levels of serum tumor necrosis factor-α in patients with hemodynamically significant pressure and volume overload. *J Am Coll Cardiol* 2000;36:208–212.

88. Oral H, Sivasubramanain N, Dyke DB, et al. Myocardial proinflammatory cytokine expression and left ventricular remodeling in patients with chronic mitral regurgitation. *Circulation* 2003;107:831–837.

89. Ling H, Enriquez-Sarano M, Seward J, et al. Clinical outcome of mitral regurgitation due to flail leaflets. *N Engl J Med* 1996;335:1417–1423.

90. Grigioni F, Enriquez-Sarano M, Ling L, et al. Sudden death in mitral regurgitation due to flail leaflet. *J Am Coll Cardiol* 1999;34:2078–2085.

91. Folland E, Kriegel B, Henderson W, et al. Implications of third heart sounds in patients with valvular heart disease: The Veterans Affairs Cooperative Study on Valvular Heart Disease. *N Engl J Med* 1992;327:458–462.

92. Desjardins V, Enriquez-Sarano M, Tajik A, et al. Intensity of murmurs correlates with severity of valvular regurgitation. *Am J Med* 1996;100:149–156.

93. Enriquez-Sarano M, Tajik A, Schaff H, et al. Echocardiographic prediction of survival after surgical correction of organic mitral regurgitation. *Circulation* 1994;90:830–837.

94. Enriquez-Sarano M, Freeman W, Tribouilloy C, et al. Functional anatomy of mitral regurgitation: Echocardiographic assessment and implications on outcome. *J Am Coll Cardiol* 1999;34:1129–1136.

95. Otto CM. Valvular regurgitation: Diagnosis, quantitation and clinical approach. In: Otto CM, ed. *Textbook of Clinical Echocardiography,* 2nd ed. Philadelphia: Saunders; 2000:265–300.

96. Bonow RO, Carabello BA, deLeon AC, et al. ACC/AHA guidelines for the management of patients with valvular heart disease: a report of the American College of Cardiology/American Heart Association task force on practice guidelines (committee on the management of patients with valvular heart disease). *J Am Coll Cardiol* 1998;32:1486–1488.

97. Leung DY, Griffin BP, Stewart WJ, et al. Left ventricular function after valve repair for mitral regurgitation: Predictive value of preoperative assessment of contractile reserve by exercise echocardiography. *J Am Coll Cardiol* 1996;28:1198–1205.

98. Enriquez-Sarano M, Klodas E, Garratt KN, et al. Secular trends in coronary atherosclerosis μ analysis in patients with valvular regurgitation. *N Engl J Med* 1996;335:316–322.

99. Duren DR, Becker AE, Sunning AJ. Long-term follow-up of idiopathic mitral valve prolapse in 300 patients: a prospective study. *J Am Coll Cardiol* 1988;11:42–47.

100. Rappaport E. Natural history of aortic and mitral valve disease. *Am J Cardiol* 1975;35:221–227.

101. Horstkotte D, Loogen F, Kleikamp G, et al. Effect of prosthetic heart valve replacement on the natural course of isolated mitral and aortic as well as multivalvular diseases: Clinical results in 783 patients up to 8 years following implantation of the Björk-Shiley tilting disc prosthesis. *Z Kardiol* 1983;72:494–503.

102. Grigioni F, Enriquez-Sarano M, Ling L, et al. Sudden death in mitral regurgitation due to flail leaflet. *J Am Coll Cardiol* 1999;34:2078–2085.

103. Rosen S, Borer J, Hochreiter C, et al. Natural history of the asymptomatic/minimally symptomatic patient with severe mitral regurgitation secondary to mitral valve prolapse and normal right and left ventricular performance. *Am J Cardiol* 1994;74:374–380.

104. Tishler M, Rowan M, LeWinter M. Effect of Enalapril on left ventricular mass and volumes in asymptomatic chronic, severe mitral regurgitation secondary to mitral valve prolapse. *Am J Cardiol* 1998;82: 242–245.

105. Marcotte F, Honos G, Walling A, et al. Effect of angiotensin converting enzyme inhibitor therapy in mitral regurgitation with normal left ventricular function. *Can J Cardiol* 1997;13:479–485.

106. Host U, Kelbaek H, Hildebrandt P, et al. Effect of Ramilpril on mitral regurgitation secondary to mitral valve prolapse. *Am J Cardiol* 1997; 80:655–658.

107. Rothlisberger C, Sareli P, Wisenbaugh T. Comparison of single dose nifedipine and captopril for chronic severe mitral regurgitation. *Am J Cardiol* 1994;73:978–981.

108. Wisenbaugh T, Sinovich V, Dullbh A, Sareli P. Six month pilot study of captopril for mildly symptomatic, severe isolated mitral and isolated aortic regurgitation. *J Heart Valve Dis* 1994;3:197–204.

109. Perry GJ, Wei CC, Su X, et al. Afterload reduction and blockade of the tissue renin angiotensin system does not improve left ventricular and cardiomyocyte remodeling in chronic mitral regurgitation. *J Am Coll Cardiol* 2002;39:1374–1379.

110. Nemoto S, Hamawaki M, DeFreitas G, Carabello BA. Differential effects of the angiotensin-converting enzyme inhibitor lisinopril versus the beta-adrenergic receptor blocker atenolol on hemodynamics and left ventricular contractile function in experimental mitral regurgitation. *J Am Coll Cardiol* 2002;40:149–154.

111. Dell'Italia LJ, Balcells E, Meng QC, et al. Volume-overload cardiac hypertrophy is unaffected by ACE inhibitor treatment in dogs. *Am J Physiol* 1997;273:(*Heart Circ Physiol* 42)H961–H970.

112. Enriquez-Sarano M, Tajik A, Schaff H, et al. Echocardiographic prediction of survival after surgical correction of organic mitral regurgitation. *Circulation* 1994;90:830–837.

113. Enriquez-Sarano M, Tajik A, Schaff H, et al. Echocardiographic prediction of left ventricular function after correction of mitral regurgitation: Results and clinical implications. *J Am Coll Cardiol* 1994;24: 1536–1543.

114. Crawford M, Souchek J, Oprian C, et al. Determinants of survival and left ventricular performance after mitral valve replacement. *Circulation* 1990;81:1173–1181.

115. Otto C. Timing of surgery in mitral regurgitation *Heart* 2003;89: 100–105.

116. Rozich JD, Carabello BA, Usher BW, et al. Mitral valve replacement with and without chordal preservation in patients with chronic mitral regurgitation. Mechanisms for differences in postoperative ejection performance. *Circulation* 1992;86:1718–1726.

117. Leung DY, Griffin BP, Stewart WJ, et al. Left ventricular function after valve repair for chronic mitral regurgitation: predictive value of preoperative assessment of contractile reserve by exercise echocardiography. *J Am Coll Cardiol* 1996;28:1198–1205.

118. Enriquez Sarano M, Schaff HV, Orszulak TA, et al. Valve repair improves the outcome of surgery for mitral regurgitation. A multivariate analysis. *Circulation* 1995;91:1022–1028.

119. Otto CM. Surgical intervention for mitral regurgitation. In: Otto CM, ed. *Valvular heart disease*. Philadelphia: Saunders, 1999.

120. Handa N, Schaff HV, Morris JJ, et al. Outcome of valve repair and the cox maze procedure for mitral regurgitation and associated atrial fibrillation. *J Thorac Cardiovasc Surg* 1999;118:628–635.

MITRAL VALVE PROLAPSE SYNDROME

Robert A. O'Rourke / Steven R. Bailey

The syndrome of mitral valve prolapse (MVP) is the most common form of valvular heart disease, occurring in 0.6 to 2.4 percent of the population, thus being more common than a bicuspid aortic valve. The incidence of MVP and risk of complications range greatly depending on the criteria used for its diagnosis[1,2] as well as the patient population studied diagnosis.[3,4] These may differ importantly in a referral population as compared with community patients.[3,4] It does not appear to differ by ethnicity. Studies of native American Indian tribes have shown the same prevalence as other general populations when screened using contemporary criteria.[5] MVP is genetically heterogenous and is inherited as an autosomal dominant trait that exhibits both sex- and age-dependent penetrance.[5a] The discovery of genes involved in the pathogenesis of this common disorder is critical to understanding its diversity in presentation.[5a,5b] Clinically, patients with MVP exhibit fibromyxomatous changes in one or both of the mitral leaflets that result in superior displacement of the leaflets into the left atrium (LA). MVP is typically a diagnosis commonly detected by cardiac auscultation with one or more systolic clicks and/or a mid-to-late systolic murmur detected on a careful physical examination. Often the auscultatory complex is the only clinical manifestation of cardiac disease, and many patients are asymptomatic. MVP is likely overdiagnosed in many patients by examiners who misidentify the auscultatory findings and/or overread the two-dimensional echocardiograms.

Midsystolic clicks were first described in the late nineteenth century and originally were attributed to a pericardial or extracardiac etiology. Subsequently, late-systolic murmurs were recognized in apparently healthy people to be associated with a benign natural history. Thus, the murmur also was considered to be extracardiac in origin.

In 1961, Reid[6] suggested that the midsystolic click and the late-systolic murmur were due to mitral regurgitation. In 1963, Barlow et al.[7] confirmed this hypothesis by left ventricular (LV) cineangiography. Subsequently, intracardiac phonocardiogram studies documented the mitral valve origin of a systolic click and late-systolic murmur.

During the past 40 years, considerable new data obtained from pathologic studies, echocardiography, and cineventriculography have demonstrated that this common syndrome is associated with prolapse of one or both mitral valve leaflets into the atrium during LV systole.

Recognition of MVP (also known as the *systolic click–late systolic murmur syndrome*) is often difficult because of the extreme variability of its clinical manifestations and the diminishing auscultatory skills of physicians who often default the physical exam in lieu of noninvasive diagnostic testing. It is, however, an important cause of incapacitating chest pain and refractory arrhythmias in certain patients. The abnormal components of the mitral valve apparatus are a potential site for endocarditis, and some patients, particularly males in their 60s and 70s, can develop severe mitral regurgitation (MR) due to ruptured chordae tendineae.

DEFINITION, ETIOLOGY, AND TIMING

MVP refers to the systolic billowing of one or both mitral leaflets into the LA, with or without MR. MVP often occurs as a clinical entity with no or only mild MR, and it is frequently associated with unique clinical characteristics when compared with the other causes of MR.[8–12] Importantly, MVP is the most common cause of significant MR and the most frequent substrate for mitral valve endocarditis in the United States.[1] The mitral valve apparatus is a complex structure composed of the mitral annulus, valve leaflets, chordae tendineae, papillary muscles, and the supporting LV, left atrium, and aortic walls[13] (Fig. 68-1). Disease processes involving any one or more of these components may result in dysfunction of the valvular apparatus and prolapse of the mitral leaflets toward the LA during systole when LV pressure exceeds LA pressure.

The complexity of the mitral valve apparatus explains the presence of secondary prolapse in many conditions that affect one or more components of the apparatus (e.g., ruptured mitral chordae). There is, however, considerable evidence that a disorder of the mitral valve leaflets exists in which there are specific pathologic changes causing redundancy of the mitral leaflets and their prolapse into the LA during systole. This is the primary form of MVP (Table 68-1).

In *primary* MVP, there is interchordal hooding due to leaflet redundancy that involves both the rough and clear zones of the involved leaflets[9] (Fig. 68-2). The height of the interchordal hooding usually exceeds 4 mm and involves at least one-half of the anterior leaflet or at least two-thirds of the posterior leaflet. The basic anatomic feature seen by microscopy in primary MVP is the marked proliferation of the *spongiosa*, the delicate myxomatous connective tissue between

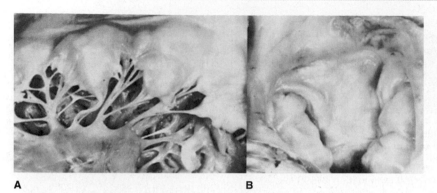

FIGURE 68-1 Myxomatous mitral valve. *A.* The opened mitral valve shows characteristic interchordal hooding and redundancy of the leaflets. *B.* The unopened mitral valve viewed from the LA side shows extensive scalloping that is characteristic of a myxomatous mitral valve. (From Guthrie and Edwards.[16] Reproduced with permission from the publisher and authors.)

TABLE 68-1 Classification of Mitral Valve Prolapse

Primary mitral valve prolapse
    Familial
    Nonfamilial
    Marfan syndrome
    Other connective tissue diseases
Mitral valve prolapse without myxomatous proliferation
    Coronary artery disease
    Rheumatic heart disease
    Cardiomyopathies
    "Flail" mitral valve leaflets
Normal variant labeled as MVP
    Inaccurate auscultation
    "Echocardiographic heart disease"

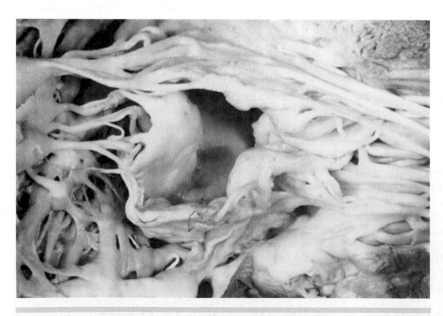

FIGURE 68-2 Myxomatous mitral valve with ruptured posterior leaflet chordae. The central part of the posterior leaflet (*lower center*) shows fragments of ruptured chordae. The intact chordae are elongated, and the leaflets show redundancy and fibrous thickening. (From Edwards F. Pathology of mitral incompetence. In: Silver MD, ed. *Cardiovascular Pathology.* New York: Churchill Livingstone; 1983. Reproduced with permission from the publisher and authors.)

the *atrialis* (a thick layer of collagen and elastic tissue forming the atrial aspect of the leaflet) and the *fibrosa,* or *ventricularis,* which is composed of dense layers of collagen and forms the basic support of the leaflet.[9] In primary MVP, myxomatous proliferation of the acid mucopolysaccharide-containing spongiosa tissue causes focal interruption of the fibrosa. Secondary effects of the primary MVP syndrome include fibrosis of the surfaces of the mitral valve leaflets, thinning and/or elongation of chordae tendineae, and ventricular friction lesions. Fibrin deposits often form at the mitral valve–LA angle.

The primary form of MVP may be familial, where it appears to be inherited as an autosomal dominant trait with varying penetrance.[5a,14,15] No *consistent* chromosomal abnormalities have yet been identified in patients with primary MVP, which also often occurs in isolated cases.[16,17] Primary MVP occurs with increasing frequency in patients with Marfan's syndrome, where it is usually present, and in other inherited connective tissue diseases such as Ehlers-Danlos syndrome,[18] pseudoxanthoma elasticum,[19] and osteogenesis imperfecta.[20] Polycystic kidney disease has been associated with a 25 percent prevalence of MVP. Marfan's syndrome is a heritable disorder of connective tissue caused by a defect in fibrillin protein encoded by the fibrillin gene on chromosome 15 at 15-q20 (see Chap. 84). Since fibrillin is diffuse, Marfan's syndrome affects skeletal,[21] ocular, cardiovascular, skin, pulmonary, and central nervous systems (see Chaps. 72 and 84). Many observers have speculated that primary MVP syndrome represents a generalized disorder of connective tissue. Thoracic skeletal abnormalities such as straight thoracic spine and pectus excavatum are commonly associated with this syndrome.[22] The mitral valve undergoes differentiation between the thirty-fifth and forty-second days of fetal life, when the vertebrae and thoracic cage are beginning chondrification and ossification.[23] Any adverse factors in this period may affect both the mitral valve and the bones of the thoracic cage. It has been postulated that the MVP syndrome is a connective tissue disorder resulting from fetal exposure to toxic substances during the early part of pregnancy.[24,25]

Others have suggested that MVP is a result of defective embryogenesis of cell lines of mesenchymal origin. The increased prevalence of primary MVP in patients with von Willebrand disease and other coagulopathies, primary hypomastia, and various connective tissue diseases has been used to support this concept.[26]

In other instances of echocardiographic excessive systolic prolapse of one or both mitral leaflets into the LA, myxomatous proliferation of the spongiosa portion of the mitral valve leaflet is absent (Table 68-1). Tei et al.[26] were able to produce de novo echocardiographic evidence of MVP, often with MR, in closed-chest dogs undergoing transient coronary artery occlusion; MVP was attributed to relative displacement of ischemic papillary muscles. Also, serial studies in patients with known ischemic heart disease occasionally have documented unequivocal MVP following an acute coronary syndrome that was documented to be absent prior to the ACS.[27] In most patients with coronary artery disease (CAD) and MVP, however, the two entities are coincident but unrelated.

Other studies[28–30] indicate that MR caused by MVP may result from postinflammatory changes, including those following rheumatic fever. In histologic studies of surgically excised valves, fibrosis with vascularization and scattered infiltration of round cells, including lymphocytes and plasmacytes, was found *without myxomatous proliferation* of the spongiosa.[28] With rheumatic carditis, the anterior mitral leaflet is more likely to prolapse.[29]

MVP has been observed in patients with hypertrophic cardiomyopathy, in whom posterior MVP may result from a disproportionately small LV cavity, altered papillary muscle alignment, or a combination of factors.[25] The mitral valve leaflet is usually normal, but occasionally, the pathologic changes of primary MVP are present. Since LV segmental wall motion abnormalities and sometimes depressed global LV function occur in certain patients with echocardiographic and auscultatory evidence of MVP and MR, nonhypertrophic cardiomyopathy has been listed as a cause of mitral prolapse.[30] This is probably not the case; the ventricular wall motion abnormalities usually disappear when the mitral valve is repaired or replaced. In MVP patients, atrial septal defects, pulmonary hypertension, anorexia nervosa, dehydration, or straight-back syndrome may be secondary to the relatively small size of the LV in this disorder, resulting in a mitral apparatus that is relatively large and redundant.[28,31] However, atrial septal defect may be associated with primary MVP.[20] Atrial septal aneurysms were considered more likely to occur in MVP patients. A review of patients from the Framingham Study did not demonstrate an increase in the prevalence of atrial septal aneurysms.[32] Patients with primary and secondary MVP must be distinguished from those with normal variations on cardiac auscultation or echocardiography. Other auscultatory findings may be misinterpreted as midsystolic clicks or late-systolic murmurs.[11,25] Patients with mild to moderate billowing of one or more nonthickened leaflets toward the LA with the leaflet coaptation point on the ventricular side of the mitral annulus and no or minimal MR by Doppler echocardiography are probably normal. Unfortunately, many such patients with neither a nonejection click nor murmur of MR are frequently overdiagnosed as having the MVP syndrome.[1,2,33]

PATHOPHYSIOLOGY

In patients with MVP, there is frequently LA and LV enlargement, depending on the presence and severity of MR.[34] The supporting apparatus is often involved, and in patients with connective tissue syndromes such as Marfan's syndrome, the mitral annulus is usually dilated, sometimes calcified, and does not decrease its circumference by the usual 30 percent during LV systole. The hemodynamic effects of mild to moderate MR are similar to those from other causes of MR.

Many studies suggest an increased prevalence of autonomic nervous system dysfunction in patients with primary MVP. In 1979, Gaffney et al.[35] reported reduced heart rate slowing with intravenous phenylephrine and an abnormal diving reflex heart rate response in patients with MVP as compared with age-matched controls. Patients with MVP had a lesser lower extremity pooling of blood in response to lower body negative pressure. Increased vagal tone and prolonged QT intervals on the electrocardiogram (ECG) are more common in patients with MVP. Measurements of serum and 24-h urine epinephrine and norepinephrine levels are often increased in patients with symptomatic MVP as compared with controls.[36] Patients with MVP often have an increased heart rate and contractility response to intravenous isoproterenol.[35] An increased incidence of high-affinity beta receptors in the lymphocytes of patients with MVP has been reported, as well as greater than usual increases in cyclic adenosine

monophosphate with isoproterenol stimulation as compared with normal individuals.[37] Patients with MVP often have postural phenomena such as orthostatic tachycardia and hypotension. Low intravascular volume and/or an abnormality in the renin-aldosterone axis may contribute to the orthostatic changes.[11,38]

ASSOCIATED CONDITIONS

Tricuspid valve prolapse, with similar interchordal hooding and histologic evidence of mucopolysaccharide proliferation and collagen dissolution, occurs in about 40 percent of patients with MVP.[9] Pulmonic valve prolapse occurs in approximately 10 percent and aortic valve prolapse in 2 percent of patients with MVP.[9] The frequent findings of thoracic skeletal abnormalities in patients with MVP were noted earlier. There is an increased incidence of secundum atrial septal defect in patients with MVP (but not of atrial septal aneurysms) and an increased incidence of MVP in patients with atrial septal defects; thus this phenomenon cannot be explained by a chance occurrence and does not represent only stretching of a patent fossa ovalis. An increased incidence of left-sided atrioventricular bypass tracts and supraventricular tachycardias also occurs in patients with MVP.[9,39]

CLINICAL MANIFESTATIONS

Symptoms

The diagnosis of MVP is most commonly made by cardiac auscultation in asymptomatic patients or by echocardiography performed for some other purpose. The patient may be evaluated because of a family history of cardiac disease or occasionally may be referred because of an abnormal resting ECG. Some patients consult their physicians because of one or more of the common symptoms that occur in patients with this syndrome. The most common presenting complaint is *palpitation*. The source of palpitation is usually ventricular premature beats, but various supraventricular arrhythmias are also frequent, and the most common sustained tachycardia is paroxysmal reentry supraventricular tachycardia (see Chap. 28). Ventricular tachycardia occurs in some patients; others have symptomatic bradyarrhythmias. Palpitation is often reported by patients at a time when continuous ambulatory ECG recordings show no arrhythmias.

Chest pain is a frequent complaint of patients with MVP. In most patients without coexisting ischemic heart disease, it is atypical (occurring at rest or exercise and is sharp, nonradiating, and prolonged in duration) and rarely resembles classic angina pectoris. In some patients it is recurrent and can be incapacitating. The etiology of the chest pain is unknown; rarely, it may represent true myocardial ischemia produced by abnormal tension on the papillary muscles and supporting ventricular wall by the prolapsing mitral leaflets.[40] Coronary artery spasm has been reported in patients with MVP, but it is unlikely to be the cause of most episodes of atypical chest pain as there rarely is ST elevation.[41]

Dyspnea and *fatigue* are frequent symptoms in patients with MVP, including many without severe MR. Objective exercise testing often fails to show impaired exercise tolerance, and some patients exhibit distinct episodes of hyperventilation. Neuropsychiatric complaints occur in certain patients with MVP. Some have panic attacks (see Chap. 91), and others have frank manic-depressive syndromes. Transient cerebral ischemic episodes occur with increased incidence in patients with MVP, and some develop stroke syndromes.[42–46] One

TABLE 68-2 Response of the Murmur of Mitral Valve Prolapse to Interventions

Intervention	Timing	Intensity
Standing upright	←	↑
Recumbent	→	↓ or 0
Squatting	→	↓ or 0
Hand-grip	←	±
Valsalva	←	±
Amyl nitrite	±	↑

NOTE: ↑ = increase; ↓ = decrease; 0 = no change; ± = variable; ← = earlier; → = later.

study showed no association between MVP and stroke.[47] Amaurosis fugax, homonymous field loss, and retinal artery occlusion have been reported; occasionally, the visual loss persists.[48] These signs likely are due to embolization of platelets and fibrin deposits that occur on the atrial side of the mitral valve leaflets.[49] *It is important to note that both MVP and panic attacks occur relatively frequently. Accordingly, the occurrence of the two syndromes in the same individual would be expected to occur frequently by chance, rather than panic attacks necessarily being part of the primary MVP syndrome.*

Physical Examination

The presence of thoracic skeletal abnormalities may suggest the diagnosis of MVP, the most common being scoliosis, pectus excavatum, straightened thoracic spine, and narrowed anteroposterior diameter of the chest.[19] Some patients with MVP may show signs, such as arachnodactyly, more typical of Marfan's syndrome.

The principal cardiac auscultatory feature of this syndrome is the midsystolic click, a high-pitched sound of short duration (see Chap. 12). The click may vary considerably in intensity and location in systole according to LV loading conditions and contractility. It results from the sudden tensing of the mitral valve apparatus as the leaflets prolapse into the LA during systole. Multiple systolic clicks may be generated by different portions of the mitral leaflets prolapsing at varying times during systole.[50] The major differentiating feature of the midsystolic click of MVP from that due to other causes (e.g., ventricular septal aneurysms, atrial myxomas, or pericarditis) is that its timing during systole may be altered by maneuvers that change hemodynamic conditions (Table 68-2).

The midsystolic click is frequently followed by a late-systolic murmur, usually medium- to high-pitched and most audible at the apex. Occasionally, the murmur has a musical or honking quality. The character and intensity of the murmur also vary with loading conditions, from brief and almost inaudible to holosystolic and loud (Fig. 68-3).

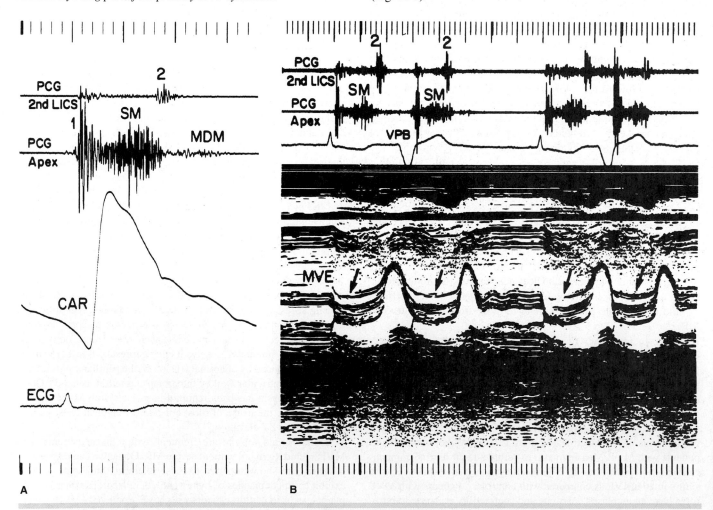

FIGURE 68-3 Phonocardiogram and echocardiogram in mitral valve prolapse. *A.* The phonocardiogram shows a high-frequency holosystolic murmur (HSM) with late-systolic accentuation. A low-frequency middiastolic murmur (MDM) is present at the apex. *B.* The echocardiogram demonstrates a hammock-shaped systolic motion of the valve leaflets. The rhythm is atrial fibrillation with bigeminy. 1, first heart sound; 2, second heart sound; MVE, mitral valve echogram. (Courtesy of Dr. Ernest Craige.)

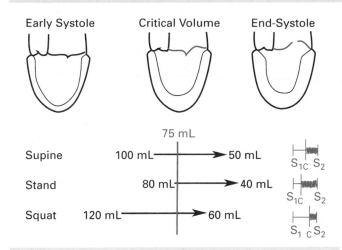

FIGURE 68-4 The effect of LV volume on the timing of MVP and the accompanying murmur. In the upper panel, three phases of LV systole are illustrated. In early systole, there is coaptation of the leaflets and no prolapse; when a critical ventricle volume of 75 mL is reached, valve prolapse commences and progresses until the end of systole. In the lower panel, three body positions are indicated; the corresponding change in volume and timing of the click-murmur are shown. The critical volume for prolapse remains constant. When the critical volume occurs earlier, the onset of the click-murmur is earlier. When the critical volume occurs later, the onset of the click-murmur is later. (From Crawford MH, O'Rourke RA. In: Isselbacher KJ et al., eds. *Harrison's Principles of Internal Medicine*, 9th ed. New York: McGraw-Hill; 1980:91–105. Reproduced with permission from the publisher, editors, and authors.)

which cause the click and murmur to move toward S_2 include squatting from the upright position and maneuvers that slow the heart rate.

Electrocardiogram

The ECG typically is normal in patients with MVP. The most common abnormality noted is the presence of ST-T-wave depression or T-wave inversion in the inferior leads (III, aV_F)[49] (Fig. 68-5). These changes may reflect ischemia of the inferior wall due to traction on the posteromedial papillary muscle by the prolapsing mitral leaflets. Sometimes ST-T-wave changes are present only during interventions that induce prolapse earlier in systole. More unusual ECG changes include prominent U waves, peaked T waves in the midprecordial leads, and QT prolongation.

MVP is associated with an increased incidence of false-positive exercise ECG results especially in females. Myocardial perfusion imaging with thallium or technetium sestamibi has been useful for differentiating false from true abnormal exercise ECG findings in patients with MVP (see Chap. 19).

Although arrhythmias may be observed on the resting ECG or during treadmill or bicycle exercise, they are detected more reliably by continuous ambulatory ECG recordings (see Chap. 33). The reported incidence of documented arrhythmias is higher in patients with MVP, ranging from 40 to 75 percent.[50] Most arrhythmias detected, however, are not life-threatening. Patients with ST-T-wave changes in the inferior ECG leads have a higher incidence of serious ventricular arrhythmias on ambulatory recordings.[24]

Dynamic auscultation is often useful for establishing the clinical diagnosis of the MVP syndrome (see Chap. 12).[25] Changes in the LV end-diastolic volume lead to changes in the timing of the midsystolic click and murmur. When end-diastolic volume is decreased, the critical LV volume is achieved earlier in systole, and the click-murmur complex occurs shortly after the first heart sound (Fig. 68-4). In general, any maneuver that decreases the end-diastolic LV volume, increases the rate of ventricular contraction, or decreases the resistance to LV ejection of blood causes prolapse to occur earlier in systole, the systolic click and murmur moving toward the first heart sound (see Table 68-2). By contrast, any maneuver that augments the LV systolic volume, reduces myocardial contractility, or increases LV afterload lengthens the time from the onset of systole to the initiation of MVP; the systolic click and/or murmur moving toward S_2. Maneuvers causing the click and/or murmur to occur earlier in systole include standing from the supine position, submaximal isometric handgrip exercise, the Valsalva maneuver, and amyl nitrite inhalation. Those

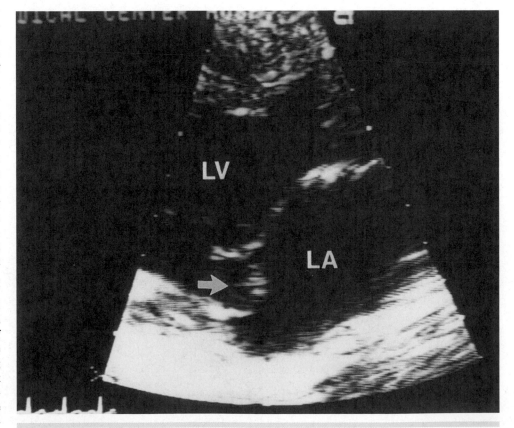

FIGURE 68-5 A parasternal two-dimensional echocardiographic view showing prolapse of a redundant posterior mitral leaflet toward the left atrium during systole. LV, left ventricle; LA, left atrium.

Echocardiography

Echocardiography (see Chap. 15) is the most useful noninvasive test for defining MVP. The M-mode echocardiographic definition of MVP includes 2 mm or more of posterior displacement of one or both leaflets or holosystolic posterior "hammocking" of more than 3 mm (see Fig. 68-3). On two-dimensional echocardiography, systolic displacement of one or both mitral leaflets, particularly when they coapt on the LA side of the annular plane, in the parasternal long-axis view indicates a high likelihood of MVP[51,52] (see Fig. 68-5). Disagreement persists concerning the reliability of an echocardiographic diagnosis of MVP when observed only in the apical four-chamber view. The diagnosis of MVP is even more certain when the leaflet thickness is greater than 5 mm during ventricular diastole. Leaflet redundancy is often associated with an enlarged mitral annulus and elongated chordae tendineae. On Doppler velocity recordings, the presence or absence of MR is an important consideration. MVP is more likely when the MR is detected as a high-velocity jet midway or more posterior in the LA.[33]

At present, there is no consensus on the two-dimensional echocardiographic criteria for MVP. Since echocardiography is a tomographic cross-sectional technique, no single view can be considered diagnostic. The parasternal long-axis view permits visualization of the medial aspect of the anterior mitral leaflet and middle scallop of the posterior leaflet. If the findings of prolapse are localized to the lateral scallop in the posterior leaflet, they would be best visualized by the apical four-chamber view.[51,52] All available echocardiographic views should be used, with the provision that anterior leaflet billowing alone in the four-chamber apical view is not diagnostic of prolapse; however, a displacement of the posterior leaflet or the coaptation point in any view including the apical views suggests the diagnosis of prolapse. The echocardiographic criteria for MVP should include structural changes such as leaflet thickening, redundancy, annular dilatation, and chordal elongation.

Patients with echocardiographic criteria for MVP but without evidence of thickened or redundant leaflets or definite MR are more difficult to classify. If such patients have auscultatory findings typical of MVP, the echocardiogram confirms the diagnosis. In contrast, a patient with typical auscultatory findings but a negative echocardiogram likely also has MVP; in the past, as many as 10 percent of patients with MVP have had a nondiagnostic echocardiographic study. Currently, this percentage is less because of more accurate studies. In clinical practice, a false diagnosis of MVP occurs too frequently. The use of echocardiography as a screening test for MVP in patients with and without symptoms who have no systolic click or murmur on serial, carefully performed auscultatory examinations *is not recommended*. The likelihood of finding MVP in such patients is extremely low. Most patients with or without symptoms who have negative dynamic cardiac auscultation and "mild mitral valve prolapse" by echocardiography should not be diagnosed as having MVP. Recommendations for echocardiography in MVP are listed in Table 68-3.[53]

Echocardiography is useful for defining LA and LV size and function and the extent of mitral leaflet redundancy, as well as for detecting associated lesions such as secundum atrial septal defect. Doppler echocardiography is helpful for the detection and *semiquantitation* of MR as well. Serial echocardiograms are often useful for following patients with murmurs, since quantitation of MR by examination alone is more difficult. In a carefully performed study comparing auscultatory findings with echocardiographic results in patients with clinical evidence of MVP, the amount of billowing of one or both mitral leaflets into the LA, the level of the leaflets' coaptation point, and the presence or absence of moderate or severe MR were each important considerations in deciding on the likelihood of MVP.[31]

Chest Roentgenogram

Posteroanterior and lateral chest x-ray films usually show normal cardiopulmonary findings. The skeletal abnormalities described earlier can be seen.[23] When severe MR is present, both LA and LV enlargement often result. Various degrees of pulmonary venous congestion are evident when failure of the left side of the heart results. Acute chordal rupture with a sudden increase in the amount of MR may present as pulmonary edema without obvious LV or LA dilatation. Calcification of the mitral annulus may be seen, particularly in adults with Marfan's syndrome (see Chap. 14).

TABLE 68-3 Recommendations for Echocardiography in Mitral Valve Prolapse

Indication	Class
1. Diagnosis, assessment of hemodynamic severity of mitral regurgitation (MR), leaflet morphology, ventricular compensation in patients with physical signs of mitral valve prolapse (MVP).	I
2. To exclude MVP in patients who have been given the diagnosis where there is no clinical evidence to support the diagnosis.	I
3. To exclude MVP in patients with first-degree relatives with known myxomatous valve disease.	IIa
4. Risk stratification in patients with physical signs of MVP with no or mild regurgitation.	IIa
5. To exclude MVP in patients in the absence of physical findings suggestive of MVP and a positive family history.	III
6. Routine repetition of echocardiography in patients with MVP with no MR and no changes in clinical signs or symptoms.	III

Class I: Conditions for which there is evidence and/or general agreement that a given procedure or treatment is useful and effective.

Class II: Conditions for which there is conflicting evidence and/or a divergence of opinion about the usefulness/efficacy of a procedure or treatment.

    Class IIa: Weight of evidence/opinion is in favor of usefulness/efficacy.

    Class IIb: Usefulness efficacy is less well established by evidence/opinion.

Class III: Conditions for which there is evidence and/or general agreement that the procedure/treatment is not useful/effective and in some cases may be harmful.

SOURCE: From ACC/AHA clinical practice guidelines for valvular heart disease. *J Am Coll Cardiol* 1998; 32:1486–1588.

Myocardial Perfusion Scintigraphy

Exercise myocardial perfusion imaging with thallium or technetium sestamibi has been recommended as an adjunct to exercise ECG for determining the presence or absence of coexistent myocardial ischemia in patients with MVP.[56] Most MVP patients *with clinical evidence of CAD* have an abnormal exercise scintigram. In comparison, a negative scintigram in these patients does not exclude ischemia as the basis for the chest pain, or does it completely exclude CAD as the etiology (see Chap. 19).

Cardiac Catheterization

Cardiac catheterization is rarely used as a diagnostic technique for MVP. Also, contrast ventriculography is unnecessary for determining LV function because it usually can be quantitated by two-dimensional echocardiogram or radionuclide ventriculography. While contrast cineventriculography is often useful for assessing the severity of MR, cardiac catheterization and angiography are used more commonly in patients with MVP to exclude CAD. Intracardiac pressures and cardiac output are usually normal in uncomplicated MVP; however, these measurements become progressively more abnormal as MR becomes more severe.

LV cineangiography usually confirms the presence of MVP.[8,11] The right anterior oblique projection is best for observing prolapse of the three scallops of the posterior leaflet. Prolapse is defined as the bowing of the leaflets beyond a line drawn from the anterior aortic prominence to the base of the heart where the posteromedial papillary muscle attaches in the right anterior oblique view. The left anterior oblique view is necessary for the adequate evaluation of prolapse of the anterior leaflet.

LV wall motion is usually normal in patients with primary MVP, but some patients show abnormal contraction patterns in the absence of CAD.[8,31] These contraction abnormalities usually represent indentation of the LV at the point of attachment of the papillary muscles; it is attributed to abnormal traction on the papillary muscles and buckling of the ventricular wall. Patients with the most severe prolapse more commonly exhibit misshapen ventricular cavities during systole, and wall motion abnormalities frequently disappear after successful mitral valve replacement or repair.[31]

Electrophysiologic Testing

The indications for electrophysiologic testing in a patient with MVP are the same as other patients (i.e., recurrent unexplained syncope, sudden death survivors, symptomatic complex ventricular ectopy, and the presence of preexcitation syndromes) (see Chap. 34). Upright tilt studies with monitoring of blood pressure and rhythm may be valuable in patients with light-headedness or syncope and in diagnosing autonomic dysfunction (see Chap. 40).

NATURAL HISTORY, PROGNOSIS, AND COMPLICATIONS

In most patient studies, the MVP syndrome is associated with a benign prognosis.[7,55–64] However, some of these

results were affected by the maxim "a disease is particularly benign if you use a false position" (Fig. 68-6). The age-adjusted survival rate for both males and females with MVP is similar to that in patients without this common clinical entity. Gradual progression of MR in patients with mitral prolapse, however, may result in progressive dilatation of the LA and LV. LA dilatation often results in atrial fibrillation, and moderate to severe MR eventually results in LV dysfunction and the development of heart failure. Pulmonary hypertension may occur with associated right ventricular dysfunction. In some patients, after a prolonged asymptomatic interval, the entire process may enter an accelerated phase as a result of LA and LV dysfunction, atrial fibrillation, and in certain instances, ruptured mitral valve chordae. The latter occurs more commonly in males and with increasing age.[9,10]

Long-term prognostic studies suggest that complications occur most commonly in patients with a mitral systolic murmur, thickened redundant mitral valve leaflets, or increased LV or LA size[54,60–65] (Fig. 68-7 and Table 68-4).

In a prospective follow-up study of 237 asymptomatic or minimally symptomatic patients with documented MVP, sudden death occurred in 6 patients.[60] In a multivariant analysis of the echocardiographic findings, the presence or absence of redundant mitral valve leaflets by M-mode echocardiography was the only variable associated with sudden death. Ten patients sustained a cerebral embolic event, 6 of whom were in atrial fibrillation with LA enlargement. These data were confirmed in a retrospective two-dimensional echocardiographic study from 456 patients with MVP.[54] Complications or a history of complications was more prevalent in those with leaflet thickening and redundancy compared with those without leaflet thickening. The incidence of stroke, however, was similar in the two groups. Long-term follow-up studies in patients with MVP associated with a floppy, myxomatous mitral valve permit several conclusions.[9] Serious complications occur in some patients with MVP, predominantly in those with diagnostic auscultatory findings. Also, redundant mitral valve leaflets and increased LV size are associated with a greater frequency of serious complications. Finally, men and people over 50 years of age are at increased risk of complications, including severe MR requiring surgery.

Sudden death is the least common complication of MVP (Table 68-5). While infrequent, the highest incidence of sudden death has been reported in the familial form of MVP. Some of these patients have been noted to have QT prolongation. Also, patients with MVP who have severe autonomic dysfunction and excessive vagotonia causing bradyarrhythmias and asystole have been reported.[67,68] Since arrhythmias are the usual cause of sudden death, it seems

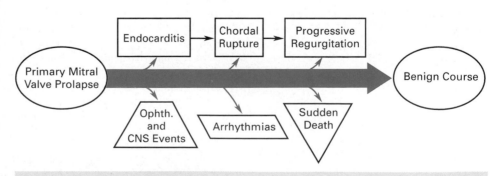

FIGURE 68-6 The course and possible complications of MVP. In most patients, the MVP syndrome is associated with a benign prognosis. CNS, central nervous system; Ophth, ophthalmologic. (From Crawford MH, O'Rourke RA. In: Isselbacher KJ et al., eds. *Harrison's Principles of Internal Medicine*, 9th ed. New York: McGraw-Hill; 1980:91–105. Reproduced with permission from the publisher, editors, and authors.)

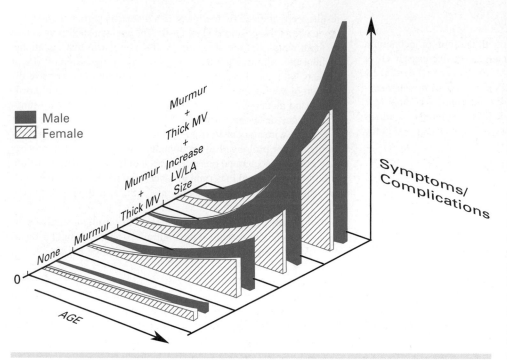

FIGURE 68-7 The relations between cardiac structure, age, and complications in the MVP syndrome. Patients with MVP, typical auscultatory findings, thickening of the valve leaflets, and LV or LA enlargement are at risk of developing complications. When two or more of these findings are present, the likelihood of complications is highest. By contrast, the absence of these features can be used to identify patients with MVP who have an exceedingly low risk. In general, complications increase with age and are more common in males than they are in females. (From Boudoulas et al.[61] Reproduced with permission from the publisher and authors.)

prudent to obtain ambulatory ECG recordings in MVP patients at highest risk. Many believe that patients with ECG ST-T-wave changes are more likely to have complex ventricular arrhythmias.[9,10] Certainly, patients with symptoms suggestive of arrhythmias or who have arrhythmias noted during physical examination or on the resting ECG should be evaluated further (see Chap. 28).

Infective endocarditis is a serious complication of MVP, and MVP is the leading predisposing diagnosis in most series of patients reported with endocarditis.[9,10,69] Since the absolute incidence of endocarditis is extremely low for the entire MVP population, there has been much debate concerning the risk of endocarditis in MVP.[70] While there is general agreement that MVP patients with murmurs and/or thickened redundant valves confirmed by echocardiography or cineangiography should receive antibiotic prophylaxis, some authorities state that patients with isolated systolic clicks and no murmurs do not need antibiotic prophylaxis for endocarditis.[71] However, the dynamic nature of MVP, with variable physical

TABLE 68-4 Use of Echocardiography for Risk Stratification in Mitral Valve Prolapse

Study	No. of Patients	Features Examined	Outcome	P
Nishimura et al., 1985[60]	237	MV leaflet ≥5 mm	↑ Sum of sudden death, endocarditis and cerebral embolus	P <0.02
		LVID ≥60 mm	↑ MVR (26 vs. 3.1%)	P <0.001
Zuppiroli et al., 1994[63]	119	MV leaflet >5 mm	↑ Complex ventricular arrhythmia	P <0.001
Babuty et al., 1994[66]	58	Undefined MV thickening	No relation to complex ventricular arrhythmias	NS
Takamoto et al., 1991[64]	142	MV leaflet ≥3 mm redundant, low echo density	↑ Ruptured chordae (48 vs. 5%)	NS
Marks et al., 1989[54]	456	MV leaflet ≥5 mm	↑ Endocarditis (3.5 vs. 0%)	P <0.02
			↑ Moderate-severe MR (11.9 vs. 0%)	P <0.001
			↑ MVR (6.6 vs. 0.7%)	P <0.02
			↑ Stroke (7.5 vs. 5.8)	NS
Chandraratna et al., 1984[65]	86	MV leaflets >5.1 mm	↑ Cardiovascular abnormalities (60 vs. 6%)	P <0.001
			(Marfan's syndrome, TVP, MR, dilated descending aorta)	

NOTE: LVID, left ventricular internal diameter; MR, mitral regurgitation; MV, mitral valve; MVR, mitral valve replacement; TVP, tricuspid valve prolapse.
SOURCE: From ACC/AHA guidelines for the clinical application of echocardiography. *Circulation* 1997;95:1686–1744 (updated 2003).

TABLE 68-5 Mitral Valve Complications in 102 Hearts with Primary Mitral Valve Prolapse

	No.	Percent
Sudden death	0	0
Primary rupture of chordae	7	7
Bacterial endocarditis	7	7
Mitral valve regurgitation	18	18
Primary rupture of chordae	(7)	—
Bacterial endocarditis	(4)	—
Severe prolapse	(4)	—
Entrapped chordae	(3)	—
Fibrin deposits	4	4

SOURCE: Modified from Lucas RV Jr, Edwards JE. The floppy mitral valve. *Curr Probl Cardiol* 1982;7:1–48.

findings on different examinations, makes it difficult to make judgments based on the presence or absence of a systolic murmur. With the increasing use of color-flow Doppler echocardiography studies, MR often has been observed in patients in whom no murmur is heard.[72] Recommendations for antibiotic endocarditis prophylaxis for patients with MVP undergoing procedures associated with bacteremia are listed in Table 68-6.

Progressive MR occurs frequently in patients with long-standing MVP. Fibrin emboli are responsible in some patients for visual problems consistent with involvement of the ophthalmic or posterior cerebral circulation. Several studies report an increased likelihood of cerebral vascular accidents of various types in patients under age 45 who have MVP than that which would would have been expected in a similar population without MVP. Therefore, it has been recommended that antiplatelet drugs such as aspirin be administered to patients who have MVP and suspected cerebral nervous system emboli. However, neither antiplatelet drugs nor anticoagulants should be prescribed routinely for patients with MVP because the incidence of embolic phenomena is very low. Recommendations for aspirin and oral anticoagulants in MVP are listed in Table 68-7.

It is important to avoid the incorrect diagnosis of MVP syndrome. This mistake is especially likely to occur in patients with neuropsychiatric symptoms, in whom an incorrect diagnosis of MVP is made

TABLE 68-6 Recommendations for Antibiotic Endocarditis Prophylaxis for Patients with Mitral Valve Prolapse Undergoing Procedures Associated with Bacteremia

Indication	Class
1. Patients with characteristic systolic click-murmur complex	I
2. Patients with isolated systolic click and echo evidence of MVP and MR	I
3. Patients with isolated systolic click, echo evidence of high-risk MVP	IIa
4. Patients with isolated systolic click and no or equivocal evidence of MVP	III

SOURCE: From ACC/AHA guidelines for the clinical application of echocardiography. *Circulation* 1997;95:1686–1744 (updated 2003).

TABLE 68-7 Recommendations for Aspirin and Oral Anticoagulants in Mitral Valve Prolapse

Indication	Class
1. Aspirin therapy for cerebral transient ischemic attacks (TIAs)	I
2. Warfarin therapy for patients in atrial fibrillation with age ≥65 yr, hypertension, mitral reguritation (MR) murmur, or history of heart failure	I
3. Aspirin therapy for patients in atrial fibrillation <65 years old with no history of MR, hypertension, or heart failure	I
4. Warfarin therapy for poststroke patients	I
5. Warfarin therapy patients for TIAs despite aspirin therapy	IIa
6. Aspirin therapy in poststroke patients with contraindications to anticoagulants	IIa
7. Aspirin therapy for patients in sinus rhythm with echocardiographic evidence of high-risk mitral valve prolapse	IIb

SOURCE: From ACC/AHA guidelines for the clinical application of echocardiography. *Circulation* 1997;95:1686–1744 (updated 2003).

from the ECG. Such an improper diagnosis can form the foundation of a chronic, often disabling cardiac neurosis. Even if the diagnosis of MVP is properly made, it is not necessarily correct to attribute neuropsychiatric symptoms to the MVP (see also Chap. 91).

TREATMENT

Most patients with MVP are asymptomatic and lack the high-risk profile described earlier. These patients with mild or no symptoms and findings of milder forms of prolapse should be assured of a benign prognosis. A normal lifestyle and regular exercise are encouraged.[8,10] For most patients in whom the *diagnosis of MVP is definite,* the authors recommend antibiotic prophylaxis for the prevention of infective endocarditis while undergoing procedures associated with bacteremia. Patients with MVP and palpitation associated with sinus tachycardia or mild tachyarrhythmias and those with chest pain, anxiety, or fatigue often respond to therapy with beta blockers.[8,10,73] However, the cessation of catecholamine stimulants such as caffeine, alcohol, cigarettes, and certain drugs may be sufficient to control symptoms.

Orthostatic symptoms are best treated with volume expansion, preferably by liberalizing fluid and salt intake. Mineralocorticoid therapy may be needed in severe cases, and wearing support stockings may be beneficial.[10] In sudden death survivors and those patients with symptomatic complex arrhythmias, specific antiarrhythmic therapy should be guided by monitoring techniques, including electrophysiologic testing when indicated[10] (see Chap. 28).

Daily aspirin therapy in a dose of 80 to 325 mg/day (see Table 68 7) is recommended for MVP patients with documented focal neurologic events. Such patients also should avoid cigarettes and oral contraceptives. Some clinicians use long-term anticoagulant therapy with warfarin in poststroke patients with prolapse, particularly when symptoms occur on aspirin therapy (see Chap. 99).

Restriction from competitive sports is recommended only when moderate LV enlargement, LV dysfunction, uncontrolled tachyarrhythmias, long QT interval, unexplained syncope, prior sudden death survival, or aortic root enlargement are present, individually or in combination.[10]

The familial occurrence of MVP should be explained to the patient and is particularly important in those with associated diseases, who are at greater risk for complications. Screening relatives can identify high-risk individuals and potentially prevent some complications. There is no contraindication to pregnancy based on the diagnosis of MVP alone.

Patients with severe MR with symptoms and/or impaired LV systolic function require cardiac catheterization studies and evaluation for mitral valve surgery.[74] The thickened, redundant mitral valve often can be repaired rather than replaced, with a low operative mortality and excellent long-term results.[75–83] Follow-up studies also suggest lower thromboembolic and endocarditis risk than with prosthetic valves.

Asymptomatic patients with MVP and no significant MR can be evaluated clinically every 2 to 3 years. Echocardiography has been suggested every 5 years in such patients to help determine the natural history and the likelihood of complications. Patients with MVP who have high-risk characteristics, including those with moderate to severe MR, should be followed more frequently, even if no symptoms are present. Avierinos et al.[3] reported a widely heterogenous natural history of asymptomatic MVP in community patients depending on the presence of risk factors that were able to separate high- from low-risk groups.

Surgical Considerations

Management of the patient with MVP may require valve surgery, particularly in those who develop a flail mitral leaflet due to rupture of the chordae tendineae or their marked elongation.[84] Most of these valves can be repaired successfully by surgeons experienced with mitral valve repair, especially when the posterior leaflet valve is predominantly affected. Symptoms of heart failure, the severity of MR, the presence or absence of atrial fibrillation, LV systolic function, LV end-diastolic and end-systolic volumes, and pulmonary artery pressure (rest and exercise) all influence the decision to recommend mitral valve surgery. Recommendations for surgery in patients with MVP and MR are the same as for those with other forms of nonischemic severe MR and include class II–IV symptoms, LV ejection fraction less than 60 percent, and/or marked increases in LV end-diastolic and end-systolic volumes.[85] If mitral valve repair is likely to be successful, severe MR with mild symptoms or atrial fibrillation is an appropriate reason for surgical referral.

References

1. Freed LA, Benjamin EJ, Levy D, et al. Mitral valve prolapse in the general population: The benign nature of echocardiographic features in the Framingham Heart Study *J Am Coll Cardiol* 2002;40(7).
2. Nishimura R, McGoon MD. Perspectives on mitral-valve prolapse. *N Engl J Med* 1999;341:48–58.
3. Avierinos J-F, Gersh BJ, Melton LJ, et al. Natural history of asymptomatic mitral valve prolapse in the community. *Circulation* 2002;106:1355–1361.
4. St. John Sutton M, Weyman AE. Mitral valve prolapse prevalence and complications. *Circulation* 2002;106:1305–1307.
5. Devereux RB, Jones EC, Roman MJ, et al. Prevalence and correlates of mitral valve prolapse in a population-based sample of American Indians: The Strong Heart Study. *Am J Med* 2001;111:679–685.
5a. Freed LA, Acierno JS Jr, Dai D, et al. A locus for autosomal dominant mitral valve prolapse on chromosome 11p15.4. *Am J Hum Genet* 2003;72(6):1551–1559.
5b. Chou HT, Shi YR, Hsu Y, Tsai FJ. Association between fibrillin-l gene exon 15 and 27 polymorphisms and risk of mitral valve prolapse. *J Heart Valve Dis* 2003;12(4):475–481.
6. Reid JV. Mid-systolic clicks. *S Afr Med J* 1961;35:353–357.
7. Barlow JB, Pocock WA, Marchand P, Denny M. The significance of late systolic murmurs. *Am Heart J* 1963;66:443–452.
8. O'Rourke RA, Crawford MH. The systolic click-murmur syndrome: Clinical recognition and management. *Curr Probl Cardiol* 1976; 1(1):1.
9. Lucas RV Jr, Edwards JE. The floppy mitral valve. *Curr Probl Cardiol* 1982;7:1–48.
10. Fontana ME, Sparks EA, Boudoulas H, Wooley CF. Mitral valve prolapse in the mitral valve prolapse syndrome. *Curr Probl Cardiol* 1991;16:315–375.
11. O'Rourke RA. The mitral valve prolapse syndrome. In: Chizner MA, ed. *Classic Teachings in Clinical Cardiology*. Cedar Grove, NJ: Laennec; 1996:1049–1070.
12. Devereux RB. Recent developments in the diagnosis and management of mitral valve prolapse. *Curr Opin Cardiol* 1995;10:107–116.
13. Perloff JK, Roberts WC. The mitral apparatus: Functional anatomy of mitral regurgitation. *Circulation* 1972;46:227–239.
14. Devereux RB, Brown WT, Kramer-Fox R, Sachs I. Inheritance of mitral valve prolapse: Effect of age and sex on gene expression. *Ann Intern Med* 1982;97:826–832.
15. Shell WE, Walton JA, Clifford ME, Willis PW III. The familial occurrence of the syndrome of mid-late systolic click and late systolic murmur. *Circulation* 1969;39:327–338.
16. Savage DD, Garrison RJ, Devereux RB, et al. Mitral valve prolapse in the general population: I. Epidemiologic features: The Framingham Study. *Am Heart J* 1983;106:571–576.
17. Procacci PM, Savran SV, Schrieter SL, Bryson AL. Prevalence of clinical mitral valve prolapse in 1169 young women. *N Engl J Med* 1976;294:1086–1088.
18. Leier CV, Call TD, Fulkerson PK, Wooley CF. The spectrum of cardiac defects in the Ehlers-Danlos syndrome, types I & III. *Ann Intern Med* 1980;92:171–178.
19. Lebwohl MG, Distefano D, Prioleau PG, et al. Pseudoxanthoma elasticum and mitral valve prolapse. *N Engl J Med* 1982;307:228–231.
20. Schwartz T, Gotsman MS. Mitral valve prolapse in osteogenesis imperfecta. *Isr J Med Sci* 1981;17:1087–1088.
21. Boulter C, Mulroy S Webb S, et al. Cardiovascular, skeletal, and renal defects in mice with a targeted disruption of the Pkd1gene. *PNAS* 2001;98(21):12174–12179.
22. Udoshi MB, Shah A, Fisher VJ, Dolgin M. Incidence of mitral valve prolapse in subjects with thoracic skeletal abnormalities: A prospective study. *Am Heart J* 1979;97:303–311.
23. Bon Tempo CP, Ronan JA Jr. Radiographic appearance of the thorax in systolic click: Late systolic murmur syndrome. *Am J Cardiol* 1975;36:27–31.
24. Crawford MH, O'Rourke RA. Mitral valve prolapse syndrome. In: Isselbacher KJ, Adams RD, Braunwald E, et al, eds. *Update I: Harrison's Principles of Internal Medicine*. New York: McGraw-Hill; 1981:91–152.
25. O'Rourke RA. The syndrome of mitral valve prolapse. In: Albert JA, ed. *Valvular Heart Disease*. New York: Lippincott-Raven; 1999:157–182.
26. Tei C, Sakamaki T, Shah PM, et al. Mitral valve prolapse in short-term experimental coronary occlusion: A possible mechanism of ischemic mitral regurgitation. *Circulation* 1983;68:183–189.
27. Crawford MH. Mitral valve prolapse due to coronary artery disease. *Am J Med* 1977;62:447–451.
28. Tomaru T, Uchida Y, Mohri N. Post-inflammatory mitral and aortic valve prolapse: A clinical and pathological study. *Circulation* 1987;76:68–76.
29. Lembo NJ, Dell'Italia LJ, Crawford MH, et al. Mitral valve prolapse in patients with prior rheumatic fever. *Circulation* 1988; 77:830–836.
30. Marcus RH, Sareli P, Pocock WA, et al. Functional anatomy of severe mitral regurgitation in active rheumatic carditis. *Am J Cardiol* 1986;63:577–584.

31. Crawford MH, O'Rourke RA. Mitral valve prolapse: A cardiomyopathic state? *Prog Cardiovasc Dis* 1984;27:133–139.

32. Lax D, Eicher M, Goldberg SJ. Mild dehydration induces echocardiographic signs of mitral valve prolapse in healthy females with prior normal cardiac findings. *Am Heart J* 1992;124:1533–1540.

33. Freed LA, Levy D, Levine RA, et al. Mitral valve prolapse and atrial septal aneurysm: An evaluation in the Framingham Heart Study. *Am J Cardiol* 2002;89:1326–1329.

34. Krivokapich J, Child JS, Dadourian BJ, Perloff JK. Reassessment of echocardiographic criteria for the diagnosis of mitral valve prolapse. *Am J Cardiol* 1988;61:131–135.

35. Fukuda N, Oki T, Iuchi A, et al. Predisposing factors for severe mitral regurgitation in idiopathic mitral valve prolapse. *Am J Cardiol* 1995;76(7):503–507.

36. Gaffney FA, Karlsson ES, Campbell W, et al. Autonomic dysfunction in women with mitral valve prolapse. *Circulation* 1979;59:894–899.

37. Boudoulas H, Reynolds JC, Mazzaferri E, Wooley CF. Metabolic studies in mitral valve prolapse syndrome. *Circulation* 1980;61:1200–1205.

38. Anwar A, Kohn SR, Dunn JF, et al. Altered beta-adrenergic receptor function in subjects with symptomatic mitral valve prolapse. *Am J Med Sci* 1991;302:89–97.

39. Santos AD, Puthenpurakal MK, Ahmad H, et al. Orthostatic hypotension: A commonly unrecognized cause of symptoms in mitral valve prolapse. *Am J Med* 1981;71:746–750.

40. Betriu A, Wigle ED, Felderhof CH, McLoughlin MJ. Prolapse of the posterior leaflet of the mitral valve associated with secundum atrial septal defect. *Am J Cardiol* 1975;35:363–369.

41. LeWinter MM, Hoffman JR, Shell WE, et al. Phuenylephrine-induced atypical chest pain in patients with prolapsing mitral valve leaflets. *Am J Cardiol* 1974;34:12–18.

42. Sabom MB, Curry RC Jr, Pepine CJ, et al. Ergonovine testing for coronary artery spasm in patients with angiographic mitral valve prolapse. *Catheter Cardiovasc Diagn* 1978;4:265–274.

43. Barnett HJM, Jones MW, Boughner DR, Kostuck WJ. Cerebral ischemic events associated with prolapsing mitral valve. *Arch Neurol* 1976;33:777–782.

44. Barletta GA, Gagliardi R, Benvenuti L, Fantini F. Cerebral ischemic attacks as a complication of aortic and mitral valve prolapse. *Stroke* 1985;16:219–223.

45. Barnett HJM, Boughner DR, Taylor DW, et al. Further evidence relating mitral valve prolapse to cerebral ischemic event. *N Engl J Med* 1980;302:139–144.

46. Petty GW, Orencia AJ, Khandheria BK, Whisnant JP. A population-based study of stroke in the setting of mitral valve prolapse: Risk factors and infarct subtype classification. *Mayo Clin Proc* 1994;69:632–634.

47. Orencia AJ, Petty GW, Khandheria BK, et al. Mitral valve prolapse and the risk of stroke after initial cerebral ischemia. *Neurology* 1995;45:1083–1086.

48. Gilon D, Buonanno FS, Jaffee MM, et al. Lack of evidence of an association between mitral valve prolapse and stroke in young patients. *N Engl J Med* 1999;341:8–13.

49. Wilson LA, Keeling PW, Malcolm AD, et al. Visual complications of mitral leaflet prolapse. *BMJ* 1977;2:86–88.

50. Chesler E, King RA, Edwards JE. The myxomatous mitral valve and sudden death. *Circulation* 1983;67:632–639.

51. Weis AJ, Salcedo EE, Stewart WJ, et al. Anatomic explanation of mobile systolic clicks: Implications for the clinical and echocardiographic diagnosis of mitral valve prolapse. *Am Heart J* 1995;129:314–320.

52. Bhutto ZR, Barron JT, Liebson PR, et al. Electrocardiographic abnormalities in mitral valve prolapse. *Am J Cardiol* 1992;70:265–266.

53. Schaal SF. Ventricular arrhythmias in patients with mitral valve prolapse. *Cardiovasc Clin* 1992;22(1):307–316.

54. Marks AR, Choong CY, Sanfilippo AJ, et al. Identification of high-risk and low-risk subgroups of patients with mitral valve prolapse. *N Engl J Med* 1989;320:1031–1036.

55. Shah PM. Echocardiographic diagnosis of mitral valve prolapse. *J Am Soc Echocardiogr* 1994;7(3 pt 1):286–293.

56. Bonow RO, Carabello B, De Leon AC Jr, et al. ACC/AHA guidelines for the management of patients with valvular heart disease. *J Am Coll Cardiol* 1998;32:1486–1588.

57. Klein GJ, Kostuck WJ, Bougher DR, Chamberlain MJ. Stress myocardial imaging in mitral leaflet prolapse syndrome. *Am J Cardiol* 1978;42:746–750.

58. Allen H, Harris A, Leatham A. Significance and prognosis of an isolated late systolic murmur: A 9- to 22-year follow-up. *Br Heart J* 1974;36:525–532.

59. Mills P, Rose J, Hollingsworth J, et al. Long-term prognosis of mitral valve prolapse. *N Engl J Med* 1977;297:13–18.

60. Nishimura RA, McGood MD, Shub C, et al. Echocardiographically documented mitral-valve prolapse: Long-term follow-up of 237 patients. *N Engl J Med* 1985;313:1305–1309.

61. Düren DR, Becker AE, Dunning AJ. Long-term follow-up of idiopathic mitral valve prolapse in 300 patients: A prospective study. *J Am Coll Cardiol* 1988;11:42–47.

62. Boudoulas H, Kolibash BH, Wooley CF. Mitral valve prolapse: A heterogenous disorder. *Prim Cardiol* 1991;17:29–43.

63. Zuppiroli A, Rinaldi M, Kramer-Fox R, et al. Natural history of mitral valve prolapse. *Am J Cardiol* 1995;75:1028–1032.

64. Takamoto T, Nitta M, Tsujibayashi T, et al. The prevalence and clinical features of pathologically abnormal mitral valve leaflets (myxomatous mitral valve) in the mitral valve prolapse syndrome: An echocardiographic and pathologic comparative study. *J Cardiol Suppl* 1991;25:75–86.

65. Chandraratna PAN, Nimalasuriya A, Kawanishi D, et al. Identification of the increased frequency of cardiovascular abnormalities associated with mitral valve prolapse by two-dimensional echocardiography. *Am J Cardiol* 1984;54:1283–1285.

66. Babuty D, Cosnay P, Breuillac JC, et al. Ventricular arrhythmia factors in mitral valve prolapse. *PACE* 1994;17:1090–1099.

67. Cheitlin MD, Armstrong WF, Aurigemma GP, et al. ACC/AHA guidelines for the clinical application of echocardiography. *Circulation* 2003;108:in press.

68. Cosgrove DM, Stewart WJ. Mitral valvuloplasty. *Curr Probl Cardiol* 1989;14:359–415.

69. Kirklin JW. Mitral valve repair for mitral incompetence. *Mod Concepts Cardiovasc Dis* 1987;56:7–11.

70. Marshall CE, Shappel SD. Sudden death and the ballooning posterior leaflet syndrome: Detailed anatomic and histochemical investigation. *Arch Pathol* 1974;98:134–138.

71. Clemens JD, Horwitz RI, Jaffe CC, et al. A controlled evaluation of the risk of bacterial endocarditis in persons with mitral valve prolapse. *N Engl J Med* 1982;307:776–781.

72. Devereux RB, Frary CJ, Kramer-Fox R, et al. Cost-effectiveness of infective endocarditis prophylaxis for mitral valve prolapse with or without a mitral regurgitant murmur. *Am J Cardiol* 1994;74:1024–1029.

73. Dajani AS, Bisno AL, Chung KJ, et al. Prevention of bacterial endocarditis: Recommendations by the American Heart Association. *JAMA* 1990;264:2919–2922.

74. Winkle RA, Lopes MG, Goodman DJ, et al. Propranolol for patients with mitral valve prolapse. *Am Heart J* 1977;93:422–427.

75. Galloway AC, Colvin SB, Baumann FG, et al. Current concepts of mitral valve reconstruction for mitral insufficiency. *Circulation* 1988;78:1087–1098.

76. Cheitlin MD. The timing of surgery in mitral and aortic valve disease. *Curr Probl Cardiol* 1987;12:75–149.

77. Cosgrove DM, Stewart WJ. Mitral valvuloplasty. *Curr Probl Cardiol* 1989;14:359–415.

78. Kirklin JW. Mitral valve repair for mitral incompetence. *Mod Concepts Cardiovasc Dis* 1987;56:7–11.

79. Cohn LH, Couper GS, Aranki SF, et al. Long-term results of mitral valve reconstruction for regurgitation of the myxomatous mitral valve. *J Thorac Cardiovasc Surg* 1994;107:143–150.

80. Eishi K, Kawazoe K, Sasako Y, et al. Comparison of repair techniques for mitral valve prolapse. *J Heart Valve Dis* 1994;3:432–438.

81. Perier P, Clausnizer B, Mistarz K. Carpentier "sliding leaflet" technique for repair of the mitral valve: Early results. *Ann Thorac Surg* 1994;57: 383–386.

82. Eishi K, Kawazoe K, Sasako Y, et al. Comparison of repair techniques for mitral valve prolapse. *J Heart Valve Dis* 1994;3:432–438.

83. Perier P, Clausnizer B, Mistarz K. Carpentier sliding leaflet technique for repair of the mitral valve: Early results. *Ann Thorac Surg* 1994;57: 383–386.

84. Ling LH, Enriquez-Sarano M, Seward JB, et al. Clinical outcome of mitral regurgitation due to flail leaflet. *N Engl J Med* 1996;335: 1417–1423.

85. Ahmed S, Nanda NC, Miller AP, et al. Usefulness of transesophageal three-dimensional echocardiography in the identification of individual segment/scallop prolapse of the mitral valve. *Echocardiography* 2003;20(2):203–209.

TRICUSPID VALVE, PULMONIC VALVE, AND MULTIVALVULAR DISEASE

Robert A. O'Rourke

DEFINITION, ETIOLOGY, AND PATHOLOGY

Tricuspid Valve Disease

Tricuspid valve dysfunction can occur with normal or abnormal valves.[1,2] The resulting hemodynamic abnormality when normal tricuspid values develop dysfunction is almost always pure regurgitation. Tricuspid regurgitation (TR) occurs when the tricuspid valve allows blood to enter the right atrium (RA) during a contraction of the right ventricle (RV).[2a] Tricuspid stenosis (TS) is caused by obstruction to flow across the valve during diastolic filling of the RV. A diagrammatic illustration of tricuspid valve disease and the prevalence of various pathologic etiologies are shown in Fig. 69-1A and B.

Many more diseases cause TR than TS. Importantly, the *normal tricuspid valve* often does not completely coapt in systole, as is shown by the frequent occurrence of TR jets as detected only by Doppler ultrasound. The volume of regurgitant blood is so small that the TR is inaudible; this finding occurs in 24 to 96 percent of normal individuals by Doppler ultrasound and thus must be considered a variant of normal.[2–4] Pathologic TR is most commonly due to diseases that cause RV dilatation and failure;[5] failure of the left ventricle (LV) and/or PH can result in TR[5a] (Table 69-1). Primary diseases of the tricuspid valve apparatus, which includes the tricuspid annulus, the leaflets, the chordae, the papillary muscle, and the RV wall, also cause TR (see Table 69-1).[6–8] The most common etiology of isolated TR is infective endocarditis in drug addicts[9] (see Chap. 83). Less common causes include myocardial infarction, trauma, carcinoid, leaflet prolapse, and such congenital abnormalities as atrial septal defect and Ebstein's anomaly[10–17] (see Chap. 73). TR also occurs in patients with rheumatoid arthritis, radiation therapy, and Marfan's syndrome.[6] Primary involvement of the tricuspid valve due to rheumatic fever results in TS, usually in association with TR (Fig. 69-2).

The most common cause of TS is rheumatic fever. This is usually associated with concomitant mitral stenosis (MS). Isolated TS can be seen with the carcinoid syndrome, infective endocarditis, endocardial fibroelastosis, endomyocardial fibrosis, and systemic lupus erythematosus, among other conditions[6–8] (Table 69-2). It has also been reported to occur in patients with Fabry's disease or Whipple's disease and in patients receiving methysergide therapy.[6] Mechanical obstruction of the valve can be due to an RA myxoma, tumor metastases, and thrombi in the RA, each resulting in the hemodynamic abnormalities of TS.[18,19] In addition, RV inflow tract obstruction can result from thrombosis endocarditis, degeneration, or calcification affecting a prosthetic tricuspid valve.

In rheumatic tricuspid valve disease, alterations in the valve are characterized by fibrosis, with contracture of the leaflets and commissural fusion. The former leads to TR and the latter to TS.[20] The stenotic component of rheumatic tricuspid valve disease is often minor and would be unrecognized clinically if it were not for the high flow across the valve caused by the coexistent TR. Whenever the tricuspid valve is affected by rheumatic disease, there is also involvement of left-sided valves.[21] Flammang and associates observed that 9.5 percent of cases requiring surgical replacement of *both* the mitral and aortic valves also had rheumatic involvement of the tricuspid valve.[22,22a]

Carcinoid heart disease occurs in up to 53 percent of patients with malignant metastatic carcinoid tumor (usually originating in the ileum; see Chap. 85). Carcinoid heart disease usually causes TR and, less often, tricuspid stenosis, pulmonic stenosis (PS), and/or pulmonic regurgitation (PR).[23,24] Changes include deposits of fibrous

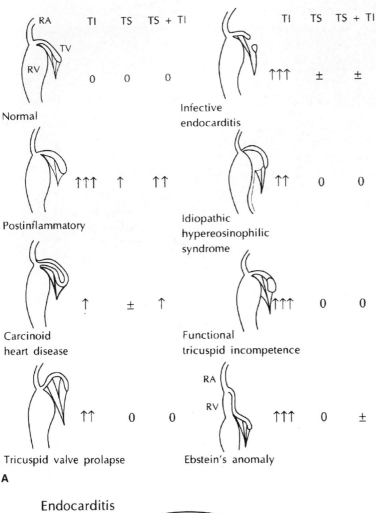

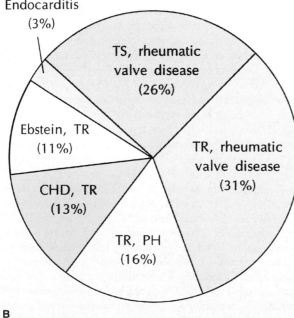

FIGURE 69-1 *A.* Tricuspid valve (TV) disease. Diagrammatic illustration of TV; RA, right atrium; RV, right ventricle; TI, tricuspid insufficiency; TS, tricuspid stenosis. *B.* Pathologic findings in TV. TR, tricuspid regurgitation; TS, tricuspid stenosis. [From Virmani R et al. Pathology of valvular heart diseases. In: Rahimtoola SH, ed. *Valvular Heart Disease.* Philadelphia: Mosby (Current Medicine, Inc.), 1997:116, with permission.]

tissue on the surfaces of these valves. Fibrous plaques can also develop on the endocardial surfaces of the RA and RV as well as on the intima of the coronary sinus and the pulmonary artery.[25] Although TS may result, the major functional abnormality is usually TR.

The most common type of TR secondary to enlargement of the orifice and annulus is caused by congestive heart failure with RV dilation due to LV disease (see Table 69-1). TR may diminish if the heart failure is treated successfully but can be permanent with long-standing dilatation of the RV.[26–28] In infective endocarditis, the TR results from improper coaptation of the leaflets because of interposed vegetations (see Table 69-1).

Myocardial infarction was not considered a common cause of TR except when secondary to chronic congestive heart failure.[29] Rare cases have been described from rupture of an RV papillary muscle.[30,31] Currently, RV infarction is recognized more often and is frequently associated with TR, as documented by echocardiography (see Chap. 52).

Various degrees of tricuspid valve prolapse are commonly present in the general population and may occur in 3 to 54 percent in patients with mitral valve prolapse (MVP)[24] (see Chap. 68). The reported incidence of *severe* TR from prolapse is low.[32]

External blunt trauma, most often in motor vehicle accidents, is a classic cause of TR. Isolated instances of rupture of a tricuspid papillary muscle have been described from external cardiopulmonary resuscitation.[33] Traumatic TR usually results from rupture of one or more of the components of the tensor apparatus, with disruption of the papillary muscle occurring more often than does rupture of the chordae.[15] Less frequently, there is a laceration of leaflet tissue.[34,35] Occasionally, traumatic TR and ruptured ventricular septum coexist.[36] TR can also occur from iatrogenic trauma produced during an endomyocardial biopsy.[37,38] Mild TR often results when a pacemaker is placed across a normally functioning tricuspid valve or after extraction of permanent pacemaker leads.[39]

Tolerance to traumatic TR varies, with up to 39 years of survival reported.[40–42] Patients with rupture of a papillary muscle tend to tolerate the TR less well than do those in whom the trauma resulted in rupture of chordae.[41] Among reported cases of TR resulting from the rupture of the chordae, a traumatic etiology is more common than is infective endocarditis.[43] Primary congenital lesions of the tricuspid valve that cause regurgitation are Ebstein's malformation and valvular dysplasia, as discussed in Chap. 64.

Pulmonic Valve Disease

Acquired lesions of the pulmonic valve generally cause PR (Table 69-3). On rare occasions, an inflammatory process can create stenosis and regurgitation of the valve. PH from any cause, such as MS, chronic lung disease, or pulmonary emboli, can produce PR. Inflammatory diseases, such as endocarditis, rheumatic fever, and, rarely, tuberculosis, can result in PR.[44–47]

PS is created by obstruction of systolic flow across the valve and is most commonly congenital (Fig. 69-3; Chaps. 63 and 64). Sarcomas and myxomas can sometimes extend to the pulmonic valve, causing PS.[48] Previous cardiac surgery on a congenital pulmonic valve lesion can result in PR. The carcinoid syndrome with cardiac involvement can create mild PS and associated PR[46]

TABLE 69-1 Diseases Causing Acquired Tricuspid Valve Regurgitation

DISEASES CAUSING PULMONARY HYPERTENSION

All left ventricular diseases with left ventricular failure
Mitral stenosis or mitral regurgitation
Pulmonary venous obstruction
Diseases causing an increase in pulmonary vascular
  resistance
  Primary pulmonary hypertension
  Acquired pulmonary vascular disease (atrial septal defects),
    ventricular septal defects, and patent ductus arteriosus
  Intrinsic pulmonary disease (chronic obstructive
    pulmonary disease, pulmonary fibrosis, and pulmonary
    resection)
  Collagen vascular diseases
Pulmonary emboli, acute and chronic

PRIMARY DISEASES OF THE TRICUSPID VALVE

Rheumatic heart disease
Rheumatoid arthritis
Trauma, penetrating and nonpenetrating
Radiation therapy
Carcinoid heart disease
Right atrial myxoma
Infective endocarditis
Eosinophilic myocarditis
Prosthetic and bioprosthetic valve malfunction, including
  thrombosis and calcification
Right ventricular myocardial infarction
Myxomatous tricuspid valve (tricuspid valve prolapse)

SOURCE: Modified from Cheitlin and MacGregor,[24] with permission.

necropsy.[49] Connective tissue diseases (see Chap. 84) can affect both the aortic and the mitral valves. For example, Marfan's syndrome MVP, resulting in mitral regurgitation (MR), often occurs together with the frequently observed changes in the aortic valve and ascending aorta. In the aging patient, calcification can develop in the aortic valve and mitral valve apparatus, as well as in the mitral annulus. Finally, infective endocarditis of the aortic or mitral valve can extend to the adjacent valve apparatus. In an autopsy series, combined aortic and mitral valve disease was observed in 33 percent of 996 patients with rheumatic fever.[50] In a 30-year follow-up of 1042 children with a history of rheumatic fever, multiple-valve involvement became apparent in 50 percent.[51] Bland and Jones followed 699 patients with cardiac involvement due to rheumatic fever for 20 years; 99 percent eventually exhibited aortic and mitral valve abnormalities.[52]

Rheumatic fever, myxomatous proliferation and prolapse, calcification in the aged, and infective endocarditis can impair both the aortic and mitral valves. The inflammatory process of rheumatic fever thickens and scars valve leaflets, which leads to fusion, fibrosis, and calcification (Fig. 69-5).

Myxomatous proliferation and valvular prolapse may affect all four valves (Fig. 69-6). Fusiform aneurysms of the aortic sinus and ascending aorta can develop in Marfan's syndrome; a dilated annulus, prolapse, ruptured chordae, and annular calcification can affect the mitral valve (Fig. 69-7). Annular dilatation, with or without prolapse, is a major cause of MR in Marfan's syndrome,[53] and most of the patients with Marfan's syndrome have MVP.

In aging patients, calcification can involve the aortic and mitral valves. Aortic stenosis is common, whereas mitral annular calcification (MAC) usually creates MR but rare cases of MS due to MAC have been documented (Fig. 69-8). Infective endocarditis can extend from either the aortic or the mitral valve to the adjacent valve through the inflammatory process (Fig. 69-9).

(Fig. 69-4). Compression of the pulmonary artery can stimulate valvular stenosis and is rarely produced by tumor, aneurysm, or even constrictive pericarditis.

Multivalvular Disease

Multivalvular disease includes mixed single valve disease [e.g., aortic stenosis (AS) plus aortic regurgitation (AR)] or combined disease affecting two or more values (e.g., MS plus TR). Rheumatic fever remains an important cause of combined disease of the mitral and aortic valves. Primary involvement of the tricuspid valve in rheumatic heart disease is unusual, and more commonly TR results from RV failure secondary to LV decompensation. A high prevalence of anatomic lesions involving two or more valves is present when the characteristic Aschoff body is observed at

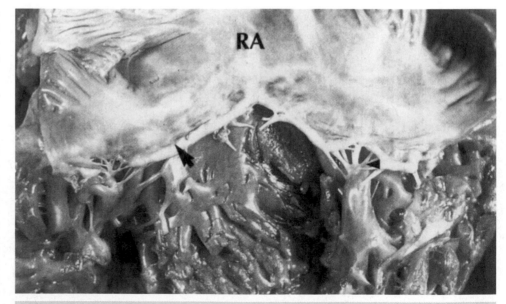

FIGURE 69-2 Heart displaying a tricuspid valve with fused, shortened chordae and rolled, thickened, fibrotic edge, consistent with chronic rheumatic heart disease. Isolated rheumatic tricuspid regurgitation or tricuspid stenosis is rare; it occurs almost always in the presence of concomitant mitral stenosis. RA, right atrium. [From Farb A, et al. Anatomy and pathology of the right ventricle (including acquired tricuspid and pulmonic valve disease). *Cardiol Clin North Am* 1993;10:1–2, with permission.]

TABLE 69-2 Diseases Causing Acquired Tricuspid Valve Stenosis

Rheumatic heart disease (usually with mitral stenosis)
Carcinoid heart disease
Fabry's disease
Whipple's disease
Endocardial fibroelastosis
Endomyocardial fibrosis
Methysergide therapy
Systemic lupus endocarditis
Right atrial myxoma or thrombus
Prosthetic valve thrombosis
Prosthetic valve infective endocarditis
Paraprosthetic valve degeneration and calcification

SOURCE: Modified from Cheitlin and MacGregor,[24] with permission.

PATHOPHYSIOLOGY

Tricuspid Valve Disease

In TR, the systolic blood flow into the RA elevates the mean RA pressure.[54] Regurgitant flow produces a prominent *cv* wave reflected through the venous system. Diastolic volume overload of the RV causes further dilatation of the RV and movement of the intraventricular septum toward the LV during diastole. RV failure further raises the mean RA and vena caval pressures and results in systemic venous congestion and signs of RV failure.[24]

TR decreases diastolic flow across the valve, elevates the RA pressure, and reduces the cardiac output.[1,55,56] With TS, stiffening of the valve by fibrosis and commissural fusion narrow the effective valvular orifice.[1,24] Flow from systemic veins or the RA into the RV is obstructed, and a pressure gradient develops in diastole between the RA and RV. The normal area of the tricuspid valve is 7 cm^2, and impairment of RV filling occurs when the valve area is reduced to less than 1.5 cm^2. Elevation of the mean RA pressure above

TABLE 69-3 Acquired Lesions of the Pulmonic Valve

Pulmonary hypertension with pulmonic regurgitation
  Mitral stenosis
  Chronic lung disease
  Pulmonary emboli
Inflammatory lesions
  Endocarditis
  Rheumatic fever
  Tuberculosis
Tumors
  Sarcoma
  Myxoma
Previous surgery or angioplasty for congenital lesions
Mediastinal lesions
  Tumor
  Aneurysm
  Constrictive pericarditis
Miscellaneous
  Carcinoid syndrome

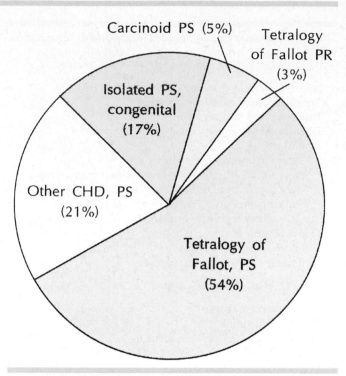

FIGURE 69-3 Pathologic findings in pulmonary valve (PV) replacement. CHD, congenital heart disease; PR, pulmonary regurgitation; PS, pulmonary stenosis. (Adapted from Altricher PM, et al. Surgical pathology of the pulmonary valve; a study of 116 cases spanning 15 years. *Mayo Clin Proc* 1989;64:1352–1360, with permission.)

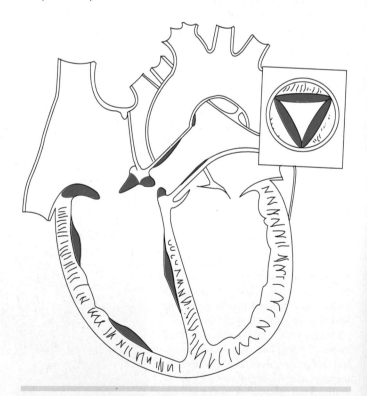

FIGURE 69-4 Carcinoid heart disease. The insert shows pulmonary stenosis. The leaflets of the tricuspid valve are thickened. The valve is predominantly incompetent and causes pulmonary regurgitation. Fibrous plaques are deposited on the lining of the right ventricle and pulmonary trunk. (From Edwards JE. Effects of malignant noncardiac tumors upon the cardiovascular system. *Cardiovasc Clin* 1971;4:282. Reproduced with permission from the publisher and author.)

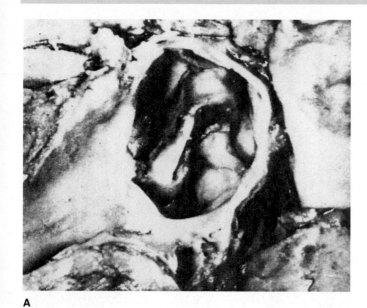

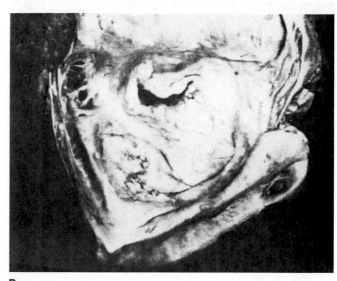

A

B

FIGURE 69-5 Rheumatic aortic stenosis and aortic regurgitation and rheumatic mitral stenosis in specimens from a 57-year-old woman. *A.* Aortic valve, unopened and viewed from above. Fusion of each of the three aortic valvular commissures, causing reduction in caliber of the orifice of the aortic valve, is apparent. The associated shortening of the cusps results in aortic regurgitation.

B. Mitral valve, unopened and viewed from above, and opened left atrium (LA). The mitral valve shows fusion at each of the commissures. The orifice is reduced in caliber. The LA is large, and calcification of the posterior part of the LA wall is present (lower part of figure).

10 mmHg usually results in peripheral edema. Development of atrial fibrillation produces a higher RA pressure in TS than when sinus rhythm is present. The hemodynamic abnormalities in TS can be further influenced by coexisting MS. Reduced RV flow in tricuspid valve obstruction has been proposed as a mechanism for protection against severe PH.

Pulmonic Valve Disease

PR is the most frequently acquired lesion of the pulmonic valve (see Table 69-3). Regurgitation may be secondary to PH or may be caused by primary abnormalities in the leaflets. PR imposes a volume overload on the RV and, if pulmonic hypertension preexists, the overload is superimposed on hypertrophied myocardium. Volume overload of the RV may cause an increase in diastolic volume of the chamber, an increase in RV stroke volume, and subsequent RV failure, resulting in TR.[1,24] Fortunately, isolated PR can usually be tolerated for a long time without cardiac decompensation.[57]

Multivalvular Disease

Multiple valve diseases affecting the mitral and aortic valves can produce a pressure overload, volume overload, or combinations of the two.[1,24] In the presence of combined valvular lesions, the pressure overload will cause concentric LV hypertrophy, even if myocardial failure develops.[1,25] An LV volume overload will result from AR and MR, and further dilatation will follow, with development of heart failure.[1,24] The combination of MS and AR usually results in a volume overload on the LV associated with LV pressure-volume work and myocardial oxygen consumption.[58,59]

Important physiologic considerations in combined valvular disease are the predominance of a single valvular lesion in altering hemodynamics and the potential failure to identify the presence of a second abnormal valve. MS produces hypertension in the left atrium

(LA) and pulmonary vein, with eventual PH and RV failure, even though AS may also be present. Despite the presence of MS, concomitant AS can create pressure overload and hypertrophy of the LV. When MR accompanies AS, the pressure and volume overloads create both LV dilatation and hypertrophy. LA enlargement and elevation of pulmonary artery pressure eventually accompany this condition. In regurgitation of both mitral and aortic valves, severe LV dilatation develops, accompanied by compensatory LV hypertrophy.[60] LV compliance increases in MR and AR, resulting in small elevations of end-diastolic pressure in the LV and LA for larger end-diastolic volumes.[61] Abnormalities in both early and late diastolic filling can accompany valvular regurgitation.[62]

In all combinations of aortic and mitral valve lesions, pulmonary congestion and elevated pulmonary capillary pressure usually follow significant depression of the contractile state of the LV. LA enlargement produced by either MS or MR is often associated with atrial fibrillation. Alterations in pulmonary blood flow and cardiac rhythm commonly accompany the LV pressure-volume overload in combined mitral and aortic valve disease.

TR usually accompanies RV dilatation secondary to PH from any combination of mitral or aortic valve diseases. Rarely, tricuspid regurgitation is due to a high-velocity jet from a VSD directed across the tricuspid valve. TS almost invariably is accompanied by disease of the mitral valve and can create significant elevations of the RA and central venous pressures.

CLINICAL MANIFESTATIONS

Symptoms

TRICUSPID VALVE DISEASE

Since TR is most frequently associated with severe LV failure or MS, presenting symptoms include dyspnea, orthopnea, and peripheral

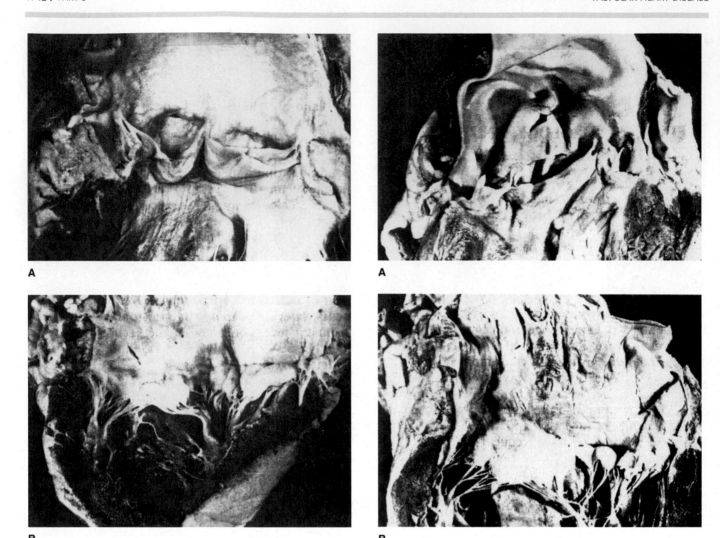

FIGURE 69-6 Prolapsed mitral valve and prolapsed aortic valve. *A.* Specimen of aortic valve from a 61-year-old man. The aortic valve shows redundance or prolapse of its right cusp. *B.* Specimen of mitral valve from a 73-year-old woman. The mitral valve shows prominent evidence of prolapse involving the posterior leaflet (right) and the posterior half of the anterior leaflet.

FIGURE 69-7 Floppy mitral valve and limited dissecting aneurysm of the ascending aorta, leading to aortic regurgitation, in a specimen from a 60-year-old man. *A.* Ascending aorta and aortic valve. The ascending aorta exhibits a laceration leading to a false channel within the aortic wall in which a hematoma is present (seen on each side of the opened aorta). Secondary distortion of the aortic valvular mechanism caused aortic regurgitation. *B.* Mitral valve, left atrium, and a portion of the left ventricle. The posterior leaflet of the mitral valve (right) shows several areas of prolapse.

edema.[63] Even though LV failure is usually present, paroxysmal nocturnal dyspnea is often absent. TR may occasionally provide a physiologic basis for the alleviation of left-sided heart failure by developing right-sided heart failure. Some patients also have less pulmonary edema due to the development of pulmonary arteriolar disease. If the TR is produced by infective endocarditis, symptoms of febrile illness may be accompanied by fatigue and peripheral edema.

The most frequent symptoms in TS are dyspnea and fatigue and peripheral edema. When MS coexists, the development of significant TS can diminish the symptoms of dyspnea, pulmonary congestion, and PH.[16,17]

PULMONIC VALVE DISEASE

Clinical manifestations of acquired pulmonic valvular lesions depend on the severity of the hemodynamic impairment as well as on the extent of the underlying disease. Isolated PR can often be tolerated without symptoms. Severe PH may cause syncope in addition to shortness of breath and fatigue. With inflammatory lesions of the pulmonic valve, febrile manifestations and pulmonary infection may be present. The carcinoid syndrome is characterized by episodes of facial flushing, increased intestinal activity, diarrhea, and bronchospasm (see Chap. 85). Tumors involving the pulmonic valve may exert pressure from expansion and metastases that affect the heart and lungs.

MULTIVALVULAR DISEASE

Dyspnea is the most frequent complaint of patients with combined mitral and aortic valve disease.[1,24,64] With combined MS and AS, chest discomfort, palpitations, and syncope are frequent clinical manifestations. Symptoms of heart failure result from pulmonary congestion and usually include fluid retention. Angina pectoris is more frequent with regurgitation of both the aortic and mitral valves. Also, syncope may develop when AR and MR coexist; palpitations are present in the majority of patients.

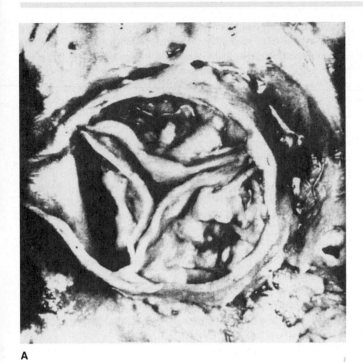

A

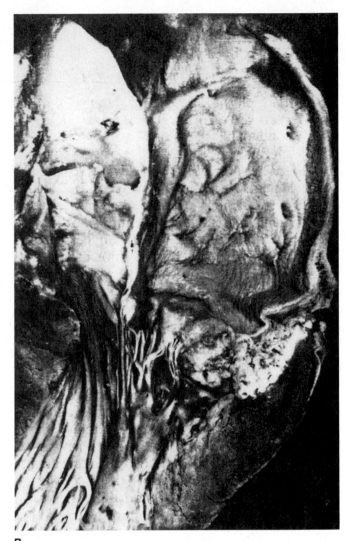

B

FIGURE 69-8 Senile calcific aortic stenosis and calcification of the mitral ring in specimens from two individuals. *A.* Aortic valve. Classic example of senile calcific aortic stenosis in the unopened aortic valve viewed from above. *B.* Left atrium (LA), mitral valve, and lateral wall of the left ventricle (LV). Sagittal section through LA and LV walls reveals a calcified mass at the junction of the LA, LV, and posterior mitral leaflet.

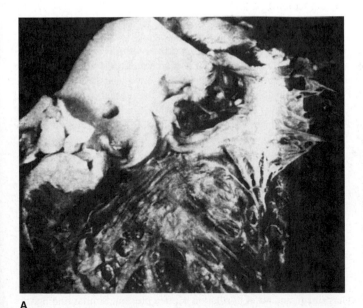

A

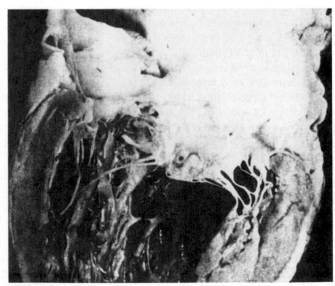

B

FIGURE 69-9 Bacterial endocarditis in specimens from a 36-year-old man. *A.* Aortic valve. The base of the aortic valve shows major destruction of a cusp with extension of inflammation onto the subjacent mitral valve. Near the free edge of the mitral valve, its ventricular aspect shows an ostium of a nonruptured mycotic aneurysm. *B.* Mitral valve, left atrium, and left ventricle. The lobulated mycotic aneurysm of the mitral valve lies near its free edge.

Angina, dizziness, syncope, and palpitations are common symptoms in AS when it is associated with MR. Angina may also be a symptom when AR and MS are the predominant lesions; but the more frequent symptoms, dyspnea and fatigue, are attributed to pulmonary congestion and heart failure (see Chaps. 66 to 68).

Physical Examination

TRICUSPID VALVE DISEASE

In patients with primary TR not due to PH, there are large *v* waves in the jugular venous pulse (JVP). There is a dilated RV with a precordial lift and right-sided third and/or fourth heart sound. There is usually a long systolic murmur in the third and fourth intercostal space at the left sternal border that increases with inspiration. The murmur is often confined to early and mid-systole or may not be heard at all when there is small gradient between the RV and RA during systole and a large regurgitant orifice (see Chap. 12). When a large amount of blood returns to the RV in diastole, a short diastolic rumble along the left sternal border may be heard. All of these findings are increased with inspiration (Rivero Carvallo's sign).[65] When RV failure occurs, the mean central venous pressure becomes elevated, and the jugular veins are pulsatile and engorged. When TR is due to PH, there is an accentuated P_2, and the high-pitched decrescendo diastolic murmur of PR is louder during inspiration in the second and third left intercostal spaces. In patients with TR and atrial fibrillation, there is a prominent *cv* wave in the jugular veins, produced by the regurgitant flow from the RV (see Chap. 12). The characteristic physical finding of TR due to PH is a holosystolic murmur at the left sternal border that increases during inspiration; there is an RV-RA pressure gradient throughout systole.

Tricuspid stenosis is frequently associated with lesions of the mitral and aortic valves. When sinus rhythm is present, the JVP will display the prominent *a* wave indicative of impaired RV diastolic filling with atrial systole. The *a* wave in the neck may be of moderate height and sometimes reaches the mandible. It is often best appreciated with the patient in the setting position. Auscultation of the heart is required to confirm that the rise of the venous *a* wave is simultaneous with the first heart sound. The *cv* wave is small, and the *y* descent is slow and insignificant (see Chap. 12).

PULMONIC VALVE DISEASE

If RV failure and TR result from PR, a prominent *cv* wave will be present in the JVP. Increased RV activity may be visible and palpable along the left sternal border. If PH is present, the pulmonic second sound will be accentuated over the left upper sternal border. The murmur of acquired PR is a high-pitched diastolic blow along the left sternal border. Thus, the murmur may be difficult to differentiate from the murmur of AR, but the absence of peripheral findings of AR is useful in identifying PR as the source of the diastolic murmur. Congenital PR characteristically is associated with a low-pitched, decrescendo murmur along the left sternal border, the peak of the murmur occurring shortly after P_2 (see Chap. 12).

MULTIVALVULAR DISEASE

In combined MS and AS, the LV apical impulse may not be displaced, but a palpable parasternal RV systolic lift is usually present. A mitral diastolic rumble is audible in most patients and can vary from grade I to III in intensity. The aortic systolic murmur is usually loud, but occasionally may be faint with severe MS. A mitral opening snap may not be audible, and in some patients the diastolic rumble of MS cannot be heard.

When both AR and MR exist, the diastolic arterial blood pressure is usually less than 70 mmHg. In those with a diastolic blood pressure above 70 mmHg, there is usually a loud holosystolic mitral murmur. If AR is the dominant lesion, the early diastolic murmur is usually prominent, whereas when MR prevails, the aortic murmur becomes less intense. MR may diminish the AR due to the increased LV diastolic filling from the enlarged LA. Depending on the contractile state of the myocardium, loud regurgitant murmurs may be associated with mild regurgitation, whereas faint murmurs may accompany severe valvular regurgitation if myocardial failure has developed. A diastolic "flow murmur" across the mitral valve is heard in the majority of patients with combined MR and AR. If AR is important, a systolic murmur produced by the large forward flow across the aortic valve often is present (see Chap. 12).

When AR and MS are both present, the LV impulse is also displaced, sustained, and forceful. The early diastolic murmur at the apex may be prominent and may be accentuated by the AR flow striking the anterior leaflet of the stenotic mitral valve. Although the low-pitched diastolic murmur of MS and the diastolic flow murmur with AR are usually reliable diagnostic parameters, neither murmur correlates with the hemodynamic measurements when the two lesions coexist.

When AR is combined with MS, the systemic pulse pressure does not necessarily reflect the severity of AR. A prominent apical impulse in apparently pure MS indicates the likelihood of associated AR but may not indicate its severity. Finally, the intensity of the aortic diastolic murmur is of little value in predicting the severity of AR in the presence of MS (see Chap. 12).

In the presence of AS and possible MR, an apical holosystolic murmur is reasonable evidence for associated MR, but its intensity is not a reliable indicator of severity.

While the murmur of TR often increases with inspiration, distinction from a concomitant MR murmur may be difficult. Identification of the rumble of TS requires careful auscultation during inspiration at the left lower sternal border.

Electrocardiogram

TRICUSPID VALVE DISEASE

Atrial fibrillation is frequent in patients with TR. When TR results from myocardial infarction, acute or chronic electrocardiographic (ECG) changes will be seen in the inferior leads, and ST-segment elevation indicating RV infarction may be present in the right-sided precordial leads. The characteristic ECG finding in TS is a large P wave of RA enlargement in the absence of RV hypertrophy[1,24,66] (see Chap. 13).

PULMONIC VALVE DISEASE

Although there are no characteristic changes with pulmonic valvular lesions, preexisting PH will produce RV hypertrophy, right-axis deviation, and changes in the *p* wave, suggesting RA enlargement. If PH is secondary to MS, P mitrale, with characteristic notches, will be present in lead II (see Chap. 13).

MULTIVALVULAR DISEASE

In combined MS and AS, ECG evidence of LV hypertrophy, LA enlargement, and atrial fibrillation is often present. Similar findings are observed in MR and AR, with a high likelihood of LA and LV enlargement along with atrial fibrillation. With AS and MR, LV hypertrophy is accompanied by a moderate incidence of atrial fibrillation. MS with severe AR also produces LV hypertrophy.

Chest Roentgenogram

TRICUSPID VALVE DISEASE

TR may produce some degree of RA enlargement, but there will usually be accompanying RV enlargement.[63] In TS, the most characteristic radiographic finding is prominence of the RA without significant pulmonary arterial enlargement or changes due to PH[1,24] (see Chap. 15).

PULMONIC VALVE DISEASE

Patients with PR have pulmonary artery prominence along with an increase in RV dimensions. If PS is acquired, there may be post-stenotic dilatation or prominence of the main pulmonary artery.

MULTIVALVULAR DISEASE

With combined MS and AS, the LA is always enlarged. LV chamber size may be significantly enlarged; however, prominent RV dimensions are usually present. Valvular calcification at either site is relatively uncommon. In AS accompanied by MR, heart size is increased, with both LV and LA enlargement. In MS with AR, marked LV enlargement is often present.

Echocardiogram

TRICUSPID VALVE DISEASE

With TR, there may be evidence of systolic prolapse, rupture of the chordae or papillary muscle, or vegetative lesions on the valve.[67] Increased RV dimensions indicate impaired RV function and the likelihood of secondary TR (see Chap. 15). Contrast echocardiography with peripheral venous injection can identify the back-and-forth flow across the valve.[68] The Doppler echocardiography technique can estimate the severity of the regurgitation and the systolic pressure in the RV[69] (Fig. 69-10). Color-flow Doppler imaging can delineate the patterns and sites of regurgitation across the valve apparatus[73] (see Chap. 15).[69a]

A characteristic pattern of TS can often be recorded with the echocardiogram. Fibrosis and calcification of the valve can be identified. Obstructive lesions, such as myxoma, thrombus, or other tumors, can be recognized by an echocardiogram. The two-dimensional echocardiogram of a patient with carcinoid syndrome with both TR and TS is shown in Fig. 69-11A and B. The Doppler echocardiography technique can be used to estimate the diastolic gradient across the valve with generally good accuracy (see Chap. 15).

PULMONIC VALVE DISEASE

Echocardiography can delineate the anatomy of the pulmonic valve as well as intrinsic or extrinsic lesions impinging on the valve apparatus. Sometimes a vegetative lesion or tumor can be detected in the pulmonic valve area. The Doppler echocardiography technique can estimate the severity of both the regurgitation and the stenosis of the valve, and analysis of Doppler echocardiography recordings can provide estimates of pulmonary artery pressure[71–73] (Fig. 69-12). Color-flow imaging can further confirm the patterns of regurgitation in the RV outflow tract (see Chap. 15).

MULTIVALVULAR DISEASE

Echocardiography provides information on valve anatomy, chamber dimensions, estimated pressure gradients, valve size, patterns of regurgitation, and estimates of ventricular function. MS and AS produce characteristic echoes (see Chap. 15). Prolapse of mitral, aortic, and tricuspid valves can be characteristically recognized with echocardiography.[74] The number of aortic cusps can be identified, as can the presence of calcium in the aortic or mitral valve apparatus. Dimensions of the LA, LV, and RV, together with LV wall-thickness measurements and determinations of mass, are useful in estimating the extent of volume and pressure overload. Two-dimensional and Doppler echocardiographic techniques can assess the orifice size of the aortic and mitral valves and estimate the valve gradients accurately.[75,76] Even in the presence of AR, appropriate modifications in the mathematical analysis of the pressure gradient can yield reasonably accurate estimates of the aortic valve gradients (see Chap. 15). Color-flow Doppler readings can identify patterns and sites of valvular-regurgitation across the aortic and mitral valves.[77,78] Also, thrombus formation in the LA and LV can be detected with various echocardiographic methods. Transesophageal echocardiography (see Chap. 15) can accurately assess prosthetic valve function and valvular repair during the operative procedures. Intracardiac echocardiography with Doppler is now available. This technology will significantly enhance our ability to interrogate mulitvalvular lesions.[79]

Nuclear Techniques

A radionuclide ventriculogram (RNV) can delineate dimensions of the RA and RV, which may help differentiate between TS and TR (see Chap. 19). RV size and function can be evaluated in stenotic and regurgitant lesions of the pulmonic valve. Myocardial perfusion imaging techniques are useful in detecting RV infarction as a cause of TR, as well as in providing estimates of RV function. RV size and function can be evaluated in stenotic and regurgitant lesions of the pulmonic valve.

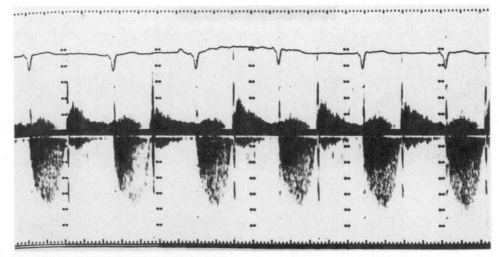

FIGURE 69-10 A continuous Doppler echocardiography recording from a patient with tricuspid valve disease illustrates tricuspid regurgitation in the lower portion and tricuspid stenosis in the upper portion of the tracing. (Reproduced with permission from and courtesy of Dr. Pamela Sears-Rogan.)

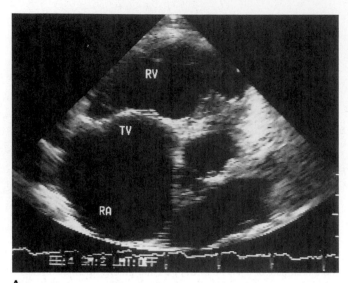

A

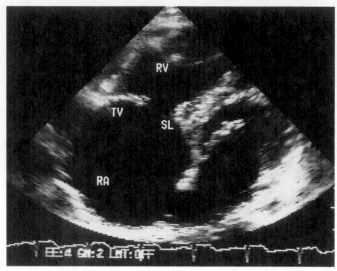

B

FIGURE 69-11 *A.* Two-dimensional echocardiogram of a 40-year-old patient, with carcinoid tumor of the testes without metastases. He presented with a testicular mass and was found to have a grade III/VI pansystolic murmur and grade III/VI diastolic murmur; both increased with inspiration. This four-chamber view shows a thickened stenotic tricuspid valve (TV) in diastole. The right atrium (RA) is enlarged, and the atrial septum bulges to the left, indicating a higher RA than left atrium (LA) pressure, which is consistent with tricuspid stenosis. The liver was normal because the humoral products of the carcinoid tumor bypassed the liver by the testicular venous drainage flowing directly to the inferior vena cava and renal veins. Carcinoid tumors arise from neuroendocrine cells known as enterochromaffin cells, which are found in or-gans derived from the embryonic gut. Because the liver detoxifies the humoral products of the carcinoid tumor, which most often arises in the ileum, it is ex-tremely rare to see carcinoid heart disease in the absence of liver metastases, making this case extremely unusual.[3,4] Only about 20 percent of patients with carcinoid tumors develop cardiovascular symptoms. RV, right ventricle. *B.* Two-dimensional echocardiogram in diastole. This is from the same patient as in (*A*). Note the thickened TV and the lack of excursion of the TV from diastole to sys-tole. This washer-like, thickened TV is characteristic of carcinoid heart disease. It is common for a carcinoid TV to be both stenotic and insufficient. With carci-noid TV disease the valve becomes thickened, and its mobility and flexibility are reduced. SL, septal leaflet. (From Cheitlin and MacGregor,[24] with permission.)

Quantitative information on LV function at rest and during exer-cise can be provided by RNV (see Chap. 19). Segmental wall motion can be assessed at rest and during exercise and may assist in the recognition of underlying coronary artery disease. Since combined lesions of the aortic and mitral valves often create PH and RV dys-function, RNV is useful in estimating the RV ejection fraction[80] (see Chap. 19).

Cardiac Catheterization

TRICUSPID VALVE DISEASE

Accurate angiographic documentation of TR is difficult to obtain be-cause the catheter overrides the tricuspid valve, and ventricular irri-tability with an RV injection can induce TR. A balloon angiographic catheter will not produce significant tricuspid regurgitation, however.

A prominent *cv* wave in the RA sug-gests TR, and an intracardiac phonocar-diogram may record a regurgitation murmur.[81]

If TS is clinically suspected, simul-taneous pressures should be recorded in the RA and RV in order to measure the gradient across the valve accurately.[62] Since the normal gradient across the tri-cuspid valve is less than 1 mmHg, small gradients may not be detected if pull-back pressure is recorded from the RV to the RA. The area of the tricuspid valve in TS is usually less than 1.5 cm^2; in severe TS, it is less than 1 cm^2.

PULMONIC VALVE DISEASE

PR can demonstrated angiographically using a straight lateral view, a right ven-tricular injection can outline the pul-monary valve as well as show post-stenotic dilatation. An aortic root injection can be helpful in the elimina-tion of AR as the etiology of a diastolic

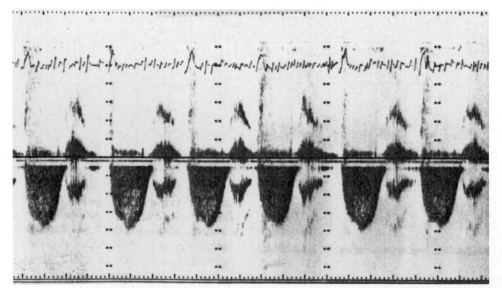

FIGURE 69-12 A Doppler echocardiography continuous tracing in a patient with TR. By employing the equation, the systolic gradient across the tricuspid valve can be calculated, and the addition of 10 mmHg yields an estimate of the pulmonary systolic pressure. Thus, in this patient, the level of PH could be estimated from the Doppler echocardiography tracing of the TR. (Reproduced with permission from and courtesy of Dr. Pamela Sears-Rogan.)

murmur along the left sternal border. Nevertheless, this distinction is usually best made by Doppler echocardiography studies.

MULTIVALVULAR DISEASE

Cardiac catheterization is appropriate for most patients with combined valvular heart disease. Gradients across the valve can be measured with precision and the valve area calculated. PH is commonly present in these patients, and LV end-diastolic pressure is often elevated despite the presence of MS (see Chap. 17).

In MR plus AR, the LV end-diastolic pressure is elevated in most patients, and the central aortic pressure is generally greater than 40 mmHg. The *v* wave of MR can be recorded in the wedge position, and capillary and pulmonary arterial pressures are abnormally elevated in most of these patients.

In AS with MR, LV end-diastolic and pulmonary artery pressures are elevated; however, the extent of pressure elevation does not necessarily reflect the severity of the MR. When it is severe, forward cardiac output may be reduced; thus, a *spuriously small* pressure gradient may be recorded across a very stenotic aortic valve. In MS with AR, the LV end-diastolic pressure is abnormal and the central aortic diastolic pressure is usually less than 70 mmHg.

In combined valvular lesions, the measurement of total angiographic LV stroke volume is useful in calculating the regurgitant volume across each valve.[1,25] When both valves are regurgitant, it is more difficult to calculate the regurgitant volume across each valve.

Assessment of ventricular function is important in patients with combined valvular lesions; yet the ejection fraction may be spuriously normal or elevated in MR and, to a lesser extent, in AR. Measurements of LV end-systolic pressure, volume, and wall thickness permit calculation of end-systolic wall stress.[82] This parameter has been particularly helpful in pressure and volume overload conditions, since the end-systolic pressure-volume wall stress calculation is relatively independent of loading conditions.

Finally, coronary arteriography should be performed at the time of cardiac catheterization in patients above the age of 35, as asymptomatic coronary artery disease may contribute to LV dysfunction. Coronary artery bypass grafting at the time of valve surgery is an important consideration.

USUAL STRATEGY OF WORKUP

Tricuspid Valve Disease

The history should identify underlying conditions, such as rheumatic fever, systemic disorders, and left-sided heart failure, as etiologies for tricuspid valve disease. The physical examination should carefully define the waveforms in the JVP. The auscultatory changes of systolic and diastolic murmurs at the left lower sternal border during the respiratory cycle should be carefully evaluated. In addition, physical findings of left-sided valvular abnormalities, particularly MS or evidence of LV failure, should be observed. Peripheral edema as evidence of impaired right-sided filling should be identified.

Echocardiography is the most useful noninvasive technique for identifying the presence, severity, and potential etiologies of TS and/or TR (see Chap. 15). If the patient undergoes cardiac catheterization for assessment of left-sided heart disease, right-sided hemodynamics should be recorded and, if clinically indicated, simultaneous pressures recorded in the RA and the RV (see Chap. 17).

Pulmonic Valve Disease

The clinical history is important in delineating causes of left-sided heart failure that can lead to PH and PR. The physical examination is important in evaluating the venous pulsations in the neck veins as well as the pulmonic murmurs. RV prominence should be carefully evaluated, as should concomitant left-sided valve lesions and evidence of heart failure. Although an ECG and chest x-ray should be obtained to assess the pulmonic artery, RV outflow tract, and body of the RV, the most useful noninvasive technique is echocardiography. The anatomy, competence of the valve, extent of regurgitation, and stenosis can be recognized and assessed by a Doppler echocardiography study. In addition, other valve lesions affecting the left side of the heart can be documented.

Multivalvular Disease

Symptoms of dyspnea, exercise intolerance, chest discomfort, or syncope should be specifically sought during a carefully taken clinical history. On physical examination, special attention should be directed to the peripheral and central arterial pulses and the JVP. Heart size, precordial movement, and auscultatory findings should be carefully noted. A 12-lead ECG and posteroanterior and lateral chest films should be obtained. Echocardiography is indicated to delineate valve anatomy, measure valve gradients, recognize regurgitant patterns, calculate orifice size, and estimate ventricular function and wall motion (see Chap. 15). A limited exercise test may help determine the exercise capacity as well as detect functional deterioration, chest pain, arrhythmias, deterioration of ventricular ejection fraction, or segmental wall motion abnormalities. If symptoms are atypical and the extent of valvular or LV function cannot be satisfactorily evaluated by noninvasive techniques, cardiac catheterization is indicated.

NATURAL HISTORY AND PROGNOSIS

Tricuspid Valve Disease

With TR due to RV hypertension, the symptoms and clinical course are primarily related to the left-sided heart conditions that produce a pressure-volume overload on the RV. TR virtually always develops with severe RV failure. In infective endocarditis of the tricuspid valve, the type of organism may significantly influence the course and the response to antibiotics (see Chap. 81).

With TS, the symptoms are usually those of MS, and the absence of pulmonary congestion in the presence of peripheral edema should raise the possibility of underlying TS. Significant TS may slow the development of characteristic symptoms of MS and result in an underestimation of the severity of mitral valve obstruction.

Pulmonic Valve Disease

In pulmonic valve lesions, the course will be more prolonged if there is chronic PH due to MS or chronic lung disease. Inflammatory conditions and tumors that affect the valve usually result in a much shorter clinical course.

Multivalvular Disease

When combined aortic and mitral valve disease are caused by rheumatic fever, 10 years or more may elapse before the development of significant murmurs, and an additional decade (or more) may elapse before symptoms become manifest. If lesions of the aortic and mitral valves are due to degenerative collagen changes, symptoms may develop later in life. When combined lesions are due to calcific changes in the aortic valve and annulus, as well as the mitral valve annulus, symptoms develop much later in life. There may, however, be rapid progression of degenerative aortic calcific stenosis over a 2- to 3-year period (see Chap. 66).

MEDICAL MANAGEMENT

Tricuspid Valve Disease

With TR, treatment of RV failure requires digitalis and diuretics, and vasodilating agents are also required for the management of LV failure. If failure of the right side of the heart is caused by MS, early intervention to enlarge or replace the mitral valve is appropriate (see Chap. 67).

In TS, the usual precautionary measures of antibiotic coverage and prevention of endocarditis apply. Peripheral edema may not respond well to administration of digitalis, diuretics, and vasodilator therapy. Tricuspid balloon valvuloplasty has been used successfully in patients with predominant TS.[83]

Pulmonic Valve Disease

Patients with congenital pulmonic valve stenosis are usually best treated by catheter balloon valvotomy (see Chaps. 73 and 74).

Prophylaxis and Medical Therapy

Antibiotic prophylaxis against endocarditis (see Chap. 81) is appropriate for patients with either tricuspid or pulmonic valve lesions. If pulmonary emboli contribute to the PH, anticoagulation is indicated (Chap. 53). Further treatment of PH may require management of left-sided heart failure, correction of MS, or the use of vasodilating agents. Vasodilating agents are often ineffective in treating primary PH (see Chap. 62).

If rheumatic fever is the likely etiology of combined aortic and mitral valve disease, prophylactic penicillin should usually be continued until age 35 years (see Chap. 64). Dental prophylaxis with antibiotic coverage, using either amoxicillin or erythromycin, should be provided in all patient groups prior to dental procedures. For genitourinary or other abdominal procedures, gram-negative antibiotic coverage should be provided (see Chap. 81).

Atrial Fibrillation

If atrial fibrillation develops, chronic anticoagulation with low-dose warfarin [International Normalized Ratio (INR) 2.0 to 3.0] is warranted, since the accompanying incidence of systemic and cerebral emboli is estimated at 10 to 20 percent (see Chap. 71).

The early development of atrial fibrillation associated with hemodynamic deterioration warrants an initial attempt at electrical cardioversion. If this is successful, digitalis as well as antiarrhythmic preparations should be administered thereafter for prophylaxis against recurrence (see Chap. 28). Chronic atrial fibrillation should be controlled with digitalis, beta blockers, and calcium blockers as indicated. The development of symptoms, particularly dyspnea, limited exercise activity, chest pain, and syncope, warrants consideration for surgery. It is usually recommended for New York Heart Association (NYHA) class II-III symptoms despite adequate medical therapy.

SURGICAL MANAGEMENT

Tricuspid Valve Disease

The decision to proceed with valvular heart surgery is usually based on the severity of the aortic and mitral valve disease, rather than on the severity of the disease of the tricuspid valve. The usual decisions to be made regarding the tricuspid valve are (1) whether a procedure should be added to the mitral and/or aortic valve procedures and, (2) if so, which procedure—annuloplasty or valve replacement—should be performed. Such patients with mild mitral disease but severe TR may require an operation on the tricuspid valve only.

The severity of the symptoms and clinical signs of tricuspid valve disease are used to determine the indications for surgery. If there are signs of TS and, particularly, if stenosis is demonstrated by cardiac catheterization and two-dimensional echocardiography, the tricuspid valve is directly visualized at operation with the anticipation of performing commissurotomy or valve replacement. Tricuspid valve balloon valvulotomy has been advocated for TS of various etiologies.[83–87] However, severe TR is a common consequence of this procedure, and results are poor when severe TR develops.

When there are signs of severe TR secondary to MS, it is important to document the duration of the regurgitation and the severity and duration of pulmonary artery hypertension. If the TR is severe and long-standing and if there is chronic pulmonary artery hypertension, tricuspid valve surgery is usually indicated. In contrast, if TR and pulmonary artery hypertension are of short duration, mitral valve replacement will usually reduce pulmonary artery pressure in the early postoperative period, and this will result in a decrease in the TR. The use of tricuspid ring valvuloplasty is being performed with increased frequency in both groups of patients.[2]

The appearance of the heart at the time of surgery is helpful in assessing the severity of tricuspid valve disease. A thinned-out RA wall together with moderate-to-marked enlargement of the RA and venae cavae are indications of significant disease. The degree of stenosis and regurgitation can be estimated by palpation through the RA appendage. Intraoperative transesophageal echocardiography (see Chap. 15) provides more precise information as to the degree of residual valvular regurgitation after repair. The American College of Cardiology/American Heart Association guidelines recommendations for surgery of TR are listed in Table 69-4. TS may be treated successfully by commissurotomy, and the procedure may be combined with annuloplasty to correct valve regurgitation. Valve replacement is occasionally necessary if the changes in the leaflets and subvalvular structures are advanced or if severe TR cannot be relieved by annuloplasty. For TR, three basic reconstructive techniques have been described. The first procedure is used widely and consists of plication of the posterior leaflet, thus converting the tricuspid valve into a functionally bicuspid valve.[87,88] De Vega described a second type of annuloplasty that narrows the annulus along the anterior and posterior leaflets with a purse-string suture.[89,90] The third major technique, described by Carpentier et al., consists of placing a carefully sized semiflexible ring along the anterior and posterior aspects of the annulus.[91] It draws in and supports the tissue evenly. Follow-up studies have shown that annular dilatation occurs in these areas rather than along the leaflets.[92]

When the leaflets and subvalvular apparatus are severely deformed, reconstruction may not be feasible. In such cases, replacement is performed with either a mechanical or tissue valve. Anticoagulation with warfarin (see Chap. 62) is generally advisable in patients with tricuspid valve replacement, and therefore the major advantage of a bioprosthetic valve is negated. If a mechanical valve is preferred and the cavity of the RV is not capacious, a low-profile, tilting disk-type prosthesis seems appropriate.

Mild TR does not seem to increase the risk of surgery involving the mitral valve or both aortic and mitral valves. When the TR is moderate to severe, however, the risk of operation is significantly increased. Although long-term improvement in TR after mitral valve replacement alone has been documented, a tricuspid procedure is generally employed in the setting of moderate-to-severe TR to enhance cardiac function in the critical early days after operation.[93] Mitral valve replacement alone does not invariably decrease TR, even several months after operation.[94]

In general, the early and late results of tricuspid annuloplasty have been superior to those of valve replacement. There is a significant incidence of thrombosis with tricuspid prostheses, and the long-term functional results have been less favorable than have been those of aortic and mitral valve replacements.[95] Good early results have been obtained with all three methods of annuloplasty.[96–100] When tricuspid valve replacement is necessary, the 30-day perioperative mortality increases to 15 to 20 percent. Two preoperative factors, severity of edema and mean pulmonary artery pressure, are important predictors of long-term survival.[101] A variety of prostheses have been used for tricuspid valve replacement with variable results.[101–106]

Infective endocarditis of the tricuspid valve is relatively common because of the increased incidence of drug abuse. In general, the treatment of tricuspid valve endocarditis is medical. When septic pulmonary embolization occurs despite intensive antibiotic treatment, tricuspid valve surgery is indicated. Excision of the valve *without replacement* has been recommended, and reinfection of the new valve in intravenous drug users is an important risk.[107] Nevertheless, since valvulectomy alone carries an important risk of heart failure, tricuspid valve replacement has been recommended by others.[108]

The cardiac output is often marginal after tricuspid valve surgery; measurements of cardiac output and pulmonary artery pressure are used to guide postoperative care. Nitroglycerin infused through a central venous catheter is a valuable adjunct in reducing pulmonary artery pressure. Prostaglandin E_1, in combination with pressor agents, may also be employed to treat severe postoperative PH.[109] Intravenous dopamine and dobutamine may be used to enhance myocardial contractility. If cardiac output remains marginal, an intraaortic balloon pump may be used to reduce left-sided pressures. Pulmonary artery balloon counterpulsation has been employed for acute RV failure.[110] The use of a temporary circulatory assist device to bypass the RV may sustain adequate circulation when RV failure is unresponsive to other measures.

Digitalis and diuretics are usually employed for several months after tricuspid valve surgery. For patients with tricuspid valve replacement, warfarin *and* dipyridamole are used as anticoagulants.[111] The additional use of antiplatelet agents in this setting may improve the long-term results.[112] A serious late complication of tilting disk valves in the tricuspid position is thrombosis. Thrombolytic therapy with streptokinase has been used successfully to restore

TABLE 69-4 Recommendations for Surgery for Tricuspid Regurgitation

Indication	Class
Annuloplasty for severe TR and pulmonary hypertension in patients with mitral valve disease requiring mitral valve surgery	I
Valve replacement for severe TR secondary to diseased or abnormal tricuspid valve leaflets not amenable to annuloplasty or repair	IIa
Valve replacement of annuloplasty for severe TR with mean pulmonary artery pressure <60 mmHg when symptomatic	IIa
Annuloplasty for mild TR in patients with pulmonary hypertension secondary to mitral valve disease requiring mitral valve surgery	IIb
Valve replacement or annuloplasty for TR with pulmonary artery systolic pressure <60 mmHg in presence of a normal mitral valve in asymptomatic patients or in symptomatic patients who have not received a trial of diuretic therapy	III

NOTE: TR, tricuspid regurgitation.
SOURCE: From Bonow et al.[1]

valve function.[113] Prophylaxis against infective endocarditis is also required (see Chap. 81).

Pulmonic Valve Disease

Pulmonic valve surgery for acquired disease is performed infrequently. PS on an acquired basis is rare. Although there are a variety of causes of PR, this hemodynamic condition is relatively well tolerated if pulmonary vascular resistance is normal. Pulmonic valve replacement may be performed for acquired conditions, such as carcinoid heart disease and infective endocarditis, but it usually is limited to cases where RV dysfunction has become severe after congenital heart disease surgery[114,115] (see Chaps. 72 and 73). In general, bioprosthetic valves have been preferred because of the tendency for mechanical valve thrombosis in this position. Pulmonic valve surgery is currently performed earlier and more commonly, since RV dysfunction may be present in asymptomatic postoperative patients with PR.[116] Percutaneously placed heart valves are now evaluated as less-invasive alternatives to surgery for treatment of PS and PR.[117]

Infective endocarditis involves the pulmonic valve in about 1 percent of cases seen at autopsy. Isolated pulmonic valve infective endocarditis is even more uncommon but may be the cause of metastatic pulmonary infections. In a review of 28 cases of this entity, the overall mortality rate was 24 percent, with all those treated by operation surviving.[118] Valvulectomy in combination with antibiotic therapy is sometimes the most effective treatment (see Chap. 85).

Multivalvular Disease

Many patients with clinical evidence of combined disease of the mitral and aortic valves have severe and progressive symptoms. Experience indicates that both valves can be replaced, with a hospital mortality rate that is now between 5 and 10 percent.

Commonly, in the presence of aortic and mitral valve disease, repair, rather than replacement, of the stenotic or regurgitant mitral valve can be accomplished (see Chap. 67). Disease of the aortic valve in adults usually requires valve replacement. The combination of aortic valve replacement with mitral valve repair probably decreases symptoms and improves long-term survival. When tricuspid valve replacement is added, the risk of the operation is higher (up to 20 percent), but even then the long-term results are considerably better than the natural history of surgically untreated patients with triple-valve disease. The use of tricuspid annuloplasty rather than replacement has greatly improved the early results of operation in this group.

When hemodynamic derangement is significant at both mitral and aortic valves, the decision to repair or replace both is easily made, and the principles of surgical treatment are the same as when one valve alone requires operation.[119,120]

MULTIVALVULAR SURGERY

Combined MS and AR When mechanical correction is anticipated in predominant MS, balloon mitral valvotomy followed by aortic valve replacement (AVR) obviates the need for double-valve replacement and its higher risk of complications.[121]

Combined MS and TR If the mitral valve anatomy is favorable for percutaneous balloon valvotomy and there is concomitant PH, valvotomy should be performed regardless of symptom status. After successful mitral valvotomy, PH and TR almost always diminish.[122]

If mitral valve surgery is performed, concomitant tricuspid annuloplasty should be considered, especially if there are preoperative signs or symptoms of right-sided heart failure, rather than risking severe, persistent TR, which may necessitate a second operation. However, TR that seems severe on echocardiography but does not cause elevation of RA or RV diastolic pressure will generally improve greatly after mitral valve replacement.

Combined MS and AS If the degree of AS appears to be mild and the mitral valve is acceptable for balloon valvotomy, this should be attempted first. If mitral balloon valvotomy is successful, the aortic valve should then be reevaluated.

Combined AS and MR Noninvasive evaluation should be performed with two-dimensional and Doppler echocardiography to evaluate the severity of both AS and MR. Attention should be paid to LV size, wall thickness and function, LA size, right-heart function, and pulmonary artery pressure. Patients with severe AS and severe MR (with abnormal mitral valve morphology) with symptoms, LV dysfunction, or PH should undergo combined AVR and mitral valve replacement or mitral valve repair. However, in patients with severe AS and lesser degrees of MR, the severity of MR may improve greatly after isolated AVR, particularly when there is normal mitral valve morphology. Intraoperative transesophageal echocardiogram and, if necessary, visual inspection of the mitral valve should be performed at the time of AVR to determine whether additional mitral valve surgery is warranted in such patients.

In patients with mild-to-moderate AS and severe MR in whom surgery on the mitral valve is indicated because of symptoms, LV dysfunction, or PH, preoperative assessment of the severity of AS may be difficult because of reduced forward stroke volume. If the mean aortic valve gradient is greater than 30 mmHg, AVR should be performed.[1] In patients with less severe aortic valve gradients, inspection of the aortic valve and its degree of opening on two-dimensional or transesophageal echocardiogram, as well as visual inspection by the surgeon, may be important in determining the need for concomitant AVR.

References

1. Bonow RO, Carabello B, de Leon AC Jr, et al. ACC/AHA guidelines for the management of patients with valvular heart disease: A report of the American College of Cardiology/American Heart Association Task Force on Practice Guidelines (Committee on Management of Patients with Valvular Heart Disease). *J Am Coll Cardiol* 1998;32:1486–1588 (updated in 2004).
2. Kostucki W, Vandenbossche JL, Friart A, Engbert H. Pulsed Doppler regurgitant flow patterns of normal valves. *Am J Cardiol* 1986;58: 309–313.
2a. Raman SV, Sparks EA, Boudoulas H, Wooley CF. Tricuspid valve disease: Tricuspid valve complex perspective. *Curr Probl Cardiol* 2002;27:103–142.
3. Sahn DJ, Maciel BC. Physiological valvular regurgitation: Doppler echocardiography and the potential for iatrogenic heart disease. *Circulation* 1988;78:1075–1077.
4. Yoshida K, Yoshikawa J, Shakudo M. Color Doppler evaluation of valvular regurgitation in normals. *Circulation* 1988;78:840–847.
5. McMichael J, Shillingford JP. The role of valvular incompetence in heart failure. *BMJ* 1957;1:537–542.
5a. Navare SM, Gemayel CY, Taub C, et al. Degree of pulmonary hypertension predicts the severity of functional tricuspid regurgitation: New findings based on invasive measurements of pulmonary artery pressure. *J Am Coll Cardiol* 2003;41(6 Suppl B): 446–447.
6. Waller BF, Howard J, Fess S. Pathology of tricuspid valve stenosis and pure TR: III. *Clin Cardiol* 1995;18:225–230.
7. Waller BF, Howard J, Fess S. Pathology of tricuspid valve stenosis and pure TR: I. *Clin Cardiol* 1995;18:97–102.
8. Waller BF, Howard J, Fess S. Pathology of tricuspid valve stenosis and pure TR: II. *Clin Cardiol* 1995;18:167–174.
9. Glancy DL, Marcus FI, Cuadra M, et al. Isolated organic tricuspid valvular regurgitation. *Am J Med* 1969;46:989–996.
10. Nishimura RA, Smith HC, Gersh BJ. TR after myocardial infarction. *Am J Cardiol* 1994;74:308.
11. Szyniszewski AM, Carson PE, Sakwa M, et al. Valve replacement for TR appearing late after healing of left ventricular posterior wall and right ventricular acute myocardial infarction. *Am J Cardiol* 1994;73:616–617.
12. Chiu WC, Shindler DM, Scholz PM, Boyarsky AH. Traumatic TR with cyanosis: Diagnosis by transesophageal echocardiography. *Ann Thorac Surg* 1996;63:992–993.
13. Chataline A, Agnew TM, Graham KJ, et al. Blunt chest trauma of the heart. *NZ Med J* 1999;112:334–336.
14. Aziz TM, Burgess MI, Rahman AN, et al. Risk factors for tricuspid valve after orthotopic heart transplantation. *Ann Thorac Surg* 1999;68:1247–1251.
15. Soga J, Yakyura Y, Osaka M. Carcinoid syndrome: A statistical evaluation of 748 reported cases. *J Exp Clin Cancer Res* 1999;18:133–141.
16. Edwards JE. The spectrum and clinical significance of tricuspid regurgitation. *Pract Cardiol* 1980;6:86–90.
17. Chockalingam A, Gnanavelu G, Elangovan S, Chockalingam V. Clinical spectrum of chronic rheumatic heart disease in India. *J Heart Value Dis* 2003;12(5):577–581.
18. Perloff JK, Harvey WP. Clinical recognition of tricuspid stenosis. *Circulation* 1960;22:346–364.
19. Kitchin A, Turner R. Diagnosis and treatment of tricuspid stenosis. *Br Heart J* 1964;26:354–379.
20. Edwards JE. The spectrum and clinical significance of TR. *Pract Cardiol* 1980;6:86–90.
21. Roguin A, Reinkerich D, Milo S, et al. Long-term follow-up of patients with severe rheumatic tricuspid stenosis. *Am Heart J* 1998;136:103–108.
22. Flammang D, Jaumin P, Kremer R. Organic tricuspid pathology in rheumatic valvulopathies. *Acta Cardiol* 1975;30:155–170.
22a. Henein MY, O'Sullivan CA, Li W, et al. Evidence for rheumatic valve disease in patients with severe tricuspid regurgitation long after mitral valve surgery: The role of 3D echo reconstruction. *J Heart Valve Dis* 2003;2:566–572.

23. Pellikka PA, Tajik AJ, Khandheria BK, et al. Carcinoid heart disease: Clinical and echocardiographic spectrum in 74 patients. *Circulation* 1993;87:1188–1196.

24. Cheitlin MD, MacGregor J. Acquired tricuspid and pulmonic valve disease. In: Rahimtoola SH, ed. *Atlas of Heart Diseases: Valvular Heart Disease.* St. Louis: Mosby;1997:11.2–1.

25. Ludwig J. Cardiac vein involvement in carcinoid syndrome: Possible evidence of retrograde blood flow in cardiac veins in tricuspid insufficiency. *Am J Clin Pathol* 1971;55:617–623.

26. McMichael J, Shillingford JP. The role of valvular incompetence in heart failure. *Br Med J* 1957;1:537–541.

27. Boucek RJ Jr, Graham TP, Morgan JP, et al. Spontaneous resolution of massive congenital tricuspid insufficiency. *Circulation* 1976;54:795–800.

28. Ajayi AA, Adigun AQ, Ojofeitim EO, et al. Arthrometric evaluation of cachexia in chronic congestive heart failure: The role of TR. *Int J Cardiol* 1999;71:79–84.

29. Collins R, Daly JJ. Tricuspid incompetence complicating acute myocardial infarction. *Postgrad Med J* 1977;53:51–52.

30. Zone DD, Botti RE. Right ventricular infarction with tricuspid insufficiency and chronic right heart failure. *Am J Cardiol* 1976;37: 445–448.

31. McAllister RG Jr, Friesinger GC, Sinclair-Smith BC. TR following inferior myocardial infarction. *Arch Intern Med* 1976;95:95–99.

32. Maranhao V, Gooch AS, Yang SS, et al. Prolapse of the tricuspid leaflets in the systolic murmur-click syndrome. *Cath Cardiovasc Diagn* 1975;1:81–90.

33. Gerry JL Jr, Bulkley BH, Hutchins GM. Rupture of the papillary muscle of the tricuspid valve: A complication of cardiopulmonary resuscitation and a rare cause of tricuspid insufficiency. *Am J Cardiol* 1977;40:825–828.

34. Jahnke EJ Jr, Nelson WP, Aaby GV, FitzGibbon GM. Tricuspid insufficiency: The result of nonpenetrating cardiac trauma. *Arch Surg* 1967;95:880–886.

35. VanGilder JE, Jain AC, Weiss RB, et al. Traumatic right ventricular aneurysm presenting as TR. *WV Med J* 1979;75:93–98.

36. Stephenson LW, MacVaugh H III, Kastor JA. Tricuspid valvular incompetence and rupture of the ventricular septum caused by nonpenetrating trauma. *J Thorac Cardiovasc Surg* 1979;77:768–772.

37. Williams MJ, Lee MY, DiSalvo TG, et al. Biopsy-induced flail tricuspid leaflet and TR following orthotopic cardiac transplantation. *Am J Cardiol* 1996;77:1339–1344.

38. Hausen B, Albes JM, Rohde R, et al. Tricuspid valve regurgitation attributable to endomyocardial biopsies and rejection in heart transplantation. *Ann Thorac Surg* 1995;59:1134–1140.

39. Marvin RF, Schrank JP, Nolan SP. Traumatic tricuspid insufficiency. *Am J Cardiol* 1973;32:723–727.

40. Brandenburg RO, McGoon DC, Campeau L, Giuliani ER. Traumatic rupture of the chordae tendineae of the tricuspid valve: Successful repair twenty-four years later. *Am J Cardiol* 1966;18:911–915.

41. Morgan JR, Forker AD. Isolated tricuspid insufficiency. *Circulation* 1971;43:559–564.

42. Croxson MS, O'Brien KP, Lowe JB. Traumatic TR: Long-term survival. *Br Heart J* 1971;33:750–755.

43. Grubier M, Denis B, Martin-Noel O. Les ruptures de cordages tricuspidiens. *Coeur Med Int* 1976;15:215–222.

44. Espino Vela J, Contreras R, Rustrian Rosa F. Rheumatic pulmonary valve disease. *Am J Cardiol* 1969;23:12–18.

45. Roberts WC, Buchbinder NA. Right-sided valvular infective endocarditis. *Am J Med* 1972;53:7–19.

46. Levitt MA, Snoey ER, Tamkin GW, Gee G. Prevalence of cardiac value anomalies in afebril injection drug users. *Acad Emerg Med* 1999; 9:911–915.

47. Seymour J, Emanuel R, Patterson N. Acquired pulmonary stenosis. *Br Heart J* 1968;30:776–785.

48. Rossignol B, Machecourt J, Denis B, et al. Cardiopathie carcinoide secondaire a une tumeur du grêle: A propos d'un cas associat insuffisance tricuspidienne et insuffisance pulmonaire. *Arch Mal Coeur Vaiss* 1977;70:1221–1226.

49. Roberts WC, Virmani R. Aschoff bodies at necropsy in valvular heart disease. *Circulation* 1978;57:803–815.

50. Clausen BJ. Rheumatic heart disease: An analysis of 796 cases. *Am Heart J* 1940;20:454–474.

51. Wilson MG, Lubschez R. Longevity in rheumatic fever. *JAMA* 1948;138:794–798.

52. Bland EF, Jones TD. Rheumatic fever and rheumatic heart disease: A twenty-year report on 1000 patients followed since childhood. *Circulation* 1951;4:836–843.

53. Roberts WC, Honig HS. The spectrum of cardiovascular disease in the Marfan's syndrome: A clinico-pathologic study of 18 necropsy patients and comparison to 151 previously reported patients. *Am Heart J* 1982;104:115–135.

54. Hansing CE, Rowe GG. Tricuspid insufficiency: A study of hemodynamics and pathogenesis. *Circulation* 1972;45:793–799.

55. Killip T, Lukas DS. Tricuspid stenosis: Physiologic criteria for diagnosis and hemodynamic abnormalities. *Circulation* 1957;16:3–13.

56. El-Sherif N. Rheumatic tricuspid stenosis: A hemodynamic correlation. *Br Heart J* 1971;33:16–31.

57. Holmes JC, Flowler NO, Kaplan S. Pulmonary valvular insufficiency. *Am J Med* 1968;44:851–862.

58. Rackley CE, Bechar VS, Whalen RE, McIntosh HD. Biplane cineangiographic determinations of left ventricular function: Pressure-volume relationships. *Am Heart J* 1967;74:766–779.

59. Baxley WA, Dodge HT, Rackley CE, et al. Left ventricular mechanical efficiency in man with heart disease. *Circulation* 1977;55:564–568.

60. Jones JW, Rackley CE, Bruce RA, et al. Left ventricular volumes in valvular heart disease. *Circulation* 1964;29:887–891.

61. Kern MJ, Aguirre F, Donohue T, Bach R. Interpretation of cardiac pathophysiology from pressure waveform analysis: Multivalvular regurgitant lesions. *Catheter Cardiovasc Diagn* 1993;28:167–172.

62. Rousseau MF, Pouleur H, Charlier AA, Bruseur LA. Assessment of left ventricular relaxation in patients with valvular regurgitation. *Am J Cardiol* 1982;50:1028–1036.

63. Salazar E, Levine HD. Rheumatic TR: The clinical spectrum. *Am J Med* 1962;33:111–129.

64. Terzaki AK, Cokkinos DV, Leachman RD, et al. Combined mitral and aortic valve disease. *Am J Cardiol* 1970; 25:588–601.

65. Rivero Carvallo JM. El diagnostica de la estenosis tricuspides. *Arch Inst Cardiol Mex* 1950;20:1–11.

66. Killip T, Lukas DS. Tricuspid stenosis: Clinical features in twelve cases. *Am J Med* 1958;24:836–852.

67. DePace NL, Ross J, Ashandrian AS, et al. TR: Noninvasive techniques for determining causes and severity. *J Am Coll Cardiol* 1984;3: 1540–1550.

68. Meltzer RS, van Hoogenhuyze D, Serruys PW, et al. Diagnosis of TR by contrast echocardiography. *Circulation* 1981;63:1093–1099.

69. Yock PG, Popp RL. Noninvasive estimation of right ventricular systolic pressure by Doppler ultrasound in patients with TR. *Circulation* 1984;70:657–662.

70. Waggoner AD, Quinones MA, Young JB, et al. Pulsed Doppler echocardiographic detection of right-sided valve regurgitation: Experimental results and clinical significance. *Am J Cardiol* 1981;47: 279–286.

71. Masuyama T, Kodama K, Kitabatake A, et al. Continuous-wave Doppler echocardiographic detection of pulmonary regurgitation and its application to noninvasive estimation of pulmonary artery pressure. *Circulation* 1986;74:484–492.

72. Isobe M, Yazaki Y, Takaku F, et al. Prediction of pulmonary arterial pressure in adults by pulsed Doppler echocardiography. *Am J Cardiol* 1986;57:316–321.

73. Chan KL, Currie PJ, Seward JB, et al. Comparison of three Doppler ultrasound methods in the prediction of pulmonary artery pressure. *J Am Coll Cardiol* 1987;9:549–554.

74. Ogawa S, Hayashi J, Sasaki H, et al. Evaluation of combined valvular prolapse syndrome by two-dimensional echocardiography. *Circulation* 1982;65:174–180.

75. Otto CM, Pearlman AS, Comens KA, et al. Determination of the stenotic aortic valve area in adults using Doppler echocardiography. *J Am Coll Cardiol* 1986;7:509–517.

76. Smith MD, Handshoe R, Handshoe S, et al. Comparative accuracy of two-dimensional echocardiography and Doppler pressure half-time methods in assessing severity of mitral stenosis in patients with and without prior commissurotomy. *Circulation* 1986;78:100–107.

77. Perry GJ, Helmcke F, Nanda NC, et al. Evaluation of aortic insufficiency by Doppler color flow mapping. *J Am Coll Cardiol* 1987;9:952–959.

78. Enriquez-Serano M, Bailey KP, Seward JB, et al. Quantitative Doppler assessment of valvular regurgitation. *Circulation* 1993;87:841–848.

79. Packer DL, Stevens CL, Curley MG, et al. Intracardiac phased-array imaging: Methods and initial clinical experience with high resolution, under blood visualization: Initial experience with intracardiac phased-array ultrasound. *J Am Coll Cardiol* 2002;39(3):509–516.

80. Winzelberg GG, Boucher CA, Pohost GM, et al. Right ventricular function in aortic and mitral valve disease: Relation of gated first-pass radionuclide angiography to clinical and hemodynamic findings. *Chest* 1981;79:520–528.

81. Cha SD, Gooch AS, Maranhao V. Intracardiac phonocardiography in TR: Relation to clinical and angiographic findings. *Am J Cardiol* 1981;48:573–583.

82. Rackley CE. Quantitative evaluation of left ventricular function by radiographic techniques. *Circulation* 1976;54:862–879.

83. Patel TM, Sani SI, Shah SC, Patel TK. Tricuspid balloon valvuloplasty: A more simplified approach using Inoue balloon. *Cath Cardiovasc Diagn* 1996;37:86–88.

84. Kratz J. Evaluation and management of tricuspid valve disease. *Cardiol Clin* 1991;9:397–407.

85. Orbe LC, Sobrino N, Arcas R, et al. Initial outcome of percutaneous balloon valvuloplasty in rheumatic tricuspid valve stenosis. *Am J Cardiol* 1993;71:353–354.

86. Onate A, Alcibar J, Inguanzo R, et al. Balloon dilatation of tricuspid and pulmonary valves in carcinoid heart disease. *Tex Heart Inst J* 1993;20:115–119.

87. Kay JH, Maselli-Campagna G, Tsuji HK. Surgical treatment of tricuspid insufficiency. *Ann Surg* 1965;162:53–58.

88. Boyd AD, Engelman RM, Isom OW, et al. Tricuspid annuloplasty: Five and one-half years' experience with 78 patients. *J Thorac Cardiovasc Surg* 1974;68:344–351.

89. De Vega NF. La annulplastia selectiva: Reguable y permanente. *Rev Esp Cardiol* 1972;25:55–60.

90. Abe T, Tsukamoto M, Morishita K, et al. 1989: De Vega's annuloplasty for acquired tricuspid disease: Early and late results in 110 patients, updated in 1996. *Ann Thorac Surg* 1996;62:1876–1877.

91. Carpentier A, Deloche A, Hanania G, et al. Surgical management of acquired tricuspid valve disease. *J Thorac Cardiovasc Surg* 1974;67:53–65.

92. Deloche A, Guerino J, Fabiani JN, et al. Étude anatomique des valvulopatheis rheumatismales tricuspidiennes. *Ann Chir Thorac Cardiovasc* 1973;44:343–349.

93. Braunwald NS, Ross J, Morrow AG. Conservative management of TR in patients undergoing mitral valve replacement. *Circulation* 1967;35(suppl 1):163–169.

94. Simon R, Oelert H, Borst HG, Lichtelen PR. Influence of mitral valve surgery on tricuspid incompetence concomitant with mitral valve disease. *Circulation* 1980;62:1152–1157.

95. Thorburn CW, Morgan JJ, Shanahan MX, Chang VP. Long-term results of tricuspid valve replacement and the problem of prosthetic valve thrombosis. *Am J Cardiol* 1983;51:1128–1132.

96. Grondin P, Meere C, Limet R, et al. Carpentier's annulus and De Vega's annuloplasty: The end of the tricuspid challenge. *J Thorac Cardiovasc Surg* 1975;70:852–861.

97. Kay JH, Mendez AM, Zubiate P. A further look at tricuspid annuloplasty. *Ann Thorac Surg* 1976;22:498–500.

98. Peterffy A, Jonasson R, Szamosi A, Henze A. Comparison of Kay's and De Vega's annuloplasty in surgical treatment of tricuspid incompetence. *Scand J Thorac Cardiovasc Surg* 1980;14:249–255.

99. Rabago G, De Vega NG, Castillon L, et al. The new De Vega technique in tricuspid annuloplasty: Results in 150 patients. *J Cardiovasc Surg* 1980;21:231–238.

100. Reed GE, Boyd AD, et al. Operative management of TR. *Circulation* 1976;54(suppl 3):III96–III98.

101. Baughman K, Kallman C, Yurchak P, et al. Predictors of survival after tricuspid surgery. *Am J Cardiol* 1984;54:137–141.

102. Breye RH, McClenathan JH, Michaelis LL, et al. TR: A comparison of nonoperative management, tricuspid annuloplasty, and tricuspid valve replacement. *J Thorac Cardiovasc Surg* 1976;72:867–874.

103. Jugdutt BI, Fraser RS, Lee SJK, et al. Long-term survival after tricuspid valve replacement: Results with seven different prostheses. *J Thorac Cardiovasc Surg* 1977;74:20–27.

104. Kouchoukos NT, Stephenson LW. Indications for and results of tricuspid valve replacement. *Adv Cardiol* 1976;17:199–206.

105. Sanfelippo PM, Giuliani ER, Danielson GK, et al. Tricuspid valve prosthetic replacement: Early and late results with the Starr-Edwards prosthesis. *J Thorac Cardiovasc Surg* 1976;71:441–445.

106. Singh AK, Christian FD, Williams DO, et al. Follow-up assessment of St. Jude medical prosthetic valve in the tricuspid position: Clinical and hemodynamic results. *Ann Thorac Surg* 1984;37:324–327.

107. Arbulu A, Asfaw I. Tricuspid valvulectomy without prosthetic replacement: Ten years of clinical experience. *J Thorac Cardiovasc Surg* 1981;82:684–691.

108. Stern H, Sisto D, Strom J, et al. Immediate tricuspid valve replacement for endocarditis. *J Thorac Cardiovasc Surg* 1986;91:163–167.

109. D'Ambra M, LaRaia P, Philbin D, et al. Prostaglandin E1: A new therapy for refractory right heart failure and PH after mitral valve replacement. *J Thorac Cardiovasc Surg* 1985;89:567–572.

110. Miller DD, Moreno-Cabral RJ, Stinson EB, et al. Pulmonary artery balloon counterpulsation for acute right ventricular failure. *J Thorac Cardiovasc Surg* 1980;80:760–763.

111. Cannegieter SC, Rosendaal FR, Wintzen AR, et al. Optimal oral anticoagulant therapy in patients with mechanical heart valves. *N Engl J Med* 1995;333:11–17.

112. Chesebro JH, Fuster V, Elveback LR, et al. Trial of combined warfarin plus dipyridamole of aspirin therapy in prosthetic heart valve replacement: Danger of aspirin compared with dipyridamole. *Am J Cardiol* 1983;51:1537–1541.

113. Boskovic D, Elezovic I, Boskovic D, et al. Late thrombosis of the Björk-Shiley tilting disc valve in the tricuspid position. *J Thorac Cardiovasc Surg* 1986;91:1–8.

114. DePace NL, Iskandrian AS, Morganroth J, et al. Infective endocarditis involving a presumably normal pulmonic valve. *Am J Cardiol* 1984;53:385–387.

115. Misbach GA, Turley K, Ebert PA. Pulmonary valve replacement for regurgitation after repair of tetralogy of Fallot. *Ann Thorac Surg* 1983;36:684–691.

116. Bonhoeffer P, Boudjemline Y, Qureshi SA, et al. Percutaneous insertion of the pulmonary valve. *J Am Coll Cardiol* 2002;39(10):1664–1669.

117. Wessel HU, Cunningham WJ, Paul MH, et al. Exercise performance in tetralogy of Fallot after intracardiac repair. *J Thorac Cardiovasc Surg* 1980;80:582–593.

118. Cassling R, Rogler W, McManus B. Isolated pulmonic valve infective endocarditis: A diagnostically elusive study. *Am Heart J* 1985;109:558–567.

119. Stephenson LW, Edic RN, Harken AH, Edmunds H Jr. Combined aortic and mitral valve replacement: Changes in practice and prognosis. *Circulation* 1984;69:640–644.

120. Kumar AS, Chander H, Trehan H. Surgical technique of multiple valve replacement with biological valves. *J Heart Valve Dis* 1995;4:45–46.

121. Blackstone EH, Kirklin JW. Death and other time-related events after valve replacement. *Circulation* 1985;72:753–767.

122. Skudicky D, Essop MR, Sareli P. Efficacy of mitral balloon valvotomy in reducing the severity of associate tricuspid valve regurgitation. *Am J Cardiol* 1994;73:209–211.

CLINICAL PERFORMANCE OF PROSTHETIC HEART VALVES

Gary L. Grunkemeier / Albert Starr / Shahbudin H. Rahimtoola

There are two classes of prosthetic heart valves (PHVs): *mechanical prostheses,* with rigid, manufactured occluders, and *biological* or *tissue valves,* with flexible leaflets of animal or human origin. There are several types of mechanical valves, depending on whether the occluding mechanism is (1) a reciprocating ball, (2) one tilting disk, or (3) two semicircular leaflets. The origin of a biological valve is from (1) the patient, (2) another human, or (3) another species. For each type there are several models available from different manufacturers.

PROSTHETIC HEART VALVES

Mechanical Valves

BALL VALVES
The first successful valve replacement devices, which led to long-term survivors, used a ball-in-cage design[1,2]; the PHV that has endured until today is the *Starr-Edwards* valve (Fig. 70-1, Plate 93).

DISK VALVES
The *Björk-Shiley* valve, introduced in 1969, has evolved through several models. One model, the Convexo-Concave (CC), introduced a structural failure mode caused by strut fracture. Results with the discontinued CC model are included because many patients are still alive with these valves. The *Medtronic Hall* valve has been used clinically since 1977 and the *OmniCarbon* valve since 1984.

BILEAFLET VALVES
The *St. Jude Medical* valve based on the bileaflet design was introduced in 1977 (Fig. 70-2A). Unlike the free-floating occluders in ball and disk valves, the two semicircular leaflets of a bileaflet valve are connected to the orifice housing by a hinge mechanism. The leaflets swing apart during opening, creating three flow areas: one central and two peripheral. Several newer bileaflet valves are available, including the *Carbomedics* valve (introduced in 1986; Fig. 70-2B), ATS Open Pivot (1992), On-X (1996), and Mira (1998).

Biological Valves

Biological valves include a wide variety of types:

1. An *autograft* valve is translocated within the same individual—the patient's pulmonary valve into the aortic valve position.
2. A *homograft* (or allograft) valve is transplanted from another human—a donor's aortic or pulmonary valve is placed into a recipient's aortic or pulmonary position.
3. A *heterograft* (or xenograft) valve is transplanted from another species—either an intact valve (a porcine aortic valve) or a valve fashioned from heterologous tissue (bovine pericardium).

The reason for using biological valves was to reduce or eliminate the need for anticoagulation, but it introduced the problem of structural valve deterioration (SVD). The first successful biological valves were homografts, pioneered by Ross[3] and Barratt-Boyes[4] in the early 1960s.

AUTOGRAFT
The pulmonary autograft procedure consists of an autotransplant of the pulmonary valve to the aortic position; the pulmonary valve is then replaced by an aortic or pulmonary homograft or bioprosthesis. It is technically a much more demanding procedure. This procedure, named after Ross who described it in 1967,[5] may be ideal for very young patients, but uses double-valve replacement to solve a single-valve problem. Ross believes the procedures performed today are very different from what he described, therefore, he feels the procedure should be called the Ross principle.[6]

HOMOGRAFT
Homograft valve replacement, is a more technically demanding operation. It achieves excellent hemodynamics, eliminates the need for anticoagulation, and has low thrombogenicity but is not free of the problem of SVD. Three surgical techniques can be used for aortic valve replacement: (1) replacement of the valve only into the subcoronary position, (2) complete aortic root replacement with reimplantation of the coronary arteries, and (3) miniroot replacement with part of the donor aortic wall inserted within the host aorta.

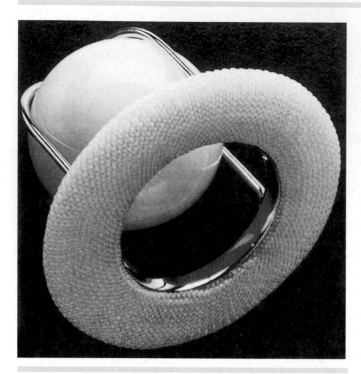

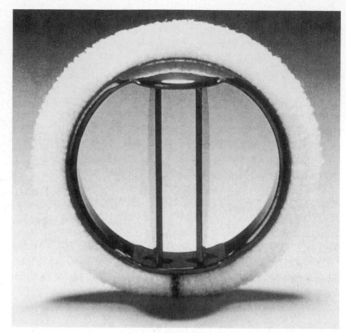

A

FIGURE 70-1 (Plate 93) Starr-Edwards caged ball valve. The ball is a silicone rubber polymer, impregnated with barium sulfate for radiopacity, which oscillates in a cage of cobalt-chromium alloy. When the valve opens, blood flows through the circular primary orifice and a secondary orifice between the ball and the housing. In the aortic position, there is a tertiary orifice between the ball and the aortic wall.

PORCINE HETEROGRAFT

Glutaraldehyde sterilizes valve tissue, renders it bioacceptable, and stabilizes the collagen cross-links for durability. The use of glutaraldehyde for tissue preservation was pioneered by Carpentier and associates,[7] who introduced the term *bioprosthesis* [8] for nonviable valves of biological origin, such as the porcine and pericardial valves.

Most porcine valves are mounted on rigid or flexible stents (Fig. 70-3, Plate 94), to which the leaflets and the sewing ring are attached. Unstented versions have also been devised by several manufacturers. Their goal was to achieve some of the potential benefit of a homograft valve, especially the hemodynamics with an easily available commercial product. They still use a porcine valve, however, which has the problem of SVD that is within the range of earlier stented valves,[9] indicating a porcine valve is a porcine valve. As with homografts, there are potentially three ways of implanting a stentless porcine valve. The stentless St. Jude Medical TSPV (Fig. 70-4A, Plate 95), Medtronic Freestyle (Fig. 70-4B, Plate 95), and Edwards Prima Plus (Plate 96) are available.

BOVINE PERICARDIAL VALVE

Biological valves that are constructed from bovine pericardium and sewn into a valvular configuration open more completely than does a porcine aortic valve, providing better hemodynamics. They also appear to be more durable, because there is extra tissue to allow for shrinkage and a higher percentage of collagen to cross-link during fixation. The first commercially available pericardial valves (Ionescu-Shiley, Hancock) had a high rate of SVD early and were taken off the market. These failures were due to design aspects rather than to an intrinsic problem with pericardial tissue. The Carpentier-Edwards Perimount pericardial valve (Fig. 70-5) uses a unique

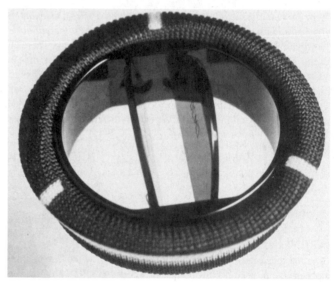

B

FIGURE 70-2 Bileaflet valves. The St. Jude Medical valve (*A*) has leaflets that open to an angle of 85° from the plane of the orifice and travel from 55° to 60° to the fully closed position, depending on valve size. The original version, whose housing did not rotate within the sewing ring, has been supplemented by a model that does rotate for intraoperative adjustment. The Carbomedics valve (*B*) has flat leaflets that open to 78° to 80° and close at an angle of 25° with the horizontal and has a carbon-coated surface on the sewing ring to inhibit thrombus formation.

method of construction that overcomes these design issues. It has been used clinically since 1982 and was approved by the Food and Drug Administration (FDA) in 1991 for the aortic position and in 2000 for the mitral position.

REPAIR

When possible, mitral valve repair[10] is generally preferable to mitral replacement.

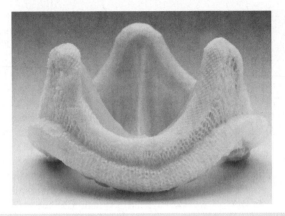

FIGURE 70-3 (Plate 94) Stented porcine valves. The Carpentier-Edwards Supra Annular Valve is designed to be implanted above rather than within the aortic annulus. It has low-pressure fixation and a cone-shaped stent, which flares out at the top to improve leaflet durability.

GUIDELINES FOR REPORTING CLINICAL RESULTS

The reporting of clinical results of heart valves has evolved since the first successful implants in 1960. As long-term experience accumulated, the need to analyze time-related events resulted in the use of actuarial analysis,[11] constant hazard ("linearized") rates,[12] Cox regression,[13] and multivariable parametric models.[14] The effectiveness of these statistical methods in comparing results from different series, however, is limited by the lack of standardization in definitions and follow-up methods.

AATS/STS Guidelines for Clinical Reporting

Standards that specified which complications should be collected and how they should be defined were proposed by a joint committee of the American Association for Thoracic Surgery (AATS) and the Society of Thoracic Surgeons (STS) in 1988, and were revised in 1996[15] as follows:

1. *Structural valvular deterioration,* or any change in function of an operated valve resulting from an intrinsic abnormality that causes stenosis or regurgitation.
2. *Nonstructural dysfunction,* a composite category that includes any abnormality that results in stenosis or regurgitation of the operated valve that is not intrinsic to the valve itself, exclusive of thrombosis and infection. This includes inappropriate sizing, which is called *valve prosthesis-patient mismatch (VP-PM).*[16]
3. *Valve thrombosis* is any thrombus, in the absence of infection, attached to or near an operated valve that occludes part of the blood flow path or that interferes with the function of the valve.
4. *Embolism* is any embolic event that occurs in the absence of infection after the immediate perioperative period. These include any new, temporary or permanent, focal or global neurologic deficits and peripheral embolic events; emboli proven to consist of nonthrombotic material are excluded.
5. *Bleeding* is any episode of major internal or external bleeding that causes death, hospitalization, or permanent injury (e.g., vision loss) or requires transfusion. This applies to all patients, whether or not they are taking anticoagulant or antiplatelet drugs.
6. *Operated valvular endocarditis* is any infection involving an operated valve. Morbidity associated with active infection—such as valve thrombosis, thrombotic embolus, bleeding event, or par-

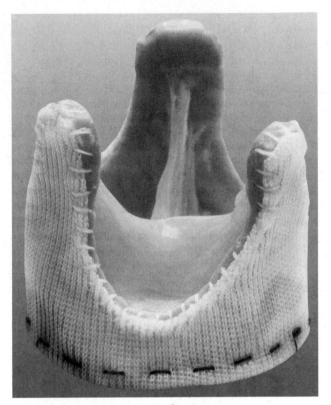

A

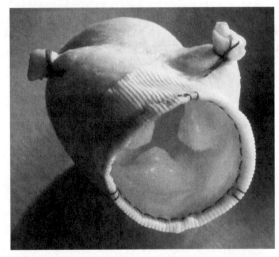

B

FIGURE 70-4 (Plate 95) St. Jude Toronto SPV (*A*) and Medtronic Freestyle (*B*) stentless porcine valves. The Toronto SPV is designed to be used as a subcoronary valve replacement. The Freestyle can be implanted using any of the methods of implantation used for homografts: subcoronary implantation of the valve alone, aortic root replacement, or cylinder (root) inclusion.

avalvular leak—is included under this category but is not included in other categories of morbidity.

The *consequences* of the preceding morbid events include reoperation, valve-related mortality, sudden unexpected unexplained death, cardiac death, total deaths, and permanent valve-related impairment.

FDA Guidelines for New Valve Approvals

In 1994, the FDA issued a guidance document for submission of premarket approval (PMA) applications for heart valves that emphasizes

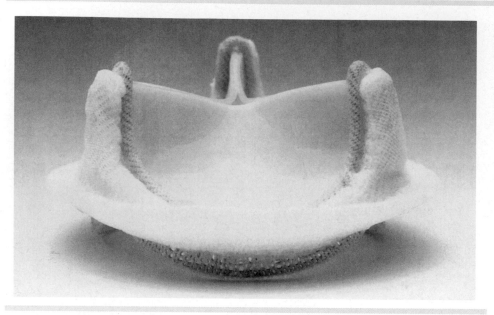

FIGURE 70-5 (Plate 96) The Carpentier-Edwards Perimount pericardial bioprosthesis uses a method of mounting the leaflets to the stent, which does not depend on retaining stitches passed through the pericardium—a design weakness of previous pericardial valves. Instead, the leaflets are anchored behind the stent pillars.

TABLE 70-1 Complications for Evaluating Clinical Performance of Replacement Heart Valves and Objective Performance Criteria (OPC) Values for Complication Rates (Percent/Year)

Definitions of Morbidity	OPC, %/YEAR	
	Mechanical	Biological
1. *Structural deterioration:* Valve deterioration, wear, stress fracture, poppet escape, clacification, leaflet tear, stent creep; *excludes* infected or thrombosed valves		
2. *Nonstructural dysfunction:* Entrapment by pannus or suture, leak, inappropriate sizing, hemolytic anemia; excludes thromboembolism and infection	(leak) 1.2 (major 0.6)	(leak) 1.2 (major 0.6)
3A. *Valve thrombosis:* Thrombosis proved by operation, autopsy, or clinical investigation; *excludes* infection	0.8	0.2
3B. *Thromboembolism:* Neurologic deficit, peripheral arterial emboli, acute myocardial infarction *after* operation in patients with known normal coronary arteries or those <40 years of age; *excludes* septic emboli, hemorrhage, immediate surgical events	3.0	2.5
4. *Anticoagulant-related hemorrhage:* Bleeding that causes death, stroke, operation, hospitalization, or transfusion in patients receiving anticoagulants and/or antiplatelet drugs	3.5 (major 1.5)	1.4 (major 0.9)
5. *Prosthetic valve endocarditis:* Based on blood cultures, clinical signs, and/or histologic evidence at reoperation or autopsy; *includes* valve thrombosis, embolus, or paravalvular leak associated with active infection	1.2	1.2

SOURCE: The complications and their definitions are adapted from Ref. 30, the OPC values are taken from Appendix K of Ref. 35.

confidence interval estimation and comparisons to objective performance criteria (OPC).[17] *OPC are complication rates for critical complications, representing averages achieved by the best currently used valves.* The OPC for complications are given in Table 70-1.

The category SVD was not included in the OPC list because the clinical PMA investigation is not designed to detect intrinsic valve failure. Structural durability should be evaluated by in vitro testing because the clinical realization of structural failure should be so small with mechanical valves that the clinical study is of insufficient size or so long-term with tissue valves that the clinical study is of insufficient duration to assess it adequately.

From the *Nonstructural dysfunction* category, the FDA included only leak, the most common and the most frequently reported subcategory, and derived OPC for major leaks and for all leaks. The FDA separated *Thromboembolism* into the separate categories of valve thrombosis and thromboembolism, and derived OPC both for major *Anticoagulant-related hemorrhage* events and for all bleeding events.

Based on the OPC values given in Table 70-1, the FDA set the minimum amount of follow-up required for a PMA study at 800 valve-years. The assumption of constant risk for heart valve complications, as embodied by the OPC formulation, is only an approximation; but if operative events are excluded and follow-up is of sufficient length, this approximation may be acceptable. However, patients with a disabling stroke and their families do not particularly care if the event occurred operatively or later; therefore, all events must be included in long-term follow-up results.

VALVE-RELATED COMPLICATIONS

In the following comparisons of literature-derived valve comparisons, actuarial valve failure-free curves are used to describe tissue valve durability, and linearized rates are used for all other complications.

Structural Valve Deterioration

There is a dual standard with regard to this serious complication, which almost always results in death or valve explant, but early SVD will remain undiagnosed unless sought for by noninvasive techniques, such as Doppler echocardiography.[18] For biological valves, SVD is probably inevitable if the patient lives long enough, whereas for mechanical valves, the acceptable rate is close to zero.

MECHANICAL VALVES

The SVD of currently used mechanical valves is extremely low and remarkable, given the harsh biological environment in which the valve must perform. For example, SVD of the Starr-Edwards valve is virtually zero after 38 years of follow-up; there were 6 cases in over 1 million patient-years of follow-up for a rate of 0.0005 percent per year.

BIOLOGICAL VALVES

Data on freedom from SVD for series of porcine and pericardial bioprostheses and homografts are shown in Fig. 70-6. The mean age of patients in the older series is about 50 years. The durability of the Carpentier-Edwards pericardial valve appears superior to that of porcine valves (see Fig. 70-6; Table 70-2). The patients in the Carpentier-Edwards pericardial valve series are older than patients in previous series of porcine valves, and it is unknown to what extent this has resulted in the improvement in their durability.

SVD was considered to be lower with *homografts* than it was with other bioprostheses. From various published reports of homografts used in the aortic position, however, it is apparent that the variation among series is wide and the results are not in general better than are those for porcine bioprostheses (see Fig. 70-6). A study from Palka et al.[18] of 570 patients age 48 ± 16 years showed the incidence of SVD detected by Doppler echocardiography at 6.8 years after aortic valve replacement was 72.1 percent.[9]

The pulmonary autograft is considered an excellent aortic valve substitute, especially for young patients and in the treatment of patients with endocarditis, however, it is technically a more difficult procedure. Data from one center which is the only one with follow-up for longer than 10 years showed 48.5 percent freedom from reoperation at 19 years[19] and, after excluding patients from three hospitals, 85 percent freedom from reoperation at 20 years.[20] To evaluate complications of this procedure fully, problems with the valve used to replace the pulmonary valve must be combined with complications of the pulmonary autograft itself. In one study of 144 patients,[21] at a mean follow-up of 4 years, 15 (10 percent) patients had

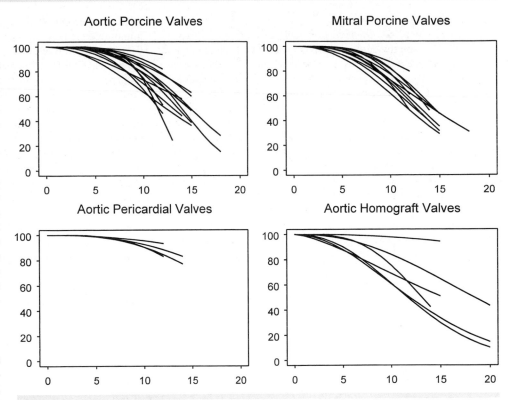

FIGURE 70-6 Structural valve deterioration with four types of biological valves. The vertical axes represent percent freedom from SVD; horizontal axes represent years after implant. These follow-up data relate to studies with minimum follow-up to 400 valve-years and conform to the FDA requirements for each location of valve. (From Grunkemeier et al.[33] Reproduced by permission of the publisher and authors.)

developed peak gradient across the homograft in the pulmonary position measured by magnetic resonance imaging (MRI) of ≥ 30 mmHg (mean 46 ± 18 mmHg) and 4 had to be reoperated. At 7 years, pulmonary homograft stenosis was 20.3 percent and reoperation rate was 3.3 percent. SVD of the pulmonary homograft is "clinically important"[21] and is an early postoperative inflammatory reaction to the pulmonary autograft that leads to extrinsic compression and/or shrinkage.[21] In small children this problem may be mitigated by use of the diseased aortic valve in the pulmonary position within a pericardial tube (unpublished data from Starr Wood Children's Cardiac Center).

TABLE 70-2 14-Year Results with Carpentier-Edwards Pericardial Valve

		FDA-Mandated Patients[a] (n = 267) Actuarial (%)
Thromboembolism/thrombosis		19 ± 4
Anticoagulant-related bleeding		6 ± 2
Endocarditis/sepsis		7 ± 2
Valve dysfunction		70 ± 4
Explant due to structural valve deterioration:	Total	15 ± 3
	≤65 years of age	24 ± 5
	>65 years of age	4 ± 2
Mortality:	Total	60 ± 3.1
	Valve-related	21 ± 3.2

[a]FDA approval was based on 719 patients at 7 years. Data from FDA-mandated longer follow-up of selected patients are from Frater et al.[61]

VALVE REPAIR

Mitral valve repair is considered preferable to replacement, when practicable. It also provides good results for treating bacterial endocarditis[22] and valve problems in elderly patients.[23] It has been suggested that it improves survival; however, there are problems associated with the comparisons (see also Chap. 67).[24]

The weakness of valve repair is durability. The 10-year actuarial reoperation rate has been reported to be 15 percent in nonrheumatic mitral disease.[25] The reoperation rate for patients with rheumatic mitral disease varies from 25 percent reoperation at 5 years[26] to 17 percent at 10 years in a large series in which calcium debridement[27] and anterior leaflet procedures were performed.[28] The reoperation rate at 10 years was 24 percent for patients less than 20 years of age and 9 percent at 10 years for patients over 20 years of age.[29]

The longest follow-up with median follow-up 17 years (range 1 to 29 years) after mitral valve repair for mitral valve prolapse performed from 1970 to 1984 is from Carpentier's group,[30] which excluded patients with ischemic heart disease and those with associated cardiac or vascular procedures. The hospital mortality was 1.9 percent [95 percent confidence interval (CI) 0.5 to 5.7 percent]. The 20 year mortality was 53 percent for the whole group (CI 45 to 61 percent); in those with posterior leaflet involvement only mortality was 54 percent, for anterior leaflet involvement was 54 percent and for involvement of both leaflets 50 percent. The reoperation rate at 20 years for posterior leaflet involvement was 3.1 percent, for anterior leaflet involvement 13.8 percent and for both leaflets involve-

ment 17.4 percent. There is another study of mitral valve repair for mitral regurgitation largely due to degenerative mitral valve.[31] At 5 years, the survival of those without atrial fibrillation was 93 percent (95 percent CI 90 to 97 percent) versus 73 percent (95 percent CI 64 to 82 percent) for patients with atrial fibrillation; patients with atrial fibrillation had many comorbid conditions.[31] However, on multivariate analysis the only predictor of inferior survival was poor left ventricular function, which was assessed *subjectively* from echocardiograms and left ventricular angiograms.

The longest follow-up (up to 29 years) after mitral valve reconstructive surgery for rheumatic mitral regurgitation performed from 1970 to 1994 is also from Carpentier's group,[32] which excluded patients with associated valve lesions, organic tricuspid valve lesions, and those with coronary artery disease. The hospital mortality was 2 percent. At 20 years, survival was 82 ± 18 percent and reoperation rate was 45 percent; the incidence of atrial fibrillation in patients who were in New York Heart Association (NYHA) Functional Classes I & II was 53 and 96 percent, respectively. Early results of aortic valve repair have been published, but further follow-up is needed to assess the long-term results.

Other Valve-Related Complications

A review[33] of a large number of published reports concerning the performance of prosthetic heart valves reveals a wide spread of results for every complication for every valve indicating that *patient-related factors* are very important determinants of complications of PHV.[9,33] In 172 series of heart valves covering 335,485 valve-years accumulated by 63,531 valves, the event rates ranged from 0 to 7.5 percent per year for thromboembolism, 0 to 0.6 percent per year for thrombosis, 0 to 9.3 percent per year for bleeding, 0 to 1.7 percent per year for infection, and 0 to 2.8 percent per year for paravalvular leak.[33] Caution must be exercised in directly comparing event rates among valves for many reasons, including the simplifications involved in the use of linearized rates, varying definitions of complications (many of these reports predate the standardized definitions), and differences in patient characteristics between series.[9,24,33,34]

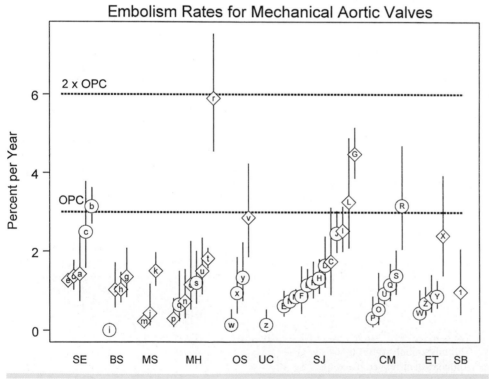

FIGURE 70-7 Embolism rates for mechanical aortic valves. Each open symbol represents a different series, and the height of the symbol is the linearized rate for the series. The vertical bar indicates the 95 percent confidence interval. There is a dashed line at the height of the FDA objective performance criteria (OPC); for approval of a new valve, the upper confidence limit should be less than twice the OPC (*upper dashed line*). Diamonds indicate that both early and late events were used to calculate the rates, circles indicate that only late events were used. Letters inside the symbols correspond to the cited references for the series in the original publication. The series are grouped by valve model, shown below the horizontal axis by two-letter abbreviations: SE, Star-Edwards caged-ball; BS, Björk-Shiley tilting disk; MS, Monostrut tilting disk; MH, Medtronic Hall tilting disk; OS, Omniscience and omnicarbon tilting disk; UC, Ultracor tilting disk; SJ, St. Jude bileaflet; CM, Carbomedics bileaflet; ET, Edwards Tekna and Duromedics bileaflet; SB, Sorin Bicarbon bileaflet. (From Grunkemeier et al.[33] Reproduced by permission of the publisher and authors.)

DIFFICULTIES IN COMPARING PUBLISHED SERIES

The wide variation previously described in reported durability of tissue valves using the same valve also occurs with other complications. Figures 70-7 to 70-10 illustrate the wide range of embolism with use of the same heart valve in different series. This variation must be due to variations between series other than the *valve model*. These include factors associated with the following:

1. *Patients*—age, ventricular function, comorbidities.
2. *Reporting center*—surgical variables, postoperative medical management, method, frequency and thoroughness of follow-up, definitions of complications.
3. Problems with *data analysis*[35,36]—many patient-related factors are known to influence thromboembolism,[24,37] stroke rates in patients with atrial fibrillation and in the elderly are equal to those observed in prosthetic valve series,[38] and standardized definitions[15] were not in effect or were not employed when many of the available series were reported.
4. *Published data*—these reports describe only a small fraction of the valves implanted and are probably not a representative subset.

Several types of bias can affect reported results. As examples, selection bias occurs in the collection and analysis of data and the decision to report them[35]; publication bias describes the fact that published series tend to be those with the best or worst, but not typical results.[39]

Major Randomized Trials

Although randomized studies provide ideal internal validity or valve-specific comparison within centers, they may lack external validity or generalizability to patients outside the study.[40] Randomized trials of heart valves can also have logistic, financial, and ethical problems.[41,42] Consequently, the number of randomized studies of valves is small, and those that exist are of necessity of small size and thus these data must be interpreted along with those from careful observational studies.

The two major randomized clinical trials that have been reported are the Edinburgh Heart Valve Trial[43] and the Veterans Administration (VA) Cooperative Study on Valvular Heart Disease.[44] Both studies compared mechanical valves to porcine bioprostheses. The Edinburgh trial compared the Björk-Shiley Standard valve to porcine valves—initially the Hancock and later the Carpentier-Edwards.[43] It contains actuarial comparisons at 5 and 12 years for the 211 aortic and 261

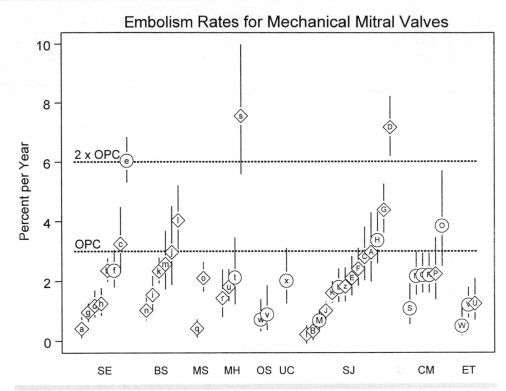

FIGURE 70-8 Embolism rates for mechanical mitral valves. For explanation of symbols and valve model abbreviations, see Fig. 70-7. (From Grunkemeier et al.[33] Reproduced by permission of the publisher and authors.)

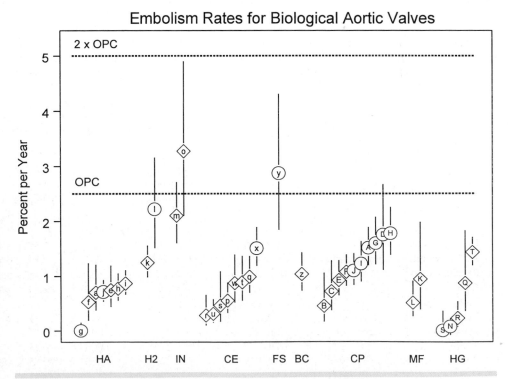

FIGURE 70-9 Embolism rates for biological aortic valves. For explanation of symbols, see Fig. 70-7. Valve model abbreviations: HA, Hancock I and Modified Orifice porcine; H2, Hancock II porcine; IN, Intact porcine; CE, Carpentier-Edwards porcine; FS, Freestyle stentless porcine; BC, Biocor stentless porcine; CP, Carpentier-Edwards Perimount pericardial; MF, Mitroflow pericardial; HG, homograft. (From Grunkemeier et al.[33] Reproduced by permission of the publisher and authors.)

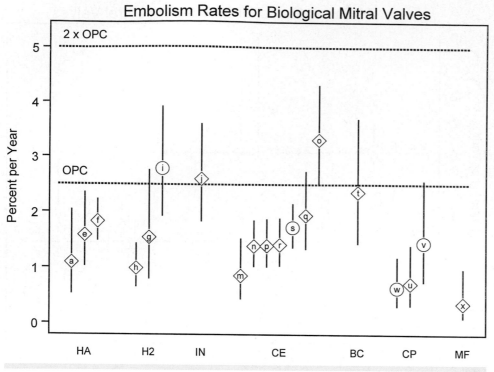

Embolism Rates for Biological Mitral Valves

FIGURE 70-10 Embolism rates for biological mitral valves. For explanation of symbols, see Fig. 70-7. Valve model abbreviations: see Fig. 70-9. (From Grunkemeier et al.[33] Reproduced by permission of the publisher and authors).

long-term findings of this randomized trial are the following: (1) Use of a mechanical valve resulted in a lower mortality and a lower reoperation rate after aortic valve replacement (AVR); (2) The mortality after mitral valve replacement (MVR) was similar with use of the two prosthetic valve types; (3) There were virtually no primary valve failures with use of a mechanical valve; (4) Primary valve failure after AVR and MVR occurred more frequently in patients with a bioprosthetic valve especially in patients aged <65 years; (5) The primary valve failure rate between the bioprosthesis and mechanical valve was not significantly different in those aged ≥65 years; (6) Use of a bioprosthetic valve resulted in a lower bleeding rate; and (7) There were no significant differences between the two valve types with regard to other valve-related complications including thromboembolism, and all complications.

Comparison of the 12- to 15-year actuarial event rates between these two trials[43, 44] showed that the bleeding and thromboembolism rates were higher in the VA study but that reoperation rates were higher in the Edinburgh study. These differences could be partially accounted for by the composition of the two patient populations. The patients in the Edinburgh trial (1) were younger and less heavily anticoagulated and minor bleeding was not recorded for the first 5 years of the trial; (2) included women and those with double-valve replacements; and (3) had a higher percentage of patients in the mitral position than in the VA study. In the VA trial late results show a better survival with mechanical valves than with bioprostheses in the aortic position

mitral valve patients. The authors concluded that survival without reoperation with a mechanical valve was better than it was with the bioprosthetic valve, but that this was somewhat offset by the increased risk of bleeding. It should be noted that bleeding during the first 5 years of follow-up was not included in the results.

The VA trial compared the standard Björk-Shiley valve to the Hancock Modified Orifice (size 21- to 23-mm aortic) or Hancock Standard (other sizes) porcine valves.[44] Table 70-3 contains actuarial comparisons of the endpoint variables at 15 years. The principal

TABLE 70-3 Probability of Death due to Any Cause, Any Valve-Related Complication and Individual Valve-Related Complications 15 Years after Randomization

Outcome Event	AORTIC VALVE REPLACEMENT			MITRAL VALVE REPLACEMENT		
	Mechanical $n = 198$	Bioprosthetic $n = 196$	p	Mechanical $n = 88$	Bioprosthesis $n = 93$	p
Death from any cause	66 ± 3%*	79 ± 3%	0.02	81 ± 4%	79 ± 4%	0.30
Any valve-related complication	65 ± 4%	66 ± 5%	0.26	73 ± 6%	81 ± 5%	0.56
Systemic embolism	18 ± 4%	18 ± 4%	0.66	18 ± 5%	22 ± 5%	0.96
Bleeding	51 ± 4%	30 ± 4%	0.0001	53 ± 7%	31 ± 6%	0.01
Endocarditis	7 ± 2%	15 ± 5%	0.45	11 ± 4%	17 ± 5%	0.37
Valve thrombosis	2 ± 1%	1 ± 1%	0.33	1 ± 1%	1 ± 1%	0.95
Perivalvular regurgitation	8 ± 2%	2 ± 1%	0.09	17 ± 5%	7 ± 4%	0.05
Reoperation	10 ± 3%	29 ± 5%	0.0004	25 ± 6%	50 ± 8%	0.15
Primary valve failure	0 ± 0%	23 ± 5%	0.0001	5 ± 4%	44 ± 8%	0.0002

n = number of patients randomized.
*Values given are actuarial percentages ± standard error.
NOTE: p values are for differences between mechanical and porcine valves.
SOURCE: From Hammermeister et al.[44]

TABLE 70-4 Recommendations for Valve Replacement with a Mechanical Prosthesis

Indication	Class
1. Patients with expected long life spans	I
2. Patients with a mechanical prosthetic valve already in place in a different position than the valve to be replaced	I
3. Patients in renal failure, on hemodialysis, or with hypercalcemia	II
4. Patients requiring warfarin therapy because of risk factors[a] for thromboembolism	IIa
5. Patients ≤65 years for AVR and ≤70 years for MVR[b]	IIa
6. Valve rereplacement for thrombosed biological valve	IIb
7. Patients who cannot or will not take warfarin therapy	III

[a]Risk factors: atrial fibrillation, severe LV dysfunction, previous thromboembolism and hypercoagulable condition.
[b]The age at which patients may be considered for bioprosthetic valves is based on the major reduction in rate of structural valve deterioration after age 65 and the increased risk of bleeding in this age group.
ABBREVIATIONS: AVR = aortic valve replacement; LV = left ventricle; MVR = mitral valve replacement.
SOURCE: ACC/AHA Guidelines,[45] with permission.

TABLE 70-5 Recommendations for Valve Replacement with a Bioprosthesis

Indication	Class
1. Patients who cannot or will not take warfarin therapy	I
2. Patients ≥65 years[a] needing AVR who do not have risk factors for thromboembolism[b]	I
3. Patients considered to have possible compliance problems with warfarin therapy	IIa
4. Patients >70 years[a] needing MVR who do not have risk factors for thromboembolism[b]	IIa
5. Valve rereplacement for thrombosed mechanical valve	IIb
6. Patients <65 years[a]	IIb
7. Patients in renal failure, on hemodialysis, or with hypercalcemia	III
8. Adolescent patients who are still growing	III

[a]The age at which patients should be considered for bioprosthetic valves is based on the major reduction in rate of structural valve deterioration after age 65 and increased risk of bleeding in this age group.
[b]Risk factors: atrial fibrillation, severe LV dysfunction, previous thromboembolism, and hypercoagulable condition.
ABBREVIATION: AVR = aortic valve replacement; LV = left ventricle; MVR = mitral valve replacement.
SOURCE: ACC/AHA Guidelines,[45] with permission.

because of the higher rate of bioprosthetic degeneration (23 versus 0 percent; $p = 0.0001$); there were also a much larger number of patients with AVR than in the Edinburgh trial.

VALVE SELECTION CRITERIA

Because of the wide variation in results among and between various valve models, it is impossible to rank valves within valve types on the basis of complication rates. Some general recommendations, however, can be made with regard to valve selection (Tables 70-4 and 70-5).[45] One review has made recommendations based on age (and therefore rate of SVD) and ability to take warfarin anticoagulant therapy (Fig. 70-11).[9]

RENAL FAILURE

The recommendation for using a mechanical PHV in patients with renal failure because of problems of increased SVD with bioprosthesis has stirred a controversy. The Renal Data System study of 5858 patients on renal dialysis[46] showed that the in-hospital mortality of valve replacement was 20 percent. The mortality with mechanical and bioprosthetic PHV was similar; at 1, 2, 3, 5 and 10 years it was approximately 45, 60, 72, 85, and 95 percent, respectively. Approximately half of the deaths were from cardiac cause, the nature of the cardiac cause is not provided or is the incidence of SVD. Furthermore, the very high mortality that is as high as or higher than that of medical therapy emphasizes that the important issue is not choice of PHV but selection of patients for PHV insertion.

Young Women   For a young woman who needs a PHV and is planning a subsequent pregnancy, the choice is between a mechanical PHV and a bioprosthesis because the incidence of SVD with a homograft is similar to that of a bioprosthesis. In addition, the results

with the autograph using the Ross procedure data beyond 10 years are conflicting. The main disadvantage with mechanical PHV is the need for warfarin and consequent warfarin embryopathy, which is low (0 to 3 percent) with close monitoring of warfarin therapy.[47] With bioprosthesis the incidence of early SVD during pregnancy and shortly after delivery is as high as 24 percent and at 10 years is 55 to 57 percent; moreover, the operative mortality of reoperation for SVD is 3.8 to 8.7 percent.[47] Discontinuing warfarin and substituting intravenous unfractionated heparin in the first 6 to 12 weeks and last 2 weeks of pregnancy reduces the incidence of warfarin embryopathy and of bleeding in the mother and baby during delivery. The data with low molecular weight heparin remains to be defined. The choice of PHV should be a joint decision by the *patient*, cardiologist, and cardiac surgeon (Fig. 70-12).[47]

MANAGEMENT OF PATIENTS WITH PROSTHETIC HEART VALVES

Patients who have undergone valve replacement are *not* cured but still have serious heart disease. They have exchanged native valvular disease for prosthetic valvular disease and must be followed with great care.[48] The clinical course of patients with prosthetic heart valves is influenced by several factors.[49]

Ventricular Dysfunction

Despite relief of valvular obstruction or regurgitation, some patients fail to improve after valve replacement or even deteriorate because of ventricular dysfunction. The cause of dysfunction may be carditis associated with rheumatic disease, myocardial degeneration and

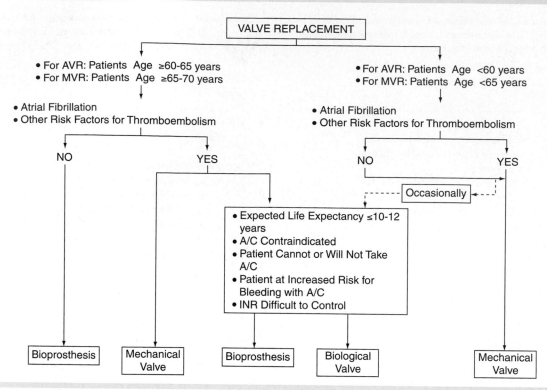

FIGURE 70-11 Suggested recommendation for choice of prosthetic heart valves based on age of the patient and the presence of risk factors. A/C, anticoagulation with warfarin; AVR, aortic valve replacement; INR, international normalized ratio; MVR, mitral valve replacement. (From Rahimtoola.[9])

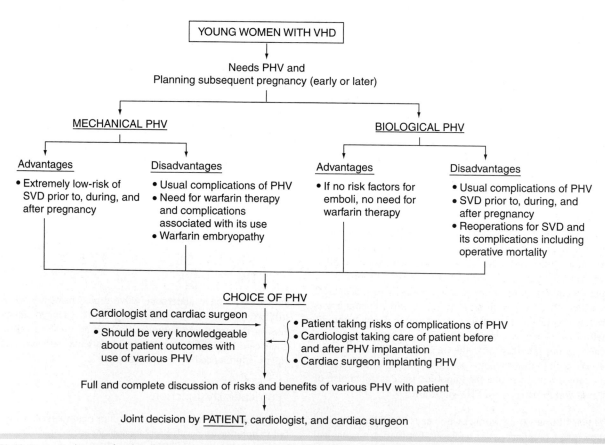

FIGURE 70-12 Factors to be considered in the choice of prosthetic heart valves (PHV) for young women with valvular heart disease (VHD). SVD, structural valve deterioration. (From Hung and Rahimtoola.[47])

fibrosis from long-standing pressure or volume overload, ischemic damage at the time of valve replacement, coronary artery disease (CAD), or other associated diseases such as systemic hypertension or idiopathic dilated cardiomyopathy. Perioperative myocardial damage is an important cause of postoperative ventricular dysfunction.

Other Cardiac Lesions

Cardiac diseases affecting primarily one valve often affect other valves, the conduction system, the coronary arteries, and the pulmonary vasculature. With the exception of pulmonary hypertension and functional tricuspid regurgitation, these disorders usually do not improve after isolated valve replacement. Rheumatic disease typically affects both mitral and aortic valves but not necessarily with the same severity at the same time. Therefore, patients who have mitral valve replacement may subsequently, years later, require aortic valve replacement, or vice versa (Chap. 69). Calcification of the aortic and mitral valve annuli may extend to the conduction system. High-degree or complete atrioventricular block may occur at the time of surgery or during the late postoperative period, requiring pacemaker implantation. CAD is very common in the age range of patients requiring valve replacement (> age 35 years); preoperative coronary arteriography is important.[50,51] Coronary bypass surgery of technically suitable vessels should be performed at the time of valve surgery if the patients have associated significant CAD.

Prosthesis-Related Problems

The incidence of problems with each prosthesis (Table 70-6) was discussed earlier. *Operative mortality* is related to advanced age of patient, NYHA Functional Classes III & IV, increased LV size, LV dysfunction, heart failure, pulmonary hypertension, low cardiac output, and presence of associated diseases. Coronary bypass surgery performed at the same time as valve replacement increases the operative mortality by 50 to 100 percent, which nevertheless is still not high, but associated CAD, if not bypassed, significantly increases both the operative and 10-year mortality.[51] Other very important factors include the occurrence of perioperative myocardial infarction, duration of the operation, aortic cross-clamp time, and whether the patient needed the operation on an elective or emergency basis.

TABLE 70-6 Major Complications of Valve Replacement

1. Operative mortality
2. Perioperative myocardial infarction
3. Prosthetic endocarditis
4. Prosthetic dehiscence
5. Prosthetic dysfunction
   a. Obstruction: Usually thrombotic, occasionally due to item 3, 4, or 8
   b. Regurgitation
   c. Hemolysis
   d. Structural failure
6. Thromboemboli
7. Hemorrhage with anticoagulant therapy
8. Valve prosthesis-patient mismatch
9. Prosthetic replacement often caused by item 3, 4, or 5, occasionally caused by item 6, 7, or 8
10. Late mortality, including sudden, unexplained death

SOURCE: Rahimtoola.[36] Reproduced with permission of the publisher and author.

The risk of *prosthetic endocarditis* is about 3 percent in the first year and 0.5 percent in subsequent years. Infections in the early postoperative period (from 2 to 12 months) are due to hospital-based organisms. Despite therapy, the infections are difficult to cure and have a high mortality (about 80 percent)[52,53]; early reoperation is usually recommended. The mortality rate from late postoperative infection (2 to 12 months or later) is approximately 40 percent[52]; about half the patients can be treated successfully with medications alone. The infected valve should be replaced in patients who do not respond to medical treatment or for other reason (see Chap. 81). The importance of adequate antibiotic prophylaxis for the prevention of endocarditis cannot be overemphasized; the prevention and treatment of prosthetic valve endocarditis are discussed in Chap. 81.

Long-term anticoagulant therapy is associated with *bleeding* episodes. The management of antithrombotic therapy is discussed in Chap. 71.

Prosthetic dehiscence is the result of sutures pulling out of the cardiac tissues. It may result from infection, inadequate surgical technique, or diseased cardiac tissue (e.g., edema, necrosis, or calcification).

Structured valve deterioration is mainly a problem with biological valves. With currently approved mechanical PHV, SVD is comparatively rare. SVD of biological PHV results from leaflet deterioration or calcification; progressive prosthetic regurgitation and/or stenosis is the rule. Bioprosthesis failure is greater in young patients, in elderly with chronic renal insufficiency, and in the mitral position. In young patients (average age <60 years), failure of mitral prostheses usually starts at 5 to 8 years and of aortic prostheses at 8 to 10 years. The incidence of SVD of aortic PHV in those aged ≥60 to 65 years[9,44,45] and of mitral PHV in those aged ≥65 to 70 years is low.[9,44,45]

Red blood cells are fractured by turbulence and contact with foreign surfaces. Some degree of *hemolysis* is present with all mechanical prostheses but not with bioprostheses. Important hemolysis, however, may occur with a perivalvular leak or severe prosthetic obstruction regardless of prosthesis type. Serum lactic dehydrogenase (LDH) is usually the simplest and most reliable index of hemolysis to follow in patients with prosthetic valves. A sudden increase in LDH may indicate prosthesis dysfunction, perivalvular leak, or cloth tear. Iron and folate therapy usually correct the anemia. Valve rereplacement may be required for severe, refractory hemolytic anemia.

Important *systemic embolization* is an unfortunate complication of prosthetic valve replacement (see Chap. 71). No prosthesis currently employed has an effective orifice as large as that of the native valve, and VP-PM[16] may occur. *Almost all patients with prosthetic heart valves have mild-to-moderate stenosis; a few have severe stenosis.* Patients with aortic valve prostheses have obstruction to left ventricular outflow (aortic stenosis), and patients with mitral valve prostheses have obstruction to left atrial emptying (mitral stenosis). This is most important in a large patient in whom a prosthesis that is considered "small" in relation to body size must be placed for technical reasons. The resulting VP-PM[16] (Table 70-7)[9] contributes to incomplete relief of symptoms. The long-term effect of VP-PM can be expected to lead to long-term effects similar to those of aortic or mitral stenosis.[16,54,55] In critically ill patients, a small prosthesis is associated with a high hospital mortality.[56] The long-term (5 to 10 year) survival in those with severe VP-PM is lower in patients with larger body size[57] than it is in patients with smaller body size and in those with associated CAD.[56,57] The more severe the VP-PM, the higher the gradient at rest and on exercise, the less reduction of LV mass, greater physical limitation and morbidity.[58] In one study,[59] at 15 years, patients who had received a 19-mm valve when compared

TABLE 70-7 Valve Prosthesis-Patient Mismatch

AORTIC VALVE		
Severity of stenosis and of VP-PM after AVR	Valve area (cm^2/m^2)	Clinical status
Mild	>0.9	Asymptomatic
Moderate	>0.6 to 0.9	Asymptomatic (symptoms with associated conditions)
Severe	≤0.6	Asymptomatic or symptomatic*

MITRAL VALVE		
Severity of mitral valve stenosis and of VP-PM after MVR	Valve area (cm^2)	Clinical status
Very mild	>2.0 cm^2	Asymptomatic
Mild	>1.5 to 2.0	Asymptomatic
Moderate	1.1 to 1.5	Usually asymptomatic, some symptomatic.
Severe	≤1.0 cm^2	Asymptomatic or symptomatic.†

*Symptoms: angina, syncope, dyspnea, heart failure; sudden death.
†Symptoms associated with left atrial and pulmonary arterial hypertension and low reduced cardiac output and their consequences.
ABBREVIATIONS: AVR, aortic valve replacement; MVR, mitral valve replacement; VP-PM, valve prosthesis-patient mismatch.
SOURCE: From Rahimtoola.[9]

to those who received a 21-mm valve had poorer functional class, less LV mass reduction, and had a higher incidence of VP-PM, heart failure, cardiac events, and valve-related death including sudden death. The presence of VP-PM must be considered when patients with prosthetic heart valves are advised concerning activity. A method to predict the expected severity of VP-PM has been described.[58]

Reoperation to replace a prosthetic heart valve is a serious complication. It is usually required for moderate-to-severe prosthetic dysfunction and dehiscence, prosthetic valve endocarditis, and occasionally recurrent thromboembolism, severe recurrent bleeding from anticoagulant therapy, or VP-PM.

Late cardiac death may result from ventricular dysfunction, other cardiac lesions, or prosthesis-related causes. Late sudden death is not uncommon. It may result from a bradyarrhythmia; a tachyarrhythmia that is often associated with ventricular dysfunction, prosthetic dysfunction, or mismatch; coronary artery disease; or a combination of these.

Management

All patients with prosthetic valves need appropriate antibiotics for prophylaxis against infective endocarditis (see Chap. 81). Patients with rheumatic heart disease continue to need antibiotics as prophylaxis against the recurrence of rheumatic carditis (see Chap. 65). Adequate antithrombotic therapy is needed for appropriate patients (see Chap. 71). During the first 4 to 6 weeks after surgery, the physician and surgeon jointly manage the patient, directing their attention toward relieving postoperative discomfort, readjusting cardiac medica-

tions, and instituting anticoagulation if not contraindicated. A graduated plan of activity is started that, usually, enables the patient to return to full activity in 4 to 6 weeks.

Several syndromes are peculiar to the postoperative period. The *postperfusion syndrome* usually appears in the third or fourth postoperative week. It is characterized by fever, splenomegaly, and atypical lymphocytes; it is benign and self-limited. The *postpericardiotomy syndrome* is characterized by fever and pleuropericarditis. It usually develops in the second or third postoperative week but can appear as late as 1 year after surgery and sometimes recurs. Although this syndrome is usually self-limited, most patients benefit from taking anti-inflammatory drugs, such as aspirin or indomethacin; a short course of glucocorticoids is also occasionally required. Even though the pericardium is left open at the end of surgery, *cardiac tamponade* has been known to occur during the first 6 weeks and needs to be relieved. Usually, anticoagulants have been given and the fluid is hemorrhagic. The *4- to 6-week postoperative visit* is critical, because by this time the patient's physical capabilities and expected improvement in functional capacity can usually be assessed. At this time, the physician should assemble essential records and data for the subsequent office follow-up, including the preoperative history, physical examination, chest roentgenogram, electrocardiogram and indication for surgery, preoperative echocardiographic/Doppler ultrasound and cardiac catheterization/angiographic reports, surgeon's operative report, postoperative complications, and hospital discharge summary. *The prosthesis model, serial number, and size should be recorded.*

The workup on this visit should include an interval or complete initial history and physical examination, electrocardiogram, chest x-ray, Doppler echocardiography, complete blood cell count, and measurement of electrolytes, LDH, and international normalized ratio (INR) if indicated (Table 70-8). The examination's main focus is on signs that relate to functioning of the prosthesis or suggest the presence of a myocardial, conduction, or valvular disorder. The auscultatory findings to expect with some normally functioning prostheses have been described.[60] Severe perivalvular mitral regurgitation can be inaudible on physical examination, a fact to remember when considering possible causes of functional deterioration in a patient.

The interval between routine follow-up visits depends on the patient's needs. Anticoagulant regulation usually does not require office visits.

Multiple noninvasive tests have emerged for assessing valvular and ventricular function. Fluoroscopy can reveal abnormal rocking of a dehiscing prosthesis or limitation of the occluder if the latter is opaque, as well as strut fracture of a Björk-Shiley valve. Radionuclide angiography, to assess ventricular function, is performed if the same data cannot be obtained by echocardiography.

TABLE 70-8 Recommendations for Follow-up Strategy of Patient with Prosthetic Heart Valves

Indication	Class
1. History, physical exam, ECG, chest x-ray, echocardiogram, complete blood count, serum chemistries, and INR (if indicated) at first postoperative outpatient evaluation[a]	I
2. Radionuclide angiography or magnetic resonance imaging to assess LV function if result of echocardiography is unsatisfactory	I
3. Routine follow-up visits at yearly intervals with earlier reevaluations for change in clinical status	I
4. Routine serial echocardiograms at time of annual follow-up visit in absence of change in clinical status	IIb
5. Routine serial fluoroscopy	III

[a]This evaluation should be performed 3 to 4 weeks after hospital discharge. In some settings, the outpatient echocardiogram may be difficult to obtain: if so, an inpatient echocardiogram may be obtained before hospital discharge.
ABBREVIATIONS: INR = international normalized ratio; LV = left ventricle.
SOURCE: ACC/AHA Guidelines,[73] with permission.

Doppler echocardiography is the most useful noninvasive test. It provides information about prosthesis stenosis or regurgitation, valve area, assessment of other valve diseases, pulmonary hypertension, atrial size, LV hypertrophy, LV size and function, and pericardial effusion or thickening. It is essential at the first postoperative visit because it allows an assessment of the effects and results of surgery and serves as a baseline for comparison should complications and/or deterioration occur later. Subsequently, it is performed as is needed; we recommend that in both symptomatic and asymptomatic patients it is performed at 1- to 2-year intervals. In patients with a bioprosthesis in the mitral position, it is essential that Doppler echocardiography is performed at 5 years and annually thereafter and in the aortic position at 8 years and annually thereafter because of the increasing incidence of bioprosthetic SVD.[61]

"Heart failure" after valve replacement may be the result of (1) preoperative LV dysfunction that improved partially or not at all, (2) perioperative myocardial damage, (3) progression of other valve disease, (4) complications of PHV, and (5) associated heart disease such as CAD and systemic arterial hypertension.

Any patient with a prosthetic heart valve who does not improve after the surgery or who later shows deterioration of functional capacity should undergo appropriate testing to determine the cause. Such studies are also usually necessary for patients who require reoperation for any cause. The indications for reoperating on a patient with prosthetic valve endocarditis have already been discussed. A patient in stable condition, without prosthetic valve endocarditis, can usually undergo reoperation with only slightly greater risk than that of the initial surgery. For the patient with catastrophic dysfunction, surgery is clearly indicated and urgent.

ACKNOWLEDGMENT

The authors wish to thank Hui-Hua Li, MD, and K. Jeanne Zerr, RN, MBA, for valuable assistance in the preparation of this chapter. We are also grateful to the heart valve manufacturers for supplying information about their products.

References

1. Harken D, Soroff HS, Taylor WJ. Partial and complete prosthesis in aortic insufficiency. *J Thorac Cardiovasc Surg* 1960;40:744–762.
2. Starr A, Edwards M. Mitral replacement: Clinical experience with a ball valve prosthesis. *Ann Surg* 1961;154:726–740.
3. Ross DN. Homograft replacement of the aortic valve. *Lancet* 1962; 2:487.
4. Barratt-Boyes BG. Homograft aortic valve replacement in aortic incompetence and stenosis. *Thorax* 1964;19:131–135.
5. Ross DN. Replacement of aortic and mitral valves with a pulmonary autograph. *Lancet* 1967;2:956–958.
6. Ross DN. The pulmonary autograft: The Ross Principle (or Ross Procedural Confusion). *J Heart Valve Dis* 2000;9:174–175.
7. Carpentier A, Lemaigre G, Robert L. Biological factors affecting long-term results of valvular homografts. *J Thorac Cardiovasc Surg* 1969; 58:467–483.
8. Carpentier A, Dubost C. From xenograft to bioprosthesis. In: Ionescu MI, Ross DN, Wooler GH, eds. *Biological Tissue in Heart Valve Replacement*. London: Butterworth;1971:515–541.
9. Rahimtoola SH. Choice of prosthetic heart valve in adult patients. *J Am Coll Cardiol* 2003;41:893–904.
10. Carpentier A. Mitral reconstruction in predominant mitral incompetence. In: Duran C, Angell WW, Johnson AD, Oury JH, eds. *Recent Progress in Mitral Valve Disease*. London: Butterworth; 1984:265–276.
11. Duvoisin GE, Brandenburg RO, McGoon DC. Factors affecting thromboembolism associated with prosthetic heart valves. *Circulation* 1967; 35,36(suppl I):70–76.
12. Stinson EB, Griepp RB, Oyer PE, et al. Long-term experience with porcine xenografts. *J Thorac Cardiovasc Surg* 1977;73:54–63.
13. Grunkemeier GL, Macmanus Q, Thomas DR, et al. Regression analysis of late survival following mitral valve replacement. *J Thorac Cardiovasc Surg* 1978;75:131–138.
14. Blackstone EH, Naftel DC, Turner ME Jr. The decomposition of time varying hazard into separate phases, each incorporating a separate stream of concomitant information. *J Am Stat Assoc* 1986;81: 615–624.
15. Edmunds LH Jr, Clark RE, Cohn LH, et al. Guidelines for reporting morbidity and mortality after cardiac valvular operations. *J Thorac Cardiovasc Surg* 1996;112:708–711.
16. Rahimtoola SH. The problem of valve prosthesis-patient mismatch. *Circulation* 1978;58:20-24.
17. *Draft Replacement Heart Valve Guidance.* Rockville, MD. Prosthetic Devices Branch, Division of Cardiovascular, Respiratory and Neurological Devices, Office of Device Evaluation, Center of Devices and Radiological Health, Food and Drug Administration. October 14, 1994.
18. Palka P, Havrocks S, Lange A, et al. Primary aortic valve replacement with cryopreserved aortic allograft. An echocardiographic follow-up study of 570 patients. *Circulation* 2002;105:61–66.
19. Matsuki O, Okita Y, Almeida RS, et al. Two decades' experience with aortic valve replacement with pulmonary autograft. *J Thorac Cardiovasc Surg* 1988;95:705–711.
20. Ross D, Jackson M, Davies J. Pulmonary autograft aortic valve replacement: Long-term results. *J Cardiac Surg* 1991;6(suppl 4):529–533.
21. Carr-White GS, Kilner PJ, Hon JFK, et al. Incidence, location, pathology, and significance of pulmonary homograft stenosis after the Ross operation. *Circulation* 2001;104[suppl. I]:16–20.
22. Hendren WG, Morris AS, Rosenkranz ER, et al. Mitral valve repair for bacterial endocarditis. *J Thorac Cardiovasc Surg* 1992;103:124–128; discussion, 128–129.
23. Jebara VA, Dervanian P, Acar C, et al. Mitral valve repair using Carpentier techniques in patients more than 70 years old: Early and late results. *Circulation* 1992;86(suppl II):53–59.
24. Rahimtoola SH. Lessons learned about the determinants of the results of valve surgery. *Circulation* 1988;78:1503–1507.
25. Aoyagi S, Tanaka K, Kawara T, et al. Long-term results of mitral valve repair for non-rheumatic mitral regurgitation. *Cardiovasc Surg* 1995; 3:387–392.

26. Skoularigis J, Sinovich V, Joubert G, et al. Evaluation of the long-term results of mitral valve repair in 254 young patients with rheumatic mitral regurgitation. *Circulation* 1994;90(suppl II):167–174.

27. Grossi EA, Galloway AC, Steinberg BM, et al. Severe calcification does not affect long-term outcome of mitral valve repair. *Ann Thorac Surg* 1994;58:685–687.

28. Grossi EA, Galloway AC, LeBoutillier M III, et al. Anterior leaflet procedures during mitral valve repair do not adversely influence long-term outcome. *J Am Coll Cardiol* 1995;25:134–136.

29. Duran CM, Gometza B, Saad E. Valve repair in rheumatic mitral disease: An unsolved problem. *J Cardiac Surg* 1994;9(suppl 2):282–285.

30. Braunberger E, Deloche A, Berrebi A, et al. Very long-term results (more than 20 years) of valve repair with Carpentier's Techniques in non-rheumatic mitral valve insufficiency. *Circulation* 2001;104[suppl I]:8–11.

31. Lim E, Barlow CW, Hosseinpour AR, et al. Influence of atrial fibrillation on outcome following mitral valve repair. *Circulation* 2001; 104[suppl I]:59–63.

32. Chaurand S, Fuzellier JF, Berrebi A, et al. Long-term (29 years) results of reconstructive surgery in rheumatic mitral insufficiency. *Circulation* 2001;104[suppl I]:12–15.

33. Grunkemeier GL, Li H-H, Starr A, et al. Long-term performance of heart valve prostheses. *Curr Probl Cardiol* 2000;25:75–154.

34. Grunkemeier GL, London MR. Reliability of comparative data from different sources. In: Butchart E, Bodnar E, eds. *Current Issues in Heart Valve Disease: Thrombosis, Embolism and Bleeding.* London: ICR; 1992:464–475.

35. Sackett DL. Bias in analytic research. *J Chronic Dis* 1979;32:51–63.

36. Rahimtoola SH. Valvular heart disease: A perspective. *J Am Coll Cardiol* 1983;3:199–215.

37. Edmunds LH Jr. Thrombotic and bleeding complications of prosthetic heart valves. *Ann Thorac Surg* 1987;44:430–445.

38. Bamford J, Warlow C. Stroke and TIA in the general population. In: Butchart EG, Bodnar E, eds. *Thrombosis, Embolism and Bleeding.* London: ICR; 1992:3–15.

39. Berlin JA, Begg CB, Louis TA. An assessment of publication bias using a sample of published clinical trials. *J Am Stat Assoc* 1989;84:381–392.

40. Kramer MS, Shapiro SH. Scientific challenges in the application of randomized trials. *JAMA* 1984;252:2739–2745.

41. Rahimtoola SH. Some unexpected lessons from large multicenter randomized clinical trials. *Circulation* 1985;72:449–455.

42. Grunkemeier GL, Starr A. Alternatives to randomization in surgical studies. *J Heart Valve Dis* 1992;1:142–151.

43. Bloomfield P, Wheatley DJ, Prescott RJ, et al. Twelve-year comparison of a Björk-Shiley mechanical heart valve with porcine bioprostheses. *N Engl J Med* 1991;324:573–579.

44. Hammermeister K, Sethi GK, Henderson WG, et al. Outcomes 15 years after valve replacement with a mechanical vs. bioprosthetic valve: Final report of the VA randomized trial. *J Am Coll Cardiol* 2000;36: 1152–1158.

45. Bonow RO, Carabello B, de Leon AC Jr, et al. ACC/AHA guidelines for the management of patients with valvular heart disease: A report of the American College of Cardiology/American Heart Association Task Force on Practical Guidelines (Committee on Management of Patients with Valvular Heart Disease). *J Am Coll Cardiol* 1998;32:1486–1588.

46. Herzog CA, Ma JZ, Collins AJ. Long-term survival of dialysis patients in the United States with prosthetic heart valves. Should ACC/AHA practice guidelines on valve selection be modified? *Circulation* 2002; 105:1336–1341.

47. Hung L, Rahimtoola SH. Prosthetic heart valve and pregnancy. *Circulation* 2003;107;1240–1246.

48. Rahimtoola SH. Valvular heart disease. In: Stein J, ed. *Internal Medicine,* 4th ed. *Cardiology,* O'Rourke RA, section ed. St. Louis: Mosby-Year Book; 1994:202–234.

49. Grunkemeier GL, Rahimtoola SH, Starr A. Prosthetic heart valves. In: Rahimtoola SH, ed. *Atlas of Heart Diseases, 11.* Philadelphia: Current Medicine; 1997:13.1–13.27.

50. Rahimtoola SH. Aortic valve stenosis. In: Rahimtoola SH, ed. *Valvular Heart Disease, II.* St. Louis: Mosby; 1997:7.02–7.26.

51. Mullany CJ, Elveback LR, Frye RL, et al. Coronary artery disease and its management: Influence on survival in patients undergoing aortic valve replacement. *J Am Coll Cardiol* 1987;10:66–72.

52. Kloster FE. Infective prosthetic valve endocarditis. In: Rahimtoola SH, ed. *Infective Endocarditis.* New York: Grune & Stratton;1978:291–305.

53. Douglas JL, Cobbs CG. Prosthetic valve endocarditis. In: Kaye D, ed. *Infective Endocarditis,* 2d ed. New York: Raven Press;1992:375–396.

54. Rahimtoola SH, Murphy E. Valve prosthesis-patient mismatch: A long-term sequela. *Br Heart J* 1981;45:331–335.

55. Rahimtoola SH. Valve prosthesis-patient mismatch: An update. *J Heart Valve Dis* 1998;7:207–210.

56. Connolly HM, Oh JK, Schaff HV, et al. Severe aortic stenosis with low transvalvular gradient and severe left ventricular dysfunction: Result of valve replacement in 52 patients. *Circulation* 2000;101:1940–1946.

57. Hé GW, Grunkemeier GL, Gately HL, et al. Up to thirty year survival after aortic valve replacement in the small aortic root. *Ann Thorac Surg* 1995;59:1056–1062.

58. Pibarot P, Dumesnil JG. Hemodynamic and clinical impact of prosthesis-patient mismatch in the aortic valve position and its prevention. *J Am Coll Cardiol* 2000;36:1131–1141.

59. Milano AD, DeCarlo M, Mecozzi G, et al. Clinical outcome in patients with 19mm and 21 aortic prosthesis. Comparison at long-term follow-up. *Ann Thorac Surg* 2002;73:37–43.

60. Vongpatawasin W, Hillis LD, Lange RA. Prosthetic heart valves. *N Engl J Med* 1996;335:407–416.

61. Frater RWM, Furlong P, Cosgrove DM, et al. Long-term durability and patient functional status of the Carpentier-Edwards Perimount pericardial bioprosthesis in the aortic position. *J Heart Valve Dis* 1998;7: 48–53.

ANTITHROMBOTIC THERAPY FOR VALVULAR HEART DISEASE

John H. McAnulty / Donogh F. McKeogh / Shahbudin H. Rahimtoola

Valve disease increases the risk of a stroke. While emboli from intracardiac thrombi are the most likely cause of the stroke in valve disease patients, other causes should be considered, particularly endocarditis.

ANTITHROMBOTIC DRUGS USED FOR VALVE DISEASE

Bleeding is a risk with all antithrombotic agents, but the frequency and consequences of a stroke make drug therapy appropriate in many patients with valve disease (Figs. 71-1 and 71-2, Table 71-1).[1,2] Warfarin, aspirin, unfractionated heparin, and thrombolytic agents are the only antithrombotic agents currently recommended for preventing thromboemboli related to valve disease. Newer drugs, such as low molecular weight heparin, the 2B–3A platelet inhibitors, the thienopyridine agents (e.g., clopidogrel), and the direct thrombin inhibitors have not yet been proved of value in preventing thromboemboli due to valve abnormalities. As these drugs are increasingly being used for other clinical syndromes occurring in patients who also require antithrombotic therapy for heart valve disease, increased bleeding is likely though not yet well defined. Individual clinical decisions will be required; some of which are addressed in this chapter.

NATIVE VALVE DISEASE

Patients with native valve disease require antithrombotic therapy only in the presence of an associated *risk factor* (Fig. 71-1, Table 71-2). The two most common associated risk factors are atrial fibrillation and left ventricular (LV) systolic dysfunction.

Risk Factors for Thromboemboli

ATRIAL FIBRILLATION
In six large prospective randomized trials assessing the value of antithrombotic therapy for primary stroke prevention in patients with nonvalvular, constant or paroxysmal, atrial fibrillation (see Chap. 29,

section on "Atrial Fibrillation"), the embolic rate (essentially a stroke) in the placebo group was 3 to 8 percent per year; warfarin therapy reduced the stroke rate to 0.5 to 2 percent per year. "Nonvalvular" is not well defined in these trials since individuals with "insignificant" valve disease were included; however, patients with mitral stenosis or prosthetic heart valves (PHV) were excluded. The Stroke Prevention in Atrial Fibrillation Investigators II Study,[3] demonstrated equal protection against an adverse neurologic event when aspirin (325 mg daily) was compared to warfarin. Aspirin was less protective if atrial fibrillation occurred in those with LV dysfunction, uncontrolled hypertension, in women over age 75, and, most importantly, patients who had had previous thromboembolic events.[4]

PREVIOUS THROMBOEMBOLI
A thromboembolic event defines patients at high risk for having a recurrent event, especially in certain clinical situations (e.g., in patients with atrial fibrillation or with a PHV).[5,6] It is unclear whether this is true in patients with native valve disease, but lifelong warfarin therapy should be considered if there are no contraindications to its use.

LEFT VENTRICULAR DYSFUNCTION
Systemic or pulmonary thromboemboli occur at a rate of over 5 percent per year in patients with LV dysfunction, but antithrombotic therapy is not of proven value in preventing or reducing the embolic rate.[7,8] Nevertheless, because the risk is sufficiently high, warfarin [international normalized ratio (INR) 2 to 3] may be used if the LV ejection fraction (EF) is ≤0.30, or aspirin (325 mg daily) may be used if warfarin use is judged to be associated with an increased risk or is impractical.

HYPERCOAGULABLE CONDITIONS
Anticoagulant therapy should be considered in the presence of any of the hypercoagulable syndromes (see Chap. 54); the most common of which are resistance to activated protein C or an associated malignancy.

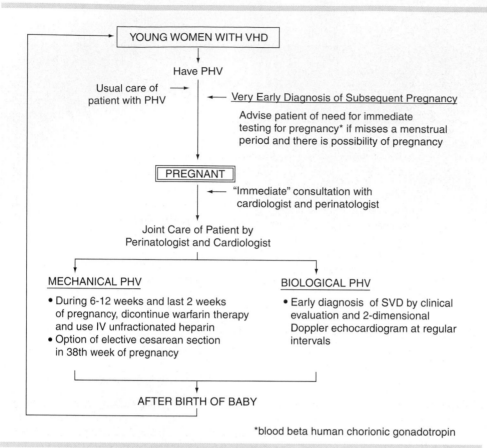

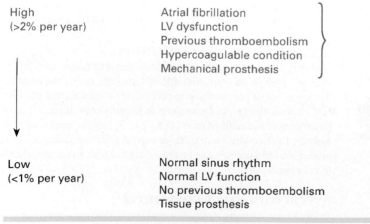

FIGURE 71-1 Management of a woman with a prosthetic heart valve (PHV) at time of pregnancy. SVD, structural valve deterioration; VHD, valvular heart disease. (From Hung and Rahimtoola.[24])

findings of concern. The value of treatment is unproven, therefore, screening is not recommended.

Antithrombotic Treatment

Without a risk factor for embolism, antithrombotic treatment is not indicated. The risk of an embolus is greater with mitral valve disease as compared to aortic valve disease because the left atrial may be larger and, therefore, there is more blood stasis and the frequency of atrial fibrillation is greater. Antithrombotic therapy is recommended *only* in the presence of *risk factors* (see Table 71-2).

- Warfarin (INR 2–3) for previous thromboemboli, LV dysfunction (LV EF ≤0.30), heart failure, hypercoagulable state
- Warfarin (INR 2–3) or aspirin (325 mg) for atrial fibrillation if lesion is other than mitral stenosis
- The just completed SPORTIF III and V clinical trials have revealed equivalency of the thromboinhibitor ximelegatron and warfarin in regard to stroke reduction and in bleeding rates in patients with nonvalvular atrial fibrillation. It is likely that this drug will soon be available for treating atrial fibrillation, including patients with valve disease. In patients with native valve disease, it would seem a reasonable option. In those with mechanical prostheses, its use cannot be recommended as there are no data available to suggest protective effects in these patients.

Screening for Patients at High Risk for Thromboemboli

The use of transthoracic (TTE) and transesophageal echocardiography (TEE) to determine which patients are at risk of thromboemboli is not yet well defined; left atrial thrombi, a patent foramen ovale, an atrial septal aneurysm, or spontaneous echo contrast are occasional

PROSTHETIC HEART VALVES

In patients with mechanical PHVs the risk of stroke exceeds 10 percent per year in patients not taking warfarin.[6] With warfarin use, the risk of thromboemboli is 1 to 3 percent per year.[9,10] In patients in sinus rhythm with biological PHVs the risk of an embolus is approximately 0.6 to 0.7 percent per year when patients are not on warfarin therapy.[9,10] While almost all studies have shown that the risk of embolism is greater with a PHV in the mitral position (mechanical or biological) than it is with a valve in the aortic position,[9,11] this was not the case in one

FIGURE 71-2 Risk of thromboembolism. Clinical variables define valve disease patients as being at high or low risk of thromboembolic events. LV, left ventricle.

TABLE 71-1 Valve Disease and Antithrombotic Therapy[a,b]

1. Prevention of thromboemboli should be addressed each time a patient with valve disease is seen.
2. Lifelong antithrombotic therapy is required in patients with atrial fibrillation (paroxysmal or persistent) (Table 71-2).
3. Warfarin therapy is required in all patients with a mechanical prothesis (Table 71-3).
4. Antithrombotic therapy should be started early after valve surgery.
5. Warfarin should be avoided in the first trimester of pregnancy.
6. Antithrombotic therapy should be individualized during noncardiac surgery and cardiovascular procedures (Table 71-5).

[a]See text for discussion.
[b]In general, whenever warfarin/aspirin therapy is recommended it is assumed that there is no specific contraindication to its use.

study.[10] With either type of PHV or valve location, the risk of emboli is probably higher in the first few days and months after valve insertion,[12] that is, before the valve is fully endothelialized.

Antithrombotic Treatment for Mechanical Prosthetic Heart Valves

It is frequently difficult to maintain a patient at a fixed or relatively fixed level of anticoagulation due to changes in the absorption of medication, the effects of various foods and medications, and

TABLE 71-2 Risk Factors for Thromboembolism

PATIENTS WITH VALVULAR HEART DISEASE

1. Atrial fibrillation
2. Previous thromboembolism
3. LV dysfunction (LV ejection fraction ≤ 0.30)
4. Mitral valve disease > aortic valve disease
5. Hypercoagulable conditions

PATIENTS WITHOUT VALVULAR HEART DISEASE[a]

In presence of atrial fibrillation risks are increased with the following comorbid conditions:[b]

	Relative Risk[c]
a. Previous TIA or stroke	2.5
b. Diabetes mellitus	1.7
c. History of hypertension	1.6
d. Coronary artery disease	1.5
e. Congestive heart failure	1.4
f. Advanced age (continuous per decade)	1.4

[a]Patients with non-valvular atrial fibrillation have about a 6-fold increased risk of thrombombolism compared with patients in normal sinus rhythm.
[b]From ACC/AHA/ESC Guidelines cited Ref. 43.
[c]Relative Risk = Comparison with atrial fibrillation in patients without these risk factors.

changes in liver function. Therefore, in clinical practice, the patient is maintained within a certain therapeutic range. This can be optimized through a program of patient education and close surveillance by an experienced health care professional.

All patients with mechanical PHV require warfarin[9,10,13] (Table 71-3). In patients with an aortic PHV without risk factors for emboli the INR should be between 2.0 and 3.0.[2] In those with one or more risk factors, low-dose aspirin is added. The INR should be between 2.5 and 3.5 in those with a previous embolus, those with multiple risk factors, and in those with a mitral prosthesis.[2] The tilting-disk valves are more thrombogenic than others and the INR may be increased to 3 and 4.5, but this is associated with an increased risk of bleeding.[14–17] There is no good evidence in patients with similar comorbid conditions that the Starr-Edwards valve models 1260/6120 have a higher rate of thromboembolism than newer high-quality mechanical PHVs.[18]

The addition of *low-dose aspirin* (50 to 100 mg/day) to warfarin therapy is suggested because it further decreases the risk of thromboembolism without increasing the incidence of major bleeds in most patients.[19–22] A metanalysis[22] showed with the addition of aspirin to anticoagulants, the odds ratio (± 95 percent confidence interval) of thromboembolic events was 0.41 (0.29 to 0.58; $p < 0.001$), the odds ratio of mortality was 0.49 (0.35 to 0.67; $p < 0.001$), and of major bleeding was 1.81 (1.21 to 1.71; $p = 0.0041$).

In a randomized trial[23] of mitral valve replacement with the St. Jude Medical valves, patients were assigned to oral anticoagulants (INR 2.5 to 3.5) or oral anticoagulants plus aspirin 200 mg/day. Patients in the aspirin-added group had a lower incidence of thrombi (4.8 vs. 13.1 percent; $p = 0.03$) and total thromboembolic events (9.1 vs. 25 percent; $p = 0.001$), but a higher incidence of major hemorrhages (19.2 vs. 8.3 percent; $p = 0.02$), which were largely due to gastrointestinal bleeding. The reduction in thromboemboli in the aspirin-added group was due to reduction in minor thromboemboli (8.2 vs. 20.8 percent; $p = 0.007$), since the reduction in major thromboembolic was not significant (0.9 vs. 4.1 percent). This study is compatible with the view that if aspirin is added to warfarin, only low-dose aspirin (80 to 100 mg) should be used and that there is a need for clinical judgment when recommending the addition of aspirin.

The thromboembolic risk is increased early after the insertion of any PHV. Heparin therapy should be initiated within the first 24 to 48 h of surgery if there is no contraindication to its use, and the *activated partial thromboplastin time* (aPTT) is maintained at a "therapeutic effect" level (Table 71-4) until warfarin therapy has achieved the recommended INR level.[12,13]

BLEEDING

Long-term anticoagulant therapy is associated with bleeding episodes. The incidence of minor bleeding is ≤ 2 to 3 percent per year. The incidence of major bleeding is ≤ 1 to ≥ 4 percent per year depending on patients' age and associated comorbid conditions; and the mortality rate is ≤ 0.5 percent per year. The incidence of these complications is lower in patients who take their medications reliably, in those in whom smooth long-term anticoagulation can be achieved, and in those who receive low-dose warfarin therapy (INR 2 to 3 vs. >3). With oral anticoagulants, low- or mid-dose warfarin therapy may be combined with low-dose aspirin, but the risk of bleeding is increased. High degrees of anticoagulation increase the incidence of bleeding without reducing the incidence of thromboembolism.

TABLE 71-3 Antithrombotic Therapy—Prosthetic Heart Valves

	MECHANICAL PROSTHETIC VALVES			BIOLOGICAL PROSTHETIC VALVES		
	Warfarin INR 2–3	Warfarin INR 2.5–3.5	Aspirin 50–100 mg	Warfarin INR 2–3	Warfarin INR 2.5–3.5	Aspirin 50–100 mg
First 3 months after valve replacement		+	±		+	±
After first 3 months						
Aortic valve						
Aortic valve	+		±			+
Aortic valve + risk factor[b]	+		+	+		
Aortic valve + embolus[c]		+	+	+		+
Mitral valve		+	±			+
Mitral valve + risk factor		+	+		+	±
Mitral valve + embolism[c]		+	+		+	+

[a]Depending on the clinical status of patient, antithrombotic therapy must be individualized (see special situations in text).
[b]Risk factors (see Fig. 71-1): atrial fibrillation, LV dysfunction, and hypercoagulable state.
[c]Embolus = previous thromboembolism
±Clinical judgment very important for addition of aspirin therapy.
NOTE: In an individual patient, there is a need for clinical judgment ± if aspirin is added to warfarin therapy.

Antithrombotic Treatment for Biological Valves

Because of an increased risk of thromboemboli during the first 3 months after implantation of a biological PHV, early anticoagulation with heparin and then warfarin is indicated.[2,12,13] After 3 months, the biological valve can be treated in the same way as that done for patients with native valve disease (see earlier) and warfarin can be discontinued in approximately two-thirds of patients with biological valves[5,14,15] if there are no associated risk factors.

SPECIAL CLINICAL SITUATIONS

Altered Native Valves

Valve disease is treated increasingly by interventional catheter techniques or surgical valve repair. The recommendations given for treatment of native valve disease would seem most applicable in such patients.

Pregnancy

The management of the woman with PHV during pregnancy has been reviewed.[18] The incidence of warfarin embryopathy is low (0 to 3.9 percent) with use of intravenous (IV) unfractionated heparin in the first 3 months (especially 6 to 12 weeks) of pregnancy,[24]. One review concluded that this strategy "eliminated the risk." IV unfractionated heparin use in the last 2 weeks of pregnancy is associated with a reduced risk of hemorrhage during delivery and the neonatal period in the mother and also the baby because warfarin crosses the placenta and, therefore, the fetus/baby is anticoagulated. To reduce the latter complication some have suggested elective cesarean section in the 38th week of pregnancy (Fig. 71-1).

Low-molecular-weight (LMW) *heparin* is currently approved *only* for prophylaxis and treatment of venous thrombosis. It has been used in pregnancy,[25] does not cross the placenta, and has other advantages. The Food and Drug Administration (FDA)[26] has issued additions to the warning and precautions sections of Lovenox (enoxaparin sodium) product labeling. These additions point out that (1) Lovenox is an LMW heparin and is *not* recommended for thrombotic prophylaxis an patients with PHVs; (2) sporatic cases of PHV

TABLE 71-4 "Therapeutic Effect" of Heparin

Unfractionated heparin	An aPTT at 8 h after a dose that has been calibrated[a] to reflect a heparin level of 0.35 to 0.70 anti-Xa units
LMW heparin	An aPTT at 8 h after a dose that has been calibrated[a] to reflect a heparin level of 0.7 to 1.1 anti-Xa units
During pregnancy	A heparin level of 0.6 to 0.7 anti-Xa units with unfractionated heparin or 0.10 to 0.11 anti-Xa units with LMW heparin[b] (aPTT measurements do not accurately reflect heparin levels during pregnancy)

[a]Calibration of aPTT to heparin levels is performed in each clinical laboratory; thus the time (number of seconds) of the aPTT reflecting the "therapeutic effect" levels will vary.
[b]*Important Note:* Although LMW heparin is increasingly being utilized in many disorders, its value in protecting against thromboemboli in patients with valve disease has *not* been proven. Therefore its use in patients with valve disease is not recommended by most experts at this time.
ABBREVIATIONS: aPTT = activated partial thromboplastin time; LMW = low molecular weight.

thrombosis and of maternal and fetal deaths have been reported with use of this drug; and (3) both teratogenic and nonteratogenic effects have been reported in women who received this drug during pregnancy. Its worth in pregnant women with PHVs needs to be evaluated in randomized trials. Thus, despite the theoretical advantages of outpatient self-administered subcutaneous LMW heparin during pregnancy, randomized studies are needed to evaluate both safety and efficacy.

Aspirin crosses the placenta and has been implicated as a cause of abortion and fetal growth retardation, but it has been used so frequently without problems that when required for valve disease, it should be continued. The direct thrombin inhibitors could also be of potential value when anticoagulation is required during pregnancy, but currently there are no available data supporting their efficacy or safety in these patients.

THROMBOSIS OF PROSTHETIC HEART VALVES

PHV obstruction may be caused by thrombus in approximately 50 percent, pannus in 10 percent, and pannus plus thrombus in 40 percent of cases. The cause may be difficult to determine and requires knowledge of the clinical presentation (result of valve obstruction) and findings on Doppler echocardiography, including transesophageal echocardiography. Pannus is tissue ingrowth; therefore, thrombolytic therapy is ineffective with obstruction or thrombosis and the PHV needs to be replaced.

Thrombotic obstruction of right-sided PHVs (tricuspid and pulmonic) treated with thrombolytics is usually successful (80 to 100 percent of the time).[27] The mortality rate is very low (close to 0 percent); embolism occurs in ≤5 percent; and stroke does not occur, but obstruction is recurrent in about 20 percent. Both streptokinase and recombinant tissue plasminogen activator (rtPA) are more effective than is urokinase. Thrombolytics are the first choice of therapy[27,28] (Table 71-5).

Left sided PHV thrombosis (aortic and mitral) is more serious. With use of thrombolytics, two reviews[27,29] documented a mortality of 6 percent, thromboembolism in 12 percent, stroke in 3 to 10 percent, major bleeding in 5 percent, and nondisabling bleeding in 14 percent. Thrombolysis was ineffective in 16 to 18 percent, and thrombosis was recurrent in 11 percent. A report of thrombolytic therapy in 110 patients with 127 thrombosed valves[28] documented complete resolution of "hemodynamic abnormalities" in 70.9 percent, partial resolution in 17.3 percent, and no change in 11 percent. The mortality was 11.8 percent; mortality in patients in New York Heart Association (NYHA) Functional Classes III & IV was 15.6 percent as compared to 2.7 percent in patients in NYHA Classes I & II ($p = 0.04$). Embolic events occurred in 15 percent and severe hemorrhagic complications in 4.7 percent. The recurrence rate was 18.9 percent.

Best results are obtained in patients who are in NYHA Functional Classes I & II and have a "small" thrombus. In a study of 36 patients[30] using streptokinase, the success rate was 53 percent initially and increased to 88 percent on repeat thrombolysis using streptokinase. All subsequent thrombolysis was with rtPA or urokinase. The success rate for NYHA Class I, II, III, & IV patients was 100, 89, 92, and 80 percent, respectively ($p = ns$). There were 5 episodes of recurrent thrombosis in 4 patients. In another study of 12 patients,[31] partial or complete success was achieved with thrombolytics in 10 patients and the remaining 2 required surgery.

Surgical replacement of the thrombosed PHV is associated with a mortality of 10 to 60 percent. Important variables determining high mortality are (1) NYHA Classes III & IV and duration in these functional classes; and (2) LV dysfunction, left atrial hypertension and pulmonary edema, pulmonary and right atrial hypertension, low cardiac output, and multisystem organ failure involving the pulmonary, hepatic, renal, and central nervous system organs and blood abnormalities. Best results are obtained in patients who are NYHA Functional Classes I & II.

Surgery and Dental Care

The risk of increased bleeding during a procedure performed with a patient on antithrombotic therapy has to be weighed against the increased risk of a thromboembolism caused by stopping the therapy.

TABLE 71-5 Prosthetic Heart Valve (PHV) Thrombosis

TRICUSPID AND PULMONARY PHV

- Thrombolytics: First Choice
- If successful:
    I.V. unfractionated heparin plus warfarin
    When INR therapeutic, substitute aspirin for heparin
- Surgery:
    Thrombolytics unsuccessful after two attempts
    Recurrent thrombosis
    Pannus

AORTIC AND MITRAL PHV

Surgery:
- Pannus or pannus plus thrombus
- "Large" thrombus
- NYHA Functional Classes III and IV
- Thrombolytic therapy unsuccessful after two attempts
- Usually for recurrent thrombosis
- Best results with "small" thrombus and patients in NYHA FC I and II

Thrombolytics:
- First choice in those with best results
- Best results with "small" thrombus and patients in NYHA FC I and II
- Patients with very severe co-morbid conditions (see text)
- Contraindications to surgery

After surgery or thrombolytics:
- I.V. Heparin plus Warfarin till INR therapeutic range
- Subsequently, warfarin *plus* aspirin

Thrombolytics unsuccessful. Contraindications to surgery
- I.V. unfractionated heparin plus warfarin for 1–3 months; then, subcutaneous heparin (aPPT 55–80s) Warfarin (INR 2.5–3.5)
- Subsequent treatment depends on clinical circumstances

The risk of stopping warfarin can be estimated and is relatively low if the drug is withheld for only a few days. As an example, and using a *worst case scenario* (e.g., a patient with a mechanical prosthesis and previous thromboemboli), the risk of a thromboembolus in a patient off warfarin could be as high as 10 to 20 percent per year. Thus, if the therapy were stopped for 3 days, the risk of an embolus would be 3/365 times 0.10 to 0.20, which equals 0.08 to 0.16 percent. There are theoretical concerns that stopping the drug and then reinstituting it might result in hypercoagulability with a thrombotic "rebound." An increase in markers for activation of thrombosis with abrupt discontinuation of warfarin therapy has been observed,[32] but it is not clear that these increase the clinical risk of thromboembolism.[32–34] In addition, when reinstituting warfarin therapy, there are theoretical concerns of a hypercoagulable state caused by suppression of proteins C and S before the drug affects the thrombotic factors. Although the risks are hypothetical, they are reasons to treat individuals at very high risk with heparin therapy until the INR returns to the desired range.

Although antithrombotic therapy must be individualized, some generalizations apply (Table 71-6). For procedures where bleeding is unlikely or would be inconsequential if it occurred, antithrombotic therapy should not be stopped. This can apply to surgery on the skin, dental prophylaxis, or simple treatment for dental caries. Eye surgery, in particular surgery for cataracts or glaucoma, is usually associated with very little bleeding.

When bleeding is likely or its potential consequences are severe, antithrombotic treatment should be altered. If a patient is taking aspirin, it should be discontinued one week before the procedure and restarted as soon as it is considered safe by the surgeon or dentist.

TABLE 71-6 Antithrombotic Therapy at the Time of Surgery

I. Usual approach
  A. If patient on warfarin
    Stop 72 h before procedure
    Restart on day of procedure or after control of active bleeding
  B. If patient on aspirin
    Stop 1 week before procedure
    Restart the day after procedure or after control of active bleeding
II. Unusual circumstances
  A. Very high risk of thrombosis if off warfarin[a]
    Stop warfarin 72 h before procedure
    Start heparin 48 h before procedure[b]
    Stop heparin 6 h before procedure
    Restart heparin within 24 h of procedure and continue until warfarin can be restarted and the INR is 2–3
  B. Surgery complicated by postoperative bleeding
    Start heparin as soon after surgery as deemed safe and maintain aPTT of 60–80 s until warfarin restarted and the INR is 2–3
  C. Very low risk from bleeding[c]
    Continue antithrombotic therapy

[a]Clinical judgment: consider this approach if recent thromboembolus or if three risk factors are present.
[b]Heparin can be given in outpatient setting before and after surgery.
[c]For example, local skin surgery, dental prophylaxis, and treatment for caries.
ABBREVIATION: aPTT = activated partial thromboplastin time.

For most patients taking warfarin, the drug should be stopped 48 to 72 h before the procedure. The INR should be ≤1.5 at the time of the procedure and restarted within 24 h after the procedure. Admission to the hospital or a delay in discharge to give heparin is usually not necessary.[32–34] Deciding who is at very high risk of thrombosis and thus should require heparin until warfarin can be reinstated may be difficult; clinical judgment is required. Heparin can usually be reserved for those who have had a recent thromboembolism (arbitrarily within 1 year), those with demonstrated thrombotic problems when previously off therapy, and those with two or more risk factors (Fig. 71-2). When used, heparin should be started 24 h after warfarin is stopped (i.e., 48 h before surgery) and stopped 6 to 12 h before the procedure. Heparin should be restarted as early after surgery as bleeding stability allows and the aPTT maintained at a "therapeutic level" (see Table 71-4) until warfarin is restarted and the desired INR can be achieved. Home administration and management of heparin (and warfarin) can be arranged to minimize time in the hospital. LMW heparin is even more easily utilized outside of the hospital (see Chap. 54).

Cardiac Catheterization and Angiography

Antiplatelet therapy or heparin need not be stopped for these procedures. Cardiac catheterization can be performed with a patient taking warfarin, but, preferably, the drug should be stopped 72 h before the procedure and restarted after the procedure on the same day.[35] If a patient is at very high risk of thromboembolism, heparin should be started 48 h before the procedure and continued until warfarin is restarted and the desired INR is achieved. If the catheterization procedure is to include a transseptal puncture (especially in a patient who has not had previous opening of the pericardium), patients should be off all antithrombotic therapy and the INR should be <1.2.[35]

Stent insertion complicates antithrombotic therapy. A thienopyridine agent, usually clopidogrel, is required for at least 30 days (3 to 12 months for a sirolimus-coated stent) for optimal prevention of in-stent thrombosis.[36,37] It has no proven efficacy in preventing thromboemboli in patients with PHV, so continuation of warfarin or aspirin is recommended.

Therapy at the Time of a Thromboembolic Event

ACUTE MANAGEMENT

An embolic event often indicates inadequate therapy for that patient's circumstances. Data and opinions about optimal timing for initiating or continuing anticoagulants in patients in whom an embolus is the presumed cause of a stroke are conflicting.[2,34–39] Ideally, treatment would be started early to prevent recurrence of an embolus, but the early use of heparin (within 72 h) is associated with a 15 to 25 percent chance of converting a nonhemorrhagic stroke into a hemorrhagic stroke.[40] The risk of early recurrent emboli is less than 5 percent.[39] On balance, it seems preferable to withhold therapy for at least 72 h (Table 71-7). If a computed tomography (CT) scan at that time reveals little or no hemorrhage, heparin should be administered to maintain an aPPT at the lower end of the therapeutic level (see Table 71-7) until warfarin, started at the same time, results in the desired INR (see Table 71-3). If the CT scan demonstrates significant hemorrhage, antithrombotic therapy should be withheld until the bleed is treated or has stabilized (7 to 14 days). Anticoagulation can then be started as just described.

TABLE 71-7 Antithrombotic Therapy at the Time of a Thromboembolic Event

I. Acute management
    A. *No* antithrombotic treatment for 72 h
    B. CT scan at 72 h
       1. *No (or little) hemorrhage* on CT:
          a. Heparin: aPTT in low "therapeutic effect" (Table 71-4)
          b. Warfarin: continue heparin until INR in desired range[a]
       2. *Hemorrhage* on CT:
          a. No treatment until bleed stabilized or treated (7–14 days), then heparin and warfarin as above
II. Chronic management
    A. If embolus occurred *off* antithrombotic therapy
       1. Treat with warfarin[a]
    B. If embolus occurred *on* antithrombotic therapy
       1. If patient was on aspirin, switch to warfarin[a]
       2. If patient was on warfarin but INR was low, increase dose until INR in high desired range[a]
       3. If patient was on warfarin and INR was in desired range, add aspirin 80–325 mg/day
       4. If recurrent embolus or bleed on warfarin plus aspirin, assess valve for possible surgery

[a]See Tables 71-2 and 71-3.
ABBREVIATIONS: CT = computed tomography; INR = international normalized ratio.

LONG-TERM MANAGEMENT

If the embolic event occurs when a patient is *off* antithrombotic therapy, long-term warfarin therapy is required (see Table 71-3). If the embolic event occurs while the patient is *on* adequate antithrombotic therapy, the dosage of antithrombotic therapy should be increased as follows:[2]

- Warfarin INR 2 to 3: Warfarin dosage increased to achieve an INR of 2.5 to 3.5.
- Warfarin INR 2.5 to 3.5: Warfarin dosage may need to be increased to achieve an INR of 3.5 to 4.5.
- Not on aspirin: Aspirin 80 to 100 mg/d should be initiated.
- Warfarin plus aspirin 80 to 100 mg/d: Aspirin dose may also need to be increased to 325 mg/d if higher dose of warfarin is not achieving the desired clinical result.
- Aspirin alone: Aspirin may need to be increased to 325 mg/d and/or warfarin added to achieve an INR of 2 to 3.

Embolism occurring after this medical approach should lead to consideration of possible valve surgery if the valve is the likely source of the thrombus.

EXCESSIVE ANTICOAGULATION

In most patients with INR above the therapeutic range, excessive anticoagulation can be managed by withholding warfarin and following the level of anticoagulation with serial INR determinations.[2] Excessive anticoagulation (INR > 5) greatly increases the risk of hemorrhage. However, rapid decreases in INR that lead to INR falling below the therapeutic level increases the risk of thromboembolism.

Patients with PHVs with an INR of 5 to 10 who are not bleeding can be managed by the following: (1) admitting the patient to the hospital; (2) withholding warfarin and administering 2.5 mg of oral vitamin K_1 (phytonadine);[2] (3) INR should be determined after 24 h and subsequently as needed; (4) additional doses of 2.5 mg of oral vitamin K_1 may be needed; (5) warfarin therapy is restarted and dose adjusted appropriately to ensure that INR is in the therapeutic range. In emergency situations, the use of fresh frozen plasma is preferable to high dose vitamin K_1, especially *parenteral vitamin K_1*, because use of the latter increases the *risk of overcorrection to a hypercoagulable state*.

Human recombinant factor (rFVIIa), dose 15 to 19 μg/kg body weight, has been used to reverse critically prolonged INR and bleeding complications safely and rapidly. Indications include an INR >10 in high-risk persons, clinical hemorrhage, and at time of diagnostic and therapeutic procedures.[41]

THERAPY AT THE TIME OF A BLEED

With significant bleeding, antithrombotic therapy should be stopped and, if the patient is at risk, drug effects should be reversed. If possible, the cause of bleeding should be corrected and antithrombotic therapy restarted as soon as possible. If this is not possible, treatment decisions are difficult. In patients with a mechanical prosthesis or multiple risk factors for thromboemboli, acceptance of intermittent bleeding with acute management for the bleeds may be necessary. In valve patients who are at lower risk of emboli or in whom the role of antithrombotic treatment is less clear (e.g., LV dysfunction), it may be optimal to withhold chronic therapy or, if a patient is on warfarin, to switch to aspirin. With mechanical PHVs, consideration should be given to replacing the mechanical valve with a biological valve in some patients (e.g., in those who have had multiple, large life- or organ-threatening bleeds).

Antithrombotic Therapy in the Patient with Endocarditis

If a patient with valve disease develops endocarditis, antithrombotic therapy should be continued[2] (see Chap. 81). If the patient presents with or develops an embolic event involving the central nervous system, therapy should be as described earlier for acute embolic events[42] (see Table 71-7). Additionally, the issue of whether or not the embolus is due to thrombus or infected vegetation should be addressed. If thrombus is likely, the chronic anticoagulation program will also require alteration.

References

1. Rahimtoola SH. Lessons learned about the determinants of the results of valve surgery. *Circulation* 1988;78:1503–1506.
2. Bonow RO, Carabello B, deLeon AC Jr, et al. ACC/AHA guidelines for the management of patients with valvular heart disease: A report of the American College of Cardiology American Heart Association Task Force on Practice Guidelines (Committee on Management of Patients with Valvular Heart Disease). *J Am Coll Cardiol* 1998;32:1486–1588.
3. Stroke Prevention in Atrial Fibrillation Investigators. Warfarin versus aspirin for prevention of thromboembolism in atrial fibrillation: Stroke Prevention in Atrial Fibrillation II Study. *Lancet* 1994;343:687–691.
4. Stroke Prevention in Atrial Fibrillation Investigators. Adjusted-dose warfarin versus low-intensity, fixed dose warfarin plus aspirin for high-risk patients with atrial fibrillation: Stroke Prevention in Atrial Fibrillation III randomized clinical trial. *Lancet* 1996;348:633–638.
5. Starr A, Grunkemeier GL. Recurrent thromboembolism: Significance and management. In: Butchart EG, Bodnar E, eds. *Thrombosis, Embolism and Bleeding.* London: ICR; 1992:402–415.

6. Blackstone EH. Analyses of thrombosis, embolism and bleeding as time-related outcome events. In: Butchart EG, Bodnar E, eds. *Thrombosis, Embolism and Bleeding*. London: ICR; 1992:445–463.

7. ACC/AHA Task Force. Guidelines for the evaluation and management of heart failure. *Circulation* 1999;92:2764–2784.

8. Al-Khadra AS, Salem DN, Rand WM, et al. Warfarin anticoagulation and survival: A cohort analysis from the Studies of Left Ventricular Dysfunction. *J Am Coll Cardiol* 1998;31:749–753.

9. Bloomfield P, Wheatley DJ, Prescott RJ, et al. Twelve-year comparison of a Bjork-Shiley mechanical heart valve with porcine bioprostheses. *N Engl J Med* 1991;324:573–579.

10. Hammermeister KE, Sethi GK, Henderson WG, et al. Outcomes 15 years after valve replacement with a mechanical versus bioprosthetic valve. *J Am Coll Cardiol* 2000;36:1152–1158.

11. Grunkemeier GL, Li H-H, Naftel DC, et al. Long-term performance of heart valve prosthesis. *Curr Probl Cardiol* 2000;25:73–156.

12. Geras M, Chesebro JH, Fuster V, et al. High risk of thromboemboli early after bioprosthetic cardiac valve replacement. *J Am Coll Cardiol* 1995; 25:1111–1119.

13. Stein PD, Alpert JS, Bussey HI, et al. Antithrombotic therapy in patients with mechanical or biological prosthetic heart valves. *Chest* 2001; 119:220S–227S.

14. Cannegieter SC, Rosendaal FR, Wintzen AR, et al. Optimal oral anticoagulant therapy in patients with mechanical heart valves. *N Engl J Med* 1995;333:11–17.

15. Saour JN, Sieck JO, Mamo LAR, et al. Trial of different intensities of anticoagulation in patients with prosthetic heart valves. *N Engl J Med* 1990;322:428–432.

16. Hylek EM, Skates SJ, Sheehan MA, et al. An analysis of the lowest effective intensity of prophylactic anticoagulation for patients with nonrheumatic atrial fibrillation. *N Engl J Med* 1996;335:540–546.

17. Acar J, Iung B, Boissel JP, et al. AREVA: Multicenter randomized comparison of low-dose versus standard-dose anticoagulation in patients with mechanical prosthetic heart valves. *Circulation* 1996;94: 2107–2112.

18. Rahimtoola SH. Choice of prosthetic heart valve in adult patients. *J Am Coll Cardiol* 2003;41:893–904.

19. Hyashi J, Nakazawa S, Oguma F, et al. Combined warfarin and antiplatelet therapy after St. Jude medical valve replacement for mitral valve disease. *J Am Coll Cardiol* 1994;23:672–677.

20. Turpie AG, Gent M, Laupacis A, et al. A comparison of aspirin with placebo in patients treated with warfarin after heart-valve replacement. *N Engl J Med* 1993;329:524–529.

21. Altman R, Rouvier J, Gurfinkel E, et al. Comparison of high-dose with low-dose aspirin in patients with mechanical heart valve replacement treated with oral anticoagulant. *Circulation* 1996;94:2113–2116.

22. Massel D, Little SH. Risks and benefits of adding anti-platelet therapy to warfarin among patients with prosthetic heart valves: A meta-analysis. *J Am Coll Cardiol* 2001;37:569–578.

23. Laffort P, Rondant R, Roques X, et al. Early and long-term (one-year) effects of the association of aspirin and oral anticoagulant on thrombi and morbidity after replacement of the mitral valve with the St. Jude Medical prosthesis. *J Am Coll Cardiol* 2000;35:739–746.

24. Hung L, Rahimtoola SH. Prosthetic heart valve and pregnancy. *Circulation* 2003;107:1240–1246.

25. Anticoagulation in Prosthetic Valves and Pregnancy Consensus Report (APPCR) Panel. Anticoagulation and enoxaparin use in patients with prosthetic heart valves and/or pregnancy. An evidenced-based review and focused analysis of current controversies and clinical strategies. *Clinical Cardiology Consensus Reports* 2002;3(9):1–20.

26. FDA Med Watch. 2002 Safety Information. http://www.fda.gov. Accessed May 22, 2003.

27. Hurrell DG, Schaff HV, Tajik AJ. Thrombolytic therapy for obstruction of mechanical prosthetic valves. *Mayo Clinic Proc* 1996;71:604–613.

28. Roudaut R, Lafitte S, Roudaut MF, et al. Fibrinolysis of mechanical prosthetic valve thrombosis: A single-center study of 127 cases. *J Am Coll Cardiol* 2003;41(4):653–658.

29. Lengyel M, Fuster V, Keltai M, et al. Guidelines for management of left-sided prosthetic valve thrombosis: A role for thrombolytic therapy. Prosthetic Valve Thrombosis. *J Am Coll Cardiol* 1997;30:1521–1526.

30. Özkan M, Kaymaz C, Kirma C, et al. Intravenous thrombolytic treatment of mechanical prosthetic valve thrombosis: A study using serial transesophageal echocardiography. *J Am Coll Cardiol* 2000;35:1881–1889.

31. Shaprina Y, Herz I, Vatini M, et al. Thrombolysis is an effective and safe therapy in stuck bileaflet mitral valves in the absence of high-risk thrombi. *J Am Coll Cardiol* 2000;35:1874–1880.

32. Tinker JH, Tarhan S. Discontinuing anticoagulant therapy in surgical patients with cardiac valve prostheses: Observations in 180 operations. *JAMA* 1978;239:738–739.

33. Bryan AJ, Butchart EG. Prosthetic heart valves and anticoagulant management during non-cardiac surgery. *Br J Surg* 1995;82:577–578.

34. Kearon C, Hirsh J. Current concepts: Management of anticoagulation before and after elective surgery. *N Engl J Med* 1997;336(21): 1506–1511.

35. Morton MJ, McAnulty JH, Rahimtoola SH, et al. Risks and benefits of postoperative cardiac catheterization in patients with ball-valve prostheses. *Am J Cardiol* 1977;40:870–875.

36. Schomig A, Neumann F, Kastrati A, et al. A randomized comparison of antiplatelet and anticoagulant therapy after the placement of coronary-artery stents. *N Engl J Med* 1998;339:1084–1089.

37. Martin L, Baim D, Jeffrey P, et al. A Clinical trial comparing three antithrombotic-drug regimens after coronary artery stenting. *N Engl J Med* 1998;339:1665–1671.

38. Chamorro A, Vila N, Saiz A, et al. Early anticoagulation after large cerebral embolic infarction: A safety study. *Neurology* 1995;45:861–865.

39. Sherman DJ, Dyken ML, Gent M, et al. Antithrombotic therapy for cerebrovascular disorders: Fourth ACCP consensus conference on antithrombotic therapy. *Chest* 1995;108(suppl):444s–456s.

40. Wijdicks E, Schievink W, Brown R, et al. The dilemma of discontinuation of anticoagulation therapy for patients with intracranial hemorrhage and mechanical heart valves. *Neurosurgery* 1998;42:769–773.

41. Deveras RAE, Kessler CM. Reversal of warfarin-induced excessive anticoagulation with recombinant human factor Vlla concentrate. *Ann Int Med* 2002;137:884–888.

42. Wilson WR, Geraci JE, Danielson GK, et al. Anticoagulant therapy and central nervous system complication in patients with prosthetic valve endocarditis. *Circulation* 1978;57:1004–1007.

43. Fuster V, Ryden LE, Asinger RW, et al. ACC/AHA/ESC Guidelines for the management of patients with atrial fibrillation: Executive Summary. *J Am Coll Cardiol* 2001;38:1231–1265.

CONGENITAL HEART DISEASE

CARDIOVASCULAR DISEASES DUE TO GENETIC ABNORMALITIES

Ali J. Marian / Ramon Brugada / Robert Roberts

ESSENTIALS OF GENETIC DISORDERS

Genetic factors play a significant role in all cardiovascular disorders (see also Chap. 5). Genetic defects are responsible for malformations of the heart and blood vessels, which account for the largest number of human birth defects, occurring in about 1 percent of all live births.[1,2] The prevalence is estimated to be tenfold higher among stillbirths.[1,2] Genetic defects are also responsible for familial cardiovascular disorders, such as cardiomyopathies and the long-QT (LQT) syndrome as well as nonfamilial and complex phenotypes, such as atherosclerosis and common forms of hypertension. Molecular genetics in conjunction with cytogenetics (the study of chromosomes and their abnormalities) provide the opportunity to decipher the genetic basis and pathogenesis of cardiovascular diseases. In view of the rapid pace of genetic discoveries, it is expected that genetic diagnosis and screening will become incorporated into standard practice in the near future. It is thus imperative that cardiologists understand the basis for genetic disorders and medical and ethical implications of genetics.

Basis for Genetic Transmission

All hereditary information is transmitted through DNA, a linear polymer composed of purine (adenine, guanine) and pyrimidine (cytosine, thymine) bases. The gene is the basic hereditary unit and consists of a distinct fragment of DNA, which encodes a specific polypeptide (protein). There are about 35,000 genes in the human genome[3] and each individual has two copies of each gene, called *alleles*. The genes are localized in a linear sequence along 23 pairs of chromosomes, including 22 pairs of autosomes (chromosomes 1 to 22) and one pair are sex chromosomes, X and Y. Females have two X chromosomes, while males carry one X and one Y chromosome. Each parent contributes one of each chromosome pair (the members of the pair are referred to as *homologous chromosomes*) and thus one copy of each gene. The site at which a gene is located on a particular chromosome is referred to as the *genetic locus*. A given gene always resides at the same genetic locus on a particular chromosome, so the loci on homologous chromosomes are identical. However, alleles residing at these loci may be identical or different, leading to homozygous (identical alleles) and heterozygous (two different alleles present at the locus) states.

The genetic information is encoded by the linear sequence of the four bases of the DNA. Translation of this information into protein is through a translational code passed on through messenger ribonucleic acid (mRNA), whereby three bases, referred to as a *codon*, encode a specific amino acid. The transcribed mRNA serves as the template that determines sequence of the amino acids in the resulting polypeptide. Both autosomal alleles are usually transcribed into mRNA and translated into protein. However, expression of a gene can be restricted to specific cells and organs or regulated during a developmental stage because of regulation by cell- and tissue-specific transcription factors. In cells that carry two X chromosomes, whether these are derived from normal females or XXY individuals with Klinefelter syndrome, only one X is active and the other X is silent after early embryogenesis.

Classification of Genetic Disorders

In general, DNA nucleotide sequences remain stable during transmission to offspring. Nonetheless, occasional base sequence changes do occur, which are referred to as *mutations*. Mutations represent stable, heritable alterations in DNA. A number of mutagenic factors—such as environmental agents, radiation, chemicals, and errors by the DNA synthetic and editing enzymes—can induce mutations. Mutations can involve a visible alteration at the level of the chromosome (chromosomal abnormalities), which can result in the deletion or translocation of a portion of the chromosome, whereby several genes are often eliminated or altered. In contrast, mutations can be restricted to minor alterations in the DNA sequence, which vary from the substitution of a single nucleotide to that of the deletion or addition of multiple nucleotides. Thus, hereditary and congenital diseases are conventionally classified into three broad categories: (1) chromosomal abnormalities, (2) single-gene or monogenic disorders, and (3) polygenic disorders or complex traits, which are due to interactions between defects in multiple genes and nongenetic factors.

CHROMOSOMAL ABNORMALITIES

Each human cell has two copies of each chromosome (*diploids*) and each chromosome has two arms, referred to as the long or "q" and the short or "p" arms. The arms of the chromosomes meet at a primary constriction referred to as the *centromere*. Mutations typically occur during meiosis when chromosomes separate; they can include large deletions, duplications, translocations, rearrangements, and aneuploidy (too few or too many chromosomes). Chromosomal abnormalities are relatively common during embryonic life and lead to spontaneous abortion, often during the first trimester of pregnancy.[1] However, a significant number of fetuses with chromosomal abnormalities survive, and such abnormalities are found in approximately 1 in 200 live-born infants. Most diseases due to chromosomal abnormalities are detected in the neonates or infants because of involvement of many genes causing phenotypes that are easily diagnosed on physical examination. Chromosomal abnormalities often lead to structural heart defects and are found in 5 to 13 percent of live-born children with congenital heart disease.[2]

The usual cause for gain of a chromosome is nondisjunction due to failure of a homologous pair of chromosomes to separate during meiosis. When an additional copy of the chromosome is added during fertilization, three copies of the same chromosome (or only one copy) are found in the new zygote instead of the chromosome pair. Two of the most common chromosomal disorders causing heart disease in the adult, namely Down's syndrome (trisomy 21) and Turner's syndrome (XO), are both due to nondisjunction. Chromosomal rearrangements occur when a chromosome breaks and rejoins within itself incorrectly, which can potentially result in an inversion of the genetic material. Inversion occurs when a chromosome breaks at two points and the intermediate segment reunites in inverted orientation. Typically there is no apparent phenotype in persons carrying an inversion, but their offspring may have severe abnormalities due to the disruption in chromosome pairing that can take place during meiosis. Isochromes are formed when two short or long arms join with loss of the other arm. Chromosomal translations occur when breaks arise in two chromosomes that are reunited after exchange of segments. Chromosome duplications or gains of chromosomal material may also be associated with phenotypic abnormality, but most commonly they cause no obvious aberration.

Chromosome deletions are large deletions (equal to or greater than 10^6 base pairs) that commonly lead to loss of a large amount of DNA and loss or disruption of multiple genes. Consequently, a series of phenotypes in a single individual may be present due to interruptions in a series of genes within the loci of a single chromosome.

SINGLE-GENE DISORDERS

A single-gene disorder is an inherited disease caused by mutations in a single gene that are necessary and sufficient for the development of the phenotype. Single-gene disorders show a Mendelian pattern of inheritance; they are classified as autosomal dominant, autosomal recessive, or X-linked (dominant or recessive). The majority of monogenic diseases exhibit an autosomal dominant mode of inheritance and therefore, in a given family, approximately half of the members are affected. Monogenic disorders with an autosomal recessive inheritance are due to mutations in both copies of the gene. Therefore, in a given family only 25 percent of the offspring exhibit the phenotype, 50 percent carry the mutation, and 25 percent are normal. In X-linked inheritance, only males exhibit the disease (in general) and females are commonly free of the phenotype but carry the mutation. However, if the mutation involves a major protein, the effect of the mutation may be dominant and females can exhibit clinical phenotype. In diseases due to mitochondrial DNA mutations, inheritance is from the mother (no male-to-male transmission), since mitochondrial DNA is predominantly inherited from the ovum.

Only a fraction of cardiovascular disorders are monogenic. The DNA mutation gives rise to a change in the corresponding amino acids of the encoded protein and exerts its deleterious effects via functional alterations, whether the proteins are enzymes, regulatory proteins, or structural elements. A change in even one amino acid located in critical domain of the protein can enhance the function (gain-of-function mutation) or impair the function (loss-of-function mutation), with a concomitant change in the phenotype. On average, a mutation occurs every 10^6 cell divisions or once every 200,000 years. Only mutations occurring in the gametes are transmitted.

In single-gene disorders, while the presence of the causal mutations is necessary for the development of the disease, other factors also affect the phenotypic expression of the disease. In particular, modifier genes or the genetic background of the affected subjects as well as environmental factors are major determinants of phenotypic expression of a single-gene disorder.

POLYGENIC DISORDERS

Polygenic or complex traits are caused by an assortment of interactions among variants of many genes and nongenetic factors. Therefore, in this setting, the presence of a single variant may not be sufficient to cause a disease, nor will its absence prevent development of the disease. Polygenic disorders account for the majority of the cardiovascular diseases, including atherosclerosis, essential hypertension, obesity, and diabetes mellitus. In polygenic diseases, multiple genes interact to induce the disorder or to provide an increased risk of developing it. Changes involving a single nucleotide are distributed throughout the human genome with a frequency of about 1 per 600 base pairs (bp).[4,5] These changes, referred to as single (or simple) nucleotide polymorphisms (SNPs) (see Chap. 5), account for most interindividual differences such as height and weight, susceptibility to disease, clinical outcome, and response to therapy (pharmacogenetics). The genes responsible for polygenic hereditary disorders are difficult to map, and the results of genetic studies are considered provisional pending proof of causality through experimentation.

Classification of Mutations

Most human diseases exhibit genetic heterogeneity, defined as being due to different genes and mutations causing the same phenotype, which may arise from multiple mutations in one gene (allele heterogeneity) or in two or more genes (locus heterogeneity). Within any one family, however, there is one causal gene and mutation in all affected members; only rarely, two different causal mutations or genes are transmitted for the same disease. A good example is familial hypertrophic cardiomyopathy (HCM), which may involve 11 different genes (locus heterogeneity) with multiple mutations in each (allelic heterogeneity). Mutations can involve a microscopically visible alteration, such as deletion or translocation of a portion of the chromosome (chromosomal abnormalities), or a minute change in the DNA sequence, such as alteration of one purine or pyrimidine base. Mutations involving only a single nucleotide are known as point mutations and are responsible for 70 percent or more of all adult single-gene disorders. A point mutation may be a substitution of one nucleotide for another, changing the amino acid sequence (missense mutation); or it may change from encoding an amino acid to become a stop codon, which will truncate the protein (truncated or nonsense mutation); or it may eliminate a stop codon so the protein is elongated (elongated mutant). Finally, it may change the codon without changing the amino acid sequence (synonomous mutation). All genes during transcription and translation are read from 5' to 3' orientation, with each triplet of bases (codon) coding for a specific amino acid. If a nucleotide is deleted (deletion) or an additional one is inserted (insertion), it will shift the reading frame; the resulting protein would be entirely different (frame-shift mutation) and usually nonfunctional. If a purine nucleotide is substituted for a pyrimidine or vice versa, the mutation is referred to as a transversion, while if purine or pyrimidine substitutes for another purine or pyrimidine, respectively, it is called a transition. Other mutations may result from the deletion or addition of several nucleotides. In myotonic dystrophy, for example, a triplet repeat several thousand nucleotides in length is inserted into the 3' end of the gene. Another type of mutation is known as a gene conversion, where two genes interact and part of the nucleotide sequence of one gene becomes incorporated into that of the other. Mutations in genes exert their deleterious effects via a structural alteration of the protein that has functional consequences, as noted.

Genetic Penetrance and Expressivity

The percentage of individuals within a family who have inherited the causal mutation and have one or more features of the disease is referred to as the penetrance. Penetrance is an all-or-none phenomenon, and any manifestation, however minute, indicates that the gene has full penetrance in that individual. Nonpenetrance refers to lack of any observable phenotype. This feature is to be distinguished from expressivity, which refers to the variable nature of the clinical phenotype, such as the severity. Thus, by definition, to have expressivity, the trait must be penetrant. Numerous genetic and environmental factors can affect expression of a gene, making it nearly impossible to determine which factor is most important in a specific individual or disease. These factors are shown in Table 72-1.

Patterns of Inheritance

Inherited disorders due to a single abnormal gene are transmitted to offspring in a predictable fashion termed Mendelian transmission. As previously noted, each individual has two copies of each gene, referred to as alleles, one transmitted from each parent. Mendel's first law states that each of the two alleles located on separate chromosomes segregates independently and is transmitted unchanged to offspring. Thus, the chance of inheriting the mother's allele versus the father's is 50 percent. Mendel's second law states that genes on the same chromosome also assert themselves independently through the process of crossover between segments of chromosomes (discussed below). Thus, the greater the distance between two loci, the more likely they are to be separated during genetic transmission.

TABLE 72-1 Factors Affecting the Phenotype in Genetic Disorders

1. Causal genes and mutations
2. Modifier genes (genetic background)
3. Age
4. Gender
5. Exogenous or environmental factors
6. Maternal factors
7. Epigenetic alterations (such as DNA methylation)
8. Posttranscriptional and posttranslation modifications
9. Gene-gene and gene-environmental interactions

Mutant genes located on any of the 22 autosomal pairs or the two sex chromosomes may produce phenotypes inherited by simple patterns classified as autosomal (dominant or recessive) or X-linked, respectively. The terms *dominant inheritance* and *recessive inheritance* refer to characteristics of the phenotype and are not characteristics of the gene per se. Dominant inheritance implies that a person with one copy of a mutant allele and one copy of the normal allele develops the phenotype associated with the mutant allele. Recessive traits, on the other hand, require both alleles to be mutant in order to produce a phenotype.

AUTOSOMAL DOMINANT INHERITANCE

Dominant disorders are those exhibiting a phenotype in heterozygous individuals, as noted. Males and females are equally affected, and offspring of an affected heterozygote have a 50 percent chance of inheriting the mutant allele. In a sporadic case, the mutation occurs de novo and in one of the germlines of parents (typically sperm) but by definition is absent in the somatic cells of parents. Autosomal dominant inheritance can be misdiagnosed as sporadic if there is low expressivity in the phenotypically normal parent carrying the mutant allele or if extramarital paternity has occurred. The following features are characteristic of autosomal dominant inheritance (Fig. 72-1): (1) each affected individual has an affected parent unless the disease occurred due to a new mutation or the heterozygous parent has low expressivity; (2) equal proportions (i.e., 50-50) of normal and affected offspring are likely to be born to an affected individual; (3) normal children of an affected individual bear only normal offspring; (4) equal proportions of males and females are affected; (5) both sexes are equally likely to transmit the abnormal allele to male and female offspring, and male-to-male transmission occurs; and (6) vertical transmission through successive generations occurs. Two other characteristic features of autosomal dominant diseases that help to differentiate this type of inheritance from autosomal recessive disorders are delayed age of onset and variable clinical expression.

AUTOSOMAL RECESSIVE INHERITANCE

Autosomal recessive phenotypes are clinically apparent when the patient carries two mutant alleles (i.e., is homozygous) at the locus responsible for the disease. The disease-causing gene is found on one of the 22 autosomes; thus both males and females will be equally affected. Clinical uniformity is typical and disease onset generally occurs early in life. Recessive disorders are more commonly diagnosed in childhood than are dominant diseases. On average, only one in four children (25 percent) will be affected. The following are characteristics of autosomal recessive disorders (Fig. 72-1): (1) parents

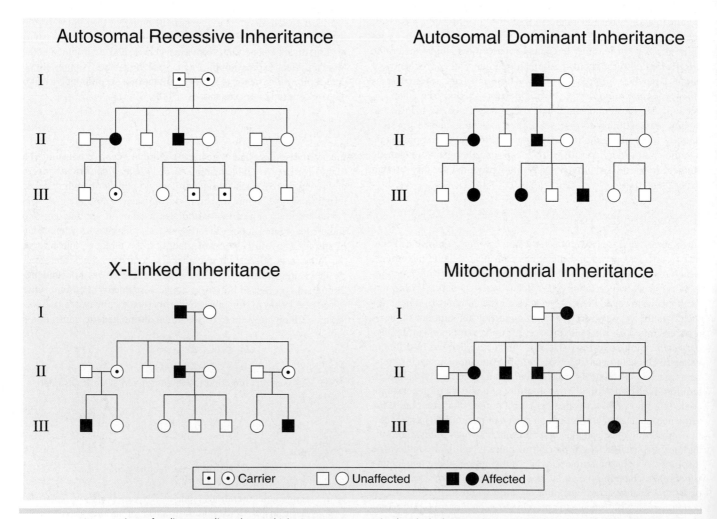

FIGURE 72-1 This typical set of pedigrees outlines the usual inheritance patterns for autosomal dominant and recessive traits, X-linked inheritance, and mitochondrial inheritance. Squares signify males and circles, females. Filled-in circles and squares are affected females and males, respectively.

are clinically normal (in alternate generations) but genetically are heterozygotes; (2) alternate generations are affected, with no vertical transmission; (3) both sexes are affected with equal frequency; and (4) each offspring of heterozygous carriers has a 25 percent chance of being affected, a 50 percent chance of being an unaffected carrier, and a 25 percent chance of inheriting only normal alleles.

X-LINKED INHERITANCE

X-linked inherited disorders are caused by defects in genes located on the X chromosome. Since females have two X chromosomes, they may carry either one mutant allele (heterozygote) or two mutant alleles (homozygote). The trait may therefore display dominant or recessive expression. Males have a single X chromosome (and one Y chromosome); therefore a male is expected to display the full syndrome whenever he inherits the abnormal gene from his mother. Hence, the terms *X-linked dominant* and *X-linked recessive* apply only to the expression of the gene in females. Since a male must pass on his Y chromosome to all male offspring, he cannot pass on a mutant X allele to his sons; therefore no male-to-male transmission in X-linked disorders can occur. On the other hand, a male must contribute his one X chromosome to all daughters. All females receiving a mutant X chromosome are known as *carriers,* and those who become affected clinically with the disease are known as *manifesting female carriers.* The characteristic features of X-linked inheritance (Fig. 72-1) include (1) no male-to-male transmission; (2) all daughters of affected males are carriers; (3) sons of carrier females have a 50 percent risk of being affected and daughters have a 50 percent chance of being carriers; (4) affected homozygous females occur only when an affected male and carrier female have children; and (5) the pedigree pattern in X-linked recessive traits tends to be oblique because of the occurrence of the trait in the sons of normal carriers but not in the sisters of affected males (i.e., uncles and nephews affected). Examples of X-linked disorders of the heart include X-linked cardiomyopathy, Barth's syndrome, and Duchenne/ Becker and Emery-Dreifuss muscular dystrophies.

MITOCHONDRIAL INHERITANCE

Spermatocytes contribute few or no mitochondria to the zygote; the entire mitochondrial DNA in a fetus is derived from the mitochondria already present in the cytoplasm of the oocyte. Thus, phenotypes due to mitochondrial DNA mutations demonstrate only maternal inheritance. The characteristic features of mitochondrial inheritance (Fig. 72-1) include (1) equal frequency and severity of disease for each sex; (2) transmission through females only, with offspring of affected males being unaffected; (3) all offspring of affected females may be affected; (4) extreme variability of expression of disease within a family (may include apparent nonpenetrance); (5) phenotype may be age-dependent; (6) organ mosaicism is common.

OVERVIEW OF GENE MAPPING AND MUTATION DETECTION

Chromosomal Mapping in Single-Gene Disorders

Until the 1980s, identification of a disease-causing gene without knowing the causal protein was nearly impossible. For the majority of diseases, neither the defect nor the protein was known. Technical advances that made chromosomal mapping feasible include (1) computerized linkage analysis, (2) development of highly informative DNA markers spanning the entire genome, and (3) detection of markers by polymerase chain reaction (PCR). The 46 chromosomes

of the human genome contain 3.2 billion bp of DNA. To locate a particular gene, one must first map the chromosomal locus, which requires knowledge of certain chromosomal landmarks, referred to as *DNA markers.* A DNA marker is a polymorphic sequence of DNA with a known chromosomal position, which can be detected by analyzing an individual's DNA (discussed in detail below). Markers are now available that span each chromosome at intervals of not more than 5 million base pairs (Mbp) on all chromosomes (a set of 700 highly polymorphic markers). Genetic distance is measured in terms of centimorgans (cM), named after the geneticist T. H. Morgan. One cM approximates 1 million bp (Mbp). Markers like genes have two alleles in a given individual and are transmitted to offspring according to Mendel's law, with the individual being heterozygous or homozygous for that marker. If a marker is homozygous, it is not informative for genetic linkage. When all of the markers are placed together on each chromosome and the genetic distance between them is estimated, a *genetic map* is produced. A map of over 5000 highly informative markers that span the entire genome has been developed.[6]

Identification of a particular locus is made possible by showing that the causal gene of interest is in close proximity to a DNA marker on the same chromosome, a method referred to as *genetic linkage analysis.* A fundamental requirement for linkage analysis is a family in which the disease of interest is transmitted to offspring over at least two and preferably three generations. At least six affected individuals are required for analyzing cosegregation of DNA markers with inheritance of the disease, although a larger number of affected individuals is preferable.

The homologous pairs of chromosomes are assorted, and one from each parent is transmitted to the offspring by chance. Each gene, allele, or marker is transmitted independently; thus the odds of any two genes (or a marker and a gene) being coinherited is by chance alone (50 percent). Even genes on the same chromosome are transmitted independently unless they are in close physical proximity to each other, in which case they cosegregate together by the mechanism of crossover between homologous chromosomes (Fig. 72-2). This provides continual mixing of the genes during every meiosis and is the predominant reason why no two individuals have the same genotype for DNA markers unless they are identical twins. Prior to meiosis, the two homologous chromosomes come together and form bridges (*chiasmata*) such that segments of equal proportion are exchanged between them, giving rise to crossover between homologous regions of various genes. The loci occupy the same chromosomal position on the homologous chromosome on which they are combined as they had on their original homologous chromosome. There is no net loss of chromosomal material or genes, but crossover leads to a constant intermixing of the chromosomes such that no two offspring will ever be identical. Crossovers occur only between homologous chromosomes. On average there are 33 crossovers between homologous chromosome pairs per meiosis. In genetic parlance, crossing over is referred to as *recombination.*

FAMILY HISTORY AND EVALUATION

The most important part of an evaluation for genetic disease is the family history. First, this may give clues to the diagnosis of a particular phenotype and inheritance patterns within an individual family. An individual's ethnic background may, for instance, suggest the need for specific types of genetic screening, such as for hemoglobinopathies in individuals of African or Mediterranean ancestry or for Tay-Sachs disease in individuals of eastern European (Ashkenazi) Jewish ancestry. The individual with the medical problem who brought the family to the attention of the physician is

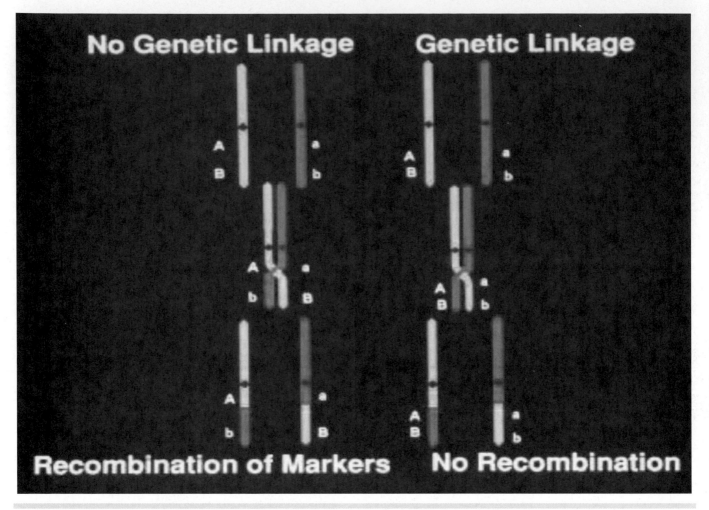

FIGURE 72-2 Linkage analysis. Loci A (disease locus) and B (DNA marker locus) are located in close proximity with minimal chance of crossover between them. Thus, even when crossover occurs between homologous segments of chromosomes during meiosis, A and B loci cosegregate together and thus are considered genetically linked.

referred to as the *proband* or *propositus* (*proposita* for females) or index case. Information should generally be collected on all individuals who are first-, second-, or third-degree relatives of the proband. First-degree relatives of the proband are the parents and children. Second-degree relatives are aunts and uncles, grandparents, and grandchildren of the proband. Third-degree relatives are first cousins, great aunts and uncles, great-grandparents, and great-grandchildren. A pedigree chart (Fig. 72-1) is then generated. This information should include medical problems and pregnancies. If relatives are deceased, the age at death and the cause of death should be recorded. With a pedigree chart and specific family information, more general questions are asked, including whether other family members have the same or similar problems. Information about various types of birth defects, mental retardation, early infant deaths, miscarriages, stillbirths, or other diseases or handicaps in the family is sought. With some disorders, there may be a variability of a particular condition (i.e., clinical heterogeneity), even within a family. For example, with a possible diagnosis of HCM, one should ask about premature death or syncope. A pregnancy history may provide information to support a possible teratogenic exposure. The date of the last menstrual period, whether the pregnancy was planned, whether contraception was used immediately prior to pregnancy, the time when the pregnancy was recognized, and when the mother sought prenatal care should be noted. Problems during the pregnancy—such as bleeding, spotting, cramping, fevers, rashes, or illnesses; drug exposures (both prescribed and nonprescribed), alcohol intake, or "recreational" drug use; and exposures to potent chemicals in the workplace or while involved in various hobbies—should be explored. Pregnancy and family histories can then be used in conjunction with the findings on physical examination to derive a potential etiologic diagnosis and to plan for further diagnostic studies. The term *etiologic diagnosis* should suggest whether a specific cardiac defect is familial (by family history), genetic but not familial (sporadic), teratogenic (by pregnancy history), or multifactorial. Prognosis and recurrence risk are linked strongly to an accurate diagnosis and its probable etiology. In sum, accurate phenotypic characterization is essential for all genetic studies.

CONCEPT OF GENETIC LINKAGE ANALYSIS

Despite the independent assortment of chromosomes and genes during meiosis, genes (alleles) on two or more loci are often coinherited because they are so close together that a chiasmatic bridge does not form between them. Two loci coinherited more than 50 percent of the time are considered genetically linked. To map the chromosomal locus responsible for a causal gene, DNA markers that are evenly distributed across the chromosomes are selected. DNA is collected from all members of a family (normal and affected) and genotyped for the selected markers. If a DNA marker is coinherited with the phenotype in the affected individuals, the chromosomal locus where the DNA marker resides is in close physical proximity to the locus of the causal gene. This is referred to as *genetic linkage* between the disease (causal gene) and the DNA marker. The concept of linkage analysis is illustrated in Fig. 72-2. Shown on the left panel is an illustration of genetic linkage between a locus for a DNA marker and that of a disease that is inherited in a Mendelian dominant fashion. The locus, designated with an "A," carries the allele responsible for the disease. The corresponding locus, "a," on the homologous chromosome has the allele that codes for the same protein but has not undergone a mutation and is thus the normal allele. The loci designated "B" and "b" represent alleles of a DNA marker of known location that has nothing to do with the disease. In the right panel, the disease and the marker loci are so close that they tend to be coinherited within the family. In contrast, in the left panel, the "A" and "b" loci are so far apart that recombination and crossover occur between the two markers; thus they segregate independently. The calculation necessary to prove definitively that genetic linkage does or does not exist between a DNA marker and a disease-related locus is sophisticated and requires advanced computer programs. The odds for and against linkage are calculated, and linkage exists if the odds in favor of linkage are at least 1000:1. Commonly the logarithm of the odds, referred to as the *LOD score* (log of the odds), is used and a LOD score of 3 or greater indicates linkage. If the LOD score is -2 (i.e., 10^{-2} or 100:1 odds against linkage), it excludes linkage. The likelihood of two genes being separated by recombination increases in proportion to the distance between them. The distance between a marker and a disease-causing gene when genetically linked is quite variable and may be anywhere from 1 to 50 Mbp but is usually within 1 to 10 Mbp. Thus, the inherent resolution of genetic linkage analysis is never better than 1 Mbp.

It is possible on the basis of linkage analysis alone to construct a chromosomal map of all of the DNA markers, with the distance between the various markers estimated in centimorgans. This is a complex calculation derived from the number of recombinations between the DNA markers during meioses. The recombination frequency between two markers, two genes, or a gene and a marker is the ratio of the number of crossover events to the total number of meioses. The lower the recombination frequency between the locus of a DNA marker and that of a disease-causing gene, the closer those two must be in physical distance on the chromosome. Even though the loci of the DNA marker and that of the disease-causing gene are in close enough proximity to be genetically linked, recombination may occur, and the extent to which recombination does occur reflects roughly the physical distance between the two loci. The recombination fraction (or *theta*) is used to develop a means of estimating the genetic distance (in centimorgans) between genetically linked loci. A recombination frequency or crossover of 1 percent between two loci, whether occupied by two genes or one gene and a DNA marker, reflects a physical distance of approximately 1 cM between them. For a marker and a gene separated by 1 cM, this means the chance of a crossover between them during meiosis is only 1 percent; thus, the chance of their being coinherited is 99 percent. This is a statistically derived genetic map, however, and the distances are only approximate.

IDENTIFICATION OF THE GENE AND MUTATION

Once the chromosomal location of a gene has been mapped, the first technique in attempting to identify the gene is referred to as the positional *candidate gene approach*. While there are only about 30,000 genes in the genome, over 100,000 expressed sequenced tags (ESTs) have been mapped. ESTs are unique DNA sequences of 100 to 200 bp, each of which is believed to represent a portion of the expressed sequences of a gene. These genes and ESTs are available through a worldwide network of databases in the United States, Europe, and Japan that is updated on a daily basis.

The known candidate genes or their representative ESTs are amplified, usually by PCR, to determine whether there is a mutation that segregates with the disease. If none of the candidate genes in the region is shown to have a mutation that cosegregates with the disease, it may be necessary to clone the region. This approach is referred to as *positional cloning*, so named because a region is cloned knowing only its position relative to the genetically linked DNA markers. Positional cloning is usually not attempted unless the region (containing the gene) between the flanking DNA markers is 1 cM or less. To reduce the region for cloning, it is necessary to expand the family with the hope of finding crossovers such that DNA markers common to all affected would span only a short distance (<1 cM). This collection of DNA markers in a region would represent the haplotype being inherited by the affected individual and contains the responsible gene. To prove that the gene causes the disease, the mutation must be identified and shown to cosegregate with the disease and not with the unaffected members in the family. The approach to chromosomal mapping of hereditary diseases by linkage analysis and subsequent isolation of the gene is summarized in Table 72-2.

Polygenic Disorders

The human genome contains over 2 million nonredundant SNPs that form the backbone of interindividual variability in susceptibility to disease, clinical outcome, and response to drug therapy (pharmacogenetics). SNPs located in regulatory and coding regions of genes can affect expression or function of the encoded proteins and therefore are considered functional, with potential biological and clinical significance. Functional variants of genes can confer salutary or harmful effect toward susceptibility to a complex phenotype. Commonly, a large number of genetic variants are involved in the etiology of a complex disease, and each particular variant accounts for a very

---

TABLE 72-2 Steps Involved in Chromosomal Mapping Gene Identification

1. Identification of a family with a familial disease
2. Collection of clinical data from the family
3. Clinical assessment to provide an accurate diagnosis of the disease using a consistent and objective criterion to separate normal individuals from those affected and from those that are indeterminate or unknown
4. Collection of blood samples for immediate DNA analysis and development of lymphoblastoid cell lines for a renewable source of DNA
5. Development of a family pedigree
6. DNA analysis for markers of known chromosomal loci that span the human genome in an attempt to find a marker locus linked to the disease
7. Identification of the gene
8. Identification of mutation(s) causing the disease
9. Demonstration of a causal relationship between the mutant gene and the disease
10. Development of a convenient test to screen for the mutation

small fraction of the risk (genotype-related risk). Since multiple gene variants, located on the same or different chromosome in the genome, are involved in the pathogenesis of a polygenic disease, inheritance of the disease does not follow a classic Mendelian pattern. Therefore there is a lack of cosegregation of a candidate gene variant (allele) with inheritance of the phenotype. Consequently it is often difficult to establish the causality of a genetic variant in susceptibility to a complex trait, and often complex in vitro and in vivo functional studies are needed.

The most commonly used technique to identify susceptibility genes for complex diseases is allelic association study with candidate genes, in which an association between a variant or a haplotype of a candidate gene with a particular phenotype is shown. The most commonly used approach is a case-control design, in which frequency of haplotypes and genotypes are compared. Prospective longitudinal studies in populations in which the phenotype is extensively and meticulously characterized are required to provide robust evidence. In general, association studies are subject to a high rate of spurious results and their results should be considered provisional pending further proof through experimentation. This is particularly problematic in retrospective case-control allelic association studies performed in a small sample size. The design of an association study, sample size, biological plausibility of the association, functional significance of the polymorphism, strength of the association, and genetic and biological gradients provide clues to the merit of an observed association between a genotype or haplotype and a complex phenotype.

A second approach to identify genes for complex traits is genomewide search to analyze segregation of polymorphic DNA markers with a phenotype. The principle behind the techniques of genomewide search is based on the likelihood of sharing a susceptibility allele between the two relatives with the phenotype. For example, two sibs with a disease are expected to share the susceptibility allele more often than by chance alone. Sib-pair analysis is often performed in more than 300 sib pairs. Several variations of this approach, such as transmission disequilibrium test (TDT), have been developed and applied to complex traits. These techniques utilize the principle of linkage disequilibrium (LD) to map the location of the susceptibility gene. LD indicates that two DNA markers that are located in close proximity in the genome are more likely to cosegregate than by chance alone. Techniques based on LD are independent of incomplete penetrance, false-positive phenotype, genetic heterogeneity, and the high frequency of the disease-related allele. According to the principle of LD, for example, in sib-pair linkage analysis it is expected that the affected sibs will share the disease-related allele more often than would be likely by chance alone. Sib-pair linkage analysis is best suited for mapping genes that denote a high genotype-related risk (approximately > 4). It is not considered a powerful technique to map the susceptibility genes that confer a modest risk for a complex trait, which is often the case. TDT is considered more powerful in mapping the susceptibility genes that confer a modest genotype-related risk. TDT examines transmission of a particular allele from heterozygous parents to their offspring. An affected offspring is more likely to inherit the disease-related phenotype from a heterozygous parent than by chance alone (50 percent per random inheritance) or as compared to the unaffected offspring. Several other variations of these allele-sharing approaches are available and have been used to map the susceptibility genes for complex traits. Currently, block-haplotype association studies assessing the inheritance of haplotypes arising from multiple SNPs are considered the desired approach.[7] Efforts are under way to develop a haplotype-map (LD map) of the human genome in order to map susceptibility genes for complex traits,

to identify the genetic determinants of clinical outcome, and for pharmacogenetic studies.[8]

GENETIC COUNSELING PRINCIPLES

Genetic counseling should provide information about the diagnosis, possible etiology, and prognosis of a disease. In addition, psychosocial issues, reproductive options, and the availability of prenatal diagnosis should be discussed. Genetic counseling should be nondirective, providing information in a nonjudgmental, unbiased manner. The family should then be able to make decisions based on medical information in the context of their religious, moral, cultural, and social backgrounds and their financial situation. Although a genetic counselor may occasionally feel frustrated with a specific couple's decision, an effective counselor does not let personal biases interfere with the counseling role. Conflicts leading to major ethical issues and disputes may arise, however, and may be particularly apparent regarding issues of nonpaternity, sex selection, pregnancy termination, and selective nontreatment of malformed infants. Couples have many potential reproductive options, but not all may be acceptable religiously or culturally. Nevertheless, potential options should be mentioned in a sensitive manner. A common misunderstanding among families in genetic counseling is the issue of prenatal diagnosis and its relationship to abortion. Prenatal diagnosis does not imply that a parent should or would terminate the pregnancy. In many circumstances the information from prenatal diagnosis may help to reassure a couple that their risk of having another handicapped child is, in fact, much lower than expected. Conversely, if defects are found, the subspecialist may use more diagnostic approaches to make rational decisions about medical management of the infant prior to or immediately after delivery.

The accelerated pace of progress in gene discovery, molecular medicine, and molecular diagnostics has begun to allow for improved genetic counseling and portends the possibility of future genetic therapy. As knowledge about the genetic basis of disease grows, however, so does the potential for discriminative health insurance policies to exclude individuals at risk or to charge prohibitively high rates on the basis of predetermined illness. For this reason planners of the Human Genome Project recognized the need to protect individuals who volunteer for genetic study as well as those diagnosed by molecular methods in the future. Also for this reason, the National Institutes of Health—Department of Energy (NIH-DOE) Working Group on Ethical, Legal, and Social Implications (ELSI) of the Human Genome Project was developed. Congress has passed a bill prohibiting companies from using DNA analysis to assess genetic risk as a basis for hiring. Only 11 states, however, prohibit the use of DNA analysis to determine who should get medical insurance or whether they qualify for high- or low-risk premiums.

CARDIOVASCULAR ABNORMALITIES DUE TO CHROMOSOMAL DEFECTS

A list of chromosomal defects causing cardiovascular abnormalities is provided in Table 72-3. The most common chromosomal defects are described briefly below.

Turner's Syndrome (45X)

Turner syndrome is the most common chromosomal abnormality in females, with an incidence of 1 per 2500 live births, corresponding to approximately 1.5 million cases worldwide.[9] It results from partial or complete monosomy of the X chromosome and is characterized by cardiovascular anomalies, short stature, low-set ears, excess nuchal skin, broad chest with widely spaced nipples, peripheral lymphedema, and ovarian dysgenesis. Cardiac abnormalities are common, with a prevalence estimated to be between 23 and 40 percent.[9] The most common cardiovascular abnormalities are bicuspid aortic valve, which is present in 10 to 20 percent, and coarctation of aorta, present in 10 percent of the adult cases. The prevalence of these abnormalities is higher in children. Less common cardiovascular anomalies include aortic stenosis, partial anomalous venous drainage, and ventricular septal defect (VSD). Aortic dilatation and dissection, partly because of concomitant hypertension, also occur in patients with Turner's syndrome (see also Chap. 12).

Turner's syndrome is caused by the absence of an X chromosome, and 50 percent of the cases have the 45X karyotype and 13 percent mosaic monosomes (45X/46XX, 45X/47XXX). The pathogenesis of Turner's syndrome entails haploinsufficiency of genes (located on the X chromosome) that, under normal conditions, escape inactivation. As discussed earlier, in females with a normal XX karyotype, one copy of the X chromosome becomes inactivated during early embryogenesis. However, inactivation is partial and expression of both copies of genes is required for normal development. Specific genes that account for cardiovascular phenotype in Turner's syndrome are unknown. However, *SHOX* (short stature homeobox-containing gene) or *PHOG* (pseudoautosomal homeobox-containing osteogenic gene) are considered responsible for the short stature in Turner's syndrome.[9]

Trisomy 21 (Down's Syndrome)

Down's syndrome is a major cause of mental retardation and congenital heart disease, with a characteristic set of facial and physical features. The prevalence of Down's syndrome is approximately 20 in 10,000 live births, affecting more than 300,000 individuals in the United States alone.[10] The risk of having a liveborn with Down's syndrome increases with maternal age and is 1 in 1000 at age 30 and 10-fold higher at age 40. The recurrence rate is about 1 to 2 percent in the offspring. Clinical manifestations include congenital anomalies of the heart and gastrointestinal tract; epicanthal folds; flattened facial profile; small, rounded ears; upslanted palpebral fissures; excess nuchal skin; and brachycephaly. An increased risk of leukemia, immune system defects, and an Alzheimer-like dementia are associated with Down's syndrome. Cardiac abnormalities are present in approximately half of the cases; the most common of these include atrioventricular canal defect and isolated VSD, which occur in 45 and 35 percent of cases, respectively. Isolated secundum atrial septal defect (ASD) is present in 8 percent and tetralogy of Fallot in 5 percent of cases (see also Chap. 12).[11]

TABLE 72-3 Partial List of Chromosomal Abnormalities Associated with Heart Disease

Chromosome Defects	Syndromes	Cardiac Phenotype
45X	Turner's syndrome	Coarctation of the aorta, ASD, aortic stenosis
Trisomy 5		Interrupted aortic arch
Trisomy 13	Patau's syndrome	CHD, VSD
Trisomy 18	Edwards' syndrome	CHD, VSD
Partial trisomy 20q		Dextrocardia
Trisomy 21	Down's syndrome	CHD, ASD, VSD, PDA
Trisomy 22		VSD
Partial tetrasomy 22	Schmid-Fraccaro syndrome	CHD
		Anomalous pulmonary venous return
Deletion 4p	Wolf-Hirschhorn syndrome	CHD
Deletion 7q11.23	Williams syndrome	CHD, supravalvular aortic stenosis, hypertension, MVP
Deletion paternal 15q11	Prader-Willi syndrome	CHD
Deletion 17p	Miller Dieker syndrome	CHD, ASD
Deletion 22q11	CATCH-22, Di George, and velocardiofacial syndromes	CHD
Rearrangement 5p15.1-3	Cri du Chat	CHD
Recombination chromosome 8	San Luis Valley syndrome	Tetralogy of Fallot

ABBREVIATIONS: CHD = congenital heart disease; ASD = atrial septal defect; VSD = ventricular septal defect; PDA = patent ductus arteriosus; MVP = mitral valve prolapse.

Down's syndrome is caused by trisomy 21, which is full trisomy in 95 percent, chromosomal translocation in 2 percent, and mosaic in 3 percent. The vast majority of errors in meiosis leading to trisomy 21 are of maternal origin and occur during meiosis I in two-thirds and during meiosis II in one-fifth of the cases of free trisomy 21. The exact causal genes for the cardiovascular defects are unknown. However, the Down's Critical Region (DCR) has been mapped to an area of approximately 5 million bp that is associated with mental retardation and most of the facial features of the syndrome. Among the candidate genes is *DSCR1*, which is abundantly expressed in the heart and brain and is a candidate for cardiac anomalies and mental retardation.[12]

The pathogenesis of Down's syndrome is unknown but is likely to involve increased expression of multiple contiguous genes. As such, overexpression of *DSCR1*, which interacts with calcineurin A, the catalytic subunit of the Ca^{2+} calmodulin-dependent protein phosphatase, is shown in the brains of patients with Down's syndrome.[13]

Trisomy 18 (Edwards' Syndrome)

Edwards' syndrome is the second most common trisomy, with a prevalence of approximately 1 in 3000 to 7000 live births. The majority of infants die within a couple of weeks and approximately 10 percent survive more than a year. The syndrome is characterized by anomalies of the heart and microcephaly with a prominent occiput, a narrow forehead, low-set and malformed ears, micrognathia, clefting of the lip and palate, clenched hand with overlapping digits, rocker-bottom feet, and various hernias. Approximately 90 percent of the cases exhibit cardiovascular anomalies, which are diverse and include VSD, ASD, patent ductus arteriosus, pulmonary stenosis, tetralogy of Fallot, transposition of the great arteries, bicuspid aortic valve, dysplastic valves, and coarctation of the aorta.[11] Full trisomy occurs in more than 90 percent of cases, chromosomal translocation in 3 percent, and mosaicism in 1 percent of the cases. The causal gene(s) for the cardiovascular anomalies remain unknown.

Trisomy 13 (Patau's Syndrome)

Trisomy 13 is a rare disorder with an incidence of 1 per 5000 live births and a high early mortality, with approximately 50 percent of the affected infants dying within the first month of life. It is characterized by cardiac, urogenital, craniofacial, and central nervous system anomalies. Specific anomalies include microcephaly with sloping forehead, microophthalmia, cleft lip and palate, overlapping fingers with postaxial polydactyly, and renal abnormalities including polycystic kidney disease. Cardiac abnormalities are present in approximately 80 percent of the cases and include VSD, ASD, patent ductus arteriosus, pulmonary stenosis, coarctation of the aorta, dextrocardia, and truncus arteriosus.[11]

Patau's syndrome is caused by nondisjunction of chromosome 13 during meiosis in the vast majority of cases and rarely by translocation. Five percent of the cases are mosaic. The causal genes for cardiovascular anomalies in trisomy 13 are unknown.

DiGeorge (CATCH-22) and Velocardiofacial Syndromes

DiGeorge and velocardiofacial (VCSF) syndromes are autosomal dominant congenital anomalies caused by hemizygous deletion of a large segment of the long arm of chromosome 22 (22q11), leading to anomalies of multiple organs including the heart and facial bones. The prevalence in the general population is approximately 1 in 4000, accounting for approximately 15 percent of all congenital heart defects.[14] The term *CATCH-22* denotes *c*ardiac, *a*bnormal facies, *t*hymic hypoplasia, *c*left palate, *h*ypocalcemia (due to parathyroid hypoplasia), and the *22*nd chromosome. A diverse array of congenital heart defects including tetralogy of Fallot, interrupted aortic arch, truncus arteriosus, and patent ductus arteriosus have been described. Patients with VCSF exhibit craniofacial anomalies, cleft palate, and a variety of cardiac abnormalities, such as aortic arch anomalies, tetralogy of Fallot, and VSD. Cardiac valves and the myocardium are usually spared.

The deletion is typically large and involves approximately 32 million bp of DNA containing multiple genes. However, linkage analysis has restricted the causal genes to a critical segment of approximately 300 to 600 kbp, referred to as the DiGeorge critical region (*DGCR*) and containing approximately 25 to 30 candidate genes.[14] A major candidate gene is *UFD1L*, which encodes a protein involved in degradation of ubiquitinated proteins and is expressed during the embryogenesis of cell lines typically associated with DiGeorge syndrome. Identification of a large deletion in human transcription factor *UFD1L* in a single patient with a phenotype similar to that of DiGeorge syndrome provides further support. Furthermore, *UFD1L* is expressed in association with the conotruncus and the 4th embryologic aortic arch. Thus, deletion of *UFD1L* is expected to lead to the development of an interrupted aortic arch, a characteristic lesion of the DiGeorge syndrome. Moreover, deletion of *UFD1L* in mice produced some of the typical cardiac phenotypes that result from defective development of the 4th branchial arch.[15] Thus the pathogenesis of cardiac anomalies in DiGeorge syndrome appears to involve decreased expression levels of *UFD1L* during embryogenesis (haploinsufficiency). Additional genes, such as *ZNF74*, which encodes a zinc-finger transcription factor, are expected to be involved in the pathogenesis of other features of DiGeorge syndrome that arise from abnormal development of the 3d and 4th pharyngeal pouches.

GENETIC BASIS OF SPECIFIC CONGENITAL HEART DISEASES

A significant number of congenital heart diseases occur in isolation and are not part of complex phenotypes as observed in chromosomal abnormalities. Recently, the causal genes for several congenital heart diseases have been identified. Preliminary studies depict a common theme in the pathogenesis of isolated congenital heart defects, which implicate deficiency of several transcriptional factors that regulate cardiac gene expression during embryogenesis. However, there is considerable phenotypic, locus, and allelic heterogeneity. The genetic causes of several specific phenotypes are discussed.

Supravalvular Aortic Stenosis

Supravalvular aortic stenosis (SVAS) is an autosomal dominant disease characterized by discrete narrowing of the ascending aorta above the level of the sinus of Valsalva. It commonly occurs as a phenotype of Williams syndrome (or Williams-Bueren syndrome) in conjunction with mental retardation in some and exceptional talents in others, hypercalcemia, characteristic facial appearance, and stenosis of other major arteries. The prevalence of SVAS is estimated to be 1 in 25,000 live births.

The gene responsible for SVAS was initially mapped to chromosome 7q11.23 and subsequently identified as *ELN*, encoding elastin.[16] Almost all cases of isolated SVAS are due to *ELN* mutations, which comprise a variety of point and deletion mutations. Mutations result in elastin deficiency, which in the vascular system leads to inelasticity of the vessel wall and subsequent fibrosis due to altered stress-strain relation (elastin arteriopathy). Thus, haploinsufficiency underlies the pathogenesis of SVAS.

Patients with Williams syndrome may exhibit additional cardiovascular phenotypes including pulmonary arterial stenosis, aortic and mitral valve abnormalities, and tetralogy of Fallot. In 98 percent of cases of Williams syndrome there is a 1.5 million–bp deletion mutation that comprises *ELN* and another 17 contiguous genes. Contribution of these genes to pathogenesis of specific phenotypes in Williams syndrome remains unknown.

Familial Atrial Septal Defect

Atrial septal defect (ASD) is among the most common congenital heart diseases, with an estimated prevalence of 1 in 10,000. ASD is usually sporadic; however, familial cases of ASD disease with an autosomal dominant mode of inheritance also have been described. Individuals with ASD are commonly asymptomatic in early life until the third and fourth decades. Common symptoms are palpitations, commonly due to supraventricular arrhythmias, and symptoms associated with pulmonary hypertension and right-sided volume overload resulting in left-to-right shunt. Uncorrected ASD can lead to heart failure and premature death in the fourth and fifth decades of life.

The first gene identified for familial ASD is *CSX1*, which is the human homologue of *Nkx2.5* in mouse and *tinman* in *Drosophila melanogaster*.[17] The gene is located on 5q35 and encodes *CSX1*, which is a predominantly cardiac-specific transcription factor that regulates expression of a variety of cardiac genes. A multiplicity of mutations have been described in patients with secundum ASD and conduction defects.[17,18] Mutations often result in haploinsufficiency, and point mutations in the DNA binding domain reduce the affinity of CSX1 for the promoter regions, resulting in decreased expression of cardiac-specific genes.[19] The spectrum of clinical phenotypes caused by mutations in CSX1 extends beyond secundum ASD and comprises other congenital heart diseases, including VSDs, tetralogy of Fallot, subvalvular aortic stenosis, and pulmonary atresia.

Holt-Oram Syndrome

Holt-Oram Syndrome is a rare autosomal dominant inherited disorder characterized by anomalies of the heart and upper extremities, hence the name *hand-heart syndrome* (see also Chap. 12). The most common congenital heart defects are atrial and VSDs as well as conduction system abnormalities and atrial fibrillation. Anomalies of the upper limb vary from mild malformation of the carpal bones to phycomyelia, but upper limb preaxial radial abnormalities are commonly present.

Mutations in *TBX5* on chromosome 12q24, which codes for transcription factor TBX5, are responsible for the cardiac and skeletal abnormalities in Holt-Oram syndrome.[20] A number of mutations have been described and most are nonsense, frameshift, or splice-junction abnormalities. The proposed molecular mechanism is haploinsufficiency, which results in reduced expression level of *TBX5* and thus abnormal morphogenesis. Haploinsufficiency due to truncation or frameshift mutations results in severe birth defects in the heart and hands, while point mutations predominantly affect either hand or heart development.[21] Mutations in the 5′ end of the gene exhibit a preponderance of cardiac abnormalities with mild skeletal abnormalities, and those in the 3′ end lead to severe skeletal and mild cardiac abnormalities.

Ellis–van Creveld Syndrome

Ellis–van Creveld syndrome is an autosomal recessive skeletal dysplasia, which is associated with congenital heart disease in the majority of cases. Skeletal anomalies include short limbs, short ribs, postaxial polydactyly, and dysplastic nails and teeth. ASD and common atrium are the typical cardiac anomalies present in two-thirds of the cases (see also Chap. 12).

The gene responsible for Ellis–van Creveld syndrome was mapped to chromosome 4p16.1[22] near an area proximal to the *FGFR3* gene, which is known to cause hypochondroplasia and achondroplasia. Subsequently splice donor, truncation, and missense mutations in a novel gene, *EvC*, were identified.[23] The pathogenesis of Ellis–van Creveld syndrome remains unknown.

Familial Patent Ductus Arteriosus (Char Syndrome)

Patent ductus arteriosus (PDA) can occur as a sole cardiac anomaly or in conjunction with other congenital heart disease. PDA as a familial disease with an autosomal dominant inheritance has been described in patients with Char syndrome. Char syndrome is a congenital disease first described by Florence Char in 1978 and characterized by a constellation of facial dysmorphism, fifth-finger middle phalangeal hypoplasia, and PDA. Variation of this syndrome is associated with bicuspid aortic valve, distinctive facial appearance, polydactyly, and fifth-finger clinodactyly. The predominant clinical features are those of PDA, which include symptoms and signs of left heart failure and pulmonary hypertension.

The gene responsible for Char syndrome was recently mapped to chromosome 6p12-21.[24] Subsequently mutations in the *TFAP2B*, which encodes a neural crest–related helix-span-helix transcription factor, were identified.[25] These findings suggest that Char syndrome results from derangement of neural crest–cell derivatives.[25]

Noonan's and Leopard Syndromes

Noonan's syndrome is an uncommon autosomal dominant disorder characterized by dysmorphic facial features, HCM, pulmonic steno-sis, mental retardation, and bleeding disorders. Leopard syndrome (*l*entigines, *e*lectrocardiographic conduction abnormalities, *o*cular hypertelorism, *p*ulmonic stenosis, *a*bnormal genitalia, *r*etardation of growth, and *d*eafness) is an allelic variant of the Noonan syndrome. Pulmonic stenosis and HCM are the primary cardiac phenotypes; endocardial and myocardial fibroelastosis have also been reported. Noonan's syndrome is also seen in conjunction with cardiofaciocutaneous syndrome and other congenital abnormalities, such as neurofibromatosis (see also Chap. 12).

Noonan's syndrome is sporadic in half of the cases and an autosomal dominant disease in the other half. The gene responsible for autosomal dominant Noonan's and Leopard syndromes was mapped to chromosome 12q22 and subsequently identified as encoding protein-tyrosine-phosphatase, nonreceptor type 11 (*PTPN11*).[26,27] Mutations in *PTPN11* are missense mutations located in interacting portions of the amino-terminal src-homology 2 (N-SH2) and protein-tyrosine-phosphatase (PTP) domains.[26,27] The proposed mechanism for the pathogenesis of Noonan's syndrome is a gain-of-function effect on the phosphotyrosine phosphatase domains. Other causal genes for Noonan's syndrome are unknown.

Familial Myxoma Syndrome (Carney Complex)

Myxomas are the most common cardiac tumors and are generally sporadic. In approximately 7 percent of cases, myxomas are familial and exhibit an autosomal dominant mode of inheritance (see also Chap. 85). Familial myxoma commonly occurs as a part of Carney complex with the constellation of cardiac myxoma, endocrine disorders, and skin pigmentation. LAMB (*l*entigines, *a*trial myxoma, *m*ucocutaneous myxoma, *b*lue nevi) and NAME (*n*evi, *a*trial myxoma, *m*yxoid neurofibromata, *e*phelides) syndromes are considered variants of Carney complex. Atrial, ventricular, and skin myxomas; endocrine tumors and disorders such as Cushing's syndrome; and skin lesions such as lentiginosis are part of the phenotypic expression of Carney complex. Clinical features of atrial myxoma may include fever, arthralgia, dyspnea, diastolic rumble, tumor plop, and systemic embolisms.

Carney complex exhibits locus heterogeneity, and at least two loci on chromosome 17q24 and 2p have been mapped.[28,29] The majority of familial cardiac myxomas (Carney complex) are caused by mutations in the *PRKRA1A* gene on chromosome 17q24, which codes for the alpha-regulatory subunit of cyclic adenosine monophosphate (cAMP)-dependent protein kinase.[30] Frameshift mutations in *PRKRA1A* result in haploinsufficiency, which suggest that the *PRKRA1A* functions as a tumor-suppressor gene.

Situs Inversus

Situs inversus is a reversal of the asymmetric anatomic position of visceral organs. In situs inversus totalis, all visceral organs are reversed in a mirror-image manner. It is part of the immotile cilia syndrome (primary ciliary dyskinesia). Kartagener syndrome is situs inversus, bronchiectasis, and male sterility. Most cases of situs inversus are sporadic. Autosomal recessive, autosomal dominant, and X-linked forms have been reported.

Situs inversus, as a component of immotile cilia syndrome, such as that in Kartagener syndrome, is caused by mutations in dyneins.[31] Dyneins are large proteins with adenosine triphosphatase (ATPase) activity that interact with intermediary filaments to produce energy and motion. Mutations in dynein axonemal intermediate chain 1 (*DNAI1*) on chromosome 9p13-p21,[32] dynein axonemal heavy chain 5 (*DNAH5*) on chromosome 5p,[33] and axonemal heavy chain dynein type 11 (*DNAH11*) on chromsome 7p21[31] have been found in patients with primary ciliary dyskinesia (and situs inversus).

Situs inversus has also been mapped to chromosome Xq26.2 and mutations in *ZIC3*, encoding a zinc-finger protein of the cerebellum, which are associated with situs ambiguus in male and situs solitus or inversus in females.[34] Other causal genes for right-left axis abnormality include *CFC1* on chromosome 2, *LEFTB* (also known as *LEFTY2*),[35] and *ACVR2B*, encoding activin receptor IIB.[36]

Alagille Syndrome (Arteriohepatic Dysplasia)

This is an autosomal dominant disorder characterized by anomalies of the right side of the heart and developmental abnormalities of eyes, skeleton, and kidney. Cardiac abnormalities are present in approximately 70 percent of cases; the most common is diffuse pulmonary artery stenosis. Others include hypoplastic pulmonary circulation, pulmonary atresia, tetralogy of Fallot, coarctation of aorta, secundum ASD, PDA, and VSD.[37] The causal gene is *JAG1*, located on chromosome 20p12.[38,39] JAG1 is a cell surface protein that is a ligand for the Notch receptor. The Notch intercellular signaling pathway mediates cell fate decisions during development. Mutations include deletion or point mutations that result in haploinsufficiency and defective cell adhesions.

GENETIC DISEASES OF CARDIAC MUSCLE

The term *cardiomyopathy* denotes an exclusive group of disorders in which the primary defect is in the myocardium, affecting cardiac myocyte structure and/or function. Cardiomyopathies are caused by mutations in contractile sarcomeric proteins. The primary defect, however, may involve not only the heart but also other tissues and organs, as in cardiomyopathies arising from metabolic disorders and mitochondrial myopathies. Myocardial dysfunction can also occur as a consequence of systemic, infiltrative, toxic, and endocrine disorders; coronary atherosclerosis; and valvular pathologies. In such conditions, the primary defect is not in the myocardium; thus myocardial involvement is considered secondary and not referred to as cardiomyopathy.

Cardiomyopathies are classified on the basis of their phenotypic characteristics into four groups: hypertrophic, dilated, restrictive, and arrhythmogenic right ventricular. Phenotypic classification, while clinically convenient and useful, does not sufficiently reflect the molecular and genetic bases of cardiomyopathies, because significant phenotypic overlap exists among mutations in identical genes.[40]

Genetic Basis of Hypertrophic Cardiomyopathy

Hypertrophic cardiomyopathy (HCM) is a relatively common autosomal dominant disease diagnosed clinically by the presence of cardiac hypertrophy (wall thickness of 13 mm or greater) in the absence of an increased external load (unexplained hypertrophy). The prevalence of HCM is approximately 1 in 500[41] in young adults and likely higher in the elderly population because of age-dependent penetrance (see Chap. 77).

Cardiac hypertrophy, the clinical hallmark of HCM, is asymmetric in approximately two-thirds of the cases with predominant involvement of the interventricular septum (Fig. 72-3). Hence the term *asymmetric septal hypertrophy* is used to describe this condi-

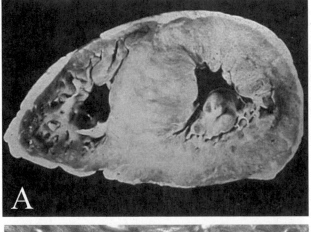

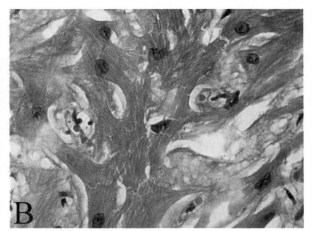

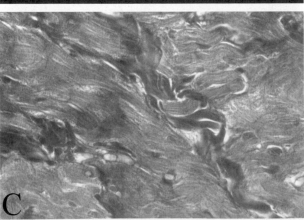

FIGURE 72-3 Main pathologic features of hypertrophic cardiomyopathy. *A.* Gross cardiac hypertrophy with predominant involvement of the interventric-ular septum and a small left ventricular cavity. *B.* Myocyte disarray and hypertrophy. *C.* Interstitial fibrosis.

tion. Rarely, hypertrophy is restricted to the apex of the heart (apical HCM). Morphologically, the left ventricular cavity is small and left ventricular ejection fraction, a measure of global systolic function, is increased. However, more sensitive indices of myocardial function show impaired contraction and relaxation.[42] Diastolic function is commonly impaired, leading to an increased left ventricular end-diastolic pressure and thus, frequently, to symptoms of heart failure.

Patients with HCM exhibit protean clinical manifestations that range from minimal or no symptoms to severe heart failure. The clinical manifestations often do not develop until the third or fourth decade of life, but the onset is variable. The majority of patients are asymptomatic or mildly symptomatic. Predominant symptoms include dyspnea, chest pain, palpitations, and/or syncope. Cardiac arrhythmias, in particular atrial fibrillation and nonsustained ventricular tachycardia, are relatively common, whereas associated Wolff-Parkinson-White (WPW) syndrome occurs but is uncommon. Sudden cardiac death (SCD) and severe systolic heart failure are relatively uncommon. SCD may occur, however, as the first manifestation of HCM in the young, asymptomatic, and apparently healthy individual.[43,44] Indeed, HCM is considered the most common cause of SCD in the young competitive athlete, accounting for approximately one-third of all such cases.[43] Nonetheless, HCM is a relatively benign disease with an estimated annual mortality rate of < 0.7 percent in the adult population.[45,46]

The pathologic hallmark of HCM is myocyte disarray, which often occupies > 20 to 30 percent of the myocardium,[47,48] as opposed to < 5 percent in normal hearts. Myocyte hypertrophy and interstitial fibrosis are also common, as is thickening of the media of intramural coronary arteries; abnormal positioning of the mitral valve apparatus is less common. Hypertrophy and myocyte disarray are more prominent in the interventricular septum, but scattered myocyte disarray is often present throughout the myocardium.[48] Cardiac hypertrophy, myocyte disarray, and interstitial fibrosis are considered major determinants of mortality and morbidity in HCM.[49–52]

MOLECULAR GENETICS OF HYPERTROPHIC CARDIOMYOPATHY

HCM is a genetically heterogeneous disease with an autosomal dominant mode of inheritance. Approximately two-thirds of patients have a family history of HCM, and in the remainder the disease is sporadic. Familial and sporadic cases both are caused by mutations in contractile sarcomeric proteins.[53] In sporadic cases, mutations arise de novo and could be transmitted to the offspring of the index cases.[54,55] Since hypertrophy is a common response of the heart to all forms of injury or stimuli, a phenotype of hypertrophy in the absence of an increased external load could also occur due to mutations other than those in sarcomeric proteins. As such, unexplained cardiac hypertrophy, which clinically denotes HCM, could also occur in metabolic disorders,[56] mitochondrial diseases,[57] and triplet repeat syndromes [58] as well as congenital heart diseases.[26] While the gross phenotype is similar, the pathogenesis of HCM caused by different classes of mutant proteins, at least in part, could differ.

Causal Genes and Mutations The pioneering work of Christine and Jonathan Seidman has led to elucidation of the molecular genetic basis of HCM. In 1990, an arginine-to-glutamine substitution at codon 403 (R403Q) in the beta-myosin heavy chain (MyHC) was identified as the first causal mutation.[59] Since then, over 150 different mutations in genes encoding 11 different contractile sarcomeric proteins and a few nonsarcomeric proteins have been identified[53] (Table 72-4). Consequently, HCM is considered primarily a disease of contractile sarcomeric proteins (Fig. 72-4, Plate 30).[60] Systematic screening of sarcomeric genes suggests that mutations in *MYHC* and *MYBPC3*, which encode beta-MyHC and myosin binding protein C (MyBP-C), respectively, are the most common causes of human HCM, accounting for approximately half of all cases.[53,61] Mutations in *TNNT2* and *TNNI3*, encoding cardiac troponin T and I, respectively, are also relatively common, each accounting for approximately 5 to 10 percent of all HCM cases.[61] Thus mutations in *MYH7*, *MYBPC3*, *TNNT2*, and *TNNI3* collectively account for approximately two-thirds of all HCM cases.[53,62,63] A small fraction of HCM cases are caused by mutations in genes encoding alpha-tropomyosin (*TPM1*),[55,60,64,65] cardiac troponin C (*TNNC1*),[66] titin (*TTN*),[67] cardiac alpha-actin (*ACTC*),[68,69] and essential and regulatory light chains (*MYL3* and *MYL2*, respectively).[70,71] In addition, rare mutations in alpha-MyHC, myosin light chain kinase, SERCA2A, and phospholamban have been reported in patients with HCM. Overall, the causal genes and mutations for approximately 80 percent of HCM cases have been identified; the remainder are yet to be identified or are due to genes inducing a phenocopy (diseases mimicking HCM).

Over 100 different mutations in the beta-MyHC, a major component of thick filaments in sarcomeres, have been identified, and the majority are missense mutations localized in the globular head of the myosin molecule.[53] Codons 403 and 719 are considered hot spots for mutations.[72,73] Missense, deletion, and insertion/deletion mutations

---

TABLE 72-4 Causal Genes for Hypertrophic Cardiomyopathy (Sarcomeric Genes)

Gene	Symbol	Locus	Frequency	Predominant Mutations
β-Myosin heavy chain	*MYH7*	14q12	~35%	Missense
Myosin binding protein-C	*MYBPC3*	11p11.2	~20%	Splice-junction and insertion/deletion
Cardiac troponin T	*TNNT2*	1q32	~20%	Missense
Cardiac troponin I	*TNNI3*	19p13.2	~5%	Missense and deletion
α-Tropomyosin	*TPM1*	15q22.1	~5%	Missense
Essential myosin light chain	*MYL3*	3p21.3	<5%	Missense
Regulatory myosin light chain	*MYL2*	12q23-24.3	<5%	Missense and 1 truncation
Cardiac α-actin	*ACTC*	15q11	<5%	Missense mutations
Titin	*TTN*	2q24.1	<5%	Missense mutation
α-Myosin heavy chain	*MYH6*	14q1	Rare	Missense and rearrangement mutations
Cardiac troponin C	*TNNC1*	3p21.3-3p14.3	Rare	Missense mutation

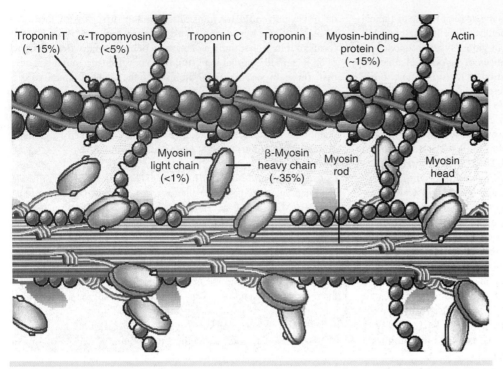

FIGURE 72-4 (Plate 30) Schematic representation of sarcomeric proteins involved in cardiomyopathies.

than causal genes. One such factor is the genetic background, which comprises DNA polymorphisms including SNPs. SNPs located in coding or regulatory regions of genes can affect gene expression and function and thus impose biological effects. Genes with functional polymorphisms can affect expression of the cardiac phenotype in HCM and thus are considered "modifier" genes. Modifier genes are neither necessary nor sufficient to cause HCM but can influence the severity of cardiac hypertrophy, risk of SCD, and expression of other cardiac phenotypes. The identity of the modifier genes for HCM and the magnitude of their effects remain largely unknown, but several have been implicated (reviewed in Ref. 26). In view of the complexity of the cardiac phenotype in HCM, a large number of genes and their functional variants can affect expression of HCM, each exerting only a modest effect.

in the rod and tail regions have also been described.[74–77] Overall, the frequency of each particular *MYHC* mutation is relatively low and a founder effect (sharing of a common ancestor) is uncommon.

Mutations in *MYBPC3* account for approximately 20 percent of all HCM cases, and over 40 mutations scattered throughout the gene have been described.[78–84] Unlike mutations in *MYHC*, a significant proportion of *MYBPC3* mutations are deletion/insertion or splice junction mutations,[79] which could result in frameshift or truncation of the MyBP-C protein, harboring severe structural and functional defects or immediate degradation of the expressed proteins. The frequency of each particular mutation is relatively low and a founder effect is uncommon.

Mutations in *TNNT2* are relatively common causes of human HCM, accounting for approximately 10 percent of all cases.[53,60,85] More than 20 mutations in *TNNT2* have been described, and codon 92 is considered a hot spot for mutations.[60,85] The majority of the mutations are missense, but deletion mutations that involve splice donor sites and could lead to truncated proteins also have been described.[60]

Mutations in *TNNI3* are also relatively uncommon and are estimated to account for about 5 to 10 percent of all HCM cases.[86,87] Mutations in other components of thin and thick filaments are uncommon causes of HCM and collectively account for approximately 5 to 10 percent of all HCM cases. Mutations in other sarcomeric genes, namely *TPM1, TNNC1, TTN, ACTC, MYL3,* and *MYL2,* are very uncommon, and those in *MYH6,* myosin light chain kinase, SERCA2A, and phospholamban are rare.

Modifier Genes and Polymorphisms A remarkable feature of HCM is the presence of a significant degree of variability in its phenotypic expression, whether it is the degree of cardiac hypertrophy or the risk of SCD. The variability is in part due to the diversity of the causal genes and mutations, which can impart a spectrum of functional and structural defects. However, the presence of a significant degree of phenotypic variability among affected members of a single family, who share identical mutations, indicates involvement of factors other

GENE EXPRESSION IN HYPERTROPHIC CARDIOMYOPATHY

The diversity of cardiac phenotypes in HCM suggests induction of expression of a variety of genes in response to the mutant protein. Since the main cellular components of hearts are fibroblasts and myocytes, phenotypic expression of HCM is expected to entail changes in expression of a large number of genes in these cells. Expression-profiling studies have identified changes in expression of genes encoding contractile sarcomeric proteins, cytoskeletal proteins, ion channels, intracellular signaling transducers, proteins maintaining the redox state, and those involved in transcriptional and translation machinery.[88,89] Among the genes upregulated are those considered the markers of "secondary" cardiac hypertrophy, such as skeletal alpha-actin, isoforms of myosin light chain, and brain natriuretic factor, which are also upregulated in conditions such as pressure overload–induced hypertrophy. The findings of upregulation of markers of secondary cardiac hypertrophy suggest that hypertrophy in HCM is also a "secondary" phenotype and that common pathways are involved in induction of cardiac hypertrophy in genetic and acquired forms. The diversity of molecular phenotype is in accord with the diversity of pathologic and clinical phenotypes in HCM that encompass not only hypertrophy and disarray but also interstitial fibrosis and others.

DETERMINANTS OF CARDIAC PHENOTYPE IN HYPERTROPHIC CARDIOMYOPATHY

A characteristic feature of HCM is the presence of a significant degree of variability in the phenotypic expression of the disease among affected individuals. A significant part of the variability is due to the diversity of the causal genes and mutations and their effects on cardiac myocyte structure and function. Nevertheless, affected individuals within a family sharing the same causal mutations and affected individuals from different families with identical causal mutations exhibit significant degrees of variability in phenotype. Collective data from genotype-phenotype correlation studies indicate that mutations exhibit highly variable clinical, ECG, and echocardiographic manifestations and that no particular phenotype is mutation-specific.[80] Thus it is clear that factors other than the causal genes and mutations, such as modifier genes and probably environmental factors, account for the variability of the clinical manifestations of HCM. It is notable that cardiac hypertrophy accelerates during puberty and adolescence in patients with HCM,[90] suggesting contribution of growth factors to expression of hypertrophy. Similarly, experimental and clinical studies suggest that cardiac hypertrophy, the clinical hallmark of HCM, is a compensatory phenotype and likely to be modulated by a large number of genetic and nongenetic factors.[91] Thus, the final phenotype in HCM is determined not only by the causal mutations but also by the effects of modifier genes, environmental factors, epigenetic and epistatic factors, and posttranscriptional and posttranslational modifications of the proteins.

Impact of Causal Genes and Mutations Causal genes and mutations are the primary determinant of expressivity of cardiac phenotype, including the severity of hypertrophy and the risk of SCD.[50,61,74,79,92–96] Collectively, these data suggest gene- and mutation-specific effects. In general, mutations in *MYH7* are associated with an early-onset, extensive hypertrophy and a high incidence of SCD, which are variable among different *MYH7* mutations.[92,93,95,97] *MYH7* mutations are considered major prognosticators in HCM (Fig. 72-5). However, there is a significant degree of variability, which is partly independent of the causal mutations and reflects the effects of modifier genes and others. Topography of the mutations and their impact on beta-MyHC function are likely to be important determinants of the severity of cardiac hypertrophy as well as the risk of SCD. However, given the relatively low frequency of each causal mutation, results of genotype-phenotype correlation studies have had limited utility and consistent correlations have been observed for only a few mutations, such as R403Q and R719W, which have been associated with a high incidence of SCD and severe hypertrophy (Fig. 72-5).[92] In contrast, G256Q and L908V are associated with a benign and Q930L with an intermediate prognosis.[92,93,98]

The phenotype in the majority of patients with *MYBPC3* mutations is mild, as the onset of clinical symptoms is late, the degree of cardiac hypertrophy is relatively mild, and the incidence of SCD is low.[78,79,97] Accordingly, the penetrance is low and a normal physical examination, electrocardiogram (ECG), and echocardiogram have low negative predictive value in early life. The clinical phenotype often develops in the fifth and sixth decades of life and is often unmasked by the presence of concomitant hypertension. Indeed, hypertensive HCM of the elderly could be a form of HCM caused by mutations in *MYBPC3* and unmasked by hypertension.[78] There is also a significant degree of variability in the phenotypic expression of HCM caused by *MYBPC3*, as "malignant" mutations, associated with severe hypertrophy and a high incidence of SCD, also have been described.[79]

In general, the risk of SCD in HCM caused by mutations in *MYH7* and *MYBPC3* is reflective of the severity of hypertrophy.[99] Mutations associated with mild hypertrophy generally carry a relatively benign prognosis and those with severe hypertrophy indicate a high incidence of SCD. This is in contrast to HCM caused by mutations in *TNNT2*, which is characterized by mild cardiac hypertrophy, a high incidence of SCD, and extensive myocyte disarray.[52,61] Inadequate genotype-phenotype correlation data are available regarding mutations in *TNNI3, TPM1, TNNC1, TTN, ACTC, MYL3*, and *MYL2*.

The results of genotype-phenotype correlation studies are subject to a large number of confounding factors, including the small size of the families; small number of families with identical mutations due to low frequency of each mutation; variability in the phenotypic expression within the same family or among families with identical mutations; influence of modifier genes (reviewed in Ref. 100); influence of nongenetic factors; and, rarely, homozygosity for causal mutations or compound mutations.[101,102] Collective data indicate that mutations exhibit highly variable clinical, ECG, and echocardiographic manifestations, and no particular phenotype is mutation-specific.[80]

Impact of Modifier Genes and Polymorphisms Cardiac hypertrophy in HCM is a compensatory phenotype, as noted, and its expression is modulated by a large number of genetic and nongenetic factors.[91] The final phenotype is a product of the interactions between the causal mutations, modifier genes, environmental factors, and epigenetic elements as well as posttranscriptional and posttranslational modifications of proteins.

Modifier genes are considered important determinants of phenotypic expression of HCM, including risk of SCD.[100] Specific modifier genes in HCM are largely unknown, but several have been implicated and a locus has been mapped in a genetically engineered mouse model.[103] Functional variants of genes coding for the components of the renin-angiotensin-aldosterone system are biologically

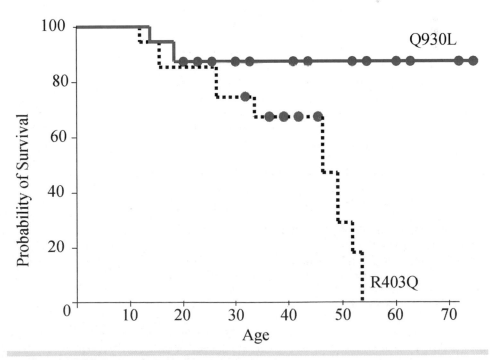

FIGURE 72-5 Kaplan-Meier survival curves in patients with hypertrophic cardiomyopathy. Survival curves in two families with two different mutations, namely arginine to glutamine substitution at amino acid 403 (R403Q) and glutamine to lysine change at amino acid 930 (Q930L) in the *MYH7* are shown.

plausible candidates and have been associated with expression of cardiac hypertrophy and SCD in HCM. Angiotensin I–converting enzyme 1 (ACE-1) gene (*ACE*) was the first gene implicated as a modifier of cardiac phenotype in human HCM.[104] ACE-1 catalyzes conversion of angiotensin I to angiotensin II and inactivates bradykinin, both of which are biologically active agents with opposing effects on cardiac growth and cellular proliferation.[105] *ACE* contains over 28 different polymorphisms, some of which are major determinants of interindividual variability in plasma, tissue, and cellular levels of ACE-1.[106] The most commonly studied *ACE* polymorphism is an insertion (I) or deletion (D) of a 287-bp Alu repeat in intron 16. The direct functional significance of the I/D polymorphism is unknown. Nonetheless, perhaps because of linkage disequilibrium with other functional SNPs, the I/D polymorphism is associated with variation in plasma, cellular, and tissue levels of ACE-1 in a codominant manner (DD > ID > II).[106]

ACE I/D polymorphism has been associated with the severity of cardiac hypertrophy and risk of SCD in HCM in most but not all studies.[104,107–112] The DD genotype is more common in HCM families with a high incidence of SCD as compared to those with a low incidence[104] and is associated with the severity of cardiac hypertrophy.[107,108,111,112] The observed association is gene-dose dependent, consistent with the biological effect of the I/D variants on plasma and tissue levels of ACE (DD > ID > II).[107] Overall, the I/D genotypes accounted for 3 to 5 percent of the variability of hypertrophic expression in genetically unrelated populations and for approximately 10 to 15 percent of the variability of expression of hypertrophy in members of the same family.[107] In addition, an interaction between the modifying effect of the I/D genotypes and the underlying causal mutations also has been reported.[108]

Variants of endothelin-1 (*EDN1*), tumor necrosis factor alpha (*TNF-α*), angiotensinogen (*AGT*), angiotensin II receptor 1 (*AGTR1*) and platelet activating factor acetylhydrolase (*PLA2G7*) have been associated with the severity of the cardiac hypertrophy.[113–115] The results, however, have been inconsistent, partly because of the small sample size of the studies, population characteristics, and presence of confounders that are common in SNP-association studies.[116]

Impact of Environmental Factors Evidence for the effect of environmental factors on cardiac phenotypes in HCM in humans, while expected, is circumstantial. Experimental data in animal models of HCM suggest worsening of phenotype with exercise.[117] Because hypertrophy is considered a secondary phenotype, one could speculate that heavy physical exercise, particularly isometric exercise, could stimulate the development of a more severe phenotype in the presence of causal mutations for HCM. While there is no direct evidence in humans, the common finding of HCM in young competitive athletes who succumb to SCD suggests heavy physical exercise may worsen the cardiac phenotypes.

PATHOGENESIS OF HYPERTROPHIC CARDIOMYOPATHY

As the diversity of the causal mutations would suggest, there is no single initial defect common to all mutations (Table 72-5). The diversity of the clinical phenotypes, such as hypertrophic, dilated, or arrhythmogenic right ventricular cardiomyopathy arising from mutations in the same gene further adds to the complexity. Topography of the causal mutation is likely to be important and the initial defect conferred by the mutation is likely to be domain- but not protein-specific. As such, mutations located in each functional domain of a given protein are expected to confer similar initial defects. Thus, the dogma of "one protein: one function" is not very applicable consid-

TABLE 72-5 Initial Defects Caused by Mutations in Sarcomeric Proteins

1. Mechanical defect
   Impaired actomyosin interaction
   Impaired cardiac myocyte, skeletal myoblasts, and
     myofibril contractile performance
2. Biochemical defects
   Impaired Ca^{+2} affinity, force, and myofibril sensitivity
3. Bioenergetics
   Impaired ATPase activity
4. Structural defects
   Impaired sarcomere assembly
   Impaired subcellular localization of sarcomeric
     proteins
   Altered stoichiometry

ering the pathogenesis of cardiomyopathies. Proteins could have multiple functions usually due to having multiple domains, and mutations in certain domains could induce certain phenotypes.

The causal mutation initiates a series of molecular events, which begins with alteration of the molecular structure and function of the protein, whether it is a gain or a loss of function (Table 72-5). Since the majority of mutant sarcomeric proteins differ from the wild type only by a single amino acid (missense mutations), the mutant proteins incorporate into the sarcomere, albeit sometimes inefficiently. Following incorporation, mutant sarcomeric proteins exert diverse functional defects including altered myofibrillar Ca^{+2} sensitivity and trafficking and reduced ATPase activity.[118] Functional phenotypes lead to activation of secondary molecules, which ultimately mediate induction of the final HCM phenotypes. The intermediary molecules in HCM are largely unknown but include those activating many intracellular signaling pathways. Accordingly, structural phenotypes, such as hypertrophy and fibrosis, are considered secondary phenotypes due to activation of intermediary molecular phenotypes (Fig. 72-6).

Many HCM mutations involve deletions or truncations that are considered null alleles because of the possible expression of unstable mRNA and proteins.[76,119] It is unclear whether genetic haploinsufficiency could lead to HCM by altering the stoichiometry of interaction of sarcomeric proteins. In addition, myocyte dropout secondary

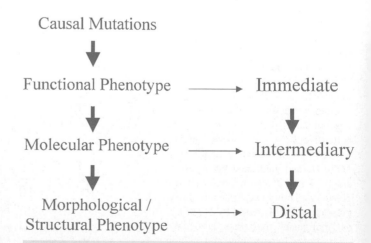

FIGURE 72-6 Sequence of phenotype characterization in the pathogenesis of cardiomyopathies.

to apoptosis has been implicated in animal models, although the significance of this in human HCM remains to be established.[120] Regardless of the initial primary defect, cardiac hypertrophy, the clinical hallmark of HCM, is considered a compensatory phenotype. Evidence suggesting the compensatory nature of cardiac hypertrophy includes upregulation of expression of molecular markers of secondary cardiac hypertrophy, such as atrial and brain natriuretic peptides,[121,122] endothelin-1,[123] transforming growth factor beta$_1$ (TGF-β_1), and insulin-like growth factor 1 (IGF-1).[124] The predominant involvement of the left ventricle and its frequent absence in the low-pressure right ventricle, despite equal expression of mutant sarcomeric protein in both, suggest a contribution of the environment to the development of hypertrophy. Furthermore, variation in hypertrophic response because of the genetic background, its absence early on in life, and its attenuation through pharmacologic interventions, at least in animal models, supports the secondary nature of hypertrophy. The primary impetus for hypertrophy is not well defined. Myocyte functional abnormalities and/or altered Ca^{+2} homeostasis are likely causes.

POTENTIAL NEW THERAPEUTIC INTERVENTIONS

Current pharmacologic interventions in HCM are empiric[125] and none has been shown to induce regression of hypertrophy, fibrosis, or disarray—major predictors of mortality and morbidity.[49,50] Absent the ability to correct the underlying genetic defect, the emphasis of pharmacologic interventions has focused on blockade of intermediary molecular mediators to prevent the development of hypertrophy and fibrosis. Studies suggest potential clinical utility of angiotensin II receptor blockers and HMG-CoA reductase inhibitors in the attenuation and reversal of cardiac hypertrophy and fibrosis in animal models of HCM.[126,127] Blockade of angiotensin II receptor 1 in cardiac troponin T-Q92 transgenic mice reduced interstitial collagen volume, expression levels of collagen alpha$_1$ (I) mRNA, and TGF-β1 protein, the latter a known mediator of profibrotic effects of angiotensin II, by approximately 50 percent to the normal levels.[126] Perhaps more attractive therapeutic agents are HMG-CoA reductase inhibitors, which have been shown in a series of experimental models to prevent or attenuate cardiac hypertrophy and fibrosis.[128–130] Simvastatin, a pleiotropic HMG-CoA reductase inhibitor, reduced left ventricular mass by 37 percent, wall thickness by 20 percent, and collagen volume fraction by 50 percent in the β-MyHC-Q403 transgenic rabbit model of human HCM.[127] In addition, indices of left ventricular filling pressure were improved significantly. There has been significant controversy regarding the utility of calcineurin inhibitors in treatment and prevention of cardiac hypertrophy in pathologic conditions. Pretreatment with diltiazem, an L-type Ca^{+2} channel blocker, prevented the exaggerated cardiac hypertrophic response to inhibitors of calcineurin. The results suggest altered calcium handling in the heart of α-MyHC-Q403$^{+/-}$ mice.[118] Collectively, the results in genetically engineered animal models suggest the need for clinical trials in humans to determine whether treatment with HMG-CoA reductase inhibitors or angiotensin II blockade induces regression or provides salutary effects in patients with HCM.

Genetic Basis of Dilated Cardiomyopathy

Dilated cardiomyopathy (DCM) is a primary disease of the myocardium that is manifest by dilatation of the left ventricular along with a gradual decline in contractility. The diagnosis is based on a left ventricular ejection fraction of < 0.45 and a left ventricular end-diastolic diameter > 2.7 cm/m^2. Patients with DCM are often asymptomatic in early stages but gradually develop symptoms and signs of heart failure, syncope, cardiac arrhythmias, and SCD. Thus, a normal history and physical examination in a subject at risk, particularly in the early decades of life, does not exclude DCM. A significant number of affected relatives of patients with DCM are asymptomatic and are diagnosed for the first time upon additional testing (such as an echocardiogram).[131] A family history of DCM is present in approximately half of all index cases with idiopathic DCM.[131,132] In the remainder, DCM is considered sporadic. Familial DCM is commonly inherited as an autosomal dominant disease,[131] which clinically manifests during the third and fourth decades of life.

An X-linked DCM is suspected when only male members of a family exhibit symptoms and signs of DCM and there is no male-to-male transmission. Three common forms of X-linked DCM have been identified, including Duchenne/Becker muscular dystrophy, Emery-Dreifuss syndrome, and Barth's syndrome.

Duchenne/Becker muscular dystrophy, a disease characterized by progressive degeneration of muscle function, commonly manifests itself as mild but progressive skeletal myopathy, early contractures, and cardiomyopathy. The incidence of Duchenne/Becker muscular dystrophy is 1 in 3500 newborn males. Duchenne muscular dystrophy is a severe form and Becker muscular dystrophy a milder form of the disease. The disease commonly manifests itself during the first and second decades of life in male patients; female family members are commonly spared or exhibit a mild phenotype later in life. Cardiac involvement includes progressive atrioventricular block, arrhythmia, loss of P-wave amplitude on the ECG, atrial standstill, DCM, akinesis/dyskinesis of the posterobasal wall of the left ventricle, and SCD. Often, DCM is the primary feature of Duchenne/Becker muscular dystrophy, and approximately 90 percent of patients will eventually develop DCM.[133] Death often occurs by the third decade.

Emery-Dreifuss muscular dystrophy is an X-linked degenerative disorder characterized by mild but progressive skeletal and cardiac myopathy. Clinical features include muscle weakness and atrophy, flexion deformities of the elbows, and mild pectus excavatum. Cardiac phenotypes include cardiomyopathy, arrhythmia, SCD, conduction defects, loss of P-wave amplitude on the ECG, and atrial standstill. DCM is also a major phenotypic component of the Barth syndrome, another X-linked disorder caused by mutations in the gene encoding taffazin.[134] The characteristic phenotype of Barth's syndrome includes skeletal and cardiac myopathy, neutropenia, and abnormal mitochondria.

DCM also occurs in multiorgan disorders, such as mitochondrial DNA mutations, triplet repeat syndromes, and metabolic disorders.

MOLECULAR GENETICS OF DILATED CARDIOMYOPATHY

DCM is an extremely heterogeneous disease, as indicated by the heterogeneity of the mapped loci and genes for familial DCM (Table 72-6). The predominant mode of inheritance is autosomal dominant; however, autosomal recessive and X-linked DCM also occur. Several causal genes for autosomal dominant DCM have been identified and the vast majority encode sarcomeric proteins, identical to the causal genes for HCM.[135] Thus, despite the contrasting phenotypes of HCM and DCM, mutations in sarcomeric genes can induce either (as well as restrictive cardiomyopathy). Since many of the known causal genes for DCM involve the myocyte cytoskeleton, DCM has been considered to be a disease of cytoskeletal proteins. However, a significant number of causal genes remain unknown; thus, designation of DCM as a cytoskeletal disease may prove to be premature.

TABLE 72-6 Causal Genes for Dilated Cardiomyopathy (DCM)

Gene	Symbol	Locus	Inheritance	Mutations/Frequency/Context
SARCOMERIC/CYTOSKELETAL				
Cardiac α-actin	ACTC	15q11-14	Autosomal dominant	Missense/uncommon; also causes HCM
β-Myosin heavy chain	MYH7	14q11-13	Autosomal dominant	Missense/uncommon; also causes HCM
Cardiac troponin T	TNNT2	1q32	Autosomal dominant	Missense/uncommon; also causes HCM
α-Tropomyosin	TPM1	15q22.1	Autosomal dominant	Missense/rare; also causes HCM
Titin	TTN	2q24.1	Autosomal dominant	Missense/uncommon; also causes HCM
CYTOSKELETAL				
α-Sarcoglycan	SGCA	17q21	Autosomal dominant	Limb-girdle muscular dystrophy
β-Sarcoglycan	SGCB	4q12	Autosomal dominant	
δ-Sarcoglycan	SGCD	5q33-34	Autosomal dominant Autosomal recessive	
Dystrophin	DMD	Xp21	X-linked	Muscular dystrophy
Muscle LIM protein	MLP (CSRP3)	11q15.1	Autosomal dominant	Rare, founder effect in families described
INTERMEDIARY FILAMENTS				
Desmin	DES	2q35	Autosomal dominant	Also causes RCM and desminopathies
αB-crystallin	CRYAB	11q35		Desminopathy
NUCLEAR PROTEINS				
Lamin A/C	LMNA	1q21.2	Autosomal dominant	DCM, conduction defect, muscular dystrophy, lipodystrophy, insulin resistance
Emerin	EMD	Xq28	X-linked	
CELL JUNCTION MOLECULES				
Desmoplakin	DSP	6p23-25	Autosomal recessive	Also causes ARVC
UNKNOWN				
Taffazin (G4.5)	TAZ	Xq28 1q32 2q14-22 2q31 3p22-25 6q23-24 9q13-22 10q21-23	X-linked	Ventricular noncompaction

ABBREVIATIONS: ARVC = arrhythmogenic right ventricular dysplasia; DCM = dilated cardiomyopathy; HCM = hypertrophic cardiomyopathy; RCM = restrictive cardiomyopathy.

Causal Genes and Mutations The gene encoding cardiac alpha-actin (*ACTC*) was the first causal gene identified for autosomal dominant DCM.[136] Subsequently, mutations in genes encoding additional components of the sarcomere, namely *MYH7, TNNT2,* and *TTN,* were found in patients with DCM.[137] Since mutations in *ACTC, MYH7,* and *TNNT2* are also known to cause HCM, these findings point to the commonality of the genetic basis of DCM and HCM and suggest that the topography of the causal mutations on the protein is the primary determinant of the ensuing clinical phenotype.

Mutations in cytoskeletal proteins—namely, delta sarcoglycan,[138] beta sarcoglycan,[139] metavinculin,[140] and dystrophin[141]—are also important causes of DCM. Mutations in alpha sarcoglycan (adhalin) cause an autosomal recessive form of DCM that occurs in conjunction with limb-girdle muscular dystrophy.[139] Recently, a mutation in muscle LIM protein (MLP) was identified in several related families with DCM.[140] MLP interacts with telethonin, a titin-interacting protein, and colocalizes with it to the Z disk. This finding, along with studies in the LIM-deficient mouse model, suggest that the Z disk is a mechanosensor that plays a major role in maintaining myocardial integrity.

An intriguing causal gene for familial DCM is the lamin A/C gene,[142,143] which encodes a nuclear envelope protein. The observed phenotype resulting from mutations in the rod domain of lamin A/C is progressive conduction disease, atrial arrhythmias, heart failure, and SCD. Finally, mutations in the intermediary filament desmin and its associated protein alphaB-crystallin have been identified in patients with DCM.[144,145] Often such mutations lead to a phenotype of cardiac and skeletal myopathy that is referred to as *desmin-related myopathy.*[145] Collectively, these findings suggest that mutations affecting the integrity of the cystoskeleton and Z disk can cause DCM.

The gene responsible for Duchenne/Becker muscular dystrophy is dystrophin, located on Xp21, which encodes a large cytoskeletal protein.[146] A variety of point, deletion, and insertion mutations or gene rearrangements in dystrophin have been described.[133,141] Approximately two-thirds of the mutations are either deletions or duplications. DCM can also occur in the absence of skeletal myopathy. Mutations leading to a frameshift induce a severe form, while missense mutations often lead to a mild form of the disease. Mutations in the 5′ region of the dystrophin gene can cause DCM without skeletal involvement.[147]

X-linked Emery-Dreifuss muscular dystrophy is caused by mutations in *EMD,* which encodes emerin, located along the nuclear rim of many cell types, and is a member of the nuclear lamina–associated protein family.[148] Barth syndrome is caused by point, deletion, and splice-junction mutations in the tafazzin (*TAZ*) or G4.5 gene, located on Xq28.[134]

Modifier Genes and Mutations As in HCM, the phenotype of DCM is affected not only by the causal mutations but also by modifier genes and environmental factors. Genetic studies to identify the modifier genes for DCM have limitations similar to those described for HCM. While SNP-association studies have identified several potential candidates, including *ACE,* none has been established to modify cardiac phenotypes in DCM. A modifier locus in a calsequestrin mouse model of DCM has been mapped.[149]

GENOTYPE-PHENOTYPE CORRELATION IN DILATED CARDIOMYOPATHY

There is no large-scale systematic study to delineate the impact of causal and modifier genes and their mutations on the DCM phenotype. Therefore the available genotype-phenotype data may be specific to a family or small number of families. Nevertheless, a diverse array of phenotypes caused by mutations in different genes is observed in DCM families. For example, mutations in cardiac alpha-actin, beta-MyHC, and cTnT cause DCM without other phenotypes, such as conduction defects or deafness.[135] In contrast, mutations in the rod domain of lamin A/C cause DCM in conjunction with progressive conduction defects, atrial arrhythmias, and SCD.[142] Mutations in the lamin A/C gene can also cause an autosomal-dominant form of Emery-Dreifuss syndrome.[150] Mutations in desmin and alphaB-crystallin genes are commonly associated with skeletal myopathy as well as DCM with unique pathologic features, a phenotype referred to as the *desmin-related myopathy.*[151] Mutations in the dystrophin gene commonly lead to skeletal and cardiac myopathy, and the severity of the myopathic phenotype is partly determined by the type of mutation. Those that are frameshift mutations—for example, insertion or deletion of a single base—cause a severe form, while missense mutations often lead to a mild form of DCM and muscular dystrophy. Mutations in the 5′ region of the dystrophin gene can cause DCM without skeletal involvement.[147]

Cardiac involvement is quite common in triplet repeat syndromes and includes DCM, conduction disorders, and arrhythmia. Prevalence of cardiac involvement increases with advancing age, and approximately three-quarters of adult patients exhibit conduction defects, such as first-degree atrioventricular block and intraventricular conduction defects.[152] There is also a direct relationship between the severity of the disease and the severity of cardiac involvement and the number of CTG repeats.[153]

PATHOGENESIS OF DILATED CARDIOMYOPATHY

Mutations in cardiac alpha-actin, beta-myosin heavy chain, cardiac troponin T, and cytoskeletal proteins impart a dominant-negative effect on transmission of the contractile force to the extracellular matrix proteins.[135,136] Identification of mutations in MLP and experiments in MLP-deficient mice suggest that impaired integrity of the Z disk plays a major role in the pathogenesis of DCM. Similarly, identification of mutations in the dystrophin-associated protein complex as causes of DCM signifies the role of sarcolemma in the pathogenesis of DCM.[138] Also, mutations in the dystrophin gene lead to decreased expression levels of dystrophin, a major cytoskeletal protein in skeletal and cardiac muscles, thus impairing mechanical coupling and myocyte shortening.[147] The molecular pathogenesis of other X-linked DCMs due to mutations in *EMD* and *TAZ* is unknown.

Pathogenesis of DCM resulting from mutations in desmin and alphaB-crystallin involves deposition of desmin and alphaB-crystallin aggregates in the myocardium.[154] Molecular pathogenesis of DCM caused by mutations in lamin A/C or emerin remain largely unknown but are likely to involve disruption of integrity of the cytoskeleton. The pathogenesis of cardiomyopathies in patients with the triplet repeat syndromes is also unclear. Expansion of the CTG (CUG in mRNA) repeats in the genes responsible for triplet repeat syndromes could indirectly affect transcription, transport, splicing, and translation of mRNAs of cardiac genes.[155]

Genetic Basis of Arrhythmogenic Right Ventricular Cardiomyopathy/Dysplasia

Arrhythmogenic right ventricular cardiomyopathy (ARVC) is a primary disorder of the myocardium characterized by progressive loss of myocytes, fatty infiltration, and replacement fibrosis (Fig. 72-7).[156] The predominant site of involvement is the right ventricle; however, the left ventricle and the interventricular septum may be involved in advances cases. ARVC is often manifest by ventricular arrhythmias originating from the right ventricle and less commonly

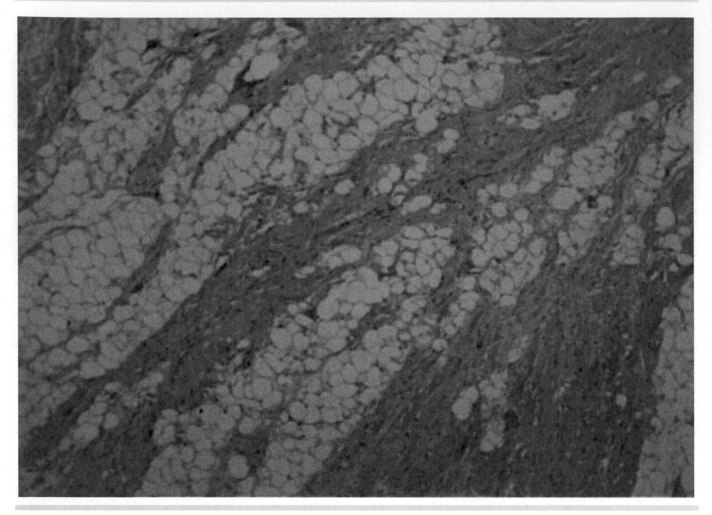

FIGURE 72-7 Histologic features of arrhythmogenic right ventricular dysplasia. Fibrofatty infiltrate in the right ventricle is shown.

with heart failure. A characteristic finding is the presence of an epsilon wave on an ECG. Other ECG findings include depolarization and repolarization abnormalities in the right precordial leads. Arrhythmogenic right ventricular dysplasia (ARVD) commonly manifests itself with minor arrhythmias during adolescence, progressing to serious ventricular arrhythmias during the third and fourth decades of life. ARVC is a relatively common cause of SCD in the young in Italy and less commonly in United States.[157] Gradual fibrofatty infiltration of the myocardium leads to regional and global right ventricular dysfunction and, less frequently, left ventricle failure. In advanced stages, both ventricles are involved and heart failure is the predominant manifestation.

ARVC is a genetic disorder, and approximately half of the index cases have a family history of ARVC. The most common mode of inheritance is autosomal dominant, but an autosomal recessive form in conjunction with keratoderma and woolly hair (Naxos disease) has been reported.[158] It is also likely that familial polymorphic ventricular tachycardia and stress-induced (or catecholaminergic) polymorphic ventricular tachycardia are phenotypic variants of ARVC.[159]

MOLECULAR GENETICS OF ARRHYTHMOGENIC RIGHT VENTRICULAR DYSPLASIA

At least eight loci for autosomal dominant ARVC have been mapped and three genes have been identified (Table 72-7). The three causal genes are *RYR2*,[159] which encodes the cardiac

TABLE 72-7 Chromosomal Loci and Causal Genes for ARVD

	Chromosome	Symbol	Protein	Function
ARVC1	14q24.3	*RYR2*	Ryanodine receptor 2	Calcium channel
ARVC2	1q42			
ARVC3	14q11-q12			
ARVC4	2q32			
ARVD5	3p23			
ARVD6	10p12-p14			
ARVD7	10q22			
ARVC8	6p28	*DSP*	Desmoplakin	Adherens junction protein
Naxos disease	17q21	*JUP*	Plakoglobin	Cell junction

ryanodine receptor; *DSP*,[160] which codes for desmoplakin; and *JUP* encoding junction plakoglobin.[158] Mutations in RYR2 are also known to cause catecholaminergic (stress-induced) ventricular tachycardia, which may be a phenotypic variant of ARVC in which myocardial structure is intact.[161] The ryanodine receptor is a tetrameric protein comprising four RYR2 polypeptides and four FK506-binding proteins. It is located on the sarcoplasmic reticulum and is the major source of calcium required for cardiac muscle excitation-contraction coupling. The activity of the channel is regulated through phosphorylation by protein kinase A, and its hyperphosphorylation inactivates the channel.[162]

Recently, a mutation in exon 7 of *DSP*, which modifies a putative phosphorylation site in the N-terminal domain binding plakoglobin, was identified in an Italian family with ARVC.[160] Desmoplakin is a large protein comprising 2871 amino acids and is a major component of desmosomes at cell-cell junctions, in particular in epidermal cells and cardiac myocytes. Domains of desmoplakin protein anchor intermediate filaments to desmosomes.

The causal gene for autosomal recessive ARVC, palmoplantar keratoderma, and peculiar woolly hairs (Naxos syndrome), is *JUP*, which encodes plakoglobin.[158] Plakoglobin is also a desmosome protein and, along with desmoplakin, anchors intermediate filaments to desmosomes. The phenotype was described first in a family from the island Naxos in Greece and was mapped to 17q21. Mutational analysis detected a 2-bp deletion in *JUP*, which encodes a major component of desmosomes and adherens junctions.

PATHOGENESIS OF ARRHYTHMOGENIC RIGHT VENTRICULAR DYSPLASIA

The pathogenesis of ARVD remains largely unknown. Identification of associated mutations in desmoplakin and plakoglobin, key components of desmosomes, suggests that ARVC is due to defective intercellular connections. Defective cell-to-cell adhesion at adherens junctions could affect stretch-sensitive calcium-permeability channels and release of calcium from ryanodine receptor release channels.[160] In addition, identification of *RYR2* as a causal gene for ARVD emphasizes the key role of intracellular calcium homeostasis in the pathogenesis of ARVC. The RYR2 protein is regulated by its gating protein FKBP12.6 and activated by Ca^{2+}, which induces the release of calcium from the sarcoplasmic reticulum into the cytosol.[162] Mutations occur in domains considered critical for the regulation of the calcium channel and binding of its gating protein FKBP12.6 to RYR2.[160] Thus mutations perturbing Ca^{2+} homeostasis lead to activation of a variety of signaling molecules that induce apoptosis and cardiac arrhythmias. An impaired response of Ca^{+2} homeostasis to defective intercellular adhesion could not only affect the excitation-contraction coupling but also induce programmed cell death and replacement fibrosis. Similarly, delayed afterdepolarizations resulting from a defective cardiac ryanodine receptor and its binding to its gating protein FKBP12.6 may be responsible for the stress-induced ventricular tachycardia.[163] Thus the underlying phenotypic differences between ARVC and catecholaminergic ventricular tachycardia, which are allelic variants caused by mutations in *RYR2*, are due to differential effects of each set of causal mutations on RyR2-mediated calcium release to the cytoplasm.[163]

Genetic Basis of Restrictive Cardiomyopathy

Restrictive cardiomyopathy (RCM) is a heart muscle disease characterized by severely enlarged atria due to elevated right and left ventricular filling pressures, normal or reduced ventricular volumes, and, usually, preserved global systolic function.[164] The clinical manifestations are those of heart failure, often with predominance of right-sided signs and symptoms. The age of onset of the disease is variable and the prognosis is relatively poor. RCM can occur as a result of systemic infiltrative disorders, such as amyloidosis and sarcoidosis, and storage diseases, such as Fabry's disease.[164] While such disorders are also genetic in etiology, RCM in such disorders is an indirect consequence and not a primary myocardial abnormality.

MOLECULAR GENETICS OF RESTRICTIVE CARDIOMYOPATHY

Familial RCM with an autosomal dominant form of inheritance in conjunction with skeletal myopathy and atrioventricular conduction defects have been described.[165–167] Two causal genes for RCM—*DES*,[168,169] encoding desmin, and *TNNI3*,[40] encoding cardiac troponin I—have been identified. Desmin is an intermediary filament that is also involved in desminopathies involving skeletal muscles as well as the heart. Mutations in *TNNI3*, which are known to cause HCM, also appear to be common causes of RCM.[40] RCM also occurs in patients with Noonan's syndrome,[170] which is caused by mutations in the protein tyrosine phosphatase, nonreceptor type II.[26] The pathogenesis of RCM remains largely unknown.

Genetic Basis of Cardiomyopathies in Trinucleotide Repeat Syndromes

Trinucleotide repeat syndromes are a group of genetic disorders caused by expansion of naturally occurring GC-rich triplet repeats in genes. The group comprises more than 10 different diseases, including myotonic muscular dystrophy (DM) and Huntington's disease.[155] Cardiac involvement is common in several forms of triplet repeat syndromes and is a major determinant of morbidity and mortality.[155,171] The phenotype commonly includes DCM, HCM, conduction disorders, and arrhythmias. Average life expectancy is about 30 to 40 years.

GENETIC BASIS OF CARDIOMYOPATHIES IN MYOTONIC DYSTROPHY

Myotonic dystrophy (DM) is an autosomal dominant disorder with highly variable penetrance and an estimated prevalence of approximately 1 in 8000 in the North American population.[58,152] It is perhaps the most common neuromuscular disorder and the most common form of muscular dystrophy in adults. DM commonly manifests itself as progressive degeneration of muscles and myotonia, cardiomyopathy, conduction defects, male-pattern baldness, infertility, premature cataracts, mental retardation, and endocrine abnormalities.[58,152] Cardiomyopathy is a common phenotypic manifestation of myotonic DM, and cardiac conduction defects, such as first-degree atrioventricular block and intraventricular conduction defects, are present in approximately three-quarters of adult patients.[152]

Mutations in two genes have been identified for DM, including expansion of CTG (CUG in mRNA) trinucleotide repeats in the 3′ untranslated region of DM protein kinase (*DMPK*), located on chromosome 19q3.[172–174] The number of CTG repeats in normal individuals varies between 5 and 37. It expands from 50 to more than several thousand in patients with DM.[58] Expansion of the repeats can interfere with DMPK transcription, RNA processing, and/or translation, resulting in decreased levels of expression of DMPK protein. The length of the CTG repeats often correlates with the severity of clinical phenotypes, including conduction defects and cardiomyopathy.[175] In addition, proteins that bind to CTG (CUG-binding proteins) have been identified that are part of the RNA processing factors regulating alternative splicing.[176] CUG-binding proteins have been shown to affect splicing of cardiac troponin T.[177]

The second gene implicated in DM is *DMWD* (gene 59), which is located immediately upstream of *DMPK*.[155] The protein is a member of a large family of eukaryotic WD-repeat (Trp-Asp)–containing proteins with a diverse array of function. The mechanisms by which mutations in *DMWD* could cause DM remain unknown, but loss of function has been implicated.[155] In addition, the expression of several others genes—namely *SIX5, SYMPLEKIN, RSHL1, 20D7,* and *GIPR*—is affected in patients with DM, implicating a role for these genes in the pathogenesis of diverse phenotypes of DM (reviewed in Ref. 178).

GENETIC BASIS OF CARDIOMYOPATHIES IN FRIEDREICH'S ATAXIA

Friedreich' ataxia (FRDA) is an autosomal recessive neurodegenerative disease that primarily involves the central and peripheral nervous system and less frequently manifests as cardiomyopathy and occasionally as diabetes mellitus.[179] FRDA is caused by the expansion of the GAA trinucleotide repeats in intron 1 of *FRDA*.[179] The encoded protein is frataxin, which is a soluble mitochondrial protein with 210 amino acids.[179] Cardiac involvement can manifest as either DCM or HCM. The severity of clinical manifestations of Friedreich's ataxia also correlates with the size of the repeats.[153]

The pathogenesis of cardiac involvement in triplet repeat syndromes and whether pathways similar to those involved in the pathogenesis of sarcomeric cardiomyopathies play a role is largely unknown.

Genetic Basis of Cardiomyopathies in Metabolic Disorders

Metabolic cardiomyopathies encompass a group of disorders in which there is a primary metabolic abnormality in the heart (Table 72-8). This metabolic abnormality also may involve other organs; however, cardiac involvement is direct and not a consequence of secondary changes in other organs. Therefore secondary involvement of the myocardium in systemic metabolic disorders is not considered a metabolic cardiomyopathy.

A prototype of metabolic cardiomyopathies is glycogen storage disease type II (glycogenosis type II or Pompe's disease). Pompe's disease is an autosomal recessive disorder caused by deficiency of alpha-1,4-glucosidase (acid maltase), which degrades alpha-1,4 and alpha-1,6 linkages in glycogen, maltose, and isomaltose.[180] Deficiency of the enzyme leads to storage of glycogen in lysosomal membranes. Phenotypic expression of Pompe's disease includes HCM, DCM, conduction defects, and muscular hypotonia.[181] The

cause is the acid maltase gene, which is mutated, leading to deficiency of acid alpha-glucosidase. A high-protein diet and recombinant acid alpha-glucosidase have been used effectively to treat this disorder.[182]

Mutations in the gene encoding AMP-activated gamma 2 noncatalytic subunit of protein kinase A (*PRKAG2*), a biosensor of the cellular energy state, have been identified in families with HCM and WPW syndrome.[183–185] Cardiac involvement varies from a predominant phenotype of preexcitation and conduction abnormalities[183] to a predominant phenotype of cardiac hypertrophy.[184] Nonetheless, the primary phenotype appears to be a deposit of glycogen in the myocardium, which is responsible for cardiac enlargement as well as facilitated atrioventricular (AV) conduction.[186]

Refsum disease is an autosomal recessive disorder characterized clinically by a tetrad of retinitis pigmentosa, peripheral neuropathy, cerebellar ataxia, and elevated protein levels in the cerebrospinal fluid.[187] ECG abnormalities are common, but cardiac hypertrophy and heart failure are not. Refsum disease is caused by mutations in the gene encoding phytanoyl-CoA hydroxylase (*PAHX* or *PHYH*).[188] Mutations reduce the enzymatic activity, leading to accumulation of phytanic acid, an unusual branched-chain fatty acid in tissues and body fluids.[56]

Cardiac involvement in patients with mucopolysaccharidosis, Niemann-Pick disease, Gaucher's disease, hereditary hemochromatosis, and CD36 deficiency have also been described (reviewed in Ref. 189).

Genetic Basis of Cardiomyopathies in Mitochondrial Disorders

Cardiomyopathies are common phenotypes associated with mitochondrial disorders, which exhibit matrilineal transmission. Since nuclear genes encode for proteins that pimarily regulate mitochondrial function, mutations in nuclear DNA can also cause mitochondrial myopathies. Mitochondrial DNA is a circular double-stranded genome of approximately 16.5 kb encoding 13 polypeptides of the respiratory chain complexes I, III, IV, and V subunits; 28 ribosomal RNAs; and 22 tRNAs. Mutations in mitochondrial oxidative phosphorylation pathways often result in a complex phenotype involving multiple organs including the heart.[190] Cardiac involvement can lead to hypertrophy as well as dilatation. Each mitochondrion has multiple copies of its own DNA and each cell contains thousands of mitochondria. Therefore mutations result in a significant degree of heteroplasmy, which increases over time as mitochondria multiply. In general, approximately 80 to 90 percent of mitochondrial DNA must mutate in order to affect mitochondrial function and lead to a clinical phenotype.[191]

Kearns-Sayre syndrome (KSS) is a mitochondrial disease caused by sporadically occurring mutations in mitochondrial DNA.[57] KSS is characterized by a triad of progressive external ophthalmoplegia, pigmentary retinopathy, and cardiac conduction defects.[57] The classic cardiac abnormality in KSS is conduction defects; however, DCM and HCM are also often observed, but a lower frequency.

L-Carnitine deficiency is a cause of mitochondrial myopathy resulting from mutations in nuclear DNA. The

---

TABLE 72-8 Examples of Causal Genes for Metabolic Cardiomyopathies

Protein	Symbol	Locus	Frequency	Mutations/Phenotype
AMP-activated protein kinase, γ2 regulatory subunit	*PRKAG2*	7q35-q36	Rare	Point and insertion mutations, HCM, WPW, and conduction defect
Acid maltase gene			Rare	Pompe's disease, DCM, HCM, conduction defects
Phytanoyl-CoA hydroxylase	*PAHX* or *PHYH*		Rare	DCM, HCM, and conduction defects

ABBREVIATIONS: DCM = dilated cardiomyopathy; HCM = hypertrophic cardiomyopathy; WPW = Wolff-Parkinson-White syndrome.

phenotype is characterized by skeletal myopathy, congestive heart failure, abnormalities of the central nervous system and liver, and, rarely, HCM.[189] Carnitine is an important component of fatty acid metabolism and is necessary for the entry of long-chain fatty acids into mitochondria. Mutations in the chromosomal gene encoding solute carrier family 22, member 5 (SLC22A5), or OCTN2 transporter impair transport of carnitine to mitochondria and cause systemic carnitine deficiency. Similarly, mutations in genes encoding enzymes involved in the transfer and metabolism of carnitine including carnitine mitochondrial carnitine palmitoyltransferase I (CATI), located in the outer mitochondrial membrane, and translocase (SLC25A20), located in the inner membrane, can lead to defective carnitine uptake and decreased tissue levels of carnitine. Treatment with high doses of oral carnitine alleviates the symptoms.

Mutations in acyl-CoA dehydrogenase also impair mitochondrial fatty acid oxidation and can lead to cardiomyopathy.[189,192] The clinical manifestations are remarkable for cardiac hypertrophy with diminished systolic function, fasting hypoglycemia, inadequate ketotic response to hypoglycemia, hepatic dysfunction, skeletal myopathy, and sudden death.[189,192] The majority of cases of medium-chain acyl-CoA dehydrogenase deficiency are caused by substitution of glutamic acid for lysine in the mutant protein, while the molecular genetic basis of short-chain acyl-CoA dehydrogenase deficiency is more heterogeneous.

Ion Channelopathies as the Basis for Cardiac Arrhythmias and Conduction Defects

Ion channels, crucial units in cardiac excitability, are glycoproteins embedded in the membrane of the cardiac myocytes through which ions selectively allow flux in and out of the cell to modulate the electrical gradient. Many different ion channels are precisely activated to give rise to the electrical current that will ultimately be responsible for the development of myocyte excitability. This is a complex process that requires a very well controlled ionic balance to prevent arrhythmogenesis.

The alpha subunit of the cardiac sodium channel gene SCN5A, responsible for phase 0 of the cardiac action potential, has recently been studied extensively. SCN5A was first cloned and characterized in 1995 and localized to 3p21.[195] The gene comprises 28 exons that code for a 2016–amino acid protein. It contains four homologous domains (DI to DIV), each of which contains six membrane-spanning segments (S1 to S6).[193] Wang et al. were first to link mutations in the SCN5A to LQT syndrome,[196] a disease characterized by prolongation of the QT interval and sudden death at a young age. Subsequently, mutations in SCN5A were linked to idiopathic ventricular fibrillation,[197] the Brugada syndrome,[194] progressive conduction defect,[198] sudden infant death syndrome (SIDS),[199] and sudden unexpected death syndrome (SUDS).[200] The last of these is a phenotype

GENETIC DISEASES OF CARDIAC RHYTHM AND CONDUCTION

Cardiac rhythm and conduction abnormalities occur as the primary phenotypes of genetic disorders or as secondary phenotypes resulting from genetic diseases that primarily affect the structure of the heart. In general, cardiac arrhythmias and conduction defects result from abnormalities in three main families of proteins: contractile sarcomeric proteins, as in HCM; the cytoskeletal proteins responsible for DCM; and ion channels and their regulators.[193] As discussed above, there is also significant phenotypic overlap, as mutations in the same gene can cause a variety of cardiac rhythm and conduction disorders. This overlap is best exemplified by mutations in the sodium channel gene SCN5A, which cause the long-QT (LQT) syndrome, Brugada syndrome, and progressive cardiac conduction defect, also known as Lenègre's or Lev's disease.[194] Therefore a simplistic classification of genetic disorders is considered preliminary, and some of the key genetic findings used to stratify patients for risk of sudden death or arrhythmias are based on studies in only a few families. Table 72-9 summarizes the list of genetic disorders in which the primary phenotype is cardiac arrhythmias and conduction defects.

TABLE 72-9 Genetic Disorders Causing Cardiac Arrhythmias in the Absence of Structural Heart Disease (Primary Rhythm Disorders)

	Rhythm	Inheritance	Locus	Gene
Supraventricular				
Atrial fibrillation	AF	AD	10q22	—
		AD	11p15	KCNQ1
Atrial standstill	SND, AF	AD	3p21	SCN5A
Absent sinus rhythm	SND, AF	AD	—	—
WPW	AVRT	AD	—	—
Familial PJRT	AVRT	AD	—	—
Conduction disorders				
PCCD	AVB	AD	19q13	—
			3p21	SCN5A
Ventricular				
LQT syndrome (RW)	TdP	AD		
LQT1			11p15	KCNQ1
LQT2			7q35	HERG
LQT3			3p21	SCN5A
LQT4			4q25	ANKB
LQT5			21q22	minK
LQT6			21q22	MiRP1
LQT7			17q23	KCNJ2
LQT syndrome (JLN)	TdP	AR	11p15	KCNQ1
			21q22	minK
Catecholaminergic PVT	VT	AD	1q42	RYR2
		AR	1p13-p11	CASQ2
Brugada syndrome	VT/VF	AD	3p21	SCN5A

ABBREVIATIONS: AD = autosomal dominant; AF = atrial fibrillation; AR = autosomal recessive; AVB = atrioventricular block; AVRT = atrioventricular reentrant tachycardia; JLN = Jervell and Lange–Nielsen; LQT = long-QT; PCCD = progressive cardiac conduction defect; PJRT = paroxysmal junctional reentrant tachycardia; RW = Romano-Ward; SND = sinus node dysfunction; TdP = torsades de pointes; VF = ventricular fibrillation; VT = ventricular tachycardia; WPW = Wolff-Parkinson-White syndrome.

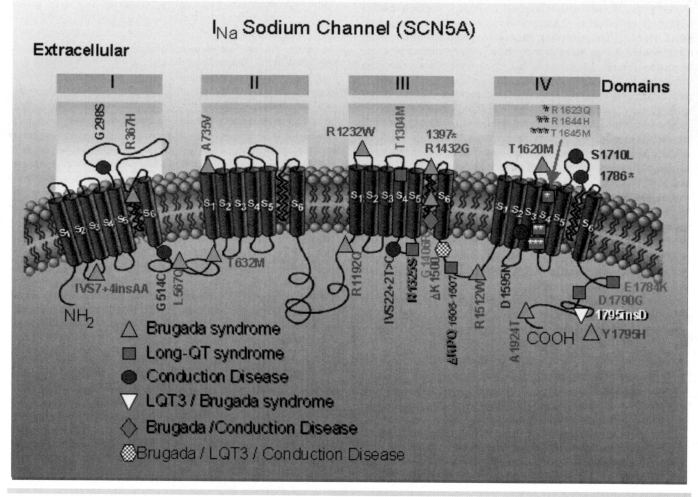

FIGURE 72-8 Schematic structure of I_{Na} sodium channel (SCN5A) and phenotypes arising from mutations in *SCN5A*.

identified some two decades ago in Southeast Asia, causing sudden death in males, usually at night.[200] Phenotypes arising from mutations in *SCN5A* are shown in Fig. 72-8.

Brugada Syndrome and Its Variants

Brugada syndrome is identified by a characteristic ECG pattern consisting of right bundle branch block and ST-segment elevation in V_1 to V_3 (Fig. 72-9) and sudden death at a young age (see also Chap. 41).[201] It was described originally in 1992 based on its ECG pattern and the occurrence of syncope or sudden death episodes in patients with structurally normal hearts.[201] The episodes of syncope and sudden death are caused by fast polymorphic ventricular tachycardia.[201,202]

Brugada syndrome often manifests itself in the third and fourth decades of life and occasionally in infants as SIDS.[199] Recent studies suggest that SUDS, which is prevalent in Southeast Asia, is a form of Brugada syndrome. SUDS has been estimated to affect up to 1 percent of the population and is the most common cause of death in young males in Thailand.[203] Death often occurs at night and more commonly in male subjects (the male-to-female ratio is 10 to 1). Electrocardiographically, the disease is identical to Brugada syndrome. As in Brugada syndrome, mutations in *SCN5A* are responsible for SUDS and biophysical data indicate a nonworking *SCN5A* or accelerated inactivation.[200]

CELLULAR BASIS OF BRUGADA SYNDROME

The electrical function of the ventricular myocardium is progressively being understood. What was once thought to be a homogeneous tissue consisting of myocyte and connective tissues is now recognized as being a heterogeneous milieu with multiple cellular subtypes having different functional and electrophysiologic properties. These electrophysiologic distinctions are due to variations in the expression of ionic currents, especially between epicardium and endocardium. These differences contribute to the development of ST-segment elevation and are the substrate for reentrant arrhythmias. Experiments involving the arterially perfused right ventricular wedge preparation have shown that the epicardial action potential notch is responsible for the inscription of the ECG J wave and that accentuation of the notch leads to amplification of the J wave, resulting in an apparent elevation of the ST segment. This has been shown in pathophysiologic states like hypothermia, where an increase in the notch in epicardium but not endocardium causes an elevation of the J point and ST segment in the ECG. Further accentuation of the pathophysiologic state will accentuate the notch and prolong the epicardial action potential, so that it repolarizes after the endocardial response. This will eventually lead to loss of the action potential dome and marked abbreviation of the epicardial response. The end result will be the creation of a transmural gradient between epicardium and endocardium and thus the substrate for reentrant arrhythmias.[204]

Experimental models of Brugada syndrome created by exposing right ventricular wedge preparations to a variety of pharmacologic agents have highlighted the importance of the potassium transient outward current (I_{to}). The high expression of I_{to} during phase 1 of the action potential plays a pivotal role in the ECG pattern of Brugada syndrome. It is the balance of currents active during phase 1 that determines the degree of ST-segment elevation. The higher expression of I_{to} in males and in the right versus the left ventricle could explain why the disease shows in the right precordial leads and the prevalence of the phenotype in males.[204]

Sodium channel blockers also increase the notch of the epicardial action potential and thus give rise to an ST-segment elevation in the wedge preparation. This has also proved useful in clinical practice as a form of diagnostic tool to unmask the ECG pattern in individuals suspected of having Brugada syndrome.[205] Sodium blockers like ajmaline, procainamide, flecainide, and pilsicainide are now being used to identify the individuals at risk.

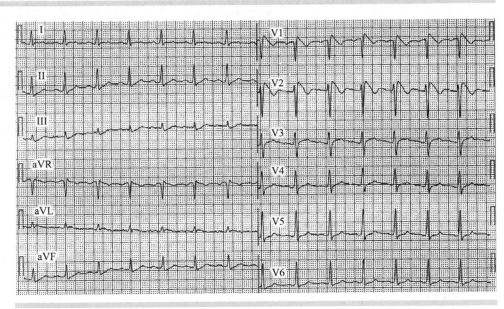

FIGURE 72-9 Typical electrocardiogram of Brugada syndrome. Note the pattern resembling a right bundle branch block and the ST elevation in leads V_1 to V_2.

GENETICS OF BRUGADA SYNDROME

SCN5A was identified as the first and thus far the only causal gene for Brugada syndrome in 1998.[197] Over 60 different mutations in SCN5A have been identified that collectively account for approximately 25 percent of all cases with Brugada syndrome. As in many other genetic disorders, Brugada syndrome also exhibits locus heterogeneity, and a second locus on chromosome 3 has been mapped.[206] However, the causal gene has not yet been identified.

SCN5A mutations induce a large spectrum of phenotypes, including Brugada syndrome, long-QT syndrome (LQT3), isolated progressive cardiac conduction defect, idiopathic ventricular fibrillation, and SUDS.[194] The phenotypes are considered allelic variants caused by mutations in SCN5A. ECG, clinical, genetic, and biophysical data have clarified the relationships among these phenotypes. The distinction between the LQT3 and Brugada syndromes is difficult to ascertain in some cases, and one family has been described manifesting the phenotype of both Brugada and LQT3 syndromes.[207] Likewise, progressive conduction disease and Brugada syndrome have been described in members of a single family.[208] Furthermore, compound heterozygosity in SCN5A leading to severe cardiac conduction disturbances and severe degeneration of the specialized conduction system has been described.[209] Collectively, these data suggest that mutations in SCN5A cause variable phenotypic manifestations that span Brugada syndrome, LQT3, and progressive conduction defects (Fig. 72-8).

PATHOGENESIS OF BRUGADA SYNDROME

The identification of mutations in SCN5A in patients with Brugada syndrome suggested that a decrease in the availability of sodium ions could shift the ionic balance in favor of I_{to} during phase 1 of the action potential. Biophysical characterization of mutations in SCN5A suggests that mutations decrease the availability of Na^{+1} current by two main mechanisms: decreased expression of the mutant channel or acceleration of inactivation of the channel. In addition, an alteration in ionic currents enhanced at higher temperatures has been implicated for certain mutations, such as the T1620M.[210] The clinical relevance of this mechanism is corroborated by the observation of several cases of ventricular fibrillation during febrile illnesses in patients with Brugada syndrome. Compared to LQT3, the pathogenesis of the Brugada syndrome could be considered a mirror image. Biophysical data indicate that LQT3 mutations cause a delayed inactivation of the channel,[193] which is exactly the opposite in Brugada syndrome, where there is an accelerated inactivation.[210]

GENOTYPE-PHENOTYPE CORRELATION IN BRUGADA SYNDROME

Limited data are available regarding the correlation between genotypes and phenotypes in patients with Brugada syndrome. This may in part be due to its recent identification, the phenotypic variability of SCN5A, and allelic and locus heterogeneity of Brugada syndrome. It has been suggested that ECG parameters, such as longer conduction intervals (PQ and HV) on the baseline ECG, could distinguish carriers of sodium channel mutations from noncarriers.[211]

Long-QT Syndrome

Long-QT (LQT) syndrome is a disease of ventricular repolarization identified by prolongation of the QT interval on the ECG.[193] It is characterized by syncopal episodes, malignant ventricular arrhythmias, and ventricular fibrillation. The majority of patients with LQT syndrome are asymptomatic. However, approximately one-third present with syncope or aborted malignant ventricular arrhythmias including torsades de pointes, which is the most typical ventricular arrhythmia in LQT syndrome. SCD is relatively common. The prognosis of untreated symptomatic cases is poor. Approximately one-fifth of untreated patients presenting with syncope die within 1 year and 50 percent die within 10 years.

The LQT syndrome is either acquired or congenital. The former is iatrogenic and commonly induced by drugs. A common cause of the acquired disease is the use of medications such as antiarrhythmics, antidepressants, and phenothiazides (Table 72-10). In addition, electrolyte imbalance such as hypokalemia, hypomagnesemia, and

TABLE 72-10 Selected Medications Associated with Prolonged QT Interval

Antiarrhythmic drugs
  Quinidine
  Procainamide hydrochloride
  Disopyramide phosphate
  Sotalol hydrochloride
  Amiodarone
  Ibutilide fumarate
  Dofetilide
  Propafenone
Anesthetics/antiasthmatics
  Droperidol
  Adrenaline
Antibiotics
  Clarithromycin
  Erythromycin
  Pentamidine
  Trimethoprim-sulfamethoxazole
  Ketoconazole
  Fluconazole
Antihistamines
  Terfenadine
  Diphenhydramine
Antihyperlipidemic
  Probucol
Central nervous system-active drugs
  Droperidol
  Haloperidol
  Pimozide
  Risperidone
Gastrointestinal stimulants
  Cisapride

hypocalcemia, especially in the presence of predisposing medications, can cause LQT syndrome.

Two patterns of inheritance have been described in the congenital LQT syndrome: (1) autosomal recessive disease, described by Jervell and Lange-Nielsen in 1957, which is associated with deafness and (2) autosomal dominant disease, described by Romano and Ward, which is not associated with deafness and is more common than the recessive form.

The pathogenesis of LQT syndrome due to mutations in the K^{+1} channel results from inadequate opening and decreased potassium outward current. Mutations in Na^{+1} channels lead to inadequate closure of the channels and excessive sodium inward currents. The result is inadequate maintenance of the electrical gradient (loss of function) during an action potential and prolongation of the QT interval.

AUTOSOMAL DOMINANT LONG-QT SYNDROME (ROMANO-WARD SYNDROME)

The first locus for the autosomal dominant disease was mapped to chromosome 11 in 1991.[212] Since then, seven loci have been mapped and six genes identified (Table 72-9). All encode proteins that are responsible for automaticity of electrical activity in cardiac cells. Mutations cause a disruption in the formation of the channels, altering the cardiac action potential and creating a voltage gradient espe-

cially at the ventricular level, which is responsible for reentrant arrhythmias.

LQT Syndrome 1   The causal gene for LQT1 is *KVLQT1* (or *KCNQ1*), which encodes a voltage-gated potassium channel alpha subunit strongly expressed in the heart.[213] It consists of 16 exons spanning 400 kb, which form six transmembrane segments. It coassembles with the beta subunit minK (KCNE1) to form the slow activating potassium current I_{Ks}. Mutations in this gene disrupt the normal function of the protein, causing a decrease in the potassium current. Several mutations have been described in *KCNQ1*.

LQT Syndrome 2   The LQT2 gene is *HERG*, which was isolated in 1994 from the hippocampus and named human *ether-a-go-go–related* gene due to its homology to the *ether-a-go-go* gene in *Drosophila*. The gene is localized on chromosome 7q35-q36 and contains 16 exons spanning an approximately 55 kb of genomic sequence. It encodes a protein that forms six transmembrane segments[214] and is responsible for the rapidly activating delayed rectifier potassium current I_{Kr} after coassembly with MIRP1 (KCNE2). As in the case of LQT1, mutations in *HERG* cause an abnormal protein with a resulting loss of potassium current.

LQT Syndrome 3   The causal gene is *SCN5A*, located on chromosome 3; it encodes for the cardiac sodium channel.[196] Mutations in *SCN5A* also cause Brugada syndrome and progressive conduction system disease, as discussed above. Electrophysiologic studies following expression of the mutant proteins in *Xenopus* oocytes indicate gain-of-function mutations evidenced by delayed inactivation and persistent leaking of sodium ions after phase 0 of the action potential.

LQT Syndrome 4   A locus for a French family with 65 affected members having LQT and sinus node dysfunction was mapped to 4q25-q27 in 1995.[215] Very recently, the causal gene was identified as *ANKB* (also known as *ANK2*), which encodes ankyrin B.[216] Mutations in ankyrin B disrupt cellular localization of the sodium pump, the sodium/calcium exchanger, and the inositol-1,4,5-triphosphate receptors, reducing their expression levels and affecting Ca^{+2} signaling in adult cardiac myocytes.[216] This finding suggests not only that mutations in ion channels cause cardiac arrhythmias but also that mutations in proteins associated with ion channels, such as ankyrin B, could induce a similar phenotype.

LQT Syndrome 5   *MinK* (minimal potassium ion channel), located on chromosome 21q22.1-q22.2, is the causal gene and contains three exons. MinK coassembles with KVLQT1 to form the cardiac I_{Ks} channel.[213] Mutations in this gene have been identified as causing both the autosomal dominant and autosomal recessive diseases.

LQT Syndrome 6   LQT6 is caused by mutations in *KCNE2* or MirP1 (minK-related peptide). It is mapped to 21q22.1, next to *MinK*, arrayed in the opposite direction. KCNE2 assembles with HERG to form the I_{Kr} current.[217] Mutations in *KCNE2* decrease potassium current availability, with slower activation.

LQT Syndrome 7   Andersen's syndrome is a rare autosomal dominant inherited disorder characterized by the constellation of periodic paralysis, cardiac arrhythmias, LQT syndrome, and dysmorphic features such as short stature, scoliosis, clinodactyly, hypertelorism, low-set or slanted ears, micrognathia, and broad forehead.[218] The causal gene is *KCNJ2*, located on chromosome 17q23; it encodes the inward rectifier potassium channel Kir2.1, expressed in skeletal and cardiac muscles. Kir2.1 is a strong inward rectified channel that prevents passage of any current at potential greater than −40 mV. Electrophysiologic studies indicate that the mutant protein exerts a dominant negative effect on Kir2.1 function, with an ultimate decrease in potassium current.

AUTOSOMAL RECESSIVE LONG-QT SYNDROME (JERVELL AND LANGE-NIELSEN SYNDROME)

The autosomal recessive forms of the LQT syndrome have been linked to mutations in the genes encoding I_{Ks} current, namely *KVLQT1* and *minK*.[219] For the LQT phenotype, which is also associated with sensorineural deafness, to be expressed, the patients must inherit a mutation from both parents. Therefore it is less common than the Romano-Ward syndrome but is associated with a more malignant course and a longer QT interval. The phenotype can also arise in recessive forms if different mutations in the same gene are inherited from the parents (compound heterozygote).

GENOTYPE-PHENOTYPE CORRELATION IN LONG-QT SYNDROME

Given the availability of a large number of families with the LQT syndrome, several genotype-phenotype correlation studies have been performed to identify the genetic determinants of triggering events, ECG phenotype, and response to therapy. The studies predominantly encompass the three most common forms of LQT syndrome—LQT 1, LQT2, and LQT3—and have significant limitations inherent to genotype-phenotype correlation studies, described above. Despite their limitations, characteristic features have emerged that could guide the analysis of patients toward a specific genetic defect (Table 72-11).[220] In general, individuals with LQT1 exhibit symptoms during physical activity, such as swimming, and have a T wave of long duration on the ECG. Individuals with LQT2 usually develop symptoms related to auditory stimuli, and the T wave is small or notched. In contrast, subjects with LQT3 are symptomatic during sleep and the ECG shows a very late T wave with a prolonged ST segment.

Mutations also carry prognostic significance; in all three groups (LQT1, 2, and 3), there is a correlation between cardiac events and the QTc interval. In general, patients with LQT1 and LQT2 have a higher risk of cardiac events than patients with LQT3. The latter, despite having fewer events, have a relatively higher mortality, which indicates that events in the LQT3 are more likely to be lethal.[221] In addition, response to drug therapy seems to correlate with the genotype. While beta blockers are considered the first line of therapy in patients with LQT1, they have not shown to be beneficial in those with LQT3, who have a slower heart rate. Preliminary data suggest LQT3 patients might benefit from Na^{+1} channel blockers, such as mexiletine, but long-term data are not yet available.[222]

Induced or Acquired Long-QT Syndrome

Induced or acquired LQT is iatrogenic, caused by a long list of medications (Table 72-10) and electrolyte abnormalities. A large number of factors determine the risk of developing LQT syndrome in an individual in response to drug therapy, including bioavailability of the drug, the interaction with other medications that affect the same

repolarizing current, and the presence of SNPs. SNPs play a major role in determining the pharmacodynamics and pharmacokinetics of drugs and thus the risk of LQT syndrome. The final effect on the repolarization will depend on the so-called repolarizing reserve, or the degree of alteration that the ionic currents can sustain before repolarization is compromised. Any combination of genetic and environmental factors (drug, electrolyte abnormalities) that decrease this "repolarization reserve" below a safe threshold will place the individual at risk for arrhythmia.[223]

Epidemiologic studies have led to the identification of mutations and SNPs in genes known to cause LQT syndrome. These SNPs are typically silent until unmasked by the use of I_{Kr} blockers. Thus, one may consider these subjects as those with unexpressed congenital LQT syndrome.[224] Recent identification of a common SNP that predisposes to induced arrhythmias in the African-American population serves as an example.[224] Nonetheless, the results of SNP-association studies are considered provisional and require support through mechanistic studies, as discussed above.

Progressive Familial Heart Block

Familial heart block is an autosomal dominant progressive disease of the cardiac conduction system characterized by initial development of bundle branch block with subsequent gradual progression to complete heart block. Two forms have been recognized. In type I, the onset is early and the disease is rapidly progressive. In type II, the onset is later in life; commonly the QRS complex is narrow and AV-nodal block predominates. Clinical features of the disease include syncope, SCD, and Stokes-Adams attacks. A locus was identified in a large family of Portuguese descent on chromosome 19q13. As discussed earlier, mutations in *SCN5A* have been identified in some families with familial heart block.[208,225] Functional studies suggest haploinsufficiency as the underlying mechanism, as the mutant allele exhibits complete loss of function.[225] In addition, AV block in conjunction with congenital heart disease, such as ASD (CSX1 mutations), and DCM (lamin A/C mutations) have been described, as discussed earlier.

Catecholaminergic Polymorphic Ventricular Tachycardia

Calcium is a key ion in excitation-contraction coupling of the heart. Calcium intervenes in the depolarizing current, creating the plateau or phase 2 of the action potential; it triggers the release of calcium from the sarcoplasmic reticulum (SR) and activates the cardiac contractile apparatus. The SR functions primarily as an intracellular store of calcium in cardiac muscle cells. Ryanodine receptors are responsible for release of the calcium from the SR and are activated by the incoming calcium; therefore they are Ca^{+2}-activated Ca^{+2} channels. Mutations in ryanodine receptors (*RYR2*) have been shown to

TABLE 72-11 Genotype-Phenotype Correlation in Long-QT Syndromes

Phenotype	Gene	T wave	Trigger
LQT1	*KCNQ1*	Early onset, broad-base T	Emotion, swimming
LQT2	*HERG*	Low amplitude	Auditory
LQT3	*SCN5A*	Late T, normal amplitude	Sleep

cause ARVC type 2 (ARVD2),[226] as discussed earlier, and familial polymorphic ventricular tachycardia (FPVT).[226]

FPVT is an autosomal dominant inherited disease with a mortality rate of approximately 30 percent by the age of 30 years. Phenotypically, it is characterized by runs of bidirectional and polymorphic ventricular tachycardia in response to vigorous exercise in the absence of evidence of structural myocardial disease.

A recessive form of FPVT also has been described and mapped to 1p13.3-p11.[227] Mutation screening has identified a missense mutation in calsequestrin 2 (*CASQ2*) as responsible for the disease. *CASQ2* is involved in the same pathway as *RYR2* to control calcium release from the SR.

Familial Atrial Fibrillation

Atrial fibrillation in the absence of known causes of secondary atrial fibrillation may be a familial disorder. The mode of inheritance is autosomal dominant. The first gene was localized to chromosome 10q22-24[228]; subsequently, genetic heterogeneity was established. Recently, the first causal gene for familial atrial fibrillation was identified as the *KCNQ1*, which is also responsible for LQT1 syndrome. The mutation for atrial fibrillation is a gain-of-function mutation, in contrast to the loss-of-function mutations observed in patients with LQT1.[229]

Monomorphic Ventricular Tachycardia

Recently a somatic point mutation (F200L) in the inhibitory subunit 2 of G protein alpha was identified in a patient with sustained monomorphic ventricular tachycardia that was unresponsive to vagal maneuvers and adenosine.[230] The mutation was present in cardiac tissue at the arrhythmogenic locus and was shown to increase intracellular cAMP concentration and to inhibit suppression of cAMP by adenosine.

Familial Wolff-Parkinson-White Syndrome

Familial Wolff-Parkinson-White (WPW) syndrome is a rare syndrome with an autosomal dominant mode of inheritance that occurs in isolation or in conjunction with other disorders, such as HCM and Pompe's disease. It is characterized by evidence of preexcitation on the ECG, palpitation, and syncope due to supraventricular arrhythmias. The phenotype of WPW syndrome in conjunction with HCM and conduction defect was found in patients with mutations in *PRKAG2*, as discussed earlier.[183–185] It has also been reported in patients with Pompe's disease, caused by mutations in α-1,4-glucosidase,[180] in those with HCM caused by mutations in *TNNI3* and *MYBPC3*, and in Leber's hereditary optic neuropathy, which is caused by mutations in mitochondrial DNA.[231]

GENETIC BASIS OF CARDIAC DISEASE IN CONNECTIVE TISSUE DISORDERS

Marfan's Syndrome

Marfan's syndrome is a primary disorder of connective tissue characterized by cardiovascular, ocular, and skeletal abnormalities.[232] There is significant variability in the clinical manifestations of Marfan's syndrome, but the predominant features are progressive dilatation of the aortic root, aortic aneurysm, dissection, and aortic and mitral valve regurgitation. The estimated prevalence of Marfan's syndrome is 1 per 10,000. The age of onset of clinical manifestations of Marfan's syndrome is variable, but cardiac phenotypes commonly occur in the third and fourth decades of life. Aortic dissection is the leading cause of premature death in patients with Marfan's syndrome. In addition to cardiovascular abnormalities, marfanoid habitus (increased height, disproportionately long limbs and digits), lens dislocation or subluxation, arachnodactyly, thoracic abnormalities, and increased joint laxity are common clinical features (see also Chap. 84).

GENETIC BASIS OF MARFAN'S SYNDROME

Marfan's syndrome is an autosomal dominant disease that exhibits locus and allelic heterozygosity. The first causal gene to be identified is the *FBN1*, encoding fibrillin, located on 15q15.23.[233,234] Fibrillin is a cysteine-rich protein with a molecular mass of 350 kDa; it is the major component of extracellular microfibrils in both elastic and nonelastic connective tissues. Over 300 nonrecurring unique mutations in *FBN1* have been described that encompass missense, nonsense, and deletion mutations, as well as abnormal splicing or exon skipping.[235] Mutations are spread throughout most of the gene, and the frequency of each particular mutation is relatively low, which makes screening for mutations tedious.

There is a significant variability in the phenotypic expression of Marfan's syndrome, which may be partly due to locus and allelic heterogeneity of the disease and partly to the effect of modifier genes and perhaps environmental factors. The clinical spectrum varies from ectopia lentis in the absence of any other phenotype to neonatal Marfan's syndrome and premature death, often within the first 2 years of life. Mutations inducing premature termination of the protein result in approximately a 50 percent reduction in the level of fibrillin, accompanied by more frequent ocular manifestations. A phenocopy of Marfan's syndrome is congenital "contractural arachnodactyly," which is characterized by severe kyphoscoliosis, generalized osteopenia, flexion contractures of the fingers, abnormally shaped ears, and, less frequently, mitral regurgitation and congenital heart disease. Recently, point mutations in the *FBN2* gene have been described as causes of contractural arachnodactyly.[236] *FBN2* mutations clustered in limited regions alter amino acids in the calcium-binding consensus sequence in the EGF-like domains. Mutations affect either the conserved cysteine residues or residues of the calcium-binding consensus sequence of the cbEGF motifs and often result in premature termination of the protein.

The pathogenesis of Marfan's syndrome entails decreased expression levels of the fibrillin protein and reduced deposition of fibrillin in vascular adventitia, resulting in weakening of the adventitia and aneurysm formation.

Ehlers-Danlos Syndrome

Ehlers-Danlos syndrome, a relatively uncommon disorder, encompasses a group of conditions characterized by increased elasticity of the skin and connective tissue diseases (see also Chap. 84).[232] The classic form of Ehlers-Danlos syndrome is characterized by joint hypermotility and fragile, bruisable skin that heals with peculiar "cigarette-paper" scars. Other clinical features include translucent elasticity of the skin, mitral valve prolapse, spontaneous rupture and aneurysm of large arteries, kyphoscoliosis, atrophic scars, and hematomas in the joint areas, especially in the knees and elbows. In the severe form, spontaneous rupture of the intestines and arteries is common. In the benign form, the only manifestations may be hyperextensibility of joints and easy bruisability. The age of onset of clinical manifestations is variable and ranges from in childhood to late adulthood.

GENETIC BASIS OF EHLERS-DANLOS SYNDROME

Ehlers-Danlos syndrome has nine different forms that are inherited in three different patterns of transmission, autosomal dominant, autosomal recessive, and X-linked recessive. Cardiovascular abnormalities are more common in forms I and IV and include congenital malformations, such as tetralogy of Fallot, atrial septal defects, and valvular abnormalities such as mitral and tricuspid valve prolapse.[232]

Mutations in genes encoding collagen components lead to Ehlers-Danlos syndrome. For example, Ehlers-Danlos type IV, which is considered the most malignant form because of proneness to spontaneous rupture of the bowel and large arteries and a high incidence of pregnancy-related complications, is caused by mutations in COL3A1.[237] The gene is located on 2q31 and encodes type III procollagen. Cardiac manifestations include aortic and coronary artery aneurysms with a high incidence of rupture. Some case of Ehlers-Danlos syndrome type I are caused by mutations in COL5A2, coding for collagen α–2 (V), and COL1A1, encoding collagen α-1(I).[232] Ehlers-Danlos syndrome is considered a primary disorder of collagen deficiency. Point and deletion mutations result in decreased collagen synthesis and consequently loss of connective tissue resiliency.

Ellis–van Creveld Syndrome

This syndrome is discussed above, in the text concerning congenital heart diseases.

Cutis Laxa

Cutis laxa comprises a heterogeneous group of acquired and genetic disorders characterized by redundant, wrinkled, loose, sagging skin that slowly returns to normal after stretching. Cardiac manifestations include pulmonic stenosis, aortic aneurysms, and right-sided heart failure. Vessels are very tortuous, resembling corkscrews on the angiogram.

Autosomal dominant and recessive and X-linked forms have been described, and mutations in the elastin gene (ELN) have been identified in the autosomal dominant form.[238] A homozygous missense mutation in the fibulin-5 (FBLN5) gene has been identified as responsible for the recessive form.[239]

Pseudoxanthoma Elasticum

Pseudoxanthoma elasticum is a genetic disorder characterized by dermatologic, ocular, and cardiovascular abnormalities resulting from degeneration of the elastic fibers. Manifestations include pseudoxanthoma, especially in areas of the neck and axillae; angioid streaks in the optic fundus; and gastrointestinal hemorrhagic and occlusive disease. Cardiovascular abnormalities include calcification of the peripheral arteries, with resulting intermittent claudication, coronary artery disease, mitral valve prolapse, and hypertension.

Recently, mutations in the ATP-binding cassette (ABC) transporter gene (ABCC6) on chromosome 16p13 were identified as the cause of psuedoxanthoma elasticum.[240] The exact biological function of ABCC6 protein and the mechanism(s) by which mutations in ABCC6 cause psuedoxanthoma elasticum are unknown.

Osteogenesis Imperfecta

Osteogenesis imperfecta (OI) comprises a heterogeneous class of connective tissue disorders characterized by bone fragility. Bone fragility results from defective collagen synthesis, which leads to decreased bone mass, disturbed organization of bone tissue, and al-

tered bone geometry (size and shape). Cardiovascular abnormalities include valvular lesions, such as mitral and aortic regurgitation, and an increased fragility of the blood vessels.

Mutations in one of the two genes encoding type I collagen, namely COL1A1 and COL1A2, have been identified as the cause.[241]

GENETIC DISORDERS OF THE PULMONARY CIRCULATION

Familial Primary Pulmonary Hypertension

Primary pulmonary hypertension (PPH) is diagnosed when mean resting pulmonary artery blood pressure is greater than 25 mmHg in the absence of known secondary causes such as lung disease or pulmonary venous congestion secondary to heart failure (see also Chap. 62). Clinical manifestations include exercise intolerance, fatigue cyanosis, syncope, and sudden cardiac death. Clinical manifestations often start in the third and fourth decades of life and are at least twice as common in females. Median survival is about 3 years. Prevalence is 1 to 2 per 100,000 individuals.

This is an autosomal dominant disease in 6 percent of all cases of PPH. A causal gene is bone morphogenic protein receptor type II (BMPR2) on chromosome 2q31-33, which encodes a transforming growth factor beta (TGF-β) receptor.[242–245] The spectrum of mutations includes nonsense and frameshift mutations, expected to produce dysfunctional protein. Bone morphogenic protein (BMP) receptor is a cell-surface receptor that belongs to the TGF-β family.[246] Mutations in another component of the TGF-β receptor family, activin-receptor–like kinase 1 (ALK1), have also been described.[247] Finally, an association between serotonin transporter (5-HTT) SNPs and pulmonary hypertension has been documented.[248]

The pathogenesis of pulmonary hypertension caused by mutations in BMPR2, ALK1, and serotonin transporter entails smooth muscle cell proliferation and apoptosis, known biological functions of these proteins. Mutations inhibit BMP/Smad-mediated signaling by diverse molecular mechanisms, leading to dysfunctional protein and promoting the proliferation of smooth muscle cells.[246,249,250]

MONOGENIC LIPID DISORDERS

The majority of common dyslipidemias are complex traits caused by interaction of multiple genes and environmental factors. SNPs in a variety of genes encoding protein components of cholesterol and fatty acid biosynthesis have been implicated in susceptibility to dyslipidemia; these are discussed elsewhere (see Chap. 43) and reviewed in Ref. 251. Monogenic forms of dyslipidemias are described briefly below.

Familial Hypercholesterolemia

Familial hypercholesterolemia (FH) is an autosomal dominant disorder with a prevalence of 1 in 500 in the mild form and in 1 in 100,000 in its severe form. It is characterized by severely elevated plasma levels of low-density lipoprotein cholesterol (LDL-C) (type IIa hyperlipidemia) and premature atherosclerosis. Plasma levels of total cholesterol are in the range of 300 to 400 mg/dL in affected heterozygous individuals and over 500 mg/dL in homozygous subjects. The affected individuals develop severe atherosclerosis involving multiple vascular territories, tendon xanthomata, and corneal arcus. Subjects homozygous for the causal mutation exhibit clinical atherosclerosis in the first and second decades of life and heterozygous subjects in the fourth and fifth decades. These patients often suffer from ischemic symptoms and/or cardiac events requiring revascularization procedures very early in life (see also Chap. 43).

The causal gene is *LDLR* located on chromosome 19p13, which encodes LDL-C receptors.[252] Over 1000 point, deletion, and splice mutations have been identified and approximately 60 percent of the mutations are missense mutations, 20 percent minor rearrangements, 13 percent major rearrangements, and 7 percent splice-junction mutations.[253] Mutations by a variety of mechanisms perturb the function of LDL-C receptors, including affecting synthesis and targeting to the cell membrane, binding to LDL-C, internalization after binding, and recycling of the receptors to the cell surface after internalization, all of which impair removal of apolipoprotein B (apoB) and apoE from the circulation.[252] Mutations affect LDL-C receptor function to variable degrees, leading to variable clinical manifestations.[254] Frameshift mutations that markedly alter the structure of the LDL-C receptors cause severely affected phenotypes; those that completely inactivate the receptors lead to severe premature atherosclerosis in childhood. In contrast, mutations that partially inactivate the receptors cause mild to moderate hypercholesterolemia. Thus the development and severity of coronary atherosclerosis vary according to causal mutations, genetic background, diet, environmental factors, and epigenetic factors.

A phenocopy of FH is familial defective apolipoprotein B100, which results in a similar phenotype (discussed below).

Familial Defective Apolipoprotein B100

Familial defective apolipoprotein B100 (FDB) is autosomal dominant, resulting in increased plasma levels of LDL-C and very low-density lipoprotein C (VLDL-C).[255,256] It is a relatively common disorder, with an estimated frequency of 1 in 500, but the prevalence varies worldwide. Clinical features of FDB include hypercholesterolemia and premature atherosclerosis. The frequency of the mutation varies in different regions of the world. The phenotype is largely similar to that of FH.

The causal gene is *APOB,* located on chromosome 2q24, and the causal mutation involves amino acid 3500 in > 99 percent of the cases, with the predominant mutation being R3500Q and rarely R3500W.[255,256] Mutations lead to increased LDL-C levels by decreasing the affinity of LDL-C receptors for apolipoprotein B, thus augmenting the accumulation of VLDL-C and LDL-C in the plasma and blood vessels.

Hypobetalipoproteinemia

Hypobetalipoproteinemia, or abetalipoproteinemia, is a rare disease characterized by extremely low plasma levels of apolipoprotein B, total cholesterol, and LDL-C.[257] HDL-C levels are high and atherosclerosis is very uncommon. Clinical features are poorly defined; they include ataxia and demyelination of the central nervous system. Sporadic and familial cases have been reported. Familial cases exhibit an autosomal dominant mode of inheritance. A causal gene is *MTP* on chromosome 4q22-24, which encodes the microsomal triglyceride transfer protein.[258] MTP is a heterodimer of a unique large subunit and the protein disulfide isomerase, which catalyzes the transport of triglyceride, cholesteryl ester, and phospholipid from phospholipid surfaces. Mutations encode truncated nonfunctional protein, thus leading to very low levels of apolipoprotein B, LDL-C, and total cholesterol.[258]

Fish-Eye Disease

Fish-eye disease is a rare autosomal dominant condition due to deficiency of lecithin:cholesterol acyltransferase (LCAT).[259] The *LCAT* gene is located on chromosome 16q22.1 and codes for a protein involved in the synthesis from prealphalipoprotein A1 and conversion of HDL_3 to HDL_2 cholesterol. A deficiency of LCAT leads to premature coronary atherosclerosis, proteinuria, anemia, renal failure, and corneal opacification.

Tangier Disease

Tangier disease (TD) is an autosomal codominant disease characterized by a virtual absence of HDL-C and very low plasma levels of apolipoprotein AI. Deposition of cholesteryl esters results in characteristic hypertrophic orange-colored tonsils, hepatosplenomegaly, and premature coronary artery disease.[260] Mutations in the ATP-binding cassette transporter (*ABCA1*) gene in patients with Tangier disease and familial hypoalphalipoproteinemia (HA), its allelic variant, are responsible for Tangier disease.[261–263] The *ABCA1* gene is located on chromosome 9q31 and codes for an mRNA of 6783 bp and a protein of 2261 amino acids.[261,263,264] ABCA1 is a transmembrane protein with 12 transmembrane domains. It acts as a flippase at the plasma membrane, stimulating cholesterol and phospholipid efflux to apolipoprotein AI and HDL-C.[260] Normally, ABCA1 transports free cholesterol to the extracellular space where it binds to apolipoprotein AI synthesized by the liver and forming nascent HDL particles from VLDL. In the absence of ABCA1, free cholesterol is not transported extracellularly and lipid-poor apolipoprotein AI rapidly degrades. Recently, common polymorphisms in the *ABCA1* gene have been associated with coronary atherosclerosis in the general population.[265,266]

MONOGENIC FORMS OF HYPERTENSION

The predominant form of hypertension is essential hypertension, which accounts for 95 percent of all cases. Hypertension is a complex phenotype caused by the interactions of multiple genes and environmental factors. Several genes, in particular those coding for the components of the renin-angiotensin-aldosterone system, have been implicated in essential hypertension[267–269]; these are discussed in Chap. 61. Only monogenic forms of hypertension are described briefly here.[270]

Glucocorticoid-Remediable Aldosteronism

Glucocorticoid-remediable aldosteronism (GRA) is a rare autosomal dominant disorder and the first described familial form of hyperaldosteronism.[269] It is caused by a chimeric mutation that joins the promoter region of the 11β-hydroxylase (*CYP11B1*) gene to the coding region of the aldosterone synthase (*CYP11B2*) gene.[271] The new chimeric gene, located on chromosome 8q24, has lost the negative feedback regulation imparted by angiotensin II. The promoter of the fusion gene, which is made up of the 5′ fragment of *CYP11B1* gene, is responsive to adrenocorticotropic hormone (ACTH). Thus expression of aldosterone remains unchecked, and excess aldosterone synthesis leads to the retention of sodium and salt and consequent hypertension. GRA responds to treatment with glucocorticoids, which suppress the production of ACTH. Alternatively, treatment with mineralocorticoid receptor blockers also controls the hypertension.

Apparent Mineralocorticoid Excess

Apparent mineralocorticoid excess (AME) is a rare autosomal recessive disease of peripheral metabolism of cortisol. Clinical manifestations of AME, in addition to hypertension, include hypokalemia, low plasma renin activity, and responsiveness to spironolactone. There are two types of AME, defined on the basis of severity of the biochemical phenotype. Both clinical variants are caused by mutations in the *HSD11B2* gene on chromosome 16q22, which encodes 11β-hydroxysteroid dehydrogenase II.[272,273] The enzyme is responsible for the peripheral conversion of biologically active cortisol to inactive cortisone. Point mutations in *HSD11B2* reduce or abolish the activity of 11β-hydroxysteroid dehydrogenase in the conversion of cortisol to cortisone. Thus, cortisol accumulates, leading to retention of salt and fluid through activation of mineralocorticoid receptors and hypertension.[273] Accordingly, patients with AME respond to blockade of mineralocorticoid receptors.

Liddle's Syndrome

Liddle's syndrome is a rare autosomal dominant disease characterized by hypertension, hypokalemic metabolic alkalosis, low plasma renin activity, and suppressed aldosterone secretion.[274] The phenotype usually develops early in life and hypertension is frequently severe. The first gene identified was the *SCNN1B*, located on locus 16p12, which encodes the beta subunit of the amiloride-sensitive Na^{+1} channel.[274] The renal epithelial Na^{+1} channel has three subunits: alpha, beta, and gamma. Subsequently mutations in the gamma subunit of epithelial sodium channels were also identified. The mutations activate the channel (gain-of-function mutations) and lead to sodium retention and hypertension.

Pseudohypoaldosteronism Type II

Pseudohypoaldosteronism type II (PHA 2), also known as the Gordon hyperkalemia-hypertension syndrome, is a rare autosomal dominant disorder characterized by hypertension and hyperkalemia early in life, mild hyperchloremia, metabolic acidosis, and suppressed plasma renin activity. Two causal genes for *PHA2—WNK4* on chromosome 17q21 and *WNK1* on chromosome 12p—have been identified.[275] *WNK4* and *WNK1* encode serine-threonine kinases expressed in the distal nephron.[275] Missense and deletion mutations exert a gain-of-function effect, increasing the expression levels of the proteins in the kidney and leading to increased renal salt reabsorption and reduced renal K^+ excretion.[275]

References

1. Hoffman JI. Incidence of congenital heart disease: II. Prenatal incidence. *Pediatr Cardiol* 1995;16:155–165.
2. Hoffman JI. Incidence of congenital heart disease: I. Postnatal incidence. *Pediatr Cardiol* 1995;16:103–113.
3. Venter JC, Adams MD, Myers EW, et al. The sequence of the human genome. *Science* 2001;291:1304–1351.
4. Wang DG, Fan JB, Siao CJ, et al. Large-scale identification, mapping, and genotyping of single-nucleotide polymorphisms in the human genome. *Science* 1998;280:1077–1082.
5. Cargill M, Altshuler D, Ireland J, et al. Characterization of single-nucleotide polymorphisms in coding regions of human genes. *Nat Genet* 1999;22:231–238.
6. Murray JC, Buetow KH, Weber JL, et al. A comprehensive human linkage map with centimorgan density. Cooperative Human Linkage Center (CHLC). *Science* 1994;265:2049–2054.
7. Gabriel SB, Schaffner SF, Nguyen H, et al. The structure of haplotype blocks in the human genome. *Science* 2002;296:2225–2229.
8. Dawson E, Abecasis GR, Bumpstead S, et al. A first-generation linkage disequilibrium map of human chromosome 22. *Nature* 2002;418:544–548.
9. Elsheikh M, Dunger DB, Conway GS, Wass JA. Turner's syndrome in adulthood. *Endocrinol Rev* 2002;23:120–140.
10. Korenberg JR, Chen XN, Schipper R, et al. Down syndrome phenotypes: The consequences of chromosomal imbalance. *Proc Natl Acad Sci USA* 1994;91:4997–5001.
11. Hyett J, Moscoso G, Nicolaides K. Abnormalities of the heart and great arteries in first trimester chromosomally abnormal fetuses. *Am J Med Genet* 1997;69:207–216.
12. Fuentes JJ, Pritchard MA, Planas AM, et al. A new human gene from the Down syndrome critical region encodes a proline-rich protein highly expressed in fetal brain and heart. *Hum Mol Genet* 1995;4:1935–1944.
13. Fuentes JJ, Genesca L, Kingsbury TJ, et al. DSCR1, overexpressed in Down syndrome, is an inhibitor of calcineurin-mediated signaling pathways. *Hum Mol Genet* 2000;9:1681–1690.
14. De Decker HP, Lawrenson JB. The 22q11.2 deletion: From diversity to a single gene theory. *Genet Med* 2001;3:2–5.
15. Lindsay EA, Botta A, Jurecic V, et al. Congenital heart disease in mice deficient for the DiGeorge syndrome region. *Nature* 1999;401:379–383.
16. Morris CA, Mervis CB. Williams syndrome and related disorders. *Annu Rev Genomics Hum Genet* 2000;1:461–484.
17. Schott JJ, Benson DW, Basson CT, et al. Congenital heart disease caused by mutations in the transcription factor NKX2-5. *Science* 1998;281:108–111.
18. Benson DW, Silberbach GM, Kavanaugh-McHugh A, et al. Mutations in the cardiac transcription factor NKX2.5 affect diverse cardiac developmental pathways. *J Clin Invest* 1999;104:1567–1573.
19. Kasahara H, Lee B, Schott JJ, et al. Loss of function and inhibitory effects of human CSX/NKX2.5 homeoprotein mutations associated with congenital heart disease. *J Clin Invest* 2000;106:299–308.
20. Basson CT, Bachinsky DR, Lin RC, et al. Mutations in human TBX5 [corrected] cause limb and cardiac malformation in Holt-Oram syndrome. *Nat Genet* 1997;15:30–35.
21. Basson CT, Huang T, Lin RC, et al. Different TBX5 interactions in heart and limb defined by Holt-Oram syndrome mutations. *Proc Natl Acad Sci USA* 1999;96:2919–2924.
22. Polymeropoulos MH, Ide SE, Wright M, et al. The gene for the Ellis-van Creveld syndrome is located on chromosome 4p16. *Genomics* 1996;35:1–5.
23. Ruiz-Perez VL, Ide SE, Strom TM, et al. Mutations in a new gene in Ellis-van Creveld syndrome and Weyers acrodental dysostosis. *Nat Genet* 2000;24:283–286.
24. Satoda M, Pierpont ME, Diaz GA, et al. Char syndrome, an inherited disorder with patent ductus arteriosus, maps to chromosome 6p12-p21. *Circulation* 1999;99:3036–3042.
25. Satoda M, Zhao F, Diaz GA, et al. Mutations in TFAP2B cause Char syndrome, a familial form of patent ductus arteriosus. *Nat Genet* 2000;25:42–46.
26. Tartaglia M, Mehler EL, Goldberg R, et al. Mutations in PTPN11, encoding the protein tyrosine phosphatase SHP-2, cause Noonan syndrome. *Nat Genet* 2001;29:465–468.
27. Tartaglia M, Kalidas K, Shaw A, et al. PTPN11 mutations in Noonan syndrome: Molecular spectrum, genotype-phenotype correlation, and phenotypic heterogeneity. *Am J Hum Genet* 2002;70:1555–1563.
28. Casey M, Mah C, Merliss AD, et al. Identification of a novel genetic locus for familial cardiac myxomas and Carney complex. *Circulation* 1998;98:2560–2566.
29. Stratakis CA, Carney JA, Lin JP, et al. Carney complex, a familial multiple neoplasia and lentiginosis syndrome. Analysis of 11 kindreds and linkage to the short arm of chromosome 2. *J Clin Invest* 1996;97:699–705.

30. Casey M, Vaughan CJ, He J, et al. Mutations in the protein kinase A R1alpha regulatory subunit cause familial cardiac myxomas and Carney complex. *J Clin Invest* 2000;106:R31–R38.

31. Bartoloni L, Blouin JL, Pan Y, et al. Mutations in the DNAH11 (axonemal heavy chain dynein type 11) gene cause one form of situs inversus totalis and most likely primary ciliary dyskinesia. *Proc Natl Acad Sci USA* 2002;99:10282–10286.

32. Pennarun G, Escudier E, Chapelin C, et al. Loss-of-function mutations in a human gene related to *Chlamydomonas reinhardtii* dynein IC78 result in primary ciliary dyskinesia. *Am J Hum Genet* 1999;65: 1508–1519.

33. Olbrich H, Haffner K, Kispert A, et al. Mutations in DNAH5 cause primary ciliary dyskinesia and randomization of left-right asymmetry. *Nat Genet* 2002;30:143–144.

34. Gebbia M, Ferrero GB, Pilia G, et al. X-linked situs abnormalities result from mutations in ZIC3. *Nat Genet* 1997;17:305–308.

35. Kosaki K, Bassi MT , Kosaki R, et al. Characterization and mutation analysis of human LEFTY A and LEFTY B, homologues of murine genes implicated in left-right axis development. *Am J Hum Genet* 1999;64:712–721.

36. Kosaki R, Gebbia M, Kosaki K, et al. Left-right axis malformations associated with mutations in ACVR2B, the gene for human activin receptor type IIB. *Am J Med Genet* 1999;82:70–76.

37. McElhinney DB, Krantz ID, Bason L, et al. Analysis of cardiovascular phenotype and genotype-phenotype correlation in individuals with a JAG1 mutation and/or Alagille syndrome. *Circulation* 2002;106: 2567–2574.

38. Li L, Krantz ID, Deng Y, et al. Alagille syndrome is caused by mutations in human Jagged1, which encodes a ligand for Notch1. *Nat Genet* 1997;16:243–251.

39. Oda T, Elkahloun AG, Pike BL, et al. Mutations in the human Jagged1 gene are responsible for Alagille syndrome. *Nat Genet* 1997;16:235–242.

40. Mogensen J, Kubo T, Duque M, et al. Idiopathic restrictive cardiomyopathy is part of the clinical expression of cardiac troponin I mutations. *J Clin Invest* 2003;111:209–216.

41. Maron BJ, Gardin JM, Flack JM, et al. Prevalence of hypertrophic cardiomyopathy in a general population of young adults. Echocardiographic analysis of 4111 subjects in the CARDIA Study. Coronary Artery Risk Development in (Young) Adults. *Circulation* 1995;92: 785–789.

42. Nagueh SF, Bachinski L, Meyer D, et al. Tissue Doppler imaging consistently detects myocardial abnormalities in patients with familial hypertrophic cardiomyopathy and provides a novel means for an early diagnosis before and independently of hypertrophy. *Circulation* 2001; 104:128–130.

43. Maron BJ, Shirani J, Poliac LC, et al. Sudden death in young competitive athletes. Clinical, demographic, and pathological profiles. *JAMA* 1996;276:199–204.

44. McKenna W, Deanfield J, Faruqui A, et al. Prognosis in hypertrophic cardiomyopathy: Role of age and clinical, electrocardiographic and hemodynamic features. *Am J Cardiol* 1981;47:532–538.

45. Maron BJ, Olivotto I, Spirito P, et al. Epidemiology of hypertrophic cardiomyopathy-related death: Revisited in a large non-referral-based patient population. *Circulation* 2000;102:858–864.

46. Cannan CR, Reeder GS, Bailey KR, et al. Natural history of hypertrophic cardiomyopathy. A population-based study, 1976 through 1990. *Circulation* 1995;92:2488–2495.

47. Maron BJ, Roberts WC. Quantitative analysis of cardiac muscle cell disorganization in the ventricular septum of patients with hypertrophic cardiomyopathy. *Circulation* 1979;59:689–706.

48. Maron BJ, Anan TJ, Roberts WC. Quantitative analysis of the distribution of cardiac muscle cell disorganization in the left ventricular wall of patients with hypertrophic cardiomyopathy. *Circulation* 1981;63: 882–894.

49. Shirani J, Pick R, Roberts WC, Maron BJ. Morphology and significance of the left ventricular collagen network in young patients with hypertrophic cardiomyopathy and sudden cardiac death. *J Am Coll Cardiol* 2000;35:36–44.

50. Spirito P, Bellone P, Harris KM, et al. Magnitude of left ventricular hypertrophy and risk of sudden death in hypertrophic cardiomyopathy. *N Engl J Med* 2000;342:1778–1785.

51. Varnava AM, Elliott PM, Baboonian C, et al. Hypertrophic cardiomyopathy: Histopathological features of sudden death in cardiac troponin T disease. *Circulation* 2001;104:1380–1384.

52. Varnava AM, Elliott PM, Mahon N, et al. Relation between myocyte disarray and outcome in hypertrophic cardiomyopathy. *Am J Cardiol* 2001;88:275–279.

53. Marian AJ, Roberts R. The molecular genetic basis for hypertrophic cardiomyopathy. *J Mol Cell Cardiol* 2001;33:655–670.

54. Watkins H, Thierfelder L, Hwang DS, et al. Sporadic hypertrophic cardiomyopathy due to de novo myosin mutations. *J Clin Invest* 1992; 90:1666–1671.

55. Watkins H, Anan R, Coviello DA, et al. A de novo mutation in alpha-tropomyosin that causes hypertrophic cardiomyopathy. *Circulation* 1995;91:2302–2305.

56. Jansen GA, Ofman R, Ferdinandusse S, et al. Refsum disease is caused by mutations in the phytanoyl-CoA hydroxylase gene. *Nat Genet* 1997;17:190–193.

57. Ashizawa T, Subramony SH. What is Kearns-Sayre syndrome after all? *Arch Neurol* 2001;58:1053–1054.

58. Korade-Mirnics Z, Babitzke P, Hoffman E. Myotonic dystrophy: Molecular windows on a complex etiology. *Nucleic Acids Res* 1998; 26:1363–1368.

59. Geisterfer-Lowrance AA, Kass S, Tanigawa G, et al. A molecular basis for familial hypertrophic cardiomyopathy: A beta cardiac myosin heavy chain gene missense mutation. *Cell* 1990;62:999–1006.

60. Thierfelder L, Watkins H, MacRae C, et al. Alpha-tropomyosin and cardiac troponin T mutations cause familial hypertrophic cardiomyopathy: a disease of the sarcomere. *Cell* 1994;77:701–712.

61. Watkins H, McKenna WJ, Thierfelder L, et al. Mutations in the genes for cardiac troponin T and alpha-tropomyosin in hypertrophic cardiomyopathy. *N Engl J Med* 1995;332:1058–1064.

62. Arad M, Seidman JG, Seidman CE. Phenotypic diversity in hypertrophic cardiomyopathy. *Hum Mol Genet* 2002;11:2499–2506.

63. Seidman CE. Hypertrophic cardiomyopathy: From man to mouse. *J Clin Invest* 2000;106:S9–S13.

64. Coviello DA, Maron BJ, Spirito P, et al. Clinical features of hypertrophic cardiomyopathy caused by mutation of a "hot spot" in the alpha-tropomyosin gene. *J Am Coll Cardiol* 1997;29:635–640.

65. Karibe A, Tobacman LS, Strand J, et al. Hypertrophic cardiomyopathy caused by a novel alpha-tropomyosin mutation (V95A) is associated with mild cardiac phenotype, abnormal calcium binding to troponin, abnormal myosin cycling, and poor prognosis. *Circulation* 2001;103: 65–71.

66. Hoffmann B, Schmidt-Traub H, Perrot A, et al. First mutation in cardiac troponin C, L29Q, in a patient with hypertrophic cardiomyopathy. *Hum Mutat* 2001;17:524.

67. Satoh M, Takahashi M, Sakamoto T, et al. Structural analysis of the titin gene in hypertrophic cardiomyopathy: Identification of a novel disease gene. *Biochem Biophys Res Commun* 1999;262:411–417.

68. Mogensen J, Klausen IC, Pedersen AK, et al. Alpha-cardiac actin is a novel disease gene in familial hypertrophic cardiomyopathy. *J Clin Invest* 1999;103:R39–R43.

69. Olson TM, Doan TP, Kishimoto NY, et al. Inherited and de novo mutations in the cardiac actin gene cause hypertrophic cardiomyopathy. *J Mol Cell Cardiol* 2000;32:1687–1694.

70. Poetter K, Jiang H , Hassanzadeh S, et al. Mutations in either the essential or regulatory light chains of myosin are associated with a rare myopathy in human heart and skeletal muscle. *Nat Genet* 1996;13:63–69.

71. Flavigny J, Richard P, Isnard R, et al. Identification of two novel mutations in the ventricular regulatory myosin light chain gene (MYL2) associated with familial and classical forms of hypertrophic cardiomyopathy. *J Mol Med* 1998;76:208–214.

72. Anan R, Greve G, Thierfelder L, et al. Prognostic implications of novel beta cardiac myosin heavy chain gene mutations that cause familial hypertrophic cardiomyopathy. *J Clin Invest* 1994;93:280–285.

73. Dausse E, Komajda M, Fetler L, et al. Familial hypertrophic cardiomyopathy. Microsatellite haplotyping and identification of a hot spot for mutations in the beta-myosin heavy chain gene. *J Clin Invest* 1993;92: 2807–2813.

74. Tesson F, Richard P, Charron P, et al. Genotype-phenotype analysis in four families with mutations in beta-myosin heavy chain gene responsible for familial hypertrophic cardiomyopathy. *Hum Mutat* 1998;12:385–392.

75. Nakajima-Taniguchi C, Matsui H, Eguchi N, et al. A novel deletion mutation in the beta-myosin heavy chain gene found in Japanese patients with hypertrophic cardiomyopathy. *J Mol Cell Cardiol* 1995; 27:2607–2612.

76. Marian AJ, Yu QT, Mares A Jr, et al. Detection of a new mutation in the beta-myosin heavy chain gene in an individual with hypertrophic cardiomyopathy. *J Clin Invest* 1992;90:2156–2165.

77. Cuda G, Perrotti N , Perticone F, Mattioli PL. A previously undescribed de novo insertion-deletion mutation in the beta myosin heavy chain gene in a kindred with familial hypertrophic cardiomyopathy. *Heart* 1996;76:451–452.

78. Niimura H, Bachinski LL, Sangwatanaroj S, et al. Mutations in the gene for cardiac myosin-binding protein C and late-onset familial hypertrophic cardiomyopathy. *N Engl J Med* 1998;338:1248–1257.

79. Erdmann J, Raible J, Maki-Abadi J, et al. Spectrum of clinical phenotypes and gene variants in cardiac myosin-binding protein C mutation carriers with hypertrophic cardiomyopathy. *J Am Coll Cardiol* 2001; 38:322–330.

80. Marian AJ. On genetic and phenotypic variability of hypertrophic cardiomyopathy: Nature versus nurture. *J Am Coll Cardiol* 2001;38: 331–334.

81. Seidman CE, Seidman JG. Molecular genetic studies of familial hypertrophic cardiomyopathy. *Basic Res Cardiol* 1998;93(suppl 3): 13–16.

82. Bonne G, Carrier L, Bercovici J, et al. Cardiac myosin binding protein-C gene splice acceptor site mutation is associated with familial hypertrophic cardiomyopathy. *Nat Genet* 1995;11:438–440.

83. Carrier L, Bonne G , Bahrend E, et al. Organization and sequence of human cardiac myosin binding protein C gene (MYBPC3) and identification of mutations predicted to produce truncated proteins in familial hypertrophic cardiomyopathy. *Circ Res* 1997;80: 427–434.

84. Watkins H, Conner D, Thierfelder L, et al. Mutations in the cardiac myosin binding protein-C gene on chromosome 11 cause familial hypertrophic cardiomyopathy. *Nat Genet* 1995;11:434–437.

85. Forissier JF, Carrier L, Farza H, et al. Codon 102 of the cardiac troponin T gene is a putative hot spot for mutations in familial hypertrophic cardiomyopathy. *Circulation* 1996;94:3069–3073.

86. Kimura A, Harada H, Park JE, et al. Mutations in the cardiac troponin I gene associated with hypertrophic cardiomyopathy. *Nat Genet* 1997; 16:379–382.

87. Kokado H, Shimizu M, Yoshio H, et al. Clinical features of hypertrophic cardiomyopathy caused by a Lys183 deletion mutation in the cardiac troponin I gene. *Circulation* 2000;102:663–669.

88. Lim DS, Roberts R, Marian AJ. Expression profiling of cardiac genes in human hypertrophic cardiomyopathy: insight into the pathogenesis of phenotypes. *J Am Coll Cardiol* 2001;38:1175–1180.

89. Hwang JJ, Allen PD, Tseng GC, et al. Microarray gene expression profiles in dilated and hypertrophic cardiomyopathic end-stage heart failure. *Physiol Genomics* 2002;10:31–44.

90. Maron BJ, Spirito P, Wesley Y, Arce J. Development and progression of left ventricular hypertrophy in children with hypertrophic cardiomyopathy. *N Engl J Med* 1986;315:610–614.

91. Marian AJ. Pathogenesis of diverse clinical and pathological phenotypes in hypertrophic cardiomyopathy. *Lancet* 2000;355:58–60.

92. Watkins H, Rosenzweig A, Hwang DS, et al. Characteristics and prognostic implications of myosin missense mutations in familial hypertrophic cardiomyopathy. *N Engl J Med* 1992;326:1108–1114.

93. Fananapazir L, Epstein ND. Genotype-phenotype correlations in hypertrophic cardiomyopathy. Insights provided by comparisons of

kindreds with distinct and identical beta-myosin heavy chain gene mutations. *Circulation* 1994;89:22–32.

94. Epstein ND, Cohn GM, Cyran F, Fananapazir L. Differences in clinical expression of hypertrophic cardiomyopathy associated with two distinct mutations in the beta-myosin heavy chain gene. A 908Leu–Val mutation and a 403Arg–Gln mutation. *Circulation* 1992;86:345–352.

95. Marian AJ, Mares A, Jr., Kelly DP, et al. Sudden cardiac death in hypertrophic cardiomyopathy. Variability in phenotypic expression of beta-myosin heavy chain mutations. *Eur Heart J* 1995;16:368–376.

96. Charron P, Dubourg O, Desnos M, et al. Clinical features and prognostic implications of familial hypertrophic cardiomyopathy related to the cardiac myosin-binding protein C gene. *Circulation* 1998;97:2230–2236.

97. Charron P, Dubourg O, Desnos M, et al. Genotype-phenotype correlations in familial hypertrophic cardiomyopathy. A comparison between mutations in the cardiac protein-C and the beta-myosin heavy chain genes. *Eur Heart J* 1998;19:139–145.

98. Marian AJ, Roberts R. Recent advances in the molecular genetics of hypertrophic cardiomyopathy. *Circulation* 1995;92:1336–1347.

99. Abchee A, Marian AJ. Prognostic significance of beta-myosin heavy chain mutations is reflective of their hypertrophic expressivity in patients with hypertrophic cardiomyopathy. *J Invest Med* 1997;45: 191–196.

100. Marian AJ. Modifier genes for hypertrophic cardiomyopathy. *Curr Opin Cardiol* 2001;17:242–252.

101. Ho CY, Lever HM, DeSanctis R, et al. Homozygous mutation in cardiac troponin T: Implications for hypertrophic cardiomyopathy. *Circulation* 2000;102:1950–1955.

102. Jeschke B, Uhl K, Weist B, et al. A high risk phenotype of hypertrophic cardiomyopathy associated with a compound genotype of two mutated beta-myosin heavy chain genes. *Hum Genet* 1998;102:299–304.

103. Semsarian C, Healey MJ, Fatkin D, et al. A polymorphic modifier gene alters the hypertrophic response in a murine model of familial hypertrophic cardiomyopathy. *J Mol Cell Cardiol* 2001;33:2055–2060.

104. Marian AJ, Yu QT, Workman R, et al. Angiotensin-converting enzyme polymorphism in hypertrophic cardiomyopathy and sudden cardiac death. *Lancet* 1993;342:1085–1086.

105. Yamazaki T, Komuro I, Yazaki Y. Role of the renin-angiotensin system in cardiac hypertrophy. *Am J Cardiol* 1999;83:53H–57H.

106. Rigat B, Hubert C, Alhenc-Gelas F, et al. An insertion/deletion polymorphism in the angiotensin I–converting enzyme gene accounting for half the variance of serum enzyme levels. *J Clin Invest* 1990;86: 1343–1346.

107. Lechin M, Quinones MA, Omran A, et al. Angiotensin–I converting enzyme genotypes and left ventricular hypertrophy in patients with hypertrophic cardiomyopathy. *Circulation* 1995;92:1808–1812.

108. Tesson F, Dufour C, Moolman JC, et al. The influence of the angiotensin I converting enzyme genotype in familial hypertrophic cardiomyopathy varies with the disease gene mutation. *J Mol Cell Cardiol* 1997;29:831–838.

109. Pfeufer A, Osterziel KJ, Urata H, et al. Angiotensin-converting enzyme and heart chymase gene polymorphisms in hypertrophic cardiomyopathy. *Am J Cardiol* 1996;78:362–364.

110. Yoneya K, Okamoto H, Machida M, et al. Angiotensin-converting enzyme gene polymorphism in Japanese patients with hypertrophic cardiomyopathy. *Am Heart J* 1995;130:1089–1093.

111. Yamada Y, Ichihara S, Fujimura T, Yokota M. Lack of association of polymorphisms of the angiotensin converting enzyme and angiotensinogen genes with nonfamilial hypertrophic or dilated cardiomyopathy. *Am J Hypertens* 1997;10:921–928.

112. Osterop AP, Kofflard MJ, Sandkuijl LA, et al. AT1 receptor A/C1166 polymorphism contributes to cardiac hypertrophy in subjects with hypertrophic cardiomyopathy. *Hypertension* 1998;32:825–830.

113. Brugada R, Kelsey W, Lechin M, et al. Role of candidate modifier genes on the phenotypic expression of hypertrophy in patients with hypertrophic cardiomyopathy. *J Invest Med* 1997;45:542–551.

114. Patel R, Lim DS, Reddy D, et al. Variants of trophic factors and expression of cardiac hypertrophy in patients with hypertrophic cardiomyopathy. *J Mol Cell Cardiol* 2000;32:2369–2377.

115. Yamada Y, Ichihara S, Izawa H, et al. Association of a G994 → T (Val279 → Phe) polymorphism of the plasma platelet-activating factor acetylhydrolase gene with myocardial damage in Japanese patients with nonfamilial hypertrophic cardiomyopathy. *J Hum Genet* 2001;46: 436–441.

116. Marian AJ. On genetics, inflammation, and abdominal aortic aneurysm: Can single nucleotide polymorphisms predict the outcome? *Circulation* 2001;103:2222–2224.

117. Geisterfer-Lowrance AA, Christe M, Conner DA, et al. A mouse model of familial hypertrophic cardiomyopathy. *Science* 1996;272:731–734.

118. Fatkin D, McConnell BK, Mudd JO, et al. An abnormal Ca²⁺ response in mutant sarcomere protein-mediated familial hypertrophic cardiomyopathy. *J Clin Invest* 2000;106:1351–1359.

119. Rottbauer W, Gautel M, Zehelein J, et al. Novel splice donor site mutation in the cardiac myosin-binding protein-C gene in familial hypertrophic cardiomyopathy. Characterization of cardiac transcript and protein. *J Clin Invest* 1997;100:475–482.

120. Tardiff JC, Factor SM, Tompkins BD, et al. A truncated cardiac troponin T molecule in transgenic mice suggests multiple cellular mechanisms for familial hypertrophic cardiomyopathy. *J Clin Invest* 1998;101:2800–2811.

121. Derchi G, Bellone P, Chiarella F, et al. Plasma levels of atrial natriuretic peptide in hypertrophic cardiomyopathy. *Am J Cardiol* 1992;70:1502–1504.

122. Hasegawa K, Fujiwara H, Doyama K, et al. Ventricular expression of brain natriuretic peptide in hypertrophic cardiomyopathy. *Circulation* 1993;88:372–380.

123. Hasegawa K, Fujiwara H, Koshiji M, et al. Endothelin-1 and its receptor in hypertrophic cardiomyopathy. *Hypertension* 1996;27:259–264.

124. Li RK, Li G, Mickle DA, et al. Overexpression of transforming growth factor-beta1 and insulin-like growth factor-I in patients with idiopathic hypertrophic cardiomyopathy. *Circulation* 1997;96:874–881.

125. Marian AJ. Hypertrophic cardiomyopathy. In: Rackel RE, ed. *Conn's Current Therapy*. Philadelphia: Saunders; 2000:286–287.

126. Lim DS, Lutucuta S, Bachireddy P, et al. Angiotensin II blockade reverses myocardial fibrosis in a transgenic mouse model of human hypertrophic cardiomyopathy. *Circulation* 2001;103:789–791.

127. Patel R, Nagueh SF, Tsybouleva N, et al. Simvastatin induces regression of cardiac hypertrophy and fibrosis and improves cardiac function in a transgenic rabbit model of human hypertrophic cardiomyopathy. *Circulation* 2001;104:317–324.

128. Oi S, Haneda T, Osaki J, et al. Lovastatin prevents angiotensin II–induced cardiac hypertrophy in cultured neonatal rat heart cells. *Eur J Pharmacol* 1999;376:139–148.

129. Park HJ, Galper JB. 3-Hydroxy-3-methylglutaryl CoA reductase inhibitors up-regulate transforming growth factor-beta signaling in cultured heart cells via inhibition of geranylgeranylation of RhoA GTPase. *Proc Natl Acad Sci USA* 1999;96:11525–11530.

130. Su SF, Hsiao CL, Chu CW, et al. Effects of pravastatin on left ventricular mass in patients with hyperlipidemia and essential hypertension. *Am J Cardiol* 2000;86:514–518.

131. Mestroni L, Rocco C, Gregori D, et al. Familial dilated cardiomyopathy: Evidence for genetic and phenotypic heterogeneity. Heart Muscle Disease Study Group. *J Am Coll Cardiol* 1999;34:181–190.

132. Kasper EK, Agema WR, Hutchins GM, et al. The causes of dilated cardiomyopathy: A clinicopathologic review of 673 consecutive patients. *J Am Coll Cardiol* 1994;23:586–590.

133. Finsterer J, Stollberger C. The heart in human dystrophinopathies. *Cardiology* 2003;99:1–19.

134. D'Adamo P, Fassone L, Gedeon A, et al. The X-linked gene G4.5 is responsible for different infantile dilated cardiomyopathies. *Am J Hum Genet* 1997;61:862–867.

135. Kamisago M, Sharma SD, DePalma SR, et al. Mutations in sarcomere protein genes as a cause of dilated cardiomyopathy. *N Engl J Med* 2000;343:1688–1696.

136. Olson TM, Michels VV, Thibodeau SN, et al. Actin mutations in dilated cardiomyopathy, a heritable form of heart failure. *Science* 1998; 280:750–752.

137. Kamisago M, Sharma SD, DePalma SR, et al. Mutations in sarcomere protein genes as a cause of dilated cardiomyopathy. *N Engl J Med* 2000;343:1688–1696.

138. Tsubata S, Bowles KR, Vatta M, et al. Mutations in the human delta-sarcoglycan gene in familial and sporadic dilated cardiomyopathy. *J Clin Invest* 2000;106:655–662.

139. Barresi R, Di Blasi C, Negri T, et al. Disruption of heart sarcoglycan complex and severe cardiomyopathy caused by beta sarcoglycan mutations. *J Med Genet* 2000;37:102–107.

140. Olson TM, Illenberger S, Kishimoto NY, et al. Metavinculin mutations alter actin interaction in dilated cardiomyopathy. *Circulation* 2002; 105:431–437.

141. Arbustini E, Diegoli M, Morbini P, et al. Prevalence and characteristics of dystrophin defects in adult male patients with dilated cardiomyopathy. *J Am Coll Cardiol* 2000;35:1760–1768.

142. Fatkin D, MacRae C, Sasaki T, et al. Missense mutations in the rod domain of the lamin A/C gene as causes of dilated cardiomyopathy and conduction-system disease. *N Engl J Med* 1999;341:1715–1724.

143. Bonne G, Di Barletta MR, Varnous S, et al. Mutations in the gene encoding lamin A/C cause autosomal dominant Emery-Dreifuss muscular dystrophy. *Nat Genet* 1999;21:285–288.

144. Li D, Tapscoft T, Gonzalez O, et al. Desmin mutation responsible for idiopathic dilated cardiomyopathy. *Circulation* 1999;100:461–464.

145. Perng MD, Muchowski PJ, van Den IJ, et al. The cardiomyopathy and lens cataract mutation in alphaB-crystallin alters its protein structure, chaperone activity, and interaction with intermediate filaments in vitro. *J Biol Chem* 1999;274:33235–33243.

146. Malhotra SB, Hart KA, Klamut HJ, et al. Frame-shift deletions in patients with Duchenne and Becker muscular dystrophy. *Science* 1988;242:755–759.

147. Muntoni F, Wilson L, Marrosu G, et al. A mutation in the dystrophin gene selectively affecting dystrophin expression in the heart. *J Clin Invest* 1995;96:693–699.

148. Bione S, Maestrini E, Rivella S, et al. Identification of a novel X-linked gene responsible for Emery-Dreifuss muscular dystrophy. *Nat Genet* 1994;8:323–327.

149. Suzuki M, Carlson KM, Marchuk DA, Rockman HA. Genetic modifier loci affecting survival and cardiac function in murine dilated cardiomyopathy. *Circulation* 2002;105:1824–1829.

150. Bonne G, Mercuri E, Muchir A, et al. Clinical and molecular genetic spectrum of autosomal dominant Emery-Dreifuss muscular dystrophy due to mutations of the lamin A/C gene. *Ann Neurol* 2000;48: 170–180.

151. Dalakas MC, Park KY, Semino-Mora C, et al. Desmin myopathy, a skeletal myopathy with cardiomyopathy caused by mutations in the desmin gene. *N Engl J Med* 2000;342:770–780.

152. Phillips MF, Harper PS. Cardiac disease in myotonic dystrophy. *Cardiovasc Res* 1997;33:13–22.

153. Bit-Avragim N, Perrot A, Schols L, et al. The GAA repeat expansion in intron 1 of the frataxin gene is related to the severity of cardiac manifestation in patients with Friedreich's ataxia. *J Mol Med* 2001; 78:626–632.

154. Bova MP, Yaron O, Huang Q, et al. Mutation R120G in alphaB-crystallin, which is linked to a desmin-related myopathy, results in an irregular structure and defective chaperone-like function. *Proc Natl Acad Sci USA* 1999;96:6137–6142.

155. Cummings CJ, Zoghbi HY. Trinucleotide repeats: Mechanisms and pathophysiology. *Annu Rev Genomics Hum Genet* 2000;1:281–328.

156. Corrado D, Fontaine G, Marcus FI, et al. Arrhythmogenic right ventricular dysplasia/cardiomyopathy: Need for an international registry. Study Group on Arrhythmogenic Right Ventricular Dysplasia/Cardiomyopathy of the Working Groups on Myocardial and Pericardial Disease and Arrhythmias of the European Society of Cardiology and of the Scientific Council on Cardiomyopathies of the World Heart Federation. *Circulation* 2000;101:E101–E106.

157. Corrado D, Basso C, Thiene G, et al. Spectrum of clinicopathologic manifestations of arrhythmogenic right ventricular cardiomyopathy/dysplasia: A multicenter study . *J Am Coll Cardiol* 1997;30:1512–1520.

158. McKoy G, Protonotarios N, Crosby A, et al. Identification of a deletion in plakoglobin in arrhythmogenic right ventricular cardiomyopathy with palmoplantar keratoderma and woolly hair (Naxos disease). *Lancet* 2000;355:2119–2124.

159. Tiso N, Stephan DA, Nava A, et al. Identification of mutations in the cardiac ryanodine receptor gene in families affected with arrhythmogenic right ventricular cardiomyopathy type 2 (ARVD2). *Hum Mol Genet* 2001;10:189–194.

160. Rampazzo A, Nava A, Malacrida S, et al. Mutation in human desmoplakin domain binding to plakoglobin causes a dominant form of arrhythmogenic right ventricular cardiomyopathy. *Am J Hum Genet* 2002;71:1200–1206.

161. Priori SG, Napolitano C, Tiso N, et al. Mutations in the cardiac ryanodine receptor gene (hRyR2) underlie catecholaminergic polymorphic ventricular tachycardia. *Circulation* 2001;103:196–200.

162. Marx SO, Reiken S, Hisamatsu Y, et al. PKA phosphorylation dissociates FKBP12.6 from the calcium release channel (ryanodine receptor): Defective regulation in failing hearts. *Cell* 2000;101: 365–376.

163. Tiso N, Salamon M, Bagattin A, et al. The binding of the RyR2 calcium channel to its gating protein FKBP12.6 is oppositely affected by ARVD2 and VTSIP mutations. *Biochem Biophys Res Commun* 2002;299:594–598.

164. Kushwaha SS, Fallon JT, Fuster V. Restrictive cardiomyopathy. *N Engl J Med* 1997;336:267–276.

165. Arbustini E, Morbini P, Grasso M, et al. Restrictive cardiomyopathy, atrioventricular block and mild to subclinical myopathy in patients with desmin-immunoreactive material deposits. *J Am Coll Cardiol* 1998;31:645–653.

166. Fitzpatrick AP, Shapiro LM, Rickards AF, Poole-Wilson PA. Familial restrictive cardiomyopathy with atrioventricular block and skeletal myopathy. *Br Heart J* 1990;63:114–118.

167. Aroney C, Bett N, Radford D. Familial restrictive cardiomyopathy. *Aust N Z J Med* 1988;18:877–878.

168. Zhang J, Kumar A, Stalker HJ, et al. Clinical and molecular studies of a large family with desmin-associated restrictive cardiomyopathy. *Clin Genet* 2001;59:248–256.

169. Zachara E, Bertini E, Lioy E, et al. Restrictive cardiomyopathy due to desmin accumulation in a family with evidence of autosomal dominant inheritance. *G Ital Cardiol* 1997;27:436–442.

170. Cooke RA, Chambers JB, Curry PV. Noonan's cardiomyopathy: A non-hypertrophic variant. *Br Heart J* 1994;71:561–565.

171. Marian AJ. *Genetics for Cardiologists*. London: Remedica Publishing; 2000:1–53.

172. Mahadevan M, Tsilfidis C, Sabourin L, et al. Myotonic dystrophy mutation: an unstable CTG repeat in the 3′ untranslated region of the gene. *Science* 1992;255:1253–1255.

173. Brook JD, McCurrach ME, Harley HG, et al. Molecular basis of myotonic dystrophy: Expansion of a trinucleotide (CTG) repeat at the 3′ end of a transcript encoding a protein kinase family member. *Cell* 1992;68:799–808.

174. Fu YH, Pizzuti A, Fenwick RG Jr, et al. An unstable triplet repeat in a gene related to myotonic muscular dystrophy. *Science* 1992;255: 1256–1258.

175. Groh WJ, Lowe MR, Zipes DP. Severity of cardiac conduction involvement and arrhythmias in myotonic dystrophy type 1 correlates with age and CTG repeat length. *J Cardiovasc Electrophysiol* 2002;13: 444–448.

176. Timchenko LT, Miller JW, Timchenko NA, et al. Identification of a (CUG)n triplet repeat RNA-binding protein and its expression in myotonic dystrophy. *Nucleic Acids Res* 1996;24:4407–4414.

177. Philips AV, Timchenko LT, Cooper TA. Disruption of splicing regulated by a CUG-binding protein in myotonic dystrophy. *Science* 1998;280:737–741.

178. Larkin K, Fardaei M. Myotonic dystrophy—A multigene disorder. *Brain Res Bull* 2001;56:389–395.

179. Palau F. Friedreich's ataxia and frataxin: Molecular genetics, evolution and pathogenesis. *Int J Mol Med* 2001;7:581–589.

180. Raben N, Plotz P, Byrne BJ. Acid alpha-glucosidase deficiency (glycogenosis type II, Pompe disease). *Curr Mol Med* 2002;2:145–166.

181. Raben N, Plotz P, Byrne BJ. Acid alpha-glucosidase deficiency (glycogenosis type II, Pompe disease). *Curr Mol Med* 2002;2: 145–166.

182. Amalfitano A, McVie-Wylie AJ, Hu H, et al. Systemic correction of the muscle disorder glycogen storage disease type II after hepatic targeting of a modified adenovirus vector encoding human acid-alpha-glucosidase. *Proc Natl Acad Sci USA* 1999;96:8861–8866.

183. Gollob MH, Green MS, Tang AS, et al. Identification of a gene responsible for familial Wolff-Parkinson-White syndrome. *N Engl J Med* 2001;344:1823–1831.

184. Blair E, Redwood C, Ashrafian H, et al. Mutations in the gamma(2) subunit of AMP-activated protein kinase cause familial hypertrophic cardiomyopathy: Evidence for the central role of energy compromise in disease pathogenesis. *Hum Mol Genet* 2001;10:1215–1220.

185. Gollob MH, Seger JJ, Gollob TN, et al. Novel PRKAG2 mutation responsible for the genetic syndrome of ventricular preexcitation and conduction system disease with childhood onset and absence of cardiac hypertrophy. *Circulation* 2001;104:3030–3033.

186. Arad M, Benson DW, Perez-Atayde AR, et al. Constitutively active AMP kinase mutations cause glycogen storage disease mimicking hypertrophic cardiomyopathy. *J Clin Invest* 2002;109:357–362.

187. Wierzbicki AS, Lloyd MD, Schofield CJ, et al. Refsum's disease: A peroxisomal disorder affecting phytanic acid alpha-oxidation. *J Neurochem* 2002;80:727–735.

188. Mihalik SJ, Morrell JC, Kim D, et al. Identification of PAHX, a Refsum disease gene. *Nat Genet* 1997;17:185–189.

189. Guertl B, Noehammer C, Hoefler G. Metabolic cardiomyopathies. *Int J Exp Pathol* 2000;81:349–372.

190. Simon DK, Johns DR. Mitochondrial disorders: Clinical and genetic features. *Annu Rev Med* 1999;50:111–127.

191. Williams RS. Canaries in the coal mine: Mitochondrial DNA and vascular injury from reactive oxygen species. *Circ Res* 2000;86: 915–916.

192. Kelly DP, Strauss AW. Inherited cardiomyopathies. *N Engl J Med* 1994;330:913–919.

193. Roden DM, Lazzara R, Rosen M, et al. Multiple mechanisms in the long-QT syndrome. Current knowledge, gaps, and future directions. The SADS Foundation Task Force on LQTS. *Circulation* 1996;94: 1996–2012.

194. Brugada R, Roberts R. Brugada syndrome: Why are there multiple answers to a simple question? *Circulation* 2001;104:3017–3019.

195. George AL, Jr., Varkony TA, Drabkin HA, et al. Assignment of the human heart tetrodotoxin-resistant voltage-gated Na$^+$ channel alpha-subunit gene (SCN5A) to band 3p21. *Cytogenet Cell Genet* 1995;68:67–70.

196. Wang Q, Shen J, Splawski I, et al. SCN5A mutations associated with an inherited cardiac arrhythmia, long QT syndrome. *Cell* 1995;80:805–811.

197. Chen Q, Kirsch GE, Zhang D, et al. Genetic basis and molecular mechanism for idiopathic ventricular fibrillation. *Nature* 1998;392: 293–296.

198. Schott JJ, Alshinawi C, Kyndt F, et al. Cardiac conduction defects associate with mutations in SCN5A. *Nat Genet* 1999;23:20–21.

199. Priori SG, Napolitano C, Giordano U, et al. Brugada syndrome and sudden cardiac death in children. *Lancet* 2000;355:808–809.

200. Vatta M, Dumaine R, Varghese G, et al. Genetic and biophysical basis of sudden unexplained nocturnal death syndrome (SUNDS), a disease allelic to Brugada syndrome. *Hum Mol Genet* 2002;11:337–345.

201. Brugada P, Brugada J. Right bundle branch block, persistent ST-segment elevation and sudden cardiac death: A distinct clinical and electrocardiographic syndrome. A multicenter report. *J Am Coll Cardiol* 1992;20:1391–1396.

202. Brugada J, Brugada R, Brugada P. Right bundle-branch block and ST-segment elevation in leads V1 through V3: A marker for sudden death in patients without demonstrable structural heart disease. *Circulation* 1998;97:457–460.

203. Nademanee K, Veerakul G, Nimmannit S, et al. Arrhythmogenic marker for the sudden unexplained death syndrome in Thai men. *Circulation* 1997;96:2595–2600.

204. Antzelevitch C. The Brugada syndrome. *J Cardiovasc Electrophysiol* 1998;9:513–516.

205. Brugada R, Brugada J, Antzelevitch C, et al. Sodium channel blockers identify risk for sudden death in patients with ST-segment elevation and right bundle branch block but structurally normal hearts. *Circulation* 2000;101:510–515.

206. Weiss R, Barmada MM, Nguyen T, et al. Clinical and molecular heterogeneity in the Brugada syndrome: a novel gene locus on chromosome 3. *Circulation* 2002;105:707–713.

207. Bezzina C, Veldkamp MW, van Den Berg MP, et al. A single Na⁺ channel mutation causing both long-QT and Brugada syndromes. *Circ Res* 1999;85:1206–1213.

208. Kyndt F, Probst V, Potet F, et al. Novel SCN5A mutation leading either to isolated cardiac conduction defect or Brugada syndrome in a large French family. *Circulation* 2001;104:3081–3086.

209. Bezzina CR, Rook MB, Groenewegen WA, et al. Compound heterozygosity for mutations (W156X and R225W) in SCN5A associated with severe cardiac conduction disturbances and degenerative changes in the conduction system. *Circ Res* 2003;92:159–168.

210. Dumaine R, Towbin JA, Brugada P, et al. Ionic mechanisms responsible for the electrocardiographic phenotype of the Brugada syndrome are temperature dependent. *Circ Res* 1999;85:803–809.

211. Smits JP, Eckardt L, Probst V, et al. Genotype-phenotype relationship in Brugada syndrome: Electrocardiographic features differentiate SCN5A-related patients from non-SCN5A-related patients. *J Am Coll Cardiol* 2002;40:350–356.

212. Keating M, Atkinson D, Dunn C, et al. Linkage of a cardiac arrhythmia, the long QT syndrome, and the Harvey ras-1 gene. *Science* 1991;252:704–706.

213. Barhanin J, Lesage F, Guillemare E, et al. K(V)LQT1 and lsK (minK) proteins associate to form the I(Ks) cardiac potassium current. *Nature* 1996;384:78–80.

214. Sanguinetti MC, Jiang C, Curran ME, Keating MT. A mechanistic link between an inherited and an acquired cardiac arrhythmia: HERG encodes the IKr potassium channel. *Cell* 1995;81:299–307.

215. Schott JJ, Charpentier F, Peltier S, et al. Mapping of a gene for long QT syndrome to chromosome 4q25-27. *Am J Hum Genet* 1995;57:1114–1122.

216. Mohler PJ, Schott JJ, Gramolini AO, et al. Ankyrin-B mutation causes type 4 long-QT cardiac arrhythmia and sudden cardiac death. *Nature* 2003;421:634–639.

217. Abbott GW, Sesti F, Splawski I, et al. MiRP1 forms IKr potassium channels with HERG and is associated with cardiac arrhythmia. *Cell* 1999;97:175–187.

218. Plaster NM, Tawil R, Tristani-Firouzi M, et al. Mutations in Kir2.1 cause the developmental and episodic electrical phenotypes of Andersen's syndrome. *Cell* 2001;105:511–519.

219. Neyroud N, Tesson F, Denjoy I, et al. A novel mutation in the potassium channel gene KVLQT1 causes the Jervell and Lange-Nielsen cardioauditory syndrome. *Nat Genet* 1997;15:186–189.

220. Schwartz PJ, Priori SG, Spazzolini C, et al. Genotype-phenotype correlation in the long-QT syndrome: Gene-specific triggers for life-threatening arrhythmias. *Circulation* 2001;103:89–95.

221. Zareba W, Moss AJ, Schwartz PJ, et al. Influence of genotype on the clinical course of the long-QT syndrome. International Long-QT Syndrome Registry Research Group. *N Engl J Med* 1998;339:960–965.

222. Roden DM. Pharmacogenetics and drug-induced arrhythmias. *Cardiovasc Res* 2001;50:224–231.

223. Camm AJ, Janse MJ, Roden DM, et al. Congenital and acquired long QT syndrome. *Eur Heart J* 2000;21:1232–1237.

224. Splawski I, Timothy KW, Tateyama M, et al. Variant of SCN5A sodium channel implicated in risk of cardiac arrhythmia. *Science* 2002;297:1333–1336.

225. Probst V, Kyndt F, Potet F, et al. Haploinsufficiency in combination with aging causes SCN5A-linked hereditary Lenegre disease. *J Am Coll Cardiol* 2003;41:643–652.

226. Laitinen PJ, Brown KM, Piippo K, et al. Mutations of the cardiac ryanodine receptor (RyR2) gene in familial polymorphic ventricular tachycardia. *Circulation* 2001;103:485–490.

227. Lahat H, Pras E, Olender T, et al. A missense mutation in a highly conserved region of CASQ2 is associated with autosomal recessive catecholamine-induced polymorphic ventricular tachycardia in Bedouin families from Israel. *Am J Hum Genet* 2001;69:1378–1384.

228. Brugada R, Tapscott T, Czernuszewicz GZ, et al. Identification of a genetic locus for familial atrial fibrillation. *N Engl J Med* 1997;336:905–911.

229. Chen YH, Xu SJ, Bendahhou S, et al. KCNQ1 gain-of-function mutation in familial atrial fibrillation. *Science* 2003;299:251–254.

230. Lerman BB, Dong B, Stein KM, et al. Right ventricular outflow tract tachycardia due to a somatic cell mutation in G protein subunitalphai2. *J Clin Invest* 1998;101:2862–2868.

231. Nikoskelainen EK, Savontaus ML, Huoponen K, et al. Pre-excitation syndrome in Leber's hereditary optic neuropathy. *Lancet* 1994;344:857–858.

232. Abdelmalek NF, Gerber TL, Menter A. Cardiocutaneous syndromes and associations. *J Am Acad Dermatol* 2002;46:161–183.

233. Dietz HC, Cutting GR, Pyeritz RE, et al. Marfan syndrome caused by a recurrent de novo missense mutation in the fibrillin gene. *Nature* 1991;352:337–339.

234. Collod-Beroud G, Boileau C. Marfan syndrome in the third millennium. *Eur J Hum Genet* 2002;10:673–681.

235. Robinson PN, Booms P, Katzke S, et al. Mutations of FBN1 and genotype-phenotype correlations in Marfan syndrome and related fibrillinopathies. *Hum Mutat* 2002;20:153–161.

236. Putnam EA, Zhang H, Ramirez F, Milewicz DM. Fibrillin-2 (FBN2) mutations result in the Marfan-like disorder, congenital contractural arachnodactyly. *Nat Genet* 1995;11:456–458.

237. Superti-Furga A, Gugler E, Gitzelmann R, Steinmann B. Ehlers-Danlos syndrome type IV: A multi-exon deletion in one of the two COL3A1 alleles affecting structure, stability, and processing of type III procollagen. *J Biol Chem* 1988;263:6226–6232.

238. Tassabehji M, Metcalfe K, Hurst J, et al. An elastin gene mutation producing abnormal tropoelastin and abnormal elastic fibres in a patient with autosomal dominant cutis laxa. *Hum Mol Genet* 1998;7:1021–1028.

239. Loeys B, Van Maldergem L, Mortier G, et al. Homozygosity for a missense mutation in fibulin-5 (FBLN5) results in a severe form of cutis laxa. *Hum Mol Genet* 2002;11:2113–2118.

240. Bergen AA, Plomp AS, Schuurman EJ, et al. Mutations in ABCC6 cause pseudoxanthoma elasticum. *Nat Genet* 2000;25:228–231.

241. Edwards MJ, Wenstrup RJ, Byers PH, Cohn DH. Recurrence of lethal osteogenesis imperfecta due to parental mosaicism for a mutation in the COL1A2 gene of type I collagen. The mosaic parent exhibits phenotypic features of a mild form of the disease. *Hum Mutat* 1992;1:47–54.

242. Newman JH, Wheeler L, Lane KB, et al. Mutation in the gene for bone morphogenetic protein receptor II as a cause of primary pulmonary hypertension in a large kindred. *N Engl J Med* 2001;345:319–324.

243. Newman JH, Wheeler L, Lane KB, et al. Mutation in the gene for bone morphogenetic protein receptor II as a cause of primary pulmonary hypertension in a large kindred. *N Engl J Med* 2001;345:319–324.

244. Machado RD, Pauciulo MW, Thomson JR, et al. BMPR2 haploinsufficiency as the inherited molecular mechanism for primary pulmonary hypertension. *Am J Hum Genet* 2001;68:92–102.

245. Lane KB, Machado RD, Pauciulo MW, et al. Heterozygous germline mutations in BMPR2, encoding a TGF-beta receptor, cause familial primary pulmonary hypertension. The International PPH Consortium. *Nat Genet* 2000;26:81–84.

246. Loscalzo J. Genetic clues to the cause of primary pulmonary hypertension. *N Engl J Med* 2001;345:367–371.

247. Trembath RC, Thomson JR, Machado RD, et al. Clinical and molecular genetic features of pulmonary hypertension in patients with hereditary hemorrhagic telangiectasia. *N Engl J Med* 2001;345:325–334.

248. Eddahibi S, Humbert M, Fadel E, et al. Serotonin transporter overexpression is responsible for pulmonary artery smooth muscle hyperplasia in primary pulmonary hypertension. *J Clin Invest* 2001;108:1141–1150.

249. Rabinovitch M. Linking a serotonin transporter polymorphism to vascular smooth muscle proliferation in patients with primary pulmonary hypertension. *J Clin Invest* 2001;108:1109–1111.

250. Rudarakanchana N, Flanagan JA, Chen H, et al. Functional analysis of bone morphogenetic protein type II receptor mutations underlying primary pulmonary hypertension. *Hum Mol Genet* 2002;11:1517–1525.

251. Marian AJ. Genetic markers: genes involved in atherosclerosis. *J Cardiovasc Risk* 1997;4:333–339.

252. Goldstein JL, Sobhani MK, Faust JR, Brown MS. Heterozygous familial hypercholesterolemia: Failure of normal allele to compensate for mutant allele at a regulated genetic locus. *Cell* 1976;9:195–203.

253. Soutar AK. Update on low density lipoprotein receptor mutations. *Curr Opin Lipidol* 1998;9:141–147.

254. Jansen AC, van Wissen S, Defesche JC, Kastelein JJ. Phenotypic variability in familial hypercholesterolaemia: An update. *Curr Opin Lipidol* 2002;13:165–171.

255. Rauh G, Keller C, Kormann B, al. Familial defective apolipoprotein B100: Clinical characteristics of 54 cases. *Atherosclerosis* 1992;92: 233–241.

256. Vrablik M, Ceska R, Horinek A. Major apolipoprotein B-100 mutations in lipoprotein metabolism and atherosclerosis. *Physiol Res* 2001;50:337–343.

257. Gregg RE, Wetterau JR. The molecular basis of abetalipoproteinemia. *Curr Opin Lipidol* 1994;5:81–86.

258. Narcisi TM, Shoulders CC, Chester SA, et al. Mutations of the microsomal triglyceride-transfer-protein gene in abetalipoproteinemia. *Am J Hum Genet* 1995;57:1298–1310.

259. Funke H, von Eckardstein A, Pritchard PH, et al. A molecular defect causing fish eye disease: an amino acid exchange in lecithin-cholesterol acyltransferase (LCAT) leads to the selective loss of alpha-LCAT activity. *Proc Natl Acad Sci USA* 1991;88:4855–4859.

260. Tall AR, Wang N. Tangier disease as a test of the reverse cholesterol transport hypothesis. *J Clin Invest* 2000;106:1205–1207.

261. Bodzioch M, Orso E, Klucken J, et al. The gene encoding ATP-binding cassette transporter 1 is mutated in Tangier disease. *Nat Genet* 1999; 22:347–351.

262. Brooks-Wilson A, Marcil M, Clee SM, et al. Mutations in ABC1 in Tangier disease and familial high-density lipoprotein deficiency. *Nat Genet* 1999;22:336–345.

263. Rust S, Rosier M, Funke H, et al. Tangier disease is caused by mutations in the gene encoding ATP-binding cassette transporter 1. *Nat Genet* 1999;22:352–355.

264. Remaley AT, Rust S, Rosier M, et al. Human ATP-binding cassette transporter 1 (ABC1): genomic organization and identification of the genetic defect in the original Tangier disease kindred. *Proc Natl Acad Sci USA* 1999;96:12685–12690.

265. Lutucuta S, Ballantyne CM, Elghannam H, et al. Novel polymorphisms in promoter region of ATP-binding cassette transporter gene and plasma lipids, severity, progression, and regression of coronary atherosclerosis and response to therapy. *Circ Res* 2001;88:969–973.

266. Brousseau ME, Bodzioch M, Schaefer EJ, et al. Common variants in the gene encoding ATP-binding cassette transporter 1 in men with low HDL cholesterol levels and coronary heart disease. *Atherosclerosis* 2001;154:607–611.

267. Jeunemaitre X, Soubrier F, Kotelevtsev YV, et al. Molecular basis of human hypertension: Role of angiotensinogen. *Cell* 1992;71:169–180.

268. Luft FC. Hypertension as a complex genetic trait. *Semin Nephrol* 2002;22:115–126.

269. Lifton RP, Gharavi AG, Geller DS. Molecular mechanisms of human hypertension. *Cell* 2001;104:545–556.

270. Toka HR, Luft FC. Monogenic forms of human hypertension. *Semin Nephrol* 2002;22:81–88.

271. Pascoe L, Curnow KM, Slutsker L, et al. Glucocorticoid-suppressible hyperaldosteronism results from hybrid genes created by unequal crossovers between CYP11B1 and CYP11B2. *Proc Natl Acad Sci USA* 1992;89:8327–8331.

272. Mune T, Rogerson FM, Nikkila H, et al. Human hypertension caused by mutations in the kidney isozyme of 11 beta-hydroxysteroid dehydrogenase. *Nat Genet* 1995;10:394–399.

273. Li A, Tedde R, Krozowski ZS, et al. Molecular basis for hypertension in the "type II variant" of apparent mineralocorticoid excess. *Am J Hum Genet* 1998;63:370–379.

274. Scheinman SJ, Guay-Woodford LM, Thakker RV, et al. Genetic disorders of renal electrolyte transport. *N Engl J Med* 1999;340:1177–1187.

275. Wilson FH, Disse-Nicodeme S, Choate KA, et al. Human hypertension caused by mutations in WNK kinases. *Science* 2001;293:1107–1112.

THE PATHOLOGY, PATHOPHYSIOLOGY, RECOGNITION, AND TREATMENT OF CONGENITAL HEART DISEASE

David R. Fulton / Michael D. Freed

INCIDENCE AND ETIOLOGY

The incidence of congenital heart disease in the United States is approximately 8 per 1000 live births.[1,2] Many infants who are born alive with cardiac defects have anomalies that do not represent a threat to life, at least during infancy. Almost one-third of those infants, or 2.6 per 1000 live births, however, have critical disease, which is defined as a malformation severe enough to result in cardiac catheterization, cardiac surgery, or death within the first year of life.[3] Today, with early detection and proper management, the majority of infants with critical disease can be expected to survive the first year of life.[3] Most who now survive infancy will join the increasingly large cohort of adults with congenital heart disease.

Estimates of the incidence of specific lesions vary, depending on whether the data are drawn from infants or older children and whether the diagnosis is based on clinical, echocardiographic, catheterization, surgical, or postmortem studies.[1–4] The incidence in other countries is remarkably similar to that reported for the United States.[5,6] Despite these differences in case material, except for bicuspid aortic valve and mitral valve prolapse, it is apparent that ventricular septal defect (VSD) is the most common malformation, occurring in 28 percent of all patients with congenital heart disease (Table 73-1).

Among 2251 infants with critical congenital heart disease in the New England Regional Infant Cardiac Program,[3] 53.7 percent were male. Certain defects, however, are considerably more common in

TABLE 73-1 Incidence of Specific Congenital Heart Defects

Defect	Percentage of Cases[a] Averaged
Ventricular septal defect	28.3
Pulmonary stenosis	9.5
Patent ductus arteriosus	8.7
Ventricular septal defect with pulmonary stenosis[b]	6.8
Atrial septal defect, secundum	6.7
Aortic stenosis	4.4
Coarctation of aorta	4.2
Atrioventricular canal[c]	3.5
Transposition of great arteries	3.4
Aortic atresia	2.4
Truncus arteriosus	1.6
Tricuspid atresia	1.2
Total anomalous pulmonary venous connection	1.1
Double-outlet right ventricle	0.8
Pulmonary atresia without ventricular septal defect	0.3

[a]Total number of cases = 103,590.
[b]Includes tetralogy of Fallot.
[c]Includes partial and complete.
SOURCE: References 1–3, 5, 6.

one sex than in the other. Aortic stenosis occurs more commonly in boys (4:1), and atrial septal defects (ASDs) occur more frequently in girls (2.5:1).

Although earlier theories concerning the etiology of congenital heart diseases suggested that most defects were multifactorial—that is, the malformations are caused by a combination of a hereditary predisposition (presumably caused by abnormalities in the genetic code) and an environmental trigger[7]—more recent advances in molecular biology suggest that a much higher percentage are caused by point mutations.[8]

Some abnormalities are caused by chromosomal aberrations (see Chap. 62). Trisomy 21 (Down's syndrome) is highly associated with complete atrioventricular (AV) canal, VSDs, and tetralogy of Fallot, and children with Turner's syndrome (XO chromosome) frequently have coarctation of the aorta. Other anomalies are caused by teratogens: VSD in fetal alcohol syndrome, Ebstein's anomaly in a fetus with prenatal exposure to lithium, and patent ductus arteriosus (PDA) in mothers who contracted rubella during the first trimester are examples.

Some syndromes are inherited as single-gene defects and have congenital heart disease as one of their manifestations. Holt-Oram syndrome, an association of radial limb abnormalities and ASDs, is caused by an abnormality of a T-box transcription factor Tbx5, and the cardiofacial syndrome, associated with abnormalities of the conotruncus, resulting in a high proportion of infants born with truncus arteriosus or interrupted aortic arch, is a result of a deletion on chromosome 22 (22 q 11).[9]

It is clear now that a higher proportion of congenital heart disease than previously thought is due to single-gene defects and that the same malformation may be caused by mutant genes at different loci.[8] With increasing knowledge of molecular mechanisms, it seems inevitable that the etiology and pathogenesis of congenital heart disease will be clarified increasingly in the years ahead.

FETAL CIRCULATION AND THE TRANSITION TO NEONATAL AND ADULT CIRCULATION

The fetus obtains all metabolic necessities, including oxygen, from the placenta. The fetal circulation is an adaptation to allow most of the right ventricular output to bypass the lungs and instead to perfuse the placenta. Most of the understanding of this adaptation comes from more than 40 years of research,[10–18] primarily on fetal lambs. The fetal circulation is arranged in parallel fashion rather than in series, with mixing at the atrial (foramen ovale) and great vessel (ductus arteriosus) levels (Fig. 73-1). Normally, systemic venous blood

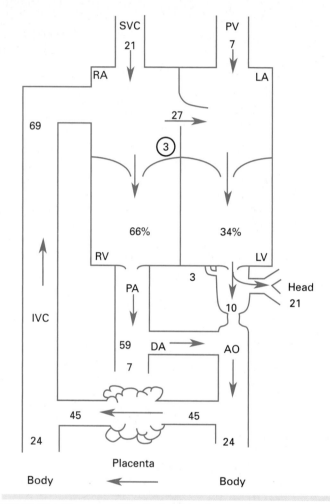

FIGURE 73-1 The course of the circulation in a late-gestation fetal lamb. *The numbers represent the percentage of combined ventricular output.* Some of the return from the inferior vena cava (IVC) is diverted by the crista dividens in the right atrium (RA) through the foramen ovale into the left atrium (LA), where it meets the pulmonary venous return (PV), passes into the left ventricle (LV), and is pumped into the ascending aorta. Most of the ascending aortic flow goes to the coronary, subclavian, and carotid arteries, with only 10 percent of combined ventricular output passing through the aortic arch (indicated by the narrowed point in the aorta) into the descending aorta (AO). The remainder of the inferior vena cava flow mixes with the return from the superior vena cava (SVC) and coronary veins, passes into the right atrium and right ventricle (RV), and is pumped into the pulmonary artery (PA). Because of the high pulmonary resistance, only 7 percent passes through the lungs (PV), with the rest going into the ductus arteriosus (DA) and then to the *descending aorta (AO),* the placenta, and the lower half of the body. (From Freed MD. Fetal and transitional circulation. In: Fyler DC, ed. *Nadas' Pediatric Cardiology.* Philadelphia: Hanley & Belfus; 1992. Reproduced with permission from the publisher and author.)

enters the right atrium via the superior or inferior vena cava. From the inferior vena cava, blood is diverted by the crista dividens through the foramen ovale into the left atrium, so that approximately 27 percent of combined ventricular output reaches the left ventricle, with the remainder passing through the tricuspid valve to the right ventricle. This left atrial flow mixes with a small volume of pulmonary venous return to enter the left ventricle and the ascending aorta. Most of this output perfuses the coronary arteries, head, and upper body vessels, with a small proportion crossing the aortic arch to the descending aorta. Right ventricular output enters the main pulmonary artery, where approximately 90 percent (59 percent of combined ventricular output) is diverted through the ductus arteriosus to the descending aorta. Thus, approximately two-thirds of the combined cardiac output passes through the right side of the heart and one-third passes through the left side of the heart.

The oxygen saturation of fetal blood is considerably lower than that in a newborn or infant because of the placenta's less efficient oxygen exchange compared with that the lungs (Fig. 73-2). The blood with the highest saturation (approximately 70 percent) is that returning from the placenta. As described above, some of this higher-saturation blood is diverted across the foramen ovale, so that saturation on the left side of the heart (65 percent) is somewhat higher than it is on the right side (55 percent). As a result, lower-saturation blood (some 55 percent) passes preferentially through the ductus arteriosus to the placenta, thus increasing the efficiency of oxygen pickup. The presence of high levels of fetal hemoglobin with a greater than normal affinity for oxygen hemoglobin promotes more efficient placental oxygen exchange related to a leftward shift of the oxygen dissociation curve.

The wide communication at the atrial level (foramen ovale) allows for near equalization of atrial and ventricular end-diastolic pressures. Similarly, at the great vessel level, the nonrestrictive ductus arteriosus allows equalization of systolic pressures in the aorta and the pulmonary artery and, in the absence of aortic or pulmonic stenosis, at the ventricular level (Fig. 73-3).

Within a few moments after birth, the circulatory physiology must switch rapidly from the placenta to the lung as the target organ for oxygen exchange. Failure of any one of a number of a complex series of pulmonary and cardiac events may result in cerebral or generalized hypoxemia, with lasting damage or death With the onset of

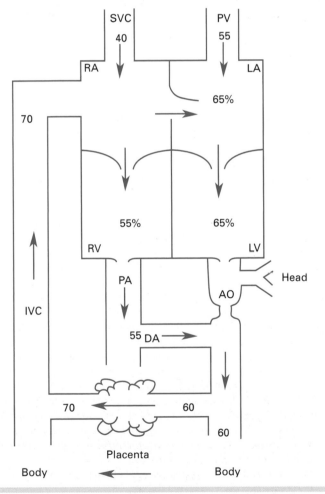

FIGURE 73-2 The numbers indicate the percent of oxygen saturation in a late-gestation lamb. The oxygen saturation is highest in the inferior vena cava, representing that primarily from the placenta. The saturation of blood in the heart is slightly higher on the left side than on the right side. The abbreviations in this diagram are the same as those in Fig. 73-1. (From Freed MD. Fetal and transitional circulation. In: Fyler DC, ed. *Nadas' Pediatric Cardiology*. Philadelphia: Hanley & Belfus; 1992. Reproduced with permission from the publisher and author.)

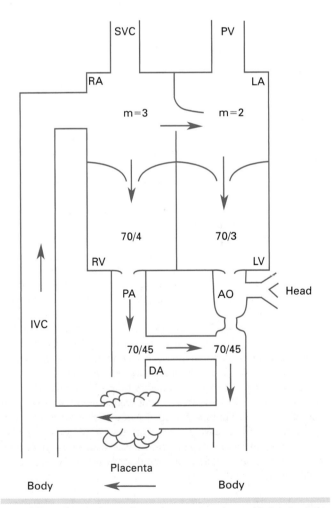

FIGURE 73-3 The numbers indicate the pressures observed in late-gestation lambs. Because large communications between the atrium and the great vessels are present, the pressures on both sides of the heart are virtually identical. The abbreviations are the same as those in Fig. 73-1. (From Freed MD. Fetal and transitional circulation. In: Fyler DC, ed. *Nadas' Pediatric Cardiology*. Philadelphia: Hanley & Belfus; 1992. Reproduced with permission from the publisher and author.)

spontaneous respiration, the lungs expand and the pulmonary arterioles, which have been vasoconstricted, dilate. The reduction in pulmonary vascular resistance results from both simple physical expansion of the lung with the onset of respiration and the vasodilation of the pulmonary resistance vessels, probably partly as a result of the high level of oxygen in alveolar gas. Simultaneously, the placenta is removed from the circulation either by clamping the umbilical cord or by constriction of the umbilical arteries. This sudden increase in systemic vascular resistance and drop in pulmonary vascular resistance causes blood leaving the right ventricle to enter the lung rather than the ductus arteriosus. The subsequent increase in pulmonary venous return to the left atrium increases left ventricular end-diastolic and left atrial pressure, shutting the flap valve of the foramen ovale against the edge of the cristae dividens, reversing the right-to-left atrial level shunt. In the presence of a lower pulmonary vascular resistance than systemic vascular resistance, some left-to-right (aorta to pulmonary artery) shunting occurs through the ductus arteriosus. The mechanism for closure of the ductus arteriosus is not completely understood. The increased level of oxygen probably causes vasoconstriction of the ductus's musculature, but there are strong suggestions that a reduction in circulating prostaglandins of the E series plays a role. Within 3 or 4 days, the biochemical closure becomes irreversible, when cellular necrosis of the endothelium leads to obliteration of the lumen. The pulmonary artery pressure drops to approximately half systemic levels within a day or so but requires another 2 to 6 weeks to decrease to adult levels.

The structure and hemodynamics of the fetal circulation have significant consequences in a neonate with congenital heart disease.[19] The parallel circulation with connections at the atrial and great vessel level allows a wide variety of congenital cardiac malformations to exist while still maintaining placental oxygen exchange and tissue delivery. For example, atresia of the tricuspid or mitral valve, while devastating after birth, does not have a significant effect in utero. Furthermore, since the right ventricle performs two-thirds of the cardiac work before birth, the left ventricle is underloaded, possibly explaining why heart failure is not uncommonly seen with congenital defects. Because the normal flow across the aortic isthmus is relatively low (only about 10 percent of combined ventricular output), this area is especially vulnerable to small changes in flow across the foramen ovale. A somewhat small foramen may result in left-sided hypoplasia, which is almost always associated with narrowing (coarctation) or atresia (interruption) at the distal transverse aorta just proximal to ductal insertion.

Since the pulmonary blood flow in utero is less than 10 percent of combined ventricular output and increases four to five times at birth, anomalies that obstruct pulmonary venous return may be masked in utero under conditions of low pulmonary venous return. Finally, the low circulating levels of oxygen before birth (Po_2 26 to 38 mmHg and saturation at 50 to 60 percent) may account for the relative level of comfort observed in infants with cyanotic heart disease. These infants may do well, at least in the short run, with a Po_2 of 30 mmHg and an aortic saturation of 50 percent—levels that would lead to cerebral and cardiac anoxia, acidosis, and death within a few minutes in an older child or adult.

Persistence of Fetal Circulation

Persistence of fetal circulation[20,21] or persistent pulmonary hypertension in a newborn results in right-to-left shunting through the patent foramen ovale and/or PDA. It occurs most commonly in full-term infants. Severe hypoxia usually is manifest in the first few hours of life with tachypnea and metabolic acidosis, and a chest roentgenogram shows diminished vascular flow but no evidence of pulmonary parenchymal disease. Physical examination may reveal a parasternal heave, a loud second heart sound, and a systolic murmur.

Polycythemia, transient myocardial ischemia from hypoglycemia, and cyanotic congenital cardiac defects must be excluded. A higher oxygen level in the right radial artery than a subdiaphragmatic site confirms right-to-left shunting through the ductus arteriosus. Echocardiography and Doppler evaluation are of the utmost importance to rule out structural heart disease, especially total anomalous pulmonary venous connection. The initial treatment[21] includes an increase in the inspired oxygen level and correction of acidosis with hyperventilation or infusion of sodium bicarbonate when necessary. Diminishing the partial pressure of carbon dioxide can lower the pulmonary resistance diminishing the right-to-left shunt. Reduction of pulmonary vascular resistance with inhaled nitric oxide is a useful adjunct to other therapies.[22] Treatment of severe disease with extracorporeal membrane oxygenation is valuable in a significant number of patients.[23] Similar hemodynamic alterations also may be seen in newborns with parenchymal lung disease.

COMPLICATIONS OF CONGENITAL HEART DISEASE

Complications associated with congenital heart disease are listed in Table 73-2.

Congestive Heart Failure

Heart failure is a potentially lethal complication of congenital heart disease and occurs in over 80 percent of infants who have malformations severe enough to require cardiac catheterization or surgery within the first year of life.[24] The onset is usually within the first 6 months of life; it is rarely found after 1 year of age without a serious intercurrent problem such as infective endocarditis, pneumonia, or anemia.

Heart failure within the first 12 to 18 h of life is usually due to malformations that involve pressure or volume overload independent of pulmonary flow, as occurs with severe valvular regurgitation or a systemic arteriovenous fistula. Rarely, myocarditis may produce failure from the time of birth, as may congenital complete heart block or supraventricular tachycardia. Other causes in this age group include primary cardiomyopathy, severe polycythemia, anemia and depressed myocardial contractility resulting from neonatal asphyxia, hypocalcemia, hypoglycemia, or sepsis. *A majority of full-term infants presenting with severe heart failure during the remainder of the first week have critical obstruction to systemic arterial flow, which in virtually all cases is unmasked by narrowing or closure of the ductus arteriosus.* Examples are aortic atresia, coarctation of the aorta, interruption of the aortic arch, and critical aortic stenosis. *During the second week of life, aortic atresia and coarctation remain the most common causes of heart failure, but left ventricular volume overload from VSD, transposition of the great arteries with a VSD, and truncus arteriosus make their appearance.* These malformations present as the pulmonary vascular resistance falls, increasing the left-to-right

TABLE 73-2 Complications of Congenital Heart Disease in Children

Congestive heart failure	Growth retardation
Hypoxemia	Pulmonary vascular disease

shunt. *Statistically, VSD is the most frequent cause of congestive failure, followed by transposition, coarctation, complete AV canal, and PDA.*

The most common symptom of congestive heart failure is tachypnea with grunting, gasping breathing or breathlessness with feeding. Observation of an undisturbed infant reveals nasal flaring and subcostal or intercostal retractions. A respiratory rate consistently above 60 is to be expected, and rates in the range of 90 to 100 are not uncommon. Poor weight gain from diminished intake and increased work of breathing is the rule. Cool, moist skin, a subdued and rapid arterial pulse, and hepatic enlargement are common accompanying signs. A gallop rhythm, pulmonary rales, and wheezing may be present. It may be difficult to distinguish the pulmonary findings of heart failure from those of pneumonia or bronchiolitis; indeed, many infants develop heart failure during an intercurrent pulmonary infection. Edema, if present, is usually found in the periorbital area and on the dorsa of the feet and hands. Cardiac enlargement is confirmed by chest roentgenography. Infants with malformations such as coarctation of the aorta and total anomalous pulmonary venous connection—abnormalities that usually are not characterized by an impressive murmur—are sometimes referred only after weeks of tachypnea and failure to thrive, when a chest roentgenogram taken to explore the possibility of lung disease has revealed cardiac enlargement.

When a sizable systemic-to-pulmonary communication exists in a premature infant, usually as a result of a PDA, signs of heart failure are often associated with signs of ventilatory failure.

Hospitalization is recommended for all infants with heart failure. Elevation of the head and chest to an angle of approximately 30 degrees and administration of humidified oxygen by techniques that do not disturb the infant help relieve tachypnea and systemic arterial hypoxia as determined by pulse oximetry. Arterial oxygen saturation levels should be monitored in newborns, particularly the premature, to avoid the risk of retrolental fibroplasia. With severe failure, oral feedings should be suspended temporarily to prevent aspiration, and fluid intake should be restricted to daily maintenance intravenously for at least the first 24 h. Anemia, acidosis, hypoxia, hypercarbia, hypoglycemia or hypocalcemia should be corrected; serum sodium, potassium, blood urea nitrogen, and creatinine concentrations should be monitored. A low threshold for the administration of antibiotics is appropriate.

Digoxin is recommended for the management of failure in infants and children, especially those with decreased ventricular systolic function, because of its excellent absorption when given orally, rapid onset of action, relatively rapid excretion, and convenience of administration. The recommended oral maintenance doses of digoxin for children, expressed in micrograms per kilogram per day, are as follows: for the premature, 5; for neonates, 10; for infants between 4 and 24 months of age, 15; for older children, 10; and for adolescents, 5. The daily maintenance dose usually is given in two divided doses approximately 12 h apart. The total digitalizing dose is four times the daily maintenance dose. Parenteral doses of digoxin are approximately 75 percent of oral doses for digitalization and maintenance. Half the digitalizing dose may be given initially, followed by the two remaining quarter doses at 4-, 8-, or 12-h intervals, depending on the desired speed of total digitalization. Maintenance therapy should be started 8 to 12 h after the last digitalizing dose. In a severely ill infant with decreased perfusion and unpredictable absorption, digitalization by the intravenous route is recommended. Impaired renal function leads to digoxin accumulation and toxicity, and so the initial and maintenance doses should be adjusted accordingly. Toxicity, if it is to occur, usually appears within the first week of therapy. If anorexia, nausea, vomiting, atrial or ventricular ectopy

or AV block appear, digoxin should be stopped and the serum digoxin level should be determined. Toxicity is probable if the level exceeds 3.0 ng/mL in an infant less than 6 months of age or 2.0 ng/mL in an older infant or child. If the need for digoxin continues, the dose is adjusted as the patient grows and gains weight.

The diuretic furosemide used intravenously in doses of 1.0 to 2.0 mg/kg or orally in doses of 1.5 to 2.0 mg/kg is very effective in the acute management of congestive heart failure. With severe failure, the dose may be increased by increments of 1.0 mg/kg intravenously if no urinary response has been achieved after 45 min. For long-term oral diuretic therapy, administration of 1.5 to 2.0 mg/kg once or twice daily is recommended. Chlorothiazide, a slightly less potent diuretic but one with a longer duration of action, may be given orally in a dose of 20 to 50 mg/kg per day. Hypokalemia and hypochloremia can be induced with these diuretics, so a daily oral supplement of potassium chloride in the range of 1.0 to 1.5 meq/kg, with adjustment depending on the serum level, may be necessary. Spironolactone, an aldosterone antagonist, has proved useful in supplementing the diuresis and preventing the hypokalemia induced by the diuretics described above. It may be given orally in a daily dose of 2 to 3 mg/kg divided bid. A regimen of spironolactone 2 to 3 mg/kg given every day and furosemide 1 mg/kg is usually adequate for long-term diuretic therapy for mild to moderate heart failure and usually does not require potassium supplementation.

In emergency situations, it may be necessary to provide an immediate inotropic stimulus in the form of intravenous sympathomimetic amines administered by constant infusion pump. Isoproterenol in a dose of 0.1 μg/kg/min exerts a powerful inotropic effect, but its usefulness may be limited by induced tachycardia and peripheral vasodilation, sometimes to the detriment of renal perfusion. Epinephrine in a dose of 0.1 to 1.0 μg/kg/min or dobutamine or dopamine in a dose of 5 to 15 μg/kg/min generally has been more helpful, with dopamine providing more adequate renal flow. The systemic arterial blood pressure, urinary output, and electrocardiogram (ECG) should be monitored continuously. Vasodilator therapy in the form of intravenous sodium nitroprusside may be of considerable help in patients with severe congestive failure that is not associated with large left-to-right shunts. The infusion rate at the start should be no higher than 0.5 μg/kg/min, but it may be increased gradually to 4.0 μg/kg/min to achieve the desired effect. Systemic arterial pressure should be monitored continuously to detect serious hypotension. The angiotensin-converting enzyme inhibitors captopril, enalapril, and lisinopril given orally have proved effective in selected patients: captopril starting at 0.1 to 0.4 mg/kg per dose in a neonate and 0.3 to 0.6 mg/kg per dose in an older child given one to four times per day, enalapril 0.16 to 0.25 mg/kg/day in two divided doses, or lisinopril 0.16 to 0.25 mg/kg/day in a single daily dose. Hypotension and/or hyperkalemia are the primary adverse effects of these agents.[25]

Infants with progressive respiratory insufficiency benefit from mechanical ventilation using a volume-controlled, positive-pressure ventilator with positive end-expiratory pressure. These measures may permit additional therapy, cardiac catheterization, and surgical intervention with a much greater margin of safety.

In newborns who have failure as a result of narrowing or closure of the ductus arteriosus in the presence of critical obstruction to flow from the left side of the heart, dramatic and lifesaving relief can be achieved with reopening of the ductus by the infusion of prostaglandin E_1 (PGE$_1$) at a dose of 0.1 μg/kg/min.

Finally, infants or children in whom medical therapy is clearly inadequate or only temporarily successful may require prompt surgical intervention for control of heart failure. *As a rule, the earlier the onset of congestive failure, the more likely the need for surgery.*

TABLE 73-3 Sequelae of Hypoxemia

Cyanosis	Exercise intolerance
Clubbing	Hypoxic spells
Polycythemia	Brain abscess
Squatting	Cerebrovascular accidents

Hypoxemia

The sequelae of hypoxemia are listed in Table 73-3. *Cyanosis,* a bluish tinge to the color of the skin caused by the presence of at least 3 to 5 g/dL of reduced hemoglobin, is frequently the initial sign of congenital heart disease in an infant. It may also be an early sign of pulmonary, central nervous system, or metabolic disease or methemoglobinemia. Prompt distinction between cardiac and noncardiac cyanosis, usually by echocardiography, is extremely important, since palliation with PGE_1 infusion followed by early surgical intervention has improved survival.

Hypoxia leading to cyanosis in congenital heart disease may be due to heart failure with pulmonary edema and pulmonary venous desaturation and/or intracardiac right-to-left shunting. The hypoxia that is due either to heart failure or to lung disease with intrapulmonary shunting usually responds dramatically to oxygen administration, whereas hypoxia that is due to cyanotic defects does not. Since many infants are relatively anemic during the first few months of life (with a hemoglobin concentration of 10.4 to 12 g/dL), cyanosis may be subtle.

When cyanosis has been present in older children for several months, the distal tips of the fingers and toes become hyperemic. Eventually, the capillary end loop dilation causes *clubbing* of the fingers and toes with a loss of the normal angle of the base of the nail and fingers. Also, with long-standing hypoxemia, the production of red blood cells increases to maintain the oxygen-carrying capacity of the blood (*polycythemia*). The increased hemoglobin concentration at any given oxygen saturation will result in more reduced hemoglobin, thus exaggerating the cyanosis.

The central nervous system may be the target organ of cerebrovascular accidents or brain abscess. *Brain abscess* is probably due to bacteremia, primarily with mouth organisms that cross from the venous system to the arterial system right to left from shunting. The incidence seems to be directly related to arterial saturation and occurs mostly in older children and adolescents.[26]

Cerebrovascular accidents are due directly to hypoxemia or indirectly in children who are polycythemic presumably secondary to sludging.[27] The former group usually consists of infants below 2 years of age who are anemic and thus may have markedly reduced oxygen levels. The latter group consists of children or young adults who are polycythemic and have sludging or in situ microthrombosis. Interestingly, iron deficiency leads to stiff red cells; therefore sludging may occur with modest levels of polycythemia (hematocrit 55 to 60 percent) in the presence of iron deficiency. With hematocrits in the range of 65 percent or higher, increased viscosity may lead to a cerebrovascular accident. Maintaining a proper level of hemoglobin has a salutory effect on hemodynamics and oxygen delivery in the presence of significant hypoxemia.[28,29] Other systems may also be affected by hypoxemia or polycythemia. In older adolescents, the increase in hemoglobin breakdown may result in hyperuricemia and can precipitate a secondary form of gout.[30]

Disturbances in hemostasis also occur with polycythemia. Coagulation factors are commonly abnormal in patients with hematocrits

in excess of 60 percent.[31] Actual platelet counts may be normal but can be increased initially in some patients, with subsequent decreases related to persistent and worsening desaturation. There is evidence of shortened platelet survival time in patients with cyanotic heart disease.[32] Laboratory evaluation of coagulation status requires that correction be made for the diminished volume of plasma and for the volume of anticoagulant used in blood samples, so as to avoid false results. Hematologic management of adults with cyanotic congenital heart disease requires special experience and knowledge.[33]

The major consequences of cyanosis can be avoided in many instances, although differences in intelligence have been demonstrated between cyanotic and acyanotic children.[34]

Retardation of Growth and Development

Children with severe cardiac malformations frequently exhibit retardation of growth and development, with height and weight near or below the third percentile or weight 20 percentile points below the mean percentile for height.[35]

Growth retardation is most severe among children with overt cyanosis and those with large left-to-right shunts that cause heart failure. Heart failure tends to cause a greater reduction of weight than of height. Skeletal retardation, reflected by bone age, usually occurs with height and weight retardation and, among children with cyanotic heart disease, correlates with the severity of hypoxemia.

Other factors contribute to growth retardation, including insufficient caloric intake, dyspnea, frequent infections, psychological disturbances, malabsorption, and hypermetabolism. Among infants with severe congenital heart disease recognized within the first year of life, there is a significantly increased incidence of subnormal birth weight, intrauterine growth retardation, and major extracardiac anomalies.[3] Finally, a relatively small number of children have associated syndromes known to be characterized by growth retardation, such as rubella and Noonan's, Turner's, and Down's syndromes. Growth retardation related primarily to congenital heart disease usually responds to surgical correction or palliation, with an impressive acceleration of growth and a return toward normal.

Although cardiac surgery is seldom recommended on the basis of growth failure alone, decelerated growth should be recognized early and, until proved otherwise, considered an index of the severity of heart disease. In general, the more successful the surgery, the less will be the retardation of growth and development, with its sequelae of physical, psychological, and intellectual problems.[36]

Pulmonary Arterial Hypertension and Pulmonary Vascular Obstructive Disease

Pulmonary arterial hypertension (PAH) and pulmonary vascular obstructive disease (PVOD) are serious complications of congenital heart disease. PAH usually results from direct transmission of systemic arterial pressure to the right ventricle or pulmonary arteries via a large communication. Less frequently, it is due to severe obstruction to blood flow through the left side of the heart at the pulmonary venous level or beyond. PVOD refers to a process involving structural and developmental changes in the smaller muscular arteries and arterioles of the lung that gradually diminishes and eventually destroys the ability of the pulmonary vascular bed to transport blood from the larger pulmonary arteries to the pulmonary veins without an abnormal elevation of proximal pulmonary arterial pressure.

Pulmonary resistance (R_p) may be as high as 8 to 10 Wood's units immediately after birth but falls rapidly throughout the first week of life. Indexed Wood's units, as a measure of resistance to flow across either the pulmonary or the systemic vascular bed, are obtained by dividing the mean pressure difference (in millimeters of mercury) across the pulmonary or systemic vascular beds by the blood flow index (expressed in liters per minute per square meter) across those respective beds. By 6 to 8 weeks, it usually has reached the normal adult level (1 to 3 Wood's units). These changes are accompanied by a gradual dilatation of the smaller followed by the larger muscular pulmonary arteries. In the weeks and months that follow, a thinning of the muscular walls occurs, with the growth of existing arteries and the development of new arteries and arterioles. The latter process contributes over 90 percent of the smaller or intraacinar pulmonary arterial vessels present in older children and adults.[37]

Increased pulmonary arterial pressure has an adverse effect on the normal maturation of the pulmonary vascular bed. Such pressure encourages a persistence of the thick muscular medial layer present in the smaller pulmonary arteries of term newborns, stimulates an extension of smooth muscle into smaller and more peripheral arteries than normal for age, and retards the growth of existing acinar arteries and the development of new ones.

In the presence of a large systemic-to-pulmonary communication, pulmonary arterial pressures remain at or near systemic levels, with the result that the diminution in pulmonary muscle mass and pulmonary resistance is less rapid and of a lesser magnitude than in a normal infant. Nevertheless, the diminution is usually sufficient to permit a large pulmonary blood flow and, as a result, congestive failure by the end of the first month. Exceptions are found among infants with a large systemic-to-pulmonary communication but with alveolar hypoxia—a stimulus for pulmonary vasoconstriction—in whom there is less than normal involution of the medial musculature and a diminution in pulmonary vascular resistance. Clinically, this is expressed by the lower incidence of congestive failure observed among infants with large VSDs born and living at high altitude. It is also seen in some children with Down's syndrome and a large VSD or AV canal who may hypoventilate or have upper airway obstruction. Rarely, an infant will maintain a very high pulmonary vascular resistance in the face of an anatomically large systemic-to-pulmonary communication without evidence of significant hypoxemia or acidemia and remain free of the signs and symptoms of congestive failure. Conversely, in a premature infant in whom the medial muscle mass is less at birth than it is in a full-term infant, the fall in pulmonary vascular resistance is usually much more rapid than normal.

Chronic PAH, increased flow, or both produce a characteristic series of histologic changes in the smaller pulmonary arteries and arterioles originally described and graded by Heath and Edwards (grades I through VI below)[38] (Fig. 73-4, Plate 97) and, more recently, by Rabinovitch[37] (grades A through C below):

- Grade I: medial hypertrophy
- Grade II: concentric or eccentric cellular intimal proliferation
- Grade III: relatively acellular intimal fibrosis with occlusion of the smaller pulmonary arteries and arterioles
- Grade IV: progressive, generalized dilatation of the distal muscular arteries and the appearance of plexiform lesions, complex vascular structures composed of a network or plexus of proliferating endothelial tissue, frequently accompanied by thrombus, within a dilated thin-walled sac
- Grade V: thinning and fibrosis of the media superimposed on the plexiform lesions
- Grade VI: necrotizing arteritis within the media
- Grade A: extension of muscle into normally nonmuscular peripheral arteries with or without a mild increase in medial wall thickness of normally muscular arteries (less than 1.5 times normal)

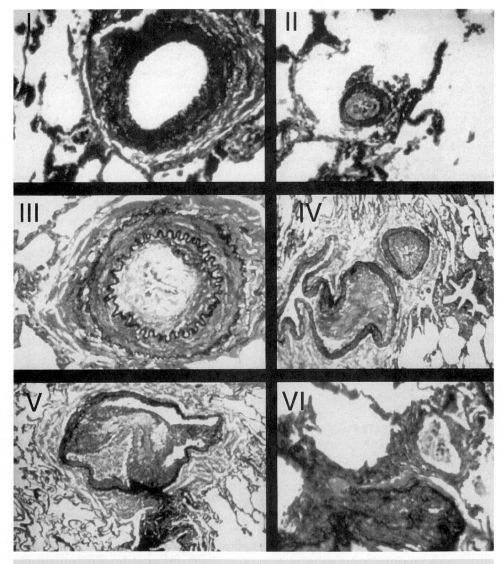

FIGURE 73-4 (Plate 97) Pulmonary vascular changes by the Heath and Edwards criteria (see text). Grades 1 to 6 are represented by panels I to VI, respectively.

- Grade B: extension of muscle as described above with an even greater increase in medial wall thickness of normally muscular arteries (mild, 1.5–2 × normal; severe, >2 × normal)
- Grade C: changes seen in grade B (severe) but with a decreased arterial concentration relative to alveoli (mild, ≥1/2 normal; severe, <1/2 normal)
- Grades A and B are partitions of Heath-Edwards grade I and may be seen with large left-to-right shunts with (B) or without increased pressure (A). Grade C criteria may be found with grades I and II, are invariable with grade III, and usually preclude a complete return to normal of pulmonary arterial pressures and resistance despite successful surgical correction of the systemic-to-pulmonary communication.

Estimation of pulmonary vascular resistance from data obtained at cardiac catheterization remains the most widely used means of assessing the state of the pulmonary vascular bed. Hypoxemia from oversedation, atelectasis, or pneumonitis at the time of study should be scrupulously avoided. If pulmonary vascular resistance is elevated, responsiveness to vasodilation induced by the inhalation of 100% oxygen, the pulmonary arterial administration of prostacyclin, or the inhalation of nitric oxide should be tested.[39]

Values of $R_p \leq 3$ Wood's units are considered normal. The status of the pulmonary vasculature also can be expressed as a ratio of pulmonary vascular resistance to systemic vascular resistance (R_p/R_s). *Pulmonary/systemic resistance ratios less than 0.2:1 are considered normal.*

As pulmonary vascular resistance increases, pulmonary blood flow generally decreases. Eventually, a point is reached where surgical closure of the defect will produce only a small diminution of blood flow, a proportionately small decrease in pulmonary arterial pressure, and no significant change in the factors contributing to the progression of vascular disease. At this point surgery usually is not recommended, since the benefits are minimal and closure of the defect may eliminate a useful "blow-off" for increasing resistance. *An R_p/R_s ratio of 0.7:1 or an R_p of 11 Wood's units with a pulmonary/systemic blood flow ratio of 1.5:1 is the criterion generally used to define this situation.* Without surgery, these patients survive as examples of the Eisenmenger syndrome, in which $R_p \geq R_s$ and at least some right-to-left shunting occurs at rest or with exercise. Some of these patients can survive for several decades and lead productive lives, with relatively mild symptoms and few limitations.[40]

The decision regarding surgery for patients with less severe PVOD is a clinical one. The higher the calculated resistance, the greater the structural changes in the pulmonary vasculature (as judged by lung biopsy or quantitative pulmonary arterial wedge angiography), and the older the patient with any given level of elevated resistance or grade of structural change, the less likely it is that the outcome of surgery will be satisfactory.[37]

The prevention of PVOD requires the identification of the patients at risk—i.e., all patients with a systemic-to-pulmonary communication and a pulmonary arterial systolic pressure higher than half the systemic arterial systolic pressure. Also included are all patients with transposition, regardless of pressure or flow, with the possible exception of those with severe pulmonary stenosis. Ideally, all patients at risk should undergo correction or pulmonary arterial banding before the end of the first year of life unless there is proof that the pulmonary arterial systolic pressure has fallen to or is less than half the systemic systolic pressure among those with normally related great arteries. Among patients with transposition with a large VSD or patent ductus arteriosus, action must be taken within the first 3 months of life.

Long-Term Problems with Surgically Corrected Defects

With advances in the surgical treatment of congenital heart defects, more patients are living to adulthood. This discussion of potential long-term problems is intended for those who follow these children after surgery and through adult life[41] (see Chap. 74). Residua, sequelae, and complications result from most surgical procedures for congenital heart defects. A residual part of the original defect, such as mitral prolapse in repaired ASD, may purposefully not have been approached surgically. Some sequelae are unavoidable consequences of the surgery, such as pulmonary regurgitation after pulmonary valvotomy. There are also complications that occur as unexpected but related events after successful surgery, such as late complete heart block. When viewed with these possibilities in mind, only surgical correction of a PDA is likely to result in no long-term problems.

Most patients have residual murmurs after surgery for congenital heart defects. Determination of the origin of these murmurs and evaluation of the severity of the hemodynamic abnormalities they represent are important. Noninvasive diagnostic tools, especially two-dimensional echocardiography and Doppler, are often useful. The risk of infective endocarditis to patients persists after surgery, with the exception of those who have undergone patent ductus ligation or division or repair of an ASD or VSD in whom there is no residual shunt. Patients in whom it has been necessary to place an artificial valve are at increased risk of endocarditis.[42,43]

There are specific problems related to some of the more common defects. For those with repaired ASDs, VSDs, and AV (canal) septal defects, a residual shunt may be present, but ordinarily it is small and not hemodynamically significance. Those with repaired AV canal defects may have important AV valve regurgitation. Repaired coarctation of the aorta can gradually become narrowed again, or patients may develop idiopathic hypertension. Surgery for valvular pulmonary stenosis usually results in mild residual stenosis and regurgitation, which are well tolerated and have little tendency to progress with time. The natural history of valvular aortic stenosis after surgery is not as benign.[44] Significant regurgitation must be avoided, so the initial results may not be as good in terms of the severity of residual stenosis. In addition, aortic stenosis tends to worsen with time; thus, proper follow-up is mandatory for these patients.

Few patients enter adulthood with the continued problem of cyanosis, since those with defects amenable to surgical correction should have had surgery well before this time. Only patients with complex and irreparable defects and those with pulmonary vascular disease should experience problems of cyanosis during the adult years. Particularly important among these patients is management of any attendant psychosocial problems (employment, insurability,[45] and learning disabilities) and difficulties related to pregnancy.[46] Those who have had surgery for cyanotic defects are more likely to have sequelae and complications. Some degree of exercise intolerance is not unusual in this group of patients, and exercise stress testing aids in their management.[47]

Dysrhythmias are particularly common among these patients. *In those who have had intraventricular repairs, most commonly for tetralogy of Fallot, late complete heart block and serious ventricular arrhythmias can occur and may result in sudden death.*[48] This risk appears to be highest in those who had transient complete heart block at the time of surgery and who develop right bundle branch block with left anterior hemiblock after surgery. Extensive intraatrial surgical procedures for transposition of the great arteries also frequently lead to dysrhythmias, most commonly sick sinus syndrome with brady-tachyarrhythmias and atrial flutter, with a high incidence of sudden death.[49] Ambulatory 24-h ECG monitoring (see Chap. 33), stress testing (see Chap. 14), and intracardiac electrophysiologic studies are important in following patients who have had complex repairs. Atrial enlargement after the Fontan operation has resulted in atrial flutter and/or fibrillation, which are frequently therapeutically challenging.[50]

Serious ventricular dysfunction[51] and venous obstruction also may occur. Despite intraatrial physiologic repairs for transposition of the great arteries, the anatomic right ventricle must perform systemic work.[52] In addition, these repairs may lead to pulmonary and/or systemic venous obstruction. Atriopulmonary connections for the repair of tricuspid atresia and many types of univentricular hearts frequently leave an anatomically abnormal ventricle as the systemic ventricle. In this group of patients, the right atrium has become the "pulmonary ventricle," with an elevated right atrial pressure that may lead to problems of systemic venous hypertension such as protein-losing enteropathy.[53]

Finally, some children have had repairs with synthetic prostheses. Since artificial valves cannot keep pace with somatic growth of the child, long-term stability is critical. Conduits with or without valves placed at surgery can degenerate or become obstructive. *Bioprosthetic valves undergo accelerated fibrosis and calcification in patients less than about 30 to 35 years of age.* In spite of these problems, the majority of patients who reach adulthood after surgical repair of congenital defects are relatively asymptomatic; they can and do lead productive lives.

INTRACARDIAC COMMUNICATIONS BETWEEN THE SYSTEMIC AND PULMONARY CIRCULATIONS, USUALLY WITHOUT CYANOSIS

Ventricular Septal Defect

PATHOLOGY AND INCIDENCE
A ventricular septal defect (VSD) is the most common congenital cardiac anomaly. It may be an isolated defect or part of a complex malformation. Approximately 80 percent of these defects are paramembranous but may extend into the inlet, trabecular, or outlet sections of the muscular septum. Less common are conal septal or subarterial doubly committed defects (5 to 7 percent), inlet defects lying beneath the septal leaflet of the tricuspid valve in the region of the atrioventricular canal (5 to 8 percent), and defects in the muscular septum that may be in the inlet, trabecular, or outlet area[54] (Fig. 73-5). Multiple muscular defects are not infrequently seen.

The incidence of VSDs is about 2 per 1000 live births, and its prevalence among school-age children has been estimated as 1 per 1000, constituting about one-quarter of the congenital cardiac malformations in combined series (Table 73-1). Males and females are affected equally.

VSDs may be isolated or associated with other congenital cardiac abnormalities. Malformations associated with VSD are, in order of decreasing frequency: (1) coarctation of the aorta, (2) additional shunts, most commonly ASD and PDA, (3) intracardiac obstructions such as subpulmonary or subaortic stenosis, mitral stenosis, and anomalous muscle bundle of the right ventricle, and (4) incompetent atrioventricular valves.

ABNORMAL PHYSIOLOGY
The consequences of a VSD depend on the size of the defect and the pulmonary vascular resistance. A small defect offers a large resistance to flow. There is no elevation of right ventricular or pulmonary

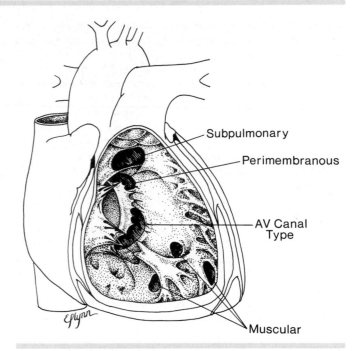

FIGURE 73-5 Different types of ventricular septal defects when viewed from the right ventricle. (From Fyler DC, ed. *Nadas' Pediatric Cardiology.* Philadelphia: Hanley & Belfus; 1992. Reproduced with permission from the publisher and author.)

Labels on figure: Subpulmonary, Perimembranous, AV Canal Type, Muscular

arterial pressure, and the left-to-right shunt may be so small that it can be detected only by two-dimensional imaging with Doppler color-flow mapping or selective left ventricular angiography. This type of defect imposes little physiologic burden on the heart, although patients are always at risk for infective endocarditis. A defect of moderate size permits a difference between the right and left ventricular systolic pressures but may allow a large left-to-right shunt with resulting left atrial hypertension and dilatation and left ventricular volume overload. The development of pulmonary vascular disease among these patients is unusual but possible.

When the effective area of the defect is large (equal to or greater than the aortic valve orifice), the defect offers virtually no resistance to flow and systolic pressures are present in the ventricles, the aorta, and the pulmonary artery. The relative resistance of the two vascular beds directly governs the proportion of blood entering the two circulations. At birth, pulmonary vascular resistance is high and there is little if any left-to-right shunt despite the presence of a large defect. This resistance to flow gradually falls over the first few weeks of life, permitting a progressively greater amount of blood to flow through the defect, through the lungs, and back to the left atrium and left ventricle. In most infants, the left ventricular volume overload eventually leads to left ventricular "failure" with elevated left ventricular end-diastolic and left atrial pressures and pulmonary congestion.

History Infants or children with a small isolated defect are asymptomatic. The murmur of a small defect may be detected within the first 24 to 36 h of life, since the very restrictive opening permits the normal rapid fall in pulmonary arterial resistance and pressures. In term infants born at sea level with a large VSD, clinical deterioration may occur at any time from about 3 to 12 weeks after birth. In premature infants, in whom the less well developed pulmonary vascular hypertrophy regresses more rapidly, failure frequently is noted at 1 to

4 weeks. Parents describe tachypnea, grunting respirations, and fatigue, particularly with feedings. Weight gain is slow, and excessive sweating is common.

Physical Examination A child with a small defect is comfortable. With moderate holes, a systolic thrill at the lower left sternal border is common. If the defect is small, the pulmonary artery pressure is normal, so the second heart sound is not accentuated. The systolic murmur along the lower left sternal border is characteristically holosystolic but may be limited to early or midsystole. This latter feature suggests a defect in the muscular septum rather than the membranous septum.

Infants with large defects, large left-to-right shunt, and PAH tend to be restless, irritable, and underweight. Moderate respiratory distress may be present. Both the right and the left ventricular systolic impulses are impressively hyperdynamic to palpation. A thrill at the lower left sternal border is common. The second heart sound is narrowly split, with a loud, frequently palpable pulmonary component. Third heart sound gallops at the apex are common. Characteristically, the systolic murmur is holosystolic at the lower left sternal border and is accompanied by a middiastolic rumble of grade 2 to 3 intensity at the apex, with the latter indicating a pulmonary/systemic blood flow ratio ($\dot{Q}_p/\dot{Q}_s$) of 2:1 or greater. Hepatic enlargement can be identified below the right costal margin. Pulmonary rales may be seen with severe failure.

With the passage of time, one may observe signs of a diminishing left-to-right shunt with an improved rate of weight gain, less dyspnea, diminution of the precordial hyperactivity, and disappearance of the apical diastolic flow rumble. This clinical improvement may be a result of the defect becoming smaller, the development of subvalvular pulmonary stenosis with little or no appreciable change in the size of the defect, or, most worrisome, the development of PVOD with continued severe PAH. With developing subpulmonary stenosis, the systolic murmur radiates more and more impressively to the upper left sternal border and the second heart sound becomes more widely split, with a progressive diminution in the intensity of the pulmonary component. Decreased flow resulting from pulmonary vascular disease is characterized by a gradual reduction in the intensity and duration of the systolic murmur, more narrow splitting of the second heart sound, and marked accentuation of the pulmonary component.

The clinical picture of advanced pulmonary vascular disease secondary to a congenital left-to-right shunt, or Eisenmenger's syndrome, is that of a relatively comfortable older child, adolescent, or young adult with mild cyanosis and clubbing in whom one finds a prominent *a* wave in the jugular venous pulse, a mild right ventricular lift, and a second heart sound that is narrowly split or virtually single with a very loud, usually palpable pulmonary component. An early pulmonary systolic ejection sound reflecting dilatation of the main pulmonary artery may be present, and there may be no systolic murmur at all. In older adolescents and adults, an early diastolic murmur of pulmonary regurgitation or a holosystolic murmur of tricuspid regurgitation may appear.

Chest Roentgenogram In the presence of a small defect, the heart's size and shape and the pulmonary blood flow are barely altered. With large defects, there is moderate to marked enlargement of the heart, with prominence of the main pulmonary arterial segment and impressive overcirculation in the peripheral lung fields. The left atrium is dilated unless an associated ASD is present, allowing decompression of the left atrium. With increasing pulmonary vascular disease, there is diminution in heart size toward normal, while the central pulmonary arteries remain dilated. The peripheral pulmonary arterial

markings become attenuated, and a "pruned" effect is produced in the outer third of the lung fields.

Electrocardiogram With a small defect, one can expect the normal progression of the mean QRS axis from right to left and the normal gradual decrease of the prominent right ventricular voltages characteristic of newborns. The left ventricular forces remain within normal limits or become slightly augmented as a reflection of the mild left ventricular volume overload. With large defects, the mean QRS axis tends to remain oriented to the right and there is little or no regression in right ventricular voltage. The left ventricular forces gradually increase, resulting in a pattern of biventricular hypertrophy within the first few weeks of life. Left atrial enlargement is usually present, as is right atrial enlargement. With the development of pulmonary vascular disease or significant pulmonary stenosis, the mean QRS axis tends to remain oriented to the right; there is no regression in right ventricular voltage, but the evidence of left ventricular and left atrial hypertrophy lessens or disappears.

Echocardiogram Two-dimensional imaging can distinguish an uncomplicated VSD from more complex malformations and is capable of imaging most defects directly when multiple transducer positions are used. The addition of pulsed-wave Doppler with color-flow mapping permits the identification of small, multiple, muscular, and other less easily visualized defects. The position and size of the opening can be determined as well as its relationships to the aorta, pulmonary artery, and AV valves. Continuous-wave Doppler echocardiography can predict the systolic right ventricular pressure from the difference between the systolic pressure measured by a blood pressure cuff, if there is no aortic stenosis, and the Doppler gradient (Fig. 73-6). In the absence of associated pulmonic stenosis, the right ventricular systolic pressure provides an estimate of the pulmonary artery pressure. Right ventricular systolic pressure also can be estimated by measuring the right ventricular to right atrial systolic pressure gradient across the tricuspid valve in the presence of tricuspid regurgitation.

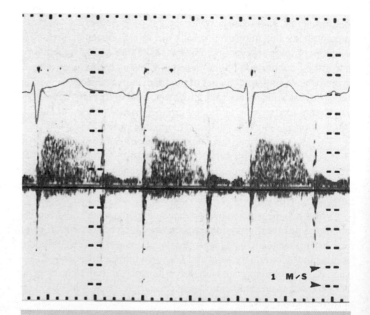

FIGURE 73-6 Continuous-wave Doppler with spectral display from the left lower sternal border of a child with a ventricular septal defect that demonstrates holosystolic turbulence with peak velocity = 2.8 m/s across the defect, compatible with an instantaneous systolic pressure difference of 31 mmHg between the right and left ventricles.

Cardiac Catheterization   Though cardiac catheterization is performed infrequently in infants with isolated VSDs, these studies show an increase in oxygen saturation at the right ventricular level, reflecting the left-to-right ventricular shunt. With small defects, the right ventricular and pulmonary arterial systolic pressures are normal. With large defects, these pressures are at or near systemic levels, and the mean left atrial pressure may be elevated to the range of 10 to 15 mmHg.

Selective left ventricular angiography in the anteroposterior, lateral, and oblique views with craniocaudal angulation are used to establish the spatial relations of the great arteries to each other, to the ventricles and also to determine the exact site, size, and number of septal defects (Fig. 73-7). Aortography is helpful in eliminating the possibility of an associated ductus arteriosus or unsuspected coarctation of the aorta if the arch cannot be well imaged by echocardiography.

NATURAL HISTORY AND PROGNOSIS

Fortunately, the majority of VSDs are small and do not present a serious clinical problem. Approximately 25 percent of these small defects close spontaneously by 18 months, 50 percent by 4 years, and 75 percent by 10 years.[55] A spontaneous closure rate approaching 45 percent within the first 12 to 14 months has been observed among infants with an uncomplicated paramembranous or muscular VSD in the neonatal period.[56] Even large defects tend to become smaller, but the likelihood of eventual spontaneous closure is much lower (probably in the range of 60 percent if judged large at 3 months of age and only 50 percent if it is still large at 6 months).[55]

Congestive failure is an almost inevitable complication of a large VSD. Approximately 80 percent of infants with large defects require hospitalization by age 4 months.[3] The risk of death with congestive failure is in the range of 11 percent. Significant subvalvular pulmonary stenosis develops in approximately 3 percent of these individuals and may progress to right-to-left shunting at the ventricular level. PVOD is seldom severe and generally reversible in the first 12 months of life; thereafter, it becomes progressively less likely to regress. Infants and children with a pulmonary systolic pressure in excess of 50 percent of the systemic arterial systolic pressure beyond the first year of life are at risk for this complication.[57] A very small number of infants with large VSDs maintain a high level of pulmonary vascular resistance throughout the first year of life and remain almost entirely free of symptoms of heart failure. In these patients, irreversible pulmonary vascular disease may develop without the usual and expected clinical signs and symptoms described above.

A small number of children, 0.6 percent in a large group of carefully followed patients, will develop aortic regurgitation as a result of prolapse of the right, the posterior, or both aortic valve leaflets into the defect.[58] This complication is more prevalent among males, in a ratio of 2:1, and seems particularly likely to occur with defects of the subpulmonary type. Shunt size appears not to be related to the development of this complication. The characteristic aortic diastolic murmur may appear at any time between ages 6 months and 20 years. Regurgitation is usually progressive, sometimes rapidly so, and predisposes these individuals to infective endocarditis.

The risk of infective endocarditis in patients with an uncomplicated VSD that is managed medically lies somewhere between 4 and 10 percent for the first 30 years of life.[59] The development of aortic regurgitation more than doubles this risk. Attempts at surgical closure of the defect with or without aortic regurgitation reduce the risk to less than half that of unoperated patients.[60]

MEDICAL MANAGEMENT

The basis of the medical management of children with VSDs is an understanding that defects frequently narrow and may close spontaneously. Approximately 70 percent of small VSDs probably close.[55] Even large muscular defects may get significantly smaller, and up to 25 percent of them will become hemodynamically insignificant if one can wait long enough. Nevertheless, significant complications can occur, and the decision whether to proceed with medical or surgical management must be reevaluated constantly.

For children with a large VSD, the first decision point usually occurs before 8 to 12 weeks of age. Infants with large septal defects generally develop significant left-to-right shunts as the pulmonary resistance drops. Congestive heart failure ensues with tachypnea, tachycardia, and difficulty feeding. Digoxin and diuretics are occasionally useful, but if the left-to-right shunt is very large, feeding may be problematic. For children who cannot gain at least 15 g per day (30 g per day is normal) in whom no other cause is found for failure to thrive, surgical repair is indicated. Occasionally, in marginal cases, increasing the caloric density of the formula from 20 calories per ounce to as much as 32 calories per ounce may promote weight gain. In children unable to take more than 10 to 12 ounces per day, however, caloric supplementation is unlikely to be sufficient and surgical repair is necessary.

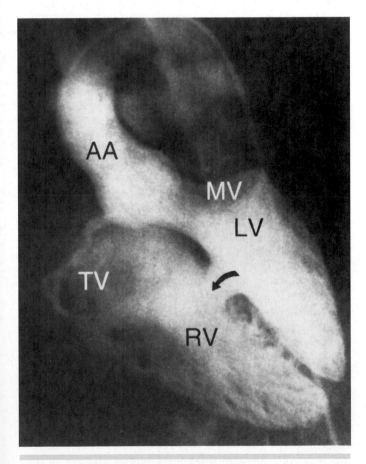

FIGURE 73-7 Multiple trabecular ventricular septal defects. Retrograde left ventriculogram, four-chamber projection, profiles the mitral and tricuspid valves and the midtrabecular VSD (*arrow*). Additional VSDs closer to the apex are more anterior in location and are not profiled in this projection. AA = ascending aorta; LV = left ventricle; MV = mitral valve; RV = right ventricle; TV = tricuspid valve. (From Lock JE, Keane JF, Perry SB. *Diagnostic and Interventional Catheterization in Congenital Heart Disease*, 2d. ed. Boston: Kluwer; 2000. Reproduced with permission from the publisher and authors.)

The second decision point in children who do not fail to thrive occurs between 9 and 12 months of age. Children with unrestrictive or mildly restrictive VSDs have pulmonary artery hypertension that may lead to irreversible pulmonary vascular obstructive disease. If the pulmonary artery pressure is elevated at 9 to 12 months of age, surgery is indicated to prevent this serious life-shortening complication. In some children, the high-pitched nature of the murmur, the normal pulmonary component of the second heart sound, the absence of right ventricular hypertension on ECG, and the large intraventricular pressure gradient on echocardiography make the estimation of normal pulmonary artery pressure firm. Occasionally in children in whom the signs, symptoms, and laboratory findings are ambiguous or conflicting, cardiac catheterization may be necessary to assure that the pulmonary artery pressure is normal and that pulmonary vascular obstructive disease is not a risk.

The third decision point occurs somewhere between 5 to 10 years of age. Though the defect has not caused failure to thrive or pulmonary hypertension, it may still produce a significant left-to-right shunt, causing a volume overload of the left ventricle. Eventually, heart failure is possible, and some recommend surgical closure during childhood if there is a significant volume overload. There is no firm number that suggests a dangerous level of left ventricular volume overload. Some centers close the VSD when the pulmonary-to-systemic flow ratio (measured by cardiac catheterization, radionuclide angiography, echocardiography, or magnetic resonance imaging) is more than 2 to 1. Others use significant left atrial and left ventricular dilation by echo. A minority of centers do not recommend surgical closure as long as the pulmonary artery pressure is normal since there are few adults with a VSD who develops late congestive heart failure.

Unfortunately, not all patients with a large defect are encountered during the first or second year of life, when it is possible to prevent injury to the pulmonary vascular bed. If significant PAH is allowed to persist, one can expect progression to irreversible pulmonary obstructive disease. For this reason, *prompt surgical closure of defects is recommended in all individuals beyond the age of 2 years if the pulmonary arterial systolic pressure is greater than half the systemic arterial systolic pressure, the mean pulmonary pressure exceeds 25 mmHg, or the R_p/R_s ratio is higher than 0.3:1.* With severe pulmonary vascular disease, a point eventually is reached where the risk of death at operation or in the months or years immediately after the operation as a result of progressive vascular disease more than offsets the possible benefits from surgical closure. At present, surgery is recommended if the calculated R_p is less than 10 Wood units/m^2 or the R_p/R_s ratio is 0.7:1, provided that the $\dot{Q}_p/\dot{Q}_s$ ratio is still 1.5:1. In adults, the upper limit of pulmonary vascular resistance for surgery is approximately 10 Wood's units. Patients in whom the defect is judged clinically to be small at 6 months of age may be reexamined at 1- or 2-year intervals to reassure the patient and family, reemphasize the importance of antibiotic protection against infective endocarditis, document further narrowing or closure of the defect, and (in a very small number of patients) detect the first signs of aortic valve prolapse.

In patients with Eisenmenger's complex,[40] stamina is limited by systemic arterial hypoxemia and, in some, right-sided heart failure. Complications to be anticipated include syncope, hemoptysis, brain abscess, hyperuricemia, and congestive failure. Pregnancy, with a maternal mortality of 30 to 60 percent, and oral contraceptives are contraindicated. Transient symptomatic relief from extreme polycythemia (usually >68 percent) may be achieved with careful erythropheresis. Travel to or living at high altitudes is poorly tolerated, and supplemental oxygen should be provided and used during air travel. A recent study reports that the average age of death for individuals with Eisenmenger's complex related to VSD is 43 years, with heart failure the cause of death in the majority.[61]

The risk of congenital heart disease for a subsequent sibling of a single affected child is on the order of 1 to 2 percent. The risk to a newborn of a parent with VSD increases to 3 percent.[62] Pregnancy in the presence of a small defect and normal pulmonary vascular resistance does not appear to carry an increased risk to the patient or infant, although precautions against infective endocarditis should be taken.

SURGICAL MANAGEMENT

Banding of the pulmonary artery to reduce pulmonary blood flow and pressures played an important role in the management of congestive heart failure and the prevention of PVOD. Now that surgical closure of VSDs in infancy is nearly uniformly successful, banding is utilized rarely. Complications of pulmonary arterial banding include deformity of the pulmonary arteries and/or pulmonary valve, progressive right ventricular hypertrophy with loss of ventricular compliance, and the development of subaortic left ventricular outflow tract obstruction.

VSDs are closed using cardiopulmonary bypass with cardioplegic arrest and moderate systemic hypothermia. Total circulatory arrest or minimal perfusion with profound hypothermia (18°C) is sometimes necessary in infants who weigh less than 5 kg.[63,64] Paramembranous VSDs may be exposed through the right atrium and the tricuspid valve orifice. A transverse or longitudinal right ventriculotomy may be necessary for closure of high conal septal defects associated with aortic valve leaflet prolapse.

Care is required to prevent injury to the AV node near the ostium of the coronary sinus and to the bundle of His as it courses inferiorly, passing on the left side of the ventricular septum near the posterocaudal margin of the septal defect. Intraoperative transesophageal echocardiography with Doppler color-flow assessment can be used for the detection of significant residual or previously unsuspected problems that may be corrected in the operating room.

Results from primary surgical closure of VSDs are generally excellent. Surgical mortality is less than 1 percent in centers with extensive experience, when surgery is performed during the early months of life prior to the evolution of PVOD. Operative risk should be even lower in older children if the pulmonary vascular resistance remains low. The pulmonary vascular bed responds favorably when the systemic-to-pulmonary shunt is eliminated before age 2 years. Normal life expectancy and functional capabilities should be anticipated postoperatively. Survival 25 years after the closure of a VSD is approximately 95 percent.[64] The mortality rate is unquestionably higher among patients who are operated on with $R_p > 7$ Wood's units.

The surgical repair of a multiple muscular VSD has been more problematic. The highly trabecular right ventricular septal surface can make the localization of all the defects difficult. A new approach has achieved successful closure from a right ventricular apical infundibulotomy.[65] Recently, devices now approved by the U.S. Food and Drug Administration (FDA) have become available to close these defects in the catheterization laboratory.[66] Other devices are now in phase 2 testing.

Between February 1989 and July 1998, 148 transcatheter closures were preformed at Children's Hospital in Boston with no deaths or late morbidity resulting from catheter-related events. By echocardiography, 83 percent of the defects were closed or had trivial residual leaks.[66] The relative role of surgery versus interventional catheterization closure remains to be determined in this subset with multiple trabeculated septal defects.

Atrial Septal Defect

DEFINITION
An ASD is a through-and-through communication between the atria at the septal level. It is to be distinguished from a patent foramen ovale, which may persist into adulthood.

PATHOLOGY
ASDs are usually sufficiently large to allow free communication between the atria. They may be subdivided according to anatomic location[67] (Fig. 73-8).

ANATOMIC TYPES

Defect at the Fossa Ovalis (Ostium Secundum) This defect classically involves the region of the fossa ovalis and is the most common type (70 percent)[67,68] (Fig. 73-8A and C). Atrial septal tissue separates the inferior edge of the defect from the AV valves. Associated partial anomalous pulmonary venous connections are not uncommon, with one or more of the right pulmonary veins draining into the right atrium or one of its tributaries. Mitral valve prolapse is present in some cases.

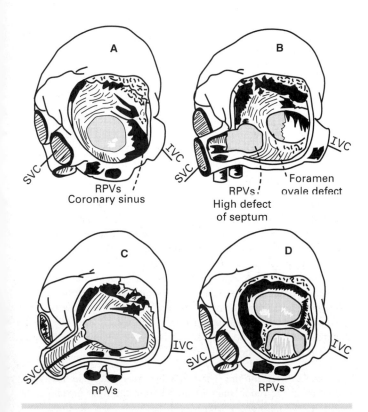

FIGURE 73-8 Types of interatrial communications. *A.* Large ostium secundum type of atrial septal defect. *B.* So-called sinus venosus type of defect—one high in the atrial septum associated with anomalous connection of the right superior pulmonary vein to the junctional area of the superior vena cava and right atrium. *C.* Very large ostium secundum type of atrial septal defect with absence of the posterior rim. *D.* Partial form of common atrioventricular canal with cleft mitral valve. SVC = superior vena cava; RPVs = right pulmonary veins; IVC = inferior vena cava. (From Lewis FJ et al.[67] Copyright 1957, American Medical Association. Reproduced with permission from the publisher and authors.)

Partial Atrioventricular Canal Defects Defects of the AV septum, which lies inferior to the fossa ovalis, constitute approximately 20 percent of ASDs and are part of a complex malformation known as *common atrioventricular canal defects*, which are considered below (Fig. 73-8D).

Sinus Venosus Defects These defects, accounting for approximately 6 percent of the total, appear to represent a biatrial connection of the superior vena cava (or, in rare instances, the inferior vena cava), which straddles the otherwise normal intact atrial septum. Also involved is an anomalous termination of one or more of the right-sided pulmonary veins either into the vena cava or into the right atrium near its junction with the vena cava (Fig. 63-8B).

Coronary Sinus Defects A coronary sinus defect is an uncommon type of ASD located in the position normally occupied by the ostium of the coronary sinus. This defect is part of a developmental complex consisting of the absence of the coronary sinus and entry of the left superior vena cava directly into the left atrium.

Conditions Common to All Anatomic Types The right atrial and ventricular chambers as well as the central pulmonary arteries become enlarged. When pulmonary hypertension intervenes, it usually does not do so before the third decade. The earliest lesion is cellular fibrous intimal thickening in the proximal segments of arterioles. The pulmonary arterial pressure then rises, followed by the development of medial hypertrophy of muscular arteries and the appearance of plexiform lesions. The right ventricular wall hypertrophies, and atherosclerosis may occur in the major pulmonary arteries. Saccular aneurysm and thrombosis with dissecting aneurysm or rupture may occur (see above, "Pulmonary Arterial Hypertension and Pulmonary Vascular Obstructive Disease"). In the final state, the pulmonary vascular bed may be difficult to distinguish from that in VSD with PVOD.

ABNORMAL PHYSIOLOGY
Usually there is no resistance to blood flow across the defect and no significant pressure difference between the two atria. A left-to-right shunt of blood occurs (Fig. 73-9) because (1) the right atrial system is more distensible than the left, (2) the tricuspid valve is normally more capacious than the mitral valve, and (3) the thinner-walled right ventricular chamber more readily accommodates a larger volume of blood at the same filling pressure than does the left ventricle. A large left-to-right shunt may be found in a neonate or young infant before the right ventricular compliance has had time to change appreciably from that of the left ventricle. Presumably, this shunt occurs because a rapid fall in pulmonary vascular resistance encourages a larger right ventricular stroke volume, a smaller end-systolic volume, and hence an increased ability of the right ventricle to accept a larger volume of blood during the diastolic filling phase of the cardiac cycle.[69] The pulmonary arterial system undergoes normal maturation after birth, with most patients tolerating the large volume load on the right ventricle and pulmonary circuit quite well for many years. With the development of pulmonary vascular disease and PAH, the left-to-right shunt decreases, largely because of the increased thickness and decreased compliance of the right ventricle. In some patients, this process continues until there is eventually shunt reversal, with arterial desaturation and cyanosis.

CLINICAL MANIFESTATIONS
ASD is found in approximately 6 percent of children who survive beyond the first year of life with congenital heart disease.[5] *If one*

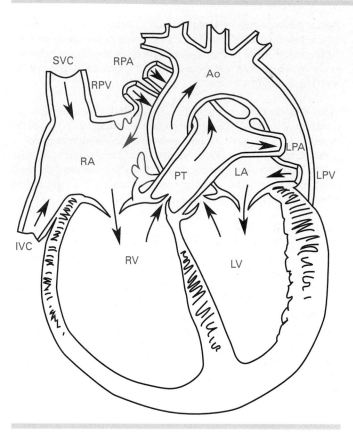

FIGURE 73-9 Atrial septal defect at fossa ovalis with left-to-right shunt. SVC = superior vena cava; IVC = inferior vena cava; RA = right atrium; RV = right ventricle; PT = main pulmonary arterial trunk; RPA = right pulmonary artery; LPA = left pulmonary artery; RPV = right pulmonary vein; LPV = left pulmonary vein; LA = left atrium; LV = left ventricle; Ao = aorta. (From Edwards JE.[68] Reproduced with permission from the publisher and author.)

excludes mitral valve prolapse and a congenitally bicuspid aortic valve, it is the most common form of congenital heart disease among adults.

ASDs are more common among females, with a female/male ratio of approximately 2:1. The mode of transmission is best explained in most instances on a multifactorial basis, in which the risk would be approximately 2.5 percent for first-degree relatives of a single affected family member. However, examples of autosomal dominant transmission are recognized[70] either as an isolated entity associated with severe AV conduction disturbances or with upper extremity malformations as in the Holt-Oram syndrome. Examples of Mendelian autosomal recessive transmission are found in the Ellis–van Creveld syndrome (see Chap. 72).

History The majority of these children are considered asymptomatic but probably most have some mild diminution of stamina, since it is not unusual for the patient or the parents to comment on the increased endurance that follows surgical correction. Symptoms of mild fatigue and dyspnea tend to be recognized in the late teens and early twenties, and at least three-quarters of these individuals will be symptomatic as adults. Congestive heart failure is rare in childhood, but a few infants, perhaps 5 percent, have heart failure in the first year of life. Failure becomes more common again in the fourth and fifth decades, usually associated with the onset of arrhythmias.[71]

Physical Examination Many of these children have a slender habitus, but normal growth and development are the rule. Prominence of the left anterior chest is common, and a hyperdynamic right ventricular systolic lift usually can be felt. Looking at the jugular venous pulse demonstrates that the *v* wave is equal to the *a* wave instead of revealing the normal *a* wave predominance. The first heart sound may be slightly accentuated at the lower left sternal border. The two components of the second heart sound are characteristically widely split, with the interval of splitting fixed despite expiration or the Valsalva maneuver. The pulmonary component of the second heart sound may be accentuated even in the absence of PAH. With increasing pulmonary arterial pressure and resistance, the interval between the aortic and pulmonary components of the second heart sound narrows and the pulmonary component becomes louder, but the lack of respiratory influence on the interval between the two components persists. A midsystolic crescendo-decrescendo murmur of grade 2 to 3 intensity is heard at the left upper sternal border, reflecting increased right ventricular stroke volume and relative pulmonary stenosis. A low- to medium-pitched early diastolic murmur over the lower left sternal border, denoting increased diastolic flow across the tricuspid valve, is present in most individuals with large shunts (see Chap. 10). Cyanosis and clubbing reflect right-to-left shunting. In this setting, the murmurs of tricuspid and pulmonary regurgitation are not uncommon.

Chest Roentgenogram Mild to moderate cardiac enlargement and prominence of the main and branch pulmonary arteries are characteristic. The absence of left atrial displacement of the barium-filled esophagus in the lateral view helps distinguish ASD from large left-to-right shunts at other levels (Fig. 73-10).

Electrocardiogram An rsR$^+$ pattern over the right precordium indicating mild right ventricular conduction delay or mild right ventricular hypertrophy is characteristic though not pathognomonic of secundum-type ASD. The mean QRS axis in the frontal plane is 90 degrees or greater in 60 percent of patients. Left-axis deviation is common in primum-type ASD. Abnormal leftward *p* axis is often present in sinus venosus–type ASD. Atrial fibrillation and atrial flutter are usually limited to adults.

Echocardiogram M-mode studies reflect volume overload of the right side of the heart with increased right atrial and right ventricular dimensions and paradoxical ventricular septal motion. Two-dimensional and Doppler echocardiography with color-flow mapping (see Chap. 75) permits identification and visualization of secundum, AV canal, and sinus venosus defects. Visualization of anomalous draining pulmonary veins is slightly more difficult. The transesophageal approach offers excellent images for those patients in whom the transthoracic approach is inadequate.[72] Recently three-dimensional (3D) echocardiograms have been shown to provide excellent images of the atrial defects[73,74] (Fig. 73-11).

Cardiac Catheterization There is a significant increase in oxygen saturation in the blood samples drawn from the right atrium, right ventricle, and pulmonary artery compared with those obtained from the superior or inferior vena cava. Pulmonary arterial and right ventricular systolic pressures are normal or only slightly elevated. A systolic pressure gradient of up to 20 mmHg across the right ventricular outflow tract is accepted as being secondary to flow rather than to organic obstruction. The right and left atrial mean and phasic pressures are virtually identical, with little if any elevation above normal (mean pressure gradient <3 mmHg) unless there are associated abnormalities.

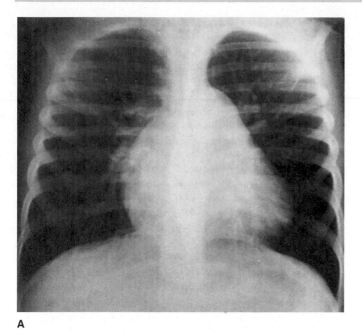

A

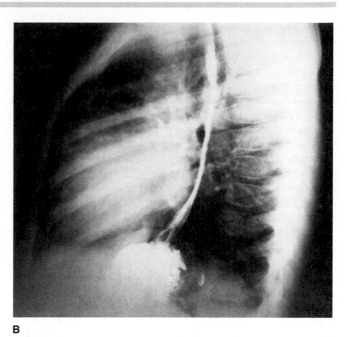

B

FIGURE 73-10 Chest roentgenogram of a 4-year-old child with a secundum atrial septal defect, a large left-to-right shunt, and normal pulmonary arterial pressures. *A.* Frontal. *B.* Lateral. Right ventricular enlargement (seen in the lateral view) accompanies prominence of the main pulmonary arterial segment and increased blood flow. No left atrial dilation is present.

NATURAL HISTORY AND PROGNOSIS

Defects of the secundum type usually go undetected in the first year or two of life because of the lack of symptoms and the unimpressive auscultatory findings. A soft systolic murmur is the usual reason for referral. Symptoms become more common in persons in their late teens and twenties, and by age 40 the majority of these individuals are symptomatic, some severely so.[75] Pulmonary vascular disease with serious pulmonary hypertension begins to make its appearance in the early twenties. *It affects approximately 15 percent of young adults, particularly women, and may be rapidly progressive, especially with pregnancy.* The incidence of atrial fibrillation or flutter also increases with each decade and is closely linked to the onset of congestive failure. Spontaneous closure of moderate and large secundum defects is unlikely beyond the first 2 years of life.[71] Heart failure is the most common cause of death among unoperated patients. Other causes of death include pulmonary embolism or thrombosis, paradoxical emboli, brain abscess, and infection.

MEDICAL MANAGEMENT

The few infants who present with symptoms of congestive failure can be treated with anticongestive therapy. If the defect is uncomplicated and the symptoms persist, surgical closure is advised without further delay. For asymptomatic infants and children, closure is recommended just before entry into school. Restrictions of activity or exercise are unnecessary. If the physical, laboratory, and echocardiographic findings are completely characteristic, preoperative catheterization is not necessary. Closure is recommended if the defect is associated with right ventricular volume overload on echocardiography. In those with pulmonary hypertension, closure is recommended for patients with $\dot{Q}_p/\dot{Q}_s$ ratios >1.5:1 by catheterization provided that the systemic arterial saturation is >92 percent and total R_p < 15 Wood's units.[76] Closure is prudent before pregnancy or the use of contraceptives in view of the tendency to develop rapidly progressive PVOD in this setting. Transcatheter closure of centrally located secundum ASDs in older infants, children, and adults using various devices appears to be an acceptable alternative to surgical closure and is now the preferred method in many centers.[77–80] *Infective endocarditis is rare, and antibiotic coverage at times of possible bacteremia is recommended only if associated mitral valve disease is suspected.*

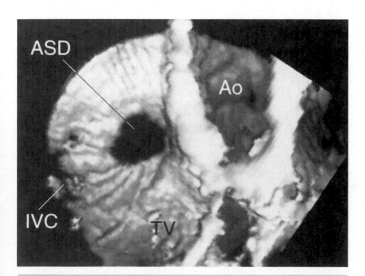

FIGURE 73-11 Three-dimensional echocardiogram of a secundum atrial septal defect (ASD). This is a right atrial en-face view that shows the size, shape, and position of the defect in relation to the right atrial septal surface. Ao = aortic valve; TV = tricuspid valve; IVC = inferior vena cava. (Courtesy of Dr. Gerry Marx.)

SURGICAL MANAGEMENT

Defects of the interatrial septum are exposed through the lateral wall of the right atrium. Ostium secundum (fossa ovalis) defects are frequently closed by direct suturing; a very large defect or one with tenuous margins is closed with a patch, usually glutaraldehyde-treated autologous pericardium. Anomalous pulmonary veins are sought along the posterolateral aspect of the superior or inferior vena cava and from within the right atrium before closure of the defect. Sutures are placed with care along the posterior rim of the inferior vena caval orifice to prevent the creation of a tunnel from the inferior vena cava into the left atrium, which would cause postoperative hypoxemia.

High ASDs of the sinus venosus type, which are often associated with anomalous drainage of one or more right pulmonary veins into the superior vena cava, are corrected by means of the placement of a pericardial or tubular Dacron patch from above the abnormally draining vein or veins down to and around the ASD (Fig. 73-12). Pulmonary venous blood thus is diverted through the ASD into the left atrium. Pericardial gusset enlargement of the superior vena cava at the cavoatrial junction may be required. Anomalous right pulmonary veins draining to the right atrium are diverted into the left atrium by placement of a patch baffle well anterior and to the right of the pulmonary vein orifices. The risks of surgery are minimal (less than 0.5 percent), with virtually all these children home by the fourth postoperative day.

In adults, clinical benefit after closure of ASDs can be anticipated even in those with significant physiologic compromise, but mortality is higher than it is in the young and the magnitude of improvement is less certain. Nonetheless, closure of ASDs is advised even when R_p approaches 15 Wood's units because of the excessive morbidity and mortality associated with a persistent interatrial communication.[81] *Morbidity in adults and the low risk of surgical closure in young children mandate closure in the preschool or preadolescent years.*

Although life-threatening complications after closure of ASDs in children are rare, transient postoperative atrial arrhythmias and postpericardiotomy syndrome with pericardial effusions occasionally are seen. The long-term prognosis for a normal life expectancy and functional capability is excellent for patients who have closure of an uncomplicated ASD during the first two decades of life.

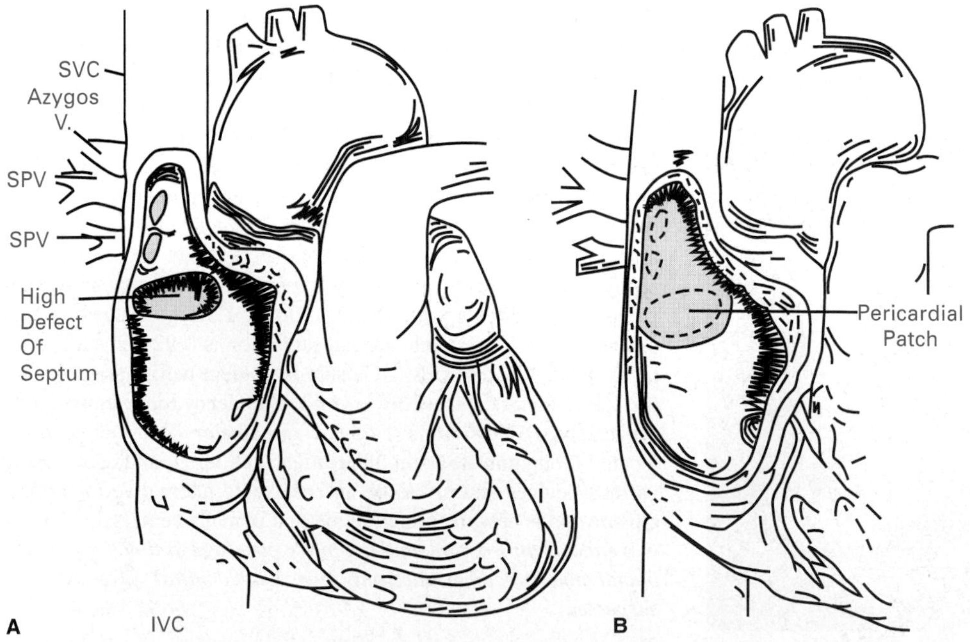

Partial Anomalous Pulmonary Venous Connection

PATHOLOGY
In partial anomalous pulmonary venous connection, one or more but not all of the pulmonary veins enter the right atrium or its venous tributaries. An ASD is usually present, but the atrial septum may rarely be intact. There are many patterns of anomalous pulmonary venous connection, but the four most common, in order of decreasing frequency, are (1) pulmonary veins from the right upper and/or middle lobe to the superior vena cava, usually with a sinus venosus ASD; (2) all the right pulmonary veins to the right atrium, usually in the polysplenia syndrome; (3) all the right pulmonary veins to the inferior vena cava, entering this systemic vein just above or below the diaphragm; and (4) the left upper or both left pulmonary veins to an anomalous vertical vein draining to the left brachiocephalic vein.

When the right pulmonary veins are connected to the inferior vena cava, the atrial septum may be intact. This venous anomaly may be isolated or may be part of the *scimitar syndrome*. That syndrome includes hypoplasia of the right lung, bronchial abnormalities, anomalous systemic pulmonary arterial supply to the right lung from branches of the descending thoracic and/or abdominal aorta, and dextroposition of the heart.

CLINICAL MANIFESTATIONS
In an old autopsy series, partial anomalous pulmonary venous connection occurred in 0.6 percent of 801 cases,[82] a much higher incidence than clinically suspected, suggesting that many cases may not be recognized during life. There is no sex predilection. Approximately 15 percent of all ASDs have this coexisting anomaly; however, in the case of the sinus venosus type, the association is in the range of 85 percent.

History When partial anomalous pulmonary venous connection coexists with an ASD, the symptoms, as well as the other clinical manifestations, are indistinguishable from those of an isolated ASD. Isolated, uncomplicated anomalous connection of a single pulmonary vein usually goes undetected clinically, since in this circumstance only about 20 percent of the pulmonary venous flow returns to the right atrium or its tributaries. When the entire venous return from one lung or two pulmonary veins is connected anomalously, approximately 65 percent of the pulmonary venous flow returns to the right side of the heart and the symptoms are similar to those of an ASD with a comparable increase in pulmonary blood flow.

Physical Examination The findings are the same as those in patients with an ASD with the exception that *the two components of the second heart sound, though usually widely split, move normally with respiration if the atrial septum is intact.*

Chest Roentgenogram Right ventricular enlargement, pulmonary arterial

FIGURE 73-12 *A.* Sinus venosus type of atrial septal defect, with its constantly accompanying anomalous pulmonary venous connection of superior pulmonary vein (SPV) to superior vena cava (SVC). *B.* Repair is accomplished with a pericardial patch placed to divert pulmonary venous blood across the defect into the left atrium and to divert superior vena caval blood to the right atrium. IVC = inferior vena cava. (This illustration appeared originally in the first edition of *The Heart,* in 1966 and again in all subsequent editions. It is reproduced here by courtesy of Dr. John W. Kirklin, Birmingham, Alabama.)

dilatation, and increased pulmonary blood flow are characteristic when more than one pulmonary vein connects anomalously. With anomalous connection of the right pulmonary veins to the inferior vena cava, the pulmonary venous pattern may assume a crescent-shaped or scimitar curve in the right lower lung field along the right lower heart border (scimitar).

Electrocardiogram   The ECG is normal (in the case of anomalous connection of a single pulmonary vein) or reflects volume overload of the right side of the heart, as was described above under "Atrial Septal Defect."

Echocardiogram   If more than one pulmonary vein drains anomalously, the volume is usually sufficient to produce the characteristic pattern of right ventricular diastolic overload. Failure to visualize an atrial septal with two-dimensional imaging and color-flow mapping from a subcostal coronal or high right-sided parasternal longitudinal view should arouse suspicion of anomalous venous return. A variety of views supplemented by color-flow mapping may be necessary to identify the anomalous connection.[83]

Cardiac Catheterization   Anomalously connected pulmonary veins may be entered directly with the venous catheter. Selective biplane angiograms in these vessels will document their site of connection. Left-to-right shunting with partial anomalous pulmonary venous connection and an intact atrial septum is usually small or moderate and may go undetected by oximetry techniques. Selective indicator dilution curves in the right and left pulmonary arteries with systemic arterial sampling can detect the lung with the anomalous pulmonary venous connection, and selective biplane angiograms in the pulmonary arterial branches will visualize these connections.

NATURAL HISTORY AND PROGNOSIS
Patients with partial anomalous pulmonary venous connection with ASD appear to follow a course similar if not identical to that of patients with an isolated ASD. When the atrial septum is intact, the course depends primarily on the volume of pulmonary venous blood returning to the right side of the heart. Rarely, PVOD may be found even in the presence of a single anomalously connected pulmonary vein and an intact atrial septum.[84]

Increasing left atrial pressure caused by mitral valve disease or diminished left ventricular compliance will, in the course of time, encourage redistribution of pulmonary arterial blood flow to the portion of the lung drained by the more compliant right atrium. Thus, patients who were initially asymptomatic with a modest volume of anomalous pulmonary venous return in youth may become symptomatic and even develop heart failure in adult life.

MEDICAL MANAGEMENT
Asymptomatic patients with small shunts require no treatment. Those with symptoms, larger pulmonary blood flows, congestive failure, or PAH require surgical correction. With an intact atrial septum, precise preoperative identification of the site of the anomalous venous connection is essential. Long-term follow-up in patients who have not had surgery is indicated to detect increasing flow or the appearance of PAH.

SURGICAL MANAGEMENT
Anomalous connection of a right pulmonary vein or veins to the superior vena cava usually is associated with a sinus venosus ASD (Fig. 73-12). (see "Atrial Septal Defect, Surgical Management," above.) Partial anomalous pulmonary veins draining to the superior vena

cava, inferior vena cava, or right atrium are repaired by diversion through the ASD into the left atrium, using a patch baffle. Isolated left-sided anomalous pulmonary veins draining to the left ascending vertical vein or the left superior vena cava are detached and anastomosed directly to the left atrial appendage. Long-term morbidity and mortality are minimal among patients with uncomplicated partial pulmonary venous connections, equivalent to those observed after closure of an ASD.

Common Atrioventricular Canal Defects

DEFINITION
AV canal defects are characterized by defects in isolation or combination including an ASD in the lowermost part of the atrial septum (ostium primum), a cleft of the mitral valve (either alone or in combination with a cleft of the tricuspid valve), or VSD. In the most severe form (complete AV canal defect), there is a large ostium primum ASD, a large VSD in the upper muscular septum and a common AV valve straddling the ventricular septum. The condition appears to result from incomplete growth of the AV endocardial cushions and the AV septum.

PATHOLOGY
The ostium primum type of ASD is characterized by a crescent-shaped upper border with no septal tissue forming the lower border. The lower aspect of the defect is bounded by the atrial surfaces of the AV valves and, in the complete type (see below), in part by the upper edge of the ventricular septum. A small amount of septal tissue separates the defect from the posterior atrial wall.

ANATOMIC TYPES
Variations occur with respect to the nature of the AV valves. Rogers and Edwards first introduced the terms *partial* and *complete* to describe these types.[85]

Partial Type   The ostium primum ASD is associated with a "cleft" in the anterior mitral leaflet or, probably more accurately, a septal commissure between the superior and inferior leaflets of the left AV valve (Figs. 73-8*D* and 73-13).[68] The tricuspid valve is not cleft or shows a minor central deficiency. The ventricular aspects of the anterior mitral valve elements are fused to the upper edge of the deficient ventricular septum, precluding an interventricular communication. If there is no atrial septal tissue or if the atrial septum is so rudimentary that it produces a common chamber involving both atria, the term *common atrium* or *single atrium* is applied.

Complete Type   The complete type of common AV canal is characterized by failure of partitioning of the primitive canal into separate AV orifices. The orifice between the atria and the ventricles is guarded by a common valve with the anterior leaflet derived from the ventral AV endocardial cushion and represents the anterior halves of the anterior mitral and septal tricuspid leaflets. The posterior leaflet originates from the dorsal AV endocardial cushion and represents the posterior halves of the anterior mitral and septal tricuspid leaflets.

Usually, considerable space exists between the anterior and posterior leaflets above and the ventricular septum below; thus, in most cases of the complete type, there is free communication between the ventricles.

Rastelli and associates[86] subdivided the complete variety into three subgroups—types A, B, and C—on the basis of the structure of the common anterior leaflet and its chordal attachments to the ventricular septum and/or papillary muscles (Fig. 73-14). Considering

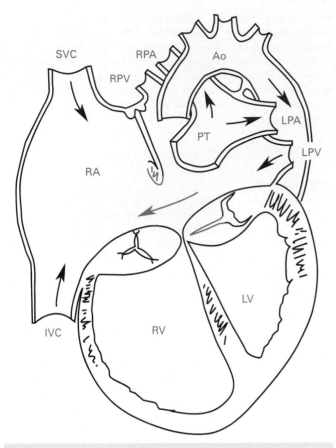

FIGURE 73-13 Common atrioventricular canal of the partial type. The mitral valve shows a cleft in its anterior leaflet, while the tricuspid valve is undisturbed. SVC = superior vena cava; IVC = inferior vena cava; RPA = right pulmonary artery; LPA = left pulmonary artery; RPV = right pulmonary vein; LPV = left pulmonary vein; LV = left ventricle; Ao = aorta. (From Edwards JE.[68] Reproduced with permission from the publisher and author.)

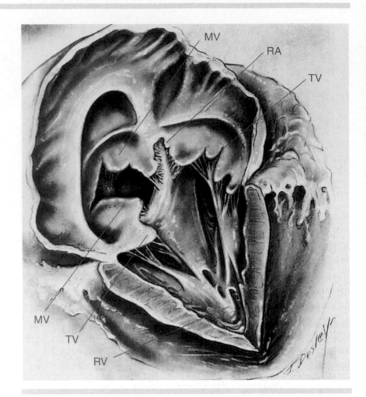

FIGURE 73-14 Complete form of common atrioventricular canal, type A. The common anterior leaflet has a recognizable mitral valve component (MV) and tricuspid valve component (TV). In type B, not illustrated, those components are attached by chordae to a papillary muscle in the right ventricle. In type C, not illustrated, the common anterior leaflet is a single unit without any attachment to the underlying ventricular septum. Type A is most amenable to repair. RV = right ventricle; RA = right atrium. (From Rastelli GC et al.[86] Reproduced with permission from the publisher and authors.)

the posterior common leaflet, there is variation among the three types in regard to the presence or absence of subdivision and whether the posterior leaflet is attached to the ventricular septum by chordae or by an imperforate membrane.

Variations from the classic types of AV canal defects are recognized, the most common being the AV canal type of isolated VSD, isolated ostium primum ASD without malformed AV valves, and isolated cleft of the anterior mitral or septal tricuspid valve leaflets.

ASSOCIATED CONDITIONS

In the asplenia syndrome, the complete variety is almost universal; with polysplenia, it occurs in about one-quarter of cases.[87] An ASD of the secundum type is present in about half of these cases. A double orifice of the mitral valve may be associated with the incomplete type, and tetralogy of Fallot may be associated with the complete type.

ABNORMAL PHYSIOLOGY

If the communication at the ventricular level is large, the right ventricular and pulmonary artery pressures will be elevated. These patients are similar to those with large VSDs. Patients with a communication at the atrial level usually have only normal or slightly elevated systolic pressures in the right side of the heart and a large pulmonary blood flow, as in the secundum type of ASD. Defects in the tricuspid

valve, mitral valve, or both may result in severe regurgitation or direct shunting of blood from the left ventricle to the right atrium.

CLINICAL MANIFESTATIONS

Approximately 3 percent of infants and children with congenital heart disease have AV canal defects. The majority, some 60 to 70 percent, have the complete form with the female/male ratio approximately 1.3:1. Well over half the patients with the complete form have associated Down's syndrome. Among children with Down's syndrome, 45 percent have some form of congenital heart disease, with malformations of the type involving the AV canal comprising approximately 50 percent of these abnormalities.[88]

History Only if the mitral valve is incompetent do the symptoms of patients with partial AV canal differ from those associated with a secundum type of ASD. The complete form of AV canal or the partial form connected with significant mitral regurgitation may be associated with poor weight gain, easy fatigue, tachypnea, repeated respiratory infections, and congestive heart failure. Patients with complete AV canal are almost invariably very sick.

Physical Examination The findings with a partial defect are those of an ASD. If the cleft anterior mitral leaflet is incompetent, the findings of mitral regurgitation also will be present. The physical findings with the complete AV canal defect are those of a very large VSD, usually with full-blown congestive failure, but the second heart sound is split and fixed. The murmur of mitral regurgitation may not be heard or recognized as such.

Chest Roentgenogram   Overall cardiac enlargement that is out of proportion to the degree of pulmonary plethora or a cardiac silhouette, suggesting combined ventricular dilatation, may serve to distinguish an uncomplicated secundum ASD from a primum defect with significant mitral regurgitation. Marked cardiac enlargement and severe pulmonary overcirculation are features of the complete AV canal defect.

Electrocardiogram   One of the most helpful diagnostic features in distinguishing individuals with AV canal defects from those with isolated ASDs or VSDs is the characteristic superior orientation of the mean QRS axis in the frontal plane, with a right bundle branch delay in the precordial leads. Between 92 and 95 percent of both types of canal have a QRS axis lying between 0 and -150 degrees. The patterns of atrial and ventricular hypertrophy reflect the underlying hemodynamic abnormalities.

Echocardiogram   Two-dimensional echo is capable of visualizing the extent of septal defects and, with Doppler study and color-flow mapping, left-to-right shunting at the atrial and/or ventricular level and associated mitral and/or tricuspid valvular regurgitation (Fig. 73-15). The anatomic features of the anterior AV leaflet and its connections may be visualized with sufficient clarity to permit subdivision of complete AV canal defects into types A, B, and C (Fig. 73-14). Straddling AV valves, a double-orifice mitral valve, single papillary muscles, and hypoplasia or outflow obstruction of the right or left ventricle also can be determined with this technique.[89]

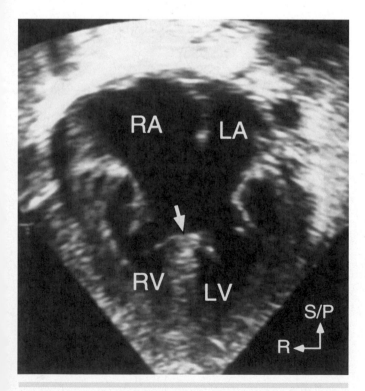

FIGURE 73-15 Apical four-chamber view of complete common atrioventricular canal. Note the large deficiency of both atrial and ventricular septa as well as apical displacement of the AV valves. The arrow points to the attachment of the inferior bridging leaflet to the ventricular septal crest. (From Levine and Geva.[89] Reproduced with permission from the publisher and authors.)

Cardiac Catheterization   Cardiac catheterization is rarely performed if the echocardiogram is characteristic and if the history, clinical examination, and echo suggest a large left-to-right shunt and low pulmonary resistance. When it is performed, a significant increase in oxygen saturation between the superior vena cava and the right atrium is present. A right ventricular or pulmonary arterial systolic pressure in excess of 60 percent of the systemic systolic pressure favors the presence of a complete canal. With a large communication between the two ventricles below the AV valves, the right ventricular, pulmonary arterial, and systemic arterial systolic pressures are virtually identical. Left ventricular angiography in the frontal view demonstrates the "gooseneck deformity" of the left ventricular outflow tract that is characteristic of AV canal malformations and allows a semiquantitative assessment of the degree of mitral regurgitation and shunting from the left ventricle to the right atrium. The left anterior oblique view with craniocaudal angulation is recommended for visualizing the interventricular defect and judging the extent of ventricular septal deficiency. Aortography is essential to eliminate the possibility of a PDA if the echocardiogram was not diagnostic.

NATURAL HISTORY AND PROGNOSIS

Partial defects without significant mitral regurgitation follow a course similar to that described for the secundum type of septal defects. An exception would be the greater likelihood of infective endocarditis because of the mitral valve deformity. Moderate or severe mitral regurgitation produces heart failure with resulting symptoms and growth retardation. Infants with a complete AV canal without protective pulmonary stenosis quickly develop and continue to have congestive failure until the course is altered by death, the development of PVOD, or surgical intervention.

MEDICAL MANAGEMENT

Children with an uncomplicated partial defect are managed in the same manner as children with an uncomplicated ASD. Those who are symptomatic should undergo early surgical closure of the primum ASD and plication of the cleft in the septal commissure of the left AV ("mitral") valve. The few patients with significant residual mitral regurgitation after surgery are managed medically until mitral valve replacement is appropriate. Those without symptoms are repaired before they start school.

The approach to an infant with complete AV canal is the same as that for an infant with a large VSD but is tempered by the knowledge that spontaneous improvement is very unlikely except at the expense of the pulmonary vascular bed. Repair is recommended by 6 months of age or earlier with intractable heart failure. Elevation of pulmonary vascular resistance in the first year of life warrants surgical intervention without delay.

With regard to genetic counseling, the risk of a subsequent sibling having heart disease in the presence of a single affected family member is in the range of 2 percent; it is probably higher for the offspring of an affected parent, particularly if that parent is the mother.[90] Concordance for AV canal defects among affected siblings or offspring is much higher than it is with other forms of congenital heart disease and approaches 90 percent.

SURGICAL MANAGEMENT

The remarkable clinical improvement that follows anatomic repair of complete common AV septal defects in infancy encourages early correction early in the first year of life.[91] Banding of the pulmonary artery in a critically ill infant with a large ventricular defect was used in the past but has been replaced by operative repair in most centers. The specifics of repair are dictated by anatomic detail: individual

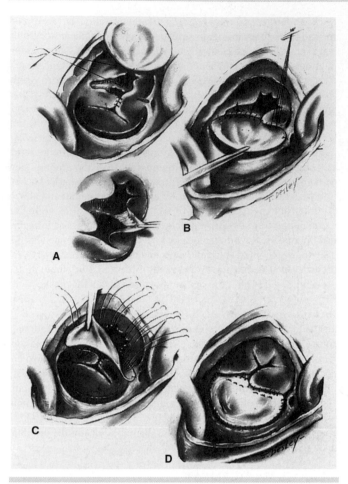

FIGURE 73-16 Steps in the repair of the complete form of common atrioventricular canal, type A. *A* and *B*. A pericardial patch is sutured to the ventricular septum. *C* and *D*. The anterior leaflet of the mitral valve is reconstructed and attached to the patch. A portion of the tricuspid leaflet is attached to the patch. (From Rastelli et al.[86] Reproduced with permission from the publisher and authors.)

variation is considerable (Fig. 73-16), but the creation of a competent, nonstenotic left-sided AV ("mitral") valve is essential for an acceptable early and long-term prognosis.

A patch is usually sutured to the right side of the ventricular septum to obliterate the interventricular communication. The anterior and posterior components of the common valve are divided, and the mitral valve is sutured to the patch at an appropriate level. The "cleft" between the left anterior and posterior leaflets is sutured to provide competence without the creation of stenosis. Prosthetic valve implantation rarely is required during primary anatomic repair.[92] The right-sided AV ("tricuspid") apparatus, although less critical to survival, is repaired using the same principles. The interatrial communication is usually closed with a separate piece of pericardium to minimize hemolysis in the presence of residual mitral regurgitation.[92] Mitral valve competence is assessed by gentle distention of the left ventricle with cold saline and more recently transesophageal echocardiography.

A partial AV canal is repaired through a right atriotomy. The cleft may be closed with a few simple interrupted sutures to encourage inversion and coaptation of the leaflet margins. The ASD usually is closed with a pericardial patch.

Permanent complete heart block once contributed substantially to early mortality and morbidity but is now rare. Patients undergoing re-

pair of a partial AV canal should be observed for the possible development of subaortic left ventricular outflow tract obstruction caused by redundant or residual endocardial cushion tissue.

In-hospital mortality after correction of a complete AV canal in infancy ranges from 3 to 10 percent[93,94]; the highest mortality is encountered during the first few months of life and in infants with severe AV valve regurgitation, elevated pulmonary vascular resistance, hypoplasia of the left or right ventricle, or other cardiac malformations. At Children's Hospital in Boston, 191 children with a median age of 4.6 months were repaired between January 1990 and December 1998, with an operative mortality of 1.5 percent. Reoperation was necessary in 22 patients (11.7 percent), a mean of 20 months later: 18 for residual mitral regurgitation and 4 for left ventricular outflow tract obstruction.[95] Successful correction of a complete AV canal can be accomplished despite associated tetralogy of Fallot, double-outlet ventricle, and other complex anomalies.[92]

EXTRACARDIAC COMMUNICATIONS BETWEEN THE SYSTEMIC AND PULMONARY CIRCULATIONS, USUALLY WITHOUT CYANOSIS

Patent Ductus Arteriosus

DEFINITION

Patent ductus arteriosus, the most common type of extracardiac shunt, represents persistent patency of the vessel that normally connects the pulmonary arterial system and the aorta in a fetus (Fig. 73-17).

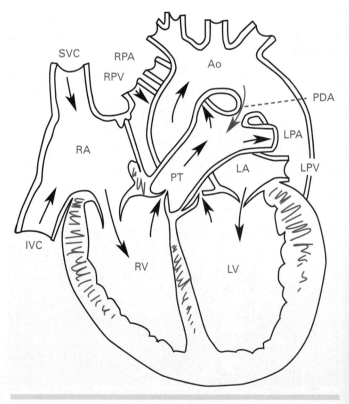

FIGURE 73-17 Patent ductus arteriosus (PDA). SVC = superior vena cava; IVC = inferior vena cava; RA = right atrium; RV = right ventricle; PT = main pulmonary arterial trunk; RPA = right pulmonary artery; LPA = left pulmonary artery; RPV = right pulmonary vein; LPV = left pulmonary vein; LA = left atrium; LV = left ventricle; Ao = aorta. (From Edwards JE.[68] Reproduced with permission from the publisher and author.)

PATHOLOGY

The ductus arteriosus usually closes within 2 or 3 days after birth and becomes the *ligamentum arteriosum*, but it may remain patent for several months prior to spontaneous closure. It courses from the origin of the left pulmonary artery below to the lower aspect of the aortic arch just beyond the level of origin of the left subclavian artery above. The recurrent branch of the left vagus nerve hooks around its lateral and inferior aspects. Constriction of the ductus postnatally involves a complex interaction of increased partial pressure of oxygen, decreased circulating PGE_2, decreased PGE_2 ductal receptors, and decreased pressure within the ductus. Subsequent vessel-wall hypoxia of the ductus promotes further closure through inhibition of prostaglandin and nitric oxide within the ductal wall.[96] Exogenous PGE_1 has been used extensively to keep the ductus open postnatally,[97] and indomethacin, a prostaglandin inhibitor, can close the ductus in many premature infants in whom persistent patency is disadvantageous.[98]

ABNORMAL PHYSIOLOGY

Patients with PDA may be divided into groups according to whether the vascular resistance through the ductus is low, moderate, or high. The resistance of the ductus is related not only to its cross-sectional area but also to its length. In patients with a very small ductus that offers high resistance, the flow across the ductus is relatively small. The extra volume of work on the left ventricle is small, and the pulmonary pressure and resistance are not elevated. Patients with only moderate resistance in the ductus have some increase in pulmonary artery pressure, with a moderately greater volume of shunting across the ductus.

In patients with a large patent ductus, the aorta and pulmonary artery are essentially in free communication; the systolic pressure in the pulmonary artery is equal to that in the aorta. Left ventricular volume overload results from recirculation through the lungs, with pulmonary congestion resulting from increased pulmonary flow and/or left ventricular failure. The left ventricle compensates by dilation followed in many cases by hypertrophy, and the pulmonary vasculature may respond to the high pressure (see "Pulmonary Arterial Hypertension," above). The right ventricle is subjected to a pressure load.

If the pulmonary resistance equals or exceeds the resistance of the systemic circulation, there is right-to-left shunting from the pulmonary artery to the aorta, resulting in hypoxemia, especially in the lower body and legs.

CLINICAL MANIFESTATIONS

History   The history of the mother's pregnancy and of perinatal events may provide clues associated with a high incidence of PDA, such as exposure to rubella in the first trimester in a nonimmunized mother. PDA is also more common in premature infants, especially those with birth asphyxia or respiratory distress.[99]

Symptoms are usually restricted to patients with large shunts that produce heart failure or with other complicating problems, such as respiratory distress in a premature infant. The symptoms related to heart failure were discussed above. Heart failure is most likely to develop in the first few weeks or months of life. If it does not appear during infancy, it is unlikely to occur before the third decade. Growth may be affected in those with large shunts and failure. The clinical presentation in a premature infant is usually very different from that in a full-term infant, particularly in one with a birth weight under 1.5 kg, who is more likely to have moderate to severe respiratory distress. In these infants, the clinical features of respiratory distress occur very early following delivery requiring mechanical ventilatory support. The inability to wean from the ventilator over the next sev-

eral days or initial improvement followed by increasing ventilatory or oxygen requirements is often the first signs that a PDA may be aggravating the clinical status.

Physical Examination   In a full-term infant or child with PDA, there is frequently a systolic thrill over the pulmonary artery and in the suprasternal notch. The peripheral pulses are generally brisk and bounding, especially with the larger shunts secondary to runoff from the aorta to the pulmonary artery in diastole. A patient with elevated pulmonary vascular resistance and a right-to-left shunt will have "differential cyanosis," with cyanosis and clubbing of the toes but not the fingers, related to shunting of hypoxemic blood from the pulmonary artery into the descending aorta. The apical impulse may be increased or displaced in those with large shunts. The right ventricular impulse is increased in a premature infant with respiratory distress and in infants and children with significant pulmonary hypertension. The typical murmur is a continuous or "machinery" murmur best heard at the left upper sternal border and below the left clavicle. It is usually a rough murmur with eddy sounds, which are helpful in making the diagnosis, and it peaks at or near the second heart sound. In patients with at least a moderate shunt, there is a mid-diastolic rumble at the apex as a result of relative mitral stenosis from increased flow across the mitral valve. The second heart sound may be difficult to hear because of the continuous murmur, but it is usually normal. The pulmonary component is accentuated in those with pulmonary hypertension.

Chest Roentgenogram   Findings on chest roentgenography are also dependent on the magnitude of the shunt. In patients with a small shunt, the chest roentgenogram is normal. With larger shunts, the left atrium and left ventricle are enlarged. Increases in pulmonary arterial flow on x-ray parallel the magnitude of the shunt. In the presence of heart failure, there are signs of pulmonary edema. In older patients who have developed Eisenmenger physiology, the only abnormality may be marked prominence of the central pulmonary arteries, with rapid tapering to the periphery of the lung fields.

Electrocardiogram   With a small shunt the ECG is normal. Left atrial hypertrophy is probably the most common abnormality found, but left ventricular hypertrophy of the volume overload type, with deep Q waves and increased R-wave voltage in the left precordial leads, is also common as the shunt's size increases and left ventricular dilation occurs. Right ventricular hypertrophy is seen with pulmonary hypertension.

Echocardiogram   In moderate to large shunts, there is left atrial enlargement, and the left ventricular end-diastolic dimension and mean velocity of circumferential fiber shortening are increased significantly. Small shunts can be detected with color-flow Doppler imaging with a typical spectral flow pattern in the pulmonary artery, while a larger ductus can be visualized with two-dimensional echocardiography. Occasionally, a trivial amount of flow is seen through the ductus as an incidental finding in those with or without associated heart disease.

Cardiac Catheterization   In those with typical, uncomplicated PDA, cardiac catheterization is not necessary unless closure in the catheterization lab is contemplated. When catheterization is performed, the catheter usually passes preferentially from the left pulmonary artery into the descending aorta except when the ductus is too small. The saturation is increased in the pulmonary artery compared with the right atrium and ventricle to a degree relative to the size of the shunt. The pulmonary arterial and right ventricular pressures are elevated in those with a large ductus. The pulmonary vascular resistance is elevated in older patients who have developed changes in the pulmonary vascular bed. These patients also have diminished saturation in the descending aorta once the pulmonary resistance reaches a level that will reverse the shunt. Aortography will opacify the ductus and pulmonary arteries.

NATURAL HISTORY AND PROGNOSIS

The complications related to PDA include infective endarteritis, heart failure, and pulmonary hypertension with vascular damage. Infection of the ductus is a risk regardless of ductal size, increasing with the length of survival. The development of a mycotic aneurysm has the potential to compress the recurrent laryngeal nerve, embolize septic material to the lungs, or rupture. Calcification of the ductal wall is common in adults. In patients with large shunts, heart failure can cause significant morbidity and mortality, particularly in a premature and young infant, and sudden death can occur. Progressive damage to the pulmonary vascular bed can occur in some, but it rarely occurs to an irreversible degree in the first year of life. Once irreversible damage occurs, premature death in late adolescence or early adulthood can be anticipated.

With improved echo technology, children without associated heart disease are identified with a trivial amount of flow through a very small (<1 mm) patent ductus. Frequently, the shunt is too small to produce an audible murmur. The natural history of this echo-Doppler-discovered ductus arteriosus without clinical findings is unknown, but most think it is benign since cardiologists have not noted patients with endarteritis in a "silent" ductus.

MEDICAL MANAGEMENT

Interruption of flow through the PDA is the ultimate goal of management. For those in heart failure, usually premature infants, medical management with diuretics and fluid restriction may play a role, but the ultimate aim is closure to prevent heart failure, reduce respiratory insufficiency, promote growth in infants, and prevent infective endarteritis and pulmonary vascular disease in older children.

For premature infants, treatment with indomethacin is usually the first-line therapy.[100] Successful closure depends on both the dosage and the timing of treatment, although the major determinants seem to be birth weight and gestational age. Because of ductal recurrence, serial treatment regimens may be necessary, especially in those weighing less than 1000 g at birth. There is increasing evidence that the administration of "prophylactic" indomethacin in infants weighing less than 1000 g at birth may be associated with a higher closure rate and a better outcome, but reopening of the ductus still occurs frequently.[101] Indomethacin therapy has been associated with an increased bleeding tendency resulting from platelet dysfunction, decreased urine output secondary to renal dysfunction, and necrotizing enterocolitis.[98] In a recent study, ibuprofen achieved closure equivalent to that of indomethacin with less renal toxicity and may prove to be a suitable alternative.[102]

For premature infants whose PDA fails to close with indomethacin or for term infants with a persistent PDA, closure has been recommended. If the PDA is large, there is usually a large left-to-right shunt with congestive heart failure. In these infants, the indication for closure is heart failure and usually failure to thrive. Even in the absence of these indications, when a large PDA is associated with PAH, closure is recommended to prevent PVOD. In children with a smaller PDA with an audible murmur but no evidence of significant hemodynamic embarrassment, closure usually is recommended because of the incidence of bacterial endarteritis, in the range of 30 percent over a lifetime. For children with a PDA without a heart murmur, which usually is discovered incidentally when an echocardiogram is performed for other reasons, closure remains controversial.

SURGICAL AND INTERVENTIONAL CATHETER CLOSURE

Surgery for a persistent PDA was first reported more than 60 years ago. The safety and efficacy of this procedure even in very young children are well established, with risks that are very low (well under 1 percent), with success of interruption almost universal. The PDA is exposed and mobilized through a small left thoracotomy in the fourth intercostal space.[103] Ductus obliteration is accomplished by division or ligation. A short, broad, or thin-walled ductus is divided between vascular clamps. The ends are closed with a continuous suture. A long, narrow, thick-walled ductus can be divided or ligated with two or three sutures spaced a few millimeters apart. The suture ligatures at each end are anchored superficially in the ductus wall to prevent migration and assure thrombosis and obliteration.

The fragile, thin-walled PDA of a premature infant is obliterated by gentle ligation with a thick suture to minimize disruption or, if small, by occlusion using metallic surgical clips. Some surgeons prefer extrapleural exposure. Ligation in the neonatal intensive care unit, avoiding transport to the operating room, is common. Transport from a remote intensive care unit to a cardiac surgical unit for ductus ligation on a "day-stay" basis is also efficacious.[104] Ductus obliteration offers clinical improvement in infants weighing as little as 500 g, with minimal operative risk, a reduced incidence of necrotizing enterocolitis, a reduced duration of intubation, and improvement in late survival.

Closure of a PDA in an adult requires particular caution; calcification and rigidity of the ductus wall complicate clamping. Placement of a Dacron patch over the aortic orifice of the ductus from within the aorta may be advisable.[105]

Recently, less invasive video-assisted thorascopic surgery has been used for PDA closure. A miniature camera is inserted into the thorax; through a separate tiny incision, a surgical stapler is inserted and a clip is placed across the PDA, interrupting flow. Among 230 patients, 1 had minimal residual flow and another had persistent dysfunction of the recurrent laryngeal nerve. There were no deaths, transfusions, or chylothoraces. The mean operating time was 20 min, and the hospital stay was 2 days.[106] At Children's Hospital in Boston, this procedure has been applied to premature infants as small as 575 g, with discharge from the hospital the day after the procedure in full-term infants and children.[107]

The PDA can be closed by interventional catheterization techniques. In 1971, Portsmann and Wierny introduced a rather complex methodology to plug a PDA by using a transarterial and transvenous approach employing very large catheters.[108] More recently, Rashkind and Cuaso introduced and others have since popularized the use of a double-umbrella device to plug a PDA,[109] but the large size of the delivery sheath of the Rashkind device makes it inapplicable to young and very small children. Gianturco coils—thin metallic wires glossed with Dacron that assume a coil configuration when released from a catheter—have become an attractive alternative (Fig. 73-18). They can be delivered through relatively small catheters and have been found to be quite effective, although their utility is limited in those <8 months of age with PDAs that are more than 3.5 or 4.0 mm at the narrowest point.[110] In the others using these coils, the results have been very promising, with a 90 percent success rate. Newer devices to occlude the ductus are continuously becoming available and will probably obviate the need for surgical closure in the not too distant future.

With several highly successful, low-risk, inexpensive, and minimally traumatic procedures available to close a persistent PDA in a neonate, child, adolescent, or adult without pulmonary vascular disease, local experience should guide the preferred option in an individual child.

Sinus of Valsalva Fistula

PATHOLOGY

Sinus of Valsalva fistula is uncommon; it also is referred to as *aortic sinus aneurysm*. Because of an assumed intrinsic weakness at the union of the aorta with the heart, the aortic media may separate from the aortic annulus and retract upward. The structure that lies between becomes aneurysmal and may rupture to form a fistula. The usual sites of the defects are the posterior (noncoronary) sinus aneurysms that rupture through the atrial septal wall into the right atrium (Fig. 73-19A) and those of the right sinus that rupture into the right ventricular infundibulum (Fig. 73-19B).[111] The aneurysm is represented by a colored pouch with multiple perforations in the wall The principal associated condition is a supracristal VSD in cases with aneurysms of the right sinus (about 50 percent).

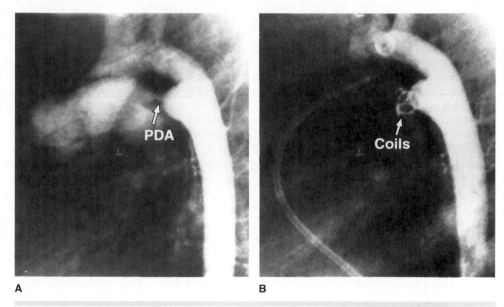

A **B**

FIGURE 73-18 Lateral angiogram showing coil occlusion of a patent ductus arteriosus. *A*. Small PDA allows shunting from descending aorta to pulmonary artery. *B*. Shunting is eliminated by a coil placed in the ductus arteriosus. (Courtesy of John F. Keane, MD.)

CLINICAL MANIFESTATIONS

Sinus of Valsalva fistulas are most common in adults.[112] When the rupture is secondary to bacterial endocarditis, evidence of a preceding infection is found. If the rupture occurs slowly, a small fistulous

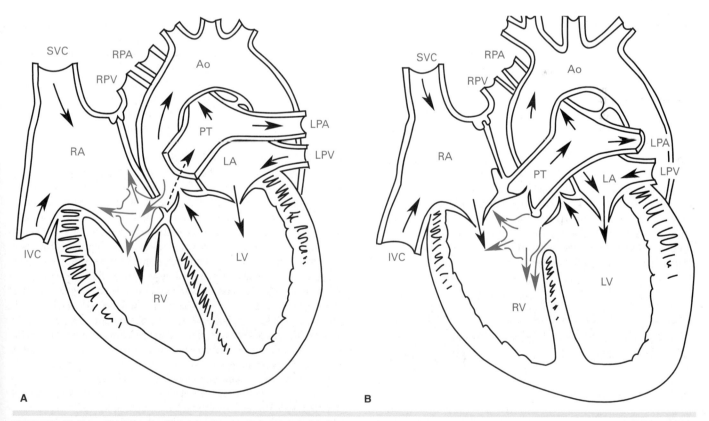

A **B**

FIGURE 73-19 Sinus of Valsalva fistula. *A*. Aneurysm involves the posterior sinus and ruptures into the right atrium. *B*. Aneurysm involves the right aortic sinus and ruptures into the right ventricle. A ventricular septal defect is commonly associated, as illustrated. SVC = superior vena cava; IVC = inferior vena cava; RA = right atrium; RV = right ventricle; PT = main pulmonary arterial trunk; RPA = right pulmonary artery; LPA = left pulmonary artery; RPV = right pulmonary vein; LPV = left pulmonary vein; I A = left atrium; LV = left ventricle; Ao = aorta. (From Edwards JE.[68] Reproduced with permission from the publisher and author.)

tract into the right atrium or ventricle develops and presents as the recent onset of a small left-to-right shunt. With sudden rupture, there is usually a tearing pain in the midchest associated with dramatically rapid development of pulmonary congestion caused by the sudden onset of a large shunt. Characteristically, the murmur is loud and continuous but is heard lower on the chest than is the murmur of PDA. A to-and-fro murmur rather than a continuous one may be heard at times. The apical impulse is hyperdynamic, and the pulse pressure is widened. VSD may complicate the clinical picture. Echocardiography or cardiac catheterization will confirm the level of the shunt. A pressure difference across the right ventricular outflow tract may be present if the right sinus is involved. Aortography or Doppler echocardiography[113] will confirm the diagnosis.

NATURAL HISTORY AND PROGNOSIS

With slow rupture and a small shunt, the major risk is infective endocarditis or extension of the rupture with an increasing shunt. With a large shunt, the heart failure is usually rapidly progressive and may result in a quick demise. A few patients seem to stabilize in this situation.

MEDICAL MANAGEMENT

Appropriate cultures should be drawn and antibiotics started if endocarditis is suspected. Treatment of heart failure should be instituted rapidly. *Because of the natural history, all patients should have this condition corrected surgically.*

SURGICAL MANAGEMENT

Aneurysms or fistulas from the noncoronary or right coronary sinuses are repaired through the aortic root while the patient is supported on total cardiopulmonary bypass with moderate hypothermia, using techniques similar to those employed for aortic valve replacement. The aortic valve leaflets, the margins of the aneurysm, and the coronary arterial orifices must be visualized precisely. Aneurysms of the noncoronary sinus can be repaired through the right atrium; those arising from the right coronary sinus are accessible through the right ventricle. In most cases, the orifice of the aneurysmal fistula is surgically obliterated using a Dacron patch. In a recent series of 129 patients, reparative methods included plication (47 percent), patch repair (40 percent), and aortic root replacement (12 percent). Sixty percent of those patients needed aortic valve replacement at the same time.[112]

A conal, or supracristal (type I), VSD must be sought and closed through either the aortic valve or the right ventricular outflow tract when an aneurysm of the right coronary sinus extends into the right ventricle. Surgical results are usually quite good. In the large series cited above, the operative survival was 96 percent, with no late deaths in an average of 5.9 years of follow-up.[112]

VALVULAR AND VASCULAR MALFORMATIONS OF THE LEFT SIDE OF THE HEART WITH RIGHT-TO-LEFT, BIDIRECTIONAL, OR NO SHUNT

Coarctation of the Aorta

PATHOLOGY

Coarctation of the aorta is a discrete narrowing of the distal segment of the aortic arch. The characteristic lesion is a deformity of the media of the aorta that involves the anterior, superior, and posterior walls and is represented by a curtain-like infolding of the wall that causes the lumen to be narrowed and eccentric.[114] In infants, the lesion lies either opposite the ductus or in a preductal location. In adolescents and adults, it is usually at the ligamentum arteriosum. An aberrant right subclavian artery may be associated. In rare cases, the narrowing lies proximal to the origin of the left common carotid artery or involves a segment of the abdominal aorta. The principal cardiac abnormality is left ventricular hypertrophy. In some infants, left ventricular endocardial fibroelastosis may be associated. Tubular hypoplasia of the distal aortic arch and isthmus is very common, especially with associated cardiac abnormalities involving left heart obstruction.[115] The proximal aorta may show a moderate degree of cystic medial necrosis. Beyond the coarctation, the lining may show a localized jet lesion. Prominent collaterals are characteristic in older infants, children, and adolescents. They may be divided into anterior and posterior systems, with the anterior system originating with the internal mammary arteries and making use of the epigastric arteries in the abdominal wall to supply the lower extremities. The posterior system involves parascapular arteries connected with the posterior intercostal arteries and carries blood to the distal aortic compartment principally for supply of the abdominal viscera. The anterior spinal artery, receiving branches from the proximal and distal compartments of the aorta, is also dilated and tortuous.

ASSOCIATED CONDITIONS

The most commonly associated defects are tubular hypoplasia of the aortic arch, PDA, VSD, and aortic stenosis (valvular and/or subvalvular). A bicuspid aortic valve is present in 46 percent of autopsy cases.[114]

ABNORMAL PHYSIOLOGY

In most instances, both the systolic and diastolic arterial pressures above the coarctation are elevated. Below the coarctation, the systolic pressure is lower than that in the upper extremities, and the diastolic pressure is usually near or only slightly below the normal range. The mechanism of upper extremity hypertension appears to involve the increased resistance to aortic flow produced by the coarctation itself, the decreased capacity and distensibility of the vessels into which the left ventricle ejects, and humoral factors.[116]

CLINICAL MANIFESTATIONS

Coarctation of the aorta occurs in approximately 4 percent of all infants and children with congenital heart disease and is the predominant lesion in approximately 8 percent of infants presenting with critical heart disease in the first year of life. It ranks behind only VSD, D-transposition of the great arteries, and tetralogy of Fallot.[3] Among all individuals born with coarctation, approximately half present within the first month or two of life with heart failure. About 50 percent of infants so admitted have uncomplicated coarctation; the remaining half can be expected to have at least one complicating cardiac abnormality. VSD is the most common (64 percent), followed by left ventricular outflow tract obstruction (31 percent).[117] The timing of ductal tissue constriction in terms of both ductal closure and perhaps aortic constriction appear to play a decisive role in the onset or worsening of symptoms in most of these patients. The male/female ratio is approximately 3:1 for isolated coarctation but is only 1.1:1 for complicated coarctation. Approximately 45 percent of children with Turner's syndrome have coarctation.

History The clinical picture in a symptomatic infant is one of dyspnea, difficulty in feeding, and poor weight gain. Older children are for the most part asymptomatic, although a few complain of mild fatigue, dyspnea, or symptoms of claudication of the lower extremities when running.

Physical Examination In a symptomatic infant, signs of congestive heart failure are characteristic. A gallop rhythm is common, and a murmur from associated defects or from the coarctation itself (posteriorly in the interscapular area) may be heard. Frequently, these murmurs are either inaudible or nondescript on admission and become characteristic only when congestive failure is brought under control. Prominent arterial pulsations may be visible in the suprasternal notch and carotid arteries, and the left ventricular impulse is forceful. An early systolic ejection click at the apex suggests the presence of a bicuspid aortic valve. The murmur from the coarctation is medium-pitched, systolic, and blowing in quality. It is best heard posteriorly in the interscapular area, usually with some degree of radiation to the left axilla, apex, and anterior precordium. Low-pitched, continuous murmurs of collateral circulation may be heard over the chest wall, particularly posteriorly, but seldom before adolescence. A short mid-diastolic rumble at the apex without clinical evidence of mitral disease is relatively common.

The characteristic systolic blood pressure difference between the upper and lower extremities may be difficult to appreciate or measure in infants with severe congestive failure or with a large VSD or PDA. With improved hemodynamic compensation, pulses in the upper extremities become readily palpable. The femoral pulses remain weak, delayed, or absent. In these very young infants, it is important to assess the brachial and carotid pulses. Weak or absent pulses in all sites are more characteristic of critical aortic stenosis or aortic atresia.

In older children and adults, the radial arterial pulses are typically strong; those in the femoral arteries are diminished, delayed, or absent. A repeatedly measured systolic or mean pressure difference between the upper and lower extremities greater than 10 mmHg is diagnostic. The pulse pressure in the leg is reduced, and in some patients no pressure can be measured by auscultation or Doppler. Approximately one-third of older children have hypertension. Some patients have only a mild pressure difference between the arms and the legs at rest but a much larger difference during treadmill exercise. A systolic pressure difference between the two arms suggests that the origin of one subclavian artery is at or below the obstruction, e.g., aberrant right subclavian from the descending aorta.

In light of the simplicity of measuring blood pressure in the upper and lower extremities of children and the importance of early detection, it is concerning that approximately 95 percent of children and adolescents with coarctation are referred by pediatricians and other health care providers to a pediatric cardiologist for evaluation of a murmur and/or hypertension.[118]

Chest Roentgenogram For a symptomatic infant, the pattern is one of impressive cardiac enlargement and venous congestion. In an older and asymptomatic child, the heart's size is generally at the upper limits of normal with a left ventricular prominence. A figure-three configuration of the left margin of the aorta at the level of the coarctation may be seen in overpenetrated films, with the upper curve formed by the slightly dilated aorta just above the coarctation, the central indentation by the coarctation itself, and the lower curve by the poststenotic dilatation below the coarctation. Notching of the inferior margin of the ribs by tortuous intercostal arteries acting as collaterals is seldom present before 7 or 8 years of age.

Electrocardiogram The ECG of a symptomatic infant reflects right or biventricular hypertrophy during the first 3 months of life. T-wave inversion in the left precordial leads is common. In older children, the ECG is usually normal or may indicate mild left ventricular and left atrial hypertrophy.

Echocardiogram Two-dimensional echocardiographic imaging of the aortic arch from the suprasternal notch permits visualization of the coarctation and detection of anatomic variations such as isthmic or transverse arch hypoplasia. The precordial and subxiphoid views are of great value in assessing the presence and severity of associated defects. Doppler flow studies are helpful for diagnostic confirmation. In infants with heart failure, left ventricular dilation and decreased contractility are common. The severity of the coarctation can be evaluated by Doppler gradients and the diminished pulsatile flow in the abdominal aorta.

Cardiac Catheterization Study of symptomatic infants characteristically reveals left atrial and left ventricular hypertension and a significant systolic pressure difference between the left ventricle and the femoral artery, particularly if the coarctation is isolated. In the presence of a large VSD and PDA, the left ventricular hypertension and the systolic pressure difference between the left ventricle and the femoral artery are less impressive and may not exist at all related to a nonrestrictive PDA supplying perfusion to the descending aorta. Every attempt should be made to define the nature and severity of associated defects. Imaging is recommended in older children to demonstrate the exact site and length of the coarctation as well as to show unusual features of the collateral circulation that may be of importance to the surgeon. Magnetic resonance imaging is an excellent and in most instances preferable alternative to angiography for demonstrating the site and length of the coarctation (Fig. 73-20).

NATURAL HISTORY AND PROGNOSIS

Approximately one-half of infants admitted with heart failure within the first weeks of life have coarctation without significant associated defects.[117] The majority of these infants respond well to medical management and, if no repair is performed, reach a stage at 2 or 3 years of age where they are indistinguishable from asymptomatic children of the same age whose coarctation is first detected during a routine physical examination. Upper extremity hypertension usually increases during the first several months of life and then tends to diminish again as collateral circulation improves, while signs of failure diminish at the same time. For infants with severe failure and any serious associated defects, balloon dilation or surgery provides virtually the only chance of survival.

The consequences of persistent hypertension in an individual who has not undergone surgery appear in the second and third decades in the form of severe hypertension, aortic rupture, or intracranial hemorrhage from an aneurysm of the circle of Willis. Heart failure often complicated by mitral or aortic valve disease, a dissecting aneurysm of the aorta, or atherosclerosis present in the fourth decade. The risk of endocarditis on the aortic or mitral valves or endarteritis at the site of coarctation appears to be spread relatively evenly over the years. The average age of death of patients who survive childhood with coarctation without surgery is 34 years.[118,119]

MEDICAL MANAGEMENT

Vigorous medical treatment is indicated for infants with severe heart failure. A newborn with severe failure may experience dramatic relief from the intravenous infusion of PGE_1 to reopen the closing ductus, which provides perfusion to the descending aorta.[97] Prompt correction of the coarctation is recommended for all infants with one or more associated defects and for all infants with isolated coarctation unless the response to medical management has been dramatic and sustained.

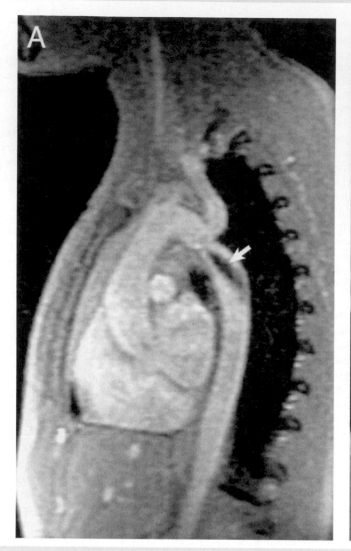
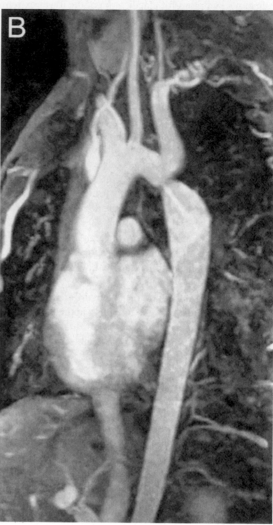

FIGURE 73-20 MRI evaluation of coarctation of the aorta. *A.* Systolic frame from a cine MR sequence showing a turbulent jet at the coarctation site (*arrow*). *B.* Gadolinium-enhanced 3D MRA subvolume maximal intensity pro-jection (MIP) image of the aorta. (From Geva T, Sahn DJ, Powell AC. Magnetic resonance imaging of congenital heart disease in adults. *Prog Pediatr Cardiol* 2003; 17: 21–39. Reproduced with permission of the authors and publisher.)

The timing and type of correction of isolated discrete coarctation of the aorta remain a topic of some dispute. There is general agreement that all children with heart failure should be repaired after a brief period of stabilization and treatment. Since heart failure is usually limited to infants in the first few months of life and balloon dilation of native coarctation in children under 6 months of age has had an unacceptable restenosis rate of up to 75 percent,[120] most cardiologists would consider surgical repair the favored approach. For infants and children without heart failure, timing has been somewhat more problematic. Historically, to minimize the possibility of recurrence among patients corrected before 12 months,[121] surgery was deferred until 1 to 4 years of age. The goal was to prevent residual or recurrent hypertension, renal disease, or significant aortic regurgitation, which appears to be related to the duration of hypertension before surgery. More recently, the reduction of the rate of restenosis has led some centers to undertake elective surgical repair between 3 and 6 months. For those in whom balloon dilation is contemplated, waiting until age 1 to 4 seems appropriate.

Currently, there is general agreement that symptomatic children under 6 months of age should be repaired surgically, and those who develop recurrent stenosis at any age should undergo balloon dilation or stent placement. The optimal therapy for the treatment of native coarctation in children older than 1 year of age remains somewhat controversial. For balloon dilation, immediate success (defined as an increase in the coarctation diameter with a residual gradient of less than 20 mmHg) occurs in a large percentage of patients.[122] However, long-term gradient relief after angioplasty has been somewhat less than that with surgery. Restenosis rates in the intermediate term seem to be directly related to the age at dilation, with 85 percent of neonates, 35 percent of infants, and 10 percent of children over 2 years of age developing restenosis.[120] Repeat dilation is almost invariably successful, and many advocate this approach even if it requires two dilations rather than a one-step surgical approach. In older children, a stent can be placed if the balloon dilation fails (Fig. 73-21). In selected older children and adults, stent deployment has been very successful, with an average reduction in the gradient from 25 to 5 mm in 32 patients at Children's Hospital in Boston.[123] Complications have usually been related to associated diseases, although small aneurysms at the site of dilation have been reported in about 5 percent of cases. Trauma to the femoral artery, related to the use of large catheters, is not uncommon.

Patients who have had coarctation repair must be followed indefinitely. Residual hypertension is prevalent in many, even when repair is completed in infancy.[124] For those with significant recoarctation expressed as a systolic pressure gradient of 20 mmHg or more at rest, balloon angioplasty and/or stent placement are recommended. Repeat surgery for recurrent coarctation is rarely necessary. Occasionally, patients with insignificant or small residual resting gradients manifest abnormal upper extremity hypertension and significant gradients with exercise.[117] These patients should probably undergo balloon angioplasty and stent placement with pharmacologic control of their hypertension if present at rest or unmasked with exercise.

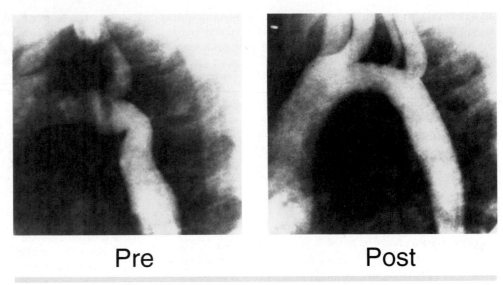

Pre   **Post**

FIGURE 73-21 Repair of coarctation with a stent. *Left panel:* coarctation caused by kink with anterior indentation. *Right panel:* narrowing eliminated with stent. (Courtesy of Audrey Marshall, MD.)

SURGICAL MANAGEMENT

The coarctation is exposed and mobilized through a left posterolateral thoracotomy. It is usually possible to resect the narrow segment and restore continuity with a direct end-to-end anastomosis (Fig. 73-22). When the narrowed segment is longer, repair by subclavian flap aortoplasty or, rarely, a tubular vascular prosthesis to bridge the gap between the two ends of the aorta may be necessary. In adults with a relatively inelastic or calcified aorta, a tubular vascular prosthesis can be used to bypass the unresected coarctation or the site of a previous repair. Dacron patch repair of coarctation has an unacceptably high incidence of late aneurysm formation and is no longer advised.[125] Tension-free suture lines are essential. Postoperative bleeding, chylothorax, paraplegia, and injury to the phrenic and recurrent laryngeal nerves remain potential complications.[126] Though long-term surgical results of those undergoing surgery in childhood are generally excellent, a large number of patients experience late hypertension.[127]

If a significant VSD is also present, some surgeons prefer to place a pulmonary arterial band at the time of coarctation repair during infancy. The VSD may then be repaired electively during the next several months, when the heart failure is well controlled. Primary repair of the VSD shortly after or simultaneously with coarctation repair is an alternative that has recently been gaining.[128]

Adequacy of collateral circulation to the spinal cord is crucial for the safe repair of coarctation. A rise in proximal systemic arterial pressure of more than 20 mmHg when the aorta is clamped above the coarctation suggests a marginal collateral circulation. Mild systemic hypothermia is a simple and useful adjunct, and monitoring of somatosensory cortical evoked potentials may warn of an impending ischemic insult to the spinal cord.[129] Postoperative paradoxical hypertension is common between the second and fifth postoperative

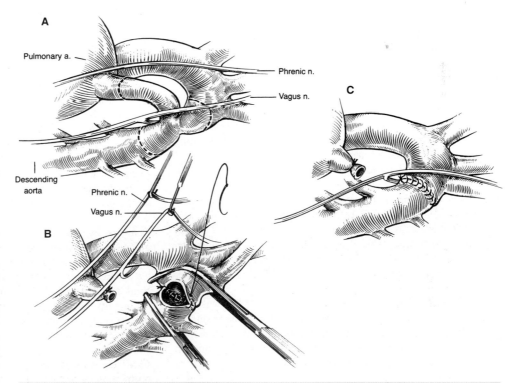

FIGURE 73-22 Repair of coarctation surgically. *A.* Discrete aortic coarctation in an infant with a small ductus arteriosus seen via left thoracotomy exposure. *B.* Repair technique using resection with end-to-end anastomosis. *C.* Complete repair. (From Castaneda AR, Jonas RA, Mayer JE Jr, Hanley FL. *Cardiac Surgery of the Neonate and Infant.* Philadelphia: Saunders; 1994:333. Reproduced with permission from the publisher and author.)

days and may contribute to the *postcoarctation syndrome,* in which ileus, abdominal pain, mesenteric vasculitis, and visceral infarction can occur. This syndrome is rarely encountered if the postoperative blood pressure is maintained within the normal range for age with sodium nitroprusside, beta blockers, or angiotensin-converting enzyme inhibitors.

Operative mortality for infants with isolated coarctation is in the range of 0 to 3 percent,[121,126,128] but it is 10 percent or higher when other cardiovascular defects are present. Excellent results have been reported among low-birth-weight infants.[130] Subsequent deaths are uncommon in surviving infants with isolated coarctation but are more likely in those with complicated associated defects.

Valvular Aortic Stenosis

DEFINITION

Aortic stenosis is defined as subtotal obstruction of varying severity in the channel of left ventricular outflow. In order of decreasing frequency, the sites of obstruction by congenital lesions are (1) valvular, (2) subvalvular, and (3) supravalvular (see Chap. 66).

PATHOLOGY

Most commonly, the aortic valve is bicuspid with two commissures, one or both of which are fused to varying degrees. A third rudimentary commissure, or raphe, is frequently present in the larger of the leaflets. The valve opening is eccentric. Less frequently encountered is a unicuspid, unicommissural, or noncommissural valve in which the orifice is often slit-like, at first glance suggesting a bicuspid valve. Uncommonly, a true dome is present, resembling the valve of congenital isolated pulmonary stenosis. Rarely, the valve is tricuspid, with fusion of one or more of the three commissures. When survival to adult life occurs, calcification may appear in the valvular tissue, leading to rigidity of the valve. Poststenotic dilation of the ascending aorta occurs in all cases to some degree. Coarctation of the aorta is the most common associated anomaly.

ABNORMAL PHYSIOLOGY

The hemodynamics of congenital valvular aortic stenosis are similar to those of acquired aortic stenosis (see Chap. 66) except that a persistent PDA or stretched foramen ovale in the immediate postnatal period may lessen the severity of pulmonary edema by diverting blood away from the left ventricle.

Severity usually is judged by the peak systolic pressure gradient (PSPG) across the aortic valve and the calculated aortic valve area determined at cardiac catheterization. In the presence of a normal cardiac output, a PSPG ≥ 75 mmHg or an aortic valve area <0.5 cm^2/m^2 is considered severe, a PSPG between 50 and 75 mmHg or a valve area between 0.5 and 0.8 cm^2/m^2 is considered moderate, and a PSPG <50 mmHg or a valve area >0.9 cm^2/m^2 is considered mild (see Chaps. 17 and 66).

CLINICAL MANIFESTATIONS

About 7 percent of infants and children with congenital heart disease have aortic stenosis in one of its several forms, approximately 80 percent of which is valvular. Valvular stenosis is much more common among males than females, with a ratio of 4:1.

History The detection of a systolic murmur leads to the discovery of this malformation in most patients, the vast majority of whom are asymptomatic. Easy fatigue, dyspnea, syncope, and angina suggest severe obstruction, but severe obstruction may exist in the absence of

any symptoms. Sudden death may occur from this malformation, but in most such cases death is preceded by either symptoms or ECG changes. Infants with critical stenosis from birth present with congestive failure within 2 weeks and represent true emergencies. A similar small number of patients with less critical but severe obstruction are detected over the course of the next 4 to 6 months.

Physical Examination The arterial blood pressure and quality of the peripheral arterial pulses of older infants and children are usually normal. A measured pulse pressure <20 mmHg suggests severe stenosis. The cardiac apical impulse may be forceful and sustained; a systolic thrill along the right upper sternal border and over the carotid arteries is present in most of these patients. The absence of a thrill suggests a PSPG below 30 mmHg. Paradoxical splitting of the second heart sound is rare and associated with very severe obstruction or coexisting myocardial disease. An early systolic ejection click at the apex is characteristic and serves to distinguish valvular aortic stenosis from other forms of left ventricular outflow tract obstruction. The classic auscultatory finding is a harsh systolic crescendo-decrescendo murmur that is loudest at the right upper sternal border, with radiation into the carotid arteries and down the left sternal border to the apex (see Chap. 12). Among infants with critical obstruction and low cardiac output, there may be no palpable peripheral pulses and no distinctive murmur until implementation of anticongestive therapy.

Chest Roentgenogram The heart's overall size is normal, but infants with failure will have generalized cardiac enlargement and varying degrees of pulmonary edema. Poststenotic dilatation of the ascending aorta is characteristic.

Electrocardiogram Left ventricular hypertrophy, as indicated by voltage criteria in the left precordial leads, is seldom helpful in distinguishing patients with severe obstruction from those with mild to moderate obstruction. However, diminished anterior forces in the right precordial leads and a deep $SV_1 \geq 30$ mm suggest severe stenosis, as does absence of the Q wave in V_6. Fifty percent of patients with severe obstruction have a flat, biphasic, or inverted T wave in V_6 (Fig. 73-23). However, severe and even critical obstruction may be present with none of the ECG abnormalities mentioned above. Monitoring of the ST segment in leads V_5 through V_7 during cautious exercise testing appears to be a reliable method of detecting children in whom a significant PSPG (>50 mmHg) has developed and in whom that gradient may represent a threat of sudden death.[131] Symptomatic infants may show right, left, or biventricular hypertrophy, frequently with T-wave inversion over the left precordium.

Echocardiogram Continuous-wave Doppler echocardiography guided by two-dimensional echocardiographic imaging predicts very accurately the peak instantaneous and mean systolic pressure gradient across discrete forms of left ventricular outflow tract obstruction (see Chap. 15) (Fig. 73-24). Two-dimensional echocardiography can distinguish the exact site of obstruction and identify hypoplasia of the left ventricle, mitral valve annulus, or aortic root to a degree that precludes survival.[132,133]

Cardiac Catheterization Infants symptomatic with severe aortic obstruction often have a left-to-right shunt through a stretched foramen ovale, PAH, and a right-to-left shunt through a PDA. A marked increase in left ventricular end-diastolic pressure is usually present. The PSPG between the left ventricle and the central aorta should be documented whenever possible. If left ventricular output is markedly diminished, this gradient may be relatively small even in the presence of severe obstruction. Left ventricular angiography will confirm the site of obstruction and outline the size of the left ventricular cavity (Fig. 73-25A).

In older infants and children, pressures on the right side of the heart are usually normal. Simultaneous recording of central aortic and left ventricular pressures or a pressure tracing upon catheter withdrawal from the left ventricle to the aorta, coupled with an accurate estimate of cardiac output, is necessary for reliable assessment of severity. Left ventricular angiography will document the site of obstruction. The aortic leaflets are typically thickened and domed, with a central or eccentric jet of contrast material entering the ascending aorta. Poststenotic dilatation is characteristic. Supravalvular aortography is recommended to assess the presence and severity of aortic regurgitation.

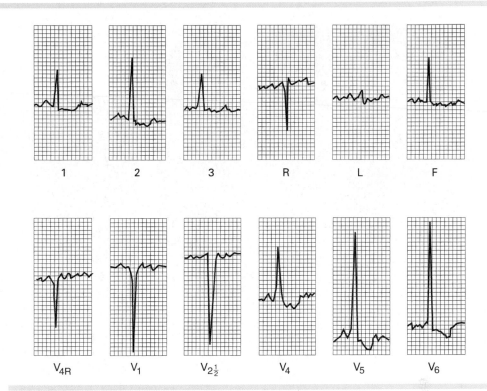

FIGURE 73-23 Electrocardiogram from an 8-year-old boy with valvular aortic stenosis and a 94-mmHg peak systolic pressure gradient. The small anterior QRS forces, abnormally large posterior forces, absent Q waves in leads V_5 and V_6, and abnormal T waves and ST segments reflect severe left ventricular systolic pressure overload with ischemia.

NATURAL HISTORY AND PROGNOSIS

About half the infants born with severe valvular aortic stenosis require hospitalization within the first week of life. Not uncommonly, the murmur is mistaken for that of a VSD. Heart failure beyond infancy and before adolescence is not seen without the presence of complicating factors. Symptomatic infants require prompt relief of obstruction by balloon or surgical valvotomy, but the mortality rate remains significant. Endocardial fibroelastosis, papillary muscle necrosis, associated intra- and extracardiac deformities, and a small left ventricular cavity contribute to this mortality rate. Survivors may have significant aortic regurgitation, but the majority can be managed medically until valve replacement is feasible.

Most infants beyond the newborn period and children with mild aortic valvular stenosis (PSPG at catheterization <25 mmHg or a Doppler mean pressure gradient <25 mmHg) remain stable, with only a 21 percent likelihood of progression in severity and the need for intervention within the subsequent 25 years. For patients with a PSPG between 25 and 49 mmHg, the likelihood of significant progression rises to 41 percent, and with a PSPG >50 mmHg, it rises to 71 percent.[44] Patients with a PSPG >50 mmHg are at risk for serious ventricular arrhythmias and sudden death. Infective endocarditis on the aortic valve (see Chap. 73) poses an extremely serious complication in the form of systemic arterial emboli and serious, even catastrophic, aortic regurgitation with congestive failure, shock, and death.[60]

MEDICAL AND SURGICAL MANAGEMENT

Infants with the characteristic murmur detected in the first weeks of life should be evaluated very carefully to be certain the obstruction is not severe and does not become severe in the next few weeks or months.[134] Those who develop heart failure should be operated on or undergo balloon valvuloplasty without delay. In a critically ill neonate, intravenous PGE_1 infusion to open the ductus may provide temporary relief of pulmonary edema en route to the operating room or catheterization laboratory. Beyond infancy, a yearly plan of

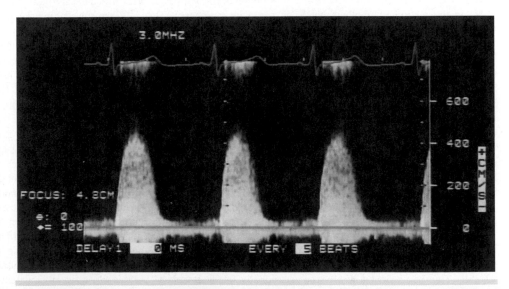

FIGURE 73-24 Doppler interrogation in the ascending aorta in a patient with valvular aortic stenosis. The peak velocity of 4.8 m/s correlates with a maximum instantaneous gradient of 92 mmHg across the aortic valve.

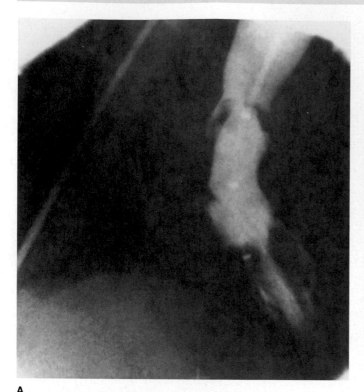

A

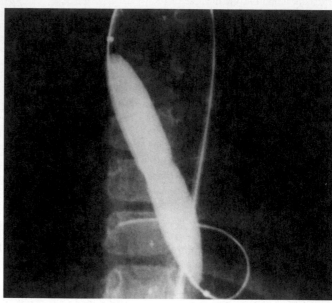

B

FIGURE 73-25 Balloon aortic valvuloplasty. *A.* Left ventricular angiogram showing a domed, thickened aortic valve with fusion of the right and left commissures. *B.* Balloon dilation using a retrograde technique. A waist is demonstrated in the midportion of the balloon before full inflation. (From Lock JE, Keane JF, Perry SB. *Diagnostic and Interventional Catheterization in Congenital Heart Disease*, 2d ed. Boston: Kluwer; 2000:151. Reproduced with permission from the publisher and authors.)

reexamination with careful questioning regarding symptoms and an ECG, an echocardiogram with Doppler assessment of the mean and maximum pressure gradient every year or two, exercise testing, and 24-h ECG monitoring about every 3 years should suffice to prevent progression from going unrecognized. Indications for cardiac catheterization for gradient assessment and possible balloon dilation include the appearance of symptoms or syncope, decreased anterior forces with an $SV_1 \geq 30$ mm or flattening or inversion of the T wave in V_6 in the resting ECG, abnormal ST–T segments on exercise testing, or a Doppler estimated maximum instantaneous gradient of >65 mmHg or mean gradient >40 mmHg.

Transluminal catheter balloon valvuloplasty has become the preferred alternative to surgery. In skilled hands, it can provide effective reduction of the transvalvular gradient while producing only a mild increment in aortic regurgitation in most instances.[135,136] Elective balloon dilation is recommended if the PSPG is >50 mmHg at catheterization with aortic regurgitation mild or nonexistent. For a neonate with critical valvular obstruction, some centers continue to rely on surgical intervention, but catheter balloon valvuloplasty has become a very competitive alternative and in the author's institution is the procedure of choice for these very sick infants.

Early studies and more recent experience suggest that the balloon diameter should not exceed that of the valve ring, and most centers now use balloons that are 85 to 90 percent of the diameter of the aortic annulus. The balloon is inflated to a pressure of 4 to 6 atm until the "waist" produced by the stenotic valve has been abolished (Fig. 73-25*B*). Transient arrhythmias are seen occasionally, but apart from creating aortic regurgitation, other complications are uncommon.

In older children, the results are usually quite good, with a reduction of the peak gradient of approximately 60 percent, a mortality rate under 2 percent, and a complication rate of about 3 percent.[135,136] In neonates, the results are more problematic, probably because of severity of disease, unstable conditions, and the size of the patient, with 12 percent early and late mortality in one series. In this center, reintervention (usually repeat balloon dilation) was necessary in 40 percent with a mean follow-up of 4.3 years.[137]

When surgical intervention is required for critical aortic stenosis during infancy, the heart is exposed through a median sternotomy and the aortic valve visualized through the ascending aorta during a brief period of low-flow perfusion with mild hypothermia. Standard cardiopulmonary bypass, mild hypothermia, and cardioplegia are used in older children.[138] The surgeon must discriminate between true commissures and abnormal raphes, because incision of the latter produces intolerable aortic valvular regurgitation. Relief of valvular stenosis is accomplished with a carefully placed incision in the middle of each fused but well-supported true commissure.

A conservative attitude is essential during operation for aortic stenosis in an infant or small child. Mild valvular regurgitation almost always occurs consequent to commissurotomy but is usually well tolerated. Moderate residual stenosis is preferred to intolerable aortic valvular regurgitation, especially in infants in whom valve implantation is technically difficult. If valve replacement is necessary in an infant or small child, use of the autograft pulmonary valve in the aortic position offers the attractive possibility of continuing growth of this neoaortic valve, which may parallel that of the patient.[139] The risk of operation is high in critically ill infants, in the range of 10 to

15 percent, particularly in those with a low ejection fraction, high left ventricular end-diastolic pressure, endocardial fibroelastosis, marked heart failure, or features of left ventricular hypoplasia.[140] Morbidity after aortic valvotomy in an older child is rare, and the likelihood of relief of left ventricular outflow tract obstruction and survival is good. The Natural History Study of Congenital Heart Defects, reporting on 133 children undergoing aortic commissurotomy after the age of 2 years, found that only 27 percent required a second operation in the subsequent 20 years, with 78 percent of those operations consisting of valve replacement. Aortic regurgitation was the indication for operation in 14 percent of those with valve replacements.[44]

Relief of aortic valve obstruction, whether by balloon valvuloplasty or surgical valvotomy, is palliative rather than curative. Gradual restenosis is the rule, with almost one-third of infants who undergo valvotomy requiring a second operation, usually valve replacement, within the next two decades. Aortic regurgitation, a well-recognized complication of valvuloplasty, valvulotomy, and/or infective endocarditis, may require surgical intervention as well. Endocarditis is a serious and lifelong hazard, with an incidence among patients followed for 20 years of approximately 5 percent, a mortality rate of just over 25 percent, and a predilection for patients in the second rather than the first decade of life and with PSPGs >50 mmHg.[44,60]

Secondary valvulotomy by balloon or surgery for recurrent or residual stenosis can be attempted, but calcification and restenosis eventually necessitate aortic valve replacement in almost all those requiring surgery on the aortic valve in infancy or childhood. A small aortic annulus severely limits the relief of left ventricular hypertension unless one resorts to Konno's operation, in which the annulus is divided; the upper ventricular septum resected, creating a VSD; patching the VSD with prosthetic material; and replacing the valve (a homograft or pulmonary autograft) into the enlarged annulus. The ascending aorta and anterior right ventricular wall are reconstructed using a prosthetic graft; in the case of an autograft, the main pulmonary artery and pulmonary valve are replaced with a cryopreserved pulmonary homograft.[141] *Children with more than mild aortic stenosis are restricted from strenuous organized athletics, isometric exercises, and activities that require a good deal of stamina and produce shortness of breath.*[142]

Supravalvular Aortic Stenosis

PATHOLOGY
The obstruction in the ascending aorta includes the following three types: (1) hourglass (discrete), (2) hypoplastic (diffuse), and (3) membranous. Associated obstructions in the pulmonary trunk, peripheral pulmonary arteries, and branches of the aortic arch are common.[143] Hypertrophy of the coronary arterial walls and premature coronary atherosclerosis have been described.[144]

CLINICAL MANIFESTATIONS
Supravalvular stenosis may be familial, associated with characteristic facies and mental retardation, sporadic, or (rarely) the result of congenital rubella. All forms may be and usually are associated with varying degrees of peripheral or branch pulmonary arterial stenosis. The familial form is transmitted as an autosomal dominant trait with variable expression (see Chap. 12). Mental retardation is not present, and there are no characteristic facial features.[145] Supravalvular aortic stenosis associated with mental retardation, frequently called *Williams syndrome,* is associated with a high and prominent forehead, epicanthal folds, underdevelopment of the bridge of the nose

and mandible, and a broad, overhanging upper lip. It is due to a deletion of the elastin gene on chromosome 7 and can now be identified by fluorescent in situ hybridization studies. It has been linked with idiopathic hypercalcemia of infancy, but hypercalcemia is not present in the majority of patients recognized beyond infancy.[146]

The symptoms of supravalvular aortic stenosis are similar to those of subvalvular aortic stenosis (see below). Patients with the familial form usually have a distinctive family history but one that seldom emerges in its entirety on initial questioning. The physical findings are also similar to those of subvalvular aortic stenosis, although a systolic blood pressure difference may be recorded between the two arms on occasion, with the right-arm pressure being greater than that of the left (Coanda effect).[147] Chest roentgenography and ECG are not distinctive unless associated pulmonary arterial stenosis leads to right ventricular hypertrophy. Echocardiography can identify the narrowed aortic lumen just above the aortic valve and provide an estimate of the severity of the obstruction by the Doppler-derived instantaneous pressure gradient.

At cardiac catheterization, a systolic pressure gradient can be demonstrated just above the aortic valve by careful pullback. Supravalvular aortography or left ventricular angiography will visualize the supravalvular narrowing (Fig. 73-26). Pressure recordings in the branch pulmonary arteries should be obtained; in the presence of any significant stenoses, pulmonary arterial angiography should be performed. Narrowing at the branch points of major arteries (coronary, carotid, mesenteric, renal, etc.) is occasionally seen.

NATURAL HISTORY AND PROGNOSIS
The sequence of progressive obstruction, the appearance of symptoms and ECG changes, and the possibility of sudden death appear to apply for supravalvular aortic stenosis as well as for valvular aortic stenosis. Infective endocarditis represents a threat to these patients throughout life.

MANAGEMENT
The indications for cardiac catheterization and follow-up are the same as those for valvular aortic stenosis. Noninvasive imaging frequently suffices, but angiography may be necessary to evaluate the gradient and rule out arterial narrowing. Surgery is usually recommended if the gradient across the narrowing exceeds 40 mmHg.

Discrete supravalvular aortic stenosis is relieved by one or more incisions through the narrow segment of the ascending aorta, usually at the level of the sinotubular ridge at the top of the commissures. Incisions are extended well down into the aortic sinuses. Ridges of obstructing fibrous tissue are excised. The aorta is enlarged by the insertion of a gusset of prosthetic vascular graft material or pericardium to increase the circumference.[138] A favorable outcome can be anticipated postoperatively in most patients with supravalvular aortic stenosis if the abnormality of the arterial wall is localized.[148] Intimal obstruction of the coronary arterial ostia may require debridement, dilation, or even saphenous vein or internal mammary bypass grafting.

Diffuse tubular hypoplasia of the ascending aorta is a technically challenging problem that is associated with a higher mortality rate and usually poor postoperative hemodynamic results.

Subvalvular Aortic Stenosis

PATHOLOGY
Three classic varieties of subvalvular aortic stenosis involve the left ventricular outflow tract: the discrete, tunnel, and muscular types.

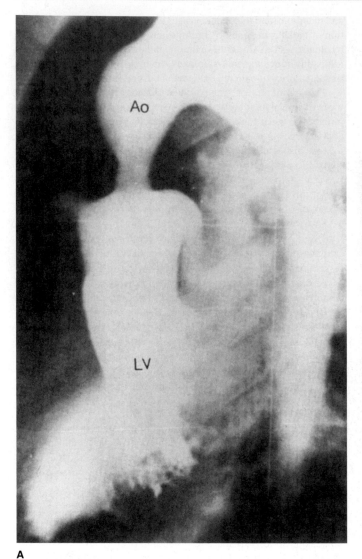

A

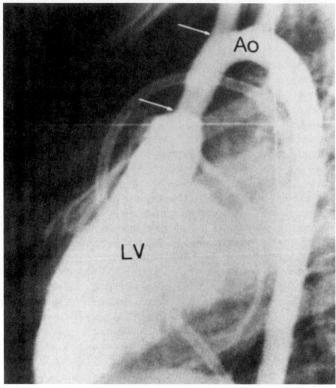

B

FIGURE 73-26 *A.* Supravalvular aortic stenosis, discrete type. The stenotic segment is located immediately above the aortic sinuses of Valsalva. The distal ascending aorta (Ao) is normal in size. LV = left ventricle. *B.* Supravalvular aortic stenosis, diffuse type. Narrowing in the ascending aorta begins above the aortic valve (*lower arrow*) and extends throughout the ascending aortic segment to the origin of the brachiocephalic vessels (*upper arrow*). In this patient, the aortic arch and descending aorta also appear hypoplastic. (Keane JF, Fellows KE, La Farge G, et al. The surgical management of discrete and diffuse supravalvular aortic stenosis. *Circulation* 1976;54:112–117. Reproduced with permission from the publisher and authors.)

The discrete type is characterized by a localized fibrous encirclement of the left ventricular outflow tract a short distance below the aortic valve (Fig. 73-27) or fibromuscular tissue that extends onto the mitral leaflet and may also attach to the aortic cusps. The tunnel type involves hypoplasia of the aortic annulus and a channel with a fibrous lining in the subjacent left ventricular outflow tract.[149,150] The muscular type also is known as *hypertrophic cardiomyopathy* (or idiopathic hypertrophic subaortic stenosis) and is discussed in Chap. 77. More than half these patients have associated malformations, of which PDA, VSD, or coarctation are the most common.

CLINICAL MANIFESTATIONS

Discrete stenosis is more common among males, with a male/female ratio of approximately 2.5:1. In the isolated forms, the majority of patients are referred because of the detection of a murmur that not uncommonly is mistaken initially for that of a VSD. The symptoms have the same implications as they do for valvular aortic stenosis. The physical examination is similar to that of valvular aortic stenosis with two exceptions: an early systolic ejection click is not heard, and an early diastolic murmur of aortic regurgitation is present in approximately one-half of these patients. The roentgenographic features and ECG are also similar to those of valvular aortic stenosis except for the absence of poststenotic dilatation of the ascending aorta. Two-dimensional echocardiography permits excellent visualization of the anatomy of the obstruction. An estimate of the systolic pressure gradient can be obtained from Doppler echocardiographic studies.

When catheterization is performed, a careful pullback pressure tracing across the left ventricular outflow tract will document the severity of the gradient and establish the site of the obstruction. Left

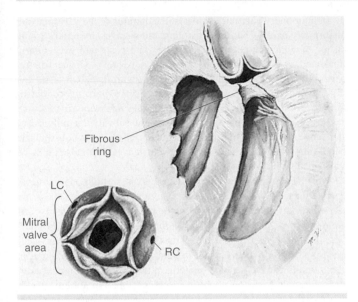

FIGURE 73-27 Localized subvalvular aortic stenosis. Obstruction is immediately upstream from the aortic valve. LC and RC = left and right coronary arteries. (From Kirklin and Ellis.[155] Reproduced with permission from the publisher and authors.)

ventricular biplane angiography will outline the nature of the obstruction. Aortography is recommended to evaluate the degree of aortic regurgitation.

NATURAL HISTORY AND PROGNOSIS
Severe heart failure in infancy is unusual and, if present, is almost invariably associated with complicating defects.[149] The obstruction is progressive in most instances, sometimes rapidly so. In one study, 75 percent of patients showed an increase of 25 mmHg or more in a 5-year period.[151] The cause of the progression is not known, but an intriguing theory suggests that distorted anatomy increases shear stress, leading to a stimulation of growth factors and cellular proliferation.[152] Associated aortic regurgitation also tends to be progressive and appears to result from damage due to the jet of blood through the obstruction, with secondary thickening and deformity of the valve leaflets. The results of surgery depend on the extent of involvement of the left ventricular outflow tract, with the best results being obtained in patients with a thin, discrete subvalvular membrane. The least satisfactory results occur in patients with tunnel obstruction.

MANAGEMENT
Medical management is similar to that of patients with valvular aortic stenosis, but surgery for the discrete type is usually recommended for pressure gradients ≥30 mmHg because of the possibility of progression of obstruction and the likelihood of progressive aortic valvular deformity and regurgitation.[153]

Continued follow-up for assessment of reobstruction and progression of aortic regurgitation and for reemphasis of the precautions against infective endocarditis is essential in all patients.[154]

Subvalvular fibromuscular (membranous) left ventricular outflow tract obstruction is exposed through the aortic root, as was described for aortic valvular stenosis (Fig. 73-27). Small half-circle needles and sutures or hooks are placed into the abnormal fibromuscular tissue, pulling it into view for precise excision from the underlying ventricular septum and the anterior mitral valve leaflet. The area of the bundle of His, which is usually just beneath the anterior commissure

between the right and noncoronary leaflets, is avoided. An additional septal myectomy or myotomy beneath and to the left of the commissure between the right and left leaflets may be required if secondary hypertrophy is significant. Immediate and early operative outcome is generally good, but *residual, recurrent, and progressive subaortic obstruction occurs in up to 25 percent of these patients, requiring long-term follow-up.*[155,156]

Diffuse tunnel obstruction in the left ventricular outflow tract poses a difficult technical problem that requires aortoseptoplasty, reconstruction of the left ventricular outflow (Konno's operation or a modification of it).[141,153]

Bicuspid Aortic Valve

PATHOLOGY
Classically, the two cusps are oriented anteriorly and posteriorly, with the anterior or conjoined cusp being the larger. A raphe, or ridge, is present along the aortic aspect of the larger cusp, running from the aortic wall to the free edge of the cusp. The most common associated condition of significance is coarctation of the aorta. The most common complication is calcification of the valve. *In about 85 percent of cases of calcific aortic stenosis in patients below age 70, the valve is congenitally bicuspid.* Aortic regurgitation from prolapse of the larger cusp is a less common complication and is usually not evident until adolescence or adult life.

CLINICAL MANIFESTATIONS
The incidence in the general population approaches 2 percent; therefore, it is the most common congenital abnormality of the heart or great vessels except possibly for mitral valve prolapse (see Chap. 68). This condition serves as the substrate for further changes including stenosis from fibrosis and deposition of calcium, regurgitation, infective endocarditis, aortic root dilatation, and dissection.[157] It is also found commonly among patients with isolated or dominant aortic regurgitation, patients with infective endocarditis with or without a history of predisposing heart disease, and in otherwise normal individuals who come to the physician's attention incidentally. Patients with uncomplicated bicuspid aortic valve are asymptomatic. The incidence among males is approximately 2.5 times that among females (see Chap. 68).

The characteristic feature is auscultatory and consists of an early systolic ejection click, which is best heard at the apex and does not vary with respiration. A soft, early, or midsystolic murmur is frequently present at the right upper sternal border. Less commonly, a soft murmur of aortic regurgitation may be heard. Two-dimensional echocardiography with adequate images can identify the bicuspid valve with a high degree of sensitivity and diagnostic accuracy.

NATURAL HISTORY AND PROGNOSIS
The majority of congenitally bicuspid aortic valves are nonobstructive at birth; but with the passage of time, a few of these valves become fibrotic, less mobile, and more obstructive, eventually becoming the site of calcium deposition, primarily among individuals between ages 15 and 65. Important calcium deposition is unusual before age 30, whereas grossly visible deposits of calcium are present in the valves of virtually all patients with severe stenosis beyond that age. A much smaller number of individuals born with a bicuspid aortic valve develop isolated aortic regurgitation. In approximately one-third, this is the result of fibrosis, prolapse, or retraction of one or both of the leaflets; in the remainder, regurgitation results from infective endocarditis on an apparently functionally normal bicuspid valve (see Chap. 81).

Congenital Mitral Regurgitation

PATHOLOGY

Mitral regurgitation may be due to a primary valve abnormality or secondary to a more complex defect (see "Common Atrioventricular Canal Defects," above). There are a variety of rare primary malformations, including isolated cleft, fenestration, and double orifice. Mitral regurgitation also occurs frequently with conditions that cause left ventricular dilatation and failure.

CLINICAL MANIFESTATIONS

Poor growth, frequent respiratory infections, and failure occur with significant mitral regurgitation. The physical findings are generally similar to those with mitral regurgitation of other causes (see Chap. 12). There may be a prominent left precordial bulge if cardiomegaly has been present from infancy. The systolic murmur may radiate to the base of the heart. Left atrial and left ventricular enlargement correlate with the degree of volume overload. Echocardiography with Doppler color-flow mapping will demonstrate these as well as left ventricular function and the severity of regurgitation. The specific defect may be outlined, such as an isolated cleft or a double-orifice valve. Findings at cardiac catheterization substantiate the hemodynamic alterations.

NATURAL HISTORY AND PROGNOSIS

Mild and even moderate mitral regurgitation may be well tolerated, but severe regurgitation leads to progressive deterioration. Endocarditis is a risk.

MANAGEMENT

Vigorous medical treatment of heart failure and infections is warranted. Every attempt should be made to control symptoms to a degree that will allow growth in infants. In infants and young children, only those with very severe and uncontrollable failure are subjected to surgery. In adolescents, continued symptoms justify surgery. Afterload reduction with an angiotensin-converting enzyme blocker may be tried. Surgery is indicated for heart failure or deteriorating left ventricular function.

At surgery, the valve and its apparatus are inspected carefully. In many cases a valvuloplasty is possible, but occasionally replacement may be necessary. Currently, the St. Jude medical prosthesis is often utilized. Lifelong anticoagulation with warfarin (see Chap. 54) is required. With body growth, replacement with a larger prosthesis may be difficult, and no good annular enlarging operation exists.

VALVULAR AND VASCULAR MALFORMATIONS OF THE RIGHT SIDE OF THE HEART WITH RIGHT-TO-LEFT, BIDIRECTIONAL, OR NO SHUNT

Pulmonary Stenosis with Intact Ventricular Septum

PATHOLOGY

Valvular pulmonary stenosis with an intact ventricular septum is usually characterized by a dome-shaped stenosis of the pulmonary valve and less commonly by dysplasia of the valve. The valve may be unicuspid, bicuspid, or tricuspid. The annulus may also be narrow. The pulmonary trunk exhibits poststenotic dilatation. In adult patients, calcification of the valve may appear.

In pulmonary valvular dysplasia, the annulus of the valve may be abnormally narrow, but the most dramatic changes are related to the cusps, of which three are identifiable. The cusps are exceedingly thickened by mucoid and dense connective tissue.[158] Concentric hypertrophy of the right ventricle is present, with its extent reflecting the degree of obstruction at the valve level. *The hypertrophy of the infundibular musculature may cause secondary infundibular stenosis.*

Less commonly, there may be isolated subvalvular pulmonary stenosis caused by infundibular narrowing or an anomalous muscle bundle across the middle of the right ventricle.[159] Both types may be associated with a VSD.

Isolated supravalvular pulmonary stenosis, or pulmonary arterial coarctations, may also occur. From angiographic studies, these are classified into four types: (1) *localized stenosis with poststenotic dilatation*, (2) *segmental stenosis*, (3) *diffuse hypoplasia*, and (4) *multiple peripheral stenoses*. The stenosis may be localized to any segment of the pulmonary arterial system. The process is unilateral in about one-third of cases and bilateral in two-thirds. Pulmonary arterial stenosis is commonly (about 75 percent) though not universally associated with other cardiovascular abnormalities, such as tetralogy of Fallot. It also may be seen as a sequela of congenital rubella or with Williams, Noonan's,[160] or Alagille's syndrome.

ABNORMAL PHYSIOLOGY

There is a pressure difference during systole between the main right ventricular cavity and the pulmonary artery. The area of the pulmonary valve orifice is normally 2 cm^2/m^2; it is about 0.5 cm^2 at birth and increases in size with body growth. In general, the effective valve area must be decreased about 60 percent before there is a hemodynamically significant obstruction to flow. PSPG may reach 150 to 240 mmHg in severe cases. The degree of obstruction is assessed by the peak and mean systolic pressure gradients and the amount of flow across the valve. In neonates, severe stenosis can be associated with a relatively small pressure difference if the flow is very low as a result of right ventricular failure. If pulmonary flow is normal, patients with PSPG at rest <40 mmHg have mild stenosis and patients with PSPG >75 mmHg have severe stenosis. When the pulmonary stenosis is severe, the right ventricle may fail and the cardiac output may be decreased at rest; this is associated with elevation of both the right ventricular end-diastolic pressure and the right atrial mean pressure. This may cause the foramen ovale to open and allow shunting of blood from the right atrium to the left atrium, resulting in arterial oxygen desaturation and cyanosis. In most adolescent or adult patients with significant pulmonary stenosis, the resting cardiac output is within normal limits but usually does not increase normally during exercise. In contrast, younger children may be able to increase cardiac output during exercise even with significant obstruction.[131,161]

CLINICAL MANIFESTATIONS

Pulmonary stenosis is one of the most common congenital heart defects and accounts for about 10 percent of patients in most large study populations (Table 73-1). The stenosis is at the level of the pulmonary valve in most instances, but it can occur within the right ventricle, in the pulmonary arteries, or in a combination of the two. Infants with severe stenosis with patency of the foramen ovale may have right-to-left shunting.

History Most infants and children are asymptomatic, but a small percentage with very severe obstruction manifest symptoms, usually mild fatigue or shortness of breath with exertion. Young infants with critical obstruction present with cyanosis if there is a patent foramen ovale or ASD. Squatting and syncope are rare in childhood.[162]

Physical Examination Patients with a dysplastic valve and occasional supravalvular stenosis have consistent noncardiac abnormalities in a familial syndrome described by Noonan,[160] with short stature, hypertelorism, ptosis, low-set ears, and mental retardation. In older patients with valvular pulmonary stenosis, cyanosis is uncommon except with severe obstruction and an atrial communication. Hepatomegaly and the murmur of tricuspid regurgitation may be present with severe obstruction. With at least moderate obstruction, a prominent *a* wave is seen on examination of the jugular venous pulse. A systolic thrill in the suprasternal notch and at the left upper sternal border is present with significant obstruction unless there is isolated subvalvular stenosis. The right ventricular parasternal impulse becomes increasingly forceful with more severe obstruction. *An early systolic click with expiration that disappears with inspiration heard at the left upper sternal border is the hallmark of valvular stenosis unless the obstruction is severe or the valve is dysplastic.* A click is not present with isolated stenosis at other levels. As the obstruction increases in severity, the pulmonary component of the second heart sound becomes progressively softer and more delayed, becoming inaudible when the right ventricular pressure reaches systemic levels or greater. The second heart sound is normal or accentuated with supravalvular stenosis. A fourth heart sound is heard if the obstruction is severe. The characteristic systolic murmur is harsh, crescendo-decrescendo in shape, and best heard at the left upper sternal border with radiation toward the left clavicle. The murmur radiates more to the axilla and back with supravalvular stenosis. The duration of the murmur and the timing of peak intensity correlate well with the severity of obstruction. With mild to moderate stenosis, the murmur peaks in midsystole and ends at or before the aortic component of the second heart sound. In patients with severe stenosis, the murmur peaks late in systole and extends beyond the aortic component of the second heart sound (see Chap. 12).[162]

Chest Roentgenogram Most patients have a normal or only slightly increased heart size, primarily of the right ventricle. Significant enlargement is seen with critical obstruction and is an ominous sign. Characteristically, the main and proximal left pulmonary arteries are prominent as a result of poststenotic dilatation when the stenosis is valvular. This finding may be absent with very severe obstructions, with a dysplastic valve, in very young infants, or with stenosis above or below the valve. The pulmonary vascular pattern is normal in most of these patients, but the vascularity is diminished in those with a right-to-left shunt at the atrial level.

Electrocardiogram Right ventricular forces in the anterior precordial leads correlate reasonably well with the degree of obstruction.[162] They are normal or demonstrate mild hypertrophy with an rsR⁺ pattern if there is mild obstruction. With severe stenosis, there is right axis deviation and right atrial hypertrophy as well as very tall pure R waves in the anterior precordial leads. The presence of a qR pattern in these leads is almost always a sign of very severe obstruction. Those with a dysplastic valve frequently have a superior QRS axis.

Echocardiogram Two-dimensional imaging allows identification of the level of obstruction, and Doppler studies provide an excellent measure of severity. Shunting at the atrial level also can be evaluated.[163]

Cardiac Catheterization Diagnostic catheterizations are rarely necessary, but data obtained before balloon dilation demonstrate an elevated right ventricular systolic pressure with a distinct systolic pressure difference across the narrowed segment, as demonstrated by slow withdrawal of the catheter from the distal pulmonary arterial branches to the proximal right ventricle. Simultaneous measurement of systemic arterial and right ventricular pressures with measurement of flow is necessary to assess severity accurately. The right ventricular end-diastolic pressure and right atrial *a* wave may be elevated. Systemic oxygen saturation is diminished only in those with more severe obstruction and a patent foramen ovale or, less commonly, a true ASD. A left-to-right shunt at the atrial level is detected in some patients with mild to moderate obstruction. With valvular stenosis, right ventricular angiography demonstrates thickened and doming valve leaflets and a jet of contrast material entering the dilated pulmonary artery (Fig. 73-28*A*). Doming is not characteristic of the dysplastic valve. Infundibular subvalvular narrowing caused by muscular hypertrophy may occur secondary to the valvular stenosis or rarely as an isolated anomaly. Isolated anomalous muscle bundles in the right ventricle also may be seen. Pulmonary arterial angiography best demonstrates the sites of obstruction with supravalvular stenoses. Ventricular volume studies have demonstrated depressed ventricular function in patients with right-to-left shunts. Balloon dilation is discussed below, under "Management."

NATURAL HISTORY AND PROGNOSIS

The clinical course of valvular stenosis is favorable in most patients with mild to moderate obstruction. In a national cooperative study,[164] 86 percent of patients had no significant increase in their pressure gradients over a 4- to 8-year interval. Those with a significant increase were less than 4 years of age and had at least moderate stenosis initially. Progression during the period of growth seems to be the likely explanation for most of the increases, but a few patients developed subvalvular muscular hypertrophy, which increased the obstruction. Even mild obstruction may progress significantly in some infants during the first year of life. The prognosis of those with severe obstruction without intervention is poor, especially in the case of infants with critical obstruction. With severe obstruction, right ventricular damage and dysfunction can ensue over the years, and heart failure or arrhythmias can cause premature death in adults.[165] Tricuspid regurgitation also may result. Obstruction of the subvalvular type frequently increases with time, while supravalvular stenosis usually does not progress. Brain abscess can occur if a right-to-left shunt is present. Infective endocarditis with vegetations on the valve, pulmonary arterial wall, or infundibular region is also a risk. The children originally followed and treated as part of the national cooperative study cited above[162,164] were reevaluated 15 to 25 years later.[166] Among the 580 patients alive at the completion of the previous study, new data were available on 464 (78.4 percent). The probability of 25-year survival was 95.7 percent compared with an expected age- and sex-matched control group survival of 96.6 percent. Ninety-seven percent were asymptomatic. Although cardiac catheterization studies were not repeated, clinical examination and echocardiography at follow-up suggested no pulmonary stenosis in 2 percent, mild stenosis in 93 percent, moderate stenosis in 3 percent, and severe stenosis in only 1 percent. Pulmonary regurgitation was present in 40 percent, usually secondary to surgical valvotomy. Endocarditis was uncommon, as were ventricular arrhythmias.

MANAGEMENT

Management obviously depends on the severity of obstruction. For those with mild to moderate valvular pulmonary stenosis, periodic reexamination is indicated to detect any evidence of progression, with more frequent evaluation for those under 1 year of age. Measures to treat heart failure should be instituted in an infant with critical stenosis, but prompt intervention is mandatory. Cyanosis or a

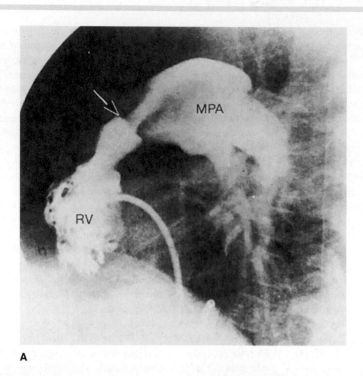

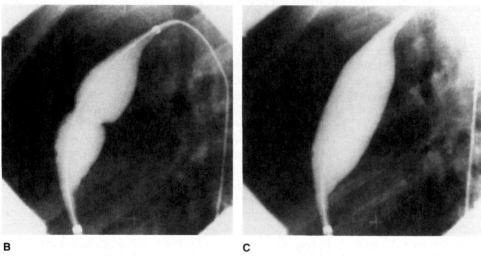

FIGURE 73-28 *A.* Lateral view of a right ventricular (RV) angiogram demonstrating the typical features of valvular pulmonary stenosis with doming of the pulmonary valve (*arrow*) and a narrow jet of contrast entering the dilated main pulmonary artery (MPA). *B.* An 18-mm balloon is inflated across the 14-mm annulus. A moderate waist is seen at 1 atm of pressure. *C.* The waist is eliminated at 4 atm. (From Lock JE, Keane JF, Perry SB. *Diagnostic and Interventional Catheterization in Congenital Heart Disease,* 2d ed. Boston: Kluwer; 2000. Reproduced with permission from the publisher and authors.)

The Valvuloplasty and Angioplasty of Congenital Anomalies Registry has published the combined results on 822 children.[156] Valvuloplasty resulted in improvement in most children with valvular obstruction, reducing the gradient from 71 ± 33 mmHg to 28 ± 24 mmHg. Valvuloplasty is, not surprisingly, less effective in children with a dysplastic pulmonary valve.[167,168] Complications were uncommon (5 in 822, or 0.6 percent), including two deaths. Valvuloplasty also has been performed in critical neonatal pulmonary stenosis with cyanosis caused by right-to-left shunting at the atrial level with a high success rate.[169,170] Subvalvular obstruction is less amenable to dilatation.

Peripheral pulmonary stenosis has also occasionally been amenable to dilatation, although the results are frequently less dramatic because of the multiple areas of stenosis and the fact that the complications, including pulmonary artery rupture, are more common.[171,172] Recently, stents have been used, with promising results,[172] in those with peripheral pulmonary artery stenosis in an attempt to keep open vessels that recoil back to normal size after the balloon is deflated. For those in whom isolated subvalvular stenosis or associated defects exist or in whom balloon dilatation has failed, surgical intervention is recommended.

The risk of death after pulmonary artery dilation is higher than that after dilatation of the valve.[160] In the large collaborative study cited above, the death rate was 3 percent, although a more recent study from the author's institution found a mortality rate less than 1 percent among 400 cases.[173]

SURGICAL MANAGEMENT

Operation rarely is indicated for isolated pulmonary valvular stenosis; balloon valvuloplasty is virtually always successful in eliminating a clinically significant obstruction. A thickened, immobile, dysplastic pulmonary valve, however, is best treated by complete surgical excision (valvectomy). A small annulus is augmented with a pericardial or Dacron gusset.[174]

Subvalvular pulmonary stenosis is relieved through a right ventriculotomy, a main pulmonary arteriotomy, or a right atriotomy. Hypertrophic parietal and septal muscle bands constituting the fibrous orifice of the os infundibulum and obstructing moderator bands or muscle bundles within the body of the right ventricle are excised. Care is exercised to avoid injury to major coronary arterial branches. Usually, the ventriculotomy can be closed either by direct suturing or by augmenting the outflow tract with a patch of pericardium or

right ventricular systolic pressure well above systemic levels also is an indication for prompt intervention. Intervention is warranted in older children when the gradient exceeds 75 mmHg and is clearly not indicated when the gradient is less than 25 mmHg. *In the intermediate group, there is still some controversy, but general practice suggests valvuloplasty when the gradient exceeds 40 mmHg, although objective data to support therapy at this level are lacking.* Balloon valvuloplasty has replaced surgical therapy as a first approach. Through the femoral vein, a balloon catheter is advanced across the valve and inflated to about 120 percent of the size of the pulmonary annulus, ripping the domed valve and thus relieving the obstruction (Fig. 73-28*B*).

Dacron to prevent constriction. A small patch that does not extend across the annulus compromises right ventricular function minimally. Larger patches to the pulmonary arterial bifurcation probably impair ventricular performance but may be necessary when there is associated annular or main pulmonary arterial hypoplasia. When possible, excision from the pulmonary artery or the right atrium is preferred to avoid ventricular injury. Excellent relief of right ventricular outflow tract obstruction can be expected after resection. Mortality and significant morbidity are rare.

Stenoses of main or extraparenchymal branch pulmonary arteries can be relieved by pericardial, synthetic, or homograft aortic or pulmonary arterial patches if the obstruction is proximal. Proximal coarctations in the larger portion of the arterial tree are more readily corrected than are those in small distal branches beyond the bifurcation of either the right or the left pulmonary artery, where results are poor.[175] In these instances, catheter balloon angioplasty, although certainly not without risk, offers nonsurgical relief of obstruction even in the small pulmonary arterial branches and should be considered the procedure of choice for distal pulmonary arterial stenoses.[171,172] Prophylaxis against infective endocarditis is recommended for all patients whether or not surgery is performed, although the risks seem to be lower than they are with many other congenital anomalies.

Tetralogy of Fallot

PATHOLOGY

Tetralogy of Fallot is characterized by biventricular origin of the aorta above a large VSD (Fig. 73-29), obstruction to pulmonary blood flow, and right ventricular hypertrophy. Fibrous continuity of the aortic origin and the anterior mitral valve is maintained.[68] The right ventricular infundibulum lies anterior to the position of the VSD and is bounded by the anterior and septal walls anteriorly and medially; the posterior wall is said to be a vertical crista supraventricularis or displaced conus septum.[176] The right ventricular infundibulum is a distinctive channel, but the caliber varies widely from only mild obstruction to atresia. Usually, it exhibits a significant degree of stenosis and is the dominant site of the obstruction to pulmonary flow that is characteristic of tetralogy. The pulmonary valve is often malformed, usually being either bicuspid or unicuspid. The valve may contribute to pulmonary stenosis, but uncommonly is it the only site of significant obstruction to pulmonary flow. Characteristically, the pulmonary trunk is thin-walled and its lumen is more narrow than normal, but usually it is wider than either the right ventricular infundibulum or the orifice of the pulmonary valve. The aorta is wider than normal, its change in caliber being roughly inversely proportional to that of the pulmonary trunk. The foramen ovale is frequently patent in patients of all ages. In all cases of tetralogy with significant pulmonary obstruction, collateral branches to the lungs arise from the aorta.

There is invariably a large malalignment VSD. Anterior, middle, or apical muscular defects are also present in up to 5 percent of children seen as infants. Many close spontaneously, but if corrective surgery is to be performed successfully, they must be evaluated.

Coronary artery abnormalities are not uncommon. The anterior descending coronary artery in the interventricular septum may arise from the right instead of the left coronary artery. Although physiologically unimportant preoperatively, the course across the right ventricular outflow tract makes the usual site of right ventriculotomy and outflow patch unavailable during reparative surgery, frequently necessitating a conduit to "jump over" the vessel. Previously, angiogra-

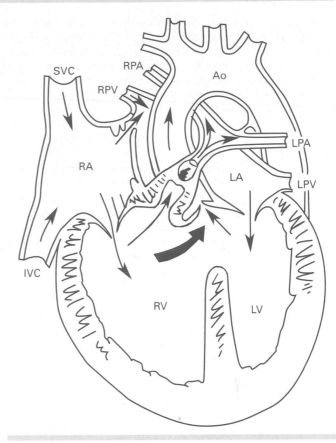

FIGURE 73-29 Classic tetralogy of Fallot. There are infundibular and pulmonary valvular stenoses. There is also right-to-left shunting at the atrial level. SVC = superior vena cava; IVC = inferior vena cava; RA = right atrium; RV = right ventricle; RPA = right pulmonary artery; LPA = left pulmonary artery; RPV = right pulmonary vein; LPV = left pulmonary vein; LA = left atrium; LV = left ventricle; Ao = aorta. (From Edwards.[68] Reproduced with permission from the publisher and author.)

phy was mandatory to establish the anatomy of the coronary circulation, but echocardiography with Doppler color flow is sufficient to detail the distribution of the proximal coronary circulation in most cases.

ASSOCIATED CONDITIONS

The condition most commonly associated with tetralogy of Fallot is right aortic arch (about 30 percent).[177] A persistent left superior vena cava has been described in 10.6 percent of cases. When an associated ASD exists, this anomaly is referred to as *pentalogy of Fallot*. The ductus arteriosus may be absent, present unilaterally on either the right or the left side, or bilateral.

ABNORMAL PHYSIOLOGY

Since the VSD is large, with an area about as great as that of the aortic valve, both ventricles and the aorta have essentially the same systolic pressures. The most important hemodynamic factor is the ratio between the resistance to flow into the aorta and the resistance to flow across the right ventricular infundibulum. If the stenosis is not severe and resistance to right ventricular outflow is not large, the pulmonary flow may be twice the systemic flow, and the arterial oxygen saturation may be normal (acyanotic tetralogy of Fallot). However, the resistance to the pulmonary flow may be increased markedly, causing right-to-left shunting, arterial desaturation, and subsequent polycythemia. When the pulmonary stenosis is very severe, collateral vessels from the systemic arteries to the distal pulmonary arteries sustain pulmonary blood flow. Drugs, heart rate, or maneuvers that increase myocardial contractility or decrease right ventricular volume increase infundibular obstruction, often partially dynamic. In addition, the infundibular hypertrophy may increase gradually over time. Since the systolic pressure in the right ventricle cannot exceed that in the left ventricle because of the large VSD, the right ventricle is "protected" from excessive pressure and work, and so heart failure is uncommon.

Hypercyanotic episodes (spells) in patients with tetralogy are of uncertain origin. It is likely that some episodes are caused by unusual hyperactivity of muscular fibers in the right ventricular outflow tract that produce or exaggerate the infundibular stenosis, increasing pulmonary resistance and thus increasing the right-to-left shunting. Some spells may be caused by a decrease in peripheral resistance and systemic arterial pressure, which also may cause the right-to-left shunt to increase and pulmonary blood flow to decrease.

CLINICAL MANIFESTATIONS

Tetralogy of Fallot is the most common congenital cardiac defect that causes cyanosis. Tetralogy with an associated ASD, or pentalogy of Fallot, is not distinguishable clinically. For a discussion on the hypoxemia and the consequences in tetralogy, see "Complications of Congenital Heart Disease, Hypoxemia" earlier in this chapter.

History   Most of these patients are diagnosed by prenatal ultrasound or present in the first days or weeks of life with a heart murmur. If the right ventricular obstruction is severe, cyanosis is present at birth and is exacerbated when the ductus closes. If the obstruction is milder, the infant may be acyanotic with left-to-right flow through the VSD and occasionally may develop heart failure. In this group, gradually increasing right ventricular obstruction may reduce the left-to-right shunt; eventually, when infundibular resistance and pulmonary resistance exceed systemic resistance, right-to-left shunting develops and cyanosis results.

Dyspnea with exertion occurs commonly in toddlers and older children with unrepaired defects. Attacks of suddenly increasing cyanosis associated with hyperpnea, or hypoxic spells,[178] are common between ages 2 months and 2 years. There are many precipitating events, including infection, exertion, and summer heat. They occur most often in the morning, with increasing irritability. The frequency and duration vary widely, but prolonged episodes can lead to syncope, seizures, and death. Squatting with exercise is common from 1.5 to 10 years of age in those who have not previously undergone repair. These problems are becoming uncommon as more and more children receive early repair.

Physical Examination   Growth is usually normal unless cyanosis is extreme. Clubbing of the fingers and toes occurs after 3 months of age and is proportional to the level of cyanosis. Signs of heart failure do not appear in tetralogy of Fallot during childhood unless there is a superimposed illness such as anemia or infective endocarditis.

Increased right ventricular activity is observed. A systolic thrill may be palpable at the left midsternal border, with a harsh midsystolic murmur in that location. Softer murmurs signal more severe obstruction and are common when presentation is in the newborn period or during hypoxic spells. The murmur ends before the second heart sound, which is characteristically single. A continuous murmur is heard if a PDA or large collateral vessels are present. An early systolic ejection sound at the left sternal border and apex is uncommon; its presence suggests primarily valvular pulmonary stenosis.

Chest Roentgenogram   The total heart size is usually normal on chest roentgenography, but right ventricular enlargement is present in the lateral view. The aorta arches to the right in many cases. Pulmonary flow is diminished. The pulmonary segment is concave and the apex is elevated, giving the *coeur en sabot* (boot-shaped) contour. A very young infant may have only diminished pulmonary flow.

Electrocardiogram   In tetralogy of Fallot, the mean QRS axis of the ECG is usually to the right, between +90 and +210 degrees. There is right ventricular hypertrophy, with a tall R wave in the right precordial leads and a deep S wave in the left leads. Some of these patients have right atrial hypertrophy.

Echocardiogram   Two-dimensional echocardiography can delineate the anatomic components of tetralogy.[179] Anomalies of the coronary arteries can be demonstrated and associated defects excluded.

Hematologic and Other Laboratory Studies   Before surgical repair, the hemoglobin and hematocrit should be measured; pulse oximetry should be performed at initial evaluation and periodically thereafter for determination of the degree of polycythemia and the early detection of anemia relative to the degree of cyanosis. The latter is common, especially in those under 2 years of age, and may predispose a patient to cerebrovascular accidents. Platelet counts and clotting studies may be advisable in older unrepaired patients with marked polycythemia, particularly if a surgical procedure is planned. Serum uric acid levels should be measured if polycythemia is severe and of long standing.

Cardiac Catheterization   In an increasing number of centers, the quality of echocardiography (especially in neonates or infants) is sufficiently diagnostic to outline the right ventricular and proximal pulmonary artery anatomy, rule out additional muscular VSDs, and establish the proximal coronary circulation. As a consequence, diagnostic cardiac catheterization and angiography are less commonly performed preoperatively than they were in the past in children with tetralogy of Fallot.

In those in whom the study is performed, the right ventricular systolic pressure is equal to the pressure in the left ventricle and aorta. If the pulmonary artery can be entered, the pressure will be normal or low. The level or levels of obstruction can be evaluated by careful pullback to the right ventricle. Caution should be observed if the pulmonary artery is entered, as the catheter may critically reduce the pulmonary flow and cause a hypoxic episode. Systemic arterial oxygen saturation is reduced because of right-to-left shunting from the right to the left ventricle. If a patent foramen ovale or ASD is present, there may be an additional right-to-left or bidirectional shunt at the atrial level. Selective biplane right ventricular angiography will demonstrate levels of obstruction, continuity and size of the pulmonary arteries, and size and position of the ventricular defect. If this is not demonstrated by echocardiography or aortography, selective coronary arteriography should be performed on all patients preoperatively to demonstrate the coronary arterial pattern.[180] Magnetic resonance imaging (MRI) provides excellent images of the pulmonary artery anatomy particularly in the case of diminutive pulmonary vessels or discontinuous pulmonary arteries (Fig. 73-30).

MEDICAL MANAGEMENT

Although the definitive treatment of tetralogy of Fallot is surgical, medical management plays a role before surgery and in the postoperative period. For a severely cyanotic newborn, prostaglandin administration is of benefit[97] to keep the ductus open until surgery can be

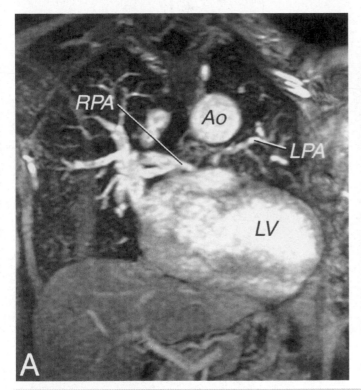

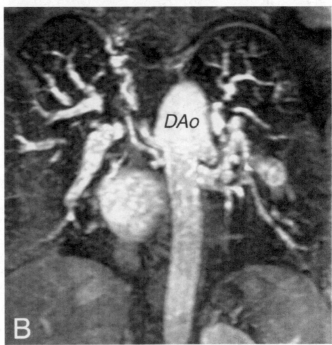

FIGURE 73-30 Preoperative MRI in a 33-year-old woman with tetraology of Fallot, pulmonary atresia, and discontinuous pulmonary arteries. *A.* gadolinium-enhanced 3D MRA subvolume maximal intensity projection (MIP) in the coronal plane showing discontinuity between the right pulmonary artery (RPA) and the left pulmonary artery (LPA). *B.* subvolume MIP image of the descending aorta (DAo) showing multiple aortopulmonary collaterals. (From Geva T, Sahn DJ, Powell AC. Magnetic resonance imaging of congenital heart disease in adults. *Prog Pediatr Cardiol* 2003; 17: 21–39. Reproduced with permission of the authors and publisher.)

done. Before surgery, the hematocrit and hemoglobin should be monitored and iron-deficiency anemia should be treated promptly to prevent strokes. Fever or other illness that would lead to dehydration and possible thrombotic complications should be treated promptly.

Hypoxic spells in an infant should be treated initially by placing the infant in the knee-chest position and administering a high concentration of oxygen and morphine sulfate. If acidosis is present and does not correct spontaneously and promptly, intravenous sodium bicarbonate and an alpha-adrenergic agonist should be given. Propranalol may be useful in preventing hypoxic spells.[181]

Bacterial endocarditis is a serious complication, especially in those who have had a systemic-to-pulmonary artery shunt. Meticulous care should be taken to maintain good dental hygiene, and prophylactic antibiotics at times of predictable risk are mandatory (see Chap. 81).

SURGICAL MANAGEMENT

Historically, the approach to tetralogy of Fallot has been either palliation or corrective surgery. The introduction of an aorta-to-pulmonary artery shunt for the treatment of tetralogy of Fallot[182] truly can be called the beginning of effective treatment for pediatric cardiovascular disease. When open heart surgery was initiated in the 1950s, tetralogy of Fallot was among the first lesions to be corrected.[183] Over the years, the age at which corrective surgery can be performed has dropped, so that in many centers primary repair is the procedure of choice at any age. Palliation, when it is now performed, almost inevitably involves a modified Blalock-Taussig shunt that interposes a graft between the subclavian artery and the ipsilateral pulmonary artery, usually on the side opposite the aortic arch.[184] Even in

the perinatal period, the placement of a 4-mm tube will result in satisfactory palliation for a year in more than 90 percent of infants.

Surgical correction for those with pulmonary stenosis involves closing the VSD, usually through a right ventriculotomy, resecting infundibular muscle, and, if the infundibulum, pulmonary valve, and main pulmonary artery are hypoplastic, using a pericardial patch to open the narrowed area. Care must be taken to avoid heart block while closing the VSD and avoid cutting a major branch of the coronary artery. If a patent foramen ovale is present, it usually is left open to allow decompression in the perioperative period. If a true ASD is present (pentalogy of Fallot), it should be closed to avoid left-to-right shunting once the right ventricle has recovered from the perioperative insult.[185] Tetralogy of Fallot and pulmonary atresia with good-sized pulmonary arteries are usually repaired by closing the VSD and interposing a conduit, frequently an aortic homograft, between the right ventricle and the pulmonary artery.[186,187] If this procedure is performed prior to 7 or 8 years of age, replacement of the conduit is to be expected secondary to somatic growth. Tetralogy of Fallot and hypoplastic and/or discontinuous pulmonary arteries call for an individualized approach that frequently involves balloon dilation of hypoplastic vessels, unifocalization of discontinuous vessels, with the intent to complete eventual repair with a conduit closing the VSD.[188] In cases where pulmonary artery stenosis has been resistant to dilation with high pressure balloons, cutting balloon therapy has been shown to increase efficacy of dilation.[189] Operative and early mortality rates for repair of tetralogy of Fallot are now quite low in most centers. Kirklin and coworkers[184] in the early 1980s reported mortality rates of 1.6 percent with operations at 5 years of age to 4.1 percent at 1 year of age. At Children's Hospital in Boston, there was a

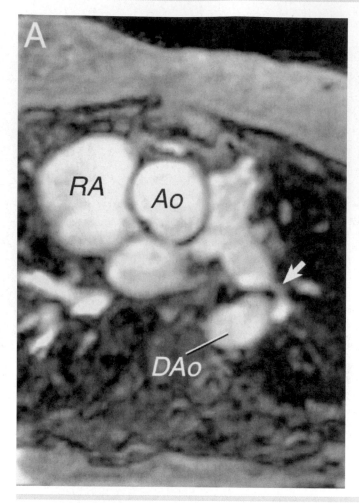

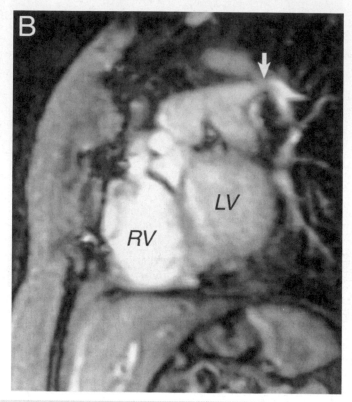

FIGURE 73-31 Postoperative MRI after tetralogy of Fallot repair in a patient with a previous Potts shunt. *A.* Gadolinium-enhanced 3D MRA subvolume maximal image projection (MIP) in the axial plane showing severe left pulmonary artery stenosis (*arrow*) at the site of the previous Potts shunt. *B.* Oblique sagittal subvolume MIP image showing the superoinferior aspect of the left pulmonary artery stenosis (*arrow*). (From Geva T, Sahn DJ, Powell AC. Magnetic resonance imaging of congenital heart disease in adults. *Prog Pediatr Cardiol* 2003; 17: 21–39. Reproduced with permission of the authors and publisher.)

4.2 percent mortality rate among 330 children under 1 year of age operated on between 1973 and 1990, with a mortality rate of only 2.5 percent in the past 6 years of the study (1984–1990).[185] Late complications have included residual peripheral pulmonary stenosis, a small incidence of residual VSDs, and, rarely, aortic regurgitation. MRI is an excellent adjunct to echocardiography for assessment of residual anatomic abnormalities, especially with respect to the distal pulmonary arterial architecture (Fig. 73-31). The long-term survivors have had atrial or, more commonly, ventricular arrhythmias and continue to be at risk for infective endocarditis.

Physicians at the Mayo Clinic, the first center to use the pump oxygenator to repair tetralogy of Fallot in the 1950s, have reported a minimum 30-year follow-up of the 162 30-day survivors of surgery.[190] The 32-year actuarial survival rate was 86 percent, with subgroup survival rates of those less then 5 years old, 5 to 7 years old, and 8 to 11 years old at the time of surgical repair being 90, 93, and 91 percent, respectively. Late sudden death from cardiac causes occurred in 10 patients during the 32-year period. The performance of some previous palliative operation (Waterston or Pott's shunts) but not a palliative Blalock-Taussig shunt was associated with higher mortality. With earlier surgery and less utilization of palliative proce-

dures, it is anticipated that the surgical results will be even better for children born in the 1980s and 1990s and beyond.

Ebstein's Anomaly

PATHOLOGY

In Ebstein's anomaly, the anterior leaflet of the tricuspid valve is attached normally to the annulus, but varying portions of the posterior and septal leaflets are displaced downward, being attached to the ventricular wall below the annulus. The proximal part of the right ventricle is thin-walled and continuous with the right atrium. The functional right ventricle is small and made up of the apical and infundibular portions of the right ventricle. An additional common finding is that the papillary muscles and chordae are highly malformed, with great variation in the manner of attachment of the two involved leaflets to the right ventricular wall. Commonly, multiple direct attachments of valvular tissue to the right ventricular mural endocardium occur.[191,192]

An interatrial communication is present in most cases, usually taking the form of a patent foramen ovale. Continuity of right atrial and right ventricular myocardial tissues, in addition to the usual connections by way of the main conduction pathways, has been observed. *The presence of Ebstein's anomaly has been associated with maternal lithium use during pregnancy, although the risk ratio remains unclear.*[193]

ABNORMAL PHYSIOLOGY

Ebstein's anomaly results in obstruction to right ventricular filling because of a decrease in the size of the right ventricle, part of which is incorporated into the huge right atrium. The deformed tricuspid valve also frequently is associated with tricuspid regurgitation with a right-to-left shunt through the foramen ovale. In the perinatal period, when the pulmonary vascular resistance is high, the tricuspid regurgitation may be severe. This results in increased right atrial pressure and, when the patent foramen ovale is open, severe cyanosis. As the pulmonary vascular resistance falls, the right-to-left shunting is decreased and hypoxemia improves. In older children, right-sided heart failure with edema and/or ascites may develop.

CLINICAL MANIFESTATIONS

History   Approximately one-half of reported patients develop symptoms of cyanosis and right-sided heart failure in early infancy. The remainder present with a murmur or abnormal chest roentgenogram, but with no symptoms, in early childhood or because of gradual progression of symptoms through late childhood or adult life.[194] The most common symptom is dyspnea on exertion. The spectrum of exercise intolerance has been described.[195] Palpitations resulting from supraventricular tachyarrhythmias occur in 20 to 30 percent of these children. Occasionally, syncope occurs as a result of arrhythmia or low cardiac output if the atrial septum is intact.

Physical Examination   A newborn with elevated pulmonary vascular resistance has severe cyanosis. In older infants and children, cyanosis and clubbing are mild. Only small percentages do not have an ASD or patent foramen ovale and thus are not cyanotic. The precordium is generally quiet even in those with striking cardiomegaly. The liver is enlarged, and the jugular venous pulse may be elevated. The holosystolic murmur of tricuspid regurgitation is heard at the lower left sternal border and may be accompanied by a "scratchy" diastolic murmur of tricuspid stenosis. The first heart sound is split and loud, and the second heart sound is widely and persistently split. Loud third and fourth heart sounds are usual, especially in older patients.

Chest Roentgenogram   Heart size, as shown by chest roentgenography, varies, but the heart is ordinarily very large because of the very dilated right atrium. In those with cyanosis, pulmonary blood flow is diminished correspondingly.

Electrocardiogram   Giant, peaked P waves are common, along with a prolonged PR interval and right ventricular conduction delay or complete right bundle branch block. In approximately 10 percent of these patients, the pattern of Wolff-Parkinson-White syndrome (with a short PR interval and slurring of the initial QRS forces or a delta wave) is seen.[194]

Echocardiogram   Two-dimensional echocardiography is very helpful in the diagnosis (Fig. 73-32), identifying the lesion, depicting the degree of displacement of the tricuspid valve into the right ventricle, and assessing the severity of the tricuspid regurgitation. In neonates, evaluation of the pulmonary valve usually allows a distinction be-

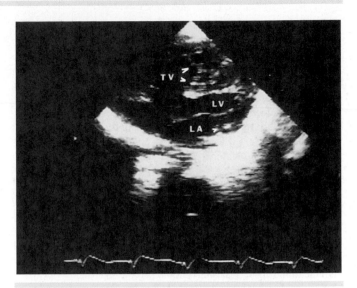

FIGURE 73-32   Two-dimensional echocardiogram in parasternal view in a patient with Ebstein's anomaly of the tricuspid valve (TV). Numerous attachments of the tricuspid valve (*arrowheads*) to the interventricular septum and right ventricular apex are seen. LV = left ventricle; LA = left atrium.

tween anatomic pulmonary atresia from absence of opening of the valve caused by severe tricuspid regurgitation and high pulmonary vascular resistance.[196]

Cardiac Catheterization   There is a higher than usual risk associated with cardiac catheterization because of the frequency of rhythm disturbances. Proper precautions and prompt use of cardioversion when necessary minimize this risk. In most cases, echocardiography and color-flow Doppler evaluation are sufficient, and catheterization is performed less commonly than it was previously.

There is usually right-to-left shunting at the atrial level. Right atrial hypertension is present. The characteristic right ventricular pressure recording is not obtained until the catheter is advanced to the apex or outflow tract. An intracardiac ECG demonstrates, on pullback from the right ventricle, an area where the ECG is ventricular but the pressure is atrial in contour.[197] This method is not infallible, but it provides good evidence of tricuspid displacement with an "atrialized" portion of the right ventricle.

NATURAL HISTORY AND PROGNOSIS

The natural history varies greatly with the severity of the abnormality. In a study of 50 patients who presented in the neonatal period, 9 (18 percent) died in the perinatal period, with late deaths in another 15 (9 from hemodynamic deterioration, 5 sudden, and 1 noncardiac), for a 10-year actuarial survival of 61 percent.[198] In a study that included more children who presented after the perinatal period, the probability of survival was 50 percent at 47 years of age.[199] Predictors of poor outcome were New York Heart Association class III or IV, cardiothoracic ratio >65 percent, and atrial fibrillation. In a review of 72 unoperated adults with isolated Ebstein's anomaly followed from the age of 25 years, 41 percent were alive 20 years later. Though parameters predicting outcome were multifactorial, the ratio of septal leaflet displacement to ventricular septal length correlated well with survival.[200]

For women who survive into adulthood without significant arrhythmias or cyanosis, successful pregnancy with good fetal outcome is possible.[201]

MEDICAL MANAGEMENT

Medical therapy varies depending on the severity of disease and the age at presentation. For those presenting with cyanosis in the perinatal period, procrastination until the pulmonary vascular resistance has decreased may be the best strategy. For those who are severely hypoxemic, maintaining the patency of the ductus with PGE₁ may be lifesaving. Reducing the pulmonary vascular resistance with nitric oxide may reduce right-to-left shunting and improve oxygenation.[202] Persistence of severe cyanosis beyond 1 week of age suggests pulmonary stenosis or pulmonary atresia in addition to Ebstein's deformity of the tricuspid valve.

For children with arrhythmias, an electrophysiologic study may be indicated. For those with disabling or life-threatening arrhythmias, radiofrequency ablation may be performed with initial success rates of about 80 percent but recurrences in 30 percent of patients.[203] In older children who develop right-sided heart failure, digoxin and diuretics may be tried, although this level of deterioration is usually an indication for surgical intervention.

SURGICAL MANAGEMENT

The surgical management of Ebstein's disease remains problematic. In the perinatal period, when the pulmonary vascular resistance is high, watchful waiting is probably the best approach. If the child remains severely hypoxemic (saturations <75%) after the pulmonary vascular resistance falls, palliation with a Blalock-Taussig shunt to improve pulmonary blood flow may be sufficient to relieve hypoxemia and should allow growth to an age at which other procedures can be considered.[204] For children in whom hypoxemia remains a significant problem, three approaches have been used. The first is a Glenn anastomosis connecting the superior vena cava to the right pulmonary artery, allowing blood from the inferior vena cava to enter the right atrium and ventricle to the pulmonary artery.[205] A more definitive procedure that eliminates hypoxemia is used primarily for children with single ventricle; however, the modified Fontan is now applied in this situation as well. In this approach, the tricuspid valve is oversewn and the patent foramen ovale closed, diverting all systemic venous return to the pulmonary arteries bypassing the right heart.[206] In a small group of patients, this has been done with success.

The more common approach has been tricuspid valve reconstruction or replacement, usually with a bioprosthesis. Among 189 patients operated on at the Mayo Clinic over a period of almost 20 years, there were 12 hospital deaths (6.3 percent) and an additional 10 late deaths. Among those followed more than 1 year after operation, more than 90 percent were in New York Heart Association class I or II.[207] More recently, other approaches have been suggested, including reconstruction of the normally shaped right ventricle with repositioning of the displaced leaflet of the tricuspid valve at the normal level[208] and reimplantation of the tricuspid valve leaflets with a vertical plication of the atrialized portion of the right ventricle to reduce its size (Fig. 73-33).[209] Intermediate-term results in severely ill neonates using improved techniques are encouraging.[210] *Although the newer approaches seem promising in small numbers of patients in the short run, many patients with the milder form of the disease can live well into adulthood[211]; therefore indications for the newer operations in patients who are asymptomatic or only mildly limited remain problematic.*

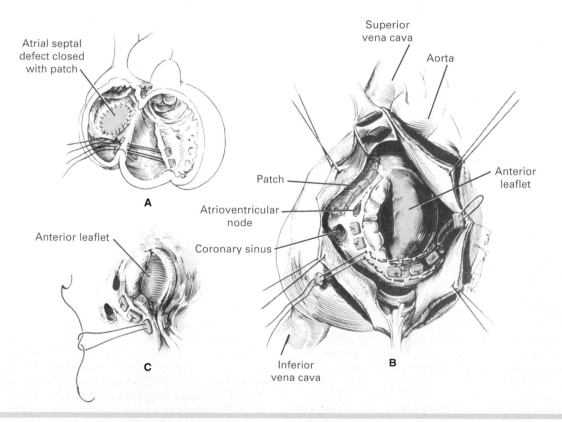

FIGURE 73-33 Danielson repair of Ebstein's malformation. *A.* Anterior cutaway drawing. The atrial septal defect is closed securely with a patch. Pledgeted sutures are placed to position the posterior leaflet at the annulus and imbricate the "atrialized" right ventricular chamber. *B* and *C.* Drawing of the right atrium showing the annuloplasty suture passed through two pledgets. Tying of this suture reduces dilation of the tricuspid valve so that the large anterior leaflet can meet the two smaller cusps and constitute a functional, essentially monocusp valve.

ABNORMALITIES OF THE PULMONARY VENOUS CONNECTIONS

Total Anomalous Pulmonary Venous Connection

PATHOLOGY

When all pulmonary veins terminate in a systemic vein or the right atrium, the term *total anomalous pulmonary venous connection* or *return* is applied (Fig. 73-34). Usually the pulmonary veins leave the lung and then join a chamber-like confluence posterior to the left atrium. From the confluence of veins, one primitive embryologic vessel persists and leads to the anomalous termination. Less commonly, two or more vessels lead to multiple sites of termination.

If the left cardinal vein persists, drainage flows superiorly into the innominate vein and then to the superior vena cava and right atrium or inferiorly into a persistent left superior vena cava and coronary sinus to the right atrium. If the right cardinal vein persists, drainage is to the superior vena cava, the azygos vein, or the right atrium directly. These types are sometimes referred to collectively as supracardiac or supradiaphragmatic drainage and are almost never associated with pulmonary venous obstruction.[212] If the site of termination is infradiaphragmatic, with connection to the portal venous system or the inferior vena cava, the anomalous vein leaves the confluence of pulmonary veins and descends into the abdomen along the esophagus to join the ductus venosus, the portal vein, or the left gastric vein. *Pulmonary venous obstruction is present in virtually all cases of infradiaphragmatic connection.*[212]

In all cases of total anomalous pulmonary venous connection, there is a patent foramen ovale. The atrium and ventricle of the left side are small in comparison with the right-sided chambers but are within normal limits in regard to absolute size. In the absence of asplenia or polysplenia syndromes, associated anomalies are not common.

ABNORMAL PHYSIOLOGY

In this anomaly, all the blood from both the pulmonary and systemic circulation eventually returns to the right atrium. In neonates with the connection below the diaphragm, the increase in pulmonary flow as the pulmonary resistance decreases after birth cannot be accommodated and the obstruction to flow causes a marked increase in pulmonary venous pressure, resulting in a very high pulmonary vascular resistance. If the ductus arteriosus is still open, the pulmonary vascular resistance exceeds systemic vascular resistance with a right-to-left shunt at the ductal level. When the ductus closes, the increased pulmonary resistance results in increased right ventricular pressure. As the right ventricle fails and right atrial pressure increases, the resulting right-to-left shunt at the atrial level may cause profound hypoxemia.

In older children with unobstructed damage above the diaphragm (supracardiac), the pulmonary resistance is usually low, facilitating a high pulmonary flow. With mixing of all pulmonary and systemic flow in the right atrium, the oxygen saturation is usually relatively high, resulting in physiology similar to that of an ASD and mild cyanosis.[213]

CLINICAL MANIFESTATIONS

Total Anomalous Pulmonary Venous Connection with Pulmonary Venous Obstruction Neonates with total anomalous venous connection below the diaphragm who have pulmonary venous obstruction present with cyanosis, which may be severe, and tachypnea.

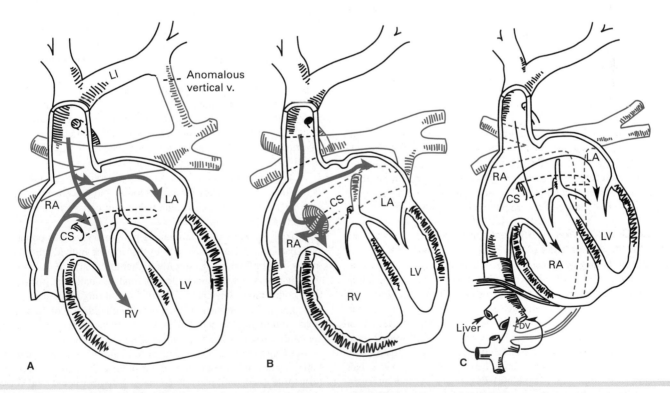

FIGURE 73-34 Three common types of total anomalous pulmonary venous connection. *A.* Total anomalous pulmonary venous connection to the left brachiocephalic (innominate) vein (LI). *B.* Total anomalous pulmonary venous connection to the coronary sinus (CS). *C.* Total anomalous pulmonary venous connection of the infradiaphragmatic type to the ductus venosus (DV). RA = right atrium; RV = right ventricle; LA = left atrium; LV = left ventricle.

Symptoms frequently develop beyond 12 h of age, allowing differentiation from respiratory distress syndrome. In addition to tachypnea, feeding difficulties and heart failure are seen.

The physical findings are usually unimpressive. The heart is not hyperactive, and thrills are absent. The second heart sound may be split, with an increased pulmonary component. Significant murmurs are uncommon.

Total Anomalous Pulmonary Venous Connection without Pulmonary Venous Obstruction These patients are usually asymptomatic at birth, although some may develop transient tachypnea. Presentation typically occurs during the first year of life. Some of these children have tachypnea and feeding difficulties, with frequent respiratory infections. Cyanosis often is mild and may not be clinically apparent. Other children may be asymptomatic and present with a heart murmur.

The cardiac examination is similar to that of an ASD with increased right-sided flow. The right ventricular impulse is usually hyperactive. The jugular venous pulse is elevated, and hepatomegaly appears early. There is a diffuse and hyperdynamic right ventricular impulse. The second heart sound is split and relatively fixed; the loudness of the pulmonary component may be increased. There is usually a grade 2 or 3 midsystolic flow murmur at the left sternal border. At the lower sternal border, there is a middiastolic rumble and prominent third and fourth heart sounds. Rales may be heard over the lung fields, and periorbital edema is common. A continuous murmur rarely may be heard over the common venous channel.

Chest Roentgenogram With the unobstructed types, the heart is enlarged with increased pulmonary flow. Pulmonary edema is uncommon. In patients with return to the left innominate vein, there may be a characteristic bulging of the superior mediastinum bilaterally, producing a "snowman" or figure-of-eight, contour. With obstructed types, the heart size is nearly normal; there is very marked pulmonary edema, which may give a granular appearance to the lungs, making differentiation from respiratory distress syndrome difficult in a newborn.

Electrocardiogram There is right axis deviation and right atrial and right ventricular hypertrophy. Commonly, there is a qR pattern in the right precordial leads.

Echocardiogram Echocardiography with color-flow Doppler is specific in defining the anomaly and the site of drainage.[214] The right side of the heart is enlarged when the venous return is unobstructed with increased flow. Although the right-sided chambers may dwarf the left heart, the left heart is usually of normal size. With obstructed return, there is evidence of severe pulmonary hypertension.

Cardiac Catheterization If echocardiography is inconclusive in delineating the site or sites of the pulmonary venous connection, catheterization may be necessary. There is an increase in oxygen saturation at the level of the abnormal connection, with similar saturations in the remainder of the chambers on both sides of the heart. Pulmonary arterial pressure is elevated to a variable degree, but it may be above systemic pressure if there is marked pulmonary venous or pulmonary vascular obstruction. Pulmonary capillary wedge pressures are elevated in proportion to the degree of venous obstruction. The atrial communication may rarely be obstructive[213]; if it is, balloon atrial septostomy may be helpful. Pulmonary arteriography usually will show the anomalous venous connection. Angiography in the common venous channel, if entered, will outline its course and any sites of obstruction optimally.

NATURAL HISTORY AND PROGNOSIS

The natural history varies depending on the degree of obstruction of egress of blood from the pulmonary veins.[213] Those who present in the perinatal period with severe cyanosis and respiratory distress, usually with pulmonary venous drainage below the diaphragm, represent a medical emergency and will die without early surgery.

Those with supracardiac drainage and some degree of obstruction and pulmonary hypertension are sufficiently tachypneic that feeding is problematic, and they fail to gain weight at a normal rate. They tolerate respiratory infections poorly and occasionally need emergency surgery for respiratory failure.

Those without pulmonary venous obstruction have large left-to-right shunts and mild cyanosis but may have no or minimal symptoms at rest or exercise. If corrective surgery is not performed, they are at risk for pulmonary vascular disease.[215]

MEDICAL MANAGEMENT

For neonates with severe cyanosis and respiratory disease, oxygen, a respirator, and PGE_1 can be used to temporize but survival is dependent on early surgery. For those with mild pulmonary hypertension and failure to thrive, surgery usually is performed semielectively. For those without pulmonary hypertension who present with murmurs and findings similar to those of an atrial septal defect, surgery is more elective but little is gained by waiting, and more centers are advocating early repair in this group as well.[216]

SURGICAL MANAGEMENT

Correction of total anomalous pulmonary venous connection requires (1) creation of a large communication between the left atrium and the pulmonary venous system, (2) obliteration of the anomalous pulmonary venous connection to the systemic circulation, and (3) closure of the associated interatrial communications.[216]

Supracardiac anomalous connection to the left brachiocephalic (vertical) vein and infracardiac connections to the portal venous system or the inferior vena cava are corrected by the creation of a wide anastomosis between the posterior aspect of the left atrium and the common transverse pulmonary vein. The stretched foramen ovale is closed. The ascending or descending anomalous pulmonary venous connection to the systemic circulation is ligated, as is the PDA.

Anomalous pulmonary venous connection to the coronary sinus is repaired by creating a large fenestration in the common wall between the coronary sinus and the left atrium. The coronary sinus is diverted into the left atrium by the placement of an intracardiac patch, which also closes the interatrial communication.

Total anomalous pulmonary venous connection to the right atrium is repaired by excision of the atrial septum and placement of a patch that diverts the opening of the anomalous pulmonary venous connection into the left atrium.

Mixed forms of total anomalous pulmonary venous connection pose particular technical difficulties that require individualized operations. Mortality rates are slightly higher after early repair of symptomatic neonates with mixed types of total anomalous pulmonary venous connections. Given the difficulty identifying pulmonary venous drainage in this setting, MRI can provide elucidation of the connections minimizing the need for or at least reducing the time required for cardiac catheterization (Fig. 73-35).

Although the results of repair of total anomalous pulmonary venous connection without obstruction in an older child have always been quite good, until recently neonates with obstructed total venous return have been problematic. In the 1960s and early 1970s, the surgical mortality rate exceeded 50 percent.[217] Between 1970 and 1980, surgical techniques improved and the mortality rate was reduced to

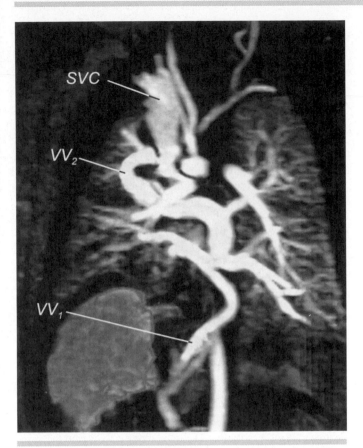

FIGURE 73-35 Maximal intensity projection coronal plane image of gadolinium-enhanced three-dimensional MRA in a newborn with obstructed mixed type total anomalous venous connection. There is infradiaphragmatic connection by means of a vertical vein (VV-1) to the portal vein, as well as supracardiac stenotic connection to the right superior vena cava (SVC) via an additional vertical vein (VV-2). (Figure courtesy of Tal Geva, M.D.)

10 to 20 percent.[218] Recent surgical results show continued improvement, with no mortality among 27 infants who underwent reparative surgery at Children's Hospital in Boston in the late 1980s.[219] Late survival has been quite good, with 98 percent surviving a median of 87 months in one study.[220]

After a satisfactory operative course, the prognosis has been excellent in those in whom a large common pulmonary vein can be attached to the back wall of the left atrium with a relatively large anastomosis. For those initially with obstructed total anomalous pulmonary venous return, the left atrium may be small and the anastomosis may be more difficult. Late obstruction of one or more pulmonary veins has been seen. When present, the obstruction can be approached by balloon dilation, stent placement, or repeat surgery.[221]

MALPOSITION OF THE CARDIAC STRUCTURES

Definition and Terminology

The *segmental approach* to the diagnosis of complex congenital heart disease[222] provides an orderly, effective method for determining the anatomic and hemodynamic interrelationships of the cardiac chambers, valves, and great vessels. For this approach to be better understood, certain definitions are helpful. Positioning of viscera is described as situs solitus, inversus, or ambiguus. In *situs solitus* (S),

the distribution of all the organs is recognized as normal—for example, a left-sided stomach and spleen, a predominantly right-sided liver, a trilobed right lung, and a bilobed left lung. In *situs inversus (totalis)* (I), the organs show a perfect mirror image in regard to left and right to that of situs solitus. Anteroposterior relations are not disturbed. When neither situs solitus nor situs inversus can be identified, *situs ambiguus* (A) is said to be present. This usually applies in cases of asplenia or polysplenia.

Almost exclusively, the *atria follow the body situs* and are so designated (morphologic right atrium to the right of the left atrium in atrial situs solitus and to the left of the left atrium in atrial situs inversus). The AV canal consists of the tricuspid valve, the mitral valve, and the septum of the AV canal and connects the atrial portion with the ventricular portion of the heart. As a rule, *each AV valve is part of the specific ventricle into which it leads*. The valve situs may be solitus, inversus, or ambiguus.

The alignment or type of AV or ventriculoarterial (VA) connection addresses the issue of what flows into what. The connection may be described at the AV or VA level as concordant (e.g., right atrium to right ventricle, left ventricle to aorta) or discordant (e.g., right atrium to left ventricle, left ventricle to pulmonary artery) or may be considered an arrangement that requires a special description. In the case of AV alignment in which the atria are not lateralized, the alignment would be ambiguous. In the univentricular heart, the designation would be double-inlet, absent right, or absent left AV connection. Special descriptions in the case of VA alignment or type of VA connection include double-outlet and single-outlet VA connection. The mode of connections, either AV or VA, addresses the structural makeup of the connecting segments: the AV canal and the infundibulum or conus. The mode of AV connection may be normal, common, stenotic, imperforate, atretic, double-orifice, overriding, straddling, or unguarded. The mode of VA connection may be expressed in terms of the position and development of the conus or infundibulum, which, although normally incorporated into the right ventricle, is not an intrinsic part of the true right ventricle. It may be described as subpulmonary, subaortic, very deficient, or bilaterally present or absent.[223]

The position of the ventricles may be described by the terms *d loop* and *l loop*. When the morphologic right ventricle lies to the right of the morphologic left ventricle, the ventricular portion of the heart is said to exhibit a d loop (D). The ventricles are said to be noninverted or in the solitus position. When the ventricular relations are reversed, l loop (L) is said to be present. The ventricles are inverted or in the inversus position. *These relationships are independent of the visceral or atrial situs as well as the position of the heart or its chambers within the chest.*

The great arteries may deviate from the usual with respect to both their anteroposterior and lateral (left-to-right) relationships. In solitus (S) or *normally related great arteries* (NRGAs), the aortic origin lies to the right of and posterior to the position of the pulmonary valve. In the inversus (I) relationship, the anteroposterior relationships are not disturbed but the aortic origin lies to the left of the pulmonary arterial origin. In *transposition of the great arteries* (TGA), the aorta arises from the anatomic right ventricle, the pulmonary artery arises from the anatomic left ventricle, and usually the aortic origin is more anterior than that of the pulmonary artery.

When the aortic origin lies to the right of the pulmonary origin, the transposition is called *dextro-* or *d-transposition* (D-TGA) (see the discussion of complete transposition of the great arteries, below). When the aortic origin lies to the left of the pulmonary origin, *levotransposition* (L-TGA) is said to be present (see the section on congenitally corrected transposition, below).

When the abnormal relationship of the great arteries is neither complete nor corrected transposition, the term *malposition of the great arteries* (MGA) may be used. Malpositions are designated as D-MGA or L-MGA, depending on the laterality in the relation between the origins of the two great arteries.[208] Within this group are found examples of the abnormal VA alignment, where one great artery arises from the appropriate ventricle and the other great artery also arises from the same (or inappropriate) ventricle. These are examples of *double-outlet right ventricle* (DORV) or *double-outlet left ventricle* (DOLV). Also included is the arterial malposition termed *anatomically corrected malposition* (ACM). This is characterized by the great arteries having a normal VA alignment (concordant), but with the aorta anterior to the pulmonary artery by virtue of an abnormal mode of VA connection: the presence of a well-developed conus lying beneath both the aorta and the pulmonary artery or only beneath the aorta. The route for the flow of blood in ACMs may be normal or abnormal, depending on the AV alignment.[223]

The Segmental Approach to Diagnosis

The segmental, or step-by-step, approach is a valuable tool for arriving at the correct diagnosis in patients with complex congenital heart disease and is independent of cardiac position. In order, one determines (1) the locations of the right and left atria and their venous connections, (2) the location of the right and left ventricles and their alignment with the atria, (3) the mode of connection of the AV valves to the ventricles, (4) the position of the great arteries and their alignment with the ventricles, and (5) the location and status of the infundibulum. In addition, one must search for associated malformations between and within each of these segments.

Determining atrial situs can be accomplished in most instances by taking advantage of the high degree of abdominal visceroatrial concordance. With abdominal situs solitus (S), the liver is on the right and the right atrium almost invariably is on the right as well; with abdominal situs inversus (I), the liver is on the left and the right atrium almost invariably is on the left. With abdominal situs ambiguus (A), the liver may be placed almost symmetrically across the midline and the atria may be located normally or inverted or both atria may have morphologic characteristics of either the right atrium or the left atrium (Fig. 12-4). A symmetric liver is found in approximately 60 percent of patients with situs ambiguus. Lateralization of the liver, which is evident in the remainder, may simulate either situs solitus or situs inversus.

When both atria have characteristics of a right atrium,[224] *dextroisomerism,* or "bilateral right-sidedness," is said to be present. This situation is usually, though not invariably, accompanied by asplenia. When both atria have characteristics of a left atrium, *levoisomerism,* or "bilateral left-sidedness," is said to exist. This usually, but again not invariably, is accompanied by polysplenia.

Bronchial situs, as determined by overpenetrated chest roentgenogram or bronchial tomography, is an excellent predictor of atrial situs, but the most accurate technique appears to be two-dimensional echocardiography with Doppler color-flow mapping. The hepatic portion of the inferior vena cava, which almost always enters the morphologic right atrium, usually can be identified easily, as can the connections and structural details of the superior vena cava, coronary sinus, pulmonary veins, atrial septum, and atrial appendages.

Additional clinical clues to atrial situs may be obtained from the ECG, where a superior and leftward orientation of the P-wave vector suggests levoisomerism and polysplenia. Howell-Heinz and Howell-Jolly bodies in the peripheral blood smear are characteristic of dextroisomerism or asplenia.

For determination of the AV, ventricular, and VA relationships, high-quality selective biplane angiography, supplemented by equally high-quality two-dimensional echocardiography with Doppler color-flow mapping, is essential.[209] Symbols used to designate the combination or sequence of segments are arranged in order as follows: (1) the visceroatrial or bronchoatrial situs, (2) the ventricular loop, and (3) the relations of the great arteries. These may be included within parentheses and preceded by abbreviations that indicate the VA alignment, for example, TGA, DORV, or single ventricle (SV). Associated malformations such as VSD, pulmonary stenosis, and straddling tricuspid valve may be listed after the parentheses. Thus, the typical or usual transposition of the great arteries with situs solitus, d-ventricular loop, and aorta arising from the right ventricle and to the right of the pulmonary artery, with an intact ventricular septum (IVS), would be designated TGA (SDD), IVS. The designation for typical corrected transposition (TGA) with situs solitus (S), l-ventricular loop (L), aorta arising from the morphologic right ventricle and lying to the left of the pulmonary artery (L), with VSD and pulmonary stenosis (PS), would be TGA (SLL), VSD, PS. This designation would apply to transposition with situs solitus, whether the heart lay in the right or left chest (dextrocardia or levocardia, respectively). It should be noted that the description of the position of the heart within the chest would offer no additional information referable to the intracardiac anatomy or great vessel alignment.[222]

Levocardia, Dextrocardia, and Mesocardia

The position of the cardiac apex indicates a condition of levocardia, dextrocardia, or mesocardia. The trend today is to discard the terms *dextroposition, dextroversion, mirror-image dextrocardia,* and *isolated dextrocardia* because they do not provide any significant information beyond what is already known—that the cardiac apex is in the right chest—and to use the broad term *dextrocardia* for all right-sided hearts, followed by a description of the visceroatrial situs. In the case of patients in whom the heart appears to have been pulled or pushed into the right chest by massive atelectasis or hypoplasia of the right lung, diaphragmatic hernia, eventration of the diaphragm, pleural effusion, obstructive emphysema, or pneumothorax, an appropriate descriptive phrase should be added. The term *isolated levocardia* is applied to all left-sided hearts with situs inversus or situs ambiguus, and a description of the visceroatrial situs should follow. Dextrocardia with complete situs inversus occurs in approximately 2 per 10,000 live births. *The incidence of congenital heart disease is relatively low among these individuals and is estimated to be about 3 percent.* Dextrocardia with situs solitus or situs ambiguus is considerably less common and occurs in perhaps 1 in 20,000 live births. The incidence of congenital heart disease is extremely high in this situation, however, probably in the range of 90 percent or greater. From these figures, one could project that approximately 12 percent of individuals found to have dextrocardia and congenital heart disease would have complete situs inversus. This estimate compares favorably with the figure of 18 percent observed in large autopsy series. About 50 percent of patients with dextrocardia and heart disease have situs solitus, and the remainder, perhaps 30 percent, have situs ambiguus.[222] An l-ventricular loop is found in the majority of patients with dextrocardia regardless of situs but is most common, as one might expect, among patients with situs inversus, in whom it approaches 80 percent. Cardiac malformations usually although not invariably are severe and complex. The most common lesions and their approximate frequency are as follows: transposition of the great arteries, 50 to 75 percent; double-outlet right ventricle, 10 to 18 percent; VSD, 60 to 80 percent; single ventricle, 15 to 40 percent; and pulmonary stenosis or atresia, 70 to 80 percent.[222] Approximately three-quarters of transposed great arteries have the segmental arrangement of corrected transposition. Tetralogy of Fallot is distinctly uncommon. Polysplenia or asplenia is found in about one-third of patients with dextrocardia and almost invariably with situs ambiguus. Kartagener's syndrome—the triad of situs inversus, sinusitis, and bronchiectasis—results from impaired ciliary movement. It is present in approximately 20 percent of patients with dextrocardia and situs inversus totalis.[225] The incidence of isolated levocardia has been estimated at approximately 0.6 per 10,000 live births. It is estimated that over 90 percent of affected individuals have associated heart disease. Situs inversus is present in approximately 15 percent, and the remainder have situs ambiguus, with the ratio of asplenia to polysplenia or accessory spleens being from 2.5:1 to 1.5:1. The associated defects are comparable in complexity and severity to those associated with dextrocardia. *Mesocardia* may exist as a variant position of the normal heart or a variant position of dextrocardia or isolated levocardia.

MEDICAL AND SURGICAL MANAGEMENT

Medical management of patients with cardiac malposition is similar to that of patients with normally located hearts, with the exceptions of continuous daily antibiotic coverage and pneumococcal vaccine for patients with asplenia and the particular attention to detail that is necessary to establish the correct diagnosis in individuals with unusual and complex malformations. Surgical management differs in the technical considerations imposed by the malposition of the heart itself, the frequency of occurrence of the l-ventricular loop, and the variability of the intracardiac conduction system.

Dextrotransposition of the Great Arteries

DEFINITION

In this condition, the aorta and the pulmonary artery are misplaced in relation to the ventricular septum, with the aorta arising from the right ventricle and the pulmonary artery arising from the left ventricle (discordant VA connection).

PATHOLOGY

In the majority of cases, there are situs solitus of the atria and viscera (S) and concordance of the AV connection and the right ventricle lies to the right of the left ventricle (d loop, D) (Fig. 73-36). The aorta lies to the right of the pulmonary arterial origin (d transposition, D) and is anterior. Of the communications between the two sides of the circulation, a narrow patent foramen and PDA are common in very young infants. The ventricular septum is intact in approximately half these patients, and another 10 percent have only a very small VSD. The remainder have a large VSD or multiple VSDs.[226]

Pulmonary stenosis of significance is very uncommon among neonates with an intact ventricular septum but develops with the passage of time in approximately one-third of patients in whom the right ventricle continues to be the systemic ventricle. In most cases it is mild and usually though not invariably the result of a bulging of the ventricular septum into the left ventricular outflow area. Approximately one-third of patients with a large VSD have significant left ventricular outflow tract obstruction (pulmonary stenosis). Causes of this obstruction include leftward malalignment of the infundibular septum, the presence of a membranous collar or ridge encircling the left ventricular outflow tract, anomalous adhesion of the anterior

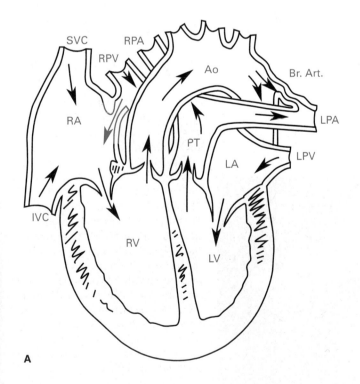

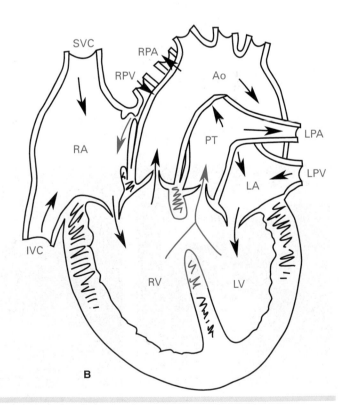

FIGURE 73-36 Complete D transposition of the great arteries. *A.* With intact ventricular septum. A patent foramen ovale and enlarged bronchial arteries (Br. Art.) are present. *B.* With ventricular septal defect and without pulmonary stenosis. SVC = superior vena cava; IVC = inferior vena cava; RA = right atrium; RV = right ventricle; Ao = aorta; LA = left atrium; LV = left ventricle.

mitral leaflet to the ventricular septum, stenotic deformity of the pulmonary valve, and, rarely, an aneurysm of endocardial tissue related to the VSD.[227]

The coronary arteries usually arise from the two aortic sinuses adjacent to the pulmonary trunk—the "facing sinuses"—with the most common arrangement being the right coronary artery arising from the rightward sinus and the left coronary artery, with its anterior descending and circumflex branches, arising from the leftward sinus. Hypertensive pulmonary vascular disease may occur at an inordinately early age, even in patients with an intact ventricular septum and initially low left ventricular pressures. Three-quarters or more of patients with d transposition, situs solitus, and d loop [TGA (SDD)] either have no significant associated cardiac defects or relatively simple malformations in the form of VSD, ASD, PDA, or pulmonary stenosis. The remainder have more complicated lesions and are not discussed in this section.

ABNORMAL PHYSIOLOGY

The systemic and pulmonary circulations are arranged so that the systemic venous return is conducted back to the systemic arterial system and the pulmonary venous return is directed to the pulmonary arterial system, with no obligatory mixing or interchange. For survival, there must be communication between the two circulations in the form of a patent foramen ovale, a PDA, or a VSD. The hemodynamics are dependent on the combination of defects present and particularly on the amount of mixing between the systemic and pulmonary circulations. The right ventricle is the systemic ventricle with concomitant pressure.

CLINICAL MANIFESTATIONS

Approximately 3 to 4 percent of children with recognized congenital heart disease have transposition of the great arteries (Table 73-1). Males are more commonly affected than females, in a ratio between 2:1 and 3:1.

History   Among infants with an intact ventricular septum, very early, severe, and progressive cyanosis is the presenting sign, making its clinical appearance within the first hour in over half and by the end of the first 24 h in over 60 percent of neonates so affected.[3] In a very few, a persistent PDA in combination with an incompetent foramen ovale or a small VSD permits survival for several weeks, but narrowing or closure of any of the three communications produces critical

hypoxemia. In infants with transposition and a sizable VSD the presentation includes severe heart failure and minimal cyanosis by the end of the first month. Infants with a large VSD and severe pulmonary stenosis present within the first days of life with cyanosis, while those with more moderate stenosis tend to show cyanosis and mild heart failure somewhat later within the first month.

Physical Examination   Among infants with an intact ventricular septum, the most prominent feature is intense cyanosis. Tachypnea and mild dyspnea are present. The right ventricular lift is forceful, and the first sound is usually loud at the lower left sternal border. In most patients, the second heart sound splits normally, confirming the presence of two semilunar valves. Murmurs are seldom impressive or distinctive. Signs of heart failure are uncommon unless the infant is beyond the first week of life and a large PDA is present. Infants with a large VSD appear thin, with mild cyanosis or a grayish pallor. Breathing is labored, and both the right and left ventricular impulses are hyperactive. A thrill is uncommon. A systolic murmur at the lower left sternal border is usually present but is seldom loud or holosystolic. A gallop rhythm and a diastolic flow rumble at the apex are typical. Infants and children with VSD and significant pulmonary stenosis are very cyanotic.

Chest Roentgenogram   With an intact ventricular septum, the size of the heart and pulmonary vascularity appear normal or at the upper limits of normal during the first week. Later, a narrow base caused by the displaced pulmonary artery may give rise to the characteristic "egg-on-side" contour. Impressive cardiomegaly, pulmonary plethora, and this characteristic contour are more common during the second week and beyond. With a large VSD, marked cardiac enlargement involving all chambers, impressive pulmonary plethora, and the egg-on-side contour are present. With significant pulmonary stenosis, the heart resembles that of a patient with tetralogy of Fallot, but it is usually slightly larger and the pulmonary vascularity is less diminished than one would expect for a comparable degree of clinical cyanosis. A right aortic arch is present in 4 to 16 percent of these patients.

Electrocardiogram   If the ventricular septum is intact, the ECG may reveal tall or peaked P waves by the second or third day of life; however, clearly abnormal right ventricular forces are usually not apparent until the latter part of the first week. The persistence of an upright T wave in leads V_1 and V_{3R} beyond 4 days of age provides an early clue that the right ventricular systolic pressure is at systemic levels. An older infant will have abnormal right axis deviation and marked right ventricular hypertrophy. A large VSD with a large pulmonary blood flow will usually produce biatrial and biventricular hypertrophy. If pulmonary blood flow is reduced toward normal—whether by significant pulmonary stenosis, pulmonary arterial banding, or severe PVOD—the pattern becomes one of right ventricular and right atrial hypertrophy.

Echocardiogram   Two-dimensional study with Doppler color-flow mapping is the diagnostic procedure of choice. The pulmonary artery can be seen arising from the left ventricle, and the aorta from the right ventricle (Fig. 73-37A).

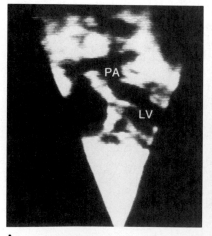

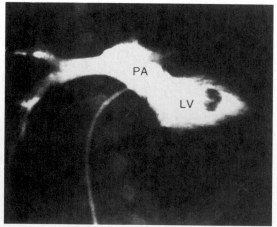

A   **B**

FIGURE 73-37 *A.* Two-dimensional echocardiogram. The left ventricle leads to a bifurcating great vessel (pulmonary artery, PA), confirming transposition. *B.* Anterolateral projection of an angiogram in the smooth-walled left ventricle (LV). The dye is ejected into the pulmonary artery.

The presence or absence of VSDs, anomalies of the AV connections, the status of the left ventricular outflow tract, and the coronary arterial pattern can be identified.

Cardiac Catheterization Systemic arterial oxygen desaturation is present in all these patients. The pulmonary arterial oxygen saturation is invariably higher than the systemic arterial saturation. The right ventricular systolic pressure will be at systemic levels; the left ventricular pressure also will be at systemic levels if a large VSD, ductus arteriosus, or marked pulmonary stenosis is present. A wide pressure difference between the two ventricles or between the two atria indicates an intact or virtually intact ventricular or atrial septum, but the lack of such a gradient certainly does not guarantee the presence of an adequate opening at either level. Selective ventricular angiography will document the diagnosis and the associated defects (Fig. 73-37*B*). The coronary arterial pattern should be established if it is not visible by echocardiography.[228] *All newborns with transposition can benefit from balloon atrial septostomy at catheterization by virtue of the increased mixing of the pulmonary and systemic venous circulations and the decompression of the left atrium.*

NATURAL HISTORY AND PROGNOSIS

Without balloon septostomy or surgical intervention, 50 percent of infants with transposition die within the first month and 90 percent die within the first year of life.[229] Those with an intact ventricular septum die very early from hypoxemia. Those with a large VSD usually live somewhat longer, but the majority die in the first months of heart failure; the few survivors have severe PVOD. Those with a large VSD and pulmonary stenosis have the best outlook, but the average life expectancy is barely 5 years even with this combination of defects. With an adequate interatrial opening—whether natural, balloon-induced, or surgically created—infants with an intact ventricular septum do relatively well during the first year. Increasing cyanosis during the first year in these patients may be due to a gradual diminution of the size of the atrial septal opening, narrowing or closure of a persistent PDA or small VSD, the gradual development of subvalvular pulmonary stenosis, or the development of PVOD. Before age 2 years, cerebrovascular accidents are a hazard to these hypoxemic infants and occur almost invariably in a setting of relative anemia rather than extreme polycythemia. The appearance of PVOD is unusual but can occur within the first 12 months of life. It becomes more common, approaching 40 percent, in the second year of life and thereafter. Infants with a large VSD and no significant pulmonary stenosis will develop PVOD and become prohibitive risks for corrective surgery by the end of the first year and possibly earlier. Those with a VSD and severe pulmonary stenosis usually become progressively more cyanotic.

Palliative and subsequent corrective operations have enabled a relatively large group of patients to survive beyond infancy and early childhood. Survivors of the atrial switch operations, such as the Mustard and Senning procedures, are prone to residual abnormalities such as pulmonary stenosis and PVOD as well as complications that result from surgery, including residual intraatrial baffle leaks, systemic and/or pulmonary venous obstruction, and arrhythmias. Late sudden death has been described in about 3 percent of survivors, probably from arrhythmias. Finally, right ventricular dysfunction with or without progressive tricuspid regurgitation has been documented in many of the somewhat older survivors of atrial inversion operations and raises the question of whether the right ventricle can function adequately as the systemic arterial ventricle beyond adolescence and early adult life.

While complications have been problematic for some, long-term follow-up of the group as a whole has been good. The Toronto experience is the oldest and largest. Among 534 children who underwent a "Mustard" procedure since 1962, there were 52 early deaths (9.7 percent). Survival at 5 years was 89 percent and 76 percent at 20 years.[49] In a study from New Zealand of 113 hospital survivors of surgery performed between 1964 and 1982, survival at 10, 20, and 28 years was 90, 80, and 80 percent, respectively, with 76 percent of survivors being New York Heart Association class I.[230] There has been less long-term follow-up of survivors of the "Senning" type of atrial repair. In a recent study of 100 patients, the actuarial survival at 13 years was 90 percent for those with simple transposition and 78 percent survival for those with complex disease.[231]

MEDICAL MANAGEMENT

The first step in the treatment of infants with an intact ventricular septum is to provide adequate systemic arterial oxygen saturation. This endpoint is reached by creating a large interatrial opening with balloon atrial septostomy and augmenting systemic-to-pulmonary arterial shunting via the ductus using intravenous PGE$_1$ infusion.[97] The latter maneuver is supported by intubation in anticipation of prostaglandin-related apnea. An adequate atrial septostomy is marked by a sustained increase in the systemic arterial oxygen saturation above 60 percent and verified by two-dimensional echocardiography. If the response PGE$_1$ is unsatisfactory and if the interatrial opening is small by echocardiography, the alternatives are to perform a balloon atrial septectomy or to proceed directly with corrective surgery in the form of the arterial switch operation.

SURGICAL MANAGEMENT

Arterial switch repair is now the preferred surgical alternative to the atrial inversion procedures for a neonate with an intact ventricular septum and for a slightly older infant with a large VSD and without significant structural pulmonary stenosis (Fig. 73-38). Arterial switching should be performed within the first 2 to 3 weeks of life, before left ventricular systolic pressure falls significantly below that of the right ventricle. For infants beyond 3 weeks of age, if the ratio of left ventricular to right ventricular pressure has fallen below 0.60, a pulmonary arterial band may be applied with or without a systemic-to-pulmonary arterial shunt. The arterial switch operation may be performed approximately 1 week later. Most patterns of coronary arterial origin and course appear to be amenable to the operation, and infants as small as 2.0 kg may be repaired successfully. In some centers, the surgical risks have been reduced to 5 to 10 percent,[232,233] although the surgical mortality continues to be higher in other centers.[234] Short- and medium-term prognosis is good,[235] but longer-term studies are awaited. Exercise performance analyzed in a small group of patients following arterial switch has shown excellent cardiopulmonary capacity.[236] The most common problem has been stenosis at the pulmonary artery anastomotic site.[237] When severe, it has usually been amenable to balloon dilation or stenting.[238] Though aortic regurgitation related to the neoaortic root has been viewed as a long-term potential problem, an intermediate follow-up study has shown a small likelihood for development of hemodynamically significant regurgitation.[239]

For infants with transposition, a large VSD, and pulmonary hypertension, the arterial switch technique with VSD closure must be carried out within the first 2 months of life to prevent severe PVOD. Infants with a large VSD and severe pulmonary stenosis may be palliated with a systemic-to-pulmonary arterial shunt and repaired in later infancy or early childhood,[186] although some centers are doing reparative surgery in infancy.[240] Finally, the severe hypoxemia present in children with a large VSD and severe PVOD may be reduced by an intraatrial repair performed as a palliative procedure, with no attempt at closure of the VSD.[241]

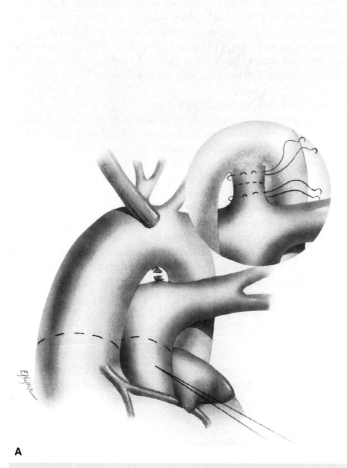

A

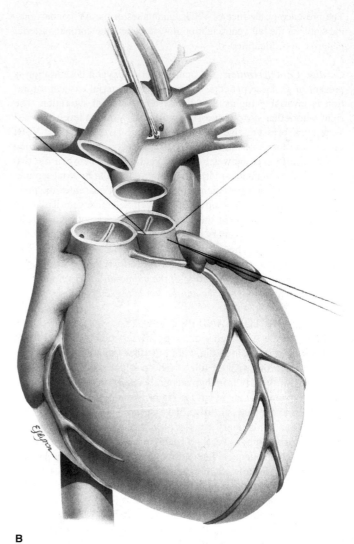

B

FIGURE 73-38 Surgical technique of the arterial switch operation. *A*. Aortic cannula is positioned distally in the ascending aorta, the ductus arteriosus is divided between suture ligatures, and the branch pulmonary arteries are dissected out to the hilum to provide adequate mobility for anterior translocation. The broken lines represent the levels of transection of the aorta and the main pulmonary artery. Marking sutures are placed in the anticipated sites of coronary transfer. *B*. Transection of the great arteries. The left ventricular outflow tract, neoaortic valve, and coronary arteries are inspected thoroughly. *C*. The coronary arterial buttons are excised from the free edge of the aorta to the base of the sinus of Valsalva. *D*. The coronary buttons are anastomosed to

V-shaped excisions made in the neoaorta. *E*. The pulmonary artery is brought anterior to the aorta (Lecompte maneuver). Anastomosis of the proximal neoaorta is shown. *F* and *G*. The coronary donor sites are filled with autologous pericardial patches. A single U-shaped patch (*F*) or two separate patches (*G*) may be used. *H*. Completed anastomosis of the proximal neopulmonary artery and the distal pulmonary artery. (Modified from Castaneda AR. Anatomic correction of transposition of the great arteries at the arterial level. In: Sabiston DC Jr, Spencer FC, eds. *Surgery of the Chest,* 5th ed. Philadelphia: Saunders; 1990. Reproduced with permission from the publisher and authors.)

Double-Outlet Right Ventricle

PATHOLOGY

In this malformation, more than 50 percent of the semilunar valve orifices of both great arteries arise from the morphologic right ventricle. In most cases, the ventricles display a d loop, and the pulmonary arterial origin is normally positioned, arising from a conus above the right ventricle. The aorta also arises from the right ventricle above conal tissue. The two semilunar valves are at about the same level, and there is no fibrous continuity between the semilunar and mitral valves (Fig. 73-39).

In most cases, the aortic origin is to the right (d malposition) of the pulmonary arterial origin, with the two vessels in a side-by-side relationship. Uncommonly, the aortic origin is distinctly anterior to

the pulmonary origin or the aorta arises to the left (l malposition) of the pulmonary artery.[242] With rare exceptions, there is a VSD. The condition may be subdivided further on the basis of the relation of the VSD to the origin of the great arteries. The VSD is subaortic in approximately two-thirds of patients, subpulmonary (*Taussig-Bing heart*) in 18 percent, related to both great arteries (*doubly committed*) in 3 percent, and remote or unrelated to either great artery in about 7 percent.[242]

ASSOCIATED CONDITIONS

Pulmonary stenosis occurs in over half these cases, with the condition usually resulting from a narrow subpulmonary conus. ASD, subaortic stenosis, and coarctation of the aorta are also relatively common, with the latter particularly associated with the subpul-

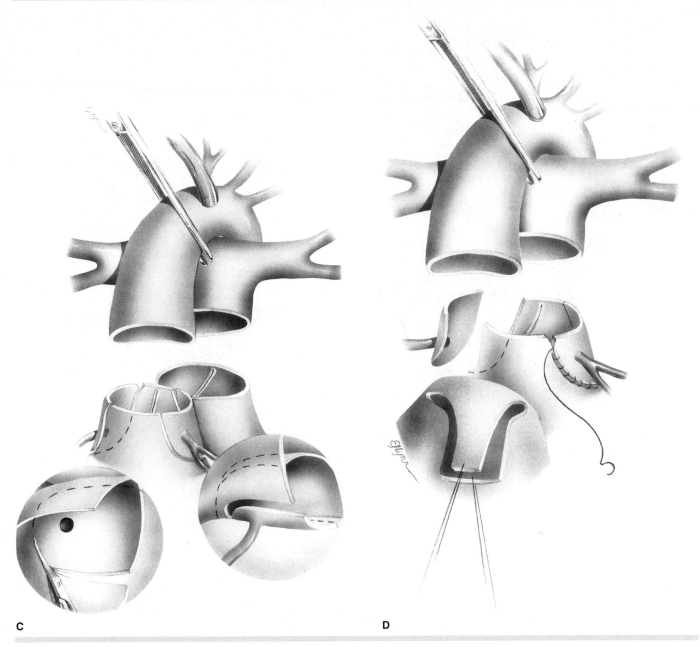

C

D

FIGURE 73-38 (*Continued*)

monary defect. Obstruction at the mitral valve may be observed in about one-fifth of cases of double-outlet right ventricle. Mitral valve straddling of the VSD and varying degrees of left ventricular hypoplasia also are encountered.

CLINICAL MANIFESTATIONS

Double-outlet right ventricle, or origin of both great arteries from the right ventricle, is a relatively rare malformation that is found in only 0.8 percent of patients with congenital heart disease. It is of considerable importance, however, because its clinical and laboratory features frequently resemble those of more common and more easily correctable malformations. Double-outlet right ventricle reflects the relationship of the great vessels to the ventricular septum; the presentation and treatment of children with this condition depend on the associated anomalies.

History and Physical Examination   Patients with a subaortic VSD without pulmonary stenosis (Fig. 73-39A) have clinical findings mimicking a large isolated VSD. Heart failure appears within a few weeks of birth; cyanosis is seldom described. Those with a subaortic VSD and pulmonary stenosis (Fig. 73-39B) usually present after the newborn period and follow a course similar to that of patients with tetralogy of Fallot. Patients with a subpulmonary defect without pulmonary stenosis (Fig. 73-39C), the Taussig-Bing malformation, resemble patients with transposition of the great arteries and a large VSD without pulmonary stenosis. The findings are those of severe heart failure without cyanosis.

Chest Roentgenogram   Cardiomegaly with pulmonary overperfusion is characteristic of all types of this anomaly without pulmonary stenosis. Double-outlet right ventricle with subaortic VSD and

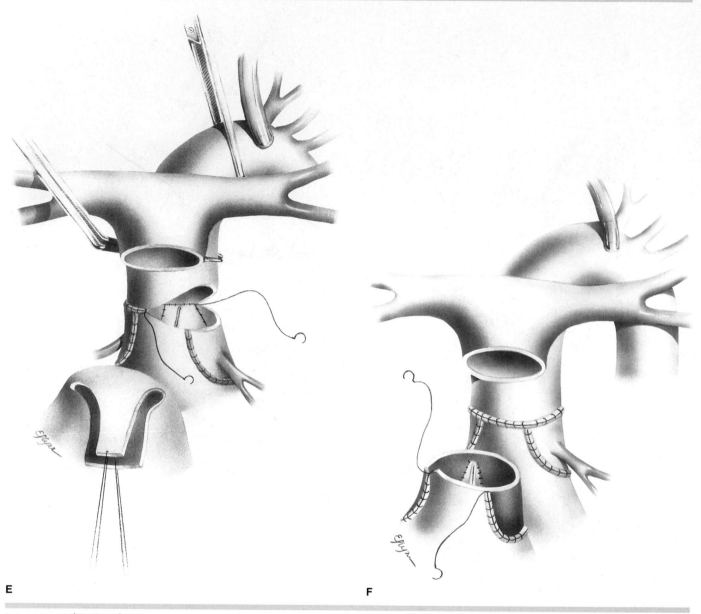

E

F

FIGURE 73-38 (*Continued*)

pulmonary stenosis resembles tetralogy of Fallot. In the case of sub-pulmonary VSD without pulmonary stenosis, the pulmonary artery usually lies beside rather than posterior to the aorta; this clearly visible, dilated main pulmonary artery may permit distinction of this malformation from transposition, which it mimics so closely.

Electrocardiogram Right axis deviation and right atrial and right ventricular hypertrophy are characteristic of double-outlet right ventricle.

Echocardiogram Two-dimensional echocardiography is very useful in demonstrating the anatomic components and associated defects.[242,243]

Cardiac Catheterization There is an increase in oxygen saturation at the right ventricular level. The pulmonary arterial saturation is lower than that of the aorta in patients with a subaortic VSD and is invariably higher than that of the aorta in those with a subpulmonary

septal defect and transposition physiology. Left ventricular systolic pressure may be higher than right pressure if the VSD is small and restrictive. Selective right and left ventricular biplane angiography and an aortogram are recommended.

NATURAL HISTORY AND PROGNOSIS

The clinical course of each variety of double-outlet right ventricle is determined by the associated defects. Without surgical intervention, those with an unguarded pulmonary artery either die in infancy with congestive failure or develop PVOD. Spontaneous narrowing or closure of the VSD may occur and is life-threatening. Increasing dyspnea, increasing intensity of the systolic murmur, and progressive left ventricular hypertrophy suggest this complication. Patients with pulmonary stenosis tend to have progressive obstruction and cyanosis.

MEDICAL MANAGEMENT

Vigorous treatment of heart failure is required for those without pulmonary stenosis. Almost all cases are best treated with surgical palli-

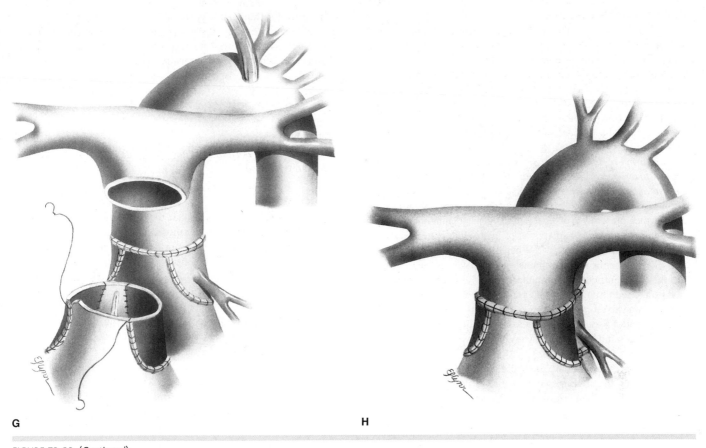

G   H

FIGURE 73-38 (*Continued*)

ation or correction in infancy. If there is pulmonary hypertension, banding or correction should be done by 2 to 3 months of age. Patients with ventricular hypoplasia, mitral stenosis, straddling AV valve, or a remote VSD are usually not candidates for biventricular repair, and initial palliation should prepare the child for a mod-ification of the Fontan operation. Whether or not corrective surgery has been performed, all patients with the left ventricular output passing through the VSD should be observed carefully for the possibility of spontaneous narrowing and obstruction at that site.

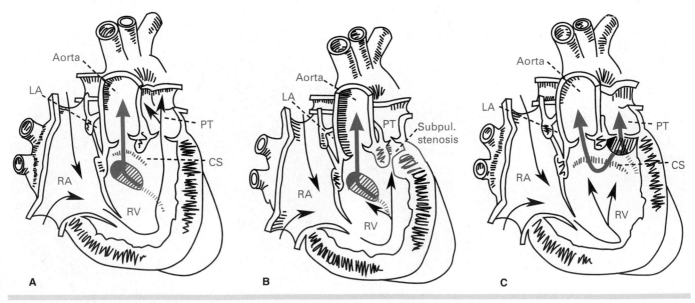

A   B   C

FIGURE 73-39 Double-outlet right ventricle. *A.* With subaortic ventricular septal defect without pulmonary stenosis. *B.* With subaortic ventricular septal defect and subpulmonary stenosis (Subpul. stenosis). *C.* With subpulmonary, supracristal ventricular septal defect. The so-called Taussig-Bing complex. RA = right atrium; RV = right ventricle; CS = crista supraventricularis; LA = left atrium; PT = main pulmonary arterial trunk.

SURGICAL MANAGEMENT

Great variability exists in the morphologic spectrum of double-outlet right ventricle. Although primary total repair of most forms of double-outlet right ventricle is now performed and preferred in infancy, palliation (pulmonary arterial banding, repair of aortic coarctation, atrial septal excision, or the creation of a systemic arterial-to-pulmonary arterial or systemic venous-to-pulmonary arterial shunt) to adjust pulmonary blood flow and thus preserve the pulmonary vascular bed, ventricular function, and AV valve competence may be considered in complex variants.

In all forms of double-outlet ventricle, the relation of the VSD to the great arteries and the magnitude of ventricular outflow tract obstruction dictate management. Surgical correction requires (1) obliteration of the interventricular communication, (2) relief of pulmonary stenosis when present, (3) diversion of oxygenated pulmonary venous blood to the aorta, and (4) diversion of hypoxemic systemic venous blood to the pulmonary artery.[244] When the VSD is committed to the aorta, a Dacron semiconduit or tunnel-shaped patch is placed to obliterate the interventricular communication while the left ventricular blood is diverted through the VSD to the aorta. Pulmonary stenosis is corrected by a valvotomy, with excision of obstructive muscle bundles and placement of a transannular patch when necessary. Otherwise, an extracardiac conduit is placed between the right ventricle and the pulmonary artery.[245,246]

When the great arteries are transposed or the VSD is not committed to the aorta, the arterial switch operation, using the concepts of Jatene and Le Compte, permits patch closure of the VSD, directing left ventricular blood into the neoaorta.[247] Further consideration of repair of double-outlet right ventricle associated with more complex defects is beyond the scope of this discussion. For a patient who is not a candidate for biventricular repair because of hypoplasia of a ventricle or a straddling AV valve, initial palliation should prepare the child for a modification of the Fontan operation.

In a 10-year review of repair of double-outlet right ventricle in 73 patients,[245] early mortality was 11 percent, with an overall actu-arial survival estimate at 8 years of 81 percent. Twenty-six percent required reoperation, and there was one death; 79 percent of the operative survivors required no restriction of physical activity, and 83 percent required no cardiac medications.

Corrected Transposition of the Great Arteries

DEFINITION

AV discordance and VA discordance form the characteristics of corrected transposition.

PATHOLOGY

Usually situs solitus is present, but the ventricles are inverted (an l loop). The great arteries are transposed and in the l position, so that the pulmonary artery arises posteriorly from the right-sided morphologic left ventricle and the l-transposed aorta arises anteriorly from the left-sided right ventricle (SLL) (Fig. 73-40). If situs inversus is present, the segmental pattern is IDD. Along with the ventricular inversion, there is AV valvular inversion. The two coronary arteries arise from the right and left (posteriorly facing) sinuses, with the right-sided coronary artery giving off the anterior descending and circumflex branches.[248]

ASSOCIATED CONDITIONS

Rarely, no associated conditions are present and the circulation is normal. In the majority of cases (about 75 percent), a VSD is present. It may be in any location, but a perimembranous subpulmonary defect is most common.

The inverted left-sided systemic tricuspid valve frequently shows some degree of abnormality, usually leading to incompetence. The most common abnormality is an Ebstein-like displacement of the septal and posterior leaflets, but dysplasia, clefts, and straddling of the ventricular septum have also been described.

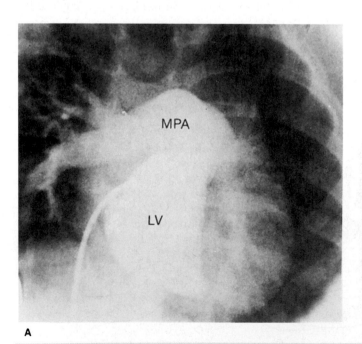

A

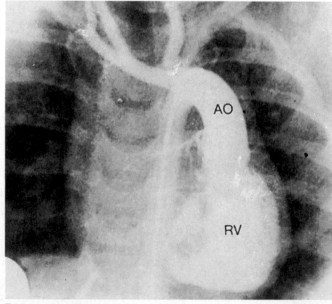

B

FIGURE 73-40 *A.* Posteroanterior view of the left ventricular (LV) angiogram in a child with corrected transposition of the great arteries. The main pulmonary artery (MPA) arises from the smooth-walled left ventricle, which receives the systemic venous blood. *B.* Posteroanterior view of the right ventricular angiogram (RV). The ascending aorta (AO) arises to the left of the pulmonary artery from the more heavily trabeculated right ventricle, which receives the pulmonary venous blood. The ventricular septum, seen here perpendicular to the frontal plane, is intact.

Pulmonary atresia or stenosis is present in about 40 percent of cases, usually associated with a VSD.[248] This obstruction is usually subvalvular, is only rarely valvular, and may characteristically result from attachments of accessory mitral valve tissue.

CLINICAL MANIFESTATIONS

Corrected transposition is an uncommon malformation, occurring in slightly fewer than 1 percent of children with congenital heart disease. The importance of this anomaly lies in its frequent association with serious AV conduction disturbances, the intracardiac malformations, and the medical and surgical implications of the ventricular inversion. The clinical picture is determined primarily by the associated anomalies. At least one-third of these patients can be expected to develop complete AV block if followed for a 20-year period.[249]

History   A slow, irregular heart rate often is detected in utero, and 10 percent of patients with congenital complete block prove to have corrected transposition. Patients with a large VSD without pulmonary stenosis usually present within the first month or so of life with symptoms indistinguishable from those of infants with a large VSD. Patients with VSD and pulmonary stenosis may present with cyanosis similar to tetralogy of Fallot.

Physical Examination   The murmur of left AV valve regurgitation may be best heard either at the apex or at the lower left sternal border. Most of these patients have a murmur of VSD or pulmonary stenosis. Occasionally, an inordinately accentuated second heart sound at the upper left sternal border suggests the presence of PAH, although in reality it represents a loud aortic valve closure resulting from the anterior and superior displacement of the aorta valve.

Chest Roentgenogram   A straight or gently curved convex upper left heart border representing the contour of the transposed ascending aorta is characteristic and is most easily recognized in patients with a VSD and pulmonary stenosis.

Electrocardiogram   Varying degrees of AV conduction delay are present in almost one-third of these patients. The initial forces of ventricular depolarization are characteristically oriented anteriorly and to the left, with Q waves in the right precordial leads and not in leads I, V_5, and V_6 resulting from depolarization of the septum from the left side (right ventricle) to the right side (left ventricle). With normal or nearly normal pressure in the systemic venous morphologic left ventricle, a QS pattern in the right and an RS pattern in the left precordial leads are usual.

Echocardiogram   Using a segmental approach, two-dimensional echocardiography permits identification of the anatomic components and associated defects.[250]

Cardiac Catheterization   When diagnostic catheterization is performed, the morphologic left ventricle is entered from the right atrium; in the presence of a VSD, the catheter may cross the defect, traverse the morphologic right ventricle, and enter the ascending aorta in the position normally occupied by the pulmonary artery. Entry into the medially placed pulmonary artery with the use of flow-guided catheters permits successful entry for the measurement of pressure. Selective angiography in both ventricles will outline the defects. The ventricular septum usually lies in the anteroposterior plane, and frequently a VSD may be imaged best angiographically in the frontal view (Fig. 73-40). Gentle manipulation of the catheter within the heart is indicated, since the production of varying degrees

of transient AV block is not uncommon; in rare instances, the block may prove permanent.

NATURAL HISTORY AND PROGNOSIS

The clinical course is determined primarily by the severity of the associated defects. It is estimated that only about 1 percent of individuals with corrected transposition have an otherwise normal heart. Even with complicating anomalies, survival to adulthood is possible,[251,252] though exercise performance is markedly abnormal.[253] A number of affected females have carried pregnancies to term, but the potential for concurrent cardiac complications suggests the need for care delivery by physicians familiar with the condition.[254] Heart failure associated with a large VSD has been the most common cause of death, with most fatalities occurring within the first year of life. AV conduction abnormalities tend to be progressive, and complete AV block may appear at any age. Similarly, left AV valve regurgitation may present at any age and significantly alters the long-term outcome.[255] Finally, the morphologic right ventricle may not be capable of sustaining adequate cardiac output over a normal life span.[252,256]

MEDICAL MANAGEMENT

Management of corrected transposition includes the treatment of heart failure, cyanosis, and AV block and the prevention of infective endocarditis. Patients with severe pulmonary hypertension or congestive heart failure should undergo early banding of the pulmonary artery or repair of the defect. Patients with a VSD, severe pulmonary stenosis, and cyanosis benefit from systemic-to-pulmonary artery shunting procedures or total correction. Those with congenital block may require prompt pacemaker therapy. Patients with significant left AV valve regurgitation require valve replacement. Regularly scheduled follow-up examinations are recommended to detect progressive AV conduction disorders and the progression or late appearance of left AV valve incompetence. Antibiotic coverage as protection against infective endocarditis is recommended, as is the introduction of an afterload reduction agent for AV valve regurgitation.[257]

SURGICAL MANAGEMENT

The conventional approach has been correction of the underlying lesion, closure of an isolated VSD, or closure of the VSD and a conduit from the left (pulmonary) ventricle to the pulmonary artery in those with L-TGA, VSD, and PS.[258] Unfortunately, this approach has led to suboptimal results because of the high incidence of complete heart block, increasing left AV valve regurgitation, and right systemic ventricular dysfunction and heart failure.[255] Despite recent advances, operative mortality rates for VSD or VSD and pulmonary stenosis or atresia remain in the range of 4 to 15 percent, with postoperative heart block in 14 to 33 percent.[259,260] The 10-year actual survival was 83 percent in one study[259] and 55 percent in the other.[260] Replacement of the regurgitant left AV valve at the first sign of progressive ventricular dysfunction has been recommended to preserve ventricular function but has been of limited utility.[261]

In view of the suboptimal results with the standard procedures, more innovative approaches have been suggested.[262] The "double-switch" procedure, an arterial switch procedure creating transposition physiology followed by concomitant atrial switch reversing the flow again, is a much more complex operation but has the advantage of using the left ventricle as the systemic ventricle and converting the problematic tricuspid valve to a systemic venous AV valve.

For those with corrected transposition, a VSD, and pulmonary stenosis, the VSD can be closed in a way that diverts the left ventricle into the aorta and the right ventricle via a conduit into the pulmonary artery. Since this also would create transposition physiology, an atrial switch is also performed. Although the early mortality for this approach is about 10 percent,[263,264] it is anticipated that the long-term results will be superior to those of the more conventional approach.

Single Ventricle

DEFINITION

The univentricular heart, or single ventricle, is characterized by the entire flow from the two atria being carried directly through the left and/or right AV valves into the single ventricular chamber. The double-inlet type of AV connection may take the form of either one common or two separate AV valves; straddling of one AV valve sometimes is included. The VA connections may be concordant (pulmonary artery from right ventricle and aorta from left ventricle), discordant (pulmonary artery from left ventricle and aorta from right ventricle), double-outlet (both great arteries from either the left or the right ventricle), or single-outlet (atresia of one great artery). Alternatively, one of the AV valves may be atretic. This is associated with normally related great vessels or transposition of the great arteries.

PATHOLOGY

A common type of single ventricle is associated with triscupid atresia in which the ventricle has the morphology of a left ventricle. There may be normally related great vessels (type I), D transposition of the great arteries (type II), or L transposition (type III). Depending on the size of the ventricular communication with the hypoplastic right ventricle, there may be pulmonary atresia (A), pulmonary stenosis (B), or no pulmonary stenosis (C).

In a large series,[265] about two-thirds were type I, and of these about two-thirds had pulmonary stenosis (I B). Among the one-third with transposition, the most common variety is without pulmonary outflow obstruction (II C). L transposition accounts for less than 5 percent in almost all series of children with tricuspid valve atresia.

When the mitral valve is severely stenotic or atretic, the left ventricle and aorta are usually hypoplastic or atretic (hypoplastic left heart syndrome). In this situation, the right ventricle is the predominant ventricle. Depending on the severity of the left-sided hypoplasia, the ascending aorta and aortic arch are usually hypoplastic as well. When there is one large atrioventricular valve or when both AV valves are present, the valve may straddle the ventricular septum, producing one large ventricle and one small ventricle (Fig. 73-41). The most common situation (65 to 70 percent of cases) is that in which the dominant ventricular chamber has the trabecular pattern of a left ventricle and communicates through an opening, the bulboventricular foramen, with a rudimentary right ventricle.[266] The VA connection is discordant (transposition of the great arteries) in about 90 percent of these patients. In about 20 percent of cases, the dominant ventricle shows the trabecular features of a right ventricle and the rudimentary chamber shows those of a left ventricle. The majority of these patients have a double-outlet VA connection from the main chamber, and a smaller number have a single-outlet connection with pulmonary atresia.[266] In 10 to 14 percent, neither ventricular sinus can be identified; this is the so-called primitive ventricle.

The term *Holmes' heart,* which is of historical interest, refers to a double-inlet left ventricle with situs solitus, normally related great arteries (SDS), an absent right ventricular sinus, and a subpulmonary infundibular outlet chamber communicating with the left ventricle via a restrictive bulboventricular foramen.[267]

ASSOCIATED CONDITIONS

Pulmonary stenosis or atresia is common. Subaortic stenosis and coarctation of the aorta occurs in association with l transposition and

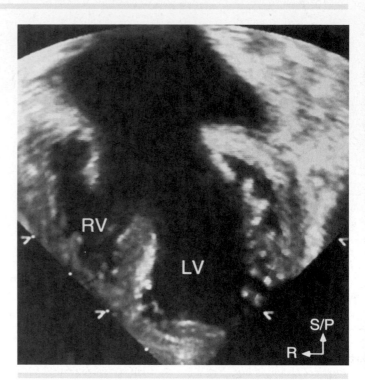

FIGURE 73-41 A malaligned atrioventricular canal with a large left ventricle (LV) and small right ventricle (RV). This would be repaired by a single ventricle approach (Fontan). (From Levine and Geva.[89] Reproduced with permission from the publisher and authors.)

may result from a narrow bulboventricular foramen. In those with tricuspid or mitral atresia, an atrial communication is present.

CLINICAL MANIFESTATIONS

This complex and challenging malformation is relatively rare. The clinical picture is determined largely by the associated defects, among which pulmonary stenosis or atresia, which is present in a little over half of the patients, and obstruction to aortic flow are the most important.

All these patients have some degree of systemic hypoxemia because of mixing of the two sides of the circulation. If pulmonary stenosis or atresia is present, the presenting symptom is usually cyanosis. Without pulmonary stenosis, the presentation is usually heart failure at 2 to 6 weeks of age as the pulmonary resistance falls. For those with subaortic stenosis and/or coarctation of the aorta, failure can occur within the first days of life as the ductus arteriosus closes. Physical examination depends on the combination of lesions present, but systolic ejection murmurs and a single second heart sound are very common.

Chest Roentgenogram Almost all these patients have at least some degree of cardiac enlargement. Those with little or no pulmonary stenosis generally have very large hearts with marked pulmonary plethora. Only patients with very severe pulmonary stenosis or atresia show a nearly normal heart size and diminished pulmonary arterial blood flow.

Electrocardiogram Evidence of right or left ventricular hypertrophy is common, depending on which ventricle predominates.

Echocardiography Two-dimensional echocardiography with Doppler color-flow studies can identify the morphologic and functional features of this malformation that are necessary to establish the diagnosis and formulate a plan for clinical management.[268]

Cardiac Catheterization   A degree of systemic arterial oxygen desaturation is present in all these patients, although the severity appears to be related mainly to the volume of pulmonary blood flow. Careful recording of intracardiac and arterial pressures is essential to detect significant or potentially significant obstruction to blood flow across either AV valve, across the atrial septum, or between the ventricle and the aorta or pulmonary artery. The morphologic features of the ventricle, the relation of the aorta and the pulmonary artery, and other features can be established with high-quality selective ventricular angiography, using specially angled views to supplement conventional views.[269]

NATURAL HISTORY AND PROGNOSIS

Since by definition only one ventricle is "usable," treatment must be aimed at preserving the anatomy, physiology, and function allowing this single ventricle to support the circulation and establishing diversion of the systemic venous return directly to the lungs without a second ventricular chamber.

These patients usually present as newborns with cyanosis, congestive failure, or a combination of both. Those in whom pulmonary arterial pressure and blood flow are increased require surgery to prevent death from congestive heart failure or progressive PVOD. Patients with severe pulmonary stenosis or atresia require systemic-to-pulmonary arterial shunting procedures. Among patients with univentricular heart, there is a propensity for the development of subaortic obstruction[270] and AV valve regurgitation.[271] Both threaten ventricular compliance and diminish the likelihood of successful long-term palliation.[272] Survivors are subject to the threats of infective endocarditis, brain abscess, and progressive PVOD.

Medical Management   Early recognition and identification of patients with these complex defects are important so that successful palliative surgical procedures can be carried out for the relief of congestive failure or cyanosis. PGE_1 is useful in neonates with ductal-dependent defects.[97] An adequate interatrial communication is essential for those with mitral or tricuspid atresia. For those with pulmonary stenosis or atresia, a Blalock-Taussig shunt can be lifesaving. Ventricular function and AV valvular competence are preserved by early creation of a bidirectional modified Glenn anastomosis (superior vena cava to undivided pulmonary artery).[273] Subaortic stenosis or obstruction at the bulboventricular foramen can be bypassed by anastomosis of the proximal pulmonary artery to the lateral aspect of the ascending aorta while pulmonary blood flow is delivered to the distal pulmonary arterial tree through a systemic arterial or systemic venous shunt.[274,275] Digitalis and diuretics may be necessary for patients with continuing heart failure. Care should be taken that anemia or severe polycythemia does not develop and that these patients are protected adequately against infective endocarditis. The pulmonary vascular bed must be protected and ventricular function and compliance carefully preserved if more definitive procedures are to be considered.

SURGICAL MANAGEMENT

Long-term palliation of children with a single ventricle is usually a three-stage approach: (1) initial palliation in the perinatal period, (2) a bidirectional Glenn at 6 to 18 months of age, and (3) a modified Fontan at 1 to 3 years of age. For complex problems, a heart transplant soon after birth has been suggested.[276]

Initial palliation for patients with univentricular AV connections requires adjustment of pulmonary blood flow with a pulmonary arterial band when it is excessive or the creation of a shunt when it is diminished. The modified Blalock-Taussig shunt is preferred in neonates. Relief of aortic stenosis and the creation of an adequate atrial communication are frequently necessary as well. The prognosis is affected adversely by a single ventricle of the right ventricular type,[277] the evolution of AV valvular regurgitation,[271] or subaortic obstruction.[278]

Ventricular function and AV valvular competence are preserved by early creation of a bidirectional modified Glenn anastomosis, in which the superior vena cava is divided with the caudad portion patched closed; the cephalad portion is sutured to the top of the right pulmonary artery. If pulmonary atresia is not present, the main pulmonary artery is closed.[279] Subaortic stenosis or obstruction at the bulboventricular foramen can be palliated by anastomosis of the proximal pulmonary artery to the lateral aspect of the ascending aorta, while pulmonary blood flow is delivered to the distal pulmonary arterial tree through a systemic arterial or systemic venous shunt (the Damus-Kaye-Stansel operation). Other surgical options for the relief of subaortic obstruction are direct enlargement of the bulboventricular foramen (VSD), the modified Norwood operation,[275] and the arterial switch operation.[274] Initially some types of single ventricle were repaired by dividing the common chamber into the right and left ventricles. This approach has largely been abandoned because of unacceptably high initial mortality resulting from problems in connecting the ventricles to the appropriate great vessels without interfering with the atrioventricular valves and the high incidence of complete heart block. The current approach is a modification of the principle suggested by Fontan and Baudet[280]—to bypass the right side of the heart, directing systemic venous blood directly to the pulmonary arteries and allowing the single functioning ventricular chamber to pump blood to the systemic circulation. First, if it has not been done already, a bidirectional Glenn anastomosis is constructed (see above), and then an intraatrial tunnel is constructed to divert the inferior vena caval blood to the caudad portion of the superior vena cava, which then is connected to the underside of the right pulmonary artery (Figs. 73-42 and 73-43). A fenestration in the baffle is sometimes used to decompress the right side in the perioperative period. Recently, instead of tunneling within the atrium, an external conduit has been used between the inferior vena cava (IVC) and the right pulmonary artery ligating the IVC–right atrial junction. The single ventricle is thus relieved of the burden of the volume overload and ventricular hypertrophy required to maintain the pulmonary circulation and is asked only to deliver systemic cardiac output.[280]

The surgical risks depend on patient selection. For those with complex forms of single ventricle and patients with elevated pulmonary pressure or resistance, ventricular dysfunction, or atrioventricular valve regurgitation, the risks are increased. For those without risk factors and with tricuspid atresia or double-inlet left ventricle, the risks are less than 5 percent.[281] Even for those with some risk factors or with more complex disease, the mortality at some centers is under 10 percent.[281,282]

For children with hypoplastic left heart syndrome, the survival from the three-stage procedure (initial Norwood, bidirectional Glenn, and Fontan) is approximately 50 percent,[283] although some centers are reporting a survival rate as high as 76 percent.[284] Birth weight less than 2.5 kg and the presence of cardiac or noncardiac anomalies are risk factors associated with early mortality.[285] There does not seem to be any significant difference in survival in centers that use the three-stage anatomic "repair" from primary heart transplantation in the perinatal period at 36 months of age.[283]

Quality and length of life are clearly improved, but persistent problems (AV valvular regurgitation, systemic embolization, limitation

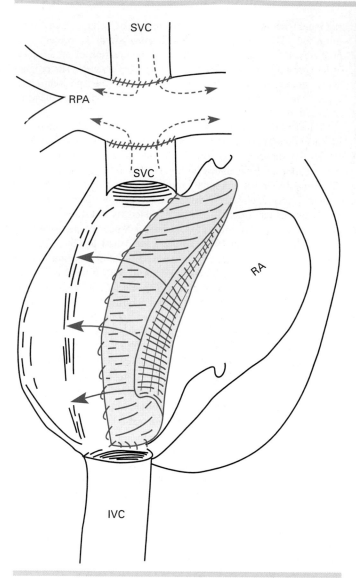

FIGURE 73-42 The modified Fontan operation. The superior vena cava (SVC) is divided. The cephalad portion is anastomosed to the superior aspect of the right pulmonary artery (RPA), and an intraatrial baffle is constructed from the inferior vena cava (IVC) to the superior vena cava along the lateral wall of the right atrium (RA). The caudad portion of the SVC then is connected to the inferior aspect of the right pulmonary artery.

of exercise tolerance, protein-losing enteropathy, atrial arrhythmias, and deterioration of ventricular function) occur with a frequency of about 1 percent per year.[281] For patients with progressive deterioration, cardiac transplantation is recommended.

CONGENITAL ABNORMALITIES OF THE CORONARY ARTERIAL CIRCULATION

Coronary Arteriovenous Fistula

PATHOLOGY

A coronary arteriovenous fistula is a fistulous communication between a coronary artery and a cardiac chamber, the coronary sinus, or the pulmonary trunk (Fig. 73-44). The site of origin may involve any of the epicardial coronary arteries. *The right coronary artery is the*

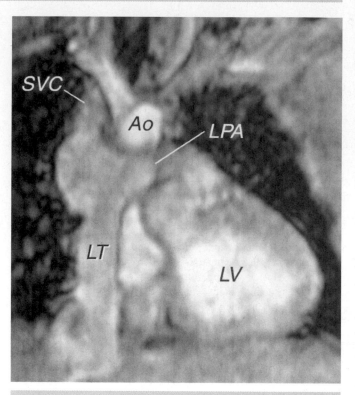

FIGURE 73-43 Cine MRI in a patient with a lateral tunnel (LT) and total cavopulmonary anastomosis. (From Geva T, Sahn DJ, Powell AC. Magnetic resonance imaging of congenital heart disease in adults. *Prog Pediatr Cardiol* 2003; 17: 21–39. Reproduced with permission of the authors and publisher.)

site of origin in somewhat over half the cases, and the two most common sites into which the fistula feeds are a cardiac vein (usually the coronary sinus) and the right ventricle. Although solitary communication is the rule, there may be multiple sites of termination. A fistula into the pulmonary trunk is usually characterized by one or more vessels opening into the pulmonary trunk and connecting with branches of each of the two main coronary arteries. The artery or arteries feeding the fistula are grossly enlarged and tortuous. Saccular aneurysms may develop in segments of dilated vessels; such aneurysms usually are observed in adults and frequently show calcification of the wall.

CLINICAL MANIFESTATIONS

Many patients with a coronary arteriovenous fistula are asymptomatic.[286,287] In some, the magnitude of the shunt into the right side of the heart is great enough to cause congestive heart failure, with a tendency for this to occur in early infancy or after 40 years of age. The classic finding is that of a continuous murmur with an unusual location, since it is loudest over the fistula. It may have a louder diastolic component, especially if communication is with the right ventricle. In those with large shunts, there may be cardiomegaly and increased pulmonary flow shown by chest roentgenography and right ventricular hypertrophy shown by ECG. Transthoracic echocardiography is usually diagnostic in children[288]; transesophageal studies may be necessary in adults. At cardiac catheterization, an increase in oxygen saturation may be encountered, usually in the right atrium or right ventricle, if the shunt is large enough. Selective coronary arteriography will demonstrate the involved coronary artery and the site of entry of the fistula. The most common complication is infective endocarditis, but thrombosis, myocardial ischemia, and rupture may occur.

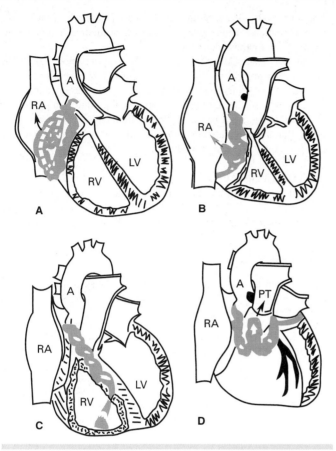

FIGURE 73-44 Anomalous communications of coronary arteries. *A.* Right coronary artery communicates with coronary sinus. *B.* Right coronary artery communicates with right atrium (RA). *C.* Anomalous communication of right coronary artery with right ventricle (RV). *D.* Two coronary arteries arise from the aorta (A) and make collateral communication with accessory coronary artery arising from pulmonary trunk (PT). LV = left ventricle.

SURGICAL MANAGEMENT

Except for very small fistulas, closure is recommended, since the flow tends to increase with age and these patients are at risk for infective endocarditis, congestive heart failure, and myocardial ischemia. Until relatively recently, closure was invariably surgical. Occasionally, closure was done without a coronary bypass by placing obliterating mattress sutures across the fistula beneath the coronary artery as it passes over the surface of the heart.[289] More commonly, cardiopulmonary bypass is preferred for safe exposure of large or multiple fistulas, such as those entering the right atrium near the junction of the superior vena cava and the right atrium, those arising from the artery to the sinoatrial node, and those between the left coronary artery and the left ventricle.[290] The orifice of the fistula is obliterated by direct suture or the placement of a Dacron or pericardial patch. Fistulas have been closed from within the open coronary artery; the artery is then repaired by direct suturing. Surgical mortality should be minimal[290]; the long-term results have been favorable.[291]

Fistulas have been closed by interventional catheterization techniques. Perry and associates[292] attempted to close fistulas in nine patients: four from the left circumflex artery, three from the left anterior descending artery, and two from the right coronary artery. Gianturco coils were used in six patients and a double-umbrella in two, with coils and an umbrella used in one. All were completely occluded. In three patients with multiple fistulas, no attempt at closure was made in the catheterization laboratory and the patients were referred for surgery. This "noninvasive" technique seems to be applicable to some children and adults with coronary AV fistulas, although long-term follow-up is necessary to be certain that the fistulas do not recur.

Origin of the Left Coronary Artery from the Pulmonary Artery

PATHOLOGY AND PATHOPHYSIOLOGY

In this anomaly, the left coronary artery arises from the pulmonary artery rather than from the aorta (Fig. 73-45). In the perinatal period, the pulmonary artery pressure is high and the left coronary is perfused with venous blood. Problems arise when the pulmonary resistance and pulmonary artery pressure fall and the diastolic pressure is insufficient to perfuse the left ventricular myocardium. In the absence of collateral vessels from the right coronary, left ventricular ischemia and eventually infarction of the left ventricular wall and papillary muscles occur. This in turn leads to congestive heart failure, usually by 3 to 8 weeks of age.

In a small group of children, extensive collaterals between the right coronary (arising normally from the aorta) and the left system develop. Perfusion via the right may be sufficient to oxygenate the left ventricular myocardium so that no ischemia develops. Over time, the higher perfusion pressure in the aorta may allow a left-to-right shunt into the pulmonary artery through the right and then the left coronary system. Eventually this may lead to a "steal" of blood from the myocardium into the lower-resistance pulmonary circuit.

CLINICAL MANIFESTATIONS

The clinical spectrum and mode of presentation in patients with this abnormality vary.[293,294] The majority present at 6 to 12 weeks of age.

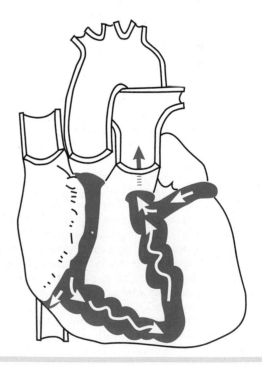

FIGURE 73-45 Anomalous origin of the left coronary artery from the pulmonary trunk. With time, wide collaterals develop between the two coronary systems so that right coronary arterial blood is shunted into the left coronary system and then into the pulmonary trunk.

Acute episodes of irritability, profuse cold sweating, pallor (possibly due to angina), and respiratory distress occur, with evidence of heart failure. Less often, these patients present at an older age with mitral regurgitation and heart failure. A few reach adolescence or adulthood with no or relatively few symptoms other than occasional exertional angina or palpitations. Sudden death may be the first and only sign of this condition.

On physical examination, the heart is enlarged, with an abnormal left ventricular apex impulse. Other signs of failure are usually present. Pallor and clammy skin are common. In some patients, a soft, continuous murmur is heard at the upper left sternal border. This murmur is more prominent in older patients, presumably because of the development of a more extensive collateral circulation. The murmur of mitral regurgitation may be heard at the apex, radiating to the axilla; however, in young infants with heart failure, there can be a surprising degree of regurgitation without a distinctive murmur.

In those with heart failure, the chest roentgenogram typically shows marked enlargement of the heart with posterior displacement of the esophagus by a large left atrium. There is pulmonary edema, and there may be atelectasis of the left lower lobe because of bronchial compression. Those with good collaterals and no left ventricular failure may have a normal x-ray.

In the infant group, the ECG demonstrates the pattern of anterolateral infarction, with deep Q wave in leads I and aV_L and abnormal R-wave progression across the precordium. Arrhythmias are common. The horizontal loop of the vectorcardiogram is clockwise and posteriorly oriented. The echocardiogram shows marked enlargement of the left atrium and ventricle with little or no left ventricular wall motion. The origin of the coronary artery can be imaged, and flow can be seen toward the pulmonary artery instead of toward the heart.[295] Myocardial perfusion imaging with thallium 201 can help distinguish an anomalous coronary artery from congestive cardiomyopathy.[296]

At cardiac catheterization, there may be an increase in saturation in the pulmonary artery if there is enough retrograde flow. There is usually some pulmonary hypertension, with very elevated pulmonary wedge pressure. Aortography or selective right coronary arteriography demonstrates the collateral circulation filling the left coronary artery retrograde, with at least faint opacification of the main pulmonary artery.

MANAGEMENT

The natural history and prognosis are related by the modes of presentation. Those who present in infancy die without surgical intervention. Medical management is aimed at control of congestive heart failure and arrhythmias before a surgical procedure.

Four approaches have been used for surgical repair. The first, which is of historical interest only, is ligation of the left coronary artery to eliminate the coronary artery–to–pulmonary artery shunt that acts as a coronary artery steal. Many children benefited from this procedure, but there continued to be myocardial ischemia and late sudden death was not eliminated. The second approach was to tunnel the coronary artery inside the pulmonary artery to the wall of the aorta and create an aortopulmonary window.[297] This usually required an external roofing of the pulmonary artery to allow egress of flow from the right ventricle. Although this surgical approach has the advantage of making a two-coronary system, a high proportion of children developed supravalvular pulmonary stenosis at the site of the intrapulmonary artery tunnel. This procedure is now used rarely. More recently, as coronary artery reimplantation has become more common in the arterial switch operation for transposition of the great arteries, surgeons have removed the anomalous coronary artery with a button

of pulmonary artery and reimplanted it onto the aorta.[298] Finally, in a few older patients, saphenous vein grafting or internal mammary artery implantation has been used.[299]

The late results after surgery have been quite good.[298,300] The congestive heart failure frequently improves, the heart becomes smaller, the left ventricular shortening fraction improves, and mitral regurgitation tends to regress. Interestingly, the infarction pattern on ECG with deep anterolateral Q waves frequently disappears, suggesting that the poor function is due to extreme ischemia rather than infarction (hibernating myocardium).[301]

ACKNOWLEDGMENTS

The authors would like to thank previous authors of this chapter including Dr. Jesse Edwards, Dr. Willis Williams, and Dr. William Plauth for their contributions, some of which appear in this edition.

References

1. Mitchell SC, Korones SB, Berendes HW. Congenital heart disease in 56,109 births. Incidence and natural history. *Circulation* 1971;43: 323–332.

2. Hoffman JI, Christianson R. Congenital heart disease in a cohort of 19,502 births with long-term follow-up. *Am J Cardiol* 1978;42:641–647.

3. Fyler DC. Report of the New England Regional Infant Cardiac Program. *Pediatrics* 1980;65:375–461.

4. Perry LW, Neill CA, Ferencz C, et al. Infants with congenital heart disease: The cases. In: Ferencz C, Rubin JD, Loffredo CA, Magee CA, eds. *Epidemiology of Congenital Heart Disease: The Baltimore-Washington Infant Study 1981–1989.* Mount Kisco, NY: Futura; 1993: 33–61.

5. Fyler DC. *Nadas' Pediatric Cardiology.* Philadelphia: Hanley & Belfus; 1992.

6. Keith JD. Prevalence, incidence and epidemiology. In: Keith JD, Rowe RD, Vlad P, eds. *Heart Disease in Infancy and Childhood,* 3d ed. New York: Macmillan; 1978:3.

7. Nora JJ. Causes of congenital heart diseases: Old and new modes, mechanisms, and models. *Am Heart J* 1993;125:1409–1418.

8. Belmont JW. Recent progress in the molecular genetics of congenital heart defects. *Clin Genet* 1998;54:11–19.

9. Hall JG. Catch 22. *J Med Genet* 1993;30:801–802.

10. Dawes GS. *Foetal and Neonatal Physiology: A Comparative Study of the Changes at Birth.* Chicago: Year Book; 1968.

11. Lind J, Wegelius C. Human fetal circulation: Changes in the cardiovascular system at birth and disturbances in the postnatal closure of the foramen ovale and ductus arteriosus. *Cold Spring Harb Symp Quant Biol* 1954;19:109–125.

12. Rudolph AM, Heymann MA. The circulation of the fetus in utero. Methods for studying distribution of blood flow, cardiac output and organ blood flow. *Circ Res* 1967;21:163–184.

13. Rudolph AM, Heymann MA. Circulatory changes during growth in the fetal lamb. *Circ Res* 1970;26:289–299.

14. Rudolph AM, Heymann MA. Cardiac output in the fetal lamb: The effects of spontaneous and induced changes of heart rate on right and left ventricular output. *Am J Obstet Gynecol* 1976;124:183–192.

15. Teitel DF, Iwamoto HS, Rudolph AM. Effects of birth-related events on central blood flow patterns. *Pediatr Res* 1987;22:557–566.

16. Coceani F, Olley PM. Role of prostaglandins, prostacyclin, and thromboxanes in the control of prenatal patency and postnatal closure of the ductus arteriosus. In: Heymann MA, ed. *Prostaglandins in the Perinatal Period.* New York: Grune & Stratton; 1980:109.

17. Rudolph AM. Fetal and neonatal pulmonary circulation. *Annu Rev Physiol* 1979;41:383–395.

18. Fineman JR, Soifer SJ, Heymann MA. Regulation of pulmonary vascular tone in the perinatal period. *Annu Rev Physiol* 1995;57:115–134.

19. Heymann MA, Rudolph AM. Effects of congenital heart disease on fetal and neonatal circulations. *Prog Cardiovasc Dis* 1972;15:115–143.

20. Levin DL, Heymann MA, Kitterman JA, et al. Persistent pulmonary hypertension of the newborn infant. *J Pediatr* 1976;89:626–630.

21. Fox WW, Duara S. Persistent pulmonary hypertension in the neonate: Diagnosis and management. *J Pediatr* 1983;103:505–514.

22. Kinsella JP, Abman SH. Recent developments in inhaled nitric oxide therapy of the newborn. *Curr Opin Pediatr* 1999;11:121–125.

23. UK collaborative randomised trial of neonatal extracorporeal membrane oxygenation. UK Collaborative ECMO Trail Group. *Lancet* 1996;348:75–82.

24. Talner NS. Heart failure. In: Emmanouilides GC, Riemenschneider TA, Gutgesell HP, eds. *Moss and Adams Heart Disease in Infants, Children and Adolescents,* 5th ed. Baltimore: Williams & Wilkins;1995:1746.

25. Seguchi M, Nakazawa M, Momma K. Effect of enalapril on infants and children with congestive heart failure. *Cardiol Young* 1992;2:14–19.

26. Fischbein CA, Rosenthal A, Fischer EG, et al. Risk factors of brain abscess in patients with congenital heart disease. *Am J Cardiol* 1974;34: 97–102.

27. Phornphutkul C, Rosenthal A, Nadas AS, Berenberg W. Cerebrovascular accidents in infants and children with cyanotic congenital heart disease. *Am J Cardiol* 1973;32:329–334.

28. Beekman RH, Tuuri DT. Acute hemodynamic effects of increasing hemoglobin concentration in children with a right to left ventricular shunt and relative anemia. *J Am Coll Cardiol* 1985;5:357–362.

29. Gidding SS, Stockman JA III. Effect of iron deficiency on tissue oxygen delivery in cyanotic congenital heart disease. *Am J Cardiol* 1988; 61:605–607.

30. Ross EA, Perloff JK, Danovitch GM, et al. Renal function and urate metabolism in late survivors with cyanotic congenital heart disease. *Circulation* 1986;73:396–400.

31. Henriksson P, Varendh G, Lundstrom NR. Haemostatic defects in cyanotic congenital heart disease. *Br Heart J* 1979;41:23–27.

32. Waldman JD, Czapek EE, Paul MH, et al. Shortened platelet survival in cyanotic heart disease. *J Pediatr* 1975;87:77–79.

33. Territo MC, Rosove MH, Perloff JK. Cyanotic congenital heart disease: Hematologic management, renal function, and urate metabolism. In: Perloff JK, Child JS, eds. *Congenital Heart Disease in Adults.* Philadelphia: Saunders; 1991:93.

34. Aram DM, Ekelman BL, Ben Shachar G, Levinsohn MW. Intelligence and hypoxemia in children with congenital heart disease: Fact or artifact? *J Am Coll Cardiol* 1985;6:889–893.

35. Cameron JW, Rosenthal A, Olson AD. Malnutrition in hospitalized children with congenital heart disease. *Arch Pediatr Adolesc Med* 1995;149:1098–1102.

36. Schuurmans FM, Pulles-Heintzberger CF, Gerver WJ, et al. Long-term growth of children with congenital heart disease: A retrospective study. *Acta Paediatr* 1998;87:1250–1255.

37. Rabinovitch M. Pathophysiology of pulmonary hypertension. In: Emmanouilides GC, Riemenschneider TA, Allen HD, Gutgesell HP, eds. *Moss and Adams Heart Disease in Infants, Children, and Adolescents,* 5th ed. Baltimore: Williams & Wilkins, 1995:1659.

38. Heath D, Edwards JE. The pathology of hypertensive pulmonary vascular disease: A description of six grades of structural changes in the pulmonary arteries with special reference to congenital cardiac septal defects. *Circulation* 1958;18:533.

39. Turanlahti MI, Laitinen PO, Sarna SJ, Pesonen E. Nitric oxide, oxygen, and prostacyclin in children with pulmonary hypertension. *Heart* 1998;79:169–174.

40. Nihill MR. Clinical management of patients with pulmonary hypertension. In: Emmanouilides GC, Riemenschneider TA, Allen HD, Gutgesell HP, eds. *Moss and Adams Heart Disease in Infants, Children and Adolescents,* 5th ed. Baltimore: Williams & Wilkins; 1995:1695.

41. Gersony WM. Long-term follow-up of operated congenital heart disease. *Cardiol Clin* 1989;7:915–923.

42. Freed MD. Infective endocarditis in the adult with congenital heart disease. *Cardiol Clin* 1993;11:589–602.

43. Morris CD, Reller MD, Menashe VD. Thirty-year incidence of infective endocarditis after surgery for congenital heart defect. *JAMA* 1998; 279:599–603.

44. Keane JF, Driscoll DJ, Gersony WM. Second natural history study of congenital heart defects: Results of treatment of patients with aortic valvular stenosis. *Circulation* 1993;87:I16–I27.

45. Hart EM, Garson A Jr. Psychosocial concerns of adults with congenital heart disease. Employability and insurability. *Cardiol Clin* 1993;11: 711–715.

46. Schmaltz AA, Neudorf U, Winkler UH. Outcome of pregnancy in women with congenital heart disease. *Cardiol Young* 1999;9:88–96.

47. Strong WB. Introduction: Pediatric cardiology exercise testing. *Pediatr Cardiol* 1999;20:1–3.

48. Chandar JS, Wolff GS, Garson A Jr, et al. Ventricular arrhythmias in postoperative tetralogy of Fallot. *Am J Cardiol* 1990;65:655–661.

49. Gelatt M, Hamilton RM, McCrindle BW, et al. Arrhythmia and mortality after the Mustard procedure: A 30-year single-center experience. *J Am Coll Cardiol* 1997;29:194–201.

50. Fishberger SB, Wernovsky G, Gentiles TL, et al. Factors that influence the development of atrial flutter after the Fontan operation. *J Thorac Cardiovasc Surg* 1997;113:80–86.

51. Moreau GA, Graham TP Jr. Clinical assessment of ventricular function after surgical treatment of congenital heart defects. *Cardiol Clin* 1989; 7:439–452.

52. Turina MI, Siebenmann R, von Segesser L, et al. Late functional deterioration after atrial correction for transposition of the great arteries. *Circulation* 1989;80:I162–I167.

53. Mertens L, Hagler DJ, Sauer U, et al. Protein-losing enteropathy after the Fontan operation: An international multicenter study. PLE study group. *J Thorac Cardiovasc Surg* 1998;115:1063–1073.

54. Graham TP, Gutgesell HP. Ventricular septal defects. In: Emmanouilides GC, Riemenschneider TA, Allen HD, Gutgesell HP, eds. *Moss and Adams Heart Disease in Infants, Children, and Adolescents,* 5th ed. Baltimore: Williams & Wilkins; 1995:724.

55. Alpert BS, Cook DH, Varghese PJ, Rowe RD. Spontaneous closure of small ventricular septal defects: Ten-year follow-up. *Pediatrics* 1979; 63:204–206.

56. Trowitzsch E, Braun W, Stute M, Pielemeier W. Diagnosis, therapy, and outcome of ventricular septal defects in the 1st year of life: A two-dimensional colour-Doppler echocardiography study. *Eur J Pediatr* 1990;149:758–761.

57. Weidman WH, Blount SG Jr, DuShane JW, et al. Clinical course in ventricular septal defect. *Circulation* 1977;56:I56–I69.

58. Rhodes LA, Keane JF, Keane JP, et al. Long follow-up (to 43 years) of ventricular septal defect with audible aortic regurgitation. *Am J Cardiol* 1990;66.340–345.

59. Gersony WM, Hayes CJ. Bacterial endocarditis in patients with pulmonary stenosis, aortic stenosis, or ventricular septal defect. *Circulation* 1977;56:I84–I87.

60. Gersony WM, Hayes CJ, Driscoll DJ, et al. Bacterial endocarditis in patients with aortic stenosis, pulmonary stenosis, or ventricular septal defect. *Circulation* 1993;87:I121–I126.

61. Cantor WJ, Harrison DA, Moussadji JS, et al. Determinants of survival and length of survival in adults with Eisenmenger syndrome. *Am J Cardiol* 1999;84:677–681.

62. Driscoll DJ, Michels VV, Gersony WM, et al. Occurrence risk for congenital heart defects in relatives of patients with aortic stenosis, pulmonary stenosis, or ventricular septal defect. *Circulation* 1993;87:I114–I120.

63. Castaneda AR, Jonas RA, Mayer JE, Hanley FL. *Cardiac Surgery of the Neonate and Infant.* Philadelphia: Saunders; 1994.

64. Moller JH, Patton C, Varco RL, Lillehei CW. Late results (30 to 35 years) after operative closure of isolated ventricular septal defect from 1954 to 1960. *Am J Cardiol* 1991;68:1491–1497.

65. Stellin G, Padalino M, Milanesi O, et al. Surgical closure of apical ventricular septal defects through a right ventricular apical infundibulotomy. *Ann Thorac Surg* 2000;69:597–601.

66. Rocchini A, Lock JE. Defect closure: Umbrella devices. In: Lock JE, Keane JF, Perry SB, eds. *Diagnostic and Interventional Catherization in Congenital Heart Disease.* Boston: Kluwer; 2000:179.

67. Lewis FJ, Winchell P, Bashour FA. Open repair of atrial septal defects: Results in sixty-three patients. *JAMA* 1957;165:922.

68. Edwards JE. Classification of congenital heart disease in the adult. In: Roberts WC, ed. *Congenital Heart Disease in Adults.* Philadelphia: Davis; 1979:1.

69. Mahoney LT, Truesdell SC, Krzmarzick TR, Lauer RM. Atrial septal defects that present in infancy. *Am J Dis Child* 1986;140:1115–1118.

70. Benson DW, Sharkey A, Fatkin D, et al. Reduced penetrance, variable expressivity, and genetic heterogeneity of familial atrial septal defects. *Circulation* 1998;97:2043–2048.

71. Murphy JG, Gersh BJ, McGoon MD, et al. Long-term outcome after surgical repair of isolated atrial septal defect. Follow-up at 27 to 32 years. *N Engl J Med* 1990;323:1645–1650.

72. Seward JB, Tajik AJ. Transesophageal echocardiography in congenital heart disease. *Am J Card Imaging* 1990;4:215–222.

73. Dall'Agata A, McGhie J, Taams MA, et al. Secundum atrial septal defect is a dynamic three-dimensional entity. *Am Heart J* 1999;137:1075–1081.

74. Acar P, Dulac Y, Roux D, et al. Comparison of transthoracic and transesophageal three-dimensional echocardiography for assessment of atrial septal defect diameter in children. *Am J Cardiol* 2003;91:500–502.

75. Hamilton WT, Hattajee CE, Dalen JE, et al. Atrial septal defect secundum: Clinical profile with physiologic correlates. In: Roberts WC, ed. *Adult Congenital Heart Disease.* Philadelphia: Davis; 1987:395.

76. Steele PM, Fuster V, Cohen M, et al. Isolated atrial septal defect with pulmonary vascular obstructive disease—Long-term follow-up and prediction of outcome after surgical correction. *Circulation* 1987;76:1037–1042.

77. Prieto LR, Foreman CK, Cheatham JP, Latson LA. Intermediate-term outcome of transcatheter secundum atrial septal defect closure using the Bard Clamshell Septal Umbrella. *Am J Cardiol* 1996;78:1310–1312.

78. Masura J, Lange PE, Wilkinson JL, et al. US/International multicenter trial of atrial septal catheter closure using the Amplatzer Septal Occluder: Initial results (abstr). *Am J Cardiol* 1998;31:57A.

79. Zamora R, Rao PS, Lloyd TR, et al. Intermediate-term results of phase I Food and Drug Administration trials of buttoned device occlusion of secundum atrial septal defects. *J Am Coll Cardiol* 1998;31:674–676.

80. Omeish A, Hijazi ZM. Transcatheter closure of atrial septal defects in children & adults using the Amplatzer Septal Occluder. *J Intervent Cardiol* 2001;14:37–44.

81. John Sutton MG, Tajik AJ, McGoon DC. Atrial septal defect in patients ages 60 years or older: Operative results and long-term postoperative follow-up. *Circulation* 1981;64:402–409.

82. Healy JE Jr. An anatomic survey of anomalous pulmonary veins: Their clinical significance. *J Thorac Cardiovasc Surg* 1952;23:433–444.

83. Silverman NH. Anomalous pulmonary venous connections. In: Silverman NH, ed. *Pediatric Echocardiography.* New York: Williams & Wilkins; 1993:179.

84. Saalouke MG, Shapiro SR, Perry LW, Scott LP III. Isolated partial anomalous pulmonary venous drainage associated with pulmonary vascular obstructive disease. *Am J Cardiol* 1977;39:439–444.

85. Rogers HM, Edwards JE. Incomplete division of the atrioventricular canal with patent interatrial foramen primum (persistent common cardioventricular ostium): Report of five cases and review of the literature. *Am Heart J* 1948;36:28.

86. Rastelli GC, Ongley PA, Kirklin JW, McGoon DC. Surgical repair of the complete form of persistent common atrioventricular canal. *J Thorac Cardiovasc Surg* 1968;55:299–308.

87. Rose V, Izukawa T, Moes CA. Syndromes of asplenia and polysplenia. A review of cardiac and non-cardiac malformations in 60 cases with special reference to diagnosis and prognosis. *Br Heart J* 1975;37:840–852.

88. Lacro RV. Dysmorphology. In: Fyler DC, ed. *Nadas' Pediatric Cardiology.* Philadelphia: Hanley & Belfus; 1992:37.

89. Levine J, Geva T. Echocardiographic assessment of common atrioventricular canal. *Prog Pediatr Cardiol* 1999;10:137–151.

90. Nora JJ, Nora AH. Maternal transmission of congenital heart diseases: New recurrence risk figures and the questions of cytoplasmic inheritance and vulnerability to teratogens. *Am J Cardiol* 1987;59:459–463.

91. Stellin G, Vida VL, Milanesi O, et al. Surgical treatment of complete A-V canal defects in children before 3 months of age. *Eur J Cardiothorac Surg* 2003;23:187–193.

92. Kirklin JW. Atrioventricular canal defect. In: Kirklin JW, Barratt-Boyes BG, eds. *Cardiac Surgery,* 2d ed. New York: Churchill Livingstone, 1993:693.

93. Hanley FL, Fenton KN, Jonas RA, et al. Surgical repair of complete atrioventricular canal defects in infancy. Twenty-year trends. *J Thorac Cardiovasc Surg* 1993;106:387–394.

94. Alexi-Meskishvili V, Ishino K, Dahnert I, et al. Correction of complete atrioventricular septal defects with the double-patch technique and cleft closure. *Ann Thorac Surg* 1996;62:519–524.

95. Daebritz S, del Nido PJ. Surgical management of common atriventricular canal. *Prog Pediatr Cardiol* 1999;10:161–171.

96. Clyman RI. Ibuprofen and patent ductus arteriosus. *N Engl J Med* 2000;343:728–730.

97. Freed MD, Heymann MA, Lewis AB, et al. Prostaglandin E1 infants with ductus arteriosus-dependent congenital heart disease. *Circulation* 1981;64:899–905.

98. Gersony WM, Peckham GJ, Ellison RC, et al. Effects of indomethacin in premature infants with patent ductus arteriosus: Results of a national collaborative study. *J Pediatr* 1983;102:895–906.

99. Siassi B, Blanco C, Cabal LA, Coran AG. Incidence and clinical features of patent ductus arteriosus in low-birthweight infants: A prospective analysis of 150 consecutively born infants. *Pediatrics* 1976;57:347–351.

100. Varvarigou A, Bardin CL, Beharry K, et al. Early ibuprofen administration to prevent patent ductus arteriosus in premature newborn infants. *JAMA* 1996;275:539–544.

101. Narayanan M, Cooper B, Weiss H, Clyman RI. Prophylactic indomethacin: Factors determining permanent ductus arteriosus closure. *J Pediatr* 2000;136:330–337.

102. Van Overmeire B, Smets K, Lecoutere D, et al. A comparison of ibuprofen and indomethacin for closure of patent ductus arteriosus. *N Engl J Med* 2000;343:674–681.

103. Castaneda AR, Jonas RA, Mayer JE, Hanley FL. *Cardiac Surgery of the Neonate and Infant.* Philadelphia: Saunders; 1994.

104. Satur CR, Walker DR, Dickinson DF. Day case ligation of patent ductus arteriosus in preterm infants: A 10 year review. *Arch Dis Child* 1991;66:477–480.

105. Bell Thomson J, Jewell E, Ellis FH Jr, Schwaber JR. Surgical technique in the management of patent ductus arteriosus in the elderly patient. *Ann Thorac Surg* 1990;30:80–83.

106. Laborde F, Folliguet T, Batisse A, et al. Video-assisted thoracoscopic surgical interruption: The technique of choice for patent ductus arteriosus. Routine experience in 230 pediatric cases. *J Thorac Cardiovasc Surg* 1995;110:1681–1684.

107. Burke RP, Wernovsky G, van der Valde M, et al. Video-assisted thoracoscopic surgery for congenital heart disease. *J Thorac Cardiovasc Surg* 1995;109:499–507.

108. Portsmann W, Wierny L. Percutaneous transfemoral closure of the patent ductus arteriosus—An alternative to surgery. *Semin Roentgenol* 1981;16:95–102.

109. Rashkind WJ, Cuaso CC. Transcatheter closure of patent ductus arteriosus. *Pediatr Cardiol* 1979;1:3–7.

110. Shim D, Fedderly RT, Beekman RH III, et al. Follow-up of coil occlusion of patent ductus arteriosus. *J Am Coll Cardiol* 1996;28:207–211.

111. Sakakibara S, Konno S. Congenital aneurysm of the sinus of Valsalva: Anatomy and classification. *Am Heart J* 1962;63:405–424.

112. Takach TJ, Reul GJ, Duncan JM, et al. Sinus of Valsalva aneurysm or fistula: Management and outcome. *Ann Thorac Surg* 1999;68:1573–1577.

113. Shaffer EM, Snider AR, Beekman RH, et al. Sinus of Valsalva aneurysm complicating bacterial endocarditis in an infant: Diagnosis with two-dimensional and Doppler echocardiography. *J Am Coll Cardiol* 1987;9:588–591.

114. Clagett OT, Kirklin JW, Edwards JE. Anatomic variations and pathologic changes in 124 cases of coarctation of the aorta. *Surg Gynecol Obstet* 1954;98:103.

115. Bharati S, Lev M. The surgical anatomy of the heart in tubular hypoplasia of the transverse aorta (preductal coarctation). *J Thorac Cardiovasc Surg* 1986;91:79–85.

116. Gardiner HM, Celermajer DS, Sorensen KE, et al. Arterial reactivity is significantly impaired in normotensive young adults after successful repair of aortic coarctation in childhood. *Circulation* 1994;89:1745–1750.

117. Beekman RH. Coarctation of the aorta. In: Emmanouilides GC, Riemenschneider TA, Allen HD, Gutgesell HP, eds. *Moss and Adams Heart Disease in Infants, Children, and Adolescents,* 5th ed. Baltimore: Williams & Wilkins; 1995:1111.

118. Ing FF, Starc TJ, Griffiths SP, Gersony WM. Early diagnosis of coarctation of the aorta in children: A continuing dilemma. *Pediatrics* 1996;98:378–382.

119. Campbell M. Natural history of coarctation of the aorta. *Br Heart J* 1970;32:633–640.

120. Fletcher SE, Nihill MR, Grifka RG, et al. Balloon angioplasty of native coarctation of the aorta: Midterm follow-up and prognostic factors. *J Am Coll Cardiol* 1995;25:730–734.

121. Zehr KJ, Gillinov AM, Redmond JM, et al. Repair of coarctation of the aorta in neonates and infants: A thirty-year experience. *Ann Thorac Surg* 1995;59:33–41.

122. Ovaert C, McCrindle BW, Nykanen D, et al. Balloon angioplasty of native coarctation: Clinical outcomes and predictors of success. *J Am Coll Cardiol* 2000;35:988–996.

123. Kreutzer J, Perry SB. Stents. In: Lock JE, Keane JF, Perry SB, ed. *Diagnostic and Interventional Catheterization in Congenital Heart Disease,* 2d ed. Boston: Kluwer; 2000:221.

124. O'Sullivan JJ, Derrick G, Darnell R. Prevalence of hypertension in children after early repair of coarctation of the aorta: A cohort study using casual and 24 hour blood pressure measurement. *Heart (British Cardiac Society)* 2002;88:163–166.

125. Parks WJ, Ngo TD, Plauth WH Jr, et al. Incidence of aneurysm formation after Dacron patch aortoplasty repair for coarctation of the aorta: Long-term results and assessment utilizing magnetic resonance angiography with three-dimensional surface rendering. *J Am Coll Cardiol* 1995;26:266–271.

126. Kirklin JW, Barratt-Boyes BG. Coarctation of the aorta and interrupted aortic arch. In: Kirklin JW, Barratt-Boyes BG, eds. *Cardiac Surgery,* 2d ed. New York: Churchill Livingstone; 1993:1263.

127. Toro-Salazar OH, Steinberger J, Thomas W, et al. Long-term follow-up of patients after coarctation of the aorta repair. *Am J Cardiol* 2002; 89:541–547.

128. Quaegebeur JM, Jonas RA, Weinberg AD, et al. Outcomes in seriously ill neonates with coarctation of the aorta. A multiinstitutional study. *J Thorac Cardiovasc Surg* 1994;108:841–851.

129. Pollock JC, Jamieson MP, McWilliam R. Somatosensory evoked potentials in the detection of spinal cord ischemia in aortic coarctation repair. *Ann Thorac Surg* 1986;41:251–254.

130. Bacha EA, Almodovar M, Wessel DL, et al. Surgery for coarctation of the aorta in infants weighing less than 2 kg. *Ann Thorac Surg* 2001; 71:1260–1264.

131. Driscoll DJ, Wolfe RR, Gersony WM, et al. Cardiorespiratory responses to exercise of patients with aortic stenosis, pulmonary stenosis, and ventricular septal defect. *Circulation* 1993;87:I102–I113.

132. Silverman NH. *Pediatric Echocardiography.* New York: Williams & Wilkins; 1993.

133. Rhodes LA, Colan SD, Perry SB, et al. Predictors of survival in neonates with critical aortic stenosis. *Circulation* 1991;84:2325–2335.

134. Yetman AT, Rosenberg HC, Joubert GI. Progression of asymptomatic aortic stenosis identified in the neonatal period. *Am J Cardiol* 1995;75:636–637.

135. McCrindle BW. Independent predictors of immediate results of percutaneous balloon aortic valvotomy in children. Valvuloplasty and Angioplasty of Congenital Anomalies (VACA) Registry Investigators. *Am J Cardiol* 1996;77:286–293.

136. Moore P, Egito E, Mowrey H, et al. Midterm results of balloon dilation of congenital aortic stenosis: Predictors of success. *J Am Coll Cardiol* 1996;27:1257–1263.

137. Egito ES, Moore P, O'Sullivan J, et al. Transvascular balloon dilation for neonatal critical aortic stenosis: Early and midterm results. *J Am Coll Cardiol* 1997;29:442–447.

138. Kirklin JW, Barratt-Boyes BG. Congenital aortic stenosis. In: Kirklin JW, Barratt-Boyes BG, eds. *Cardiac Surgery,* 2d ed. New York: Churchill Livingstone; 1993:1195.

139. Elkins RC, Knott-Craig CJ, Ward KE, Lane MM. The Ross operation in children: 10-year experience. *Ann Thorac Surg* 1998;65:496–502.

140. Hawkins JA, Minich LL, Tani LY, et al. Late results and reintervention after aortic valvotomy for critical aortic stenosis in neonates and infants. *Ann Thorac Surg* 1998;65:1758–1762.

141. Najm HK, Coles JG, Black MD, et al. Extended aortic root replacement with aortic allografts or pulmonary autografts in children. *J Thorac Cardiovasc Surg* 1999;118:503–509.

142. Graham TP Jr, Bricker JT, James FW, Strong WB. 26th Bethesda conference: Recommendations for determining eligibility for competition in athletes with cardiovascular abnormalities. Task Force 1: Congenital heart disease. *J Am Coll Cardiol* 1994;24:867–873.

143. Fyler DC. Aortic outflow abnormalities. In: Fyler DC, ed. *Nadas' Pediatric Cardiology.* Philadelphia: Hanley & Belfus; 1992:506.

144. van Son JA, Edwards WD, Danielson GK. Pathology of coronary arteries, myocardium, and great arteries in supravalvular aortic stenosis. Report of five cases with implications for surgical treatment. *J Thorac Cardiovasc Surg* 1994;108:21–28.

145. Ensing GJ, Schmidt MA, Hagler DJ, et al. Spectrum of findings in a family with nonsyndromic autosomal dominant supravalvular aortic stenosis: A Doppler echocardiographic study. *J Am Coll Cardiol* 1989; 13:413–419.

146. Zalzstein E, Moes CA, Musewe NN, Freedom RM. Spectrum of cardiovascular anomalies in Williams-Beuren syndrome. *Pediatr Cardiol* 1991;12:219–223.

147. French JW, Guntheroth WG. An explanation of asymmetric upper extremity blood pressures in supravalvular aortic stenosis: The Coanda effect. *Circulation* 1970;42:31–36.

148. van Son JA, Danielson GK, Puga FJ, et al. Supravalvular aortic stenosis. Long-term results of surgical treatment. *J Thorac Cardiovasc Surg* 1994;107:103–114.

149. Wright GB, Keane JF, Nadas AS, et al. Fixed subaortic stenosis in the young: Medical and surgical course in 83 patients. *Am J Cardiol* 1983; 52:830–835.

150. Choi JY, Sullivan ID. Fixed subaortic stenosis: Anatomical spectrum and nature of progression. *Br Heart J* 1991;65:280–286.

151. Freedom RM, Pelech A, Brand A, et al. The progressive nature of subaortic stenosis in congenital heart disease. *Int J Cardiol* 1985;8:137–148.

152. Cape EG, Vanauker MD, Sigfusson G, et al. Potential role of mechanical stress in the etiology of pediatric heart disease: Septal shear stress in subaortic stenosis. *J Am Coll Cardiol* 1997;30:247–254.

153. Drinkwater DC, Laks H. Surgery for subvalvular aortic stenosis. *Prog Pediatr Cardiol* 1994;3:189–201.

154. Maginot KR, Williams RG. Fixed subaortic stenosis. *Prog Pediatr Cardiol* 1994;3:141–149.

155. Kirklin JW, Ellis FH Jr. Surgical relief of diffuse subvalvular aortic stenosis. *Circulation* 1961;24:739.

156. de Vries AG, Hess J, Witsenburg M, et al. Management of fixed subaortic stenosis: A retrospective study of 57 cases. *J Am Coll Cardiol* 1992;19:1013–1017.

157. Braverman AC. Bicuspid aortic valve and associated aortic wall abnormalities. *Curr Opin Cardiol* 1996;11:501–503.

158. Koretzky ED, Moller JH, Korns ME, et al. Congenital pulmonary stenosis resulting from dysplasia of valve. *Circulation* 1969;40:43–53.

159. Li MD, Coles JC, McDonald AC. Anomalous muscle bundle of the right ventricle. Its recognition and surgical treatment. *Br Heart J* 1978; 40:1040–1045.

160. Noonan JA. Hypertelorism with Turner phenotype. A new syndrome with associated congenital heart disease. *Am J Dis Child* 1968;116: 373–380.

161. Stone FM, Bessinger FB Jr, Lucas RV Jr, Moller JH. Pre- and postoperative rest and exercise hemodynamics in children with pulmonary stenosis. *Circulation* 1974;49:1102–1106.

162. Ellison RC, Freedom RM, Keane JF, et al. Indirect assessment of severity in pulmonary stenosis. *Circulation* 1977;56:I14–I20.

163. Lima CO, Sahn DJ, Valdes-Cruz LM, et al. Noninvasive prediction of transvalvular pressure gradient in patients with pulmonary stenosis by quantitative two-dimensional echocardiographic Doppler studies. *Circulation* 1983;67:866–871.

164. Nugent EW, Freedom RM, Nora JJ, et al. Clinical course in pulmonary stenosis. *Circulation* 1977;56:I38–I47.

165. Mody MR. The natural history of uncomplicated valvular pulmonic stenosis. *Am Heart J* 1975;90:317–321.

166. Hayes CJ, Gersony WM, Driscoll DJ, et al. Second natural history study of congenital heart defects. Results of treatment of patients with pulmonary valvular stenosis. *Circulation* 1993;87:I28–I37.

167. Stanger P, Cassidy SC, Girod DA, et al. Balloon pulmonary valvuloplasty: Results of the Valvuloplasty and Angioplasty of Congenital Anomalies Registry. *Am J Cardiol* 1990;65:775–783.

168. Marantz PM, Huhta JC, Mullins CE, et al. Results of balloon valvuloplasty in typical and dysplastic pulmonary valve stenosis: Doppler echocardiographic follow-up. *J Am Coll Cardiol* 1988;12:476–479.

169. Ali Khan MA, al Yousef S, Huhta JC, et al. Critical pulmonary valve stenosis in patients less than 1 year of age: Treatment with percutaneous gradational balloon pulmonary valvuloplasty. *Am Heart J* 1989;117:1008–1014.

170. Ladusans EJ, Qureshi SA, Parsons JM, et al. Balloon dilatation of critical stenosis of the pulmonary valve in neonates. *Br Heart J* 1990;63:362–367.

171. Kan JS, Marvin WJ Jr, Bass JL, et al. Balloon angioplasty—Branch pulmonary artery stenosis: Results from the Valvuloplasty and Angioplasty of Congenital Anomalies Registry. *Am J Cardiol* 1990;65:798–801.

172. O'Laughlin MP. Catheterization treatment of stenosis and hypoplasia of pulmonary arteries. *Pediatr Cardiol* 1998;19:48–56.

173. Baker C, McGowen F, Lock J, Keane J. Management of pulmonary artery trauma due to balloon dilation. *J Am Coll Cardiol* 1998;31:57A.

174. Vancini M, Roberts K, Silove E, Singh S. Surgical treatment of congenital pulmonary stenosis due to dysplastic leaflets and small valve annulus. *J Thorac Cardiovasc Surg* 1980;79:464–468.

175. McGoon MD, Fulton RE, Davis GD, et al. Systemic collateral and pulmonary artery stenosis in patients with congenital pulmonary valve atresia and ventricular septal defect. *Circulation* 1977;56:473–479.

176. Becker AE, Connor M, Anderson RH. Tetralogy of Fallot: A morphometric and geometric study. *Am J Cardiol* 1975;35:402–412.

177. Rao BN, Anderson RC, Edwards JE. Anatomic variations in the tetralogy of Fallot. *Am Heart J* 1971;81:361–371.

178. Morgan B, Guntheroth W, Bloom R, Fyler D. A clinical profile of paroxysmal hyperpnea in cyanotic congenital heart disease. *Circulation* 1965;31:66–69.

179. Hagler DJ, Tajik AJ, Seward JB, et al. Wide-angle two-dimensional echocardiographic profiles of conotruncal abnormalities. *Mayo Clin Proc* 1980;55:73–82.

180. Formanek A, Nath PH, Zollikofer C, Moller JH. Selective coronary arteriography in children. *Circulation* 1980;61:84–95.

181. Ponce FE, Williams LC, Webb HM, et al. Propranolol palliation of tetralogy of Fallot: Experience with long-term drug treatment in pediatric patients. *Pediatrics* 1973;52:100–108.

182. Blalock A, Taussig H. The surgical treatment of malformations of the heart in which there is pulmonary stenosis or pulmonary atresia. *JAMA* 1945;128:129.

183. Lillehei C, Cohen M, Warden H. Direct vision intracardiac surgical correction of the tetralogy of Fallot, pentalogy of Fallot, and pulmonary atresia defects: Report of the first 10 cases. *Ann Surg* 1955;142:418–442.

184. Kirklin JW, Blackstone EH, Kirklin JK, et al. Surgical results and protocols in the spectrum of tetralogy of Fallot. *Ann Surg* 1983;198:251–265.

185. Castaneda A, Jonas R, Mayer J, Hanley F. Tetralogy of fallot. In: Castaneda A, Jonas R, Mayer J, Hanley F, eds. *Cardiac Surgery of the Neonate and Infant*. Philadelphia: Saunders; 1994:215.

186. Rastelli GC, Wallace RB, Ongley PA. Complete repair of transposition of the great arteries with pulmonary stenosis. A review and report of a case corrected by using a new surgical technique. *Circulation* 1969;39:83–95.

187. Perron J, Moran AM, Gauvreau K, et al. Valved homograft conduit repair of the right heart in early infancy. *Ann Thorac Surg* 1999;68:542–548.

188. Kreutzer J, Perry SB, Jonas RA, et al. Tetralogy of Fallot with diminutive pulmonary arteries: preoperative pulmonary valve dilation and transcatheter rehabilitation of pulmonary arteries. *J Am Coll Cardiol* 1996;27:1741–1747.

189. Bergersen LJ, Perry SB, Lock JE. Effect of cutting balloon angioplasty on resistant pulmonary artery stenosis. *Am J Cardiol* 2003;91:185–189.

190. Murphy JG, Gersh BJ, Mair DD, et al. Long-term outcome in patients undergoing surgical repair of tetralogy of Fallot. *N Engl J Med* 1993;329:593–599.

191. Lev M, Liberthson RR, Joseph RH, et al. The pathologic anatomy of Ebstein's disease. *Arch Pathol Lab Med* 1970;90:334–343.

192. Schreiber C, Cook A, Ho SY, et al. Morphologic spectrum of Ebstein's malformation: Revisitation relative to surgical repair. *J Thorac Cardiovasc Surg* 1999;117:148–155.

193. Cohen LS, Friedman JM, Jefferson JW, et al. A reevaluation of risk of in utero exposure to lithium. *JAMA* 1994;271:146–150.

194. Watson H. Natural history of Ebstein's anomaly of tricuspid valve in childhood and adolescence. An international co-operative study of 505 cases. *Br Heart J* 1974;36:417–427.

195. Driscoll DJ, Mottram CD, Danielson GK. Spectrum of exercise intolerance in 45 patients with Ebstein's anomaly and observations on exercise tolerance in 11 patients after surgical repair. *J Am Coll Cardiol* 1988;11:831–836.

196. Roberson DA, Silverman NH. Ebstein's anomaly: Echocardiographic and clinical features in the fetus and neonate. *J Am Coll Cardiol* 1989;14:1300–1307.

197. Hernandez F, Richkind R, Cooper H. The intracavitary electrocardiogram in the diagnosis of Ebstein's anomaly. *Am J Cardiol* 1958;1:181–190.

198. Celermajer DS, Cullen S, Sullivan ID, et al. Outcome in neonates with Ebstein's anomaly. *J Am Coll Cardiol* 1992;19:1041–1046.

199. Gentles TL, Calder AL, Clarkson PM, Neutze JM. Predictors of long-term survival with Ebstein's anomaly of the tricuspid valve. *Am J Cardiol* 1992;69:377–381.

200. Attie F, Rosas M, Rijlaarsdam M, et al. The adult patient with Ebstein anomaly. Outcome in 72 unoperated patients. *Medicine* 2000;79:27–36.

201. Donnelly JE, Brown JM, Radford DJ. Pregnancy outcome and Ebstein's anomaly. *Br Heart J* 1991;66:368–371.

202. Kulik TJ. Inhaled nitric oxide in the management of congenital heart disease. *Curr Opin Cardiol* 1996;11:75–80.

203. Reich JD, Auld D, Hulse E, et al. The Pediatric Radiofrequency Ablation Registry's experience with Ebstein's anomaly. Pediatric Electrophysiology Society. *J Cardiovasc Electrophysiol* 1998;9:1370–1377.

204. Starnes VA, Pitlick PT, Bernstein D, et al. Ebstein's anomaly appearing in the neonate. A new surgical approach. *J Thorac Cardiovasc Surg* 1991;101:1082–1087.

205. Marianeschi SM, McElhinney DB, Reddy VM, et al. Alternative approach to the repair of Ebstein's malformation: Intracardiac repair with ventricular unloading. *Ann Thorac Surg* 1998;66:1546–1550.

206. van Son JA, Falk V, Black MD, et al. Conversion of complex neonatal Ebstein's anomaly into functional tricuspid or pulmonary atresia. *Eur J Cardiothorac Surg* 1998;13:280–284.

207. Danielson GK, Driscoll DJ, Mair DD, et al. Operative treatment of Ebstein's anomaly. *J Thorac Cardiovasc Surg* 1992;104:1195–1202.

208. Carpentier A, Chauvaud S, Mace L, et al. A new reconstructive operation for Ebstein's anomaly of the tricuspid valve. *J Thorac Cardiovasc Surg* 1988;96:92–101.

209. Quaegebeur JM, Sreeram N, Fraser AG, et al. Surgery for Ebstein's anomaly: The clinical and echocardiographic evaluation of a new technique. *J Am Coll Cardiol* 1991;17:722–728.

210. Knott-Craig CJ, Overholt ED, Ward KE, et al. Repair of Ebstein's anomaly in the symptomatic neonate: An evolution of technique with 7-year follow-up. *Ann Thorac Surg* 2002;73:1786–1792.

211. Radford DJ, Graff RF, Neilson GH. Diagnosis and natural history of Ebstein's anomaly. *Br Heart J* 1985;54:517–522.

212. Lucas RV Jr, Lock JE, Tandon R, Edwards JE. Gross and histologic anatomy of total anomalous pulmonary venous connections. *Am J Cardiol* 1988;62:292–300.

213. Gathman GE, Nadas AS. Total anomalous pulmonary venous connection: Clinical and physiologic observations of 75 pediatric patients. *Circulation* 1970;42:143–154.

214. Chin AJ, Sanders SP, Sherman F, et al. Accuracy of subcostal two-dimensional echocardiography in prospective diagnosis of total anomalous pulmonary venous connection. *Am Heart J* 1987;113:1153–1159.

215. Newfeld EA, Wilson A, Paul MH, Reisch JS. Pulmonary vascular disease in total anomalous pulmonary venous drainage. *Circulation* 1980;61:103–109.

216. Castaneda AR, Jonas RA, Mayer JE, Hanley FL. *Cardiac Surgery in the Neonate and Infant.* Philadelphia: Saunders; 1994.

217. Behrendt DM, Aberdeen E, Waterson DJ, Bonham-Carter RE. Total anomalous pulmonary venous drainage in infants. I. Clinical and hemodynamic findings, methods, and results of operation in 37 cases. *Circulation* 1972;46:347–356.

218. Norwood WI, Hougen TJ, Castaneda AR. Total anomalous pulmonary venous connection: Surgical considerations. *Cardiovasc Clin* 1981;11:353–364.

219. van der Velde ME, Parness IA, Colan SD, et al. Two-dimensional echocardiography in the pre- and postoperative management of totally anomalous pulmonary venous connection. *J Am Coll Cardiol* 1991;18:1746–1751.

220. Bando K, Turrentine MW, Ensing GJ, et al. Surgical management of total anomalous pulmonary venous connection. Thirty-year trends. *Circulation* 1996;94:II12–II26.

221. Lacour-Gayet F, Zoghbi J, Serraf AE, et al. Surgical management of progressive pulmonary venous obstruction after repair of total anomalous pulmonary venous connection. *J Thorac Cardiovasc Surg* 1999;117:679–687.

222. Van Praagh R, Weinberg P, Smith S. Malpositions of the heart. In: Adams F, Emmanouilides G, Riemenschneider T, eds. *Moss' Heart Disease in Infants, Children, and Adolescents.* Baltimore: Williams & Wilkins; 1989:530.

223. Van Praagh R. Segmental approach to diagnosis. In: Fyler D, ed. *Nadas' Pediatric Cardiology.* Philadelphia: Hanley & Belfus; 1992:27.

224. Van Praagh S, Santini F, Sanders S. Cardiac malpositions with special emphasis on visceral heterotaxy (asplenia and polysplenia syndromes). In: Fyler D, ed. *Nadas' Pediatric Cardiology.* Philadelphia: Hanley & Belfus; 1992:589.

225. Rooklin AR, McGeady SJ, Mikaelian DO, et al. The immotile cilia syndrome: A cause of recurrent pulmonary diseases in children. *Pediatrics* 1980;66:526–531.

226. Fyler D. D-transposition of the great arteries. In: Fyler D, ed. *Nadas' Pediatric Cardiology.* Philadelphia: Hanley & Belfus; 1992:557.

227. Paul M, Wernovsky G. Transposition of the great arteries. In: Emmanouilides G, Riemenschneider T, Allen H, Gutgesell H, eds. *Moss and Adams Heart Disease in Infants, Children, and Adolescents,* 5th ed. Baltimore: Williams & Wilkins; 1995:1154.

228. Yoo S, Burrows P, Moes C. Evaluation of coronary arterial patterns in complete transposition by laidback aortography. *Cardiol Young* 1996;6:149–155.

229. Liebman J, Cullum L, Belloc NB. Natural history of transposition of the great arteries. Anatomy and birth and death characteristics. *Circulation* 1969;40:237–262.

230. Wilson NJ, Clarkson PM, Barratt-Boyes BG, et al. Long-term outcome after the mustard repair for simple transposition of the great arteries. 28-year follow-up. *J Am Coll Cardiol* 1998;32:758–765.

231. Kirjavainen M, Happonen JM, Louhimo I. Late results of Senning operation. *J Thorac Cardiovasc Surg* 1999;117:488–495.

232. Wernovsky G, Mayer JE Jr, Jonas RA, et al. Factors influencing early and late outcome of the arterial switch operation for transposition of the great arteries. *J Thorac Cardiovasc Surg* 1995;109:289–301.

233. Pretre R, Tamisier D, Bonhoeffer P, et al. Results of the arterial switch operation in neonates with transposed great arteries. *Lancet* 2001;357:1826–1830.

234. Gutgesell HP, Massaro TA, Kron IL. The arterial switch operation for transposition of the great arteries in a consortium of university hospitals. *Am J Cardiol* 1994;74:959–960.

235. Wernovsky G, Freed M. Transposition of the great arteries: Results and outcome of the arterial switch operation. In: Freedom R, ed. *Atlas of Heart Diseases.* Philadelphia: Current Medicine; 1997:116.1.

236. Mahle WT, McBride MG, Paridon SM. Exercise performance after the arterial switch operation for D-transposition of the great arteries. *Am J Cardiol* 2001;87:753–758.

237. Williams WG, Quaegebeur JM, Kirklin JW, Blackstone EH. Outflow obstruction after the arterial switch operation: A multiinstitutional study. Congenital Heart Surgeons Society. *J Thorac Cardiovasc Surg* 1997;114:975–987.

238. Nakanishi T, Matsumoto Y, Seguchi M, et al. Balloon angioplasty for postoperative pulmonary artery stenosis in transposition of the great arteries. *J Am Coll Cardiol* 1993;22:859–866.

239. Hutter PA, Thomeer BJ, Jansen P, et al. Fate of the aortic root after arterial switch operation. *Eur J Cardiothorac Surg* 2001;20:82–88.

240. Castaneda AR, Jonas RA, Mayer JE, Hanley FL. *Cardiac Surgery of the Neonate and Infant.* Philadelphia: Saunders; 1994.

241. Sagin-Saylam G, Somerville J. Palliative Mustard operation for transposition of the great arteries: Late results after 15–20 years. *Heart* 1996;75:72–77.

242. Hagler D. Double-outlet right ventricle. In: Emmanouilides G, Riemenschneider T, Allen H, Gutgesell H, eds. *Moss and Adams Heart Disease in Infants, Children, and Adolescents,* 5th ed. Baltimore: Williams & Wilkins; 1995:1246–1270.

243. Snider AR, Serwer G. *Echocardiography in Pediatric Heart Disease.* Chicago: Year Book; 1990.

244. Kirklin J, Barratt-Boyes B. Double outlet right ventricle. In: Kirklin J, Barratt-Boyes B, eds. *Cardiac Surgery,* 2d ed. New York: Churchill Livingstone; 1993:1469.

245. Aoki M, Forbess JM, Jonas RA, et al. Result of biventricular repair for double-outlet right ventricle. *J Thorac Cardiovasc Surg* 1994;107:338–349.

246. Belli E, Serraf A, Lacour-Gayet F, et al. Surgical treatment of subaortic stenosis after biventricular repair of double-outlet right ventricle. *J Thorac Cardiovasc Surg* 1996;112:1570–1578.

247. Mavroudis C, Backer CL, Muster AJ, et al. Taussig-Bing anomaly: Arterial switch versus Kawashima intraventricular repair. *Ann Thorac Surg* 1996;61:1330–1338.

248. Freedom R. Congenitally corrected transposition of the great arteries: Definitions and pathologic anatomy. *Pediatr Cardiol* 1999;10:3–16.

249. Fischbach P, Law I, Serwer G. Congenitally corrected I-transposition of the great arteries: Abnormalities of atrioventricular conduction. *Prog Pediatr Cardiol* 1999;10:37–43.

250. Snider A, Serwer G, Ritter S. Abnormalities in ventricular connection. In: Snider A, Serwer G, Ritter S, eds. *Echocardiography in Pediatric Heart Disease.* St. Louis: Mosby; 1990:317–323.

251. Connelly MS, Liu PP, Williams WG, et al. Congenitally corrected transposition of the great arteries in the adult: Functional status and complications. *J Am Coll Cardiol* 1996;27:1238–1243.

252. Graham TP Jr, Bernard YD, Mellen BG, et al. Long-term outcome in congenitally corrected transposition of the great arteries: A multiinstitutional study. *J Am Coll Cardiol* 2000;36:255–261.

253. Fredriksen PM, Chen A, Veldtman G, et al. Exercise capacity in adult patients with congenitally corrected transposition of the great arteries. *Heart (British Cardiac Society)* 2001;85:191–195.

254. Therrien J, Barnes I, Somerville J. Outcome of pregnancy in patients with congenitally corrected transposition of the great arteries. *Am J Cardiol* 1999;84:820–824.

255. Lundstrom U, Bull C, Wyse RK, Somerville J. The natural and "unnatural" history of congenitally corrected transposition. *Am J Cardiol* 1990;65:1222–1229.

256. Cowley C, Rosenthal A. Congenitally corrected transposition of the great arteries: The systemic right ventricle. *Prog Pediatr Cardiol* 1999;10:31–35.

257. Warnes CA. Congenitally corrected transposition: The uncorrected misnomer. *J Am Coll Cardiol* 1996;27:1244–1245.

258. Kirklin J, Barratt-Boyes B. Congenitally corrected transposition of the great arteries. In: Kirklin J, Barratt-Boyes B, eds. *Cardiac Surgery.* New York: Churchill Livingstone; 1993:1511.

259. Sano T, Riesenfeld T, Karl TR, Wilkinson JL. Intermediate-term outcome after intracardiac repair of associated cardiac defects in patients with atrioventricular and ventriculoarterial discordance. *Circulation* 1995;92:II272–II278.

260. Termignon JL, Leca F, Vouhe PR, et al. "Classic" repair of congenitally corrected transposition and ventricular septal defect. *Ann Thorac Surg* 1996;62:199–206.

261. van Son JA, Danielson GK, Huhta JC, et al. Late results of systemic atrioventricular valve replacement in corrected transposition. *J Thorac Cardiovasc Surg* 1995;109:642–652.

262. Ilbawi MN, DeLeon SY, Backer CL, et al. An alternative approach to the surgical management of physiologically corrected transposition with ventricular septal defect and pulmonary stenosis or atresia. *J Thorac Cardiovasc Surg* 1990;100:410–415.

263. Imai Y. Double-switch operation for congenitally corrected transposition. *Adv Card Surg* 1997;9:65–86.

264. Reddy VM, McElhinney DB, Silverman NH, Hanley FL. The double switch procedure for anatomical repair of congenitally corrected transposition of the great arteries in infants and children. *Eur Heart J* 1997;18:1470–1477.

265. Rosenthal A, Dick M. Tricuspid atresia. In: Emmanouilides G, Riemenschneider T, Allen H, Gutgesell H, eds. *Moss and Adams Heart Disease in Infants, Children, and Adolescents,* 5th ed. Baltimore: Williams & Wilkins; 1995:902.

266. Hagler D, Edwards W. Univentricular atrioventricular connection. In: Emmanouilides G, Riemenschneider T, Allen H, Gutgesell H, eds. *Moss and Adams Heart Disease in Infants, Children and Adolescents,* 5th ed. Baltimore: Williams & Wilkins; 1995:1278.

267. Dobell AR, Van Praagh R. The Holmes heart: Historic associations and pathologic anatomy. *Am Heart J* 1996;132:437–445.

268. Silverman N. *Pediatric Echocardiography.* Baltimore: Williams & Wilkins; 1993.

269. Freedom R, Culham J, Moes C. *Angiocardiography of Congenital Heart Disease.* New York: Macmillan; 1989.

270. George B, Kaplan S. Single ventricle and subaortic obstruction. *Prog Pediatr Cardiol* 1994;3:167–176.

271. Moak JP, Gersony WM. Progressive atrioventricular valvular regurgitation in single ventricle. *Am J Cardiol* 1987;59:656–658.

272. Donofrio MT, Jacobs ML, Norwood WI, Rychik J. Early changes in ventricular septal defect size and ventricular geometry in the single left ventricle after volume-unloading surgery. *J Am Coll Cardiol* 1995;26:1008–1015.

273. Mainwaring R, Lamberti J, Moore J. The bidirectional Glenn and Fontan procedures: Integrated management of the patient with a functionally single ventricle. *Cardiol Young* 1996;6:198–207.

274. van Son JA, Reddy VM, Haas GS, Hanley FL. Modified surgical techniques for relief of aortic obstruction in [S,L,L] hearts with rudimentary right ventricle and restrictive bulboventricular foramen. *J Thorac Cardiovasc Surg* 1995;110:909–915.

275. Norwood WI, Lang P, Hansen DD. Physiologic repair of aortic atresia-hypoplastic left heart syndrome. *N Engl J Med* 1983;308:23–26.

276. Bailey LL, Nehlsen-Cannarella SL, Doroshow RW, et al. Cardiac allotransplantation in newborns as therapy for hypoplastic left heart syndrome. *N Engl J Med* 1986;315:949–951.

277. Mayer JE Jr, Bridges ND, Lock JE, et al. Factors associated with marked reduction in mortality for Fontan operations in patients with single ventricle. *J Thorac Cardiovasc Surg* 1992;103:444–451.

278. Matitiau A, Geva T, Colan SD, et al. Bulboventricular foramen size in infants with double-inlet left ventricle or tricuspid atresia with transposed great arteries: Influence on initial palliative operation and rate of growth. *J Am Coll Cardiol* 1992;19:142–148.

279. Jacobs ML, Rychik J, Rome JJ, et al. Early reduction of the volume work of the single ventricle: The hemi-Fontan operation. *Ann Thorac Surg* 1996;62:456–461.

280. Fontan F, Baudet E. Surgical repair of tricuspid atresia. *Thorax* 1971;26:240–248.

281. Cetta F, Feldt RH, O'Leary PW, et al. Improved early morbidity and mortality after Fontan operation: The Mayo Clinic experience, 1987 to 1992. *J Am Coll Cardiol* 1996;28:480–486.

282. Petrossian E, Reddy VM, McElhinney DB, et al. Early results of the extracardiac conduit Fontan operation. *J Thorac Cardiovasc Surg* 1999;117:688–696.

283. Jacobs ML, Blackstone EH, Bailey LL. Intermediate survival in neonates with aortic atresia: A multi-institutional study. The Congenital Heart Surgeons Society. *J Thorac Cardiovasc Surg* 1998;116:417–431.

284. Bove EL. Surgical treatment for hypoplastic left heart syndrome. *Jpn J Thorac Cardiovasc Surg* 1999;47:47–56.

285. Gaynor JW, Mahle WT, Cohen MI, et al. Risk factors for mortality after the Norwood procedure. *Eur J Cardiothorac Surg* 2002;22:82–89.

286. Tkebuchava T, Von Segesser LK, Vogt PR, et al. Congenital coronary fistulas in children and adults: Diagnosis, surgical technique and results. *J Cardiovasc Surg (Torino)* 1996;37:29–34.

287. Vavuranakis M, Bush CA, Boudoulas H. Coronary artery fistulas in adults: Incidence, angiographic characteristics, natural history. *Cathet Cardiovasc Diagn* 1995;35:116–120.

288. Velvis H, Schmidt KG, Silverman NH, Turley K. Diagnosis of coronary artery fistula by two-dimensional echocardiography, pulsed Doppler ultrasound and color flow imaging. *J Am Coll Cardiol* 1989;14:968–976.

289. Urrutia-S CO, Falaschi G, Ott DA, Cooley DA. Surgical management of 56 patients with congenital coronary artery fistulas. *Ann Thorac Surg* 1983;35:300–307.

290. Mavroudis C, Backer CL, Rocchini AP, et al. Coronary artery fistulas in infants and children: A surgical review and discussion of coil embolization. *Ann Thorac Surg* 1997;63:1235–1242.

291. Blanche C, Chaux A. Long-term results of surgery for coronary artery fistulas. *Int Surg* 1990;75:238–239.

292. Perry SB, Rome J, Keane JF, et al. Transcatheter closure of coronary artery fistulas. *J Am Coll Cardiol* 1992;20:205–209.

293. Hurwitz RA, Caldwell RL, Girod DA, et al. Clinical and hemodynamic course of infants and children with anomalous left coronary artery. *Am Heart J* 1989;118:1176–1181.

294. Wesselhoeft H, Fawcett JS, Johnson AL. Anomalous origin of the left coronary artery from the pulmonary trunk. Its clinical spectrum, pathology, and pathophysiology, based on a review of 140 cases with seven further cases. *Circulation* 1968;38:403–425.

295. Schmidt KG, Cooper MJ, Silverman NH, Stanger P. Pulmonary artery origin of the left coronary artery: Diagnosis by two-dimensional echocardiography, pulsed Doppler ultrasound and color flow mapping. *J Am Coll Cardiol* 1988;11:396–402.

296. Gutgesell HP, Pinsky WW, DePuey EG. Thallium-201 myocardial perfusion imaging in infants and children. Value in distinguishing anomalous left coronary artery from congestive cardiomyopathy. *Circulation* 1980;61:596–599.

297. Takeuchi S, Imamura H, Katsumoto K, et al. New surgical method for repair of anomalous left coronary artery from pulmonary artery. *J Thorac Cardiovasc Surg* 1979;78:7–11.

298. Cochrane AD, Coleman DM, Davis AM, et al. Excellent long-term functional outcome after an operation for anomalous left coronary artery from the pulmonary artery. *J Thorac Cardiovasc Surg* 1999;117:332–342.

299. el Said GM, Ruzyllo W, Williams RL, et al. Early and late result of saphenous vein graft for anomalous origin of left coronary artery from pulmonary artery. *Circulation* 1973;48:2–6.

300. Rein AJ, Colan SD, Parness IA, Sanders SP. Regional and global left ventricular function in infants with anomalous origin of the left coronary artery from the pulmonary trunk: Preoperative and postoperative assessment. *Circulation* 1987;75:115–123.

301. Rahimtoola SH. Concept and evaluation of hibernating myocardium. *Annu Rev Med* 1999;50:75–86.

CONGENITAL HEART DISEASE IN ADULTS

Carole A. Warnes / John E. Deanfield

Congenital heart disease of moderate or severe degree occurs in about 6 per 1000 live births.[1] Without early treatment, the majority of patients would die in infancy or childhood, with only 5 to 15 percent surviving until puberty.[2] The advent of surgical procedures, as well as advances in medical treatment, has transformed the outlook for children with even complex defects. The majority now survive into adolescence and adult life. This success story has radically altered both the size and complexity of the population of young adults with congenital heart disease. In the United States alone, well over one-half million patients with functionally important congenital cardiac malformations have reached adulthood in the past four decades.[3] Since most patients now surviving to adult life will have undergone surgery during childhood, "total correction" is not the rule.[4] The term *total correction* is itself a misnomer, perhaps with the exception of the successfully ligated ductus arteriosus without residua. The misperception of "cure" leads adults not to seek understanding of their anomaly, to fail to follow endocarditis prophylaxis, and to fail in pursuing continued cardiac care.[5] The majority, if not all, require long-term surveillance, and many need reoperation. Other adults may require their first operation for congenital heart lesions that were well tolerated during childhood.

Both the "natural" survivors and the postoperative patients require specialized medical care. Arrhythmia is common, as are residual or deteriorating hemodynamic problems and endocarditis. Although cardiologists specializing in the care of adults may be expert in one or more of these areas, the critical relationship between rhythm and hemodynamic status in hearts with complex circulations (as after Fontan's operation or after intraatrial repair for transposition) may lead to treatment errors by those inexperienced in the treatment of congenital heart defects. Patients with cyanosis require special care because of erythrocytosis, bleeding, renal problems, and arthropathy; moreover, they require specific counsel-

ing and management regarding pregnancy. In addition to the medical problems, psychosocial problems such as the search for employment, life and health insurance, participation in sports, sexual activity, and contraception are of great importance to adolescents and young adults with congenital heart disease. Many of the "normal" ordeals of growing up are more difficult for this group, in whom chronic illness, embarrassing scars, and/or exercise limitation may inhibit normal social intercourse and maturation.

Over the last few years, the specialist needs of this growing population have begun to be appreciated. In addition to the challenge of continuing the expert care of their complex cardiac problems, from the pediatric environment into the much wider adult medical community, knowledge of the long-term fate of patients with congenital heart disease is essential for pediatric cardiologists in order to refine initial management strategy. A rather short-term view of "success" or "failure" has been encouraged by rapid changes in medical and surgical policies over the last four decades. Nevertheless, there are clear examples, such as the management of transposition of the great arteries, where awareness of long-term problems has altered the primary surgical approach. The Mustard or Senning procedures (see later) provide a physiologic repair at acceptably low risk but may result in long-term systemic ventricular dysfunction, arrhythmias, and sudden death. This has enabled the introduction of anatomic repair by the arterial-switch procedure, despite high surgical mortality in the early series, with the expectation of a more satisfactory long-term outcome.

The optimal solutions for delivery of care to the adult with congenital heart disease will depend on the different medical systems in operation around the world. The common requirements include collaboration between pediatric and adult cardiologists, the establishment of a few specialist centers with appropriate medical, surgical, anesthetic, and nonmedical staff together with investigational facilities, and the establishment of treatment guidelines, and centralization of accumulating knowledge.[6] The report of a consensus conference on adult congenital heart disease, commissioned by the Canadian Cardiovascular Society, represents an important step forward.[7] This includes recommendations for training and a hierarchy of care from the community to the specialist center. Similar training guidelines have been published in the United States.[8]

MEDICAL CONSIDERATIONS

Many young adults with congenital heart disease have mild lesions that have not required and may not ever require surgery. The most common defects in this category are small ventricular septal defect, mild pulmonary valve stenosis, mild aortic valve stenosis, and mitral valve prolapse (Table 74-1). Such patients need infrequent follow-up (e.g., biannual) to assess any progression in severity of the lesion, to reinforce the need for antibiotic prophylaxis against infective endocarditis (see Chap. 81), and to obtain psychosocial advice. Other patients reach adult life with more complex defects that are still unrepaired. Some may still be candidates for palliative or definitive surgery, whereas in others surgery may no longer be possible, often because of the presence of irreversible pulmonary vascular disease. More and more survivors of surgery in childhood are now reaching adult life; they now form the largest group of patients (Table 74-2). The majority need continuing medical surveillance, as late cardiovascular problems may result from hemodynamic disturbances, arrhythmia, and endocarditis. Such patients can also develop noncardiac problems as a consequence of their heart disease (e.g., secondary to cyanosis) and are, of course, susceptible to all the potential acquired "medical problems" of adulthood.

Hemodynamics

Study of the hemodynamic consequences of repaired and unrepaired congenital heart disease is a crucial aspect of long-term follow-up.

TABLE 74-1 Common Congenital Heart Defects Compatible with Survival to Adult Life without Surgery or Interventional Catheterization

Mild pulmonary valve stenosis
Peripheral pulmonary stenosis
Bicuspid aortic valve
Mild subaortic stenosis
Mild supravalvar aortic stenosis
Small atrial septal defect
Small ventricular septal defect
Small patent ductus arteriosus
Mitral valve prolapse
Ostium primum atrial septal defect (atrioventricular septal defect)
Marfan's syndrome
Ebstein's anomaly
Corrected transposition (atrioventricular-ventriculo-arterial discordance)
Balanced complex lesions (e.g., double-inlet ventricle with pulmonary stenosis)
Defects with pulmonary vascular obstructive disease (Eisenmenger's syndrome)

TABLE 74-2 Common Congenital Heart Defects Surviving to Adult Life after Surgery/Interventional Catheterization

Aortic valve disease, valvotomy or replacement
Pulmonary stenosis, valvotomy
Tetralogy of Fallot
Atrial septal defect
Ventricular septal defect
Atrioventricular septal defect
Transposition of the great arteries, atrial redirection
Complex transposition of the great arteries
Total anomalous pulmonary venous connection
Pulmonary atresia/ventricular septal defect
Fontan operation for complex congenital heart disease
Ebstein's anomaly
Coarctation of the aorta
Mitral valve disease

Progressive congestive cardiac failure secondary to myocardial deterioration is the most common cause of disability and death in patients whose ventricles may have been subjected to many years of volume and pressure loading, often with chronic hypoxia. A significant number of the adult postoperative patients with congenital heart disease have been repaired at older ages than is the current practice. This may result in greater preoperative damage and pulmonary vascular disease, which may persist postoperatively. In the early era of open-heart surgery, myocardial protection was sometimes less than optimal, resulting in myocardial damage.

It should also be appreciated that postoperative circulations created by the repair of many congenital heart defects result in an adequate physiologic repair (e.g., deoxygenated blood to lungs and oxygenated blood to the body) but often have far from normal anatomy. For example, after the Mustard and Senning operation for transposition of the great arteries, the right ventricle remains on the systemic side of the circulation. Some of these patients have evidence of deteriorating right ventricular function, and there is increasing concern that this will become a major life-threatening problem with longer follow-up.[9] Similar concerns have been expressed for systemic ventricular function after Fontan's operation.[10] The different morphology and loading conditions for these ventricles suggest that standard indices of ventricular function, derived from studies of structurally normal hearts, may be inappropriate for such patients (see also Chap. 24).[11] Prospective serial studies are beginning to define "normal ranges" for congenital heart defects and to examine their "natural" and "unnatural" history.[12]

Residual hemodynamic defects are often present in repaired patients and may cause problems even many years after surgery. These may be amenable to further surgery (see later) or require long-term medical treatment. Medical management of cardiac failure in patients with congenital heart disease is adopting therapies shown to be of benefit with heart failure from cardiomyopathy or ischemic heart disease.[13–16] Appreciation of ventricular "remodeling" and the effect of neurohumoral responses on symptoms and disease progression has led to increasing and earlier use of angiotensin-converting enzyme inhibitors and, in some cases, beta blockers in addition to standard therapy with digoxin and diuretics. These may also slow the rate of progressive deterioration in ventricular function reported in certain congenital heart diseases even when they have been adequately "corrected."

Cyanosis

Adults with congenital heart disease may have central cyanosis from right-to-left shunting secondary to their unrepaired cardiac defect or to pulmonary vascular disease (Eisenmenger's syndrome) (see Chap. 73). The latter complication should be seen less frequently in years ahead as a result of the trend to early recognition and repair of congenital heart disease in infancy. Currently, however, a significant number of patients reach adult life with pulmonary vascular disease as a result of lesions such as large ventricular septal defect, atrioventricular septal defect, truncus arteriosus, and double-outlet right ventricle. Their pulmonary vascular resistance may already have been too high for surgical repair at the time of diagnosis; in others, pulmonary vascular disease may have progressed despite repair of the congenital heart defect.

Chronic cyanosis may lead to erythrocytosis and hyperviscosity. Many patients with cyanotic congenital heart disease establish a stable high hematocrit but few symptoms of hyperviscosity.[17] They have a low risk of stroke and do not require venesection.[18] In others, the hemoglobin concentration may rise progressively. Once it exceeds 20 g/dL, they are at risk from thromboembolic complications and may suffer from headache, dizziness, and fatigue. Symptoms may be improved with judicious venesection by the removal of 500 mL of blood and volume replacement with normal saline or dextrose.[18] Overzealous venesection, however, may result in both acute and chronic problems, including cardiovascular collapse in patients with Eisenmenger's syndrome, iron depletion, microcytosis, and hyperviscosity in its own right.[19] The paradoxical anemia of erythrocytotic patients with iron deficiency due to repeated phlebotomy may be missed and indeed has been shown to increase the risk of stroke.[20] This study demonstrated that phlebotomies and microcytosis were strongly associated with stroke, perhaps because iron-deficient red blood cells are less deformable than are normal red blood cells and do not pass through the microcirculation as readily as iron-replete cells.

Patients with chronic cyanosis also develop defective hemostasis from abnormalities in platelet function and in the coagulation and fibrinolytic systems,[19,20] especially in patients with marked erythrocytosis. The risk of hemorrhage, especially at surgery, is well recognized and may be fatal. Hyperuricemia is common because of increased red blood cell turnover and renal dysfunction. Arthralgia is well recognized, but gouty arthritis is rare and may be misdiagnosed. Renal impairment is common[21] and can deteriorate to renal failure as a result of relatively minor interventions, such as injection of contrast medium at angiography or the injudicious use of nonsteroidal antiinflammatory agents or gentamycin.[22,23] Patients with right-to-left shunts are at risk of paradoxic embolus, which may cause a cerebrovascular accident or renal infarction. Air filters must be utilized with all intravenous lines. A cerebral abscess is a well-known complication of a septic embolus and must always be considered in the cyanotic patient with low-grade fever, or any neurologic symptoms, however transient. Facial and truncal acne is common, and is not only a cosmetic problem but a potential source of sepsis. A specific concern has been the safety of air travel in adults with cyanotic congenital heart disease, as in-flight atmospheric conditions on commercial jets approach altitude equivalents of 6000 to 8000 ft (1829 to 2438 m). In a one report, however, only modest (approximately 6 percent) decreases in systemic arterial oxygen saturation were found, with no adverse effects.[24]

Progressive kyphoscoliosis has been recognized for many years as a complication of congenital heart disease.[25] This is common in cyanotic patients and in those with previous thoracotomy. The degree of deformity, if left untreated, may become profound and compromise pulmonary function. Treatment with bracing or insertion of a Harrington rod may be indicated, since the kyphoscoliosis may significantly reduce both the quality and quantity of life. Surgical repair is not possible, however, in those with Eisenmenger's syndrome since the surgical risk is too high.

The prognosis for patients with Eisenmenger's syndrome depends on the site of the lesion and the medical and cardiac care they receive.[26–28] Death may result from right-sided heart failure, pulmonary hemorrhage, or arrhythmia. It can also occur prematurely due to potentially avoidable complications such as inappropriate drug therapy or injudicious general anesthesia. Special care must be employed during noncardiac surgery, utilizing cardiac anesthesia, maintenance of preload, and cardiac monitoring.[29] Data suggest promise for chronic prostacyclin therapy in reducing pulmonary artery pressure, but this is preliminary.[30]

Infective Endocarditis

Patients with both unoperated and operated congenital heart disease are at risk from infective endocarditis. Lifelong antibiotic prophylaxis is recommended, but the specific indications and optimal regimens are still debated.[31,32] The American Heart Association (AHA) Special Report on Prevention of Infective Endocarditis has stratified risk groups for the various lesions.[32] Prophylaxis is advocated for all lesions except isolated secundum atrial septal defect and repaired secundum atrial septal defect, ventricular septal defect, or patent ductus arteriosus without residua beyond 6 months (see Chap. 81). The wide variety of portals of entry include dental work, skin sepsis, obstetric and gynecologic procedures, genitourinary and gastrointestinal interventions, and surgery. There is also a risk of bacteremia and infective endocarditis in young adults who have their ears pierced or acquire a tattoo.[33] Patients must be educated and preferably should carry an information card with them. The symptoms of endocarditis may be subtle, and the diagnosis must be considered in any patient who experiences unexplained malaise or fever. Injudicious prescription of antibiotics without previous blood culture may mask the problem and make bacteriologic diagnosis and appropriate treatment difficult. Both general measures such as oral hygiene as well as skin and nail care and appropriate antibiotic treatment are important. Among 102 patients with congenital heart disease who completed a questionnaire, there was a disturbing lack of knowledge about endocarditis prevention measures and indeed about their cardiac lesion in general.[34]

Electrophysiologic Problems

Arrhythmias and conduction defects have a major impact on the prognosis and management of both unoperated and operated patients and have been linked to sudden death in a number of conditions.[35] The principles of diagnosis and treatment are similar to those employed in patients with arrhythmia due to other causes, with some important exceptions. Rhythm disturbances that may be benign in a structurally normal heart may be life-threatening in congenital heart disease. Restoration of sinus rhythm is usually much more important, and rate control of atrial arrhythmias is usually not a good treatment option. Special consideration must be given before the use of therapies that may have negative inotropic properties. In unoperated patients, chamber dilatation, myocardial hypertrophy, and fibrosis may all contribute to the genesis of arrhythmia. In operated patients, additional sinus or atrioventricular (AV) node damage and atrial and/or ventricular scarring may cause electrophysiologic problems. The etiology is multifactorial, and the clinical significance of arrhythmia depends very much on the hemodynamic context in which it occurs.

Supraventricular arrhythmia and sinus node injury, not surprisingly, occur most often in conditions with "atrial defects" or those requiring atrial surgery.[36,37] Abnormalities of sinus node function are common in patients with atrial septal defect, particularly the sinus venosus type,[38] and are often seen after Mustard's or Senning's operation for transposition of the great arteries.[39] Sinus node dysfunction has also been reported after surgery for tetralogy of Fallot, Fontan's procedure, and many other operations for congenital heart lesions.[40] Clinical manifestations include sinus bradycardia, sinoatrial block, sinus arrest, and occasionally the tachybradycardia syndrome with paroxysmal atrial flutter and fibrillation. Although bradycardia has been postulated as the cause of sudden death in some conditions, current evidence indicates that tachyarrhythmia is usually a more likely explanation.

Indications for pacemaker implantation in asymptomatic individuals are still controversial, since the arrhythmia is benign in many cases. It should be noted that pacing may be difficult because of the complex underlying anatomy and lack of a suitable site for endocardial lead fixation.[41] The choice of pacemaker will depend on the precise indication. The simplest VVI pacemaker may be adequate prophylaxis against bradycardia-related sudden death. In general, however, rate-responsive pacemakers are preferable and dual-chamber pacing may provide the best hemodynamics (see also Chap. 32).[42]

Injury to the AV node and proximal conduction tissue may result from surgery for lesions such as ventricular septal defect, AV septal defect, or tetralogy of Fallot. Transient complete AV block in the postoperative period has been shown to have prognostic significance in some reports, particularly if the site of damage is below the bundle of His. Whether transient perioperative AV block warrants permanent pacing and whether an invasive electrophysiologic study can help stratify risk are unresolved.[36] Postoperative right bundle branch block is frequent after ventriculotomy and may be due to injury related to closure of a ventricular septal defect or to interruption of distal Purkinje fibers by ventriculotomy or muscle resection.[35,36]

Tachyarrhythmias can be life-threatening. Late sudden death has been reported in several lesions, both before and after repair. In general, the worse the disease (i.e., more complex anatomy and/or more extensive surgery), the greater the incidence of sudden death, although aortic stenosis and coarctation are also represented in this group. Studies suggest that the risk increases incrementally 20 years after surgical repair.[43] The identification of patients at risk and their management are important but controversial issues. After the Mustard and Senning operation, atrial flutter with a rapid ventricular response is dangerous, especially when it occurs in association with right ventricular dysfunction or venous pathway obstruction.[44] Medical or electrical cardioversion should be promptly used to restore sinus rhythm, and drug therapy may need to be accompanied by pacemaker insertion. Ablation (surgical or catheter) has been advocated for certain cases of atrial flutter (see Chap. 36). Atrial tachyarrhythmias are also common after Fontan's operation; sinus node injury, atrial suturing, and a dilated hypertensive right atrium probably contribute.[40,43] Modification of the operation to exclude the right atrium from the Fontan circuit—the total cavopulmonary connection—may reduce the incidence of potentially serious early and late rhythm disturbances.[45]

Ventricular arrhythmias are known to occur after open heart surgery, particularly repair of tetralogy of Fallot.[46,47] Studies using ambulatory electrocardiographic (ECG) monitoring in postoperative patients have documented asymptomatic complex ectopy and nonsustained ventricular tachycardia in up to 50 percent of patients,[47,48]

and more than 20 percent have inducible ventricular tachycardia at electrophysiologic study.[49] Experimental and clinical studies have shown that the electrical substrate for reentry arrhythmia is present in the right ventricle.[50] In several reports, advanced age at surgery is a predisposing factor,[48,51] an observation that suggests factors present at the time of repair may be involved in the genesis of postoperative arrhythmia in addition to the myocardial damage occurring at the time of surgery or during postoperative follow-up.[52] This is consistent with morphologic studies that have documented increasing fibrosis of the right ventricle as part of the natural history of defects such as tetralogy of Fallot.[53] The current practice of early surgical repair for tetralogy of Fallot may reduce the incidence of such postoperative ventricular arrhythmia. Other postulated risk factors include elevated right ventricular systolic pressure, reduced right ventricular ejection fraction, pulmonary regurgitation, and a ventriculotomy scar.[54] The clinical significance of nonsustained ventricular tachycardia and especially the indications for prophylactic antiarrhythmic therapy remain unclear.[44] There is a disparity between the high frequency of ventricular arrhythmia and the much lower incidence of sudden death.[55,56] The predictive value of an abnormal ambulatory ECG or of electrophysiologic study has not been established.[57] Furthermore, prophylactic antiarrhythmic therapy has not been shown to be of value in asymptomatic patients with congenital heart defects. Such therapy may have proarrhythmic potential, be negatively inotropic, or have serious extracardiac side effects. As a result, there is insufficient evidence to advocate prophylactic treatment for asymptomatic individuals with nonsustained arrhythmia. In contrast, there are a few cases of sudden death, out-of-hospital ventricular fibrillation, and/or sustained ventricular tachycardia in almost all large series of patients after repair of tetralogy of Fallot. Identification of "at risk" individuals and appropriate treatment remains a challenge. Reports have indicated a link between the electrical and mechanical properties of the right ventricle, which may have clinical relevance.[58] The QRS duration on the surface ECG correlates with cardiothoracic ratio and, in a retrospective review, a QRS of >180 ms was a marker for sudden death or out-of-hospital cardiac arrest.[59,60] Others have reported that, while a trend toward QRS prolongation and sudden death may emerge when large groups of patients are evaluated, this marker has a low predictive accuracy in the individual patient.[61,62] Further refinements in risk stratification in adults with tetralogy of Fallot or other congenital heart lesions are necessary and may involve hemodynamic and electrophysiologic testing both at rest and after exercise, evaluation of ventricular late potentials, and heart rate variability.[63] It should be remembered, however, that despite the attention given to ventricular arrhythmia after repair of tetralogy of Fallot, a major source of morbidity in such patients is from atrial arrhythmia.[64]

Radiofrequency ablation, so successfully used to treat arrhythmia in patients with structurally normal hearts (see Chap. 36), is applied to patients with congenital heart disease. These represent some of the most challenging electrophysiologic procedures because of the complex cardiac anatomy, enlarged chamber size, abnormal localization of the underlying conduction system, and multiple reentry circuits. Nevertheless, ablation may have a role, not merely in subjects with accessory pathways or AV reentry tachycardia but also in intraatrial reentry arrhythmias that may be present after operations such as the Fontan and Mustard or Senning procedures.[65,66]

Pregnancy

An increasing number of women with complex and postoperative congenital heart defects are reaching childbearing age. Advice is sought on both maternal and fetal risk, as well as on the incidence of congenital heart disease in the offspring. In the United States, most maternal cardiac disease is congenital in origin. Data are accumulating regarding outcomes of pregnancy in many complex anomalies.[67-72] Prepregnancy counseling is mandatory for all patients whether operated or unoperated. The evaluation should include a detailed history, physical exam, ECG, and chest x-ray along with a comprehensive echocardiogram to evaluate ventricular function, all valve lesions and defects, and pulmonary artery pressure. If pulmonary artery pressure and resistance is in doubt following noninvasive testing, a cardiac catheterization may be necessary. An exercise test may facilitate a detailed assessment of functional capacity.

There are profound changes in the maternal cardiovascular system during pregnancy, including a large (30 to 40 percent) increase in blood volume, a fall in peripheral vascular resistance, and an increase in cardiac output (approximately 40 percent) (see also Chap. 92). In general, women with left-to-right shunts or valvular regurgitation tolerate pregnancy well, whereas those with right-to-left shunts or valvular stenosis do less well.[73,74] Asymptomatic young women with small or moderate left-to-right shunts and normal pulmonary artery pressures can expect an uncomplicated pregnancy and labor. In the presence of a large left-to-right shunt, however, heart failure may be provoked or aggravated by pregnancy. Patients with cyanosis have the most problems in carrying a fetus to term and have a high incidence of early spontaneous abortion. Early studies showed that with higher degrees of cyanosis (as reflected by the maternal hemoglobin), the incidence of spontaneous abortion increased and the handicap to fetal growth became more pronounced. Infants are unlikely to survive if the maternal hemoglobin is >18 g/dL.[75] A study from Presbitero et al. demonstrated a clear relation between the degree of hypoxia and fetal loss.[76] (Table 74-3). When the maternal oxygen saturation was 85 percent, only 2 out of 17 pregnancies (12 percent) resulted in live-born infants. Only 41 of 96 pregnancies (43 percent) produced a live birth in 45 cyanosed mothers. There were 49 spontaneous abortions and 6 stillbirths in this series, again reflecting the high risk that maternal cyanotic congenital heart disease poses for the fetus. Meticulous care during pregnancy and delivery lessened the maternal complication rate, but this was still considerable. Such patients require rest and a short labor as well as avoidance of dehydration and sepsis. In such situations, the decision as to whether or not to continue with the pregnancy depends on an assessment of the risk to the mother and fetus as compared with the patient's desire to have children.

An elevated pulmonary vascular resistance, from either Eisenmenger's syndrome or primary pulmonary hypertension, is a clear contraindication to pregnancy. Pregnancy for women with Eisenmenger's syndrome carries approximately a 50 percent mortality.[77] Termination of pregnancy is always preferable; ideally, this should be done with cardiac anesthesia. If such patients are seen late in pregnancy and termination is not feasible, management should concentrate on maintenance of adequate preload and avoidance of vasodilation. The ideal management around the time of delivery for these patients is controversial because individual experience is small. Vaginal delivery is usually associated with less blood loss than cesarean section. The latter, however, can be done quickly with all medical personnel in attendance. One report has suggested an approach of elective delivery by cesarean section under general anesthesia.[78] The use of prophylactic heparin before and after delivery is also controversial, and there is no established consensus.[78,79] Even after successful delivery, however, death frequently occurs within the few days following from deteriorating hemodynamics or pulmonary infarction.[77] Patients with Marfan's syndrome and aortic root dilation (>40 mm) are at greater risk of aortic dissection and rupture, and while those without preexisting cardiovascular disease whose aortic root is smaller often tolerate pregnancy well, the risk is unpredictable.[80,81] Patients with severe aortic stenosis are also at increased risk because of the fall in afterload which accompanies pregnancy and exaggerates the valve gradient.[82,83] While early reports suggested a high risk of aortic rupture and cerebral hemorrhage in patients with aortic coarctation,[84] more recent data have been more encouraging.[85] Fetal risk is increased, however, presumably as a result of compromised placental blood supply.

The management of pregnant women with mechanical prosthetic cardiac valves is a special problem because of the risk to the mother of thromboembolism and the risk to the fetus of anticoagulants (warfarin crosses the placenta and is teratogenic).[86,87] Depending on the condition involved and the mother's motivation and compliance, the use of unfractionated heparin, administered intravenously or subcutaneously in the first and third trimesters, and warfarin in the midtrimester is one treatment option. Heparin, however, is a poor anticoagulant during pregnancy; even with meticulous control of anticoagulation, there is still an increased risk of valve thrombosis.[88] In addition, there is also an increased risk of fetal loss with this approach. No control studies exist with regard to low-molecular-weight heparin. Because of the poor results with heparin, some clinicians have advocated the use of warfarin throughout pregnancy despite the risk of fetal teratogenicity.[89] This risk may be less if the dose of warfarin is <5 mg/day.[90] Nonetheless, this approach is still very controversial despite the fact that fetal teratogenicity with warfarin may have been overemphasized.[91] Before prescribing any cardiovascular drug during pregnancy, the effects on both mother and fetus must be considered.

Management of labor should be specifically directed toward avoidance of rapid changes in the circulatory volume, blood pressure, or cardiac output. In most cases vaginal delivery is recommended, with careful attention to maternal position and analgesic agents. The AHA no longer recommends endocarditis prophylaxis for vaginal delivery.[32] This, however, is not based on controlled data, and most cardiologists recommend antibiotics under these circumstances for almost all congenital heart defects.

TABLE 74-3 Fetal Outcome in Cyanotic Congenital Heart disease and its Relation with Maternal Cyanosis

Hemoglobin, g/dL[a]	Pregnancy, no.	Live Births, no.	Live Born, %
≤16	28	20	71
17–19	40	18	45
≥20	26	2	8
Arterial Oxygen Saturation, %[b]	Pregnancy, no.	Live Births, no.	Live Born, %
≤85	17	2	12
85–89	22	10	45
≥90	13	12	92

[a]Hemoglobin level unknown in two pregnancies.
[b]Arterial oxygen saturation unknown in 44 pregnancies.
SOURCE: From Presbitero P, Somerville J, Stone S, et al. Pregnancy in cyanotic congenital heart disease: Outcome of mother and fetus. *Circulation* 1994; 89:2673–2676. Reproduced with permission from the publisher and authors.

Genetic Counseling

The risk of recurrence is an important issue , and genetic counseling should be provided for all potential parents. It has been estimated that the cause of congenital heart disease is genetic in approximately 8 percent of cases (e.g., velocardiofacial syndrome and Holt-Oram syndrome with autosomal dominant transmission) and environmental in 2 percent (e.g., congenital rubella syndrome).[92] In the remainder, genetic and environmental factors are thought to interact.[93] The greater the number of affected first-degree relatives within the family, the greater the recurrence risk. Recurrence risks in siblings of patients with congenital heart disease are well documented and range between 1 and 8 percent.[94] For the affected potential parents, however, the risk of recurrence in offspring is the key information, and fewer data exist. Early reports suggested that recurrence risks were considerably higher in offspring compared to siblings. Studies, such as the Second Natural History of Congenital Heart Defects (NHS-2), have suggested a low risk (1.2 percent for aortic stenosis, 2.8 percent for pulmonary stenosis, and 2.9 percent for ventricular septal defects).[95] There is considerable variation in recurrence risks in reported series, and factors inherent in study design, ascertainment bias, and follow-up account for many of the differences. In addition, certain forms of congenital heart disease recur more frequently than do others (e.g., left ventricular outflow tract obstruction), and the recurrence risk appears to be higher in pregnancies with affected mothers rather than with fathers. Accumulation of further information will be invaluable for patient counseling. Fetal cardiac ultrasound at approximately 18 weeks of pregnancy facilitates early diagnosis.

Investigation and Imaging

Transthoracic echocardiography and cardiac catheterization with angiocardiography are the principal investigations in pediatric cardiology. Transthoracic echocardiography is an invaluable tool in adults also, although image acquisition is more challenging because of body habitus and chest wall abnormalities as a result of previous surgeries.[96] Transesophageal echocardiography is becoming increasingly important for the definition of cardiac structure and function,[96–98] and multiplane probes with color-flow Doppler allow simultaneous assessment of anatomy and physiology. Specific areas of the heart that are well imaged in this way include systemic and pulmonary venous drainage, atrial lesions (including baffle function), AV valve morphology and function, left ventricular outflow tract lesions (including the ascending aorta in Marfan's syndrome), as well as intracavity thrombus or vegetations (Fig. 74-1).[98,99] Intraoperative transesophageal echocardiography is particularly helpful during repair of congenital heart defects when new information may alter the planned procedure or lead to a revision of the initial repair.[100]

Magnetic resonance imaging (MRI) can also provide valuable anatomic information, which in some cases is superior to that from ultrasound even via a transesophageal approach. Rapid technologic advances—including three-dimensional image reconstruction, software to study hemodynamics such as velocity mapping, and cinemagnetic resonance imaging—may reduce the need for invasive investigation (Fig. 74-2).[101–103] The expertise required both to acquire and interpret MRI information is likely to be confined to specialized regional centers, but access to the MRI facility should be available to all units managing adult patients with congenital heart disease.

In parallel with the decreasing need for diagnostic cardiac catheterization, there has been a dramatic rise in the indications for and scope of interventional procedures in adult patients with congen-

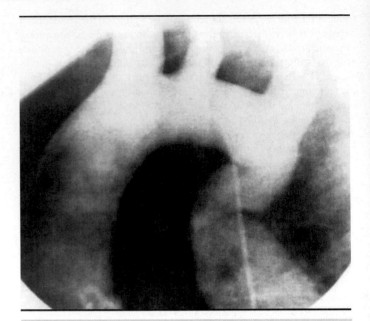

FIGURE 74-1 Transesophageal echocardiogram of a patient with Marfan's syndrome and dilated sinuses of Valsalva. The intimal flap (arrows) of an aortic dissection is visualized superior to the aortic valve leaflets.

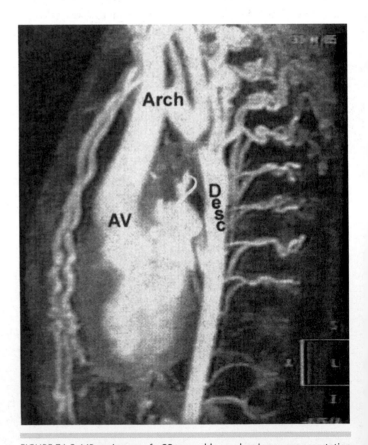

FIGURE 74-2 MR angiogram of a 33-year-old man showing severe coarctation and development of extensive collateral vessels involving the intercostal and internal mammary arteries. AV, aortic valve; Desc, descending aorta. (From Oh JK, Seward JB, Tajik AJ: Congenital heart disease. In: Oh JK, Seward JB, Tajik AJ (eds): *The Echo Manual*, 2nd ed. Philadelphia-New York: Lippincott-Raven, 1999; 233. Reproduced with permission from the publisher and authors.)

ital heart disease.[104] Residual defects after repair that are amenable to treatment in the catheterization laboratory include coronary fistulas, paravalvular leaks, and pulmonary artery stenoses. Optimum management of patients with complex congenital heart disease can often be achieved by planned collaboration between surgeon and interventional cardiologist. In other patients with a range of relatively simple lesions—including patent ductus arteriosus, pulmonary valve stenosis, atrial septal defect/patent foramen ovale, and certain forms of ventricular septal defect—definitive treatment avoiding surgery may be achieved by interventional catheterization.

PSYCHOSOCIAL ASPECTS

During adolescence, a crucial transition occurs for the patient with congenital heart disease. By the end of the teenage years, the young adult must understand the nature and implications of his or her heart problem. Sensible advice and guidance must be available regarding employment, insurance, socialization, contraception, exercise, and sports.

Employment

Most patients can work and should have access to employment appropriate to their physical and intellectual capabilities. The report of the Natural History Study of Congenital Heart Defects suggested that among patients with ventricular septal defect, pulmonary stenosis, and aortic stenosis, in comparison with national normal standards, a greater percentage achieved higher levels of education (college and beyond).[105] No similar data are yet available for large groups of patients with more complex defects, although their situation will undoubtedly prove worse.

Despite the excellent potential of many adults with congenital heart disease, job discrimination is frequently encountered, even when a patient has been cleared by a cardiologist. In the United States, the National Rehabilitation Act of 1973 seeks to prevent job discrimination by employers with ≥10 employees by obliging them to consider only the present capacity of applicants to perform a given job and not projections of future deterioration. In other countries, employers frequently take into account future prospects for absenteeism or premature career curtailment. In these circumstances, young adults with congenital heart defects are often at a disadvantage, particularly if they apply for jobs with long training periods.

Restrictions for employment exist for jobs in which the safety of others is the direct responsibility of an individual, such as driving a bus or truck. Most armed services exclude applicants with a cardiac history. The regulations for commercial airline pilots are clearer and subject to regular review. In Europe, a risk of sudden cardiac death or acute disability below 1 percent per annum is the maximum considered acceptable for multicrew flights, and it is 0.1 percent for solo flights. The number of congenital heart defects in which low-risk rates are clearly defined remains small.[106]

Insurance

Life insurance is difficult to obtain for many young adults in the absence of adequate long-term survival data for their congenital heart lesions. Most of the data used to assess risk do not apply to currently performed medical or surgical procedures. In 1986, a survey in the United States recorded that only patients with very simple lesions were insured at regular rates.[107] These included mild pulmonary valve stenosis, uncomplicated repaired atrial septal defect, ventricu-

lar septal defect, and patent ductus arteriosus. A similar survey in the United Kingdom in 1993 evaluated both employment status and insurability of young adults with congenital heart disease.[108] In general, policies were as restrictive as those in the earlier survey, with most lesions either insurable at higher rates or not insurable at all. Marked inconsistencies were found, making "shopping around" mandatory. This situation is likely to improve when health care professionals are able to provide high-quality follow-up data on morbidity and mortality relevant to current treatment protocols (see Chap. 104).

Despite surgical repair, long-term cardiac care into adult life is usually required for patients with congenital heart disease and, in many countries, health care costs are spiraling dramatically.[109] Medical expenses incurred during childhood are usually reimbursed as part of the parents' policy. This coverage often ceases to be available once the patient reaches the age of maturity. A new policy sought at this stage often excludes benefits for medical or surgical treatment of the cardiac condition itself. As a result, the level of medical surveillance of the adult patient with congenital heart disease drops dramatically after age 21 years. This is a major problem as, with adequate regular follow-up, costs for adults with congenital heart disease are considerably lower than they are for those with other chronic diseases.

Psychosocial Development

Large controlled longitudinal studies of the psychosocial consequences of congenital heart disease are rare and difficult to interpret.[110] Most patients with congenital heart disease appear well adjusted but have subtle feelings of "difference" from their peers. Lack of self-esteem and fear of isolation are common.[111,112] These feelings are often compounded by reminders such as exercise limitation, presence of scars, cardiac symptoms, hospital visits, and family anxiety with parental overprotection. As a result, patients should be encouraged to lead as normal a life as possible and to discuss their heart disease openly. Anxieties about sexual activity, marriage, and childbirth are common, but patients often find these aspects difficult to discuss, particularly with the doctor in a regular clinic.[112,113] Often, such issues are best handled by the team caring for the patient, which may include a nurse, social worker, and psychologist. Resentment and rebellion against all adult authority figures may occur, including the doctor. Compliance with medical treatment and advice can be affected.

The impact of congenital heart disease on intellectual development is controversial. Interpretation of testing must take into account the very abnormal childhood experienced by many patients, with absences from school for medical reasons as well as decreased social interaction. All studies of intellect exclude patients with genetic syndromes and other dysmorphic, somatic, or neurologic defects, but subtle abnormalities are easily missed.[114] Certain aspects of development appear to be more specifically affected by congenital heart disease. For example, walking is delayed in cyanotic children, but speech is not. This will affect the relevance of early IQ testing on later performance. Data suggest that cyanosis is associated with mild intellectual impairment.[115,116] This is reduced by early corrective surgery even involving cardiopulmonary bypass.

Contraception

Sexually active adolescents and young adults should be given appropriate advice about contraception.[117] In general, the low-dose estrogen oral contraceptive pill is safe for young women with congenital heart disease.[118] Exceptions include women with hypertension (e.g., associated with coarctation of the aorta) and those with pulmonary vascular disease or cyanosis with associated erythrocytosis. Progesterone preparations are alternatives, although they have a lower contraceptive efficacy.[119] They are, however, inappropriate for patients with cardiac failure because of the tendency for fluid retention. Barrier methods, either using condom or diaphragm, are safe and effective, but intrauterine devices should probably not be used because of the risk of endocarditis and of increased bleeding, particularly in cyanotic women.[120] In women with severe pulmonary vascular disease or with lesions in which pregnancy would result in high maternal risk, laparoscopic sterilization should be considered.

Exercise and Sports

Exercise is of both physical and psychological benefit. It leads to improved cardiovascular fitness and decreased likelihood of obesity, hypertension, and ischemic heart disease.[121,122] Furthermore, participation in exercise and sports is part of normal socialization in adolescent and adult life. In many adults with congenital heart disease, exercise capacity is diminished, even after surgery. Reduced performance may also reflect lack of regular exercise in protected individuals with congenital heart defects. This is often reinforced by doctors who, if in doubt, tend to limit exercise.

The 26th Bethesda Conference provided recommendations for competition in athletics by patients with cardiovascular abnormalities.[123] An important consideration is the danger of bodily injury from collision or the consequences of syncope. Another consideration is whether prolonged long-term exercise might contribute to progressive hemodynamic deterioration (e.g., left ventricular hypertrophy and aortic stenosis). In some cases, exercise capacity is clearly normal and the risk is minimal, as after closure of a small patent ductus arteriosus. In others, exercise capacity is limited and the risk is high, as in severe pulmonary hypertension. Between these extremes the recommendations must take into account the individual, the underlying cardiac defect, hemodynamic status, and the type of sport and form of exercise contemplated (e.g., social or competitive, contact or noncontact). Formal testing should be performed (preferably including measurement of oxygen uptake), both as a measure of the effects of submaximal and maximal exercise and also as a reassurance to the patient. A 12-minute walking test gives a good guide to functional capacity, whereas a treadmill protocol with more strenuous effort is employed to assess risk by revealing occult arrhythmia, ischemia, or fall in blood pressure (see Chap. 16). Subjective estimates of exercise capacity are often inaccurate.

In general, volume overload, valve regurgitation, and left-to-right shunts are associated with good exercise tolerance, whereas pressure overload, valve stenosis, and right-to-left shunt are not. The recommendations provided by the Bethesda Conference should be considered as guidelines only. The physician with knowledge of the severity of the patient's lesion and physiologic and psychologic response to training and competition may choose to modify these recommendations.[123] Those patients with a history of symptomatic arrhythmia, syncope, pulmonary hypertension, or myocardial dysfunction deserve special attention since they are probably at higher risk. Patients with fixed, elevated pulmonary vascular resistance have limited exercise capacity, and for them exercise has considerable risk. Walking should be encouraged, but strenuous exercise avoided. The most controversial recommendations are those for aortic stenosis and Marfan's syndrome. It could be argued that exercise has an adverse effect on sudden death or the progression of left ventricular hypertrophy in the former, and may increase the risk of progressive

aortic dilatation in the latter. Thus patients with more than mild aortic stenosis should be counseled against moderate to strenuous activities. Patients with Marfan's syndrome, particularly those with aortic root dilatation, should be counseled against isometric exercise and activities with the potential for bodily collision. While many adults with repaired congenital heart lesions have impaired exercise capacity,[124] supervised training programs can improve aerobic fitness and increase the safe level at which they can participate in sports. Such programs also improve psychological adjustment and self-esteem.

SURGICAL CONSIDERATIONS

Reoperations

Reoperations in adults with congenital heart disease provide a particular challenge.[125,126] The risks are often higher than they are for primary procedures. Careful preoperative planning should include complete understanding of the cardiac anatomy and its relations and study of previous operative reports. Sternal reentry is particularly risky when the ventricle immediately beneath the sternum is a high-pressure chamber or when an extracardiac conduit lies in this position. Postoperative hemodynamic and respiratory problems are particularly common after reoperation because of the increased duration of surgery, previously scarred myocardium and/or lung disease, and greater use of blood products. The need for reoperation may come as a shock to patients and relatives who may have believed that childhood surgery was curative. As a result, resentment is frequent and tact is required. Indications for reoperation are shown in (Table 74-4).

Inevitable Reoperation

Early repair of congenital heart defects that have involved insertion of a prosthetic valve or extracardiac conduit commonly results in a need for reoperation to replace prostheses that are either too small or have undergone degeneration. Extracardiac conduits are commonly used for repair of pulmonary atresia with ventricular septal defect, truncus arteriosus, transposition with left ventricular outflow tract

TABLE 74-4 Indications for Reoperation in Adults with Congenital Heart Disease

1. Inevitable reoperation after definitive repair prosthetic valves, extracardiac conduits placed at an early age that become of inadequate size because of body growth.
2. Residual defects after definitive repair: ventricular septal defect after tetralogy of Fallot and left AV valve regurgitation after AV septal defect repair
3. New/recurrent defects after definitive repair: subaortic stenosis, restenosis of aortic valve, pulmonary regurgitation in tetralogy of Fallot
4. Staged repair of complex defects: pulmonary atresia with ventricular septal defect
5. Unexpected complications: infective endocarditis
6. Heart/heart-lung transplantation for uncorrectable congenital heart disease
7. Patient operated on for congenital heart disease with new acquired heart disease: coronary disease

obstruction and/or ventricular septal defect, congenitally corrected transposition with left ventricular outflow tract obstruction, and/or ventricular septal defect and were used in early Fontan's operations. Development of obstruction is influenced by the type and size of conduit, technique of insertion, and timing of the original operation. In one series of 143 survivors of heterograft conduit insertion, all had to be replaced in 10 years.[127] A homograft aorta or pulmonary artery and valve have also been used for the repair of pulmonary atresia with ventricular septal defect.[128] For all conduits, calcification and obstruction remain significant complications. Besides the conduit itself, improved operative technique and the use of a large conduit have clear beneficial influence on the need for early replacement. This may be facilitated by utilizing a prosthetic roof of pericardium placed over the fibrous tissue bed of the explanted conduit, thus permitting a large tissue valve to be inserted.[129] Patients with right-sided conduits need careful follow-up, particularly toward the end of the expected life of the conduit, since the signs of severe obstruction may be subtle and may be missed. As a result, replacement may be performed too late. The consequent major deleterious effects on right ventricular function increase the risk of surgery and may not be fully reversible. Regular, noninvasive evaluation by echocardiography or MRI is indicated in selected patients and may provide the information usually obtained by cardiac catheterization and angiography. Reoperation is usually indicated if the right ventricular pressure is 75 percent of the systemic or if there is evidence of deteriorating ventricular function.[130]

Residual and Recurrent Defects

Residual or recurrent defects may have a major impact on morbidity and mortality but may be difficult to distinguish unless careful assessment after the original repair has been performed.

The reported need for reoperation after the commonly performed reparative operation for tetralogy of Fallot varies between 1.8 and 13 percent over a follow-up of up to 31 years.[131,132] Ventricular septal defect and right ventricular outflow tract obstruction are common residual abnormalities. Pulmonary regurgitation is extremely common and inevitable after transannular patching as part of the original repair. This represents the most common indication for reoperation in adults.[133] The hemodynamic consequences of pulmonary regurgitation for the right ventricle are greater in the presence of other defects such as residual obstruction and/or ventricular septal defect. Pulmonary valve replacement has not been frequently required in the first two decades after repair but is increasingly performed because of the late deleterious effects of pulmonary regurgitation on the right ventricle.[134] Indications include progressive right ventricular dilatation and a decrease in exercise tolerance.[135] This is often accompanied by progressive tricuspid regurgitation and atrial arrhythmias. When surgery is performed before the development of right ventricular failure, both clinical status and right ventricular function improve.[136] The optimal method for assessing pulmonary regurgitation in serial follow-up has not been determined; therefore appropriate guidelines for intervention are still not established.

Several studies have emphasized the palliative nature of aortic valvotomy in childhood.[137,138] Isolated aortic stenosis most frequently results from a bicuspid aortic valve, although in neonates and infants the structural abnormality of the aortic valve is more severe and the results of surgery even worse (see Chap. 73). In a series of 59 patients who underwent open aortic valvotomy >1 year of age, actuarial survival was 94 percent at 5 years but only 77 percent at 22 years. Reoperation was carried out in 36 percent, and the actuarial probability of reoperation was 44 percent at 22 years. When serious

events comprising death, reoperation, and endocarditis were grouped together, 92 percent were free of events at 5 years but only 39 percent at 22 years. Others have reported a similar long-term outcome.[137] The causes of restenosis have not been studied in detail but appear to be related to the degree of residual obstruction.

Staged Repair

For complex congenital heart disease, definitive repair may not be possible until the anatomy and physiology of the circulation have been improved by one or more palliative procedures as part of a staged approach to "correction." This course is often necessary for patients with pulmonary atresia and ventricular septal defect, hypoplastic pulmonary arteries, and multifocal pulmonary blood supply. Palliative procedures to increase flow to the central pulmonary arteries and unifocalization of pulmonary flow by anastomosis (direct or indirect) of collateral vessels to the pulmonary arteries may eventually result in the ability to perform a repair (conduit insertion between the right ventricle and pulmonary artery and ventricular septal defect closure) with an acceptable postoperative right ventricular/left ventricular pressure ratio.[139,140] Good surgical results have been reported from such an approach, but the long-term outcome is not yet available.[141]

Other situations in which definitive repair may be indicated in the young adult include complex congenital heart defects with one functioning ventricle palliated by a systemic-pulmonary shunt or pulmonary artery banding in childhood. In selected patients who fulfill the stringent criteria for Fontan's operation, it is likely that long-term results will be better after Fontan's operation than when the ventricle is left with a chronically increased load secondary to a systemic pulmonary shunt.[12] Fontan's operation, however, should be considered palliative rather than curative: long-term problems are frequent.

Unexpected Reoperations

Indications for unexpected reoperation include thrombosis in a low-flow circulation such as the Fontan, prosthetic valve failure or thrombosis, and infective endocarditis. The latter may be particularly difficult to diagnose in complex congenital heart disease where the site of vegetations may not be easy to image (e.g., in a Blalock-Taussig shunt). Reoperation in the patient with uncontrolled endocarditis carries a particularly high risk.

Heart and Heart-Lung Transplantation

Despite the major successes of the last three decades, an increasing number of patients survive to adult life with deteriorating clinical status. Their only remaining prospect may be a heart or heart-and-lung transplant (see Chap. 26), despite the surgical problems of multiple previous chest incisions, complex venous anatomy, and borderline pulmonary vascular resistance. Nonetheless, the results in this patient group may be excellent.[142] The shortage of donors and the ability to monitor rejection in a single organ have stimulated great interest in single-lung transplantation for patients with primary pulmonary hypertension and Eisenmenger's syndrome (in conjunction with closure of the shunt).[143]

First Operations for Congenital Heart Disease in Adults

The first surgical repair of a congenital heart defect may be required in the teenager or adult. This may be because the lesion has been mild and of little hemodynamic significance in childhood but has progressed in severity with time. Examples include a bicuspid aortic valve with progressive stenosis, Marfan's syndrome with aortic root dilatation, and Ebstein's anomaly with worsening symptoms. Alternatively, lesions such as small-to-moderate atrial septal defects may have been missed or misdiagnosed until adult life. In certain complex congenital heart defects, the combination of lesions produces a balanced hemodynamic state compatible with prolonged survival without intervention. Patients with double-inlet ventricle and pulmonary stenosis, complex pulmonary atresia, and tetralogy of Fallot may remain well until the second and even third decades of life before deteriorating.[144] The contemplation of heart surgery in an adolescent or young adult is often terrifying. The scar on the chest may cause embarrassment, and the patient may be discriminated against both socially and at work. All these issues need to be dealt with sympathetically by the physician.

Noncardiac Surgery

When performed without adequate preparation, noncardiac surgery in adults with congenital heart disease is a major cause of avoidable morbidity and mortality. All the anesthetic risks encountered for cardiac reoperation apply equally to noncardiac surgery, but in the latter the patient may be managed by medical staff who may be unfamiliar with the significance of the congenital heart disease. Many patients with congenital heart defects are at increased risk for arrhythmia and from agents that depress ventricular function. The surgeon must be aware of the presence of a pacemaker or pacing leads that may affect the safe use of diathermy. Prophylaxis against infective endocarditis is usually indicated, and the choice of antibiotic regimen is dictated by the surgical procedure and intervention being undertaken (see Chap. 81). In patients with pulmonary vascular disease, general anesthesia may have disastrous consequences, with a sudden fall in systemic vascular resistance.[29] Similar hemodynamic changes may induce a severe hypercyanotic spell in a patient with unrepaired tetralogy of Fallot, and meticulous pre-, intra-, and postoperative hemodynamic monitoring is mandatory together with the avoidance of vasodilating anesthetic agents, hypoxia, hypoventilation, and blood or volume loss. Cyanotic patients also have impaired hemostasis, and some patients may be taking anticoagulants. Intravenous lines, drugs, and infusions must be managed carefully in patients with intracardiac shunts, as air or emboli may reach the systemic circulation. The safety of noncardiac surgery in adults with congenital heart disease is greatly increased when physicians, anesthesiologists, and surgeons familiarize themselves with these issues, seek specialized advice, and, if necessary, refer the patient to a team with more experience.

SPECIFIC LESIONS

General Considerations

Some lesions that are commonly seen in adult congenital heart disease, both as a result of natural and unnatural survival, are listed in Tables 74-1 and 74-2.

The relatively short era of open-heart surgery, the evolution and refinement of surgical techniques, and myocardial protection along with the trend toward earlier definitive repair means that long-term outcome data relevant to current practice are not available.

Correct application of survival analysis is essential for interpretation of follow-up data. In particular, the use of hazard functions providing an estimate of instantaneous risk is particularly valuable. The

following section deals with some specific defects seen in adults with congenital heart disease.

Atrial Septal Defect

Atrial septal defects are among the most common congenital anomalies in adolescents and adults, accounting for up to 30 percent of congenital heart disease in this age group.[145,146] Approximately 75 percent of defects are ostium secundum defects, 20 percent are ostium primum defects (discussed later), and 5 percent are sinus venosus defects; defects at other sites are rare.[147,148] Associated lesions include pulmonary stenosis, mitral valve prolapse, and mitral regurgitation. Atrial septal defects may be associated with other syndromes, including the Holt-Oram syndrome[149] (see Fig. 12-2) and may be familial.[150] In the latter, conduction disease manifesting as prolongation of the PR interval and, rarely, heart block have been described.[150] Lutembacher's syndrome (atrial septal defect coexisting with mitral stenosis) is now rare.

NATURAL HISTORY

Survival into adulthood is the rule, and patients living into their 80s and 90s have been reported.[145] Life expectancy, however, is not normal. Death during the first 20 years of life is infrequent, but after the age of 40 years, the mortality increases to about 6 percent per year.[151,152] Defects may go unrecognized for many years because symptoms are rare until later life and physical signs may be subtle. Later, the natural history is characterized by progressive symptoms and cardiomegaly, the development of atrial arrhythmias, right ventricular hypertrophy, and pulmonary hypertension. The mechanisms for the development of symptoms are multifactorial[145] and include the following:

1. Change in left ventricular compliance from superimposed hypertension or coronary artery disease that increases the shunt with age. Long-standing right ventricular volume overload, although relatively well tolerated, ultimately leads to right ventricular dysfunction and progression of tricuspid regurgitation.
2. Supraventricular arrhythmias, particularly atrial fibrillation and flutter, increase with time and may cause symptoms and cardiac failure (Fig. 74-3).

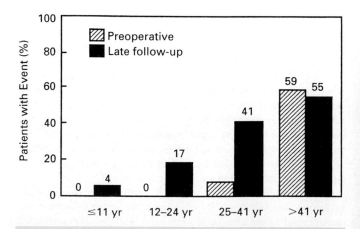

FIGURE 74-3 Incidence of atrial flutter or atrial fibrillation preoperatively and at late follow-up according to the age at operation after repair of atrial septal defect. (From Murphy JG, Gersh BJ, McGoon MD, et al. Long-term outcome after surgical repair of isolated atrial septal defects: Follow-up at 27–32 years. *N Engl J Med* 1990;323:1645. Reproduced with permission from the publisher and authors.)

3. Progressive pulmonary hypertension after the third decade of life.
4. Rarer complications, including systemic and pulmonary emboli, recurrent chest infections, and infective endocarditis (in patients with coexisting mitral valve disease).

MANAGEMENT

Surgical closure either by direct suture or use of a patch has been performed for more than 40 years. Surgery carries a low risk (<1 percent operative mortality) provided that the pulmonary vascular resistance is not significantly elevated.[148] In older patients (≥40 years of age), the indication for closure is a little more controversial. Shah et al. compared the outcome of patients treated medically and surgically when diagnosed after the age of 25 years.[153] This unrandomized study followed patients for more than 20 years and concluded that there was no difference in survival or symptoms between the two groups and no difference in the incidence of new arrhythmia, stroke, or other embolic phenomena in the follow-up period. Notably, however, more than 70 percent of patients in both the medical and surgical groups were asymptomatic at presentation, which may partly explain the favorable outcome of the medically treated group, who had a 91 percent survival. Konstantinides et al. evaluated 179 patients with secundum atrial septal defect ≥40 years of age and compared the outcome of medically and surgically treated groups.[154] They demonstrated a reduced mortality after surgical closure with a 95 percent surgical survival versus an 84 percent medical survival at 10 years. Nonfatal cardiovascular complications, however, were similar with atrial fibrillation and flutter occurring with a similar incidence in both groups. The functional status of the medically treated group deteriorated in 34 percent of patients and improved in many of the surgical patients, particularly those in class III or IV.

A randomized study compared the outcomes of 232 patients >40 years old having surgical closure of their secundum atrial septal defect with an age-matched population of 241 patients treated medically.[155] New York Heart Association (NYHA) classification was I or II for all patients. The survival analysis (median follow-up 7.3 years) revealed no difference in overall mortality between the surgical and medical treatments, but the incidence of nonfatal complications was reduced by surgical closure of the defect. Thus it seems reasonable to conclude that symptomatic adult patients will improve after surgical repair, and the only real contraindication is severe pulmonary vascular disease. When surgery is delayed, symptoms are likely to be progressive and surgical repair is less likely to prevent problems with atrial fibrillation and thromboembolic events. For those with preexisting atrial fibrillation, a concomitant right-sided maze procedure may facilitate restoration and maintenance of sinus rhythm.[156] The management of the asymptomatic adult patient is less clear, but certainly closure of the defect halts progression of right ventricular volume overload, tricuspid regurgitation, and progression of pulmonary vascular disease, and it can be accomplished with low surgical risk. The standard surgical approach remains a midline sternotomy, but patients should be made aware of the alternatives of thoracotomy or inframammary incision. Although morbidity may be higher, the resulting scar may be less offensive, especially to young women.

Closure of an atrial septal defect has been achieved in selected patients by use of a variety of occlusion devices inserted at cardiac catheterization.[157–161] A multicenter nonrandomized trial reported that success rates of device closure compared favorably to surgical closure but appropriate patient selection is an important factor for successful device closure.[162] Eventually, the transcatheter technique may supplant surgery as the method of closure for atrial septal defects of appropriate size, morphology, and location. In addition, the presence of a patent foramen ovale has been suggested as a risk factor for cerebral embolus. Determining the risk of clinical events in asymptomatic subjects with patent foramen ovale and indications for treatment are highly controversial areas. Catheter treatment may become the method of choice for patients who have a clear indication for intervention.

LATE RESULTS

In a study of patients undergoing surgical repair of an atrial septal defect between 1956 and 1960, late survival of patients undergoing operation at below 24 years of age was not significantly different from an age- and sex-matched control population. Late survival in patients aged 25 to 41 years was good but less than that of the control population, whereas repair after age 41 years was associated with significantly poorer late survival (see Fig. 74-3). The combination of older age at operation and pulmonary hypertension had an additive effect on late mortality.[163] In this and other series, the propensity for atrial fibrillation and flutter increased as a function of age both before and after the operation (Fig. 74-4).[163,164] Of late deaths, 22 percent were due to stroke, and all occurred in patients with postoperative atrial fibrillation or flutter. These data support the current policy of repair at a preschool age. A separate study of 66 patients who underwent closure of atrial septal defect between 60 and 78 years of age implied a benefit in survival in patients discharged from the hospital compared with unoperated historical age- and sex-matched controls.[165] A study of patients over 70 years of age showed improved survival of patients in NYHA Class II and III when treated surgically compared to medical treatment. Patients in NYHA Class IV did poorly with medical or surgical treatment.

The near-normal survival and low morbidity in patients undergoing repair within the first two decades of life have important implications for employment and insurance recommendations. Such patients should be encouraged to lead a normal life, and competitive sports should not be restricted in the absence of hemodynamic or electrophysiologic sequelae. Patients who have undergone repair in the third decade of life or later require careful regular surveillance. Although late survival is good, the development of supraventricular arrhythmia and risk of cerebrovascular accident are of concern. Anticoagulation is indicated in patients with atrial fibrillation and should be considered in those with supraventricular tachycardia or atrial flutter in the

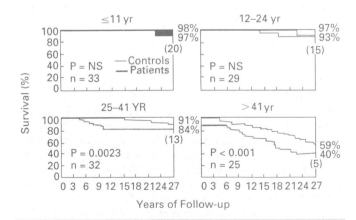

FIGURE 74-4 Long-term survival of perioperative survivors of atrial septal defect repair by age at time of operation. Controls are survival in an age- and sex-matched population. (From Murphy JG, Gersh BJ, McGoon MD, et al. Long-term outcome after surgical repair of isolated atrial septal defects: Follow-up at 27–32 years. *N Engl J Med* 1990;323:1645. Reproduced with permission from the publisher and authors.)

absence of other contraindications. Long-term follow-up is recommended for patients repaired in adult life who have increased pulmonary artery pressure at the end of operation, pre- and postoperative arrhythmia, ventricular dysfunction, or coexisting heart disease.

Ventricular Septal Defect

Isolated ventricular septal defect, although one of the most common congenital abnormalities in infants and children, is far less frequent in the adolescent and adult for several reasons.[145] First, most patients with a hemodynamically significant defect will have undergone repair in childhood; second, spontaneous decrease in size and closure are common for small or moderate perimembranous or muscular defects (this decreases in frequency with increasing age); last, patients with large, unoperated defects may die earlier in life.[166] The spectrum of isolated ventricular septal defects in the adult is thus limited to the following four groups of patients: (1) those with small, restrictive defects that were either small to begin with or have partially closed; (2) those with Eisenmenger's syndrome and a predominant right-to-left shunt with cyanosis[167] who need to be distinguished from those who develop secondary infundibular pulmonary stenosis, which can also decrease the left-to-right shunt and may result in cyanosis with shunt reversal[168] (see Chap. 73); (3) the occasional patient with a moderately restrictive defect in whom the diagnosis has been overlooked or who has not had closure in childhood; and (4) those who have had their defects closed in childhood.[169]

NATURAL HISTORY

The natural history of small, restrictive ventricular septal defects is very favorable, but lifelong endocarditis prophylaxis is required. A subset of patients with perimembranous defects or defects in the outlet septum may develop aortic cusp prolapse and aortic regurgitation. This may be progressive and is often severe by the end of the second decade of life. As incompetence increases, the ventricular septal defect may become "closed" by the prolapsing cusp; if it is left to develop, however, aortic valve replacement may be necessary.[170] Such defects are associated with a high risk of infective endocarditis. Severe and progressive pulmonary vascular disease is a feature of older patients with nonrestrictive large defects. Eisenmenger's syndrome is compatible with survival into young adult life, but the complications of right-sided heart failure, paradoxical emboli, and erythrocytosis usually result in death by the third decade. Occasionally, patients with moderate-sized ventricular septal defects and left-to-right shunts who did not develop pulmonary vascular disease present in adolescence and young adult life with symptoms of fatigue, effort intolerance, and respiratory infections.

MANAGEMENT

Patients with small ventricular septal defects are asymptomatic and should be managed conservatively. Continued medical follow-up is, however, helpful to remind patients about the need for prophylaxis against infective endocarditis and to minimize inappropriate discrimination during the search for employment and insurance. Ventricular septal defects associated with aortic cusp prolapse and aortic regurgitation should be repaired even when the shunt is small in an effort to prevent progressive deterioration of the aortic valve. Surgical repair is indicated in the rare adult with a significant left-to-right shunt (pulmonary to systemic flow ratio exceeding 2:1) and a low pulmonary vascular resistance. The management of patients with large defects and infundibular narrowing causing right-to-left shunting and cyanosis is similar to that for tetralogy of Fallot (see later).

Unfortunately, adults are still seen with a large ventricular septal defect and pulmonary vascular disease. In those with borderline pulmonary vascular resistance (7 to 10 U/m^2), surgery may be attempted, but the benefits are unpredictable as the pulmonary vascular disease may progress despite closure of the defect.[171] Medical management and consideration for heart-lung or single-lung transplantation are the only realistic options for patients with established severe pulmonary vascular disease, although prostacyclin may hold some promise.[30]

LATE RESULTS

Late results of surgery are good, but the life expectancy for the whole group is not normal. In a study of 179 operative survivors between 1956 and 1959, 30-year survival was 82 percent, compared with 97 percent in age- and sex-matched controls.[168] Only 25 percent of patients in the series were over 10 years of age at surgery, and their 30-year survival of 70 percent was substantially lower than the 88 percent in patients under 2 years of age at operation. Thirty-year survival was 83 percent for patients aged 3 to 10 years at surgery. Older age at repair and preoperative pulmonary vascular disease are important predictors of late outcome. Postoperative conduction defects, especially right bundle branch block, are common, but complete heart block, which was seen in the early surgical experience, is now rare. Late ventricular arrhythmia has been reported, as after repair of tetralogy of Fallot,[172] but the incidence of late sudden death is extremely low.

Certain selected ventricular septal defects may be closed with transcatheter devices. One report described successful closure of 21 muscular ventricular septal defects in 12 patients, half of whom had complex heart defects.[173] Subsequent cardiac surgery for associated lesions was performed in 11 of 12 patients.

In postoperative patients, the risk of late infective endocarditis is very small provided that the defect is isolated and is completely closed. Antibiotic prophylaxis, however, is often advised, particularly for 6 months postoperatively. Recommendations regarding physical activity and competitive sports require detailed evaluation, which may include exercise testing, cross-sectional echocardiography, and ambulatory electrocardiographic monitoring. The presence of abnormal left ventricular function, a more than trivial residual shunt, arrhythmia, or any degree of pulmonary hypertension mandates some restriction of physical activity.

Atrioventricular Septal Defect

The term AV septal defect describes the spectrum of lesions that involve a defect at the site of the normal AV septum, resulting in an abnormality involving the AV valves, ventricular architecture, and left ventricular outflow tract. A variety of different classifications have been used (see Chap. 73), but the defects are usefully divided into "partial" and "complete" forms. In the former, there is a defect in the primum or inferior part of the atrial septum but no direct intraventricular communication (ostium primum defect). In the latter, there is a large ventricular component beneath either or both the superior or inferior bridging leaflets of the AV valve. The deficiency of the ventricular septum together with the abnormal AV valves produces an elongated left ventricular outflow tract characteristically described as having a "goose neck" appearance at angiography. The morphologic and functional features, together with the associated cardiac and noncardiac abnormalities, determine the natural history. Subaortic stenosis is a common association and may occur de novo even after surgical repair.[174]

NATURAL HISTORY

In the New England Regional Cardiac Registry, 5 percent of newborns with cardiac disease had AV septal defects, with two-thirds being the "complete" form.[175] Down's syndrome is very frequently associated, especially with complete defects. The noncardiac features, especially mental retardation, have a major influence on management in adolescence and adult life.

The natural history of partial AV septal defects with little left AV valve regurgitation is similar to that of large secundum atrial septal defects (see earlier). A small number develop pulmonary vascular disease, and symptomatic deterioration in unoperated adults is often due to the onset of supraventricular arrhythmia. If the left AV valve is more than mildly regurgitant, the natural history is much worse, with a large left-to-right shunt, often with at least moderate pulmonary hypertension and early symptoms of cardiac failure. Patients with complete defects do even worse. Their course is characterized by the early development of pulmonary vascular disease (especially in patients with Down's syndrome who may have irreversible damage before their first birthday) with consequent right-to-left shunting and all the problems of patients with Eisenmenger's syndrome. As a result, surgery needs to be undertaken early if it is to be successful, and most uncorrected patients seen in adolescence or young adulthood will have a pulmonary vascular resistance that is too high for repair (greater than 8 to 10 U/m^2). Their outcome is poor, but survival into their thirties is possible. Uncorrected patients with partial AV septal defects may present to the adult cardiologist for consideration of surgery, which should be recommended for those with a significant left-to-right shunt in the absence of other contraindications.

MANAGEMENT

Surgical repair involves closure of the atrial and ventricular septal defects and restoration of a competent left AV valve as far as is possible. Surgical mortality in experienced centers is approximately 10 percent for complete defects and less than 5 percent for partial defects.[148]

LATE RESULTS

Patients with repair of both partial and complete forms of AV septal defect have now been followed for more than 20 years. Late results are good in the absence of pulmonary vascular disease and significant residual left AV valve regurgitation. Some patients with complete defects who were corrected later in childhood, before the need for correction in early infancy was appreciated, have developed progressive pulmonary vascular disease. This late complication should be greatly reduced in patients undergoing repair in the first 6 months of life, as is now technically feasible. After repair of partial AV septal defect, a 20-year survival of 87 percent has been reported.[176] Closure of the left AV valve cleft and age less than 20 years at operation were associated with better survival. Reoperation was needed in 11 percent of patients, most commonly for residual or recurrent left AV valve regurgitation or stenosis. Even patients who are repaired late in adult life ($\geq$40 years of age) can have excellent results with an early mortality of only 6 percent and a good chance of left AV valve repair in experienced hands.[177]

During long-term follow-up, careful attention must be paid to the status of the left AV valve. If the regurgitation increases in severity, mitral valve replacement may be necessary. Monitoring for arrhythmia at intervals is also currently recommended; in general, little intervention is usually required apart from lifelong infective endocarditis prophylaxis. Surgically repaired non-Down's patients without pulmonary vascular disease can often enjoy life without cardiovascular disability and should not be discouraged from competitive sports, pregnancy, or employment. Restrictions are clearly required for those with pulmonary vascular disease, left AV valve regurgitation, or mitral valve replacement on anticoagulants. The recurrence risk of congenital heart disease in offspring of mothers with AV septal defect is higher than average, and potential parents should be counseled.

Tetralogy of Fallot

Tetralogy of Fallot is the most common form of cyanotic congenital heart disease seen in the adult. Nonetheless, in the developed world the unoperated patient with tetralogy of Fallot has fortunately become a rarity since the overwhelming majority of patients will have undergone palliation or, more usually, repair in childhood. From an anatomic and pathophysiologic standpoint, the manifestations of tetralogy of Fallot are similar in all age groups, although hypercyanotic spells, which are often seen in infants and young children, are rare in adults. The development of systemic hypertension with age is a problem as this increases the afterload to both ventricles.[145] Although pulmonary blood flow may improve, this occurs at the expense of right ventricular failure. Acquired calcific aortic stenosis has similar effects. Aortic regurgitation may occur as a result of cusp prolapse into the subaortic ventricular septal defect, and the aorta itself may be dilated. The aortic regurgitation may also be exacerbated by infective endocarditis. The volume overload is transmitted to both ventricles, so patients may present with right ventricular failure as a consequence of aortic regurgitation. The development of chronic obstructive lung disease is another manifestation of an acquired cardiopulmonary disease that may place the adult patient with tetralogy of Fallot at particular risk.

NATURAL HISTORY

Survival into the seventh decade is described,[178] but the natural history in the unoperated patient, which is determined by the severity of obstruction of the right ventricular outflow tract and pulmonary vasculature, is poor. Only 25 percent of patients reach the age of 10 years, and only 3 percent reach the age of 40 years.[145,148] Complications of right-to-left shunting and erythrocytosis, which include stroke and cerebral abscess, are common and, in many instances, fatal. Patients are at continuing risk of infective endocarditis; the development of congestive heart failure in adolescence or early adult life is a major cause of death, as is arrhythmia. Myocardial fibrosis resulting from long-standing right ventricular pressure overload and hypoxemia are postulated mechanisms.[179] Prior palliative surgery with a Cooley or Waterston shunt (between the ascending aorta and right pulmonary artery) or a Potts shunt (between the descending aorta and the left pulmonary artery) can lead to the late development of pulmonary vascular disease.[180]

MANAGEMENT

The focus of medical treatment in unoperated patients is on the elevated hematocrit, bleeding disorders, and abnormal uric acid metabolism and the complications of pregnancy. Repair is indicated in all suitable patients, and the principles and techniques are not significantly different in adults than they are in children,[147] (see Chap. 73). Most adults are suitable for repair, but the occasional patient with an underdeveloped pulmonary vascular bed may require a palliative shunt procedure. Intracardiac repair consists of closure of the ventricular septal defect and relief of right ventricular outflow tract obstruction. In some patients, this may require excision of the pulmonary valve and patch reconstruction of the annulus and outflow tract. In the occasional patient with an anomalous origin of the left coronary artery from the right coronary artery, a conduit between the right ventricle and pulmonary artery may be required.[148]

LATE RESULTS

Late survival is excellent, even in patients who underwent repair during the very early years of open heart surgery.[148] At the Mayo Clinic, the cumulative 30-year survival for patients undergoing successful surgery between 1956 and 1960 was 86 percent compared to 95 percent in age- and sex-matched controls (see Fig. 74-4).[181] In a previous series of 396 hospital survivors of repair between 1955 and 1962 at the same institution, 91 percent were alive at 20 years. At 30 years, 77 percent of the initial cohort of 106 patients undergoing surgery between 1954 and 1960 by Lillehei and associates were alive, including one patient who was 45 years of age at the time of operation.[182] Surgery cannot be considered "curative" as survival even in excellent series is slightly but significantly worse than for a matched control population. The risk factors for an adverse late outcome include older age at surgery (>5 years), preoperative congestive heart failure, a previous Potts shunt, persistent right ventricular systolic hypertension, and a residual ventricular septal defect.[180,181] Late death may be sudden, due to tachyarrhythmia or, very rarely in the current era, due to conduction disease[183] (see earlier). Left and right ventricular failure due to right ventricular pressure overload or left ventricular volume overload is another important cause of late mortality in older patients.[145]

The late functional outcome is excellent for the majority of patients. Most lead normal lives, but the results appear to be better in those undergoing surgery at a younger age.[184] Persistent or recurrent symptoms may be the result of incomplete relief of right ventricular systolic hypertension or recurrent or residual ventricular septal defects. These problems are often manifest within the first few years after surgery and may require reoperation. Progressive aortic dilatation and aortic regurgitation may also occur requiring aortic valve replacement.[185] In adult life the most common problem is pulmonary regurgitation, which may be well tolerated for decades but may be associated with late impairment of exercise capacity and frequently atrial arrhythmias.[133] Right ventricular volume overload may also be well tolerated for years but ultimately results in right ventricular failure and progressive tricuspid regurgitation. Pulmonary valve replacement can be accomplished with a low risk.[134,136] Late referral is common, however, and many patients have already developed advanced right ventricular dysfunction and secondary tricuspid regurgitation requiring additional tricuspid valve annuloplasty at the time of pulmonary valve replacement.[134,186]

Current information links pulmonary regurgitation, cardiomegaly, QRS duration, with potentially life-threatening ventricular arrhythmia.[58-60] This may be important for identification of risk of late sudden death, which has been a rare event in most long-term follow-up series. Asymptomatic ventricular arrhythmia is very common during long-term follow-up. It is again related to older age at repair, but the link between nonsustained ventricular arrhythmia and adverse clinical outcome is uncertain (see earlier).[51,52] Objective testing has emphasized the effects of older age at operation on subsequent exercise performance. This is essentially normal for children repaired at <5 years of age but is usually impaired when surgery is undertaken in adolescence or adulthood.[124]

Before unrestricted physical activity after repair of tetralogy of Fallot can be recommended, careful evaluation—including echocardiography, ECG monitoring, and exercise testing—should be undertaken. Normal activity including competitive sports seems reasonable if surgery has been performed at a young age, right and left ventricular function and size are normal, and there is no residual ventricular septal defect or significant right ventricular outflow tract obstruction and no worrisome arrhythmia. In those who do not fulfill these stringent criteria, the degree to which physical activity should be restricted must be individualized. Long-term follow-up of all patients with tetralogy of Fallot is recommended.

Pulmonary Stenosis

Isolated pulmonary valve stenosis is a common form of adult congenital heart disease and is characterized typically by a trileaflet valve with fused commissures. A dysplastic valve without commissural fusion occurs infrequently in otherwise normal children, but more commonly in patients with Noonan's syndrome[145] (see Fig. 12-18). Subvalvar stenosis due to infundibular hypertrophy is usually a secondary phenomenon in response to obstruction to right ventricular outflow but may occur as a rare isolated entity. Supravalvular or peripheral pulmonary artery stenosis is also extremely uncommon as an isolated entity but is associated with tetralogy of Fallot and supravalvar aortic stenosis in Williams' syndrome (see Fig. 12-36).

NATURAL HISTORY

Prolonged survival into adult life is common and depends upon the severity of obstruction. In patients with severe pulmonary stenosis, symptoms of right-sided heart failure increase with time because of progressive obstruction and alterations in right ventricular compliance.[187] In the Joint Study of the Natural History of Congenital Heart Disease, 19 percent of patients with severe stenosis aged 2 to 11 years and 37 percent aged 12 to 21 years were symptomatic. The natural history of moderate pulmonary stenosis in older patients is more favorable, with less tendency to progression.

MANAGEMENT

Patients with mild stenosis are asymptomatic and require no intervention other than antibiotic prophylaxis against infective endocarditis, although infective endocarditis is rare, with an incidence of 0.94 per 10,000 patient years.[188] In patients with more severe stenosis (>40-mm gradient between the right ventricle and pulmonary artery), intervention to reduce severity should be considered even if there are no symptoms.[189]

Surgical valvotomy for isolated pulmonary stenosis has been successfully performed for more than 40 years. Perioperative morbidity and mortality are minimal beyond the neonatal period in patients without severe congestive cardiac failure or right ventricular dysplasia.[148] Late results are also excellent. In a study from the Mayo Clinic of patients undergoing surgery between 1956 and 1957, late survival for those undergoing valvotomy who are over 21 years of age was similar but not identical to that of an age- and sex-matched control population (Fig. 74-5). Among patients undergoing surgery at an older age, late survival, although still good, was less than that of the control population. (Fig. 74-6).[190] This effect of age on late outcome, which was independent of the use of ventriculotomy, outflow patches, and pulmonary regurgitation, is likely the result of long-standing pressure overload on the right ventricle. Late functional results are excellent, and pulmonary regurgitation is well tolerated in the short and medium term. More severe pulmonary regurgitation may result when a pulmonary valvectomy or transannular patch is required, as may be the case for a small or dysplastic valve; the long-term consequences on the right ventricle and functional capacity are not yet well documented (see "Tetralogy of Fallot," earlier).

Surgical valvotomy is now rarely required after infancy because of the advent of catheter balloon pulmonary valvotomy. In most in-

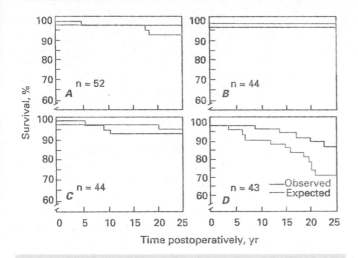

FIGURE 74-5 Long-term survival of perioperative survivors of surgical repair of pulmonary valve stenosis by age at time of operation. *A.* Ages 0 to 4 years. *B.* Ages 5 to 10 years. *C.* Ages 11 to 20 years. *D.* Ages 21 to 68 years. Survival is expected in an age- and sex-matched population. Values of *p* for comparison between the expected and observed survivals: .07, .34, .16, and <.002 for panels *A, B, C,* and *D,* respectively. (From Kopecky SL, Gersh BJ, McGoon MD, et al. Long-term outcome of patients undergoing surgical repair of isolated pulmonary valve stenosis: Follow-up at 20–30 years. *Circulation* 1988;78:1150. Reproduced with permission from the publisher and authors.)

stitutions, balloon valvotomy is the initial procedure of choice at all ages, although gradient reduction is less in patients with dysplastic valves.[191] Interventional catheter procedures should be confined to centers with experienced operators.

Although long-term data are not yet available, the midterm results (up to 10 years) suggest results similar to surgical valvotomy—that is, little or no recurrence over a 22- to 30-year period.[192] The late effects of pulmonary regurgitation resulting from the use of large balloons need to be determined. The risk of infective endocarditis in patients with mild pulmonary stenosis or in those with mild gradients after surgical or balloon valvotomy is low. Long-term follow-up is

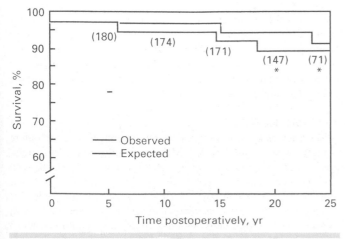

FIGURE 74-6 Long-term survival of perioperative survivors following surgical repair of isolated pulmonary stenosis and expected survival of age- and sex-matched control populations. Difference between expected and observed *p* < .002. (From Kopecky SL, Gersh BJ, McGoon MD, et al. Long-term outcome of patients undergoing surgical repair of isolated pulmonary valve stenosis: Follow-up at 20–30 years. *Circulation* 1988;78:1150. Reproduced with permission from the American Heart Association and authors.)

recommended to evaluate not only the right ventricular outflow tract gradient but also pulmonary regurgitation, right ventricular function, and exercise performance. In patients with good relief of pulmonary stenosis, no restriction of physical activities, including competitive sports, is required. In those with moderate residual obstruction or right ventricular dysfunction, exercise intensity should be reduced (see also Chap. 95).

Left Ventricular Outflow Tract Obstruction

Congenital left ventricular outflow tract obstruction may occur at valvular, subvalvular, and supravalvular levels. Aortic valve stenosis is a common abnormality in adults with congenital heart disease. It may either be an isolated defect or be associated with other lesions, such as coarctation or ventricular septal defect. It is usually due to a bicuspid aortic valve, which may be present in 1 to 2 percent of the total adult population and is 3 to 4 times more common in males than it is in females.[193] Unicuspid and tricuspid stenotic valves are less common.[148] Subvalvar stenosis encompasses a morphologic spectrum of fibrous or fibromuscular obstructions; either a discrete "membrane" below the aortic valve, a discrete fibromuscular ridge, or a diffuse narrowing extending well into the left ventricular cavity forming a "tunnel."[194] The condition occurs more commonly in patients with long and narrow left ventricular outflow tracts,[195] and perhaps this morphology promotes turbulence and shear stresses, which stimulate cellular proliferation.[196] Abnormal ventricular bands or chords may also contribute to obstruction along with abnormal chordal attachments of the anterior mitral valve leaflet. A dynamic component of obstruction may also occur as left ventricular hypertrophy progresses. Common associated anomalies include ventricular septal defect and coarctation of the aorta. Supravalvar stenosis is the least common variety of left ventricular outflow tract obstruction except in the context of Williams' syndrome.[197]

NATURAL HISTORY

The natural history of congenital valvar aortic stenosis in adults is variable but is characterized by progressive stenosis over time (Fig. 74-7[145]). By the age of 45 years, approximately half of all bicuspid aortic valves have some degree of narrowing. The severity of obstruction at the time of diagnosis correlates with the pattern of progression (see Fig. 64-7).[198] Bacterial endocarditis is relatively uncommon (1.8 to 2.7 cases per 100 patient-years),[199] but antibiotic prophylaxis is necessary, even for functionally normal valves. Slowly progressive aortic regurgitation is well recognized in young adulthood, but sudden deterioration is rare except as a sequel to infection.[200,201] Associated abnormalities of the aorta are not uncommon, and aneurysmal dilatation and dissection of the ascending aorta may be seen even with functionally normal valves. Fragmentation of the elastic fibers in the media has been noted histologically, and premature smooth muscle cell apoptosis has been implicated. These findings suggest a common genetic abnormality involving both the aortic valve and ascending aortic wall.[202]

Discrete subaortic stenosis may cause rapidly progressive obstruction in childhood and young adulthood. Progressive aortic regurgitation is common, and infective endocarditis is considered to be a particular hazard.[201] Some patients with mild subaortic stenosis, however, show little progression in their gradient over several years.[203] The natural history of supravalvular aortic stenosis is poor and survival to adulthood is exceptional.[145] The presence of associated congenital abnormalities and possibly premature coronary artery disease with systolic hypertension is likely a contributory factor to this adverse outcome.

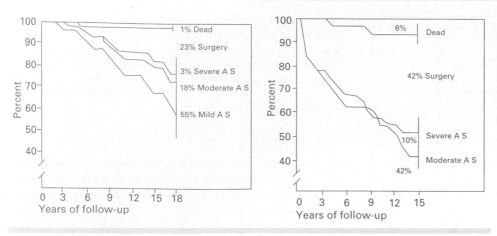

FIGURE 74-7 Left: Cumulative actuarial curves of 153 patients presenting with mild aortic stenosis. Bars show ±1 standard error in age at presentation 6.5 years (range 1 to 25 years); mean follow-up 8.8 years (range, 1 to 26 years). Right: Cumulative actuarial curves of 54 patients presenting with moderate aortic stenosis. Conventions as in left-hand figure. Mean age at presentation 11.8 years (range, 1 to 25 years). Mean follow-up 8.5 years (range, 1 to 24 years). (From Hossack KF, Neutze JM, Lowe JB, Barratt-Boyes BG. Congenital valvar aortic stenosis: Natural history and assessment for operation. *Brit Heart J* 1980;43:561. Reproduced with permission from the publisher and authors.)

MANAGEMENT

The development of symptoms (e.g., angina, exertional dyspnea, and syncope) mandates prompt intervention in aortic valve stenosis. In asymptomatic younger individuals (<40 years), however, the documentation of severe aortic stenosis may in itself be considered an indication for intervention.[189,204] Mild aortic stenosis in asymptomatic patients with gradients below 50 mmHg warrants careful surveillance. The management of patients in the intermediate group (gradients 50 to 75 mmHg) is more controversial, but evidence argues in favor of elective intervention. Calculation of aortic valve area is important as left ventricular–aortic gradients may be misleading if there is reduced cardiac output.

Surgery in the young adult with congenital aortic stenosis must be considered as palliative.[138,205] In the absence of calcification, young patients (<21 years of age) may be candidates for aortic valvotomy. Perioperative mortality in adolescents and adults is extremely low, and late survival is excellent. A large proportion (35 to 45 percent), however, will require reoperation, including aortic valve replacement, over a follow-up period of 20 to 25 years.[137,138] Catheter balloon valvotomy has been utilized in adolescents and young adults with mobile noncalcified valves, but the results are also palliative.[206,207]

Valve replacement is the only option for valves unsuitable for valvotomy, including those with significant calcification and regurgitation. The pulmonary autograft ("Ross") operation represents an attractive surgical alternative to prosthetic or homograft aortic valve replacement. The choice of operation is discussed elsewhere (see Chap. 66), but the age and size of the patient are major considerations, as well as individual characteristics that determine the safety of anticoagulation, such as the desire for future pregnancies.

Subaortic stenosis is usually amenable to more definitive surgical repair. This fact, in conjunction with the potential for progressive aortic regurgitation, justifies a more aggressive approach even in asymptomatic patients with lesser gradients.[208,209] Excision of the obstructive membrane together with a myectomy or myotomy is usually required. Subaortic stenosis occasionally recurs, and persistent or progressive aortic regurgitation may develop. Operative mortality is low, but the risks are greater in patients with "tunnel" forms of obstruction and in patients with obstruction at several levels. This usually requires a more aggressive surgical intervention with exten-

sive myectomy, Konno procedure's, or modification thereof.[210]

Hospital mortality for repair of supravalvular aortic stenosis is low, and late morbidity and mortality rates are also excellent. Nevertheless, residual abnormality such as aortic regurgitation or stenosis may persist after aortoplasty.

Medical follow-up of patients who have undergone surgical or balloon valvotomy should focus on the development of restenosis, the severity and progression of aortic regurgitation, and the constant hazard of infective endocarditis. Echocardiography has facilitated serial evaluation of gradients, valve areas, ventricular dimensions, function, and mass. The acceptable level of physical activity in patients with left ventricular outflow tract obstruction remains controversial. It is debatable whether any patient who has had significant obstruction should be allowed to participate in competitive sports. A residual mean gradient greater than 20 mmHg or persistent left ventricular hypertrophy is considered to be a contraindication to vigorous physical activity. Before one approves strenuous activity in others, evaluation should include ECG monitoring and maximal exercise testing (see Chap. 16).

Coarctation of the Aorta

Although coarctation of the aorta is a congenital malformation, nearly 20 percent of the cases presenting at the Mayo Clinic over a 20-year period were diagnosed initially in adolescence or adulthood. Most commonly, coarctation diagnosed at ages beyond childhood was discovered in asymptomatic patients in whom a routine physical examination for athletic participation or employment disclosed upper limb hypertension with diminished or absent femoral pulses. Coarctation of the aorta may occur anywhere along the descending aorta, even below the diaphragm, but in more than 95 percent of cases it is located below the origin of the left subclavian artery and may involve the origin of this vessel. Usually, there is a discrete infolding of the aortic wall causing eccentric narrowing of the lumen. Frequently there is secondary aortic dilatation proximal and distal to the coarcted area (Fig. 74-8).

NATURAL HISTORY

Isolated, severe aortic coarctation may cause congestive heart failure as early as the neonatal period. More frequently, however, coarctation producing symptoms during early infancy is associated with other congenital cardiovascular abnormalities such as ventricular septal defect, left ventricular outflow tract obstruction, or mitral valve abnormality. Many patients with undetected coarctation will remain symptom-free until adolescence or early adulthood, when symptoms such as headaches related to hypertension, leg fatigue, or leg cramps may develop. Occasionally, a major catastrophic event such as a cerebrovascular accident, infective endocarditis, or even rupture of the aorta is the first recognized symptom. A bicuspid aortic valve is found in approximately 25 to 50 percent of patients with coarctation, and these abnormal valves have a tendency to calcify in early or middle adult life, producing aortic stenosis. Aortic stenosis

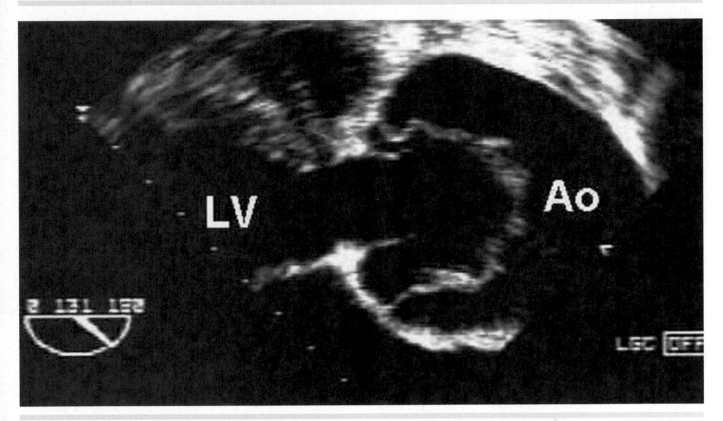

FIGURE 74-8 Aortic angiogram of a 40-year-old man with mild coarctation of the aorta (peak gradient 18 mmHg). Note the entire aorta, including the arch vessels, is dilated consistent with a diffuse arteriopathic process. Just distal to the coarctation, the aorta measures 40 mm.

may be the presenting condition, and subsequent investigation may disclose an additional coarctation of the aorta. In the era before surgical intervention, approximately 50 percent of patients with coarctation died within the first three decades, and 75 percent were dead by age 50.[211] Death was most frequently caused by a complication of hypertension, such as stroke or aortic dissection, but other causes included endocarditis, endarteritis, and congestive heart failure.

MANAGEMENT

Infrequently, a mild degree of coarctation may be present which would not justify intervention. In the great majority of cases, however, symptoms or the presence of significant upper-body hypertension mandates surgical repair. On occasion, an asymptomatic adolescent or adult patient with a severe coarctation will be normotensive at rest because of well-developed collaterals around the coarctation site. Such patients have inappropriate hypertension with exercise, however, and should be repaired. There is evidence that residual hypertension and late complications are directly related to age at the time of repair.[212]

Surgery for coarctation has been available since 1945.[213] Various techniques have been used, including end-to-end anastomosis, patch grafting, and the use of the subclavian flap technique.[214] Aneurysmal or atherosclerotic changes in the aorta found in adolescents or adults may occasionally mandate the use of an interposition prosthetic graft. Surgery is performed without cardiopulmonary bypass, and the risk of death from operation is small, although it is higher in adults than it is in children. Serious morbidity is rare, but occasionally paraplegia secondary to spinal cord ischemia and bowel ischemia or infarction occur.[215] For patients who require concomitant surgical procedures such as aortic valve replacement, an ascending-to-descending aortic bypass may be utilized through a median sternotomy.[216,217] Some patients require antihypertensive medication because of transient postoperative hypertension for a short period, whereas in others hypertension may persist, requiring long-term treatment.

Balloon angioplasty was originally used for recurrent coarctation after surgical repair, but is being increasingly utilized for native coarctation. Immediate reduction of the degree of obstruction and gradient is usually possible but is achieved at the price of tearing both the aortic intima and media. Dissection and rupture are more of a risk than with recoarctation, where scarring and adhesions from previous surgery may better support the aortic wall.[218] Late aneurysm formation, presumably secondary to the disruption of the media, has been observed.[219] Balloon-expandable stents have also been utilized with the rationale that overdilatation of the coarctation segment is unnecessary, thus avoiding major transmural tears. In addition, elastic recoil of the segment is reduced thereby relieving obstruction better than with balloon dilatation alone.[220] Intermediate term results are good, although long-term follow-up is not available.[221]

LATE RESULTS

The Mayo Clinic has published late results in 646 patients with coarctation operated upon between 1946 and 1981.[212] The median age at operation was 16 years (range, 1 week to 72 years) with 72 patients (11 percent) over age 35. Although survival was good (91 percent at 10 years, 72 percent at 30 years), the mean age of death was 38 years, confirming the previous finding that life expectancy is reduced, even after repair. In this and other series reporting long-term follow-up, the most common cause of death was premature coronary artery disease with secondary myocardial infarction.[222] Other causes included congestive heart failure, stroke, and ruptured aortic aneurysm. Age at operation was a powerful prognostic factor. The older the patient at the time of repair, the greater the probability of premature death, making it highly likely that the duration of preoperative obstruction and hypertension is important in the etiology of arterial disease and subsequent cardiovascular events.

The incidence of recoarctation with all surgical techniques is low for repairs performed after infancy, but surgery in later years for associated abnormalities such as aortic and mitral valve disease may be required, and are more common indications for reoperation than recoarctation.[223] The majority of survivors are asymptomatic, but there is a high incidence of late hypertension, despite satisfactory early fall in blood pressure after surgery and good relief of obstruction. In one series, only 32 percent of patients were normotensive 30 years after repair and 25 percent were significantly hypertensive.[222] Long-term blood pressure surveillance including blood pressures with exercise is therefore mandatory as hypertension is directly related to many of the late vascular complications.[212,222] This incidence may decline significantly as more patients are diagnosed and repaired during infancy or early childhood. Long-term regular follow-up should also include surveillance of the repaired aorta (MRI is very suitable), assessment of the aortic valve, and endocarditis prophylaxis.

Transposition of the Great Arteries

In complete transposition of the great arteries, the aorta arises from the right ventricle and the pulmonary artery from the left ventricle (discordant ventriculoarterial connection). As a result, the systemic and arterial circulations run "in parallel" rather than "in series" and predominantly desaturated blood enters the aorta. Oxygenation and survival depend on mixing between the systemic and pulmonary circulations at the atrial level in simple transposition (via a patent foramen ovale or atrial septal defect. In approximately half the cases, there are associated anomalies: ventricular septal defect (30 percent), left ventricular outflow tract obstruction (5 to 10 percent), ventricular septal defect with left ventricular outflow tract obstruction (10 percent), patent ductus arteriosus, and, more rarely, coarctation of the aorta or AV valve anomalies.[224] These associated conditions affect both the natural history and surgical management.

NATURAL HISTORY

Transposition of the great arteries is relatively common, but the natural history is so poor that very few patients survive past childhood without intervention. Death is usually due to profound hypoxia and its hematologic consequences. In transposition of the great arteries with large ventricular septal defect, severe hypoxia is rare, but patients do badly as a result of heart failure from excessive pulmonary flow and early pulmonary vascular disease.[118] Transposition, with ventricular septal defect and left ventricular outflow tract obstruction, presents with early hypoxia. Occasionally, prolonged survival into adult life may occur with a large atrial septal defect, ventricular septal defect, and/or patent ductus arteriosus with the development of pulmonary vascular disease (Eisenmenger's syndrome) or with associated ventricular septal defect and left ventricular outflow tract obstruction.

MANAGEMENT

The outlook has been transformed by the use of catheter balloon atrial septostomy.[225] In the late 1950s and early 1960s, the Senning[226] and Mustard[227] operations involving atrial redirection of the systemic and pulmonary venous returns were introduced. These operations are usually performed between 3 and 12 months of age,

with a trend over the years to earlier surgery. Both procedures have been undertaken with excellent early mortality (approximately 2 percent operative mortality). Long-term follow-up for both procedures is now available, with comparable late results apart from a lower incidence of baffle obstruction after Senning's operation.[228] Follow-up now extends to 30 years in some patients.[229] One study reported an actuarial survival of 90 percent at 10 years, 80 percent at 20 years, and 80 percent at 28 years after the Mustard repair.[39,230] Seventy-six percent of the survivors were in NYHA Class I. Late problems, however, are now recognized, with sudden death, arrhythmia, tricuspid regurgitation, and right (systemic) ventricular dysfunction the major concerns.[230] These late complications have led to the increasing acceptance of the arterial switch operation as the operation of choice.[231] This procedure involves transection and reanastomosis of the great arteries (aorta to left ventricle, pulmonary artery to right ventricle) with coronary artery transfer. The mortality for this procedure has decreased, but the long-term results into adult life are not yet available. For transposition with ventricular septal defect, the mortality for atrial repair with ventricular septal defect closure has always been higher than it has been for simple transposition, and arterial switch is the operation of choice. Transposition with ventricular septal defect and left ventricular outflow tract obstruction is usually palliated in infancy with a systemic-to-pulmonary shunt followed by repair by Rastelli's procedure in later childhood.[232] This involves closure of the ventricular septal defect to connect the left ventricle to the aorta and insertion of a valved conduit from the right ventricle to the pulmonary artery. Long-term results are good, but further surgery to replace the extracardiac conduit in adolescent and adult life is inevitable (see "Surgical Considerations" earlier).

LATE RESULTS

There are two specific problems after atrial redirection have caused concern during long-term follow-up: arrhythmia and systemic ventricular dysfunction. Loss of sinus rhythm is progressive and has not been prevented by modification of surgical technique for either Mustard's or Senning's operation.[233,234] In most cases, it is asymptomatic, but occasionally profound bradycardia may necessitate pacemaker insertion. There appears, however, to be no relation between loss of sinus rhythm and risk of sudden death. More worrisome is the development of atrial tachyarrhythmias, including atrial flutter. This arrhythmia has profound hemodynamic consequences after intraatrial repair and is a risk factor for sudden death, especially in the presence of right ventricular dysfunction. Deteriorating performance of the right ventricle supporting the systemic circulation is seen in many patients, but the precise basis for this problem remains unclear and the time frame extremely variable.[9]

Risk stratification for sudden death remains a clinical challenge. Assessment should include evaluation of cardiac performance at rest and exercise and evaluation of systemic and venous pathways. Transesophageal echocardiography is particularly useful in this situation. Heart transplantation should be considered in the patient who has severe right ventricular failure or disabling arrhythmias. An alternative approach is to perform pulmonary artery banding as preparation for conversion of the atrial repair to an arterial switch. Published results have indicated a significant surgical mortality for this approach. As a result, case selection and timing, as well as optimal surgical strategy, remain unclear.[235] The rather limited information after arterial switch operation suggests that electrophysiologic problems are much less prevalent[236] with better preservation of sinus node function and lower prevalence of clinically relevant tachyarrhythmias.[237] The systemic left ventricle after the switch is at risk from the surgical procedure itself, potential myocardial ischemia from coronary distortion, as well as aortic regurgitation. Early results, however, are encouraging, but few patients have yet reached adult life. Because of the high incidence of observed and potential medical problems, all patients who have had both atrial or arterial repair of transposition of the great arteries should have lifelong follow-up by a cardiologist at a center specializing in adult congenital heart disease.

Congenitally Corrected Transposition (Atrioventricular and Ventriculoarterial Discordance)

In congenitally corrected transposition of the great arteries, there is a discordant AV connection (right atrium to left ventricle and left ventricle to right atrium) and a discordant ventriculoarterial connection (left ventricle to pulmonary artery and right ventricle to aorta). As a result of this "double discordance," the systemic and pulmonary venous returns flow to the appropriate great arteries, hence the potentially confusing term *corrected transposition*.[238]

NATURAL HISTORY
In a small proportion of cases (approximately 10 percent in reported series, but this is probably an underestimate) there are no associated cardiac defects.[239] Such individuals are pink and asymptomatic, and survival to the ninth decade has been reported.[68] The only specific difference from normal hearts is the tendency to develop AV conduction problems and complete heart block. Complete heart block may be present from birth ($\approx$10 percent) and is said to develop in about 2 percent of patients per year.[240] The majority of cases have a ventricular septal defect (90 percent) and/or pulmonary stenosis (80 percent).[241] The combination of these lesions may cause cyanosis. Abnormalities of the tricuspid valve (systemic AV valve) are common and may be due to an intrinsic tricuspid valve abnormality such as Ebstein's malformation. These defects influence the natural history and surgical strategy required. In adult patients the diagnosis of congenitally corrected transposition is often overlooked. Late referral with severe systemic AV valve regurgitation and advanced systemic ventricular dysfunction is common.[242] Aortic regurgitation of some degree is present in more than 25 percent of adults but seldom requires surgical attention.[243]

MANAGEMENT
Strategies and indications for surgery differ from those in patients with normal connections because of the potential for the operation to aggravate systemic ventricular dysfunction, systemic AV valve incompetence, or conduction problems. Palliative surgery in childhood is sometimes performed, as definitive repair may involve insertion of an extracardiac conduit. In a large retrospective study of 111 patients managed over a 20-year period, it was concluded that patients with symptomatic heart failure should be repaired before the systemic ventricle dilates and the tricuspid regurgitation becomes severe.[239] Patients with more than mild tricuspid regurgitation whose valves were not replaced did poorly. In contrast, the patients with cyanosis did much better, and the timing of intracardiac surgery can be delayed and determined by the patient's symptoms. In one series of surgical repair of 127 patients, 56 percent required reoperation within 20 years for AV valve regurgitation, pulmonary stenosis, or both.[244] Systemic AV valve regurgitation is common in adults with congenitally corrected transposition[245] and tends to be progressive.[246] It may be related to an Ebstein-like malformation of the left AV valve, but these valves, in contrast to Ebstein's anomaly of the right AV valve, cannot be repaired adequately and always need to be replaced. Systemic AV valve replacement should always be performed before there is compromise of systemic (morphologic right)

ventricular function. In one series of 40 patients, systemic AV valve replacement was accomplished without surgically induced complete heart block, an early mortality of 10 percent ($n = 4$), and 8 late deaths.[247] The principal cause of death in all 12 patients was systemic ventricular failure. Survival correlated with preoperative systemic ventricular ejection fraction of $\geq$44 percent. It thus seems appropriate to refer these patients for valve replacement at the earliest signs of ventricular dysfunction.

Alternative surgical strategies involving a "double switch" have been adopted by some units. These involve an atrial repair by Mustard's or Senning's operation, together with connection of the left ventricle to the aorta (via a patch through the ventricular septal defect) or an arterial switch.[248,249] The advantage of these approaches is that the morphologic left ventricle (with mitral valve) supports the systemic circulation. While this is an attractive option, it should be stressed that few patients who have received double-switch procedures have reached adolescence, and long-term follow-up data are not yet available for comparison with the conventional surgical approach.

LATE RESULTS
The long-term outcome for well-repaired patients is good, whereas those with symptomatic heart failure preoperatively do badly. Atrial arrhythmias are common in long-term follow-up and in one series occurred in 36 percent of survivors.[250] Since repairs may involve insertion of an extracardiac conduit, prosthetic AV valve, and pacemaker, careful long-term follow-up is mandatory.

Complex Lesions

A number of complex congenital heart defects involve structural abnormalities that preclude the creation of a biventricular circulation. The changing nomenclature and classification that has been applied to these defects over the years is a major source of confusion (see Chap. 73). This group of patients includes those with double-inlet ventricle (single ventricle), absent right or left AV connection (tricuspid or mitral atresia), some cases of pulmonary atresia or intact ventricular septum, and cases with straddling of an AV valve and hypoplastic left or right ventricles. The natural history of these defects is highly variable and depends to a large extent on the impact of the associated defects. In a report of 191 patients with double-inlet ventricle presenting in the first year of life, actuarial survival before definitive repair for the whole group was 57 percent at 1 year and 42 percent at 10 years.[144] On multivariate analysis, pulmonary stenosis, balanced pulmonary flow, and older age at presentation were factors favoring survival, whereas right atrial isomerism, common AV orifice, pulmonary atresia, obstruction to systemic output, and anomalous pulmonary venous return were detrimental. Despite the complex morphologic defects, prolonged natural survival is possible, particularly if the physiology is well balanced.[251] The patients with double-inlet left ventricle with discordant ventriculoarterial connection and pulmonary stenosis with balanced pulmonary flow do best, with predicted actuarial survivals of 96 percent at 1 year and 91 percent at 10 years.

MANAGEMENT
For most patients with complex congenital heart disease prolonged survival into adult life is possible only with one or more palliative operations (such as systemic to pulmonary shunt, Glenn shunt, pulmonary artery banding, and relief of systemic outflow obstruction) or after a Fontan-type procedure. With palliative surgery alone, clinical deterioration usually begins in the second decade of life and

TABLE 74-5 Indications for Hospitalizations after Fontan Procedure for 215 Surviving Patients Who Returned a Questionnaire

Indication	Patients Hospitalized (No.)[a]
Cardiac operation	62
Other	57
Arrhythmia	52
Pacemaker insertion or replacement	22
Heart failure	14
Abdominal swelling	10
Leg edema	9
Endocarditis	7
Protein-losing enteropathy	6
Hypoproteinemia	4
Stroke	4
Liver problems	1
Brain abscess	1

[a]A patient may have provided multiple indications for one hospitalization.
SOURCE: Driscoll DJ, Offord KP, Feldt RH, et al. Five- to fifteen-year follow-up after Fontan operation. *Circulation* 1992;85:469–496. Reproduced with permission from the publisher and authors.

is often due to progressive ventricular dysfunction and/or AV valve regurgitation.[252,253]

The goals of management during childhood have been to maintain suitable anatomy and physiology for the Fontan circulation. A number of modifications of Fontan's original operation have been introduced[254–256] (see Fig. 74-8). The basic principle is to separate the systemic and pulmonary circuits by returning systemic venous blood to the pulmonary artery without incorporating a subpulmonary ventricle. This circulation is less "flexible" than one with two function-

ing ventricles; the operative risk and postoperative status are largely dependent on the patient's suitability. Most important are a low pulmonary vascular resistance and adequate ventricular function (both systolic and diastolic), allowing the circulation to operate with an acceptably low systemic venous pressure. Careful preoperative hemodynamic assessment is vital to optimize patient selection. The operative risk varies considerably between institutions.

LONG-TERM RESULTS

The early and medium-term results of the successful Fontan's operation are excellent when compared to the preoperative status of the patients. Improvement in arterial saturation and exercise tolerance has been confirmed by objective testing.[256] With longer follow-up, however, increasing problems develop[10,257](Table 74-5). Fontan's own analysis of 334 patients revealed a premature decline in survival and functional status and a late rise in hazard for which no risk factors could be identified other than the Fontan state per se.[10] Arrhythmia is a particularly common problem and occurs in approximately 20 percent at 10-year follow-up[257] (Table 74-6). Other problems include thrombus in the atria and declining ventricular function.[10,257] Anticoagulation policy differs widely even between specialist centers. The increasing concerns regarding stasis of blood in the right atrium and thrombus formation has led to wider routine use of long-term anticoagulants, but this is not standard practice. Patients with a history of documented atrial arrhythmias, a fenestration in the Fontan connection, and "smoke" in the right atrium on echocardiography have the strongest indications for anticoagulation. Protein-losing enteropathy (PLE) is another important complication and probably results from elevated systemic venous pressure, which subsequently causes lymphangiectasia. PLE is associated with fluid accumulation, such as pleural effusion, ascites, and peripheral edema. The diagnosis can be confirmed by quantifying gastrointestinal protein loss utilizing alpha$_1$ antitrypsin clearance. The cumulative risk for the development of PLE in 10 years in one reported large series was approximately 13 percent[258]; once this complication had developed, the 5-year survival was approximately 50 percent. Therapy includes sodium restriction, dietary modification, and anticongestive measures such as diuretics and afterload-reducing agents. Many patients require periodic albumin infusion, but medical management of PLE is usually only partially successful. Obstruction in the Fontan circuit should always be ruled out as a potential cause, since reoperation may result in resolution of the PLE. Chronic subcutaneous heparin therapy may also resolve the PLE,[259,260] as may percutaneous atrial fenestration.[261,262] Occasional reports suggest improvement with steroid therapy.[263] Cardiac transplantation appears to pose a high risk and does not always resolve the protein loss.[259] Other concerns are the effects of nonpulsatile pulmonary flow favoring the development of pulmonary arteriovenous malformations as seen after the Glenn anastomosis.[264] Extrapolation of these data to current practice is difficult, but Fontan's procedure should be considered to be palliative, not curative.

TABLE 74-6 Arrhythmias in 215 survivors of the Fontan Operation

Results from Follow-up Questionnaire	5 YEARS POSTOP PATIENTS		CURRENT PATIENTS	
	No.	%	No.	%
Syncope	18	8	17	8
Rapid heart rate (tachycardia)	44	20	45	21
Slow heart rate (bradycardia)	17	8	15	7
Palpitations	51	24	60	28
Atrial flutter or fibrillation	26	12	41	19
Premature ventricular contractions	13	6	15	7
Ventricular tachycardia	9	4	13	6
Pacemaker	[b]	[b]	22	10
Number of antiarrhythmic medications[a]				
0	179	83	167	78
1	31	13	40	19
2	5	2	8	4

[a]Excluding digitalis.
[b]"Presence of a pacemaker" asked only for patient's current status.
SOURCE: From Driscoll DJ, Offord KP, Feldt RH, et al. Five-to-fifteen-year follow-up after Fontan operation. *Circulation* 1992;85:469–496. Reproduced with permission from the publisher and authors.

Despite these complications, more and more modifications of Fontan's operation are performed, and more long-term data are necessary to see whether important complications can be reduced in this way. Much interest has involved conversion of the Fontan to a more "hydrodynamically efficient" circuit to improve atrial arrhythmias and PLE.[265] A high mortality rate, however, is associated with PLE surgery, and in one series only 50 percent of the survivors were cured.[259] Atrial arrhythmias may also persist after the Fontan conversion,[266,267] even though hydrodynamics are improved. Perhaps concomitant arrhythmia circuit cryoablation may improve the results.[268]

Some surgical modifications which have been introduced may improve early and late hemodynamics and the functional results. Perforation of the patch at surgery (fenestrated Fontan) allows a hypertensive right atrium to decompress via a right-to-left shunt at the atrial level.[269] These holes may be closed later with an occlusion device at catheterization. Other "Fontan" operations have excluded the right atrium from the circulation, creating a total cavopulmonary connection (superior vena cava to right pulmonary artery via a bidirectional Glenn anastomosis and inferior vena cava blood channeled to the pulmonary artery.[270] Data suggest improved flow and energy characteristics compared to the standard atriopulmonary connection[271] and fewer early supraventricular arrhythmias.[272] Other modifications have created an extracardiac Fontan connection using a tube graft in the hope of preventing atrial distension and atrial arrhythmias.[273,274]

All patients who have complex congenital heart defects palliated by systemic to pulmonary shunt, cavopulmonary anastomosis (bidirectional Glenn), or Fontan's procedure should have lifelong regular cardiac follow-up at a specialist center. Particular attention should be paid to ventricular function, detection of thrombus in the right atrium,[275] residual shunts, systemic AV valve regurgitation, AV malformations in the lung, obstruction at the Fontan anastomosis (especially in early operations involving a right atrium to pulmonary artery conduit), and PLE (see earlier).

Ebstein's Anomaly of the Tricuspid Valve

Ebstein's anomaly is characterized by displacement of the proximal attachments of the tricuspid valve from the AV ring into the right ventricle (see Chap. 73). This structural abnormality divides the right ventricle into an "atrialized" portion and distal "ventricularized" portion. The severity is variable and accounts for the broad clinical spectrum, from severe disease causing fetal or neonatal death to mild disease compatible with natural survival as late as the eighth decade of life. Ebstein's anomaly is an uncommon defect occurring in less than 1 percent of patients with congenital heart disease, but it is disproportionately represented in the adult congenital heart disease population because of its favorable natural history.

The diagnosis of Ebstein's anomaly is now much easier with echocardiography, which has altered our understanding of the natural history. In a large collaborative study of Ebstein's anomaly reported in 1974, only 7 percent of patients were under 1 year of age.[276] Neonates presenting with Ebstein's anomaly represent, not surprisingly, the worst end of the spectrum, with a severe anatomic defect and a high incidence of associated abnormalities, particularly right ventricular outflow tract obstruction. Their poor outcome is predictable from their anatomy.[277] Those who survive this period with or without surgery may live into adult life, although there is continued morbidity and mortality throughout childhood. Many patients are minimally symptomatic in childhood and do not present until adolescence or adult life. Symptoms and signs, when they develop, include cyanosis due to right-to-left shunting at the atrial level,

dyspnea and fatigue secondary to hypoxia and low cardiac output, and palpitation due to supraventricular arrhythmia. Ebstein's anomaly is often associated with ventricular preexcitation, which may involve one or more, usually right-sided, accessory pathways. Approximately 25 to 30 percent of adults will have symptomatic arrhythmias that may be difficult to treat and can result in sudden death.[278] Progressive heart failure may develop with time and may be related not only to right-sided problems but also to left-sided abnormalities. Excessive fibrosis has been reported in the left ventricle, and left ventricular dysfunction may be induced on exercise.[277,279] Early cyanosis is an adverse risk factor for survival, as is congestive cardiac failure

MANAGEMENT

Surgery may consist of repair or replacement of the tricuspid valve together with closure of the atrial septal defect to prevent cyanosis[280] (Fig. 74-9). In 189 patients aged 11 months to 64 years (mean 19.1 years), a tricuspid valve reconstruction was possible in 58.2 percent, and in 36.5 percent a prosthetic valve, usually a bioprosthesis, was inserted. In the occasional patient, the atrial septal defect may be responsible for a left-to-right shunt and can be closed as the sole procedure. In others, the functioning right ventricle is too small for a biventricular circulation, and Fontan's procedure may be the only option. Cross-sectional echocardiography is very useful in determining whether the tricuspid valve is amenable to repair, delineating the mobility or tethering of the elongated anterior leaflet and the presence or absence of fenestration. The results of surgery are affected by the presence of arrhythmia. Uncontrolled preoperative supraventricular arrhythmia is a risk factor for early postoperative rhythm problems that may have serious hemodynamic consequences. It is usually recommended that division of an accessory pathway be performed at

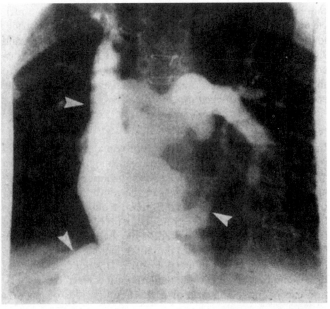

A

FIGURE 74-9 Angiograms showing (A) Fontan conduit from right atrium to pulmonary artery. There is dilatation of the right atrium with filling of the inferior vena cava, superior vena cava, and coronary sinus. (B) Total cavopulmonary connection. The superior vena cava is connected to the right pulmonary artery ("bidirectional Glenn"), and the inferior vena cava is baffled to the pulmonary artery. (Courtesy of Dr ID Sullivan, Great Ormond Street Hospital for Children, London.)

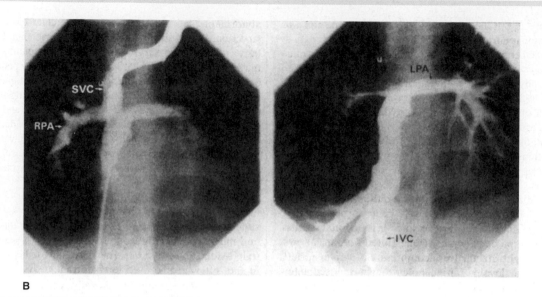

B

FIGURE 74-9 (*Continued*)

the time of tricuspid valve surgery. The pathways are usually in the posteroseptal or right free wall position and may be multiple. An alternative approach is to perform catheter radiofrequency ablation of the accessory pathway before surgery. In hearts with marked enlargement of the right atrium, catheter ablation is challenging and, in the setting of an atrial communication, poses the additional risk of a paradoxical embolus and stroke. If there are no accessory pathways, a right-sided maze procedure at the time of tricuspid valve surgery may successfully control supraventricular arrhythmia.[156]

LATE RESULTS

The long-term outlook for well-repaired patients is good; reduction in heart size is usual (Fig. 74-10), and atrial arrhythmias are reduced.

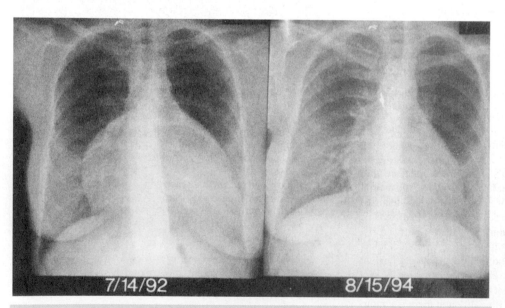

FIGURE 74-10 The chest radiograph on the left shows severe cardiac enlargement associated with Ebstein's anomaly in a 32-year-old woman. She had had a right Blalock-Taussig shunt at age 12. Following tricuspid valve repair and closure of a secundum atrial septal defect, there has been dramatic reduction in the size of the heart, shown on the right.

Exercise capacity improves postoperatively, particularly in those who are cyanotic before surgery.[281] Of 149 patients receiving a porcine bioprosthesis in the Mayo Clinic series, the 10-year survival was 92.5 percent, and 92 percent of them were NYHA Class I or II. Bioprosthesis durability in the tricuspid position performs favorably, with freedom from bioprosthesis replacement being 80.6 percent at 10 and 15 years.[282]

Marfan's Syndrome

Although this autosomal dominant syndrome is congenital in the sense that the patient is born with an abnormal gene (genes), the heart defect is usually acquired. Mutations of fibrillin 1, the main constituent of extracellular microfibrils, are the cause of the pleiotropic manifestations of Marfan's syndrome.[283] The typical phenotypic features—tall, thin stature, pectus deformities, arachnodactyly—by which the condition is currently diagnosed, may be obvious, subtle, or absent (see Fig. 10-7).The clinical features have been codified into the so-called Ghent nosology,[284] as the clinical variability of the condition can make diagnosis difficult.[285] Cardiovascular complications occur in 30 to 60 percent of patients and are the cause of a decreased life expectancy.[286] Mitral valve prolapse is the most common finding in the pediatric population,[287] but aortic root dilation with a potential for aortic dissection or severe aortic valve regurgitation is the most serious later complication.[288] In a review of 257 patients seen between 1939 and 1972, the median age of death was reported to be about 45 years, with aortic root problems accounting for three-fourths of the deaths (see also Chap. 84).[286] By 1995 a multicenter study reported that the median survival had improved to 72 years.[289]

MANAGEMENT

The risk of dissection is broadly related to the degree of dilation of the aortic root. Dilation can be followed serially by regular cross-sectional echocardiography, which should be performed at least annually. Particularly close monitoring is necessary during puberty and the rapid-growth phase of adolescence. Emphasis has been placed on the use of nomograms to relate the aortic measurements to the patients' age and body surface area. Treatment with beta blockade has been advocated for patients with evidence of aortic root enlargement. Elective aortic root replacement has a low operative mortality, but in contrast, emergency repair, usually for acute aortic dissection, carries a much higher early mortality. In a multicenter study of 675 patients having aortic root replacement, the 30-day mortality rate was 1.5 percent for those having elective repair, 2.6 percent for urgent repair (within 7 days of a surgical consult), and 11.7 percent for patients having emergency repair (within 24 h of a surgical consult).[290] Of the 158 patients, 46 percent with aortic dissection had an aneurysm with a diameter of 6.5 cm or less. Elective aortic root surgery therefore is generally recommended when the aorta exceeds 5.5 cm in diameter.[291] Consideration should be given to earlier surgery if there is a family history of aortic disssection or a rapid change in the size of the aortic root is observed.[292] The aortic valve itself may also need to be replaced, although preliminary results from valve-sparing procedures, which eliminate the need for long-term anticoagulants necessary for conventional mechanical valve replacements, suggest cautious optimism.[290,293] Importantly, more than 10 percent of patients in the multicenter study had problems with the residual aorta, emphasizing the need for continued vigilance of the aorta with MRI or CT imaging and meticulous control of blood pressure. As regular long-term follow-up visits are required, patients with the Marfan's syndrome are not uncommon in adult "congenital" heart clinics. In addition to their cardiac care, patients need expert help with skeletal and ocular problems, genetic counseling, advice on physical activity (see earlier), and general psychosocial support.

References

1. Hoffman JI Kaplan S. The incidence of congenital heart disease. *J Am Coll Cardiol* 2002;39(12):1890–1900.
2. MacMahon B, McKeown T, Record R. The incidence and life expectation of children with congenital heart disease. *Brit Heart J* 1953; 15:121–129.
3. Warnes CA, Liberthson R, Danielson GK, et al. Task force 1: The changing profile of congenital heart disease in adult life. *J Am Coll Cardiol* 2001;37(5):1170–1175.
4. Stark J. Do we really correct congenital heart defects? *J Thorac Cardiovasc Surg*, 1989;97:109.
5. Moons P, De Volder E, Budts W, et al. What do adult patients with congenital heart disease know about their disease, treatment, and prevention of complications? A call for structured patient education. *Heart* 2001;86(1):74–80.
6. Warnes C. Establishing an adult congenital heart disease clinic. *Am J Cardiovasc Imaging* 1995;9(1):11–14.
7. 1996 Consensus Conference on Adult Congenital Heart Disease. *Can Cardiovascul Soc* Montreal.
8. Child JS, Collins-Nakai RL, Alpert JS, et al. Task force 3: Workforce description and educational requirements for the care of adults with congenital heart disease. *J Am Coll Cardiol* 2001;37(5):1183–1187.
9. Graham T, Arwood G, Boucek R, et al. Abnormalities of right ventricular function following Mustard's operation for transposition of the great arteries. *Circulation* 1975;52:678–684.
10. Fontan F, Kirklin J, Fernandez G, et al. Outcome after a "perfect" Fontan operation. *Circulation* 1990;81:152–1536.
11. Redington A. Functional assessment of the heart after corrective surgery for complete transposition. *Cardiol Young* 1991;1:84–90.
12. Gewillig M, Lundstrom U, Deanfield J, et al. Impact of the Fontan operation on left ventricular size and contractility. *Circulation* 1990;81: 118–127.
13. CIBIS I.aC. A randomized trial of beta-blockade in heart failure: The Cardiac Insufficiency Bisprolol Study (CIBIS). *Circulation* 1994;90: 1765–1773.
14. Pfeffer M, Braunwald E, Moye L, et al. Effect of captopril on mortality and morbidity in patients with left ventricular dysfunction after myocardial infarction: Results of the survival and ventricular enlargement trial. *N Engl J Med* 1992;327:669–677.
15. Packer M, O'Connor C, Ghali J, et al. Effect of amlodipine on morbidity and mortality in severe chronic heart failure. *N Engl J Med* 1996;335:1107–1114.
16. Packer M, Coats AJ, Fowler MB. Effect of carvedilol on survival in severe chronic congestive heart failure. *N Engl J Med* 2001;344: 1651–1658.
17. Territo M, Rosove M, Perloff J. Cyanotic congenital heart disease: Haematologic management, renal function, and urate metabolism. In: Perloff J, Child J, eds. *Congenital Heart Disease in Adults.* Saunders: Philadelphia, 1991:94–95.
18. Perloff J, Rosove M, Child J, et al. Adults with cyanotic congenital heart disease: Haematological management. *Ann Intern Med* 1988; 109:406–413.
19. Rosove M, Hocking W, Canobbio M, et al. Chronic hypoxaemia and decompensated erythrocytosis in cyanotic congenital heart disease. *Lancet* 1986;313–315.
20. Ammash N, Warnes CA. Cerebrovascular events in adult patients with cyanotic congenital heart disease. *J Am Coll Cardiol* 1996; 28(3):768–772.
21. Perloff JK, Latta H, Barsotti P. Pathogenesis of the glomerular abnormality in cyanotic congenital heart disease. *Am J Cardiol* 2000; 86(11):1198–1204.
22. Ross E, Perloff J, Danovitch G, et al. Renal function and urate metabolism in late survivors with cyanotic congenital heart disease. *Circulation* 1986;73:396–400.
23. Dittrich S, Haas NA, Buhrer C, et al. Renal impairment in patients with long-standing cyanotic congenital heart disease. *Acta Paediatr* 1998;87(9):949–954.
24. Harinck E, Hutter P, Hoorntje T, et al. Air travel and adults with cyanotic heart disease. *Circulation* 1996;93:272–276.
25. Jordan C, White R Jr, Fischer K, et al. The scoliosis of congenital heart disease. *Am Heart J* 1972;84:463–469.
26. Niwa K, Perloff J, Kaplan S, et al. Eisenmenger syndrome in adults: Ventricular septal defect, truncus arteriosus, univentricular heart. *J Am Coll Cardiol* 1999;34:223–232.
27. Daliento L, Somerville J, Presbitero P, et al. Eisenmenger syndrome: Factors relating to deterioration and death. *Eur Heart J* 1998; 19(12):1845–1855.
28. Somerville J. How to manage the Eisenmenger syndrome. *Int J Cardiol* 1997;63:1–8.
29. Ammash NM, Connolly HM, Abel MD, et al. Noncardiac surgery in Eisenmenger syndrome. *J Am Coll Cardiol* 1999;33(1):222–227.
30. Rosenzweig EB, Kerstein D, Barst RJ. Long-term prostacyclin for pulmonary hypertension with associated congenital heart defects. *Circulation* 1999;99(14):1858–1865.
31. Working Party of the British Society for Antimicrobial Chemo. The antibiotic prophylaxis of infective endocarditis. *Lancet* 1982;2:1323–1326.
32. Dajani A, Talbert K, Wilson W, et al. Prevention of bacterial endocarditis. *JAMA* 1997;277:1794–1801.
33. Cetta F, Graham LC, Lichtenberg RC, et al. Piercing and tattooing in patients with congenital heart disease: Patient and physician perspectives. *J Adolesc Health* 1999;24(3):160–162.
34. Cetta F, Warnes CA. Adults with congenital heart disease: Patient knowledge of endocarditis prophylaxis. *Mayo Clin Proc* 1995;70(1):50–54.

35. Vetter V, Horowitz L. Electrophysiologic residua and sequelae of surgery for congenital heart defects. *Am J Cardiol* 1982;50:588–604.

36. Garson A Jr. Chronic postoperative arrhythmia. In: *Pediatric Arrhythmia: Electrophysiology and Pacing,* Gillette P, Garson A Jr, eds. Philadelphia: Saunders, 1990:667–678.

37. Dodo H, Gow R, Hamilton R, et al. Chaotic atrial rhythm in children. *Am Heart J* 1995;129:990–995.

38. Boelens M, Friedli B. Sinus node function and conduction system before and after surgery for secundum atrial septal defect: An electrophysiologic study. *Am J Cardiol* 1984;53:1415–1420.

39. Puley G, Siu S, Connelly M, et al. Arrhythmia and survival in patients >18 years of age after the Mustard procedure for complete transposition of the great arteries. *Am J Cardiol* 1999;83(7):1080–1084.

40. Gewillig M, Wyse R, de Leval M, et al. Early and late arrhythmia after the Fontan operation: Predisposing factors and clinical consequences. *Br Heart J* 1992;67:72–79.

41. Warfield DA, Hayes DL, Hyberger LK, et al. Permanent pacing in patients with univentricular heart. *Pacing Clin Electrophysiol* 1999; 22(8):1193–1201.

42. Stewart W, DiCola V, Hawthorne J. Doppler ultrasound measurement of cardiac output in patients with physiologic pacemakers: Effects of left ventricular function and retrograde ventriculoatrial conduction. *Am J Cardiol* 1984;54:308–312.

43. Silka MJ, Hardy BG, Menashe VD, et al. A population-based prospective evaluation of risk of sudden cardiac death after operation for common congenital heart defects. *J Am Coll Cardiol* 1998;32(1): 245–251.

44. Gewillig M, Cullen S, Mertens B, et al. Risk factors for arrhythmia and death after Mustard operation for simple transposition of the great arteries. *Circulation* 1991;84(suppl IV):187–192.

45. Gardiner H, Dhillon R, Bull C, et al. Prospective study of the incidence and determinants of arrhythmia after total cavopulmonary connection. *Circulation* 1996;94(suppl II):II-17–II-21.

46. Deanfield J, McKenna W, Hallidie-Smith K. Detection of late arrhythmia and conduction disturbance after correction of tetralogy of Fallot. *Brit Heart J* 1980;44:577–583.

47. Garson A, Nihill M, McNamara D, et al. Status of the adult and adolescent after repair of tetralogy of Fallot. *Circulation* 1979;59:1232–1240.

48. Vaksmann G, Fournier A, Davignon A, et al. Frequency and prognosis of arrhythmias after operative "correction" of tetralogy of Fallot. *Am J Cardiol* 1990;66:346–349.

49. Lucron H, Marcon F, Bosser G, et al. Induction of sustained ventricular tachycardia after surgical repair of tetralogy of Fallot. *Am J Cardiol* 1999;83:1369–1373.

50. Deanfield J, McKenna W, Rowland E. Local abnormalities of right ventricular depolarization after repair of tetralogy of Fallot: A basis for ventricular arrhythmia. *Am J Cardiol* 1985;55:522–526.

51. Deanfield J, McKenna W, Presbitero P, et al. Ventricular arrhythmia in unrepaired and repaired tetralogy of Fallot: Relation to age, timing of repair and haemodynamic status. *Brit Heart J* 1984;52:77–86.

52. Sullivan I, Presbitero P, Gooch V, et al. Is ventricular arrhythmia in repaired tetralogy of Fallot an effect of operation or a consequence of the course of the disease? *Brit Heart J* 1987;58:40–44.

53. Jones M, Ferrans V. Myocardial degeneration in congenital heart disease: Comparison of morphologic findings in young and old patients with congenital heart disease associated with muscular obstruction to right ventricular outflow. *Am J Cardiol* 1977;39:1051–1063.

54. Kobayashi J, Hirose H, Nakano S, et al. Ambulatory electrocardiographic study of the frequency and cause of ventricular arrhythmia after correction of tetralogy of Fallot. *Am J Cardiol* 1984;54:1310–1313.

55. Quattlebaum T, Varghese J, Neill C, et al. Sudden death among postoperative patients with tetralogy of Fallot: A follow-up study of 243 patients for an average of twelve years. *Circulation* 1976;54:289–293.

56. Dunnigan A, Pritzker M, Benditt D, et al. Life-threatening ventricular tachycardias in later survivors of surgically corrected tetralogy of Fallot. *Brit Heart J* 1984;52:198–206.

57. Alexander ME, Walsh EP, Saul JP, et al. Value of programmed ventricular stimulation in patients with congenital heart disease. *J Cardiovasc Electrophysiol* 1999;10(8):1033–1044.

58. Gatzoulis M, Clark A, Newman C, et al. Right ventricular diastolic function 15–35 years after repair of tetralogy of Fallot: Restrictive physiology predicts superior exercise performance. *Circulation* 1995; 91:1775–1781.

59. Gatzoulis M, Till J, Somerville J, et al. Mechanoelectrical interaction in tetralogy of Fallot: QRS prolongation relates to right ventricular size and predicts malignant ventricular arrhythmias and sudden death. *Circulation* 1995;92:231–237.

60. Gatzoulis MA, Balaji S, Webber SA, et al. Risk factors for arrhythmia and sudden cardiac death late after repair of tetralogy of Fallot: A multicentre study. *Lancet* 2000;356(9234):975–981.

61. Larson M, Warnes C. Repaired tetralogy of Fallot: ECG predictors of death and ventricular tachycardia (abst). *J Am Coll Cardiol* 1998; 31(no. 2 suppl A):355A.

62. Kugler JD. Predicting sudden death in patients who have undergone tetralogy of fallot repair: Is it really as simple as measuring ECG intervals? *J Cardiovasc Electrophysiol* 1998;9(1):103–106.

63. McLeod K, Hillis W, Houston A, et al. Reduced heart rate variability following repair of tetralogy of Fallot. *Heart* 1999;81:656–660.

64. Roos-Hesselink J, Perlroth J, McGhie J, et al. Atrial arrhythmias in adults after repair of tetralogy of Fallot: Correlations with clinical, exercise, and echocardiographic findings. *Circulation* 1995;91: 2214–2219.

65. Rodefeld M., Gandhi S, Huddleston C, et al. Anatomically based ablation of atrial flutter in an acute canine model of the modified Fontan operation. *J Thorac Cardiovasc Surg* 1996;112:898–907.

66. Kalman J, VanHare G, Olgin J, et al. Ablation of "incisional" reentrant atrial tachycardia complicating surgery for congenital heart disease: Use of entrainment to define a critical isthmus of conduction. *Circulation* 1996;93:502–512.

67. Canobbio MM, Mair DD, van der Velde M, et al. Pregnancy outcomes after the Fontan repair. *J Am Coll Cardiol* 1996;28(3):763–767.

68. Connolly HM, Grogan M. Warnes CA. Pregnancy among women with congenitally corrected transposition of the great arteries. *J Am Coll Cardiol* 1999;33(6):1692–1695.

69. Connolly HM, Warnes CA. Outcome of pregnancy in patients with complex pulmonic valve atresia. *Am J Cardiol* 1997;79(4):519–521.

70. Zuber M, Gautschi N, Oechslin E, et al. Outcome of pregnancy in women with congenital shunt lesions. *Heart* 1999;81(3):271–275.

71. Genoni M, Jenni R, Hoerstrup SP, et al. Pregnancy after atrial repair for transposition of the great arteries. *Heart* 1999;81(3):276–277.

72. Connolly, HM, Warnes CA. Ebstein's anomaly: Outcome of pregnancy. *J Am Coll Cardiol* 1994;23(5):1194–1198.

73. Warnes C, Cyanotic congenital heart disease in pregnancy. In: Oakley C, ed. *Heart Disease in Pregnancy*. London: BMJ Publishing Group, 1997:83–96.

74. Warnes C. Congenital heart disease and pregnancy. In: Elkayam U, Gleicher N, eds. *Cardiac Problems in Pregnancy*. New York: Wiley, 1998:39–53.

75. Neill C, Swanson S. Outcome of pregnancy in congenital heart disease. *Circulation* 1961;24:1003.

76. Presbitero P, Somerville J, Stone S, et al. Pregnancy in cyanotic congenital heart disease: Maternal complications and factors influencing successful fetal outcome. *J Am Coll Cardiol* 1992;19(suppl A):288A.

77. Gleicher N, Midwall J, Hochberger D, et al. Eisenmenger's syndrome and pregnancy. *Obst Gynecol* 1975;34:721–741.

78. Avila W, Grinberg M, Snitcowsky R, et al. Maternal and fetal outcome in pregnant women with Eisenmenger's syndrome. *Eur Heart J* 1995;16:460–464.

79. Pitts J, Crosby W, Basta L. Eisenmenger's syndrome in pregnancy: Does heparin prophylaxis improve the maternal mortality rate? *Am Heart J* 1977;93:321–326.

80. Rossiter R, Repke J, Morales A, et al. A prospective longitudinal evaluation of pregnancy in the Marfan syndrome. *Am J Obstet Gynecol* 1995;173:1599–1606.

81. Elkayam U, Ostrzega E, Shotan A, et al. Cardiovascular problems in pregnant women with the Marfan syndrome. *Ann Intern Med* 1995;123(2):117–122.

82. Siu SC, Sermer M., Harrison D.A., et al. Risk and predictors for pregnancy-related complications in women with heart disease. *Circulation* 1997;96(9):2789–2794.

83. Lao T, Sermer M, Magee L, et al. Congenital aortic stenosis and pregnancy—A reappraisal. *Am J Obstet Gynecol* 1993;169:540–545.

84. Mendelson C. Pregnancy and coarctation of the aorta. *Am J Obstet Gynecol* 1940;39:1014–1021.

85. Connolly H, Ammash N, Warnes C. Pregnancy in women with coarctation of the aorta. *J Am Coll Cardiol* 1996;43A.

86. Hall J, Pauli R, Wilson K. Maternal and fetal sequelae of anticoagulation during pregnancy. *Am J Med* 1980;68:122–140.

87. Iturbe-Alessio I, Del Carmen Fonseca M, Mutchinik O, et al. Risks of anticoagulant therapy in pregnant women with artificial heart valves. *N Engl J Med* 1986;315:1390–1393.

88. Salazar E, Izaguirre R, Verdejo J, et al. Failure of adjusted doses of subcutaneous heparin to prevent thromboembolic phenomena in pregnant patients with mechanical cardiac valve prostheses. *J Am Coll Cardiol* 1996;27:1698–1703.

89. Sbarouni E, Oakley C. Pregnancy and prosthetic heart valves. *Brit Heart J* 1994;71:196–201.

90. Cotrufo M, deLuca T, Calabro R, et al. Coumadin anticoagulation during pregnancy in patients with mechanical valve prostheses. *Eur J Cardiothorac Surg* 1991;5:300–305.

91. Elkayam U. Anticoagulation in pregnant women with prosthetic heart valves. *J Am Coll Cardiol* 1996;27:1704–1706.

92. Nora J, Nora A. The evolution of specific genetic and environmental counseling in congenital heart disease. *Circulation* 1978;57:205–213.

93. Burn J. The aetiology of congenital heart disease. In: Anderson R, et al, eds. *Paediatric Cardiology*. Edinburgh: Churchill Livingstone. 1987:15–63.

94. Allan L, Crawford D, Chita S, et al. Familial recurrence of congenital heart disease in a prospective series of mothers referred for fetal echocardiography. *Am J Cardiol* 1986;58:334–337.

95. Driscoll D, Michels V, Gersony W, et al. Occurrence risk for congenital heart defects in relatives of patients with aortic stenosis, pulmonary stenosis, or ventricular septal defect. *Circulation* 1993;87(suppl I):I-114–I-120.

96. Houston A, Hillis S, Lilley S, et al. Echocardiography in adult congenital heart disease. *Heart* 1998;80(suppl 1):12–26.

97. Tworetzky W, McElhinney DB, Brook MM, et al. Echocardiographic diagnosis alone for the complete repair of major congenital heart defects. *J Am Coll Cardiol* 1999;33(1):228–233.

98. Stumper O. Imaging the heart in adult congenital heart disease editorial. *Heart* 1998;80(6):535–536.

99. Ammash NM, Seward JB, Warnes CA, et al. Partial anomalous pulmonary venous connection: Diagnosis by transesophageal echocardiography. *J Am Coll Cardiol* 1997;29(6):1351–1358.

100. Randolph GR, Hagler DJ, Connolly HM, et al. Intraoperative transesophageal echocardiography during surgery for congenital heart defects. *J Thorac Cardiovasc Surg* 2002;124(6):1176–1182.

101. Choe YH, Ko JK, Lee HJ, et al. MR imaging of non-visualized pulmonary arteries at angiography in patients with congenital heart disease. *J Korean Med Sci* 1998;13(6):597–602.

102. Hartnell GG, Notarianni M. MRI and echocardiography: How do they compare in adults? *Semin Roentgenol* 1998;33(3):252–261.

103. Wimpfheimer O, Boxt LM. MR imaging of adult patients with congenital heart disease. *Radiol Clin North Am* 1999;37(2):421–438, vii.

104. Harrison D, McLaughlin P. Interventional cardiology for the adult patient with congenital heart disease: The Toronto Hospital experience. *Can J Cardiol* 1996;12:965–971.

105. Weidman W, Lenfant C, Hayes C, et al. Symposium: The report of the natural history study of congenital heart defects: A 20-year follow-up. In: *61st Scientific Session of the American Heart Association,* Washington, DC, 1988.

106. Deanfield J. Adult congenital heart disease with special reference to the data on long-term follow-up of patients surviving to adulthood with or without surgical correction. *Eur Heart J* 1992;13(suppl H):111–116.

107. Truesdell S. Life insurance for children with cardiovascular disease. *Pediatrics* 1986;77:687.

108. Celermajer D, Deanfield J. Employment and insurance for young adults with congenital heart disease. *Brit Heart J* 1993;69:539–543.

109. Garson A, Allen H, Gersony W, et al. Cost of congenital heart disease in children and adults: Sources of variation assessed by multicenter study. *Circulation* 1991;84(suppl II):II–385.

110. Mahoney L, Truesdell S, Hamburgen M, et al. Insurability, employability, and psychosocial considerations. In: Perloff J, Child J, eds. *Congenital Heart Disease in Adults*, Saunders: Philadelphia. 1991:178–189.

111. Brandhagen D, Feldt R, Williams D. Long-term psychologic implications of congenital heart disease: A 25-year follow-up. *Mayo Clin Proc* 1991;66:474–479.

112. Utens EM, Bieman HJ, Verhulst FC, et al. Psychopathology in young adults with congenital heart disease. Follow-up results. *Eur Heart J* 1998;19(4):647–651.

113. Gupta S, Giuffre RM, Crawford S, et al. Covert fears, anxiety and depression in congenital heart disease. *Cardiol Young* 1998;8(4):491–499.

114. Myers-Vando R, Steward M, Folkins C, et al. The effects of congenital heart disease on cognitive development, illness causality concepts, and vulnerability. *Am J Orthopsychiatry* 1979;49:617–625.

115. Aram D, Ekelman B, Ben-Shachae G, et al. Intelligence and hypoxemia in children with congenital heart disease. *J Am Coll Cardiol* 1985;6:889–893.

116. Newburger J, Silbert A, Buckley L, et al. Cognitive function and age at repair of transposition of the great arteries in children. *N Engl J Med* 1984;310:1495–1499.

117. Swan L, Hillis WS, Cameron A. Family planning requirements of adults with congenital heart disease editorial. *Heart* 1997;78(1):9–11.

118. Bonnar J. Coagulation effects of oral contraception. *Am J Obstet Gynecol* 1987;157:1042–1048.

119. Fraser I. Progestogens for contraception. *Austr Fam Physician* 1988;17:882–885.

120. Whittemore R. Pregnancy and congenital heart disease. In: Adams F, Emmanoulides G, Riemenschneider T, eds. *Heart Disease in Infants, Children, and Adults*, Baltimore:Williams & Wilkins, 1989:684–690.

121. Rocchini A, Katch V, Anderson J, et al. Blood pressure in obese adolescents: Effects of weight loss. *Pediatrics* 1988;82:16–23.

122. Powell K, Thompson P, Casperen C, et al. Physical activity and the incidence of coronary heart disease. *Annu Rev Public Health* 1987;8:281–287.

123. 26th Bethesda Conference: Recommendations for determining eligibility for competition in athletes with cardiovascular abnormalities. *J Am Coll Cardiol* 1994;24:845–899.

124. Fredriksen PM, Veldtman G, Hechter S, et al. Aerobic capacity in adults with various congenital heart diseases. *Am J Cardiol* 2001;87(3):310–314.

125. Stark J, Pacifico A. eds. *Reoperations in Cardiac Surgery,*. Berlin: Springer-Verlag, 1989.

126. Dore A, Glancy DL, Stone S, et al. Cardiac surgery for grown-up congenital heart patients: Survey of 307 consecutive operations from 1991 to 1994. *Am J Cardiol* 1997;80(7):906–913.

127. Jonas R, Freed M, Mayer J Jr, et al. Long-term follow-up of patients with synthetic right heart conduits. *Circulation* 1985;72(suppl II):77–83.

128. Ross D, Somerville J. Correction of pulmonary atresia with a homograft aortic valve. *Lancet* 1966;2:1446–1447.

129. Cerfolio R, Danielson G, Warnes C, et al. Results of an autologous tissue reconstruction for replacement of obstructed extracardiac conduits. *J Thorac Cardiovasc Surg* 1995;110:1359–1366.

130. Stark J. Reoperations in patients with extracardiac valved conduits. In: Stark J, Pacifico A, eds. *Reoperations in Cardiac Surgery,* Berlin: Springer-Verlag, 1989:271–290.

131. Poirier R, McGoon D, Danielson G, et al. Late results after repair of tetralogy of Fallot. *J Thorac Cardiovasc Surg* 1977;73:900–908.

132. Zhao H, Miller D, Reitz B, et al. Surgical repair of tetralogy of Fallot: Long-term follow-up with particular emphasis on late death and reoperation. *J Thorac Cardiovasc Surg* 1985;89:204–220.

133. Oechslin EN, Harrison DA, Harris L, et al. Reoperation in adults with repair of tetralogy of fallot: Indications and outcomes. *J Thorac Cardiovasc Surg* 1999;118(2):245–251.

134. Discigil B, Dearani JA, Puga FJ, et al. Late pulmonary valve replacement after repair of tetralogy of Fallot. *J Thorac Cardiovasc Surg* 2001;121(2):344–351.

135. Wessel H, Cunningham W, Paul M, et al. Exercise performance in tetralogy of Fallot after intracardiac repair. *J Thorac Cardiovasc Surg* 1980;80:582–593.

136. Yemets I, Williams W, Webb G, et al. Pulmonary valve replacement late after repair of tetralogy of Fallot. *Ann Thorac Surg* 1997;64:526–530.

137. Presbitero P, Somerville J, Revel-Chion R, et al. Open aortic valvotomy for congenital aortic stenosis: Late results. *Brit Heart J* 1982; 47:26–34.

138. Hsieh K, Keane J, Nadas A, et al. Long-term follow-up of valvulotomy before 1968 for congenital aortic stenosis. *Am J Cardiol* 1986; 58:338–341.

139. Puga F, Leoni F, Julsrud P, et al. Complete repair of pulmonary atresia, ventricular septal defect, and severe peripheral arborization abnormalities of the central pulmonary arteries: Experience with preliminary unifocalization procedures in 38 patients. *J Thorac Cardiovasc Surg* 1989;6:1018–1029.

140. Sullivan I, Wren C, Stark J, et al. Surgical unifocalisation in pulmonary atresia and ventricular septal defect: A realistic goal? *Circulation* 1988;78(suppl III):5–13.

141. Watterson K, Wilkinson J, Kari T, et al. Very small pulmonary arteries: The central end-to-side shunt. *Ann Thorac Surg* 1991;52:1132–1137.

142. Speziali G, Driscoll DJ, Danielson GK, et al. Cardiac transplantation for end-stage congenital heart defects: The Mayo Clinic experience. Mayo Cardiothoracic Transplant Team (see comments). *Mayo Clin Proc* 1998;73(10):923–928.

143. Mendeloff EN, Huddleston CB. Lung transplantation and repair of complex congenital heart lesions in patients with pulmonary hypertension. *Semin Thorac Cardiovasc Surg* 1998;10(2):144–151.

144. Franklin R, Spiegelhalter D, Anderson R, et al. Double inlet ventricle presenting in infancy: Survival without definitive repair. *J Thorac Cardiovasc Surg* 1991;101:767–776.

145. Child J, Perloff J. Natural survival patterns: A narrowing base. In: Child J, Perloff J, eds. *Congenital Heart Disease in Adults,* Philadelphia: Saunders, 1991:21–59.

146. Borow K, Braunwald E. Congenital heart disease in the adult. In: Braunwald E, ed. *Heart Disease,* Philadelphia:Saunders, 1988: 976–1002.

147. Warnes C, Fuster V, Dirscoll D, et al. Atrial septal defect, In: Giuliani E, et al, ed. *Cardiology Fundamentals and Practice,* St. Louis: Mosby-Year Book, 1991:1622–1638.

148. Kirklin J, Barratt-Boyes B, ed. *Cardiac Surgery,* New York: Wiley, 1986:463–497.

149. Massumi R, Nutter D. The syndrome of familial defects of the heart and upper extremities (Holt-Oram syndrome). *Circulation* 1966;34:65–76.

150. Nora J, McNamara D, Fraser F. Hereditary factors in atrial septal defect. *Circulation* 1967;35:448–456.

151. Perloff J. Ostium secundum atrial septal defect—survival for 87–94 years. *Am J Cardiol* 1984;53:388–389.

152. Campbell M. Natural history of atrial septal defect. *Brit Heart J* 1970; 32:820–826.

153. Shah D, Azhar M, Oakley C, et al. Natural history of secundum atrial septal defect in adults after medical or surgical treatment: A historical prospective study. *Brit Heart J* 1994;71:224–228.

154. Konstantinides S, Geibel A, Olschewski M, et al. A comparison of surgical and medical therapy for atrial septal defects in adults. *N Engl J Med* 1995;333:469–473.

155. Attie F, Rosas M, Granados N, et al. Surgical treatment for secundum atrial septal defects in patients >40 years old. A randomized clinical trial. *J Am Coll Cardiol* 2001;38(7):2035–2042.

156. Theodoro DA, Danielson GK, Porter CJ, et al. Right-sided maze procedure for right atrial arrhythmias in congenital heart disease. *Ann Thorac Surg* 1998;65(1):149–153; discussion 153–144.

157. Lock J. The adult with congenital heart disease: Cardiac catheterization as a therapeutic intervention. *J Am Coll Cardiol* 1991;18:330–331.

158. Hellenbrand W, Fahey J, McGowan F, et al. Transesophageal echocardiographic guidance of transcatheter closure of atrial septal defect. *Am J Cardiol* 1990;66:207–213.

159. Banerjee A, Bengur AR, Li JS, et al. Echocardiographic characteristics of successful deployment of the Das Angel Wings atrial septal defect closure device: Initial multicenter experience in the United States. *Am J Cardiol* 1999;83(8):1236–1241.

160. Thanopoulos BD, Laskari CV, Tsaousis GS, et al. Closure of atrial septal defects with the Amplatzer occlusion device: Preliminary results see comments. *J Am Coll Cardiol* 1998;31(5):1110–1116.

161. Walsh KP, Tofeig M, Kitchiner DJ, et al. Comparison of the Sideris and Amplatzer septal occlusion devices. *Am J Cardiol* 1999;83(6): 933–936.

162. Du Z, Hijazi Z, Kleinman CS. Comparison between transcatheter and surgical closure of secundum atrial septal defect in children and adults. *J Am Coll Cardiol* 2002;39:1836–1844.

163. Murphy J, Gersh B, McGoon M, et al. Long-term outcome after surgical repair of isolated atrial septal defect. *N Engl J Med* 1990;323: 1645–1697.

164. Brandenburg R. Jr, Holmes D Jr, Brandenburg R, et al. Clinical follow-up study of paroxysmal supraventricular arrhythmias after operative repair of a secundum type atrial septal defect in adults. *Am J Cardiol* 1983;51:273–276.

165. St. John Sutton M, Tajik A, McGoon D. Atrial septal defect in patients aged 60 or older: Operative results and long-term postoperative follow-up. *Circulation* 1981;64:402–409.

166. Engle M, Kline S, Borer J. Ventricular septal defect, In: Roberts W, ed. *Adult Congenital Heart Disease,* Philadelphia:Davis, 1987:409–441.

167. Wood P. The Eisenmenger syndrome or pulmonary hypertension with reversed central shunt. *BMJ* 1958:2:701–709.

168. Warnes C, Fuster V, Driscoll D, et al. Ventricular septal defect, In: Guiliani E, et al., eds. *Cardiology: Fundamentals and Practice,* St. Louis: Mosby-Year Book, 1991:1639–1652.

169. Ammash NM, Warnes CA. Ventricular septal defects in adults. *Ann Intern Med* 2001;135(9):812–824.

170. Tatsuno K, Konno S, Sakakibara S. Ventricular septal defect with aortic insufficiency: Angiocardiographic aspects and a new classification. *Am Heart J* 1973;85:13–21.

171. Cartmill T, DuShane J, McGoon D, et al. Results of repair of ventricular septal defect. *J Thorac Cardiovasc Surg* 1966;52:486–499.

172. Blake R, Chung E, Wesley H, et al. Conduction defects, ventricular arrhythmias and late death after surgical closure of ventricular septal defect. *Brit Heart J* 1982;47:305–315.

173. Bridges N, Perry S, Keane J, et al. Preoperative transcatheter closure of congenital muscular ventricular septal defects. *N Engl J Med* 1991; 324:1312–1317.

174. Reeder G, Danielson G, Seward J, et al. Fixed subaortic stenosis in atrioventricular canal defect: A Doppler echocardiographic study. *J Am Coll Cardiol* 1992;20:386–394.

175. Report of the New England Regional Infant Cardiac Program. *Pediatrics* 1980;65(suppl):441–444.

176. El-Nadjdawi E, Driscoll D, Puga F, et al. Operation for partial atrioventricular septal defect : A forty-year review. *J Thorac Cardiovasc Surg* 2000;121:398–399.

177. Bergin M, Warnes C, Tajik A, et al. Partial atrioventricular canal defect: Long-term follow-up after initial repair in patients greater than or equal to 40 years old. *J Am Coll Cardiol* 1995;25:1189–1194.

178. Phadke A, Phadke S, Handy M, et al. Acyanotic Fallot's tetralogy with survival to the age of 70 years: Case report. *Indian Heart J* 1977; 29:46–49.

179. Deanfield J, Ho S, Anderson R, et al. Late sudden death after repair of tetralogy of Fallot: A clinicopathological study. *Circulation* 1983;67: 636–641.

180. Katz N, Blackstone E, Kirklin J, et al. Late survival and symptoms after repair of tetralogy of Fallot. *Circulation* 1982;65:403–410.

181. Murphy J, Gersh B, Mair D, et al. Long-term outcome in patients undergoing surgical repair of tetralogy of Fallot. *N Engl J Med* 1993; 329:593–599.

182. Lillehei C, Varco R, Cohen M, et al. The first open heart corrections of tetralogy of Fallot: A 26-31 year follow-up of 106 patients. *Ann Surg,* 1986;204:490–501.

183. Deanfield J. Late ventricular arrhythmias occurring after tetralogy of Fallot: Do they matter? *Int J Cardiol* 1991;30:143–150.

184. Wennevold A, Rygg I, Lauridsen P, et al. Fourteen- to nineteen-year follow-up after corrective repair of tetralogy of Fallot. *Scand J Thorac Cardiovasc Surg* 1982;16:41–45.

185. Dodds GA 3rd, Warnes CA, Danielson GK. Aortic valve replacement after repair of pulmonary atresia and ventricular septal defect or tetralogy of Fallot. *J Thorac Cardiovas Surg* 1997;113(4):736–741.

186. Therrien J, Siu SC, McLaughlin PR, et al. Pulmonary valve replacement in adults late after repair of tetralogy of Fallot: Are we operating too late? *J Am Coll Cardiol* 2000;36(5):1670–1675.

187. Nugent E, Freedom R, Nora J, et al. Clinical course in pulmonary stenosis. *Circulation* 1977;56(suppl I):I-38–I-47.

188. O'Fallon WM, Crowson CS, Rings LJ, et al. Second natural history study of congenital heart defects. Materials and methods. *Circulation* 1993;87(2 Suppl):I4–15.

189. Bonow RO, Carabello B, de Leon AC, et al. ACC/AHA Guidelines for the Management of Patients with Valvular Heart Disease. Executive Summary. A report of the American College of Cardiology/ American Heart Association Task Force on Practice Guidelines (Committee on Management of Patients with Valvular Heart Disease). *J Heart Valve Dis* 1998;7(6):672–707.

190. Kopecky S, Gersh B, McGoon M, et al. Long-term outcome of patients undergoing surgical repair of isolated pulmonary valve stenosis: Follow-up at 20 to 30 years. *Circulation* 1988;78:1150–1156.

191. Chen CR, Cheng TO, Huang T, et al. Percutaneous balloon valvuloplasty for pulmonic stenosis in adolescents and adults. *N Engl J Med* 1996;335(1):21–25.

192. McCrindle BW. Independent predictors of long-term results after balloon pulmonary valvuloplasty. Valvuloplasty and Angioplasty of Congenital Anomalies (VACA) Registry Investigators. *Circulation* 1994;89(4):1751–1759.

193. Friedman W, Johnson A, Congenital aortic stenosis. In: Roberts W, ed. *Adult Congenital Heart Disease*, Philadelphia:Davis, 1987:357–374.

194. Kelly D, Wulfsberg B, Rowe R. Discrete subaortic stenosis. *Circulation* 1972;46:309–322.

195. Kleinert S, Geva T, Echocardiographic morphometry and geometry of the left ventricular outflow tract in fixed subaortic stenosis. *J Am Coll Cardiol* 1993;22:1501–1508.

196. Freedom R. The long and short of it: Some thoughts about the fixed forms of left ventricular outflow tract obstruction. *J Am Coll Cardiol* 1997;30:1843–1846.

197. Williams J, Barratt-Boyes B, Lowe J. Supravalvular aortic stenosis. *Circulation* 1961;24:1311–1318.

198. Mills P, Leech G, Davies M, et al. The natural history of a nonstenotic bicuspid aortic valve. *Brit Heart J* 1978;40:951–957.

199. Gersony W, Hayes C. Bacterial endocarditis in patients with pulmonary stenosis, aortic stenosis, or ventricular septal defect. *Circulation* 1977;56(suppl I):I-84–I-87.

200. Fontana R, Edwards J. *Congenital Cardiac Disease: A Review of 357 Cases Studied Pathologically.* Philadelphia: Saunders, 1962.

201. Muna W, Ferrans V, Pierce J, et al. Discrete subaortic stenosis in Newfoundland dogs: Association of infective endocarditis. *Am J Cardiol* 1978;41:746–754.

202. Bonderman D, Gharehbaghi-Schnell E, Wollenek G, et al. Mechanisms underlying aortic dilatation in congenital aortic valve malformation. *Circulation* 1999;99(16):2138–2143.

203. Rohlicek CV, del Pino S Font, Hosking M, et al. Natural history and surgical outcomes for isolated discrete subaortic stenosis in children. *Heart* 1999;82: 708–713.

204. Wagner H, Ellison R, Keane J, et al. Long-term follow-up of valvotomy before 1968 for congenital aortic stenosis. *Am J Cardiol* 1986; 58:338–341.

205. Kugelmeier J, Egloff L, Real F, et al. Congenital aortic stenosis: Early and late results of aortic valvotomy. *Thorac Cardiovasc Surg* 1982; 30:91–95.

206. Sandhu S, Lloyd T, Crowley D, et al. Effectiveness of balloon valvuloplasty in the young adult with congenital aortic stenosis. *Catheter Cardiovasc Diagn* 1995;36:122–127.

207. McCrindle BW. Independent predictors of immediate results of percutaneous balloon aortic valvotomy in children. Valvuloplasty and Angioplasty of Congenital Anomalies (VACA) Registry Investigators. *Am J Cardiol* 1996;77(4):286–293.

208. Somerville J, Stone S, Ross D. Fate of patients with fixed subaortic stenosis after surgical removal. *Brit Heart J* 1980;43:629–647.

209. Brauner R, Laks H, Drinkwater D Jr, et al. Benefits of early surgical repair in fixed subaortic stenosis. *J Am Coll Cardiol* 1997;30:1835–1842.

210. van Son J, Schaff H, Danielson G, et al. Surgical treatment of discrete and tunnel subaortic stenosis. Late survival and risk of reoperation. *Circulation* 1993;88(5 Pt 2):II59–69.

211. Campbell M. Natural history of coarctation of the aorta. *Brit Heart J* 1970;32:633–640.

212. Cohen M, Fuster V, Steele P, Coarctation of the aorta: Long-term follow-up and prediction of outcome after surgical correction. *Circulation* 1989;80:840–845.

213. Gross R, Hufnagel C, Coarctation of the aorta: Experimental studies regarding its surgical correction. *N Engl J Med* 1945;233:287–293.

214. Waldhausen J, Shitman V, Werner J, et al. Surgical intervention in infants with coarctation of the aorta. *J Thorac Cardiovasc Surg* 1981; 81:323–325.

215. Keen G. Spinal cord damage and operations for coarctation of the aorta: Aetiology, practice, and prospects. *Thorax* 1987;42:11–18.

216. Morris R, Samuels L, Brockman S. Total simultaneous repair of coarctation and intracardiac pathology in adult patients. *Ann Thorac Surg* 1998;65:1698–1702.

217. Connolly HM, Schaff HV, Izhar U, et al. Posterior pericardial ascending-to-descending aortic bypass: An alternative surgical approach for complex coarctation of the aorta. *Circulation* 2001;104(12 suppl 1): I133–I137.

218. McCrindle BW, Jones TK, Morrow WR, et al. Acute results of balloon angioplasty of native coarctation versus recurrent aortic obstruction are equivalent. Valvuloplasty and Angioplasty of Congenital Anomalies (VACA) Registry Investigators. *J Am Coll Cardiol* 1996; 28(7):1810–1817.

219. Shaddy RE, Boucek MM, Sturtevant JE, et al. Comparison of angioplasty and surgery for unoperated coarctation of the aorta. *Circulation* 1993;87(3):793–799.

220. Rosenthal E. Stent implantation for aortic coarctation: The treatment of choice in adults? *J Am Coll Cardiol*, 2001;38(5):1524–1527.

221. Hamdan MA, Maheshwari S, Fahey JT, et al. Endovascular stents for coarctation of the aorta: Initial results and intermediate-term follow-up. *J Am Coll Cardiol* 2001;38(5):1518–1523.

222. Presbitero P, Demarie D, Villani M, et al. Long-term results (15-30 years) of surgical repair of aortic coarctation. *Brit Heart J* 1987;57: 462–467.

223. Attenhofer Jost, CH, Schaff HV, Connolly HM, et al. Spectrum of reoperations after repair of aortic coarctation: Importance of an individualized approach because of coexistent cardiovascular disease. *Mayo Clin Proc* 2002;77(7):646–653.

224. Fyler D. Report of the New England regional cardiac infant program. *Pediatrics* 1980;65:375–460.

225. Rashkind W, Miller W. Creation of an atrial septal defect without thoractomy: A palliative approach to complete transposition of the great arteries. *JAMA* 1966;196:991–992.

226. Senning A. Surgical correction of transposition of the great vessels. *Surgery* 1959;45:966–980.

227. Mustard W. Successful two-stage correction of transposition of the great vessels. *Surgery* 1964;55:469–472.

228. Turina M, Seibenmann R, Segesser L, et al. Late functional deterioration after atrial correction for transposition of the great arteries. *Circulation* 1989;80(suppl I):162–167.

229. Gelatt M, Hamilton R, McCrindle B, et al, Arrhythmia and mortality after the Mustard procedure: A 30-year single-center experience. *J Am Coll Cardiol* 1997;29:194–201.

230. Wilson NJ, Clarkson PM, Barratt-Boyes BG, et al. Long-term outcome after the Mustard repair for simple transposition of the great arteries. 28-year follow-up. *J Am Coll Cardiol* 1998;32(3):758–765.

231. Jatene A, Fontes V, Paulista P, et al. Successful anatomic correction of transposition of the great vessels: A preliminary report. *Arg Braz Cardiol* 1975;28:461–464.

232. Rastelli G, Wallace R, Ongley P. Complete repair of transposition of the great arteries with pulmonary stenosis: A review and report of a case corrected by using a new surgical technique. *Circulation* 1969; 39:83–95.

233. Deanfield J, Camm J, Macartney F, et al. Arrhythmia and late mortality after Mustard and Senning operation for transposition of the great arteries: An eight year prospective study. *J Thorac Cardiovasc Surg* 1988;96:569–576.

234. Flinn C, Wolff G, Dick M, et al. Cardiac rhythm after the Mustard operation for complete transposition of the great arteries. *N Engl J Med* 1984;310:1635–1638.

235. Mee R. Two-stage repair: Pulmonary artery banding and switch. *J Thorac Cardiovasc Surg* 1986;92:385–390.

236. Wernovsky G, Hougen T, Walsh E, et al. Mid-term results after the arterial switch operation for transposition of the great arteries with intact ventricular septum: Clinical, hemodynamic, echocardiographic, and electrophysiologic data. *Circulation* 1988;77:1333–1344.

237. Rhodes L, Wernovsky C, Keane J, et al. Arrhythmias and intracardiac conduction after the arterial switch operation. *J Thorac Cardiovasc Surg* 1995;19:303–310.

238. Warnes CA. Congenitally corrected transposition: The uncorrected misnomer. *J Am Coll Cardiol* 1996;27(5):1244–1245.

239. Lundstrom U, Bull C, Wyse R, et al. The natural and "unnatural" history of congenitally corrected transposition. *Am J Cardiol* 1990;65: 1222–1229.

240. Huhta J, Maloney J, Ritter D, et al. Complete atrioventricular block in patients with atrioventricular discordance. *Circulation* 1983;67: 1374–1377.

241. Allwork S, Bentall H, Becker A, et al. Congenitally corrected transposition of the great arteries: Morphologic study of 32 cases. *Am J Cardiol* 1976;38:910–923.

242. Beauchesne LM, Warnes CA, Connolly HM, et al. Outcome of the unoperated adult who presents with congenitally corrected transposition of the great arteries. *J Am Coll Cardiol* 2002;40(2):285–290.

243. Graham T, Bernard Y, Mellen B, Long-term outcome in congenitally corrected transposition of the great arteries. *J Am Coll Cardiol* 2000; 36:255–261.

244. Yeh T, Connelly M, Coles J, et al. Atrioventricular discordance: Results of repair in 127 patients. *J Thorac Cardiovasc Surg* 1999;117: 1190–1203.

245. Prieto LR, Hordof AJ, Secic M, et al. Progressive tricuspid valve disease in patients with congenitally corrected transposition of the great arteries. *Circulation* 1998;98(10):997–1005.

246. Voskuil M, Hazekamp MG, Kroft LJ, et al. Postsurgical course of patients with congenitally corrected transposition of the great arteries. *Am J Cardiol* 1999;83(4):558–562.

247. van Son J, Danielson G, Huhta J, et al. Late results of systemic atrioventricular valve replacement in corrected transposition. *J Thorac Cardiovasc Surg* 1995;109:642–653.

248. Yagihari T, Kishimoto H, Isobe F, et al. Double switch operation in cardiac anomalies with atrioventricular and ventriculoarterial discordance. *J Thorac Cardiovasc Surg* 1994;107:351–358.

249. Ilbawi M, DeLeon S, Backer C, et al. An alternative approach to the surgical management of physiologically corrected transposition with ventricular septal defect and pulmonary stenosis or atresia. *J Thorac Cardiovasc Surg* 1990;100:410–415.

250. Connelly M, Piu P, Williams W, et al. Congenitally corrcted transposition in the adult: Functional status and complications. *J Am Coll Cardiol* 1996;27:1238–1243.

251. Ammash NM; Warnes CA. Survival into adulthood of patients with unoperated single ventricle. *Am J Cardiol* 1996;77(7):542–544.

252. Moodie D, Ritter D, Tajik A, et al. Long-term follow-up in the unoperated univentricular heart. *Am J Cardiol* 1984;53:1124–1128.

253. Moodie D, Ritter D, Tajik A, et al. Long-term follow-up after palliative operation for univentricular heart. *Am J Cardiol* 1984;53:1648–1651.

254. Fontan F, Baudet E. Surgical repair of tricuspid atresia. *Thorax* 1971; 26:240–248.

255. Choussat A, Fontan E, Besse P, et al. Selection criteria for Fontan's procedure. In: Anderson R, Shineborune E, eds. *Paediatric Cardiology*, Edinburgh: Churchill Livingstone, 1978.

256. Fontan F, Deville C, Quagebeur J, et al. Repair of tricuspid atresia in 100 patients. *J Thorac Cardiovasc Surg* 1983;85:647–660.

257. Driscoll D, Offord K, Felot R, et al. Five to fifteen year follow-up after Fontan operation. *Circulation* 1992;81:1520–1536.

258. Feldt R, Driscoll D, Offord K, et al. Protein-losing enteropathy after the Fontan operation. *J Thorac Cardiovasc Surg* 1991;112: 672–680.

259. Mertens L, Hagler DJ, Sauer U, et al. Protein-losing enteropathy after the Fontan operation: An international multicenter study. PLE study group. *J Thorac Cardiovasc Surg* 1998;115(5):1063–1073.

260. Kelly AM, Feldt RH, Driscoll DJ, et al. Use of heparin in the treatment of protein-losing enteropathy after Fontan operation for complex congenital heart disease. *Mayo Clin Proc* 1998;73(8):777–779.

261. Mertens L, Dumoulin M, Gewillig M. Effective percutaneous fenestration of the atrial septum in protein-losing enteropathy after the Fontan operation. *Brit Heart J* 1994;72:591–592.

262. Warnes C, Feldt R, Hagler D. Protein-losing enteropathy after the Fontan operation: Successful treatment by percutaneous fenestration of the atrial septum. *Mayo Clin Proc* 1996;71:378–379.

263. Zellers T, Brown K. Protein-losing enteropathy after the modified Fontan operation: Oral prednisone treatment with biopsy and laboratory proved improvement. *Pediatr Cardiol* 1996;17:115–117.

264. Mathur M, Glenn W. Long-term evaluation of cavopulmonary artery anastomosis. *Surgery* 1973;74:889–916.

265. Marcelletti CF, Hanley FL, Mavroudis C, et al. Revision of previous Fontan connections to total extracardiac cavopulmonary anastomosis: A multicenter experience. *J Thorac Cardiovasc Surg* 2000;119(2): 340–346.

266. Kreutzer J, Keane J, Lock J, et al. Conversion of modified Fontan procedure to lateral atrial tunnel cavopulmonary anastomosis. *J Thorac Cardiovasc Surg* 1996;111:1169–1176.

267. van Son J, Mohr F, Hambsch J, et al. Conversion of atriopulmonary or lateral atrial tunnel cavopulmonary anastomosis to extracardiac conduit Fontan modification. *Eur J C-T Surg* 1999;15:150–157.

268. Deal B, Mavrousid C, Backer C, et al. Impact of arrhythmia circuit cryoablation during Fontan conversion for refractory atrial tachycardia. *Am J Cardiol* 1999;83:563–568.

269. Bridges N, Lock J, Castaneda A. Baffle fenestration with subsequent transcatheter closure: Modifications of the Fontan operation for patients at higher risk. *Circulation* 1990;82:1681–1689.

270. de Leval M, Kilner P, Gewillig M, et al. Total cavopulmonary connection: A logical alternative to atriopulmonary connection for complex Fontan operations. *J Thorac Cardiovasc Surg* 1988;96:682–695.

271. Be'eri E, Maier SE, Landzberg MJ, et al. In vivo evaluation of Fontan pathway flow dynamics by multidimensional phase-velocity magnetic resonance imaging. *Circulation* 1998;98(25):2873–2882.

272. Fishberger SB, Wernovsky G, Gentles TL, et al. Factors that influence the development of atrial flutter after the Fontan operation. *J Thorac Cardiovasc Surg* 1997;113(1):80–86.

273. Laschinger J, Redmond J, Cameron D, et al. Intermediate results of the extracardiac Fontan procedure. *Ann Thorac Surg* 1996;62:1261–1267.

274. Petrossian E, Reddy V, McElhinney D, et al. Early results of the extracardiac conduit Fontan operation. *J Thorac Cardiovasc Surg* 1999. 117:688–696.

275. Balling G, Vogt M, Kaemmerer H, et al. Intracardiac thrombus formation after the Fontan operation. *J Thorac Cardiovasc Surg* 2000;119(4 Pt 1):745–752.

276. Watson H. Natural history of Ebstein's anomaly of the tricuspid valve in childhood and adolescence: An internation cooperative study of 505 cases. *Brit Heart J* 1974;36:417–427.

277. Celermajer D, Dodd S, Greenwald S, et al. Morbid anatomy in neonates with Ebstein's anomaly of the tricuspid valve: Pathophysiologic and clinical implications. *J Am Coll Cardiol* 1992;19:1049–1053.

278. Till J, Celermajer D, Deanfield J, The natural history of arrhythmias in Ebstein's anomaly. *J Am Coll Cardiol* 1992;19(suppl A):273A.

279. Saxena A, Fong L, Tristram M, et al. Late noninvasive evaluation of cardiac performance in mildly symptomatic older patients with Ebstein's anomaly of the tricuspid valve: Role of radionuclide imaging. *J Am Coll Cardiol* 1991;17:182–186.

280. Danielson G, Driscoll D, Mair D, et al. Operative treatment of Ebstein's anomaly. *J Thorac Cardiovasc Surg*, 1992;104:1195–1202.

281. MacLellan-Tobert S, Driscoll D, Mottram C, et al. Exercise tolerance in patients with Ebstein's anomaly. *J Am Coll Cardiol* 1997;29: 1615–1622.

282. Kiziltan H, Theodoro D, Warnes C, et al. Late results of bioprosthetic tricuspid valve replacement in Ebstein's anomaly. *Ann Thorac Surg* 1998;66:1539–1545.

283. Ramirez F, Gayraud B, Pereira L, Marfan syndrome: New clues to genotype-phenotype correlations. *Ann Med* 1999;31:202–207.

284. De Paepe A, Devereux RB, Dietz HC, et al. Revised diagnostic criteria for the Marfan syndrome. *Am J Med Genet* 1996;62(4):417–426.

285. Dean JC. Management of Marfan syndrome. *Heart* 2002;88(1): 97–103.

286. Murdoch J, Walker B, Halpern B, et al. Life expectancy and causes of death in the Marfan syndrome. *N Engl J Med* 1972;286:804–808.

287. Pyeritz Rl Wappel M. Mitral valve dysfunction in the Marfan syndrome. *Am J Med* 1983;74:797–807.

288. Gott VL, Cameron DE, Alejo DE, et al. Aortic root replacement in 271 Marfan patients: A 24-year experience. *Ann Thorac Surg* 2002; 73(2):438–443.

289. Silverman D, Burton K, Gray J, et al. Life expectancy in the Marfan syndrome. *Am J Cardiol* 1995;75:157–160.

290. Gott VL, Greene PS, Alejo DE, et al. Replacement of the aortic root in patients with Marfan's syndrome. *N Engl J Med* 1999;340(17): 1307–1313.

291. Coady M, Rizzo J, Hammond G, et al. What is the appropriate size criterion for resection of thoracic aortic aneurysms? *J Thorac Cardiovasc Surg* 1997;113(3):476–491.

292. Legget ME, Unger TA, O'Sullivan CK, et al. Aortic root complications in Marfan's syndrome: Identification of a lower risk group. *Heart* 1996;75(4):389–395.

293. Yacoub M, Gehle P, Chandrasekaran V, et al. Late results of a valve-preserving operation in patients with aneurysms of the ascending aorta and root. *J Thorac Cardiovasc Surg* 1998;115(5):1080–1090.

CARDIOMYOPATHY AND SPECIFIC HEART MUSCLE DISEASES

CLASSIFICATION OF CARDIOMYOPATHIES

Jay W. Mason

Despite controversy in classifying the cardiomyopathies, there is general agreement on the definition. Cardiomyopathy is a primary disorder of the heart muscle that causes abnormal myocardial performance and is not the result of disease or dysfunction of other cardiac structures. Thus, in most classifications the term *cardiomyopathy* excludes cases of myocardial failure due to myocardial infarction, systemic arterial hypertension, and valvular stenosis or regurgitation. Although *cardiomyopathy* is easily defined, classification of its various forms is difficult. This difficulty results because the great majority of cases of cardiomyopathy are associated with generalized cardiac dilatation and ventricular systolic dysfunction, in which the etiology is unknown.

CLASSIFICATION SCIENCE

Physicians and biomedical scientists use classification schemes to draw relations and distinctions between diseases. This process promotes understanding and aids recollection. Even disorders we know little about can be understood if appropriately placed in a class with other disorders we do know about.

The science of classification requires that all items within the classified domain be included and that each item appear in only one class. Inability to make clear distinctions between biological systems makes this latter requirement the most demanding. Classification must be based on those features of the individual units within the domain that are understood or recognizable and that permit a useful distinction between groups.

Thus, the classification of cardiomyopathies should be based on an extensive, current category of knowledge about heart diseases and should be as useful as possible to physicians and scientists.

CATEGORIES OF KNOWLEDGE ABOUT CARDIOMYOPATHIES

Knowledge about cardiomyopathies falls into several categories: etiology, gross anatomy, histology, genetics, biochemistry, immunology, hemodynamic function, prognosis, treatment, and others. No single classification scheme can utilize all of these areas of knowledge because there is so much overlap between them.

The best classifications use a single category of knowledge with which to separate items in the domain. However, the most useful knowledge category differs among users of the classification. A histologic classification will be useful to the pathologist, while a functional categorization is more valuable to the treating physician. If only one classification is to be used by both clinicians and scientists, etiologic categorization seems to be most successful. It must be recognized, however, that no single classification can serve all users and all purposes.

Several commonly employed classifications of cardiomyopathy are discussed later. For clarity, the primary categories of each classification are displayed in Tables 75-1 to 75-7, but only a few representative diseases are mentioned within each category. The exceptions are the etiologic classification (see Table 75-3) and the *International Classification of Disease* (see Tables 75-5 and 75-6), in which more nearly complete listings are provided.

THE WORLD HEALTH ORGANIZATION CLASSIFICATION

The only currently used clinical classification of cardiomyopathy that was developed by consensus is that of the *World Health Organization* (WHO) and the International Society and Federation of Cardiology[1,2]. This scheme is outlined in Table 75-1. Because it was developed by a panel of experts and has the implied backing of the WHO, it is widely recognized and frequently used. Although it has been in existence since 1980, it has not gained general acceptance.

The 1980 WHO committee[1] reserved the term *cardiomyopathy* for myocardial disease of unknown cause. This somewhat restricted usage was not adopted widely and is not adhered to in this text. The more common usage includes all forms of heart disease in which the myocardium is primarily involved, as defined at the start of this chapter, but excludes valvular heart disease, systemic arterial hypertension, and coronary atherosclerosis. In its 1995 classification, the WHO committee (entirely new except for one member) moved

TABLE 75-1 World Health Organization Classifications of Cardiomyopathies

I. Former WHO classification[a]
  A. Heart muscle diseases of unknown cause
    1. Dilated cardiomyopathy
    2. Hypertrophic cardiomyopathy
    3. Restrictive cardiomyopathy
    4. Unclassified cardiomyopathy
  B. Specific heart muscle disease
    1. Infective
    2. Metabolic
      a. Endocrine
      b. Familial storage diseases and infiltrations
      c. Deficiency
      d. Amyloid
    3. General system disease
      a. Connective tissue disorders
      b. Infiltrations and granulomas
    4. Heredofamilial
      a. Muscular dystrophies
      b. Neuromuscular disorders
    5. Sensitivity and toxic reactions
II. New WHO classification[b]
  A. Functional classification of cardiomyopathy
    1. Dilated cardiomyopathy
    2. Hypertrophic cardiomyopathy
    3. Restrictive cardiomyopathy
    4. Arrhythmogenic right ventricular cardiomyopathy
    5. Unclassified cardiomyopathies
  B. Specific cardiomyopathies
    1. Ischemic cardiomyopathy
    2. Valvular cardiomyopathy
    3. Hypertensive cardiomyopathy
    4. Inflammatory cardiomyopathy
      a. Idiopathic
      b. Autoimmune
      c. Infectious
    5. Metabolic cardiomyopathy
      a. Endocrine
      b. Familial storage diseases and infiltrations
      c. Deficiency
      d. Amyloid
    6. General system disease
      a. Connective tissue disorders
      b. Infiltrations and granulomas
    7. Muscular dystrophies
    8. Neuromuscular disorders
    9. Sensitivity and toxic reactions
    10. Peripartal cardiomyopathy

[a]This dates from 1980; see Reference 1.
[b]This dates from 1995; see Reference 2.
NOTE: These are listings of major categories only; specific disorders are not listed.

TABLE 75-2 Functional Classification of Cardiomyopathies

I. Cardiac dilatation
  A. With systolic failure
    1. Idiopathic dilated cardiomyopathy
    2. Late cardiac amyloidosis
    3. Tachycardia-induced congestive failure
  B. Without systolic failure
    1. High cardiac output state
    2. Bradycardia-induced congestive failure
II. Cardiac hypertrophy
  A. With obstruction
    1. Hypertrophic obstructive cardiomyopathy
  B. Without obstruction
    1. Hypertrophic cardiomyopathy
    2. Left ventricular hypertrophy due to systemic hypertension
III. Cardiac restriction
  A. Early cardiac amyloidosis
  B. Endomyocardial fibrosis

NOTE: This is a complete listing of primary categories, but only a few specific examples are provided for illustration.

separate categorizations in series, one based primarily on left ventricular morphology and function and the other based on etiology. A resultant disadvantage is that diseases are placed in two schema that overlap.

The WHO designation of ischemic cardiomyopathy as a specific cardiomyopathy "with impaired contractile performance not explained by the extent of coronary artery disease or ischemic damage" has led to confusion. If ischemia is thought not to be the cause for the impairment, perhaps the adjective *ischemic* should be replaced by one describing the perceived cause, or by *idiopathic*. Most clinicians use *ischemic cardiomyopathy* to describe dilatation and dysfunction, which they believe *is* caused by an ischemic insult. It might be best to eliminate this ambiguous term, since, for the most part, it defines a primary vascular disorder.

FUNCTIONAL CLASSIFICATION OF CARDIOMYOPATHIES

The most widely used functional classification of cardiomyopathy recognizes three disturbances of function: dilatation, hypertrophy, and restriction (Table 75-2). *Dilatation* is dominated by left ventricular cavity enlargement and systolic failure. *Hypertrophy* includes both obstructive and nonobstructive forms. *Restriction* is characterized by inadequate compliance causing restriction of diastolic filling. The value of this scheme is that virtually all cardiomyopathies are readily placed in one of the three categories, and the therapeutic approaches to each category are distinctly different. For example, left ventricular afterload reduction is a cornerstone of therapy for dilated cardiomyopathies with systolic failure, but is of little benefit in the restrictive forms. There are some shortcomings of the functional classification, however. Many diseases are physiologically heterogeneous. Almost all hypertrophic conditions have an element of diastolic restriction. Most dilated ventricles display myocyte hypertrophy. Some diseases change from one category to another during their course; the best example is cardiac amyloidosis, which initially exhibits diastolic stiffness, with complete preservation of systolic performance, followed years later by dilatation and systolic failure.

toward this more common usage, stating, "With increasing understanding of etiology and pathogenesis, the difference between cardiomyopathy and specific heart muscle disease has become indistinct."[2] Examination of the 1980 and 1995 WHO classifications reveals that they are, in fact, somewhat awkward schemes that employ two

TABLE 75-3 Etiologic Classification of Cardiomyopathies

I. Infective/inflammatory
  Idiopathic lymphocytic
    myocarditis
  Peripartum myocarditis
  Eosinophilic myocarditis
  Giant-cell myocarditis
  Viral myocarditis
  Rickettsial myocarditis
  Bacterial myocarditis
  Mycobacterial heart disease
  Spirochetal heart disease
  Fungal myocarditis
  Protozoal myocarditis
  Metazoal myocarditis
  Helminthic myocarditis
  Chemical or drug hypersensitivity
  Autoimmune myocarditis
II. Metabolic
  A. Endocrine
    1. Thyroid disease
      Thyrotoxicosis
      Hypothyroidism
    2. Pheochromocytoma
    3. Acromegaly
    4. Diabetes mellitus
    5. Carcinoid heart disease
  B. Uremia
  C. Hyperoxaluria
  D. Gout
  E. Storage diseases and infiltrative
    processes
    1. Lysosomal storage diseases
      GM1 gangliosidosis
      Tay-Sachs disease and
        variants
      Sandhoff's disease
      Niemann-Pick disease
      Gaucher's disease
      Fabry's disease
      Farber's disease
      Fucosidosis
      Hurler's syndrome
      Scheie's syndrome
      Hunter's syndrome
      Sanfilippo's syndrome
      Morquio's syndrome
      Maroteaux-Lamy syndrome
    2. Glycogen storage diseases
      Pompe's disease
      Cori's disease
      Andersen's disease
      Dominantly inherited
        cardioskeletal myopathy
        with lysosomal
        glycogen storage and
        normal acid maltase
        levels
    3. Refsum's disease

    4. Hand-Schüller-Christian
      syndrome
    5. Adipositos cordis
    6. Hemochromatosis
  F. Deficiencies
    1. Electrolyte
      Hypocalcemia
      Hypophosphatemia
    2. Nutritional
      Kwashiorkor
      Beriberi
      Pellagra
      Scurvy
      Selenium
      Carnitine
III. Amyloid
  AL (primary amyloid, myeloma-
    associated amyloid)
  AA (secondary amyloid, familial
    Mediterranean fever-associated
    amyloid)
  AF (familial amyloid)
  SSA (senile cardiac amyloid,
    senile systemic amyloid)
  IAA (atrial amyloid)
IV. General system disorders
  A. Collagen vascular
    (connective tissue)
    Systemic lupus erythematosus
    Polyarteritis nodosa
    Rheumatoid arthritis
    Scleroderma
    Dermatomyositis
    Whipple's disease
    Kawasaki's disease
  B. Sarcoidosis
  C. Neoplastic
V. Muscular dystrophies, myopathies,
    and neuromuscular disorders
  A. Muscular dystrophies
    Duchenne's muscular
      dystrophy
    Becker's muscular dystrophy
    Myotonic dystrophy
    Facioscapulohumeral
      muscular dystrophy
    Limb girdle dystrophy
    Scapuloperoneal dystrophy,
      including Emery-Dreifuss
      muscular dystrophy
    Congenital muscular
      dystrophy
    Distal muscular dystrophy
  B. Congential myopathies
    Central-core disease
    Desmin myopathy
    Multicore myopathy
    Nemaline myopathy

    Myotubular myopathy
      (centronuclear)
    Congenital fiber-type
      disproportion
    Barth's syndrome
    McLeod's syndrome
    Bethlem's syndrome
  C. Mitochondrial myopathies,
    including
    Kearns-Sayre syndrome
  D. Neuromuscular disorders,
    Friedreich's ataxia
VI. Toxicity, hypersensitivity,
    and physical agent effects
  A. Toxic effects
    1. Caused by drugs, heavy
      metals, and chemical
      agents
      Alcohol (ethyl)
      Amphetamine/
        methamphetamine
      Anthracyclines
      Antidepressants
      Antimony
      Arsenic
      Arsine gas
      Carbon monoxide
      Catecholamines
      Chloroquine
      Cobalt
      Cocaine
      Cyclophosphamide
      Emetine
      5-Fluorouracil
      Hydrocarbons
      Interferon
      Lead
      Lithium
      Mercury
      Methysergide
      Paracetamol
      Phenothiazines
      Phosphorus
      Reserpine
    2. Caused by scorpions,
      spiders, arthropods,
      and snakes
      Scorpions
      Arthropods
      Black widow spider
      Snakes
  B. Hypersensitivity reactions
    Acetazolamide
    Amitriptyline
    Amphotericin B
    Ampicillin
    Carbamazepine
    Chlorthalidone

(Continued)

TABLE 75-3 Etiologic Classification of Cardiomyopathies (*Continued*)

Hydrochlorothiazide	Sulfonylureas	Idiopathic endocardial fibrosis
Indomethacin	Tetracycline	Endocardial fibroelastosis
Isoniazid	C. Physical agents	Infantile cardiomyopathy
Methyldopa	Heat	Arrhythmogenic right ventricular
Oxyphenbutazone	Hypothermia	dysplasia
Para-aminosalicylic acid	Radiation	Carbohydrate-deficient blood
Penicillin	VII. Miscellaneous	glycoprotein syndrome
Phenindione	Peripartum heart disease	Simpson-Golabi-Behmel syndrome
Phenylbutazone	Tachycardia-induced	Isolated ventricular noncompaction
Phenytoin	cardiomyopathy	syndrome
Streptomycin	Ectodermal dysplasia–associated	Myoadenylate deaminase deficiency
Sulfadiazine	cardiomyopathy	
Sulfisoxazole		

NOTE: This is an essentially complete listing of cardiomyopathies of known cause.

TABLE 75-4 Endomyocardial Biopsy Histology Classification of Cardiomyopathies

  I. Inflammatory/immune cardiomyopathy
      Lymphocytic myocarditis
      Rheumatic carditis
      Sarcoidosis
      Giant cell myocarditis
      Cardiac allograft rejection
      Chagas cardiomyopathy
      Hypersensitivity myocarditis
 II. Infectious cardiomyopathy
      Toxoplasmosis
      Lyme carditis
      Cytomegalovirus
III. Infiltrative cardiomyopathy
      Glycogen storage
      Hemochromatosis
      Right ventricular lipomatosis
      Amyloidosis
 IV. Cardiac tumors
      Cardiac origin
      Noncardiac origin
  V. Miscellaneous specific cardiomyopathies
      Anthracycline cardiotoxicity
      Endocardial fibrosis
      Endocardial fibroelastosis
      Fabry's disease
      Carcinoid disease
      Irradiation injury
      Kearns-Sayre syndrome
      Henoch-Schonlein purpura
      Chloroquine cardiomyopathy
      Carnitine deficiency
      Hypereosinophilic syndrome
 VI. Nonspecific abnormalities
      Idiopathic dilated cardiomyopathy
      Other cardiomyopathies of unknown cause
VII. No histologic abnormality

NOTE: This represents a relatively complete listing of diagnoses that have been made by endomyocardial biopsy and reported in the literature.

TABLE 75-5 ICD-9 Classification of Heart Disease

ICD-9 Code	Description
402.00	Hypertensive heart disease, malignant, w/o CHF
402.01	Hypertensive heart disease, malignant, w CHF
402.10	Hypertensive heart disease, benign, w/o CHF
402.11	Hypertensive heart disease, benign, w CHF
402.90	Hypertensive heart disease, unspecified, w/o CHF
402.91	Hypertensive heart disease, unspecified, w CHF
422.90	Acute myocarditis, unspecified
422.91	Idiopathic myocarditis
425.0	Endomyocardial fibrosis
425.1	Hypertrophic obstructive cardiomyopathy
425.2	Obscure cardiomyopathy of Africa
425.3	Endomyocardial fibroelastosis
425.4	Idiopathic cardiomyopathy
425.5	Alcoholic cardiomyopathy
425.7	Nutritional and metabolic cardiomyopathy
425.8	Cardiomyopathy in other diseases classified elsewhere
425.9	Secondary cardiomyopathy, unspecified
428.0	Congestive heart failure
428.1	Left heart failure
428.9	Heart failure, unspecified
429.0	Myocarditis, unspecified
429.1	Myocardial degeneration
429.3	Cardiomegaly
429.82	Hyperkinetic heart disease
674.84	Postpartum cardiomyopathy

ABBREVIATION: CHF = congestive heart failure.

TABLE 75-6 "Cardiomyopathy" Cited in ICD-10

I25.5	Ischemic cardiomyopathy
I42	Cardiomyopathy
I42.0	Dilated cardiomyopathy
I42.1	Obstructive hypertrophic cardiomyopathy
I42.2	Other hypertrophic cardiomyopathy
I42.5	Other restrictive cardiomyopathy
I42.6	Alcoholic cardiomyopathy
I42.7	Cardiomyopathy due to drugs and other external agents
I42.8	Other cardiomyopathies
I42.9	Cardiomyopathy, unspecified
O90.3	Cardiomyopathy in the puerperium

The functional scheme also associates diseases that have vastly different causes, some of which require special therapeutic interventions. For example, the primary therapy for cardiac hemochromatosis, often an initially restrictive disease, is removal of excessive iron stores; this would not, of course, be effective treatment for other diseases similarly classified. Despite its shortcomings, the functional classification of cardiomyopathy remains the most popular among clinicians because it is based on easily understood physiology and is relevant to therapy.

TABLE 75-7 Therapeutic Classification of Cardiomyopathies

I. Reduce ventricular afterload
   Idiopathic dilated cardiomyopathy
   Late cardiac amyloidosis
II. Reduce ventricular preload
   Endocardial fibrosis
   Early cardiac amyloidosis
III. Increase ventricular compliance
   Hypertrophic cardiomyopathy
IV. Relieve ventricular obstruction
   Hypertrophic obstructive cardiomyopathy
V. Improve cardiac rhythm
   Cardiomyopathy of persistent tachycardia
VI. Specific therapy
   A. Replace deficiency
      Carnitine deficiency cardiomyopathy
   B. Remove toxic agent
      Hemochromatosis
      Hypersensitivity
   C. Immunosuppression
      Giant-cell myocarditis
      Lymphocyte myocarditis(?)
   D. Correct systemic disease
      Uremic cardiomyopathy
      Cardiomyopathy of cancer
      Systemic lupus erythematosus
   E. Modulate neurohormonal environment
      Idiopathic dilated cardiomyopathy
      Most causes of congestive heart failure

NOTE: This is a complete listing of primary categories with a few specific examples for illustration.

ETIOLOGIC CLASSIFICATION

This scheme utilizes knowledge about cardiomyopathies more extensively than all the others. It has the most primary categories because there are numerous known causes that are not interrelated. Table 75-3 categorizes the diseases covered in Chaps. 69, 73 to 80, 85, 86, and 91 to 94. The general outline established by WHO in 1980 is followed roughly. In many cases the etiologic agent is poorly understood (e.g., uremic cardiomyopathy), or the cardiomyopathy is associated with another disease, but the mechanism responsible for heart failure is unknown (e.g., cardiomyopathy of systemic neoplasia).

While this classification has the advantage of being inclusive, it has the disadvantage of being awkwardly long. It has 7 primary and 42 secondary categories. In addition, most similarly classified disorders are anatomically, physiologically, and therapeutically unrelated. Thus, this classification is not used routinely by clinicians. It has been used most frequently as an organizational scheme in textbooks and reviews concerning heart muscle disease and cardiomyopathy.

ENDOMYOCARDIAL BIOPSY CLASSIFICATION

Because the heart can be safely biopsied, antemortem histologic diagnosis can be used to classify cardiomyopathies. Dozens of specific myocardial diseases can be detected by biopsy (Table 75-4). The great strength of histologic diagnosis is that it is definitive and unequivocal when a specific disease is observed. In contrast, numerous deficiencies make this method of classification relatively restricted in use. The foremost problem is that, although the number of specific histologic diagnoses is large, they represent a small proportion of all cases—certainly fewer than 15 percent. The histology in most patients with cardiomyopathy is nonspecific and nondiagnostic. Hypertrophy, or fiber attenuation, and fibrosis may be seen in varying degrees in almost any disorder and are the only findings in most cases of idiopathic dilated cardiomyopathy and hypertrophic cardiomyopathy (as well as in many instances of heart failure due to myocardial infarction and valvular dysfunction). Furthermore, completely normal histology may occasionally be seen on biopsy in cases of severe dilatation and systolic failure.

Myocardial biopsy samples can be subjected to several additional analytic techniques that expand the potential for classification using endomyocardial biopsy. While at present these analyses are only investigational and none can be generally applied, it is likely that one or more of them will become clinically useful in the future and could form the basis of a classification with wide appeal.

INTERNATIONAL CLASSIFICATION OF DISEASE

The International Classification of Disease was developed by WHO in 1948 for registering disease incidences. In 1977, the United States National Center for Health Statistics (NCHS) modified the ICD-9 code to allow coding of medical records. That modification was labeled "ICD-9-CM," which stands for *International Classification of Disease*, Ninth Revision, Clinical Modification. In 1989 it became mandatory for physicians in the United States to include an ICD-9-CM code on their Medicare claims. It is fascinating to see how utterly different a classification system intended for governmental statistics and claims payment is in comparison to those intended for scientific or clinical purposes. The code is a remarkable hodgepodge, combining multiple categories of knowledge into one classification system. Diseases are variously defined according to one or more features such as etiology, anatomy, physiology, comorbidity, symptoms, and even method and extent of diagnosis. It is no wonder that this code is impossible to remember and notoriously ambiguous and difficult to use. In Table 75-5, the codes describing cardiomyopathies have been extracted from the 1999 version of the ICD-9-CM, where they appear in several groups scattered throughout the listing. Relatively few— 25—cardiomyopathy diagnoses are coded, and these represent only 9 specific entities. Some well-recognized myocardial diseases are completely ignored, such as arrhythmogenic right ventricular dysplasia. The new revision of the code, ICD-10, has not yet come into general use for medical coding, but was used by the NCHS for its 1999 mortality statistics report. The revision includes minor changes in terminology for the cardiomyopathies and has added a leading letter, resulting in an alphanumeric code. Arrhythmogenic right ventricular dysplasia is still absent from the listing. Table 75-6 shows all instances of "cardiomyopathy" in ICD-10. This classification system and the method of classification it represents are certainly not recommended to physicians and scientists.

THERAPEUTIC CLASSIFICATION

A classification based on specific therapies borrows heavily from the functional and the etiologic classifications of cardiomyopathy. This classification adds information regarding treatment that is not available in other schemes and therefore may be useful to clinicians.

Nevertheless, this classification has several shortcomings. First, often more than one class of therapy is appropriate for a disease. Therefore, the classification must categorize diseases on the basis of their *primary* therapy. This introduces some instability to the classification, since therapeutic preferences are subject to variance in opinion and to change with new research. The greatest fault of therapeutic categorization is that when new therapies are introduced, the existing classification becomes obsolete. The therapeutic classification shown in Table 75-7 illustrates the sensitivity of this approach to opinion. Some might argue, for example, that diuretic therapy remains the primary treatment for dilated cardiomyopathy.

Note that some commonly employed therapies, such as inotropic agents and cardiac transplantation, do not appear in Table 75-7 because they are often not the initial or primary therapies.

GENE-BASED CLASSIFICATION

Aside from traumatic, iatrogenic, infectious, and certain other secondary cardiac disorders, most heart diseases result from an abnormality of gene function. Even among the previous exceptions, genetic influences often determine outcomes. For example, infectious myocardial processes critically depend on and are modified by gene expression. Many diseases caused by adverse gene behavior are due to inherited or acquired genetic mutations and others result from more common gene variants. Several diseases are now defined genetically, including hypertrophic cardiomyopathy, long QT syndrome, forms of dilated cardiomyopathy, muscular dystrophies involving the heart, arrhythmogenic right ventricular dysplasia, and Brugada syndrome. A genetic classification of cardiomyopathies would specify the type of genetic disorder (chromosomal, single genic, polygenic, mitochondrial, or somatic cellular) and the mode of inheritance (autosomal or X-linked, and dominant or recessive), the chromosomes or chromosomal locations, and the genes involved. A classification system based upon genetic derangements is diagnostically and therapeutically useless unless the biochemical and resultant physiologic aberrations are understood. Thus, complete genetic classification should also identify the specific mutation or the regional location of the mutation within the gene, since phenotype and therapy often vary with each specific mutation or region of mutation.

In the future, many cardiac diseases will be shown to be caused by genes functioning at the extremes of normal behavior, and these behavior abnormalities could be classified in much the same way as inherited mutations. Gene-based classification will become the best classification system for cardiomyopathies, because it will at once precisely and uniquely define the disease and make evident the necessary diagnostic and therapeutic actions.[3]

Since the clinical course of many cardiomyopathies is the result not only of genetic defects but also of the responses of normal genes to abnormal pathophysiology imposed by those defects, cardiomyopathies can also be characterized dynamically by their RNA expression, using complimentary DNA arrays. This extension of genetic classification to include a point-in-time assessment of gene expression could become an important tool allowing the treating physician to provide highly individualized therapy, tailored to the immediate state of the disease process.[4]

SUMMARY

No single classification of cardiomyopathy is generally accepted within the biomedical community. An attempt to gain a consensus for one of the many classifications in current use is not likely to succeed because we are unable to subdivide meaningfully cases of idiopathic dilated cardiomyopathy, which constitute the large majority of all cases. At present, the individual health practitioner or scientist should use the classification scheme that best serves his or her purpose. For clinicians, this will often be the functional classification.

In the future, a widely acceptable classification may develop that is based on the molecular genetics of myocardial disease. Although this field is only beginning to develop, it is the discipline most likely to contribute to the understanding of causes and the development of new treatments for myocardial disease.

References

1. Report of the WHO/ISFC task force on the definition and classification of cardiomyopathies. *Br Heart J* 1980;44:672–673.
2. Richardson P, McKenna W, Bristow M, et al. Report of the 1995 World Health Organization/International Society and Federation of Cardiology Task Force on the Definition and Classification of cardiomyopathies. *Circulation* 1996;93:841–842.
3. Keating MT, Sanguinetti MC. Molecular genetic insights into cardiovascular disease. *Science* 1996;272:681–685.
4. Chien KR. Genomic circuits and the integrative biology of cardiac diseases. *Nature* 2000;407:227–232.

DILATED CARDIOMYOPATHIES

Luisa Mestroni / Edward M. Gilbert / Teresa J. Bohlmeyer / Michael R. Bristow

BACKGROUND AND HISTORICAL PERSPECTIVE

This chapter describes the phenotypic and clinical characteristics of the primary and secondary dilated cardiomyopathies, the most common cause of the clinical syndrome of chronic heart failure.[1] Heart failure is an enormously important clinical problem, which, if not contained or solved, may ultimately overwhelm health care resources.[2] The clinical syndrome of heart failure is a complex process where the primary pathophysiology is quickly obscured by a variety of superimposed secondary adaptive, maladaptive, and counterregulatory processes (see also Chap. 24). Heart failure is best understood and approached from the vantage point of *myocardial failure*, most commonly associated with a dilated cardiomyopathy phenotype.[3] As an indication of the importance of the problems of cardiomyopathy and heart failure, the cardiomyopathies have been reclassified by a World Health Organization/International Society and Federation of Cardiology (WHO/ISFC) task force[3] (and elaborated on further below).

Importance of Heart Failure

Due to its high prevalence (1 to 1.5 percent of the adult population) and high morbidity, including frequent hospitalizations, the clinical syndrome of heart failure is among the most costly medical problems in the United States.[2] Despite improvements in the treatment of heart failure introduced in the last 10 years, including the general availability of cardiac transplantation and better medical treatment, clinical outcome following the onset of symptoms has not changed substantially.[1] That is, mortality remains high (median survival of 1.7 years for men and 3.2 years for women),[1] the natural history progressive,[1] the cost excessive,[2] and disability[2] and morbidity[2,4] among the highest of any disease or disease syndrome.

Relationship of Myocardial Failure and Dilated Cardiomyopathies to the Clinical Syndrome of Heart Failure

The vast majority of the cases of heart failure are caused by heart muscle disease (cardiomyopathy). Within the WHO categorization[3] of cardiomyopathy (Table 76-1), the most common cause of the clinical syndrome of heart failure is a secondary (ischemic, valvular, hypertensive, etc.) or a primary (e.g., idiopathic or familial) *dilated cardiomyopathy,* defined as a ventricular chamber exhibiting increased diastolic and systolic volumes and a low (<40 percent) ejection fraction. The natural history of the clinical syndrome of heart failure depends on the course of myocardial failure, since (1) the most powerful single predictor of outcome is the degree of left ventricular (LV) dysfunction as assessed by the LV ejection fraction[5]; (2) treatment that improves intrinsic ventricular function improves the natural history of heart failure[6]; and (3) treatment that ultimately worsens intrinsic function, such as many types of positive inotropic agents, is associated with an adverse effect on outcome.[6]

THE WHO/ISFC CLASSIFICATION OF CARDIOMYOPATHIES

The WHO/ISFC classification of cardiomyopathies was revised in 1996[3] to accommodate several rapidly emerging realities. The first was that the molecular genetic basis of previously unknown types of heart muscle disease is rapidly being elucidated, so it really makes no sense to reserve the classification for "unknown etiologies" of cardiomyopathy.[7] The second consideration was that many of the mechanisms responsible for the natural history of myocardial dysfunction are qualitatively similar in primary versus secondary dilated cardiomyopathies,[8] which accurately predicted a qualitatively similar

TABLE 76-1 The World Health Organization//International Society and Federation of Cardiology Classification of the Cardiomyopathies

Category	Definition

I. Dilated (DCM)
  1. Primary
  2. Secondary
	↑ EDV, ↑ ESV; low EF

II. Restrictive (RCM)
  1. Primary
  2. Secondary
	↓ EDV, ↔ ESV; ↑ FP, ↔ EF

III. Hypertrophic (HCM)	↑↑ septal and ↑ posterior wall thickness, myofibrillar disarray Mutation in sarcomeric protein, autosomal dominant inheritance
IV. Arrhythmogenic RV (ARVC)	Fibrofatty replacement of RV myocardium Autosomal dominant (most) and recessive inheritance

V. Unclassified
  1. Primary
  2. Secondary
	Not meeting criteria for other categories
	Features of > one category

ABBREVIATIONS: EDV = end-diastolic volume, ESV = end-systolic volume, EF = LV ejection fraction, FP = LV filling pressure; CM = cardiomyopathy.
SOURCE: From Richardson et al.[3]

response to treatment targeted at these mechanisms.[9,10] This made the exclusion of secondary or "known cause"[7] cardiomyopathies gratuitous, and their inclusion in the new classification allows all cardiomyopathies to be classified under one scheme.

As shown in Table 76-1, the WHO/ISFC classification of cardiomyopathy uses two separate methods to define the individual categories. The first is based on the global anatomic description of chamber dimensions in systole and diastole. Thus the dilated and restrictive categories have definitions based on left ventricular dimensions or volume, which also define function via calculated ejection fraction (see Table 76-1). The justification for this is that these two groups have distinct natural histories and respond distinctly differently to medical treatment. The second method of creating individual categories within the WHO/ISFC classification is for cardiomyopathies that are genetically based, have unique myocardial phenotypic features, and do not exhibit extracardiac phenotypes. Thus hypertrophic cardiomyopathy (HCM), caused by mutations in contractile proteins manifesting as a unique phenotype, merits a separate category. The same is true for arrhythmogenic right ventricular dysplasia (ARVC), which also has a unique phenotype and likely will turn out to be completely genetic in basis, as has been the case with HCM. On the other hand, genetic cardiomyopathies without unique phenotypes, such as the dilated cardiomyopathy of Becker-Duchenne, are included as one form of the anatomic/chamber dimension category (category I).

The WHO/ISFC classification includes another assignment of nomenclature in "secondary" cardiomyopathies, i.e., those associated with known cardiac or systemic processes.[3] These are referred to as *specific cardiomyopathies,* named for the disease process with which they are associated. Thus an ischemic cardiomyopathy would be a specific cardiomyopathy related to previous myocardial infarction (MI) and the subsequent remodeling process, which usually would fall within the dilated class. On the other hand, a hypertensive cardiomyopathy might be classified as either dilated or restrictive depending on the chamber dimensions. Therefore the correct term for

these cardiomyopathies would be *ischemic dilated cardiomyopathy* and *hypertensive dilated* (or *restrictive*) *cardiomyopathy.*

Molecular Mechanisms in Cardiomyopathies and Myocardial Failure: Disease Phenotype Produced by Alterations in Gene Expression

As shown in Table 76-2, there are three general categories of mechanisms whereby altered gene expression can lead to a phenotypic change in cardiac myocytes.[11] These are (1) a single gene defect, e.g., as present in β-myosin heavy-chain codon 403 in familial HCM[12] and in an analogous region of α-MHC in HCM transgenic mouse models[13,14]; (2) polymorphic variation in modifier genes, such as is present in many components of the renin-angiotensin system[15–17]; and (3) maladaptive regulated expression of completely normal genes, such as for the mechanisms responsible for progressive myocardial dysfunction and remodeling in secondary dilated cardiomyopathies.[6,11]

GENETIC CAUSES OF CARDIOMYOPATHIES IN HUMANS AND ANIMAL MODELS

The ability to genetically manipulate the cardiovascular system has made it possible to investigate the role of a number of genes in the developing and adult mouse heart (for a review, see Ikeda and Ross[18]). The discovery that mutations in sarcomeric proteins lead to HCM has made it possible to generate animal models for this disease.[13,14] In the case of myosin mutations, a single genetic defect initiates a pathway which ultimately leads to hypertrophy and then, in males, may result in late decompensation and ventricular

TABLE 76-2 Three General Mechanisms by which Alterations in Gene Expression Can Influence the Development or Progression of a Dilated Cardiomyopathy

Type of Process	Examples
Gene mutation	• Cytoskeletal genes • Sarcomeric genes • Signaling pathway genes
Polymorphic variation in modifier genes	Angiotensin-converting enzyme (ACE),[16,54,55] β₂-adrenergic receptor,[57] endothelin type A receptor[59]
Altered expression of a completely normal, wild-type gene	Decreased expression: β₁-adrenergic receptors,[8] α-MyHC,[60,61] SERCA-2[62] Increased expression: ANP,[63] β-MyHC,[60] ACE,[64,65] TNF-α,[66] endothelin,[67] βARK[68]

dilatation.[14] Multiple gene mutations have now been associated causally with familial dilated cardiomyopathies, as discussed further on in this chapter.

A serendipitous genetic model of dilated cardiomyopathy and heart failure (*myf 5* mice) has been generated by activation of a skeletal muscle genetic program in the heart.[19] These mice have a dilated cardiomyopathy phenotype characterized by progressive myocardial dysfunction and dilatation. They develop the clinical syndrome of heart failure, and they have an extraordinarily high (>90 percent at 260 days) heart failure–related mortality.[19] Another serendipitous genetic model of dilated cardiomyopathy is the muscle LIM protein (MLP) knockout mouse.[20] MLP is a positive regulator of muscle differentiation, which is ordinarily expressed at high levels in the heart and may be involved in myofibrillar protein assembly along the actin-based cytoskeleton.[20] MLP knockout mice exhibit typical features of dilated cardiomyopathy, including decreased systolic and diastolic function and β-adrenergic receptor pathway desensitization.[20]

These characteristics make this model very useful in assessing the mechanisms which lead to the development and progression of myocardial failure. Thus, in transgenic mouse models, both altered expression of contractile proteins and perturbation of myocyte cytoarchitecture can lead to the dilated cardiomyopathy phenotype.

There are several additional transgenic mouse models of cardiomyopathy that may be more relevant to the production of a dilated phenotype in humans. Several of them involve overexpression of components of the adrenergic receptor pathway, the heterodimeric G-protein α_s subunit ($G\alpha_s$)[21]; the α_2-,[22] β_1-,[23,24] and β_2-adrenergic receptors,[25] and protein kinase A.[26] These β-adrenergic pathway transgenic mouse models exhibit similar histopathology, consisting of myocyte hypertrophy and increased fibrosis, evidence of apoptosis, systolic and diastolic dysfunction, and ultimately development of left ventricular dilatation.[21–25,27] Other transgenic mice that ultimately develop a dilated phenotype include those with cardiac restricted overexpression of activated MEK5,[28] CaM kinase IV,[29] activated calcineurin,[30] and calsequestrin.[31] Still another mouse model of dilated cardiomyopathy includes mitochondrial transcription factor A gene knockout.[32]

Several transgenic models of concentric or symmetric left ventricular hypertrophy have now been reported, including overexpression of *ras*,[33] *myc*,[34] α_1-adrenergic receptors,[35] the heterodimeric G-protein α_q subunit ($G_{\alpha q}$),[36] and the protein kinase C (PKC).[37] The mechanisms for the induction of increased ventricular wall thickness are diverse, inasmuch as the *ras*, α_1-receptor, $G_{\alpha q}$, and PKC overexpressors exhibit true cellular hypertrophy with an increase in cell size,[33,35–37] whereas the *myc* animal exhibits cardiac myocyte hyperplasia.[34] The HCM phenotypes discussed earlier illustrate the principle that apparently diverse signals can culminate in the same phenotype, presumably by converging on final common pathways.

Multiple gene defects have been identified that can produce a dilated cardiomyopathy in humans, as discussed in more detail in the section on familial forms of dilated cardiomyopathy. As listed in Table 76-2, these include mutations in cytoskeletal genes, such as desmin,[38] dystrophin,[39,40] delta-sarcoglycan,[41] metavinculin,[42] and lamin[43,44] as well as sarcomeric genes, such as cardiac α-actin,[45] cardiac beta-myosin heavy chain, cardiac troponin T,[46] α-tropomyosin,[47] and titin.[48] Likewise, cytoskeletal and sarcomeric gene mutations may cause the naturally occurring dilated cardiomyopathy in animals: in the Syrian hamster, the disease is caused by mutations in the delta-sarcoglycan gene,[49] whereas in turkeys, it is due to mutations in cardiac troponin T.[50] Recently, a mutation of the phospholamban gene has been identified in idiopathic dilated cardiomyopathy (IDC),[51] indicating that altered signaling pathways may lead to the same IDC phenotype.

POLYMORPHIC VARIATION IN MODIFIER GENES

Genes exhibit polymorphic variation; i.e., normal variants of genes exist in the population that are of slightly different size or sequence.[52] Some gene polymorphisms are associated with differences in function of the expressed protein gene product, and some of these differences in function likely account for the "biological variation" routinely encountered in population studies of disease susceptibility or clinical response to treatment.

Examples of modifier genes that may have an impact on the natural history of a dilated cardiomyopathy (Table 76-2) include the angiotensin-converting enzyme (ACE) *DD* genotype,[15–17] where individuals are homozygous for the "deletion" variant, which is associated with increased circulating[15] and cardiac tissue[53] ACE activity. The *DD* genotype appears to be a risk factor for early remodeling after MI[54] and for the development of end-stage ischemic and idiopathic dilated cardiomyopathy.[16,17,55] Other potentially important polymorphic variants that may influence the natural history of a cardiomyopathy involve the angiotensin AT$_1$ receptor,[56] β_2-adrenergic receptors,[57] the α_{2C}-adrenergic receptor with or without a β_1-receptor polymorphism,[58] and the endothelin receptor type A.[59]

Finally, recent pharmacogenomic studies have shown that polymorphic variations can influence the response to medications. Patients with the DD genotype, who were found to have a worse prognosis, at the same time appeared to respond significantly better to beta-blocker therapy compared to the other genotypes (*II* and *ID*).[17]

ALTERED, MALADAPTIVE EXPRESSION OF A COMPLETELY NORMAL GENE

The third way in which altered gene expression can contribute to the development of a cardiomyopathy is altered, maladaptive expression of a completely normal "wild-type" gene.[11] This occurs most commonly in the context of progression of heart muscle disease and myocardial failure, which is the natural history of virtually all cardiomyopathies once they are established. Examples in this category (see Table 76-2) include downregulation of β_1-adrenergic receptors,[8] α-myosin heavy chain (α-MHC),[60,61] and the sarcoplasmic reticulum Ca^{2+} ATPase[62] genes and upregulation in the atrial natriuretic peptide (ANP),[63] β-myosin heavy chain (β-MHC),[60] ACE,[64,65] tumor necrosis factor alpha (TNF-α),[66] endothelin,[67] and β-adrenergic receptor kinase (βARK)[68] genes. These concepts are discussed further below.

Recent data have shown that, in patients who respond to treatment by increasing left ventricular ejection fraction, beta-blocker therapy may restore some aspects of altered gene expression, increasing the expression of sarcoplasmic-reticulum calcium ATPase and of α-myosin heavy chain, and decreasing β-myosin heavy chain.[69]

PATHOPHYSIOLOGIC PROCESSES INVOLVED IN MYOCARDIAL DYSFUNCTION/REMODELING AND THEIR PROGRESSION

Tissue preparations and myocytes isolated from failing human hearts exhibit evidence of decreased contractile function.[70] Assuming that loading conditions and ischemia are not adversely affecting cardiac myocyte function, in the setting of chronic systolic dysfunction from a dilated cardiomyopathy, progressive myocardial failure is most likely caused by myocardial cell loss or changes in the gene expression of proteins which regulate or produce muscle contraction. Figures 76-1 and 76-2 summarize these general points and emphasize the central roles of the renin-angiotensin system (RAS) and adrenergic nervous system (ANS) in promoting cell loss, growth and remodeling, and altered gene expression.[6]

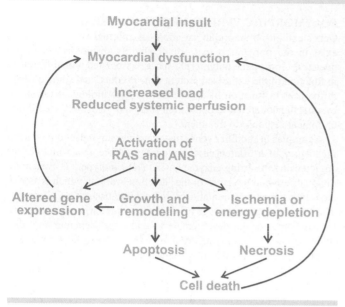

FIGURE 76-1 Relationship of neurohormonal activation and production of cardiac myocyte loss due to apoptosis and necrosis and altered gene expression. Cell loss and altered gene expression result in more myocardial dysfunction, and a vicious cycle is established. RAS = renin-angiotensin system; ANS = adrenergic nervous system.

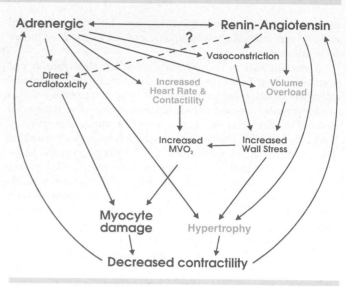

FIGURE 76-2 Heart failure compensatory mechanisms that are activated to support the failing heart. Light-colored areas indicate physiologic mechanisms that stabilize pump function.

MYOCARDIAL DYSFUNCTION AND REMODELING DUE TO ALTERED EXPRESSION OF CONTRACTILITY-REGULATING GENES AND CHANGES IN SARCOMERIC ASSEMBLY

Gene expression can be defined broadly as the expression of a fully or normally functioning protein gene product or, more narrowly (and commonly), as the steady-state abundance of a gene's mRNA transcript. Using either definition, numerous abnormalities of gene expression of normal, wild-type genes have been demonstrated in the failing human heart as discussed earlier, with examples listed in Table 76-2. In order to characterize the abnormalities that may account for progressive myocardial dysfunction and remodeling, it is useful to subdivide them into two general categories,[71] as shown in Table 76-3. The first category encompasses mechanisms that subserve *intrinsic* function, or the mechanisms responsible for contraction and relaxation of the heart in the basal or resting state. *Intrinsic function* is defined as myocardial contraction and relaxation in the absence of extrinsic influences, such as neurotransmitters or hormones. The second general category is *modulated* function, which comprises the mechanisms responsible for the remarkable ability of the heart to increase or decrease its performance dramatically (by two- to tenfold) and rapidly in response to various physiologic or physical stimuli. Other critical organs such as the brain, kidney, and liver do not exhibit this quality. *Modulated function* is defined as stimulation or inhibition of myocardial contraction or relaxation by endogenous bioactive compounds, including neurotransmitters, cytokines, autocrine/paracrine substances, and hormones.

In the failing human heart, changes are present in the expression of genes potentially responsible for both general types of myocardial function depicted in Table 76-2.[6,71] Abnormalities of intrinsic function include the factors responsible for an altered length-tension relation,[72–74] a blunted force-frequency response,[75,76] and/or the signals responsible for abnormal cellular and chamber remodeling.[77,78] In the case of the abnormal force frequency and length-tension responses, the evidence favors abnormal contractile function of individual cardiac myocytes.[70] As shown in Table 76-3, these abnormalities likely reside in the contractile proteins or their regulatory elements,[60,61,79,80] mechanisms involved in excitation-contraction coupling,[62] or the cytoskeleton.[20,81–83] However, within these possibilities for altered intrinsic function, there is not currently a consensus as to which specific abnormalities are present in IDC, the most common form of heart failure studied in humans. For cellular remodeling, in both human ventricles[84] and animal models[78,85] the assembly of sarcomeres in series leads to a myocyte that is markedly increased in length but not in diameter, which contributes to remodeling at the chamber level. Such remodeling places the chamber and the myocyte at an energetic disadvantage because of the attendant increase in wall stress,[86] which is one of the major determinants of myocardial oxygen consumption. Inadequate myocyte energy production, particularly associated with key subcellular ion flux mechanisms or the myosin ATPase cycle,[87] in turn would contribute to myocyte contractile dysfunction. Moreover, the hypertrophy process itself leads to a qualitative change in contractile protein gene expression (induction of a "fetal" gene program), which reduces contractile function.[11,60,61,79] On the other hand, cardiac myocyte contractile dysfunc-

TABLE 76-3 General Categorization of Myocardial Function

INTRINSIC (*function in the absence of neural or hormonal influence*)	MODULATED (*Function that may be stimulated or inhibited by extrinsic factors including neurotransmitters, cytokines, or hormones*)
• Contractile proteins	• R-G-adenylyl cyclase pathways
• E-C coupling mechanisms	• R-G-phospholipase C pathways
• R-G-adenylyl cyclase pathways	
• Bioenergetics	
• Cytoskeleton	
• Sarcomere and cell remodeling	

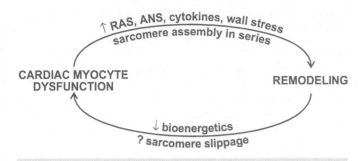

FIGURE 76-3 Relationship between progressive myocardial dysfunction and remodeling. RAS = renin-angiotensin system; ANS = adrenergic nervous system.

tion likely plays a role in the remodeling process, inasmuch as medical treatment which improves intrinsic myocardial function can reverse remodeling.[6,69] Thus contractile dysfunction and remodeling at the cellular level are intimately related to the progressive contractile dysfunction and chamber enlargement that define the natural history of myocardial failure.[88] These concepts are summarized in Fig. 76-3.

In contrast to abnormalities of intrinsic function, a consensus has been reached on several specific abnormalities in the stimulation component of modulated function. Most of these changes concern β-adrenergic signal transduction.[8,11,71] The ability of β-adrenergic stimulation to increase heart rate and contractility is markedly attenuated in the failing heart due to multiple changes at the level of receptors, G proteins, and adenylyl cyclase. This produces a major abnormality in the stimulation component of modulated function. In addition, the inhibition component of modulated function is also abnormal in the failing heart due to a reduction in parasympathetic drive.[89]

There is obviously overlap between the two major subdivisions of myocardial function. Recent data indicate that even in the absence of adrenergic stimulation, β-adrenergic receptors have intrinsic activity.[90–93] That is, a small percentage of receptors are in an activated state without agonist occupancy and, as such, can support intrinsic myocardial function.[91,92] Thus overexpression of human β_2-adrenergic receptors can markedly increase intrinsic myocardial function,[92] as can enhancement of sarcoplasmic reticulum calcium uptake and release by genetic ablation of the phospholamban gene.[94] The recent realization that active-state, agonist-unoccupied β-adrenergic receptors can modulate intrinsic myocardial function is the reason why the "R-G-adenylyl cyclase" mechanism appears in both categories in Table 76-3.

PROGRESSIVE MYOCARDIAL DYSFUNCTION AND REMODELING DUE TO LOSS OF CARDIAC MYOCYTES

The second general mechanism by which myocardial function may be adversely affected is by loss of cardiac myocytes, which may also play a role in the progression of ventricular dysfunction in dilated cardiomyopathies. Cardiac myocyte loss can occur via toxic mechanisms producing necrosis, or by "programmed cell death," producing apoptosis. Apoptosis, which is likely due to a combination of growth signaling and cell cycle dysregulation, has been described in end-stage IDC[95] as well as in the β_1-adrenergic receptor,[23] the $G_{\alpha s}$ overexpressor transgenic mice,[27] and in models of hypertrophy.[96] However, data from human studies refer to a very late stage of IDC or ischemic dilated cardiomyopathy, treated with multiple powerful intravenous inotropic medications[95]; it is therefore not clear whether apoptosis plays a significant role in remodeling and/or chamber systolic dysfunction before this point is reached in the natural history of the dilated cardiomyopathies.

Importance of "Compensatory" Mechanisms in the Progression of Myocardial Failure

As depicted in Figs. 76-1 and 76-2, there is now a large body of information supporting the idea that *activation of the ANS and RAS compensatory mechanisms contributes to, or is responsible for, the progressive nature of both myocardial failure and the natural history of the heart failure clinical syndrome.*[6] This evidence includes the observations that activation of both these systems is associated with progression of myocardial dysfunction and the heart failure syndrome, and clinical trial data that consistently demonstrate that inhibition of these systems can prevent deterioration in or improve myocardial function as well as reduce mortality.[6,10] Although we now know that chronic activation of the ANS and RAS contributes to the progressive nature of myocardial dysfunction in human heart failure, we know virtually nothing about how these systems adversely affect the biology of the cardiac myocyte. What we do know is that mechanisms within both general categories outlined in Table 76-3 must be involved in the adverse myocardial effects mediated by the ANS and RAS. This is so because modulated function may be improved by treatment with ACE inhibitors or beta-blocking agents. Progressive myocardial dysfunction and remodeling are attenuated by both beta-blocking agents and ACE inhibitors; in cardiomyopathies, intrinsic myocardial function is improved and remodeling is reversed by chronic treatment with beta-blocking agents.[6,69] Additionally, mortality in chronic heart failure is directly related to activation of the ANS[97,98] and RAS[99] and may be related to the activation of other neurohormonal or autocrine/paracrine systems as well.

Regardless of the type or cause of dilated cardiomyopathy, an initial myocardial insult resulting in this phenotype exhibits common pathophysiologic features that are summarized in Fig. 76-1. That is, a myocardial insult that produces systolic dysfunction will be followed by the initiation of processes designed to temporarily stabilize pump function. The possible mechanisms available for such stabilization are in fact limited. As shown in Fig. 76-2, in chronological order of their action, they are an increase in heart rate and contractility mediated by an increase in cardiac β-adrenergic signaling (produced within seconds of the onset of pump dysfunction), volume expansion in order to use the Frank-Starling mechanism to increase stroke volume (evident within hours of the onset of pump dysfunction), and cardiac myocyte hypertrophy to increase the number of contractile elements (evident within days or weeks of the onset of pump dysfunction). As shown in Fig. 76-2, these compensatory adjustments are largely accomplished by activation of the RAS and adrenergic nervous ANS systems. However, despite the short-term (days to months) stability achieved via these mechanisms, they ultimately prove harmful.[6] The best evidence that chronic, continued activation of the RAS and ANS contributes to progressive myocardial dysfunction and remodeling comes from clinical trials where both inhibitors of the RAS (ACE inhibitors) and ANS (β-adrenergic receptor–blocking agents) prevent these two phenomena, and beta-blocking agents actually may reverse remodeling and progressive systolic dysfunction.[6]

Much current work is focused on the precise pathophysiologic mechanisms by which activation of the RAS and ANS produces remodeling and adverse effects on myocardial function. Some of the possibilities are given in Fig. 76-1; they include an exacerbation of ischemia and/or energy depletion, leading to cell loss via necrosis, cell loss by programmed cell death, direct promotion of hypertrophy and remodeling through stimulation of cell growth, and alterations in cardiac myocyte gene expression.[6] A key feature of the schema shown in Fig. 76-1 is the process of remodeling, which is discussed in more detail in Chap. 26. Virtually all dilated cardiomyopathies undergo this process, which is characterized by progressive dilatation, progressive myocardial systolic dysfunction in viable segments, and a change in chamber shape whereby the ventricle becomes less elliptical and more round.[6,77] As shown in Fig. 76-3, this places the ventricle at an energetic disadvantage,[6,77,86] which likely contributes to further myocardial dysfunction, which then contributes to progressive remodeling. The latter observation is based on data with β-adrenergic blocking agents, which produce an improvement in systolic dysfunction that can be detected prior to a reversal in remodeling.[6] As emphasized by Fig. 76-3, each myocardial degenerative process likely begets the other, leading to an inexorably progressive deterioration in myocardial performance and clinical condition.

SCOPE OF DILATED CARDIOMYOPATHIES

The number of cardiac or systemic processes that can produce a dilated cardiomyopathy or are associated with it is plentiful and remarkably varied, as shown in Table 76-4. The dilated phenotype is by far the most common form of cardiomyopathy, comprising over 90 percent of subjects referred to specialized centers.[100] In the United States, the most common dilated cardiomyopathy is ischemic dilated cardiomyopathy,[1] or the cardiomyopathy that follows myocardial infarction (MI). Other common secondary dilated cardiomyopathies are hypertensive and valvular dilated cardiomyopathies, both produced in part by chronically increased wall stress. The primary cardiomyopathy, IDC, is another relatively common dilated phenotype,[101,102] as discussed below.

Selected Common Types of Dilated Cardiomyopathies

ISCHEMIC CARDIOMYOPATHY

Definition/Diagnosis Ischemic cardiomyopathy is defined as a dilated cardiomyopathy in a subject with a history of MI or evidence of clinically significant (i.e., ≥ 70 percent narrowing of a major epicardial artery) coronary artery disease, in whom the

TABLE 76-4 Types of Dilated Cardiomyopathies

Ischemic insult (ischemic cardiomyopathy)
Valvular disease (mitral regurgitation, aortic regurgitation, aortic stensosis); (valvular cardiomyopathy)
Chronic hypertension (hypertensive cardiomyopathy)
Tachyarrhythmias (supraventricular, ventricular, atrial flutter)
Familial (autosomal dominant, autosomal recessive, X-linked)
Idiopathic
Toxins
    Ethanol
    Chemotherapeutic agents (anthracyclines such as doxorubicin and daunorubicin)
    Cobalt
    Antiretroviral agents (zidovudine, didanosine, zalcitabine)
    Phenothiazines
    Carbon monoxide
    Lithium
    Lead
    Cocaine
    Mercury
Metabolic abnormalities
    Nutritional deficiencies (thiamine, selenium, carnitine, protein)
    Endocrinologic disorders (hypothyroidism, acromegaly, thyrotoxicosis, Cushing's disease, pheochromocytoma, catecholamines, diabetes mellitus)
    Electrolyte disturbances (hypocalcemia, hypophosphatemia)
Infectious
    Viral (coxsackievirus, cytomegalovirus, HIV)
    Rickettsial
    Bacterial
    Mycobacterial
    Spirochetal
    Fungal
    Parasitic (toxoplasmosis, trichinosis, Chagas' disease)
Systemic disorders
    Systemic lupus erythematosis
    Juvenile rheumatoid arthritis
    Polyarteritis nodosa
    Kawasaki disease
    Collagen vascular disorders (scleroderma, lupus erythematosus, dermatomyositis)
    Hemochromatosis
    Amyloidosis
    Sarcoidosis
    Pseudoxanthoma elasticum
    Hypereosinophilic syndrome
Hypersensitivity myocarditis
Peri/postpartum dysfunction
Arrhythmogenic right ventricular dysplasia or cardiomyopathy
Infantile histiocytoid
Neuromuscular dystrophies
    Becker or Duchenne's muscular dystrophy, X-linked cardioskeletal myopathy
Facioscapulohumoral muscular dystrophy
Erb's limb-girdle dystrophy
Myotonic dystrophy
Friedreich's ataxia
Emery-Dreifuss muscular dystrophy
Inborn errors of metabolism
Mitochondrial cardiomyopathies
Keshan cardiomyopathy

coronary arteries. In most cases, the degree of fibrosis does not appear to be extensive enough to cause changes in systolic or diastolic function. Intracardiac thrombi and mural endocardial plaques (from the organization of thrombi) are present at necropsy in more than 50 percent of patients with IDC.[146,147] The effect of anticoagulation on the incidence of thrombi has not been carefully studied, but systemic and pulmonary emboli are more frequent in patients with ventricular thrombi or plaques.[148]

The characteristic findings of IDC on microscopy are marked myocyte hypertrophy, very large, bizarrely shaped nuclei,[149–151] (Fig. 76-4), increased interstitial fibrosis (Fig. 76-4), myocyte atrophy, and myofilament loss.[147,152] In isolated cardiac myocytes, the major cellular phenotypic change is a marked increase in cell length without a concomitant increase in diameter.[84] As described earlier, this cellular lengthening or remodeling contributes to the chamber remodeling/dilatation that characterizes IDC and other cardiomyopathies. These morphologic changes in IDC are not specific and are generally found in secondary cardiomyopathies such as in the noninfarcted regions of ischemic dilated cardiomyopathy.[105] Also, the morphometric changes in IDC do not correlate with the severity of illness.[151,152] Ultrastructural abnormalities such as mitochondrial changes, T-tubular dilatation, and intracellular lipid droplets may be observed in IDC but can also be seen in other forms of heart disease.[151] There may be interstitial parenchymal and perivascular focal infiltrates of small lymphocytes.[150–154] The lymphocytic infiltrates that are present on histologic examination in IDC are not associated with adjacent myocyte damage, in contrast to myocarditis where adjacent myocyte necrosis is observed. Fibrosis is nearly always present in IDC,[150–154] and its pattern is quite variable, from a fine perimyocytic distribution to coarse scars indistinguishable from those present in chronic ischemia. However, small intramural arteries and capillaries are structurally normal in IDC.[151]

A number of immune regulatory abnormalities have been identified in IDC, including humoral[155] and cellular autoimmune reactivity against myocytes,[156] decreased natural killer cell activity,[157] and abnormal suppressor cell activity.[158,159] These abnormalities suggest that immune defects may be important etiologic factors in the development of IDC. These findings, however, are not universally present in patients with IDC, and some abnormalities are also present in other types of heart muscle disease. For example, an increase in the cardioselective M7 antimitochondrial antibodies is found in both IDC and hypertrophic cardiomyopathy but not in heart failure from coronary artery disease.[160] The incidence of some autoreactive antibodies, such as antinuclear and antifibrillary antibodies, increases with the severity of heart failure.[161] It is likely that many of the antibodies detected in IDC and other myocardial diseases do not have pathogenic relevance but rather are secondary to the primary degenerative process. However, it is possible that certain antibodies present in IDC may have important functional implications. For example, anti-β_1-adrenergic receptor antibodies[162,163] could modify β-adrenergic receptor activity[164] and produce

chronic increases in signal transduction that are harmful to the failing heart. Disturbed energy metabolism from antibodies to the ADP/ATP carrier of the inner mitochondrial membrane is another potential pathogenetic autoimmune mechanism[165,166]; these antibodies are present in some individuals with idiopathic dilated cardiomyopathy[165] and have been shown to impair metabolism and myocardial function.[166]

There has been great interest in histocompatibility locus antigens (HLAs) in IDC, since these antigens are known to be associated with immune regulatory functions, and many autoimmune diseases are found to have positive HLA antigenic associations. HLA associations have also been identified in IDC; the frequency of HLA-B27, HLA-A2, HLA-DR4, and HLA-DQ4 is increased compared to controls, and the frequency of HLA-DRw6 is decreased compared to controls.[167,168] Genetic abnormalities in the HLA region potentially could alter immune response and thereby increase disease susceptibility to infectious agents such as enteroviruses. Thus, the association of IDC with specific HLAs suggests a possible immunologic etiology for this disease. However, these specific HLAs are present in less than 50 percent of patients with IDC, and the heterogeneity of these antigens does not point to a unique site for a putative disease-associated gene. Thus, while the autoimmune hypothesis is an attractive candidate for the etiology of some cases of IDC, it remains unproved.

A clinical and pathologic syndrome that is similar to IDC may develop after resolution of viral myocarditis in animal models and biopsy-proven myocarditis in human subjects.[169] This has led to speculation that IDC may develop in some individuals as a result of subclinical viral myocarditis. Theoretically, an episode of myocarditis could initiate a variety of autoimmune reactions that injure the myocardium and ultimately result in the development of IDC. The abnormalities in immune regulation and the variety of antimyocardial antibodies present in IDC are consistent with this hypothesis. However, it is generally not possible to isolate an infectious virus or to demonstrate the presence of viral antigens in the myocardium of patients with IDC. Enteroviral ribonucleic acid (RNA) sequences

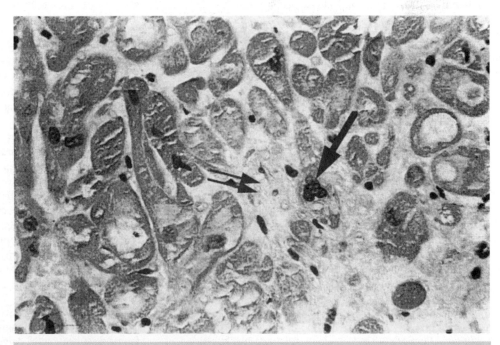

FIGURE 76-4 Right ventricular endomyocardial biopsy from a subject with IDC. Note the increased nuclear size (*large arrow*) and the increased interstitial fibrosis.

may be found in heart biopsy samples in IDC, but with a very variable frequency (0 to 30 percent).[170–172] Furthermore, active myocardial inflammation is usually not detected in IDC,[153,154] and, in controlled trials, corticosteroid therapy of patients with IDC does not result in significant clinical improvements.[173] More recent experimental data have shown in vitro and in vivo that the enteroviral protease 2A is able to cleave dystrophin and disrupt the cytoskeleton in cardiac myocytes, providing a potential link between viral infection and a genetic model of the disease.[174] Furthermore, analysis of human viruses other than enteroviruses suggests that adenoviruses, herpes, and cytomegalovirus can also cause myocarditis and potentially IDC, particularly in children and young subjects.[175,176] Further investigation will be necessary to understand the significance of these findings, particularly in the adult population.

As also discussed in Chap. 26, endomyocardial biopsy of the right or left ventricle may be a valuable diagnostic adjunct for diagnosing specific myocardial processes that can produce a dilated phenotype, such as myocarditis and infiltrative cardiomyopathies. Since several of these other dilated cardiomyopathies may have specific treatments and/or a different prognosis than IDC, endomyocardial biopsy may be warranted in many individuals presenting with a dilated cardiomyopathy. In the future, biopsy may be used more frequently to identify genetic disorders resulting in abnormal gene or protein expression,[63] such as can now be done to diagnose Becker-Duchenne cardiomyopathy.[134,135] Since special staining, electron microscopy, or molecular analysis of the biopsy material may be necessary, endomyocardial biopsy is best performed in specialized cardiomyopathy/heart failure centers.

Prognosis   Several studies of the natural history of IDC have been conducted.[108,177,178] The prognosis is generally better than for ischemic cardiomyopathy[106–108]; prior to the routine use of ACE inhibitors, the survival was approximately 50 percent in 5 years.[177] The prognosis has been substantially improved since then,[108] inasmuch as ACE inhibition,[179] β-adrenergic blockade,[10] and cardiac transplantation (in the high-risk group)[180,181] are all effective treatments in this condition.

Treatment   The treatment of IDC is similar to that discussed above for ischemic cardiomyopathy except there is no issue of revascularization. The risk of thromboembolic complications may be higher than in ischemic cardiomyopathy, resulting in a lower threshold for anticoagulation. β-Adrenergic blockade produces a quantitatively greater degree of improvement in LV function compared to ischemic cardiomyopathy,[182] either because there is a greater degree of adrenergic activation[8] or there is more viable myocardium to work with in IDC. Approximately 10 percent of IDC subjects treated with β-adrenergic blockade will normalize their myocardial function, and this form of treatment should be offered to all IDC subjects who do not have a contraindication before cardiac transplantation is considered.[183]

SELECTED SPECIFIC DILATED CARDIOMYOPATHIES WITH UNIQUE MANAGEMENT ISSUES

Anthracycline Cardiomyopathy

Definition/Diagnosis   The commonly used and highly efficacious anthracycline antibiotic anticancer agents doxorubicin and daunorubicin produce a dose-related cardiomyopathy[184–189] that may limit

their clinical application. Within the WHO/ISFC classification, an anthracycline cardiomyopathy would most likely be in the "dilated" category, but because the extent of dilatation may initially be minimal (see below), it could also be in the "unclassified" category. The cardiomyopathy produced by these agents depends on the total cumulative dose; for the more widely used compound doxorubicin (Adriamycin), the incidence of heart failure due to cardiomyopathy dramatically increases above total cumulative doses of 450 mg/m^2 in subjects without underlying cardiac problems or other risk factors.[185] *Prior mediastinal radiation involving the heart is a powerful risk factor for anthracycline cardiomyopathy,*[186] *and the risk is also evident if radiation treatment follows chemotherapy.*[188,189] In subjects with risk factors, anthracycline cardiomyopathy can present at lower cumulative doses than 450 mg/m^2.[186–188]

Although the diagnosis of anthracycline cardiomyopathy can be made clinically, the definitive diagnosis depends on the demonstration of a substantial number of cardiac myocytes exhibiting the characteristic anthracycline effect.[184,186–189] Tissue sampling is best done by endomyocardial biopsy, which allows for thin-section electron microscopic processing of the sample and more definitive resolution of the anthracycline effect with light microscopy.[184,186–189]

Distinct Pathophysiology   In the absence of a tissue diagnosis, anthracycline cardiomyopathy may be diagnosed clinically by exclusion of other causes of cardiomyopathy in a subject who has had at least 350 mg/m^2 of doxorubicin or the equivalent amount of another anthracycline. As shown in Fig. 76-5, the anthracycline cardiac myocytic lesion consists of cell vacuolization progressing to cell dropout, and when 16 to 25 percent of the total number of sampled cells exhibit this morphology, myocardial dysfunction results.[186]

There are some distinguishing clinical features of anthracycline cardiomyopathy that may relate to its pathophysiology. These include a relative absence of hypertrophy and dilatation and a higher heart rate (110 to 130 beats per minute) than is usually encountered in ambulatory heart failure. The reasons for these features are that the onset of symptoms may be relatively acute (remodeling takes time to develop) and the anthracycline inhibits contractile protein synthesis,[190] thus reducing the amount of compensatory dilatation and remodeling. In this situation, the only option available for stabilizing cardiac output is increasing the heart rate, since increasing stroke volume via a larger end-diastolic volume has been precluded. The increased heart rate is produced by a greater than expected hyperadrenergic state; therefore these subjects may be exceptionally dependent on adrenergic support.

Prognosis   The prognosis of anthracycline cardiomyopathy is poor[108] and depends on numerous factors, including the age and underlying prechemotherapy cardiac status of the patient and the time of presentation relative to the last dose of drug. Subjects who present late (several months) or very late (years) after the last dose have a better prognosis because the anthracycline myocardial effect takes at least 60 days to become fully manifest.[191] That is, subjects who develop heart failure within a few days of the last dose of drug have an additional cardiomyopathic burden to face, as the last one to two doses produce their full morphologic effect over the next 1 to 2 months.

Treatment/Prevention   Subjects who develop anthracycline cardiomyopathy should be aggressively treated with conventional heart failure treatment, since some degree of reversibility is likely. Conventional treatment consists of ACE inhibitors, digoxin, and diuretics. β-Adrenergic blockade has been used successfully in some subjects,[192,193] but because of the high adrenergic drive, it may be difficult to administer. On the other hand, the heightened adrenergic mechanism may be producing a commensurate amount of adverse effect on the myocardium, and so the potential for a favorable response may be even greater than in other kinds of cardiomyopathy. In severe refractory cases, cardiac transplantation may be performed provided that the patient's cancer is in complete remission and is not likely to recur (~70 percent chance of cure).

Several strategies have been shown to lower the risk of developing anthracycline cardiomyopathy without compromising the chemotherapy response rate. These include using endomyocardial biopsy and right-sided catheterization with exercise to assess risk, which virtually eliminates clinical cardiomyopathy and allows more anthracycline to be administered to less susceptible subjects[194]; using serial radionuclide angiography with[195] or without[196] exercise as a monitoring strategy, which may be somewhat helpful but because of a low specificity reduces the total amount of chemotherapy that can safely be administered to some subjects[194,195]; giving the agents at low doses weekly[197] or as 48- to 72-h infusions[198] rather than as boluses every 3 to 4 weeks; using a liposomal formulation[199]; or concomitantly administering a second agent that reduces toxicity.[200] Unfortunately, none of these strategies completely eliminates the risk of developing a clinical cardiomyopathy.

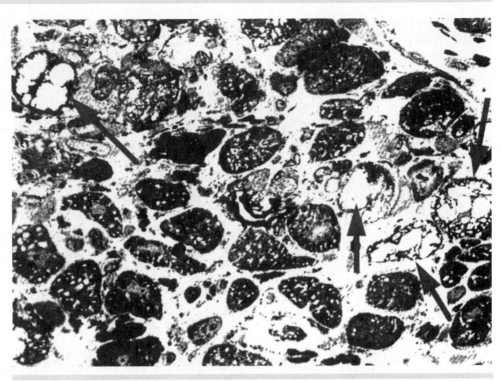

FIGURE 76-5 Cardiac myocyte vacuolization in cases of Adriamycin cardiomyopathy classified on endomyocardial biopsy as grade 3 by the Billingham classification.[186,187,194]

Postpartum Cardiomyopathy

Definition/Diagnosis Postpartum or *peripartum cardiomyopathy* is defined as the presentation of systolic dysfunction and clinical heart failure during the last trimester of pregnancy or within 6 months of delivery.[201] Given the extreme hemodynamic load produced by pregnancy, it is perhaps surprising that postpartum cardiomyopathy is not more common.

Distinct Pathophysiology Postpartum cardiomyopathy will most likely be classified within the "dilated" WHO/ISFC category, but occasionally it will be "unclassified" because dilatation and remodeling has not had time to occur. Postpartum cardiomyopathy is likely a heterogeneous group of disorders, consisting of the addition of the hemodynamic load of pregnancy to a variety of underlying myocardial processes including hypertensive heart disease, familial or idiopathic dilated cardiomyopathy, and myocarditis.[202]

Prognosis Postpartum cardiomyopathy has a better prognosis than other causes of dilated cardiomyopathy.[108] Approximately half of subjects who develop postpartum cardiomyopathy will recover completely,[203] and the majority of the rest will improve. Subjects who have developed a postpartum cardiomyopathy should never become pregnant again, even if myocardial function has recovered fully.[204]

Treatment Treatment should be aggressive, as for idiopathic dilated cardiomyopathy. Cardiac transplantation may be required in severely compromised patients who do not improve.

Amyloid Cardiomyopathy

Definition/Diagnosis As discussed in Chap. 79, amyloidosis comprises a group of diseases characterized by extracellular deposition of proteins characterized by their unique β-pleated sheet conformation and recognized electron microscopically as randomly arranged nonbranching fibers ranging from 8 to 14 nm in length. Amyloidosis is classified according to the type of amyloid protein involved.[205] Amyloidosis involving the heart is not rare and accounts for up to 10 percent of all nonischemic cardiomyopathies in autopsy studies.[206,207]

Amyloid cardiomyopathy may present in the WHO/ISFC "restrictive," "dilated," or "unclassified" categories. Most commonly it presents as a restrictive cardiomyopathy with conduction system abnormalities. In the setting of systemic amyloidosis (secondary or primary forms) the presence of increased wall thickness on echocardiogram plus low electrocardiographic voltage is highly suggestive of cardiac involvement.[208] In primary systemic amyloidosis, a monoclonal immunoglobulin spike is detectable in urine or serum in approximately 80 percent of subjects.[209] The definitive diagnosis of amyloid cardiomyopathy is made by tissue examination, ideally premortem by endomyocardial biopsy.[208] In systemic forms, the tissue diagnosis may be made by rectal, skin or tongue biopsy of any abnormal tissue in these locations coupled with an unexplained myocardial process. As shown in Fig. 76-6, the characteristic histologic signature of amyloid is extracellular deposition of a fibrillar protein with a characteristic periodicity on electron microscopy.[210] Although a Congo Red stain can identify most cases, electron microscopy is more sensitive and specific and should be routinely used when amyloid is suspected. A recent study of cycle-dependent variation of

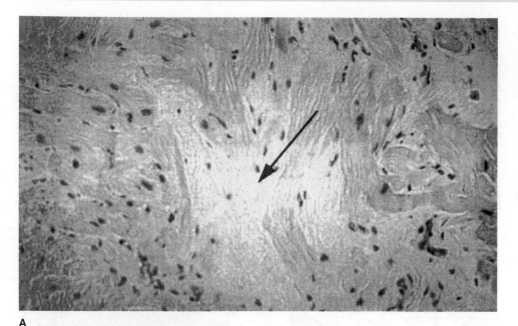

A

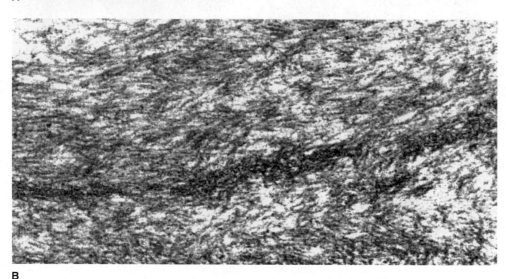

B

FIGURE 76-6 *A.* Right ventricular biopsy demonstrating interstitial amyloid deposition (H&E stain, ×100). *B.* Electron micrograph of the same biopsy specimen illustrating the characteristic 8- to 14-nm, nonbranching, randomly oriented amyloid fibrils.

are thought by some to be curable and other forms are characterized by slow progression of disease.[214]

Treatment There is no definitive treatment of amyloid cardiomyopathy. Treatment is generally empiric and consists of diuretics when needed, pacemaker treatment of bradyarrhythmias, and the avoidance of digoxin, which may be arrhythmogenic in any infiltrative cardiomyopathy. There is limited evidence that chemotherapy directed at amyloid secretion by abnormal β-lymphocytes can produce favorable effects in some patients.[215] Cardiac transplantation should be avoided even in primary localized amyloid cardiomyopathy, because it will invariably recur in the heart or in other organs. The exception may be familial forms of amyloidosis where the abnormal protein is a transthyretin, or prealbumin, variant synthesized in the liver. Combined liver and heart transplantation can be curative in this situation.[216]

Alcohol Cardiomyopathy

Definition/Diagnosis An *alcohol cardiomyopathy* is said to be present when other causes of a dilated cardiomyopathy have been excluded and there is a history of heavy, sustained alcohol intake. The requirement in terms of alcohol amount is 80 g of alcohol per day for males and 40 g for females,[217] typically over several years. However, in susceptible individuals it is likely that lower amounts of intake can produce a cardiomyopathy. The histologic features of alcohol cardiomyopathy are nonspecific and do not differ from IDC. Other than

myocardial integrated backscatter (CV-IB) at the left ventricular posterior wall showed that it was a strong predictor of cardiac death and all-cause death in patients with cardiac amyloidosis.[211]

Distinct Pathophysiology Although the source and chemical nature of amyloid protein differ among the various types of amyloidosis, the tissue/organ pathophysiology is the same—i.e., the slow destruction of the heart by the inexorable deposition of a β-pleated sheet fibril that is insoluble and impervious to proteolytic digestion.[207] Recently, mutations in the transthyretin gene[212] and apolipoprotein A1 gene[213] have been described in cardiac amyloid.

Prognosis The prognosis is uniformly bad regardless of the type of amyloidosis,[108] and the majority of subjects with amyloid cardiomyopathy are dead within 2 years of diagnosis. However, it is important to classify the subtype of amyloidosis, as some forms of this disease

history, the only potentially distinguishing feature between IDC and alcohol cardiomyopathy is that the latter may present with a relatively high cardiac output.

Distinct Pathophysiology The pathophysiology of alcohol cardiomyopathy is thought to be related to the toxic effects of alcohol, plus, in some subjects, nutritional components such as thiamine deficiency. Genetic factors may predispose to alcoholic cardiomyopathy, like the angiotensin-converting enzyme (ACE) DD polymorphism.[218]

Prognosis The prognosis depends on the degree of impairment of myocardial function and the extent of abstinence from alcohol and, in an extremely compromised patient, the administration of thiamine. There is evidence that the prognosis is somewhat better for alcohol cardiomyopathy than for IDC.[219]

Treatment The treatment of alcohol cardiomyopathy does not differ from that of IDC except for the need for total abstinence from alcohol. Obviously these subjects are not good candidates for cardiac transplantation because of their high relapse rate to alcoholism.

Chagas' Cardiomyopathy

Definition/Diagnosis Chagas' disease is discussed in Chap. 79 as a cause of myocarditis. In addition, Chagas' disease is the most common cause of nonischemic cardiomyopathy in South and Central America, with over 10 million people affected.[220] It is caused by a parasite, the leishmanial or tissue form of the protozoan *Trypanosoma cruzi*. Although in the United States the vector (*Triatoma*, or kissing bug) is found only in the Southwest, Chagas' disease may be transmitted by blood transfusions; as a result, it could become relatively more important in this country. The natural history consists of an initial myocarditis most commonly presenting in childhood, associated with acute myocardial infection followed by recovery, and, in some individuals, the development of a dilated cardiomyopathy 10 to 30 years later.

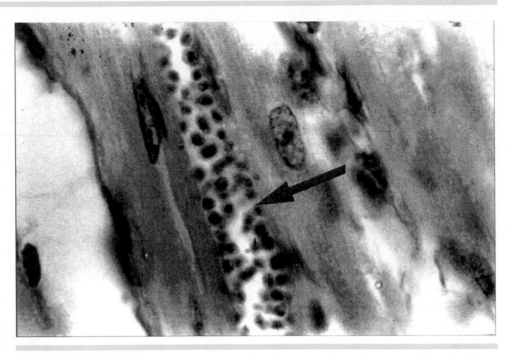

FIGURE 76-7 Leishmanial forms of *T. cruzi* within the swollen cytoplasm of a cardiac myocyte (Chagas' cardiomyopathy). (H&E stain, ×250). (Courtesy of Dr. Elmer Koneman).

The diagnosis of Chagas' cardiomyopathy is based on clinical (history, LV functional and electrocardiographic) criteria and a positive serologic test for *T. cruzi*.[221] Electrocardiographic abnormalities consist of bundle branch or hemiblocks (indeed, hemiblocks were first described by Rosenbaum et al.[222] in Chagas' afflicted hearts with discrete foci of involvement), LV hypertrophy, and first- or second-degree atrioventricular (AV) block.[223] Recently Doppler tissue imaging has been presented as being a more sensitive technique for the study of diastolic function in Chagas' disease than conventional Doppler echocardiography.[224,225] The histologic lesion of chronic Chagas' consists of mononuclear infiltrates, fibrosis, and, as shown in Fig. 76-7, foci of the leishmanial form of *T. cruzi* in myocardial fibers. The LV functional abnormalities may initially be segmental and may include an apical aneurysm; later, they become more global.[221,223]

Distinct Pathophysiology The basis for Chagas' cardiomyopathy is unknown but may be immunologic, whereby antibodies generated against *T. cruzi* cross-react with cardiac myocyte antigens including myosin.[226]

Prognosis The prognosis is relatively good for a dilated cardiomyopathy and similar to that for IDC; the 5-year survival in Chagas' cardiomyopathy with heart failure is around 50 percent.[221,227] Compared to IDC, death likely occurs more commonly due to an arrhythmic mechanism.[221] However, as for IDC and most other dilated cardiomyopathies, mortality risk depends directly on the degrees of ventricular dysfunction and exercise intolerance.[221]

Treatment There is no definitive treatment for Chagas' cardiomyopathy; nonspecific treatment includes pacemaker implantation for heart block and heart failure treatment as for IDC. Verapamil has been recently demonstrated to attenuate the extent of myocardial injury in murine models of chronic *T. cruzi* infection.[228] Also, amiodarone appears to be particularly effective in treating arrhythmias associated with Chagas' cardiomyopathy; in one study it reduced mortality compared to standard treatment.[229] The role of cardiac transplantation is still somewhat uncertain, but it can be done at acceptable risk,[230] especially when coupled with trypanocidal agents.[231]

SUMMARY

Dilated cardiomyopathies are important because they are the most common cause of heart failure, which is the single most costly medical problem in the adult U.S. population. Cardiomyopathies in general are a heterogeneous group of diseases, but they can be classified under a newly modified WHO/ISFC classification system, which, although imperfect, should be of great value in standardizing the terminology and encouraging systematic investigative and clinical approaches to diagnosis and treatment. Within this classification system, primary and secondary dilated cardiomyopathies comprise the single largest and most important group. Current diagnosis and treatment of dilated cardiomyopathies varies somewhat among the various types, but the cornerstones of medical management are similar in most cases.

Genetic causes and influences on the natural history of dilated cardiomyopathies are the new frontier in this field, and their elucidation is almost certain to lead to new therapeutic and diagnostic approaches. In the near future, molecular genetic testing will be routinely done for many cardiomyopathies that may have a single gene defect as the cause. As we learn more about the influence of polymorphic genetic variation on the natural history and selection of specific medical therapy, genetic testing will be performed in most patients with cardiomyopathies.

References

1. Ho KKL, Anderson KM, Kannel WB, et al. Survival after the onset of congestive heart failure in Framingham Heart Study subjects. *Circulation* 1993;88:107–115.

2. O'Connell JB, Bristow MR. Economic impact of heart failure in the United States: Time for a different approach. *J Heart Lung Transplant* 1994;13:S107–S112.

3. Richardson P, McKenna WJ, Bristow MR, et al. Report of the 1995 World Health Organization/International Society and Federation of Cardiology. Task Force on the definition and classification of cardiomyopathies. *Circulation* 1996;93:841–842.

4. Guccione AA, Felson DT, Anderson JJ, et al. The effects of specific medical conditions on the functional limitations of elders in the Framingham Study. *Am J Public Health* 1994;84:351–358.

5. Cohn JN, Johnson GR, Shabetai R, et al. Ejection fraction, peak exercise oxygen consumption, cardiothoracic ratio, ventricular arrhythmias, and plasma norepinephrine as determinants of prognosis in heart failure. *Circulation* 1993;87(suppl VI):VI-5–VI-16.

6. Eichhorn EJ, Bristow MR. Medical therapy can improve the biologic properties of the chronically failing heart: A new era in the treatment of heart failure. *Circulation* 1996;94:2285–2296.

7. WHO/ISFC. Task Force on Cardiomyopathies. Report of the WHO/ISFC Task Force on the definition and classification of cardiomyopathies. *Br Heart J* 1980;44:672–673.

8. Bristow MR, Anderson FL, Port JD, et al. Differences in β-adrenergic neuroeffector mechanisms in ischemic versus idiopathic dilated cardiomyopathy. *Circulation* 1991;84:1024–1039.

9. Packer M, Bristow MR, Cohn JN, et al. Effect of carvedilol on morbidity and mortality in patients with chronic heart failure. *N Engl J Med* 1996;334:1349–1355.

10. Bristow MR. β-adrenergic receptor blockade in chronic heart failure. *Circulation* 2000;101:558–569.

11. Bristow MR. Why does the myocardium fail? New insights from basic science. *Lancet* 1998;352 (suppl):8–14.

12. Geisterfer-Lawrence AA, Kass S, Tanigawa G, et al. A molecular basis for familial hypertrophic cardiomyoapthy: A beta-cardiac myosin heavy chain missense mutation. *Cell* 1990;62:999–1006.

13. Geisterfer-Lawrence AA, Christe M, Conner DA, et al. A mouse model of familial hypertrophic cardiomyopathy. *Science* 1996;272:731–735.

14. Vikstrom KL, Factor SM, Leinwand LA. Mice expressing mutant myosin heavy chains are a model for familial hypertrophic cardiomyopathy. *Mol Med* 1996;2:556–567.

15. Tiret L, Rigat B, Visvikis S, et al. Evidence, from combined segregation and linkage analysis, that a variant of the angiotensin I–converting enzyme (ACE) gene controls plasma ACE levels. *Am J Hum Gen* 1992;51:197–205.

16. Raynolds MV, Bristow MR, Bush E, et al. Angiotensin-converting enzyme DD genotype in patients with ischæmic or idiopathic dilated cardiomyopathy. *Lancet* 1993;342:1073–1075.

17. McNamara DM, Holubkov R, Janosko K, et al. Pharmacogenetic interactions between beta-blocker therapy and the angiotensin-converting enzyme deletion polymorphism in patients with congestive heart failure. *Circulation* 2001;103:1644–1648.

18. Ikeda Y, Ross JJ. Models of dilated cardiomyopathy in the mouse and the hamster. *Curr Opin Cardiol 2000*. 2000;15:197–201.

19. Edwards JG, Lyons GE, Micales BK, et al. Cardiomyopathy in transgenic myf5 mice. *Circ Res* 1996;78:379–387.

20. Arber S, Hunter JJ, Ross JJ, et al. MLP-deficient mouse exhibit a disruption of cardiac cytoarchitectural organization, dilated cardiomyopathy and heart failure. *Cell* 1997;88:393–403.

21. Iwase M, Bishop SP, Uechi M, et al. Adverse effects of chronic endogenous sympathetic drive induced by cardiac $G_{s\alpha}$ overexpression. *Circ Res* 1996;78:517–524.

22. Hein L, Altman JD, Kobilka KB. Two functionally distinct α_2-adrenergic receptors regulate sympathetic neurotransmission. *Nature* 1999;402:181–184.

23. Bisognano JD, Weinberger HD, Knudson OA, et al. Myocardial directed over-expressing the human beta(1)-adrenergic receptor in transgenic mice. *J Mol Cell Cardiol* 2000;32:817–830.

24. Engelhardt S, Hein L, Wiesman F, Lohse MJ. Progressive hypertrophy and heart failure in β_1-adrenergic receptor transgenic mice. *Proc Natl Acad Sci USA* 1999;96:7059–7064.

25. Liggett SB, Tepe NM, Lorenz JN, et al. Early and delayed consequences of β_2-adrenergic receptor overexpression in mouse hearts: Critical role for expression level. *Circulation* 2000;101:1707–1714.

26. Antos CL, Frey N, Marx SO, et al. Dilated cardiomyopathy and sudden death resulting from constitutive activation of protein kinase A. *Circ Res* 2001;89:997–1004.

27. Geng Y-J, Ishikawa Y, Vatner DE, et al. Apoptosis of cardiac myocytes in Gs alpha transgenic mice. *Circ Res* 1999;84:34–42.

28. Nicol RL, Frey N, Pearson G, et al. Activated MEK5 induces serial assembly of sarcomeres and eccentric cardiac hypertrophy. *EMBO J* 2001;20:2757–2567.

29. Passier R, Zeng H, Frey N, et al. CaM kinase signaling induces cardiac hypertrophy and activates the MEF2 transcription factor in vivo. *J Clin Invest* 2000;105:1395–1406.

30. Molkentin JD, Lu JR, Antos CL, et al. A calcineurin-dependent transcriptional pathway for cardiac hypertrophy. *Cell* 1998;93:215–228.

31. Cho MC, Rapacciuolo A, Koch WJ, et al. Defective beta-adrenergic receptor signaling precedes the development of dilated cardiomyopathy in transgenic mice with calsequestrin overexpression. *J Biol Chem* 1999;274:22251–22256.

32. Li H, Wang J, Wilhelmsson H, et al. Genetic modification of survival in tissue-specific knockout mice with mitochondrial cardiomyopathy. *Proc Natl Acad Sci USA* 2000;97:3467–3472.

33. Hunter JJ, Tanaka N, Rockman HA, et al. Ventricular expression of a MLC-2v-ras fusion gene induces cardiac hypertrophy and selective diastolic dysfunction in transgenic mice. *J Biol Chem* 1995;270:23173–23178.

34. Robbins RJ, Swain JL. C-myc protooncogene modulates cardiac hypertrophic growth in transgenic mice. *Am J Physiol* 1992;62:H590–H597.

35. Milano CA, Dolber PC, Rockman HA, et al. Myocardial expression of a constitutively active α_{1B}-adrenergic receptor in transgenic mice induces cardiac hypertrophy. *Proc Natl Acad Sci USA* 1994;91:10109–10113.

36. D'Angelo DD, Sakatra Y, Lorenz JN, et al. Transgenic $G_{\alpha q}$ over-expression induces cardiac contractile failure in mice. *Proc Natl Acad Sci* 1997;94:8121–8126.

37. Wakasaki H, Koya D, Schoen FJ, et al. Targeted overexpression of protein kinase C beta2 isoform in myocardium causes cardiomyopathy. *Proc Natl Acad Sci USA* 1997;94:9320–9325.

38. Li D, Tapscoft T, Gonzalez O, et al. Desmin mutation responsible for idiopathic dilated cardiomyopathy. *Circulation* 1999;100:461–464.

39. Towbin JA, Hejtmancik F, Brink P, et al. X-linked cardiomyopathy (XLCM): Molecular genetic evidence of linkage to the Duchenne muscular dystrophy (dystrophin) gene at the Xp21 locus. *Circulation* 1993;87:1854–1865.

40. Muntoni F, Cau M, Ganau A, et al. Deletion of the dystrophin muscle-promoter region associated with X-linked dilated cardiomyopathy. *N Engl J Med* 1993;329:921–925.

41. Tsubata S, Bowles KR, Vatta M, et al. Mutations in the human delta-sarcoglycan gene in familial and sporadic dilated cardiomyopathy. *J Clin Invest* 2000;106:655–662.

42. Olson T, Illenberger S, Kishimoto N, et al. Metavinculin mutations alter actin interaction in dilated cardiomyopathy. *Circulation* 2002;105:431–437.

43. Fatkin D, MacRae C, Sasaki T, et al. Missense mutations in the rod domain of the lamin A/C gene as causes of dilated cardiomyopathy and conduction-system disease. *N Engl J Med* 1999;341:1715–1724.

44. Brodsky GL, Muntoni F, Miocic S, et al. A lamin A/C gene mutation associated with dilated cardiomyopathy with variable skeletal muscle involvement. *Circulation* 2000;101:473–476.

45. Olson TM, Michels VV, Thibodeau SN, et al. Actin mutation in dilated cardiomyopathy: A heritable form of heart failure. *Science* 1998;280: 750–752.

46. Kamisago M, Sharma SD, DePalma SR, et al. Mutations in sarcomere protein genes as a cause of dilated cardiomyopathy. *N Engl J Med* 2000;343:1688–1696.

47. Olson T, Kishimoto NY, Withby FG, Michels V. Mutations that alter the surface charge of alpha-tropomyosin are associated with dilated cardiomyopathy. *J Mol Cell Cardiol* 2001;33:723–732.

48. Gerull B, Gramlich M, Atherton J, et al. Mutations of TTN, encoding the giant muscle filament titin, cause familial dilated cardiomyopathy. *Nat Genet* 2002;30:201–204.

49. Nigro V, Okazaki Y, Belsito A, et al. Identification of the Syrian hamster cardiomyopathy gene. *Hum Mol Genet* 1997;6:601–607.

50. Biesiadecki BJ, Jin JP. Exon skipping in cardiac troponin T of turkeys with inherited cardiomyopathy. *J Biol Chem* 2002;277: 18459–18468.

51. Schmitt JP, Kamisago M, Asahi M, et al. Dilated cardiomyopathy and heart failure caused by a mutation in phospholamban. *Science* 2003; 299:1410–1413.

52. Lander E, Kruglyak L. Genetic dissection of complex traits: Guidelines for interpreting and reporting linkage results. *Nat Genet* 1995;11: 241–247.

53. Jan Danser AH, Maarten ADH, Schalekamp MD, et al. Angiotensin-converting enzyme in the human heart: Effect of the deletion/insertion polymorphism. *Circulation* 1995;92:1387–1388.

54. Pinto YM, van Gilst WH, Kingma JH, et al. Deletion-type allele of the angiotensin-converting enzyme gene is associated with progressive ventricular dilatation after anterior myocardial infarction. *J Am Coll Cardiol* 1995;25:1622–1626.

55. Andersson B, Sylven C. The DD genotype of the angiotensin-converting enzyme gene is associated with increased mortality in idiopathic dilated cardiomyopathy. *J Am Coll Cardiol* 1996;28:162–167.

56. Bonnardeaux A, Davies E, Jeunemaitre X, et al. Angiotensin II type 1 receptor gene polymorphisms in human essential hypertension. *Hypertension* 1994;24:63–69.

57. Liggett SB, Wagoner LE, Craft LL, et al. The Ile164 beta2-adrenergic receptor polymorphism adversely affects the outcome of congestive heart failure. *J Clin Invest* 1998;102:1534–1539.

58. Small KM, Wagoner LE, Levin AM, et al. Synergistic polymorphism of β_1- and α_{2C}-adrenergic receptors and the risk of congestive heart failure. *N Engl J Med* 2002;347:1135–1142.

59. Charron P, Tesson F, Poirier O, et al. Identification of a genetic risk factor for idiopathic dilated cardiomyopathy. Involvement of a polymorphism in the endothelin receptor type A gene. CARDIGENE group. *Eur Heart J* 1999;20:1587–1591.

60. Lowes BD, Minobe WA, Abraham WT, et al. Changes in gene expression in the intact human heart: Down-regulation of α-myosin heavy chain in hypertrophied, failing ventricular myocardium. *J Clin Invest* 1997;100:2315–2324.

61. Miyata S, Minobe WA, Bristow MR, Leinwand LA. Myosin isoform expression in the failing and non-failing human heart. *Circ Res* 2000; 86:386–390.

62. Mercadier JJ, Lompre AM, Duc P, et al. Altered sarcoplasmic reticulum Ca-ATPase gene expression in the human ventricle during end-stage heart failure. *J Clin Invest* 1990;85:305–309.

63. Feldman AM, Ray PE, Silan CM, et al. Selective gene expression in failing human heart. Quantification of steady-state levels of messenger RNA in endomyocardial biopsies using the polymerase chain reaction. *Circulation* 1991;83:1866–1872.

64. Studer R, Reinecke H, Muler B, et al. Increased angiotensin-I converting enzyme gene expression in the failing human heart. Quantification by competitive RNA polymerase chain reaction. *J Clin Invest* 1994;94: 301–310.

65. Zisman LS, Asano K, Dutcher DL, et al. Differential regulation of cardiac angiotensin converting enzyme binding sites and AT1 receptor density in the failing human heart. *Circulation* 1998;98:1735–1741.

66. Torre-Amione G, Kapadia S, Lee J, et al. Tumor necrosis factor-α and tumor necrosis factor receptors in the failing human heart. *Circulation* 1996;93:704–711.

67. Zolk O, Quattek J, Sitzler G, et al. Expression of endothelin-1, endothelin-converting enzyme, and endothelin receptors in chronic heart failure. *Circulation* 1999;99:2118–2123.

68. Ungerer M, Böhm M, Elce JS, et al. Altered expression of β-adrenergic receptor kinase and β_1-adrenergic receptors in the failing human heart. *Circulation* 1993;87:454–463.

69. Lowes BD, Gilbert EM, Abraham WT, et al. Myocardial gene expression in dilated cardiomyopathy treated with beta-blocking agents. *N Engl J Med* 2002;346:1357–1365.

70. Davies CH, Davia K, Bennett JG, et al. Reduced contraction and altered frequency response of isolated ventricular myocytes from patients with heart failure. *Circulation* 1995;92:2540–2549.

71. Bristow MR, Gilbert EM. Improvement in cardiac myocyte function by biologic effects of medical therapy: A new concept in the treatment of heart failure. *Eur Heart J* 1995;16(suppl F):20–31.

72. Ross J, Braunwald E. Studies on Starling's law of the heart IX. The effects of impeding venous return on performance of the normal and failing ventricle. *Circulation* 1964;30:719–727.

73. Schwinger RHG, Bohm M, Koch A, et al. The failing human heart is unable to use the Frank-Starling mechanism. *Circ Res* 1994;74: 959–969.

74. Holubarsch C, Thorsten R, Goldstein DJ, et al. Existence of the Frank-Starling mechanism in the failing human heart: Investigations on the organ, tissue, and sarcomere levels. *Circulation* 1996;94:683–689.

75. Feldman MD, Gwathmey JK, Phillips P, et al. Reversal of the force-frequency relationship in working myocardium from patients with end-stage heart failure. *J Appl Cardiol* 1988;3:273–283.

76. Muleiri LA, Hasenfuss G, Leavitt B, et al. Altered myocardial force-frequency relationship in the human heart failure. *Circulation* 1992; 85:1743–1750.

77. Cohn JN. Structural basis for heart failure: Ventricular remodeling and its pharmacological inhibition. *Circulation* 1995;91:2504–2507.

78. Gerdes AM, Capasso JM. Structural remodeling and mechanical dysfunction of cardiac myocytes in heart failure. *J Mol Cell Cardiol* 1995; 27:849–856.

79. Nadal-Ginard B, Mahdavi V. Molecular basis of cardiac performance. *J Clin Invest* 1989;84:1693–1700.

80. Hirzel HO, Tuchschmid CR, Schneider J, et al. Relationship between myosin isoenzyme composition, hemodynamics, and myocardial structure in various forms of human cardiac hypertrophy. *Circ Res* 1985;57:729–740.

81. Tsutsui H, Ishihara K, Cooper GIV. Cytoskeletal role in the contractile dysfunction of hypertrophied myocardium. *Science* 1993;260: 682–687.

82. Yoshida K, Ikeda S, Nakamura A, et al. Molecular analysis of the Duchenne muscular dystrophy gene in patients with Becker muscular dystrophy presenting with dilated cardiomyopathy. *Muscle Nerve* 1993;16:1161–1166.

83. Maeda M, Holder E, Lowes BD, et al. Dilated cardiomyopathy associated with deficiency of the cytoskeletal protein metavinculin. *Circulation* 1997;95:17–20.

84. Gerdes AM, Kellerman SE, Schocken DD. Implications of cardiomyocyte remodeling in heart dysfunction. In: Dhalla NS, Beamish RE, Takeda N, Nagano N, eds. *The Failing Heart*. New York: Raven Press; 1995:197–205.

85. Gerdes AM, Odera T, Wang X, McCune SA. Myocyte remodeling during progression to failure in rats with hypertension. *Hypertension* 1996;28:609–614.

86. Zhang J, McDonald KM. Bioenergetic consequences of left ventricular remodeling. *Circulation* 1995;92:1011–1019.

87. Sata M, Sugiura S, Yamashita H, et al. Coupling between myosin ATPase cycle and creatine kinase cycle facilitates cardiac actomyosin sliding in vitro: A clue to mechanical dysfunction during myocardial ischemia. *Circulation* 1996;93:310–317.

88. Cintron C, Johnson G, Francis G, et al. Prognostic significance of serial changes in left ventricular ejection fraction in patients with congestive heart failure. *Circulation* 1993;87(suppl VI):17–23.

89. Binkley PF, Nunziata E, Haas GH, et al. Parasympathetic withdrawal is an integral component of autonomic imbalance in congestive heart failure: Demonstration in human subjects and verification in a paced canine model of ventricular failure. *J Am Coll Cardiol* 1991;18: 464–472.

90. Chidiac P, Hebert TE, Valiquette M, et al. Inverse agonist activity of β-adrenergic antagonists. *Mol Pharm* 1994;45:490–499.

91. Mewes T, Dutz S, Ravens U, Jakobs KH. Activation of calcium currents in cardiac myocytes by empty β-adrenoceptors. *Circulation* 1993;88:2916–2922.

92. Milano CA, Allen LF, Rockman HA, et al. Enhanced myocardial function in transgenic mice overexpressing the β₂-adrenergic receptor. *Science* 1994;264:562–566.

93. Bond RA, Leff P, Johnson TD, et al. Physiological effects of inverse agonists in transgenic mice with myocardial overexpression of the β₂-adrenoceptor. *Nature* 1995;374:272–276.

94. Luo W, Grupp IL, Harrer J, et al. Targeted ablation of the phospholamban gene is associated with markedly enhanced myocardial contractility and loss of β-agonist stimulation. *Circ Res* 1994;75:401–409.

95. Narula J, Haider N, Virmani R, et al. Apoptosis in myocytes in end-stage heart failure. *N Engl J Med* 1996;335:1182–1189.

96. Teiger E, Than VD, Richard L, et al. Apoptosis in pressure overload–induced heart hypertrophy in the rat. *J Clin Invest* 1996;97:2891–2897.

97. Cohn JN, Levine TB, Olivari MT, et al. Plasma norepinephrine as a guide to prognosis in patients with chronic congestive heart failure. *N Engl J Med* 1984;311:819–823.

98. Kaye DM, Lefkovits J, Jennings GL, et al. Adverse consequences of high sympathetic nervous activity in the failing human heart. *J Am Coll Cardiol* 1995;26:1257–1263.

99. Swedberg K, Eneroth P, Kjekshus J, Wilhelmsen L. Hormones regulating cardiovascular function in patients with severe congestive heart failure and their relation to mortality. *Circulation* 1990;82:1730–1736.

100. Bristow MR, O'Connell JB, Mestroni L. Myocardial diseases. In: *Kelley's Textbook of Internal Medicine,* 4th ed. Philadelphia: Lippincott, Williams & Wilkins; 2000:464–474.

101. Codd MB, Sugrue DD, Gersh BJ, Melton LJ. Epidemiology of idiopathic dilated and hypertrophic cardiomyopathy: A population based study in Olmstead County, MN 1975–1984. *Circulation* 1989; 80:564–572.

102. Rakar S, Sinagra G, Di Lenarda A, et al. Epidemiology of dilated cardiomyopathy. A prospective post-mortem study of 5252 necropsies. *Eur Heart J* 1997;18:117–123.

103. McKay RG, Pfeffer MA, Pasternak RC, et al. Left ventricular remodeling after myocardial infarction: A corollary to infarct expansion. *Circulation* 1986;74:693–702.

104. Mitchell GF, Lamas GA, Vaughan DE, Pfeffer MA. Left ventricular remodeling in the year after myocardial infarction: A quantitative analysis of contractile segment lengths and ventricular shape. *J Am Coll Cardiol* 1992;19:1136–1144.

105. Gerdes AM, Kellerman SE, Moore JA, et al. Structural remodeling of cardiac myocytes from patients with chronic ischemic heart disease. *Circulation* 1992;86:426–430.

106. Franciosa JA, Willen M, Ziesche S, Cohn JN. Survival in men with severe chronic left ventricular failure due to either coronary heart disease or idiopathic dilated cardiomyopathy. *Am J Cardiol* 1983; 51:831–836.

107. Likoff MJ, Chandler SL, Kay HR. Clinical determinants of mortality in chronic congestive heart failure secondary to idiopathic dilated or to ischemic cardiomyopathy. *Am J Cardiol* 1987;59:634–638.

108. Felker GM, Thompson RE, Hare JM, et al. Underlying causes and long term survival in patients with initially unexplained cardiomyopathy. *N Engl J Med* 2000;342:1077–1084.

109. CIBIS-II, Investigators and Committees. The cardiac insufficiency bisoprolol study II: (CIBIS-II): A randomised trial. *Lancet* 1999;353: 9–13.

110. MERIT-HF Study Group. Effect of metoprolol CR/XL in chronic heart failure: Metoprolol CR/XL Randomized Intervention Trial in Congestive Heart Failure (MERIT-HF). *Lancet* 1999;353:2001–2006.

111. Packer M, Fowler MB, Roecker EB, et al. Effect of carvedilol on the morbidity of patients with severe chronic heart failure: Results of the carvedilol prospective randomized cumulative survival (COPERNICUS) study. *Circulation* 2002;106:2164–2166.

112. Moss AJ, Zareba W, Hall WJ, et al. Prophylactic implantation of a defibrillator in patients with myocardial infarction and reduced ejection fraction. *N Engl J Med* 2002;346:877–883.

113. Bristow MR, Feldman AM, Saxon LA. Heart failure management using implantable devices for ventricular resynchronization: Comparison of Medical Therapy, Pacing, and Defibrillation in Chronic Heart Failure (COMPANION) trial. COMPANION Steering Committee and COMPANION Clinical Investigators. *J Card Failure* 2000;6: 276–285.

114. Rathore SS, Curtis JP, Wang Y, et al. Association of serum digoxin concentration and outcomes in patients with heart failure. *JAMA* 2003; 289:871–878.

115. Levy D, Larson MG, Vasan RS, et al. The progression from hypertension to congestive heart failure. *JAMA* 1996;275:1557–1562.

116. Quaife RA, Lynch D, Badesch DB, et al. Right ventricular phenotypic characteristics in subjects with primary pulmonary hypertension or idiopathic dilated cardiomyopathy. *J Cardiac Failure* 1999;5:46–54.

117. Devereux RB, Roman MJ. Left ventricular hypertrophy in hypertension: Stimuli, patterns, and consequences. *Hypertens Res.* 1999;22:1–9.

118. Bristow MR. Mechanisms of development of heart failure in the hypertensive patient. *Cardiology* 1999;92:3–6.

119. Nielsen I. The natural history of hypertensive heart disease as suggested by echocardiography. *Acta Med Scand Suppl* 1986;714:165–169.

120. Grossman W. Cardiac hypertrophy: Useful adaptation or pathologic process. *Am J Med* 1980;69:576–584.

121. Moreno PR, Jang IK, Block PC, Palacios IF. The role of percutaneous balloon valvuloplasty in patients with cardiogenic shock. *Amer J Med* 1994;23:1071–1075.

122. Packer M, O'Conner CM, Ghali JK, et al. Effect of Amlodipine on morbidity and mortality in severe chronic heart failure. *N Engl J Med* 1996;335:1107–1114.

123. Scognamiglio R, Rahimtoola SH, Fasoli G, et al. Nifedipine in asymptomatic patients with severe aortic regurgitation and normal left ventricular function. *N Engl J Med* 1994;331:689–694.

124. Gregori D, Rocco C, Miocic S, Mestroni L. Estimating the frequency of familial dilated cardiomyopathy in the presence of misclassification errors. *J Appl Statistics* 2001;28:53–62.

125. Grünig E, Tasman JA, Kucherer H, et al. Frequency and phenotypes of familial dilated cardiomyopathy. *J Am Coll Cardiol* 1998;31: 186–194.

126. Baig MK, Goldman JH, Caforio ALP, et al. Familial dilated cardiomyopathy: Cardiac abnormalities are common in asymptomatic relatives and may represent early disease. *J Am Coll Cardiol* 1998;31:195–201.

127. D'Adamo P, Fassone L, Gedeon A, et al. The X-linked gene G4.5 is responsible for different infantile dilated cardiomyopathies. *Am J Hum Genet* 1997;61:862–867.

128. Mestroni L, Rocco C, Gregori D, et al. Familial dilated cardiomyopathy: Evidence for genetic and phenotypic heterogeneity. *J Am Coll Cardiol* 1999;34:181–190.

129. Muntoni F, Di Lenarda A, Porcu M, et al. Dystrophin gene abnormalities in two patients with idiopathic dilated cardiomyopathy. *Heart* 1997;78:608–612.

130. Milasin J, Muntoni F, Severini GM, et al. A point mutation in the 5' splice site of the dystrophin gene first intron responsible for X-linked dilated cardiomyopathy. *Hum Mol Genet* 1996;5:73–79.

131. Taylor MRG, Fain P, Sinagra G, et al. Natural history of dilated cardiomyopathy due to lamin A/C gene mutations. *J Am Coll Cardiol* 2003;41:771–780.

132. Ortiz-Lopez R, Li M, Su J, et al. Evidence for a dystrophin missense mutation as a cause of X-linked dilated cardiomyopathy. *Circulation* 1997;95:2434–2440.

133. Arbustini E, Pilotto A, Repetto A, et al. Autosomal dominant dilated cardiomyopathy with atrioventricular block: A lamin A/C defect-related disease. *J Am Coll Cardiol* 2002;39:981–990.

134. Bies RD, Maeda M, Roberds SL, et al. A'5 dystrophin duplication mutation causes membrane deficiency of alpha-dystroglycan in a family with X-linked cardiomyopathy. *J Mol Cell Cardiol* 1997;29:31175–31188.

135. Maeda M, Nakao S, Miyazato H, et al. Cardiac dystrophin abnormalities in Becker muscular dystrophy assessed by endomyocardial biopsy. *Amer Heart J* 1995;129:702–707.

136. Melacini P, Fanin M, Duggan DJ, et al. Heart involvement in muscular dystrophies due to sarcoglycan gene mutations. *Muscle Nerve*. 1999;22:473–479.

137. Fatkin D, Christe ME, Aristizabal O, et al. Neonatal cardiomyopathy in mice homozygous for the Arg403Gln mutation in the alpha cardiac myosin heavy chain gene. *J Clin Invest* 1999;103:147–153.

138. McConnell BK, Jones KA, Fatkin D, et al. Dilated cardiomyopathy in homozygous myosin-binding protein-C mutant mice. *J Clin Invest* 1999;104:1235–1244.

139. Daehmlow S, Erdmann J, Knueppel T, et al. Novel mutations in sarcomeric protein genes in dilated cardiomyopathy. *Biochem Biophys Res Commun* 2002;289:116–120.

140. Iwase M, Uechi M, Vatner DE, et al. Dilated cardiomyopathy induced by cardiac Gs-alpha overexpression. *Circulation* 1996;94:I-16.

141. Tiranti V, Jaksch M, Hofmann S, et al. Loss-of-function mutations of SURF-1 are specifically associated with Leigh syndrome with cytochrome *c* oxidase deficiency. *Ann Neurol* 1999;46:161–166.

142. Grasso M, Diegoli M, Brega A, et al. The mitochondrial DNA mutation T12297C affects a highly conserved nucleotide of tRNA [Leu(CUN)] and is associated with dilated cardiomyopathy. *Eur J Hum Genet* 2001;9:311–315.

143. Mestroni L, Maisch B, McKenna WJ, et al. Guidelines for the study of familial dilated cardiomyopathies. *Eur Heart J* 1999;20:93–102.

144. Crispell KA, Hanson EL, Coates K, et al. Periodic rescreening is indicated for family members at risk of developing familial dilated cardiomyopathy. *J Am Coll Cardiol* 2002;39:1503–1597.

145. Crispell KA, Wray A, Ni H, et al. Clinical profiles of four large pedigrees with familial dilated cardiomyopathy: Preliminary recommendations for clinical practice. *J Am Coll Cardiol* 1999;34:837–847.

146. Silver MA. Anatomy of the failing heart in dilated cardiomyopathy. In: Engelmeier RS, O'Connell JB, eds. *Drug Therapy in Dilated Cardiomyopathy and Myocarditis.* New York: Marcel Dekker; 1988:1–12.

147. Roberts WC, Siegel RJ, McManus BM. Idiopathic dilated cardiomyopathy: Analysis of 152 necropsy patients. *Am J Cardiol* 1987;60:1340–1355.

148. Falk RH, Foster E, Coats MH. Ventricular thrombi and thromboembolism in dilated cardiomyopathy. *Am Heart J* 1992;123:136–142.

149. Rowan R, Maesk MA, Billingham ME. Ultrastructural morphometric analysis of endomyocardial biopsies. *Am J Cardiovasc Pathol* 1988;2:137–144.

150. Baandrup U, Olsen EG. Critical analysis of endomyocardial biopsies from patients suspected of having cardiomyopathy. *Br Heart J* 1981;45:475–486.

151. Arbustini E, Pucci R, Pozzi R, et al. Ultrastructural changes in myocarditis and dilated cardiomyopathy. In: Baroldi G, Camerini F, Goodwin JF, eds. *Advances in Cardiomyopathies.* Berlin: Springer Verlag; 1990:274–289.

152. Schwarz F, Mall G, Zebe H, et al. Determinants of survival in patients with congestive cardiomyopathy: Quantitative morphologic findings and left ventricular hemodynamics. *Circulation* 1984;70:923–928.

153. Tazelaar HD, Billingham ME. Leukocytic infiltrates in idiopathic dilated cardiomyopathy. *Am J Surg Pathol* 1986;10:405–412.

154. Hammond EH, Anderson JL, Menlove RL. Diagnostic and prognostic value of immunofluorescence and electronmicroscopic findings in idiopathic dilated cardiomyopathy. In: Baroldi G, Camerini F, Goodwin JF, eds. *Advances in Cardiomyopathies.* Berlin: Springer Verlag; 1990:290–301.

155. Caforio ALP, Keeling PJ, Zachara E, et al. Evidence from family studies for autoimmunity in dilated cardiomyopathy. *Lancet* 1994;344:773–777.

156. Kawai C, Takatsu T. Clinical and experimental studies on cardiomyopathy. *N Engl J Med* 1975;293:592–597.

157. Anderson JL, Carlquist JF, Hammond EH. Deficient natural killer cell activity in patients with idiopathic dilated cardiomyopathy. *Lancet* 1982;2:1124–1127.

158. Fowles RE, Bieker CP, Stinson EB. Defective in vitro suppressor cell function in idiopathic congestive cardiomyopathy. *Circulation* 1979;59:483–491.

159. Gerli R, Rambotti P, Spinozzi F, et al. Immunologic studies of peripheral blood from patients with idiopathic dilated cardiomyopathy. *Am Heart J* 1986;112:350–355.

160. Klein R, Maisch B, Kochsiek K, Berg PA. Demonstration of organ specific antibodies against heart mitochondria (anti-M) in sera from patients with some forms of heart disease. *Clin Exp Immunol* 1984;58:283–292.

161. Maisch B, Deeg P, Liebau G, Kochsiek K. Diagnostic relevance of humoral and cytotoxic immune reactions in primary and secondary dilated cardiomyopathy. *Am J Cardiol* 1983;52:1071–1078.

162. Limas CJ, Goldenberg IF, Limas C. Autoantibodies against β-adrenoreceptors in human idiopathic dilated cardiomyopathy. *Circulation* 1989;64:97–103.

163. Magnusson Y, Marullo S, Hoyer S, et al. Mapping of a functional autoimmune epitope on the β_1-adrenergic receptor in patients with idiopathic dilated cardiomyopathy. *J Clin Invest* 1990;86:1658–1663.

164. Magnusson Y, Wallukat G, Waagstein F, et al. Autoimmunity in idiopathic dilated cardiomyopathy. Characterization of antibodies against the beta 1-adrenoceptor with positive chronotropic effect. *Circulation*. 1994;89:2760–2767.

165. Schultheiss H-P, Bolte HD. Immunological analysis of autoantibodies against the adenine nucleotide translocator in dilated cardiomyopathy. *J Mol Cell Cardiol* 1985;17:603–617.

166. Schultheiss HP. Disturbance of the myocardial energy metabolism in dilated cardiomyopathy due to autoimmunological mechanisms. *Circulation* 1993;87(suppl IV):43–48.

167. Anderson JL, Carlquist JF, Lutz JR, et al. HLA A, B, and DR typing in idiopathic dilated cardiomyopathy: A search for immune response function. *Am J Cardiol* 1984;33:1326–1330.

168. Carlquist JF, Menlove RL, Murray MB, et al. HLA class II (DR and DQ) antigen associations in idiopathic dilated cardiomyopathy. Validation study and meta-analysis of published HLA association studies. *Circulation* 1991;83:515–522.

169. Gilbert EM, Mason JW. Immunosuppressive therapy of myocarditis. In: Engelmeier RS, O'Connell JB, eds. *Drug Therapy in Dilated Cardiomyopathy and Myocarditis.* New York: Marcel Dekker; 1987:233–263.

170. Bowles NE, Richardson PJ, Olsen ECJ, Archard LC. Detection of coxsackie-B virus specific RNA sequences in myocardial biopsy samples from patients with myocarditis and dilated cardiomyopathy. *Lancet* 1986;1:1120–1128.

171. Archard LC, Bowles NE, Cunningham L, et al. Enterovirus RNA sequences in hearts with dilated cardiomyopathy: A pathogenetic link between virus infection and dilated cardiomyopathy. In: Baroldi G, Camerini F, Goodwin JF, eds. *Advances in Cardiomyopathies.* Berlin: Springer-Verlag; 1990:194–198.

172. Giacca M, Severini GM, Mestroni L, et al. Low frequency of detection by nested polymerase chain reaction of enterovirus ribonucleic acid in endomyocardial tissue of patients with idiopathic dilated cardiomyopathy. *J Am Coll Cardiol* 1994;24:1033–1040.

173. Parrillo JE, Cunnion RE, Epstein SE, et al. A prospective, randomized, controlled trial of prednisone for dilated cardiomyopathy. *N Engl J Med* 1989;321:1061–1067.

174. Badorff C, Lee GH, Lamphear BJ, et al. Enteroviral protease 2A cleaves dystrophin: Evidence of cytoskeletal disruption in an acquired cardiomyopathy. *Nat Med* 1999;5:320–326.

175. Pauschinger M, Doerner A, Kuehl U, et al. Enteroviral RNA replication in the myocardium of patients with left ventricular dysfunction and clinically suspected myocarditis. *Circulation* 1999;99:889–895.

176. Martin AB, Webber S, Fricker FJ, et al. Acute myocarditis: Rapid diagnosis by PCR in children. *Circulation* 1994;90:330–339.

177. Fuster V, Gersh BJ, Giuliani ER, et al. The natural history of idiopathic dilated cardiomyopathy. *Am J Cardiol* 1981;47:525–531.

178. Redfield MM, Gersh BJ, Bailey KR, et al. Natural history of idiopathic dilated cardiomyopathy: Effect of referral bias and secular trend. *J Am Coll Cardiol* 1993;22:1921–1926.

179. The SOLVD Investigators. Effect of angiotensin converting enzyme inhibition with enalapril on survival in patients with reduced left ventricular ejection fraction and congestive heart failure: Results of the Treatment Trial of the Studies of Left Ventricular Dysfunction (SOLVD); a randomized double blind trial. *N Engl J Med* 1991;325:293–302.

180. Hosenpud JD, Novick RJ, Bennett LE, et al. The registry of the international society for heart and lung transplantation: Thirteenth official report-1996. *J Heart Lung Transplant* 1996;15:655–674.

181. Deng MC, De Meester JM, Smits JM, et al. Effect of receiving a heart transplant: Analysis of a national cohort entered on to a waiting list, stratified by heart failure severity. *BMJ* 2000;321:540–545.

182. Woodley SL, Gilbert EM, Anderson JL, et al. β-Blockade with bucindolol in heart failure due to ischemic vs idiopathic dilated cardiomyopathy. *Circulation* 1991;84:2426–2441.

183. Waagstein F, Bristow MR, Swedberg K, et al. Beneficial effects of metoprolol in idiopathic dilated cardiomyopathy. *Lancet* 1993;342:1441–1446.

184. Bristow MR, Mason JW, Billingham ME, Daniels JR. Doxorubicin cardiomyopathy: Evaluation by phonocardiography, endomyocardial biopsy, and cardiac catheterization. *Ann Intern Med* 1978;88:168–175.

185. Von Hoff DD, Layard MW, Basa P, et al. Risk factors for doxorubicin-induced congestive heart failure. *Ann Intern Med* 1979;91:710–717.

186. Bristow MR, Mason JW, Billingham ME, Daniels JR. Dose-effect and structure function relationships in doxorubicin cardiomyopathy. *Am Heart J* 1981;102:709–718.

187. Bristow MR, Billingham ME, Mason JW, Daniels JR. The clinical spectrum of anthracycline antibiotic cardiotoxicity. *Cancer Treat Rep* 1978;62:873–879.

188. Billingham ME, Bristow MR, Glatstein J, et al. Adriamycin cardiotoxicity: Endomyocardial biopsy evidence of enhancement by irradiation. *Am J Surg Pathol* 1977;1:17–23.

189. Kantrowitz NE, Bristow MR. Cardiotoxicity of antitumor agents. *Prog Cardiovasc Dis* 1984;27:195–200.

190. Lewis W, Kleinerman J, Puszkin S. Interaction of Adriamycin in vitro with myofibrillar proteins. *Circ Res* 1982;50:547–553.

191. Jaenke RS. Delayed and progressive myocardial lesions after Adriamycin administration in rabbits. *Cancer* 1976;36:2958–2966.

192. Shaddy RE, Olsen SL, Bristow MR, et al. Efficacy and safety of metoprolol in the treatment of doxorubicin-induced cardiomyopathy in pediatric patients. *Am Heart J* 1995;129:197–199.

193. Shaddy RE, Tani LY, Gidding SS, et al. Beta-blocker treatment of dilated cardiomyopathy with congestive heart failure in children: A multi-institutional experience. *J Heart Lung Transplant* 1999;18:269–274.

194. Bristow MR, Lopez MB, Mason JW, et al. Efficacy and cost of cardiac monitoring in patients receiving doxorubicin. *Cancer* 1982;50:32–41.

195. McKillop JH, Bristow MR, Goris ML, et al. Sensitivity and specificity of radionuclide ejection fractions in doxorubicin cardiotoxicity. *Am Heart J* 1983;105:1048–1056.

196. Alexander J, Dainiak N, Berger HJ, et al. Serial assessment of doxorubicin cardiotoxicity with quantitative radionuclide angiocardiography. *N Engl J Med* 1979;300:278–283.

197. Torti FM, Bristow MR, Howes AE, et al. Endomyocardial biopsy evidence of reduced cardiotoxicity of doxorubicin delivered on a weekly schedule. *Ann Intern Med* 1983;99:745–749.

198. Legha SS, Benjamin RS, Mackay B, et al. Reduction of doxorubicin cardiotoxicity by prolonged continuous intravenous infusion. *Ann Intern Med* 1982;96:133–139.

199. Rahman A, More N, Schein PS. Doxorubicin-induced chronic cardiotoxicity and its prevention by liposomal administration. *Cancer* 1982;42:1817–1825.

200. Speyer JL, Green MD, Kramer E, et al. Protective effect of the bispiperazinedione ICRF-187 against doxorubicin-induced cardiac toxicity in women with advanced breast cancer. *N Engl J Med* 1988;319:745–752.

201. Pearson GD, Veille JC, Rahimtoola S, et al. Peripartum cardiomyopathy: National Heart, Lung, and Blood Institute and Office of Rare Diseases (National Institutes of Health) workshop recommendations and review. *JAMA* 2000;283:1183–1188.

202. Midei MG, DeMent SH, Feldman AM, et al. Peripartum myocarditis and cardiomyopathy. *Circulation* 1990;81:922–928.

203. O'Connell JB, Costanzo-Nordin MR, Subramanian R, et al. Peripartum cardiomyopathy: Clinical, hemodynamic histologic and prognostic characteristics. *J Am Coll Cardiol* 1986;8:52–56.

204. Elkayam U, Tummala PP, Rao K, et al. Maternal and fetal outcomes of subsequent pregnancies in women with peripartum cardiomyopathy. *N Engl J Med* 2001;344:1567–1571.

205. Jacobson DR, Busbaum JN. Genetic aspects of amyloidosis. *Adv Hum Genet* 1991;20:69–75.

206. Kyle RA, Griepp PR. Amyloidosis (AL): Clinical and laboratory feature in 229 cases. *Mayo Clin Proc* 1983;58:665–672.

207. Glenner GG. Amyloid deposits and amyloidosis. *N Engl J Med* 1980;302:1283–1292.

208. Hamer JP, Janssen S, van Rijswik MH, Lie KI. Amyloid cardiomyopathy in systemic non-hereditary amyloidosis. Clinical, echocardiographic and electrocardiographic findings in 30 patients with AA and 24 patients with AL amyloidosis. *Eur Heart J* 1992;13:623–627.

209. Stone MJ. Amyloidosis: A final common pathway for protein deposition in tissues. *Blood* 1990;75:531–545.

210. Schroeder JS, Billingham ME, Rider AK. Cardiac amyloidosis: Diagnosis by transvenous endomyocardial biopsy. *Am J Med* 1975;59:269–273.

211. Koyoma J, Ray-Sequin PA, Falk RH. Prognostic significance of ultrasound myocardial tissue characterization in patients with cardiac amyloidosis. *Circulation* 2002;106:556–561.

212. McCarthy RE, Kasper EK. A review of the amyloidoses that infiltrate the heart. *Clin Cardiol* 1998;21:547–552.

213. Hamidi AL, Liepnieks JJ, Hamidi AK, et al. Hereditary amyloid cardiomyopathy caused by a variant apolipoprotein A1. *Am J Pathol* 1999;154:221–227.

214. Kingman A, Pereira NL. Cardiac amyloidosis. *J S C Med Assoc* 2001;97:201–206.

215. Kyle RA, Gertz MA, Greipp PR, et al. A trial of three regimens for primary amyloidosis—Colchicine alone, melphalan and prednisone, and melphalan, prednisone, and colchicine. *N Engl J Med* 1997;336:1202–1207.

216. Holmgren G, Ericzon BG, Groth CG. Clinical improvement and amyloid regression after liver transplantation in hereditary transthyretin amyloidosis. *Lancet* 1993;341:1113–1116.

217. Maisch B. Alcohol and the heart. *Hertz* 1996;21:207–212.

218. Fernandez-Sola J, Nicolas JM, Oriola J, et al. Angiotensin-converting enzyme gene polymorphism is associated with vulnerability to alcoholic cardiomyopathy. *Ann Intern Med* 2002;137:321–326.

219. Prazak P, Pfisterer M, Osswald S, et al. Differences of disease progression in congestive heart failure due to alcoholic as compared to idiopathic dilated cardiomyopathy. *Eur Heart J* 1996;17:251–257.

220. World Health Organization Expert Committee. Chagas' disease. In: *World Health Organ Tech Rep Ser* 1984:50–55.

221. Mady C, Cardoso RHA, Barretto ACP, et al. Survival and predictors of survival in patients with congestive heart failure due to Chagas' cardiomyopathy. *Circulation* 1994;90:3098–3102.

222. Rosenbaum MB. The hemiblocks: Diagnostic criteria and clinical significance. *Mod Concepts Cardiovasc Dis* 1970;39:141–146.

223. Laranja FS, Dias E, Nobrega G, Miranda A. Chagas' disease: A clinical, epidemiological, and pathological study. *Circulation.* 1956;14:1035–1060.

224. Barros MV, Rocha MO, Ribeiro AL, Machado FS. Doppler tissue imaging to evaluate early myocardium damage in patients with

undetermined form of Chagas' disease and normal echocardiogram. *Echocardiography* 2001;18:131–136.

225. Barros MV, Rocha MO, Ribeiro AL, Machado FS. Tissue Doppler imaging in the evaluation of the regional diastolic function in Chagas' disease. *J Am Soc Echocardiogr* 2001;14:353–359.

226. Tibbetts RS, McCormick TS, Rowland EC, et al. Cardiac antigen-specific autoantibody production is associated with cardiomyopathy in *Trypanosoma cruzi*–infected mice. *J Immunol* 1994;152:1493–1499.

227. Bestetti RM, Muccillo G. Clinical course of Chagas' heart disease: A comparison with dilated cardiomyopathy. *Int J Cardiol* 1997;60: 187–193.

228. Chandra M, Shirani J, Shtutin M, et al. Cardioprotective effects of verapamil on myocardial structure and function in a murine model of chronic *Trypanosoma cruzi* infection (Brazil strain): An echocardiographic study. *Int J Parasitol* 2002;32:207–215.

229. Nul DR, Grancelli HO, Perrone SV, et al. Randomised trial of low-dose amiodarone in severe congestive heart failure. *Lancet* 1994; 344:493–498.

230. Bocchi EA, Bellotti G, Mocelin AO, et al. Heart transplantation for chronic Chagas' heart disease. *Ann Thorac Surg* 1996;61:1727–1733.

231. Blanche C, Aleksic I, Takkenberg JJM, et al. Heart transplantation for Chagas' cardiomyopathy. *Ann Thorac Surg* 1995;60:1406–1499.

HYPERTROPHIC CARDIOMYOPATHY

Rick A. Nishimura / Steven R. Ommen / A. Jamil Tajik

Hypertrophic cardiomyopathy (HCM) is an inheritable autosomal dominant disease of the heart muscle, characterized by a small left ventricular cavity and marked hypertrophy of the myocardium with myofibril disarray.[1-7] There may or may not be a dynamic left ventricular outflow tract obstruction. The prevalence is approximately 1:500 to 1:1000 persons.[4,8,8a,8b]

The etiology of the hypertrophy was unclear in the past. The basis of the disease was ascribed to multiple etiologies, such as an abnormality of calcium metabolism, a neural crest disorder, or an abnormal response to catecholamine stimulation.[9,10] However, in 1989, investigators first mapped the genetic mutation for HCM to chromosome 14.[11,12] This mutation later was shown to affect the encoding of beta-myosin heavy chain protein, which is a major component of the sarcomere and contractile apparatus in the cardiomyocytes.[13,14] Subsequently, over 100 mutations have been found in patients with HCM in the genes encoding sarcomere proteins. Thus, HCM is felt to be a disease of the sarcomere, whose alteration in structure and/or function underlines the pathology and pathophysiology in affected individuals.[15-25]

HCM subsequently has been shown to be a highly heterogeneous disease, with a diverse pathology, pathophysiology, and clinical course.[4-7] The pathophysiology of HCM is complex, consisting of one or more multiple interrelated processes including dynamic left ventricular outflow tract obstruction, mitral regurgitation, diastolic dysfunction, myocardial ischemia, and cardiac arrhythmias.[1,2] Some patients may present with severe limiting symptoms of dyspnea, angina, and syncope, yet other patients remain completely asymptomatic throughout life. HCM is the most common cause of sudden cardiac death in young people, including trained athletes.[26-32] However, the overall prognosis of patients with HCM in nonreferral centers is comparable to that of an age-matched, sex-matched control population.[4,33-39] Treatment, therefore, may vary from reassurance only to implantation of an automatic defibrillator to creation of a localized myocardial infarction.

HISTORICAL PERSPECTIVE

The first anatomic description of this entity was by Teare in 1958, when he reported the pathologic findings in 8 young patients, 7 of whom had died suddenly.[40] He found massive hypertrophy of the ventricular septum with a small ventricular cavity. The gross picture was associated with microscopic evidence of myocardial disarray of the individual muscle fibers, which was speculated to be due to either a benign tumor or hamartoma. At the same time, Sir Russell Brock reported on patients with functional subvalvular left ventricular outflow tract gradients confirmed by pressure gradients.[41] Patients had been diagnosed as having aortic valvular stenosis with associated hypertension, and the gradient was attributed to secondary left ventricular hypertrophy, which developed from the pressure overload. Braunwald et al. in the 1960s defined the specific disease process, in which asymmetric septal hypertrophy, myofibril disarray, and a dynamic subvalvular pressure gradient was documented.[42,43] This entity was considered to be a primary process with no known cause. A genetic connection was suggested when a familial link was shown to be associated with this entity in an autosomal dominant fashion.[44]

Since these initial descriptions, the disease process has come to be known by a wide variety of names. This disease has been called asymmetric septal hypertrophy (ASH), idiopathic hypertrophic subaortic stenosis, muscle subaortic stenosis, and hypertrophic obstructive cardiomyopathy. The World Health Organization has designated the term *hypertrophic cardiomyopathy* to describe this unique process of primary muscle hypertrophy, which may exist with or without a dynamic left ventricular outflow tract gradient.[45]

The evolution of M-mode and two-dimensional echocardiography resulted in a noninvasive diagnostic tool to identify patients with HCM. M-mode echocardiography was used to define ASH, which was present if the ratio of septal to posterior wall thickness exceeded 1.3.[46,47] Systolic anterior motion (SAM) of the mitral valve on M-mode echocardiography was found to correlate with the dynamic left ventricular outflow tract obstruction.[48] Two-dimensional echocardiography showed that hypertrophy in patients with HCM could involve areas other than the ventricular septum and further led to the understanding of the complex pathophysiology of HCM.[1,49] It is now recognized that some patients with HCM may not have gross hypertrophy yet still be at risk for disease complications such as sudden death.[31,50,51]

Initial descriptions of patients with HCM originated from several large referral centers.[3–5,52–54] These were selected younger patients, children and young adults, usually less than 50 years old, who had been referred because they had been judged to have either a high-risk status or severe symptoms requiring highly specialized care. Those patients who were asymptomatic or older patients were underrepresented in these studies. There were high-mortality rates of 3 to 7 percent per year reported from these tertiary centers, and many patients died suddenly. These numbers grossly overestimated the overall risk and impact of the disease. More recent reports from nontertiary centers with less selected, regional, or community base cohorts have been reported.[4,33–39] These studies include many asymptomatic patients who had their diagnosis made by echocardiography, as well as older patients. In these studies, the overall mortality of HCM is similar to control populations. It is now well accepted that although there still remains a select group of patients who are identified at high risk for sudden catastrophic events, the majority of patients with HCM live an uneventful, asymptomatic life.[4]

ETIOLOGY

The characteristic pathologic and pathophysiologic features of HCM have intrigued physicians for decades, and a multitude of causes have been postulated for the disorder. It was speculated that HCM develops as a response to an increase in catecholamine stimulation.[9,10] Histochemical studies of resected myocardium from patients with HCM revealed an increased sympathetic nerve supply and a high norepinephrine content of the muscle.[55] HCM has been associated with neural crest disorder, such as pheochromocytoma, multiple lentiginosis, and neurofibromatosis.[9,10,56]

Investigators now believe that hypertrophic cardiomyopathy is due to a mutation in any one of at least 10 genes, each encoding proteins of the cardiac sarcomere.[15–18,22,25] Thus, the full clinical spectrum of HCM can be looked upon as a single unified disease entity and a primary disorder of the sarcomere. Affected genes thus far encode beta-myosin heavy chain, myosin-binding protein C, cardiac troponins T and I, alpha-tropomyosin, actin, titin, and myosin light chains.[50,51,57–70] These known mutations are inherited in an autosomal dominant manner.

Several types of mutations have been identified in these genes, including deletions, insertions, and missense and splice site mutations.[24,25] Mutant peptides that are encoded affect function of the contractile unit of the sarcomere by becoming incorporated into the sarcomere itself.[15,16,71] Different mutations may result in a different biophysical consequence. Some defects may alter the actin-myosin cross-bridge formation, and others may affect the movement and force generation of the thick and thin filaments. It has been hypothesized that the sarcomeric dysfunction can lead to "compensatory" myocardial hypertrophy, though the precise impetus for hypertrophy has not yet been identified.[15,16,71–73] Studies of polymorphisms within the renin-angiotensin-aldosterone system have supported a role for modifying genes in the degree of hypertrophy.[74] Phenotypic expression of HCM is probably not only the product of the mutations, but also of modifier genes and environmental factors.[75,76]

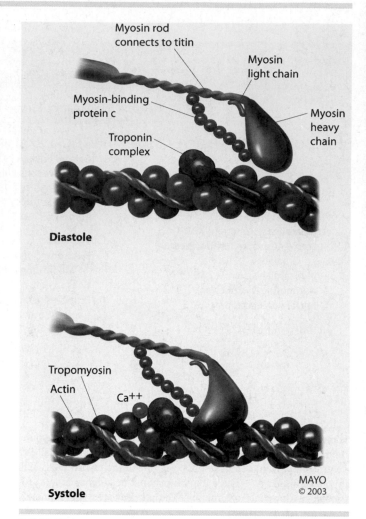

FIGURE 77-1 Schematic diagram of the sarcomere. Hypertrophic cardiomyopathy is a disease of the sarcomere, with mutations found of at least 10 genes coding for various parts of the sarcomere.

There may be a large number of genes that ultimately influence the expression of the phenotype of HCM.

The multiple different genes that are affected and the multiple mutations that occur within each gene likely contribute to the variable presentation and prognosis of patients with HCM. The age of phenotypic expression, degree of hypertrophy, and prognosis have all been associated with specific gene mutations. (Fig. 77-1)

Another genetic locus has been mapped to chromosome 7 in patients with cardiac hypertrophy and electrophysiologic abnormalities such as Wolff-Parkinson-White syndrome.[77–79] This is not a gene encoding the sarcomere but rather a mutation in the γ2 regulatory subunit (PRKAG2) of adenosine monophosphate activated protein kinase, an enzyme that modulates glucose metabolism. Histopathologic and biochemical studies of the myocardium have shown myocyte enlargement with glycogen-filled vacuoles, suggesting that these patients who in the past were diagnosed as having HCM may have a different disease process similar to a glycogen storage disease.

PATHOLOGY

Gross examination of the heart in HCM demonstrates asymmetric septal hypertrophy with a small left ventricular cavity (Fig. 77-2).[80–82] The mural endocardium may be thickened by fibrous tissue and there

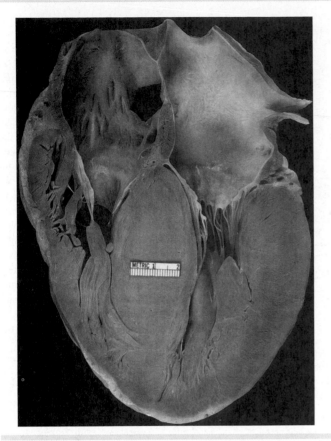

FIGURE 77-2 Pathologic specimen of a patient who died suddenly with hypertrophic cardiomyopathy. There is massive hypertrophy of the myocardium and a small left ventricular cavity. The left atrium is enlarged. (Courtesy of Dr. W. D. Edwards.)

fibers. This disorganization results in a "whorling" of muscle fibers that are characteristic of HCM (Fig. 77-3). Myocardial disarray is noted not only in the ventricular septum but also in the left ventricular free wall. This disarray is not specific to HCM and can be seen in any pressure-overloaded ventricle, although the proportion of myocardial disarray is much greater in patients with HCM.[85,86]

PATHOPHYSIOLOGY

The pathophysiology of patients with HCM is complex and consists of multiple interrelated abnormalities.[1,2,4,6,7] These include diastolic dysfunction, left ventricular outflow tract obstruction, mitral regurgitation, myocardial ischemia, and arrhythmias. The varying combination and degrees of these abnormalities account for the wide spectrum of presentation by patients with HCM.

Diastolic Dysfunction

The major pathophysiologic abnormality in patients with HCM is diastolic dysfunction (Fig. 77-4).[1,2,87–89] Diastolic dysfunction arises from multiple factors, which ultimately affect both ventricular relaxation and chamber stiffness. An impairment of ventricular relaxation results from the high systolic contraction load caused by an outflow tract obstruction, and nonuniformity of ventricular contraction and relaxation, as well as delayed inactivation caused by abnormal intracellular calcium reuptake. The severe hypertrophy of the myocardium results in an increase in chamber stiffness. Diffuse myocardial ischemia may further affect both relaxation and chamber stiffness. Associated with these alterations is a compensatory increase in the contribution of late diastolic filling during atrial systole. With exercise or any other type of catecholamine stimulation, the decrease in the diastolic filling period as well as myocardial ischemia will further lead to severe abnormalities of diastolic filling of the heart, with an increase in pulmonary venous pressure causing symptoms of dyspnea.

is often a plaque located on the upper septal area where the mitral valve has been opposed to the septum during systole. The mitral valve itself is usually intrinsically normal. However, there may be elongation of the mitral chordae and anterior displacement of hypertrophied papillary muscles. Abnormal attachments of the mitral valve chordal apparatus to the septum and attachments of the papillary muscle head directly into the leaflets may be found. The left atrium is usually dilated at autopsy. Although the epicardial coronary arteries are normal, the intramural coronary arterioles in the septum are small because of intimal hyperplasia and are increased in number.[83,84]

In the original report by Teare,[40] bizarre arrangements of the muscle fiber bundles separated by clefts lined with endothelin were described. The myocardial disarray consists of short runs of severely hypertrophied fibers interrupted by connective tissue. There are large and bizarre nuclei and fibrosis present, with degenerating muscle

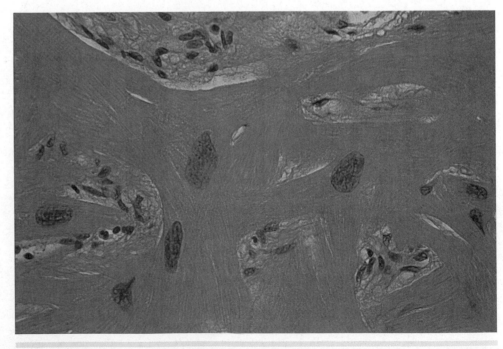

FIGURE 77-3 Microscopic section of the myocardium from a patient with hypertrophic cardiomyopathy. There is myofiber disarray present. (Courtesy of Dr. W. D. Edwards.)

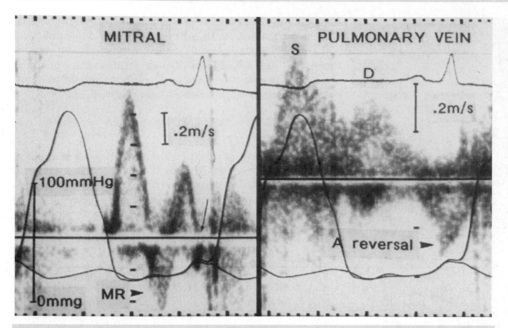

FIGURE 77-4 Evidence of severe diastolic dysfunction in a patient with hypertrophic cardiomyopathy. The left ventricular and left atrial pressures are shown in both the left and right panel. The mean left atrial pressure is severely elevated to 30 mm of mercury. Left: the mitral flow velocity curve is shown, demonstrating a high E:A ratio and a short deceleration time. Diastolic mitral regurgitation (MR) is present. There is abrupt cessation of the "a" duration (arrow). Right: the pulmonary vein velocity curve is shown, with a high velocity at atrial reversal of long duration. The systolic forward flow (S) and diastolic forward flow (D) is shown.

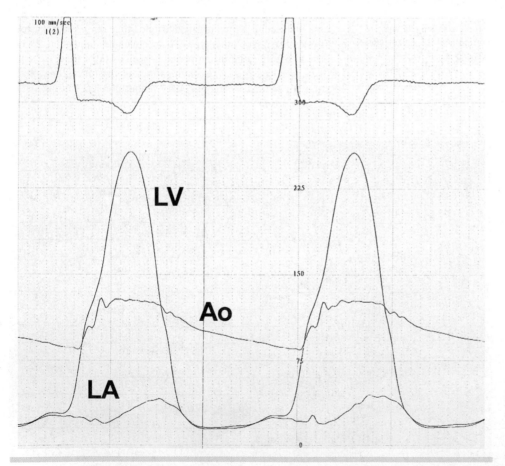

FIGURE 77-5 Cardiac catheterization pressure curves showing a severe left ventricular outflow tract obstruction. The gradient between the left ventricle (LV) and aorta (Ao) is nearly 100 mm of mercury. The left atrial (LA) pressure is also elevated. There is a "spike and dome" pattern on the aortic pressure curve.

Left Ventricular Outflow Pressure Gradient

The original description by Brock in 1957 emphasized the functional subvalvular left ventricular outflow tract gradient (Fig. 77-5).[41] This obstruction was further characterized by Braunwald et al. who described the dynamic nature of the gradient related to alterations in the load and contractility of the left ventricle.[43] The obstruction itself causes an increase in left ventricular systolic pressure, which leads to a complex interplay of abnormalities including prolongation of ventricular relaxation, elevation of left ventricular diastolic pressure, mitral regurgitation, myocardial ischemia, and a decrease in forward cardiac output.[1,2]

In the past, the significance of the outflow tract gradient was controversial. It was proposed that the intraventricular pressure gradient does not actually signify outflow obstruction but instead is the result of rapid and early emptying of a hyperdynamic ventricle.[90–92] However, subsequent studies have shown that aortic flow continues throughout systole, indicating that a true obstruction does exist.[1,2]

The mechanism of obstruction is multifactorial. The obstruction was initially thought to be due to systolic contraction of the hypertrophied basal ventricular septum, which would then encroach into the left ventricular outflow tract with a resultant Venturi effect on the mitral valve leaflets.[1,2,93] The Venturi effect would "suck" the mitral valve leaflets into the left ventricular outflow tract and produce further obstruction. The interplay of the mitral valve leaflets and the obstruction may also be secondary to a structural abnormality of the mitral valve apparatus. In patients with HCM, there may be elongated mitral valve leaflets and chordae with abnormally positioned papillary muscles. During ventricular systole, flow against the abnormally positioned mitral valve apparatus will result in a drag force on a portion of the mitral valve leaflets and actually "push" the leaflets into the outflow tract.[94–97] Obstruction can also be present in the mid-cavitary region due to hypertrophied papillary muscles abutting against the septum.[98]

The obstruction to left ventricular outflow is dynamic, varying with

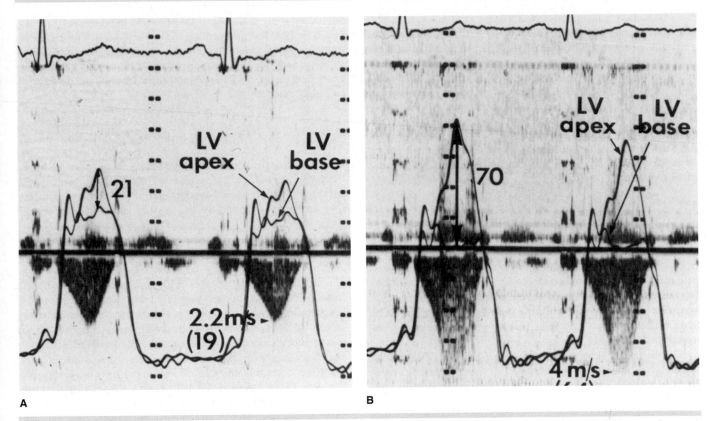

A

B

FIGURE 77-6 The dynamic nature of the left ventricular outflow tract obstruction is shown by simultaneous Doppler echocardiography and cardiac catheterization. The cardiac catheterization is performed with a pressure measurement of the left ventricular apex and left ventricular base. The gradient occurs during systole between the left ventricular apex and left ventricular base. The continuous wave Doppler velocities through the left ventricular outflow tract is shown. The calculated gradient from the Doppler echocardiogram is shown in parenthesis. Left: The gradient in the baseline state is 21 mm of mercury as assessed by both cardiac catheterization and Doppler echocardiography. Right: During inhalation of amyl nitrite, the gradient increases to 70 mm of mercury.

loading conditions and contractility of the ventricle (Fig. 77-6).[43] There is also spontaneous variability in the gradient.[99] An increase in myocardial contractility, a decrease in ventricular volume, or a decrease in afterload will increase the degree of subaortic obstruction. Patients may have little or no obstruction to left ventricular outflow at rest but will generate large left ventricular outflow tract gradients under conditions such as the strain phase of the Valsalva maneuver, exercise, or during pharmacologic provocation. It has been well established that this dynamic left ventricular outflow tract obstruction contributes in part to the debilitating symptoms that may occur in these patients.

Myocardial Ischemia

Severe myocardial ischemia and even infarction may occur in patients with HCM.[83,100,101] The myocardial ischemia is frequently unrelated to the atherosclerotic epicardial coronary artery disease. Patients with HCM have compromised coronary blood flow to the left ventricular myocardium because of abnormally small and partially obliterated intramural coronary arteries.[83,84,102] There may also be myocardial oxygen demand–supply mismatch, in which the severely hypertrophied myocardium creates a myocardial oxygen demand that exceeds the capacity of the coronary circulation.[1] Elevations of myocardial wall tension from abnormal diastolic dysfunction and the high left ventricular pressure gradient may also contribute to myocardial ischemia.[100]

Autonomic Dysfunction

During exercise, approximately 25 percent of patients with HCM will have an abnormal blood pressure response defined by either a failure of systolic blood pressure to rise greater than 20 mmHg or a fall in systolic blood pressure.[103,104] This inability to augment and sustain systolic blood pressure occurs despite an appropriate rise in cardiac output and is due to systemic vasodilatation during exercise. It is speculated that there is a high degree of abnormal autonomic tone in patients with HCM. The presence of this finding is associated with a poorer prognosis.[103,105]

Mitral Regurgitation

Mitral regurgitation is common in patients with left ventricular outflow tract obstruction and may play a primary role in producing symptoms of dyspnea in patients with HCM.[1,2,106] The temporal sequence of events of "eject-obstruct-leak" supports the concept that mitral regurgitation in most patients is a secondary phenomenon.[1,2,106] Mitral regurgitation is usually caused by the distortion of the mitral valve apparatus from the SAM secondary to the left ventricular outflow tract obstruction. The jet of mitral regurgitation is directed laterally and posteriorly and predominates during mid and late systole (see Fig. 77-6). The severity of mitral regurgitation is proportional to the left ventricular outflow tract obstruction. Changes in ventricular load and contractility that affect the severity of outflow tract obstruction will similarly affect the degree of mitral regurgitation. Thus, an increase in afterload or an increase in preload will decrease mitral regurgitation, which is secondary to SAM of the mitral valve, and this response does not occur when there is a primary abnormality of the mitral valve apparatus.

In patients who have severe limiting symptoms of dyspnea, mitral regurgitation is usually the primary cause of symptoms. There may be patients who have a concomitant primary abnormality of the mitral valve leaflet such as an unsupported segment due to ruptured chordae.[107] It is important to identify these patients who have intrinsic disease of the mitral valve apparatus, since this finding will influence subsequent treatment.

CLINICAL PRESENTATION

There is a wide variability in the clinical presentation of patients with HCM.[3,4] The majority of patients who have HCM are asymptomatic, with the disease diagnosed on the basis of an abnormal electrocardiogram (ECG), heart murmur, or screening echocardiogram. When symptoms are present, a triad of dyspnea, angina, and syncope occur. Sudden death may occur, particularly in the young population, of patients less than 50 years old.

Dyspnea is a common symptom, occurring in up to 90 percent of symptomatic patients with HCM. The stiff noncompliant hypertrophied ventricle causes elevated left ventricular filling pressures. Abnormalities of ventricular relaxation decrease early diastolic filling, which is worsened with exercise. The diastolic filling abnormalities are enhanced by the occurrence of a dynamic left ventricular outflow tract obstruction or concomitant mitral regurgitation.[1,2] However, dyspnea may occur in the absence of outflow tract obstruction or mitral regurgitation, if there is severe diastolic dysfunction.

Angina occurs in 70 to 80 percent of patients with symptomatic HCM, and 15 percent of all patients at autopsy have associated myocardial infarction.[83] The angina may frequently occur in the absence of epicardial coronary disease, related to a number of mechanisms including small artery narrowing, intramural compression of small arteries from myocardial hypertrophy, abnormal diastolic filling, oxygen supply–demand mismatch, and abnormal coronary flow reserve.

Complete syncope occurs in approximately 20 percent of patients with HCM and over one half of all patients with this disorder will have presyncopal symptoms. Syncope can be due to either a hemodynamic abnormality or rhythm abnormality. It has been speculated that activation of left ventricular baroreceptors result in a reflex vasodilatation as a cause of syncope, and that mechanism is worsened by a dynamic left ventricular outflow tract gradient. The syncope in this case occurs either during or immediately after exercise. In other instances, cardiac arrhythmia is the most likely cause of syncope.

Patients with HCM often describe an increase in symptoms during hot humid weather, presumably due to fluid loss and a decrease in preload. Symptoms also may be more prominent after eating a large meal or after drinking alcohol. Other concomitant problems such as anemia or fever may result in an exacerbation of symptoms.

Older patients, in their seventh, eighth, and ninth decades, may present differently than do younger patients.[4,5,108–111] Many of these patients will have had a history of hypertension, thus presenting on medications such as diuretics or vasodilators that exacerbate an outflow tract obstruction. Moderate symptoms of dyspnea are present in most older patients due to their diastolic dysfunction. If severe mitral regurgitation or outflow tract obstruction is present, these patients may have debilitating symptoms of dyspnea. Atrial fibrillation occurs

not uncommonly in older patients (up to 25 to 30 percent) and may herald further clinical deterioration.[33,37] Embolic events may occur in the setting of atrial fibrillation.[112] Older patients may also have manifestations of other concomitant cardiac disease, such as coronary artery disease, degenerative valvular aortic stenosis, and mitral annular calcification.

PHYSICAL EXAMINATION

The classic physical findings of HCM apply to patients who have a left ventricular outflow tract gradient. The majority of patients with HCM may not have an outflow tract gradient but do have findings of left ventricular hypertrophy on physical examination (see also Chap. 12).

Carotid Pulse

The classic carotid pulsation is brisk and bifid with a "spike and dome" pattern, characterized by a rapid rise (percussion wave) followed by a midsystolic drop that is in turn followed by a secondary wave (tidal wave). The mid-systolic drop in amplitude of the carotid pulse contour is associated with premature closure of the aortic valve and coincides with SAM of the mitral valve. The upstroke is brisk, and in the presence of pronounced obstruction, there is a longer ejection time. The carotid pulsation with dynamic left ventricular outflow tract obstruction differs from that of a fixed obstruction, such as seen with valvular or discrete subvalvular aortic stenosis. In these latter two instances, there is a decrease in rate of rise and decrease in amplitude of the carotid pulsation.

Jugular Venous Pulse

The jugular venous pressure is normal in most patients with HCM. The "a" wave, however, may be prominent indicating a decrease in compliance ventricle due to the hypertrophy of the right ventricular free wall or septum, pulmonary hypertension from left-sided diastolic pressure elevation, or right ventricular outflow obstruction.

Apical Impulse

The apical impulse is almost always abnormal in patients with HCM and reflects the myocardial hypertrophy. The apical impulse is a sustained systolic thrust, which continues throughout most of the systole. There is frequently a bifid impulse due to a forceful atrial systole. There may be a "triple-ripple" with a third component occurring near the end of systole if outflow tract obstruction is present. A systolic thrill may be palpable at the apex from severe mitral regurgitation or the lower left sternal border from outflow tract obstruction.

Cardiac Sounds

Auscultation usually reveals a normal or loud first heart sound. The second heart sound is usually split physiologically, although about 20 percent of patients may have a paradoxical split due to either a concomitant left bundle branch block or severe left ventricular outflow tract obstruction. A fourth heart sound is usually present, especially if there is severe hypertrophy. In young patients, in their second and third decades, an early diastolic filling sound is frequently heard, indicating early rapid filling. A diastolic flow rumble may also be present if there is severe concomitant mitral regurgitation.

Murmurs

The classic murmur from left ventricular outflow tract obstruction is a crescendo–decrescendo murmur located primarily at the left sternal border. The murmur usually ends before the second heart sound. The murmur can radiate to the base of the heart as well as to the apex, but unlike valvular aortic stenosis, there is seldom radiation to the carotid arteries. Mitral regurgitation may be a separate murmur audible at the apex and is more holosystolic in nature. The presence of an aortic diastolic decrescendo murmur should suggest another disease, such as aortic valve disease or a discrete subvalvular stenosis.

Dynamic auscultation should be performed to differentiate the murmur of HCM from that of valvular aortic stenosis and mitral regurgitation. Maneuvers that decrease the left ventricular volume will increase the dynamic gradient and increase the intensity of the murmur (Fig. 77-7). The change in murmur intensity during the strain phase of the Valsalva maneuver has been proposed as a method to diagnose the dynamic murmur of HCM. Due to the variability in the patient performance of this maneuver, however, this classic response of the murmur to the Valsalva maneuver may not occur in all patients. The most reliable method for diagnosing a dynamic left ventricular outflow tract obstruction is the response of the murmur to the stand-squat-stand position. From the standing position to a prompt squat, the murmur will markedly decrease in intensity, due to an increase in afterload and an increase in preload. From the squatting to standing position, there will be an increase in intensity of the murmur immediately as afterload is reduced. A progressive increase in intensity of the murmur will continue for the next four to five beats as preload to the left side of the heart is reduced. Other maneuvers that are used to change the intensity of the murmur include leg raising to increase preload or the inhalation of amyl nitrite to decrease afterload and increase heart rate (see also Chap. 12).

The change in the intensity of the murmur for a beat after premature ventricular contraction or following any long pause is useful. There will be an increase in left ventricular contractility and decrease in afterload for the beat after a long pause. There will thus be an increase in intensity of the systolic murmur after a pause in hypertrophic obstructive cardiomyopathy while the murmur of organic mitral regurgitation will remain unchanged or decrease in intensity.

DIAGNOSTIC TESTING

Electrocardiogram and Holter Monitoring

The ECG is abnormal in the majority of patients with HCM.[42] A normal axis is present in 60 to 70 percent of patients and a left axis in 30 percent. Seventy to eighty percent of patients will demonstrate left ventricular hypertrophy on the resting 12-lead ECG (Fig. 77-8). Although bundle branch blocks and atrioventricular blocks are unusual, more than 80 percent of patients undergoing electrophysiologic studies actually demonstrate a prolonged H-V interval.[113] Abnormal Q-waves simulating myocardial infarction are seen in 25 percent of patients, due to a disturbance of activation of ventricular septum. The ECG in patients with a variant of HCM involving primarily the apex (apical HCM) will show a distinctive pattern of diffuse symmetric T-wave inversions across the precordium (Fig. 77-9).

The basic rhythm in most patients is normal sinus rhythm, but ambulatory monitoring will demonstrate a high incidence of supraventricular tachycardia (46 percent), premature ventricular contractions (43 percent), and nonsustained ventricular tachycardia (26 percent).[114–116] Atrial fibrillation may occur in up to 25 to 30 percent of the older population. Preexcitation has also been associated with HCM, and a rapid ventricular response with atrial fibrillation may lead to deterioration and sudden death.

Chest X-Ray

The chest x-ray usually shows mild to moderate enlargement of the cardiac silhouette. The left ventricular contour is rounded, consistent with concentric left ventricular hypertrophy. There is usually enlargement of the left atrium, and the right-sided chambers are usually normal. The presence of aortic valvular calcification or a dilated ascending aorta should raise the question of aortic valvular disease.

Echocardiography

Two-dimensional and Doppler echocardiography has become the gold standard for diagnosing HCM.[1,2] The finding of increased wall thickness with two-dimensional echocardiography in the absence of another etiology is the basis for the diagnosis of HCM (Fig. 77-10). Initially, the diagnosis of HCM was made on M-mode echocardiography by the finding of ASH, in which the ratio of septal-to-posterior

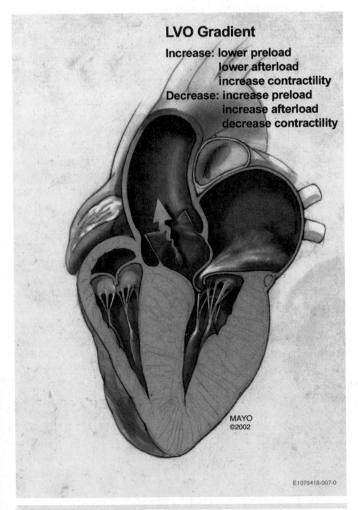

LVO Gradient

Increase: lower preload
lower afterload
increase contractility

Decrease: increase preload
increase afterload
decrease contractility

MAYO
©2002

E1078418-007-0

FIGURE 77-7 Schematic diagram of the left ventricle in hypertrophic cardiomyopathy during systole. There is projection of the basal septum into the outflow tract with systolic anterior motion of the mitral valve, which results in left ventricular outflow tract obstruction. The obstruction is dynamic, dependent upon the preload, afterload, and contractility of the heart.

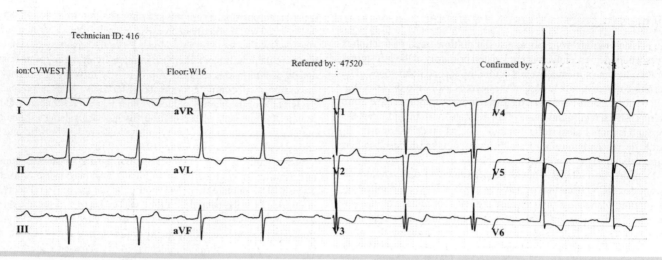

FIGURE 77-8 A 12-lead electrocardiogram from a patient with hypertrophic cardiomyopathy. There is severe left ventricular hypertrophy present. There is high voltage as well as secondary ST-T wave abnormalities.

wall thickness exceeded 1.3:1.[46] However, two-dimensional echocardiography subsequently has shown that the hypertrophy can be distributed throughout the myocardium.[49,117,118] The most common distribution is diffuse involvement of the entire ventricular septum. Hypertrophy, however, can be localized to the basal septum, localized to the lateral wall, localized to the cardiac apex, or can involve the entire myocardium (Fig. 77-11). No phenotypic expression can be considered "classic" or particularly typical of this disease. The average maximal wall thickness of the left ventricular wall in a popula-

tion of patients with HCM is usually 20 to 22 mm. Wall thickness may be markedly increased in some patients, up to 30 to even 50 mm.

The hypertrophy of the myocardium is different morphologically in the younger versus the older age group.[111] In the young population, less than 50 years old, there is classically diffuse hypertrophy of the entire septum, with a convex septal contour. In the old population, greater than 60 years old, there is the appearance of a "sigmoid" septum, in which the hypertrophy is localized to the basal and midseptum. The remaining septum is concave in contour, and there is

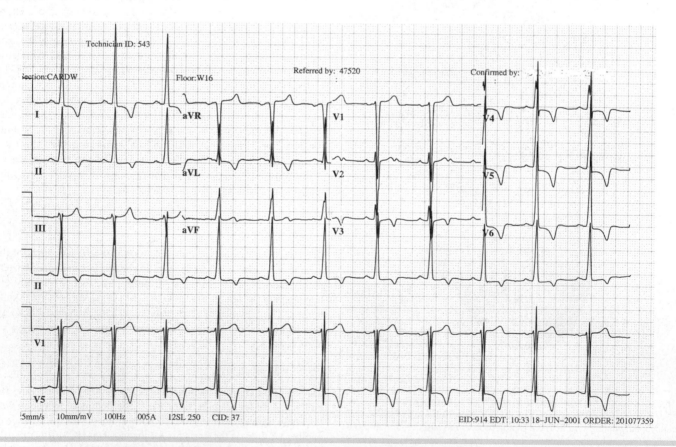

FIGURE 77-9 A 12-lead electrocardiogram from a patient with the apical variant of hypertrophic cardiomyopathy. There are diffuse T-wave inversions across the precordium as well as left ventricular hypertrophy by voltage.

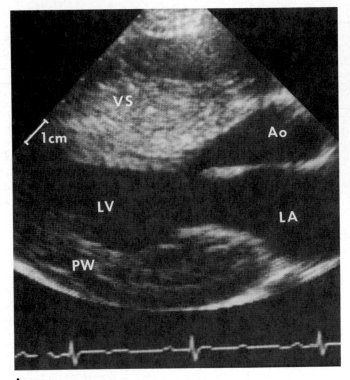

A

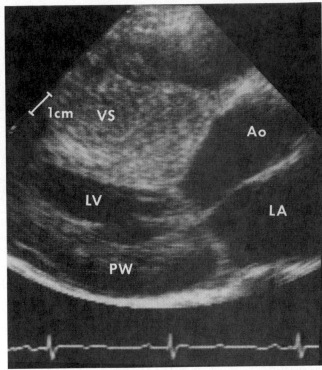

B

FIGURE 77-10 A two-dimensional echocardiogram from a patient with severe hypertrophic cardiomyopathy. There is a severe increase in left ventricular wall thickness, with a much greater increase in thickness of the ventricular septum (VS). The ratio of ventricular septal thickness to posterior wall (PW) thickness is 2.5:1. Left: Parasternal long axis view during diastole. Right: Parasternal long axis view during systole. There is systolic anterior motion of the mitral valve causing left ventricular outflow tract obstruction. Ao, aorta; LA, left atrium; LV, left ventricle.

also a sharp angle of the septum with the long axis of the aorta. Dynamic left ventricular outflow obstruction associated with SAM of the mitral valve may be present in both types of morphologies. The older patients with the sigmoid septum will frequently have systemic hypertensions, and it is speculated that the hypertrophy may be an abnormal response to the pressure overload.

Genetic studies examining patients with the genotypic diagnosis of HCM have shown that the phenotype is not always expressed as severe thickening of the left ventricle.[50,51,69,70,119] These findings may be related to the variability in the degree of penetrance and age of penetrance in this disorder. There are some genotype-affected patients who may only show a mild increase of 15 to 18 mm. There are other genotype-affected individuals who have been observed with normal wall thickness of less than 12 mm. The phenotypic expression of myocardial hypertrophy may not be evident at a young age. There are some gene mutations, such

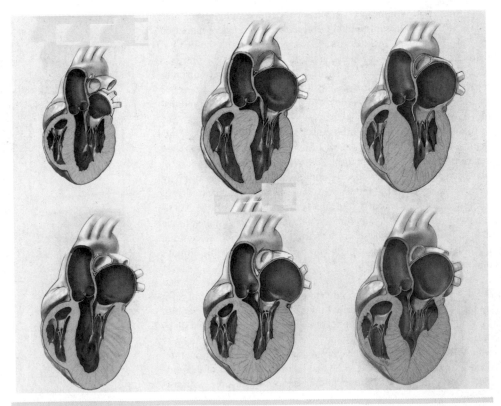

FIGURE 77-11 Schematic diaphragm of the different variants of hypertrophic cardiomyopathy. Upper left is the normal heart for comparison. Shown are variants of the location and degree of hypertrophy.

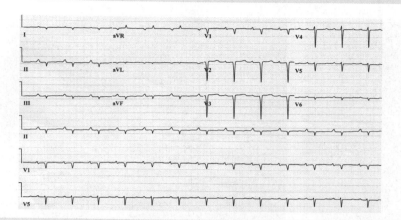

FIGURE 77-12 A 12-lead electrocardiogram (ECG) from a patient with amyloid heart disease. The two-dimensional echocardiogram in this patient showed a severe increase in left ventricular wall thickness, simulating hypertrophic cardiomyopathy. However, the low voltage and loss of forces on the ECG indicates that an infiltrative disease is responsible for the increased left ventricular wall thickness.

as the myosin-binding protein C mutation, in which the phenotypic expression of hypertrophy may not appear until middle-age.[50,51,69,70,119] Doppler tissue imaging of the intrinsic myocardial contraction and relaxation properties may be useful in identifying a positive genotype with subclinical morphologic features.[120,121]

The finding of increased wall thickness on echocardiography can be seen in other abnormalities. Increased afterload on the left ventricle from either hypertension or valvular aortic stenosis may cause an increase in the left ventricular wall thickness. Patients with chronic renal failure, especially those on dialysis, will also present with increased wall thickness on echocardiography. Infiltrative and glycogen storage diseases such as cardiac amyloidosis, Fabry's disease, and Friedreich's ataxia may present with increased wall thickness and thus will mimic HCM on echocardiography (see also Chap. 15).[122–124] It is important to correlate the findings of increased left ventricular wall thickness on echocardiography with the ECG. If there are relatively low voltages on the 12-lead ECG in the presence of increased wall thickness, then suspicion of an infiltrative disorder (amyloidosis) should be raised (Fig. 77-12).

In young athletes, a physiologic form of left ventricular hypertrophy may occur, which is an adaptation to intense training.[125,126] The resultant findings on echocardiography in these athletes may be difficult to differentiate from HCM. Elite athletes who have a dilated ventricular cavity with septal thickness less than 14 to 15 mm most likely have athlete's heart, but the combination of these findings may not always be present. A reduction in wall thickness after cessation of training is useful to identify the athletic heart but may not be practical in all patients.[125,126] Future investigations with Doppler tissue imaging and myocardial strain, which examine intrinsic myocardial systolic and diastolic function, may provide insight into this difficult diagnostic challenge.[127]

ASH is a normal feature in embryonic life, having been recorded in 94 percent of embryos, 65 percent of fetuses, 25 percent of term infants, and 12 percent of normal infants more than two weeks old. This finding has particular implications for prenatal ultrasound diagnosis of HCM. There is a subset of newborns of diabetic mothers who will have both asymmetric septal hypertrophy and outflow tract obstruction. This is thought to be due to a manifestation of generalized organomegaly, and these findings normally resolve within 6 months.[128]

Two-dimensional echocardiography is also useful for defining the presence and severity of left ventricular outflow tract obstruction.[129,130] If true dynamic obstruction is present, there will be SAM of the mitral valve apparatus. Most patients will have SAM of the anterior leaflet, but this may also occur with the posterior leaflet.[131] There are frequently abnormalities of the papillary muscle consisting of severe hypertrophy and anterior displacement.[129,132] The mitral valve leaflets and chordae may be elongated. The exact site of the obstruction may be determined on two-dimensional echocardiography by visualizing the region of the SAM-septal contact.[133] In the classic form of HCM, the obstruction will occur at the most basal portion of the septum as it projects into the left ventricular outflow tract. However, the obstruction may also extend into the left ventricle from SAM of the chordal apparatus. There may be patients with mid-ventricular obstruction in whom a hypertrophied papillary muscle abuts against the ventricular septum.[98] Two-dimensional echocardiography is useful for ruling out other causes of left ventricular outflow tract obstruction, such as discrete subaortic stenosis or tunnel subaortic stenosis.[134]

Doppler echocardiography can be used to define the pathophysiologic processes that are present in patients with HCM. In the presence of a dynamic left ventricular outflow tract obstruction, there will be a high-velocity "dagger-shaped" signal on continuous wave Doppler interrogation of the left ventricular outflow tract[135] (Fig. 77-13). The peak velocity is proportional to the gradient and can be

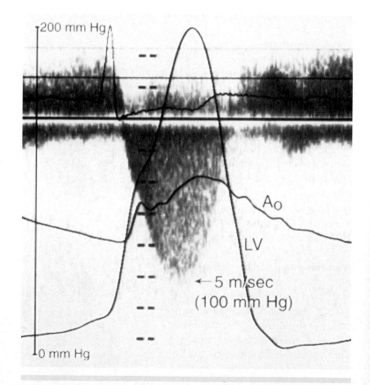

FIGURE 77-13 Simultaneous Doppler echocardiogram and cardiac catheterization demonstrating the presence of severe left ventricular outflow tract obstruction. The gradient between the left ventricle (LV) and aorta (Ao) at catheterization is 100 mm of mercury. A continuous wave Doppler across the left ventricular outflow tract reveals a peak velocity of 5 m/s, which is consistent with a calculated left ventricular outflow tract gradient of 100 mm of mercury.

directly converted to a pressure gradient by the modified Bernoulli's equation (pressure gradient $= 4 \times$ velocity^2). In patients with low outflow tract velocities (less than 3 m/s), provocation with maneuvers should be performed during the Doppler study to determine if there is a labile or latent obstruction. These maneuvers could be the strain phase of the Valsalva maneuver, inhalation of amyl nitrite, or exercise.

Mitral regurgitation frequently is present and associated with dynamic outflow tract obstruction. Color flow Doppler imaging can be used to determine the presence of mitral regurgitation and provide a semiquantitative estimate of the severity.[136] If the mitral regurgitation is secondary to distortion of the mitral valve apparatus from the SAM, the color jet will be directed laterally and posteriorly (Fig. 77-14, Plate 98). In addition, the regurgitation will predominate in mid to late systole. If there is a holosystolic signal of mitral regurgitation that is directed centrally or anteriorly, then a primary abnormality of the mitral valve apparatus should be suspected. The mitral regurgitation signal by continuous wave Doppler may contaminate the lower velocity outflow tract velocity signal, and care must be taken to differentiate the true outflow tract velocity from the mitral regurgitation jet (Fig. 77-15).

Diastolic function can be assessed noninvasively by Doppler echocardiography. The transmitral flow velocity curves alone cannot be used for analysis of diastolic function due to the complex interplay of relaxation and compliance abnormalities that are present in patients with HCM.[137] However, pulmonary vein flows and Doppler tissue imaging together with the transmitral flow velocity curves can accurately determine the left ventricular filling pressures.[138]

Transesophageal echocardiography is usually not necessary in the evaluation of the patient with HCM. In most patients, the clinically necessary anatomic and hemodynamic information can be obtained by transthoracic echocardiography. However, patients in whom discrete subvalvular stenosis or a primary abnormality of the mitral valve is suspected may benefit from transesophageal echocardiography.

Cardiac magnetic resonance imaging provides high-resolution moving images of the myocardium and accurately determines the site and extent of hypertrophy in patients with HCM. Areas of myocardial ischemia can be detected and abnormal blood flow velocities can be evaluated. The clinical utility of this imaging modality remains to be determined.

Cardiac Catheterization

Cardiac catheterization is not required in the routine assessment of most patients with HCM, as the diagnosis and determination of outflow tract obstruction can usually be made

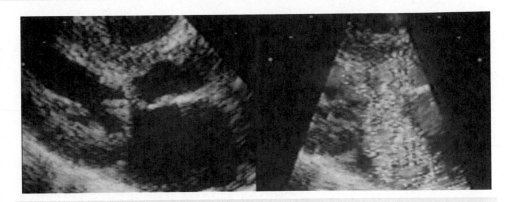

FIGURE 77-14 (Plate 98) Color flow Doppler imaging of a patient with hypertrophic cardiomyopathy, severe systolic anterior motion of the mitral valve, and secondary mitral regurgitation. Left: A still frame two-dimensional echocardiogram from the parasternal view showing systolic anterior motion of the mitral valve. Right: Color flow imaging demonstrating a large mosaic jet of mitral regurgitation directed posteriorly.

by two-dimensional and Doppler echocardiography. In those uncommon circumstances in which there is a discrepancy between the echocardiogram and the clinical presentation, cardiac catheterization may be of benefit in demonstrating the presence and severity of a left ventricular outflow tract obstruction.

The outflow tract obstruction has been assessed by a "pull-back" pressure tracing, placing an end-hole catheter at the left ventricular apex, pulling back to the base and then into the aorta. The systolic gradient will be between the apex and base (Fig. 77-16). Cavity obliteration may occur, however, due to the small left ventricular cavity with hyperdynamic systolic function. This results in catheter "entrapment," and a falsely increased left ventricular systolic pressure is measured. The gradient is ideally assessed by a simultaneous left ventricular inflow and left ventricular outflow (or aortic) pressure.[1,2] The left ventricular inflow position avoids the problem of catheter entrapment and is best obtained by a transseptal approach.

When there is little resting obstruction, provocation of the gradient should be performed. In the catheterization laboratory, the strain phase of the Valsalva maneuver or infusion of isoproterenol can be

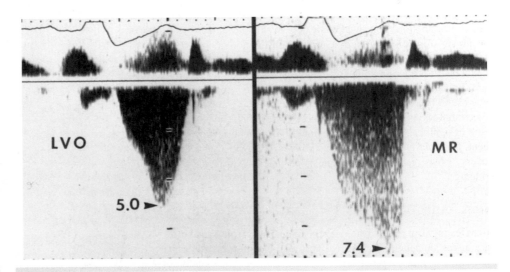

FIGURE 77-15 Continuous wave Doppler echocardiogram from a patient with both left ventricular outflow tract obstruction and mitral regurgitation. The continuous wave Doppler jet has a similar contour for both the left ventricular outflow tract velocity (LVO; left panel) and the mitral regurgitation (MR; right panel) jet. The mitral regurgitation signal is of higher velocity and the signal is holosystolic.

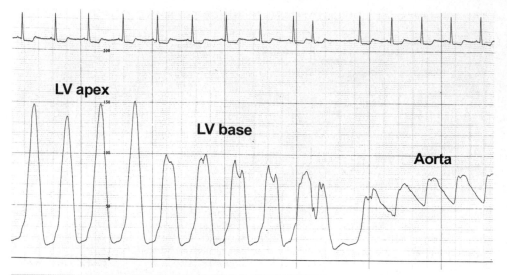

FIGURE 77-16 Cardiac catheterization traces from a patient with hypertrophic cardiomyopathy. An end-hole catheter is placed in the left ventricular apex, pulled back to the left ventricular base, and finally pulled into the ascending aorta. The systolic gradient of 50 mm of mercury is between the left ventricular apex and left ventricular base. Note the marked decrease in pulse pressure on the first beat after the catheter has been pulled into the aorta, which is a beat following a premature contraction. There is a "spike and dome" pattern on the aortic pressure curve.

Exercise testing, however, is of value in patients with HCM. Several parameters from exercise testing are adverse prognostic factors, including a drop in blood pressure with exercise and the appearance of ventricular arrhythmias.[104,141] In addition, exercise testing, particularly using metabolic measures of oxygen consumption, is useful in obtaining an objective measurement of exercise tolerance.[142]

NATURAL HISTORY

The natural history of patients with HCM is highly variable.[3,4,6,7] The prior published literature was based on studies performed at tertiary referral centers.[53,54,114,143] Therefore, the overall clinical impression of HCM has been influenced by the biases created by these highly selected patient referral patterns. The annual mortality from such centers has been high with

used. The Brockenbrough phenomenon is useful for determining the presence of a latent obstruction and can be assessed at the time of catheterization (Fig. 77-17). After a premature contraction, there will be an increase in the contractility of the ventricle resulting in a marked increase in the degree of dynamic obstruction. Thus there will be an increase in gradient as well as a decrease in the aortic pulse pressure after the pause. This is in contradistinction to a fixed obstruction in which there will be an increase in gradient from the increase in stroke volume but an increase in aortic pulse pressure will also occur.

Left ventriculography will usually reveal a small left ventricular cavity size with hypertrophied papillary muscles further impinging into the cavity. Hyperdynamic systolic function will cause complete obliteration of the mid and apical cavity in systole (Fig. 77-18). In the apical variant of HCM, there will be a fixed obliteration of the apex by the hypertrophied muscle, causing a "spade-like" configuration. There may be an apical akinetic or dyskinetic pouch with "aneurysm" formation and mid-ventricular obstruction.

Coronary angiography may be indicated if there are symptoms of angina out of proportion to the degree of obstruction or other symptoms. Epicardial coronary disease is seen in up to 25 percent of older patients.[139] The combination of the epicardial disease and the high myocardial oxygen demand from the hypertrophied muscle may result in significant symptoms of angina. Myocardial bridging is frequent, particularly in young patients with severe hypertrophy. Controversy exists regarding the prognosis of patients with myocardial bridging.[140]

Stress Testing

Stress testing is of limited value for the diagnosis of epicardial coronary disease in patients with HCM. The combination of the myocardial oxygen supply and demand mismatch and the small coronary arteriolar disease will result in findings of myocardial ischemia on ECG and nuclear imaging, even in the absence of epicardial coronary disease.

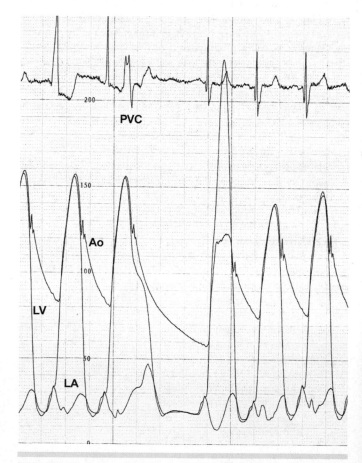

FIGURE 77-17 Cardiac catheterization from a patient with no resting left ventricular outflow tract obstruction. However, following a premature ventricular contraction (PVC), there is a left ventricular outflow tract gradient of near 100 mm of mercury. The pulse pressure of the ascending aorta (Ao) is decreased on the beat following the PVC. This phenomenon is termed the *Brockenbrough phenomenon*. LA, left atrium; LV, left ventricle.

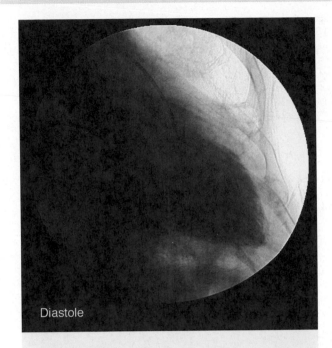

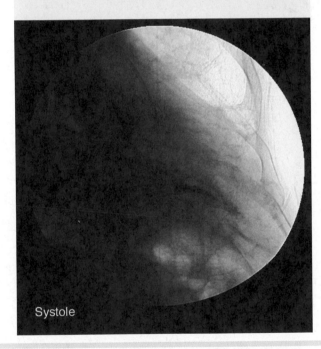

FIGURE 77-18 Left ventriculography from a patient with hypertrophic cardiomyopathy. There is near complete systolic obliteration of the left ventricular cavity. Top: diastole. Bottom: systole.

several reports indicating an annual mortality of 3 percent per year. Children with HCM had a poorer prognosis, with 30 percent showing deterioration and 30 percent experiencing sudden death over a 7-year follow-up, with an annual mortality of up to 6 to 7 percent per year. The perception that HCM is associated with high mortality has been refuted by more recently reported mortality rates, from unselected regional populations, of about 1 percent per year.[4,33–39] HCM in the elderly has been shown to have an annual mortality similar to control populations.[108]

Nonetheless, there are clearly patient subgroups at high risk for death.[3–5] Death can be sudden and unexpected, usually in the young

patients.[26,28,144,145] Progressive heart failure, especially associated with atrial fibrillation, will occur in the older patients. Sudden death is most frequent in young adults but may also occur in the older population.[38] Reports of sudden death in infants and very young children are extremely rare. Sudden death usually occurs in patients who have no symptoms or those that are mild. A substantial proportion of patients will die during or just after vigorous physical activity. HCM has been shown to be the most common of sudden death among young competitive athletes.[26,27,29,30,146,147] Thus, young athletes with HCM should be prevented from engaging in competitive sports (see also Chap. 41).[148]

The mechanism of sudden death has been established from patients experiencing implantable defibrillator discharges.[149–151] Ventricular tachycardia and fibrillation appear to be the primary mechanism responsible to sudden death. However, other mechanisms may also play a role, including asystole, rapid atrial fibrillation, and electrical mechanical dissociation.

There are several parameters that have been associated with an increased risk of sudden death.[28,52,53,115,116,144,145,152] These include (1) a prior cardiac arrest or sustained ventricular tachycardia, (2) a family history of premature sudden death due to HCM, (3) repetitive nonsustained ventricular tachycardia on ambulatory Holter monitoring, (4) massive degree of ventricular hypertrophy (wall thickness greater than 30 mm), and (5) hypotensive response to exercise. Other findings such as myocardial bridging in young patients or severe ischemia on radionuclide imaging have been associated with an increased risk of sudden death.[153] Electrophysiologic studies have not been shown to be of benefit and risk stratification in these patients. Monomorphic ventricular tachycardia is seldom induced at the time of electrophysiologic studies. Frequently, polymorphic ventricular tachycardia or ventricular fibrillation is induced during stimulation studies, but this is a nonspecific finding.[154,155]

Other complications of HCM include infective endocarditis, systemic embolism, and atrial fibrillation. Infective endocarditis may occur in 4 to 5 percent of patients with HCM.[42,156] The lesions are usually located at the point of opposition of the mitral valve against the septum but can involve the mitral valve and less often the aortic valve. Atrial fibrillation itself will occur in up to 30 percent of older patients.[37,157] It usually indicates advanced disease and is associated with clinical deterioration. Acute atrial fibrillation should be regarded as a medical emergency especially in the presence of hemodynamic deterioration, and immediate cardioversion to normal sinus rhythm is indicated. Systemic embolism occurs in 6 percent of patients and is usually associated with atrial fibrillation. Anticoagulation is recommended for patients with atrial fibrillation and HCM but will not fully eliminate the risk of stroke.

Less than 5 percent of patients in a referral-based population will develop an "end-stage" phase of HCM.[158,159] In these patients, there are progressive congestive heart failure symptoms with a significant limitation of exercise tolerance and atrial arrhythmias. The left ventricular cavity will enlarge and the dynamic outflow tract gradient will disappear. Eventually, the morphologic appearance of the ventricle will be similar to that of a dilated cardiomyopathy. These patients have a poor outlook with a high risk of death due to heart failure or arrhythmias.

TREATMENT

Treatment (Table 77-1) of HCM has been challenging due to the relatively small number of patients with this disease. There are no randomized trials for analysis of treatment regimens. Data regarding

TABLE 77-1 Treatment of Hypertrophic Cardiomyopathy

Ref	Author	Year	Number of Patients	Length of Follow-up (months*)	Gradient 1	Gradient 2	NYHA 1	NYHA 2	Complications (%)	Mortality (%)	Comment
				DUAL-CHAMBER PACING							
262	McDonald et al.	1988	9	3–24	—	—	3	1.5	—	—	Improved exercise capacity
263	Jeanrenaud et al.	1992		82	47	3					
264	Cannon et al.	1994	12	4	—	—	3.3	—	—	8	Symptoms improved by 1–2 classes
207	Fananapazir et al.	1994	84	28	96	27	3.2	1.6	—	—	
265	Posma et al.	1996	6	3	65	19	3.5	2	—	—	Improved homogeneity of perfusion with pacing
215	Slade et al.	1996	56	11	78	36	2.75	1.69	—	—	Only patients responding to temporary pacing were entered
211	Gadler et al.	1997	19 (<40 mmHg)	6	22	—	3	1.9	—	0	Comparison of outcome of minimal versus significant resting gradient
			22 (>40 mmHg)		86	26	2.8	1.8			
208	Kappenberger et al.	1997	83	3 AAI	59	33	2.6	2.4	36	0	Randomized crossover
				3 DDD	59	30	2.6	1.7			
214	Nishimura et al.	1997	21	3 DDD	76	55	2.9	2.4	—	—	Double-blind crossover study demonstration placebo effect to AAI pacing
				3 AAI	76	83		2.6	—	—	
266	Rishi et al.	1997	10	23	53	16	—	—	—	—	Pediatric-aged patients
210	Gadler et al.	1999	80	3 DDD			2.54	1.7			Randomized crossover with 1 year of follow-up in preferred mode
				3 AAI				2.2			
				12				1.62			
212	Linde et al.	1999	81	3 DDD	70	33	2.6	1.7	—	—	Subjective symptom reporting disportionate to objective parameters in inactive pacing mode (PIC)
				3 AAI	71	52	2.5	2.2			
213	Maron et al.	1999	48	3 DDD	82	48					Double-blind crossover with 6 additional months of active pacing3/4 objective exercise data obtained

(continued)

TABLE 77-1 Treatment of Hypertrophic Cardiomyopathy (*Continued*)

Ref	Author	Year	Number of Patients	Length of Follow-up (months*)	Gradient 1	Gradient 2	NYHA 1	NYHA 2	Complications (%)	Mortality (%)	Comment
267	Pavin et al.	1999	23	3 AAI / 6 unblinded / 16	82 / 82 / 93	76 / 48 / 31	— / — / 2.9	— / — / 1.6	—	—	Mitral regurgitation significantly improved with pacing
				SURGERY							
268	Tajik et al.	1974	43	84	77		3	1.7	—	16	
176	Morrow et al.	1975	83	72	96	0	3.3	1.5	10	7	Mitral valve replacement
194	Cooley et al.	1976	27	8–61	74	7	—	72% improved	10	4	
269	Agnew et al.	1977	49	89	85	<10	2.8	1.4	10	4	
270	Maron et al.	1978	124	62	73	23	3	1.7	—	8	Improved cardiac output and hemodynamics
271	Redwood et al.	1979	41	6	37–118	—	—	—	5	—	
272	Maron et al.	1983	240	60	—	—	≥3	70% improved	—	8	All patients age > 65
273	Cooper et al.	1987	11 HCM +CAD	54	65	3	3.2	1.9	—	27	
			41 HCM no CAD		95	17				8	Improved O$_2$ supply/demand
274	Cannon et al.	1989	20	6	64	4	≥3	—	—	—	
188	Krajcer et al.	1989	127 Myectomy	118	69	10	3.2	2.1	3	5	
			58 Mitral valve replacement		75	10	3.4	2.2	3	7	
275	McIntosh et al.	1989	58	6	66	4	3.1	1.8	~ 20	9	Mitral valve replacement
276	Mohr et al.	1989	115	61	70	9	2.3	1.4	11	5	
200	Mohr et al.	1989	47	60	70	10	1.9	1.3	13	0	Mean age 21.5 years; range 0–38 years
277	Siegman et al.	1989	28	58	86	3	3.3	2	21	14	HCM and CAD
177	Cohn et al.	1992	31	78	96	5	3.1	1.7	6	0	
278	Diodati et al.	1992	30	6	79	15	—	—	—	—	Improved exercise capacity
193	McIntosh et al.	1992	36	6–12	81	16	2.9	1.8	—	3	Myectomy plus mitral valve plication
185	Schulte et al.	1993	364	98	54	9	3	1.6	—	5	
189	Schoendube et al.	1994	58	84	85	—	91% Class III-IV	23% Class III-IV	21	0	
186	ten Berg et al.	1994	38	82	72	6	3	1.5	5	0	Myectomy
279	Heric et al.	1995	178	44	93	21	2.8	1.4		6	
191	Schoendube et al.	1995	58	84	79	5	3.1	1.8	7	0	Myectomy
192	Kofflard et al.	1996	8		95	18	2.6	1	0	0	Myectomy + mitral leaflet extension
			12		87	23	2.8	1.7	0	0	Myectomy alone
181	McCully et al.	1996	65	20	73	9	3.2	1.6	6	4.6	0% mortality in isolated myectomy
280	Robbins & Stinson	1996	158	72	64	10	2.8			3.2	0% mortality in patients <60 years old; 95% of patients with improved symptoms
281	Theodoro et al.	1996	25	77	100	14	2.2	1.1	4	0	Pediatric-aged patients

(continued)

TABLE 77-1 **Treatment of Hypertrophic Cardiomyopathy** (*Continued*)

Ref	Author	Year	Number of Patients	Length of Follow-up (months*)	Gradient 1	Gradient 2	NYHA 1	NYHA 2	Complications (%)	Mortality (%)	Comment
183	Merrill et al.	2000	22	79	78	12	—	—	9	0	
187	Yu et al.	2000	104	5 days							Mitral regurgitation related to severity of obstruction and relieved with myectomy
282	Ommen et al.	2002	73		57	4	2.6		*	0	29% of patients developed transient postoperative atrial fibrillation
196	Ommen et al.	2002	256		68	10	2.7		1	0	Intraoperative transesophageal echocardiography detected secondary cardiac anomalies
				ABLATION							
223	Sigwart	1995	3	3	27	8	—	—	—	4.40	
221	Knight et al.	1997	18	3	67	22	2.6	1.1	11	0	
233	Kuhn et al.	1997									
226	Faber et al.	1998	91	3	74	15	2.8	1.1	15	1	
283	Seggewis et al.	1998	25	3	62	18	2.8	1.2	28	4	
230	Gietzen et al.	1999	37	7	45	5	3	1.7	38	4	
284	Henein et al.	1999	20	6	60	22	—	—	—	—	
285	Kim et al.	1999	20	3	58	14	2.7	1.6	10	0	Improved exercise capacity
235	Kuhn et al.	1999	62	6	54	6	—	—	—	—	
138	Nagueh et al.	1999	29	6	54	6	3.1	1.2	—	—	Improved parameters of diastolic function following ablation
225	Faber et al.	2000	25	3	60	20	2.8	1.4	20	4	3 patients required repeat ablation
				12	60	9	2.8	1.4			
				30	60	3	2.8	1.2			
228	Faber et al.	2000	162	3	77	12	2.8	1.3	9	2	Use of echocardiographic myocardial contrast
238	Lakkis et al.	2000	50	12	74	6	3	1.1	22	4	Improved exercise capacity
286	Ruzyllo et al.	2000	25	3	85	36	2.8	—	28	0	
				6	85	32	2.8	1.2			
287	Boekstegers et al.	2001	50	4–6	80	18	2.8	1.9	10	0	
				12–18	80	17	2.8	—			
288	Flores-Ramirez et al.	2001	30	6	66	12	—	—	—	—	
289	Mazur et al.	2001	26	24	36	0	3	1	27	0	LVH regression demonstrated

(*continued*)

TABLE 77-1 Treatment of Hypertrophic Cardiomyopathy (*Continued*)

Ref	Author	Year	Number of Patients	Length of Follow-up (months*)	Gradient 1	Gradient 2	NYHA 1	NYHA 2	Complications (%)	Mortality (%)	Comment
						COMPARISONS					
290	Ommen et al.	1999	19 Pacing	3	77	55	2.9	2.4	—	—	Exercise time and oxygen consumption better in surgical group
291	Nagueh et al.	2001	20 Myectomy	14	76	9	2.8	1.3	—	—	
			41 Ablation	12	76	8	3.4	1.1	22	2	9 new pacemakers, 1 death
			41 Myectomy	13	78	4	3.1	1.2		0	1 new pacemaker, 8 transient AFs, no deaths
244	Qin et al.	2001	25 Ablation	3	64	24	3.5	1.9	24	0	Similar outcomes between the two procedures
245	Firoozi et al.	2002	26 Myectomy		62	11	3.3	1.5	7	0	
			20 Ablation		91	21	2.3	1.6	15	5	Surgical patients with better objective measures of exercise capacity
			24 Myectomy		83	12	2.4	1.5	4	5	

ABBREVIATIONS: AAI, atrial sense atrial inhibit; AF, atrial fibrillation; CAD, coronary artery disease; DDD, dual-chamber pacemaker; HCM, hypertrophic cardiomyopathy; LVH, left ventricular hypertrophy; NYHA, New York Heart Association; PIC, pacing in cardiomyopathy.
*Unless otherwise noted.

treatment have been mainly derived from retrospective, observational, and nonrandomized studies of a small number of patients.

Treatment has also been mainly directed at patients with dynamic left ventricular outflow tract obstruction, and there has been little to offer to patients who are symptomatic in the absence of left ventricular outflow tract obstruction. The nonobstructive variant of HCM is more common (50 to 70 percent) than is the obstructive variant (30 to 50 percent).

General Guidelines for Therapy

General guidelines should be prescribed for all patients with HCM. Screening of all first-degree relatives by echocardiography is recommended, since HCM is due to an autosomal dominant gene disorder. Screening of first-degree relatives should be performed every 3 years for children and young adults and then every 5 years thereafter. All patients with HCM should be prohibited from engaging in strenuous activity and competitive athletics.[148] Low-to-moderate levels of aerobic exercise is permitted. Those patients with a dynamic left ventricular outflow tract obstruction should be given infective endocarditis prophylaxis.[156] Patients should be instructed to keep themselves well hydrated at all times.

Medical Therapy

Medical therapy should be considered the initial therapeutic approach to relieving symptoms of patients with HCM. The medical therapy is mainly directed at those patients with a dynamic left ventricular outflow tract obstruction.

Beta-adrenergic blocking agents are the initial drug of choice for patients with symptomatic hypertrophic obstructive cardiomyopathy.[6,7,42,143,160–162] Theoretic advantages of beta blockers include (1) decreased heart rate response to exercise; (2) decreased outflow tract gradient with exercise; (3) relief of angina by a decrease in myocardial oxygen demand; and (4) improvement in diastolic filling. Acute hemodynamic studies have shown that beta-blocking agents obstruct the increase in gradient that occurs with isoproterenol and exercise but have no effect on the resting gradient. Clinical studies of the effect of beta blockers result in an improvement in angina, exercise tolerance, and syncope in 60 to 80 percent of patients. Only about 40 percent of patients, however, would continue to have sustained symptomatic improvement.[160,161,163] There has been no proven reduction in the incidence of sudden death with beta blockade. Doses much larger than that used for patients with coronary disease are often required to treat optimally the symptoms of patients with HCM. The dosage of beta blocker should be titrated to obtain a resting heart rate of 60 beats/min and may require up to 480 mg equivalent of propranolol.

Calcium channel blockers are of value in the treatment of HCM.[88,164–169] Experimental work with calcium blockers as modifiers of ischemia-induced diastolic abnormalities prompted investigation of their use in HCM. By preventing calcium influx, they theoretically not only decrease inotropy and chronotropy but also improve abnormal diastolic relaxation.[88,167–169] Verapamil has been the calcium channel blocker used most frequently due to its minimal effect on afterload.Clinical studies have shown a decrease in both basal and provoked gradients during acute drug intervention with verapamil. In contrast to beta-blocking drugs, an improvement in diastolic filling occurred with verapamil as judged by radionuclide angiographic studies.[88,167–169] Verapamil has been shown to improve exercise tolerance by 20 to 30 percent in short-term follow-up. As with beta blockers, verapamil will result in sustained symptomatic improvement in less than 50 percent of patients at long-term follow-up. Calcium channel blockers may improve angina to a greater degree than do beta blockers. Large doses of calcium channel blockers are often required to treat the symptoms of patients with HCM. The dosage of verapamil should be titrated to obtain a resting heart rate of 60 beats/ min and may require up to 480 mg/d.

There is a subset of patients who will undergo hemodynamic deterioration with calcium channel blocking agents, presumably due to a lowering of the afterload.[170] This deterioration particularly occurs in the presence of large outflow tract gradients and high diastolic filling pressures. Death from pulmonary edema has been reported after therapy with verapamil.

Disopyramide has also been used to treat patients with hypertrophic obstructive cardiomyopathy.[171–174] The negative inotropic effect will decrease the gradient and improve symptoms. The dose of disopyramide required to produce symptomatic benefit is between 300 to 600 mg/d. The anticholinergic side effects of this approach may limit the efficacy of disopyramide in older patients.

The standard clinical practice for patients with symptomatic hypertrophic obstructive cardiomyopathy is to start beta-blockade as the initial therapy. The beta-blocker should be gradually increased to optimal dosages, with a goal of a resting heart rate of 60 bpm. If patients cannot tolerate beta-blockers due to either fatigue or other side effects, a calcium channel blocker, usually verapamil, should then be started. If there is a severe outflow tract obstruction and symptoms, the calcium blocker should be started under monitored condition in the hospital. If a patient does tolerate large dosages of either a beta-blocker or calcium channel blocker and continues to be severely symptomatic, there is no data to show that the combination of two drugs is better than one drug alone. Disopyramide may be added to either the beta blocker or verapamil if symptoms persist. In those patients in whom medical therapy is ineffective, these patients should be considered for other treatment options, such as septal myectomy, dual-chamber pacing, or septal ablation.

Septal Myectomy

Surgical therapy for HCM has been performed for over four decades and currently consists of myotomy–myectomy, known as the Morrow procedure.[175,176] This operation is now established as a proven approach for relieving outflow tract obstruction and has become the "gold standard" therapy for patients with obstruction and severe drug refractory symptoms.[177–186]

This procedure consists of a transaortic resection of a small amount of muscle from the proximal to mid-septal region. This enlarges the left ventricular outflow tract and significantly decreases or totally abolishes the left ventricular outflow tract obstruction. In patients with concomitant mitral regurgitation secondary to SAM of the mitral valve, the mitral regurgitation also disappears as a result of the myectomy.[187,188] In some institutions, a more extensive myectomy procedure is performed in which the septal resection is wide and ex-

tended to the level of the papillary muscles. In those patients with abnormalities of the papillary muscle, dissection and reduction of the anomalous papillary muscle apparatus may also be performed at the time.[189,190] Mitral valvuloplasty or plication in combination with myectomy has been proposed for some patients with particularly deformed or elongated mitral valve leaflets.[191–193]

Mitral valve replacement had been recommended in patients with HCM on the assumption that the anterior leaflet of the mitral valve contributes to the outflow tract obstruction.[194] However, this should be performed only when there is associated severe unrepairable organic disease of the mitral valve. It is highly unusual that a carefully performed septal myectomy cannot be done in patients with severe obstruction, even when there is only a modest increase in septal thickness (16 to 19 mm).

The operative mortality for septal myectomy is now less than 5 percent overall.[177–186] In experienced centers, the operative risk in patients younger than 50 years old or in patients who have isolated septal myectomy is less than 1 percent. The risk is higher in elderly patients who require other procedures, such as aortic valve replacement, mitral valve repair, Maze procedure, or coronary artery bypass grafting. Complications of the surgery are rare. Heart block, ventricular septal defect, and aortic regurgitation have been reported. However, with increasing experience and newer surgical techniques, these complications occur in less than 1 percent of patients undergoing operation. These results are dependent not only on surgical expertise but also related to the use of intraoperative transesophageal echocardiography, which guides the surgeon as to adequacy of resection. The presence of residual mitral regurgitation or other cardiac structural abnormalities can be detected by transesophageal echocardiography.[195–197]

The results of an adequately performed septal myectomy are complete abolition of gradient, reduction in secondary mitral regurgitation, and a marked improvement in symptoms. Many patients are able to achieve near normal exercise capacity and return to a normal lifestyle. Long-term follow-up over several decades is now available for patients who have had septal myectomy.[177,183–185,188,191,198,199] Patients who undergo this procedure have been shown to maintain long-lasting improvement in symptoms and exercise capacity. If outflow tract obstruction is relieved after the surgery, adult patients will not redevelop an outflow tract obstruction. There is some evidence from cohort studies that mortality may be improved after septal myectomy, particularly in younger patients with severe outflow tract obstruction,[200] but there are no randomized trials to confirm this.

Dual-Chamber Pacing

Implantation of a dual-chamber pacemaker has been proposed as a less invasive therapeutic modality for treatment of symptomatic patients with hypertrophic obstructive cardiomyopathy.[201–203] Pacing the right ventricular apex in a subset of patients can decrease the outflow tract gradient, presumably due to alteration of ventricular contraction with a decrease in systolic projection of the basal septum into the left ventricular outflow tract. There may also be a chronic remodeling effect during continuous pacing with enlargement of the left ventricular cavity and further decrease in outflow tract obstruction.

There are technical considerations when using pacemaker therapy for treatment of patients with hypertrophic obstructive cardiomyopathy.[201–203] Pacing or sensing atrium in addition to pacing the ventricle is necessary in order to maintain the important hemodynamic

HOCM Pacing Study

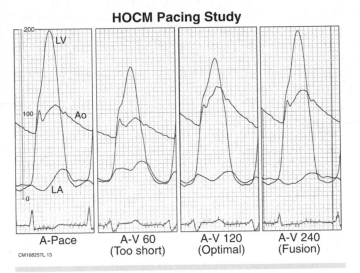

| A-Pace | A-V 60 (Too short) | A-V 120 (Optimal) | A-V 240 (Fusion) |

CM168257L.13

FIGURE 77-19 Cardiac catheterization study during atrioventricular sequential pacing in a patient with hypertrophic obstructive cardiomyopathy, demonstrating the effect of the differing atrioventricular (AV) intervals. The left ventricular (LV) pressure, aortic (Ao) pressure, and left atrial (LA) pressures are shown. In the baseline state (A pace), the patient is undergoing atrial pacing with native antegrade atrioventricular conduction. There is a left ventricular outflow tract obstruction of 100 mm of mercury. Left center panel: The patient is undergoing atrioventricular pacing with an atrioventricular interval of 60 ms. This interval is too short, as atrial contraction is now occurring on top of a closed mitral valve, causing an elevation of left atrial pressure. Although the gradient is decreased, there is also a drop in aortic pressure due to the decreased preload in the left ventricle. Right center panel: This is the optimal atrioventricular interval of 120 ms. The gradient has been decreased to 35 mm of mercury. Right panel: The atrioventricular delay is 240 ms. There is fusion between the antegrade conduction and the paced QRS complex with incomplete preexcitation. The gradient across the left ventricular outflow tract is 60 mm of mercury.

contribution of atrial contraction. There is an optimal atrioventricular delay for most advantageous hemodynamic performance (Fig. 77-19).[204,205] Too short an atrioventricular interval will cause abnormal diastolic filling, an increase in left atrial pressure, and a reduction in preload. Too long an atrioventricular delay will result in incomplete preexcitation of the right ventricle with suboptimal reduction in the gradient. It is necessary to have the pacemaker tip placed in the apex of the right ventricle to achieve the greatest reduction in gradient.

There was initial enthusiasm for dual-chamber pacing in HCM when several cohort trials emerged, which demonstrated improvement in the gradient and relief of symptoms in over 90 percent of patients.[206,207] However, subsequent more rigorous studies have shown that dual-chamber pacing is less efficacious than it was in the prior observational studies.[208–215] In the trials that have used a "randomization process" with the incorporation of a blinded placebo arm, symptomatic improvement assessed by quality of life score was reported with a similar frequency by patients after a period of pacing versus a period of no pacing. The subjectively reported symptomatic benefit during pacing in patients with HCM frequently occurs without objective evidence of improved exercise capacity. Objective measurements of exercise capacity did not differ significantly during periods with or without continuous pacing. An overall decrease in outflow tract gradient did occur during pacing, but the reduction was

25 to 40 percent of baseline, as compared to 80 to 90 percent with septal myectomy. Thus, the average outflow tract gradient after continuous pacing in many studies still remains at or over 50 mmHg.

Despite the less than optimal results, there is a subset of patients who will respond to dual-chamber pacing. About 40 percent of patients will have continued symptomatic improvement with dual-chamber pacing.[201,211] This degree of symptomatic improvement is significantly less than that achieved with other therapeutic invasive modalities.[216] About 10 to 20 percent of patients will achieve a combination of symptomatic improvement, a decrease in outflow tract gradient, and an objective improvement in exercise tolerance.[213] However, there are no known parameters at the present time that can identify patients who will uniformly respond to dual-chamber pacing. Thus, the role of dual-chamber pacing should be limited to those patients who are at high risk for other therapeutic modalities, such as the elderly patient with multiple comorbidities. Other candidates for dual-chamber pacing might be those who have significant bradycardia in which pacing may allow an increased dosage of medication or in those patients who need an automatic defibrillator as a primary treatment.

Septal Ablation

Alcohol septal ablation is a new investigative therapeutic modality in which 100 percent alcohol is infused in a first septal perforator artery, producing a controlled myocardial infarction of the proximal septum.[217–224] The subsequent remodeling of the basal septum region will then result in reduction or even abolition of the outflow tract obstruction. The technique is a percutaneous coronary artery intervention that uses the standard balloons used for treatment of epicardial coronary disease (Figs. 77-20 and 77-21).

The initial results from several centers have shown impressive short-term outcomes following septal ablation.[221,225–239] The outflow tract gradient is reduced from a mean of 60 to 70 mm of mercury to less than 20 mm of mercury. The majority of patients are improved from the symptomatic standpoint. There have also been documented significant increases in objective measurements of exercise tolerance. Symptomatic improvement after septal ablation has been documented in patients presenting with resting left ventricular outflow tract obstruction as well as in patients with provocable gradients.[229,236]

The major complication of septal ablation has been complete heart block. In the early experience, heart block occurred in 30 to 40 percent of patients undergoing septal ablation. However, as the procedure evolved, the complication of complete heart block has decreased. The evolution of the technique involves using small doses of alcohol selectively and using guidance by myocardial contrast echocardiography.[226,240,241] In some studies, the incidence of complete heart block requiring a permanent pacemaker has dropped to less than 15 percent.

Other complications of septal ablation include have included coronary dissections, large myocardial infarctions from "spillage" of the alcohol into other coronary arteries, ventricular septal defects, and myocardial perforations. Intractable ventricular fibrillation has occurred during the time of the procedure. The true incidence of these complications is unknown, as they most likely occur in centers with little or moderate experience or in those with low volumes and thus are not reported in the literature. Late complications of complete heart block or ventricular arrhythmias may occur as late as 10 to 12 days following the procedure. The true incidence of these later complications is unclear.

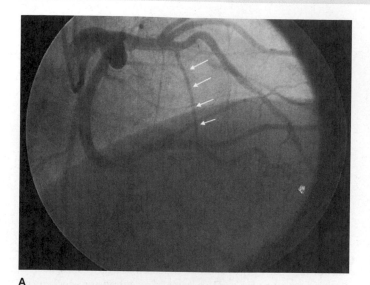

A

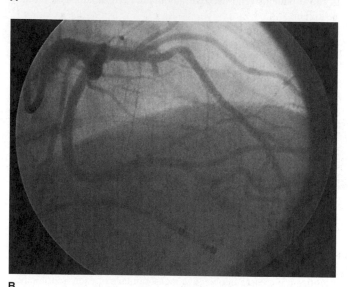

B

FIGURE 77-20 Coronary angiogram of a patient undergoing septal ablation. A large first septal perforator artery is shown by the white arrows. In the right panel, following the septal ablation, there has been complete cessation of flow in the first septal perforator artery.

Although septal ablation has been an attractive catheter-based alternative to septal myectomy, the ultimate role of this procedure in the treatment of HCM is unclear.[4,224,242,243] Whether the results of septal ablation are comparable to septal myectomy remains controversial.[244,245] There has been the concern that the production of a myocardial infarction may have detrimental long-term outcome. Patients with HCM are already prone to ventricular arrhythmias and whether a myocardial infarction may increase the susceptibility to arrhythmia is unclear. In addition, adverse ventricular remodeling after myocardial infarction is another potential concern. There is now limited follow-up of less than 5 years, and this may not be long enough for long-term detrimental effects to have emerged.

There is concern that this procedure is performed at centers that do not have knowledge of this complex underlying disease process. Patients may be presenting for consideration of septal ablation but may have other anatomic or pathophysiologic abnormalities that would make them unsuitable for the procedure, such as fixed subaor-

tic stenosis, concomitant primary mitral valve disease, or anomalous papillary muscle apparatus. The large number of procedures that have been performed in recent years has raised concerns that the threshold for intervention has been lowered as a result of the less invasive nature of septal ablation. There are no data that this procedure should be performed for any indication other than severe symptoms unresponsive to optimal medical management.

Treatment of Nonobstructive Cardiomyopathy

The previously mentioned treatments apply to patients with left ventricular outflow tract obstruction. Less is known about treatment of patients without obstruction, in whom the major pathophysiologic abnormality is severe diastolic dysfunction. Diuretics are used to decrease elevated filling pressures. Both beta blockers and calcium channel blockers have been used to improve diastolic filling. Verapamil may have a greater effect on improving relaxation abnormalities. Cardiac transplantation remains the only therapy for those patients who have severe symptoms unresponsive to conventional treatments. Promising new therapies with angiotensin-converting enzyme inhibitors, angiotensin II receptor blockers, statins, and calcium channel blockers may be of benefit based upon animal models of HCM and await human trials.[15,16,18,24,25,246,247]

Pregnancy

All patients with HCM who wish to become pregnant should be given prenatal counseling about the risk of transmission of disease to their offspring and be followed at a tertiary center with expertise in high-risk pregnancies and cardiac disease. Patients with HCM usually tolerate pregnancy well, if they are not severely symptomatic prior to conception. This is due in part to the increase in blood volume that occurs during pregnancy. If patients have been on treatment with beta blockers or calcium channel blockers, these drugs should be continued throughout the pregnancy. Additional low-dose diuretics may be required if pulmonary congestion occurs. There is no evidence that pregnancy will increase the risk of sudden death. Labor and delivery should be done in a high-risk center with meticulous attention to the cardiac disease throughout, given the fluid shifts that occur.

Prevention of Sudden Death

Sudden unexpected death is the most devastating complication of HCM.[4–7,26–32,52,53,114,116,146,147,248,249] Sudden death occurs most frequently in the asymptomatic or mildly symptomatic patient and mainly in the young population. However, patients who are prone to sudden death constitute only a minority of the overall disease population. Therefore, a major focus of investigation has been to identify patients at high risk for sudden death.

There are several clinical features associated with a high risk for sudden death in patients with HCM.[4,6,7,52,53,114–116,144,145,152,250–252] Those patients who have had a prior cardiac arrest or spontaneous sustained ventricular tachycardia are at highest risk. A family history of premature sudden death in a patient with HCM portends a high risk, particularly if there are multiple occurrences. Other less predictive parameters include unexplained syncope, nonsustained ventricular tachycardia, abnormal blood pressure response to exercise, and extreme left ventricular hypertrophy.

It has been proposed that genotype analysis might be used as a stratifying marker for prognosis, particularly since specific mutations have been shown to convey either favorable or adverse progno-

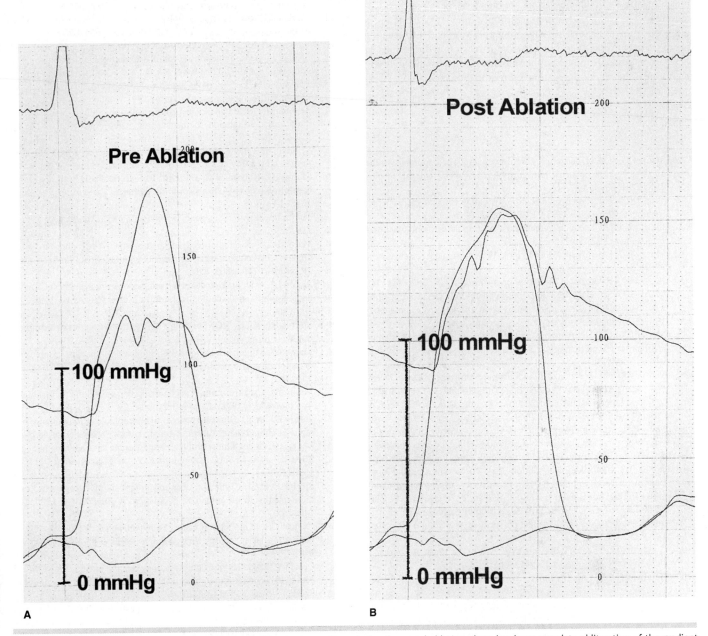

A

B

FIGURE 77-21 Left: Cardiac catheterization before ablation, demonstrating left ventricular outflow tract obstruction of 60 mm of mercury. Right: Follow-ing the septal ablation, there has been complete obliteration of the gradient across the left ventricular outflow tract.

sis.[15,16,18,253–256] These studies, however, are based upon relatively a small number of genotype families. Extrapolating these conclusions about risk based upon genotype to an overall HCM population is not proven.[257,258]

At the present time, there are no antiarrhythmic agents that have been shown to improve survival in patients with HCM. Amiodarone has been shown in retrospective nonrandomized trials to be associated with improved survival in young patients with HCM.[259,260] However, due to the potential toxicity of taking amiodarone for long periods in these young patients, the risk may outweigh the benefit.[261] Implantation of an automatic defibrillator is the most effective and reliable treatment option at the present time for protecting patients against sudden death due to ventricular arrhythmias.[149] Those patients deemed at high risk for sudden death should have placement of

an automatic defibrillator. This is strongly warranted for patients with prior cardiac arrest or sustained spontaneous ventricular tachycardia. In other patients, clinical judgment must be made for an individual patient, taking into consideration the overall clinical profile and other risk factors.

CONCLUSION

HCM is a fascinating disease entity that has intrigued cardiologists for decades. It is now well accepted that HCM is a genetic disorder of the sarcomere. It is a highly heterogeneous disease, with a diverse pathology, pathophysiology, and clinical course. Therapies have been introduced for treatment of obstruction, and the long-term follow-up of each of these is required to determine the optimal therapy for individual patients. The genetic discoveries have raised important questions about the diagnosis and prognosis of these patients. Genetic models have provided the opportunity to identify therapies to inhibit the growth factor or its signaling pathways and attenuate the extent of hypertrophy and fibrosis. The extension of the results of these animal models to human therapy and ultimately the ability to manipulate the abnormal genome are the basis of future therapy.[15,16,18,24,25,246,247]

References

1. Wigle ED, et al. Hypertrophic cardiomyopathy: The importance of the site and the extent of hypertrophy. A review. *Prog Cardiovasc Dis* 1985;28:1–83.
2. Wigle ED, et al. Hypertrophic cardiomyopathy: Clinical spectrum and treatment. *Circulation* 1995;92:1680–1692.
3. Spirito P, et al. The management of hypertrophic cardiomyopathy. *N Engl J Med* 1997;336:775–785.
4. Maron BJ. Hypertrophic cardiomyopathy: A systematic review. *JAMA* 2002;287(10):1308–1320.
5. Maron BJ. Hypertrophic cardiomyopathy. *Lancet* 1997;350:127–133.
6. Maron BJ, et al. Hypertrophic cardiomyopathy: Interrelations of clinical manifestations, pathophysiology, and therapy. *N Engl J Med* 1987;316:780–789.
7. Maron BJ, et al. Hypertrophic cardiomyopathy: Interrelatons of clinical manifestations, pathophysiology, and therapy. *N Engl J Med* 1987;316:844–852.
8. Maron BJ, et al. Prevalence of hypertrophic cardiomyopathy in a general population of young adults: Echocardiographic analysis of 4111 subjects in the CARDIA Study. Coronary Artery Risk Development in (Young) Adults. *Circulation* 1995;92:785–789.
8a. Maron BJ, McKenna WJ, Danielson GK, et al. American College of Cardiology/European Society of Cardiology clinical expert consensus document on hypertrophic cardiomyopathy. A report of the American College of Cardiology Foundation Task Force on Clinical Expert Consensus Documents and the European Society of Cardiology Committee for Practice Guidelines. *J Am Coll Cardiol* 2003;42:1687–1713.
8b. Nishimura RA, Ommen SR, Tajik AJ. Cardiology patient page. Hypertrophic cardiomyopathy: A patient perspective. *Circulation* 2003;108:133–135.
9. Goodwin JF. ?IHSS. ?HOCM. ?ASH. A plea for unity. *Am Heart J* 1975;89(3):269–77.
10. Goodwin JF. The frontiers of cardiomyopathy. *Br Heart J* 1982;48:1–18.
11. Hejtmancik JF, et al. Localization of gene for familial hypertrophic cardiomyopathy to chromosome 14q1 in a diverse US population. *Circulation* 1991;83(5):1592–1597.
12. Jarcho JA, et al. Mapping a gene for familial hypertrophic cardiomyopathy to chromosome 14q1. *N Engl J Med* 1989;321(20):1372–1378.
13. Geisterfer-Lowrance AA, et al. A molecular basis for familial hypertrophic cardiomyopathy: A beta cardiac myosin heavy chair gene missense mutation. *Cell* 1990;62:999–1006.
14. Rosenzweig A, et al. Preclinical diagnosis of familial hypertrophic cardiomyopathy by genetic analysis of blood lymphocytes. *N Engl J Med* 1991;325:1753–1760.
15. Roberts R, Sigwart U. New concepts in hypertrophic cardiomyopathies, Part I. *Circulation* 2001;104(17):2113–2116.
16. Roberts R, Sigwart U. New concepts in hypertrophic cardiomyopathies, Part II. *Circulation* 2001;104(18):2249–2252.
17. Marian AJ, Roberts R. Molecular genetics of hypertrophic cardiomyopathy. *Annu Rev Med* 1995;46:213–222.
18. Marian AJ, Roberts R. Recent advances in the molecular genetics of hypertrophic cardiomyopathy. *Circulation* 1995;92(5):1336–1347.
19. Marian AJ, et al. Detection of a new mutation in the beta-myosin heavy chain gene in an individual with hypertrophic cardiomyopathy. *J Clin Invest* 1992;90(6):2156–2165.
20. Marian AJ. Pathogenesis of diverse clinical and pathological phenotypes in hypertrophic cardiomyopathy. *Lancet* 2000;355:58–60.
21. Marian AJ, Roberts R. The molecular genetic basis for hypertrophic cardiomyopathy. *J Mol Cell Cardiol* 2001;33(4):655–670.
22. Watkins H, et al. Characteristics and prognostic implications of myosin missense mutations in familial hypertrophic cardiomyopathy. *N Engl J Med* 1992;326:1108–1114.
23. Watkins H, et al. Sporadic hypertrophic cardiomyopathy due to de novo myosin mutations. *J Clin Invest* 1992;90:1666–1671.
24. Seidman JG, Seidman C. The genetic basis for cardiomyopathy: From mutation identification to mechanistic paradigms. *Cell* 2001;104:557–567.
25. Seidman C. Genetic causes of inherited cardiac hypertrophy: Robert L. Frye Lecture. *Mayo Clin Proc* 2002;77(12):1315–1319.
26. Maron BJ, Roberts WC, Epstein SE. Sudden death in hypertrophic cardiomyopathy: A profile of 78 patients. *Circulation* 1982;65:1388–1394.
27. Maron BJ, et al. Sudden death in young athletes. *Circulation* 1980;62:218–229.
28. Maron BJ, et al. Sudden death in patients with hypertrophic cardiomyopathy: Characterization of 26 patients with functional limitation. *Am J Cardiol* 1978;41:803–810.
29. Maron BJ, et al. Sudden death in young competitive athletes. Clinical, demographic, and pathological profiles. *J Am Med Assoc* 1996;276:199–204.
30. Maron BJ, Klues HG. Surviving competitive athletics with hypertrophic cardiomyopathy. *Am J Cardiol* 1994;73:1098–1104.
31. Maron BJ, Kragel AH, Roberts WC. Sudden death in hypertrophic cardiomyopathy with normal left ventricular mass. *Br Heart J* 1990;63:308–310.
32. Maron BJ. Cardiovascular risks to young persons on the athletic field. *Ann Intern Med* 1998;129:379–386.
33. Maron BJ, et al. Clinical course of hypertrophic cardiomyopathy in a regional United States cohort. *J Am Med Assoc* 1999;281:650–655.
34. Maron BJ, et al. Clinical profile of hypertrophic cardiomyopathy identified de novo in rural communities. *J Am Coll Cardiol* 1999;33:1590–1595.
35. Spirito P, et al. Clinical course and prognosis of hypertrophic cardiomyopathy in an outpatient population. *N Engl J Med* 1989;320:749–755.
36. Cannan CR, et al. Natural history of hypertrophic cardiomyopathy. A population-based study, 1976 through 1990. *Circulation* 1995;92:2488–2495.
37. Cecchi F, et al. Hypertrophic cardiomyopathy in Tuscany: Clinical course and outcome in an unselected regional population. *J Am Coll Cardiol* 1995;26:1529–1536.
38. Maron BJ, et al. Epidemiology of hypertrophic cardiomyopathy-related death: Revised in a large non-referral-based patient population. *Circulation* 2000;102:858–864.
39. Maron BJ, Spirito P. Impact of patient selection biases on the perception of hypertrophic cardiomyopathy and its natural history. *Am J Cardiol* 1993;72:970–972.
40. Teare D. Asymmetrical hypertrophy of the heart in young adults. *Br Heart J* 1958;20:1–18.
41. Brock RC. Functional obstruction of the left ventricle. *Guy's Hosp Rep* 1957;106:221–238.
42. Frank S, Braunwald E, Idiopathic hypertrophic subaortic stenosis. Clinical analysis of 126 patients with emphasis on the natural history. *Circulation* 1968;37(5):759–788.
43. Braunwald E, et al. Idiopathic hypertrophic subaortic stenosis: I. A description of the disease based upon an analysis of 64 patients. *Circulation* 1964;30(suppl IV):3–217.
44. Clark CE, Henry WL, Epstein SE. Familial prevalence and genetic transmission of idiopathic hypertrophic subaortic stenosis. *N Engl J Med* 1973;289(14):709–14.
45. Brandenburg RO, Chazov E, Cherian G. Report of the WHO/ISFC task force on definition and classification of cardiomyopathies. *Circulation* 1981;64:437a–438a.

46. Henry WL, Clark CE, Epstein SE. Asymmetric septal hypertrophy. Echocardiographic identification of the pathognomonic anatomic abnormality of IHSS. *Circulation* 1973;47(2):225–233.

47. Menge H, Brandenburg RO, Brown AL Jr. The clinical, hemodynamic, and pathologic diagnosis of muscular subvalvular aortic stenosis. *Circulation* 1961;24:1126–1136.

48. Shah PM, Gramiak R, Kramer DH. Ultrasound localization of left ventricular outflow obstruction in hypertrophic obstructive cardiomyopathy. *Circulation* 1969;40:3–11.

49. Maron BJ, Gottdiener JS, Epstein SE. Patterns and significance of distribution of left ventricular hypertrophy in hypertrophic cardiomyopathy. A wide angle, two dimensional echocardiographic study of 125 patients. *Am J Cardiol* 1981;48:418–428.

50. Charron P, et al. Clinical features and prognostic implications of familial hypertrophic cardiomyopathy related to the cardiac myosin-binding protein C gene. *Circulation* 1998;97:2230–2236.

51. Charron P, et al. Diagnostic value of electrocardiography and echocardiography for familial hypertrophic cardiomyopathy in genotyped children. *Eur Heart J* 1998;19:1377–1382.

52. McKenna WJ, Deanfield JE. Hypertrophic cardiomyopathy: An important cause of sudden death. *Arch Dis Child* 1984;59:971–975.

53. McKenna W, et al. Prognosis in hypertrophic cardiomyopathy: Role of age and clinical, electrocardiographic and hemodynamic features. *Am J of Cardiol* 1981;47:532–538.

54. Shah PM, et al. The natural (and unnatural) history of hypertrophic obstructive cardiomyopathy. *Circ Res* 1974;(suppl II):179–195.

55. Van Noorden S, Olsen EG, Pearse AG. Hypertrophic obstructive cardiomyopathy, a histological, histochemical, and ultrastructural study of biopsy material. *Cardiovasc Res* 1971;5(1):118–131.

56. St John Sutton MG, et al. Hypertrophic obstructive cardiomyopathy and lentiginosis: A little known neural ectodermal syndrome. *Am J Cardiol* 1981;47(2):214–217.

57. Yu B, et al. Molecular pathology of familial hypertrophic cardiomyopathy caused by mutations in the cardiac myosin binding protein C gene. *J Med Genet* 1998;35:205–210.

58. Watkins H, et al. Mutations in the cardiac myosin binding protein-C gene on chromosome 11 cause familial hypertrophic cardiomyopathy. *Nat Genet* 1995;11:434–437.

59. Watkins H, et al. Mutations in the genes for cardiac troponin T and alpha-tropomyosin in hypertrophic cardiomyopathy. *N Engl J Med* 1995;332:1058–1064.

60. Thierfelder L, et al. Alpha-tropomyosin and cardiac troponin T mutations cause familial hypertrophic cardiomyopathy: A disease of the sarcomere. *Cell* 1994;77:701–712.

61. Charron P. et al. Diagnostic value of electrocardiography and echocardiography for familial hypertrophic cardiomyopathy in a genotyped adult population. *Circulation* 1997;96:214–219.

62. Kimura A, et al. Mutations in the cardiac troponin I gene associated with hypertrophic cardiomyopathy. *Nat Genet* 1997;16:379–382.

63. Karibe A, et al. Hypertrophic cardiomyopathy caused by a novel alpha-tropomyosin mutation (V95A) is associated with mild cardiac phenotype, abnormal calcium binding to troponin, abnormal myosin cycling, and poor prognosis. *Circulation* 2001;103(1):65–71.

64. Ho CY, et al. Homozygous mutation in cardiac troponin T: Implication for hypertrophic cardiomyopathy. *Circulation* 2000;102:1950–1955.

65. Flavigny J, et al. Identification of two novel mutations in the ventricular regulatory myosin light chain gene (MYL2) associated with familial and classical forms of hypertrophic cardiomyopathy. *J Mol Med* 1998;76:208–214.

66. Erdmann J, et al. Spectrum of clinical phenotypes and gene variants in cardiac myosin-binding protein C mutation carriers with hypertrophic cardiomyopathy. *J Am Coll Cardiol* 2001;38:322–330.

67. Mogensen J, et al. Alpha-cardiac actin is a novel disease gene in familial hypertrophic cardiomyopathy. *J Clin Invest* 1999;103:R39–R43.

68. Moolman JC, et al. Sudden death due to troponin T mutations. *J Am Coll Cardiol* 1997;29:549–555.

69. Niimura H, et al. Sarcomere protein gene mutations in hypertrophic cardiomyopathy of the elderly. *Circulation* 2002;105:446–451.

70. Niimura H, et al. Mutations in the gene for cardiac myosin-binding protein C and late-onset familial hypertrophic cardiomyopathy. *N Engl J Med* 1998;338(18):1248–1257.

71. Marian AJ, et al. Expression of a mutation causing hypertrophic cardiomyopathy disrupts sarcomere assembly in adult feline cardiac myocytes. *Circ Res* 1995;77(1):98–106.

72. Perryman MB, et al. Expression of a missense mutation in the messenger RNA for beta-myosin heavy chain in myocardial tissue in hypertrophic cardiomyopathy. *J Clin Invest* 1992;90(1):271–277.

73. Marian AJ, et al. Expression of a mutant (Arg92Gln) human cardiac troponin T, known to cause hypertrophic cardiomyopathy, impairs adult cardiac myocyte contractility. *Circ Res* 1997;81(1):76–85.

74. Lechin M, et al. Angiotensin-I converting enzyme genotypes and left ventricular hypertrophy in patients with hypertrophic cardiomyopathy. *Circulation* 1995;92(7):1808–12.

75. Marian AJ, et al. Angiotensin-converting enzyme polymorphism in hypertrophic cardiomyopathy and sudden cardiac death. *Lancet* 1993; 342(8879):1085–1086.

76. Osterop AP, et al. AT1 receptor A/C1166 polymorphism contributes to cardiac hypertrophy in subjects with hypertrophic cardiomyopathy. *Hypertension* 1998;32:825–830.

77. Gollob MH, et al. Identification of a gene responsible for familial Wolff-Parkinson-White syndrome. *N Engl J Med* 2001;344:1823–1831.

78. Blair E, et al. Mutations in the gamma(2) subunit of AMP-activated protein kinase cause familial hypertrophic cardiomyopathy: Evidence for the central role of energy compromise in disease pathogenesis. *Hum Mol Genet* 2001;10:1215–1220.

79. Arad M, et al. Constitutively active AMP kinase mutations cause glycogen storage disease mimicking hypertrophic cardiomyopathy. *J Clin Invest* 2002;109:357–362.

80. Olsen EG. The pathology of cardiomyopathies. A critical analysis. *Am Heart J* 1979;98(3):385–392.

81. Davies MJ, McKenna WJ. Hypertrophic cardiomyopathy-pathology and pathogenesis. *Histopathology* 1995;26:493–500.

82. Davies MJ, Pomerance A, Teare RD, Pathological features of hypertrophic obstructive cardiomyopathy. *J Clin Pathol* 1974;27(7):529–535.

83. Maron BJ, Epstein SE, Roberts WC. Hypertrophic cardiomyopathy and transmural myocardial infarction without significant atherosclerosis of the extramural coronary arteries. *Am J Cardiol* 1979;43:1086–1102.

84. Maron BJ, et al. Intramural ("small vessel") coronary artery disease in hypertrophic cardiomyopathy. *J Am Coll Cardiol* 1986;8:545–557.

85. Maron BJ, Roberts WC, Quantitative analysis of cardiac muscle cell disorganization in the ventricular septum of patients with hypertrophic cardiomyopathy. *Circulation* 1979;59:689–706.

86. Maron BJ, Anan TJ, Roberts WC, Quantitative analysis of the distribution of cardiac muscle cell disorganization in the left ventricular wall of patients with hypertrophic cardiomyopathy. *Circulation* 1981;63: 882–894.

87. Nihoyannopoulos P, et al. Diastolic function in hypertrophic cardiomyopathy: Relation to exercise capacity. *J Am Coll Cardiol* 1992;19:536–540.

88. Bonow RO, et al. Verapamil-induced improvement in left ventricular diastolic filling and increased exercise tolerance in patients with hypertrophic cardiomyopathy: Short-and long-term effects. *Circulation* 1985;72:853–864.

89. Bonow RO, et al. Regional left ventricular asynchrony and impaired global left ventricular filling in hypertrophic cardiomyopathy: Effect of verapamil. *J Am Coll Cardiol* 1987;9:1108–1116.

90. Criley JM. Unobstructed thinking (and terminology) is called for in the understanding and management of hypertrophic cardiomyopathy. *J Am Coll Cardiol* 1997;29:741–743.

91. Criley JM, Siegel RJ. Has "obstruction" hindered our understanding of hypertrophic cardiomyopathy? *Circulation* 1985;72:1148–1154.

92. Criley JM, Siegel RJ. Obstruction is unimportant in the pathophysiology of hypertrophic cardiomyopathy. *Postgrad Med J* 1986;62:515–529.

93. Shah PM, Taylor RD, Wong M. Abnormal mitral valve coaptation in hypertrophic obstructive cardiomyopathy: Proposed role in systolic anterior motion of mitral valve. *Am J Cardiol* 1981;48:258–262.

94. Sherrid MV, et al. Systolic anterior motion begins at low left ventricular outflow tract velocity in obstructive hypertrophic cardiomyopathy. *J Am Coll Cardiol* 2000;36:1344–1354.

95. Sherrid MV, et al. An echocardiographic study of the fluid mechanics of obstruction in hypertrophic cardiomyopathy. *J Am Coll Cardiol* 1993;22:816–825.

96. Sherrid MV. Dynamic left ventricular outflow obstruction in hypertrophic cardiomyopathy revisited: significance, pathogenesis, and treatment. *Cardiol Rev* 1998;6(3):135–145.

97. Jiang L, et al. An integrated mechanism for systolic anterior motion of the mitral valve in hypertrophic cardiomyopathy based on echocardiographic observations. *Am Heart J* 1987;113:633–644.

98. Falicov RE, et al. Mid-ventricular obstruction: A variant of obstructive cardiomyopathy. *Am J Cardiol* 1976;37:432–437.

99. Kizilbash AM, Heinle SK, Grayburn PA. Spontaneous variability of left ventricular outflow tract gradient in hypertrophic obstructive cardiomyopathy. *Circulation* 1998;97:461–466.

100. Cannon RO III, et al. Myocardial ischemia in patients with hypertrophic cardiomyopathy: Contribution of inadequate vasodilator reserve and elevated left ventricular filling pressures. *Circulation* 1985;71:234–243.

101. Cannon RO III, et al. Differences in coronary flow and myocardial metabolism at rest and during pace between patients with obstructive and patients with nonobstructive hypertrophic cardiomyopathy. *J Am Coll Cardiol* 1987;10:53–62.

102. Tanaka M, et al. Quantitative analysis of narrowings of intramyocardial small arteries in normal hearts, hypertensive hearts, and hearts with hypertrophic cardiomyopathy. *Circulation* 1987;75:1130–1139.

103. Sadoul N, et al. Prospective prognostic assessment of blood pressure response during exercise in patients with hypertrophic cardiomyopathy. *Circulation* 1997;96:2987–2991.

104. Frenneaux MP, et al. Abnormal blood pressure response during exercise in hypertrophic cardiomyopathy. *Circulation* 1990;82:1995–2002.

105. Olivotto I, et al. Prognostic value of systemic blood pressure response during exercise in a community-based patient population with hypertrophic cardiomyopathy. *J Am Coll Cardiol* 1999;33:2044–2051.

106. Wigle ED, et al. Mitral regurgitation in muscular subaortic stenosis. *Am J Cardiol* 1969;24:698–706.

107. Zhu WX, et al. Mitral regurgitation due to ruptured chordae tendineae in patients with hypertrophic obstructive cardiomyopathy. *J Am Coll Cardiol* 1992;20(1):242–7.

108. Fay WP, et al. Natural history of hypertrophic cardiomyopathy in the elderly. *J Am Coll Cardiol* 1990;16:821–826.

109. Lewis JF, Maron BJ. Elderly patients with hypertrophic cardiomyopathy: A subset with distinctive left ventricular morphology and progressive clinical course late in life. *J Am Coll Cardiol* 1989;13:36–45.

110. Lewis JF, Maron BJ. Clinical and morphologic expression of hypertrophic cardiomyopathy in patients greater than 65 years of age. *Am J Cardiol* 1994;73:1105–1111.

111. Lever HM, et al. Hypertrophic cardiomyopathy in the elderly. Distinctions from the young based on cardiac shape. *Circulation* 1989;79:580–589.

112. Maron BJ, et al. Clinical profile of stroke in 900 patients with hypertrophic cardiomyopathy. *J Am Coll Cardiol* 2002;39:301–307.

113. Ingham RE, et al. Electrophysiologic findings in patients with idiopathic hypertrophic subaortic stenosis. *Am J Cardiol* 1978;41(5):811–816.

114. McKenna WJ, et al. Arrhythmia and prognosis in infants, children and adolescents with hypertrophic cardiomyopathy. *J Am Coll Cardiol* 1988;11:147–153.

115. McKenna WJ, et al. Arrhythmia in hypertrophic cardiomyopathy. I: Influence on prognosis. *Br Heart J* 1981;46:168–172.

116. McKenna WJ, et al. Arrhythmia in hypertrophic cardiomyopathy: Exercise and 48 hour ambulatory electrocardiographic assessment with and without beta adrenergic blocking therapy. *Am J Cardiol* 1980;45(1):1–5.

117. Shapiro LM, McKenna WJ. Distribution of left ventricular hypertrophy in hypertrophic cardiomyopathy: A two-dimensional echocardiographic study. *J Am Coll Cardiol* 1983;2:437–444.

118. Klues HG, Schiffers A, Maron BJ. Phenotypic spectrum and patterns of left ventricular hypertrophy in hypertrophic cardiomyopathy: Morphologic observations and significance as assessed by two-dimensional echocardiography in 600 patients. *J Am Coll Cardiol* 1995;26:1699–1708.

119. Maron BJ, et al. Development of left ventricular hypertrophy in adults in hypertrophic cardiomyopathy caused by cardiac myosin-binding protein C gene mutations. *J Am Coll Cardiol* 2001;38:315–321.

120. Ho CY, et al. Assessment of diastolic function with Doppler tissue imaging to predict genotype in preclinical hypertrophic cardiomyopathy. *Circulation* 2002;105:2997.

121. Nagueh SF, et al. Tissue Doppler imaging consistently detects myocardial abnormalities in patients with hypertrophic cardiomyopathy and provides a novel means for an early diagnosis before and independently of hypertrophy. *Circulation* 2001;104(2):128–30.

122. Sachdev B, et al. Prevalence of Anderson-Fabry disease in male patients with late onset hypertrophic cardiomyopathy. *Circulation* 2002;105:1407–1411.

123. Chandrasekaran K, et al. Feasibility of identifying amyloid and hypertrophic cardiomyopathy with the use of computerized quantitative texture analysis of clinical echocardiographic data. *J Am Coll Cardiol* 1989;13(4):832–40.

124. Alboliras ET. et al. Spectrum of cardiac involvement in Friedreich's ataxia: Clinical, electrocardiographic and echocardiographic observations. *Am J Cardiol* 1986;58(6):518–524.

125. Pelliccia A, et al. Remodeling of left ventricular hypertrophy in elite athletes after long-term deconditioning. *Circulation* 2002;105(8):944–949.

126. Pelliccia A, et al. The upper limit of physiologic cardiac hypertrophy in highly trained elite athletes. *N Engl J Med* 1991;324:295–301.

127. Palka P, et al. Differences in myocardial velocity gradient measured throughout the cardiac cycle in patients with hypertrophic cardiomyopathy, athletes and patients with left ventricular hypertrophy due to hypertension. *J Am Coll Cardiol* 1997;30:760–768.

128. Gutgesell HP, Speer ME, Rosenberg HS. Characterization of the cardiomyopathy in infants of diabetic mothers. *Circulation* 1980;61(2):441–450.

129. Klues HG, et al. Diversity of structural mitral valve alterations in hypertrophic cardiomyopathy. *Circulation* 1992;85:1651–1660.

130. Klues HG, Roberts WC, Maron BJ. Morphological determinants of echocardiographic patterns of mitral valve systolic anterior motion in obstructive hypertrophic cardiomyopathy. *Circulation* 1993;87:1570–1579.

131. Maron BJ, et al. Systolic anterior motion of the posterior mitral leaflet: A previously unrecognized cause of dynamic subaortic obstruction in patients with hypertrophic cardiomyopathy. *Circulation* 1983;68:282–293.

132. Klues HG, Roberts WC, Maron BJ. Anomalous insertion of papillary muscle directly into anterior mitral leaflet in hypertrophic cardiomyopathy. Significance in producing left ventricular outflow obstruction. *Circulation* 1991;84:1188–1197.

133. Schwammenthal E, et al. Prediction of the site and severity of obstruction in hypertrophic cardiomyopathy by color flow mapping and continuous wave Doppler echocardiography. *J Am Coll Cardiol* 1992;20:964–972.

134. Bruce, C.J., et al. Fixed left ventricular outflow tract obstruction in presumed hypertrophic obstructive cardiomyopathy: Implications for therapy. *Ann Thorac Surg* 1999;68(1):100–104.

135. Sasson Z, et al. Doppler echocardiographic determination of the pressure gradient in hypertrophic cardiomyopathy. *J Am Coll Cardiol* 1988;11:752–756.

136. Nishimura RA, et al. Evaluation of hypertrophic cardiomyopathy by Doppler color flow imaging: Initial observations. *Mayo Clin Proc* 1986;61(8):631–639.

137. Nishimura RA, et al. Noninvasive doppler echocardiographic evaluation of left ventricular filling pressures in patients with cardiomyopathies: A simultaneous Doppler echocardiographic and cardiac catheterization study. *J Am Coll Cardiol* 1996;28(5):1226–1233.

138. Nagueh SF, et al. Changes in left ventricular diastolic function 6 months after nonsurgical septal reduction therapy for hypertrophic obstructive cardiomyopathy. *Circulation* 1999;99:344–347.

139. Stewart S, Schreiner B. Coexisting idiopathic hypertrophic subaortic stenosis and coronary artery disease. Clinical implication and operative management. *J Thorac Cardiovasc Surg* 1981;82(2):278–280.

140. Yetman AT, et al. Myocardial bridging in children with hypertrophic cardiomyopathy—A risk factor for sudden death. *N Engl J Med* 1998; 339:1201–1209.

141. Frenneaux MP, et al. Determinants of exercise capacity in hypertrophic cardiomyopathy. *J Am Coll Cardiol* 1989;13:1521–1526.

142. Sharma S, et al. Utility of cardiopulmonary exercise in the assessment of clinical determinants of functional capacity in hypertrophic cardiomyopathy. *Am J Cardiol* 2000;86:162–168.

143. Frank MJ, et al. Long-term medical management of hypertrophic obstructive cardiomyopathy. *Am J Cardiol* 1978;42:993–1001.

144. Elliott PM, et al. Relation between severity of left ventricular hypertrophy and prognosis in patients with hypertrophic cardiomyopathy. *Lancet* 2001;357:420–424.

145. Elliott PM, et al. Sudden death in hypertrophic cardiomyopathy: Identification of high risk patients. *J Am Coll Cardiol* 2000;36:2212–2218.

146. Maron BJ, Epstein SE, Roberts WC. Causes of sudden death in competitive athletes. *J Am Coll Cardiol* 1986;7:204–214.

147. Maron BJ, Pelliccia A, Spirito P. Cardiac disease in young trained athletes. Insights into methods for distinguishing athlete's heart from structural heart disease, with particular emphasis on hypertrophic cardiomyopathy. *Circulation* 1995;91:1596–1601.

148. Maron BJ, Isner JM, McKenna WJ. 26th Bethesda conference: Recommendations for determining eligibility for competition in athletes with cardiovascular abnormalities. Task force 3: hypertrophic cardiomyopathy, myocarditis and other myopericardial diseases and mitral valve prolapse. *J Am Coll Cardiol* 1994;24:880–885.

149. Maron BJ, et al. Efficacy of implantable cardioverter-defibrillators for the prevention of sudden death in patients with hypertrophic cardiomyopathy. *N Engl J Med* 2000;342:365–673.

150. Elliott PM, et al. Survival after cardiac arrest or sustained ventricular tachycardia in patients with hypertrophic cardiomyopathy. *J Am Coll Cardiol* 1999;33:1596–1601.

151. Silka MJ, et al. Sudden cardiac death and the use of implantable cardioverter-defibrillators in pediatric patients. The pediatric electrophysiology society. *Circulation* 1993;87:800–807.

152. Spirito P, et al. Magnitude of left ventricular hypertrophy and risk of sudden death in hypertrophic cardiomyopathy. *N Engl J Med* 2000; 342:1778–1785.

153. Dilsizian V, et al. Myocardial ischemia detected by thallium scintigraphy is frequently related to cardiac arrest and syncope in young patients with hypertrophic cardiomyopathy. *J Am Coll Cardiol* 1993;22: 796–804.

154. Fananapazir L, et al. Prognostic determinants in hypertrophic cardiomyopathy. Prospective evaluation of a therapeutic strategy based on clinical, Holter, hemodynamic, and electrophysiological findings. *Circulation* 1992;86:730–740.

155. Fananapazir L, et al. Electrophysiologic abnormalities in patients with hypertrophic cardiomyopathy. A consecutive analysis in 155 patients. *Circulation* 1989;80:1259–1268.

156. Spirito P, et al. Infective endocarditis in hypertrophic cardiomyopathy: Prevalence, incidence, and indications for antibiotic prophylaxis. *Circulation* 1999;99:2132–2137.

157. Olivotto I, et al. Impact of atrial fibrillation on the clinical course of hypertrophic cardiomyopathy. *Circulation* 2001;104:2517–2524.

158. Spirito P. et al. Occurrence and significance of progressive left ventricular wall thinning and relative cavity dilatation in hypertrophic cardiomyopathy. *Am J Cardiol* 1987;60:123–129.

159. ten Cate FJ, Roelandt J. *Am Heart J* 1979;97:762–765.

160. Flamm MD, Harrison DC, Handock EW. Muscular subaortic stenosis. Prevention of outflow obstruction with propranolol. *Circulation* 1968;38:846–858.

161. Adelman AG, et al. Long-term propranolol therapy in muscular subaortic stenosis. *Br Heart J* 1970;32:804–811.

162. Shah PM, et al. Echocardiographic assessment of the effects of surgery and propranolol on the dynamics of outflow obstruction in hypertrophic subaortic stenosis. *Circulation* 1972;45:516–521.

163. Kaltenbach M, et al. Treatment of hypertrophic obstructive cardiomyopathy with verapamil. *Br Heart J* 1979;42:35–42.

164. Rosing DR, et al. Verapamil therapy: A new approach to the pharmacologic treatment of hypertrophic cardiomyopathy: III. Effects of long-term administration. *Am J Cardiol* 1981;48:545–553.

165. Rosing DR, et al. Verapamil therapy: A new approach to the pharmacologic treatment of hypertrophic cardiomyopathy. I. Hemodynamic effects. *Circulation* 1979;60:1201–1207.

166. Rosing DR, et al. Verapamil therapy: A new approach to the pharmacologic treatment of hypertrophic cardiomyopathy. II. Effects on exercise capacity and symptomatic status. *Circulation* 1979;60:1208–1213.

167. Bonow RO, et al. Atrial systole and left ventricular filling in hypertrophic cardiomyopathy: Effect of verapamil. *Am J Cardiol* 1983;51:1386–1391.

168. Bonow RO, et al. Effects of verapamil on left ventricular systolic and diastolic function in patients with hypertrophic cardiomyopathy: Pressure-volume analysis with a nonimaging scintillation probe. *Circulation* 1983;68:1062–1073.

169. Bonow RO, et al. Effects of verapamil on left ventricular systolic function and diastolic filling in patients with hypertrophic cardiomyopathy. *Circulation* 1981;64:787–796.

170. Epstein SE, Rosing DR. Verapamil: Its potential for causing serious complications in patinets with hypertrophic cardiomyopathy. *Circulation* 1981;64:437–441.

171. Matsubara H, et al. Salutary effect of disopyramide on left ventricular diastolic function in hypertrophic obstructive cardiomyopathy. *J Am Coll Cardiol* 1995;26:768–775.

172. Pollick C, et al. Disopyramide in hypertrophic cardiomyopathy. I. Hemodynamic assessment after intravenous administration. *Am J Cardiol* 1988;62:1248–1251.

173. Pollick C. Muscular subaortic stenosis: Hemodynamic and clinical improvement after disopyramide. *N Engl J Med* 1982;307:997–999.

174. Sherrid M, Delia E, Dwyer E. Oral disopyramide therapy for obstructive hypertrophic cardiomyopathy. *Am J Cardiol* 1988;62:1085–1088.

175. Morrow AG. Operative methods utilized to relieve left ventricular outflow obstruction. *J Thorac Cardiovasc Surg* 1978;76:423–430.

176. Morrow AG, et al. Operative treatment in hypertrophic subaortic stenosis. Techniques, and the results of pre and postoperative asessments in 83 patients. *Circulation* 1975;52:88–102.

177. Cohn LH, Trehan H, Collins JJ Jr. Long-term follow-up of patients undergoing myotomy/myectomy for obstructive hypertrophic cardiomyopathy. *Am J Cardiol* 1992;70:657–660.

178. Havndrup O, et al. Outcome of septal myectomy in patients with hypertrophic obstructive cardiomyopathy. *Scand Cardiovasc J* 2000; 34(6):564–569.

179. Williams WG, et al. Results of surgery for hypertrophic obstructive cardiomyopathy. *Circulation* 1987;76:V104–V108.

180. McCully RB, et al. Hypertrophic obstructive cardiomyopathy: Preoperative echocardiographic predictors of outcome after septal myectomy. *J Am Coll Cardiol* 1996;27:1491–1496.

181. McCully RB, et al. Extent of clinical improvement after surgical treatment of hypertrophic obstructive cardiomyopathy. *Circulation* 1996; 94:467–471.

182. McIntosh CL, Maron BJ. Current operative treatment of obstructive hypertrophic cardiomyopathy. *Circulation* 1988;78:487–495.

183. Merrill WH, et al. Long-lasting improvement after septal myectomy for hypertrophic obstructive cardiomyopathy. *Ann Thorac Surg* 2000;69(6):1732–1735; discussion 1735–1736.

184. Schulte HD, et al. Management of symptomatic hypertrophic obstructive cardiomyopathy–long-term results after surgical therapy. *Thorac Cardiovasc Surg* 1999;47:213–218.

185. Schulte HD, et al. Prognosis of patients with hypertrophic obstructive cardiomyopathy after transaortic myectomy. Late results up to twenty-five years. *J Thorac Cardiovasc Surg* 1993;106:709–717.

186. ten Berg JM, et al. Hypertrophic obstructive cardiomyopathy. Initial results and long-term follow-up after Morrow septal myectomy. *Circulation* 1994;90:1781–1785.

187. Yu EH, et al. Mitral regurgitation in hypertrophic obstructive cardiomyopathy: Relationship to obstruction and relief with myectomy. *J Am Coll Cardiol* 2000;36:2219–2225.

188. Krajcer Z, et al. Septal myotomy-myomectomy versus mitral valve replacement in hypertrophic cardiomyopathy. Ten-year follow-up in 185 patients. *Circulation* 1989;80:157–164.

189. Schoendube FA, et al. Surgical correction of hypertrophic obstructive cardiomyopathy with combined myectomy, mobilisation and partial excision of the papillary muscles. *Europ J Cardiothorac Surg* 1994;8:603–608.

190. Maron BJ, Nishimura RA, Danielson GK. Pitfalls in clinical recognition and a novel operative approach for hypertrophic cardiomyopathy with severe outflow obstruction due to anomalous papillary muscle. *Circulation* 1998;98:2505–2508.

191. Schoendube FA, et al. Long-term clinical and echocardiographic follow-up after surgical correction of hypertrophic obstructive cardiomyopathy with extended myectomy and reconstruction of the subvalvular mitral apparatus. *Circulation* 1995;92:II122–II127.

192. Kofflard MJ, et al. Initial results of combined anterior mitral leaflet extension and myectomy in patients with obstructive hypertrophic cardiomyopathy. *J Am Coll Cardiol* 1996;28:197–202.

193. McIntosh CL, et al. Initial results of combined anterior mitral leaflet plication and ventricular septal myotomy-myectomy for relief of left ventricular outflow tract obstruction in patients with hypertrophic cardiomyopathy. *Circulation* 1992;86:II60–II67.

194. Cooley DA, Wukasch DC, Leachman RD. Mitral valve replacement for idiopathic subaortic stenosis. Results in 27 patients. *J Cardiovasc Surg (Torino)* 1976;17:380–387.

195. Grigg LE, et al. Transesophageal Doppler echocardiography in obstructive hypertrophic cardiomyopathy: Clarification of pathophysiology and importance in intraoperative decision making. *J Am Coll Cardiol* 1992;20:42–52.

196. Ommen SR, et al. Impact of intraoperative transesophageal echocardiography in the surgical management of hypertrophic cardiomyopathy. *Am J Cardiol* 2002;90(9):1022–1024.

197. Marwick TH, et al. Benefits of intraoperative echocardiography in the surgical management of hypertrophic cardiomyopathy. *J Am Coll Cardiol* 1992;20:1066–1072.

198. Beahrs MM, et al. Hypertrophic obstructive cardiomyopathy: Ten- to 21-year follow-up after partial septal myectomy. *Am J Cardiol* 1983;l51(7):1160–1166.

199. Mohr R, et al. The outcome of surgical treatment of hypertrophic obstructive cardiomyopathy. Experience over 15 years. *J Thorac Cardiovasc Surg* 1989;l97:666–674.

200. Mohr R, et al. Results of operation for hypertrophic obstructive cardiomyopathy in children and adults less than 40 years of age. *Circulation* 1989;80:II91–II96.

201. Erwin JP III, et al. Dual chamber pacing for patients with hypertrophic obstructive cardiomyopathy: A clinical perspective in 2000. *Mayo Clin Proc* 2000;75(2):173–180.

202. Nishimura RA, et al. Dual-chamber pacing for cardiomyopathies: A 1996 clinical perspective. *Mayo Clin Proc* 1996;l71(11):1077–1087.

203. Symanski JD, Nishimura RA. The use of pacemakers in the treatment of cardiomyopathies. *Curr Probl Cardiol* 1996;21(6):385–443.

204. Nishimura RA, et al. Effect of dual-chamber pacing on systolic and diastolic function in patients with hypertrophic cardiomyopathy. Acute Doppler echocardiographic and catheterization hemodynamic study. *J Am Coll Cardiol* 1996;27(2):421–430.

205. Betocchi S, et al. Effects of dual-chamber pacing in hypertrophic cardiomyopathy on left ventricular outflow tract obstruction and on diastolic function. *Am J Cardiol* 1996;77:498–502.

206. Fananapazir L, et al. Impact of dual-chamber permanent pacing in patients with obstructive hypertrophic cardiomyopathy with symptoms refractory to verapamil and beta-adrenergic blocker therapy. *Circulation* 1992;85(6):2149–2161.

207. Fananapazir L, et al. Long-term results of dual-chamber (DDD) pacing in obstructive hypertrophic cardiomyopathy. Evidence for progressive symptomatic and hemodynamic improvement and reduction of left ventricular hypertrophy. *Circulation* 1994;90:2731–2742.

208. Kappenberger L, et al. Pacing in hypertrophic obstructive cardiomyopathy. A randomized crossover study. PIC study group. *Eur Heart J* 1997;18:1249–1256.

209. Kappenberger LJ, et al. Clinical progress after randomized on/off pacemaker treatment for hypertrophic obstructive cardiomyopathy. Pacing in cardiomyopathy (PIC) study group. *Europace,* 1999;1:77–84.

210. Gadler, F., et al., Significant improvement of quality of life following atrioventricular synchronous pacing in patients with hypertrophic obstructive cardiomyopathy. Data from 1 year of follow-up. PIC study group. Pacing in Cardiomyopathy. *Eur Heart J* 1999;20:1044–1050.

211. Gadler F, et al. Long-term effects of dual chamber pacing in patients with hypertrophic cardiomyopathy without outflow tract obstruction at rest. *Eur Heart J* 1997;18:636–642.

212. Linde C, et al. Placebo effect of pacemaker implantation in obstructive hypertrophic cardiomyopathy. PIC study group. Pacing in Cardiomyopathy. *Am J Cardiol* 1999;83:903–907.

213. Maron BJ, et al. Assessment of permanent dual-chamber pacing as a treatment for drug-refractory symptomatic patients with obstructive hypertrophic cardiomyopathy. A randomized, double-blind, crossover study (M-PATHY). *Circulation* 1999;99(22):2927–2933.

214. Nishimura RA, et al. Dual-chamber pacing for hypertrophic cardiomyopathy: A randomized, double-blind, crossover trial. *J Am Coll Cardiol* 1997;29(2):435–441.

215. Slade AK, et al. DDD pacing in hypertrophic cardiomyopathy: A multicentre clinical experience. *Heart* 1996;75:44–49.

216. Ommen SR, et al. Comparison of dual-chamber pacing versus septal myectomy for the treatment of patients with hypertropic obstructive cardiomyopathy: A comparison of objective hemodynamic and exercise end points. *J Am Coll Cardiol* 1999;34(1):191–196.

217. Braunwald E. A new treatment for hypertrophic cardiomyopathy? *Eur Heart J* 1997;18(5):709–710.

218. Braunwald E. Induced septal infarction: a new therapeutic strategy for hypertrophic obstructive cardiomyopathy. *Circulation* 1997;95(8):1981–1982.

219. Braunwald E. Hypertrophic cardiomyopathy—the benefits of a multidisciplinary approach. *N Engl J Med* 2002;347(17):1306–1307.

220. Braunwald E, Seidman CE, Sigwart U. Contemporary evaluation and management of hypertrophic cardiomyopathy. *Circulation* 2002;106(11):1312–1316.

221. Knight C, et al. Nonsurgical septal reduction for hypertrophic obstructive cardiomyopathy: Outcome in the first series of patients. *Circulation* 1997;95:2075–2081.

222. Seggewiss H, et al. Percutaneous transluminal septal myocardial ablation in hypertrophic obstructive cardiomyopathy: Acute results and 3-month follow-up in 25 patients. *J Am Coll Cardiol* 1998;31(2):252–258.

223. Sigwart U. Non-surgical myocardial reduction for hypertrophic obstructive cardiomyopathy. *Lancet* 1995;346:211–214.

224. Wigle ED, et al. To ablate or operate? That is the question (editorial). *J Am Coll Cardiol* 2001;15:1707–1710.

225. Faber L, et al. Percutaneous transluminal septal myocardial ablation for hypertrophic obstructive cardiomyopathy: Long term follow up of the first series of 25 patients. *Heart* 2000;83(3):326–331.

226. Faber L, Seggewiss H, Gleichmann U. Percutaneous transluminal septal myocardial ablation in hypertrophic obstructive cardiomyopathy: Results with respect to intraprocedural myocardial contrast echocardiography. *Circulation* 1998;l98:2415–2421.

227. Faber L, et al. Intraprocedural myocardial contrast echocardiography as a routine procedure in percutaneous transluminal septal myocardial ablation: detection of threatening myocardial necrosis distant from the septal target area. *Catheter Cardiovasc Interv* 1999;47(4):462–466.

228. Faber L, Ziemssen P, Seggewiss H, Targeting percutaneous transluminal septal ablation for hypertrophic obstructive cardiomyopathy by intraprocedural echocardiographic monitoring. *J Am Soc Echocardiogr* 2000;13:1074–1079.

229. Gietzen FH, et al. Role of transcoronary ablation of septal hypertrophy in patients with hypertrophic cardiomyopathy, New York Heart Association functional class III or IV, and outflow obstruction only under provocable conditions. *Circulation* 2002;106(4):454–459.

230. Gietzen FH, et al. Acute and long-term results after transcoronary ablation of septal hypertrophy (TASH). Catheter interventional treatment

for hypertrophic obstructive cardiomyopathy. *Eur Heart J* 1999; 20(18):1342–1354.

231. Knight CJ. Five years of percutaneous transluminal septal myocardial ablation. *Heart* 2000;83(3):255–256.

232. Kuhn H. Transcoronary ablation of septal hypertrophy (TASH): A 5-year experience. *Z Kardiol* 2000;89:559–564.

233. Kuhn H, et al. Induction of subaortic septal ischaemia to reduce obstruction in hypertrophic obstructive cardiomyopathy. Studies to develop a new catheter-based concept of treatment. *Eur Heart J* 1997;18:846–851.

234. Kuhn H, et al. Transcoronary ablation of septal hypertrophy (TASH): A new treatment option for hypertrophic obstructive cardiomyopathy. *Z Kardiol* 2000;89(suppl 4):IV41–IV54.

235. Kuhn H, et al. Changes in the left ventricular outflow tract after transcoronary ablation of septal hypertrophy (TASH) for hypertrophic obstructive cardiomyopathy as assessed by transoesophageal echocardiography and by measuring myocardial glucose utilization and perfusion. *Eur Heart J* 1999;20(24):1808–1817.

236. Lakkis N, et al. Efficacy of nonsurgical septal reduction therapy in symptomatic patients with obstructive hypertrophic cardiomyopathy and provocable gradients. *Am J Cardiol* 2001;88(5):583–586.

237. Lakkis N. New treatment methods for patients with hypertrophic obstructive cardiomyopathy. *Curr Opin Cardiol* 2000;15(3):172–177.

238. Lakkis NM, et al. Nonsurgical septal reduction therapy for hypertrophic obstructive cardiomyopathy: One-year follow-up. *J Am Coll Cardiol* 2000;36:852–855.

239. Shamim W, et al. Nonsurgical reduction of the interventricular septum in patients with hypertrophic cardiomyopathy. *N Engl J Med*, 2002;347(17): 1326–1333.

240. Lakkis NM, et al. Echocardiography-guided ethanol for hypertrophic obstructive cardiomyopathy. *Circulation* 1998;98:1750–1755.

241. Nagueh SF, et al. Role of myocardial contrast echocardiography during nonsurgical septal reduction therapy for hypertrophic obstructive cardiomyopathy. *J Am Coll Cardiol* 1998;32(1):225–229.

242. Spirito P, Rubartelli P. Alcohol septal ablation in the management of obstructive hypertrophic cardiomyopathy. *Ital Heart J* 2000;1(11):721–725.

243. Maron BJ. Role of alcohol septal ablation in treatment of obstructive hypertrophic cardiomyopathy. *Lancet* 2000;355:425–426.

244. Qin JX, et al. Outcome of patients with hypertrophic obstructive cardiomyopathy after percutaneous transluminal septal myocardial ablation and septal myectomy surgery. *J Am Coll Cardiol* 2001;38(7): 1994–2000.

245. Firoozi S, et al. Septal myotomy-myectomy and transcoronary septal alcohol ablation in hypertrophic obstructive cardiomyopathy. A comparison of clinical, haemodynamic and exercise outcomes. *Eur Heart J* 2002;23(20):1617–1624.

246. Patel R, et al. Simvastatin induces regression of cardiac hypertrophy and fibrosis and improves cardiac function in a transgenic rabbit model of human hypertrophic cardiomyopathy. *Circulation* 2001;104(3): 317–324.

247. Roberts R. A perspective: The new millennium dawns on a new paradigm for cardiology—molecular genetics. *J Am Coll Cardiol* 2000; 36(3):661–667.

248. Maron BJ. Hypertrophic cardiomyopathy and sudden death: New perspectives on risk stratification and prevention with the implantable carioverter-defibrillator. *Eur Heart J* 2000;21:1979–1983.

249. Maron BJ, et al. "Malignant" hypertrophic cardiomyopathy: Identification of a subgroup of families with unusually frequent premature death. *Am J Cardiol* 1978;41:1133–1140.

250. Spirito P, Maron BJ. Relation between extent of left ventricular hypertrophy and occurrence of sudden cardiac death in hypertrophic cardiomyopathy. *J Am Coll Cardiol* 1990;15:1521–1526.

251. Maron BJ, Cecchi F, McKenna WJ. Risk factors and stratification for sudden cardiac death in patients with hypertrophic cardiomyopathy. *Br Heart J* 1994;72:S13–S18.

252. Maron BJ, et al. Prognostic significance of 24 hour ambulatory electrocardiographic monitoring in patients with hypertrophic cardiomyopathy: A prospective study. *Am J Cardiol* 1981;48:252–257.

253. Watkins H. Sudden death in hypertrophic cardiomyopathy. *N Engl J Med* 2000;342:422–424.

254. Anan R, et al. Prognostic implications of novel beta cardiac myosin heavy chain gene mutations that cause familial hypertrophic cardiomyopathy. *J Clin Invest* 1994;93:280–285.

255. Anan R, et al. Patients with familial hypertrophic cardiomyopathy caused by a Phe110IIe missense mutation in the cardiac troponin T gene have variable cardiac morphologies and a favorable prognosis. *Circulation* 1998;98:391–397.

256. Marian AJ, et al. Sudden cardiac death in hypertrophic cardiomyopathy. Variability in phenotypic expression of beta-myosin heavy chain mutations. *Eur Heart J* 1995;16(3):368–76.

257. Ackerman MJ, et al. Prevalence and age-dependence of malignant mutations in the beta-myosin heavy chain and troponin T genes in hypertrophic cardiomyopathy: A comprehensive outpatient perspective. *J Am Coll Cardiol* 2002;39(12):2042–2048.

258. Van Driest SL, et al. Prevalence and severity of "benign" mutations in the beta-myosin heavy chain, cardiac troponin T, and alpha-tropomyosin genes in hypertrophic cardiomyopathy. *Circulation* 2002;106(24):3085–3090.

259. McKenna WJ, et al. Amiodarone for long-term management of patients with hypertrophic cardiomyopathy. *Am J Cardiol* 1984;54:802–810.

260. McKenna WJ, et al. Improved survival with amiodarone in patients with hypertrophic cardiomyopathy and ventricular tachycardia. *Br Heart J* 1985;53:412–416.

261. Cecchi F, et al. Prognostic value of non-sustained ventricular tachycardia and the potential role of amiodarone treatment in hypertrophic cardiomyopathy assessment in an unselected non-referral based patient population. *Heart* 1998;79:331–336.

262. McDonald K, et al. Functional assessment of patients treated with permanent dual chamber pacing as a primary treatment for hypertrophic cardiomyopathy. *Eur Heart J* 1988;9:893–898.

263. Jeanrenaud X, Goy JJ, Kappenberger L. Effects of dual-chamber pacing in hypertrophic obstructive cardiomyopathy. *Lancet* 1992;339: 1318–1323.

264. Cannon RO III, et al. Results of permanent dual-chamber pacing in symptomatic nonobstructive hypertrophic cardiomyopathy. *Am J Cardiol* 1994;73:571–576.

265. Posma JL, et al. Effects of permanent dual-chamber pacing on myocardial perfusion in symptomatic hypertrophic cardiomyopathy. *Heart* 1996;76:358–362.

266. Rishi F, et al. Effects of dual-chamber pacing for pediatric patients with hypertrophic obstructive cardiomyopathy. *J Am Coll Cardiol*, 1997;29:734–740.

267. Pavin D, et al. Effects of permanent dual-chamber pacing on mitral regurgitation in hypertrophic obstructive cardiomyopathy. *Eur Heart J* 1999;20:203–210.

268. Tajik AJ, et al. Idiopathic hypertrophic subaortic stenosis. Long-term surgical follow-up. *Am J Cardiol* 1974;34(7):815–822.

269. Agnew TM, et al. Surgical resection in idiopathic hypertrophic subaortic stenosis with a comined approach through aorta and left ventricle. *J Thorac Cardiovasc Surg* 1977;74:307–316.

270. Maron BJ, et al. Long-term clinical course and symptomatic status of patients after operation for hypertrophic subaortic stenosis. *Circulation* 1978;57:1205–1213.

271. Redwood DR, et al. Exercise performance after septal myotomy and myectomy in patients with obstructive hypertrophic cardiomyopathy. *Am J Cardiol* 1979;44:215–220.

272. Maron BJ, Epstein SE, Morrow AG. Symptomatic status and prognosis of patients after operation for hypertrophic obstructive cardiomyopathy: Efficacy of ventricular septal myotomy and myectomy. *Eur Heart J* 1983;4(suppl F):175–185.

273. Cooper MM, et al. Operation for hypertrophic subaortic stenosis in the aged. *Ann Thorac Surg* 1987;44:370–378.

274. Cannon RO III, et al. Effect of surgical reduction of left ventricular outflow obstruction on hemodynamics, coronary flow, and myocardial metabolism in hypertrophic cardiomyopathy. *Circulation* 1989;79: 766–775.

275. McIntosh CL, et al. Clinical and hemodynamic results after mitral valve replacement in patients with obstructive hypertrophic cardiomyopathy. *Ann Thorac Surg* 1989;47:236–246.

276. Mohr R, et al. The outcome of surgical treatment of hypertrophic obstructive cardiomyopathy. Experience over 15 years. *J Thorac Cardiovasc Surg* 1989;97(5):666–674.

277. Siegman IL, et al. Results of operation for coexistent obstructive hypertrophic cardiomyopathy and coronary artery disease. *J Am Coll Cardiol* 1989;13:1527–1533.

278. Diodati JG, et al. Predictors of exercise benefit after operative relief of left ventricular outflow obstruction by the myotomy-myectomy procedure in hypertrophic cardiomyopathy. *Am J Cardiol* 1992;69:1617–1622.

279. Heric B, et al. Surgical management of hypertrophic obstructive cardiomyopathy. Early and late results. *J Thorac Cardiovasc Surg* 1995;110:195–206.

280. Robbins RC, Stinson EB. Long-term results of left ventricular myotomy and myectomy for obstructive hypertrophic cardiomyopathy. *J Thorac Cardiovasc Surg* 1996;111:586–594.

281. Theodoro DA, et al. Hypertrophic obstructive cardiomyopathy in pediatric patients: Results of surgical treatment. *J Thorac Cardiovasc Surg* 1996;112:1589–1597.

282. Ommen SR, et al. Clinical predictors and consequences of atrial fibrillation after surgical myectomy for obstructive hypertrophic cardiomyopathy. *Am J Cardiol* 2002;89:242–244.

283. Seggewiss H, et al. Percutaneous transluminal septal myocardial ablation in hypertrophic obstructive cardiomyopathy: Acute results and three-month follow-up in 25 patients. *J Am Coll Cardiol* 1998;31:252–258.

284. Henein MY, et al. Electromechanical left ventricular behavior after nonsurgical septal reduction in patients with hypertrophic obstructive cardiomyopathy. *J Am Coll Cardiol* 1999;34:1117–1122.

285. Kim JJ, et al. Improvement in exercise capacity and exercise blood pressure response after transcoronary alcohol ablation therapy of septal hypertrophy in hypertrophic cardiomyopathy. *Am J Cardiol* 1999;83(8):1220–1223.

286. Ruzyllo W, et al. Left ventricular outflow tract gradient decrease with non-surgical myocardial reduction improves exercise capacity in patients with hypertrophic obstructive cardiomyopathy. *Eur Heart J* 2000;21:770–777.

287. Boekstegers P, et al. Pressure-guided nonsurgical myocardial reduction induced by small septal infarctions in hypertrophic obstructive cardiomyopathy. *J Am Coll Cardiol* 2001;38:846–853.

288. Flores-Ramirez R, et al. Echocardiographic insights into the mechanisms of relief of left ventricular outflow tract obstruction after nonsurgical septal reduction therapy in patients with hypertrophic obstructive cardiomyopathy. *J Am Coll Cardiol* 2001;37:208–214.

289. Mazur W, et al. Regression of left ventricular hypertrophy after nonsurgical septal reduction therapy for hypertrophic obstructive cardiomyopathy. *Circulation* 2001;103(11):1492–1496.

290. Ommen SR, et al. Comparison of dual-chamber pacing versus septal myectomy for the treatment of patients with hypertrophic obstructive cardiomyopathy: A comparison of objective hemodynamic and exercise end point. *J Am Coll Cardiol* 1999;34:191–196.

291. Nagueh SF, et al. Comparison of ethanol septal reduction therapy with surgical myectomy for the treatment of hypertrophic obstructive cardiomyopathy. *J Am Coll Cardiol* 2001;38(6):1701–1706.

RESTRICTIVE, OBLITERATIVE, AND INFILTRATIVE CARDIOMYOPATHIES

Brian D. Hoit / Darryl Miller

RESTRICTIVE CARDIOMYOPATHY

Definition of Restrictive Cardiomyopathy

The most recent report from the 1995 World Health Organization/ International Society and Federation of Cardiology (WHO/IFSFC) Task Force classifies cardiomyopathies by the dominant pathophysiology or, whenever possible, by etiologic and pathogenetic factors.[1] Although this definition differentiates primary cardiomyopathies from other pathologic processes that disturb myocardial function— such as ischemic, hypertensive, valvular, and congenital heart diseases—the WHO/IFSFC classification remains controversial. The clinicopathologic classification scheme initially proposed by Goodwin is similar and includes dilated or congestive, hypertrophic, and restrictive forms.[2] *Restrictive cardiomyopathy* refers to either an idiopathic or systemic myocardial disorder characterized by restrictive filling, normal or reduced left ventricular (LV) and right ventricular (RV) volumes, and normal or nearly normal systolic (LV and RV) function. Thus, the clinical and hemodynamic picture (i.e., elevated venous pressure with prominent X and Y descents, a small or normal-sized LV, and pulmonary congestion) simulates constrictive pericarditis. Restrictive cardiomyopathy may be noninfiltrative or infiltrative and occurs with or without obliteration; infiltration may be interstitial (e.g., amyloidosis, sarcoidosis) or cellular (e.g., hemochromatosis).

Restrictive cardiomyopathy has assumed importance in clinical cardiology for several reasons. First, these myocardial disorders epitomize diastolic heart failure; thus, abnormal ventricular diastolic compliance and impaired ventricular filling constitute their central pathophysiologic components and congestion and elevated diastolic pressure are their major clinical and hemodynamic manifestations. Second, the hemodynamic and clinical manifestations may mimic those produced by constrictive pericarditis, which, in contrast to restrictive cardiomyopathy, is a surgically curable disorder. Accordingly, its lack of recognition may have dire consequences. Third, restrictive cardiomyopathy may present with interventricular conduction delays, heart block, or skeletal muscle disease, often making the diagnosis difficult. Fourth, diagnostic criteria for restriction are not universally accepted, and the morphologic spectrum overlaps with hypertrophic cardiomyopathy, challenging our traditional concepts of classification.[3,3a] Finally, a comprehensive echo Doppler assessment has become an important, noninvasive means of detecting the pathophysiology, morphology, and prognosis of the restrictive cardiomyopathies.[4]

Clinical Features of Restrictive Cardiomyopathy

Involvement of the myocardium (or endomyocardium) and ventricular obliteration may occur either in isolation or in the setting of systemic or iatrogenic disease (Table 78-1). Thus, in the strictest sense, restrictive cardiomyopathy is not necessarily a primary disease of heart muscle. Irrespective of the etiology, terminology, or nature of the myocardial process, the ventricles are small (generally <110 mL/m²), and stiff, restricting ventricular filling. Despite normal (or near normal) systolic function, ventricular diastolic, jugular, and pulmonary venous pressures are increased. Typically, LV filling pressures exceed RV filling pressures by more than 5 mmHg, but equalization of the diastolic pressures and a "square root" dip and plateau of early diastolic pressures of the RV and LV may be seen if the compliances of these chambers are similarly affected. Importantly, the hemodynamics of constrictive pericarditis may be simulated. Moreover, elevated atrial pressures produce symptoms of systemic and pulmonary venous congestion (dyspnea, orthopnea, edema, abdominal discomfort), and relatively underfilled ventricles are responsible for reduced cardiac output and fatigue. In patients with restrictive cardiomyopathy as part of a systemic disorder, cardiac symptoms may dominate or overshadow symptoms referable to other organ systems. Patients with constrictive cardiomyopathy generally have lower RV systolic pressures (<40 mmHg) and an RV end-diastolic pressure greater than one-third of the pressure RV systolic pressure, as opposed to patients with restrictive cardiomyopathy, but these differences are far from absolute.

Physical Findings

Patients with advanced restrictive cardiomyopathy present with signs and symptoms suggestive of heart failure in the absence of cardiomegaly. Physical examination reflects the elevated systemic and pulmonary venous pressure. Striking elevation of the jugular venous pulse and prominent X and especially Y descents are characteristic. A low pulse volume, owing to a reduced stroke volume and tachycardia,

TABLE 78-1　Classification of the Restrictive Cardiomyopathies

Myocardial
1. Noninfiltrative cardiomyopathies
    Idiopathic
    Familial
    Pseudoxanthoma elasticum
    Scleroderma
2. Infiltrative cardiomyopathies
    Amyloidosis
    Sarcoidosis
    Gaucher's disease
3. Storage disease
    Hemochromatosis
    Fabry's disease
    Glycogen storage diseases
Endomyocardial
1. Obliterative
    Endomyocardial fibrosis
    Hypereosinophilic syndrome
2. Nonobliterative
    Carcinoid
    Malignant infiltration
    Iatrogenic (radiation, drugs)

may be seen in severe cases. The apical impulse is not displaced and systolic murmurs of atrioventricular regurgitation and filling sounds marking the abrupt cessation of rapid early diastolic filling may be present; an S_4 may also be present. Hepatomegaly, ascites, and peripheral edema are also common clinical findings.

Diagnostic/Imaging Studies

Electrocardiographic (ECG) abnormalities such as abnormal voltage, atrial and ventricular arrhythmias, and conduction disturbances are

frequent, particularly in infiltrative disease; when restrictive cardiomyopathy is due to amyloid infiltration, low voltage is usual (Fig. 78-1). Atrial fibrillation is common in idiopathic restrictive cardiomyopathy and cardiac amyloidosis.

The chest radiograph usually reveals normal-sized ventricles, although atrial enlargement and pericardial effusion may produce an enlarged cardiac silhouette. Pleural effusions and signs of pulmonary congestion may also be present.

Echocardiographic findings are nonspecific but in many cases are useful to exculpate other, more common causes of heart failure. Although ventricular systolic function is usually preserved, abnormal diastolic function that progresses through the patterns of abnormal relaxation to a restrictive filling may be identified.

Cardiac MRI can help distinguish between the cardiomyopathies.[3b] For example, the cardiomyopathy associated with hemochromatosis produces very low signal intensity due to deposition of iron. MRI is also excellent for differentiating between restrictive and constrictive disease (see below).

Endomyocardial biopsy is occasionally useful in patients with severe constrictive/restrictive physiology as it may identify the subset of patients with specific forms of restrictive cardiomyopathy in whom thoracotomy should be avoided.

DIFFERENTIATION FROM CONSTRICTIVE PERICARDITIS

The differentiation of restrictive cardiomyopathy and constrictive pericarditis remains a challenge. It is important to make the distinction as the treatments differ considerably. Constrictive pericarditis requires surgical treatment and is usually curable, while restrictive cardiomyopathy is treated medically. Although several clinical, imaging, and hemodynamic features are helpful in distinguishing restrictive cardiomyopathy from constrictive pericarditis (Table 78-2), considerable overlap and diagnostic confusion exist. The pathophysiologic basis for this distinction includes (1) transmission of intrathoracic pressure to the ventricles (limited by the stiff pericardium in constrictive pericarditis but not in restrictive cardiomyopathy); (2) the principal determinant of the diastolic ventricular pressure-volume relation (ventricular versus pericardial compliance in restrictive cardiomyopathy versus constrictive pericarditis); and (3) involvement of the ventricular septum in restrictive cardiomyopathy versus the capacity for ventricular interdependence in constrictive pericarditis.

Recently, Doppler techniques (spectral Doppler, color M-mode, and Doppler tissue imaging) have assumed an important role in characterizing the nature of transvalvular filling and in clinically distinguishing between constrictive pericarditis and restrictive cardiomyopathy.[4–6] These Doppler flow patterns and the associated respiratory changes are illustrated in Fig. 78-2. In the *normal subject*, the early filling wave (E) of mitral flow is greater than the late, atrial systolic wave (A), and neither change significantly with respiration. In contrast, the E and A velocities of tricuspid valve flow increase slightly with inspiration.

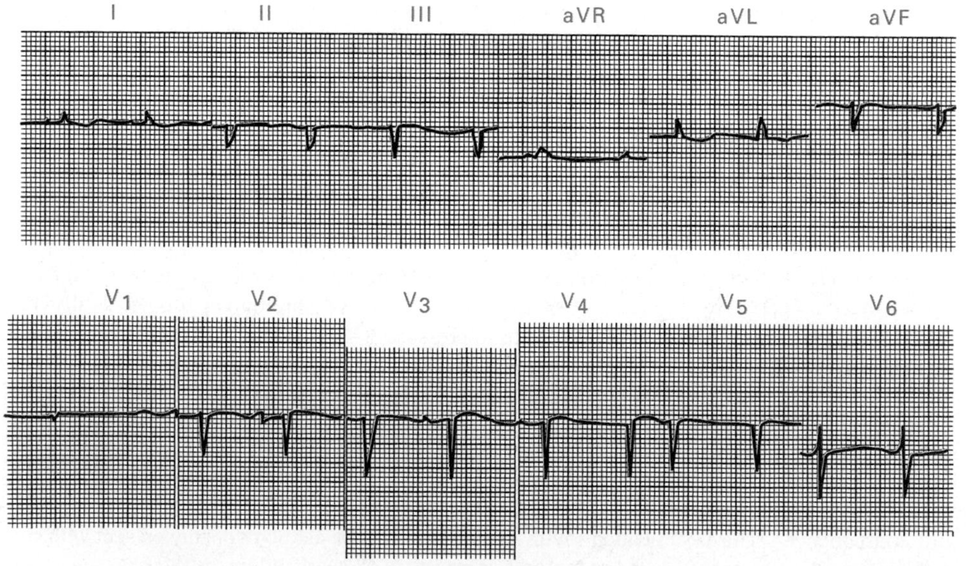

FIGURE 78-1　Electrocardiogram of a patient with amyloidosis. Note the low voltage, which is in striking contrast to the increased left ventricular wall thickness shown echocardiographically. (From Shabetai R. Restrictive, obliterative, and infiltrative cardiomyopathies. In: Alexander WA, Schlant R, Fuster V, et al., eds. *Hurst's The Heart*, 9th ed. New York: McGraw-Hill; 1998:2077. Reproduced with permission.)

The deceleration time of the LV early diastolic wave ranges from 150 to 240 ms, and the LV isovolumic relaxation time ranges from 70 to 110 ms. Pulmonary venous flow is generally biphasic, with a dominant wave during systole (S) and a smaller wave during diastole (D); respiratory changes are minimal and atrial systolic reversals are generally small. Hepatic vein flow consists of a larger S and smaller D wave with small reversals (V_r and A_r) after each wave, respectively. With expiration, S and D waves decrease and V_r and A_r increase. Doppler tissue imaging (DTI) shows a prominent longitudinal axis velocity in early diastole (E_a >8 cm/s) and a smaller velocity after atrial contraction (A_a). The slope of early diastolic LV filling on color M-mode (Vp) is >45 cm/s. In the patient with *restrictive cardiomyopathy,* mitral valve flow shows an increased E/A ratio ($\geq$2) with a short (<150 ms) deceleration time and a short (<70 ms) isovolumic relaxation time (a "restrictive" pattern of filling) without respiratory variation. The tricuspid valve flow shows an increased E/A ratio without respiratory variation, a shortened deceleration time, and a short isovolumic relaxation time that shortens further with inspiration. The S/D ratio of pulmonary venous flow is <1, atrial reversals are increased (not shown in Fig. 78-1), and there is little respiratory variation. The S/D ratio of hepatic venous flow is <1 and prominent reversals are seen during inspiration. Doppler tissue imaging shows a striking decrease in E_a (<8 cm/s) and the propagation velocity on color M-mode is <45 cm/s.

In *constrictive pericarditis,* mitral and tricuspid valve flows are also "restrictive," but unlike those in restrictive cardiomyopathy, they display marked respiratory variation. The isovolumic relaxation time shortens during expiration. The S/D of pulmonary venous flow is <1, with increased velocities (especially diastolic) in expiration, resulting in a further decrease in the S/D ratio. In contrast to restrictive cardiomyopathy, hepatic venous flow reversals occur in expiration, early diastolic tissue velocities (E_a) are normal on DTI, and the transmitral propagation velocity is >45 cm/s.

Despite the considerable interest and potential clinical value in the ability to discriminate restrictive

TABLE 78-2 Clinical and Hemodynamic Features That Help Distinguish Restrictive Cardiomyopathy from Constrictive Pericarditis

	Restrictive Cardiomyopathy	Constrictive Pericarditis
History	Systemic disease that involves the myocardium, multiple myeloma, amyloidosis, cardiac transplant	Acute pericarditis, cardiac surgery, radiation therapy, chest trauma, systemic disease involving the pericardium.
Chest radiogram	Absence of calcification, massive atrial enlargement	Helpful when calcification persists, moderate atrial enlargement
ECG	Bundle branch blocks, AV block	Abnormal repolarization
CT/MRI	Normal pericardium	Helpful if thickened (>4mm) pericardium
Hemodynamics	Helpful if unequal diastolic pressures; concordant effect of respiration on diastolic pressures	Diastolic equilibration Dip and plateau
Biopsy	Fibrosis, hypertrophy, infiltration	Normal

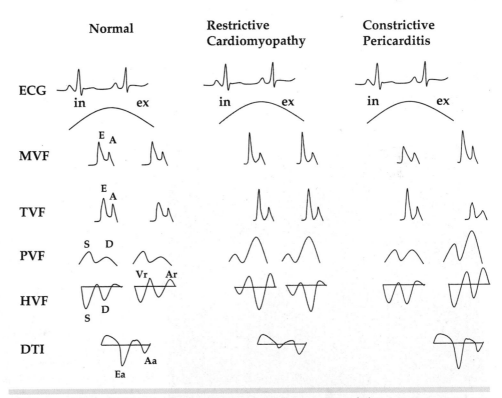

FIGURE 78-2 Schematic of Doppler flows during inspiration (in) and expiration (ex) in normals, restrictive cardiomyopathy, and constrictive pericarditis. See text for details. E, early diastolic filling; A, atrial systolic filling; S, systolic flow; D, diastolic flow; Vr, V-wave reversals; Ar, atrial systolic reversals; Ea, early diastolic tissue velocities; Aa, late diastolic tissue velocites; MVF, mitral valve flow; TVF, tricuspid valve flow; PVF, pulmonary venous flow; HVF, hepatic venous flow; DTI, Doppler tissue imaging. (From Hoit BD. Restrictive cardiomyopathy, In: Pohost G, O'Rourke R, Shah P, Berman D, eds. *Imaging in Cardiovascular Disease.* New York: Lippincott Williams & Wilkins; 2000:60–70. Reproduced with permission.)

cardiomyopathy from constrictive pericarditis, there is no uniform agreement regarding the characteristic features of the Doppler indices, especially those of venous flows. Moreover, rigorous studies of the sensitivity and specificity of these Doppler findings are lacking and relatively few patients have been examined. Thus, the diagnostic certainty is related to the number of "pathognomonic" findings in concert with clinical information and additional imaging studies.

Although radionuclide ventriculographic indices of LV diastolic function may differentiate constrictive pericarditis and restrictive cardiomyopathy, measurements of LV filling such as the peak filling rate, time to peak filling, and various filling fractions require careful attention to technical detail. The need for stable heart rates, the lack of venous flows, and the inability to observe the influence of respiration on cardiac blood flows are important limitations of the radionuclide ventriculographic technique. MRI and computed tomography (CT) are useful for accurately assessing pericardial thickness (Fig. 78-3); a pericardium >4.0 mm thick can distinguish the two entities.

Recent preliminary data suggest that constrictive pericarditis is associated with severe autonomic dysfunction that involves all segments of the autonomic nervous system, whereas in restrictive cardiomyopathy the autonomic dysfunction is localized to the parasympathetic efferent pathway.[7] Invasive hemodynamics may be helpful (see below), and occasionally a histologic diagnosis is necessary.

It is important to remember that clinical and laboratory testing, including imaging and pathologic studies, may produce results consistent with mixed constrictive pericarditis and restrictive cardiomyopathy; indeed, the two entities may coexist [for example, after mediastinal irradiation or after coronary artery bypass grafting (CABG)]. In these cases, a decision to treat conservatively or surgically explore a patient requires experienced clinical judgment.

Cardiac Catheterization

Most patients in whom restrictive cardiomyopathy is a serious consideration should undergo right- and left-sided heart catheterization to document the diagnosis, assess severity, and, in some patients, establish the etiology by means of endomyocardial biopsy. As in pa-

tients with constrictive pericarditis, extra care must be taken to obtain high-quality pressure recordings with appropriate gain and optimal damping conditions, and to attend to details such as the transducer height and system calibration. The venous pressure is elevated and the deep and rapid fall of the right atrial Y descent is striking. During inspiration, the descent of the V wave in the right atrium becomes deeper, steeper, and more pointed, whereas the other waves of the venous pulse and the mean atrial pressure do not vary throughout the respiratory cycle. The RV systolic pressure is often within the range of 35 to 45 mmHg, and the early portion of diastole is characterized by a deep, sharp dip followed by a plateau, during which no further increase in RV pressure occurs (Fig. 78-4). These hemodynamic features are identical to those of constrictive pericarditis and may cause diagnostic confusion. There is usually only modest pulmonary hypertension and the pulmonary arterial diastolic pressure is a few millimeters of mercury higher than the pulmonary wedge pressure, which is often quite elevated. The pulmonary wedge and the right atrial pressures may be identical and simulate further the hemodynamics of constrictive pericarditis; however, a higher LV than RV filling pressure strongly favors the diagnosis of restrictive cardiomyopathy rather than constrictive pericarditis. LV systolic pressure is normal, while the LV diastolic pressure tracing shows the same abnormalities as those of the RV (Fig. 78-4).

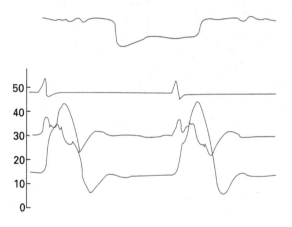

LV and RV

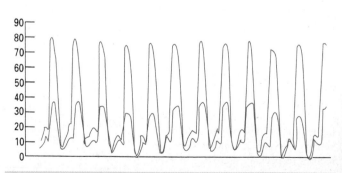

FIGURE 78-4 *Top:* Right-sided heart hemodynamic data from a patient with amyloidosis recorded with a high-fidelity catheter. From the top tracing down is a respirometer, electrocardiogram, right ventricular (RV) dP/dt, and RV pressure. Note the characteristic dip-and-plateau configuration. *Bottom:* Simultaneous RV and LV pressure tracings from another patient with cardiac amyloidosis. In this patient, the typical dip-and-plateau pattern was not present, but during inspiration LV and RV diastolic pressures equilibrated. (From Shabetai R. Restrictive, obliterative, and infiltrative cardiomyopathies. In: Alexander WA, Schlant R, Fuster V, et al., eds. *Hurst's The Heart,* 9th ed. New York: McGraw-Hill; 1998:2079. Reproduced with permission.)

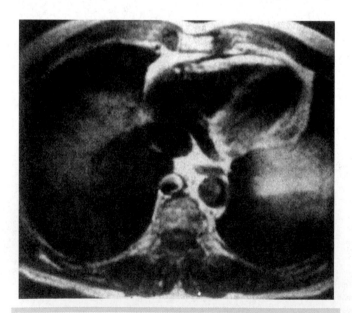

FIGURE 78-3 Magnetic resonance image showing normal pericardium as a low-intensity (*black*) line anterior to the right ventricle between high-intensity (*white*) epicardial and mediastinal fat. (From Hoit BD. Imaging the pericardium. *Cardiol Clin* 1990;8:588. Reproduced with permission.)

Left ventriculography usually shows a normal ejection fraction and the absence of major regional wall motion abnormalities. Endomyocardial biopsy is an integral part of the workup of many patients with restrictive cardiomyopathy. When distinction from constrictive pericarditis is particularly difficult, the biopsy may furnish proof of myocardial disease and establish the cause of restrictive cardiomyopathy (e.g., amyloidosis), or (by virtue of unremarkable histology) suggest the need for surgical exploration, even in the absence of a thickened pericardium.

Differences and similarities in coronary flow dynamics between restrictive cardiomyopathy and constrictive pericarditis have also been described. Patients with either restrictive cardiomyopathy or constrictive pericarditis have rapid deceleration of diastolic flow velocity, reduction of peak hyperemic flow velocity, and restriction of coronary flow reserve. The differences are characterized by rapid acceleration and more rapid deceleration of diastolic flow velocity in constrictive pericarditis compared to restrictive cardiomyopathy.[6]

Treatment of Restrictive Cardiomyopathy (General Considerations)

Except in certain instances described below ("Specific Restrictive Cardiomyopathic Diseases"), the treatment of restrictive cardiomyopathy is empiric and directed toward the treatment of diastolic heart failure. Reduction in the elevated ventricular diastolic pressures produces substantial improvement in pulmonary and systemic congestion, but judicious use of diuretics is warranted in view of the steep pressure-volume relation of the ventricles and the need to maintain a relatively high filling pressure. Vasodilators may also jeopardize ventricular filling and should be used cautiously. Calcium channel blockers are used by some because of their beneficial effect in hypertrophic cardiomyopathies, but improvement in ventricular compliance with their use has not been demonstrated in restrictive cardiomyopathy. Atrial fibrillation potentially worsens ventricular filling and therefore maintenance of normal sinus rhythm is essential; however, digoxin should be used with caution because of its potential arrhythmogenicity, especially in amyloidosis. Anticoagulation with warfarin may be indicated in patients with atrial fibrillation, valvular regurgitation, and low cardiac output, because of the high incidence of thromboembolic complications.

SPECIFIC RESTRICTIVE CARDIOMYOPATHIC DISEASES

A useful classification of the restrictive cardiomyopathies is shown in Table 78-1. This scheme is based on the cardiac compartment predominantly involved (i.e., myocardial versus endomyocardial); the myocardial diseases are divided into the noninfiltrative, infiltrative, and the storage diseases, and the endomyocardial diseases are divided into obliterative (i.e., endomyocardial fibrosis and the hypereosinophilic syndrome), and the nonobliterative (carcinoid, infiltrative, and iatrogenic).

Myocardial Diseases

NONINFILTRATIVE CARDIOMYOPATHIES

Idiopathic and Familial Restrictive Cardiomyopathy Although idiopathic restrictive cardiomyopathy is not generally recognized to have a familial predisposition, several small families have recently been reported.[8,9] The phenotypes have been variable with both auto-

somal dominant and recessive patterns of inheritance. No genetic linkage studies of large families with idiopathic restrictive cardiomyopathy have been described. Only one disease-causing gene, the desmin gene (*DES*), located on chromosome 2q35, has been identified.[9,10] The desmin-related myopathies are a heterogeneous group of autosomal dominant myopathies characterized by skeletal myopathy and cardiac conduction abnormalities with accumulation of desmin deposits in skeletal and cardiac muscle.[11] Restrictive cardiomyopathy is a relatively uncommon manifestation of desmin-related myopathy and mutations in the *DES* gene may also cause a dilated cardiomyopathy.[9] Myocyte hypertrophy and fibrosis on endomyocardial biopsy characterize idiopathic restrictive cardiomyopathy, and the absence of myocyte disarray is an important pathologic distinction from hypertrophic cardiomyopathy. However, overlap syndromes characterized by physiologic evidence of restriction and myocyte hypertrophy but without myocyte disarray or LV hypertrophy on echocardiography are reported.[12] Moreover, it was recently postulated that primary restrictive and hypertrophic cardiomyopathies may represent different phenotypic expressions of the same genetic disease.[13] An echocardiographic feature distinguishing primary restrictive cardiomyopathy from cardiac amyloidosis (in addition to the associated clinical features) is the increased LV wall thickness in the latter. In both disorders (and restrictive cardiomyopathies in general), ventricular dimensions are normal or reduced, systolic function is variable, and atrial dimensions are increased.

Two-dimensional and Doppler echocardiography is a reliable, noninvasive technique for diagnosing primary restrictive cardiomyopathy. A dominant mitral early diastolic "E" velocity, an increased pulmonary venous atrial systolic "A" reversal velocity and duration, and shortened mitral deceleration time are present in both children and adults with primary restrictive cardiomyopathy (Fig. 78-5). On CT or MRI scans, evidence of restrictive filling (e.g., right atrial and caval enlargement) is common in both restrictive cardiomyopathy and constrictive pericarditis. MRI may differentiate primary restrictive cardiomyopathy from amyloidosis based on tissue characterization.[14]

The prognosis of true idiopathic restrictive cardiomyopathy is difficult to establish because prior studies have included patients with hypertension, coronary artery disease, and ventricular enlargement and hypertrophy.[15] Although idiopathic restrictive cardiomyopathy initially may have a protracted course,[15] the prognosis is poor in older patients (particularly males) with increasing signs of systemic and pulmonary venous congestion, atrial fibrillation, and marked left atrial enlargement (>60 mm); in that group, the Kaplan-Meier 5-year survival is 64 percent, compared with the expected 85 percent survival.

Pseudoxanthoma Elasticum Pseudoxanthoma elasticum is a rare, genetically heterogeneous disorder characterized by fragmentation and calcification of elastic fibers involving the skin, eyes, and gastrointestinal and cardiovascular systems. Although endocardial fibroelastosis uncommonly causes restrictive cardiomyopathy (Fig. 78-6), coronary artery disease with premature death is a major problem in these patients.

Progressive Systemic Sclerosis Myocardial fibrosis, which may have a patchy distribution and be present in both ventricles, is found in the majority of patients with scleroderma at autopsy. On echocardiography, LV wall thickening in the absence of hypertension and evidence of LV dysfunction may be seen, but heart failure due to either restrictive or dilated cardiomyopathy is rare. Pericardial involvement and electrocardiographic abnormalities (heart block, supraventricular and ventricular tachycardia, and pseudoinfarction patterns) are

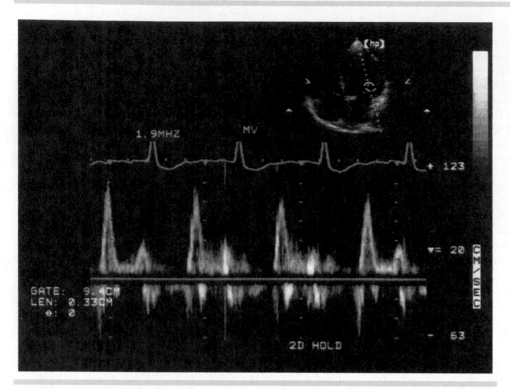

FIGURE 78-5 Doppler record of mitral inflow velocity from a patient with idiopathic restrictive cardiomyopathy. Note the dominant early diastolic wave. (From Shabetai R. Restrictive, obliterative, and infiltrative cardiomyopathies. In: Alexander WA, Schlant R, Fuster V, et al., eds. *Hurst's The Heart*, 9th ed. New York: McGraw-Hill; 1998:2077. Reproduced with permission.)

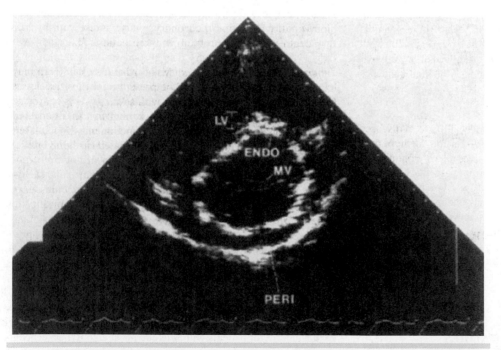

FIGURE 78-6 Short-axis view of the left ventricle (LV) at the mitral valve (MV) level in a patient with pseudoxanthoma elasticum. Note the calcified endomyocardium (ENDO) and echodense pericardium (PERI). The endocardial calcification was clearly visible by fluoroscopy. (From Shabetai R. Restrictive, obliterative, and infiltrative cardiomyopathies. In: Alexander WA, Schlant R, Fuster V, et al., eds. *Hurst's The Heart*, 9th ed. New York: McGraw-Hill; 1998:2085. Reproduced with permission.)

common. Pulmonary hypertension is a leading cause of morbidity and mortality in patients with scleroderma.

INFILTRATIVE CARDIOMYOPATHIES

Amyloidosis   Amyloidosis is a systemic disorder characterized by interstitial deposition of linear, rigid, nonbranching amyloid protein fibrils in multiple organs (e.g., heart, kidney, liver, nerve). Although there are four types of amyloidosis, cardiac involvement is most common in the first type, primary amyloidosis (AL type), which is caused by plasma cell production of immunoglobulin light chains; primary amyloidosis occurs often in association with multiple myeloma. Multiple myeloma is also reported to cause diastolic heart failure in the absence of amyloidosis.[14,14a,16] Cardiac deposition of amyloid protein (protein A, a nonimmunoglobin) may also occur in the second type, secondary amyloidosis, which is due to chronic infections (such as tuberculosis) or autoimmune disease (such as rheumatoid arthritis). Amyloidosis may also be familial (the third type) and commonly presents (especially at postmortem examination) in the elderly as senile amyloidosis (the fourth type). Mutations of the protein transthyretin (formerly called prealbumin) are usually inherited as an autosomal dominant trait and produce peripheral and autonomic neuropathy in addition to cardiac disease; over 50 mutations have been described.[17] Cardiac involvement occurs late in the disease and, although present in less than one-third of cases, it is responsible for over half of the deaths.[18] A transthyretin mutation at isoleucine 122 was recently reported as a cause of late-onset cardiac amyloidosis in African Americans.[19]

CLINICAL FEATURES   Amyloid deposits may be interstitial and widespread, resulting in restrictive cardiomyopathy, or localized to (1) conduction tissue, resulting in heart block and ventricular arrhythmias (especially familial amyloid); (2) the cardiac valves, causing valvular regurgitation; (3) the pericardium, producing constriction; and (4) the coronary arteries, resulting in ischemia. Amyloid may be isolated to the subendocardium in senile amyloid and amyloid secondary to chronic disease. Deposition of amyloid and atrial natriuretic factor (ANF) in the atria is frequent in aged hearts.[20] Despite sinus rhythm, atrial mechanical failure and thrombus formation may result due to electromechanical dissociation.[21] Atrial and brain natriuretic peptide are expressed in ventricular myocytes in patients with cardiac amyloidosis.[22] In some cases, the clinical picture is dominated by autonomic neuropathy (orthostatic hypotension, syncope, diarrhea, lack of sweating, and impotence) and nephropathy and cardiac involvement are unrecognized. Cardiac manifestations define a spectrum, often progressive through stages of severity, from the asymptomatic to biventricular failure.

DIAGNOSTIC/IMAGING STUDIES The cardiac silhouette on the chest radiograph may be normal or moderately enlarged. The ECG typically shows decreased voltage, a pseudoinfarction pattern, left axis deviation; arrhythmias and conduction disturbances may predominate the clinical course.

The M-mode echocardiogram may reveal symmetrical wall thickness involving the right and left ventricles, a small or normal LV cavity, variable (but often depressed) systolic function, left atrial enlargement, and a small pericardial effusion (Fig. 78-7). Digitized M-mode tracings may reveal decreased rates of systolic wall thickening and diastolic wall thinning and increased isovolumic relaxation time, especially in the early stages.

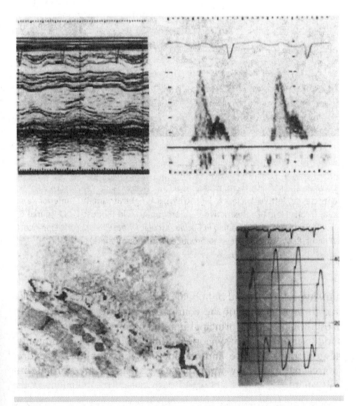

FIGURE 78-7 Amyloidosis. *Top left:* M-mode echocardiogram showing increased thickness of the left ventricular myocardium (calibration mark = 1 cm). *Top right:* Doppler tracing of mitral inflow velocity. Note that the atrial contribution to mitral blood flow velocity is markedly reduced (calibration mark = 20 cm/s). *Bottom left:* Electromicrograph showing extensive replacement of myocardium by amyloid. *Bottom right:* Right ventricular pressure tracing. A diastolic dip-plateau pattern is absent because of tachycardia. (From Shabetai R. Restrictive, obliterative, and infiltrative cardiomyopathies. In: Alexander WA, Schlant R, Fuster V, et al., eds. *Hurst's The Heart,* 9th ed. New York: McGraw-Hill; 1998:2083. Reproduced with permission.)

Two-dimensional echocardiographic findings include thickening of the ventricular myocardium, the interatrial septum and valves (especially the AV valves), enlarged papillary muscles, and dilated atria and inferior vena cava (Fig. 78-8). LV wall thickness is an important prognostic variable; in one study, patients with biopsy-proven amyloidosis having a mean wall thickness ≥15 mm had a median survival of 0.4 years, whereas patients with a mean wall thickness ≤12 mm had a median survival of 2.4 years.[23] Highly reflective echoes producing a granular or sparkling appearance and occurring in a patchy distribution are characteristic echocardiographic findings but are neither sensitive nor specific; concentric hypertrophy, as occurs in hypertension or aortic stenosis, may produce a uniformly speckled or echolucent appearance of the myocardium; and idiopathic hypertrophic cardiomyopathy may display a patchy, granular sparkling. Although they correlate with wall thickness, granular echoes may not be seen. Importantly, their recognition is subjective and is affected by ultrasound instrument settings. Thus, granular sparkling alone is an unreliable finding. The infiltrative pathology associated with amyloidosis may be detected by tissue characterization using MRI.[14] Amyloid cardiomyopathy may exist despite the absence of echocardiographic evidence of infiltration (see also Chap. 15).[24]

Doppler studies may show the restrictive pattern of LV filling—i.e., a transmitral E/A ratio ≥2 without respiratory variation, transmitral diastolic deceleration time <150 ms, and an isovolumic relaxation time ≤70 ms (Fig. 78-7). The RV filling pattern is often abnormal. The systolic-to-diastolic pulmonary venous flow ratio is <1 and atrial reversals increase with inspiration in the pulmonary and hepatic veins. However, the *earliest sign* of amyloid cardiomyopathy is impaired LV relaxation, manifest by an E/A ratio <1, and increased isovolumic relaxation and transmitral diastolic deceleration times. The severity of combined systolic and diastolic abnormalities can be determined with an echo Doppler index using isovolumic contraction and relaxation and ejection times.[25] In addition, Doppler has shown utility in prognosis; a deceleration time <150 ms and an increased E/A transmitral ratio are strong predictors of cardiac death.[26]

Abnormalities of LV filling are also demonstrated with the LV time-activity curve from radionuclide ventriculography.[27] Moreover, radionuclide imaging using technetium-99m pyrophosphate or indium-111 antimyosin may be useful in diagnosis. The variable clinical, diagnostic, and prognostic features reflect the location, nature, and extent of amyloid deposition and the temporal course of the disease. Serum and urine protein electrophoresis is diagnostic in most cases of primarily amyloidosis, but monoclonal protein is not secreted in 10 percent of cases.[18] Endomyocardial biopsy of the RV (most helpful if an abdominal fat aspirate is negative) provides the diagnosis, establishes the histochemistry, and quantifies myocardial damage and atrophy.[28]

Treatment of Amyloidosis The treatment of amyloidosis is unrewarding and symptomatic therapy is fraught with hazard; patients are sensitive to digoxin and calcium channel blockers, and hypotension with vasodilators and diuretics is a threat due to the steep LV pressure-volume relation. It is important to distinguish between familial and primary amyloidosis because the former carries a better prognosis than the latter, with a median survival of 5.8 years.[29] Immunosuppressive therapy with melphalan and prednisone is the established treatment regimen for primary (AL) amyloidosis. In a recent study, multiple alkylating agents failed to increase the response rate or survival time over this conventional regimen.[30] Autologous stem cell infusion reduces the monoclonal gammopathy, but has little effect on existing infiltrative amyloid.[29] Orthotopic cardiac transplantation

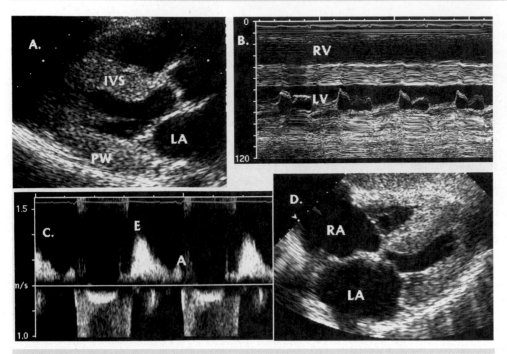

FIGURE 78-8 M-mode two-dimension, and Doppler echocardiogram from a patient with biopsy-proven amyloidosis causing hemodynamic restriction. LV systolic function is mildly impaired, wall thickness is increased, and there is biatrial enlargement. A. parasternal long axis view; B. M-mode through the thickened mitral valve; C. Doppler of restrictive diastolic mitral inflow and systolic mitral regurgitation; D. subcostal 4-chamber view. RV, right ventricle; LV, left ventricle; LA, left atrium; RA, right atrium; IVS = interventricular septum; PW = LV posterior wall; E = early diastolic transmitral velocity; A = late diastolic transmitral velocity.

Echocardiographic findings include evidence of systolic and diastolic LV dysfunction, LV aneurysm formation, abnormal ventricular wall thickness, pericardial effusion, regional wall motion abnormalities in the basal septum with apical sparing, and evidence of cor pulmonale. Thallium 201 has been used to indicate areas of myocardial involvement although the defects are relatively nonspecific for sarcoidosis. Patients with gallium-67 uptake have been shown to respond better to corticosteroids.[33] MRI may detect mass lesions due to sarcoid granuloma or scar.[34] Endomyocardial biopsy is useful but may be falsely negative. An important entity in the differential diagnosis is giant-cell myocarditis, which is characterized by a more aggressive and fatal course than cardiac sarcoid.[35] Treatment with prednisone for symptomatic patients is warranted in highly suspicious or proven cases because the cardiac granuloma may be sensitive. High-grade AV nodal block usually requires a permanent pacemaker, and in patients at high risk for sudden cardiac death, an automatic implantable cardioverter defibrillator (AICD) is appropriate. Calcium channel blockers may ameliorate diastolic dysfunction in patients with restrictive cardiomyopathy; patients with dilated cardiomyopathy are treated for congestive heart failure.[36] Cardiac transplantation is an appropriate consideration for intractable heart failure or arrhythmia.[36]

is generally not recommended because of the systemic nature of amyloidosis and the possibility of recurrence in the transplant, but successful cases have been reported.[31] Liver transplantation may be lifesaving in patients with familial amyloidosis,[32] since the liver is the site of transthyretin production. The use of alkylating agents in familial amyloidosis can be leukemogenic, and it is therefore important to differentiate primary from familial amyloidosis.[29]

Sarcoidosis   Sarcoidosis is a disorder of unknown etiology characterized by the presence of noncaseating granulomas that involve many organs (e.g., lung, skin, lymph nodes, liver, spleen). Granulomas involve the heart in sarcoidosis in as many as 25 percent of patients but are frequently subclinical. Nevertheless, in approximately half of the fatalities, cardiac involvement is responsible. Rarely, sarcoid is confined to the heart. The combination of extracardiac manifestations and cardiac abnormalities favors a presumptive diagnosis of sarcoidosis without biopsy. It is important to suspect cardiac sarcoidosis early, as aggressive treatment improves the prognosis. Interstitial granulomatous inflammation initially produces diastolic dysfunction, but later, when the disease is more extensive, it may produce systolic (at times focal) abnormalities. Localized thinning and dilatation of the basilar LV resembling ischemic heart disease are characteristic. Restrictive cardiomyopathy is uncommon. However, sarcoid pulmonary involvement is frequent and produces echo and Doppler findings of pulmonary hypertension and right heart failure. High-grade AV block, due to involvement of the conduction system, and ventricular arrhythmias are the principal manifestations and may result in sudden cardiac death; syncope is common. The ECG commonly demonstrates T-wave and conduction abnormalities. Pseudoinfarct patterns may appear with extensive myocardial involvement.

Gaucher's Disease   Gaucher's disease is the most common lysosomal storage disease. It is due to an inherited deficiency of the enzyme β-glucocerebroside, which results in accumulation of cerebroside in the reticuloendothelial system, brain, and heart. Diffuse interstitial infiltration of the left ventricle occurs, with reduced LV wall compliance and cardiac output, but is often subclinical. LV and left-sided valvular thickening and pericardial effusion are seen on echo.[37] Enzyme replacement therapy with alglucerase (the placental derivative) and imiglucerase (the recombinant form) has revolutionized the treatment of Gaucher's disease but its high cost still limits its availability in many countries.[38]

STORAGE DISEASES

Hemochromatosis   Type 1 or hereditary hemochromatosis is an autosomal recessive iron-storage disease caused by mutations in the HLA-linked *HFE* gene (the first hemochromatosis gene identified). It is seen mostly in men and almost entirely in people of northern European descent. Type 2 or juvenile hemochromatosis is a rare, autosomal recessive disease caused by an unidentified locus on chromosome 1q. It presents in the second and third decades of life, and equally affects men and women. Type 3 hemochromatosis is autosomal recessive and is caused by mutations in TFR2 (which encodes a transferring receptor isoform). Type 4 hemochromatosis is autosomal dominant, with mutations in the gene *ferroportin 1*, which encodes an intestinal iron transport molecule. Type 5 hemochromatosis is also autosomal dominant, with mutations in the H subunit of the iron storage molecule ferritin.[39]

The clinical features of hemochromatosis are due to accumulation of iron in the heart, pancreas, skin, liver, anterior pituitary and gonads. Myocardial iron deposition in hemochromatosis, either primary or secondary (e.g., resulting from multiple transfusions, ineffective erythropoiesis), usually produces dilated cardiomyopathy but may cause restrictive cardiomyopathy. Arrhythmia and conduction disturbances are common; indeed, congestive heart failure, conduction abnormalities, and supraventricular and ventricular arrhythmias occur in one-third of patients. Interstitial fibrosis is variable and unrelated to the extent of iron deposition, which occurs in the myocyte; secondarily, myocardial fibrosis may develop. Bronze diabetes and hepatic dysfunction, reflecting iron deposition in the skin, pancreas and liver are frequent associated manifestations.

Findings consistent with either dilated or restrictive cardiomyopathy may be seen; the presence of systolic dysfunction indicates a poor prognosis (Fig. 78-9). Granular sparkling and atrial enlargement may be observed, but these are nonspecific signs. Quantitative ultrasonic analysis of integrated backscatter has been used experimentally to detect changes in the echo reflectivity of the myocardium due to iron deposition in thalassemia major.[40] CT and MRI may demonstrate subclinical cardiac involvement, and tissue characterization may be possible with MRI. Endomyocardial biopsy is confirmatory; in selected instances, it may be useful in excluding the diagnosis.

Repeated phlebotomy is recommended for primary hemochromatosis, and the chelating agent desferrioxamine is often beneficial in secondary hemochromatosis. Cardiac transplantation (with or without liver transplantation) may be considered in selected cases.

Fabry's Disease Fabry's disease is an X-linked, genetically heterogeneous disorder of glycosphingolipid metabolism caused by lysosomal ceramide (α-galactosidase) deficiency that leads to accumulation of glycolipid in the heart, skin, and kidneys. Glycolipid accumulation in the myocardium and vascular and valvular endothelium may present with a restrictive, hypertrophic, or dilated cardiomyopathy, mitral regurgitation, ischemic heart disease, or aortic degeneration. Echocardiographic findings in restrictive cardiomyopathy mimic those seen in amyloid, and LV mass correlates with the severity of disease. Hypertension, mitral valve prolapse, and heart failure are common clinical presentations. Definitive diagnosis may require endomyocardial biopsy. Enzyme replacement therapy has proven effective but is limited by cost and the availability of the enzyme.[41]

Pompe's Disease Pompe's disease (glycogen storage type II) is due to an inherited (autosomal recessive) metabolic abnormality due to

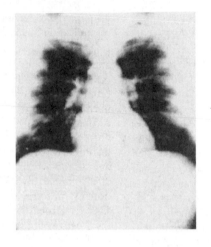
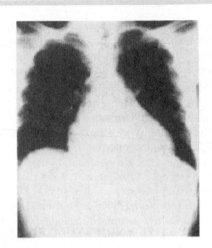
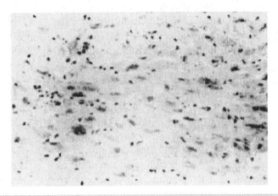

FIGURE 78-9 Chest radiograph of a patient with cardiac hemochromatosis before (*top right*) and after (*top left*) several months of treatment with phlebotomy. *Bottom:* Endomyocardial biopsy that established the diagnosis. (From Shabetai R. Restrictive, obliterative, and infiltrative cardiomyopathies. In: Alexander WA, Schlant R, Fuster V, et al., eds. *Hurst's The Heart*, 9th ed. New York: McGraw-Hill; 1998:2084. Reproduced with permission.)

acid maltase deficiency that causes massive amounts of glycogen deposition in the heart and skeletal muscles. A hypertrophied, hypokinetic LV in an infant with muscle hypotonia, hyperreflexia, and failure to thrive are characteristic findings. The echocardiographic manifestations may be indistinguishable from hypertrophic obstructive cardiomyopathy. The diagnosis can be made by absence of α-1,4-glucosidase activity on skeletal muscle biopsy. Adults with glycogen storage type III disease (debranching enzyme deficiency) may have marked LVH on echocardiography.[42]

Endomyocardial Diseases

OBLITERATIVE ENDOMYOCARDIAL DISEASE

Endomyocardial Fibrosis and Hypereosinophilic Syndrome Endomyocardial diseases that cause restrictive obliterative cardiomyopathies include endomyocardial fibrosis (EMF) and hypereosinophilic (Loeffler's) syndrome. The former accounts for 10 to 20 percent of deaths due to heart disease in equatorial Africa but is seen throughout the world. In contrast, Loeffler's endocarditis is seen mainly in countries with a temperate climate. Although it shares similar pathologic features with EMF, it affects mainly men; is usually related to parasitic infections, leukemia, and immunologic reactions; and is characterized by intense eosinophila and thromboembolic phenomena. The two conditions may represent different forms of the same disease (Loeffler's endocarditis representing an early and EMF an advanced stage), but considerable differences exist. Moreover, the endemic variety EMF may be related to high levels of cerium and low levels of magnesium, and may be pathophysiologically distinct from Loeffler's.[43]

Hypereosinophilic Syndrome   Cardiac involvement occurs in the majority of patients with the hypereosinophilic syndrome (unexplained eosinophilia exceeding 1500 eosinophils per cubic milliliter for at least 6 months and symptoms of organ involvement) and often has a biventricular distribution. Cardiotoxic eosinophils (abnormal cells containing vacuoles and having fewer than the normal number of granules) are central to the pathogenesis. The disease is characterized by organ damage from eosinophilic infiltration and mediator release. The cardiac pathology consists of an acute eosinophilic myocarditis, fibrinoid myocarditis, fibrinoid vasculitis of the intramural coronary arteries, mural thrombosis formation along damaged endocardium (often with eosinophils), fibrotic endocardial thickening and endomyocardial fibrosis with ventricular obliteration. In addition to symptoms due to cardiac involvement, patients have skin rash and constitutional symptoms. The disease is aggressive and rapidly progressive. ECG abnormalities (especially involving the T wave) are common but nonspecific. Hemodynamic findings are typical of restrictive cardiomyopathy.

Endomyocardial Fibrosis   In contrast to Loeffler's syndrome, EMF has a more insidious onset, has no gender predilection, and most often affects children and young adults. The disease is more indolent than Loeffler's, and biventricular involvement occurs in only about half the cases. LV involvement produces symptoms due to pulmonary congestion, whereas the less common isolated RV involvement (about 10 percent) may simulate constrictive pericarditis. Atrioventricular valve regurgitation and embolic episodes are frequent complications, and atrial fibrillation is common.

ECHOCARDIOGRAPHIC FEATURES   Echocardiography may be normal in the acute necrotic stage and endomyocardial biopsy may be needed to make the diagnosis if cardiac disease is suspected. Endomyocardial disease is characterized by endocardial fibrosis of the apex and subvalvular regions of one or both ventricles, resulting in restriction to inflow to the affected ventricle. Although their clinical presentations differ, the pathology, and therefore the cardiac imaging studies, are generally similar in the endomyocardial diseases. M-mode echo findings are nonspecific and digitized M-mode studies reveal a decreased peak filling rate and a decreased duration of the peak filling. On two-dimensional echocardiography, apical obliteration of the right and/or left ventricle, apical thrombus, preservation of ventricular systolic function with thickening of the posterior atrioventricular valve apparatus and posterobasilar LV wall, echo densities in the endocardium, and small ventricular and large atrial cavities are noted (Fig. 78-10). Involvement of the posterior mitral and tricuspid valve leaflets results in mitral and tricuspid regurgitation; less commonly, restricted motion may produce stenosis. Sparing of the outflow tracts is characteristic. Doppler interrogation yields typical patterns of restriction (increased E/A, decreased IVRT, decreased deceleration time), mitral and tricuspid regurgitation, and, less often, stenosis. Not surprisingly, the location, extent, and severity of involvement determine the clinical picture.

TREATMENT OF THE OBLITERATIVE RESTRICTIVE CARDIOMYOPATHIES   Medical therapy of Loeffler's syndrome is often ineffective and frustrating. Treatment consists of symptomatic relief, anticoagulants, corticosteroids, hydroxyurea, and most recently, interferon alpha, and palliative surgery in the late, fibrotic stage.[44] Surgical excision of fibrotic endocardium and valve replacement may offer symptomatic improvement, but at the expense of high (15 to 25 percent) operative mortality; thrombosis of mechanical valves can occur despite adequate anticoagulation. The prognosis of advanced disease is grim (50 percent 2-year mortality), but it is considerably better in those with milder disease.

NONOBLITERATIVE ENDOMYOCARDIAL DISEASES

Carcinoid Syndrome   Carcinoid syndrome results from metastatic carcinoid tumors (most commonly arising in the small bowel and appendix but also the bronchus and other sites) and consists of cutaneous flushing, diarrhea, and bronchoconstriction; involvement of the heart occurs as a late complication of carcinoid syndrome in approximately 50 percent of patients. Hepatic metastases produce serotonin, bradykinin, and other substances that affect right heart structures. As these substances are inactivated in the lungs, LV involvement is distinctly uncommon and when present, suggests a right-to-left intracardiac shunt. Fibrous

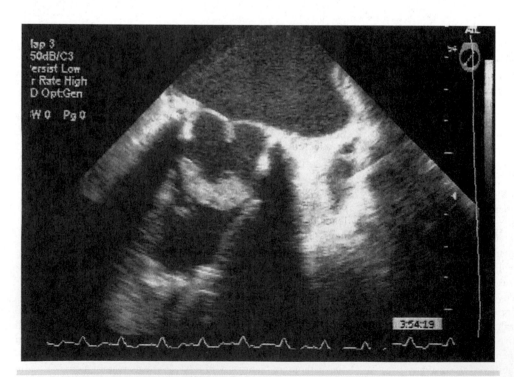

FIGURE 78-10 Transesophageal echocardiogram from a patient with eosinophilic endocarditis and prosthetic mitral valve replacement. Thrombus is noted below the valve struts, which at the the time of surgery was found to be adherent to the posterior LV wall. Note the apical obliteration and the apical endocardial thickening and calcification.

endocardial plaque comprising smooth muscle cells in a stroma of collagen and acid mucopolysaccharide on the tricuspid and pulmonic valves and right heart endocardium is characteristic. Although tricuspid and pulmonic stenosis and regurgitation dominate the clinical picture, restrictive cardiomyopathy may occur.

The chest radiograph is often normal, but cardiomegaly, pleural effusions, and nodules may be evident; unlike the case with congenital pulmonic stenosis, poststenotic dilatation of the pulmonary artery trunk does not occur.[45] Electrocardiographic abnormalities are common, but nonspecific; a low-voltage QRS complex may be seen in advanced disease. Two-dimensional echocardiography reveals thickened, retracted, immobile tricuspid and pulmonic valves, and right atrial and ventricular enlargement; right atrial wall thickening may be seen on transesophageal echocardiography. Pulmonary outflow tract obstruction can occur due to pulmonary annular constriction. Low-velocity tricuspid and pulmonic regurgitation on Doppler indicates normal pulmonary arterial pressures, which is typical of carcinoid heart disease. Echocardiographic findings are detected in approximately two-thirds of patients with carcinoid. In one study, cardiac involvement was associated with a reduced 3-year survival as compared with those without cardiac involvement.[45] Metastatic carcinoid tumor to the heart is uncommon, intramyocardial, occurring with roughly equal frequency in the right and left ventricles, and can be recognized on echocardiography if the tumor size is at least 1 cm.[46] Catheterization findings are usually those of tricuspid regurgitation and/or pulmonic stenosis.

Therapy is symptomatic, usually with a somatostatin analog such as octreotide. Despite a decrease in 5-HIAA excretion, the valvular lesions do not regress. Valvular replacement (usually mechanical) or repair is warranted in patients with severe valve dysfunction. Premature degeneration of a bioprosthetic valve may be caused by the carcinoid process.

MALIGNANT INFILTRATION

Malignant Infiltration   Infiltrating tumors of the heart are generally metastatic (lung, breast, melanoma, lymphoma, leukemia) and rarely produce restriction to ventricular filling unless the pericardium is involved. Infiltration on echocardiography is suggested by a localized increase in wall thickness, often associated with abnormal wall motion and pericardial effusion. CT and MRI scans are also useful.

Iatrogenic Disease   Pericardial disease frequently complicates radiation therapy to the chest and may produce constrictive pericarditis; however, endo- and myocardial involvement may produce restrictive cardiomyopathy, at times presenting years after radiation therapy has been completed. Anthracyclines and methysergide can cause endomyocardial fibrosis. Oils containing L-tryptophan were withdrawn from the market when they were implicated in the genesis of the eosinophilia-myalgia syndrome; this syndrome was associated with restrictive cardiomyopathy.[47] Finally, a restrictive pattern of LV filling is common soon after orthotopic cardiac transplantation and may persist for at least 1 year in as many as 15 percent.[48]

References

1. WHO/ISFC Task Force. Richardson P (Chairman). Report of the 1995 World Health Organization/International Society and Federation of Cardiology Task Force on the Definition and Classification of Cardiomyopathies. *Circulation* 1996;93:841–842.
2. Goodwin J, Oakley C. The cardiomyopathies. *Br Heart J* 1972;44:672–673.
3. Angelini A, Calzolari V, Thiene G, et al. Morphologic spectrum of primary restrictive cardiomyopathy. *Am J Cardiol* 1997;80:1046–1050.
3a. Chatterjee K, Alpert J. Constrictive pericarditis and restrictive cardiomyopathy: Similarities and differences. *Heart Fail Monit.* 2003;3:118–126.
3b. Soler R, Rodriguez E, Remuinan C, et al. Magnetic resonance imaging of primary cardiomyopathies. *J Comput Assist Tomogr.* 2003;27:724–734.
4. Klein A, Cohen G, Pietrolungo J, et al. Differentiation of constrictive pericarditis from restrictive cardiomyopathy by Doppler transesophageal echocardiographic measurements of respiratory variations in pulmonary venous flow. *J Am Coll Cardiol* 1993;22:1935–1943.
5. Garcia M, Rodriguez L, Ares M, et al. Differentiation of constrictive pericarditis from restrictive cardiomyopathy: Assessment of left ventricular diastolic velocities in longitudinal axis by doppler tissue imaging. *J Am Coll Cardiol* 1996;27:108–114.
6. Akasaka T, Yoshida K, Yamamuro A, et al. Phasic coronary flow characteristics in patients with constrictive pericarditis: Comparison with restrictive cardiomyopathy. *Circulation* 1997;96:1874–1881.
7. Singh M, Juneja R, Bali HK, et al. Autonomic functions in restrictive cardiomyopathy and constrictive pericarditis: A comparison. *Am Heart J* 1998;136:443–448.
8. Kushuwaha SS, Fallon JT, Fuster V. Restrictive Cardiomyopathy. *N Engl J Med* 1997;336(4):267–276.
9. Fatkin D, Graham RM. Molecular mechanisms of inherited cardiomyopathies. *Physiol Rev* 2002;82:945–980.
10. Goldfarb LG, Park KY, Cervenakova L, et al. Missense mutations in desmin associated with familial cardiac and skeletal myopathy. *Nat Genet* 1998;19:402–403.
11. Dalakas MC, Park K, Semina-Mora C, et al. Desmin myopathy, a skeletal myopathy with cardiomyopathy caused by mutations in the desmin gene. *N Engl J Med* 2000;342:770–780.
12. Cooke R, Chambers J, Curry P. Noonan's cardiomyopathy: A non-hypertrophic variant. *Br Heart J* 1994;71:561–565.
13. Angelini A, Calzolari V, Thiene G, et al. Morphologic spectrum of primary restrictive cardiomyopathy. *Am J Cardiol* 1997;80:1046–1050.
14. Celetti F, Fattori R, Napoli G, et al. Assessment of restrictive cardiomyopathy of amyloid or idiopathic etiology by magnetic resonance imaging. *Am J Cardiol* 1999;83:798–801.
14a. Wald DS, Gray HH. Restrictive cardiomyopathy in systemic amyloidosis. *QJM.* 2003;96:380–382.
15. Ammash NM, Seward JB, Bailey KR, et al. Clinical profile and outcome of idiopathic restrictive cardiomyopathy. *Circulation* 2000;101:2490–2496.
16. Schattner A, Epstein M, Berrebi A, et al. Case report: Multiple myeloma presenting as a diastolic heart failure with no evidence of amyloidosis. *Am J Med Sci* 1995;310:256–257.
17. Saraiva MJ. Transthyretin mutations in health and disease. *Hum Mutat* 1995;5:191–196.
18. Kyle RA. Amyloidosis. *Circulation* 1995;91:1269–1271.
19. Jacobson DR, Pastore RD, Yaghoubian R, et al. Variant-sequence transthyretic (isoleucine 122) in late-onset cardiac amyloidosis in black Americans. *N Engl J Med* 1997;336:466–473.
20. Kawamura S, Takahashi M, Ishihara T, et al. Incidence and distribution of isolated atrial amyloid: Histologic and immunohistochemical studies of 100 aging hearts. *Pathol Int* 1995;45:335–342.
21. Dubrey S, Pollak A, Skinner M, et al. Atrial thrombi occurring during sinus rhythm in cardiac amyloidosis: Evidence for atrial electromechanical dissociation. *Br Heart J* 1995;74:541–544.
22. Takemura G, Takatsu Y, Doyama K, et al. Expression of atrial and brain natriuretic peptides and their genes in hearts of patients with cardiac amyloidosis. *J Am Coll Cardiol* 1998;4:754–765.
23. Cueto-Garcia L, Reeder G, Kyle R, et al. Echocardiographic findings in systemic amyloidosis: Spectrum of cardiac involvement and relation to survival. *J Am Coll Cardiol* 1985;6:737–743.
24. Gertz MA, Grogan M, Kyle RA, et al. Endomyocardial biopsy-proven light chain amyloidosis (AL) without echocardiographic features of infiltrative cardiomyopathy. *Am J Cardiol* 1997;80:93–95.

25. Tei C, Dujardin KS, Hodge DO, et al. Doppler index combining systolic and diastolic myocardial performance: Clinical value in cardiac amyloidosis. *J Am Coll Cardiol* 1996;28:658–664.

26. Klein AL, Hatle LK, Taliercio CP, et al. Prognostic significance of Doppler measures of diastolic function in cardiac amyloidosis: A Doppler echocardiography study. *Circulation* 1991;83:808–816.

27. Lenihan DJ, Gerson MC, Hoit BD, et al. Mechanisms, diagnosis, and treatment of diastolic heart failure. *Am Heart J* 1995;130:153–166.

28. Arbustini E, Merlini G, Gavazzi A, et al. Cardiac immunocyte-derived (AL) amyloidosis: An endomyocardial biopsy study in 11 patients. *Am Heart J* 1995;130:528–536.

29. Zieman SJ, Fortnum NJ. Hypertrophic and restrictive cardiomyopathies in the elderly. *Cardiol Clin* 1999;17(1):159–172.

30. Gertz MA, Lacy MQ, Lust JA, et al. Prospective randomized trial of melphalan and prednisone versus vincristine, carmustine, melphalan, cyclophosphamide, and prednisone in the treatment of primary systemic amyloidosis. *J Clin Oncol* 1999;17:262–267.

31. Pelosi F Jr, Capehart J, Roberts WC. Effectiveness of cardiac transplantation for primary (AL) cardiac amyloidosis. *Am J Cardiol* 1997;79: 532–535.

32. Skinner M, Lewis WD, Jones LA, et al. Liver transplantation as a treatment for familial amyloidotic polyneuropathy. *Ann Intern Med* 1994; 15:133–134.

33. Okayama K, Kurata C, Tawarchara K, et al. Diagnostic and prognostic value of myocardial scintigraphy with thallium-201 and gallium-67 in cardiac sarcoidosis. *Chest* 1995;107:330–334.

34. Chandra M, Silverman ME, Oshinski J, et al. Diagnosis of cardiac sarcoidosis aided by MRI. *Chest* 1996;110:562–565.

35. Cooper LH, Berry G, Rizeq M, et al. Giant cell myocarditis. *J Heart Lung Transplant* 1995;14:394–401.

36. Shabetai R. Sarcoidosis and the heart. *Curr Treat Options Cardiovasc Med* 2000;2:385–398.

37. Saraclar M, Atalay S, Kocak N, et al. Gaucher's disease with mitral and aortic involvement: Echocardiographic findings. *Pediatr Cardiol* 1991; 13:56–58.

38. Elstein D, Abrahamov A, Hadas-Halpern I, et al. Gaucher's disease. *Lancet* 2001;358:324–327.

39. Bomford A. Genetics of haemachromatosis. *Lancet* 2002;360:1673–1681.

40. Lattanzi F, Bellotti P, Picano E, et al. Quantitative ultrasonic analysis of myocardium in patients with thalassemia major and iron overload. *Circulation* 1993;87:748–754.

41. Peters FPJ, Vermeulen A, Kho TL. Anderson-Fabry's disease:α-galactosidase deficiency. *Lancet* 2001;357:138–140.

42. Coleman R, Winter H, Wolf B, et al. Glycogen storage disease type III (glycogen debranching enzyme deficiency): Correlation of biochemical defects with myopathy and cardiomyopathy. *Ann Intern Med* 1992;116: 896–900.

43. Shaper A. What's new in endomyocardial fibrosis? *Lancet* 1993;342: 255–256.

44. Baratta L, Afeltra A, Delfino M, et al. Favorable response to high-dose interferon-alpha in idiopathic hypereosinophilic syndrome with restrictive cardiomyopathy—Case report and literature review. *Angiology* 2002;53:465–470.

45. Pellikka P, Tajik A, Khandheria B, et al. Carcinoid heart disease: Clinical and echocardiographic spectrum in 74 patients. *Circulation* 1993; 87:1188–1196.

46. Pandya UH, Pellika PA, Enriquez-Sarano M, et al. Metastatic carcinoid tumor to the heart: Echocardiographic-pathologic study of 11 patients. *J Am Coll Cardiol* 2002;40:1328–1332.

47. Berger PB, Duffy J, Reeder GS, et al. Restrictive cardiomyopathy associated with eosinophilia-myalgia syndrome. *Mayo Clin Proc* 1994;69: 162–165.

48. Valantine HA, Fowler MB, Hunt SA, et al. Changes in Doppler echocardiographic indexes of left ventricular function as potential markers of acute cardiac rejection. *Circulation* 1987;76:V86–V92.

MYOCARDITIS AND SPECIFIC CARDIOMYOPATHIES—ENDOCRINE DISEASE AND ALCOHOL

Sean P. Pinney / Donna M. Mancini

The diagnosis of cardiomyopathy encompasses a wide spectrum of diseases with widely divergent pathogenic mechanisms that have as their final common pathway the syndrome of congestive heart failure. A list of etiologies associated with the development of cardiomyopathy is presented in Fig. 79-1.

Coronary artery disease, hypertension, valvular heart disease, and cardiomyopathy are the most common causes of heart failure for both sexes. Comparison of the Framingham[1] and SOLVD[2] (Study of Left Ventricular Dysfunction) registries demonstrates a shift in the predominant etiology of heart failure from hypertension to ischemic heart disease. This probably reflects recent intensified efforts to control high blood pressure.

Inflammatory cardiomyopathies, particularly viral myocarditis, have served as a model to understand the development of heart failure. More than 70 different specific cardiomyopathies associated with general systemic disease, neuromuscular disorders, hypersensitivity and toxic reactions, and the peripartum state have been described. When they are considered as a group, these disorders are infrequent; considered individually, they are rare.

This chapter reviews the inflammatory cardiomyopathies and specific cardiomyopathies with an emphasis on endocrine and infiltrative disorders. Cardiac disorders caused by pulmonary hypertension and congenital cardiac anomalies are not addressed.

MYOCARDITIS

Infective

VIRAL

In its most literal sense, *myocarditis* means inflammation of the myocardium. As early as 1806, a relationship between infection and chronic heart disease (diphtheria) was postulated, but it was not until the 1970s, with the advent of endomyocardial biopsy, that the diagnosis of myocarditis could be established during life. Multiple infectious etiologies (Table 79-1)[3] have been implicated as the cause of myocarditis, the most common being viral, specifically, the enterovirus coxsackie B. In the majority of patients, active myocarditis remains unsuspected because the cardiac dysfunction is subclinical, asymptomatic, and self-limited. The discovery of myocarditis in 1 to 9 percent of routine postmortem examinations suggests that myocarditis is a major cause of sudden, unexpected death.[4]

Pathogenesis Infection by cardiotropic viruses prompted the initial hypothesis that the viral infection was responsible for myocardial injury. However, several investigators noted that cardiac dysfunction increased after the eradication of the infective agent and speculated

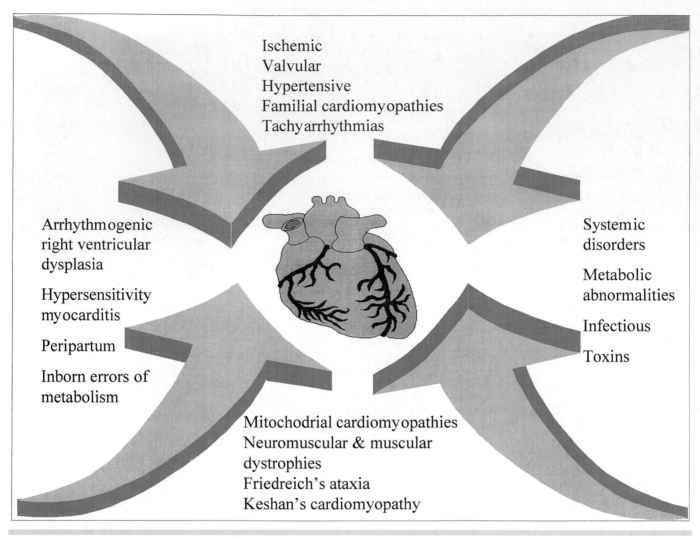

FIGURE 79-1 Various etiologies that can lead to cardiomyopathy.

TABLE 79-1 Causes of Myocarditis

Infectious
  Viruses
    Coxsackievirus, echovirus, HIV, Epstein-Barr virus,
      influenza, cytomegalovirus, adenovirus, hepatitis
      (A and B), mumps, poliovirus, rabies, respiratory
      synctial virus, rubella, vaccinia, varicella zoster,
      arbovirus
  Bacteria
    *Cornyebacterium diptheriae, Streptococcus pyogenes,
      Staphylococcus aureus, Haemophilus pneumoniae,
      Salmonella* spp., *Neisseria gonorrhoeae, Leptospira,
      Borrelia burgdorferi, Treponema pallidum, Brucella,
      Mycobacterium tuberculosis,* Actinomyces, *Chlamydia*
      spp., *Coxiella burnetti, Mycoplasma pneumoniae,
      Rickettsia* spp.
  Fungi
    Candida spp., *Aspergillus* spp., *Histoplasma,
      Blastomyces, Cryptococcus, Coccidioidomyces*

Parasites
  Trypanosoma cruzii, Toxoplasma, Schistosoma, Trichina
Noninfectious
  Drugs causing hypersensitivity reactions
    Antibiotics: sulfonamides, penicillins,
      chloramphenicol, amphotericin B, tetracycline,
      streptomycin
    Antituberculous: isoniazid, para-aminosalicylic acid
    Anticonvulsants: phenindione, phenytoin,
      carbamazepine
    Anti-inflammatories: indomethacin, phenylbutazone
    Diuretics: acetazolamide, chlorthalidone,
      hydrochlorothiazide, spironolactone
    Others: amitriptyline, methyldopa, sulfonylureas
  Drugs not causing hypersensitivity reactions
    Cocaine, cyclophosphamide, lithium, interferon alpha
  Nondrug causes
    Radiation, giant-cell myocarditis

that the pathogenesis of myocarditis may be due to two distinct phases of myocardial cell damage—the first due to direct viral infection and the second due to the host's immune response (Fig. 79-2). Support for this theory comes initially from the work of Woodruff, who noted that the histologic evidence of cardiac injury in coxsackie B infection appeared only after the virus was no longer detectable in the myocardium.[5] Subsequently, demonstration of T-lymphocyte and macrophage infiltration,[6] perforin granules,[7] and a variety of cytokines known to depress myocardial contractility[8] in endomyocardial biopsies of patients with active carditis strengthened the concept of immune-mediated injury.

Our understanding of the specific immune responses that lead to myocardial injury is derived largely from animal models of myocarditis induced by cardiotropic viruses.[9] A time line for experimental viral myocarditis is shown in Fig. 79-3. After gaining entry to the body from the gastrointestinal tract (enterovirus) or through the respiratory tract (adenovirus and enterovirus), these cardiotropic viruses bind to the coxsackie-adenoviral receptor (CAR), which, in turn allows for the incorporation of the viral genome into the myocyte.[10] In the acute phase of viral myocarditis (days 0 to 3), mice injected with coxsackievirus show evidence of direct viral cytotoxicity, with myocyte necrosis in the absence of an inflammatory cell infiltrate.[11] Activated macrophages begin to express interleukin (IL)-1β, IL-2, tumor necrosis factor alpha (TNF-α), and interferon gamma (IFN-γ).[12,13]

This ushers in the second or subacute phase (days 4 to 14) of myocarditis, which is characterized by the infiltration of natural killer (NK) cells, production of neutralizing antibody, and cell-mediated immune pathogenicity. The first wave of infiltrating cells consists mainly of NK cells that play a dual role.[9] By limiting viral replication, NK cells can be protective. However, NK cells release perforin and granzymes, which form circular pore lesions on the membrane surface of virus-infected cells.[14] While this activity produces cardiomyocyte damage, uninfected cells are spared from injury.[15]

Cytokines are a major mediator of immune activation and its maintenance.[16] Circulating levels of IL-1, IL-2, and IL-6 are elevated in patients with acute myocarditis,[17] as is TNF-α mRNA and protein expression.[18] In animal models, overexpression of TNF-α produces florid myocarditis,[19] whereas mice deficient in the TNF p55 receptor (TNF-R1$^{-/-}$) experience milder autoimmune myocarditis.[20] However, a recent study by Wada et al.

suggests that TNF-α may actually play a protective role in the acute stage of viral myocarditis.[21] The observed full recovery of some patients with severe left ventricular dysfunction may be the result of short-term exposure to these inflammatory cytokines.[16] Nitric oxide, which has a beneficial role in maintaining vascular tone, may have a deleterious effect in acute myocarditis, contributing to the progression of myocyte damage in animal models of myocarditis.[22]

Host resistance to virus-mediated damage occurs through the combined actions of NK cells, infiltrating mononuclear cells, and the expression of neutralizing antibody. After invading the myocardium, coxsackievirus increases its expression, becoming maximal on day 4.[23] Almost no neutralizing antibody is present until day 4, after

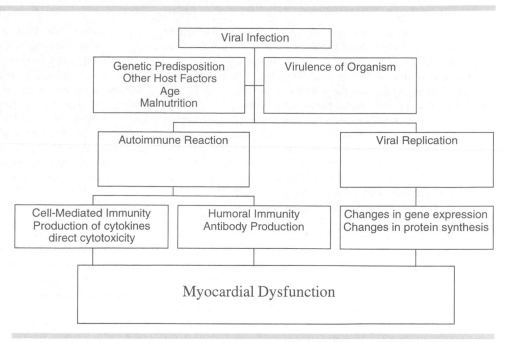

FIGURE 79-2 Flow diagram illustrating various factors that contribute to the development of myocardial dysfunction after viral infection.

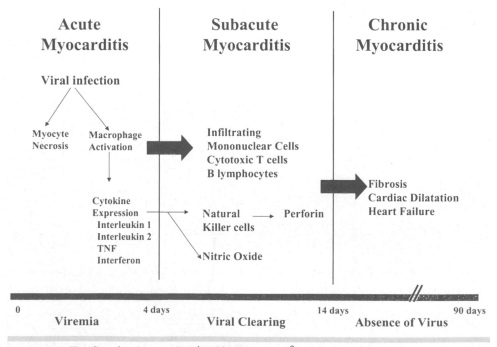

FIGURE 79-3 Time line of viral myocarditis. (Modified from Kawai,[9] with permission.)

which titers quickly rise, becoming maximal on day 14. The rise in antibody titer is closely related to the elimination of virus from the heart. Infiltrating mononuclear cells appear in the myocardium between 5 and 10 days following viral infection.[5,24] In combination with neutralizing antibodies, these mononuclear cells help to suppress viral infection and limit cardiomyocyte damage.

T lymphocytes are attracted to the myocardium through classic cell-mediated immunity. Within the cytoplasm of infected myocytes, viral particles are broken down into peptide fragments and then placed on the cell surface in association with major histocompatibility-complex class 1 antigen.[25] Through their T-cell receptor (TCR), cytotoxic T-cells recognize virus-infected cells and destroy them by either cytokine production or perforin-mediated cell cytolysis.[9] In spite of the damage done to the myocardium in the process of eliminating infected cells, were it not for cell-mediated immunity in combination with neutralizing antibodies and NK cells, viral replication could continue unchecked. Indeed, when host defense mechanisms are inadequate, chronic viral infection produces widespread cardiac damage and eventual cardiac dilation and failure.[26] On the other hand, continuous exuberant T-cell activation can be equally destructive. This occurs when antigens intrinsic to the myocardium cross-react with viral peptides, leading to sustained T-cell activation (so called molecular mimicry), which can ultimately lead to dilated cardiomyopathy.[9,16,27]

A third or chronic phase of viral myocarditis (days 15 to 90) occurs following the elimination of virus and is typified by insidious ongoing myocardial damage.[9] Hearts from infected mice are hypertrophied and myocardial fibrosis is prominent. Inflammatory cells are no longer seen. The mechanisms involved in the transition from this stage to the development of dilated cardiomyopathy are not fully understood, but three mechanisms seem likely—persistent viral infection, ongoing autoimmune destruction, and apoptosis.

Attempts to culture virus from human myocardial tissue have generally been unsuccessful. However, identification of viral genomic fragments in myocardial samples by in situ hybridization and polymerase chain reaction from patients with myocarditis and dilated cardiomyopathy has been reported.[28–30] These genomic fragments may not be capable of replicating as intact cardiotropic virus but probably serve as a persistent source of antigen to drive the deleterious immune responses.[31]

Autoimmune-mediated heart disease results from a process of molecular mimicry whereby antibodies to viral proteins cross-react with structural elements of the heart. For example, injection of myosin into susceptible mice produces active myocarditis.[32] One reason for this may lie in the fact that myosin shares about 40 percent identity with the amino acid sequence of CVB3 capsid protein.[33] Several other circulating heart-specific autoantibodies have been identified, including antisarcolemma antibody, which also exhibits cross-reactivity with CVB3 capsid protein.[34] Further investigation with this virus-free model of myocarditis will help in elucidating the pathogenesis of molecular mimicry.

Apoptosis, or programmed cell death, may be a third pathogenic mechanism leading from myocarditis to dilated cardiomyopathy. While this association is currently speculative, certain viruses have been identified as triggers of apoptosis.[35] Cytokines may activate death-domain sequences or ceramide-mediated signaling pathways as part of the remodeling process.[36] Although animal models of myocarditis can progress to dilated cardiomyopathy, as can patients with clinically suspected or biopsy-proven myocarditis, the percentage of patients with idiopathic dilated cardiomyopathy representing the end stage of an active myocarditis is unknown.

Clinical Presentation The clinical manifestations of myocarditis are variable, ranging from an asymptomatic or self-limited disease in some to profound cardiogenic shock in others. Cardiac involvement typically occurs 7 to 10 days following a systemic illness. The most obvious symptom suggesting myocarditis is an antecedent viral syndrome with fever, myalgias, and malaise. The majority of patients have no specific cardiovascular complaints but may have ST-segment and T-wave abnormalities on the electrocardiogram (ECG) suggesting myocarditis.[37] Chest pain may occur in up to 35 percent of patients and may be typically ischemic, somewhat atypical, or pericardial in character. Chest pain usually reflects associated pericarditis but occasionally may result from myocardial ischemia.[38]

Acute dilated cardiomyopathy from lymphocytic myocarditis can produce mild, moderate, or fulminant heart failure. The vast majority of patients with mild symptoms have spontaneous recovery in ventricular function and normalization of heart size. Patients with New York Heart Association (NYHA) class III or IV heart failure typically have greater degrees of ventricular dilation and dysfunction. While some recover spontaneously, it is estimated that half will be left with residual myocardial dysfunction and a quarter will either die or require cardiac transplantation.[38] Biopsy-proven relapses have occurred in some patients and recurrent myocarditis should be suspected if ventricular function subsequently deteriorates.[39] Fulminant myocarditis is often dramatic and accompanied by a rapid onset of symptoms.[40] Patients are severely ill, with circulatory collapse and evidence of end-organ dysfunction. They frequently have fever, severe global myocardial dysfunction, and a minimal increase in left ventricular end-diastolic dimension. Mechanical circulatory support has been required, as a bridge to either cardiac transplantation or recovery.[41,42]

Occasionally patients will present with a clinical syndrome identical to an acute myocardial infarction, with ischemic chest pain and ST-segment elevations on the ECG[43,44] (Fig. 79-4). Left ventricular dysfunction may be present in less than half of patients and

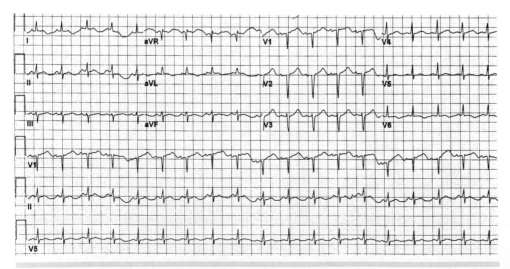

FIGURE 79-4 Electrocardiographic tracing consistent with an anteroseptal myocardial infarction and lateral ischemia in a patient with acute myocarditis and normal coronary arteries.

tends to be diffuse rather than segmental.[45] At autopsy, the coronary arteries are usually widely patent, although viral coronary arteritis has been reported.[46] Coronary vasospasm has also been associated with acute myocarditis.[47]

Patients may present with syncope or palpitations with atrioventricular (AV) block or ventricular arrhythmia. Complete AV block is common, with some patients presenting with Stokes-Adams attacks. The complete heart block is generally transient and rarely requires a permanent pacemaker.[48] Sudden cardiac death can be the initial presentation of myocarditis in some patients, presumably from complete heart block or ventricular tachycardia. In a 20-year review of sudden death among Air Force recruits, 20 percent had myocarditis documented at autopsy.[49] In some patients with refractory ventricular arrhythmias, endomyocardial biopsy or autopsy has revealed myocarditis. Systemic or pulmonary thromboembolic disease is also associated with myocarditis.[50]

A familial tendency for the development of myocarditis may be present. In one report, a suppressor cell defect was detected, predisposing to development of active myocarditis.[51] Patients with peripartum cardiomyopathy have a high frequency of myocarditis on endomyocardial biopsy.[52] The immunoregulatory changes during and following pregnancy may heighten susceptibility to viral myocarditis, and exposure to trophoblastic antigens may predispose to immune-mediated myocardial injury.

Diagnosis Laboratory findings are generally not diagnostic. Leukocytosis, eosinophilia, and an elevated erythrocyte sedimentation rate are sometimes present, as are elevated titers to cardiotropic viruses. A fourfold rise in IgG titer over a 4- to 6-week period is required to document acute infection. Elevated IgM antibody titer may denote an acute infection more specifically than a rise in IgG antibody titer. Unfortunately, a rise in antibody titer documents only the response to a recent viral infection and does not indicate active myocarditis. Abnormalities in peripheral T- and B-lymphocyte counts have been reported, but these findings have not been consistent and cannot be used as diagnostic adjuncts. An increase in the MB band of creatine phosphokinase (CPK) is observed in approximately 10 percent of patients, but newer troponin assays are proving to be more sensitive for detecting myocardial injury in suspected myocarditis.[53,54] The classic clinical triad of preceding viral illness, pericarditis, and associated laboratory abnormalities used to diagnose coxsackie B–induced myocarditis is present in fewer than 10 percent of histologically proven cases.[39]

The ECG most frequently shows sinus tachycardia.[55] Diffuse ST-T-wave changes, prolongation of the QTc interval, conduction delay, low voltage, and even an acute myocardial infarct pattern have been noted in patients with myocarditis. Cardiac arrhythmias are frequently observed, including complete heart block, ventricular tachycardia and supraventricular arrhythmias—especially in the presence of congestive heart failure or pericardial inflammation.[56]

Echocardiography can reveal left ventricular systolic dysfunction in patients with a normal-sized left ventricular cavity. Segmental wall motion abnormalities may be observed.[57] Wall thickness may be increased, particularly early in the course of the disease, when inflammation is fulminant.[58] Ventricular thrombi are detected in 15 percent of those studies.[59] Echocardiographic findings in active myocarditis can mimic restrictive, hypertrophic, or dilated cardiomyopathy.

Endomyocardial biopsy is the critical test to confirm the diagnosis. Endomyocardial biopsy techniques enable the repetitive sampling of the human myocardium with minimal discomfort, minor morbidity and a mortality rate of 0.2 percent.[52] Right ventricular myocardial specimens can be obtained by accessing the right internal jugular or femoral vein.[60] Intravascular biopsy of the left ventricle is

TABLE 79-2 Diagnoses That Can Be Made by Endomyocardial Biopsy

1. Myocarditis
   Giant-cell myocarditis
   Cytomegalovirus
   Toxoplasmosis
   Chagas
   Rheumatic
   Lyme
2. Infiltrative
   Amyloid
   Sarcoid
   Hemochromatosis
   Carcinoid
   Hypereosinophilic
   Glycogen storage
   Cardiac tumors
3. Toxins
   Doxorubicin
   Chloroquine
   Radiation injury
4. Genetic
   Fabry
   Kearns-Sayre syndrome
   Right ventricular dysplasia

infrequently performed due to the higher morbidity associated with this approach. The right ventricular bioptome is positioned under fluoroscopy or echocardiography to sample the interventricular septum. As the myocarditis can be focal, a minimum of four to six fragments are obtained. Using the Stanford bioptome, typical samples are 2 to 3 mm in maximal diameter and 5 mg in wet weight. Samples are processed, paraffin-imbedded, sectioned, and stained with hematoxylin-eosin and trichrome. Special stains are employed if other diagnoses are considered. Diagnoses that can be made or confirmed by endomyocardial biopsy are listed in Table 79-2.

Several investigators have performed endomyocardial biopsies in patients with unexplained congestive heart failure and/or ventricular arrhythmia.[4,39,52,61] The percentage of patients with biopsies interpreted as myocarditis varied widely, primarily owing to the different diagnostic criteria for active myocarditis used by the investigators. This variability of endomyocardial biopsy criteria prompted a meeting of cardiac pathologists to reach a consensus on the pathologic definition of myocarditis, now known as the *Dallas criteria*.[62] These criteria separate initial biopsies into myocarditis, borderline myocarditis, or no myocarditis. Active myocarditis was defined as "an inflammatory infiltrate of the myocardium with necrosis and/or degeneration of adjacent myocytes not typical of the ischemic damage associated with coronary artery disease" (Fig. 79-5). Examination of a minimum of four to six fragments from each patient is required for interpretation. The term *borderline* myocarditis is applied when the inflammatory infiltrate is too sparse or myocyte injury is not demonstrated. Repeat biopsy is then suggested. A high frequency of active myocarditis is confirmed by repeat biopsy in patients whose initial histologic samples demonstrated borderline myocarditis.[63] When right ventricular endomyocardial biopsy has failed to establish the diagnosis, sampling the left ventricle may improve diagnostic yield.

Although the Dallas criteria standardize the description of biopsy samples, histopathology alone may be inadequate to identify the presence of active myocarditis. Alternative classification schemes

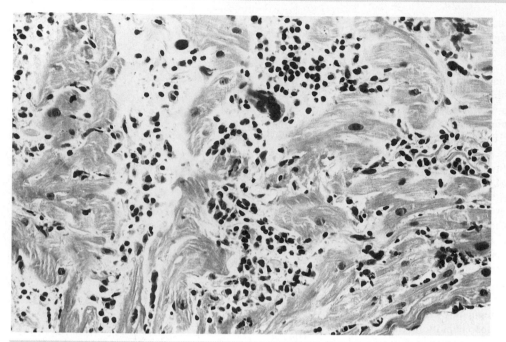

FIGURE 79-5 Photomicrograph showing extensive interstitial infiltrates of lymphocytes and myocytes with focal myocyte necrosis. (H&E, ×40.)

have been proposed, including one that combines histopathologic and clinical criteria.[64] Myocarditis is divided into four subgroups—fulminant, acute, chronic active, and chronic persistent. These categories provide prognostic information and suggest which patients may or may not benefit from immunosuppressive therapy (Table 79-3). Additionally, use of immunohistologic markers of inflammation, such as upregulation of histocompatibility leukocyte antigens (HLAs) on myocytes or detection of autoantibodies, may aid diagnosis as these changes are generalized and not focal.

Endomyocardial biopsy must be applied as quickly as possible to maximize the diagnostic yield. Resolution of active myocarditis has been documented within 4 days of initial biopsy, with progressive clearing over several weeks on serial biopsy.[65] Progression of active myocarditis to dilated cardiomyopathy has been documented when serial biopsies are performed.[66]

Noninvasive Studies Although technetium 99m–pyrophosphate scintigraphy has proved useful in the detection of myocarditis in a murine model, it has not been effective in diagnosing myocarditis in humans. Imaging with gallium 67, an inflammation-avid radioisotope, has shown promise as a screening method for active myocarditis, with a specificity and sensitivity of 83 percent and a negative predictive value of 98 percent in biopsy-proven myocarditis.[67] Indium 111–labeled antimyosin antibody scans can be used to detect myocyte necrosis. Application of this technique in patients with myocarditis has demonstrated a sensitivity of 83 percent, a specificity of 53 percent, and a negative predictive value of a normal scan of 92 percent.[68] In those patients who were antimyosin antibody–positive and biopsy-negative, the possibility of inflammation undetected by biopsy has been considered. Antimyosin imaging, however, detects myocyte injury independent of etiology, and noninflammatory causes of heart muscle injury in young patients may cause false-positive scans. The usefulness of scintigraphy in diagnosing myocarditis is limited by low specificity, radiation exposure, and expense.

Tissue alterations associated with myocarditis may be identifiable using magnetic resonance imaging (MRI).[69] Preliminary results suggest that myocardial inflammation may induce abnormal signal intensity of the myocardial walls. Use of T_2-weighted images to

TABLE 79-3 Clinicopathologic Classification of Myocarditis

	Fulminant	Acute	Chronic Active	Chronic Persistent
Symptom onset	Distinct	Indistinct	Indistinct	Indistinct
Clinical presentation	Cardiogenic shock, severe LV dysfunction	CHF, LV dysfunction	CHF, LV dysfunction	Non-CHF symptoms, normal LV function
Initial biopsy	Multifoci of active myocarditis	Active or borderline myocarditis	Active or borderline myocarditis	Active or borderline myocarditis
Clinical natural history	Complete recovery or death	Incomplete recovery or dilated CM	Dilated CM	Non-CHF symptoms, normal LV function
Histologic natural history	Complete resolution of myocarditis	Complete resolution of myocarditis	Ongoing or resolving myocarditis, fibrosis	Ongoing or resolving myocarditis
Immunosuppressive therapy	No benefit	Sometimes beneficial	No benefit	No benefit

KEY: CHF, congestive heart failure; LV, left ventricular; CM, cardiomyopathy.
SOURCE: Modified Lieberman et al.,[64] with permission.

visualize tissue edema has been described in several case reports of patients with active myocarditis. More recently, contrast medium–enhanced MRI has been used to characterize myocardial changes in myocarditis.[70] The MRI imaging contrast agent gadopentetate dimeglumine accumulates in inflammatory lesions. It is a hydrophilic agent that accumulates in the extracellular space of water-containing tissues. Gadolinium increases the signal of T_1-weighted images. A total of 19 patients with clinically suspected myocarditis and 18 normal subjects underwent contrast-enhanced MRI. Global relative enhancement was higher in patients than controls. Contrast MRI and echocardiographic digital image processing can visualize the area of inflammation and the extent of inflammation and may prove to be valuable techniques in both the diagnosis and monitoring of disease activity.[71]

Despite the promise of noninvasive techniques, endomyocardial biopsy remains the diagnostic standard.

Treatment The cornerstone of therapy for patients with acute myocarditis is supportive care. Diuretics, angiotensin-converting enzyme inhibitors, beta blockers, and aldosterone antagonists should be given in the proper clinical context. Because digoxin has been shown to increase the expression of inflammatory cytokines in an animal model, it should be used cautiously and at a low dose.[72]

When acute myocarditis presents with profound hemodynamic collapse, mechanical circulatory support devices may be used to bridge patients either to cardiac transplantation or to recovery.[41,42] Although improvement in cardiac function has been reported to parallel the clearance of the inflammatory infiltrate, the duration of necessary device support has ranged from 7 to 70 days.[73,74] Serial endomyocardial biopsy, echocardiography, right heart catheterization, and exercise testing with simultaneous hemodynamic and echocardiographic measurements are all employed to determine native cardiac reserve and the suitability for device explantation.

Acceptance of the hypothesis of immune-mediated injury has led many to question whether anti-inflammatory therapy could provide additional clinical benefit to patients with inflammatory dilated cardiomyopathy treated with conventional heart failure regimens. Parillo studied 102 patients with dilated cardiomyopathy and classified them as being "reactive," with endomyocardial or laboratory evidence of ongoing inflammation, or "nonreactive."[75] The study's primary endpoint was an increase in left ventricular ejection fraction equal to or greater than 5 percent. At 3 months follow-up, 67 percent of reactive patients receiving prednisone reached this endpoint, as compared to only 28 percent in the reactive control group. After 9 months of follow-up, the prednisone-induced improvement in left ventricular ejection fraction was no longer present. Nonreactive patients did not improve with prednisone. In spite of these negative results, the authors concluded that prednisone therapy could provide modest improvements in clinical endpoints, but only in certain reactive subpopulations.

Anecdotal success with immunosuppression in active viral myocarditis led to the large multicenter Myocarditis Treatment Trial.[76] In this study, 111 patients with biopsy-proven myocarditis and left ventricular ejection fraction less than 45 percent were randomized to receive conventional therapy alone versus immunosuppressive therapy with prednisone in combination with either azathioprine or cyclosporine. The primary endpoint of the study was change in ejection fraction over 28 weeks. For all patients, the average increase in ejection fraction over baseline was 9 percent.

Treatment assignment was not predictive of improvement in left ventricular ejection fraction, attenuation of clinical disease, or mortality (Fig. 79-6).

A more recent study examined the selected use of immunosuppressive therapy in patients with dilated cardiomyopathy and immunohistochemical evidence of inflammation.[77] Eighty-four patients with dilated cardiomyopathy for at least 6 months who had increased HLA expression on endomyocardial biopsy specimens were randomized to receive standard heart failure therapy alone or in combination with prednisone and azathioprine. After 2 years follow-up, there was no difference in the composite primary endpoint of death, transplantation, or hospital readmission. Those patients treated with immunosuppressive therapy, however, experienced a significant increase in ejection fraction at 3 and 24 months.

High-dose intravenous immune globulin (IVIG) has both immune modulatory and antiviral effects. Administration of IVIG to children with new-onset cardiomyopathy and to women with peripartum cardiomyopathy was associated with significant improvements in ventricular function.[78,79] Subsequently, a small open-label study was performed in 10 adult patients with new-onset heart failure.[80] Significant improvement in left ventricular function was observed in 9 of 10 patients. Unfortunately, when IVIG was tested in a prospective placebo-controlled trial in 62 patients with recent-onset dilated cardiomyopathy and left ventricular ejection fraction less than 40 percent, the results were disappointing.[81] Although ejection fraction improved by 16 percent at 1 year in the IVIG-treated group, this increase was essentially equaled by those taking placebo. Thus no benefit of immunomodulation could be demonstrated.

Taken as a whole, these trials do not support the routine use of immunosuppressive therapy in myocarditis. However, present data suggest that subgroups with ongoing myocarditis may be more likely to benefit from immunosuppression, although no uniform methodology yet exists to identify them.[82]

Last, use of antiviral therapy is currently being assessed in the European Study of Epidemiology and Treatment of Cardiac Inflammatory Disease.[83] Patients with positive enteroviral titers are being

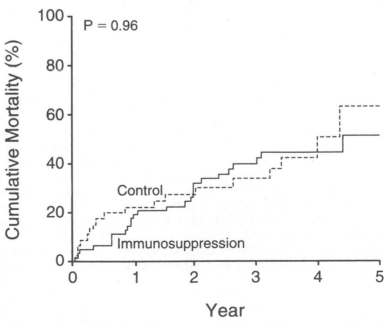

FIGURE 79-6 Actuarial mortality curves from the Myocarditis Treatment Trial illustrating no difference in survival between the treatment groups. (From Mason et al.,[76] with permission.)

randomized to treatment with interferon alpha versus placebo, while those with cytomegalovirus (CMV) myocarditis will receive either intravenous immunoglobulin or placebo. The primary endpoint of this trial is an increase in ejection fraction equal to or greater than 5 percent.

Prognosis   About one-third of those who present with clinical carditis and recover will be left with some cardiac abnormality, ranging from mild changes on ECG to significant heart failure. Approximately 40 percent of all patients will completely recover.[39] Currently there are no clinical criteria that reliably predict who will recover, although the vast majority of patients with mild reductions in left ventricular ejection fraction and NYHA class I or II heart failure recover completely. Paradoxically, patients with fulminant myocarditis have an excellent long-term prognosis despite their experience of circulatory collapse. In one study, long-term transplant-free survival was 93 percent, as compared to only 45 percent for those with acute myocarditis.[40]

The prognosis of myocarditis depends to some extent on the causative agent, but if clinical heart failure develops, 5-year mortality rates are in the range of 50 to 60 percent, comparable to the figures seen in idiopathic cardiomyopathy.[84] Chronic inflammation, viral persistence, or both may affect disease progression and prognosis. Future therapies will need to identify the predominant factor to target treatment and hopefully improve survival.

Human Immunodeficiency Virus   Human immunodeficiency virus (HIV) is increasingly recognized as a cause of dilated cardiomyopathy. In some inner-city hospitals, it may represent a very common diagnosis. The relatively recent emergence of this virus in the early 1980s has provided a unique opportunity to prospectively monitor the development of heart failure to chronic viral infection. The etiology of this cardiomyopathy may be from infection of myocardial cells with HIV or coinfection with other cardiotropic viruses, postviral autoimmune response, or cardiotoxicity from illicit drugs or drug therapy. Barbaro et al.[85] studied the development of dilated cardiomyopathy in 952 asymptomatic HIV-positive patients. Patients with a history of illicit drug use, prior cardiac disease, previous treatment with antiretroviral or immunomodulating drugs, or an ejection fraction less than 50 percent were excluded from prospective study. In the 60 months of follow up, 8 percent of the patients developed cardiomyopathy, with annualized incidence rate of 16 cases per 1000 patients. A predisposing factor to the development of cardiomyopathy was a CD4± cell count below 400/mL. In 83 percent of the patients, a histologic diagnosis of myocarditis was made. In 92 percent of these positive biopsies, HIV nucleic acid sequences were detected by in situ hybridization. Coexistent infection with coxsackievirus group B, CMV, and Epstein-Barr virus was detected in a small segment of this cohort. Other studies suggest disease duration and illicit drug use as factors contributing to the development of this disease.[86]

As the symptoms of heart failure and HIV can be very similar (i.e., fatigue, wasting, etc.), careful cardiologic follow-up of these patients is probably indicated to detect early development of left ventricular dysfunction. Conventional heart failure management can then be instituted to alleviate cardiac-related symptoms (see also Chap. 88).

Cytomegalovirus   CMV may lead to myocarditis in the general population, but ordinarily the myocarditis is self-limited and asymptomatic. In the cardiac transplant recipient, however, CMV myocarditis may become a more serious disease, resulting in cardiac dysfunction.[87] The treatment of CMV myocarditis is intravenous ganciclovir, which effectively eradicates the virus. Early CMV infection correlates with the development of allograft coronary artery disease, the major cause of death beyond the first year after cardiac transplantation. It is proposed that infection of either subintimal fibroblasts or endothelial cells results in immunologic injury that predisposes to this potentially fatal condition.

NONVIRAL

Chagas' Disease   American trypanosomiasis, or Chagas' disease, is the most common cause of congestive heart failure in the world. This condition results from the bite of the reduviid bug, leading to infection with *Trypanosoma cruzi,* and is endemic to rural South and Central America.

Pathogenesis   The pathogenesis of chronic chagasic cardiomyopathy is controversial because the parasite is rarely present in the myocardium. As in the viral cardiomyopathy model, the cardiac injury is thus thought to be immunologically mediated.[88] Both cellular and humoral immune responses have been implicated in the myocardial injury. Myocardial biopsies demonstrate that the inflammatory infiltrate in chronic Chagas' disease consists mainly of CD8+ T cells, with a low number of CD4+ T cells.[89] This suggests some degree of immunologic depression in the host, since the activation of T-helper cells is known to be the most effective mechanism of defense against the parasites.[90] Some have postulated that the diminished expression of CD4+ T cells during acute *T. cruzi* infection may be related to a mechanism of tolerance induced by the parasite. Evidence for this comes from studies showing that the addition of IL-1 in vitro restores helper T-cell function, thus implicating a macrophage defect in this process.[91] Furthermore, IL-2 and the IL-2 receptor are absent or scarce in the inflammatory infiltrate,[92] attesting to the attenuated role of the T-helper subset in this disease.

Clinical Presentation   This parasitic disease has an acute phase, where hematogenous spread of the parasite leads to invasion of various tissues and organ systems. The invasion is accompanied by an intense inflammatory reaction with mononuclear cells and is characterized by fever, sweating, myalgias, myocarditis, hepatosplenomegaly, and a case fatality rate of about 5 percent. Most patients recover from the acute illness and enter an asymptomatic latent phase, but 20 to 30 percent will develop a chronic form of the disease up to 20 years after the initial infection.

The chronic stage is a result of gradual tissue destruction. The gastrointestinal tract and heart are the most common sites of involvement, with the primary cause of death being cardiac failure. In the gut, the destruction of the myenteric plexus is responsible for the development of megaesophagus and megacolon. In the heart, the myofibrils and the Purkinje fibers are replaced by fibrous tissue, leading to cardiomegaly, congestive heart failure, heart block, and arrhythmia. The microscopic findings are those of extensive fibrosis, but a chronic cellular infiltrate composed of lymphocytes, plasma cells, and macrophages is often present and parasites are found in about one-quarter of the patients.

Diagnosis of the acute disease depends on the discovery of trypomastigotes in the blood of the infected individual. In chronic infection, direct diagnosis is less useful because there are fewer circulating trypomastigotes. Xenodiagnosis (where the patient is bitten by reduviid bugs bred in the laboratory and the parasite is subsequently identified in the intestine of the insect) is the most useful test, which will detect infection in about half the patients. The complement-fixation test (Machado-Guerreiro test) also has high sensitivity and specificity for identification of chronic Chagas' disease. In the other lab tests, it is necessary to rely on positive serologic tests (such as the indirect immunofluorescent antibody, enzyme-linked immunosorbent assay, and hemagglutination tests) together with symptoms and signs compatible with Chagas' disease.

Endomyocardial biopsy may show active myocarditis using the Dallas criteria.[93] Noninvasive assessment commonly shows segmental wall motion abnormalities, specifically apical aneurysms. ECG findings include complete heart block, atrioventricular block, or right bundle branch block with or without fascicular block in 11 percent of infected individuals.[94] Ventricular arrhythmias may require antiarrhythmic drugs.

The treatment of chronic Chagas' disease is symptomatic and includes a pacemaker for complete heart block, an implantable cardioverter-defibrillator for recurrent ventricular arrhythmia, and standard therapy for congestive heart failure as outlined for other forms of myocarditis. Antiparasitic agents such as Nifurtimox and benzimidazole eradicate parasitemia during the acute phase and are typically curative. They should be administered if the disease has not previously been treated and may be used as prophylaxis if there is a high likelihood of recurrence, such as following immunosuppressive therapy. The role of immunosuppression therapy for chagasic myocarditis is controversial, and heart transplantation is effective for end-stage refractory cardiac disease.

Lyme Carditis Lyme disease results from infection with the spirochete *Borrelia burgdorferi*, introduced by a tick bite. The initial presenting symptom in patients with the disease who progress to cardiac involvement is frequently complete heart block. Left ventricular dysfunction may be seen but is unusual.[95] Endomyocardial biopsy may show active myocarditis. Rarely are spirochetes seen on biopsy. Corticosteroid administration is helpful in treating Lyme carditis following therapy with tetracycline.

Other Infectious Causes of Cardiomyopathy Among other infectious etiologies is *Toxoplasma gondii*, which is curable by pyrimethamine and sulfadiazine and occurs most commonly in the immune-deficient host.[96] Leptospirosis is yet another common cause in fatal cases of myocarditis. Fifty percent of cases have ST- and T-wave changes on the ECG.

Rheumatic Carditis One form of myocarditis that has declined dramatically in the latter half of the twentieth century is rheumatic carditis.[97] The availability of antibiotics and changes in the virulence and serotypes of group A streptococcus may explain the decreasing frequency of this disease.[98]

Acute rheumatic fever can occur in children and young adults. It generally follows a group A streptococcal pharyngitis, but only indirect evidence linking the two has been found. Rheumatic carditis may result from a direct toxic effect of some streptococcal product versus an immunologic mechanism.[99] Group A streptococci have a number of structural components similar to those of human tissue. Antibodies to streptococci cross-react with the glycoproteins of heart valves. The serum of patients with rheumatic fever contains autoantibodies to myosin and sarcolemma. The Aschoff body, pathognomic for this disorder, represents persistent focal inflammatory lesions in the myocardium. These nodules can persist for years after an acute attack. Macrophages containing myosin have been identified in these nodules.

Clinical diagnosis is made using the Jones criteria.[100] The major manifestations are carditis, polyarthritis, chorea, erythema marginatum, subcutaneous nodules, and evidence of preceding streptococcal infection (i.e., positive throat culture, history of scarlet fever, elevated antistreptolysin titers). Minor criteria are nonspecific findings such as fever, arthralgia, previous rheumatic fever or rheumatic heart disease, elevated ESR or C-reactive protein, and prolonged PR inter-

val. Diagnosis is made by the presence of two major criteria or one major and two minor criteria. Debate as to whether the Jones criteria should be modified to incorporate Doppler-echo indices is ongoing.[101]

Two-thirds of patients present with an antecedent pharyngitis, followed by the symptoms of rheumatic fever in 1 to 5 weeks, with a mean presentation of 18.6 days. Severe carditis resulting in death can occur, but is unusual. Congestive heart failure (CHF) is observed in only 5 to 10 percent of cases. Usually the carditis is mild, the predominant effect being scarring of the heart valves. Physical examination is notable for fever and heart murmurs, reflecting the acute valvulitis. The mitral valve is involved three times as frequently as the aortic valve; therefore mitral murmurs are more common. Mitral regurgitation is the most common finding. A middiastolic murmur over the apical area can frequently be heard. This is called the Carey Coombs murmur, and its presence almost certainly confirms mitral valvulitis. Aortic insufficiency can be auscultated with aortic valvulitis.

There are no characteristic ECG findings, though PR prolongation and nonspecific ST-T-wave changes are frequently described. Endomyocardial biopsy demonstrates the Aschoff nodules as well as a diffuse cellular interstitial infiltrate including lymphocytes, polymorphonuclear cells, histiocytes, and eosinophils. Laboratory tests suggestive of rheumatic fever include antibodies to antistreptolysin O and anti-DNAase B, an elevated ESR rate, and elevated C-reactive protein. Extracardiac manifestations generally present with an acute migratory polyarthritis of the large joints.

Aspirin and penicillin are the mainstays of therapy. Corticosteroids can also provide symptomatic relief. Treatment with intravenous immunoglobulin produces no detectable clinical or echocardiographic improvements.[102] Mitral valve repair during acute carditis is associated with an increased mortality risk and should be undertaken only when heart failure is refractory to optimal anti-inflammatory therapy.[103]

Once rheumatic fever is diagnosed, antibiotic prophylaxis is required to prevent recurrent episodes. The most effective method is a single monthly intramuscular injection of 1.2 million units of benzathine penicillin G until age 21.

Noninfective

HYPERSENSITIVITY

Hypersensitivity myocarditis is an example of the early phase of eosinophilic myocarditis and is thought to be due to an allergic reaction to a variety of drugs (Table 79-4). Methyldopa, the penicillins,

TABLE 79-4 Drugs Causing Eosinophilic Myocarditis

Acetazolamide	Oxyphenylbutazone
Amitriptyline	Para-aminosalicylic acid
Amphotericin B	Penicillin
Ampicillin	Phenindione
Carbamazepine	Phenobarbital
Cefaclor	Phenylbutazone
Chloramphenicol	Phenytoin
Chlorthalidone	Spironolactone
Desipramine	Streptomycin
Hydrochlorothiazide	Sulfadiazine
Indomethacin	Sulfisoxazole
Interleukin-4	Sulfonylureas
Isoniazid	Tetanus toxoid
Methyldopa	Tetracycline

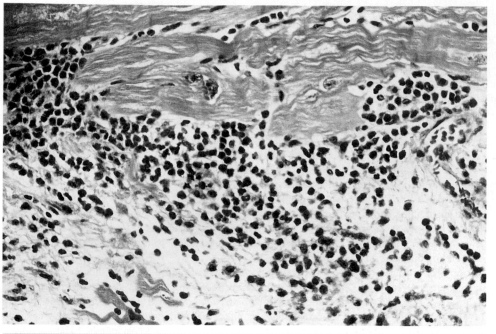

FIGURE 79-7 Photomicrograph showing interstitial infiltrates rich in eosinophils. (H&E, ×40.)

sulfonamides, tetracycline, and the antituberculous drugs are the pharmaceuticals most commonly associated with this entity. It is characterized by peripheral eosinophilia and infiltration into the myocardium by eosinophils, multinucleated giant cells, and leukocytes (Fig. 79-7).[104] The major basic protein of the eosinophil granule may be detected in the presence of acute necrotizing myocarditis, suggesting toxicity of the granule contents.[105] Good success has been reported with stopping the offending agent and treatment with corticosteroids.[106] Unfortunately, the presence of this condition often goes unnoticed and the first manifestation of cardiac involvement is sudden death due to arrhythmia.

GIANT-CELL MYOCARDITIS

Giant-cell myocarditis is an extremely rare but aggressive form of myocarditis, typically progressive and unresponsive to medical therapy.[107] This disease is most prevalent in young adults, with a mean age at onset of 42 years (and a range of 16 to 69 years). Association with other autoimmune disorders is reported in approximately 20 percent of cases. Diagnosis is made by endomyocardial biopsy. Widespread or multifocal necrosis with a mixed inflammatory infiltrate including lymphocytes and histiocytes is required for histologic diagnosis. Eosinophils are frequently noted, as are multinucleated giant cells in the absence of granuloma (Fig. 79-8). Immunophenotyping of the cellular infiltrate has shown lymphocyte populations composed of T-helper or in some cases T-suppressor cells.

The clinical course is usually characterized by progressive CHF and is frequently associated with refractory ventricular arrhythmia. This condition is almost uniformly and rapidly fatal. Comparison of survival of patients with giant-cell myocarditis with that of patients with lymphocytic myocarditis demonstrates significantly worse survival in those patients with giant-cell disease (Fig. 79-9). Case reports and the Giant Cell Myocarditis Registry suggest that treatment with certain immunosuppressive regimens, but not steroids alone, can extend transplant-free survival by a few months.[108] Some patients may require mechanical circulatory support as a bridge to transplant.[109] Rare cases of complete recovery have been described; for example, one patient treated with OKT3 and high-dose steroids had complete resolution of giant cell myocarditis and was able to be successfully weaned off a biventricular support device.[110] However, cardiac transplantation represents the best treatment option despite the possibility of recurrence in the transplanted heart.[107] Giant cells can be detected on routine surveillance biopsies up to 9 years posttransplant. This cellular infiltrate may respond to an increase in immunosuppressive therapy.

PERIPARTUM CARDIOMYOPATHY

Peripartum cardiomyopathy is an uncommon form of CHF first described by Virchow in 1870.[111] Estimates of its incidence vary from 1 to 1300 to 1

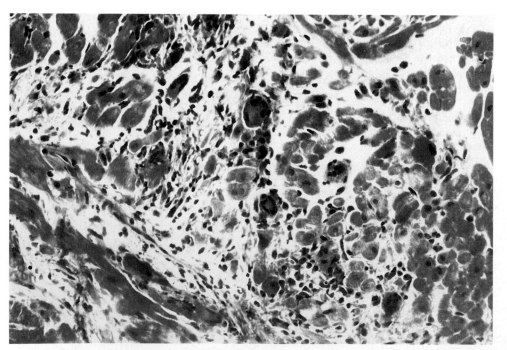

FIGURE 79-8 Photomicrograph showing extensive myocyte damage and infiltrates of mononuclear cells and numerous multinucleated giant cells. (H&E, ×60.)

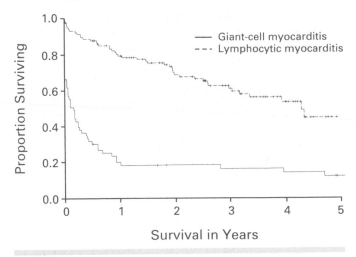

FIGURE 79-9 Kaplan-Meier survival curves for patients with giant-cell myocarditis versus lymphocytic myocarditis. (From Cooper et al.,[107] with permission.)

in 15,000 pregnancies. The disease occurs more commonly in obese multiparous black females over age 30. Twin pregnancies, preeclampsia, and long-term use of tocolytic agents are other predisposing factors.[112] Patients present with heart failure in the last trimester of pregnancy or in the first 5 months postpartum. Absence of a demonstrable cause of heart failure and structural heart disease is required to make the diagnosis. Indeed, the hemodynamic stress of pregnancy can frequently unmask previously unknown cardiac disease.

Pathogenesis

The etiology of this disorder is unclear. Proposed mechanisms include nutritional deficiencies, genetic disorders, viral or autoimmune etiologies, hormonal problems, volume overload, alcohol, physiologic stress of pregnancy, or unmasking of latent idiopathic dilated cardiomyopathy. Several lines of evidence suggest that peripartum cardiomyopathy may be the result of myocarditis due to a viral illness or an autoimmune etiology.[113–115] Given the relatively immunosuppressed state of pregnancy, susceptibility to cardiotropic viruses is higher.[116] Additionally, several studies have demonstrated histologic evidence of myocarditis on endomyocardial biopsy samples obtained from patients with peripartum cardiomyopathy.[52,113,114] Other investigators have postulated an autoimmune etiology to peripartum cardiomyopathy, specifically immunologic responses to fetal and endometrial antigens that cross-react with the patient's myocytes. In one case report, a patient with peripartum cardiomyopathy had antibodies to smooth muscle and actin produced in response to actin and myosin released during uterine degeneration after delivery. These antibodies later cross-reacted with the myocardium and induced cardiomyopathy.[117]

Clinical Presentation

The presentation is that of heart failure. Symptoms include shortness of breath, dyspnea on exertion, edema, palpitations, syncope, sudden death, and thromboembolic phenomena. The incidence of thromboembolism is high due to the hypercoagulability of pregnancy.[112] Physical findings are notable for S_3, S_4, tricuspid or mitral insufficiency murmurs, edema, rales, ascites, hepatomegaly, jugular venous

distension. The ECG frequently shows left ventricular hypertrophy. Echocardiographic findings can range from single-chamber left ventricular enlargement to four-chamber dilatation. Endomyocardial biopsy may reveal myocarditis in as many as 50 percent of these women, but generally the findings are nonspecific.[52] Biopsies in patients with peripartum cardiomyopathy have the highest yield when performed early after onset of symptoms.[118]

Prognosis and Treatment

Too few patients with peripartum cardiomyopathy have been studied to fully analyze the natural history of the disease. In a small series of 27 patients, left ventricular size was analyzed at 6 months; 14 patients (50 percent) had normal dimensions. None of these patients died of CHF—compared with 85 percent of those patients with persistent cardiomegaly, who died from CHF within 5 years.[119] The authors concluded, therefore, that if the congestive cardiomyopathy persists for more than 6 months, it is likely to be irreversible and associated with a worse prognosis. Similar findings were published in another series by O'Connell et al.[118] These authors noted that those patients with higher ejection fractions and smaller ventricular diastolic dimensions at the time of diagnosis have a better long-term prognosis. Recovery of left ventricular function correlates with resolution of myocarditis with or without immunosuppressive therapy.[113] The use of corticosteroids in the treatment of this disorder is controversial and should be reserved for patients with endomyocardial evidence of myocarditis and persistent ventricular dysfunction.[52,113,115] The incidence of thromboembolism is high due to the hypercoagulability of pregnancy; therefore anticoagulation is recommended.[112]

Patients with refractory heart failure referred for transplant have a posttransplant survival comparable with that of patients with idiopathic dilated cardiomyopathy, though higher early rejection rates are noted.

Questions still remain regarding the safety of subsequent pregnancy for patients with stable heart failure or recovery of left ventricular function. There are several case reports of women with this diagnosis who went on to subsequent pregnancies. The outcomes of these patients are variable, with a few having uneventful pregnancies and others developing an exacerbation or recurrence of fulminant heart failure. Dobutamine echocardiography has detected impaired contractile reserve in some women with peripartum cardiomyopathy who apparently had recovered normal ventricular function.[120] Subsequent pregnancy should be viewed as posing a high risk, and all patients with this disorder should be counseled about birth control and contraceptive methods.

NEUROMUSCULAR DISEASES

Several heritable neuromuscular dystrophies may be associated with cardiomyopathy. Included in this category are diseases such as Becker's, Duchenne's, and X-linked cardioskeletal myopathy, myotonic dystrophy (Steinert's disease), congenital myotonic dystrophy, limb-girdle muscular dystrophy (Erb's disease), familial centronuclear myopathy, Kugelberg-Welander syndrome, Friedreich's ataxia, and Barth's syndrome. The myocardial involvement, natural history, and prognosis of each of these disorders are variable.

Duchenne's dystrophy is an X-linked disease with proximal muscle weakness and cardiomyopathy. A dystrophin gene mutation is responsible. Death usually results from respiratory and/or cardiorespiratory failure. Patients with myotonic dystrophy present between age 20 and 50 years, usually with arrhythmias.

Several mitochondrial myopathies have also been described.[121] Mitochondria are essential cellular organelles that convert oxygen to biochemically useful energy. Additionally, mitochondria function as calcium storage sites and modulators of cellular pH. As such, mitochondrial function affects muscle and ventricular function. Mitochondria are unique organelles with their own maternally inherited DNA, which encodes several respiratory chain proteins. Genetic defects in the mitochondrial respiratory chain enzymes—specifically complexes I, III, and IV—have been recognized as the cause in some cardiomyopathies. The presentation in mitochondrial myopathies is extremely heterogeneous, as each cell will contain a mixture of normal and mutant DNAs. Deletion mutations in DNA can occur and are frequently observed in these myopathies.

Mitochondrial myopathies include such disorders as Kearns-Sayre syndrome, chronic ophthalmoplegia, myoclonic epilepsy, ragged-red-fiber disease, and mitochondrial encephalomyopathy. The MELAS syndrome—(mitochondrial encephalopathy, lactic acidosis, and stroke-like episodes) is associated with cardiomyopathy and generalized microangiopathy. Kearns-Sayre syndrome results from a deletion mutation in mitochondrial DNA. This ocular myopathic disease is associated with dilated or hypertrophic cardiomyopathy with cardiac conduction defects.

Defects in transport of molecules from the cytoplasm into the mitochondria have also been associated with cardiac and skeletal myopathy. One example is that of carnitine deficiency, discussed further on in this chapter.

INFILTRATIVE CARDIOMYOPATHIES

The infiltrative cardiomyopathies comprise several acquired and heritable conditions; these include amyloidosis, hemochromatosis, carcinoid, sarcoidosis, glycogen storage disease, endocardial fibroelastosis, and endomyocardial fibrosis due to hypereosinophilic syndromes or other collagen vascular disorders such as scleroderma or Churg-Strauss syndrome.

Amyloid

CLASSIFICATION AND PATHOGENESIS

The most commonly encountered of the infiltrative cardiomyopathies is amyloidosis, leading to an overproduction of a monoclonal immunoglobulin protein that is deposited throughout the body. Secondary amyloidosis results from the deposition of a protein other than immunoglobulin. Whereas no systemic diseases are associated with primary amyloid, other chronic diseases are present in the secondary form. Secondary amyloidosis may result from familial, senile, or chronic inflammatory processes (rheumatoid arthritis, juvenile rheumatoid arthritis, ankylosing spondylitis, Crohn's disease, tuberculous paraplegia associated with decubitus ulcers, cystic fibrosis, and heroin use with chronically infected cutaneous injection sites). Familial Mediterranean fever is an autosomal recessive inherited disease of Sephardic Jews, Armenians, and other Mediterranean peoples associated with amyloid deposition. In the familial diseases, more than 40 different genetic mutations of the plasma protein transthyretin (prealbumin) have been associated with amyloid deposition. Inheritance is autosomal dominant, with the genetic defect being confined to a single amino acid substitution in the mature protein (see also Chap. 78).[122,123]

The frequency of cardiac involvement varies with the different etiologies. Of patients with primary amyloid, one-third to one-half have cardiac involvement and more than one-fourth have sympto-

matic heart failure. Cardiac involvement in patients with secondary amyloidosis is much less frequent. Indeed, in amyloid due to chronic inflammatory processes, amyloid protein deposition is usually limited to the intima and media of arterioles and not the heart. Familial amyloidosis is the rarest form of systemic amyloidosis, affecting only about 4 percent of cases; however, cardiomyopathy is present in 68 percent of those affected. Familial amyloidosis can manifest initially with progressive neuropathy, cardiomyopathy, or renal involvement. In some of the families, cardiac amyloidosis is not even symptomatic, while in others cardiac symptoms predominate. Senile cardiac amyloidosis is common in the elderly but often does not lead to a clinical cardiac syndrome and is detected only postmortem.[124]

CLINICAL PRESENTATION

Amyloid fibrils are rigid and as such lead primarily to relaxation abnormalities and diastolic dysfunction; however, when myocardial replacement occurs, systolic dysfunction becomes a prominent feature.[125] The cardiomyopathy may be restrictive or congestive in nature. Systolic left ventricular function deteriorates late in the disease process, only after marked amyloid deposition. The clinical presentation is that of congestive heart failure, with a more frequent occurrence of right-sided symptoms. Sudden death and myocardial infarction may result from vascular involvement. Atrial arrhythmias, especially atrial fibrillation, are common and associated with a high risk for thromboembolism.

DIAGNOSIS

Diagnosis is made by characteristic echocardiographic features and endomyocardial biopsy.[126] Echocardiography can demonstrate symmetrical thickening of the left ventricular wall with a diffuse hyperrefractile, granular, sparkling appearance of the myocardium (Fig. 79-10A). Abnormal left ventricular diastolic filling, manifest by reduction in the rate and volume of rapid diastolic filling with enhanced atrial contraction, can be seen very early in the disease process.[127] The ECG typically demonstrates low voltage despite marked hypertrophy on echo (Fig. 79-10B). A pseudoinfarct or postinfarct anterior wall pattern is often present.[128] Cardiac involvement is generally seen when mean left ventricular wall thickness on the echocardiogram is greater than 11 mm in the absence of a history of hypertension or valvular heart disease, with unexplained low voltage (<0.5 mV) on the ECG. The majority of patients presenting with cardiac involvement have a monoclonal protein spike in the serum or urine, reflecting the primary nature of the disease.

Amyloid is detected easily in endomyocardial biopsy specimens using Congo red staining and is observed in the interstitium in a pericellular or nodular pattern, in the endocardium, or in myocardial blood vessels. Sulfated alcian blue, methyl violet, and thioflavine T are other histochemical stains used to detect cardiac amyloid (Fig. 79-10C). Immunoperoxidase stains for kappa and lambda light chains and for prealbumin may categorize the type of cardiac amyloid. Electron microscopic examination of biopsy specimens is likely the most sensitive method of recognizing amyloidosis (Fig. 79-10D).

Radionuclide imaging using technetium-99m pyrophosphate and indium-111 antimyosin showing increased diffuse uptake, can also be used to diagnose cardiac amyloidosis.

TREATMENT

Symptoms of congestive heart failure often improve after diuresis, but increasing doses of diuretics are often required as cardiac and renal disease progress. Increased myocardial concentrations of digoxin may occur from binding of the drug to amyloid fibrils, thus increasing the propensity for digoxin toxicity. Digoxin should therefore be used with caution in these patients. Beta blockers and calcium channel antagonists are contraindicated.

Prognosis depends on the extent of myocardial involvement, but once heart failure is present, the prognosis is poor, with a 5-year survival below 5 percent. Indeed, patients with primary amyloidosis who fall into NYHA class III or have recurrent cardiac syncope rarely survive for more than 6 months. Echocardiography with Doppler assessment can provide prognostic information. A shortened deceleration time and an increased ratio of early diastolic filling velocity to the atrial filling velocity were more powerful predictors of mortality from cardiac causes than left ventricular wall thickness or fractional shortening.[129]

Chemotherapeutic regimens consisting of oral melphalan and prednisone have prolonged survival of amyloid patients in clinical trials.[130,131] However, patients with cardiac involvement usually do not survive long enough to receive enough cycles of melphalan to prolong their survival or cannot safely tolerate treatment. Treatment with high-dose melphalan followed by stem-cell transplant as treatment for primary amyloidosis is now being investigated.

Because of recurrence in the transplanted heart, results following heart transplantation have proved disappointing.[132] The immediate and early postoperative outcomes are similar to those in patients undergoing transplantation for other cardiac diseases; however, late survival is reduced (39 percent at 48 months) owing to recurrence of the disease in the transplanted organ and progressive disease in other organ systems. With the continuing donor shortage, the outcome associated with primary amyloidosis is unacceptable to the majority of cardiac transplant centers. Use of combined sequential cardiac and bone marrow transplant is now being actively investigated.

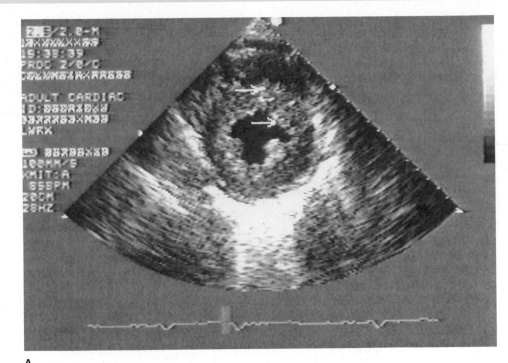

A

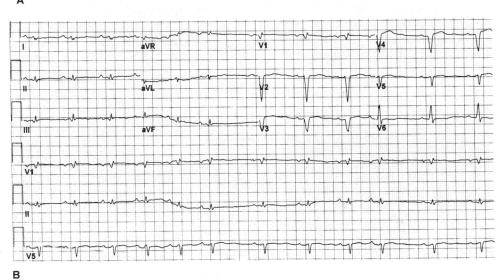

B

FIGURE 79-10 Cardiac amyloidosis. *A.* Two-dimensional echocardiographic parasternal short-axis view demonstrating symmetrical thickening of the left ventricular wall and granular sparkling appearance of the myocardium. *B.* 12-lead electrocardiogram demonstrating low voltage and a pseudoinfarct pattern. *C.* Photomicrograph showing diffuse interstitial accumulations of waxy homogeneous material. (H&E, ×60.) *D.* Electron microscopy of an amyloid deposit (*asterisk*) in a cardiac biopsy.

Sarcoidosis

PATHOGENESIS

Sarcoidosis is a systemic granulomatous disease of unknown etiology characterized by enhanced cellular immune responses. The pathologic hallmark of this disease is the noncaseating granuloma (Fig. 79-11). The initial lesion is an inflammatory infiltrate consisting of activated helper-inducer T lymphocytes and abundant macrophages that secrete cytokines. The macrophages aggregate and differentiate into epithelioid and multinucleated giant cells. Fibroblasts, mast cells, collagen fibers, and proteoglycans encase the inflammatory cells into a ball-like cluster. The fibrotic response results in end-organ damage.

Clusters of cases have been observed, suggesting spread by person-to-person exposure or environmental agents/pathogens. Genetic factors may also play a role in the development of the disease, as an exaggerated cellular immune response and the formation of granulomas may develop in genetically predisposed hosts after exposure to the offending antigen.

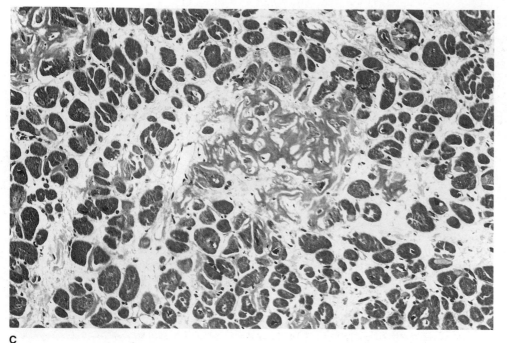

C

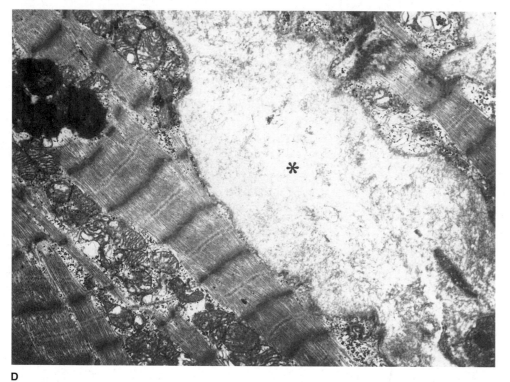

D

FIGURE 79-10 *(Continued)*

Cardiac sarcoid is more common than previously recognized. In an autopsy study of 38 patients with sarcoidosis, 76 percent had cardiac involvement, accounting for 50 percent of the deaths.[134] Cardiac sarcoid is more likely fatal and less likely to be diagnosed antemortem than pulmonary sarcoid. In another autopsy series, myocardial granulomas were present in 27 percent of patients with sarcoidosis.[135] However, there was no clinical evidence of sarcoidosis in over one-third of these patients during life. Frequently the initial presentation is that of sudden death. Myocardial involvement peaks between the third and sixth decades of life. Less than 10 percent of patients with sarcoid have symptoms referable to the cardiovascular system.

In myocardial sarcoid, portions of the myocardial wall are replaced by sarcoid granulomas, which preferentially involve the cephalad portion of the ventricular septum or the left ventricular papillary muscles.[136] Myocardial involvement is much more common than pericardial involvement.[137] Cor pulmonale due to extensive pulmonary sarcoidosis with interstitial fibrosis may occur.

Because of the varied extent and location of the myocardial granulomas, presenting signs and symptoms range from first-degree heart block to fulminant heart failure.[138] First-degree AV block, bundle-branch block, complete heart block, ventricular arrhythmias, sudden death, and heart failure occur with a frequency of 10 to 20 percent.[138] Heart failure can present as a cardiomyopathy with restrictive hemodynamics or systolic dysfunction. Some 25 percent of the deaths due to cardiac sarcoid are from heart failure, while sudden death accounts for one-third to one-half of the deaths.

DIAGNOSIS

In diagnosing cardiac sarcoid, evidence of other organ system involvement—including lymphadenopathy, hepatomegaly, splenomegaly, or pulmonary findings—should be sought. In cases where the heart is involved to a much greater degree than are other organs, little or no evidence of extracardiac sarcoidosis may be found. Chest x-ray, ECG, and echocardiography findings will depend on the extent and location of involvement. Due to the scattered nature of the granulomas, endomyocardial biopsy lacks sensitivity and seldom makes the diagnosis despite high specificity. Magnetic resonance imag-

CLINICAL PRESENTATION

The clinical manifestations of sarcoidosis are protean. The disease may be widespread or limited to a single organ. Virtually any organ except the adrenal gland may be involved. The lymphoid, pulmonary, cardiovascular, hepatobiliary, and hematologic systems are most commonly involved, with the lungs being affected in over 90 percent of patients.[133]

ing has been useful in diagnosing scars or lesions in the myocardium due to sarcoid.[139]

TREATMENT

Although no controlled trials have been performed, high-dose corticosteroids are usually given in the hope that the course of disease may be altered. Administration of corticosteroids can improve cardiac symptoms and reverse ECG changes in over half of the treated patients.[140] Antiarrhythmic drugs should be used as necessary, although drug therapy of ventricular tachycardia in patients with sarcoidosis, even when guided with programmed ventricular stimulation, is associated with a high rate of arrhythmia recurrence or sudden death.[141] Automatic internal cardioverter/defibrillators have been advocated. Prognosis after the diagnosis of cardiac sarcoid is variable but can be poor. In one series of 247 patients, survival was 41 percent at 5 years and 15 percent at 10 years.[142,143] Transplantation is also a successful treatment, as the recurrence of sarcoid in the allograft is low, possibly due to posttransplant steroid therapy.[144]

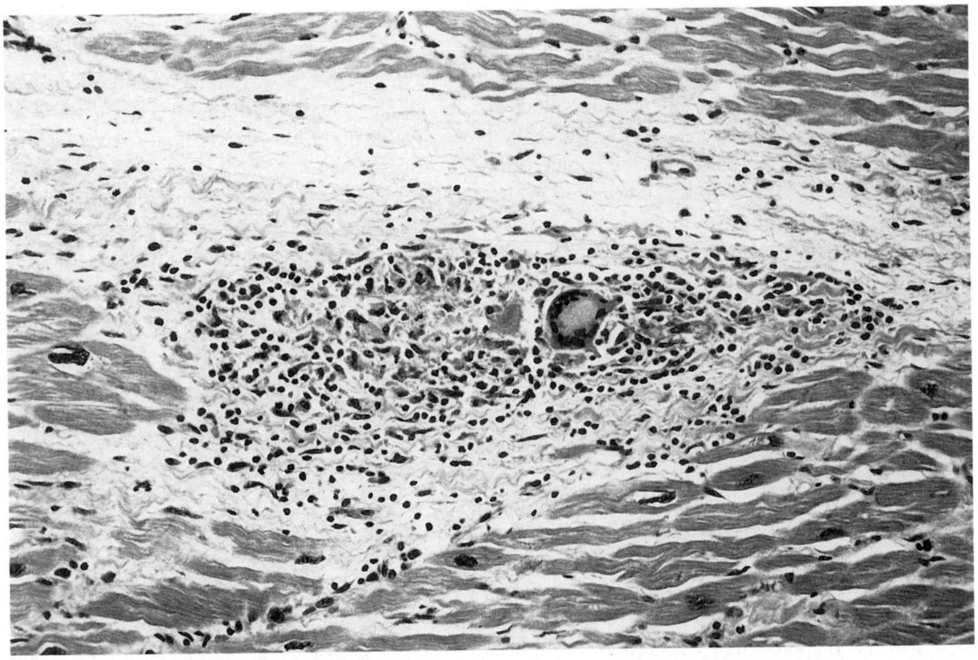

Hemochromatosis

Primary hemochromatosis is an inborn error of metabolism leading to iron deposition in a variety of organs, including the heart, and resultant secondary myocardial fibrosis. Both restrictive and dilated presentations can occur.[145,146] Treatment with phlebotomy is highly effective. In the secondary forms of hemochromatosis due to multiple blood transfusions for blood dyscrasias, chelation therapy is highly effective. Diagnosis is made by symptom constellation in the presence of an elevated serum iron and ferritin. Endomyocardial biopsy is diagnostic (Fig. 79-12).

Carcinoid and Other Infiltrative Cardiomyopathies

Carcinoid heart disease typically leads to a restrictive pattern and often has asymmetrical involvement due to the predilection of the carcinoid for the tricuspid valve apparatus.[147,148] Diagnosis is generally made with right-sided heart findings in the setting of systemic features of carcinoid syndrome. Cardiac involvement responds favorably to control of the primary tumor with chemotherapy or catheter

FIGURE 79-11 Photomicrograph showing interstitial noncaseating granulomas with a multinucleated giant cell. (H&E, ×40.)

embolization.[148] Tricuspid valve replacement and/or pulmonary valvulotomy and outflow tract enlargement have been recommended when hemodynamically indicated.[148] Alternatively, balloon valvuloplasty for tricuspid or pulmonary stenoses has been used successfully.[149]

There are other heritable lesions leading to infiltrative cardiomyopathy. Pseudoxanthoma elasticum (also known as endocardial

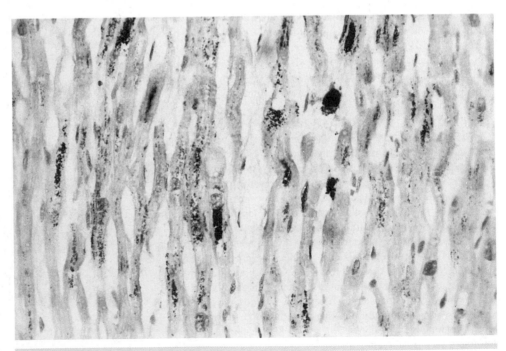

FIGURE 79-12 Photomicrograph showing Perls' stain of hemochromatosis with deposits scattered throughout the myocyte. (×100.)

fibroelastosis) is an inherited disorder of elastic tissue metabolism that leads to a thickening and calcification of the endocardium.[150] Similarly, a number of metabolic inherited disorders cause massive infiltration of the myocardium in infancy and childhood. The best known is Pompe's disease, which is an autosomal recessive disorder caused by a deficiency of the enzyme α-glucosidase, leading to massive glycogen deposition in the cardiac and skeletal musculature. Interestingly, the pathophysiology resembles that of hypertrophic rather than restrictive cardiomyopathy.[151] Prognosis is poor, with no known therapy. Death typically ensues within the first year of life.

Eosinophilic Heart Disease

Eosinophilic heart disease was originally described several decades ago by Löffler, who reported the observation of endocardial lesions, termed "endocarditis parietalis fibroplastica," in association with blood eosinophilia.[152] Although initially thought to represent an isolated disease, Löffler's syndrome is now recognized to be only one manifestation of a spectrum of hypereosinophilic syndromes. Recently cases of isolated eosinophilic myocarditis without signs of endocardial involvement, with or without vasculitis, have been described.[153] Hypereosinophilic syndromes are characterized by peripheral eosinophilia and endocardial disease consisting of eosinophilic infiltration, fibrosis, and eventual occlusion of the ventricular cavity by scar and thrombus. This leads to a very severe form of restrictive myocardial disease referred to as *obliterative myocardial disease*.[154]

PATHOGENESIS

Löffler's endomyocardial disease is considered to be an immunologic disorder caused by clones of abnormal eosinophils infiltrating both sides of the heart. This group of diseases may begin with myocarditis due to the direct toxic effects of the eosinophils and their granules.[155] Indeed, hypersensitivity myocarditis, discussed earlier in this chapter, may be an early variant of this disease. Chronic disease culminates in endomyocardial fibrosis after the disappearance of the initial eosinophilia. The eosinophilic endocardial disease has since been well described and is characterized by intense endocardial fibrotic thickening of the apex and subvalvular regions of one or both ventricles.[156] These changes lead to inflow obstruction and restrictive physiology.

CLINICAL PRESENTATION

Löffler's syndrome was initially described primarily in men from temperate climates in their fourth decade of life with a hypereosinophilic syndrome. Diffuse organ involvement may be observed (lungs, bone marrow, brain), with cardiac involvement in more than 75 percent of patients. The typical clinical presentation includes weight loss, fever, cough, skin rash, and CHF. Overt cardiac dysfunction occurs in about half the patients and is the leading cause of death. Chest x-ray reveals cardiomegaly. ECG findings most commonly include nonspecific ST- and T-wave changes, atrial fibrillation, and right bundle branch block. Echocardiography commonly demonstrates localized thickening of the left ventricle with valvular leaflet abnormalities and atrial enlargement due to atrioventricular valvular regurgitation and restrictive physiology.[157] In cases of advanced endomyocardial fibrosis, there may be apical obliteration by thrombus but normal systolic function.[155]

Diagnosis is easily established in the acute phase by endomyocardial biopsy. Variable degrees of acute inflammatory eosinophilic myocarditis are observed. Marked changes can be seen histologically

in the coronary vessels, including inflammatory, fibrotic, and thrombotic changes typically containing eosinophils. Fibrotic thickening of up to several millimeters can be observed.[155] Mural thrombosis is common.

Medical therapy with corticosteroids and cytotoxic drugs in the early stages of disease may substantially improve survival.[105,158] Routine therapy for heart failure with digitalis, diuretics, afterload reduction, and anticoagulation are adjuncts in the management of these patients. Surgical therapy offers palliation once the later fibrotic stages have been reached.[159]

CARDIOMYOPATHY DUE TO ENDOCRINE DISORDERS

Thyroid

Thyroid hormone has long been recognized to affect the heart and the peripheral vasculature.[160] Changes in cardiac function are mediated by T3 regulation of cardiac-specific genes.[161] Thyroid hormone metabolism is frequently abnormal in patients with CHF. In a study of 84 patients with advanced heart failure, T3 levels were found to be low.[162] Furthermore, a low T3/reverse T3 ratio was the only independent predictor of prognosis when a multivariate regression analysis was performed with known predictors of poor outcome such as ejection fraction, serum sodium, or hemodynamic variables. The low conversion to T3 was postulated to be an adaptive mechanism to decreased catabolism. In a subsequent study, Hamilton et al. studied the effects of intravenous T3 infusion to patients with class III or IV heart failure.[163] Cardiac output increased without a change in left ventricular ejection fraction or filling pressures. This was thought to be secondary to the effects of T3, causing vascular smooth muscle dilatation and therefore peripheral vasodilation. In another study of thyroid hormone replacement in heart failure, 20 patients with class II and III idiopathic dilated cardiomyopathy were given L-thyroxine orally.[164] Cardiac output improved, peripheral vascular resistance decreased, and exercise performance increased. The higher oxygen consumption at peak exercise may be due to improved oxygen uptake by skeletal muscle, increased perfusion of the musculature, or improved muscle metabolism by local action of L-thyroxine. Similar results were obtained in a study by Moruzzi and colleagues.[165] In this series of 20 patients, ejection fraction, cardiac output, and left ventricular diastolic dimensions all increased. Functional capacity and peak exercise cardiac output also improved. The beneficial effects were sustained with chronic therapy.

Like thyroid deficiency, thyroid toxicity can lead to the development of both high- and low-output cardiac failure. A prolonged tachycardia and high-output state caused by thyrotoxicosis is thought eventually to produce left ventricular dilatation. A consequent progressive decline in systolic function leads to low-output heart failure. This process can often be reversed by reduction of excess hormone levels. In a study of seven patients with a dilated cardiomyopathy and hyperthyroidism, Umpierrez et al. demonstrated echocardiographic normalization of left ventricular function after treatment with propylthiouracil or methimazole.[166]

Pheochromocytoma

Hypertension and its sequelae are the major cardiovascular manifestations of pheochromocytoma. However, there have been reports of a specific catecholamine-induced myocarditis and/or cardiomyopathy.[167,168] Degenerative and fibrotic myocardial changes have been described in autopsy specimens of patients dying of suprarenal tumors.[167] Although progression to cardiac involvement is unusual, when the presentation of the tumor is aggressive, pheochromocytoma patients typically die of cardiovascular causes, most commonly congestive heart failure or malignant ventricular arrhythmias. In the largest series, 15 of the 26 patients with proven pheochromocytomas had a pathologic diagnosis of myocarditis at autopsy.[168] Hemodynamic stabilization is generally obtained with alpha and beta blockers, and prompt adrenalectomy is required to eliminate catecholamine-induced cardiotoxicity. The cardiac abnormalities can be reversed with tumor resection.[169,170]

Acromegaly

It is not clear whether acromegalic cardiomyopathy is a specific entity or is secondary to the hypertension or atherosclerosis associated with this condition. However, 10 to 20 percent of patients with acromegaly develop CHF.[171] The CHF that develops in these patients is particularly resistant to conventional therapy owing to higher collagen content in the acromegalic heart.[171,172] Histopathologically, the myocytes display cellular hypertrophy, patchy fibrosis, and myofibrillar degeneration. Inflammatory and degenerative damage to the sinoatrial and AV nodes can lead to sudden death. Surgery and irradiation remain the mainstays of therapy, but often the cardiopathic manifestations persist despite a fall in growth hormone levels.[173] Treatment of acromegalic patients without clinical heart failure decreases left ventricular mass and improves diastolic function.[174]

Diabetes

Analysis of the Framingham data showed that the risk of developing heart failure was substantially increased among diabetic patients. Even after exclusion of patients with prior coronary or rheumatic disease and controlling for age, hypertension, obesity, and hypercholesterolemia, the diabetic patients have a fivefold increased risk of developing congestive heart failure.[175] This increased incidence suggested that the metabolic abnormalities associated with diabetes may contribute to myocyte dysfunction and produce a diabetes-induced cardiomyopathy. Histologically, this cardiomyopathy shows no evidence of epicardial atherosclerotic disease or abnormalities in myocardial capillary basal lamina.[176] Typically, interstitial fibrosis and arteriolar hyalinization are present. Clinically both systolic and diastolic dysfunction can occur, and the severity of the dysfunction is related to the degree of metabolic control (see Chap. 86).[177]

TOXINS

Alcohol

Although moderate alcohol consumption on a regular basis is associated with an inverse risk of myocardial infarction,[178] chronic alcohol abuse is a major risk factor for the development of congestive cardiomyopathy accounting for up to 45 percent of all dilated cardiomyopathies.[179] In one observational study completed over a 5-year period, 20 percent of chronic alcoholic women and 26 percent of chronic alcoholic men developed dilated cardiomyopathy.[180] As an estimated 10 percent of the adult population are heavy alcohol users, cardiac toxicity from alcohol is a major problem.

PATHOGENESIS

The cardiodepressant effects of alcohol have been demonstrated following acute and chronic ingestion in animal models and in normal and alcoholic human subjects. Chronic excessive alcohol use can result in CHF, hypertension, and arrhythmias. Cardiac damage results from direct toxic effects of alcohol or one of its metabolites. Nutritional deficiencies, toxic cofactors, sympathetic stimulation, or coexistent hypertension may also contribute to disease development.

Orally ingested alcohol is converted in the liver to acetaldehyde by the alcohol dehydrogenase enzyme system. Acetaldehyde is then converted into acetic acid by oxidation via acetaldehyde dehydrogenase. The activity of these enzyme systems varies greatly between individuals and in particular between races. Thus, depending on individual enzyme system activity, there are varying levels of alcohol and acetaldehyde concentrations after ingestion of an alcoholic beverage. Alcohol and acetaldehyde are both potent vasodilators. Additionally, acetaldehyde results in marked catecholamine release. Both alcohol and acetaldehyde interfere with a variety of cellular metabolic functions, including calcium transport and binding, lipid metabolism and fatty acid composition of the sarcolemma, protein synthesis, myofibrillar ATPase, and mitochondrial respiration.[179,181] Although ethanol can interfere with a number of myocardial metabolic steps, no predominant factor has been identified. Recently a nonoxidative pathway for the metabolism of alcohol in several organ systems including the heart has been described.[182] Nonesterified fatty acids are esterified with ethanol to produce fatty acid ethyl esters (FAEE). These molecules can accumulate in mitochondria and impair cellular function. Fatty acid ethyl esters are synthesized at high rates in the heart owing to the lack of oxidative ethanol metabolism in this organ. Other studies have demonstrated interference with lipid metabolism leading to triglyceride accumulation and alteration of the fatty acid composition of the sarcolemma.[179] Increased levels of acyl-CoA from enhanced glycerol acyltransferase activity may lead to triglyceride accumulation. The cellular membrane changes result in decreased calcium uptake by the sarcolemma. Alcohol also is found to be an inhibitor of the sodium-potassium ATPase.

For many years, alcoholic cardiomyopathy was believed to be due to nutritional deficiencies. Indeed, subjects with heavy beer consumption could develop thiamine deficiency. As beer contains no thiamine, the consumption of this high-calorie, high-carbohydrate beverage can exhaust existing thiamine stores, particularly in the presence of a deficient diet. Thus, a small percentage of patients with alcohol cardiomyopathy may have coexistent thiamine deficiency.

Contamination of alcoholic beverages with heavy metals has resulted in heart failure. In the nineteenth century, an epidemic of heart failure occurred in Manchester, England, following accidental contamination of the beer with arsenic. More recently, in the 1960s, a new variant of alcoholic cardiomyopathy was described.[183] Patients presented with massive pericardial effusion, low cardiac output, elevated venous pressure, and polycythemia. After considerable medical detective work, the syndrome was linked to cobaltous chloride that was added to the beer as a foaming agent to increase and stabilize the beer head. Removal of the additive resulted in the resolution of this miniepidemic.

CLINICAL PRESENTATION

Although approximately 10 percent of the adult population are heavy drinkers, the prevalence of cardiac disease in this group is low—significantly lower than the prevalence of liver disease in the same population. Although patients with alcoholic cirrhosis may have evidence of asymptomatic myocardial disease, compensated liver disease per se does not adversely effect cardiac function.[184]

The disease is observed most frequently in males age 30 to 55 years with a greater than 10-year history of heavy alcohol use. The disease is extremely rare in premenopausal women. The amount and duration of alcohol use is frequently difficult to establish. Criteria used to define heavy chronic alcohol use have included such estimates as the use of 125 mL/day of alcohol and/or 30 to 50 percent of daily calories derived from alcohol for a minimum of 10 years. In a study of 50 asymptomatic alcoholic men, Rubin et al. demonstrated that cardiomyopathy, as well as abnormalities of skeletal muscle, are common among persons with chronic alcoholism, and that alcohol is toxic to striated muscle in a dose-dependent manner.[185]

Presenting symptoms include dyspnea on exertion, orthopnea, paroxysmal nocturnal dyspnea, fatigue, weakness, arrhythmias, or embolic phenomena. Atrial fibrillation is extremely common, followed by atrial flutter and ventricular premature contractions. Sudden death can be the initial presentation. ECG findings include first-degree heart block, left ventricular hypertrophy, nonspecific interventricular conduction defects, bundle branch blocks and prolongation of the QT interval. The echocardiogram frequently shows left ventricular hypertrophy, single- to four-chamber enlargement, and mural thrombi.

In animal studies, left ventricular biopsies from dogs that developed alcoholic cardiomyopathy showed an accumulation of glucoprotein-like material in the interstitium on light microscopy as well as a dilatation of the intercalated disks on electron microscopic evaluation. These studies also demonstrated abnormalities of the sarcoplasmic reticulum and swelling of subsarcolemma regions.[186,187] The severity of these changes related to the duration and extent of alcohol use. Several histologic changes have been described on endomyocardial biopsies in alcoholic cardiomyopathy, but none of these changes are pathognomonic. Changes include myocyte loss, increased fibrosis, loss of sarcolemmal integrity, myofibrillar degeneration, mitochondrial swelling, and intercellular edema.[188] Electron microscopy shows mitochondrial swelling with dense intramitochondrial inclusions, swollen vesiculated sarcoplasmic reticulum, and myofibrillar disruption.

TREATMENT

The mainstay of treatment is abstinence from alcohol. Alcohol withdrawal may have a remarkable impact on disease manifestation and progression, especially in the milder forms of the disease.[189] In animal models, following cessation of alcohol use, the hearts recover. In humans, the duration and extent of abuse is correlated with outcome.[190] Prognosis is extremely poor in those patients who continue to drink in excess of 100 g of ethanol daily as compared to patients who moderate their alcohol consumption.[191] In 1 year of follow-up, men with alcoholic cardiomyopathy who became abstinent or curtailed their drinking to 60 g of ethanol per day experienced an average improvement in ejection fraction of approximately 13 percent, with sustained improvement over 4 years. In contrast, those who continued to drink heavily suffered a progressive deterioration in cardiac function.

Although, early in the disease process, abstinence can result in recovery, there is a point at which cessation of alcohol is no longer effective, and this correlates with the development of structural histologic abnormalities.[189] Survival of patients with alcoholic dilated cardiomyopathy who become abstinent was believed to be significantly better than the long-term survival of patients with a comparable class of CHF due to idiopathic cardiomyopathy.[189] These observations tended to be made at a time before the widespread use of angiotensin-converting enzyme (ACE) inhibitors and

beta blockers for the treatment of dilated cardiomyopathy, when 5-year survival rates were less than 50 percent. A recent study of 338 men with dilated cardiomyopathy treated with ACE inhibitors found that 7-year transplant-free survival was greatest in the group with idiopathic dilated cardiomyopathy and poorest for those with alcoholic cardiomyopathy who continued to drink heavily.[192] Patients with alcoholic cardiomyopathy who abstained from alcohol had a significant improvement in ejection fraction and 7-year survival, which paralleled that of the idiopathic dilated cardiomyopathy group.

Cocaine

Myocardial ischemia, infarction, coronary spasm, cardiac arrhythmias, sudden death, myocarditis, and dilated cardiomyopathy are all reported cardiovascular complications of cocaine abuse.[193] Clinical and experimental evidence suggests a variety of theories for the cardiotoxic effects of cocaine (see Chap. 50).

The pharmacologic effects of cocaine on the heart partly explain its toxic effects.[193] By blocking the reuptake of norepinephrine, cocaine induces tachycardia, vasoconstriction, hypertension, cardiomyopathy, and ventricular arrhythmias. Cardiomyopathy may then result from secondary changes in the heart due to tachycardia or sustained increased ventricular afterload.

Cocaine has also been shown to exert a direct toxic effect on the heart. In vitro studies with isolated rabbit ventricular tissue[194] or isolated blood-perfused dog preparations[195] showed that high-dose cocaine depressed myocardial contractile force. Acute ventricular dilatation and reversible systolic dysfunction after intravenous cocaine administration have been documented in vivo in dogs.[196]

Dilated cardiomyopathy in the absence of coronary abnormalities and myocarditis has been reported.[197] In these cases, myocardial depression is global and is generally reversible; it is attributed to a direct myocardial depressant effect of cocaine.[198]

There are no clinical or histologic features specific for cocaine-induced myocardial damage. Endomyocardial biopsy and autopsy studies confirm the presence of myocyte necrosis and a diffuse inflammatory cellular infiltrate in cocaine users.[199] "Contraction-band necrosis" has been seen in a patient presenting with a clinical course similar to that of catecholamine cardiomyopathy, but this is not characteristic.[200] Although eosinophilic infiltrates can be seen, cocaine is not included in the list of typical drugs associated with a hypersensitivity syndrome. Thus the diagnosis is usually presumptive and is one of exclusion. The treatment of cocaine-related myocarditis and cardiomyopathy is nonspecific and focuses on abstinence and heart failure therapy.

Chemotherapeutic Agents

Several chemotherapeutic agents can cause an acute and/or chronic cardiomyopathy. Among them, the anthracycline group (doxorubicin) and cyclophosphamide are the most common agents associated with heart failure.

Doxorubicin has been used as single or combination therapy for treatment of many different tumors including breast and esophageal tumors as well as sarcomas and lymphomas from the late 1960s. Its use is limited by its cardiotoxicity. The cause of the cardiotoxicity is unknown, but it is suspected to be due to increased oxidative stress from the generation of free radicals by doxorubicin. Moreover, endogenous antioxidants are reduced by treatment with doxorubicin. Increased oxidative stress results in the loss of myofibrils and cellular vacuolization, similar to what is observed with doxorubicin administration.[201]

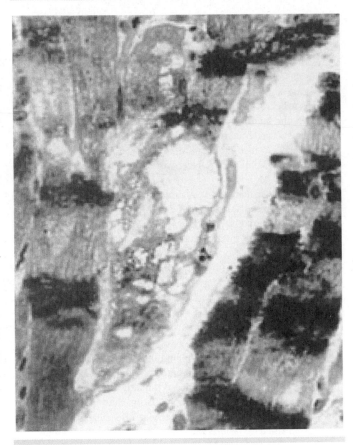

FIGURE 79-13 Loss of myofibrils and vacuolization of cytoplasm (toluidine blue stain, ×40) in a patient with doxorubicin cardiotoxicity. (From Singal et al.,[202] with permission.)

Doxorubicin can be associated with early or late cardiotoxicity. Risk factors for the development of doxorubicin cardiomyopathy include age greater than 70 years, combination chemotherapy, mediastinal irradiation, prior cardiac disease, hypertension, and liver disease. The early or acute cardiotoxicity manifests as a pericarditis-myocarditis syndrome and is not dose-related.[202] Left ventricular dysfunction is rarely seen, but arrhythmias, abnormalities of conduction, decreased QRS voltage, and nonspecific ST-segment and T-wave abnormalities are commonly observed. The prognosis is good, with quick resolution of the abnormalities upon discontinuation of therapy.

In contrast, late or chronic cardiotoxicity is due to the development of a dose-dependent degenerative cardiomyopathy[203] (Fig. 79-13). This syndrome generally occurs at doses above 550 mg/m^2. Serial assessment of nuclear ejection fractions is used clinically to monitor for adverse effects.[204] However, histopathologic grading is most useful in delineating the safety of continued doxorubicin administration. Cardiotoxicity may occur during therapy within a year of the last dose of anthracycline or as late as 6 to 10 years after its cessation. Therefore a course of this chemotherapy commits patients to prolonged cardiac surveillance.

The best management of anthracycline cardiotoxicity is prevention by limiting dosage. Lowering the peak blood levels of the drug by giving a continuous rather than bolus infusion also appears to significantly decrease drug-related damage.[202] Coadministration of doxorubicin with agents that would block free radical formation and not decrease its antineoplastic effects has been studied. Dexrazoxane, an iron chelating agent, has been used in clinical trials of patients with breast cancer or small-cell lung cancer to limit the cardiotoxicity of doxorubicin. The incidence of heart failure and the decrease in ejection fraction is lower in those patients receiving combined therapy. Unfortunately, dexrazoxane is a potent myelosuppressive agent and may also interfere with cancer therapy. Studies with probucol, an alternative antioxidant, are ongoing.

Heart failure due to doxorubicin has been very difficult to treat and is typically refractory to conventional therapy. In children with doxorubicin-induced cardiomyopathy, recent reports have described diminished symptoms and improved left ventricular function after treatment with beta blockers. Further studies on the use of these agents are needed.

In contrast to the anthracyclines, cyclophosphamide leads to an acute cardiotoxicity that is not related to cumulative dose.[205] Pericarditis, systolic dysfunction, arrhythmias, and myocardial edema make up the spectrum of cardiac abnormalities. Prior left ventricular dysfunction is a risk factor for development of significant cardiomyopathy with cyclophosphamide. Although mortality is not trivial, survivors exhibit no residual cardiac abnormalities.[206]

Chemical Toxins

A variety of compounds can lead to a spectrum of cardiotoxicity, including cardiomyopathy. They include interferon alpha,[207] IL-2,[208] phenothiazines,[209] emetine,[210] methysergide,[211] chloroquine,[212] lithium,[213] hydrocarbons,[214] lead,[215] and carbon monoxide.[216] A summary of the cardiotoxicity seen with each compound is outlined in Table 79-5.

TABLE 79-5 Major Cardiovascular Complications of Chemical Toxins

Agent	Cardiac Toxicity
Cobalt	Congestive heart failure
Cocaine	Coronary abnormalities, arrhythmias, myocarditis, myocardial depression
Interferon alpha	Arrhythmias, dilated cardiomyopathy, congestive heart failure
Interleukin-2	Myocardial ischemia/infarct, arrhythmias, eosinophilic myocarditis
Phenothiazines	Electrocardiographic changes, arrhythmias, sudden death
Emetine	Mononuclear and histiocyte infiltration, electrocardiographic abnormalities
Methysergide	Left-sided valvular lesions, fibrotic endocardial and pericardial lesions, restriction and constriction
Chloroquine	Arrhythmias, cardiac dysfunction
Lithium	Arrhythmias, cardiac dilatation with myofibrillar degeneration
Hydrocarbons	Electrocardiographic changes, arrhythmias, and cardiomegaly
Lead	Electrocardiographic changes, arrhythmias, and congestive heart failure
Carbon monoxide	Arrhythmias and transient biventricular dysfunction

CARDIOMYOPATHIES ASSOCIATED WITH NUTRITIONAL DEFICIENCIES

Vitamins

Thiamine deficiency, or beriberi, produces a clinical syndrome characterized by high-output cardiac failure and severe lactic acidosis. Dramatic hemodynamic improvements are seen after bolus infusion of thiamine.[217] Untreated, beriberi may be fatal. Vitamin D deficiency, or rickets, and vitamin D excess are associated with cardiovascular morbidity and mortality as well. There are about 25 reported cases of hypocalcemic cardiomyopathy in the adult population caused mostly by idiopathic hypoparathyroidism.[218] Similarly in children, cardiomyopathy has been documented in cases of hypocalcemia caused by vitamin D deficiency rickets.[219] Excess doses of vitamin D in humans have been associated with calcium deposition in the heart and QT shortening but not frank cardiomyopathy. Similarly, vitamin A, vitamin B_6, vitamin C, and niacin deficiency are not directly associated with overt cardiac dysfunction in humans but can be associated with ECG abnormalities.

Selenium

Interest in the role of selenium deficiency in cardiovascular diseases originated from observations of cardiomyopathy and sudden cardiac death in animals with dietary selenium deficiency.[220] Cardiomyopathy associated with inadequate dietary intake of selenium, termed Keshan's disease, has also been described in humans. This syndrome was discovered in regions of China with a low soil content of selenium.[221] Whether the cardiomyopathy results from the actual selenium deficiency or the selenium deficiency increases susceptibility to cardiotropic viruses is unclear. Coxsackievirus B3 (CVB 3/20), which causes no pathology in hearts of selenium-adequate mice, induces extensive myocarditis in selenium-deficient mice.[222] Furthermore, coxsackievirus B3 recovered from the hearts of selenium-

deficient mice and inoculated into selenium-adequate mice induced significant heart damage, suggesting mutation of the virus to a virulent genotype.[223] These findings may underlie the seasonal variation characteristic of Keshan's disease.

This disease is typically seen in children and pregnant women. Both acute and chronic forms of Keshan's disease exist.[224] In the acute form, cardiogenic shock, severe arrhythmias, and pulmonary edema are the manifestations of the systolic impairment. The chronic type shows a moderate to severe heart enlargement with varying degrees of cardiac insufficiency; often patients are asymptomatic. Its incidence is dramatically reduced with supplementation of sodium selenite.

Other than Keshan's disease, circumstantial evidence supports an association between selenium deficiency and cardiomyopathy. Congestive cardiomyopathy with low selenium levels has been reported in patients receiving total parenteral nutrition.[225] Patients with congestive cardiomyopathy have significantly lower serum selenium concentrations than healthy control subjects. Left ventricular ejection fraction is positively correlated with the selenium concentration in patients with cardiomyopathies.[225]

Carnitine

L-Carnitine is an essential compound in the transport of long chain fatty acids into mitochondria, where they undergo beta oxidation. Since the normal heart obtains approximately 60 percent of its total energy production from fatty acid oxidation, this function of carnitine is thought to be of major importance.[226] Because of this function of carnitine and case reports that have shown that some patients with carnitine deficiency exhibit cardiomyopathy, it is believed that adequate levels of carnitine are required for normal energy metabolism and contractile function of the heart.[227] Interestingly, not all patients with carnitine deficiency exhibit cardiomyopathy. This may be explained perhaps by the degree of carnitine deficiency or by how cardiac performance is assessed.[228]

Deficiencies of carnitine can be either primary or secondary. Primary deficiencies arise from several genetic disorders involving carnitine synthesis or handling. These rare conditions are severe and are associated with muscle and plasma carnitine levels as low as 10 percent of normal (Fig. 79-14). Several case reports have established that primary carnitine deficiency is associated with cardiomyopathy.[229,230] The cardiomyopathy that ensues presents within 3 to 4 years of birth and is profound[231]; clinically, however, it responds to carnitine supplementation.

Secondary carnitine deficiencies are much more common and arise from a large number of genetic diseases associated with defects in acyl-CoA metabolism. In patients with long-chain or short-chain acyl-CoA dehydrogenase deficiency, carnitine levels are reduced to 25 to 50 percent of normal and a depression in cardiac contractile performance has been found.[232] Secondary carnitine deficiencies can also be acquired as a result

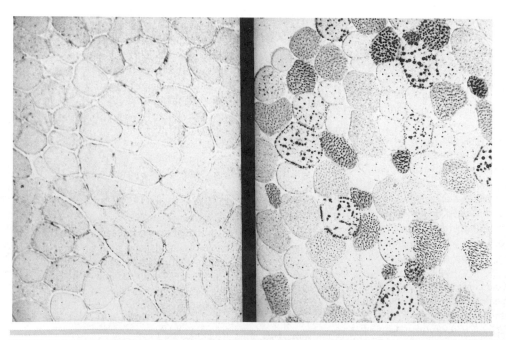

FIGURE 79-14 Photomicrograph of oil red O stain demonstrating lipid deposits in type I and II fibers in normal (*right*) and carnitine-deficient (*left*) skeletal muscle.

of liver disease, renal disease[233] (Fanconi's syndrome, renal tubular acidosis), dietary insufficiencies[234] (chronic total parenteral nutrition, malabsorption), diabetes mellitus, and heart failure.[235] Many of these types of secondary carnitine deficiency are often associated with cardiomyopathy. In cases of secondary carnitine deficiency, however, it has been difficult to determine whether the symptoms are due to carnitine deficiency or to the underlying genetic metabolic disorder. Based on this observation and the inconsistent reports of cardiomyopathy with these secondary deficiencies, it appears that a clear and strong association can be made only between cardiomyopathy and primary carnitine deficiency.

Coenzyme Q

Coenzyme Q (2,3-dimethoxy-5 methyl-6-decapreyl-1,4-benzoquinone) is another important factor involved in oxidative phosphorylation in mitochondria of the heart.[236] It has been postulated that its depletion, when found in myocardial biopsies of patients with cardiomyopathy, may contribute to heart failure. Several studies have claimed subjective and objective improvement in patients with heart failure after oral therapy with coenzyme Q.[237–239] These studies were small, unblinded, uncontrolled trials. Recently two placebo-controlled double-blind randomized trials of coenzyme Q were performed in heart failure patients stabilized on conventional therapy.[240,241] In these studies, treatment with oral coenzyme Q failed to improve resting left ventricular systolic function or quality of life despite an increase in plasma levels of coenzyme Q to more than twice basal values. Thus, given the lack of convincing and consistent data, coenzyme Q supplementation is not included in the basic repertoire of heart failure medications.

CARDIOMYOPATHIES ASSOCIATED WITH ALTERED METABOLISM

Hyperoxaluria

Both primary and secondary oxalosis are characterized by excessive deposition of calcium oxalate crystals in various body tissues, including the heart.[242] Oxalate crystals are frequently deposited in the conduction system, leading to heart block, and occasionally in the myocardium and the coronary arteries. On histology, variable degrees of cellular reaction—including fibrosis, necrosis, and mononuclear cell infiltration—can be seen, as well as foreign-body giant cells and myocardial granulomas. Cases of primary oxalosis can be reversed after combined kidney/liver transplantation.[243]

Hyperuricemia

Atheroselerosis and coronary artery disease are the most common cardiac manifestations associated with gout, but heart muscle disease is uncommon.[244] Uric acid crystals can be found in the blood vessel walls, in the myocardial interstitium, along the valve surfaces, and in the pericardium and can lead to a granulomatous response with the formation of multinucleated giant cells.

IDIOPATHIC CARDIOMYOPATHY

Idiopathic cardiomyopathy (IDC) is the term used to describe a group of myocardial diseases of unknown cause. Idiopathic dilated cardiomyopathy probably represents the end result of a number of

TABLE 79-6　Potentially Reversible Dilated Cardiomyopathies

Ischemic with viable myocardium	Endocrine
	Hyperthyroidism
Valvular without surgically correctable lesion	Pheochromocytoma
	Metabolic
Inflammatory	Hypocalcemia
CMV	Hypophosphatemia
Toxoplasmosis	Uremia
Mycoplasma	Carnitine
Lyme	Nutritional
Toxic	Selenium
Alcohol	Thiamine
Cocaine	Infiltrative
Cobalt	Hemochromatosis
	Sarcoidosis
	Hypersensitivity

disease processes involving myocyte dysfunction, myocyte loss, myocyte hypertrophy, and fibrosis. It is a diagnosis of exclusion. The prevalence of IDC is estimated to be between 7 and 13 percent of all patients with systolic dysfunction.[1,2] In 1278 patients with a dilated cardiomyopathy referred to a large tertiary care center, extensive diagnostic testing including endomyocardial biopsy failed to identify any clear etiology in 51 percent of the patients. Myocarditis and occult coronary artery disease were the most frequently identified causes. As discussed earlier in this chapter, an idiopathic dilated cardiomyopathy may be the end result of an infectious myocarditis. Endocardial biopsy in patients with dilated cardiomyopathy may reveal an inflammatory infiltrate. Surreptitious alcohol use as well as undiagnosed and untreated hypertension probably represent other etiologies of cardiomyopathy in many of these cases. Familial factors have generally been more predominant in hypertrophic cardiomyopathies than in dilated congestive cardiomyopathy. However, accumulating data suggest that genetic factors contribute to these cases as well. When one is making the diagnosis of idiopathic dilated cardiomyopathy, it is most important to exclude potentially reversible etiologies (Table 79-6).

Several studies of the natural history of IDC have concluded that the prognosis for this condition is better than that for ischemic cardiomyopathy. The clinical response to beta blockade in IDC, as gauged by improvement in ventricular function, is greater than that for the ischemic group.[245] About 10 percent of patients with IDC will normalize their ejection fraction on beta blockade[246]; therefore, if tolerated, this therapy is warranted before consideration of cardiac transplantation.

References

1. Ho K, Pinsky J, Kannel W, et al. The epidemiology of heart failure: The Framingham study. *J Am Coll Cardiol.* 1993;22:6.
2. Bourassa MG, Gurne O, Bangdiwala, et al. Natural history and patterns of current practice in heart failure. *J Am Coll Cardiol* 1993; 22:14A.
3. Brodison A, Swann J. Myocarditis: A review. *J Infect* 1998;3:99.
4. Feldman AM, McNamara D. Myocarditis. *N Engl J Med* 2000;343: 1388.
5. Woodruff J. Viral myocarditis: A review. *Am J Pathol* 1980;101:427.
6. Chow L, Ye Y, Linder J, et al. Phenotypic analysis of infiltrating cells in human myocarditis. *Arch Pathol Lab Med* 1989;113:1357.

7. Young L, Joag S, Zheng L-M, et al. Perforin-mediated myocardial damage in acute myocarditis. *Lancet* 1990;336:1019.

8. Satoh M, Tamura G, Segawa I, et al. Expression of cytokine genes and presence of enteroviral genomic RNA in endomyocardial biopsy tissues of myocarditis and dilated cardiomyopathy. *Virchows Arch* 1996; 427:503.

9. Kawai C. From myocarditis to cardiomyopathy: Mechanisms of inflammation and cell death: Learning from the past for the future. *Circulation* 1999;99:1091.

10. Bergelson JM, Cunningham JA, Droguett G, et al. Isolation of a common receptor for Coxsackie B viruses and adenoviruses 2 and 5. *Science* 1997;275:1320.

11. Wilson FM, Miranda QR, Chason JL, et al. Residual pathologic changes following murine coxsackie A and B myocarditis. *Am J Pathol* 1969;55:253.

12. Shioi T, Matsumori A, Sasayama S. Persistent expression of cytokine in the chronic stage of viral myocarditis in mice. *Circulation* 1996;94:2930.

13. Matsumori A. Molecular and immune mechanisms in the pathogenesis of cardiomyopathy: Role of viruses, cytokines, and nitric oxide. *Jpn Circ J* 1997;61:275.

14. Gebhard JR, Perry CM, Harkins S, et al. Coxsackie B3-induced myocarditis: Perforin exacerbates disease, but plays no detectable role in virus clearance. *Am J Pathol* 1998;153:417.

15. Godeny EK, Gauntt CJ. Interferon and natural killer cell activity in coxsackie virus B3-induced murine myocarditis. *Eur Heart J* 1987; 8(suppl):433.

16. Liu PP, Mason JW. Advances in the understanding of myocarditis. *Circulation* 2001;104:1076.

17. Matsumori A, Yamada T, Suzuki H, et al. Increased circulating cytokines in patients with myocarditis and cardiomyopathy. *Br Heart J* 1994;72:561.

18. Satoh M, Tamura G, Segawa I, et al. Expression of cytokine genes and presence of enteroviral genomic RNA in endomyocardial biopsy tissues of myocarditis and dilated cardiomyopathy. *Virchows Arch* 1996; 427:503.

19. Bryant D, Becker L, Richardson J, et al. Cardiac failure in transgenic mice with myocardial expression of tumor necrosis factor-α (TNF). *Circulation* 1998;97:1375.

20. Bachmaier K, Pummerer C, Kozieradzki I, et al. Low-molecular weight tumor necrosis factor receptor p55 controls induction of autoimmune heart disease. *Circulation* 1997;95:655.

21. Wada H, Saito K, Kanda T, et al. Tumor necrosis factor-α (TNF-α) plays a protective role in acute viral myocarditis in mice: A study using mice lacking TNF-α. *Circulation* 2001;103:743.

22. Ishiyama S, Hiroe M, Nishikawa T, et al. Nitric oxide contributes to the progression of myocardial damage in experimental autoimmune myocarditis in rats. *Circulation* 1997;95:489.

23. Tomioka N, Kishimoto C, Matsumori A, et al. Effects of prednisolone on acute viral myocarditis in mice. *J Am Coll Cardiol* 1986;7:868.

24. Lodge PA, Herzum M, Olszewski J, et al. Coxsackievirus B-3 myocarditis: Acute and chronic forms of the disease caused by different immunopathogenic mechanisms. *Am J Pathol* 1987;128:455.

25. Seko Y, Tsuchimochi H, Nakamura T, et al. Expression of major histocompatibility complex class I antigen in murine ventricular myocytes infected with coxsackievirus B3. *Circ Res* 1990;67:360.

26. Andreoletti L, Hober D, Becquart P, et al. Experimental CVB3-induced chronic myocarditis in two murine strains: Evidence of interrelationships between virus replication and myocardial damage in persistent cardiac infection. *J Med Virol* 1997;52:206.

27. Opavsky MA, Penninger J, Aitken K, et al. Susceptibility to myocarditis is dependent on the response of T lymphocytes to coxsackieviral infection. *Circ Res* 1999;85:551.

28. Weiss L, Movahed L, Billingham M, et al. Detection of coxsackievirus B3 RNA in myocardial tissues by the polymerase chain reaction. *Am J Pathol* 1991;138:497.

29. Nicholson F, Ajetunmobi J, Li M, et al. Molecular detection and serotypic analysis of enterovirus RNA in archival specimens from patients with acute myocarditis. *Br Heart J* 1995;74:522.

30. Fujioka S, Koide H, Kitaura Y, et al. Molecular detection and differentiation of enteroviruses in endomyocardial biopsies and pericardial effusions from dilated cardiomyopathy and myocarditis. *Am Heart J* 1996;131:760.

31. Gauntt C, Pallansch M. Coxsackievirus B3 clinical isolates and murine myocarditis. *Virus Res* 1996;41:89.

32. Neu N, Rose NR, Beisel KW, et al. Cardiac myosin induces myocarditis in genetically predisposed mice. *J Immunol* 1987;139:3630.

33. Cunningham MW, Antone SM, Gulizia JM, et al. Cytotoxic and viral neutralizing antibodies crossreact with streptococcal M protein, enteroviruses, and human cardiac myosin. *Proc Natl Acad Sci USA* 1992;89:1320.

34. Wolfgram LL, Beisel KW, Rose NR. Heart-specific autoantibodies following murine coxsackievirus B3 myocarditis. *J Exp Med* 1985;161: 1112.

35. Rao I, Debbas M, Sabbatini P, et al. The adenovirus EIA proteins induce apoptosis, which is inhibited by the EIB 19-kDa and Bcl-2 proteins. *Proc Natl Acad Sci USA* 1992;89:7742.

36. Liu P, Sole MJ. What is the relevance of apoptosis to the myocardium? *Can J Cardiol* 1999;15:8B.

37. Grist NR, Bell EJ. Coxsackie viruses and the heart (editorial). *Am Heart J* 1969;77:295.

38. Dec GW. Introduction to clinical myocarditis. In: Cooper LT, ed. *Myocarditis: From Bench to Bedside.* Totowa, NJ: Humana Press; 2003: 257–281.

39. Dec GW Jr, Palacios IF, Fallon JT, et al. Active myocarditis in the spectrum of acute dilated cardiomyopathies: Clinical features, histologic correlates, and clinical outcome. *N Engl J Med* 1985;312:885.

40. McCarthy RE III, Boehmer JP, Hruban RH, et al. Long-term outcome of fulminant myocarditis as compared with acute (nonfulminant) myocarditis. *N Engl J Med* 2000;342:690.

41. Kesler KA, Pruitt AL, Turrentine MW, et al. Temporary left-sided mechanical cardiac support during acute myocarditis. *J Heart Lung Transplant* 1994;13:268.

42. Maybaum S, Stockwell P, Naka Y, et al. Assessment of myocardial recovery in a patient with acute myocarditis supported with a left ventricular assis device—A case report. *J Heart Lung Transplant* 2003;22: 202.

43. Costanzo-Nordin MR, O'Connell JB, Subramanian R, et al. Myocarditis confirmed by biopsy presenting as acute myocardial infarction. *Br Heart J* 1985;53:25.

44. Miklozek CL, Crumpacker CS, Royal HD, et al. Myocarditis presenting as acute myocardial infarction. *Am Heart J* 1988;115:768.

45. Dec GW Jr, Waldman H, Southern J, et al. Viral myocarditis mimicking acute myocardial infarction. *J Am Coll Cardiol* 1992;20:85.

46. Burch G, Shewey L. Viral coronary arteritis and myocardial infarction. *Am Heart J* 1976;92:11.

47. Ferguson D, Farwell A, Bradley W, et al. Coronary artery vasospasm complicating acute myocarditis. *West J Med* 1988;148:664.

48. Kimby A, Sodermark T, Volpe U, et al. Stokes-Adams attacks requiring pacemaker treatment in three patients with acute nonspecific myocarditis. *Acta Med Scand* 1980;207:177.

49. Phillips M, Robinowitz M, Higgins J, et al. Sudden cardiac death in Air Force recruits: A 20-year review. *JAMA* 1986;256:2696.

50. Kojima J, Miyazaki S, Fujiwara H, et al. Recurrent left ventricular mural thrombi in a patient with acute myocarditis. *Heart Vessels* 1988;4: 120.

51. O'Connell JB, Fowles R, Robinson JA, et al. Clinical and pathologic findings of myocarditis in two families with dilated cardiomyopathy. *Am Heart J* 1984;107:127.

52. Felker GM, Hu W, Hare JM, et al. The spectrum of dilated cardiomyopathy: The Johns Hopkins experience with 1,278 patients. *Medicine* 1999;78:270.

53. Lauer B, Niederau C, Kuhl Ü, et al. Cardiac troponin T in patients with clinically suspected myocarditis. *J Am Coll Cardiol* 1997;30:1354.

54. Smith SC, Ladenson JH, Mason JW, et al. Elevations of cardiac troponin I associated with myocarditis: Experimental and clinical correlates. *Circulation* 1997;95:163.

55. Karjalainen J, Viitasalo M, Kala R, et al. 24-Hour electrocardiographic recordings in mild acute infectious myocarditis. *Ann Clin Res* 1984; 16:34.

56. Hosenpud JD, McAnulty JH, Niles NR. Unexpected myocardial disease in patients with life threatening arrhythmias. *Br Heart J* 1986; 56:55.

57. Chandraratna P, Nimalasuriya A, Reid C, et al. Left ventricular asynergy in acute myocarditis. *JAMA* 1983;250:1428.

58. Arvan S, Manalo E. Sudden increase in left ventricular mass secondary to acute myocarditis. *Am Heart J* 1988;116:200.

59. Pinamonti B, Alberti E, Cigalotto A, et al. Echocardiographic findings in myocarditis. *Am J Cardiol* 1988;62:285.

60. Murphy JG, Frantz RP. Endomyocardial biopsy in myocarditis. In: Cooper LT, ed. *Myocarditis: From Bench to Bedside.* Totowa, NJ: Humana Press, 2003:371–389.

61. Wu L, Lapeyre AC III, Cooper LT. Current role of endomyocardial biopsy in the management of dilated cardiomyopathy and myocarditis. *Mayo Clin Proc* 2001;76:1030.

62. Aretz HT, Billingham ME, Edwards WD, et al. Myocarditis: A histopathologic definition and classification. *Am J Cardiovasc Pathol* 1987;1:3.

63. Dec GW, Fallon JT, Southern JF. "Borderline" myocarditis: An indication for repeat endomyocardial biopsy. *J Am Coll Cardiol* 1990;15:283.

64. Lieberman EB, Hutchins GM, Rose NR, et al. Clinicopathologic description of myocarditis. *J Am Coll Cardiol* 1991;18:1617.

65. Keogh A, Billingham M, Schroeder J. Rapid histological changes in endomyocardial biopsy specimens after myocarditis. *Br Heart J* 1990; 64:406.

66. Billingham M, Tazelaar H. The morphological progression of viral myocarditis. *Postgrad Med J* 1986;62:581.

67. O'Connell JB, Henkin RE, Robinson JA, et al. Gallium-67 imaging in patients with dilated cardiomyopathy and biopsy-proven myocarditis. *Circulation* 1984;70:58.

68. Dec GW, Palacios I, Yasuda T, et al. Antimyosin antibody cardiac imaging: Its role in the diagnosis of myocarditis. *J Am Coll Cardiol* 1990; 16:97.

69. Gagliardi M, Bevilacqua M, Di Renzi P, et al. Usefulness of magnetic resonance imaging for diagnosis of acute myocarditis in infants and children, and comparison with endomyocardial biopsy. *Am J Cardiol* 1991;68:1089.

70. Friedrich MG, Strohm O, Schulz-Menger J, et al. Contrast media-enhanced magnetic resonance imaging visualizes myocardial changes in the course of viral myocarditis. *Circulation* 1998;97:1802.

71. Lieback E, Hardouin I, Meyer R, et al. Clinical value of echocardiographic tissue characterization in the diagnosis of myocarditis. *Eur Heart J* 1996;17:135.

72. Matsumori A, Igata H, Ono K, et al. High doses of digitalis increase the myocardial production of proinflammatory cytokines and worsen myocardial injury in viral myocarditis: A possible mechanism of digitalis toxicity. *Jpn Circ J* 1999;63:934.

73. Rockman HA, Adamson RM, Dembitsky WP, et al. Acute fulminant myocarditis: Long-term follow-up after circulatory support with a left ventricular assist device. *Am Heart J* 1991;121:922.

74. Holman WL, Bourge RC, Kirklin JK. Case report: Circulatory support for seventy days with resolution of acute heart failure. *J Thorac Cardiovasc Surg* 1991;102:932.

75. Parillo JE, Cunnion RE, Epstein SE, et al. A prospective, randomized, controlled trial of prednisone for dilated cardiomyopathy. *N Engl J Med* 1989;321:1061.

76. Mason JW, O'Connell JB, Herskowitz A, et al. A clinical trial of immunosuppressive therapy for myocarditis. *N Engl J Med* 1995; 333:269.

77. Wojnicz R, Nowalany-Kozielska E, Wojciechowska C, et al. Randomized, placebo-controlled study for immunosuppressive treatment of inflammatory dilated cardiomyopathy: Two-year follow-up results. *Circulation* 2001;104:39.

78. Drucker NA, Colan SD, Lewis AB, et al. Gammaglobulin treatment of acute myocarditis in the pediatric population. *Circulation* 1994;89:252.

79. Bozkurt B, Villanueva FS, Holubkov R, et al. Intravenous immune globulin in the therapy of peripartum cardiomyopathy. *J Am Coll Cardiol* 1999;34:177.

80. McNamara DM, Rosenblum WD, Janosko KM, et al. Intravenous immune globulin in the therapy of myocarditis and acute cardiomyopathy. *Circulation* 1997;95:2476.

81. McNamara DM, Holubkov R, Starling RC, et al. Controlled trial of intravenous immune globulin in recent-onset dilated cardiomyopathy. *Circulation* 2001;103:2254.

82. Parillo JE. Inflammatory cardiomyopathy (myocarditis): Which patients should be treated with anti-inflammatory therapy? *Circulation* 2001;104:4.

83. Maisch B, Hufnagel G, Schonian U, et al. The European Study of epidemiology and treatment of cardiac inflammatory disease (ESETCID). *Eur Heart J* 1995;16(suppl O):173.

84. Grogan M, Redfield M, Baily K, et al. Long term outcome of patients with biopsy proven myocarditis: Comparison with idiopathic dilated cardiomyopathy. *J Am Coll Cardiol* 1995;26:80.

85. Barbaro G, DiLorenzo G, Grisoris B, Barbarini G. Incidence of dilated cardiomyopathy and detection of HIV in myocardial cells of HIV-positive patients: Gruppo Italiano per lo Studio Cardiologico dei Pazienti Affetti da AIDS. *N Engl J Med* 1998;339:1093.

86. Flotats A, Domingo P, Carrio I. Dilated Cardiomyopathy in HIV-infected patients. *N Engl J Med* 1999;340:732.

87. Gonwa T, Capehart J, Pilcher J, et al. Cytomegalovirus myocarditis as a cause of cardiac dysfunction in a heart transplant recipient. *Transplantation* 1989;47:197.

88. Sadigursky M, von Kreuter B, Ling P-Y, et al. Association of elevated antisarcolemma, anti-idiotype antibody levels with the clinical and pathologic expression of chronic Chagas myocarditis. *Circulation* 1989;80:1269.

89. Higuchi M, Reis M, Aiello V, et al. Association of an increase in CD8+ T cells with the presence of *Trypanosoma cruzi* antigens in chronic, human, chagasic myocarditis. *Am J Trop Med Hyg* 1997;56: 485.

90. Sher A, Coffman R. Regulation of immunity to parasites by T cells and T cell-derived cytokines. *Annu Rev Immunol* 1992;10:385.

91. Ribeiro-dos-Santos R, Pirmez A, Savino W. Role of autoreactive immunological mechanisms in chagasic carditis. *Res Immunol* 1991; 142:134.

92. Reis M, Higuchi MdL, Benvenuti L, et al. An in situ quantitative immunohistochemical study of cytokines and IL-2R+ in chronic, human, chagasic myocarditis: Correlation with the presence of myocardial *T. cruzi* antigens. *Clin Immunol Immunopathol* 1997;83:165.

93. Higuchi M, De Morais C, Barreto A, et al. The role of active myocarditis in the development of heart failure in chronic Chagas' disease: A study based on endomyocardial biopsies. *Clin Cardiol* 1987; 10:665.

94. Maguire J, Mott K, Lehman J, et al. Relationship of electrocardiographic abnormalities and seropositivity to *Trypanosoma cruzi* within a rural community in northeast Brazil. *Am Heart J* 1983;105:287.

95. Nagi KS, Joshi R, Thakur RK. Cardiac manifestations of Lyme disease: A review. *Can J Cardiol* 1996;12:503.

96. Hofman P, Drici MD, Gibelin P, et al. Prevalence of toxoplasma myocarditis in patients with the acquired immunodeficiency syndrome. *Br Heart J* 1993;70:376.

97. Murray CJ, Lopez AD, eds. *Global Health Statistics: A Compendium of Incidence, Prevalence and Mortality Estimates for Over 200 Conditions. Global Burden of Disease and Injury Series.* Vol 2. Cambridge, MA: Harvard School of Public Health; 1996:132.

98. Massell B, Chute C, Walker A, et al. Penicillin and the marked decrease in morbidity and mortality from rheumatic fever in the United States. *N Engl J Med* 1988;318:280.

99. Krisher K, Cunningham M. Myosin: A link between streptococci and heart. *Science* 1985;227:413.

100. Dajani AS, Ayoub E, Bierman FZ, et al. Special writing group of the Committee on Rheumatic Fever, Endocarditis and Kawasaki disease of the Council of Cardiovascular Disease in the Young of the American

Heart Association. Guidelines for the diagnosis of rheumatic fever: Jones criteria: 1992 update. *JAMA* 1992;268:2069.

101. Narula J, Chandrasekhar Y, Rahimtoola S. Diagnosis of acute rheumatic carditis: The echoes of change. *Circulation* 1999;100:1576.

102. Voss LM, Wilson NJ, Neutze JM, et al. Intravenous immunoglobulin in acute rheumatic fever: A randomized controlled trial. *Circulation* 2001;103:401.

103. Skoularigis J, Sinovich V, Joubert G, et al. Evaluation of the long-term results of mitral valve repair in 254 young patients with rheumatic mitral regurgitation. *Circulation* 1994;90:II167.

104. Kounis N, Zavras G, Soufas G, et al. Hypersensitivity myocarditis. *Ann Allergy* 1989;62:71.

105. Spry C, Tai P-C. The eosinophil in myocardial disease. *Eur Heart J* 1987;8:81.

106. Kim C, Vlietstra R, Edwards W, et al. Steroid-responsive eosinophilic myocarditis: Diagnosis by endomyocardial biopsy. *Am J Cardiol* 1984;53:1472.

107. Cooper LT Jr, Berry GJ, Shabetai R. Idiopathic giant-cell myocarditis—Natural history and treatment. Multicenter Giant Cell Myocarditis Study Group Investigators. *N Engl J Med* 1997;336:1860.

108. Cooper LT Jr. Idiopathic giant cell myocarditis. In: Cooper LT, ed. *Myocarditis: From Bench to Bedside.* Totowa, NJ: Humana Press; 2003: 405–420.

109. Brilakis ES, Olson LJ, Berry GJ, et al. Survival outcomes of patients with giant cell myocarditis bridged by ventricular assist devices. *ASAIO J* 2000;46:569.

110. Pinderski LJ, Fonarow GC, Hamilton M, et al. Giant cell myocarditis in a young man responsive to T-lymphocyte cytolytic therapy. *J Heart Lung Transplant* 2002;21:818.

111. Brown CS, Bertolet BD. Peripartum cardiomyopathy: A comprehensive review. *Am J Obstet Gynecol* 1998;178:409.

112. Lampert MD, Lange RM. Peripartum cardiomyopathy. *Am Heart J* 1995;130:860.

113. Midei MG, DeMent SH, Feldman AM, et al. Peripartum myocarditis and cardiomyopathy. *Circulation* 1990;81:922.

114. Rizeq MN, Rickenbocker PR, Fowler MB, et al. Incidence of myocarditis in peripartum cardiomyopathy. *Am J Cardiol* 1994;74:474.

115. Melvin KR, Richardson PJ, Olson EG, et al. Peripartum cardiomyopathy due to myocarditis. *N Engl J Med* 1982;307:731.

116. Farber PA, Glasgow LA. Factors modulating host resistance to virus infection: II. Enhanced susceptibility of mice to encephalomyocarditis virus infection during pregnancy. *Am J Pathol* 1968;53:463.

117. Knobel B, Melamud E, Kishon Y. Peripartum cardiomyopathy. *Isr J Med Sci* 1984;20:1061.

118. O'Connell JB, Costanzo-Nordin MR, Subramanian R, et al. Peripartum cardiomyopathy: Clinical, hemodynamic, histologic and prognostic characteristics. *J Am Coll Cardiol* 1986;8:52.

119. Demakis JG, Rahimtoola SH, Sutton GC, et al. Natural course of peripartum cardiomyopathy. *Circulation* 1971;44:1053.

120. Lambert MB, Weinert L, Hibbard J, et al. Contractile reserve in patients with peripartum cardiomyopathy and recovered left ventricular function. *Am J Obstet Gynecol* 1997;176:189.

121. Hirano M, Davidson M, DiMauro S. Mitochondria and the heart. *Curr Opin Cardiol* 2001;16:201.

122. Kushwaha SS, Fallon JT, Fuster V. Medical progress: Restrictive cardiomyopathy. *N Engl J Med* 1997;336:267.

123. Carrell R, Lomas D. Conformational disease. *Lancet* 1997;350:134.

124. Hodkinson H, Pomerance A. The clinical significance of senile cardiac amyloidosis: A prospective clinico-pathological study. *Q J Med* 1977;46:381.

125. Falk RH, Comenzo RL, Skinner M. The systemic amyloidoses. *N Engl J Med* 1997;337:898.

126. Bhandari A, Nanda N. Myocardial texture characterization by two-dimensional echocardiography. *Am J Cardiol* 1982;51:817.

127. Click R, Olson L, Edwards W, et al. Echocardiography and systemic diseases. *J Am Soc Echocardiogr* 1994;7:201.

128. Gertz M, Kyle R. Primary systemic amyloidosis: A diagnostic primer. *Mayo Clin Proc* 1989;64:1505.

129. Klein AL, Hatle LK, Taliercio C, et al. Prognostic significance of Doppler measures of diastolic function in cardiac amyloidosis: A Doppler echocardiography study. *Circulation* 1991;83:808.

130. Skinner M, Anderson JJ, Simms R, et al. Treatment of 100 patients with primary amyloidosis: A randomized trial of melphalan, prednisone, and colchicines versus colchicine only. *Am J Med* 1996; 100:290.

131. Kyle RA, Gertz MA, Griepp PR, et al. A trial of three regimens for primary amyloidosis: Colchicines alone, melphalan and prednisone, and melphalan, prednisone, and colchicines. *N Engl J Med* 1997;336:1202.

132. Hosenpud J, DeMarco T, Frazier O, et al. Progression of systemic disease and reduced long-term in patients with cardiac amyloidosis undergoing heart transplantation: Follow-up results of a multicenter survey. *Circulation* 1991;84:III.

133. Newman LS, Rose CS, Maier LA. Sarcoidosis. *N Engl J Med* 1997; 336:1224.

134. Perry A, Vuitch F. Causes of death in patients with sarcoidosis: A morphologic study of 38 autopsies with clinicopathologic correlation. *Arch Pathol Lab Med* 1995;119:167.

135. Silverman K, Hutchins G, Bulkley B. Cardiac sarcoid: A clinicopathologic study of 84 unselected patients with systemic sarcoidosis. *Circulation* 1978;58:1204.

136. Shammas RL, Movahed A. Sarcoidosis of the heart. *Clin Cardiol* 1993;16:462.

137. Matsui Y, Iwai K, Tackibana T, et al. Clinicopathologic study of fatal cardiac sarcoidosis. *Ann NY Acad Sci* 1976;278:455.

138. Fleming H. Cardiac sarcoidosis. *Semin Respir Med* 1986;8:65.

139. Chandra M, Silverman ME, Oshinski J, et al. Diagnosis of cardiac sarcoidosis aided by MRI. *Chest* 1996;110:562.

140. Schaedel H, Kirsten D, Schmidt A, et al. Sarcoid heart disease: Results of follow-up investigations. *Eur Heart J* 1991;12:26.

141. Winters S, Cohen M, Greenberg S, et al. Sustained ventricular tachycardia associated with sarcoidosis: Assessment of the underlying cardiac anatomy and the prospective utility of programmed ventricular stimulation, drug therapy and an implantable antitachycardia device. *J Am Coll Cardiol* 1991;18:937.

142. Roberts W, McAllister H, Ferrans V. Sarcoidosis of the heart: A clinicopathologic study of 35 necropsy patients and review of 78 previously described necropsy patients. *Am J Med* 1977;63:86.

143. Fleming H. Sarcoidosis heart disease. *BMJ* 1986;292:1095.

144. Valentine HA, Tazelaar HD, Macoviak J, et al. Cardiac sarcoidosis: Response to steroids and transplantation. *J Heart Transplant* 1987;5:244.

145. Skinner C, Kenmure C. Hemachromatosis presenting as congestive cardiomyopathy and responding to venesection. *Br Heart J* 1973; 35:466.

146. Short E, Winkle R, Billingham M. Myocardial involvement in idiopathic hemachromatosis, morphological and clinical improvement following venesection. *Am J Med* 1981;70:1275.

147. Strickman N, Hall R. Carcinoid heart disease. In: Kapoor A, Reynolds R, eds. *Cancer and the Heart.* New York: Springer-Verlag; 1986.

148. Pellikka PA, Tajik AJ, Khandheria BK, et al. Carcinoid heart disease: Clinical and echocardiographic spectrum in 74 patients. *Circulation* 1993;87:1188.

149. Onate A, Alsibar J, Inguanzo R, et al. Balloon dilation of tricuspid and pulmonary valve in carcinoid heart disease. *Texas Heart Inst J* 1993; 20:115.

150. Rosenzweig B, Guarneri E, Kronzon I. Echocardiographic manifestations in a patient with pseudoxanthoma elasticum. *Ann Intern Med* 1993;119:487.

151. Hwang B, Meng C, Lin C, et al. Clinical analysis of 5 infants with glycogen storage disease of the heart—Pompe's disease. *JPN Heart J* 1986;27:25.

152. Löffler W. Endocarditis parietalis fibroplastica mit Bluteosinophilie, ein eigenartiges Krankheitsbild. *Schweiz Med Wochenschr* 1936; 66:817.

153. Galiuto L, Enriquez-Sarano M, Reeder G, et al. Eosinophilic myocarditis manifesting as myocardial infarction: Early diagnosis and successful treatment. *Mayo Clin Proc* 1997;72:603.

154. Acquatella H, Schiller N, Puigbo J, et al. Value of two-dimensional echocardiography in endomyocardial disease with and without eosinophilia: Clinical and pathologic study. *Circulation* 1983;67:1219.

155. Olsen E, Spry C. Relation between eosinophilia and endomyocardial disease. *Prog Cardiovasc Dis* 1985;27:241.

156. Solley G, Maldonado J, Gleich G, et al. Endomyocardiopathy with eosinophilia. *Mayo Clin Proc* 1976;51:697.

157. Hendren W, Jones E, Smith M. Aortic and mitral valve replacement in idiopathic hypereosinophilic syndrome. *Ann Thorac Surg* 1988;46:570.

158. Arnold M, McGuire L, Lee J. Löffler's fibroplastic endocarditis. *Pathology* 1988;20:79.

159. Blake D, Palmer I, Olinger G. Mitral valve replacement in idiopathic hypereosinophilic syndrome. *J Thorac Cardiovasc Surg* 1985;89:630.

160. Maitland M, Frishman W. Thyroid hormone and cardiovascular disease. *Am Heart J* 1998;135:187.

161. Dillman W. Biochemical basis of thyroid hormone action in the heart. *Am J Med* 1990;88:626.

162. Hamilton M, Stevenson L, Luu M, et al. Altered thyroid hormone metabolism in advanced heart failure. *J Am Coll Cardiol* 1990;16:91.

163. Hamilton M, Stevenson L. Thyroid hormone abnormalities in heart failure: Possibilities for therapy. *Thyroid* 1996;6:527.

164. Moruzzi P, Doria E, Agostoni P, et al. Usefulness of L-thyoxine to improve cardiac and exercise performance in idiopathic dilated cardiomyopathy. *Am J Cardiol* 1994;73:374.

165. Moruzzi P, Doria E, Agostoni P. Medium-term effectiveness of L-thyroxine treatment in idiopathic dilated cardiomyopathy. *Am J Med* 1996;101:461.

166. Umpierrez G, Challapalli S, Patterson C. Congestive heart failure due to reversible cardiomyopathy in patients with hyperthyroidism. *Am J Med Sci* 1995;310:99.

167. Van Vliet P, Rarchell H, Titus J. Focal myocarditis associated with pheochromocytoma. *N Engl J Med* 1966;274:1102.

168. Imperato-McGinley J, Cautier T, Ehlers K, et al. Reversibility of catecholamine-induced dilated cardiomyopathy in a child with a pheochromocytoma. *N Engl J Med* 1987;316:793.

169. Lam J, Shub G, Sheps S. Reversible dilatation of hypertrophied left ventricle in pheochromocytoma: Serial two-dimensional echocardiographic observations. *Am Heart J* 1985;109:613.

170. Salathe M, Wein P, Ritz R. Rapid reversal of heart failure in a patient with phaeochromocytoma and catecholamine-induced cardiomyopathy who was treated with captopril. *Br Heart J* 1992;68:527.

171. Lie J, Grossman S. Pathology of the heart in acromegaly: Anatomic findings in 27 autopsied patients. *Am Heart J* 1980;100:41.

172. Rossi L, Thiene G, Caregaro L, et al. Dysrhythmias and sudden death in acromegalic heart disease. A clinicopathologic study. *Chest* 1977;72:495.

173. Baldwin A, Cundy T, Butler J, et al. Progression of cardiovascular disease in acromegalic patients treated by external pituitary irradiation. *Acta Endocrinol* 1985;108:26.

174. Vianna CB, Vieira ML, Mady C, et al. Treatment of acromegaly improves myocardial abnormalities. *Am Heart J* 2002;143:873.

175. Abbott R, Donahue R, Kannel W, et al. The impact of diabetes on survival following myocardial infarction in men vs women. The Framingham Study. *JAMA* 1988;260:3456.

176. Sutherland C, Fisher B, Frier B, et al. Endomyocardial biopsy pathology in insulin-dependent diabetic patients with abnormal ventricular function. *Histopathology* 1989;14:593.

177. Raman M, Nesto RW. Heart disease in diabetes mellitus. *Enocrinol Metab Clin North Am* 1996;25:425.

178. Mukamal KJ, Conigrave KM, Mittleman MA, et al. Roles of drinking pattern and type of alcohol consumed in coronary heart disease in men. *N Engl J Med* 2003;348:109.

179. Waldenstrom A. Alcohol and congestive heart failure. *Alcohol Clin Exp Res* 1998;22:315s.

180. Fernandez-Sola J, Estruch R, Nicolas JM, et al. Comparison of alcoholic cardiomyopathy in women versus men. *Am J Cardiol* 1997;80:481.

181. Richardson P, Patel V, Preedy V. Alcohol and the myocardium. *Novartis Foundation Symp* 1998;216:35.

182. Beckemeier M, Bora P. Fatty acid ethyl esters: Potentially toxic products of myocardial ethanol metabolism. *J Mol Cell Cardiol* 1998;30:2487.

183. Morin Y, Daniel P. Quebec's beer drinkers cardiomyopathy: Etiologic considerations. *Can Med Assoc J* 1967;97:926.

184. Estruch R, Fernandez-Sola J, Sacanella E, et al. Relationship between cardiomyopathy and liver disease in chronic alcoholism. *Hepatology* 1995;22:532.

185. Rubin E. Alcoholic myopathy in heart and skeletal muscle. *N Engl J Med* 1979;301:28.

186. Regan T, Khan M, Ettinger P, et al. Myocardial function and lipid metabolism in the chronic alcoholic animal. *J Clin Invest* 1974;54:740.

187. Regan T, Levinson G, Oldewurtel H, et al. Ventricular function in noncardiacs with alcoholic fatty liver: The role of ethanol in the production of cardiomyopathy. *J Clin Invest* 1969;48:397.

188. Spies CD, Sander M, Stangl K, et al. Effects of alcohol on the heart. *Curr Opin Crit Care* 2001;7:337.

189. Demakis J, Proskey A, Rahimtoola S, et al. The natural course of alcoholic cardiomyopathy. *Ann Intern Med* 1974;80:293.

190. Vecchia L, Bedogni F, Bozzola L, et al. Prediction of recovery after abstinence in alcoholic cardiomyopathy: Role of hemodynamic and morphometric parameters. *Clin Cardiol* 1995;19:45.

191. Nicolas JM, Fernandez-Sola J, Estruch R, et al. The effect of controlled drinking in alcoholic cardiomyopathy. *Ann Intern Med* 2002;136:192.

192. Gavazzi A, De Maria R, Parolini M, et al. Alcohol abuse and dilated cardiomyopathy in men. *Am J Cardiol* 2000;85:1114.

193. Lange RA, Hillis D. Cardiovascular complications of cocaine use. *N Engl J Med* 2001;345:351.

194. Hauge N, Perrault C, Morgan J. Effects of cocaine on intracellular Ca++ handling in mammalian myocardium (abstr). *Circulation* 1988;78:359.

195. Herman E, Vlck J. A study of direct effect of cocaine on the heart (abstr). *Fed Proc* 1987;46:1148.

196. Franker T, Temsey-Armos P, Brewster P, et al. Mechanisms of cocaine-induced myocardial depression in dogs. *Circulation* 1990;81:1012.

197. Chakko S, Myerburg R. Cardiac complications of cocaine abuse. *Clin Cardiol* 1995;18:67.

198. Hale S, Alker K, Rezkalla S, et al. Adverse effects of cocaine in cardiovascular dynamics, myocardial blood flow, and coronary artery diameter in an experimental model. *Am Heart J* 1989;118:927.

199. Virmani R, Robinowitz M, Smialek J, et al. Cardiovascular effects of cocaine: An autopsy study of 40 patients. *Am Heart J* 1988;115:1068.

200. Chokshi S, Moore R, Pandian N, et al. Reversible cardiomyopathy associated with cocaine intoxication. *Ann Intern Med* 1989;111:1039.

201. Singal PK, Iliskovic N, Li T, et al. Adriamycin cardiomyopathy: Pathophysiology and prevention. *FASEB J* 1997;11:931.

202. Singal P, Iliskovic N. Current concepts: Doxorubicin-induced cardiomyopathy. *N Engl J Med* 1998;339:900.

203. Lipshultz S, Colan S, Gelber R, et al. Late cardiac effects of doxorubicin therapy for acute lymphoblastic leukemia in childhood. *N Engl J Med* 1991;324:808.

204. Ganz WI, Sridhar KS, Ganz SS, et al. Review of tests for monitoring doxorubicin-induced cardiomyopathy. *Oncology* 1996;53:461.

205. Goldberg M, Antin J, Guinan E, et al. Cyclophosphamide cardiotoxicity: An analysis of dosing as a risk factor. *Chem Toxins* 1986;68:1114.

206. Gottdiener J, Applebaum F, Ferrans V, et al. Cardiotoxicity associated with high dose cyclophosphamide therapy. *Arch Intern Med* 1981;141:758.

207. Deyton L, Walker R, Kovacs J, et al. Reversible cardiac dysfunction associated with interferon alpha therapy in AIDS patients with Kaposi's sarcoma. *N Engl J Med* 1989;321:1246.

208. Schuchter L, Hendricks C, Holland K, et al. Eosinophilic myocarditis associated with high-dose interleukin-2 therapy. *Am J Med* 1990;88:439.

209. Horowitz J. Drugs that induce heart problems: Which agents? What effects? *J Cardiovasc Med* 1983;8:308.

210. Khan M, Haider B, Thind L. Emetine-induced cardiomyopathy in rabbits. *J Submicrosc Cytol* 1983;15:495.

211. Harbin A, Gerson M, O'Connell J. Stimulation of acute myopericarditis by constrictive pericardial disease with endomyocardial fibrosis due to methylsergide therapy. *J Am Coll Cardiol* 1984;4:196.

212. Ratliff N, Estes M, Myles J, et al. Diagnosis of chloroquine cardiomyopathy by endomyocardial biopsy. *N Engl J Med* 1987;316:191.

213. Brafy H, Horgan J. Lithium and the heart: Unanswered questions. *Chest* 1988;93:166.

214. Cunningham S, Dalzell G, McGirr P, et al. Myocardial infarction and primary ventricular fibrillation after glue sniffing. *BMJ* 1987; 294:739.

215. Kopp S, Barron J, Tow J. Cardiovascular actions of lead and relationship to hypertension: A review. *Environ Health Perspect* 1988;78:91.

216. McMeekin J, Finegan B. Reversible myocardial dysfunction following carbon monoxide poisoning. *Can J Cardiol* 1987;3:118.

217. Gabrielli A, Caruso L, Stacpoole PW. Early recognition of acute cardiovascular beriberi by interpretation of hemodynamics. *J Clin Anesth* 2001;13:230.

218. Kudoh C, Tanaka S, Marusaki S, et al. Hypocalcemic cardiomyopathy in a patient with idiopathic hypoparathyroidism. *Intern Med* 1992; 31:561.

219. Mustafa A, Birgas J-L, McCrindle B. Dilated cardiomyopathy as a first sign of nutritional vitamin D deficiency rickets in infancy. *Can J Cardiol* 1999;15:699.

220. Burk R. Selenium in nutrition. *World Rev Nutr Diet* 1978;30:88.

221. Yang G. Keshan disease: An endemic selenium-related deficiency disease. In: Chandara R, ed. *Trace Elements in Nutrition of Children.* New York: Raven Press; 1985.

222. Beck M, Kolbeck P, Shi Q, et al. Increased virulence of a human enterovirus (coxsackievirus B3) in selenium deficient mice. *J Infect Dis* 1994;170:351.

223. Beck M, Shi Q, Morris V, et al. Rapid genomic evolution of a non-virulent Coxsackievirus B3 in selenium-deficient mice results in selection of identical virulent isolates. *Nat Med* 1995;1:433.

224. Huttunen J. Selenium and cardiovascular disease—An update. *Biomed Environ Sci* 1997;10:220.

225. Oster O, Prellwitz W. Selenium and cardiovascular disease. *Biol Trace Elem Res* 1990;24:91.

226. Neely J, Morgan H. Relationship between carbohydrate metabolism and energy balance of heart muscle. *Annu Rev Physiol* 1974;36:413.

227. Christensen E, Virke-Jorgensen J. Six years experience with carnitine supplementation in a patient with an inherited defective carnitine transport system. *J Inherit Metab Dis* 1995;18:233.

228. Paulson D. Carnitine deficiency-induced cardiomyopathy. *Mol Cell Biochem* 1998;180:33.

229. Famularo G, De Simone C. A new era for carnitine. *Immunol Today* 1995;16:211.

230. Scholte H, Rodriguez Pereira R, de Jonge P, et al. Primary carnitine deficiency. *J Clin Chem Clin Biochem* 1990;28:351.

231. Stanley C. Carnitine disorders. *Adv Pediatr* 1993;42:209.

232. Bennett M, Hale D, Pollitt R, et al. Endocardial fibroelastosis and primary carnitine deficiency due to a defect in the plasma membrane carnitine transport (clinical conference). *Clin Cardiol* 1996;19:243.

233. Ahmad S, Robertson H, Golper T, et al. Multicenter trial of L-carnitine in maintenance hemodialysis patients: II. Clinical and biochemical effects. *Kidney Int* 1990;38:912.

234. Heinonen O, Takala J. Carnitine status during prolonged total parenteral nutrition. *J Pediatr* 1993;122:503.

235. Regitz V, Bossaller C, Strasser R, et al. Metabolic alterations in end-stage and less severe heart failure—Myocardial carnitine decrease. *J Clin Chem Clin Biochem* 1990;28:611.

236. Crane F. Physiological coenzyme Q function and pharmacological reactions. In: Folkers K, Yamamura Y, eds. *Biomedical and Clinical Aspects of Coenzyme Q.* Amsterdam: Elsevier; 1986.

237. Langsjoen P, Langsjoen P, Folkers K. Long-term efficacy and safety of coenzyme Q_{10} therapy for idiopathic dilated cardiomyopathy. *Am J Cardiol* 1990;65:521.

238. Morisco C, Trimarco B, Condorelli M. Effect of coenzyme Q_{10} therapy in patients with congestive cardiac failure: A long-term multicenter randomized study. *Clin Invest* 1993;71:S134.

239. Lampertico M, Comis S. Italian multicenter study on the efficacy and safety of coenzyme Q_{10} as adjuvant therapy in heart failure. *Clin Invest* 1993;71:S129.

240. Khatta M, Alexander BS, Kritchen CM, et al. The effect of coenzyme Q_{10} in patients with congestive heart failure. *Ann Intern Med* 2000; 132:636.

241. Waton P, Scalia G, Galbraith A, et al. Lack of effect of coenzyme Q on left ventricular function in patients with congestive heart failure. *J Am Coll Cardiol* 1999;33:1549.

242. Cochat P. Primary hyperoxaluria type 1. *Kidney Int* 1999;55:2533.

243. Fyfe B, Israel D, Quish A, et al. Reversal of primary hyperoxaluria cardiomyopathy after combined liver and renal transplantation. *Am J Cardiol* 1995;75:210.

244. Rosenberg A, Bergstrom L, Troost B, et al. Hyperuricemia and neurologic deficits: A family study. *N Engl J Med* 1970;282:992.

245. Woodley S, Gilbert E, Anderson J, et al. β-blockade with bucindilol in heart failure due to ischemic vs idiopathic dilated cardiomyopathy. *Circulation* 1991;84:2426.

246. Waagstein F, Bristow M, Swedberg K, et al. Beneficial effects of metoprolol in idiopathic dilated cardiomyopathy. *Lancet* 1993;342:1441.

PART TWELVE

PERICARDIAL DISEASES AND ENDOCARDITIS

DISEASES OF THE PERICARDIUM

Brian D. Hoit / Michael D. Faulx

Anatomy of the Pericardium

The pericardium is composed of visceral and parietal components. The visceral pericardium is a mesothelial monolayer that adheres firmly to the epicardium, reflects over the origin of the great vessels, and—together with a tough, fibrous coat—envelops the heart as the parietal pericardium (Fig. 80-1). The pericardial space is enclosed between these two serosal layers and normally contains up to 50 mL of a plasma ultrafiltrate, the pericardial fluid. Pericardial reflections around the great vessels tether the pericardium superiorly and result in the formation of two potential spaces: the oblique and transverse sinuses. The left atrium is anterior to the oblique sinus and is therefore largely an extrapericardial chamber; this relationship explains why effusions generally are not seen behind the left atrium. Superior and inferior pericardiosternal and diaphragmatic ligaments limit displacement of the pericardium and its contents within the chest and neutralize the effects of respiration and change of body position. The phrenic nerves are embedded in the parietal pericardium and, for this reason, are vulnerable to injury during pericardial resection.

Histologically, the pericardium is composed predominantly of compact collagen layers interspersed with elastin fibers. The abundance and orientation of the collagen fibers are responsible for the characteristic viscoelastic mechanical properties of the pericardium. For example, the pressure-volume relation of the pericardium is nonlinear; i.e., the relation is initially flat (producing little to no change in pressure for large changes in volume) and develops a "bend" or "knee" at a critical pressure, which terminates in a steep slope (producing large changes in pressure for small changes in volume)

(Fig. 80-2). In addition, the pericardium is anisotropic; i.e., it stretches more in the short axis than in the long axis.

Physiology of the Pericardium

The pericardium is not essential for life; no adverse consequences follow congenital absence or surgical removal of the pericardium. However, the pericardium serves many important (although subtle) functions (Table 80-1). It limits distention of the cardiac chambers and facilitates interaction and coupling of the ventricles and atria.[1] Thus, changes in pressure and volume on one side of the heart can influence pressure and volume on the other side. Limitation of cardiac filling volumes by the pericardium may also limit cardiac output and oxygen delivery during exercise.[2] The pericardium also influences quantitative and qualitative aspects of ventricular filling[3]; the thin-walled right ventricle (RV) and atrium are more subject to the influence of the pericardium than is the more resistant, thick-walled left ventricle (LV).

Although the magnitude and importance of pericardial restraint of ventricular filling at physiologic cardiac volumes remain controversial, there is general agreement that pericardial reserve volume (i.e., the difference between unstressed pericardial volume and cardiac volume) is relatively small and that pericardial influences become significant when the reserve volume is exceeded. This may occur with rapid increases in blood volume and in disease states characterized by rapid increases in heart size (e.g., acute mitral and tricuspid regurgitation, pulmonary embolism, RV infarction). In contrast, chronic stretching of the pericardium results in "stress relaxation";

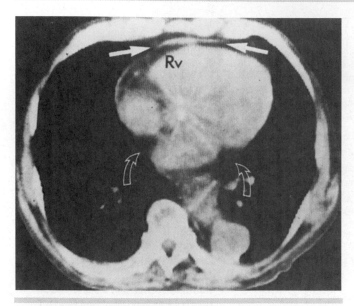

FIGURE 80-1 Computed tomographic (CT) scan shows the normal pericardium as a thin, curvilinear line (*open arrows*). The increased thickening over the anterior surface of the heart (*solid arrows*) is probably an artifact from transmitted right ventricular pulsations. (From Moncada R, Baker M. In: Higgins CB, ed. *CT of the Heart and Great Vessels*. Mt. Kisco, NY: Futura; 1983:292. Reproduced with permission.)

this explains why large but slowly developing effusions do not produce tamponade. In addition, the pericardium adapts to cardiac growth by "creep" (i.e., an increase in volume with constant stretch) and cellular hypertrophy. Pericardial thickening, which is characterized by mesothelial cell and matrix rearrangements, and the absence of diastolic abnormalities on echocardiography are features of vibroacoustic disease (morphologic and dynamic changes with exposure to large pressure amplitude and low-frequency noise).[4]

The pericardium serves a variety of other important functions. It prevents excessive torsion and displacement of the heart, minimizes friction with surrounding structures, and is an anatomic barrier to the

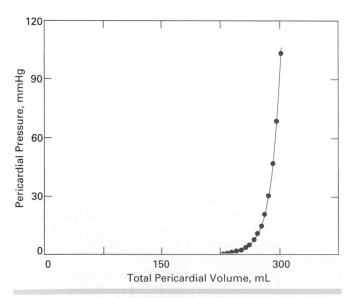

FIGURE 80-2 Pericardial pressure-volume relation in a dog. (From Holt JP. The normal pericardium. *Am J Cardiol* 1970;26:455. Reproduced with permission.)

TABLE 80-1 Functions of the Pericardium

Mechanical
  Effects on chambers
    Limits short-term cardiac distention
    Facilitates cardiac chamber coupling and interaction
    Maintains pressure-volume relation of the cardiac chambers and output from them
    Maintains geometry of left ventricle
  Effects on whole heart
    Lubricates, minimizes friction
    Equalizes gravitation and inertial, hydrostatic forces
    Mechanical barrier to infection
Immunologic
Vasomotor
Fibrinolytic
Modulation of myocyte structure and function and gene expression
Vehicle for drug delivery and gene therapy

spread of infection from contiguous structures. The thin layer of pericardial fluid reduces friction on the epicardium and equalizes gravitational, hydrostatic, and inertial forces over the surface of the heart; transmural cardiac pressures therefore do not change during acceleration or differ regionally within cardiac chambers. The pericardium also has immunologic, vasomotor, paracrine, and fibrinolytic activities.[5,6] Epicardial mesothelial cells may modulate myocyte structure and function and gene expression.[7] Finally, the pericardial space has been used as a vehicle for drug delivery and gene therapy; studies using radiolabeled growth factors indicate that substances more consistently and reproducibly gain access to the coronary arteries via pericardial fluid than via endoluminal delivery.[8,9]

PERICARDIAL MICROPHYSIOLOGY

The pericardium is richly innervated; neuroreceptors in the epicardium and fibrosa, sympathetic afferents, stretch-sensitive mechanoreceptors, and phrenic afferents monitor dynamic changes in cardiac volume and tension. Chemo- and mechanoreceptors with sympathetic afferents may be responsible for the transmission of pericardial pain.[10]

The mesothelium of the pericardium is metabolically active and produces prostaglandin E_2, eicosanoids, and prostacylin; these substances modulate sympathetic neurotransmission and myocardial contractility and may influence epicardial coronary arterial tone. The concentration of angiogenic growth factors, basic fibroblast growth factor (bFGF), and vascular endothelial growth factor (VEGF) increases in unstable angina,[11] suggesting a role for these factors in response to ischemia and injury. The level of brain natriuretic peptide (BNP) in the pericardial fluid is a more sensitive and accurate indicator of ventricular volume and pressure than is either plasma BNP or atrial natriuretic factor; it may play an autocrine/paracrine role in heart failure.[12] In addition, levels of pericardial 8-iso-prostaglandin F (PGF)-2α (a marker of oxidant stress) increase directly with increasing ventricular dilatation and severity of heart failure, suggesting a role of oxidant stress in ventricular remodeling and the development of heart failure.[13]

Pericardial Pressure

Pericardial pressure measured by a fluid-filled catheter in the pericardial space is subatmospheric and is essentially equal to pleural pressure throughout the respiratory cycle. Small fluctuations related to the events of the cardiac cycle (pericardial pressure is lowest during ventricular ejection) are superimposed on the larger fluctuations related to the events of the respiratory cycle. Although much of our understanding of pericardial physiology is based on fluid pressure, pericardial restraint is a contact force, defined as fluid pressure plus deformational force (much like the force at the knee joint that, although considerable, is negligible when measured with a needle in the joint space). Pericardial contact pressure measured with flat balloons is considerably higher than liquid pressure and varies regionally.[3]

Balloon pressure is similar to the theoretical pericardial pressure that is calculated as the difference in LV diastolic pressure before and after pericardiectomy. This theoretical pressure has important implications for understanding the role of the pericardium in states of altered ventricular loading, such as pulmonary hypertension, aortic stenosis, and congestive heart failure, but it does not explain pericardial influences on transmural pressure—for example, during acceleration and deceleration. When liquid versus contact pressure is more relevant is controversial among physiologists, but is far less relevant to clinicians, who measure pericardial pressure only when there is a pericardial effusion.

Pathology of the Pericardium

In view of the pericardium's simple structure, clinicopathologic processes involving it are understandably few; indeed, pericardial heart disease includes only pericarditis (an acute, subacute, or chronic fibrinous, "noneffusive," or exudative process) and its complications, tamponade and constriction (an acute, subacute, or chronic adhesive, fibrocalcific response), and congenital lesions. However, despite a limited number of clinical syndromes, the pericardium is affected by virtually every category of disease, including infectious, neoplastic, immune/inflammatory, metabolic, iatrogenic, traumatic, and congenital etiologies. Thus, the physician is likely to encounter patients with pericardial disease in a variety of settings, either as an isolated phenomenon or as a complication of a variety of systemic disorders, trauma, or certain drugs.

Pericardial disease often remains clinically silent, detected only during the evaluation of unrelated complaints by the electrocardiogram (ECG), chest radiography, or echocardiography. Despite exhaustive etiologic lists (Table 80-2), the cause of pericardial heart disease is often never identified. Recently, an increased prevalence of pericarditis (owing largely to therapeutic advances such as cardiovascular surgery, hemodialysis, and radiation therapy), pericardial involvement in HIV, and advances in the recognition, diagnosis, and therapy of pericarditis and its complications have resulted in a resurgence of interest in pericardial heart disease. The remainder of this chapter reviews pericarditis and its sequelae, pericardial effusions, cardiac tamponade and constrictive pericarditis, and congenital diseases of the pericardium.

ACUTE PERICARDITIS

Acute fibrinous or dry pericarditis is a syndrome characterized by typical chest pain, a pathognomonic pericardial friction rub, and specific ECG changes. A variety of conditions is associated with acute pericarditis (Table 80-2). The following description refers to viral and idiopathic pericarditis without significant effusion. Specific forms of pericardial heart disease are reviewed further on in the chapter.

TABLE 80-2 Causes of Pericardial Heart Disease

Idiopathic
Infectious
  Bacterial [*Pneumococcus, Streptococcus, Staphylococcus, Haemophilus influenzae*, gram-negative rods, *Brucella melitensis, Francisella tularensis, Legionella pneumophilia, Neisseria gonorrhoeae, Neisseria meningitidis, Borrelia burgdorferi* (Lyme disease), *Myocoplasma*]
  Viral (coxsackievirus, echovirus, adenovirus, varicella, influenza, cytomegalovirus, HIV, hepatitis B, mumps, infectious mononucleosis)
  Mycobacterial (*Mycobacterium tuberculosis, Mycobacterium avium-intracellulare*)
  Fungal (*Histoplasma, Coccidioidomycosis, Blastomyces, Candida albicans, Nocardia, Actinomyces*)
  Protozoal (*Toxoplasma, Echinococcus*, amebae)
  AIDS-associated
Neoplastic
  Primary (mesothelioma, fibrosarcoma)
  Secondary (breast, lung, melanoma, lymphoma, leukemia)
Immune/inflammatory
  Connective tissue diseases (rheumatoid arthritis, systemic lupus erythematosus, scleroderma, acute rheumatic fever, dermatomyositis, mixed connective tissue disease, Wegener's granulomatosis)
  Arteritis (temporal arteritis, polyarteritis nodosa, Takayasu's arteritis)
  Acute myocardial infarction and post-MI (Dressler's syndrome)
  Postcardiotomy
  Posttraumatic
Metabolic
  Nephrogenic
  Aortic dissection
  Myxedema
  Amyloidosis
Iatrogenic
  Radiation injury
  Instrument/device trauma (implantable defibrillators, pacemakers, catheters)
  Drugs (hydralazine, procainamide, daunorubicin, isoniazid, anticoagulants, cyclosporine, methysergide, phenytoin, dantrolene, mesalazine)
  Cardiac resuscitation
Traumatic
  Blunt trauma
  Penetrating trauma
  Surgical trauma
Congenital
  Pericardial cysts
  Congenital absence of pericardium
  Mulibrey nanism

History

Acute pericarditis typically produces sharp retrosternal pain that radiates to the trapezius ridge and is aggravated by lying down and relieved by sitting up; its onset is frequently heralded by a prodrome

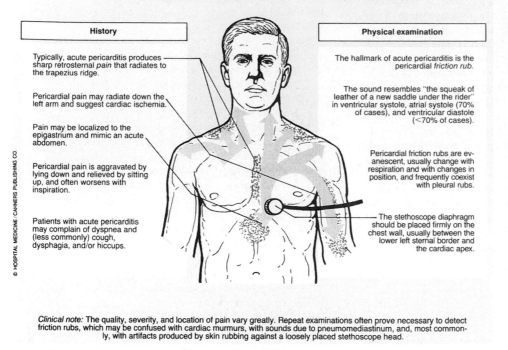

FIGURE 80-3 Clinical features of acute pericarditis: History and physical examination. (From Hoit BD. Acute pericarditis: Diagnosis and differential diagnosis. *Hosp Pract* 1991;27:23–43. Reproduced with permission.)

Physical Findings

The hallmark of acute pericarditis is the pericardial friction rub; because of its superficial, creaky, or scratchy character, it often is likened to the sound of walking on dry snow or the squeak of a leather saddle (Fig. 80-3). Rubs are heard anywhere over the precordium but most often between the lower left sternal edge and the cardiac apex; they are usually heard best with the diaphragm of the stethoscope applied firmly and with respiration suspended. Most pericardial friction rubs are independent of the respiratory cycle, but on occasion they are louder during inspiration. The pericardial rub may be confined to ventricular systole but most often includes a component during atrial systole and occasionally during ventricular diastolic filling, resulting in biphasic and triphasic rubs, respectively. Biphasic rubs must be distinguished from murmurs of mixed aortic valve disease, and monophasic rubs are often mistaken for systolic murmurs. Frequent examinations are necessary to detect a rub because of its evanescent nature; pericardial fluid does not prevent a friction rub.

of fever, malaise, and myalgia (Fig. 80-3). The pain of pericarditis is often worse with inspiration and is difficult to distinguish from pleurisy; in some cases, the pain is indistinguishable from that of myocardial infarction. The quality, severity, and location of pain vary greatly, and chest pain may be absent in acute pericarditis, especially in early pericarditis complicating myocardial infarction or cardiac surgery and in uremic pericarditis.

In uncomplicated pericarditis, the jugular venous pressure usually remains normal. Ventricular third and fourth heart sounds indicate coexisting myocardial disease. The history and physical examination are also helpful in recognizing complications and in identifying underlying diseases associated with pericarditis. Depending on the etiology, there may be fever and other signs of inflammation or systemic illness.

Electrocardiography

The ECG may either confirm the clinical suspicion of pericardial disease or first alert the clinician to the presence of pericarditis (Fig. 80-4). Serial tracings may be needed to distinguish the ST-segment elevations caused by acute pericarditis from those caused by acute myocardial infarction (MI) or normal early repolarization. The ST-T-wave changes in acute pericarditis are diffuse and have characteristic evolutionary changes. In the first stage, ST-segment elevations (which differ from ischemic ST-segment elevations by their upward concavity and seldom exceed 5 mm in height) typically occur within a few hours of the onset of chest pain and persist for hours or days. Depression of the PR segment (except in lead aVR) occurs in this stage and differentiates acute pericarditis from early

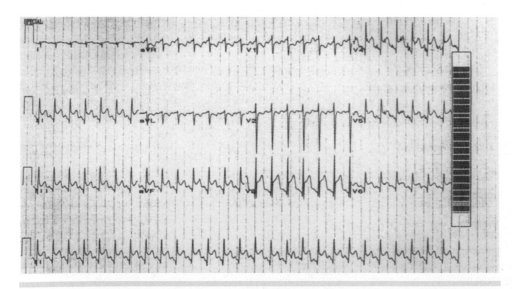

FIGURE 80-4 Twelve-lead electrocardiogram from a patient with acute pericarditis. (From Hoit BD. Pericardial disease and pericardial heart disease. In: O'Rourke RA, ed. *Stein's Internal Medicine*, 5th ed. St. Louis: Mosby-Year Book; 1998:273. Reproduced with permission.)

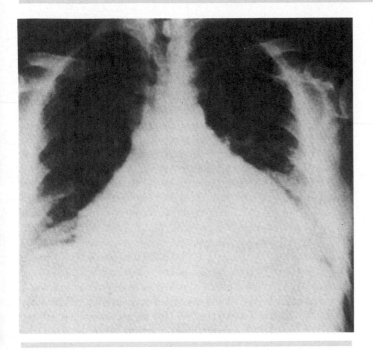

FIGURE 80-5 Chest radiograph from a patient with a large pericardial effusion. Note the "flask-shape" appearance of the cardiac silhouette. (From Hoit BD. Imaging the pericardium. *Cardiol Clin* 1990;8:588. Reproduced with permission.)

repolarization variants. In the second stage, the ST segments return to baseline; at this point, the T waves may appear normal or exhibit a loss of amplitude. In the third stage, tracings show inversion of T waves. T-wave inversions may persist indefinitely, particularly with tuberculous, uremic, or neoplastic pericarditis. The ECG normalizes in the variably present fourth stage. In a typical case of acute pericarditis, the approximate time frame for these ECG changes is 2 weeks. However, only about half of patients with acute pericarditis display all four ECG stages, and variations are very common. Atrial arrhythmias complicate 5 to 10 percent of cases of acute pericarditis.

The ST-segment elevation seen in acute pericarditis can usually be distinguished from that of acute MI by the absence of Q waves, the upwardly concave ST segments, and the absence of associated T-wave inversions. The acute ST-segment elevation of Prinzmetal's variant of angina is more transitory and is associated with ischemic pain. Although the ST-segment elevation in the early repolarization variant (common in young individuals, especially blacks, athletes, and psychiatric patients) may simulate the ECG of acute pericarditis, the former is distinguished by the absence of PR-segment depression and evolutionary ST-T-wave changes.

Imaging and Laboratory Studies

In uncomplicated acute pericarditis, the chest radiograph is generally normal. However, an enlarged cardiac silhouette may be evident because of a moderate or large pericardial effusion (Fig. 80-5). The chest radiograph may provide evidence of tuberculosis, fungal disease, pneumonia, or neoplasm.

Echocardiographic identification of pericardial effusion confirms the clinical diagnosis of acute pericarditis (Fig. 80-6), but a patient with purely fibrinous acute pericarditis often has a normal echocardiogram. Echocardiography estimates the volume of pericardial fluid, identifies cardiac tamponade, suggests the basis of pericarditis, and documents associated acute myocarditis with congestive heart failure.

Although 99m-technetium pyrophosphate scans may be positive in patients with pericarditis associated with epicarditis and gallium scans have proved useful in displaying the characteristics of purulent pericarditis, these tests are rarely used to diagnose acute pericarditis.

Nonspecific blood markers of inflammation, such as the erythrocyte sedimentation rate and the white blood cell count, usually increase in cases of acute pericarditis. Patients with extensive epicarditis occasionally have increases in serum cardiac isoenzymes suggestive of acute MI. In one series, nearly half of all patients presenting with acute, idiopathic pericarditis had increased serum troponin I levels, half of which were within the range considered diagnostic for acute myocardial infarction.[14] Although no significant

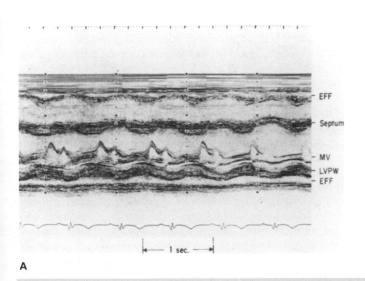

A

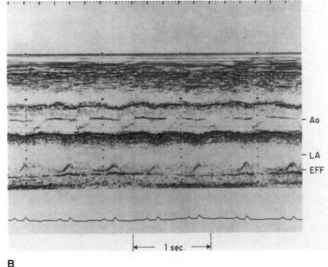

B

FIGURE 80-6 M-mode echocardiograms of pericardial effusion (EFF). *A*. The effusion appears as an echo-free space posterior to the left ventricular posterior wall (LVPW). Note that parietal pericardium has relatively flat motion throughout the cardiac cycle. MV = mitral valve. *B*. Pericardial effusion behind the left atrium (LA). Note the exaggerated motion of the posterior left atrial wall. (From Hoit BD. Imaging the pericardium. *Cardiol Clin* 1990;8:588. Reproduced with permission.)

coronary artery disease was detected in any of the patients who ultimately underwent coronary angiography, acute myocardial infarct should remain high on the differential diagnosis in this setting, as more than half of the patients with elevated troponin I presented with concurrent ST-segment elevation on ECG.

Therapy for Acute Pericarditis

Hospitalization is warranted for many patients who present with an initial episode of acute pericarditis to determine the etiology and observe for cardiac tamponade. Establishing the exact cause of acute pericarditis is an important aspect of management, but considerable judgment must be exercised in deciding whether and how to investigate the possibility of concomitant systemic disease.

An extensive evaluation is generally unnecessary in a young, previously healthy adult who presents with a viral syndrome, typical pericardial chest pain, and a pericardial friction rub. Most cases of viral pericarditis are recognized long after the period of viral activity, making a specific etiologic diagnosis and antiviral chemotherapy unnecessary. Thus, differentiating viral from idiopathic pericarditis is difficult, expensive, and generally of little practical importance. Depending on the history and symptoms at presentation, trauma, myocarditis, systemic lupus erythematosus (SLE), and/or purulent pericarditis require consideration in younger patients. In older adults, myocardial infarction, tuberculosis, and especially neoplastic disease should be considered.

Acute pericarditis usually responds to oral nonsteroidal anti-inflammatory agents [e.g., aspirin (ASA) 650 mg every 3 to 4 h or ibuprofen 600 to 800 mg every 6 h]. Indomethacin reduces coronary blood flow and theoretically should be avoided. Some data suggest that the addition of colchicine (1 mg/day) is effective for an acute episode and may prevent recurrences.[15] The intensity of therapy is dictated by the distress of the patient; narcotics may be required for severe pain. Some cases necessitate steroid therapy (prednisone 60 to 80 mg/day) for a week to control pain, with the dose tapered rapidly thereafter. Corticosteroids should be avoided unless there is a specific indication as they may enhance viral multiplication and produce recurrences when the dose is tapered; colchicine may be useful in this situation. Nevertheless, corticosteroids are useful in acute pericarditis associated with uremic pericarditis and connective tissue diseases. Importantly, tuberculous and pyogenic pericarditis should be excluded before steroid therapy is initiated.

Patients in whom pericarditis represents one manifestation of systemic illness (such as sepsis, uremia, connective tissue disease, or neoplasia) should receive therapy directed toward the primary disorder in addition to palliative and supportive treatment.

RECURRENT PERICARDITIS

Recurrent or relapsing acute pericarditis is one of the most distressing disorders of the pericardium for both patient and physician; it may occur with or without pericardial effusion and is occasionally associated with pleural effusion or parenchymal pulmonary lesions. Recurrences occur with highly variable frequency over a course of many years. The reasons for relapse are unclear, but the phenomenon suggests that acute pericarditis itself may represent or generate an autoimmune process. Recurrences may be spontaneous but more commonly are associated with discontinuation or tapering doses of anti-inflammatory drugs. When associated with pericardial effusion, relapsing pericarditis can cause cardiac tamponade; however, this is unusual.

Painful recurrences of pericarditis may respond to nonsteroidal anti-inflammatory agents but commonly require corticosteroids.

Once steroids are administered, dependency and the development of steroid-induced abnormalities are potential sequelae. Prednisone is begun at a high dose (60 to 80 mg/day), but rapid tapering should be initiated within a few days of clinical resolution. When necessary, the risks of long-term steroids should be minimized by using the lowest possible dose, alternate-day therapy, combinations with nonsteroidal drugs, or colchicine (1 to 2 mg/day). In addition to its use as an adjunct to corticosteroid therapy, colchicine may be used as monotherapy for the prevention of recurrent pericarditis. In the most difficult cases, relapse occurs every time the dose of prednisone is reduced below 5 to 20 mg/day. When this occurs, the patient should be maintained for several weeks on the lowest suppressive dose before the next taper commences. Intrapericardial administration of triamcinolone (300 mg/m^2) has been shown to relieve symptoms in patients with recurrent autoreactive myopericarditis[16]; and azathioprine (50 to 100 mg/day) has also been used to prevent recurrent episodes.[17] Two World Heart Federation studies, CIRP (Colchicine in Recurrent Pericarditis) and TRIPE (Triamcinolone in Pericardial Effusion), are presently under way to validate the effectiveness of these therapies.[18] Although encouraging results have been reported in a series of patients who underwent pericardiectomy for recurrent pericarditis, pericardiectomy may simply abbreviate rather than terminate the painful recurrences. Thus, pericardiectomy should be considered only when repeated attempts at medical treatment have clearly failed.

PERICARDIAL EFFUSION

Etiology

Accumulation of transudate, exudate, or blood in the pericardial sac, a common complication of pericardial disease, should be sought in all patients with acute pericarditis.

Pericardial effusions are reported to be associated with heart failure, valvular disease, and myocardial infarction in 14, 21, and 15 percent of cases, respectively.[19] Hydropericardium results from elevated right atrial pressure and limited venous and lymphatic drainage from the pericardium. Although this is the usual explanation for effusions associated with heart failure and LV hypertrophy, recurrent bloody effusions that can be attributed only to congestive heart failure may occur.

Pericardial effusions are very common after cardiac surgery. In 122 consecutive patients studied before and serially after cardiac surgery, effusions were present in 103 patients; the majority appeared by postoperative day 2, reached their maximum size by postoperative day 10, and usually resolved without sequelae within the first postoperative month.[20] However, large effusions or effusions causing pericardial tamponade are uncommon following cardiothoracic surgery. In one retrospective survey of over 4500 postoperative patients, only 48 were found to have moderate or large effusions by echocardiography; of those, 36 met diagnostic criteria for tamponade.[21] Use of preoperative anticoagulants, valve surgery, and female gender were all associated with a higher incidence of tamponade. Symptoms and physical findings of significant postoperative pericardial effusions are frequently nonspecific, and echocardiographic detection and echo-guided pericardiocentesis, when necessary, are safe and effective; prolonged catheter drainage reduces the recurrence rate.[22] Pericardial effusions in cardiac transplant patients are associated with an increased incidence of acute rejection.[23] Chronic effusive pericarditis is an entity of unknown etiology that may be associated with large, asymptomatic effusions. Many conditions that cause pericarditis (e.g., uremia, tuberculosis, neoplasia, connective tissue disease) produce chronic pericardial effusions.

Nature of the Pericardial Fluid

Characteristics of the pericardial fluid other than culture and cytology are usually too nonspecific to be of diagnostic value. However, in one retrospective series, one-fifth of the patients had a specific etiologic diagnosis that had implications for management and prognosis.[24] Moreover, in certain situations, it is mandatory to determine the nature of the pericardial fluid. For example, in patients with neoplastic disease, it is important to determine whether pericardial effusion indicates invasion of the pericardium or a complication of radiation therapy. Cytologic examination of the fluid is also important in cases in which the primary tumor has not been identified clearly. In cases of bacterial or other nonviral infections, it becomes necessary to discover whether the pericardial effusion is exudative and to culture pericardial fluid; this is particularly important when tuberculous or fungal pericarditis is suspected. Transudative effusions (hydropericardium) occur in heart failure and other states associated with chronic salt and water retention (including pregnancy), and exudative effusions occur in a large number of the infectious and inflammatory causes of pericarditis. Although frank hemorrhagic effusions suggest recent intrapericardial bleeding, sanguineous and serosanguineous effusions occur in many infectious and inflammatory disorders. In certain disorders, the nature of the pericardial fluid has greater diagnostic value. For example, chylous pericarditis implies injury or obstruction to the thoracic duct, and cholesterol pericarditis is either idiopathic or associated with hypothyroidism, rheumatoid arthritis, or tuberculosis.

Diagnostic Studies

The etiology of a pericardial effusion is difficult to determine on historical or clinical grounds. In one series of 322 patients admitted to a tertiary care hospital with at least moderate effusions, the cause of the effusion was attributed to a preexisting medical condition in 192 patients. In the remaining patients, those with inflammatory signs were more likely to have acute idiopathic pericarditis; those without inflammatory signs or tamponade were more likely to have chronic, idiopathic effusions; and those presenting with tamponade but without inflammatory signs were more likely to have a malignant effusion.[25]

Specific diagnoses are possible using visual, cytologic, and immunologic analysis of the pericardial effusion and pericardioscopic-guided biopsy.[19] Observations using these techniques have suggested that (1) fibrin strands and neovascularization are common in inflammatory pericardial diseases; (2) the etiology of viral pericarditis can be established by using a variety of methods, such as in situ hybridization, microneutralization, and polymerase chain reaction; (3) combined analysis of the cytology in the effusion and epicardial biopsy are most important and pericardial biopsy is often inconclusive; and (4) viral and autoreactive effusions are associated with high titers of antimy-

olemmal and antisarcolemmal antibodies and in vitro cardiocytolysis of isolated rat heart cells. Additionally, the presence of inflammatory markers such as interleukin-6, interleukin-8, and interferon gamma in pericardial fluid in the absence of these markers in the serum may help distinguish between autoreactive and lymphocytic effusions.[26] However, the clinical utility of these diagnostic methods and observations remains to be determined.

There are clinical situations in which it is unnecessary to obtain pericardial fluid for analysis. For example, when pericardial effusion is found in a patient with typical viral or idiopathic pericarditis, pericardiocentesis should not be considered unless the effusion fails to respond to anti-inflammatory treatment or cardiac tamponade develops. Similarly, when a patient undergoing chronic hemodialysis develops pericardial effusion, examination of pericardial fluid is needed only when the clinical course suggests a different etiology or when hemodynamic compromise is suspected.

IMAGING STUDIES

Echocardiography is the procedure of choice for the diagnosis of pericardial effusion. Although flask-shaped enlargement of the cardiac silhouette on chest radiography occurs with a moderate or large pericardial effusion (Fig. 80-5), differentiation of large effusions from cardiac dilatation often is difficult or impossible. In contrast, the relative contributions of cardiac enlargement and pericardial effusion to overall cardiac enlargement and the relative roles of tamponade and myocardial dysfunction to altered hemodynamics can be evaluated with echocardiography. Attention to technical detail results in excellent sensitivity and specificity. The diagnostic feature on M-mode echocardiography is the persistence of an echo-free space between parietal and visceral pericardium throughout the cardiac cycle (Fig. 80-6). Separations that are observed only in systole represent clinically insignificant accumulations. Two-dimensional (2D) echocardiography (Fig. 80-7) has superior spatial orientation and allows delineation of the size and distribution of pericardial effusion as

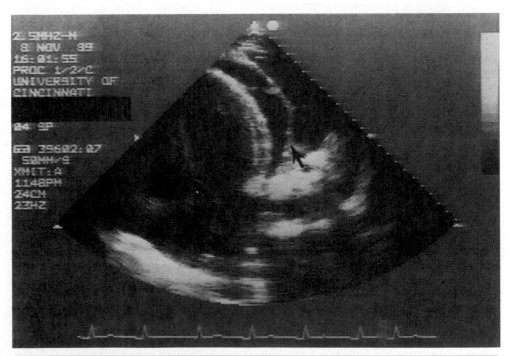

FIGURE 80-7 Two-dimensional echocardiogram from a patient with pleural and pericardial effusions. The thickness of the pericardium (*arrow*) can be appreciated in this patient. (From Hoit BD. Imaging the pericardium. *Cardiol Clin* 1990;8:596. Reproduced with permission.)

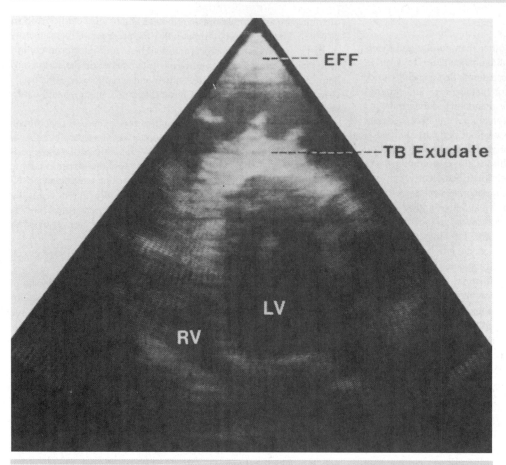

FIGURE 80-8 Two-dimensional echocardiogram from a patient with tuberculous pericarditis. Note the thickened pericardium with shaggy exudate that bridges a large pericardial effusion (EFF). (From Hoit BD. Imaging the pericardium. *Cardiol Clin* 1990;8:590. Reproduced with permission.)

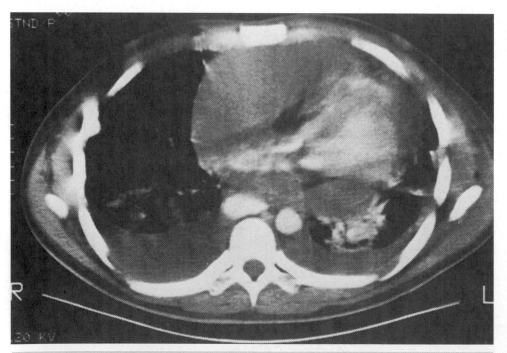

FIGURE 80-9 Computed tomographic scan from a patient with a large pericardial effusion. Note the compression of contrast-filled cardiac chambers. (From Hoit BD. Imaging the pericardium. *Cardiol Clin* 1990;8:590. Reproduced with permission.)

well as detection of loculated fluid. As the amount of pericardial fluid increases, fluid distributes from the posterobasilar LV apically and anteriorly and then laterally and posteriorly to the left atrium. Pericardial effusions are described as small, moderate, or large based on the size of the echo-free space seen between the parietal and visceral pleurae on two-dimensional echocardiography. Small effusions have an echo-free space < 5 mm, moderate sized effusions range between 5 and 10 mm, and more than 10 mm indicates a large effusion.[27] Fluid adjacent to the right atrium is an early sign of pericardial effusion. Frond-like, band-like, or shaggy intrapericardial echoes should alert one to the possibility of a difficult and potentially less therapeutic pericardiocentesis (Fig. 80-8) but have little value in identifying the cause of the effusion. Epicardial fat tissue is more prominent anteriorly but may appear circumferentially, thus mimicking effusion (lipid envelope). Fat is slightly echogenic and tends to move in concert with the heart, two characteristics that help distinguish it from an effusion, which is generally echolucent and motionless. In addition to its mimicry, pericardial fat accumulation was shown to be a coronary risk factor in a population of Japanese men.[28]

Pericardial effusions are easily detected by computed tomography (Fig. 80-9). The size, geometry, and distribution of pericardial effusions can be obtained with this technique, and the attenuation coefficients for blood, exudate, chyle, and serous fluid are generally sufficiently characteristic to identify the nature of the effusion. Computed tomography may be useful in identifying loculated and atypically loculated pericardial effusions and in guiding pericardiocentesis. Loculated and recurrent pericardial effusions can be treated safely and effectively with video-assisted thoracoscopic pericardial fenestration.[29]

Magnetic resonance imaging (MRI) detects pericardial effusion with high sensitivity and provides an estimate of pericardial fluid volume; in addition, it effectively detects loculated pericardial effusion and pericardial thickening. Inflamed pericardium and adhesions have high signal intensity relative to pericardial fluid and myocardium, providing a potential means of identifying the nature of the effusion.

Treatment of Pericardial Effusion

Drainage of a pericardial effusion is usually unnecessary unless purulent pericarditis is suspected or cardiac tamponade supervenes, although pericardiocentesis is sometimes needed to establish the etiology of a hemodynamically insignificant pericardial effusion. Persistent or progressive effusion, particularly when the cause is uncertain, also warrants pericardiocentesis. However, routine drainage of a large pericardial effusion without tamponade or suspected purulent pericarditis has a low diagnostic yield and no clear therapeutic benefit.[30] Anticoagulants should be discontinued temporarily, if possible, to reduce the risk of cardiac tamponade. In patients on chronic oral anticoagulation, heparin should be used, since its effect can be reversed rapidly. Large effusions may respond to nonsteroidal antiinflammatory drugs, corticosteroids, or colchicine.[15] Specific treatment for pericardial effusion is considered below.

CARDIAC TAMPONADE

Cardiac tamponade is a hemodynamic condition characterized by equal elevation of atrial and pericardial pressures, an exaggerated inspiratory decrease in arterial systolic pressure (pulsus paradoxus), and arterial hypotension. Arterial hypotension is generally a late sign in chronic effusions, and occasionally a heightened sympathoadrenal state produces systemic hypertension. As intrapericardial pressure rises, venous pressures increase to maintain cardiac filling and prevent collapse of the cardiac chambers. Although the absolute intracardiac pressures are elevated, the transmural pressures—i.e., cavitary diastolic pressure minus pericardial pressure—are practically zero or even negative. The greatly reduced preload is responsible for the fall in cardiac output, and when compensatory mechanisms are exhausted, arterial pressure decreases.

Clinical Features

Cardiac tamponade may be acute or chronic and should be viewed hemodynamically as a continuum ranging from mild (pericardial pressure lower than 10 mmHg) to severe (pericardial pressure higher than 15 to 20 mmHg). Mild cardiac tamponade is frequently asymptomatic, whereas moderate tamponade and especially severe tamponade produce precordial discomfort and dyspnea.

Tamponade may be so sudden that the patient does not complain of symptoms; in less drastic circumstances, patients with acute cardiac tamponade may complain of severe shortness of breath accompanied by chest tightness and dizziness. The venous pressure is greatly elevated, and the systemic arterial pressure is severely depressed. Pulsus paradoxus can usually be appreciated but may be absent when hypotension is extreme. In striking contrast to the elevation of venous pressure, arterial hypotension, and pulsus paradoxus, cardiac pulsations often are impalpable (Beck's triad). In the most severe cases, consciousness may be impaired, and except for the raised venous pressure, such patients appear to be in hypovolemic shock.

When cardiac tamponade complicates a diagnostic procedure, vague discomfort, generalized uneasiness, and precordial pain are common. Fluoroscopy shows an enlarged cardiac silhouette and diminished pulsations.

Cardiac tamponade should be suspected in a victim of recent chest trauma who appears to be in shock, especially when the venous pressure is elevated. When circumstances are deemed life-threatening, an immediate therapeutic trial of rapid infusion of fluid and diagnostic pericardiocentesis should be attempted. Otherwise, pericardiocentesis should be delayed until the presence of significant pericardial fluid can be demonstrated by prompt echocardiography. An exception to this rule occurs when tamponade complicates diagnostic procedures; in this instance, when pressures are being monitored and fluoroscopy is available, the diagnosis can safely be established without echocardiographic confirmation.

Other causes of acute tamponade are cardiac rupture complicating acute MI and rupture of a dissecting hematoma of the proximal aorta. Although successful pericardiocentesis may relieve aortic tamponade and increase hemorrhage, a limited pericardiocentesis is reasonable if cardiac tamponade is severe enough to be considered a threat to survival. Cardiac tamponade is an uncommon but potentially lethal complication of percutaneous coronary intervention. In one review of over 25,000 interventions at a single center over a 7-year period, the incidence of tamponade was only 0.12 percent, but the in-hospital mortality rate was 42 percent.[31] The use of atheroablative therapy was associated with a higher incidence of tamponade than angioplasty and stenting alone. Finally, after cardiac surgery, dyspnea and fatigue should raise the suspicion of tamponade; in these instances, the effusion is often loculated, and echocardiographic and hemodynamic findings may be unreliable.

A large number of diseases may be associated with more slowly developing cardiac tamponade. In these instances, symptoms may be due to the underlying illness, the culpable pericardial disease, and/or the tamponade itself. Many patients with inflammatory pericarditis give a history of prodromal fever, myalgia, and arthralgia, and patients with neoplastic disease may have symptoms associated with the neoplasm and its treatment. The symptoms of cardiac compression include rapidly progressive dyspnea accompanied by fullness or tightness in the chest, occasionally with dysphagia; pericardial pain is often absent. The course may be less rapid, allowing time for an increase in abdominal girth and the rapid onset and progression of edema.

Pathophysiology

Elevated intrapericardial pressure exerted on the heart throughout the cardiac cycle, with only slight momentary relief when intrapericardial pressure falls (owing to the decrease in cardiac volume during ventricular ejection), is responsible for the pathophysiologic findings of cardiac tamponade. To understand the relation between venous and pericardial pressures in cardiac tamponade, it is useful to review the normal biphasic pattern of venous return. A surge of venous return at the onset of ventricular ejection is accompanied by a small reduction in intrapericardial pressure. A second surge of venous return occurs in early diastole, when the tricuspid valve opens and atrial pressure decreases. In contrast, the venous return in cardiac tamponade is unimodal and is confined to ventricular systole; in severe cardiac tamponade, venous return is halted in diastole, at a time when cardiac volume and intrapericardial pressure are maximal. Pericardial pressure and right atrial pressure are elevated above normal and are equal to each other (Fig. 80-10). The inspiratory fall in intrathoracic pressure is transmitted to the pericardial space, which preserves the normal inspiratory increase in systemic venous return (Kussmaul's sign is absent).

Although systolic ventricular function is often supernormal, unrelieved extreme tamponade becomes fatal when venous pressure cannot increase to equal the pericardial pressure and maintain circulation. In severe cases, diminution of myocardial perfusion is aggravated by direct compression of the epicardial coronary arteries, abnormal transmyocardial distribution of blood flow, and, as a result, impaired ventricular systolic function.

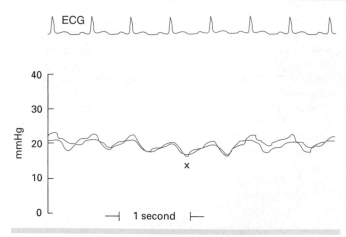

FIGURE 80-10 Simultaneous right atrial and pericardial pressures from a patient with severe cardiac tamponade. The pressures are elevated and equal to one another, and only the X descent on the right atrial tracing is present; the Y descent is absent. The pressures fall normally during inspiration. (From Shabetai R. Diseases of the pericardium. In: Alexander WA, Schlant R, Fuster V, et al., eds. *Hurst's The Heart,* 9th ed. New York: McGraw-Hill; 1998:2179. Reproduced with permission.)

PULSUS PARADOXUS

In healthy individuals, systolic blood pressure may decline by as much as 10 mmHg during quiet inspiration. Pulsus paradoxus is an exaggeration of this normal physiologic response. A number of normal and abnormal mechanisms combine to create pulsus paradoxus in cardiac tamponade. Inspiratory augmentation of systemic venous return in cardiac tamponade increases the volume of the right side of the heart at the expense of the left side. The volume of the left side of the heart is decreased, in part by bulging of the intraventricular septum from right to left (changing the size, shape, and compliance of the LV) and in part by increased transmural pericardial pressure (decreasing pulmonary venous return). However, the inspiratory expansion of the volume of the right side of the heart and the transit time of the resulting augmented right heart stroke volume are important in the genesis of pulsus paradoxus. In addition, the negative thoracic pressure produced by inspiration is transmitted to the aorta, increasing LV afterload and reducing stroke volume. LV stroke volume falls more sharply than normal in response to decreased ventricular filling in cardiac tamponade because the small ventricle is operating on the steep ascending limb of the Starling curve. Finally, inspiratory traction by the diaphragm on the taut pericardium, reflex changes in vascular resistance and cardiac contractility, and increased respiratory effort owing to pulmonary congestion contribute to the genesis of pulsus paradoxus.

Pulsus paradoxus appears when both ventricles fill against a common resistance. Therefore, when LV diastolic pressure is elevated by coexisting LV disease, pulsus paradoxus does not develop in cardiac tamponade.[32] Similarly, atrial septal defects and aortic regurgitation prevent reciprocal inspiratory changes in the filling of the two sides of the heart; therefore, in these conditions, cardiac tamponade can occur without pulsus paradoxus.[33]

Physical Findings

Physical findings are dictated by both the severity of cardiac tamponade and the time course of its development. Careful inspection of the jugular venous pulse waveform is essential for the diagnosis, although the venous pressure may be normal in early tamponade,

whereas extreme elevations of venous pressure may go unrecognized in a recumbent or semirecumbent patient. Compression of the heart by pericardial fluid results in a characteristic loss of the atrial Y descent, but because of the decrease in intrapericardial pressure that occurs during ventricular ejection, the systolic atrial filling wave and the X descent are maintained. Kussmaul's sign, a failure of venous pressure to decrease during inspiration, is a sign of constriction and is generally not seen in pure cardiac tamponade.

An inspiratory decline of systolic arterial pressure exceeding 10 mmHg (pulsus paradoxus) may be detected with palpation of an arterial pulse, such as the femoral or brachial artery, and quantified by using sphygmomanometry by subtracting the pressure at which Korotkoff's sounds are heard only during expiration from the pressure at which sounds are heard through the respiratory cycle. The origin of the paradoxical pulse is complex and multifactorial, and pulsus paradoxus is neither sensitive nor specific for cardiac tamponade.[33] Nevertheless, in the appropriate clinical setting, pulsus paradoxus is a key finding that signifies cardiac tamponade, and its presence should be sought diligently.

Diagnostic and Imaging Studies

Low voltage on the ECG and/or electrical alternans should suggest cardiac tamponade. However, electrical alternans is insensitive, occurring in only about 20 percent of instances. When effusion is massive, the heart swings freely within the pericardial sac and acquires a pendular, rotary motion that is associated with electrical alternans. When tamponade is suspected, an echocardiogram should be obtained unless even a brief delay might prove life-threatening. During inspiration, a greater than normal increase in RV dimension and decrease in LV dimension occur in many cases of tamponade. These respiratory changes also accompany other conditions associated with pulsus paradoxus, such as chronic obstructive pulmonary disease and pulmonary embolism. Diastolic collapse of the RV, which is recognized as an abnormal posterior motion of the anterior RV wall during diastole (Fig. 80-11), signifies that pericardial pressure exceeds early diastolic RV pressure—i.e., that transmural RV diastolic pressure is negative (see also Chap. 13). Although this sign is a relatively sensitive and specific marker for tamponade, RV diastolic collapse is sensitive to alterations in ventricular loading conditions and may not be seen in the presence of RV hypertrophy. In addition, collapse of the right heart chamber occurs with smaller collections of fluid and higher pericardial pressures when there is coexisting LV dysfunction.[32] Late diastolic right atrial collapse is virtually 100 percent sensitive for tamponade but is less specific (Fig. 80-12). Duration of right atrial collapse exceeding one-third of the cardiac cycle increases specificity without sacrificing sensitivity. Posterior loculated effusions after cardiac surgery have been reported to produce left atrial and LV diastolic collapse.[34] Transesophageal echocardiography may be valuable in the detection and treatment of unusual cases of cardiac tamponade. In patients with unexplained hypotension who are undergoing transesophageal echocardiography, a diagnosis of a nonventricular limitation to cardiac output was associated with improved survival in the intensive care unit compared with a diagnosis of ventricular disease or hypovolemia/low systemic vascular resistance.[35]

During cardiac tamponade, tricuspid and pulmonary flow velocities measured by Doppler echocardiography (Fig. 80-13) increase markedly with inspiration, and flow velocities in the mitral and aortic valves decrease significantly compared with normal control patients and patients with asymptomatic effusions. Changes in the pattern of venous flow (reflecting the predominance of systolic flow) and exag-

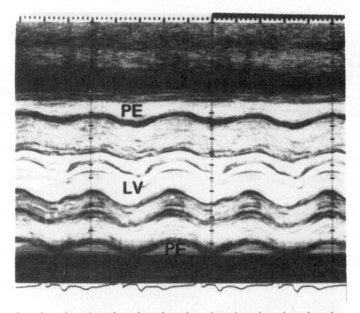

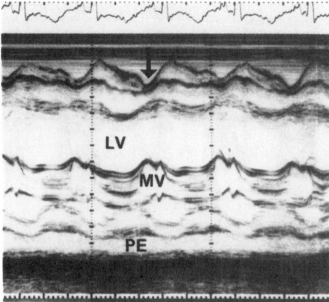

FIGURE 80-11 M-mode echocardiograms of pericardial effusion. The effusion (PE) appears as an echo-free space surrounding the heart. The effusion on the left does not cause cardiac compression. The effusion on the right demonstrates right ventricular diastolic collapse *(arrow)*, evident as abnormal motion of the anterior free wall of the right ventricle that occurs after the mitral valve (MV) opens. LV = left ventricle. (From Hoit BD. Pericardial disease and pericardial heart disease. In: O'Rourke RA, ed. *Stein's Internal Medicine*, 5th ed. St. Louis: Mosby-Year Book; 1998:273. Reproduced with permission.)

gerated respiratory variations of venous flow velocities (Fig. 80-14) are also seen in cardiac tamponade.[36] Indeed, abnormal venous flow had a good correlation with clinical tamponade, with greater sensitivity than RV diastolic collapse and greater specificity than right atrial collapse.[37]

Cardiac Catheterization

The diagnosis of cardiac tamponade is confirmed by right heart catheterization. The right atrial, pulmonary capillary wedge, and pulmonary artery diastolic pressures are elevated, usually between 10 and 30 mmHg, and are equal within 4 to 5 mmHg (Fig. 80-15). Pericardial pressure is elevated and is equal to right atrial pressure; the degree of elevation is related to both the severity of tamponade and the patient's intravascular volume status (Fig. 80-16). The right atrial and wedge pressure tracings reveal an attenuated or absent Y descent. Cardiac output is reduced, and systemic vascular resistance is elevated. Equal elevation of diastolic pressures may also be seen with dilated cardiomyopathy and with RV infarction. Neither Kussmaul's sign nor the early ventricular diastolic dip and plateau (i.e., the "square root" sign) characteristic of pericardial constriction is seen in tamponade.

Management of Cardiac Tamponade

Removal of small amounts of pericardial fluid (about 50 mL) produces considerable symptomatic and hemodynamic improvement because of the steep pericardial pressure-volume relation. Unless there is concomitant cardiac disease or coexisting constriction (i.e., effusive-constrictive pericarditis), removal of all the pericardial fluid

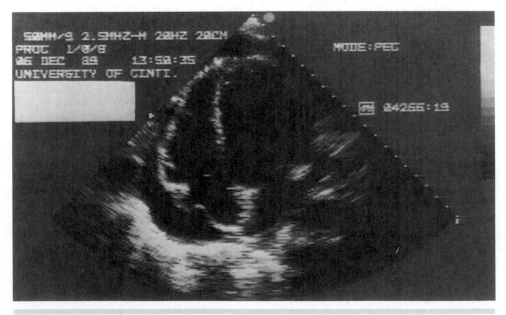

FIGURE 80-12 Two-dimensional echocardiogram in the apical four-chamber view. During late diastole, there is inversion of the lateral wall of the right atrium. (From Hoit BD. Imaging the pericardium. *Cardiol Clin* 1990;8:593. Reproduced with permission.)

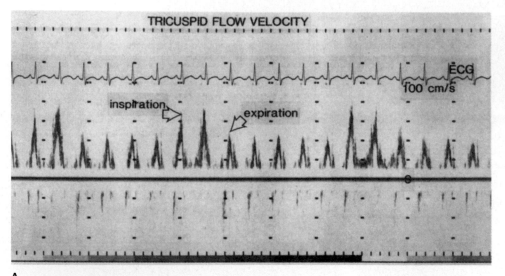

A

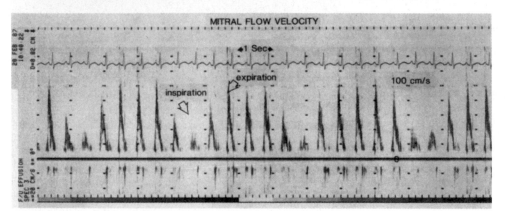

B

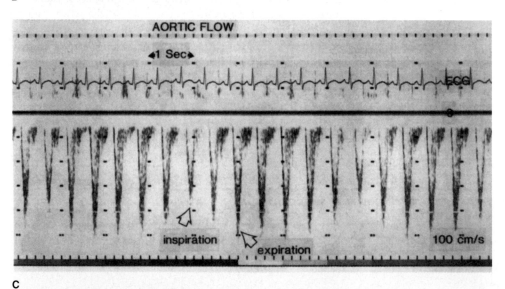

C

FIGURE 80-13 Doppler echocardiogram in a patient with cardiac tamponade. Note the inspiratory increase of tricuspid flow velocities (*A*) and the expiratory increase of mitral (*B*) and aortic (*C*) flow velocities. (From Hoit BD. Imaging the pericardium. *Cardiol Clin* 1990;8:594. Reproduced with permission.)

normalizes pericardial, atrial, ventricular diastolic, and arterial pressures and cardiac output. Unless the situation is immediately life-threatening, pericardiocentesis should be performed by experienced staff in a facility equipped for hemodynamic monitoring. The advantages of needle pericardiocentesis include the ability to perform careful hemodynamic measurements and relatively simple logistic and personnel requirements. The safety of the procedure has been improved by using 2D echo guidance, with one center reporting no significant complications in 53 cases using a probe-mounted needle.[38] A catheter can be advanced over a guidewire into the pericardial space and remain there for several days; sclerosing agents, steroids, urokinase, and specific chemotherapeutic agents may be given through the catheter. Cisplatin instillation (30 mg/m^2 for 24 h) safely prevented recurrence of pericardial effusion (93 percent at 3 months, 83 percent at 6 months) in 42 patients with neoplastic effusion; patients with lung cancer fared better than those with breast cancer.[39] Although pericardiocentesis may provide effective relief, percutaneous balloon pericardiotomy, subxiphoid pericardiotomy, or the surgical creation of a pleuropericardial or peritoneal-pericardial window [40,41] may be required. Nevertheless, in one retrospective review, pericardiocentesis with intrapericardial sclerotherapy was as effective as an open surgical drainage procedure in patients with malignant pericardial effusion.[42] The feasibility and accuracy of three-dimensional computer-assisted pericardiocentesis was recently described in the experimental laboratory.[43]

Open surgical drainage offers several advantages, including complete drainage, access to pericardial tissue for histopathologic and microbiologic diagnoses, the ability to drain loculated effusions, and the absence of traumatic injury resulting from blind placement of a needle into the pericardial sac. The choice between needle pericardiocentesis and surgical drainage depends on institutional resources and physician experience, the etiology of the effusion, the need for diagnostic tissue samples, and the prognosis of the patient. Needle pericardiocentesis is often the best option when the etiology is known and/or the

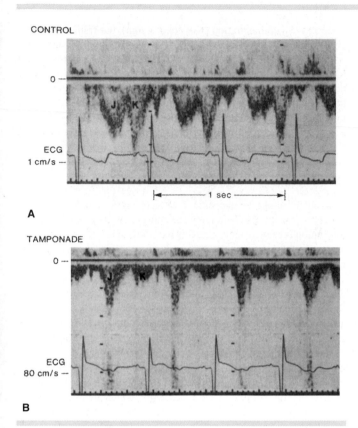

A

B

FIGURE 80-14 Doppler echocardiograms of pulmonary venous flow velocity from a dog before (A) and after (B) creation of cardiac tamponade. Note the predominance of systolic flow after tamponade. J = systolic flow; K = diastolic flow on control flow velocity (A). (From Hoit BD. Imaging the pericardium. *Cardiol Clin* 1990;8:595. Reproduced with permission.)

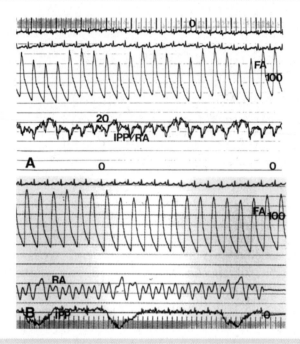

FIGURE 80-15 Hemodynamic record from a patient with cardiac tamponade before (A) and after (B) pericardiocentesis. A. Pulsus paradoxus is evident from the femoral artery (FA) pressure tracing. Note the absent Y descent on the right atrial (RA) tracing and the equal and elevated RA and pericardial (IPP) pressures. B. After removal of pericardial fluid, pericardial and right atrial pressures decrease and the pulsus paradoxus disappears. (Courtesy of Noble O Fowler, MD. From Hoit BD. Pericardial disease and pericardial heart disease. In: O'Rourke RA, ed. *Stein's Internal Medicine*, 5th ed. St. Louis: Mosby-Year Book;1998:273. Reproduced with permission.)

diagnoses of tamponade is in question, and surgical drainage is optimal when the presence of tamponade is certain but the etiology is unclear. It should be recognized that surgical approaches (subxiphoid pericardiotomy and thoracoscopic drainage) can be performed using local anesthesia with little attendant morbidity. Irrespective of the method of retrieval, pericardial fluid should be sent for smear, culture, and cytology.

Fluids should be given to patients with cardiac tamponade who are awaiting pericardial drainage, in an effort to expand the intravascular volume. Dobutamine or nitroprusside may be used to increase cardiac output after the blood volume has been expanded, but only as a temporizing measure. Vagal reflexes complicating tamponade and pericardiocentesis are treated with atropine. Positive-pressure breathing should be avoided, and metabolic acidosis, if present, should be corrected.

Recurrent effusions may be treated by repeat pericardiocentesis, sclerotherapy with tetracycline, surgical creation of a pericardial window, or pericardiectomy. A pericardial window is usually created in patients with malignant effusions, and pericardiectomy may be required for recurrent effusions in dialysis patients. The approach to surgical pericardiectomy depends on the clinical scenario.[44] In acute life-threatening situations, in high-risk patients, or for diagnostic purposes, the subxiphoid approach is generally used. For primarily effusive disease, a left anterior thoracotomy is generally performed, whereas a median sternotomy is the incision of choice with constrictive disease. Video-assisted thoracoscopic pericardiectomy (VATS) is an alternative to open thoracotomy, but it requires general anesthesia and single-lung ventilation and is therefore not suitable for patients with poor pulmonary reserve. In critically ill patients, a pericardial window may be created percutaneously with a balloon catheter.[45]

CONSTRICTIVE PERICARDITIS

Constrictive pericarditis is a condition in which a thickened, scarred, and often calcified pericardium limits diastolic filling of the ventricles. Although acute pericarditis from most causes may eventuate in constrictive pericarditis, the most common antecedents are idiopathic conditions, cardiac trauma and surgery, tuberculosis and other infectious diseases, neoplasms (particularly lung and breast), radiation therapy, renal failure, and connective tissue diseases. Rare causes include Dressler's syndrome, sarcoidosis, Whipple's disease, amyloidosis, and dermatomyositis. "Mulibrey" nanism is a hereditary form of constrictive pericarditis that is associated with abnormalities of the *mu*scle, *li*ver, *br*ain, and *ey*es.

Clinical Features

Constrictive pericarditis resembles the congestive states caused by myocardial disease and chronic liver disease. Patients generally complain of fatigue, dyspnea, weight gain, abdominal discomfort, nausea, increased abdominal girth, and edema. Although symptoms usually develop over years, they progress over a period of months in patients with subacute constrictive pericarditis after trauma, cardiac surgery, and mediastinal irradiation and may develop acutely and resolve spontaneously during the course of pericarditis.

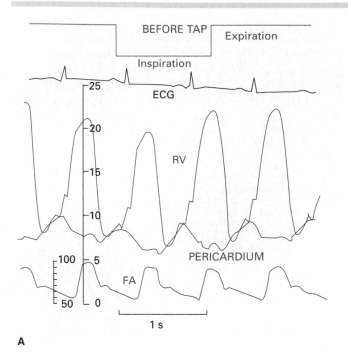

A

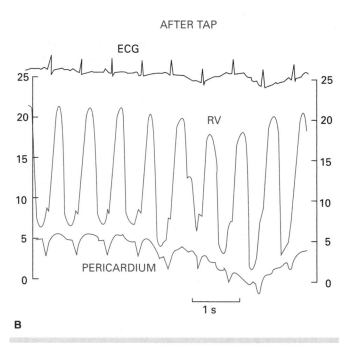

B

FIGURE 80-16 *A.* Low-pressure cardiac tamponade. Right ventricular (RV) diastolic pressure is only slightly elevated but is equal to pericardial pressure. Hypotension and pulsus paradoxus are absent. *B.* After pericardiocentesis, pericardial pressure is consistently lower than ventricular diastolic pressure. (From Shabetai R. Diseases of the pericardium. In: Alexander WA, Schlant R, Fuster V, et al, eds. *Hurst's The Heart,* 9th ed. New York: McGraw-Hill; 1998:2185. Reproduced with permission.)

Physical Findings

Physical findings include ascites, hepatosplenomegaly, edema, and, in long-standing cases, severe wasting. This general appearance often leads to an erroneous diagnosis of hepatic cirrhosis. However, misdiagnosis is avoided through a careful examination of the neck veins. In constrictive pericarditis, the venous pressure is elevated and displays deep Y and often deep X descents. The venous pressure fails

to decrease with inspiration (Kussmaul's sign), but frank inspiratory swelling of the neck veins is uncommon. Kussmaul's sign lacks specificity, as it is seen also in cases of restrictive cardiomyopathy, RV failure and infarction, and tricuspid stenosis. The heart is often normal in size; when it is not, enlargement is modest. A pericardial knock that is similar in timing to the third heart sound is pathognomonic but occurs infrequently. Pulsus paradoxus may occur with associated pericardial effusion (effusive-constrictive pericarditis). Except in severe cases, the arterial blood pressure is normal.

Diagnostic and Imaging Studies

Low QRS voltage, nonspecific T-wave changes, and P mitrale are common, but the ECG findings are nonspecific (Fig. 80-17). Atrial fibrillation is seen in approximately one-third of cases, and atrial flutter is seen less often, although the exact percentage of atrial arrhythmias depends on the duration of constriction.

The cardiac silhouette may be normal or enlarged. Pericardial calcification is present in less than half the cases seen in the United States and Europe. Pericardial calcification may be seen with chronic adhesive pericarditis in the absence of constriction, but then it is usually less dense and has a more patchy distribution (Fig. 80-18).

Pericardial thickening and calcification and abnormal ventricular filling produce characteristic changes on the M-mode echocardiogram. Increased pericardial thickness is suggested by parallel motion of the epicardium and parietal pericardium, which are separated by a relatively echo-free space at least 1 mm thick. Echocardiographic correlates of the hemodynamic abnormalities of constrictive pericarditis include flattening of the LV posterior wall endocardium, abnormal septal motion, and occasionally premature opening of the pulmonary valve (Fig. 80-19). These findings, which reflect abnormal filling of the ventricles, are insensitive and subtle and lack the specificity to be clinically useful. Although no sign or combination of signs on M-mode echocardiography is diagnostic of constrictive pericarditis, a normal study virtually rules out the diagnosis.

More recently, Doppler tissue imaging (DTI) has been used in the diagnosis of constrictive pericarditis, and may be particularly useful in differentiating between constrictive pericarditis and restrictive cardiomyopathy (see Chap. 68). The myocardial velocity gradient of the LV posterior wall is significantly lower during rapid ventricular filling and ejection in patients with restrictive cardiomyopathy than in healthy controls or in individuals with constrictive pericarditis.[46] Mitral annular velocity is also reduced in patients with restrictive cardiomyopathy compared to those with constrictive pericarditis, and this relationship is evident in the absence of significant respiratory variation in early diastolic filling—a prominent feature of constrictive pericarditis.[47] Computed tomography (CT) is a highly accurate method of evaluating pericardial thickness and therefore plays an essential role in the diagnosis and management of constrictive disease (Fig. 80-20). The normal pericardium is identified as a 1- to 2-mm curvilinear line of soft tissue density, whereas in constrictive pericarditis, the parietal pericardium is 4 to 20 mm thick. Failure to visualize the posterolateral LV wall on dynamic CT suggests myocardial fibrosis or atrophy and is associated with a poor surgical outcome. Because of the close physiologic similarities of constrictive pericarditis and restrictive cardiomyopathy, increased pericardial thickness detected by tomographic scanning is the most reliable means of distinguishing between the two disorders, as normal pericardial thickness excludes most cases of constrictive pericarditis. CT also is useful in planning pericardiectomy because of its ability to define the distribution of pericardial thickening.[48]

Accurate definition of pericardial thickness and its distribution also is possible with MRI (Fig. 80-21).[49] Unlike CT, ECG gating is necessary for adequate visualization, resolution is not quite as good, and calcification is difficult to distinguish from fibrosis. However, excellent diagnostic accuracy in identifying surgically confirmed constrictive pericarditis has been reported.[50] Preliminary studies suggest that phase velocity mapping techniques may provide additional diagnostic information, analogous to Doppler echo.

Cardiac Catheterization

Cardiac catheterization is used to confirm the clinical suspicion of pericardial disease, uncover occult constriction, diagnose effusive-constrictive disease, and identify associated coronary, myocardial, and valvular disease. Endomyocardial biopsy is sometimes necessary to exclude restrictive cardiomyopathy, which shares many hemodynamic abnormalities with constrictive pericarditis.

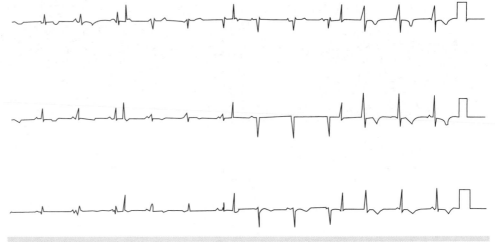

FIGURE 80-17 Electrocardiogram of a patient with tuberculous constrictive pericarditis showing widespread inversed polarity of the T waves. Leads are mounted in the conventional sequence. (From Shabetai R. Diseases of the pericardium. In: Alexander WA, Schlant R, Fuster V, et al, eds. *Hurst's The Heart,* 9th ed. New York: McGraw-Hill; 1998:2188. Reproduced with permission.)

Differences between Constrictive Pericarditis and Cardiac Tamponade

The waveform of venous pressure in constrictive pericarditis differs from that in cardiac tamponade. In constrictive pericarditis, cardiac volume is determined by the thickened, rigid pericardium, and the heart is unable to exceed this volume, which is attained near the end of the first third of diastole. During ejection, venous return commences unimpeded; therefore the normal systolic surge of venous return is preserved. Cardiac compression remains insignificant at end systole (unlike cardiac tamponade), so that when the tricuspid valve

opens, blood fills the ventricles at a supernormal rate. Thus, in constrictive pericarditis, the venous return is biphasic, but with a diastolic component greater than or equal to the systolic component.

Unlike the case in cardiac tamponade, the intrapericardial space is obliterated in constrictive pericarditis. As a result, during inspiration, the decreased intrathoracic pressure is not transmitted to the heart, venous pressure does not fall, and systemic venous return fails to increase. Another important distinction from cardiac tamponade is that early diastolic filling is faster than normal in constrictive pericarditis; consequently, the ventricular diastolic pressure is characterized by a dip in early diastole (Fig. 80-22). By the end of the rapid filling phase, the ventricles are completely filled and the ventricular diastolic pressure remains unchanged and elevated for the remainder of diastole.

In contrast to cardiac tamponade, early diastolic filling in constrictive pericarditis is unrestrained, and only at the end of the first third of diastole does the stiff pericardium abruptly restrict ventricular filling. As a result, ventricular pressure falls rapidly in early diastole and subsequently rises abruptly to an elevated level, where it remains until the next ventricular systole. End-diastolic ventricular pressures and mean atrial pressures are elevated and nearly equal (within 5 mmHg), and end-diastolic volumes and, consequently, stroke volume and cardiac output are reduced. These pathophysiologic changes are responsible for the hemodynamic and physical findings that characterize constrictive pericarditis.

Pulsus paradoxus is much less common in constrictive pericarditis than it is in cardiac tamponade because, in constrictive pericarditis, inspiratory increases in venous return and in the volume of the right side of the heart seldom occur, and the position of the ventricular septum relative to the two ventricles is not as dramatically altered. Systolic LV function is usually unimpaired in both constrictive pericarditis and cardiac tamponade. Long-standing calcific constrictive pericarditis may invade the myocardium and coronary vessels, leading to conduction disturbances and impaired ventricular function.

Syndromes of Constrictive Pericarditis

Classic *chronic constrictive pericarditis* is encountered less frequently than it was in the past, whereas *subacute constrictive pericarditis* is becoming more common. In the latter syndrome, pericardial calcification is uncommon and the course may span a matter of

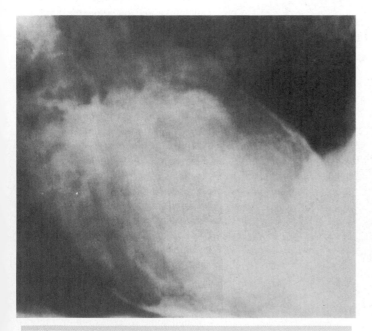

FIGURE 80-18 Calcification of the pericardium seen on a lateral chest radiograph in a patient with chronic constrictive pericarditis. (Courtesy of Ralph Shabetai, MD. From Hoit BD. Imaging the pericardium. *Cardiol Clin* 1990;8:595. Reproduced with permission.)

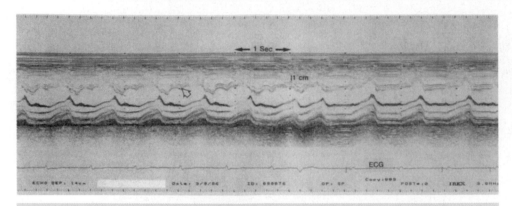

FIGURE 80-19 M-mode echocardiogram from a patient with constrictive pericarditis. An abrupt posterior motion of the septum begins after the onset of atrial systole. This atrial systolic notch is not seen on premature or paced beats. Note also the thickened pericardium and flat posterior wall in middle and late diastole. (From Tei C, Child JS, Tanaka H, et al. Atrial systolic notch on the interventricular septum echogram: An echocardiographic sign of constrictive pericarditis. *J Am Coll Cardiol* 1983;1:908. Reproduced with permission.)

weeks to a few years. *Postoperative constrictive pericarditis* is an important cause of constriction, with a reported incidence of 0.2 percent[51]; this incidence is surprisingly low considering that the pericardium is subject to cellular injury and is exposed to proinflammatory substances such as blood and local hypothermia.

Occult constrictive pericarditis requires a fluid challenge for detection. In the first series reported, the patients complained of nondescript chest pain, for which they underwent cardiac catheterization and coronary arteriography. Although hemodynamic studies revealed normal basal atrial and ventricular pressures, the right atrial pressure waveform assumed the characteristics of constrictive pericarditis and the diastolic pressures in the two ventricles became equal after a

rapid infusion (10 min) of approximately 1 L of saline solution. Histologic examination confirmed the surgical findings of a thickened and fibrosed pericardium. Rapid, large fluid challenges at cardiac catheterization should be administered with caution; furthermore, the induction of hemodynamic changes suggesting constrictive pericarditis using this technique should seldom if ever be taken alone as an indication for pericardiectomy.

Localized constrictive pericarditis is rare, but occasionally a localized band constricts the inflow or outflow region of one or more of the cardiac chambers. The clinical picture then simulates valve disease or venous obstruction. Evidence of *transient (acute) constriction* may occur in about 15 percent of patients with acute effusive pericarditis.[52] Therefore, before one proceeds with pericardiectomy, the possibility that pericardial constriction may be reversible and amenable to medical therapy should be considered.

Management of Constrictive Pericarditis

Pericardiectomy is the definitive treatment for constrictive pericarditis but is unwarranted either in very early constriction or in severe, advanced disease (functional class IV), when the risk of surgery is excessive (30 to 40 percent mortality) and the benefits are diminished.[53] Involvement of the visceral pericardium also increases the surgical risk. Symptomatic relief and normalization of cardiac pressures may take several months after pericardiectomy; they occur sooner when the operation is carried out before the disease is too chronic and when the pericardiectomy is almost complete. Complete or extensive pericardial resection is desirable, as recurrences may be seen more frequently in patients who have undergone partial versus complete resection of the pericardium. However, data suggest that in some instances, subtotal pericardiectomy may be preferred.[54] In highly selected patients, orthotopic transplantation may be considered. Constriction may be transitory with a course lasting weeks to a few months in patients recovering from acute effusive pericarditis. In these patients, the procedure should be delayed until it is clear that the constrictive process is not transitory.

Pericardiectomy is commonly carried out via a median sternotomy, although some surgeons prefer a thoracotomy. Despite a decline in the risk of mortality, it remains 5 to 15 percent. The risk is increased by heavy calcifi-

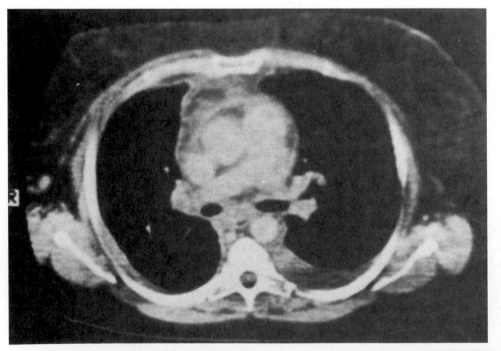

FIGURE 80-20 Computed tomogram from a patient with constrictive pericarditis. The diffusely thickened pericardium is bordered by low-intensity epicardial and mediastinal fat. (Courtesy of Dr. N. O. Fowler. From Hoit BD. Imaging the pericardium. *Cardiol Clin* 1990;8:597. Reproduced with permission.)

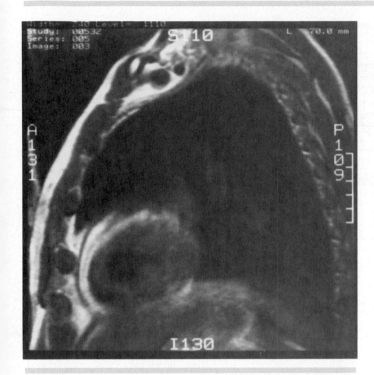

FIGURE 80-21 MRI scan (spin-echo image) from a patient with constrictive pericarditis. The pericardium is viewed as a line of low signal intensity (*black*) sandwiched between higher-intensity epicardial and pericardial fat (*white*). Note the regional variation of pericardial thickness, which is normally 1 to 2 mm. (From Hoit BD. Pericardial disease and pericardial heart disease. In: O'Rourke RA, ed. *Stein's Internal Medicine*, 5th ed. St. Louis: Mosby-Year Book; 1998:273. Reproduced with permission.)

cation and involvement of the visceral pericardium. LV systolic dysfunction may occur after decortication of a severely constricted heart. Although this condition may require treatment for several months, it usually resolves completely.

Recent data suggest that despite reduced perioperative mortality, the late survival of contemporary patients after pericardiectomy is inferior to that of an age- and sex-matched group of historical controls. The long-term outcome was predicted by three variables in a recent stepwise logistic regression analysis; specifically, the prognosis was worse with increasing age and New York Heart Association (NYHA) class and a postirradiation etiology.[55]

Medical therapy of constrictive pericarditis plays a small but important role. In some patients, constrictive pericarditis resolves either spontaneously or in response to various combinations of nonsteroidal anti-inflammatory drugs, steroids, and antibiotics. Antibiotic therapy should be initiated before surgery and continued afterward. Diuretics and digoxin (in the presence of atrial fibrillation) are useful in patients who are not candidates for pericardiectomy because of their high surgical risk. Preoperative diuretics should be used sparingly with the goal of reducing, not eliminating, elevated jugular pressure, edema, and ascites. Postoperatively, diuretics should be given if spontaneous diuresis does not occur; the central venous pressure may take weeks to months to return to normal after pericardiectomy. The LV ejection fraction may decrease postoperatively, only to return to normal months later. In the interim, digoxin, diuretics, and vasodilators may be useful.

Prevention consists of appropriate therapy for acute pericarditis and adequate pericardial drainage. Although instillation of fibrinolytics is promising, corticosteroids are often ineffective.[56]

EFFUSIVE-CONSTRICTIVE PERICARDITIS

Effusive-constrictive pericarditis occurs when pericardial fluid accumulates between the thickened, fibrotic parietal pericardium and visceral pericardium. Neoplasia, chest irradiation, infection, idiopathic pericarditis, and connective tissue diseases are common antecedents. Transient effusive-constrictive pericarditis may complicate chemotherapy.[57] The hemodynamic features are those of cardiac tamponade before, and constrictive pericarditis after, pericardiocentesis. Thus, removal of pericardial fluid fails to lower atrial and ventricular diastolic pressures, but the previously attenuated or absent atrial Y descent becomes prominent (Fig. 80-23).

SPECIFIC FORMS OF PERICARDIAL HEART DISEASE

Idiopathic Pericarditis

Acute pericarditis is most often idiopathic and is typically a self-limited disease lasting 2 to 6 weeks. Recurrence occurs in 25 percent of cases and occasionally proves resistant to therapy.[58] Small pericardial effusions occur commonly, but cardiac tamponade is unusual. Heart failure caused by associated myocarditis and constrictive pericarditis are uncommon. These complications usually can be detected by clinical and echocardiographic evaluation. The clinical course and prognosis of individuals with pericarditis are otherwise determined largely by the presence and nature of any underlying disease.

Infectious Pericarditis

VIRAL PERICARDITIS
Viral pericarditis is the most common infectious type, although a definitive diagnosis from acute and convalescent (3 weeks) viral neutralizing antibodies is generally not helpful in a sporadic case of pericarditis. Viral isolation from pericardial fluid and in situ hybridization techniques have been used to identify a specific etiology.[19] However, viral infection is often presumed rather than proved, and many cases are classified as idiopathic. Epicardial biopsy via a pericardioscope is a promising investigative technique for establishing the etiology of acute pericarditis. Common viral infections causing acute pericarditis are those resulting from echovirus and coxsackievirus; however, a great many different viruses may cause pericarditis (Table 80-2).

BACTERIAL PERICARDITIS
Bacterial (purulent) pericarditis is most often caused by streptococci, staphylococci, and gram-negative rods; *Haemophilus influenzae* is an important cause in children.[59] The increasing frequency of cardiac surgery and instrumentation, selection-induced changes in the flora responsible for hospital-acquired infections, and the prolonged survival of immunocompromised hosts (HIV, steroids) have changed the incidence and bacterial spectrum of purulent pericarditis. Pericardial involvement often is unrecognized when it complicates systemic infection; unusually high fever and white blood cell counts are clues to the presence of pericarditis. Children and immunosuppressed patients of all ages are most vulnerable, and the characteristic features of acute pericarditis are frequently absent. The course of bacterial pericarditis is fulminant, often presenting with cardiac tamponade; adhesive and constrictive pericarditis are common sequelae in survivors and may develop suddenly and early.[59] However, pericarditis

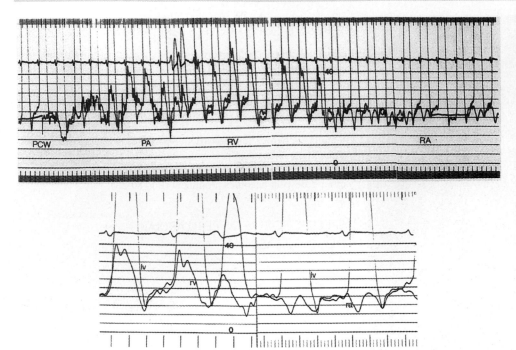

FIGURE 80-22 Hemodynamic record of a patient with surgically proven constrictive pericarditis. *Top*. Slow-paper-speed recording of high-gain left ventricular (LV) pressure and simultaneous right heart pullback from pulmonary capillary wedge (PCW) to pulmonary artery (PA), right ventricle (RV), and right atrium (RA). *Bottom*. Fast-paper-speed recording of LV and simultaneous RV and RA pressure tracings. Note the increased and equal atrial and diastolic pressures, the prominent X and Y descents on the RA tracing, and the dip and plateau on the RV and LV tracings during longer diastoles. (Courtesy of Peter J. Engel, MD. From Hoit BD. Pericardial disease and pericardial heart disease. In: O'Rourke RA, ed. *Stein's Internal Medicine*, 5th ed. St. Louis: Mosby-Year Book; 1998:273. Reproduced with permission.)

complicating systemic infection and sepsis may go unrecognized and misdiagnosed.[60] Many patients lack the typical findings of pericarditis, and the diagnosis of purulent pericarditis often is made either at autopsy or after cardiac tamponade develops; empyema is a common antecedent.[59] Purulent pericarditis is rarely caused by anaerobic bacteria, and the few reported cases resulted from contiguous infection or hematogenous seeding. Bacterial pericarditis is treated with surgical exploration and drainage and appropriate systemic antibiotics. Fibrinolytics may be used to lyse fibrous adhesions and prevent constrictive pericarditis.[61]

Legionella infections account for about 10 percent of community-acquired pneumonias and may be associated with pericarditis more often than previously was appreciated. Studies suggest that patients with pericardial involvement tend to be younger and healthier than are those without it.[62] Recurrent pericarditis, effusion, and chronic constriction occur in about 20 percent of cases. Pericarditis is an early complication of Lyme disease.[63]

MYCOBACTERIAL AND FUNGAL PERICARDITIS

Tuberculosis is a major cause of pericarditis in nonindustrialized countries but an uncommon cause in the United States. Nevertheless, its incidence is increasing because of HIV infection; therefore tuberculosis should be considered in the differential diagnosis of pericardial heart disease.[64] Tuberculous pericarditis results from hematogenous spread of primary tuberculosis or from the breakdown of infected mediastinal lymph nodes; therefore affected individuals generally lack the typical symptoms and signs of pulmonary tuberculosis. Fever, weight loss, and night sweats occur early; pericardial pain and friction rubs are often absent. Patients may present with tamponade or constriction, which may be subacute. A fibrinous pericarditis with caseating necrosis and mononuclear infiltrate gives rise to an effusive phase, which is often voluminous and hemodynamically significant. An adhesive phase follows resolution of the effusion and eventuates in dense, calcific adhesions with clinical constriction in nearly 50 percent of patients.

Mycobacteria are difficult to culture from pericardial fluid, which is diagnostic in only one-third of cases; real time polymerase chain reaction (rtPCR) was recently used to amplify and identify *Mycobacterium tuberculosis*.[65] A presumptive diagnosis generally requires a history of contact and/or purified protein derivative conversion (although the latter lacks sensitivity and specificity). Gadolinium-enhanced MRI may be useful in early diagnosis.[66] Increased adenosine deaminase activity (ADA) in pericardial fluid is supportive. In one study, a pericardial fluid ADA level of 72 U/L or greater demonstrated a sensitivity and specificity of 100 and 94 percent, respectively, for the diagnosis of tuberculous pericarditis.[67] However, the diagnosis of tuberculous pericarditis is presently based

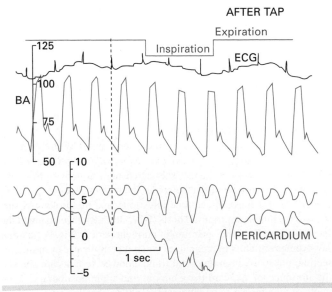

FIGURE 80-23 Recording from a patient with effusive-constrictive pericarditis caused by lung cancer. The tracings were obtained during the pericardiocentesis; right atrial pressure elevation persists, and there are prominent X and Y descents without respiratory variation. (From Shabetai R. *The Pericardium*. New York: Grune & Stratton; 1981:273. Reproduced with permission.)

on (1) histologic identification, (2) culture of *M. tuberculosis,* (3) pericarditis with proven extracardiac tuberculosis, or (4) pericardial effusion responsive to antituberculosis therapy.

Early pericardiectomy has been recommended by some researchers in all cases of tuberculous pericarditis, but the long-term (16 years) prognosis of patients without cardiac compression during the acute illness who are treated with medical therapy alone is excellent.[68] Multiple-drug therapy and corticosteroids are effective in tuberculous pericarditis, whereas atypical mycobacterial infections (especially *Mycobacterium avium-intracellulare*) may be resistant to treatment. Patients with tuberculous pericarditis should receive triple-drug therapy (isoniazid, rifampin, and streptomycin or ethambutol) for a minimum of 9 months. Corticosteroids may be useful if pericardial effusion persists or recurs during therapy; pericardiectomy may be necessary for recurrent cardiac tamponade. It is unclear whether open drainage or corticosteroid use prevents the progression to constrictive pericarditis.[69] Nevertheless, patients should be observed for constriction, as up to half these patients will require pericardiectomy.[70] In contrast, pericarditis complicating deep fungal infection (histoplasmosis, coccidioidomycosis) may be immunologic, resolve spontaneously, and not require specific therapy. Surgical decompression and specific antifungal therapy may be necessary for disseminated infection with *Candida, Aspergillus, Actinomycetes,* and *Nocardia.*

HIV PERICARDITIS

Human immunodeficiency virus (HIV) is an important cause of pericardial heart disease. HIV-associated pericardial effusions are increasingly more common, especially in urban referral centers. A retrospective survey at one inner-city medical center revealed that of 122 patients admitted with pericardial effusion over a 9-year period, 40 (33 percent) had associated HIV infection.[71] Among those patients with HIV-associated effusions, 16 (40 percent) presented with cardiac tamponade, and the presence of a pericardial effusion predicted a poor prognosis in HIV-infected individuals. Typically, pericardial effusions are small and asymptomatic in outpatients, but large effusions and tamponade are common in hospitalized patients with acquired immunodeficiency syndrome (AIDS). Indeed, in one study, a moderate or large effusion was present in more patients with symptomatic than asymptomatic HIV infection (17 vs. 2 percent), and most of these cases were clinically unsuspected.[72] The incidence and prevalence of pericardial effusion in a prospective, 5-year follow-up study of AIDS patients were high (11 percent per year and 5 percent, respectively).[73] A literature review of echocardiographic and autopsy series found an average incidence of pericardial disease of 21 percent.[74]

Pericardial involvement may be due to associated malignancies (e.g., lymphoma and Kaposi's sarcoma), viruses (including HIV), and opportunistic infections (e.g., mycobacteria, cytomegalovirus, *Nocardia,* and cryptococci) and, irrespective of its cause, predicts a poor prognosis in patients with HIV infection.[71] Large, symptomatic pericardial effusion in patients with HIV infection should be aggressively investigated, as two-thirds of these cases have an identifiable cause.[74] Tamponade in patients with HIV is mycobacterial (*M. tuberculosis* or *M. avium-intracellulare*) in origin in approximately one-third of patients.[74]

In 68 patients with HIV infection prospectively admitted to the intensive care unit, only 5 had evidence of cardiac disease, but 35 had echocardiographic abnormalities (20 effusions, 2 with tamponade, 15 cases of LV dysfunction, and 4 valvular abnormalities).[75] The presence of an effusion was associated with greater than 6-month mortality in patients with AIDS (96 vs. 36 percent); interestingly, an asymptomatic pericardial effusion may signal end-stage HIV disease independent of the CD4+ count and albumin level.[73]

Neoplastic Pericarditis

Metastatic neoplasia remains the leading cause of pericardial disease in hospitalized patients, most often in patients with lung or breast cancer, melanoma, lymphoma, and acute leukemia. Many cases are asymptomatic and are found only incidentally at autopsy, but others cause symptoms and may progress to cardiac tamponade. Primary cardiac tumors may invade the pericardium directly.

Primary mesothelioma of the pericardium is a rare and highly lethal tumor.[76] Signs and symptoms are nonspecific, and chest radiography and echocardiography are insensitive for its detection; CT and MRI are the most promising diagnostic tests. Other primary tumors of the pericardium are quite rare.

In patients with elevated jugular pressure and an intrathoracic mass, an important inclusion in the differential diagnosis is the superior vena cava syndrome. In this disorder, the characteristic pulsations of the jugular veins are not observed and pulsus paradoxus is not present. However, in a patient with respiratory distress, pulsus alternans, arrhythmia, and/or tachycardia, pulsus paradoxus may be obscured.

The pericardium may be thickened and cause constriction; less commonly, effusive-constrictive pericarditis occurs. Echocardiography rapidly and accurately detects pericardial effusion, identifies metastatic lesions, and provides evidence for cardiac compression. MRI is particularly useful in evaluating pericardial mass lesions. In many cases, neoplastic cells can be recovered from the pericardial fluid, which is usually bloody. However, it is important to remember that more than half of pericardial effusions in cancer patients are due to causes other than metastatic disease, such as infections, radiation, and drug therapy; thus, the presence of pericarditis in cancer patients does not imply imminent death.[77]

Post–Myocardial Infarction Pericarditis

Pericarditis is common in the first few days after an MI, occurring in as many as 28 to 43 percent of fatal infarctions, but it is clinically apparent in as few as 7 percent of cases.[78] When friction rub is required for diagnosis, there is an underestimation of the incidence of postinfarction pericarditis. On average, pericarditis was diagnosed by rub alone in 14 percent compared with 25 percent when classic symptoms, a rub, or both were used as diagnostic criteria. The detection of atypical T-wave evolution on ECG (i.e., either persistent positivity or temporally late positivity) may be a more sensitive and objective means of diagnosing postinfarction pericarditis.[79]

Pericardial involvement is related to infarct size and is associated with a poor prognosis.[80] An important clinical problem is the extent to which acute pericarditis in MI influences management with anticoagulants. A pericardial friction rub occurring in the first 2 or 3 days without an associated pericardial effusion should not influence clinical decisions, but pericarditis occurring later in the course or accompanied by pericardial effusion or tamponade is a contraindication to anticoagulant therapy.

In a prospective, consecutive series of 174 patients with acute MI, pericarditis occurred in 24 percent and was associated with anterior infarct location, heparin therapy, and pericardial effusion.[81] Cardiac tamponade seldom occurs except in patients who receive systemic anticoagulants or have cardiac rupture.

Thrombolytic therapy almost invariably precedes the development of pericarditis; therefore clinical decision making is usually not affected. Surprisingly, thrombolytic therapy reduces the incidence of postinfarction pericarditis by approximately half.[82] However, when acute pericarditis is mistaken for acute MI, thrombolytic therapy can have calamitous consequences. In patients treated mistakenly for myopericarditis with thrombolytics, the outcome was favorable.[83]

Dressler's syndrome (post-MI syndrome) consists of pleuropericardial chest pain, friction rub, fever, leukocytosis, and pulmonary infiltrates. It usually occurs weeks or months (>10 days to 2 weeks) after the causative infarction. Dressler's syndrome may be caused by a combination of viral activation and myocardial antibodies and is clinically and pathogenetically similar to the postpericardiotomy syndrome. Cardiac tamponade and late constriction may occur. For reasons that are not entirely clear, thrombolytic therapy has helped render post-MI pericarditis nearly extinct.

Radiation-Induced Pericardial Disease

Radiation injury to the pericardium is said to occur after exposure in excess of 4000 rads; the incidence also is dependent on the use of subcarinal blocks, the nature of the radiation source, and the duration and fractionation of the radiation regimen. For example, approximately 20 percent of Hodgkin's disease patients receiving cobalt-60 radiation with anterior weighting of the beam develop pericarditis, whereas the incidence of pericarditis after high-dose radiation for breast cancer (which includes less of the heart in the radiation field) is less than 5 percent.

Acute pericarditis occurring early during therapy is uncommon and most likely a result of the radiation-induced effects on the tumor rather than a direct toxic effect of the radiation on the pericardium. In this instance, therapy should not be disrupted, although a reduction in dose may be necessary. A delayed (usually less than 1 year but highly variable) form of pericardial injury may present as acute pericarditis or effusion (often with some degree of cardiac compression). The reaction of the pericardium to radiation is fibrinous inflammation,[84] often with an effusion. Although the acute lesion usually subsides within 2 years without sequelae, constrictive and effusive-constrictive pericarditis may become manifest only after many years.

The incompletely understood pathophysiology of radiation pericarditis involves, in part, extensive damage to the pericardial microcirculation and pericardial lymphatics with resultant ischemic injury. The incidence increases when anteriorly weighted field techniques are employed and is more common in patients who have also received adjunctive chemotherapy.

In the effusive stage, the differential diagnosis includes recurrence of the neoplasm; examination of pericardial fluid is then helpful, as the fluid is positive in about 30 percent of cases. Effusion may be due to the hypothyroid state induced by radiation therapy. Cytology is reliable in breast and lung cancer but less so in lymphoma and leukemia, where pericardial biopsy may be needed. Acute radiation-induced pericarditis can be managed symptomatically as acute idiopathic pericarditis. Hemodynamically insignificant pericardial effusion can also be managed conservatively, as spontaneous resolution is the rule; however, pericardiectomy should be offered to symptomatic patients with large, recurrent pericardial effusions. Constrictive pericarditis requires pericardiectomy unless the biopsy reveals significant endomyocardial fibrosis.

Traumatic Pericardial Disease

Blunt trauma and penetrating trauma are important causes of pericarditis, particularly among young men. Chronic constrictive pericarditis, recurrent pericardial effusion, and recurrent acute pericarditis are well-recognized complications. Traumatic pericarditis may be life-threatening. The application of echocardiography in the trauma unit rapidly and accurately diagnoses hemopericardium in patients with potentially penetrating cardiac wounds.[85] Failure to repair the injury responsible for tamponade is associated with a poor clinical outcome.[86] Constrictive pericarditis occasionally occurs and may be delayed, presenting weeks or years after the injury.[87] Chylous pericardial effusions generally follow traumatic or surgical injury to the thoracic duct but may result from neoplastic obstruction of the thoracic duct or may be idiopathic.

Nephrogenic Pericardial Disease

Pericarditis complicates both uremia and dialytic therapy (hemo- and peritoneal dialysis) and may be clinically silent. The clinical manifestation of nephrogenic pericardial disease may be acute fibrinous pericarditis, pericardial effusion, or cardiac tamponade; classic constrictive pericarditis is rare.

The pathogenesis remains unknown. The etiology of pericarditis in dialyzed patients may be different from that in end-stage renal disease. The theory that uremic pericarditis is a chemical response to retained products of metabolism fails to account for a poor relationship between the blood urea nitrogen (BUN) or other nitrogenous metabolites and the frequency of pericarditis. Since pericarditis is less common in patients undergoing peritoneal dialysis than in those receiving hemodialysis, there is a possible role for "middle molecules." Moreover, the hemorrhagic diathesis seen in the uremic syndrome may predispose to pericarditis; the resultant pericarditis is highly vascular; consequently, the uremia or dialysis-related pericardial effusion is generally bloody. Renal insufficiency is associated with increased susceptibility to infection, and therefore the possibility of viral, tuberculous, or even bacterial pericarditis must be considered. Immunologic abnormalities also have been implicated as a cause of pericardial disease in this setting. A presumptive diagnosis of dialysis-related pericarditis should be made only after other causes of pericardial heart disease (such as neoplasia and post-MI) that are common in this patient population have been excluded.

The clinical manifestations of cardiac tamponade may be atypical and difficult to distinguish from cardiovascular deterioration in patients undergoing hemodialysis. Cardiac tamponade remains one of the principal causes of hemodialysis-associated morbidity and terminates fatally in 20 percent of cases.

Although intensification of dialysis is an accepted treatment modality for hemodynamically insignificant disease, considerable controversy exists regarding the optimal management of large, persistent, or recurrent pericardial effusion and tamponade. Severe tamponade is an indication for pericardial drainage, but a conservative approach—intensification of dialysis and the use of nonsteroidal anti-inflammatory drugs—may suffice in less severe cases. The instillation of nonabsorbable steroids directly into the pericardial space has been advocated. Dialysis-associated effusive pericarditis usually responds to an intensification of dialysis and regional heparinization or to a change to peritoneal dialysis. Pericardiectomy may be necessary for intractable effusions.

Myxedema Pericardial Disease

Pericarditis with effusion (sometimes containing cholesterol) occurs in about one-third of patients with myxedema. Effusions develop slowly and may reach a prodigious size; slow resolution usually follows the institution of thyroid replacement therapy. A case of hypothyroidism and viral pericarditis in a patient presenting to the emergency room with abdominal pain and shock was reported recently.[88]

Connective Tissue Disease–Related Pericardial Disease

Pericarditis may accompany virtually any connective tissue disease and may present as either acute or chronic pericarditis with or without an effusion.[89] Although tamponade, effusive-constrictive disease, and constrictive pericarditis are recognized complications, most cases are subclinical and in many instances are recognized only at autopsy. Rheumatoid pericardial disease is more common in middle-aged men in whom the onset of arthritis is acute. Serologic tests for rheumatoid disease are usually positive, and typical rheumatoid nodules are common. Rheumatoid arthritis is one of the causes of cholesterol pericarditis. Constrictive pericarditis is usually subacute and seldom calcific. Pericardiectomy may be required within months of the first diagnosis of acute pericarditis and is almost always required within 5 years.[90]

Effusions are common in patients with systemic lupus erythematosus (SLE), and recurrent pericarditis, adhesion, and constriction may eventuate[91]; indeed, pericardial disease develops in nearly all patients with SLE when life is prolonged by steroid treatment. The pericardial fluid usually has high protein content and normal or slightly reduced glucose content; LE cells may be found. As in rheumatoid arthritis, the complement level is low.

Pericardial involvement may be found in systemic sclerosis (scleroderma), often in association with cardiomyopathy and diffuse scleroderma.[92] Dermatomyositis may be associated with pericardial involvement, including tamponade. Pericarditis is a rare complication in a wide variety of connective tissue disorders and arteritides (Table 80-2).

Iatrogenic Pericardial Disease

Iatrogenic pericardial disease results from both the calculated complications and the unanticipated misadventures of diagnostic and therapeutic procedures. Radiation pericarditis is one type of iatrogenic pericardial disease and was discussed earlier. Postcardiotomy syndrome, which complicates 5 to 30 percent of cardiac operations, usually appears in the second or third week to 2 months after cardiac surgery; affected patients frequently have high titers of antiheart and antiviral antibodies and may develop cardiac tamponade.

Cardiac perforation complicating diagnostic cardiac catheterization and pacemaker insertion, complications of endoscopic sclerotherapy of esophageal varices, and automatic defibrillator electrode placement are other causes of iatrogenic pericardial disease. Pericardial abnormalities may develop in response to a number of drugs, of which the more important are hydralazine, procainamide, and daunorubicin, although these abnormalities have been reported with a number of agents (Table 80-2). Cardiac tamponade after thrombolysis with t-PA given for stroke has been reported.

CONGENITAL PERICARDIAL HEART DISEASE

Absence and Partial Absence of the Pericardium

Congenital absence of the pericardium is an uncommon anomaly, usually involving a part or all of the left parietal pericardium. Its presence usually is suspected from the chest radiogram, which shows a leftward shift of the cardiac silhouette, elongation of the left heart border, and radiolucencies between the aortic knob and the pulmonary artery and between the left hemidiaphragm and the base of the heart (Fig. 80-24). This anomaly may be associated with congenital malformations of the heart and lungs.[94]

Although most of these patients are asymptomatic, chest pain may result from torsion of the great vessels, and recurrent pulmonary infections may be a significant feature. Physical findings are not often helpful, but a conspicuous LV heave may be found when the

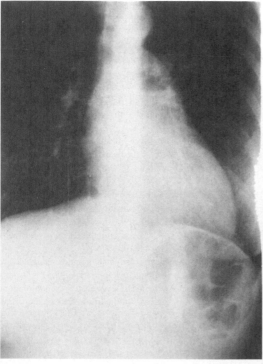

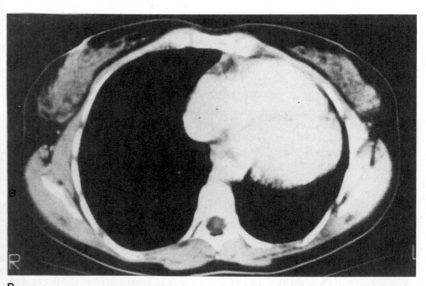

A **B**

FIGURE 80-24 *A.* Posteroanterior chest radiogram of a patient with congenital absence of the pericardium. *B.* Computed tomography scan of the same patient. (Reproduced with permission from Hoit BD. Imaging the pericardium. *Cardiol Clin* 1990;8:598.)

deficiency is substantial. Systolic and diastolic murmurs have been described.

The ECG in patients with complete absence of the left side of the pericardium usually shows an incomplete right bundle branch block. Echocardiographic changes consist of RV enlargement and paradoxical septal motion. Contrast-enhanced CT and MRI detect lesions missed by chest radiography and echocardiography and reliably establish the anatomy of the defect.[95]

Total and very small defects are not associated with pathophysiologic changes, whereas medium-size defects may allow herniation of the left atrium. Strangulation requires surgical closure or enlargement of the defect to reduce the herniation; this may be accomplished with a thoracoscope.

Pericardial Cysts

Pericardial cysts are rare remnants of defective embryologic development of the pericardium. Cysts usually present as a prominent round, sharply demarcated opacity seen on chest radiography in an asymptomatic patient. They vary greatly in size and are most commonly found in the right cardiophrenic angle, although hilar and mediastinal locations are observed occasionally. Cysts are benign and produce no local or general symptoms; their importance lies in differentiation from neoplasm. Although they can be demonstrated on echocardiography, the nature of the lesion usually is confirmed by CT. A case of video-assisted surgical excision of a recurrent pericardial cyst has been reported.[96]

References

1. Shabetai R. The pericardium: An essay on some recent developments. *Am J Cardiol* 1978;42(6):1036–1043.
2. Hammond HK, White FC, Bhargava V, et al. Heart size and maximal cardiac output are limited by the pericardium. *Am J Physiol* 1992;263 (6 part 2): H1675–H1681.
3. Hoit BD, Lew WY, LeWinter M. Regional variation in pericardial contact pressure in the canine ventricle. *Am J Physiol* 1988;255 (6 part 2):H1370–H1377.
4. Castelo Branco NA, Aguas AP, Sousa Pereira A, et al. The human pericardium in vibroacoustic disease. *Aviat Space Environ Med* 1999;70: A54–A62.
5. Soos P, Juhasz-Nagy A, Ruskoaho H, et al. Locally different role of atrial natriuretic peptide (ANP) in the pericardial fluid. *Life Sci* 2002;71: 2563–2573.
6. Spodick D. Macrophysiology, microphysiology, and anatomy of the pericardium: A synopsis. *Am Heart J* 1992;124:1046–1051.
7. Eid H, Larson DM, Springhorn JP, et al. Role of epicardial mesothelial cells in the modification of phenotype and function of adult rat ventricular myocytes in primary coculture. *Circ Res* 1992;71(1):40–50.
8. Laham RJ, Hung D, Simons M. Therapeutic myocardial angiogenesis using percutaneous intrapericardial drug delivery. *Clin Cardiol* 1999; 22:I6–I9.
9. Stoll HP, Carlson K, Keefer LK, et al. Pharmacokinetics and consistence of pericardial delivery directed to coronary arteries: Direct comparison with endoluminal delivery. *Clin Cardiol* 1999;22:I10–I16.
10. Kostreva DR, Pontus SP. Pericardial mechanoreceptors with phrenic afferents. *Am J Physiol* 1993;264:H1836–H1846.
11. Fujita M, Ikemoto M, Kishishita M, et al. Elevated basic fibroblast growth factor in pericardial fluid of patients with unstable angina. *Circulation* 1996;94:610–613.
12. Tanaka T, Hasegawa K, Fujita M, et al. Marked elevation of brain natriuretic peptide levels in pericardial fluid is closely associated with left ventricular dysfunction. *J Am Coll Cardiol* 1998;31(2):399–403.
13. Mallat Z, Philip I, Lebret M, et al. Elevated levels of 8-iso-prostaglandin F2alpha in pericardial fluid of patients with heart failure: A potential role for in vivo oxidant stress in ventricular dilatation and progression to heart failure. *Circulation* 1998;97(16):1536–1539.
14. Bonnefoy E, Godon P, Kirkorian G, et al. Serum cardiac troponin I and ST-segment elevation in patients with acute pericarditis. *Eur Heart J* 2000;21:832–836.
15. Adler Y, Finkelstein Y, Guindo J, et al. Colchicine treatment for recurrent pericarditis: A decade of experience. *Circulation* 1998;97(21): 2183–2185.
16. Maisch B, Ristic AD, Seferovic P, et al. Intrapericardial treatment of autoreactive myocarditis with triamcinolon. Successful administration in patients with minimal pericardial effusion. *Herz* 2000;25(8): 781–786.
17. Marcolongo R, Russo R, Laveder F, et al. Immunosuppressive therapy prevents recurrent pericarditis. *J Am Coll Cardiol* 1995;26(5): 1276–1279.
18. Maisch B, Ristic AD, Seferovic PM. New directions in diagnosis and treatment of pericardial disease. A project of the Taskforce on Pericardial Disease of the World Heart Federation. *Herz* 2000;25(8):769–780.
19. Maisch B. Percardial diseases, with a focus on etiology, pathogenesis, pathophysiology, new diagnostic imaging methods, and treatment. *Curr Opin Cardiol* 1994;9(3):379–388.
20. Weitzman LB, Tinker WP, Kronzon I, et al. The incidence and natural history of pericardial effusion after cardiac surgery—An echocardiographic study. *Circulation* 1984;69:506–511.
21. Kuvin JT, Harati NA, Pandian NG, et al. Postoperative cardiac tamponade in the modern surgical era. *Ann Thorac Surg* 2002;74:1148–1153.
22. Tsang TS, Barnes ME, Hayes SN, et al. Clinical and echocardiographic characteristics of significant pericardial effusions following cardiothoracic surgery and outcomes of echo-guided pericardiocentesis for management: Mayo Clinic experience, 1979–1998. *Chest* 1999;116(2): 322–331.
23. Ciliberto GR, Anjos MC, Gronda E. Significance of pericardial effusion after heart transplantation. *Am J Cardiol* 1995;76:297–300.
24. Mueller XM, Tevaearai HT, Hurni M, et al. Etiologic diagnosis of pericardial disease: The value of routine tests during surgical procedures. *J Am Coll Surg* 1997;184(6):645–649.
25. Sagrista-Sauleda J, Merce J, Permanyer-Miralda G, et al. Clinical clues to the causes of large pericardial effusions. *Am J Med* 2000;109:95–101.
26. Pankuweit S, Wadlich A, Meyer E, et al. Cytokine activation in pericardial fluids in different forms of pericarditis. *Herz* 2000;25(8):748–754.
27. Karia DH, Xing, YQ, Kuvin JT, et al. Recent role of imaging in the diagnosis of pericardial disease. *Curr Cardiol Rep* 2002;4(1):33–40.
28. Taguchi R, Takasu J, Itani Y, et al. Pericardial fat accumulation in men as a risk factor for coronary artery disease. *Atherosclerosis* 2001;157: 203–209.
29. Geissbuhler K, Leiser A, Fuhrer J, et al. Video-assisted thoracoscopic pericardial fenestration for loculated or recurrent effusions. *Eur J Cardiothorac Surg* 1998;14(4):403–408.
30. Merce J, Sagrista-Sauleda J, Permanyer-Miralda G, et al. Should pericardial drainage be performed routinely in patients who have a large pericardial effusion without tamponade? *Am J Med* 1998;105(2): 106–109.
31. Fejka M, Dixon SR, Safian RD, et al. Diagnosis, management, and clinical outcome of cardiac tamponade complicating percutaneous coronary intervention. *Am J Cardiol* 2002;90:1183–1186.
32. Hoit BD, Gabel M, Fowler NO. Cardiac tamponade in left ventricular dysfunction. *Circulation* 1990;82(4):1370–1376.
33. Hoit BD, Shaw D. The paradoxical pulse in tamponade: Mechanisms and echocardiographic correlates. *Echocardiography* 1994;11:477–487.
34. Russo AM, O'Connor WH, Waxman HL. Atypical presentations and echocardiographic findings in patients with cardiac tamponade occurring early and late after cardiac surgery. *Chest* 1993;104(1):71–78.
35. Heidenreich PA, Stainback RF, Redberg RF, et al. Transesophageal echocardiography predicts mortality in critically ill patients with unexplained hypotension. *J Am Coll Cardiol* 1995;26(1):152–158.
36. Hoit BD, Ramrakhyani K. Pulmonary venous flow in cardiac tamponade: Influence of left ventricular dysfunction and the relation to pulsus paradoxus. *J Am Soc Echocardiogr* 1991;4(6):559–570.

37. Merce J, Sagrista-Sauleda J, Permanyer-Miralda G, et al. Correlation between clinical and Doppler echocardiographic findings in patients with moderate and large pericardial effusion: Implications for the diagnosis of cardiac tamponade. *Am Heart J* 1999;138(4):759–764.

38. Maggiolini S, Bozzano A, Russo P, et al. *J Am Soc Echocardiogr* 2001; 14(8):821–824.

39. Maisch B, Ristic AD, Pankuweit S, et al. Neoplastic pericardial effusion. Efficacy and safety of intrapericardial treatment with cisplatin. *Eur Heart J* 2002;23(20):1625–1631.

40. Olson JE, Ryan MB, Blumenstock DA. Eleven years' experience with pericardial-peritoneal window in the management of malignant and benign pericardial effusions. *Ann Surg Oncol* 1995;2(2):165–169.

41. Allen KB, Faber LP, Warren WH, et al. Pericardial effusion: Subxiphoid pericardiostomy versus percutaneous catheter drainage. *Ann Thorac Surg* 1999;67(2):437–440.

42. Girardi LN, Ginsberg RJ, Burt ME. Pericardiocentesis and intrapericardial sclerosis: Effective therapy for malignant pericardial effusions. *Ann Thorac Surg* 1997;64(5):1427–1428.

43. Chavanon O, Carrat L, Pasqualini C, et al. Computer-guided pericardiocentesis: Experimental results and clinical perspectives. *Herz* 2000; 25(8):761–768.

44. Chen EP, Miller JI. Modern approaches and use of surgical treatment for pericardial disease. *Curr Cardiol Rep* 2002;4(1):41–46.

45. Ziskind AA, Pearce AC, Lemmon CC, et al. Percutaneous balloon pericardiotomy for the treatment of cardiac tamponade and large pericardial effusions: Description of technique and report of the first 50 cases. *J Am Coll Cardiol* 1993;21(1):1–5.

46. Palka P, Lange A, Donnelly JE, et al. Differentiation between restrictive cardiomyopathy and constrictive pericarditis by early diastolic Doppler myocardial velocity gradient at the posterior wall. *Circulation* 2000; 102(6):655–662.

47. Ha JW, Oh JK, Ommen SR, et al. Diagnostic value of mitral annular velocity for constrictive pericarditis in the absence of respiratory variation in mitral inflow velocity. *J Am Soc Echocardiogr* 2002;15(12): 1468–1471.

48. Oren RM, Grover-McKay M, Stanford W, et al. Accurate preoperative diagnosis of pericardial constriction using cine computed tomography. *J Am Coll Cardiol* 1993;22(3):832–838.

49. Sayad DE, Clarke GD, Peshock RM. Magnetic resonance imaging of the heart and its role in current cardiology. *Curr Opin Cardiol* 1995; 10(6):640–649.

50. Blackwell GG, Pohost GM. The usefulness of cardiovascular magnetic resonance imaging. *Curr Probl Cardiol* 1994;19(3):117–175.

51. Kutcher MA, King SB III, Alimurung BN, et al. Constrictive pericarditis as a complication of cardiac surgery: Recognition of an entity. *Am J Cardiol* 1982;50:742–748.

52. Sagrista-Sauleda J, Permanyer-Miralda G, Candell RJ, et al. Transient cardiac constriction: An unrecognized pattern of evolution in effusive acute idiopathic pericarditis. *Am J Cardiol* 1987;59:961–966.

53. Seifert FC, Miller DC, Oesterle SN, et al. Surgical treatment of constrictive pericarditis: Analysis of outcome and diagnostic error. *Circulation* 1985;72(3 part 2):II264–II273.

54. Nataf P, Cacouch P, Dorent R. Results of subtotal pericardiectomy for constrictive pericarditis. *Eur J Cardiothorac Surg* 1993;7:252–256.

55. Ling LH, Oh JK, Schaff HV, et al. Constrictive pericarditis in the modern era: Evolving clinical spectrum and impact on outcome after pericardiectomy. *Circulation* 1999;100:1380–1386.

56. Mann-Segal DD. The use of fibrinolytics in purulent pericarditis. *Intens Care Med* 1999;25:338–339.

57. Woods T, Vidarsson B, Mosher D, et al. Transient effusive-constrictive pericarditis due to chemotherapy. *Clin Cardiol* 1999;22(4):316–318.

58. Fowler NO, Harbin AD. Recurrent acute pericarditis: Follow-up study of 31 patients. *J Am Coll Cardiol* 1986;7:300–305.

59. Sagrista-Sauleda J, Barrabes JA, Permanyer-Miralda G, et al. Purulent pericarditis: Review of a 20-year experience in a general hospital. *J Am Coll Cardiol* 1993;22(6):1661–1665.

60. Arsura EL, Kilgore WB, Strategos E. Purulent pericarditis misdiagnosed as septic shock. *South Med J* 1999;92(3):285–288.

61. Mann-Segal DD. The use of fibrinolytics in purulent pericarditis. *Intens Care Med* 1999;25(3):338–339.

62. Puelo J, Matar F, McKeown P, et al. *Legionella* pericarditis diagnosed by direct fluorescent antibody staining. *Ann Thorac Surg* 1995;60: 444–446.

63. Nagi KS, Joshi R, Thakur RK. Cardiac manifestations of Lyme disease: A review. *Can J Cardiol* 1996;12(5):503–506.

64. Mastroianni A, Coronado O, Chiodo F. Tuberculous pericarditis and AIDS: Case reports and review. *Eur J Epidemiol* 1997;13(7):755–759.

65. Rana BS, Jones RA, Simpson IA. Recurrent pericardial effusion: The value of polymerase chain reaction in the diagnosis of tuberculosis. *Heart* 1999;82(2):246–247.

66. Hayashi H, Kawamata H, Machida M, et al. Tuberculous pericarditis: MRI features with contrast enhancement. *Br J Radiol* 1998;71(846): 680–682.

67. Aggeli C, Pitsavos C, Brili S, et al. Relevance of adenosine deaminase and lysozyme measurements in the diagnosis of tuberculous pericarditis. *Cardiology* 2000;94(2):81–85.

68. Long R, Younes M, Patton N, et al. Tuberculous pericarditis: Long-term outcome in patients who received medical therapy alone. *Am Heart J* 1989;117(5):1133–1139.

69. Trautner BW, Darouiche RO. Tuberculous pericarditis: Optimal diagnosis and management. *Clin Infect Dis* 2001;33:954–961.

70. Fowler N. Tuberculous pericarditis. *JAMA* 1991;266:99–103.

71. Chen Y, Brennessel D, Walters J, et al. Human immunodeficiency virus–associated pericardial effusion: Report of 40 cases and review of the literature. *Am Heart J* 1999;137(3):516–521.

72. Silva-Cardoso J, Moura B, Martins L, et al. Pericardial involvement in human immunodeficiency virus infection. *Chest* 1999;115(2):418–422.

73. Heidenreich PA, Eisenberg MJ, Kee LL, et al. Pericardial effusion in AIDS: Incidence and survival (see comments). *Circulation* 1995; 92(11):3229–3234.

74. Estok L, Wallach F. Cardiac tamponade in a patient with AIDS: A review of pericardial disease in patients with HIV infection. *Mt Sinai J Med* 1998;65(1):33–39.

75. Blanc P, Boussuges A, Souk-aloun J, et al. Echocardiography on HIV patients admitted to the ICU. *Intens Care Med* 1997;23(12):1279–1281.

76. Thomason R, Schlegel W, Luccam M. Primary malignant mesothelioma of the pericardium. *Tex Heart Inst* 1994;21:170–174.

77. Wilkes JD, Fidias P, Vaickus L, et al. Malignancy-related pericardial effusion: 127 cases from the Roswell Park Cancer Institute. *Cancer* 1995;76(8):1377–1387.

78. Widimsky P, Gregor P. Pericardial involvement during the course of myocardial infarction: A long-term clinical and echocardiographic study. *Chest* 1995;108(1):89–93.

79. Oliva P, Hammill S, Edwards W. Electrocardiographic diagnosis of postinfarction regional pericarditis: Ancillary observations regarding the effect of reperfusion on the rapidity and amplitude of T-wave inversion after acute myocardial infarction. *Circulation* 1993;88:896–904.

80. Correale E, Maggioni AP, Romano S, et al. Comparison of frequency, diagnostic and prognostic significance of pericardial involvement in acute myocardial infarction treated with and without thrombolytics: Gruppo Italiano per lo Studio della Soprav-vivenza nell'Infarto Miocardico (GISSI). *Am J Cardiol* 1993;71(16):1377–1381.

81. Madias J, Perdoncin R, Bartoszyk O. Pericarditis and pericardial effusion in patients with acute myocardial infarction. *Am J Noninvas Cardiol* 1994;8:270–277.

82. Correale E, Maggioni AP, Romano S, et al. Pericardial involvement in acute myocardial infarction in the post-thrombolytic era: Clinical meaning and value. *Clin Cardiol* 1997;20(4):327–331.

83. Millaire A, de Groote P, Decoulx E, et al. Outcome after thrombolytic therapy of nine cases of myopericarditis misdiagnosed as myocardial infarction. *Eur Heart J* 1995;16(3):333–338.

84. Benoff LJ, Schweitzer P. Radiation therapy–induced cardiac injury. *Am Heart J* 1995;129(6):1193–1196.

85. Rozycki GS, Feliciano DV, Oshsner MG, et al. The role of ultrasound in patients with possible penetrating cardiac wounds: A prospective multicenter study. *J Trauma* 1999;46(4):543–551.

86. Thakur RK, Aufderheide TP, Boughner DR. Emergency echocardiographic evaluation of penetrating chest trauma. *Can J Cardiol* 1994; 10(3):374–376.

87. Meleca MJ, Hoit BD. Previously unrecognized intrapericardial hematoma leading to refractory abdominal ascites. *Chest* 1995;108(6): 1747–1748.

88. Gupta R, Munyak J, Haydock T, et al. Hypothyroidism presenting as acute cardiac tamponade with viral pericarditis. *Am J Emerg Med* 1999;17(2):176–178.

89. Langley RL, Treadwell EL. Cardiac tamponade and pericardial disorders in connective tissue diseases: Case report and literature review. *J Natl Med Assoc* 1994;86(2):149–153.

90. Hakala M, Pettersson T, Tarkka M, et al. Rheumatoid arthritis as a cause of cardiac compression: Favourable long-term outcome of pericardiectomy. *Clin Rheumatol* 1993;12:199–203.

91. Moder KG, Miller TD, Tazelaar HD. Cardiac involvement in systemic lupus erythematosus. *Mayo Clin Proc* 1999;74(3):275–284.

92. Thompson AE, Pope JE. A study of the frequency of pericardial and pleural effusions in scleroderma. *Br J Rheumatol* 1998;37(12): 1320–1321.

93. Kasner SE, Villar-Cordova CE, Tong D, et al. Hemopericardium and cardiac tamponade after thrombolysis for acute ischemic stroke. *Neurology* 1998;50(6):1857–1859.

94. Nasser W. Congenital absence of the left pericardium. *Am J Cardiol* 1970;26:466–478.

95. Gassner I, Judmaier W, Fink C, et al. Diagnosis of congenital pericardial defects, including a pathognomonic sign for dangerous apical ventricular herniation, on magnetic resonance imaging. *Br Heart J* 1995;74: 60–66.

96. Horita K, Sakao Y, Itoh T. Excision of a recurrent pericardial cyst using video-assisted thoracic surgery. *Chest* 1998;114(4):1203–1204.

INFECTIVE ENDOCARDITIS

Jeffrey L. Anderson / Merle A. Sande / Marinka Kartalija / Joseph B. Muhlestein

Infective endocarditis (IE) is a disease caused by microbial infection of the endothelial lining of the heart. Its characteristic lesion, a *vegetation,* usually develops on a heart valve but occasionally appears elsewhere on the endocardium. *Infective endarteritis* is a variant of IE characterized by an infectious nidus on the lining of a large artery. IE remains a serious, life-threatening condition, but steady progress continues to be made in its diagnosis and management.[1–3]

DEFINITIONS AND TERMINOLOGY

Abbreviations used for the various forms of endocarditis are presented in Table 81-1.

Subacute bacterial endocarditis (SBE) refers to IE that progresses over a period of weeks to months and is usually caused by organisms of low virulence, such as *viridans* streptococci, which possess limited ability to infect other tissues.[4–7]

In contrast, *acute bacterial endocarditis* (ABE) evolves over a period of days to 1 or 2 weeks; the clinical progress is rapidly changing, complications develop earlier, and the diagnosis is usually apparent in less than 2 weeks.[7–9] ABE is usually caused by primary pathogens such as *Staphylococcus aureus,* which are capable of causing invasive infection at many other sites in the body.

Native valve endocarditis (NVE) refers to infections of both normal and previously diseased (congenital or acquired) native valves. *Prosthetic valve endocarditis* (PVE) involves infection of an artificial heart valve and may be divided into early or late (>1 year) postoperative PVE.[10]

Nonbacterial thrombotic endocarditis (NBTE) describes sterile vegetations. The term *noninfective endocarditis* is a misnomer because the lesions are primarily thrombotic rather than inflammatory in nature.[11] NBTE ranges from microscopic platelet aggregates to the large vegetations of marantic endocarditis, which sometimes develop in terminal malignancy or other chronic diseases.[12–14]

Designating IE by the infecting organism and the type of endocarditis is prognostically and therapeutically useful: for example, "*Staph. aureus* ABE" or "*Candida albicans* PVE."

TABLE 81-1 Endocarditis Abbreviations

ABE:	Acute bacterial endocarditis
IE:	Infective endocarditis
NBTE:	Nonbacterial thrombotic endocarditis
NIE:	Nosocomial infectious endocarditis
NVE:	Native valve endocarditis
PVE:	Prosthetic valve endocarditis
SBE:	Subacute bacterial endocarditis

TABLE 81-2 Temporal Trends in Infectious Endocarditis

Increasing median age of patients
Increasing ratio of males to females
Increasing proportion of acute cases
Decreasing incidence of classic signs of advanced SBE (e.g., Osler's nodes, finger clubbing, splenomegaly, Roth's spots)
Decreasing proportion due to streptococci, increased proportion due to staphylococci
Increasing diversity of etiologic organisms (gram-negative bacilli; fungi; miscellaneous rare, unusual microbes)
Increasing prevalence due to injection drug use
Increasing prevalence of prosthetic valve infections
Increasing prevalence of concomitant human immunodeficiency virus (HIV) infection and IE

EARLY STUDIES

Riviere, Lancisi, and Morgagni each described patients who died with IE in the seventeenth and eighteenth centuries.[16] Jean-Baptiste Bouillaud introduced the terms *endocardium* and *endocarditis* between 1824 and 1835. By 1846, Virchow recognized valvular vegetations at autopsy, and by 1869–1872, he had demonstrated bacteria within vegetations, indicating their microbial nature.[14]

William Osler studied IE extensively, choosing it as the subject for his Goulstonian lectures of 1885.[15,16] Further advances were made by Lenharz and associates[14] in Germany; by Horder[17] in England; and by Blumer,[4] Thayer,[5] Allen,[18] Libman and Friedberg,[19] and Beeson et al.[20] in the United States. The technique of blood culture was introduced between 1890 and 1910.[6] In 1955, Kerr published a classic monograph summarizing knowledge on IE to that date.[6]

Attempts to cure IE before the advent of antibiotics were unsuccessful. In 1939, one patient with infective endarteritis involving a patent ductus arteriosus was cured by surgical closure of the ductus.[21] The first successes in the treatment of IE are closely linked to the history of penicillin.[22–24] After initial failures, by 1944 it had been established that penicillin,[25] unlike sulfonamides,[26] could cure most cases of streptococcal endocarditis. The benefit of antibiotic treatment subsequently was clearly established.[27–31] Surgical replacement of cardiac valves was first reported in 1965.[32]

EPIDEMIOLOGY

Incidence and Prognosis

IE is a life-threatening disease. Antibiotic therapy for 4 to 6 weeks may reduce mortality to 20 to 50 percent; cardiac surgery is necessary for further reduction in 20 to 50 percent.[1,33]

The incidence of IE has been estimated to be 1.6 to 6.0 cases per 100,000 person-years.[1,33–39] The rate is higher after age 50 (15 per 100,000 person-years) and among patients with valvular heart disease, prosthetic heart valves, or congenital heart disease or users of injection drugs.[40] A population study from Delaware Valley, which included a large number of injection drug users (IDUs), reported a rate of 11.6 per 100,000 per year.[41]

Evolution of the Clinical Syndrome

IE today is a different disease from that seen in the preantibiotic era, when its salient clinical features were exhaustively reported.[4–6] Since 1961, many authors have described the "changing face" of IE,[39,42–47] identifying the trends summarized in Table 81-2. In a 2002 French study, IE was characterized by an increasing proportion without previously known heart disease (47 percent), with group D streptococcal

and staphylococcal IE, requiring early valve surgery (50 percent), and surviving hospitalization (mortality 17 vs. 22 percent).[33]

Susceptible Populations

The striking changes in the clinical features and epidemiology of IE are due to changes in susceptible populations, to earlier diagnosis and treatment of subacute disease, and to the impact of antibiotic therapy.[45,48] The prevalence of rheumatic heart disease has steadily decreased, whereas survivors of congenital heart disease have increased. Illicit drugs use has increased markedly since the 1960s, and HIV has spread widely.[49] Other increasing predisposing conditions include immunosuppression and organ transplantation, especially renal.[50,51] Still other increasing conditions include diabetes mellitus, chronic hemodialysis, and poor dental hygiene.[52]

Effect of Antibiotics

Although the advent of antibiotics revolutionized treatment of IE, its overall incidence has not changed strikingly. Rapidly effective antibiotic treatment for pneumococcal pneumonia and gonorrhea has been associated with a striking decrease in IE caused by *Streptococcus pneumoniae* and *Neisseria gonorrhoeae* since 1944, whereas the incidence caused by unusual, resistant organisms has increased during the antibiotic era.[48,53–56] However, widespread use of antimicrobials has influenced the epidemiology of IE less than have alterations in populations at risk.[45] Prophylactic antibiotics before bacteremia-causing medical procedures has not reduced the incidence of IE significantly; indeed, only a small proportion of all cases is attributable to such procedures.[57–59] Also, startling recent studies question the effectiveness of prophylactic antibiotics for dental procedures,[59,60] and some have called for a rethinking of antibiotic prophylaxis.[61] Certainly, those at clearly increased risk need to be better defined, and the overprescribing of antibiotics, with its attendant risks and costs, should be avoided.

Preexisting Heart Disease

IE may develop in the absence of known heart disease. This most commonly presents as an ABE,[60] in children less than 2 years of age,[62–68] and/or in IDUs.[69–74] However, for most cases of IE, preexisting valvular heart disease or another predisposing cardiac condition

TABLE 81-3 Approximate Frequency of Major Preexisting Cardiac Lesions in Patients with Infective Endocarditis in the United States

Lesion	Children under 2 years, %	Children 2–15 Years, %	Adults 15–50 Years, %	Adults >50 Years, %	Adults Who Are IV Drug Abusers, %
No known heart disease	50–70	10–15	10–20	10	50–60
Congenital heart disease[a]	30–50	70–80	25–35	15–25	10
Rheumatic heart disease	Rare	10	10–15	10–15	10
Degenerative heart disease	0	0	Rare	10–20	Rare
Previous cardiac surgery	5	10–15	10–20	10–20	10–20
Previous endocarditis	Rare	5	5–10	5–10	10–20

[a]Includes mitral valve prolapse.
SOURCE: Adapted from Refs. 34–39, 41–49, 53, 54, 62–74, 90, 221.

exists. Frequencies of predisposing factors in children, adults, and IDUs are given in Table 81-3. IE is much less frequently associated with mitral stenosis than with mitral regurgitation (MR) (with or without stenosis) (Chap. 67). Estimates of the relative propensity of various cardiac lesions to become infected are presented in Table 81-4.

Mitral valve prolapse (MVP) is now the most common valvular condition predisposing to IE[2,75–83] (Chap. 68). MVP underlies 15 to 30 percent or more of cases.[34,76,79,80,84] The incidence of IE with known MVP is approximately 100 per 100,000 patient-years.[83,85] Risk factors for IE across the spectrum of MVP include mitral regurgitation and thickened mitral leaflets.[83,85] However, the annual risk of complications with MVP, including IE, is small, and the need for IE prophylaxis has been controversial. The American Heart Association (AHA) has developed recommendations for IE prophylaxis of MVP.[86] Risk primarily is increased (five- to eightfold) with associated mitral regurgitation (MR),[76,77,82] and prophylactic antibiotics are cost-effective in those with auscultatory or Doppler evidence for MR.[86] In contrast, IE risk is not importantly increased in the absence of regurgitation, and prophylaxis generally is not recommended[5,76,77,86–88] (Chap. 68). Although commonly used to assess MVP, routine use of echocardiography does not appear to be cost-effective.[78]

Prosthetic heart valves are increasingly prevalent and increase the risk of IE. Risk is relatively greater early after mechanical valve placement, but late risk is equivalent for mechanical and bioprostheses.[89]

Children

IE is uncommon during childhood and rare during infancy[62–68,90,91] except in the setting of cyanotic heart disease.[92] Males predominate.[93] No predisposing cardiac disease is found in 15 percent, but the proportion is higher under 2 years of age (Table 81-3). IE in these younger children and infants is usually associated with infection elsewhere,[94] is caused by invasive pathogens, and follows an acute course. IE may complicate staphylococcal or group B streptococcal septicemia associated with pneumonia, other respiratory tract infections, osteomyelitis, severe burns,[62,66] or nosocomial catheter infections.[94]

SBE without an obvious source typically occurs in older children with congenital or acquired heart disease.[94] IE of surgically constructed systemic pulmonary shunts is most commonly due to viridans streptococci.[93]

Common underlying cardiac lesions include tetralogy of Fallot, other cyanotic congenital heart diseases, ventricular septal defects, aortic stenosis, patent ductus arteriosus, pulmonary stenosis, and coarctation of the aorta. A high proportion (77 percent) of IE complicating congenital heart disease occurs after palliative or corrective surgery.[66,93,95] Secundum atrial septal defects rarely become infected (Chap. 73). Successful repair of a ventricular septal defect and closure of a patent ductus arteriosus greatly reduces the risk of IE. In developed countries, rheumatic heart disease is now a much less common predisposing condition than in the past.

TABLE 81-4 Estimates of the Relative Risk of Infective Endocarditis Posed by Various Cardiac Lesions

Relatively High Risk	Intermediate Risk	Very Low or Negligible Risk
Prosthetic heart valves	Mitral valve prolapse with regurgitation	Mitral valve prolapse without regurgitation
Previous infective endocarditis	Pure mitral stenosis	Trivial valvular regurgitation by echocardiography without structural abnormality
Cyanotic congenital heart disease	Tricuspid valve disease	
Aortic valve disease	Pulmonary valve disease	
Mitral regurgitation	Asymmetric septal hypertrophy	Atrial septal defects, secundum type
Mitral regurgitation and stenosis	Hyperalimentation or pressure-monitoring lines that reach the right atrium	Arteriosclerotic plaques
Patent ductus arteriosus		Coronary artery disease
Ventricular septal defect	Nonvalvular intracardiac prosthetic implants	Syphilitic aortitis
Coarctation of the aorta		Cardiac pacemakers
	Degenerative valvular disease in elderly patients	Surgically corrected cardiac lesions (without prosthetic implants, more than 6 months after operation)

SOURCE: Adapted from Refs. 35, 37, 38, 43, 53, 54, 75–82, 84, 90.

The diagnosis of IE is more difficult in infants and small children, although signs and symptoms are similar, including fever (99 percent of cases) and a new or changing murmur (21 percent). Blood cultures are usually positive (>90 percent). *Viridans* streptococci (38 percent of cases), *Staph. aureus* (32 percent), and enterococci (7 percent) are the most common etiologic organisms.[93] Once IE is suspected, improved criteria are helpful in diagnosis.[94]

Antibiotic recommendations for children are generally similar to those for adults, with appropriate dose adjustment for age. As for adults, surgical intervention should not be delayed if heart failure supervenes despite medical therapy.[96] Similarly, *Staph. aureus* IE in children is more frequently complicated, requires surgery, and has a higher mortality rate.[93,97]

The Elderly

IE in the elderly is becoming more common and presents unique diagnostic and therapeutic challenges.[98–102] The median age has risen steadily, and one-fourth of IE patients now are over age 60.[34,103] The risk of IE is strongly age-related, being five times greater after age 80.[38] Males outnumber females by 1.5 to 1 overall and by as much as 8 to 1 after age 60.[31,104] Elderly patients are more likely to have degenerative or calcific valve lesions.[99] After age 70, a higher proportion of IE organisms have a gastrointestinal source (group D streptococci and enterococci in up to 50 percent),[101] and the mortality risk increases (28 versus 13 percent).[101]

Intravenous Drug Users

Illicit intravenous and other injection-site drug use poses a high risk for IE.[69–74,105] IDUs are 300 times more likely to die with IE than nonusers.[106] Addicts seldom use sterile injection techniques; bacteremias are common and arise either from direct injection of bacteria or from skin or mucosal flora or local infection at injection sites.[107]

Staph. aureus causes over 60 percent of IE cases among IDUs.[53,74] Gram-negative bacilli, especially *Pseudomonas*,[108,109]

and yeasts and other fungi[110] are also are more common in IDUs than in nonaddicts (Table 81-5). *Candida* (*Candida parapsilosis* and other species) is the most common fungal cause of drug-related IE, but a wide range of other fungi have been reported.[110,111] Polymicrobial and culture-negative IE account for less than 5 percent of IDU cases.[69,71,74,112]

Endocarditis in addicts frequently follows an acute course,[8,69,70,111] reflecting the high frequency of *Staph. aureus* infection and accounting for the modest increase over the past 25 years in the proportion of acute to subacute cases of IE.[45]

The outstanding clinical feature of IE in IDUs is the high incidence of right-sided valvular infection: the tricuspid valve is involved in 60 to 70 percent of cases[53,65,113] and the aortic and/or mitral valves in 30 to 40 percent.[53,113] More than one valve on either side of the heart may be infected simultaneously. However, pulmonic valve infection is unusual (2 percent of cases). Occasionally (3 percent of cases), endocarditis may occur on the eustachian valve, which should be interrogated during echocardiographic assessment.[114]

Tricuspid vegetations commonly embolize to the lungs, causing septic pulmonary infarcts. Multiple focal opacities may be seen on chest x-ray, sometimes with cavitation. In a drug addict with fever, this radiologic finding suggests right-sided ABE.[8,74] Mortality rates are lower (4 percent) in IDUs than in other IE populations despite the high frequency of *Staph. aureus* IE. This reflects the more benign nature of tricuspid than left-sided valvular disease and the younger age of IDUs. The presence of hematuria, proteinuria, or pyuria in a febrile IDU with no obvious infective source is predictive of definite IE.[115]

Patients Infected with Human Immunodeficiency Virus

IE is independently associated with HIV infection, although the primary risk factor is continued intravenous drug use.[116,117] Prior IE, female sex, and skin abscesses are other independent risk factors.[118] In one study, the adjusted odds ratio for IE was 2.3 for HIV-infected IDUs with CD4+ cell counts >350/mm^3 and rose to 8.3 when CD4+ cell count fell to <350.[119] *Bartonella* is opportunistic for IE in

TABLE 81-5 Frequency of Various Organisms Causing Infective Endocarditis[a]

Organism	NVE, %	IV Drug Abusers, %	Early PVE, %	Late PVE, %
Streptococci	60	15–25	5	35
Viridans, alpha-hemolytic	35	5–10	<5	25
Streptococcus bovis	10	<5	<5	<5
Enterococcus faecalis	10	10	<5	<5
Other streptococci	<5	<5	<5	<5
Staphylococci	25	50	50	30
Coagulase-positive	23	50	20	10
Coagulase-negative	<5	<5	30	20
Gram-negative aerobic bacilli	<5	5	20	10
Fungi	<5	<5	10	5
Miscellaneous bacteria	<5	5	5	5
Diphtheroids, propionibacteria	<1	<5	5	<5
Other anaerobes	<1	<1	<1	<1
Rickettsiae	<1	<1	<1	<1
Chlamydiae	<1	<1	<1	<1
Polymicrobial infection	<1	1–5	5	5
Culture-negative endocarditis	5–10	<5	<5	<5

[a]These are representative figures collated from the literature; wide local variations in frequency are to be expected. NVE = native valve endocarditis; PVE = prosthetic valve endocarditis; IV = intravenous.
SOURCE: Adapted from Refs. 43, 54, 69–74, 110–113, 118–121, 123, 124, 130, 179.

acquired immunodeficiency syndrome (AIDS).[120] Patients in earlier stages of HIV infection respond well to standard treatment for IE, but mortality rises when the CD4+ cell count falls below 200/mm³ [49,121] (Chap 88).

Postcardiac Surgery Patients

Cardiac surgery, especially valve replacement, has created a new population at risk for IE. In the 1950s, surgeons first noted that *Staph. epidermidis* endocarditis occurred fairly frequently after mitral valvulotomy.[108] Subsequently, *Staph. epidermidis,* which rarely infects native valves, was noted to be a common cause of both early and late PVE (Table 81-5).[10,87,88,105,122] Contamination of blood circulating through the pump or from operating room air may lead to early PVE. Late PVE usually originates from normal flora of the skin or gastrointestinal tract. Gram-negative bacilli and fungi cause early postoperative PVE much more frequently than they do NVE.[10,105,123] The spectrum of organisms causing late PVE more nearly resembles that of subacute NVE (Table 81-5).

Figure 81-1 shows the time-related risk of PVE after valve replacement. Onset peaks at 3 to 9 weeks after surgery and then the risk rapidly falls.[88] This time course supports the inoculation of *Staph. epidermidis* and certain other organisms at the time of surgery as a cause of early PVE. In contrast, streptococcal bacteremias cause PVE independent of the time of surgery.

Although the prevalence of postsurgical endocarditis has increased, the incidence rate has decreased in association with improved operative technique and the use of prophylactic antibiotics. Currently, rates are 0.5 percent for early PVE (range, 0.3 to 1.2 percent)[10,87,88,122] and 0.3 to 0.5 percent per year for late PVE.[10,105,123,124]

Obstetric and Gynecologic Patients

Endocarditis occurring as a complication of pregnancy is most likely to develop at the time of delivery or in the puerperium.[125] Normal delivery presents a low risk of IE even in the presence of preexisting valvular disease,[126] but bacteremias associated with perinatal infections such as endometritis, parametritis, septic thrombophlebitis in pelvic veins, or urinary tract infections can seed the mother's endocardium.[125] Septic abortion or pelvic infection related to intrauterine contraceptive devices also can provide the portal of entry for

bacteremia resulting in IE.[127] Organisms most often involved are *Enterococcus faecalis,* group B streptococci, *Staph. aureus,* and, occasionally, gram-negative enteric bacilli or anaerobes.

Nosocomial Infective Endocarditis

Hospital-acquired (nosocomial) IE is of importance because of its high mortality rate, preventable nature, and often clandestine presentation.[128] Nosocomial IE (NIE) can involve either prosthetic or native valves.[129,130] NIE is not rare and may be increasing.[129] One study[131] reported that 35 (28%) of 125 IE cases were probably nosocomial.

Intensive medical care predisposes to endocarditis in several ways. Endovascular and endocardial damage can be produced by surgery and indwelling catheters. Portals of entry are provided by wounds, biopsy sites, pacemakers, intravascular and urinary catheters,[132] and intratracheal airways. In one study, the majority (75 percent) of suspected sources were vascular access sites.[133] Nosocomial bacteremias may give rise to IE late during hospitalization, often without predisposing cardiac pathology[133] and with a high mortality rate.[134] Bacteremia persisting for 72 h or more after removal and treatment of an infected catheter should raise the question of IE, especially when a diseased or prosthetic valve is present.[134,135]

Many of these predisposing factors coexist in severely burned patients and may lead to IE.[136] A predisposition to IE has also been reported with flow-directed pulmonary catheters.[135] Because persistent bacteremia and fever are the only consistent findings with ABE following burns, an echocardiogram may be of diagnostic value.[137]

Another group at high risk of NIE are patients with prosthetic valves who develop bacteremias, especially if the organism is a *Staphylococcus.*[130] The portal of entry is most often an intravascular line or device. Delayed PVE can develop even after an appropriate course of antibiotics for the nosocomial infection.

In contrast, catheterization of the right side of the heart for brief periods, as in the coronary care unit, in patients without bacteremias presents a very low risk for IE.

IE is rare in patients with leukemia but has been observed in other immunocompromised patients—for example, after bone marrow transplantation[138] and heart transplantation.[139] After solid organ transplantation, *Aspergillus fumigatus* or *Staph. aureus* were causative in 50 percent of 46 cases in one report, whereas *viridans* streptococci were isolated in only 4 percent.[140] Of 10 cases occurring within 30 days of transplantation, 6 were fungal. No predisposing cardiac lesion was known in 80 percent. Infected venous access devices and wounds were suspected portals of entry in three-fourths. The mortality rate was 57 percent, and most infections were not diagnosed prior to death.[140]

The leading organisms causing NIE are staphylococci, enterococci, *Candida* species, and gram-negative bacilli. *Staph. aureus* is associated especially with wound infections, cellulitis, and cannula infections; *Staph. epidermidis* occurs with ventriculoatrial shunts; and *C. albicans* with parenteral alimentation.

The prognosis for nosocomial native valve endocarditis (up to 50 percent mortality) is worse than for other forms of native valve IE.[129,133] NIE patients often have serious underlying disease that may obscure and delay diagnosis, and the organisms most commonly involved are difficult to eradicate.

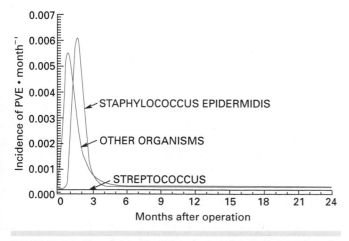

FIGURE 81-1 Incidence of prosthetic valve endocarditis (PVE) over 24 months after valve replacement. The hazard function has been stratified according to the infecting organisms. (From Ivert TSA, Dismukes WE, Cobbs CG, et al. Prosthetic valve endocarditis. *Circulation* 1984;69:223. Reproduced with permission.)

Hemodialysis

Creation of arteriovenous (AV) shunts for hemodialysis provides a ready portal for bacteremias that can cause IE. The high cardiac output associated with an AV fistula also may predispose to both local infectious arteritis and IE.[141] Clinically, IE has been reported in 2 to

6 percent of patients on long-term hemodialysis employing either AV fistulas or cannulas. *Staph. aureus* and *Staph. epidermidis* are the most common etiologic organisms, followed by *viridans* streptococci and *E. faecalis.*[142] Mortality is high (53 percent), and a high index of suspicion and echocardiography followed by aggressive treatment are necessary to improve outcome.[142] A poor 1-year prognosis in mitral valve IE is associated with low presenting hemoglobin, elevated leukocyte count, severe aortic and mitral regurgitation, and annular calcification.[143]

Pacemaker and Defibrillator Infective Endocarditis

The placement of permanent pacemaker or implantable defibrillator leads into the right ventricle may result in endocardial lead infection (0.2 to 7 percent of patients).[144–148] These infections may occur early (6 weeks to 3 months after placement) and be caused by *Staph. epidermidis* (in 90 percent) or late, when *Staph. epidermidis* or *Staph. aureus* may each account for nearly 50 percent. Gram-negative bacilli cause the remaining few. Definitive diagnosis usually requires TEE, which will detect vegetations in or around the leads in >90 percent of cases. A chest x-ray suggesting pulmonary emboli may assist diagnosis in some cases. Cure requires removal of the generator and leads and treatment with antibiotics.

Infective Endarteritis

Focal endarteritis outside of the heart can closely mimic IE, including vascular and immunologic phenomena.[53] In the past, about one-quarter of patients with an uncorrected patent ductus arteriosus developed infective endarteritis.[6] Coarctation of the aorta also presented a significant risk, although IE on an associated bicuspid aortic valve was three times more common. Endarteritis occasionally complicates traumatic arteriovenous fistulas, but arteriosclerotic aneurysms rarely become infected.[53]

The spectrum of organisms causing infective endarteritis is similar to that of those causing IE except for a higher frequency of salmonellae in infected arteriosclerotic abdominal aneurysms.[53,149] The pattern of embolization with infective endarteritis differs according to the site of infection. Thus, petechiae may occur on the skin of the lower extremities with an infected abdominal aneurysm, and infarctions may appear in the lungs with an infected dialysis fistula in the forearm.

ETIOLOGIC ORGANISMS

The range of microbes causing IE is extraordinarily wide, yet a few species account for the vast majority of cases. On native valves, streptococci or staphylococci cause >80 percent of infections.[31,37,43,131] However, the incidence of infection due to other organisms is higher among IDUs and patients with prosthetic valves. Table 81-5 summarizes representative frequencies of etiologic organisms causing IE on native valves, in IDUs, and on prosthetic valves. Note that these may vary widely by country and hospital.

Streptococci

Streptococci cause more cases of endocarditis than any other group of organisms.[31,37,150–152] Alpha-hemolytic or *viridans* streptococci account for the majority of these cases, although their relative frequency has decreased over the last 30 years. *Viridans* streptococci are ubiquitous in oropharyngeal and gastrointestinal flora. Except for *Strep. milleri,* they are generally low-grade pathogens, often recovered from clinical specimens in mixed cultures but seldom themselves pathogenic. Their prevalent role in SBE pathogenesis is explained by the frequency with which they enter the bloodstream and their ability to adhere to endocardium rather than their innate virulence. Penicillin-resistant *viridans* streptococci are increasingly common, and penicillin-resistant *viridans* streptococcal IE has been reported.[153]

The nomenclature of *viridans* streptococci is complex and subject to frequent revision.[150,154,155] Species commonly causing SBE include *Strep. sanguis, Strep. mitis, Strep. oralis,* and *Strep. gordonii.* Less commonly, *Strep. milleri* group organisms (*Strep. anginosus, Strep. intermedius,* or *Strep. constellatus*) are etiologic.[150,152,154] A few causal strains require media supplemented with L-cysteine or pyridoxine.[156–159]

Group D streptococci are the next most frequent cause of streptococcal IE.[104,160,161] The nonenterococcal group D species, *Strep. bovis,* accounts for about one-fifth of streptococcal cases. *Strep. bovis* IE tends to occur in older patients, affects multiple valves including previously normal valves, is associated with a high rate of neurologic complications, and requires surgery more often than IE caused by other species.[162,163] Gastrointestinal lesions, especially colonic polyps and cancers, are present in >50 percent with *Strep. bovis* bacteremia and/or endocarditis.[163–165] Hence recovery of *Strep. bovis* from blood cultures should prompt investigation of colonic disease.

Strains of *E. faecalis* (enterococci) cause about 10 percent of streptococcal IE. Previously, enterococcal IE was said to occur in association with infections of the genitourinary tract in women of childbearing age and of the urinary tract in older men with prostatic disease. Today, enterococcal IE also is common in drug addicts and in patients with chronic renal disease or with nosocomial endocarditis.[104] Enterococcal urinary tract, wound, or intravenous line infections are the source of NIE.[166,167] Fewer than 2 percent of nosocomial bacteremic patients develop IE, whereas one-third of community-acquired enterococcal bacteremias without a primary infectious focus are associated with IE.[166] *E. faecium* antibiotic resistance may present major difficulty in IE treatment.[104,168–170]

IE caused by any of many other species or strains of streptococci is rare compared with *viridans* and group D.

Strep. pneumoniae ABE primarily affects the aortic valve, often in the absence of valvular disease and requiring early valve replacement for aortic regurgitation and cardiac failure. However, this is uncommon since the advent of antibiotics.[171–173] In debilitated alcoholics, bacteremic pneumococcal pneumonia is occasionally complicated by endocarditis and meningitis and carries an extremely poor prognosis.[171]

Beta-hemolytic streptococci are a rare cause of IE. Among 31 cases, one-third had diabetes mellitus, three-fourths had significant complications of IE, and half required cardiac surgery.[174] In children, group A streptococcal IE may complicate varicella.[175] Group B streptococcal endocarditis is also rare; it may complicate obstetric procedures (including abortions) and intravenous drug use and involve the tricuspid valve.[176]

Staphylococci

Staph. aureus is the leading cause of acute bacterial endocarditis. Endocarditis due to *S. aureus* often originates from nosocomial sources or from the injection of recreational drugs. *S. aureus* IE has a high rate of mortality (20 to 40 percent), embolic complications, valvular destruction, and perivalvular spread with the need for surgical intervention.[40,177] The median duration of illness prior to hospitalization was 3 days in one series.[178] *Staph. aureus* is the predominant etiologic organism of IDU-related IE,[74] and it frequently causes PVE.[105]

Staph. aureus IE is often associated with diabetes mellitus (13 percent in one study), corticosteroid therapy (11 percent), cirrhosis (5 percent), malignancy (4 percent), and/or chronic renal failure (4 percent).[178] In nosocomial cases, infected intravascular devices are commonly the portals of entry.

Because *Staph. aureus* is an invasive, primary pathogen, patients with staphylococcal ABE often develop metastatic infections of skin and soft tissue, bone, joints, eye, and/or brain.[178–181] More than one-third will have central nervous system involvement.[178] Only a minority of all patients with *Staph. aureus* bacteremia develop IE (6 to 15 percent), and it is often difficult to identify this subgroup. Use of TEE in this setting is highly effective. Factors that increase the probability of IE are (1) community-acquired bacteremia, (2) absence of a primary focus of infection, and (3) metastatic staphylococcal infection. Up to two-thirds of patients with all three characteristics have IE.[181]

Staph. epidermidis is a rare cause of NVE (<5 percent), which usually has an indolent subacute or chronic course.[182] However, serious complications—including systemic embolization, heart failure, myocardial abscess, and valve destruction—are common, and mortality is high (up to 36 percent).[183] In striking contrast, *Staph. epidermidis* is a common cause of PVE (40 to 50 percent), which may follow either an acute or subacute course.[182,184]

Staph. lugdunensis, a recently described species of coagulase-negative staphylococcus, is more likely to infect native cardiac valves (about 5 percent of staphylococcal IE) than *Staph. epidermidis*[185] and is especially virulent, often leading to native valve destruction and the requirement for valve replacement.[186]

Gram-Negative Bacteria

Although most gram-negative species that colonize or infect humans can cause IE, they account for only a small proportion of NVE. Three percent of IE cases are caused by a group of nutritionally fastidious gram-negative bacilli comprising *Haemophilus* species, *Actinobacillus actinomycetemcomitans, Cardiobacterium hominis, Eikenella corrodens,* and *Kingella kingae* and referred to as *HACEK.*[187,188] Presentation may include symptoms (fever) for 2 weeks to 3 months, a new or changing murmur, splenomegaly, and emboli.[189] Blood cultures are usually positive within 3 to 4 days.[189] Prognosis with medical therapy and surgery when necessary (25 percent of patients) is good (87 percent survival).

Haemophilus is the most common etiologic HACEK organism; HACEK IE is characterized by large vegetations and arterial emboli (35 to 60 percent).[190] Etiologic species of HACEK IE include *H. parainfluenzae* (62 percent), *H. aphrophilus* (21 percent), and *H. paraphrophilus* (10 percent), but only rarely *H. influenzae.*

Common aerobic enteric gram-negative bacilli seldom cause IE. *Escherichia coli* and *Klebsiella* are notably rare causes[109] despite their frequent association with bacteremia. This disparity is probably explained by their low adhesiveness to heart valves[191] and fibrin[192] and susceptibility to complement-mediated bacteriolysis.[193] Nevertheless, gram-negative bacilli are a frequent cause of early (15 to 20 percent of cases) and late (10 percent) PVE,[10,105] and they account for about 5 percent of IE in IDUs.[69,72–74] *Pseudomonas* species, *Serratia,* and *Enterobacter* species predominate. Resistant strains such as *Stenotrophomonas* (*Xanthomonas*) *multophilia,* in association with IDUs and indwelling catheters, are becoming a recognized cause of nosocomial and prosthetic valve IE.[194] IE cases caused by species of *Salmonella, Brucella, Acinetobacter,* and other

gram-negative species also have been reported.[109] *Brucella* IE is well known in the Mediterranean basin.[195–197]

Endocarditis caused by anaerobic bacteria is rare (<1 percent of IE),[198,199] probably because of high oxygen tension at the blood/endocardial interface.

N. gonorrhoeae IE follows an acute course often involving the right heart,[5] but it has become uncommon since the introduction of penicillin.[54,55]

Yeasts and Dimorphic Fungi

Candida and *Aspergillus* genera account for the great majority of IE caused by yeasts and other fungal species.[110,111,200,201] *Candida* causes NVE in IDUs and patients receiving parenteral alimentation, whereas *Aspergillus* often involves prosthetic valves. Fungal infection of native valves in nonaddicts is being increasingly recognized (Table 81-5).[202]

Miscellaneous Organisms

Many other organisms occasionally cause IE (Table 81-6).

Q fever (*Coxiella burnetii*) is a chronic febrile illness with prominent hepatic as well as potential cardiac valvular involvement (7 percent of cases).[182–188] Most Q-fever IE cases have been reported from Europe, Canada, and Australia. Presentation typically includes intermittent fever for months to years (91 percent) and congestive heart failure (77 percent); almost all have valvular heart disease (97 percent). Diagnosis is usually based on serology or identification of the organism in cardiac tissue.[203] *Bartonella* may cause up to 3 percent of IE.[204] In the past, most of these cases were categorized as culture-negative, and some were misdiagnosed as chlamydial (cross-reacting serology).[204] When *Bartonella* is suspected (homeless patient: *Bartonella quintana;* association with cats: *Bartonella henselae*), polymerase chain reaction (PCR)–based genomic detection or antibody determination are considerably more sensitive than blood culture.[205]

Chlamydial endocarditis is rare; a few cases have been reported in bird fanciers.[206,207] Etiologic diagnosis requires specialized culture techniques, serologic studies, or examination of vegetations using

TABLE 81-6 Some Unusual or Rare Causes of Infective Endocarditis

Bacteria	Fungi
Bacillus cereus	*Blastoschizomyces*
Bartonella elizabethae	*capitatus*
Bartonella henselae	*Conidiobolus* species
Corynebacterium diphtheriae biotype *gravis*	*Curvularia lunata*
	Engyodontium album
Corynebacterium jeikeium	*Fusarium oxysporum*
Corynebacterium pseudodiphtheriticum	*Histoplasma capsulatum*
	Neosartorya fischeri
Erysipelothrix rhusiopathiae	*Phialophora richardsiae*
	Pseudallescheria boydii
Haemophilus influenzae type b	*Scedosporium inflatum*
	Scedosporium apiospermum
Lactobacillus species	
Legionella species	*Thermomyces lanuginosus tsiklinsky*
Mycoplasma hominis	
Rothia dentocariosa	*Trichosporon beigelii*
Streptobacillus moniliformis	

immunofluorescent antibodies. More than 50 cases of *Listeria mono-cytogenes* NVE or PVE have been reported; the mortality rate is high (37 percent).[208] Other unusual species occasionally infecting pros-thetic valves include *Mycoplasma hominis,*[209] *Legionella* species,[56] and mycobacteria.[210]

Culture-Negative Endocarditis

Culture-negative endocarditis refers to active IE with repeatedly negative blood cultures.[211–213] New diagnostic techniques, includ-ing PCR to identify unculturable organisms in excised vegetations or systemic emboli, have improved our understanding of culture-negative IE.[214,215] This syndrome was occasionally observed in the preantibiotic era,[216] usually in subacute cases of long duration (*Endocarditis lenta*). Today, most (but not all) culture-negative cases are caused by antibiotic treatment sufficient to suppress bacteremia but not to sterilize the vegetation. In most cases, organisms eventually reappear in the blood after antibiotics are discontinued, usually within a few days.

In a small percentage, cultures remain persistently negative.[131] *C. burnetti* and *Bartonella* species are currently the most prevalent etio-logic agents of culture-negative IE.[214] Negative blood cultures occur in about one-fifth of patients with NVE or PVE caused by *Candida* or other yeasts[111] and four-fifths with IE caused by *Aspergillus* or other molds.[111,200,217,218] Whipple's disease is a rare but increasingly seen cause of culture-negative IE[219]; the recent successful cultivation of *Tropherma whippelii*[220] may allow for the development of sero-logic testing.

Rates of culture-negative endocarditis vary widely. Among large multicenter series, up to 15 to 20 percent may be culture-negative.[31,211–213] Smaller series usually show rates of about 5 per-cent.[221,222] In some cases, a working clinical diagnosis of endocardi-tis gains support from a favorable response to empiric antibiotic treatment, but a definitive etiologic diagnosis may require detection of organisms in infected emboli or vegetations recovered at surgery or autopsy. When a patient appears to have culture-negative IE, the possibilities in Table 81-7 should be considered.

PATHOGENESIS AND PATHOLOGY

A general concept of the pathogenesis of NBTE and SBE is pre-sented in Fig. 81-2.

Noninfective Endocarditis

Sterile, thrombotic valvular lesions develop under a variety of condi-tions.[223] Small aggregates of platelets occur frequently on the sur-faces of valves damaged by congenital, rheumatic, or granlomatous disease or IE.[224] Endocardial injury exposes subendothelial connec-tive tissue (collagen), activating platelets to adhere and aggregate. Microscopic platelet thrombi may embolize harmlessly or stabilize and grow by deposition of more platelets and fibrin to form NBTE vegetations. This process can be initiated in animal models by catheter-induced endothelial damage.[225] In humans, intracardiac catheters may produce identical lesions.[135,136] Both experimental[226] and human[136,138,223] NBTE can be colonized by circulating bacteria, resulting in IE.

Vegetations of marantic endocarditis occur most often with advanced malignancy[12,13,227] but may also complicate other chronic wasting diseases, such as tuberculosis or uremia.

Sterile vegetations (*"Libman-Sacks endocarditis,"* Chap. 84) sometimes develop in patients with systemic lupus erythematosus

TABLE 81-7 Considerations for Apparent Culture-Negative IE

Antibiotic therapy already given (e.g., oral dose taken at home)
Slow-growing etiologic organism (e.g., a nutritionally variant *Streptococcus* or HACEK species, or mycobacteria)
Nutritionally fastidious organism (special procedures or supplemented media needed for nutritionally variant streptococci, *Coxiella burnetii* [Q fever], *Chlamydia, Mycoplasma, Bartonella,* and *Legionella*)
A strict anaerobe (anaerobic culture required)
Aspergillus or other molds (rarely recovered from blood; may be recovered from tissue or arterial embolus removed at surgery)
Another nonculturable organism (e.g., *C. burnetti, Bartonella* spp., Whipple's bacillus; may be diagnosed by polymerase chain reaction on tissue obtained at surgery)
Fever due to non-IE cause (e.g., rheumatic fever, tuberculosis, brucellosis, malignancy)
NBTE or marantic endocarditis (look for underlying disease such as malignancy or tuberculosis)
Libman-Sacks endocarditis (a variant of NBTE, associated with antiphospholipid antibody syndrome and/or systemic lupus erythematosus)

and/or antiphospholipid antibodies.[228] Libman-Sacks vegetations are typically small, sessile masses located on the ventricular surfaces of the mitral valve leaflets.

The vegetations of NBTE are friable white or tan masses, usually situated along the lines of valve closure (Fig. 81-3, Plate 99). They vary greatly in size, from tiny to large and exuberant, with corre-sponding tendencies to embolize to arteries supplying the myo-cardium, spleen, kidney, brain, mesentery, or extremities and cause infection. Fresh vegetations readily dislodge and embolize.[223] Histo-logically, NBTE vegetations consist of degenerating platelets inter-woven with strands of fibrin and forming a bland, featureless eosinophilic mass except for a few trapped leukocytes.[223,225]

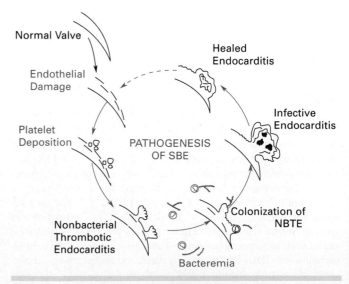

FIGURE 81-2 Main events in the pathogenesis of nonbacterial thrombotic en-docarditis (NBTE) and subacute bacterial endocarditis (SBE).

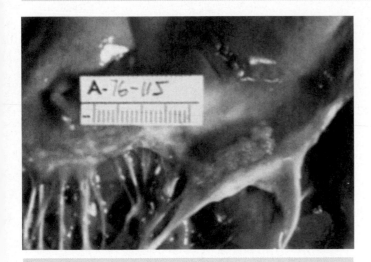

FIGURE 81-3 (Plate 99) Typical vegetation of nonbacterial thrombotic endocarditis found at necropsy in a cachectic patient who died with disseminated lung cancer.

Pathogenesis of Infective Endocarditis

For IE to develop, microbes must attach to an endocardial surface and elude local host defenses, allowing persistence and multiplication. In SBE, which usually develops on abnormal valves, circulating bacteria probably colonize preexisting platelet aggregates or NBTE.[223] It is uncertain whether ABE develops by colonization of microscopic sterile vegetations or by direct microbial invasion of normal endocardium.

Attachment of a circulating microorganism to a deposit of fibrin and platelets (NBTE) on disrupted endocardium is a critical first step in IE initiation. Virulence factors, representing a variety of surface components and receptors, give certain microbes selective adherence advantages.[53,229] Dextran production by *viridans* streptococci was identified as an important adherence factor for IE.[192] Other microbial factors include a fibronectin-binding protein,[230] enterococcal aggregation and binding substances,[231] and FimA, a surface-associated streptococcal and enterococcal protein that, when used as an antigen, induces an antibody that prevents valve adherence and endocarditis in animal models.[229,231–233] The finding of FimA in 80 percent of IE-related streptococci and enterococci raises the intriguing possibility of a protective vaccine. Fibronectin binding is a property shared by many though not all bacteria commonly causing IE.[53,229] Clumping factor produced by coagulase-positive staphylococci favors attachment to fibrinogen, adherence to platelet-fibrin thrombi, and ability to cause endocarditis in rats.[234] Extracellular slime production by coagulase-negative staphylococci may favor localization on prosthetic valves.[235]

Adherence of *Staph. aureus* to platelets is an important virulence factor for experimental IE[235–241] (Korzeniowski and Sande, Personal communication, 1999). Acetylsalicylic acid treatment reduces *Staph. aureus*–induced platelet aggregation and adherence to fibrin (with or without platelets) in vitro and vegetation size and embolic events in vivo[241] (Korzeniowski and Sande, Personal communication, 1999). *Staph. aureus* (and enterococcal) adherence to damaged valves induces tissue factor and thromboplastin and activates the clotting cascade, generating thrombin.[224,237,242] Resulting vegetations provide a protected environment for unrestricted bacterial growth. However, thrombin also elicits platelet secretion of a cationic protein with potent antimicrobial properties, thrombin-induced platelet microbicidal protein (tPMP).[238,243] *Staph. aureus* strains resistant to tPMP readily cause IE,[239] whereas strains that hypersecrete alpha toxin (which lyses platelets and releases tPMP) produce less virulent IE.[240]

Microbes that cannot adhere or elude host defenses quickly die, whereas those that adhere and survive multiply rapidly before entering a stationary phase.[226] The vegetation provides an ideal supporting stroma for growth of microbial colonies into which circulating nutrients readily diffuse. Bacteria provoke powerful stimuli to thrombosis,[242,244] including thromboplastin generated by leukocytes exposed to fibrin.[244] New fibrin layers deposit around growing bacterial colonies, enlarging the vegetations.[225] Inflammatory cytokines[245] and other leukocytes contribute to local and systemic disease manifestations.

The frequency and location of vegetations, relevant to understanding and managing endocarditis, are presented in Table 81-8. Relative IE risk is proportional to the mean blood pressure resting on individual valves[246]; thus, left-sided valves are involved much more frequently than right-sided, IE in IDUs being a notable exception. No single unifying mechanism to explain the propensity for right-sided endocarditis in IDUs has yet emerged.[247]

Vegetations are usually located on the downstream side of anatomic abnormalities. Rodbard's[248] unifying concept is that vegetations preferentially arise at a site where blood has flowed from a high-pressure source (e.g., the LV) through a narrow orifice (e.g., a stenotic aortic valve) into a low-pressure sink (e.g., the aorta). Other examples are MR, ventricular septal defect (VSD), and aortic coarctation. Experimentally, Rodbard showed that, due to Venturi effects and turbulence, bacteria carried in an aerosol flowing through a constricted tube into an area of low pressure were deposited on the walls of the tube immediately beyond the constriction.[248] These observations are consistent with the actual location of vegetations found at autopsy in cases of IE (Fig. 81-4). Vegetations may also develop on

TABLE 81-8 Approximate Frequency of Anatomic Locations of Vegetations in SBE, ABE, and Endocarditis Associated with IV Drug Abuse[a]

Location	SBE, %	ABE, %	Endocarditis in IV Drug Abusers, %
Left-sided valves	85	65	40
Aortic	15–26	18–25	15–20
Mitral	38–45	30–35	15–20
Aortic and mitral	23–30	15–20	13–20
Right-sided valves	5	20	50–70
Tricuspid	1–5	15	45–65
Pulmonary	1	Rare	2
Tricuspid and pulmonary	Rare	Rare	3
Left- and right-sided sites	Rare	5–10	5–10
Other sites (patent ductus, ventricular septal defect, coarctation, jet lesions)	10	5	5

[a]SBE = subacute bacterial endocarditis; ABE = acute bacterial endocarditis.
SOURCE: Adapted from Refs. 54, 69–74, 95, 131, 179, 246, 250.

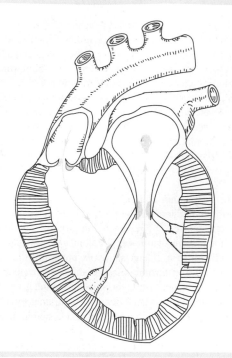

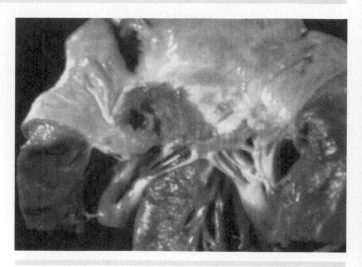

FIGURE 81-5 (Plate 100) Typical vegetation of bacterial endocarditis, complicated by perforation of the anterior mitral valve leaflet. Note that the valve shows preexisting chronic rheumatic disease, with thickening, deformity, and fusion of the chordae tendineae.

FIGURE 81-4 Sites where endocarditis occurs in aortic and mitral regurgitation. The arrows on the left indicate a high-velocity regurgitant stream passing through the orifice of an incompetent aortic valve into a low-pressure sink (left ventricle in diastole). Vegetations appear on the ventricular surface of the aortic valve. The regurgitant stream may cause a jet lesion on the chordae tendineae of the anterior leaflet of the mitral valve. The arrow on the right shows regurgitation from the high-pressure source of the left ventricle during systole into the left atrium, with vegetations developing on the atrial surface of the mitral valve. Vegetations also can occur on the jet lesion where the regurgitant stream through the mitral valve strikes the atrial endocardium, an area known as *MacCallum's patch*. (From Rodbard S. Blood velocity and endocarditis. *Circulation* 1963; 27:8. Reproduced with permission.)

Immune Response

Infected vegetations stimulate the humoral immune system to produce nonspecific antibodies. A polyclonal increase in gamma globulins, a positive rheumatoid factor, and occasionally a false-positive serologic test for syphilis may result.[253] Rheumatoid factor appears in 25 to 50 percent of SBE present for >6 weeks and can be a useful diagnostic clue; it reverts to negative after cure.[254–256] Antiendocardial and antisarcolemmal antibodies can be detected in 60 to 100 percent of cases,[257] more commonly in SBE.

Specific antibodies to commensal organisms that cause SBE may be present in low titer before infection; titers rise during active infection and fall after treatment.[6]

Hemolytic complement levels are low in about 30 percent of patients early in the course of IE, rise later, and return to normal after treatment.[258–264] The lowest levels are found in patients with immune-complex glomerulonephritis.

Circulating immune complexes have been detected in 82 to 97 percent of patients with either ABE or SBE.[263–266] Higher concentrations correlate with extracardiac manifestations, with longer duration of illness, and with hypocomplementemia. Glomerulonephritis associated with IE is mediated by immune complexes.[267,268] It is likely but unproven that arthritis, tenosynovitis, and possibly pericarditis, Osler's nodes, and Roth's spots[263,265,267] represent inflammatory responses involving immune complexes. Antibodies to teichoic acids are frequently found in the serum of patients with *Staph. aureus* IE[269] but have not proven useful diagnostically.

jet lesions, sites of endothelial roughening, and reactive fibrosis, where a swift, turbulent regurgitant stream of blood strikes the endothelium.[249] *MacCallum's patch,* located on the wall of the left atrium where an infected vegetation occasionally develops in patients with MR, is an example of a jet lesion (Fig. 81-4).

Vegetations of IE vary greatly in size and morphology, from small (<1 mm), warty nodules to large (several centimeters), cauliflower-like polypoid masses that may cause functional valve stenosis (Fig. 81-5, Plate 100). Except for the fact that fungal vegetations are often larger than bacterial ones, the etiologic organism does not predict size reliably. Color also varies widely, from white to tan to greenish-gray.[71,250] Histologically, colonies of microorganisms are found embedded in a fibrin-platelet matrix.[225,226,251,252] Vegetations characteristically contain few leukocytes (which are prevented from reaching bacteria by layers of fibrin surrounding colonies) (Fig. 81-6).

Development of an abscess occurs more frequently with ABE than with SBE.[249,251] Abscesses often develop by direct extension of infection into the fibrous cardiac skeleton, the rings of supporting connective tissue around the valves. They can further extend into adjacent myocardium and rupture into the pericardium. Hematogenous seeding occasionally leads to myocardial abscesses elsewhere.

Most patients who die with PVE have abscesses that spread around the sewing ring with partial dehiscence of the prosthetic valve.[10,105] Disturbances of the cardiac conduction system, located nearby, are also frequent.[252]

CLINICAL MANIFESTATIONS

Clinical and laboratory manifestations of IE can be grouped under evidence of systemic infection, evidence of an intravascular lesion, and evidence of an immunologic reaction to infection (Table 81-9).

History

The symptoms of SBE develop insidiously and with great variability.[6,31,43,131] Fevers, chills, rigors, and night sweats suggest systemic infection. General malaise (anorexia, fatigue, weakness) is typical. Weight loss is common, as are headaches and musculoskeletal complaints (myalgias, arthralgias, back pains).[270] The symptom complex is often described as "flu-like." The diagnosis may be delayed until symptoms persist and worsen over 4 to 8 weeks.[271,272] When present, symptoms and signs of heart failure or arterial embolism (e.g., a focal neurologic deficit; chest, flank, or left-upper-quadrant pain; hematuria; ischemia of an extremity) point to an intravascular process.

In the acute form of IE, the course is accelerated and symptoms often accentuated, with hectic fevers, rigors, and prostration leading to hospitalization within a few days.[8,31,113,273,274]

Heart failure may develop or worsen abruptly with either SBE or ABE as a consequence of sudden mechanical complications such as valve leaflet perforation, rupture of chordae tendineae or sinus of Valsalva, or functional stenosis by a large vegetation.[251,275] Alternatively, insidious development or worsening of heart failure may occur with progressive damage to cardiac valves and associated structures; myocarditis or myocardial infarction due to coronary artery embolism may also contribute.

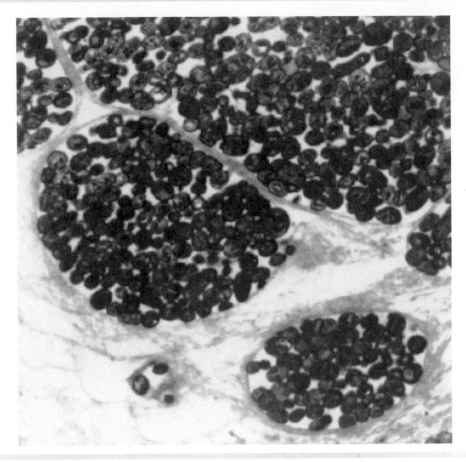

FIGURE 81-6 Electron micrograph of a vegetation of experimental streptococcal endocarditis (×7800). Note the very large number of cocci in colonies, the protective layers of fibrin, and the absence of leukocytes, all factors that may impede the efficacy of antimicrobial therapy. (From Durack DT. Experimental bacterial endocarditis: 4. Structure and evolution of very early lesions. *J Pathol* 1975;115:81. Reproduced with permission.)

Physical Examination

Astute recognition of the unique physical findings of progressive IE often allows for a bedside diagnosis (Chap. 12).

Patients with endocarditis may appear acutely or chronically ill. Intermittent chills, rigors, and sweating often provide evidence of a systemic infection. Asthenia and recent weight loss are often notable. Anemia is common.[94] The skin of some patients with long-standing SBE shows the sallow hue of uremia.[6]

VASCULAR PHENOMENA
A variety of striking physical findings of IE arise from vascular abnormalities.

Petechiae Petechiae are common in both SBE and ABE but rare in NBTE. Most are due to microembolization to small vessels in the skin or mucous membranes. They commonly occur in crops in the conjunctival sac, on the hard palate, behind the ears, and over the chest, but any area of the trunk and extremities may be affected. Some may have a pale central spot.

Splinter Hemorrhages Linear hemorrhages under the nails but not reaching the nail margin, resembling tiny splinters of wood, are found in 20 percent of patients with SBE. They are probably caused by microembolization to linear subungual capillaries. Because splinter hemorrhages are found in 5 to 8 percent of hospitalized patients without IE, they alone are of limited diagnostic value.[276]

Osler's Nodes Osler's nodes are painful, tender, erythematous nodules in the skin of the extremities, usually the pulp of the fingers, occurring in 10 to 20 percent of SBE and <10 percent of ABE patients[277] (see Fig. 12-15, Plate 34). Occasionally, the center of these pea sized, red lesions is pale, but necrosis does not occur. Their cause appears to be inflammation at the site of lodgment of small infected emboli in distal arterioles,[266] and etiologic organisms sometimes can be recovered from them.[278]

Janeway Lesions Janeway lesions—small (<5 mm), flat, irregular, nontender erythematous spots—are found on the palms and soles of a few patients with SBE and ABE. Unlike petechiae, they are not hemorrhagic, and they blanch on pressure.[6,44]

Ocular Lesions Conjunctival petechiae are small, bright-red hemorrhages that are easily seen with eyelid eversion (Chap 12). They are not specific for endocarditis, being found sometimes after cardiac surgery and with septicemia (Fig. 81-7, Plate 101). Nevertheless, the discovery of conjunctival hemorrhages in a patient with unexplained fever and a heart murmur makes the diagnosis of IE highly likely.

Retinal hemorrhages are found in 10 to 25 percent of both SBE and ABE. Their appearance is quite variable (Chap. 12). *Roth's spots* appear to represent cytoid bodies and associated hemorrhage caused by microinfarction of retinal vessels. Roth's spots are not foci of infection and are nonspecific to IE.

TABLE 81-9 Summary of the Major Clinical Manifestations of Infective Endocarditis

Manifestation	History	Examination	Investigations
Systemic infection	Fever, chills, rigors, sweats, malaise, weakness, lethargy, delirium, headache, anorexia, weight loss, backache, arthralgia, myalgia Portal of entry: oropharynx, skin, urinary tract, drug addiction, nosocomial bacteremia	Fever, pallor, weight loss, asthenia, splenomegaly	Anemia, leukocytosis (variable), raised erythrocyte sedimentation rate, positive blood culture, abnormal cerebrospinal fluid
Intravascular lesion	Dyspnea, chest pain, focal weakness, stroke, abdominal pain, cold and painful extremities	Murmurs, signs of cardiac failure, petechiae (skin, eye, mucosae), Roth's spots, Osler's nodes, Janeway lesions, splinter hemorrhages, stroke, mycotic aneurysm, ischemia or infarction of viscera or extremities	Blood in urine, chest roentgenogram, echocardiography, arteriography, liver-spleen scan, lung scan, brain scan, CT scan, histology, culture of emboli
Immunologic reactions	Arthralgia, myalgia, tenosynovitis	Arthritis, signs of uremia, vascular phenomena, finger clubbing	Proteinuria, hematuria, casts, uremia, acidosis, polyclonal increases in gamma globulins, rheumatoid factor, decreased complement, immune complexes in serum, antistaphylococcal teichoic acid antibodies

SOURCE: Adapted from Refs. 6–8, 43, 53, 54, 131.

Loss of vision during IE may be caused by embolization to the brain or retinal artery or from optic neuritis or ophthalmitis. Endophthalmitis may occur in patients with *Candida* IE and/or candidemia. The typical retinal lesions are rounded, white, cotton-like exudates.

CLUBBING OF THE FINGERS
Previously common, finger clubbing is now found in <5 percent of SBE cases (see Fig. 12-19A), presumably because of earlier diagnosis and treatment. The pathogenesis of clubbing, which usually resolves after eradication of SBE, is not understood.

SIGNS OF EMBOLIZATION
A decreased or absent pulse in an extremity may signal arterial occlusion by an embolized vegetation. Embolism to a cerebral artery may result in transient neurologic signs or progress to a completed stroke. Infarctions of the spleen, kidney, or bowel can present with abdominal pain and palpable tenderness, mimicking bowel obstruction or peritonitis. Embolic coronary artery occlusion may cause myocardial infarction, heart failure, or death and is sometimes an unexpected finding at autopsy. These complications are illustrated in Figs. 81-8 to 81-12 and Plates 102–106.

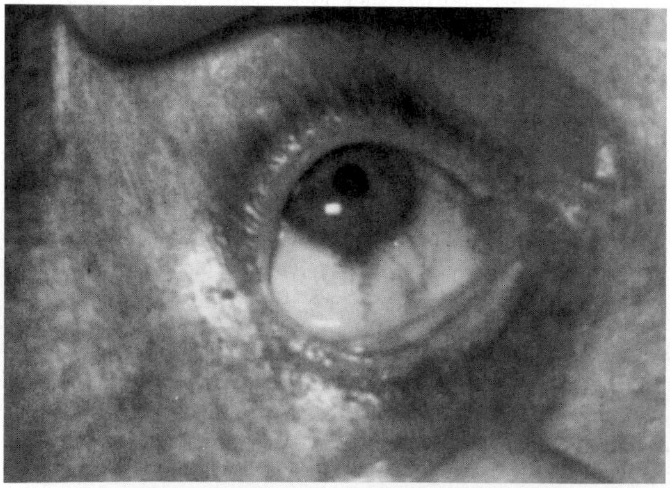

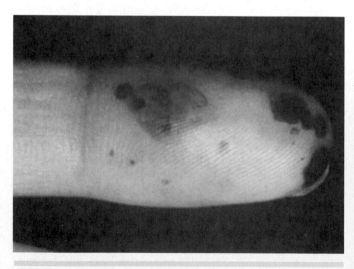

FIGURE 81-7 (Plate 101) Typical conjunctival petechiae in a patient with subacute bacterial endocarditis due to *Streptococcus sanguis*.

FIGURE 81-8 (Plate 102) Ischemic, hemorrhagic, and pustular lesions on the extremities in acute *Staphylococcus aureus* endocarditis.

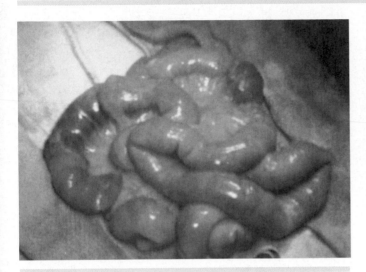

FIGURE 81-9 (Plate 103) Segmental ischemia and necrosis in the gut, presenting as acute abdomen.

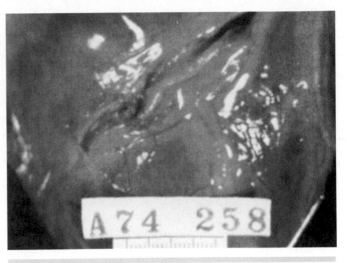

FIGURE 81-11 (Plate 105) An infected embolus in a coronary artery.

SPLENOMEGALY

Splenomegaly occurs commonly (one-quarter of ABE and one-half of SBE cases). The spleen is usually soft and only slightly tender except with recent embolic infarction, when palpation is often painful. Radionuclide scanning may reveal splenic infarction or abscess.

CARDIAC EXAMINATION

Fever or congestive failure with IE often causes a rapid pulse. Conduction system disturbances may indicate an abscess near the conduction system. Aortic regurgitation may result in a collapsing pulse (Chaps. 12 and 66).

One or more murmurs are present in most patients at some stage of IE. These murmurs may be due to preexisting cardiac disease, to the infection, or to both. The classic triad of fever, anemia, and a *new* murmur still should suggest IE even in the modern era, although these signs are nonspecific.

New or changing cardiac murmurs are an important diagnostic finding, more so in ABE than SBE. Structural damage caused by IE may lead to mitral, aortic, or tricuspid regurgitation (MR, AR, or TR). The diastolic murmur of AR developing during a febrile illness is much more likely a sign of IE than a nonspecific association with fever, anemia, and a hyperdynamic circulation.

Similarly, a new regurgitant murmur in a febrile patient with a prosthetic valve should immediately raise suspicion of PVE.

TR may be silent; only one-third of patients with tricuspid valve IE demonstrate a typical systolic murmur.[8]

COMPLICATIONS

Heart Failure

Heart failure is the most important complication of IE[31,279–281] because it exerts a critical influence on prognosis. A 1951 report noted a death rate of 37 percent for SBE without and 85 percent with heart failure.[279] Previously, heart failure occurred in up to 55 percent of cases.[280] Today, heart failure fortunately is less common because of earlier and more effective treatment, including surgery.

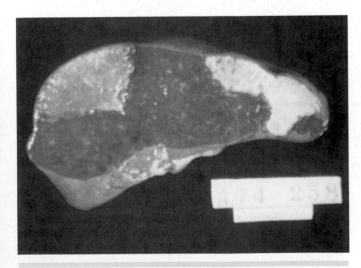

FIGURE 81-10 (Plate 104) Infarctions in the spleen.

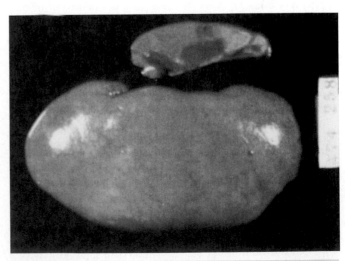

FIGURE 81-12 (Plate 106) Kidney from a patient with subacute bacterial endocarditis showing two abnormalities: (1) typical ischemic infarctions due to emboli and (2) swelling and petechiae (flea-bitten kidney) due to immune-complex glomerulonephritis.

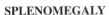

Sudden worsening of LV failure because of perforation or destruction of a valve leaflet or rupture of a chordae tendinea is an indication for immediate valve replacement. Intractable failure can also result from rupture of a sinus of Valsalva (the right sinus into the right atrium or ventricle and the left sinus into the pulmonary artery).[251] Bulky vegetations occasionally occlude a valve orifice, causing functional stenosis (e.g., during fungal PVE).[282,283]

Embolism

Arterial embolism is recognized during the course of SBE in 12 to 40 percent and ABE in 40 to 60 percent, and autopsy findings indicate many undetected events. Pelletier and Petersdorf[131] reported a 50 percent incidence of major arterial emboli among 125 IE cases affecting brain ($N = 25$), lung (17), coronary artery (8), spleen (8), extremities (8), gut (4), or eye (3). Antiphospholipid antibodies are a major risk factor for embolism.[284] Embolism before antibiotic therapy and increasing vegetation size despite antibiotic therapy are risk factors for new emboli.[285]

Conduction Abnormalities

The proximal conduction system [atrioventricular (AV) node, His-Purkinje system, proximal bundle branches] lies near the apex of the interventricular septum and the valve rings (especially aortic). A conduction abnormality occurs in 4 to 16 percent of IE cases and is more common with aortic valve infection.[252,275,286] Abnormalities occur as first- (45 percent), second- (15 percent), or third- (20 percent) degree AV block or as isolated bundle branch blocks (15 percent).[252] *A new, unstable, or changing conduction abnormality suggests extension of IE near or into the AV node or bundle of His, may indicate a valve-ring abscess, is associated with a worse prognosis, and constitutes a strong indication for TEE and consideration of surgical intervention.*[281] Patients with perivalvular abscess have a high rate of death after hospital discharge and a high incidence of complications, including pseudoaneurysms and fistulas.[287]

Neurologic Manifestations

Nervous system involvement during the course of IE is common and clinically important.[288–291] In some series, neurologic complications approach or even surpass heart failure as a determinant of mortality.[291] Significant neurologic abnormalities occur in 29 to 50 percent with IE; up to two-thirds of related embolic events involve the central nervous system.[288,291–293] IE presents as a neurologic complaint in 10 to 15 percent of cases. The wide range of syndromes includes toxic confusional states, psychiatric symptoms, minor or major strokes (Fig. 81-13), meningoencephalitis, and cranial or peripheral nerve lesions.[291] (Chap. 99).

Approximately four-fifths of cerebrovascular complications occur as infarction and one-fifth as hemorrhage.[292] Strokes tend to occur early in the course of illness, are more common with mitral valve IE, and are predicted by vegetation length.[294] Infarction is usually due to embolism, most often to a middle cerebral artery outside the circle of Willis. Hemorrhage may be a complication of emboli or mycotic aneurysms.[288–290, 295–297]

A meningeal reactive cerebritis occurs in 7 to 15 percent of patients and is prevalent especially in those with staphylococcal ABE.[43,288,290–293] Bacterial meningitis may be mistakenly diagnosed because the cerebrospinal fluid contains polymorphonuclear neutrophil leukocytes (PMNs) and may have a raised protein concentration; a minority of patients may have a positive cerebrospinal fluid culture (up to 20 percent with staphylococcal ABE). However, cere-

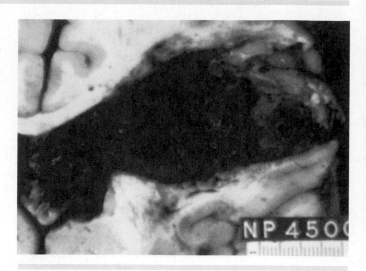

FIGURE 81-13 (Plate 107) Massive cerebral hemorrhage with intraventricular extension due to rupture of a small, peripheral mycotic aneurysm. The patient had been bacteriologically cured of *Staphylococcus epidermidis* endocarditis several weeks previously. Cultures of the blood, valve, and aneurysm taken at necropsy were negative.

brospinal glucose levels are usually normal and cultures usually negative. These abnormalities resolve with treatment of IE.

Cerebritis and associated meningoencephalitis may develop in brain tissue surrounding small infected emboli lodged in cerebral vessels.[291] Computed tomography and MRI often reveal multiple areas of cerebritis, even in patients with no central nervous system symptoms (Fig. 81-14). In patients with ABE, this inflammatory reaction may progress to a brain abscess; it resolves during antibiotic treatment of IE. Brain abscess is distinctly uncommon in SBE.[291] Bacterial meningitis occurs in some patients with pneumococcal endocarditis.[171]

Mycotic Aneurysm

Mycotic aneurysm develops in 3 to 15 percent of patients with IE and has serious consequences if expansion and rupture occur (Fig. 81-13, Plate 107). The proximal aorta, including the sinuses of Valsalva (25 percent of aneurysms), visceral arteries (24 percent), arteries to the extremities (22 percent), and cerebral arteries (15 percent) are most often involved.[295,296,298] Intracerebral aneurysms are often multiple.[296,298]

Mycotic aneurysms develop when the wall of an artery is damaged by the inflammatory response to microbes.[262,299–301] Microbes reach the arterial wall via microemboli to the vasa vasorum or by luminal impaction of larger infected emboli. The arterial wall does not readily support bacterial growth, and organisms often die spontaneously even if untreated. However, mycotic aneurysms may continue to enlarge even when organisms are gone, due to persistent inflammation and expansive remodeling under pulsatile arterial pressure (Fig. 81-9, Plate 103).[295,296,298,302]

Prolonged Fever

Fever usually abates within 2 to 3 days of beginning antibiotic therapy for less virulent organisms, and over 90 percent of patients become afebrile within 2 weeks.[2] Persistence of fever beyond 14 days should raise concern for myocardial abscess, metastatic or nosocomial infection, pulmonary embolism, or drug hypersensitivity and should prompt further diagnostic assessment.

DIFFERENTIAL DIAGNOSIS

Because the clinical manifestations of IE are numerous and often nonspecific, the differential diagnosis is broad.[6,43,131,303] Of the many conditions that may be considered, only a few leading examples can be given.

ABE shares many clinical features with other septicemias and febrile illnesses caused by invasive pathogens such as *Staph. aureus*, *Neisseria*, pneumococci, and gram-negative bacilli. Thus, differential diagnosis frequently includes sepsis, pneumonia, meningitis, brain abscess, stroke, malaria, acute pericarditis, vasculitis, and disseminated intravascular coagulopathy.

SBE must be considered during the workup of every patient with fever of unknown origin.[221,303,304]

Diagnostic Criteria

IE can be surprisingly difficult to diagnose with certainty,[221,305] and the diagnosis is suspected much more often than it is confirmed. Presenting symptoms and signs are highly variable and often consistent with other diagnoses, and the primary lesion is inaccessible to direct inspection. In this setting, the development, critical assessment, and modification of standard criteria for IE diagnosis has represented an important clinical advance.[95,221,222,306] These standards utilize major and minor criteria, somewhat analogous to the modified Jones criteria used for the diagnosis of acute rheumatic fever (Chap. 65).[307] Of proposed diagnostic schema, the original and *modified Duke criteria* have received the most attention; their usefulness is best validated prospectively.[2,221,222,306,308–310] The original Duke criteria show excellent specificity (99 percent) and negative predictive value (92 percent).[222,309,310] However, sensitivity is lower, and they should not be used to guide urgent management decisions early in the course of a suspected case.

Modified versions of the Duke criteria have been proposed to improve on sensitivity while retaining specificity. One version adds two minor criteria (new-onset heart failure and presence of conduction disturbance).[309] Another version, from Duke University, is presented in Tables 81-10 and 81-11.[306] These modified Duke criteria recognize *Staph. aureus* bacteremia and Q-fever serology as major criteria, and they emphasize the role of TEE.

LABORATORY INVESTIGATIONS

Routine Laboratory Tests

A hypoproliferative anemia usually develops during the course of SBE.[94,307] It is most often mild to moderate in degree with a normochromic, normocytic smear. Anemia occurs less often in ABE and may be due to hemolysis. Low-grade hemolysis associated with a prosthetic valve may confound interpretation when PVE is being considered.

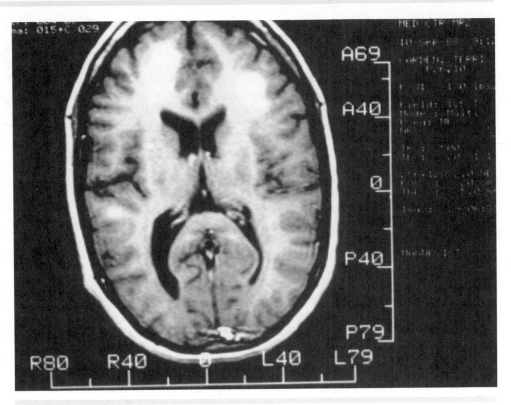

FIGURE 81-14 Magnetic resonance image of the brain in a patient with acute left-sided *Staphylococcus aureus* endocarditis, showing multiple areas of focal cerebritis. This patient had no focal central nervous system signs and recovered fully with antimicrobial therapy. (MRI by courtesy of the Department of Radiology, Duke University, Durham, NC.)

Leukocytosis is not a reliable manifestation of SBE.[94] Low-grade polymorphonuclear leukocytosis is characteristic, but the leukocyte count may be normal. Leukocytosis with an increase in bands is common with ABE, and neutrophils often show toxic granulations. Occasionally in ABE, staphylococci can be identified within neutrophils on Gram's stain of buffy coat smears.[311] In one-third of SBE cases, abnormal histiocytes may be found in smears of peripheral blood.[312]

The erythrocyte sedimentation rate (ESR) is elevated in 90 percent of IE cases and does not fall to normal until 3 to 6 months, even with successful treatment. C-reactive protein is also usually elevated (96 percent) but falls to normal more quickly during successful therapy.[313] Cryoglobulinemia also has been reported.[314] Urinalysis shows microscopic hematuria and/or slight proteinuria in 50 percent,

TABLE 81-10   Criteria for Diagnosis of IE

Major criteria (Specifically defined in Table 81-11)
   Microbiologic evidence (from blood or tissue)
   Evidence of endocardial involvement
Minor criteria (Specifically defined in Table 81-11)
   Clinical predisposition
   Fever
   Immunologic phenomena
   Microbiologic findings
Definite IE: 2 major criteria, 1 major plus 3 minor, or 5
   minor criteria
Possible IE: 1 major and 1 minor criterion or 3 minor criteria

SOURCE: From Li et al.,[306] with permission.

TABLE 81-11 Definitions of Diagnostic Criteria for IE

Major criterion: Microbiologic
  Isolation from two separate blood cultures of a typical organism: *viridans* streptococci, *Strep. bovis*, HACEK group, *Staph. aureus*, or community-acquired enterococcal bacteremia in absence of a primary focus
  Or persistently positive blood culture with recovery of a microorganism consistent with IE
  Or single positive blood culture for *Coxiella burnetii* or phase 1 IgG antibody titer to *C. burnetii* >1:800
Major criterion: Endocardial involvement
  New valvular regurgitation (increase or change in preexisting murmur not sufficient)
  Positive echocardiogram for IE (TEE for PVE):
    1. Discrete, echogenic, oscillating intracardiac mass located at a site of endocardial injury (e.g., on a valve or supporting structure, in pathway of regurgitant jet, or site of implanted material), or
    2. Periannular abscess, or
    3. New dehiscence of a prosthetic valve
Minor criterion: Predisposing cardiac condition or injection drug use
  High-risk conditions: Previous IE, aortic valve disease, rheumatic heart disease, prosthetic heart valve, coarctation of aorta, complex cyanotic congential heart diseases
  Moderate-risk conditions: Mitral valve prolapse with regurgitation or leaflet thickening, isolated mitral stenosis, tricuspid valve disease, pulmonary stenosis, hypertrophic cardiomyopathy
  Low- or no-risk conditions: Secundum atrial septal defect, ischemic heart disease, previous coronary artery bypass graft surgery, MVP with thin leaflets, no regurgitation
Minor criterion: Fever
  Temperature >38° C (>100.4° F)
Minor criterion: Vascular phenomena
  Major arterial emboli, septic pulmonary infarcts, mycotic aneurysm, intracranial hemorrhage, conjunctival hemorrhages, Janeway lesions
  Petechiae and splinter hemorrhages are excluded
Minor criterion: Immunologic phenomena
  Glomerulonephritis, Osler's nodes, Roth's spots, rheumatoid factor
Minor criterion: Microbiologic findings
  Positive blood culture(s) but not meeting major criteria
  Or serologic evidence of active infection with organisms consistent with IE
  But exclude single isolates of coagulase-negative staphylococci or organisms rarely causing IE

SOURCE: From Li et al.,[306] with permission.

even in the absence of renal complications.[6,315] Red blood cell casts and heavy proteinuria are characteristic of immune-complex glomerulonephritis, often in association with decreased total serum complement.[267] Gross hematuria suggests renal infarction.

Serologic Tests

Nonspecific serologic abnormalities are common. A polyclonal increase in gamma globulins is characteristic. Rheumatoid factor is present in >50 percent of cases of SBE with symptoms lasting longer than 6 weeks[221, 254–256] but is rarely positive in ABE. Occasional false-positive serologic tests for syphilis occur.[253]

Specific serologic tests are important for the diagnosis of IE caused by *C. burnetii* (Q fever) and *Bartonella,* which are difficult to culture. In these cases, positive serology (>1:800 phase 1 IgG antibody titer to *C. burnetii* or positive microimmunofluorescence or PCR test for *Bartonella*) or a single positive blood culture may be added as major diagnostic criteria.[204,306,316]

Blood Cultures

Isolation of a typical organism or detection of persistent bacteremia constitutes the most important diagnostic test for IE. Blood cultures

should be drawn from all patients with undiagnosed fever and a heart murmur. Cultures should also be taken from patients with other symptoms or signs consistent with IE if no other diagnosis has been made.

Bacteremia in SBE is usually continuous.[20] The number of organisms in venous blood commonly ranges from 1 to 200 per milliliter. In untreated patients, three separate blood specimens usually suffice to achieve a diagnosis by culture.[317] Blood cultures taken on the day of admission were positive in 93 percent of patients with culture-positive IE in one study.[293] In some series, somewhat lower rates have been reported (62 to 68 percent).[131,221] Additional specimens obtained over a longer period may be required if antibiotics have recently been given.

A practical approach for suspected SBE is to draw three separate samples of venous blood, each of 16 to 20 mL, on the first day, with at least 1 h between the first and last venipuncture. Half of each sample is inoculated into an aerobic broth culture medium and the other half into another (usually anaerobic) medium. These media should support growth of fastidious, nutritionally variant bacteria[156,318] and ideally should contain a resin to remove antibiotics. As soon as a culture turns positive, Gram's stain and subculture should be performed. If all three samples (six bottles) are negative by the second or third day but the diagnosis of IE still seems likely, two more venous blood samples should be drawn. With prior antibiotic exposure, several further samples may be taken over a few weeks to identify late recrudescence of bacteremia.

For ABE, three venous blood samples are drawn for culture and empiric antibiotic therapy is begun immediately. Over 95 percent of *Staph. aureus* IE cultures become positive, usually within 24 h.[8]

Because *Staph. epidermidis*[274] and diphtheroids[319] can cause IE, special care must be taken during venipuncture to avoid contamination with these common skin organisms. If all cultures are positive, IE is likely, whereas if only one of three grow one of these organisms, contamination should be suspected.

If cultures are negative but the diagnosis of IE remains likely, incubation should be extended for 3 weeks and Gram's stains made at 5 days, 2 weeks, and 3 weeks even if no growth is apparent. HACEK organisms, pyridoxyl-requiring *viridans* streptococci, some fungi, *Bartonella,* and some others may require longer than the standard 3 to 5 days to grow.[320] Hopefully, new serologic and PCR-based techniques will help to clarify diagnosis in culture-negative cases.[215,321,322] In a recent study of 51 febrile IDUs, PCR had a sensitivity and specificity of 87 percent compared to blood cultures, and 8 of 8 with IE were PCR-positive.[323]

Electrocardiography

Electrocardiography (ECG) should be performed initially and repeated at intervals. A new disturbance of conduction or onset of arrhythmia suggests possible myocardial extension of infection.[124] Thus, development of even asymptomatic PR-interval prolongation can have major implications: a worsening prognosis and probable need for cardiac surgery.[96] ECG can also lead to a diagnosis of myocardial infarction due to coronary artery embolism. Continuous ECG monitoring may be appropriate when disease progression is a concern or when changes in conduction or rhythm are noted.

Echocardiography

Both transthoracic (TTE) and transesophageal (TEE) echocardiographic studies play a key role in diagnosis, prognosis, and management of IE.[300–304] Positive findings, properly interpreted, constitute important diagnostic criteria (Tables 81-10 and 81-11) and, in the setting of positive blood cultures, essentially establish the diagnosis.[221,306] TTE combined with color-flow Doppler imaging (Chap. 15) may provide considerable information about the presence, location, and properties of vegetations, perforations, and other valvular abnormalities; abscesses; pericarditis; and the state of cardiac function (Fig. 81-15A to D).[324–328] Sensitivity of TTE for detection of vegetations today is 50 to 75 percent.[306] With TEE, this sensitivity increases to >95 percent (Chap. 15).[286,326] TEE also detects abscesses and valve perforations with much greater sensitivity[328–330] and is better than TTE for evaluation of PVE, especially of mitral valves.[331,332]

Current recommendations are to *use TTE* for initial evaluation of patients with native valves and a relatively low probablility (<4 percent) of IE.[333] *Initial TEE* becomes more cost-effective and efficient for patients with higher prior probabilities (4 to 60 percent).[334] TEE is also superior for the assessment of suspected myocardial abscess or perivalvular extension of IE. Color-flow Doppler technology is useful to demonstrate abnormal flow patterns created by valve perforations, fistulas, and pseudoaneurysms.[329] TEE assessment may better determine the appropriate duration of antibiotic therapy (2 or 4 weeks) for catheter-associated *Staph. aureus* bacteremia than standard risk-factor assessment alone.[178,335–337]

Echocardiography has some limitations.[338] It is not cost-effective in patients with a low pretest probability.[335,339] With higher probability, a negative study (especially if TEE) does have negative predictive value, but it can never exclude the diagnosis of IE.[190,221,335,339] Sensitivity for detection of vegetations is somewhat lower on the right side (about 70 percent) than on the left (>95 percent).[286,338] Prosthetic valves reduce the sensitivity, but findings are still usually informative. Occasionally, echocardiography provides a false-positive reading for "vegetation." This possibility should be particularly considered in patients with myxomatous degeneration or other preexisting focal valve pathology and when surgery is contemplated.

Serial echocardiography can guide decision making on the progress of therapy and the need and timing for surgery.[207] Detection of an abscess, perforation of a valve, or rupture of a chorda tendinea or sinus of Valsalva[251] may indicate the need for surgical intervention. Successful antimicrobial treatment may result in the disappearance, decrease, or persistence (without change) of vegetations; therefore, serial echocardiography *should not be used* as a "test of cure."[338] However, progressive enlargement of a vegetation indicates possible treatment failure and constitutes a relative indication for surgical intervention. In a study of *Staph. aureus* IE, visualization of vegetation by TTE carried a higher risk of embolization or death (68 percent) than by TEE only (16 percent, $p < 0.01$).[337] A metanalysis concluded that large vegetations (>10 mm) increased the odds ratio for embolization (2.8, $p < 0.01$) but not for death.[341] Overall, the value of echocardiography for predicting outcomes remains uncertain.[341,342]

Other Imaging Studies

The most important contribution of the chest x-ray is to provide evidence of congestive heart failure. The radiographic presence of multiple small, patchy pulmonary infiltrates in a febrile IDU may indicate septic emboli arising from right-sided IE.[69–71] Valvular calcification may identify a predisposing substrate to IE. Widening of the aorta may be caused by a mycotic aneurysm. Fluoroscopy can demonstrate abnormal motion of a prosthetic valve and suggest partial dehiscence.

Computed tomography[149,343] (Chap. 28) and magnetic resonance imaging (MRI)[291] (Chap. 21) can be useful in assessing focal neurologic lesions[344] and aortic widening. Angiographic studies can demonstrate mycotic aneurysms in the brain or elsewhere[296,298]; MRI now offers a noninvasive diagnostic alternative.

Cardiac Catheterization with Cineangiography

Cardiac catheterization is not usually necessary for IE patients who respond well to antimicrobial therapy without complications. When surgical intervention is considered, additional information provided by cardiac catheterization and cineangiography (Chap. 17) is often needed.[345] Coronary angiography should be performed in adults over 40 years of age so that coronary bypass can be performed, if indicated, at the time of valve replacement. Hemodynamic and angiographic evaluation of valvular and other cardiac pathology may be additive to echocardiography. Occasionally, a previously unsuspected diagnosis is made. Physiologic measurements, including cardiac output, right and left heart pressures, and the degree of valvular regurgitation may help determine the need and timing of surgery. In older series, cardiac catheterization was shown to improve clinical assessment of IE.[345] With increasingly accurate noninvasive imaging, the role of catheterization in younger IE patients for noncoronary indications is decreasing.

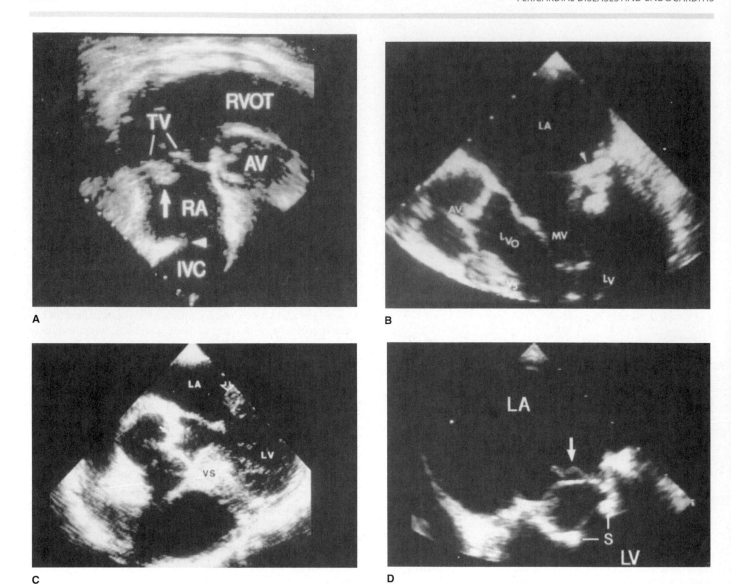

FIGURE 81-15 *A–D*. Echocardiograms from 4 patients with infective endocarditis showing vegetations located at different sites. *A*. Transesophageal echocardiogram (TEE) showing a large vegetation (*arrow*) on the tricuspid valve (TV). IVC = inferior vena cava; RA = right atrium; AV = aortic valve; RVOT = right ventricular outflow tract. *B*. Large vegetation (*arrowhead*) involving both the atrial and ventricular surfaces of the posterior mitral valve leaflet. LA = left atrium; MV = anterior leaflet of the mitral valve; LVO = left ventricular outflow tract; AV = aortic valve. *C*. TEE showing vegetations on both the mitral (*open arrow*) and aortic valve (*arrow*) in a patient with acute *Staphylococcus aureus* endocarditis. LA = left atrium; LV = left ventricle; VS = ventricular septum. *D*. TEE showing a vegetation on the cusp of a bioprosthetic valve (*arrow*). LA = left atrium; LV = left ventricle; S = artificial valve struts. (Kindly provided by Dr. B. Khanderia and Dr. J. Steckelberg, Mayo Clinic, Rochester, MN.)

Radionuclide Imaging

In animals, experimental vegetations have been located by scanning for radiolabeled platelets deposited onto a growing endocardial lesion.[346] Gallium-67 scans have shown increased uptake in the heart in some patients with IE. Scintigraphic studies following injection of indium 111–labeled leukocytes have been used to detect intracardiac abscesses.[81,347] Single photon emission computed tomography immunoscintigraphy using antigranulocyte antibody also has been described to diagnose IE. However, no radionuclide technique has sufficient sensitivity, specificity, or incremental value over echocardiography to justify its routine use for the detection of vegetations. In selected cases, scintigraphy using indium 111–labeled leukocytes can be used to detect mycotic aneurysms and extracardiac foci of infection.[348] Liver-spleen imaging may reveal splenic infarctions, confirming embolization.

TREATMENT

General Principles

IE management aims to eradicate the infecting organism as soon as possible so as to operate with optimal timing if surgery is required and to treat complications effectively. Treatment must be continued long enough to ensure that relapse will not occur. However, patients with the more easily cured forms of IE should not be subjected to unnecessarily long, expensive, and potentially toxic in-hospital treatment.[349] Many patients can be cured in 2[350–352] or 4 weeks,[353] but others require treatment for 6 weeks or longer.

Guidelines for preventive therapy are limited by the paucity of clinical trials in humans (which raise ethical and statistical issues). Questions about which subject, which antibiotic, what dosage, and for what duration remain incompletely answered. Experimental studies in animals have helped improve our understanding of conditions facilitating IE and the mode of action and potential utility of antibiotics in IE prevention as well as in devising recommendations for prophylaxis.[354]

Microbiologic Tests

For group A streptococcal IE, nothing more than positive identification is necessary, because these organisms are usually still sensitive to low concentrations of penicillin. For most other bacteria, the minimal inhibitory concentration (MIC) of relevant antibiotics should be determined. Many organisms are resistant to intermediate or even high concentrations of penicillin.[355,356] Many strains are tolerant (that is, inhibited but not killed by achievable antibiotic levels).[357,358] Since there is no definitive evidence that tolerance determines treatment outcome, measurement of minimal bactericidal concentrations (MBC) is not necessary in most cases.

The serum bactericidal titer (SBT or Schlichter test) has frequently been used to monitor IE treatment.[31,359] The infecting organism is exposed in vitro to the patient's serum, drawn during antibiotic therapy, and the maximal dilution that will inhibit and kill the organism is determined. On the basis of empiric clinical experience, desirable SBT should be 1:8 or higher at intervals during each day. For streptococcal IE, SBTs are often 1:128 to 1:1024. However, SBT is technically difficult to perform and standardize and is now regarded as obsolete by most experts.[359,360] Rarely, SBT might be informative, as in treating unusual organisms or when treatment appears to be failing.

Dosing regimens that result in widely fluctuating serum antibiotic concentrations are often employed for treating IE, and they are usually effective. Whether regimens maintaining continuous therapeutic serum concentrations offer any therapeutic benefits over intermittent regimens is unknown.

Choice of Antibiotics

Whenever possible, bactericidal antibiotics are chosen for the treatment of IE.[31,353] Some cures have been achieved with bacteriostatic drugs, but results are unreliable.[26,361,362] Bactericidal action is generally needed, because host defense mechanisms are inadequate within vegetations: protective layers of fibrin surrounding the colonies of bacteria allow relatively few phagocytes to enter (Fig. 81-6). Thus, to reliably effect a cure, antibiotic therapy must eradicate organisms completely without the help of phagocytes to eliminate subpopulations that are resistant or in a resting phase. Nevertheless, in treating unusual organisms, it may occasionally be necessary to use a bacteriostatic antibiotic in combination with other drugs to achieve optimal antibacterial effect.

For the common forms of bacterial endocarditis caused by gram-positive organisms, specific therapeutic regimens can be recommended with confidence based on extensive published experience.[350,363] Some of these are listed in Table 81-12.

Antibiotic resistance is increasingly threatening traditional treatment regimens. Penicillin resistance is rising among *viridans* streptococci, the majority of which have previously been fully sensitive.[364,365] In 1996, some 13 percent of blood culture isolates showed high-level resistance (MIC >4.0 mg/mL) and 42 percent, intermediate resistance (MIC 0.25 to 2.0 mg/mL).[365] Use of combined antibiotic regimens such as beta-lactam plus aminoglycoside or even vancomycin plus aminoglycoside should be considered for the treatment of resistant strains.[364] Enterococcal IE requires a synergistic bactericidal combination. Synergistic combinations of a beta-lactam

and an aminoglycoside have treated enterococci successfully for many years, but increasing resistance, especially to vancomycin, presents new problems.[366] The most resistant species is *Enterococcus faecium,* which may exhibit high-level resistance to vancomycin as well as intrinsic resistance to beta-lactam antibiotics and imipenem.[104] The optimal treatment for IE with these strains is unknown. Animal models have demonstrated comparable efficacy in MRSA endocarditis with linezolid as compared with vancomycin.[367,368]

Several antibiotic combinations have been tried with some success. These include high-dose ampicillin plus imipenem plus or minus a fluoroquinolone,[104,369] ampicillin plus imipenem plus vancomycin,[370] ampicillin plus a fluoroquinolone,[371] and quinupristin/dalfopristin plus doxycycline plus rifampin.[372] Because sensitivity and "cidal" versus "static" responses differ markedly among isolates, in vitro time-kill testing to various drugs alone and in combination may be needed to help with drug selection. An infectious disease consultation is recommended.[104,369–374]

Staph. epidermidis PVE is difficult to eradicate with antibiotics alone.[184] *Staph. epidermidis* is frequently resistant to semisynthetic penicillins, cephalosporins, and other antibiotics. A regimen combining vancomycin, rifampin, and an aminoglycoside, chosen according to sensitivity tests, is most likely to succeed. Rifampin resistance may develop during treatment.

Right-sided endocarditis in drug abusers due to *Staph. aureus* is a common, difficult management problem. A short course of therapy (2 weeks) was more successful with gentamicin combined with cloxacillin in a recent randomized clinical trial.[375]

Treatment of IE due to less common organisms must be chosen on the basis of limited published experience,[53,54,353,376] microbiologic testing, and individual considerations. Generally, a beta-lactam antibiotic should be included in the regimen. Combinations of two or more antibiotics are often employed. Potentially useful regimens for these rarer forms of IE are too numerous to detail here. Eradication of Q fever is difficult and usually requires valve replacement. Relapse rates may be lower with doxycycline combined with hydroxychloroquine for at least 18 months than combined with fluoroquinolone.[220,377]

Empiric Therapy

When the etiologic organism is unknown, empiric therapy should depend on whether the patient has acute or subacute disease. ABE requires broad-spectrum therapy that covers *Staph. aureus* as well as many species of streptococci and gram-negative bacilli. SBE requires a regimen that treats most streptococci, including *E. faecalis.* To meet these requirements, the following suggestions are offered:

- For ABE: nafcillin 2.0 g IV q 4 h plus ampicillin 2.0 g IV q 4 h plus gentamicin 1.5 mg/kg IV q 8 h. If methicillin-resistant *Staph. aureus* is considered likely (for example, in a hospital-acquired case), vancomycin 1.0 g IV q 12 h should be substituted for nafcillin until antibiotic sensitivity is known.
- For SBE: ampicillin 2.0 g IV q 4 h plus gentamicin 1.5 mg/kg IV q 8 h.

Therapy may include vancomycin and gentamicin for culture-negative PVE occurring within 1 year of valve surgery; ceftriaxone or cefotaxime may be added to cover HACEK organisms if PVE begins more than 1 year postoperatively.[2]

Treatment should be adjusted when the etiologic organism is identified and again when antibiotic sensitivity is known. In those few cases where empiric therapy is administered as a therapeutic trial to help confirm a diagnosis, treatment should be continued without interruption or unnecessary change for at least 2 weeks.

TABLE 81-12 Treatment Regimens for Infective Endocarditis[a, b, c]

Organism	Treatment Regimen: Dose and Route	Duration in Weeks	Comments
Fully penicillin-sensitive streptococci: MIC ≤ 0.1 μg/mL *viridans* (α-hemolytic) streptococci; *Strep. bovis; Strep. pneumoniae; Strep. pyogenes* group A, C, etc.; *Strep. agalactiae* group B	1. Penicillin G[c] 4 million units every 6 h IV alone (4 weeks) *or* 2. Penicillin G[c] 4 million units every 6 h IV with gentamicin (2 weeks) 3. Ceftriaxone 2 g IV or IM once daily alone (2 weeks) *or* 4. Ceftriaxone 2 g IV or IM once daily *or* with gentamicin 1 mg/kg twice a day or 3 mg/kg 4 times a day (2 weeks) 5. Vancomycin 15 mg/kg IV every 12 h (4 weeks)[a,b]	4 4 4	Suitable for hospitalized patients but less convenient for outpatient therapy For patients allergic to penicillins but not cephalosporins or for outpatient therapy in selected patients For patients allergic to penicillins and cephalosporins
Relatively penicillin-resistant streptococci: MIC > 0.1 < 1.0 μg/mL, some *viridans* (α-hemolytic) streptococci; some *S. pneumoniae;* etc.	1. Penicillin G[c] 4 million units IV every 4 h *plus* gentamicin 1.0 mg/kg every 12 h IV or IM (for first 2 weeks only)[a] *or* 2. Vancomycin 15 mg/kg IV every 12 h[b]	4(2) 4	For outpatient therapy in selected patients, ceftriaxone 2 g IV once daily may be substituted for penicillin if ceftriaxone MIC ≤ 4 μg/mL, *plus* gentamicin 2.0 mg/kg given once daily. For patients allergic to penicillins
Penicillin-resistant streptococci: MIC ≥ 1.0 μg/mL, *E. faecalis, E. faecium,* other enterococci; some other streptococci	1. Penicillin G[c] 18–30 million units/day IV continuously or in divided doses *plus* gentamicin 1mg/kg IV or IM every 8 h *or* 2. Ampicillin 12 g/day IV continuously or in divided doses *plus* gentamicin 1.0 mg/kg IV every 8 h, *or* 3. Vancomycin 15 mg/kg IV every 12 h *plus* gentamicin 1.0 mg/kg IV every 8 h[a,b]	4–6 4–6 4–6	Susceptibility testing needed; do not use penicillin- or ampicillin-containing regimen if strain produces β-lactamase 4-week regimen recommended for most cases with symptoms for <3 months, otherwise 6 weeks For patients allergic to penicillin; 4 weeks should be adequate for most cases; serum levels should be monitored
Staphylococci (in the absence of prosthetic material)	Methicillin-susceptible staphylococci: 1. Nafcillin 2 g IV every 4 h IV 4–6 weeks *or* 2. Nafcillin 2 g IV every 4 h IV × 4–6 wks *plus* gentamicin 1.0 mg/kg every 8 h IV × 3–5 days 3. Vancomycin 15 mg/kg IV every 12 h 4–6 weeks[b]	 4–6 4–6 4–6	β-lactam-containing regimens preferred over vancomycin unless patient is definitely hypersensitive to penicillins and cephalosporins; for patients with severe disseminated staphylococcal infection, antimicrobial synergy may be advantageous during early stages of treatment; therefore, gentamicin 1.0 mg/kg IV every 8 h for first 3–5 days only may be added to any of these regimens
In right-sided uncomplicated tricuspid endocarditis	Nafcillin 2 g IV every 4 h and gentamicin 1 mg/kg twice a day or 3 mg/kg 4 times a day Methicillin-resistant staphylococci: Vancomycin 15 mg/kg IV every 12 h[b]	2 4–6	
Staphylococci (associated with prosthetic valve or other prosthetic material)	Methicillin-susceptible staphylococci: Nafcillin 2 g IV every 4 h *plus* gentamicin 1.0 mg/kg IV every 8 h[a] *plus* rifampin 600 mg orally 4 times a day	≥6	Cefazolin or vancomycin may be substituted for nafcillin if necessary due to drug hypersensitivity

(continued)

TABLE 81-12 Treatment Regimens for Infective Endocarditis[a, b, c] (*Continued*)

Organism	Treatment Regimen: Dose and Route	Duration in Weeks	Comments
	Methicillin-resistant staphylococci: Vancomycin 15 mg/kg IV every 12 h *plus* gentamicin 1.0 mg/kg IV or IM every 8 h *plus* rifampin 300 mg orally every 8 h[a,b]	≥6	
HACEK group organisms: *Haemophilus* species *Actinobacillus actinomycetemcomitans* *Cardiobacterium hominis* *Eikenella* species *Kingella kingae*	1. Ceftriaxone 2 g IV or IM once daily *or* 2. Ampicillin 12 g/day IV continuously or in divided doses *plus* gentamicin 1.0 mg/kg every 12 h IV or IM[a]	4 4	Other third-generation cephalosporins may be substituted, using appropriate dose adjustment Less convenient for outpatient therapy
Pseudomonas aeruginosa, other gram-negative bacilli *Neisseria* species	Extended-spectrum penicillin *or* third-generation cephalosporin *or* imipenem *plus* aminoglycoside 1. Penicillin G[c] 2 million units IV every 6 h *or* 2. Ceftriaxone 1 g IV or IM once daily	4–6 3–4 3–4	Combination therapy recommended; final choice of antibiotic regimen to be made after sensitivity results available Organisms often highly sensitive to penicillin, but must be tested for β-lactamase production; 3 weeks should be adequate for most patients without complication

[a]All gentamicin- and vancomycin-containing regimens require monitoring for potential toxicity; monitoring of serum concentrations will usually be required.
[b]Vancomycin dose not to exceed 2.0 g/day.
[c]May substitute ampicillin 2 g/day by continuous infusion or in divided doses (2 g IV q 4 h).
SOURCE: Adapted from Scheld and Sande[53] and from Wilson et al.[352] and Sanford JP, Modlering RC, Gilbert DN: *The Sanford Guide to Antimicrobial Therapy 2000.* Portland, OR: Health Sciences University; 2000.

Duration of Therapy

Extensive experience with the common forms of IE provides the basis for recommendations on duration of therapy (Table 81-12). The response of *Staph. aureus* IE to treatment can be variable; some patients (e.g., young IDUs) recover swiftly and can often be cured within 2 weeks.[74,351] In contrast, others remain febrile for 10 to 14 days with abscesses or extracardiac manifestations of disseminated infection. Although 4 weeks of therapy is adequate in most cases of *Staph. aureus* IE, some require treatment for 6 weeks or longer to achieve a cure. For *E. faecalis* IE, 4 weeks is usually adequate. Relapse rates are higher in patients with mitral valve infection and in those with symptoms for >3 months,[160] in whom treatment should continue for 6 weeks. When optimal treatment duration is uncertain, relatively more prolonged treatment is advisable to provide a reasonable margin of safety.

Outpatient Therapy

Although hospitalization is generally indicated for initiation, treatment can often be completed on an outpatient basis if defervescence has occurred, blood cultures are negative, and indications for surgery are absent.[378] In these cases, parenteral treatment may be completed at home or in an appropriate outpatient clinic setting. Supervised parenteral treatment outside the hospital should be fully effective in achieving a microbiologic cure and offers obvious benefits: patient convenience and cost containment.[374,379,380] The risks posed by possible late complications (e.g., an embolic stroke or sudden heart failure) must be balanced against benefits in selecting candidates for outpatient parenteral therapy. Although further studies are needed, current experience suggests that more than half of IE patients could receive at least some of their treatment as outpatients.

Role of Surgery

Combining cardiac surgery with medical therapy has resulted in reduced mortality in complicated IE patients (i.e., those with heart failure or uncontrolled infection). Valve replacement optimally should be undertaken before hemodynamic deterioration or perivalvular extension occurs, which leads to a sharp rise in perioperative mortality and adverse late outcomes.[330,381–383] Indications for operative intervention occur during the course of about one-third of IE cases.[96,384] Both correct selection of patients and optimal timing of surgery are critical.[385]

Major indications for surgery are moderate or severe heart failure not responding to medical treatment, valvular obstruction, periannular or myocardial abscess, prosthetic valve dehiscence, persistent bacteremia despite appropriate antibiotics, and fungal infection. In most such cases, surgery should proceed promptly even if the infection is still active.

Relative indications for surgery include recurrent emboli, staphylococcal and gram-negative bacillary infections (especially involving prosthetic valves), persistent fever despite treatment, and vegetations that enlarge during treatment.[10,124,281,385] A recent echocardiographic study suggested that early surgery also be considered in patients with highly mobile vegetations >15 mm in size regardless of the degree of valve destruction, heart failure, or response to antibiotic therapy.[386] IE due to *Pseudomonas aeruginosa, Brucella* species, *C. burnetii, Candida* and other fungi, and drug-resistant enterococci is usually resistant to medical therapy[387,388]; in such cases surgery is generally advised. PVE is an indication for surgical evaluation and frequently requires intervention; late-onset (>1 year) PVE with a sensitive organism affords the best chance for a medical cure. Combined surgical and medical therapy results in reduced mortality (relative risk, 0.18) compared with medical therapy alone for *Staph. aureus* PVE, suggesting that this may be another indication for valve replacement.[177]

Correct timing is essential to optimal surgical management.[384,389] Surgery undertaken too early exposes patients to the risks of operative mortality and the early and late morbidity associated with valve replacement, which may be unnecessary for those who respond well to medical therapy. If surgery can be delayed safely, antibiotic therapy can eradicate or reduce infective burden and complications, increasing the surgical success rate and reducing the risk of postoperative IE recurrence.[343] In contrast, if surgery is delayed too long, sudden death may occur or hemodynamic status deteriorate so seriously that surgery is no longer feasible. This is tragic, because long-term survival improves with earlier operation even if endocardial infection is still active.[281,390,391] Careful, frequent reexamination, together with serial echocardiography and sometimes cardiac catheterization, is indicated when operation is a consideration. The natural history of the specific IE should influence decision making: penicillin-sensitive streptococcal IE can almost always be cured bacteriologically (Table 81-13), and the immediate prognosis is usually good. Therefore surgery may be reserved only for those with heart failure that do not respond well to medical treatment. Similarly, young IDUs with acute staphylococcal IE have a good prognosis,[8,351] and surgery can be reserved for those with intractable heart failure or definite signs of treatment failure. In contrast, the likelihood that fungal PVE will be eradicated is remote (Table 81-13), and these cases should usually undergo surgery early.[392] The development of severe AR, especially when accompanied by heart failure, usually requires urgent surgery. Other cases likely to require operation are those with early-onset PVE, valve-ring abscess, or gram-negative bacillary PVE.[10] In one retrospective study of 181 patients with cerebral complications, the risk of postoperative neurologic deterioration and death depended on the interval between the prior neurologic event and surgery (44 percent event rate for <1 week interval versus 2 percent for >1 month).[393] In contrast, other experience has indicated little added risk in the absence of intracranial hemorrhage.[394,395] Indeed, stroke is usually not viewed as a contraindication for urgent valve replacement. Piper et al. suggested that when IE is complicated by stroke, cardiac surgery be performed within 72 h of cerebral embolism, when the risk of secondary cerebral hemorrhage appears to be low.[395] Computed tomography (CT) is obligatory prior to surgery in order to identify patients with early reperfusion hemorrhage, which would predispose to a worse outcome with cardiac surgery and anticoagulation.

Over the past decade, surgical approaches have evolved toward increasingly radical debridement of infected tissue and more extensive use of reconstructive materials.[281,392] For example, an aortic root homograft instead of a standard prosthetic valve is now often inserted after debridement of a valve-ring abscess.[396] The Ross operation (Chap. 70) has been advocated for patients with complicated aortic root infections.[397,398]

Several surgical procedures other than valve replacement may be useful for selected cases of IE.[347] Debridement of vegetations ("vegetectomy"), often combined with valvuloplasty, can allow cure of IE while sparing the native valve.[282,283,399]

The sudden onset of AR or MR with acute LV failure can occur without warning, even in the most favorable forms of IE. Thus, early consultation with the surgical service should be sought for most pa-

TABLE 81-13 Estimate of Microbiologic Cure Rates for Various Forms of Endocarditis[a]

Native Valve Endocarditis	Antimicrobial Therapy Alone	Antimicrobial Therapy Plus Surgery
Viridans streptococci, group A streptococci, *S. bovis,* pneumococci, gonococci	98	98
Enterococcus faecalis	90	>90
Staph. aureus (in young intravenous drug users)	90	>90
Staph. aureus (in elderly patients with chronic underlying diseases)	50	70
Gram-negative aerobic bacilli[b]	40	65
Fungi	<5	50

Prosthetic Valve Endocarditis	Early PVE	Late PVE	Early PVE	Late PVE
Viridans streptococci, group A streptococci, *S. bovis,* pneumococci, gonococci	c	80	c	90
Enterococcus faecalis	c	60	c	75
Staph. aureus	25	40	50	60
Staph. epidermidis	20	40	60	70
Gram-negative aerobic bacilli[b]	<10	20	40	50
Fungi	<1	<1	30	40

[a]Morbidity and mortality are significantly greater than these figures for microbiologic cure indicate.
[b]Excluding HACEK species.
[c]Insufficient data to estimate rates.
SOURCE: Adapted from Refs. 9, 11, 32, 33, 110, 116, 259, 323, 324, 350, 365, in *Hurst's The Heart,* 10th ed., Chap. 73.

tients with IE so that appropriate surgery can be performed without delay if necessary.

After valve-replacement surgery, antimicrobial therapy should be continued to a total duration at least as long as recommended for nonsurgical cases (Table 81-12).[2]

Anticoagulant Therapy

Even though the infected vegetation is a thrombotic lesion, there is *no evidence that anticoagulation benefits* the course of IE. On the contrary, early experience showed that simultaneous treatment with penicillin and heparin carried an increased risk of fatal intracerebral hemorrhage.[400] Further experience suggested that warfarin could usually be given safely to patients with PVE.[401–403] However, in a recent series of 21 patients with *Staph. aureus* PVE, 11 had hemorrhagic cerebrovascular events. All 11 died, and all had been on oral anticoagulants.[403] The cumulative experience suggests the anticoagulation guidelines summarized in Table 81-14.

Fibrinolytic agents could theoretically promote lysis or resolution of vegetations. Recombinant tissue plasminogen activator decreased vegetation size and improved the results of penicillin therapy in rabbits with fresh vegetations.[11] Similarly, aspirin therapy reduces the size of experimental vegetations and improves rates of sterilization by antibiotics.[404] No clinical value of these antithrombotic therapies has been shown, however.

Management of Complications

HEART FAILURE

The development of moderate or severe heart failure due to structural valvular damage is usually an indication for *prompt surgical intervention*, even if infection is still active.[384,390] With mild heart failure, the decision should be individualized, remembering that lives may be lost if cardiac function suddenly worsens.

EMBOLI

The occurrence of one or more major arterial embolic events is a relative indication for surgery. The predictable early and long-term mortality and morbidity of valve replacement must be weighed against the unpredictable likelihood of further emboli, making embolization a weaker indication for valve replacement than heart failure.[385,390] Because the frequency of emboli declines rapidly after 1 to 2 weeks of antibiotic therapy,[405] the most logical time to operate for the purpose of preventing further emboli would be early, within 1 week of diagnosis. The authors' opinion is that operative intervention during antibiotic treatment should seldom be undertaken *solely* because of a single embolic event.

RENAL FAILURE

In the antibiotic era, the incidence and importance of renal failure have greatly diminished.[6] However, one recent series found that acute renal insufficiency (creatinine >2 mg/dL) developed in one-third of 204 IE patients and increased mortality risk fivefold.[406] Independent risk factors for renal insufficiency were increased age and thrombocytopenia. Less than 5 to 10 percent of SBE patients now develop severe renal failure due to immune-complex glomerulonephritis, but they may benefit by timely dialysis until antibiotic treatment results in clearance of bacterial antigens and associated immune-complex nephritis. Renal function usually improves once infection has been controlled, but full recovery may take weeks to months. Occasionally, creatinine clearance worsens for a time despite a favorable treatment response, perhaps reflecting persistence of bacterial antigen after bacteriologic cure. Corticosteroids may be of value in a few cases.[406]

Some ABE patients with septicemia, shock, or disseminated intravascular coagulopathy develop severe acute renal failure and require dialysis as part of their intensive care.

MYCOTIC ANEURYSM

Mycotic aneurysm is diagnosed in less than 5 percent of IE patients, but the consequences of aneurysm expansion and rupture are serious, especially in the brain (Chap. 99).[295,298,299] Small aneurysms often thrombose or resolve spontaneously during or after antibiotic therapy. Once aneurysms exceed 0.5 to 2 cm in diameter, they are likely to continue to enlarge and eventually rupture despite cure of infection.[302] Prophylactic surgery is indicated for large, accessible aneurysms.

Intracranial mycotic aneurysms are difficult to diagnose and manage. They may be multiple and/or located in inaccessible sites. They may present with headaches, subarachnoid hemorrhage, or stroke, but many are asymptomatic. The therapeutic dilemma is whether to treat conservatively with antibiotics and hope for resolution, risking serious or fatal hemorrhage, or operate, risking operative neurologic damage. Symptoms or signs consistent with an intracranial aneurysm indicate the need for prompt CT and/or MRI. Cerebral angiography is now less often required. In general, large (over 0.5 cm diameter) or expanding aneurysms, or aneurysms that have already leaked or begun to bleed, should be clipped if a surgical approach is feasible. Endovascular coiling generally compares favorably with neurosurgical clipping for therapy of subarachnoid aneurysms, but it has not been tested for mycotic aneurysms.[407]

PROGNOSIS

IE is one of the few infectious diseases that is virtually always fatal if untreated. Spontaneous recovery, reported occasionally in the preantibiotic era,[6] may have represented false-positive diagnosis. The interval to death with untreated SBE varied widely, with a median of about 6 months.[6] Almost all patients with ABE died within less than 4 weeks.

Heart failure has traditionally been the leading adverse prognostic factor.[279] Because current surgical techniques usually afford effective treatment for heart failure, neurologic complications now approach or exceed heart failure as the most important adverse prognostic factor.[291] Other adverse factors include—among others—renal failure, fungal infection, prosthetic valve infection, and development of abscesses of the valve ring or myocardium.[408] PVE also

TABLE 81-14 Recommendations for Anticoagulation During IE

Avoid heparin except for urgent indications (e.g, massive pulmonary embolism).

Discontinue or avoid oral anticoagulants if possible, especially with intracranial complications and *Staph. aureus* IE.

Anticoagulate with warfarin for clear-cut indications only, such as a mechanical prosthetic heart valve; carefully regulate prothrombin time [e.g., to therapeutic International Normalized Ratios (INRs) of 2.5–3.5]. Avoid overanticoagulation.

Choose antibiotic regimens not requiring intramuscular injections if anticoagulation is instituted.

has a poor prognosis; survival at 6 months in one series was only 54 percent[409] (early-onset PVE 37 percent; late-onset PVE, 65 percent).

IE in hemodialysis patients has a 1-year mortality of 56 percent.[143] Favorable prognostic factors include youth (age <55), early diagnosis and treatment (early surgical intervention), IE complicating MVP, absence of congestive heart failure, and penicillin-sensitive streptococcal infection.[410,411] Prognosis also is good with *Staph. aureus* infection of the tricuspid valve in young IDUs.[8,363]

With early diagnosis and appropriate therapy, including surgery, the prognosis for elderly patients can be improved.[99] Bacterial eradication can be achieved in a high proportion of patients with IE.[9,350,374,379] Approximate cure rates are listed in Table 81-13. Nevertheless, a significant number of late deaths occur despite microbiologic cure,[88,412] perhaps the result of IE-related damage on top of preexisting disease.

RECURRENT ENDOCARDITIS

Recurrent endocarditis is a term encompassing both relapses and reinfections. *Relapse* refers to recurrence of infection with the same organism, the result of treatment failure. The frequency of relapse can be predicted for various forms of IE (Table 81-13). Relapses occasionally occur even after completion of optimal treatment, so meticulous clinical follow-up is indicated for at least 2 months. Any clinical suspicion of relapse should lead to blood cultures. Most relapses occur within a few weeks, but organisms can persist in seemingly healed vegetations and cause late relapse. Positive valve cultures at the time of surgery increase the risk of relapse and reoperation, particularly for *Staph. aureus* IE.[413] Variables predicting recurrence in a large Italian study were positive valve culture, prosthetic valve IE, and persistence of fever at the seventh postoperative day.[414]

Reinfection refers to a new episode of IE occurring after cure of a previous episode.[415] Usually a different organism is involved; when the new isolate is similar to the initial organism, molecular typing can be used to diffentiate reinfection from relapse. IE patients remain at permanent risk of reinfection (see Tables 81-3 and 81-4). Recurrent episodes occur in 2 to 31 percent of cases,[6,46,48,412,415] the wide variation being due in part to variable durations of follow-up. Occasionally, a patient may suffer two or more reinfections.[415] IDUs and those with severe periodontitis are at increased risk. Patients with prior NVE treated with valve replacement are at high risk to develop PVE.[88]

THE CHALLENGE OF PROPHYLAXIS

Because various invasive procedures induce bacteremias with species that often cause IE,[416–418] prophylactic antibiotics are frequently given to susceptible patients in an attempt to prevent IE. Although antibiotics prevent IE in experimental animals, their clinical effectiveness has not been evaluated in prospective randomized trials, leaving many questions unanswered (Table 81-15). Indeed, the low risk of IE after procedures practically precludes definitive study.[58,390]

Less than 15 percent of SBE and even fewer of ABE cases follow identifiable medical procedures that cause transient bacteremias.[57,416,417,419] However, because IE poses serious morbidity and mortality risk, the AHA and the practicing medical community have accepted the practice of using antibiotic prophylaxis. This practice requires that an antibiotic regimen be administered before certain dental and surgical procedures in patients with known heart lesions that pose a significant risk of IE.

TABLE 81-15 Outstanding Questions regarding IE Prophylaxis

Is antibiotic prophylaxis effective?
Does the prophylactic benefit outweigh potential adverse effects of the antibiotic, drug cost, and risk of selecting drug-resistant organisms?
Which operations and diagnostic procedures should be covered?
Which patients should receive antibiotics?
What antibiotic regimens are most effective?

Because several hundred cases of streptococcal IE following dental and genitourinary tract procedures have been recorded, the potential causative role of these procedures seems likely.[416,417] A short "incubation period" is typically reported, with symptoms developing within 2 weeks of the procedure.[271] Indeed, when 273 cases of IE were examined retrospectively, their histories within 3 months prior to IE yielded no overall correlation with dental procedures.[59,416]

In the absence of prospective controlled trials, empiric recommendations for prophylaxis of bacterial endocarditis have been made on the basis of indirect information.[58,419,420] This includes the risk of bacteremia after various procedures (Table 81-16), the relative risk posed by the cardiac lesion (Table 81-4), reports of prophylaxis failures,[79] in vitro susceptibility studies (i.e., on streptococci), studies in laboratory animals,[354,421] and retrospective clinical reports.[37,422,423]

Prevention is most likely to be effective and recommended for high-risk individuals (i.e., those with previous IE or with prosthetic valves) undergoing high-risk procedures (i.e., tooth extractions).[419,424] On the basis of existing data, the case for prophylaxis is strongest prior to dental extractions or gingival surgery (including implant placement but not routine dental care, filling of cavities, root canal, cleaning and sealing of teeth) and for patients with prosthetic valves or a history of prior IE. If any of these four conditions are present, antibiotic prophylaxis seems reasonable.[59] In many situations, uncertainties exist, and the patient's and physician's preferences influence the decision. *Updated consensus recommendations* by the AHA may aid in guiding decision making.[86,420] These guide-

TABLE 81-16 Caveats for Antibiotic Prophylaxis

1. Most cases are not attributable to an invasive procedure.
2. Cardiac conditions should be stratified into high-, moderate-, and low/negligible-risk categories; these are primarily based on potential outcomes if endocarditis occurs.
3. There are specific procedures that may cause high-grade bacteremia and for which prophylaxis is most likely to be effective.
4. There is an algorithm for deciding on prophylaxis in patients with mitral valve prolapse.
5. The initial dose of amoxicillin is reduced to 2 g for oral and dental procedures; a follow-up dose is no longer recommended. Clindamycin (not erythromycin) is recommended as an alternative therapy in penicillin-allergic individuals.
6. Prophylactic recommendations for gastrointestinal and genitourinary procedures have been simplified.[86,420]

TABLE 81-17 Suggested Regimens for Prophylaxis of Infective Endocarditis[a]

STANDARD REGIMEN	
For dental procedures and oral or upper respiratory tract surgery	Amoxicillin 2.0 g orally 1 h before procedure[b]
SPECIAL REGIMENS	
Parenteral regimen for high-risk patients; also for gastrointestinal (GI) or genitourinary (GU) tract procedures	Ampicillin 2.0 g IM or IV *plus* gentamicin 1.5 mg/kg IM or IV, 0.5 h before procedure,[b] 6 h later, ampicillin 1 g IM or IV or amoxicillin 1 g orally
Parenteral regimen for penicillin-allergic patients	Vancomycin 1.0 g IV *slowly* over 1–2 h *plus* gentamicin 1.5 mg/kg IM or IV[b]; complete within 30 min of starting the procedure
Oral regimen for penicillin-allergic patients (oral and respiratory tract only)	Clindamycin 600 mg orally 1 h before procedure[b]
Oral regimen for minor GI or GU tract procedures	Amoxicillin 2.0 g orally 1 h before procedure[b]
Parenteral regimen for cardiac surgery including valve replacement	Cefazolin 2.0 g IV on induction of anesthesia, repeated 8 and 16 h later[c] *or* Vancomycin 1.0 g IV *slowly* over 1 h starting on induction of anesthesia, then 0.5 g IV 8 and 16 h later[c]

[a]Note that (1) these regimens are empiric suggestions, no regimen has been proved effective for prevention of endocarditis, and prevention failures may occur with any regimen; (2) these regimens are not intended to cover all clinical situations, and the practitioner should use his or her own judgment on safety and cost-benefit issues in each individual case; (3) one or two additional doses may be given if the period of risk for bacteremia is prolonged.
[b]Pediatric dosages: ampicillin 50 mg/kg; gentamicin 1.5 mg/kg; amoxicillin: for children who weigh more than 60 lb, use same as for adults; for children less than 60 lb, use one-half the adult dose; vancomycin 20 mg/kg; clindamycin 20 mg/kg; cefazolin 30 mg/kg. Do not exceed 2.0 g ampicillin, 120 mg gentamicin.
[c]Vancomycin is preferred if *S. epidermidis* is an important cause of postoperative infection in that hospital. Gentamicin 1.5 mg/kg IV or IM may be added to each dose, only if postoperative gram-negative infections have occurred with significant frequency.
SOURCE: Durack DT. Nine controversies in the management of infective endocarditis. In: Petersdorf RG, et al., eds. *Update V: Harrison's Principles of Internal Medicine.* New York: McGraw-Hill; 1984:35; and Dajani et al.[86] Adapted and reproduced with permission of the publisher and author.

lines emphasize the points summarized in Table 81-16. Specific regimens suggested for prophylaxis of IE are listed in Table 81-17.

Prophylaxis does not always succeed. Of 52 apparent failures in one series, 42 had heart disease and received oral penicillin or erythromycin, usually to cover dental procedures.[79] Common errors in prophylaxis are starting antibiotics too early, continuing too long, using low doses, and covering tooth extractions but not lesser dental procedures in high-risk patients.[58]

In the absence of pelvic infection, prophylaxis for IE in patients with heart lesions is not recommended to cover normal delivery, therapeutic abortion, dilatation and curettage, and insertion or removal of intrauterine contraceptive devices. Similarly, antibiotics are not recommended before many common medical procedures, such as cardiac catheterization, insertion of temporary pacemakers, endotracheal intubation, bronchoscopy, endoscopy, or radiographic contrast studies of the upper and lower gastrointestinal tract. In comparison, some physicians choose to cover even these low-risk procedures in patients with prosthetic valves because such patients are at higher risk for IE.

Surgeons currently administer antibiotics to virtually all patients undergoing cardiac surgery, attempting to prevent both wound infections and IE, although the efficacy of this for the prevention of IE has not been proved.[58] Current recommendations call for parenteral administration of an antistaphylococcal antibiotic just prior to operation, followed by one or two further doses (Table 81-17). The regimen may be modified if local experience shows a significant frequency of early PVE caused by *Staph. epidermidis* or gram-negative bacilli (Table 81-17).

In summary, prophylactic antibiotic paradigms for IE have been developed over time by various expert bodies (including the AHA) but are based on indirect evidence. Therefore, it seems prudent for expert committees to continue to reassess and update recommendations on the benefit/risk of IE prophylaxis.

ADHERENCE TO MANAGEMENT GUIDELINES

Practical application often lags behind management guidelines. Delahaye and colleagues assessed the quality of management of IE in France (Rhone-Alpes region).[425] A surprisingly high rate of failure to comply with key components of IE management guidelines was found. A high percentage of patients at risk did not receive mandated antibiotic prophylaxis. A further concern was the relative reluctance to proceed to surgery when indicated.

Potential reasons for lack of adherence to guidelines are given in Table 81-18.[426] Information gathering in each geographic region

TABLE 81-18 Potential Reasons for Failure to Adhere to IE Management Guidelines

Infrequent management of IE by individual physicians
Inadequate education regarding IE during medical training
Inadequate availability of continuing medical education offerings regarding IE
Inadequate dissemination (and emphasis) of guidelines to potential treating physicians
Disagreement regarding importance of adherence to current guidelines (e.g., for dental prophylaxis)
Lack of medical care system programs to assess and assure compliance with practice guidelines

SOURCE: From Muhlestein,[426] with permission.

about compliance with guidelines is to be strongly encouraged. Determining the extent of compliance will be critical to further improvements in the quality of care for this important, high-risk group of patients.[426]

ACKNOWLEDGMENT

This chapter is a modification of the chapter by David Durack in previous editions of this book.

References

1. Alestig K, Hogevik H, Olaison L. Infective endocarditis: A diagnostic and therapeutic challenge for the new millennium. *Scand J Infect Dis* 2000;32:343–356.
2. Mylonakis E, Calderwood SB. Infective endocarditis in adults. *N Engl J Med* 2001;3445:1318–1330.
3. Mauri L, De Lemos JA, O'Gara PT. Infective endocarditis. *Curr Probl Cardiol* 2001;26:562–610.
4. Blumer G. Subacute bacterial endocarditis. *Medicine* 1923;2:105–170.
5. Thayer WS. Studies on bacterial (infective) endocarditis. *Johns Hopkins Hosp Rep* 1926;22:1–185.
6. Kerr AJ. *Subacute Bacterial Endocarditis.* Springfield, IL: Charles C Thomas; 1955.
7. Hermans PE. The clinical manifestations of infective endocarditis. *Mayo Clin Proc* 1982;57:15–21.
8. Chambers HF, Korzeniowski OM, Sande MA, National Collaborative Endocarditis Study group. *Staphylococcus aureus* endocarditis: Clinical manifestations in addicts and nonaddicts. *Medicine* 1983;62: 170–177.
9. Korzeniowski OM, Kaye D. Infective endocarditis. In: Braunwald E, ed. *The Heart: A Textbook of Cardiovascular Medicine.* Philadelphia: Saunders, 1992:1078–1105.
10. Douglas JL, Cobbs CG. Prosthetic valve endocarditis. In: Kaye D, ed. *Infective Endocarditis.* New York: Raven Press; 1992:375–396.
11. Meyer MW, Witt AR, Krishnan LK, et al. Therapeutic advantage of recombinant human plasminogen activator in endocarditis: Evidence from experiments in rabbits. *Thromb Haemost* 1995;73:680–682.
12. MacDonald RA, Robbins SL. The significance of nonbacterial thrombotic endocarditis: An autopsy and clinical study of 78 cases. *Ann Intern Med* 1957;46:255–273.
13. Barry WE, Scarpelli D. Nonbacterial thrombotic endocarditis. *Arch Intern Med* 1962;109:79–84.
14. Major RM. Notes on the history of endocarditis. *Bull Hist Med* 1945; 17:351–359.
15. Osler W. Chronic infectious endocarditis. *Q J Med* 1909;2:219–230.
16. Osler W. The Goulstonian lectures, on malignant endocarditis. *Br Med J* 1885;1:467–579.
17. Horder TJ. Infective endocarditis: With an analysis of 150 cases and with special reference to the chronic form of the disease. *Q J Med* 1909;2:289–329.
18. Allen AC. Nature of vegetations of bacterial endocarditis. *Arch Pathol* 1939;27:661–671.
19. Libman E, Friedberg CK. *Subacute Bacterial Endocarditis.* New York: Oxford University Press, 1947.
20. Beeson PB, Brannon ES, Warren JV. Observations of the sites of removal of bacteria from the blood in patients with bacterial endocarditis. *J Exp Med* 1945;81:9–23.
21. Touroff ASW, Vesell H. Subacute *Streptococcus viridans* endocarditis complicating patent ductus arteriosus: Recovery following surgical treatment. *JAMA* 1940;115:1270–1272.
22. Durack DT. Review of early experience in treatment of bacterial endocarditis, 1940–1955. In: Bisno AL, ed. *Treatment of Infective Endocarditis.* New York: Grune & Stratton; 1981:1–14.
23. Dawson MH, Hunter TH. The treatment of subacute bacterial endocarditis with penicillin: Results in twenty cases. *JAMA* 1945;127: 129–137.
24. Abraham EP, Chain E, Fletcher CM, et al. Further observations on penicillin. *Lancet* 1941;2:177–189.
25. Loewe L, Rosenblatt P, Greene HJ, Russell M. Combined penicillin and heparin therapy of subacute bacterial endocarditis: Report of seven consecutive successfully treated patients. *JAMA* 1944;124: 144–149.
26. Galbreath WR, Hull E. Sulfonamide therapy of bacterial endocarditis: Results in 42 cases. *Ann Intern Med* 1943;18:201–203.
27. Bloomfield AL, Armstrong CD, Kirby WMM. The treatment of subacute bacterial endocarditis with penicillin. *J Clin Invest* 1945;24: 251–267.
28. Hunter TH. The treatment of some bacterial infections of the heart and pericardium. *Bull NY Acad Med* 1952;28:213–228.
29. Finland M. Treatment of bacterial endocarditis (concluded). *N Engl J Med* 1954;250:419–428.
30. Geraci JE. The antibiotic therapy of infective endocarditis: Therapeutic data on 172 patients seen from 1951 through 1957: Additional observations on short-term therapy (two weeks) for penicillin-sensitive streptococcal endocarditis. *Med Clin North Am* 1958;42:1101–1148.
31. Weinstein L, Schlesinger J. Treatment of infective endocarditis 1973. *Prog Cardiovasc Dis* 1973;26:275–296.
32. Wallace AG, Young GJ, Osterhout S. Treatment of acute bacterial endocarditis by valve excision and replacement. *Circulation* 1965;31: 450–453.
33. Hoen B, Alla F, Selton-Suty C, et al. Changing profile of infective endocarditis: Results of a 1-year survey in France. *JAMA* 2002;288: 75–81.
34. Harris SL. Definitions and demographic characteristics. In: Kaye D, ed. *Infective Endocarditis.* New York: Raven Press; 1992:1–18.
35. Steckelberg JM, Wilson WR. Risk factors for infective endocarditis. *Infect Dis Clin North Am* 1993;7:9–19.
36. Smith RH, Radford DJ, Clark RA, Julian DG. Infective endocarditis: A survey of cases in the southeast of Scotland 1969–72. *Thorax* 1976;31: 373–379.
37. van der Meer JTM, Van Wijk W, Thompson J, et al. Efficacy of antibiotic prophylaxis for prevention of native-valve endocarditis. *Lancet* 1992;339:135–140.
38. Hogevik H, Olaison L, Andersson R, et al. Epidemiologic aspects of infective endocarditis in an urban population: A 5-year prospective study. *Medicine* 1995;74:324–339.
39. Uwaydah MM, Weinberg AN. Bacterial endocarditis—A changing pattern. *N Engl J Med* 1965;273:1231–1235.
40. Tak T, Reed KD, Haselby RC, et al. An update on epidemiology, pathogenesis and management of infective endocarditis with emphasis on *Staphylococcus aureus*. *WMJ* 2002;101:24–33.
41. Berlin JA, Abrutyn E, Strom BL, et al. Incidence of infective endocarditis in the Delaware Valley, 1988–1990. *Am J Cardiol* 1995;76: 933–936.
42. Kaye D, McCormack RC, Hook EW. The changing pattern since the introduction of penicillin therapy. *Antimicrob Agents Chemother* 1961: 37–46.
43. Lerner PI, Weinstein L. Infective endocarditis in the antibiotic era. *N Engl J Med* 1966;274:199–206; 259–266; 323–331; 388–393.
44. Finland M, Barnes MW. Changing etiology of bacterial endocarditis in the antibiotic era: Experiences at the Boston City Hospital 1933–1965. *Ann Intern Med* 1970;72:341–348.
45. Durack DT, Petersdorf RG. Changes in the epidemiology of endocarditis. In: Kaplan EL, Taranta AV, ed. *Infective Endocarditis: An American Heart Association Symposium.* Dallas: American Heart Association; 1977:3–8.
46. Baddour LM. Twelve-year review of recurrent native-valve infective endocarditis: A disease of the modern antibiotic era. *Rev Infect Dis* 1988;10:1163–1170.
47. Dysson C. Infective endocarditis: An epidemiological review of 128 episodes. *J Infect* 1999;38:87–93.
48. Garvey GJ, Neu HC. Infective endocarditis—An evolving disease: A review of endocarditis at the Columbia-Presbyterian Medical Center, 1968–1973. *Medicine* 1978;57:105–127.

49. Pulvirenti JJ, Kerns E, Benson C, et al. Infective endocarditis in injection drug users: Importance of human immunodeficiency virus serostatus and degree of immunosuppression. *Clin Infect Dis* 1996;22:40–45.

50. Mouly S, Ruimy R, Launay O, et al. The changing clinical aspects of infective endocarditis: Descriptive review of 90 episodes in a French teaching hospital and risk factors for death. *J Infect* 2002;45:246–256.

51. Abbott KC, Duran M, Hypolite I, et al. Hospitalizations for bacterial endocarditis after renal transplantation in the United States. *J Nephrol* 2001;14:353–360.

52. Strom BL, Abrutyn E, Berlin JA. Risk factors for infective endocarditis: Oral hygiene and nondental exposures. *Circulation* 2000;102:2842–2848.

53. Scheld WM, Sande MA. Endocarditis and intravascular infections. In: Mandell GL, Douglas RG Jr, Dolin R, eds. *Principles and Practice of Infectious Diseases.* New York: Churchill Livingstone; 1995:740–783.

54. Weinstein L, Rubin RH. Infective endocarditis 1973. *Prog Cardiovasc Dis* 1973;16:239–273.

55. Tunkel AR, Mandell GL. Infecting microorganisms. In: Kaye D, ed. *Infective Endocarditis.* New York: Raven Press; 1992:85–97.

56. Tompkins LS, Roessler BJ, Redd SC. *Legionella* prosthetic-valve endocarditis. *N Engl J Med* 1988;318:530–534.

57. Bayliss R, Clarke C, Oakley C, et al. The teeth and infective endocarditis. *Br Heart J* 1983;50:506–512.

58. Durack DT. Prophylaxis of infective endocarditis. In: Mandell GL, Douglas RG Jr, Dolin R, eds. *Principles and Practice of Infectious Diseases.* New York: Churchill Livingstone; 1995:793–813.

59. Strom BL, Abrutyn E, Berlin JA, et al. Dental and cardiac risk factors for infective endocarditis. *Ann Intern Med* 1998;129:761–769.

60. Mansur AJ, Grinberg M, da Luz PL, Bellotti G. The complications of infective endocarditis: A reappraisal in the 1980s (see comments). *Arch Intern Med* 1992;152:2428–2432.

61. Seymour RA, Lowry R, Whitworth JM, Martin MV. Infective endocarditis, dentistry and antibiotic prophylaxis: Time to rethink? *Br Dent J* 2000;189:610–616.

62. Johnson DH, Rosenthal A, Nadas AS. A forty-year review of bacterial endocarditis in infancy and childhood. *Circulation* 1975;51:581–588.

63. Hansen D, Schmiegelow K, Jacobsen JR. Bacterial endocarditis in children: Trends in its diagnosis, course, and prognosis. *Pediatr Cardiol* 1993;13:198–203.

64. Saiman L, Prince A, Gersony WM. Pediatric infective endocarditis in the modern era. *J Pediatr* 1993;122:847–853.

65. Awadallah SM, Kavey RW, Byrum CJ, et al. The changing pattern of infective endocarditis in childhood. *Am J Cardiol* 1991;68:90–94.

66. Stull TL, LiPuma JJ. Endocarditis in children. In: Kaye D, ed. *Infective Endocarditis.* New York: Raven Press; 1992:313–327.

67. Ifere OAS, Masokano KA. Infective endocarditis in children in the Guinea savannah of Nigeria. *Ann Trop Paediatr* 1991;11:233–240.

68. Saitoh M, Hishi T, Tamura M, Komoshita S. Forty year review of bacterial endocarditis in infants and children. *Acta Paediatr Jpn* 1991; 33:613–616.

69. El-Khatib MR, Wilson FM, Lerner AM. Characteristics of bacterial endocarditis in heroin addicts in Detroit. *Am J Med Sci* 1976;271:197–201.

70. Reisberg BE. Infective endocarditis in the narcotic addict. *Prog Cardiovasc Dis* 1979;22:193–204.

71. Dressler FA, Roberts WC. Infective endocarditis in opiate addicts: Analysis of 80 cases studied at necropsy. *Am J Cardiol* 1989;63:1240–1257.

72. Weisse AB, Heller DR, Schimenti RJ, et al. The febrile parenteral drug user: A prospective study in 121 patients. *Am J Med* 1993;94:274–280.

73. Carrel T, Schaffner A, Vogt P, et al. Endocarditis in intravenous drug addicts and HIV infected patients: Possibilities and limitations of surgical treatment. *J Heart Valve Dis* 1993;2:140–147.

74. Sande MA, Lee BL, Mills J, Chambers HFI. Endocarditis in intravenous drug users. In: Kaye D, ed. *Infective Endocarditis.* New York: Raven Press; 1992:345–359.

75. Corrigall D, Bolen J, Hancock EW, Popp RP. Mitral valve prolapse and infective endocarditis. *Am J Med* 1977;63:215–222.

76. Clemens JD, Horwitz RI, Jaffe CC, et al. A controlled evaluation of the risk of bacterial endocarditis in persons with mitral-valve prolapse. *N Engl J Med* 1982;307:776–781.

77. Beton DC, Brear SG, Edwards JD, Leonard JC. Mitral valve prolapse: An assessment of clinical features, associated conditions and prognosis. *Q J Med* 1983;52:150–164.

78. Heidenreich PA. The clinical impact of echocardiography on antibiotic prophylaxis use in patients with suspected mitral valve prolapse. *Am J Med* 1997;102:337–343.

79. Durack DT, Kaplan EL, Bisno AL. Apparent failures of endocarditis prophylaxis: Analysis of 52 cases submitted to a national registry. *JAMA* 1983;250:2318–2322.

80. Clemens JD, Ransohoff DF. A quantitative assessment of predental antibiotic prophylaxis for patients with mitral-valve prolapse. *J Chronic Dis* 1984;37:531–544.

81. Devereux RB, Hawkins I, Kramer-Fox R, et al. Complications of mitral valve prolapse: Disproportionate occurrence in men and older patients. *Am J Med* 1986;81:751–758.

82. MacMahon SW, Hickey AJ, Wilcken DEL, et al. Risk of infective endocarditis in mitral valve prolapse with and without precordial systolic murmurs. *Am J Cardiol* 1986;58:105–108.

83. Bonow RO, Carabello B, de Leon ACJ, et al. Guidelines for the management of patients with valvular heart disease: Executive summary: A report of the American College of Cardiology/American Heart Association Task Force on Practice Guidelines (Committee on Management of Patients with Valvular Heart Disease). *Circulation* 1998;98:1949–1984.

84. MacMahon SW, Roberts K, Kramer-Fox R, et al. Mitral valve prolapse and infective endocarditis. *Am Heart J* 1987;113:1291–1298.

85. Zuppiroli A, Rinaldi M, Kramer-Fox R, et al. Natural history of mitral valve prolapse. *Am J Cardiol* 1995;75:1028–1032.

86. Dajani AS, Taubert KA, Wilson W, et al. Prevention of bacterial endocarditis. Recommendations by The American Heart Association. *JAMA* 1997;277:1794–1801.

87. Baumgartner WA, Miller DC, Reitz BA, et al. Surgical treatment of prosthetic valve endocarditis. *Ann Thorac Surg* 1983;35:87–104.

88. Ivert TSA, Dismukes WE, Cobbs CG, et al. Prosthetic valve endocarditis. *Circulation* 1984;69:223–232.

89. Kassai B, Gueyffier F, Cucherat M, Boissel JP. Comparison of bioprosthesis and mechanical valves: A meta-analysis of randomised clinical trials. *Cardiovasc Surg* 2000;8:477–483.

90. Dhawan A, Grover A, Marwaha RK, et al. Infective endocarditis in children: Profile in a developing country. *Ann Trop Paediatr* 1993;13:189–194.

91. Elward K, Hruby N, Christy C. Pneumococcal endocarditis in infants and children: Report of a case and review of the literature. *Pediatr Infect Dis J* 1990;9.652 657

92. Brook MM. Pediatric bacterial endocarditis: Treatment and prophylaxis. *Pediatr Clin North Am* 1999;46:275–287.

93. Martin JM, Neches WH, Wald ER, et al. Infective endocarditis: 35 years of experience at a children's hospital. *Clin Infect Dis* 1997;24:669–675.

94. Del Pont JM, De Cicco LT, Vartalitis C, et al. Infective endocarditis in children: Clinical analyses and evaluation of two diagnostic criteria. *Pediatr Infect Dis* 1995;14:1079–1086.

95. Kaplan EL, Rich H, Gersony W, Manning J. A collaborative study of infective endocarditis in the 1970s: Emphasis on infections in patients who have undergone cardiovascular surgery. *Circulation* 1979;59:327–335.

96. Jung JY, Saab SB, Almond CH. The case for early surgical treatment of left-sided primary infective endocarditis. *J Thorac Cardiovasc Surg* 1975;70:509–518.

97. Picarelli D, Leone R, Duhagon P, et al. Active infective endocarditis in infants and childhood: Ten-year review of surgical therapy. *J Cardiovasc Surg* 1997;12:406–411.

98. Bayliss R, Clarke C, Oakley CM, et al. Incidence, mortality and prevention of infective endocarditis. *J R Coll Phys Lond* 1986;20:15–20.

99. Werner GS, Schulz R, Fuchs FB, et al. Infective endocarditis in the elderly in the era of transesophageal echocardiography: Clinical

features and prognosis compared with younger patients. *Am J Med* 1996;100:90–97.

100. Felder RS, Nardone D, Palac R. Prevalence of predisposing factors for endocarditis among an elderly institutionalized population. *Oral Surg Oral Med Oral Pathol* 1992;73:30–34.

101. Selton-Suty C, Hoen B, Grentzinger A, et al. Clinical and bacteriological characteristics of infective endocarditis in the elderly. *Heart* 1997;77:260–263.

102. Dhawan VK. Infective endocarditis in elderly patients. *Clin Infect Dis* 2002;34:806–812.

103. Steckelberg JM, Melton LJ, Ilstrup DM, et al. Influence of referral bias on the apparent clinical spectrum of infective endocarditis. *Am J Med* 1990;88:582–588.

104. Eliopoulos GM. Enterococcal endocarditis. In: Kaye D, ed. *Infective Endocarditis*. New York: Raven Press; 1992:209–229.

105. Threlkeld MG, Cobbs CG. Infectious disorders of prosthetic valves and intravascular devices. In: Mandell GL, Bennett JE, Dolin R, eds. *Principles and Practice of Infectious Diseases*. New York: Churchill Livingstone; 1995:783–793.

106. Burke AP, Kalra P, Li L, et al. Infectious endocarditis and sudden unexpected death: incidence and morphology of lesions in intravenous addicts and non-drug abusers. *J Heart Valve Dis* 1997;6:198–203.

107. Tuazon CU, Sheagren JN. Increased rate of carriage of *Staphylococcus aureus* among narcotic addicts. *J Infect Dis* 1974;129:725–727.

108. Reyes MP, Lerner AM. Current problems in the treatment of infective endocarditis due to *Pseudomonas aeruginosa*. *Rev Infect Dis* 1983;5: 314–321.

109. Cohen PS, Maguire JH, Weinstein L. Infective endocarditis caused by gram-negative bacteria: A review of the literature, 1945–1977. *Prog Cardiovasc Dis* 1980;22:205–242.

110. Rubinstein E, Noriega ER, Simberkoff MS, et al. Fungal endocarditis: Analysis of 24 cases and review of the literature. *Medicine* 1975;54: 331–344.

111. Moyer DV, Edwards JEJ. Fungal endocarditis. In: Kaye D, ed. *Infective Endocarditis*. New York: Raven Press; 1992:299–312.

112. Baddour LM, Meyer J, Henry B. Polymicrobial infective endocarditis in the 1980s. *Rev Infect Dis* 1991;13:963–970.

113. Faber M, Frimodt-Moller N, Espersen F, et al. *Staphylococcus aureus* endocarditis in Danish intravenous drug users: High proportion of left-sided endocarditis. *Scand J Infect Dis* 1995;27:483–487.

114. San Roman JA, Vilacosta I, Sarria C, et al. Eustachian valve endocarditis: Is it worth searching for? *Am Heart J* 2001;142:1037–1040.

115. Palepu A, Cheung SS, Montessori V, et al. Factors other than the Duke criteria associated with infective endocarditis among injection drug users. *Clin Invest Med* 2002;25:118–125.

116. Cicalini S, Forcina G, De Rosa FG. Infective endocarditis in patients with human immunodeficiency virus infection. *J Infect* 2001;42: 267–271.

117. Wilson LE, Thomas DL, Astemborski J, et al. Prospective study of infective endocarditis among injection drug users. *J Infect Dis* 2002;185: 1761–1766.

118. Spijkerman IJ, van Ameijden EJ, Mientjes GH, et al. Human immunodeficiency virus infection and other risk factors for skin abscesses and endocarditis among injection drug users. *J Clin Epidemiol* 1996;49: 1149–1154.

119. Manoff SB. Human immunodeficiency virus infection and infective endocarditis among injecting drug users. *Epidemiology* 1996;7:566–570.

120. Drancourt M, Birtles R, Chaumentin G, et al. New serotype of *Bartonella henselae* in endocarditis and cat-scratch disease. *Lancet* 1996; 347:441–443.

121. Ribera E, Miro JM, Cortes E, et al. Influence of human immunodeficiency virus 1 and degree of immunosuppression in the clinical characteristics and outcome of infective endocarditis in intravenous drug users. *Arch Intern Med* 1998;158:2043–2050.

122. Braimbridge MV, Eykyn SJ. Prosthetic valve endocarditis. *J Antimicrob Chemother* 1987;20:173–180.

123. Watanakunakorn C. Prosthetic valve infective endocarditis. *Prog Cardiovasc Dis* 1979;22:181–192.

124. Karchmer AW, Dismukes WE, Buckley MJ, Austen WG. Late prosthetic valve endocarditis: Clinical features influencing therapy. *Am J Med* 1978;64:199–206.

125. Seaworth BJ, Durack DT. Infective endocarditis in obstetric and gynecologic practice. *Am J Obstet Gynecol* 1986;154:180–188.

126. Sugrue D, Blake S, Troy P, MacDonald D. Antibiotic prophylaxis against infective endocarditis after normal delivery—Is it necessary? *Br Heart J* 1980;44:499–502.

127. Cobbs CG. IUD and endocarditis. *Ann Intern Med* 1973;78:451.

128. Gilleece A, Fenelon L. Nosocomial infective endocarditis. *J Hosp Infect* 2000;46:83–88.

129. Fernandez-Guerrero ML, Verdejo C, Azofra J, de Gorgolas M. Hospital-acquired infectious endocarditis not associated with cardiac surgery: An emerging problem. *Clin Infect Dis* 1995;20:16–23.

130. Fang G, Keys TF, Gentry LO, et al. Prosthetic valve endocarditis resulting from nosocomial bacteremia: A prospective, multicenter study. *Ann Intern Med* 1993;119:560–567.

131. Pelletier LL, Petersdorf RG. Infective endocarditis: A review of 125 cases from the University of Washington Hospitals, 1963–72. *Medicine* 1977;56:287–313.

132. Raad II, Bodey GP. Infectious complications of indwelling vascular catheters. *Clin Infect Dis* 1992;15:197–210.

133. Lamas CC. Hospital acquired native valve endocarditis: Analysis of 22 cases presenting over 11 years. *Heart* 1998;79:442–447.

134. Gouello JP, Asfar P, Brenet O, et al. Nosocomial endocarditis in the intensive care unit: An analysis of 22 cases. *Crit Care Med* 2000;28: 377–382.

135. Rowley KM, Clubb KS, Smith GJW, Cabin HS. Right-sided infective endocarditis as a consequence of flow-directed pulmonary artery catheterization: A clinicopathological study of 55 autopsied patients. *N Engl J Med* 1984;311:1152–1156.

136. Ehrie M, Morgan AP, Moore FD, O'Connor NE. Endocarditis with the indwelling balloon-tipped pulmonary artery catheter in burn patients. *J Trauma* 1978;18:665–666.

137. Cartotto RC. Acute bacterial endocarditis following burns: Case report and review. *Burns* 1998;24:369–373.

138. Martino P, Micozzi A, Venditti M, et al. Catheter-related right-sided endocarditis in bone marrow transplant recipients. *Rev Infect Dis* 1990;12:250–257.

139. Khoo DE, Zebro TJ, English TAH. Bacterial endocarditis in a transplanted heart. *Pathol Res Pract* 1989;185:445–447.

140. Paterson DL. Infective endocarditis in solid organ transplant recipients. *Clin Infect Dis* 1998;26:689–694.

141. Lillehei CW, Bobb JRR, Visscher MB. The occurrence of endocarditis with valvular deformities in dogs with arteriovenous fistulas. *Ann Surg* 1950;132:577–590.

142. Cross AS, Steigbigel RT. Infective endocarditis and access site infections in patients on hemodialysis. *Medicine* 1976;55:453–465.

143. Maraj S, Jacobs LE, Kung SC, et al. Epidemiology and outcome of infective endocarditis in hemodialysis patients. *Am J Med Sci* 2002;324: 254–60.

144. Klug D, Lacroix D, Savoye C, et al. Systemic infection related to endocarditis on pacemaker leads: Clinical presentation and management. *Circulation* 1997;95:2098–2107.

145. Cacoub P. Pacemaker infective endocarditis. *Am J Cardiol* 1998; 82:480–484.

146. Victor F. Pacemaker lead infection: Echocardiographic features, management, and outcome. *Heart* 1999;81:82–87.

147. Voet JG. Pacemaker lead infection: Report of three cases and review of the literature. *Heart* 1999;81:88–91.

148. Brown LA, Baddley JW, Sanchez JE, Bachmann LH. Implantable cardioverter-defibrillator endocarditis secondary to *Candida albicans*. *Am J Med Sci* 2001;322:160–162.

149. Gomes MN, Choyke PL, Wallace RB. Infected aortic aneurysms: A changing entity. *Ann Surg* 1992;215:435–442.

150. Brennan RO, Durack DT. The *viridans* streptococci in perspective. In: Remington JS, Schwartz MN, eds. *Current Clinical Topics in Infectious Diseases*. New York: McGraw-Hill, 1984:253–289.

151. Sussman JI, Baron EJ, Tenenbaum MJ, et al. *Viridans* streptococcal endocarditis: Clinical, microbiological, and echocardiographic correlations. *J Infect Dis* 1986;154:597–603.

152. Watanakunakorn C, Pantelakis J. Alpha-hemolytic streptococcal bacteremia: A review of 203 episodes during 1980–1991. *Scand J Infect Dis* 1993;25:403–408.

153. Levy CS, Kogulan P, Gill VJ, et al. Endocarditis caused by penicillin-resistant *viridans* streptococci: 2 cases and controversies in therapy. *Clin Infect Dis* 2001;33:577–579.

154. Facklam RR. Physiological differentiation of *viridans* streptococci. *J Clin Microbiol* 1977;5:184–201.

155. Douglas CWI, Heath J, Hampton KK, Preston FE. Identity of viridans streptococci isolated from cases of infective endocarditis. *J Med Microbiol* 1993;39:179–182.

156. Carey RB, Gross KC, Roberts RB. Vitamin B6-dependent *Streptococcus mitor (mitis)* isolated from patients with systemic infections. *J Infect Dis* 1975;131:722–726.

157. Rouff KL. Nutritionally variant streptococci. *Clin Microbiol Rev* 1991; 4:184–190.

158. Bouvet A, Grimont F, Grimont PAD. *Streptococcus defectivus* sp nov and *Streptococcus adjacens* sp nov: Nutritionally variant streptococci from human clinical specimens. *Int J Syst Bacteriol* 1989;39:290–294.

159. Bouvet A. Human endocarditis due to nutritionally variant streptococci: *Streptococcus adjacens* and *Streptococcus defectivus*. *Eur Heart J* 1995;16(suppl B):24–27.

160. Wilson WR, Wilkowske CJ, Wright AJ, et al. Treatment of streptomycin-susceptible and streptomycin-resistant enterococcal endocarditis. *Ann Intern Med* 1984;100:816–823.

161. Moellering RCJ, Watson BK, Kunz LJ. Endocarditis due to group D streptococci: Comparison of disease caused by *Streptococcus bovis* with that produced by the enterococci. *Am J Med* 1974;57:239–250.

162. Kupferwasser I. Clinical and morphological characteristics in *Streptococcus bovis* endocarditis: A comparison with other causative microorganisms in 177 cases. *Heart* 1998;80:276–280.

163. Duval X, Papastamopoulos V, Longuet P, et al. Definite *Streptococcus bovis* endocarditis: Characteristics in 20 patients. *Clin Microbiol Infect* 2001;7:3–10.

164. Murray HW, Roberts RB. *Streptococcus bovis* bacteremia and underlying gastrointestinal disease. *Arch Intern Med* 1978;138:1097–1099.

165. Klein RS, Catalano MT, Edberg SC, et al. *Streptococcus bovis* septicemia and carcinoma of the colon. *Ann Intern Med* 1979;91: 560–562.

166. Maki DG, Agger WA. Enterococcal bacteremia: Clinical features, the risk of endocarditis, and management. *Medicine* 1988;67:248–269.

167. Murray BE. The life and times of the enterococcus. *Clin Microbiol Rev* 1990;3:46–65.

168. Megran DW. Enterococcal endocarditis. *Clin Infect Dis* 1992;15: 63–71.

169. Eliopoulos GM. Increasing problems in the therapy of enterococcal infections. *Eur J Clin Microbiol Infect Dis* 1993;12:409–412.

170. Frieden TR, Munsiff SS, Low DE, et al. Emergence of vancomycin-resistant enterococci in New York City. *Lancet* 1993;342:76–79.

171. Bruyn GAW, Thompson J, Van Der Meer JWM. Pneumococcal endocarditis in adult patients. A report of five cases and review of the literature. *Q J Med* 1990;74:33–40.

172. Aronin SI. Review of pneumococcal endocarditis in adults in the penicillin era. *Clin Infect Dis* 1998;26:1341–1342.

173. Lindberg J. Pneumococcal endocarditis is not just a disease of the past: An analysis of 16 cases diagnosed in Denmark 1986–1997. *Scand J Infect Dis* 1998;30:469–472.

174. Baddour LM. Infective endocarditis caused by beta-hemolytic streptococci. The Infectious Diseases Society of America's Emerging Infections Network. *Clin Infect Dis* 1998;26:66–71.

175. Winterbotham A. Endocarditis caused by group A beta-hemolytic streptococcus in an infant: Case report and review. *Clin Infect Dis* 1999;29:196–198.

176. Azzam ZS. Group B streptococcal tricuspid valve endocarditis: A case report and review of literature. *Int J Cardiol* 1998;64:259–263.

177. John MD, Hibberd PL, Karchmer AW, et al. *Staphylococcus aureus* prosthetic valve endocarditis: Optimal management and risk factors for death. *Clin Infect Dis* 1998;26:1302–1309.

178. Roder BL. Clinical features of *Staphylococcus aureus* endocarditis: A 10-year experience in Denmark. *Arch Intern Med* 1999;159:462–469.

179. Pankey GA. Acute bacterial endocarditis at the University of Minnesota Hospitals, 1939–1959. *Am Heart J* 1962;64:583–591.

180. Watanakunakorn C, Tan JS, Phair JP. Some salient features of *Staphylococcus aureus* endocarditis. *Am J Med* 1973;54:473–481.

181. Bayer AS, Lam K, Gintzon L, et al. *Staphylococcus aureus* bacteremia: Clinical, serologic, and echocardiographic findings in patients with and without endocarditis. *Arch Intern Med* 1987;147:457–462.

182. Keys TF, Hewitt WL. Endocarditis due to micrococci and *Staphylococcus epidermidis*. *Arch Intern Med* 1973;132:216–220.

183. Huebner J. Coagulase-negative staphylococci: Role as pathogens. *Ann Res Med* 1999;50:223–236.

184. Karchmer AW, Archer GL, Dismukes WE. *Staphylococcus epidermidis* causing prosthetic valve endocarditis: Microbiologic and clinical observations as guides to therapy. *Ann Intern Med* 1983;98:447–455.

185. Borgert SJ. Destructive native valve endocarditis caused by *Staphylococcus lugdunensis*. *South Med J* 1999;92:812–814.

186. Patel R, Piper KE, Rouse MS, et al. Frequency of isolation of *Staphylococcus lugdunensis* among stapylococcal isolates causing endocarditis: A 20-year experience. *J Clin Microbiol* 2000;38:4262–4263.

187. Chen YC, Chang SC, Luh KT, Hsieh WC. *Actinobacillus actinomycetemcomitans* endocarditis: A report of four cases and review of the literature. *Q J Med* 1992;81:871–878.

188. Geraci JE, Wilson WR. Endocarditis due to gram-negative bacteria: Report of 56 cases. *Mayo Clin Proc* 1982;57:145–148.

189. Badley AD. Infective endocarditis caused by HACEK microorganisms. *Annu Rev Med* 1997;48:25–33.

190. Darras-Joly C. *Haemophilus* endocarditis: Report of 42 cases in adults and review: *Haemophilus* Endocarditis Study Group. *Clin Infect Dis* 1997;24:1087–1094.

191. Gould K, Ramirez-Ronda CH, Holmes RK, Sanford JP. Adherence of bacteria to heart valves in vitro. *J Clin Invest* 1975;56:1364–1370.

192. Scheld WM, Valone JA, Sande MA. Bacterial adherence in the pathogenesis of endocarditis: Interaction of bacterial dextran, platelets, and fibrin. *J Clin Invest* 1978;61:1394–1404.

193. Durack DT, Beeson PB. Protective role of complement in experimental *E. coli* endocarditis. *Infect Immun* 1977;16:213–217.

194. Gutierrez RF. Endocarditis caused by *Stenotrophomas maltophilia*: Case report and review. *Clin Infect Dis* 1996;23:1261–1265.

195. Al-Kasab S, Al-Fagih MR, Al-Yousef S, et al. *Brucella* infective endocarditis: Successful combined medical and surgical therapy. *J Thorac Cardiovasc Surg* 1988;95:862–867.

196. Delvecchio G, Fracassetti O, Lorenzi N. *Brucella* endocarditis. *Int J Cardiol* 1991;33:328–329.

197. Uddin MJ. The role of aggressive medical therapy along with early surgical intervention in the cure of *Brucella* endocarditis. *Ann Thorac Cardiovasc Surg* 1998;4:209–213.

198. Felner JM, Dowell VR. Anaerobic bacterial endocarditis. *N Engl J Med* 1970;283:1188–1192.

199. Nastro LJ, Finegold SM. Endocarditis due to anaerobic gram-negative bacilli. *Am J Med* 1973;54:482–496.

200. Kammer RB, Utz JP. *Aspergillus* species endocarditis: The new face of a not so rare disease. *Am J Med* 1974;56:506–521.

201. Aspesberro F. Fungal endocarditis in critically ill children. *Eur J Pediatr* 1999;158:275–280.

202. Pierrotti LC, Baddour LM. Fungal endocarditis, 1995–2000. *Chest* 2002;122:302–310.

203. Siegman-Igra Y. Q fever endocarditis in Israel and a worldwide review. *Scand J Infect Dis* 1997;29:41–49.

204. Raoult D, Brouqui P, Marchou B, Gastaut JA. Acute and chronic Q fever in patients with cancer. *Clin Infect Dis* 1992;14:127–130.

205. La Sacola B. Culture of *Bartonella quintana* and *Bartonella henselae* from human samples: A 5-year experience (1990 to 1998). *J Clin Microbiol* 1999;37:1899–1905.

206. Ward C, Ward AM. Acquired valvular heart disease in patients who keep pet birds. *Lancet* 1974;2:734–736.

207. van der Bel-Kahn J, Watanakunakorn C, Menefee MG, et al. *Chlamydia trachomatis* endocarditis. *Am Heart J* 1978;95:627–636.

208. Spyrou N, Anderson M, Foale R. *Listeria* endocarditis: Current management and patient outcome: World literature review. *Heart* 1997;77:380–383.

209. Cohen JI, Sloss LJ, Kundsin R, Golightly L. Prosthetic valve endocarditis caused by *Mycoplasma hominis. Am J Med* 1989;86:819–821.

210. Malinverni R, Bille J, Glauser MP. Single-dose rifampin prophylaxis for experimental endocarditis induced by high bacterial inocula of *viridans* streptococci. *J Infect Dis* 1987;156:151–157.

211. Cannady PBJ, Sanford JP. Negative blood cultures in infective endocarditis: A review. *South Med J* 1976;69:1420–1424.

212. Pesanti EL, Smith IM. Infective endocarditis with negative blood cultures: An analysis of 52 cases. *Am J Med* 1979;66:43–50.

213. Hoen B, Selton-Suty C, Lacassin F, et al. Infective endocarditis in patients with negative blood cultures: Analysis of 88 cases from a one-year nationwide survey in France. *Clin Infect Dis* 1995;20:501–506.

214. Brouqui P, Raoult D. Endocarditis due to rare and fastidious bacteria. *Clin Microbiol Rev* 2001;14:177–207.

215. Goldenberger D, Kunzli A, Vogt P, et al. Molecular diagnosis of bacterial endocarditis by broad-range PCR amplification and direct sequencing. *J Clin Microbiol* 1997;35:2733–2739.

216. Libman E. The clinical features of cases of subacute bacterial endocarditis that have spontaneously become bacteria-free. *Am J Med Sci* 1913;146:626–645.

217. Gubler JG. Whipple endocarditis without overt gastrointestinal disease: Report of four cases. *Ann Intern Med* 1999;131:144–146.

218. Roux JP, Koussa A, Cajot MA, et al. Primary *Aspergillus* endocarditis: Apropos of a case and review of the international literature. *Ann Chir* 1992;46:110–115.

219. Fenollar F, Lepidi H, Raoult D. Whipple's endocarditis: Review of the literature and comparisons with Q fever, *Bartonella* infection, and blood culture–positive endocarditis. *Clin Infect Dis* 2001;33:1309–1316.

220. Raoult D, Birg ML, La Scola B, et al. Cultivation of the bacillus of Whipple's disease. *N Engl J Med* 2000;342:620–625;1538.

221. Durack DT, Bright DK, Lukes AS, Service DE. New criteria for diagnosis of infective endocarditis: Utilization of specific echocardiographic findings. *Am J Med* 1994;96:200–209.

222. Cecchi E, Parrini I, Chinaglia A, et al. New diagnostic criteria for infective endocarditis. A study of sensitivity and specificity. *Eur Heart J* 1997;18:1149–1156.

223. Angrist A, Oka M, Nakao K. Vegetative endocarditis. *Pathol Annu* 1967;2:155–212.

224. Grant RT, Wood JEJ, Jones TD. Heart valve irregularities in relation to subacute bacterial endocarditis. *Am Heart J* 1928;14:247–261.

225. Durack DT. Experimental bacterial endocarditis: IV. Structure and evolution of very early lesions. *J Pathol* 1975;115:81–89.

226. Durack DT, Beeson PB. Experimental bacterial endocarditis: I. Colonization of a sterile vegetation. *Br J Exp Pathol* 1972;53:44–49.

227. Bryan CS. Nonbacterial thrombotic endocarditis in patients with malignant tumors. *Am J Med* 1969;46:787–793.

228. Hojnik M, George J, Ziporen L, Shoenfeld Y. Heart valve involvement (Libman-Sacks endocarditis) in the antiphospholipid syndrome. *Circulation* 1996;93:1579–1587.

229. Livornese LLJ, Korzeniowski O. Pathogenesis of infective endocarditis. In: Kaye D, ed. *Infective Endocarditis.* New York: Raven Press; 1992:19–35.

230. Campbell KM, Johnson CN. Identification of *Staphylococcus aureus* binding proteins on isolated porcine cardiac valve cells. *J Lab Clin Med* 1990;115:217–223.

231. Schlievert PM. Aggregation and binding substances enhance pathogenicity in rabbit models of *Enterococcus faecalis* endocarditis. *Infect Immun* 1998;66:218–223.

232. Burnette-Curley D, Wells V, Viscount H, et al. FimA, a major virulence factor associated with *Streptococcus parasanguis* endocarditis. *Infect Immun* 1995;63:4669–4674.

233. Viscount HB, Munro CL, Burnette-Curley D, et al. Immunization with FimA protects against *Streptococcus parasanguis* endocarditis in rats. *Infect Immun* 1997;65:994–1002.

234. Moreillon P, Entenza JM, Francioli P, et al. Role of *Staphylococcus aureus* coagulase and clumping factor in pathogenesis of experimental endocarditis. *Infect Immun* 1995;63:4738–4743.

235. Baddour LM, Christensen GD, Hester MG, Bisno AL. Production of experimental endocarditis by coagulase-negative staphylococci: Variability in species virulence. *J Infect Dis* 1984;150:721–727.

236. Sullam PM. Diminished platelet binding in vitro by *Staphylococcus aureus* is associated with reduced virulence in a rabbit model of infective endocarditis. *Infect Immunol* 1996;64:4915–4921.

237. Drake T, Pang M. *Staphylococcus aureus* induces tissue factor expression in cultured human cardiac valve endothelium. *J Infect Dis* 1988;66:3476–3479.

238. Dhawan VK, Yeaman MR, Cheung AL, et al. Phenotypic resistance to thrombin-induced platelet microbicidal protein in vitro is correlated with enhanced virulence in experimental endocarditis due to *Staphylococcus aureus. Infect Immun* 1997;65:3293–3299.

239. Dhawan VK, Bayer AS, Yeaman MR. In vitro resistance to thrombin-induced platelet microbicidal protein is associated with enhanced progression and hematogenous dissemination in experimental *Staphylococcus aureus* infective endocarditis. *Infect Immun* 1998;66:3476–3479.

240. Bayer AS, Ramos MD, Menzies BE, et al. Hyperproduction of alpha-toxin by *Staphylococcus aureus* results in paradoxically reduced virulence in experimental endocarditis: A host defense role for platelet microbicidal proteins. *Infect Immun* 1997;65:4652–4660.

241. Kupferwasser LI, Yeaman MR, Shapiro SM, et al. Acetylsalicylic acid reduces vegetation bacterial density, hematogenous bacterial dissemination, and frequency of embolic events in experimental *Staphylococcus aureus* endocarditis through antiplatelet and antibacterial effects. *Circulation* 1999;99:2791–2797.

242. Drake TA, Rogers GM, Sande MA. Tissue factor is a major stimulus for vegetation formation in enterococcal endocarditis in rabbits. *J Clin Invest* 1984;73:1750–1753.

243. Yeaman MR, Puentes SM, Norman DC, Bayer AS. Partial characterization and staphylocidal activity of thrombin-induced platelet microbicidal protein. *Infect Immun* 1992;60:1202–1209.

244. van Ginkel CJW, Thorig L, Thompson J, et al. Enhancement of generation of monocyte tissue thromboplastin by bacterial phagocytosis: Possible pathway for fibrin formation on infected vegetations in bacterial endocarditis. *Infect Immun* 1979;25:388–395.

245. Capo C, Zugun F, Stein A, et al. Upregulation of tumor necrosis factor alpha and interleukin-1 beta in Q fever endocarditis. *Infect Immun* 1996;64:1638–1642.

246. Lepeschkin E. On the relation between the site of valvular involvement in endocarditis and the blood pressure resting on the valve. *Am J Med Sci* 1952;224:318–319.

247. Frontera JA, Gradon JD. Right-side endocarditis in injection drug users: Review of proposed mechanisms of pathogenesis. *Clin Infec Dis* 2000;30:374–379.

248. Rodbard S. Blood velocity and endocarditis. *Circulation* 1963;27:18–28.

249. Edwards JE, Burchell HB. Endocardial and intimal lesions (jet impact) as possible sites of origin of murmurs. *Circulation* 1958;18:946–960.

250. Buchbinder NA, Roberts WC. Left-sided valvular active infective endocarditis: A study of forty-five necropsy patients. *Am J Med* 1972;53:20–35.

251. Scully RE, Mark EJ, McNeely WF, McNeely BU. Case records of the Massachusetts General Hospital. *N Engl J Med* 1996; 334:105–111.

252. DiNubile MJ, Calderwood SB, Steinhaus DM, Karchmer AW. Cardiac conduction abnormalities complicating native valve active endocarditis. *Am J Cardiol* 1986;58:1213–1217.

253. Phair JP, Clarke J. Immunology of infective endocarditis. *Prog Cardiovasc Dis* 1977;22:137–144.

254. Williams RC, Kunkel HG. Rheumatoid factor, complement, and conglutinin aberrations in patients with subacute bacterial endocarditis. *J Clin Invest* 1962;41:666–675.

255. Messner RP, Laxdal T, Quie PG, Williams RCJ. Rheumatoid factors in subacute bacterial endocarditis—Bacterium, duration of disease or genetic predisposition? *Ann Intern Med* 1968;68:746–754.

256. Sheagren JN, Tuazon CU, Griffin C, Padmore N. Rheumatoid factor in acute bacterial endocarditis. *Arthritis Rheum* 1976;19:887–890.

257. Maisch B, Eichstadt H, Kochsick K. Immune reactions in infective endocarditis: I. Clinical data and diagnostic relevance of antimyocardial antibodies. *Am Heart J* 1983;106:329–337.

258. Weinstein L, Schlesinger JJ. Pathoanatomic, pathophysiologic and clinical correlations in endocarditis. (First of two parts.). *N Engl J Med* 1974;291:832–837.

259. Wadsworth AB. A study of the endocardial lesions developing during *Pneumococcus* infection in horses. *J Med Res* 1919;34:280–291.

260. Mair W. Pneumococcal endocarditis in rabbits. *J Pathol Bacteriol* 1923;26:426–428.

261. Durack DT, Gilliland BC, Petersdorf RG. Effect of immunization on susceptibility to experimental *Streptococcus mutans* and *Streptococcus sanguis* endocarditis. *Infect Immun* 1978;22:52–56.

262. Durack DT, Beeson PB. Pathogenesis of infective endocarditis. *Infective Endocarditis*. New York: Grune & Stratton; 1978:1–53.

263. Bayer AS, Theofilopoulos AN, Eisenberg R, et al. Circulating immune complexes in infective endocarditis. *N Engl J Med* 1976;295:1500–1505.

264. Bayer AS, Theofilopoulos AN, Tillman DB, et al. Use of circulating immune complex levels in the serodifferentiation of endocarditic and nonendocarditic septicemias. *Am J Med* 1979;66:58–62.

265. Maisch B, Mayer E, Schubert U, et al. Immune reactions in infective endocarditis: II. Relevance of circulating immune complexes, serum inhibition factors, lymphocytotoxic reactions, and antibody-dependent cellular cytotoxicity against cardiac target cells. *Am Heart J* 1983;106: 338–344.

266. Cabane J, Godeau P, Hereeman A, et al. Fate of circulating immune complexes in infective endocarditis. *Am J Med* 1979;66:277–282.

267. Gutman RA, Striker GE, Gilliland BC, Cutler RE. The immune complex glomerulonephritis of bacterial endocarditis. *Medicine* 1972;51: 1–25.

268. Levy RL, Hong R. The immune nature of subacute bacterial endocarditis (SBE) nephritis. *Am J Med* 1973;54:645–652.

269. Nagel JG, Tuazon CU, Cardella TA, Sheagren JN. Teichoic acid serologic diagnosis of staphylococcal endocarditis: Use of gel diffusion and counterimmunoelectrophoretic methods. *Ann Intern Med* 1975;82:13–17.

270. Churchill MAJ, Geraci JE, Hunder GG. Musculoskeletal manifestations of bacterial endocarditis. *Ann Intern Med* 1977;87:754–759.

271. Starkebaum MK, Durack DT, Beeson PB. The "incubation period" of subacute bacterial endocarditis. *Yale J Biol Med* 1977;50:49–58.

272. Karchmer AW. Staphylococcal endocarditis. In: Kaye D, ed. *Infective Endocarditis*. New York: Raven Press; 1992:225–249.

273. Khan MY, Hall WH, Gerding DN. Infective endocarditis in narcotic addicts. *Minn Med* 1975;58:83–84.

274. Freedman LR, Valone JJ. Experimental infective endocarditis. *Prog Cardiovasc Dis* 1979;22:169–180.

275. Steckelberg JM, Murphy JG, Wilson WR. Cure rates and long-term prognosis. In: Kaye D, ed. *Infective Endocarditis*. New York: Raven Press; 1992:435–453.

276. Kilpatrick ZM, Greenberg PA, Sanford JP. Splinter hemorrhages— Their clinical significance. *Arch Intern Med* 1965;115:730–735.

277. Howard EJ. Osler's nodes. *Am Heart J* 1960;59:633–634.

278. Alpert JS, Krous HF, Dalen JE, et al. Pathogenesis of Osler's nodes. *Ann Intern Med* 1976;85:471–473.

279. Cates JE, Christie RV. Subacute bacterial endocarditis: A review of 442 patients treated in 14 centres appointed by the Penicillin Trials Committee of Medical Research Council. *Q J Med* 1951;20:93–130.

280. Mills J, Utley J, Abbott J. Heart failure in infective endocarditis. *Chest* 1974;66:151–159.

281. Lytle BW, Priest BP, Taylor PC, et al. Surgical treatment of prosthetic valve endocarditis. *J Thorac Cardiovasc Surg* 1996;111:198–207.

282. Tanaka M, Abe T, Hosokawa S, et al. Tricuspid valve *Candida* endocarditis cured by valve-sparing debridement. *Ann Thorac Surg* 1989; 48:857–858.

283. Pruett TL, Rotstein OD, Anderson RW, Simmons RL. Tricuspid valve endocarditis: Successful treatment with valve-sparing debridement and antifungal chemotherapy in a multiorgan transplant recipient. *Am J Med* 1986;80:116–118.

284. Kupferwasser LI, Hafner G, Mohr-Kahaly S, et al. The presence of infection-related antiphospholipid antibodies in infective endocarditis determines a major risk factor for embolic events. *J Am Coll Cardiol* 1999;33:1365–1371.

285. Vilacosta I, Graupner C, San Roman JA, et al. Risk of embolization after institution of antibiotic therapy for infective endocarditis. *J Am Coll Cardiol* 2002;39:1489–1495.

286. Sokil AB. Cardiac imaging in infective endocarditis. In: Kaye D, ed. *Infective Endocarditis*. New York: Raven Press; 1992:125–150.

287. Chan KL. Early clinical course and long-term outcome of patients with infective endocarditis complicated by perivalvular abscess. *CMAJ* 2002;167:19–24.

288. Ziment I. Nervous system complications in bacterial endocarditis. *Am J Med* 1969;47:593–607.

289. Pruitt AA, Rubin RH, Karchmer AW, Duncan GW. Neurologic complications of bacterial endocarditis. *Medicine* 1978;57:329–343.

290. Jones HRJ, Siekert RG. Neurological manifestations of infective endocarditis: Review of clinical and therapeutic challenges. *Brain* 1989;112: 1295–1315.

291. Francioli P. Central nervous system complications of infective endocarditis. In: Scheld WM, Durack DT, eds. *Infections of the Central Nervous System*. New York: Lippincott-Raven; 1997:523–553.

292. Jones HR, Siekert RG, Geraci JE. Neurologic manifestations of bacterial endocarditis. *Ann Intern Med* 1969;71:21–28.

293. Heiro M, Nikoskelainen J, Engblom E, et al. Neurologic manifestations of infective endocarditis: A 17-year experience in a teaching hospital in Finland. *Arch Intern Med* 2000;160:2781–2787.

294. Cabell CH, Pond KK, Peterson GE, et al. The risk of stroke and death in patients with aortic and mitral valve endocarditis. *Am Heart J* 2001; 142:75–80.

295. Stengel A, Wolferth CC. Mycotic (bacterial) aneurysms of intravascular origin. *Arch Intern Med* 1923;31:527–554.

296. Brust JCM, Dickinson PCT, Hughes JEO, Holtzman RNN. The diagnosis and treatment of cerebral mycotic aneurysms. *Ann Neurol* 1990; 27:238–246.

297. Chukwudelunzu FE, Brown RDJ, Wijdicks EF, Steckelberg JM. Subarachnoid haemorrhage associated with infectious endocarditis: Case report and literature review. *Eur J Neurol* 2002;9:423–427.

298. Salgado AV, Furlan AJ, Keys TF. Mycotic aneurysm, subarachnoid hemorrhage, and indications for cerebral angiography in infective endocarditis. *Stroke* 1987;18:1057–1060.

299. Nakata Y, Shionoya S, Kamiya K. Pathogenesis of mycotic aneurysm. *Angiology* 1968;19:593–601.

300. Masuda J, Yutani C, Waki R, et al. Histopathological analysis of the mechanisms of intracranial hemorrhage complicating infective endocarditis. *Stroke* 1992;23:843–850.

301. McFarland MM. Pathology of infective endocarditis. In: Kaye D, ed. *Infective Endocarditis*. New York: Raven Press; 1992:57–83.

302. Bamford J, Hodges J, Warlow C. Late rupture of a mycotic aneurysm after "cure" of bacterial endocarditis. *J Neurol* 1986;233:51–53.

303. Bush LM, Johnson CC. Clinical syndrome and diagnosis. In: Kaye D, ed. *Infective Endocarditis*. New York: Raven Press; 1992: 99–115.

304. Durack DT, Street AC. Fever of unknown origin: Reexamined and redefined. *Curr Clin Top Infect Dis* 1991;11:35–51.

305. von Reyn CF, Levy BS, Arbeit RD, et al. Infective endocarditis: An analysis based on strict case definitions. *Ann Intern Med* 1981;94: 505–517.

306. Li JS, Sexton DJ, Mick N, et al. Proposed modifications to the Duke criteria for the diagnosis of infective endocarditis. *Clin Infect Dis* 2000;30:633–638.

307. Dajani AS, Ayoub E, Bierman FZ, et al. Guidelines for the diagnosis of rheumatic fever: Jones criteria, 1992 update. *JAMA* 1992;268: 2069–2073.

308. Habib G, Derumeaux G, Avierinos JF, et al. Value and limitations of the Duke criteria for the diagnosis of infective endocarditis. *J Am Coll Cardiol* 1999;33:2023–2029.

309. Perez-Vazquez A, Farinas MC, Garcia-Palomo JD, et al. Evaluation of the Duke criteria in 93 episodes of prosthetic valve endocarditis: Could sensitivity be improved? *Arch Intern Med* 2000;160:1185–1191.

310. Dodds GA, Sexton DJ, Durack DT, et al. Negative predictive value of the Duke criteria for infective endocarditis. *Am J Cardiol* 1996;77:403–407.

311. Powers DL, Mandell GL. Intraleukocytic bacteria in endocarditis patients. *JAMA* 1974;227:312–313.

312. Engle RL, Koprowska I. The appearance of histiocytes in blood in subacute bacterial endocarditis. *Am J Med* 1959;26:965–973.

313. Hogevik H, Olaison L, Andersson R, et al. C-reactive protein is more sensitive than erythrocyte sedimentation rate for diagnosis of infective endocarditis. *Infection* 1997;25:82–85.

314. Agarwal A, Clements J, Sedmak DD, et al. Subacute bacterial endocarditis masquerading as type III essential mixed cryoglobulinemia. *J Am Soc Nephrol* 1997;8:1971–1976.

315. Kaye MM, Kaye D. Laboratory findings including blood cultures. In: Kaye D, ed. *Infective Endocarditis*. New York: Raven Press; 1992: 117–124.

316. Fournier PE, Casalta JP, Habib G, et al. Modification of the diagnostic criteria proposed by the Duke Endocarditis Service to permit improved diagnosis of Q fever endocarditis. *Am J Med* 1996;100:629–633.

317. Belli J, Waisbren BA. The number of blood cultures necessary to diagnose most cases of bacterial endocarditis. *Am J Med Sci* 1956;232: 284–288.

318. Ellner JJ, Rosenthal MS, Lerner PI, McHenry M. Infective endocarditis caused by slow-growing, fastidious, gram-negative bacteria. *Medicine* 1979;58:145–158.

319. Gerry JL, Greenough WB. Diphtheroid endocarditis: Report of nine cases and review of the literature. *Johns Hopkins Med J* 1976;139:61–68.

320. Zbinden R, Hany A, Luthy R, et al. Antibody response in six HACEK endocarditis cases under therapy. *APMIS* 1998;106:547–552.

321. Patel R, Newell J, Procop GW, et al. Use of polymerase chain reaction for citrate synthase gene to diagnose *Bartonella quintana* endocarditis. *Am J Clin Pathol* 1999;112:36–40.

322. Das I, De Giovanni JV, Gray J. Endocarditis caused by *Haemophilus parainfluenzae* identified by 16s ribosomal RNA sequencing. *J Clin Pathol* 1997;50:72–74.

323. Rothman RE, Majmudar MD, Kelen GD, et al. Detection of bacteremia in emergency department patients at risk for infective endocarditis using universal 16S rRNA primers in a decontaminated polymerase chain reaction assay. *J Infect Dis* 2002;186:1677–1681.

324. De Castro S, d'Amati G, Cartoni D, et al. Valvular perforation in left-sided infective endocarditis: A prospective echocardiographic evaluation and clinical outcome. *Am Heart J* 1997;134:656–664.

325. Aly AM, Simpson PM, Humes RA. The role of transthoracic echocardiography in the diagnosis of infective endocarditis in children. *Arch Pediatr Adolesc Med* 1999;153:950–954.

326. Mugge A, Daniel WG, Frank G, Lichtlen PR. Echocardiography in infective endocarditis: Reassessment of prognostic implications of vegetation size determined by the transthoracic and transesophageal approach. *J Am Coll Cardiol* 1989;14:631–638.

327. Pavlides GS, Hauser AM, Stewart JR, et al. Contribution of transesophageal echocardiography to patient diagnosis and treatment: A prospective analysis. *Am Heart J* 1990;120:910–914.

328. Daniel WG, Mugge A, Martin RP, et al. Improvement in the diagnosis of abscesses associated with endocarditis by transesophageal echocardiography. *N Engl J Med* 1991;324:795–800.

329. De Castro S, Cartoni D, d'Amati G, et al. Diagnostic accuracy of transthoracic and multiplane transesophageal echocardiography for valvular perforation in acute infective endocarditis: correlation with anatomic findings. *Clin Infect Dis* 2000;30:825–826.

330. Baumgartner FJ, Omari BO, Robertson JM, et al. Annular abscesses in surgical endocarditis: Anatomic, clinical, and operative features. *Ann Thorac Surg* 2000;70:442–447.

331. Morguet AJ, Werner GS, Andreas S, Kreuzer H. Diagnostic value of transesophageal compared with transthoracic echocardiography in suspected prosthetic valve endocarditis. *Herz* 1995;20:390–398.

332. Lengyel M. The impact of transesophageal echocardiography on the management of prosthetic valve endocarditis: Experience of 31 cases and review of the literature. *J Heart Valv Dis* 1997;6:204–211.

333. Cheitlin MD, Alpert JS, Armstrong WF, et al. ACC/AHA guidelines for the clinical application of echocardiography: Executive summary: A report of the American College of Cardiology/American Heart Association Task Force on Practice Guidelines (Committee on Clinical Application of Echocardiography): Developed in collaboration with the American Society of Echocardiography. *J Am Coll Cardiol* 1997; 29:862–879.

334. Heidenreich PA, Masoudi FA, Maini B, et al. Echocardiography in patients with suspected endocarditis: A cost-effective analysis. *Am J Cardiol* 1999;107:198–208.

335. Fowler VG, Li J, Corey GR, et al. Role of echocardiography in evaluation of patients with *Staphylococcus aureus* bacteremia: Experience in 103 patients. *J Am Coll Cardiol* 1997;30:1072–1078.

336. Rosen AB, Fowler VG, Corey GR, et al. Cost-effectiveness of transesophageal echocardiography to determine the duration of therapy for intravascular catheter-associated *Staphylococcus aureus* bacteremia. *Ann Intern Med* 1999;130:810–820.

337. Fowler VG, Sanders LL, Kong LK, et al. Infective endocarditis due to *Staphylococcus aureus:* 59 prospectively identified cases with follow-up. *Clin Infect Dis* 1999;28:106–114.

338. Stewart JA, Silimperi D, Harris P, et al. Echocardiographic documentation of vegetative lesions in infective endocarditis: Clinical implications. *Circulation* 1980;61:374–380.

339. Lindner JR, Case RA, Dent JM, et al. Diagnostic value of echocardiography in suspected endocarditis: An evaluation based on the pretest probability of disease. *Circulation* 1996;93:730–736.

340. Tischler MD, Vaitkus PT. The ability of vegetation size on echocardiography to predict clinical complications: A meta-analysis. *J Echocardiogr* 1997;10:562–568.

341. Lancellotti P, Galiuto L, Albert A, et al. Relative value of clinical and transesophageal echocardiographic variables for risk stratification in patients with infective endocarditis. *Clin Cardiol* 1998;21: 572–578.

342. De Castro S, Magni G, Beni S, et al. Role of transthoracic and transesophageal echocardiography in predicting embolic events in patients with active infective endocarditis involving native cardiac valves. *Am J Cardiol* 1997;80:1030–1034.

343. Gillinov AM, Shah RV, Curtis WE, et al. Valve replacement in patients with endocarditis and acute neurologic deficit. *Ann Thorac Surg* 1996;61:1125–1129.

344. Moriarty JA, Edelman RR, Tumeh SS. CT and MRI of mycotic aneurysms of the abdominal aorta. *J Comput Assist Tomogr* 1992;16: 941–943.

345. Welton DE, Young JB, Raizner AE, et al. Value and safety of cardiac catheterization during active infective endocarditis. *Am J Cardiol* 1979;44:1306–1310.

346. Riba AL, Thakur ML, Gottschalk A, et al. Imaging experimental infective endocarditis with indium-111–labeled blood cellular components. *Circulation* 1979;59:336–343.

347. Campeau RJ, Ingram C. Perivalvular abscess complicating infective endocarditis: Complementary role of echocardiography and indium-111–labeled leukocytes. *J Clin Nucl Med* 1998;23:582–584.

348. Ben-Haim S, Seabold JE, Hawes DR, Rooholamini SA. Leukocyte scintigraphy in the diagnosis of mycotic aneurysm. *J Nucl Med* 1992; 33:1486–1493.

349. Olaison L, Belin L, Hogevik H, et al. Incidence of beta-lactam–induced delayed hypersensitivity and neutropenia during treatment of infective endocarditis. *Arch Intern Med* 1999;159:607–615.

350. Wilson WR, Karchmer A, Dajani A, et al. Antibiotic treatment of adults with infective endocarditis due to *viridans* streptococci, enterococci, staphylococci and HACEK microorganisms. *JAMA* 1995;274: 1706–1713.

351. Chambers HF, Miller RT, Newman MD. Right-sided *Staphylococcus aureus* endocarditis in intravenous drug abusers: Two-week combination therapy. *Ann Intern Med* 1988;109:619–624.

352. Wilson WR, Geraci JE, Wilkowske CJ, Washington JA. Short-term intramuscular therapy with procaine penicillin plus streptomycin for infective endocarditis due to *viridans* streptococci. *Circulation* 1978; 57:1158–1161.

353. Baldassare JS, Kaye D. Principles and overview of antibiotic therapy. In: Kaye D, ed. *Infective Endocarditis.* New York: Raven Press; 1992: 169–190.

354. Glauser MP, Francioli P. Relevance of animal models to the prophylaxis of infective endocarditis. *J Antimicrob Chemother* 1987;20(suppl A):87–93.

355. Blount JG. Bacterial endocarditis. *Am J Med* 1965;38:909–922.

356. Pulliam L, Inokuchi S, Hadley WK, Mills J. Penicillin tolerance in experimental streptococcal endocarditis. *Lancet* 1979;2:957.

357. Denny AE, Peterson LR, Gerding DN, Hall WH. Serious staphylococcal infections with strains tolerant to bactericidal antibiotics. *Arch Intern Med* 1979;139:1026–1031.

358. Brennan RO, Durack DT. Therapeutic significance of penicillin tolerance in experimental streptococcal endocarditis. *Antimicrob Agents Chemother* 1983;23:273–277.

359. Reller LB. The serum bactericidal test. *Rev Infect Dis* 1986;8:803–808.

360. MacGowan A, McMullin C, James P, et al. External quality assessment of the serum bactericidal test: Results of a methodology/interpretation questionnaire. *J Antimicrob Chemother* 1997;39:277–284.

361. Kane LW, Finn JJ. The treatment of subacute bacterial endocarditis with aureomycin and chloromycetin. *N Engl J Med* 1951;244:623–628.

362. Schein J, Baehr G. Sulfonamide therapy of subacute bacterial endocarditis. *Am J Med* 1948;4:66–72.

363. Korzeniowski O, Sande MA. Combination antimicrobial therapy for *Staphylococcus aureus* endocarditis in patients addicted to parenteral drugs and in nonaddicts: A prospective study. *Ann Intern Med* 1982; 97:496–503.

364. Martinez F, Martin-Luengo F, Garcia A, Valdes M. Treatment with various antibiotics of experimental endocarditis caused by penicillin-resistant *Streptococcus sanguis. Eur Heart J* 1995;16:687–691.

365. Doern GV, Ferraro MJ, Brueggmann AB, Ruoff KL. Emergence of high rates of antimicrobial resistance among *viridans* group streptococci in the United States. *Antimicrob Agents Chemother* 1996;40:891–894.

366. Johnson AP, Warner M, Woodford N, et al. Antibiotic resistance among enterococci causing endocarditis in the UK: Analysis of isolates referred to a reference laboratory. *BMJ* 1998;317:629–630.

367. Dailey CF, Dileto-Fang CL, Buchanan LV, et al. Efficacy of linezolid in treatment of experimental endocarditis caused by methicillin-resistant *Staphylococcus aureus. Antimicrob Agents Chemother* 2001;45: 2304–2308.

368. Oramas-Shirey MP, Buchanan LV, Dileto-Fang CL, et al. Efficacy of linezolid in a staphylococcal endocarditis rabbit model. *J Antimicrob Chemother* 2001;47:349–352.

369. Brandt CM, Rouse MS, Laue NW, et al. Effective treatment of multidrug-resistant enterococcal experimental endocarditis with combinations of cell wall–active agents. *J Infect Dis* 1996;173:909–913.

370. Antony SJ, Ladner J, Stratton CW, et al. High-level aminoglycoside-resistant *Enterococcus* causing endocarditis successfully treated with a combination of ampicillin, imipenem and vancomycin. *Scand J Infec Dis* 1997;29:628–630.

371. Tripodi MF, Locatelli A, Adinolfi LE, et al. Successful treatment with ampicillin and fluoroquinolones of human endocarditis due to high-level gentamicin-resistant enterococci. *Eur J Clin Microbiol Infect Dis* 1998;17:734–736.

372. Matsumura S, Simor AE. Treatment of endocarditis due to vancomycin-resistant *Enterococcus faecium* with quinupristin/dalfopristin, doxycycline, and rifampin: A synergistic drug combination. *Clin Infect Dis* 1998;27:1554–1556.

373. Landman D, Quale JM. Management of infections due to resistant enterococci: A review of therapeutic options. *Antimicrob Chemother* 1997;40:161–170.

374. Francioli P, Etienne J, Hoigne R, et al. Treatment of streptococcal endocarditis with a single daily dose of ceftriaxone sodium for 4 weeks: Efficacy and outpatient treatment feasibility. *JAMA* 1992;267: 264–267.

375. Fortun J, Nava E, Martinez-Beltran J, et al. Short-course therapy for right-side endocarditis due to *Staphylococcus aureus* in drug abusers: Cloxacillin versus glycopeptides in combination with gentamicin. *Clin Infect Dis* 2001;33:120–125.

376. Resnekov L. Staphylococcal endocarditis following mitral valvotomy with special reference to coagulase-negative *Staphylococcus albus. Lancet* 1959;2:597–600.

377. Raoult D, Houpikian P, Tissot Dupont H, et al. Treatment of Q fever endocarditis: Comparison of 2 regimens containing doxycycline and ofloxacin or hydroxychloroquine. *Arch Intern Med* 1999;159:167–173.

378. Andrews MM, von Reyn CF. Patient selection criteria and management guidelines for outpatient parenteral antibiotic therapy for native valve infective endocarditis. *Clin Infect Dis* 2001;33:203–209.

379. Stamboulian D, Bonvehi P, Arevalo C, et al. Antibiotic management of outpatients with endocarditis due to penicillin-susceptible streptococci. *Rev Infect Dis* 1991;13:S160–S163.

380. Rehm SJ. Outpatient intravenous antibiotic therapy for endocarditis. *Infect Dis Clin North Am* 1998;12:879–901.

381. Reinhartz O, Herrman M, Redling F, Zerkowski HR. Timing of surgery in patients with acute infective endocarditis. *J Cardiovasc Surg (Torino)* 1996;37:397–400.

382. Alexiou C, Langley SM, Stafford H, et al. Surgery for active culture-positive endocarditis: Determinants of early and late outcome. *Ann Thorac Surg* 2000;69:1448–1454.

383. Alexiou C, Langley SM, Stafford H, et al. Surgical treatment of infective mitral valve endocarditis: Predictors of early and late outcome. *J Heart Valve Dis* 2000;9:327–334.

384. Aranki SF, Adams DH, Rizzo RJ, et al. Determinants of early mortality and late survival in mitral valve endocarditis. *Circulation* 1995;92: 143–149.

385. Douglas JL, Dismukes WE. Surgical therapy of infective endocarditis on natural valves. In: Kaye D, ed. *Infective Endocarditis.* New York: Raven Press; 1992:397–411.

386. Di Salvo G, Habib G, Pergola V, et al. Echocardiography predicts embolic events in infective endocarditis. *J Am Coll Cardiol* 2001;37: 1069–1076.

387. Rex JH, Walsh TJ, Sobel JD, et al. Practice guidelines for the treatment of candidiasis. *Clin Infect Dis* 2000;30:662–678.

388. Ellis ME, AL-Abdely H, Sandridge A, et al. Fungal endocarditis: Evidence in the world literature, 1965–1995. *Clin Infect Dis* 2001;32: 50–62.

389. Chamoun AJ, Conti V, Lenihan DJ. Native valve infective endocarditis: What is the optimal timing for surgery? *Am J Med Sci* 2000;320: 255–262.

390. Durack DT. Nine controversies in the management of endocarditis. In: Petersdorf RG, Adams RD, Braunwald E, et al, eds. *Harrison's Principles of Internal Medicine,* 10th ed. New York: McGraw-Hill; 1983: 35–45.

391. Vlessis AA, Hovaguimian H, Jaggers J, et al. Infective endocarditis: Ten year review of medical and surgical therapy. *Ann Thorac Surg* 1996;61:1217–1222.

392. Muehrcke D, Lytle BW, Cosgrove DMI. Surgical and long-term antifungal therapy for fungal prosthetic valve endocarditis. *Ann Thorac Surg* 1996;60:538–543.

393. Eishi K, Kawazoe K, Kuriyama Y, et al. Surgical management of infective endocarditis associated with cerebral complications: Multicenter retrospective study in Japan. *J Thorac Cardiovasc Surg* 1995; 110:1745–55.

394. Parrino PE, Dron IL, Ross SD, et al. Does a focal neurologic deficit contraindicate operation in a patient with endocarditis? *Ann Thorac Surg* 1999;67:59–64.

395. Piper C, Wiemer M, Schulte HD, Horstkotte D. Stroke is not a contraindication for urgent valve replacement in acute infective endocarditis. *J Heart Valve Dis* 2001;10:703–711.

396. Glazier JJ, Verwilghen J, Donaldson RM, Ross DN. Treatment of complicated prosthetic aortic valve endocarditis with annular abscess formation by homograft aortic root replacement. *J Am Coll Cardiol* 1991; 17:1177–1182.

397. Joyce F, Tingleff J, Pettersson G. Expanding indications for the Ross operation. *J Heart Valve Dis* 1995;4:352–363.

398. Joyce F, Tingleff J, Pettersson G. The Ross operation: Results of early experience including treatment for endocarditis. *Eur J Cardiothorac Surg* 1989;9:384–392.

399. Hughes CF, Noble N. Vegetectomy: An alternative surgical treatment for infective endocarditis of the atrioventricular valves in drug addicts. *J Thorac Cardiovasc Surg* 1988;95:857–861.

400. Katz LN, Elek SR. Combined heparin and chemotherapy in subacute bacterial endocarditis. *JAMA* 1944;124:149–152.

401. Wilson WR, Geraci JE, Danielson GK, et al. Anticoagulant therapy and central nervous system complications in patients with prosthetic valve endocarditis. *Circulation* 1978;57:1004–1007.

402. Kanis JA. The use of anticoagulants in bacterial endocarditis. *Postgrad Med J* 1974;50:312–313.

403. Tornos P, Almirante B, Mirabet S, et al. Infective endocarditis due to *Staphylococcus aureus:* Deleterious effect of anticoagulant therapy. *Arch Intern Med* 1999;159:473–475.

404. Nicolau DP, Marangos MN, Nightingale CH, Quintiliani R. Influence of aspirin on development and treatment of experimental *Staphylococcus aureus* endocarditis. *Antimicrob Agents Chemother* 1995;39: 1748–1751.

405. Steckelberg JM, Murphy JG, Ballard D, et al. Emboli in infective endocarditis: The prognostic value of echocardiography. *Ann Intern Med* 1991;114:635–640.

406. Conlon PJ, Jefferies F, Krigman HR, et al. Predictors of prognosis and risk of acute renal failure in bacterial endocarditis. *Clin Nephrol* 1998; 49:96–101.

407. International Subarachnoid Aneurysm Trial (ISAT) Collaborative Group. International subarachnoid aneurysm trial (ISAT) of neurosurgical clipping versus endovascular coiling in 2143 patients with ruptured intracranial aneurysms: A randomized trial. *Lancet* 2002;360: 1267–1274.

408. Ahern H. Cellular responses to oxidative stress: Extensively studied bacterial systems provide insights into more complex systems and, potentially, human diseases. *ASM News* 1991;57:627–630.

409. Lu VL, Fang GD, Keys TF, et al. Prosthetic valve endocarditis: Superiority of surgical valve replacement versus medical therapy only. *Ann Thorac Surg* 1994;58:1073–1077.

410. Netzer RO, Altwegg SC, Zollinger E, et al. Infective endocarditis: Determinants of long-term outcome. *Heart* 2002;88:61–66.

411. Wallace SM, Walton BI, Kharbanda RK, et al. Mortality from infective endocarditis: clinical predictors of outcome. *Heart* 2002;88:53–60.

412. Ormiston JA, Neutze JM, Agnew TM, et al. Infective endocarditis: A lethal disease. *Aust NZ J Med* 1981;11:620–629.

413. Renzulli A, Carozza A, Marra C, et al. Are blood and valve cultures predictive for long-term outcome following surgery for infective endocarditis? *Eur J Cardiothorac Surg* 2000;17:228–233.

414. Renzulli A, Carozza A, Romano G, et al. Recurrent infective endocarditis: A multivariate analysis of 21 years of experience. *Ann Thorac Surg* 2001;72:39–43.

415. Welton DE, Young JB, Gentry WO, et al. Recurrent infective endocarditis: Analysis of predisposing factors and clinical features. *Am J Med* 1979;66:932–938.

416. Everett ED, Hirschmann JV. Transient bacteremia and endocarditis prophylaxis: A review. *Medicine* 1977;56:61–77.

417. Sullivan NM, Sutter VL, Mims MM, et al. Clinical aspects of bacteremia after manipulation of the genitourinary tract. *J Infect Dis* 1973; 127:49–55.

418. Shorvon PJ, Eykyn SJ, Cotton PB. Gastrointestinal instrumentation, bacteraemia, and endocarditis. *Gut* 1983;24:1078–1093.

419. Durack DT. Prevention of infective endocarditis. *N Engl J Med* 1995; 332:38–44.

420. Dajani AS, Taubert KA, Wilson WR, et al. Prevention of bacterial endocarditis: Recommendations by the American Heart Association. *Circulation* 1997;96:358–366.

421. Durack DT. Experience with prevention of experimental endocarditis. In: Kaplan EL, Taranta AV, ed. *Infective Endocarditis.* American Heart Association Monograph No. 52. Dallas: American Heart Association; 1977:28–32.

422. Horstkotte D, Friedrichs W, Pippert H, et al. Nutzen der Endokarditisprophylaxe bei Patienten mit Prothetischen Herzklappen. *Z Kardiol* 1986;75:8–11.

423. Imperiale TF, Horwitz RI. Does prophylaxis prevent postdental infective endocarditis? A controlled evaluation of protective efficacy. *Am J Med* 1990;88:131–136.

424. Gould IM, Buckingham JK. Cost effectiveness of prophylaxis in dental practice to prevent infective endocarditis. *Br Heart J* 1993;70: 79–83.

425. Delahaye F, Rial M-O, de Gevigney G, et al. A critical appraisal of the quality of the management of infective endocarditis. *J Am Coll Cardiol* 1999;33:788–793.

426. Muhlestein JB. Infective endocarditis: How well are we managing our patients? *J Am Coll Cardiol* 1999;33:794–795.

PART THIRTEEN

ANESTHESIA, SURGERY, AND THE HEART

PERIOPERATIVE EVALUATION AND MANAGEMENT OF PATIENTS WITH KNOWN OR SUSPECTED CARDIOVASCULAR DISEASE WHO UNDERGO NONCARDIAC SURGERY

Debabrata Mukherjee / Kim A. Eagle

Each year in the United States, approximately 25 million patients undergo noncardiac surgery. Of these, approximately 50,000 suffer perioperative myocardial infarction, and more than half of 40,000 perioperative deaths are caused by cardiac events.[1-3] As the population of the United States continues to age over the next several decades, both the total number and the percentage of patients who are over 65 years of age will increase. These patients represent the largest group in whom surgeries are performed, a group in whom approximately a quarter of surgeries are associated with significant risk of cardiac morbidity and death, and a group at increased risk for the presence of cardiac disease. As such, the number of patients with significant perioperative risk undergoing noncardiac surgery can be expected to increase.

Most perioperative cardiac morbidity and deaths are related to myocardial ischemia, congestive heart failure, or arrhythmias. Therefore, preoperative evaluation and perioperative management to reduce morbidity and mortality rates emphasize the detection, characterization, and treatment of coronary artery disease, left ventricular systolic dysfunction, and significant arrhythmias. However, not all patients with underlying cardiac disease are at significantly increased perioperative risk of a morbid cardiac event. The purpose of preoperative evaluation is not to clear patients for surgery but to assess medical status, cardiac risks posed by the surgery planned, and recommend strategies to reduce risk. Evaluation must be tailored to the circumstances that have prompted the consultation and to the nature of the surgical illness. There are two goals of the preoperative evaluation: first, to identify patients at increased risk of an adverse peri-operative cardiac event and, second, to identify patients with a poor long-term prognosis due to cardiovascular disease who come to medical attention only because of the problem requiring noncardiac surgery. In this sense, the preoperative evaluation represents an opportunity to identify and treat patients, thereby affecting long-term prognosis, even though their risk at the time of noncardiac surgery may not be prohibitive.

Preoperative evaluation can identify many patients at increased risk of an adverse cardiac event, and appropriate perioperative management can reduce that risk. The internist and cardiologist play a vital role in the evaluation and management of patients before, during, and after noncardiac surgery. This chapter reviews available data and recommendations for the preoperative evaluation and perioperative management of patients with known or suspected cardiovascular disease undergoing noncardiac surgery. The nature of preoperative evaluation and perioperative management should be individualized to the patient and the clinical scenario surrounding surgery. Patients presenting with an acute surgical emergency mandate only a rapid preoperative assessment, with subsequent management directed at preventing or minimizing cardiac morbidity and death. Among such patients, a more thorough evaluation can often be performed after surgery. In contrast, patients undergoing an elective procedure with no surgical urgency can undergo a more thorough preoperative evaluation. Among patients presenting for cardiac evaluation prior to "same-day" elective surgery, perioperative risk to the patient must be weighed against the impact of additional testing and cancellation or delay of the surgical procedure.

CLINICAL DETERMINANTS OF PERIOPERATIVE CARDIOVASCULAR RISK

The majority of patients at increased risk of adverse perioperative cardiac events can be identified using a simple bedside or office assessment. A careful history, physical examination, and review of the resting 12-lead electrocardiogram (ECG) are usually sufficient to allow stratification of most patients into low, intermediate, or high risk for an adverse perioperative cardiac event. A number of investigators have established readily accessible clinical markers that predict increased perioperative risk of myocardial infarction, congestive heart failure, or death.[4–14] Some investigators have used a quantitative scoring system to rank the importance of individual risk factors.[4,12,14] The advantage of such systems rests with the observation that some clinical features are stronger predictors of perioperative risk than are others. Current recommendations of the American College of Cardiology (ACC) and the American Heart Association (AHA)[15] designate risks factors as belonging to three groups: major, intermediate, and minor (Table 82-1). In the guidelines, greater weight is given to active than to quiescent disease, and the severity of disease is used to modify its importance.

History

Historical features are important in the identification of patients at increased perioperative cardiac risk. Because most perioperative morbidity and deaths are related to myocardial ischemia, congestive heart failure, and arrhythmias, the assessment of historical risk factors relies heavily on the recognition of coronary artery disease, left ventricular dysfunction, and significant arrhythmias. Risk factors recognized as predictive of increased perioperative risk[15] include advanced age, poor functional capacity, and prior history of coronary artery disease, congestive heart failure, arrhythmia, valvular heart disease, diabetes mellitus, uncontrolled systemic hypertension, renal insufficiency, and stroke. Coronary artery disease is a major risk factor in the setting of recent myocardial infarction or unstable or severe angina pectoris and an intermediate risk factor in the setting of mild stable angina pectoris or remote myocardial infarction. Similarly, congestive heart failure is a major risk factor if decompensated and an intermediate risk factor if compensated. A history of arrhythmias may be a major, intermediate, or minor risk factor, depending on the nature and severity of the arrhythmia as well as the presence of underlying heart disease.

A patient's preoperative functional capacity significantly influences the assessment of perioperative cardiac risk. Good functional capacity in an asymptomatic patient predicts low perioperative risk despite the presence of other risk factors. Impaired functional capacity is important in three regards in the assessment of perioperative cardiac risk. First, among patients with chronic coronary artery disease and among those who have experienced an acute cardiac event, poor functional capacity is associated with an increased risk of subsequent cardiac morbidity and death.[16] Second, many of the historical features that predict increased perioperative risk assume physical activity. Because most symptoms of cardiac disease are either associated exclusively with or exacerbated by increased physical activity, significant noncardiac limitations in physical capacity are associated with inherent problems in the ability to detect symptoms of underlying cardiac diseases and thereby to diagnose them. Finally, poor functional capacity is associated with impaired conditioning and therefore a lesser ability to accommodate the cardiovascular stresses that may accompany noncardiac surgery. Because the ability to perform tasks in daily activities correlates well with maximal oxygen uptake on treadmill testing, the assessment of functional capacity on preoperative history is an important feature in the assessment of perioperative risk.

Physical Examination

Features on physical examination may be useful in assessing perioperative risk. Patients with uncontrolled systemic hypertension should be identified and treated. Because congestive heart failure[4,15,17] and valvular heart disease[4,15,17] are associated with increased risk, physical findings suggestive of these diagnoses should be sought. The physical examination should include general appearance (cyanosis, pallor, dyspnea during conversation/minimal activity, Cheyne-Stokes respiration, poor nutritional status, obesity, skeletal deformities, tremor and anxiety), blood pressure in both arms, carotid pulses, extremity pulses, and ankle-brachial indices. Jugular venous pressure and positive hepatojugular reflex are reliable signs of hypervolemia in chronic heart failure; pulmonary rales and chest x-ray evidence of pulmonary congestion correlate better with acute heart failure. Patients with aortic stenosis can be identified by a typical murmur with diminished and delayed upstroke of the carotid or brachial pulse. Patients with mitral stenosis, mitral regurgitation, or aortic regurgitation may be at increased perioperative risk of developing congestive heart failure in the setting of sufficiently severe disease as well as at increased risk of infective endocarditis. Finally, the presence of carotid or other vascular bruits helps identify patients at increased risk of occult coronary artery disease.

TABLE 82-1 Clinical Predictors of Increased Perioperative Cardiovascular Risk

Major predictors
    Acute or recent myocardial infarction[a] with evidence of
       ischemia based on symptoms or noninvasive testing
    Unstable or severe[b] angina (Canadian class III or IV)
    Decompensated heart failure
    High-grade atrioventricular block
    Symptomatic ventricular arrhythmias with underlying
       heart disease
    Supraventricular arrhythmias with uncontrolled ventricular
       rate
    Severe valvular heart disease
Intermediate predictors
    Mild angina pectoris (class 1 or 2)
    Prior MI by history or Q waves on ECG
    Compensated or prior heart failure
    Diabetes mellitus (particularly insulin-dependent)
    Renal insufficiency (creatinine ≥ 2.0 mg/dL)
Minor predictors
    Advanced age
    Abnormal ECG (left ventricular hypertrophy, left bundle
       branch block, ST-T abnormalities)
    Rhythm other than sinus (e.g., atrial fibrillation)
    Low functional capacity (inability to climb one flight of
       stairs with a bag of groceries)
    History of stroke
    Uncontrolled systemic hypertension

[a]Recent myocardial infarction is defined as greater than 7 days but less than or equal to 1 month; acute myocardial infarction is within 7 days.
[b]May include stable angina in patients who are usually sedentary.
SOURCE: Adapted from Eagle et al.,[15] with permission.

Comorbid Diseases

A patient's overall health affects perioperative cardiovascular risk; associated medical conditions may exacerbate risk or complicate perioperative cardiac management. Patients with diabetes mellitus have an increased risk of concomitant coronary artery disease, and the possibility of silent ischemia complicates both the preoperative recognition of coronary artery disease and the perioperative recognition of ischemia. Patients with either restrictive or obstructive pulmonary disease are at increased risk of perioperative respiratory complications, and the associated hypoxemia, hypercapnea, acidosis, and increased work of breathing can exacerbate cardiac stress and precipitate myocardial ischemia. Patients with preexisting renal dysfunction may be predisposed to volume retention in the perioperative period, and hypovolemia may lead to renal hypoperfusion and thereby can exacerbate renal dysfunction. Patients with anemia of any cause are at increased risk of myocardial ischemia and congestive heart failure, mediated by increased cardiac stress and increased cardiac work. Optimal management of noncardiac conditions may therefore reduce the risk of cardiac morbidity in the perioperative period.

Surgery-Specific Risks

Perioperative cardiac risk is related in two ways to the type of noncardiac surgery being performed. First, some types of noncardiac surgery identify a group of patients at increased risk for concomitant cardiac disease based on shared risk factors that predispose patients to both noncardiac and cardiac disease. The most notable example of this relationship is seen with vascular surgery and coronary artery disease. In this case, the same factors that result in clinical peripheral arterial occlusive disease also predispose to the development of coronary artery disease. Among such patients, coronary artery disease may be known or occult, with no symptoms because of the physical limitations associated with significant peripheral vascular disease. Second, the nature of noncardiac surgery may be associated with variable degrees of cardiac stress, mediated by fluctuations in heart rate, blood pressure, intravascular volume, and oxygenation as well as the cardiac stresses associated with the duration of the procedure, pain, and neurohumoral activation.[4,5,11,12,18–21] Emergency procedures are associated with a two- to fivefold increase in perioperative cardiac risk compared with elective procedures.[1,17] Other types of noncardiac surgery associated with high perioperative risk include aortic and peripheral vascular surgery and prolonged abdominal, thoracic, or head and neck procedures with large fluid shifts. The ACC/AHA Task Force Report on Perioperative Cardiac Evaluation[15] stratifies noncardiac surgical procedures as involving high, intermediate, and low cardiac risk (Table 82-2).

The perioperative administration of anesthesia may also affect perioperative cardiac risk. Although there is no one best myocardial protective anesthetic technique,[22–26] differences in anesthetic techniques may favor the use of one over another for individual patients. Opioid-based general anesthesia generally does not affect cardiovascular function, although the commonly employed inhalational agents cause afterload reduction and decreased myocardial contractility. Spinal anesthesia results in sympathetic blockade, with decreases in both preload and afterload and the potential for shifts in both systemic blood pressure and intravascular volume. In general, hemodynamic effects are minimal when spinal anesthesia is used for infrainguinal procedures, whereas higher dermatomal levels of spinal anesthesia, as required for abdominal procedures, may be associated with significant hemodynamic effects, including hypotension and reflex tachycardia. No study has clearly demonstrated any beneficial

TABLE 82-2 Cardiac Risk Stratification for Different Types of Surgical Procedures

High risk (reported cardiac risk[a] >5%)
 Emergency major operations, particularly in the elderly
 Aortic, major vascular, and peripheral vascular surgery
 Extensive operations with large volume shifts/and or blood loss
Intermediate risk (reported cardiac risk <5%)
 Intraperitoneal and intrathoracic
 Carotid endarterectomy
 Head and neck surgery
 Orthopedic
 Prostate
Low risk[a] (reported cardiac risk <1%)
 Endoscopic procedures
 Superficial biopsy
 Cataract
 Breast surgery

[a]Combined incidence of cardiac death and nonfatal myocardial infarction.
[b]Does not generally require further preoperative cardiac testing.
Source: Adapted from Eagle et al.,[15] with permission.

change in outcome from the use of pulmonary artery catheters, ST-segment monitoring, or transesophageal echocardiography. Decisions regarding specific anesthetic technique and intraoperative monitoring are best left to the anesthesiologists involved in the patient's care.

PREOPERATIVE TESTING

Patients at very low risk and those at high risk of an adverse perioperative cardiac event can typically be identified using clinically available features described above. Patients at low risk generally require no additional testing prior to noncardiac surgery. Among patients undergoing elective noncardiac surgery in whom risk is determined to be intermediate or high, additional testing may be useful to better define risk.[15] It is well to employ a stepwise approach to the preoperative assessment of cardiac risk (Fig. 82-1). Testing may include coronary angiography or noninvasive testing to assess for the presence and significance of coronary artery disease, left ventricular function, and/or valvular heart disease.

Resting Left Ventricular Function

Impaired left ventricular systolic or diastolic function is predictive of perioperative congestive heart failure. The greatest risk of complications occurs among patients with left ventricular ejection fraction of less than 35 percent; among critically ill patients, severely impaired left ventricular systolic function is associated with a higher risk of death. Preoperative left ventricular systolic function can be assessed noninvasively using radionuclide ventriculography or echocardiography, or it may be assessed invasively using contrast ventriculography. Unless recently defined, preoperative assessment of left ventricular systolic function should be performed among patients with poorly controlled congestive heart failure and should be considered among patients with prior congestive heart failure and among patients with dyspnea of unknown cause.

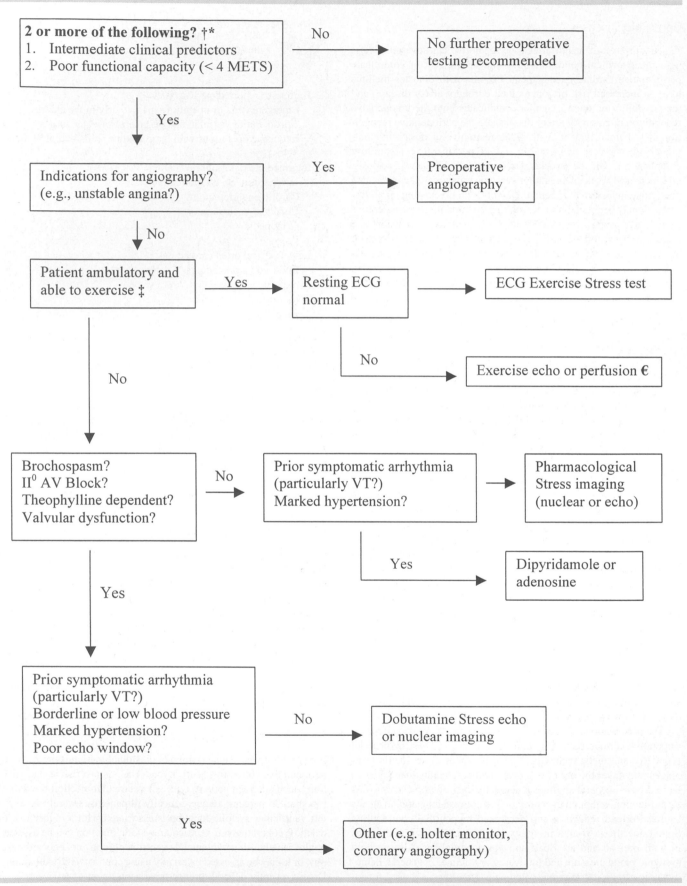

FIGURE 82-1 Supplemental preoperative evaluation: When and which test? ECG = electrocardiogram; VT = ventricular tachycardia; METS = metabolic equivalents. (Adapted from Eagle et al.,[15] with permission.) *Testing is indicated only if the results will affect care. †Refer to Table 82-1 for a list of clinical predictors and Table 82-2 for the definition of high-risk surgical procedures. ‡Able to achieve more than or equal to 85 percent maximum predicted heart rate (MPHR). ¢In the presence of left bundle branch block, vasodilator perfusion imaging is preferred.

Functional Testing and Risk of Coronary Artery Disease

EXERCISE TESTING

Preoperative cardiac stress testing is useful in the objective assessment of functional capacity, to help identify patients at risk of perioperative myocardial ischemia or cardiac arrhythmias, and to aid in the assessment of long-term as well as perioperative prognosis. In general, poor functional capacity may be due to advanced age, deconditioning, myocardial ischemia or other causes of reduced cardiac reserve, or poor pulmonary reserve. Reduced functional capacity identifies patients at increased risk of subsequent cardiac morbidity and death.[16] Clinical history can be used to estimate functional capacity. In addition, preoperative exercise testing is a useful tool to objectively assess functional capacity as well as to assess hemodynamic response to stress and the potential for stress-induced myocardial ischemia or cardiac arrhythmias.

In a general population, the mean sensitivity and specificity of exercise electrocardiographic studies for the detection of coronary artery disease are 68 and 77 percent, respectively, with reported ranges of sensitivity from 23 to 100 percent and specificity from 17 to 100 percent.[27] The accuracy of exercise electrocardiographic studies for the detection of coronary artery disease is influenced by the prevalence of disease in the population studied, the degree of exercise achieved, and the number, location, and severity of diseased vessels. The mean sensitivity and specificity for the detection of multivessel disease is 81 and 66 percent, respectively.[28] In addition to assessment for the presence of coronary artery disease, exercise testing is useful for the assessment of prognosis. In a large cohort of 4083 medically treated patients in the Coronary Artery Surgery Study (CASS),[29] exercise testing was useful for identifying both high- and low-risk subgroups of patients. The mortality rate was 5 percent per year or more among a high-risk subset comprising 12 percent of the total population who were unable to achieve an exercise work load greater than Bruce stage I and had an abnormal exercise electrocardiogram. In contrast, mortality was less than 1 percent per year among a low-risk subset comprising 34 percent of the total population who were able to achieve at least Bruce stage III with a normal exercise electrocardiogram. Preoperative exercise testing has been shown to be useful in the prediction of perioperative cardiac risk among patients undergoing peripheral vascular surgery, abdominal aortic aneurysm repair, or other major noncardiac surgery.[30–40] In these published reports, the negative predictive value for perioperative death or myocardial infarction was 91 to 100 percent, with a positive predictive value of 0 to 81 percent.

NONEXERCISE STRESS TESTING

Many patients undergoing noncardiac surgery are unable to exercise. Approximately 30 to 50 percent of patients undergoing noncardiac surgery are unable to achieve an adequate exercise workload for a diagnostic study. This is especially problematic among patients with peripheral vascular occlusive disease, in whom the same factors that cause peripheral disease predispose to coronary atherosclerosis; significant peripheral vascular disease severely limits exercise tolerance and therefore the ability to perform diagnostic exercise stress testing. For this reason, pharmacologic stress testing may offer advantages in the preoperative testing of some patients undergoing peripheral vascular surgery as well as of other patients who are not able to perform adequate physical exercise due to noncardiac limitations.

Pharmacologic stress testing for the detection of coronary artery disease can be performed using one of two general methods. Infusion of the adrenergic agonist dobutamine leads to increases in heart rate, myocardial contractility, and, to a lesser degree, blood pressure, resulting in increased myocardial oxygen demand. In the setting of a limited oxygen supply, increased demand causes myocardial ischemia. Dobutamine infusion is typically used in conjunction with echocardiographic imaging, and the failure of wall motion to augment with dobutamine or for it to become frankly dyskinetic indicates of ischemia. Alternatively, pharmacologic "stress" can be achieved using the coronary vasodilators dipyridamole or adenosine. Nuclear perfusion imaging, such as thallium scintigraphic imaging, is typically used in conjunction with dipyridamole and adenosine. Coronary artery disease is detected as heterogeneity of perfusion in response to maximal coronary vasodilation.

Dipyridamole thallium scintigraphy has been extensively studied for the assessment of coronary artery disease and perioperative risk among patients undergoing vascular[11,41–56] and other noncardiac surgery.[57–62] Published reports found a uniformly high negative predictive value for perioperative morbidity associated with normal dipyridamole thallium scintigraphic results, with values ranging from 95 to 100 percent and an average value of approximately 99 percent. The positive predictive value of dipyridamole thallium redistribution for myocardial infarction or death from cardiac causes has been reported to be from 4 to 20 percent among studies including more than 100 patients. There is also important long-term prognostic value associated with preoperative nuclear perfusion imaging,[46,50,63] suggesting that late postoperative risk after uncomplicated noncardiac surgery can also be predicted by preoperative testing. Although any abnormality on dipyridamole thallium scintigraphy is suggestive of coronary artery disease and is associated with a higher perioperative cardiac risk compared with patients with a normal scan, perioperative cardiac risk associated with a fixed perfusion defect is substantially lower than that associated with perfusion redistribution. In addition, the size of a perfusion defect is directly related to perioperative cardiac risk.[50,51,53]

Dobutamine stress echocardiography is well established for the noninvasive detection and characterization of coronary artery disease,[64–69] with an overall predictive accuracy equivalent to that of dipyridamole thallium scintigraphy. Several studies have evaluated the utility of dobutamine stress echocardiography for preoperative assessment of patients undergoing vascular or other noncardiac surgery.[70–75] Negative predictive values for perioperative events ranged from 93 to 100 percent. Positive predictive values were 17 to 43 percent for any cardiac event and 7 to 23 percent for predicting myocardial infarction or death. As was seen with studies using nuclear perfusion imaging, most studies of dobutamine stress echocardiography did not blind treating physicians to stress test results, and subsequent alteration of patient management based on abnormal noninvasive test results presumably contributed to a low event rate despite a positive test result. A metanalysis of preoperative pharmacologic stress tests[76] demonstrated similar power of dobutamine stress echocardiography and dipyridamole thallium scintigraphy in predicting adverse cardiac events after noncardiac surgery.

Because clinical factors are usually able to identify patients at low or high risk of an adverse cardiac event after noncardiac surgery,[15,21] preoperative stress testing typically has the greatest utility among patients at intermediate risk. Exercise electrocardiographic study allows assessment of functional capacity as well as evaluation for evidence of coronary artery disease based on ST-segment analysis and hemodynamics. Performance of exercise echocardiographic testing or exercise nuclear perfusion imaging should be considered in the presence of significant resting ECG abnormalities that preclude diagnostic testing for coronary artery disease, such as left bundle branch block, left ventricular hypertrophy with strain, or digitalis effect. Nonexercise stress testing, such as dobutamine stress echocardiographic or dipyridamole thallium scintigraphic studies, should be considered among patients who are unable to perform adequate physical exercise.

FINANCIAL IMPLICATIONS OF NONINVASIVE TESTING

The performance of preoperative noninvasive testing should be based on an assessment of risk and benefit to the patient. In this setting, benefit is defined as the likelihood that testing may alter management and improve outcome because of an adverse perioperative or long-term prognosis. Risk to the patient should include risk associated with additional procedures precipitated by noninvasive testing as well as any risk associated with the noninvasive testing. With the high costs associated with many evaluation strategies, development and implementation of evidence-based guidelines may lead to more efficient and cost-effective use of appropriate noninvasive testing.

As noted above, clinical features can be used to identify patients at very low risk of an adverse perioperative cardiac event, including asymptomatic patients having undergone coronary revascularization within 5 years as well as those without specific clinical markers for increased risk. Additional testing of selected patients at intermediate or higher risk can potentially reduce the cost of testing without affecting patients' outcomes. Based on a previous study validating the use of selective noninvasive testing before major aortic surgery,[77] the cost implications of selective testing were assessed in the ACC/AHA Task Force report.[15] In the previous study, the application of a clinical algorithm resulted in only 29 percent of 201 patients undergoing noninvasive testing prior to aortic surgery, with an associated 0.5 percent perioperative cardiac mortality rate. Using estimated costs, the use of selected testing was associated with a total cost of $32,886 for 58 patients, compared with an estimated total cost of $113,967 if all 201 had undergone noninvasive screening. Froehlich et al. recently demonstrated that implementation of the ACC/AHA cardiac risk-assessment guidelines appropriately reduced resource use and costs in patients who underwent elective aortic surgery without affecting outcomes.[78] Preoperative stress testing (88 to 47 percent; $p < 0.00001$), cardiac catheterization (24 to 11 percent; $p < 0.05$), and coronary revascularization (25 to 2 percent; $p < 0.00001$) were all significantly reduced with appropriate use of the ACC/AHA guidelines.[78] The low perioperative mortality rate associated with the use of a clinical algorithm and selected noninvasive testing suggest that substantial cost can be avoided without compromising patients' safety.

PREOPERATIVE THERAPY FOR CORONARY ARTERY DISEASE

Coronary artery disease is responsible for the majority of adverse perioperative cardiac events. Once disease is recognized, specific therapy should be instituted to minimize the risk of perioperative myocardial ischemia, myocardial infarction, or death.

Coronary Revascularization

There are no prospective trials testing the impact of either preoperative coronary artery bypass grafting or percutaneous coronary intervention on perioperative cardiac morbidity and mortality rates. However, several retrospective studies suggest that patients with successful prior coronary revascularization have a low risk of perioperative cardiac events during noncardiac surgery and that the risk of death is comparable to that among patients with no clinical evidence of coronary artery disease.[79–82]

Although these data support the theory that coronary artery bypass surgery lowers the risk of adverse cardiac events associated with noncardiac surgery, they do not address the overall effect on morbidity and mortality rates associated with the surgical coronary revascularization. In the assessment of patients undergoing noncardiac surgery, the well-established long-term benefits of coronary artery bypass surgery should be considered, as should any impact on noncardiac surgical morbidity and mortality rates. There may be some patients for whom coronary artery bypass grafting should be performed prior to noncardiac surgery only because of an otherwise prohibitive perioperative cardiac risk. However, there are many more patients with advanced coronary artery disease who are candidates for surgical coronary revascularization, based on long-term prognosis, who are identified only during preoperative cardiac assessment. Among such patients, elective noncardiac surgery of intermediate or high risk should generally be postponed for the performance of coronary artery bypass surgery.

Several small, retrospective studies[83–85] have suggested that there is a low risk of perioperative myocardial infarction or death following preoperative percutaneous coronary intervention. One study of 1049 noncardiac surgeries performed among 1829 patients enrolled in the Bypass Angioplasty Revascularization Investigation (BARI) trial demonstrated a low incidence of myocardial infarction or death among patients having undergone either coronary artery bypass surgery or percutaneous coronary intervention, with event rate of 1.6 percent among patients in both groups.[86] The absence of any evident difference between groups suggests that previous percutaneous coronary intervention confers protection from perioperative cardiac events that is equivalent to that conferred by surgical revascularization, assuming that patients have been followed closely and that recurrent ischemia has been effectively treated. Overall, indications for revascularization among patients undergoing preoperative evaluation should be considered the same as for the general population.[15] These include patients who have poorly controlled angina pectoris despite maximal medical therapy and patients with one of several high-risk coronary characteristics—i.e., clinically significant stenosis (>50 percent) of the left main coronary artery, severe two- or three-vessel coronary artery disease (>70 percent stenosis) with involvement of the proximal left anterior descending coronary artery, easily induced myocardial ischemia on preoperative stress testing, and left ventricular systolic dysfunction at rest.

Coronary stents are now used in more than 80 percent of coronary interventions and use of stents presents unique challenges because of the risk of coronary thrombosis and bleeding during the initial recovery phase. In a cohort of 40 patients who received stents within 30 days of noncardiac surgery, all 8 deaths and 7 myocardial infarctions, as well as 8 of 11 bleeding episodes, occurred in patients who had undergone surgery within 14 days after stent placement.[87] The complications appeared to be related to serious bleeding resulting from postprocedural antiplatelet therapy or to coronary thrombosis in those who did not receive 4 full weeks of dual antiplatelet therapy after stenting. These results suggest that it is prudent to wait at least 2 weeks, and preferably 4 weeks, after coronary stenting to perform noncardiac surgery in order to allow complete endothelization and a full course of antiplatelet therapy to be given. Poststenting therapy currently includes a combination of aspirin and clopidogrel for at least 4 weeks, followed by aspirin for an indefinite period.

Medical Therapy for Coronary Artery Disease

Several nonrandomized studies have addressed the effect of anti-ischemic medical therapy on perioperative prognosis.[88–95] Although data are lacking to support the empiric use of nitroglycerin or calcium channel blockers, there is increasing evidence that the use of perioperative beta blockers may reduce the risk of an adverse cardiac event. Three small retrospective studies suggest that perioperative therapy with beta blockers may result in fewer episodes of myocardial ischemia detectable on ECG[93,94] and of acute myocardial infarction.[92] One randomized study among 112 high-risk patients undergoing vascular surgery demonstrated a reduction in risk of perioperative myocardial infarction or death from 34 to 3 percent with the use of empiric beta blocker therapy.[96] Another randomized, placebo-controlled study used atenolol in 200 high-risk patients scheduled to undergo noncardiac surgery.[97] Atenolol was administered either intravenously or orally 2 days preoperatively and continued for 7 days postoperatively. The incidence of perioperative ischemia was significantly lower in the atenolol group than in the placebo group.[98,99] There was no difference in the incidence of perioperative myocardial infarction or death from cardiac causes, but the rate of event-free survival at 6 months was higher in the atenolol group.

Poldermans et al. reported on the perioperative use of bisoprolol in elective major vascular surgery.[100] Bisoprolol was started at least 7 days preoperatively, the dose being adjusted to achieve a resting heart rate of less than 60 beats per minute, and it was continued for 30 days postoperatively. The study was confined to patients who had at least one risk factor for an adverse cardiac event in the perioperative period (a history of congestive heart failure, prior myocardial infarction, diabetes, angina pectoris, heart failure, age >70 years, or poor functional status) and evidence of inducible myocardial ischemia on dobutamine echocardiography. Patients with extensive regional wall motion abnormalities were excluded. Bisoprolol was associated with a 91 percent reduction in the perioperative risk of myocardial infarction or death from cardiac causes in this high-risk population. Urban et al. evaluated the role of prophylactic beta blockers in patients undergoing elective total knee arthroplasty.[101] A total of 107 patients were preoperatively randomized into two groups, control and beta blockers, who received postoperative esmolol infusions on the day of surgery and metoprolol for the next 48 h to maintain a heart rate less than 80 beats per minute. The number of ischemic events and total ischemic time were significantly lower with esmolol than in the control group.[101] These data support the empiric use of beta-blocker therapy among patients undergoing intermediate or high-risk noncardiac surgery. It is important to recall that beta blockers are indicated for patients with angina pectoris or its equivalent, recent MI, distant MI, dilated cardiomyopathy, and/or hypertension. Thus, when one or more of these conditions are identified for the first time in a preoperative assessment, initiation of beta-blocker therapy is warranted.

MANAGEMENT OF SPECIFIC CONDITIONS

Patients with a variety of medical conditions known to increase cardiovascular risk may require noncardiac surgery. For these patients, appropriate perioperative medical management may prevent the occurrence or minimize the impact of an adverse cardiovascular event. Factors that contribute to increased perioperative risk include interruptions in routine medical therapy as well as physical and mental stresses associated with the surgical procedure and convalescent period. As such, cardiovascular stresses include alteration in normal medications during the preoperative period; fluctuation in heart rate, blood pressure, intravascular volume, and oxygenation during surgery; dynamic fluid shifts; pain; and limitations in the use of oral medications in the postoperative period. It is important to note that the period of maximum cardiac risk appears to occur in the postoperative period.[102] Because, cardiovascular risk is not limited to the intraoperative period, appropriate emphasis should be placed on the treatment of specific conditions throughout all phases of the perioperative period.

Coronary Artery Disease

Among patients with known coronary artery disease undergoing noncardiac surgery, perioperative management should include monitoring for evidence of myocardial ischemia, therapy to prevent and treat ischemia, and postoperative surveillance to ensure that the patient did not experience an ischemic event that could mandate an alteration in therapy.

Monitoring can be accomplished with surveillance of ECG ST segments,[9,97] transesophageal echocardiographic assessment of regional and global left ventricular wall motion,[49] and invasive measurement of pulmonary arterial and pulmonary capillary wedge pressures. Therapy to prevent ischemia should be individualized to the patient and the surgical procedure but should include beta-adrenergic antagonists. Among many patients with known coronary artery disease, the prevention of ischemia can involve the simple continuation of a routine anti-ischemic regimen or conversion of a regimen to a similar one available for topical or intravenous delivery during periods in which the patient is unable to take medications orally. Nitroglycerin compounds can be administered topically or via intravenous infusion. Several beta-adrenergic antagonists and calcium channel blocking agents are available for administration via intravenous bolus or infusion. In some patients, oral medications can be crushed and delivered through a nasogastric tube that is then clamped for 30 min to allow absorption in the upper intestine. Because of the adverse effects associated with rapid withdrawal of beta-blocking medications as well as the demonstrated benefit associated with their perioperative use,[92,93,96–99] every effort should be made to continue these medications during the perioperative period among patients who receive them preoperatively. Current data suggest that attempts to keep the patient's resting heart rate between 50 and 60 beats per minute and a stress-related heart rate after surgery under 80 is particularly effective.

At a minimum, an anti-ischemic regimen used prior to surgery should be continued during the perioperative period. Additional anti-ischemic medications can be used empirically and should be used in the event that ischemia is detected during the perioperative period. Intravenous nitroglycerin and/or beta blockers can be titrated to specific endpoints of heart rate or blood pressure or to resolution of the observed ischemia. In addition, pain relief and correction of any underlying anemia are helpful in reducing tendencies to postoperative ischemia.

Because patients with known coronary artery disease or risk factors for disease are at risk of acute myocardial infarction complicating noncardiac surgery, assessment for change in status is appropriate following a surgical procedure. A simple 12-lead ECG preoperatively, immediately postoperatively, and daily for 2 days is generally sufficient to evaluate for change if there has been no evidence of perioperative ischemia or infarction. Alternative means of assessing for perioperative infarction include assessment of serum creatine kinase (CPK), creatine kinase MB isoenzyme (CPK-MB) fractions, and troponin; echocardiographic assessment of left ventricular wall motion; and nuclear perfusion studies.

At the conclusion of the perioperative period, it is important to resume anti-ischemic medications used by the patient prior to undergoing noncardiac surgery. In addition, antiplatelet agents such as aspirin, which may have been temporarily discontinued prior to surgery, should be reinitiated when no longer contraindicated.

Hypertension

Among patients who are treated for hypertension, preoperative evaluation should include a review of present medications and any history of intolerance to previous antihypertensive medications as well as assessment for adequacy of antihypertensive therapy. Brief evaluation for rare but potentially treatable causes of secondary hypertension should include assessment for an abdominal bruit, suggestive of renal artery stenosis; for radial-femoral delay, indicative of aortic coarctation; and for hypokalemia in the absence of diuretic use, which could suggest hyperaldosteronism.

Blood pressure should be well controlled prior to elective surgery,[102–104,106] and antihypertensive medications should be continued throughout the perioperative period. If there is a period in which the patient is unable to receive oral medications, topical or intravenous equivalents should be substituted. Rapid withdrawal of beta-blocking medications has associated adverse effects on heart rate and blood pressure, may precipitate myocardial ischemia, and should be avoided.

Mild or moderate preoperative hypertension in the absence of associated cardiovascular or metabolic abnormalities should not necessitate delay of surgery.[103,105] However, severe hypertension (e.g., diastolic blood pressure of 110 mmHg or greater) should be controlled prior to an elective surgical procedure. If surgery is urgent, then preoperative blood pressure control can usually be achieved rapidly with the use of intravenous beta blockers, calcium channel blockers, nitroglycerin, or nitroprusside. Finally, patients with preoperative hypertension appear to be predisposed to the development of intraoperative hypotension.[106] A potential for blood pressure lability, with associated ischemia and hypoperfusion, exists among patients with preoperative hypertension; therefore blood pressure should be carefully monitored and treated if necessary.[107,108]

Congestive Heart Failure

Congestive heart failure is associated with increased cardiovascular risk during noncardiac surgery.[4,5,9,12,14,109] A careful history and physical examination should include efforts to identify evidence of congestive heart failure, and every effort should be made to treat it prior to surgery.

Congestive heart failure may be the result of a variety of cardiac abnormalities, including left ventricular systolic dysfunction, diastolic dysfunction, and valvular heart disease. Although congestive heart failure is an independent risk factor for adverse perioperative cardiac outcome, specific underlying causes of congestive heart failure may each be associated with specific independent risks, and the specific nature of the risk may be determined by the nature of the underlying disease. For these reasons, the cause of the underlying process responsible for congestive heart failure should be identified when possible. If left ventricular systolic function is not known, it is generally prudent to establish whether it is normal or abnormal prior to surgery. Similarly, evaluation of left ventricular diastolic dysfunction or valvular heart disease may help in perioperative management. If there are risk factors for coronary artery disease, further evaluation for coronary disease as a cause of left ventricular systolic dysfunction may be appropriate (see also Chap. 25).

Cardiomyopathy

Patients with dilated and hypertrophic cardiomyopathies are predisposed to develop perioperative congestive heart failure. Among patients with preoperative signs or symptoms of congestive heart failure, preoperative evaluation should include assessment of left ventricular systolic and diastolic function as well as valve function. Systolic function can be determined noninvasively using either echocardiographic or radionuclide techniques. Echocardiographic imaging offers additional information reflecting diastolic function and valvular function, which could also contribute to congestive heart failure. If not previously performed, preoperative echocardiographic imaging should be strongly considered among patients with congestive heart failure.

Patients with hypertrophic cardiomyopathy require special consideration during the perioperative period. Hypertrophic cardiomyopathy can affect hemodynamics by means of dynamic left ventricular outflow obstruction or may precipitate congestive heart failure mediated by diastolic dysfunction. Left ventricular noncompliance can make patients with hypertrophic cardiomyopathy extremely sensitive to even small amounts of excess intravascular volume, while an underfilled left ventricle can exacerbate dynamic left ventricular outflow obstruction, with a resulting decrease in stroke volume and systemic hypotension. Therefore perioperative management should be directed at maintaining intravascular volume within a potentially narrow range and controlling periprocedural heart rate. These maneuvers reduce the likelihood of congestive heart failure and minimize left ventricular outflow obstruction. Catecholamines as a class should be avoided because of their potential to exacerbate dynamic left ventricular outflow obstruction (see also Chap. 77).

Valvular Heart Disease

Most valvular heart disease in an adult population is acquired and therefore increasingly common among older patients undergoing noncardiac surgery. Although most elective noncardiac surgery need not be delayed, some types of valvular heart disease can pose excessive risk to the patient and should be addressed prior to an elective surgical procedure.

Antibiotic prophylaxis should be used to reduce the risk of infective endocarditis among patients with organic valvular heart disease whenever noncardiac surgery involves a risk of bacteremia. Such procedures include oral, dental, gastrointestinal, and genitourologic procedures, in which normal bacterial flora may gain transient access to the bloodstream. Specific recommendations for prophylactic antibiotic regimens are published for specific types of noncardiac surgery in which there exists an increased risk of infective endocarditis.[110]

AORTIC STENOSIS

Severe aortic stenosis presents the greatest valve-associated cardiovascular risk for patients undergoing noncardiac surgery.[4] The presence of fixed obstruction to left ventricular outflow dramatically limits functional cardiac reserve and may be associated with intracavitary left ventricular pressures in excess of 300 mmHg. Accompanying left ventricular hypertrophy predisposes the patient to diastolic dysfunction and pulmonary congestion. In general, severe or symptomatic aortic stenosis should be addressed prior to the initiation of elective noncardiac surgery. In most cases, aortic valve replacement is indicated as the definitive therapy of choice.[111–113] If cardiac surgery is contraindicated, percutaneous aortic balloon valvotomy can be used to mitigate left ventricular outflow obstruction, even if only as a temporizing measure (see Chap. 66). When neither surgery nor percutaneous aortic valvotomy is considered feasible, noncardiac surgery with careful hemodynamic assessment may still be appropriate, albeit with a heightened risk of perioperative death. In such patients, avoidance of intraoperative or postoperative hypotension is particularly important.

MITRAL STENOSIS

The hemodynamic impact associated with mitral stenosis is affected by heart rate. The central problem with tachycardia in mitral stenosis is that increases in heart rate are associated with shortening of the diastolic portion of the cardiac cycle and a resultant rise in left atrial pressure. As a result, pulmonary congestion can be precipitated by tachycardia of even moderate degree. For this reason, heart rate should be well controlled in the perioperative period among patients with mitral stenosis of any severity. Patients with severe mitral stenosis undergoing high-risk noncardiac surgery may benefit from surgical or percutaneous intervention.[114] The relative risks and benefits and the likelihood of success associated with percutaneous balloon mitral valvotomy, surgical commissurotomy, or mitral valve replacement must be weighed in the context of mitral valve anatomy and other patient-specific factors (see Chap. 67).

AORTIC REGURGITATION AND MITRAL REGURGITATION

Patients with significant aortic regurgitation are predisposed to volume overload in the perioperative period, and volume status should be carefully monitored to prevent pulmonary congestion. In addition, patients with severe aortic regurgitation may benefit from afterload reduction in the form of angiotensin-converting enzyme inhibitors, calcium channel blockers, nitroglycerin, or hydralazine.[115,116] Just as patients with mitral stenosis are sensitive to tachycardia, patients with significant aortic regurgitation are sensitive to excessive bradycardia. Prolongation of the diastolic interval associated with bradycardia increases the time during which aortic regurgitation occurs and increases total regurgitant volume.

Mitral regurgitation can be due to a variety of underlying causes. As for patients with congestive heart failure, establishing the cause of mitral regurgitation may help define other associated perioperative risks, especially if mitral regurgitation occurs as a manifestation of coronary artery disease. Patients with significant mitral regurgitation may develop volume overload and pulmonary congestion. Diuretics and afterload-reducing therapy should be used to optimize hemodynamic status preoperatively in patients with severe mitral regurgitation who are undergoing major noncardiac surgery.

Special attention should be paid to left ventricular function in patients with severe mitral regurgitation. The left atrium and pulmonary venous system serve as a low-impedance system that effectively "afterload-reduces" the left ventricle in the setting of significant mitral regurgitation. Because of this, even a mild decrease in left ventricular ejection fraction in the setting of severe mitral regurgitation should be taken as evidence of significant impairment in systolic function and reduced left ventricular functional reserve.

PROSTHETIC HEART VALVES

Patients with either tissue or mechanical heart valve prostheses should receive appropriate antibiotic prophylaxis when undergoing noncardiac surgery with an accompanying potential for bacteremia.[110] Patients with mechanical heart valve prostheses also require careful management of anticoagulation in the perioperative period. As a general rule, anticoagulation can be discontinued when necessary for safe performance of noncardiac surgery and should be reinstituted when it is no longer contraindicated for hemostasis. The risk of valve thrombosis or thromboembolism is related to the location and type of valve prosthesis, the length of time during which the patient is not fully anticoagulated, and the level of anticoagulation maintained during that period. A mechanical prosthesis in the mitral position is at greater risk of thrombus formation than is a similar valve in the aortic position due to the larger cross-sectional area of the mitral prosthesis and associated lower velocities of flow.

Similarly, anticoagulation titrated to a subtherapeutic level maintains more protection against thrombus formation than does no anticoagulation. Finally, the risk of thrombus formation is cumulative and increases with time as the patient receives less than therapeutic anticoagulation.

Patients who require minimally invasive procedures with a low hemorrhagic risk may be managed by allowing long-term anticoagulation to decrease to a subtherapeutic range and resuming the normal dose of warfarin immediately following the procedure.[117] Among patients with mechanical heart valves who are undergoing major noncardiac surgery and in whom anticoagulation is contraindicated at the time of surgery, it is usually prudent to discontinue oral anticoagulation several days prior to surgery and to administer intravenous heparin to maintain anticoagulation until the time of surgery. The short half-life of heparin allows the patient to safely undergo surgery within a few hours of its discontinuation. Reestablishing therapeutic anticoagulation usually requires several days after warfarin is initiated; the patient should therefore receive heparin in the postoperative period until oral anticoagulation is fully therapeutic. Heparin should be reinitiated when the risk of bleeding is no longer prohibitive and may be started with either a bolus followed by intravenous infusion or with intravenous infusion alone, dictated by the risk of postoperative hemorrhage (see Chap. 71). Low-molecular-weight heparins are being increasingly utilized in this situation.

Arrhythmia and Conduction Disturbances

Supraventricular and ventricular arrhythmias typically do not represent a serious risk to the patient undergoing noncardiac surgery. However, the arrhythmia may herald the presence of underlying cardiopulmonary disease, and any increased perioperative risk associated with ventricular and supraventricular arrhythmias[4] is most likely related to the underlying disease. The finding of an arrhythmia in the perioperative period should prompt a search for underlying cardiopulmonary disease, drug toxicity, or metabolic derangement that could be both responsible for the arrhythmia and present a risk to the patient.

An otherwise benign arrhythmia can present risk if it unmasks an otherwise silent cardiac disease. For example, a rapid supraventricular tachycardia can provoke myocardial ischemia in the presence of minimal coronary artery disease and similarly can precipitate significant pulmonary congestion in the setting of only mild or moderate mitral stenosis. Ventricular ectopy—including isolated ventricular premature complexes, complex ectopy, and nonsustained ventricular tachycardia—usually does not require specific therapy unless there is evidence of associated hypoperfusion. Thus, hypotension or ongoing myocardial ischemia associated with an arrhythmia warrants therapy directed at the arrhythmia more than would the presence of the arrhythmia alone.

Perioperative atrial fibrillation is common, especially following intrathoracic surgical procedures (where there can be direct atrial irritation) as well as among patients with underlying cardiac or pulmonary diseases. Because of the high-catecholamine state early following major surgery, it may not be possible to establish and maintain normal sinus rhythm in the setting of postoperative atrial fibrillation, and therapy should first be directed at rate control and anticoagulation when feasible. Cardioversion of atrial fibrillation in the early postoperative period should be limited to patients with evidence of hemodynamic compromise and hypoperfusion associated with the arrhythmia. For most patients, rate control can be accomplished with the use of beta-adrenergic antagonists or calcium channel blocking agents administered orally or intravenously. Although digoxin can also be administered, it is typically not as effective for rate control in patients with a high-catecholamine state. Because of the risk of atrial thrombus formation and associated thromboembolic events, patients with atrial fibrillation, including postoperative atrial fibrillation, should be anticoagulated when feasible. Many patients with postoperative atrial fibrillation spontaneously revert to sinus rhythm when perioperative stresses have sufficiently decreased. If a patient does not spontaneously return to sinus rhythm, elective cardioversion should be performed prior to discharge. Any form of cardioversion from atrial fibrillation—whether chemical, electrical, or spontaneous—carries an associated risk of subsequent thromboembolism ascribed to a period of atrial mechanical dysfunction following cardioversion.[118,119] For this reason, patients should receive therapeutic anticoagulation for 3 to 4 weeks following successful cardioversion.

Patients with evidence of intraventricular conduction delay on ECG but without a history of symptoms or electrical evidence of advanced heart block do not appear to be at substantial risk of progressing to complete heart block in the perioperative period. If high-grade conduction block develops, treatment can usually be managed in the short term with transthoracic pacing units. Special note should be made of the presence of a left bundle branch block among patients undergoing right heart catheterization for hemodynamic monitoring. Because of the risk of inducing transient right bundle branch block during catheter manipulation through the right ventricle, the possibility of complete heart block exists, and measures to provide temporary pacing should be available.

SUMMARY OF KEY ELEMENTS OF ACC/AHA GUIDELINES

- It is important to determine the urgency of noncardiac surgery. In many cases patient- or surgery-specific factors dictate immediate surgery and may not allow further cardiac assessment or treatment. Perioperative medical management, surveillance, and postoperative risk stratification is appropriate in these cases.
- Patients with bypass surgery in the past 5 years or percutaneous coronary intervention from 6 months to 5 years previously and remaining free of clinical evidence of ischemia generally have low risk of cardiac complications from surgery and may proceed without further testing, particularly if they are functionally very active and asymptomatic.
- Patients with favorable invasive/noninvasive testing in the past 2 years generally require no further cardiac workup if they have been asymptomatic since the test and are functionally active.
- Patients with an unstable coronary syndrome, decompensated heart failure, symptomatic arrhythmias, or severe valvular heart disease scheduled for elective noncardiac surgery should have surgery cancelled or delayed until the cardiac problem is clarified and treated.
- Patients with <1 intermediate clinical predictors of cardiac risk for adverse perioperative events (Table 82-1) and moderate or excellent functional capacity can generally undergo low- or intermediate-risk surgery with low event rates.
- Poor functional capacity or a combination of high-risk surgery and moderate functional capacity in a patient with intermediate clinical predictors of cardiac risk for adverse perioperative events (Table 82-1) (especially if ≥2) often requires further noninvasive cardiac testing.
- Patients with minor or no clinical predictors of risk and moderate or excellent functional capacity can safely undergo noncardiac surgery.

- Results of noninvasive testing can be used to define further management, including intensified medical therapy or proceeding directly with surgery or cardiac catheterization. Cardiac catheterization may lead to coronary revascularization and is especially justifiable when it is likely to improve the patient's long-term prognosis.

CONCLUSIONS

Appropriate preoperative evaluation and therapy may significantly improve periprocedural and long-term outcomes. Successful management of high-risk patients requires an integrated team approach between surgeons, anesthesiologists, cardiologists, and internists. In general, indications for further cardiac testing and revascularization are the same as in the nonoperative setting. In the absence of contraindications, beta-blocker therapy should be considered in all patients at high risk for coronary events who are scheduled to undergo noncardiac surgery. For many patients, evaluation prior to noncardiac surgery may be the first comprehensive assessment of their short- and long-term cardiac risk and provides an opportunity not only to decrease their immediate periprocedural risk but also to improve their long-term outcomes with appropriate evidence-based therapies.

References

1. Mangano DT. Perioperative cardiac morbidity. *Anesthesiology* 1990;72:153–184.
2. National Center for Health Statistics. *Vital Statistics of the United States: 1980,* vol 2, *Mortality,* part A. DHHS pub no (PHS) 85-1101. Hyattsville, MD: NCHS U.S. Public Health Services; 1985.
3. National Center for Health Statistics. *Vital Statistics of the United States: 1988,* vol 3. DHHS pub no (PHS) 89-1232. Washington, DC: NCHS U.S. Public Health Services; 1989:10–17,66,67,100,101.
4. Goldman L, Caldera DL, Nussbaum SR, et al. Multifactorial index of cardiac risk in noncardiac surgical procedures. *N Engl J Med* 1977;297:845–850.
5. Ashton CM, Petersen NJ, Wray NP, et al. The incidence of perioperative myocardial infarction in men undergoing noncardiac surgery. *Ann Intern Med* 1993;118:504–510.
6. Hollenberg M, Mangano DT, Browner WS, et al. Predictors of postoperative myocardial ischemia in patients undergoing noncardiac surgery: The study of perioperative ischemia research group. *JAMA* 1992;268:205–209.
7. Hubbard BL, Gibbons RJ, Lapeyre AC III, et al. Identification of severe coronary artery disease using simple clinical parameters. *Arch Intern Med* 1992;152:309–312.
8. Lette J, Waters D, Bernier H, et al. Preoperative and long-term cardiac risk assessment: Predictive value of 23 clinical descriptors, 7 multivariate scoring systems, and quantitative dipyridamole imaging in 350 patients. *Ann Surg* 1992;216:192–204.
9. Mangano DT, Browner WS, Hollenberg M, et al. Association of perioperative myocardial ischemia with cardiac morbidity and mortality in men undergoing noncardiac surgery: The study of perioperative ischemia research group. *N Engl J Med* 1990;323:1781–1788.
10. Michel LA, Jamart J, Bradpiece HA, et al. Prediction of risk in noncardiac operations after cardiac operations. *J Thorac Cardiovasc Surg* 1990;100:595–605.
11. Eagle KA, Coley CM, Newell JB, et al. Combining clinical and thallium data optimizes preoperative assessment of cardiac risk before major vascular surgery. *Ann Intern Med* 1989;110:859–866.
12. Detsky AS, Abrams HB, McLaughlin JR, et al. Predicting cardiac complications in patients undergoing non-cardiac surgery. *J Gen Intern Med* 1986;1:211–219.
13. Foster ED, Davis KB, Carpenter JA, et al. Risk of noncardiac operation in patients with defined coronary disease: The coronary artery surgery study (CASS) registry experience. *Ann Thorac Surg* 1986;41:42–50.

14. Cooperman M, Pflug B, Martin EW Jr, et al. Cardiovascular risk factors in patients with peripheral vascular disease. *Surgery* 1978;84:505–509.

15. Eagle KA, Berger PB, Calkins H, et al. ACC/AHA guideline update for perioperative cardiovascular evaluation for noncardiac surgery-executive summary. A report of the American College of Cardiology/American Heart Association Task Force on Practice Guidelines (Committee to Update the 1996 Guidelines on Perioperative Cardiovascular Evaluation for Noncardiac Surgery). *J Am Coll Cardiol* 2002;39(3):542–553.

16. Morris CK, Ueshima K, Kawaguchi T, et al. The prognostic value of exercise capacity: A review of the literature. *Am Heart J* 1991;122:1423–1431.

17. Detsky AS, Abrams HB, Forbath N, et al. Cardiac assessment for patients undergoing noncardiac surgery: A multifactorial clinical risk index. *Arch Intern Med* 1986;146:2131–2134.

18. Tarhan S, Moffitt EA, Taylor WF, et al. Myocardial infarction after general anesthesia. *JAMA* 1972;220:1451–1454.

19. Steen PA, Tinker JH, Tarhan S. Myocardial reinfarction after anesthesia and surgery. *JAMA* 1978;239:2566–2570.

20. Rao TL, Jacobs KH, El-Etr AA. Reinfarction following anesthesia in patients with myocardial infarction. *Anesthesiology* 1983;59:499–505.

21. Hertzer NR. Fatal myocardial infarction following peripheral vascular operations: A study of 951 patients followed 6 to 11 years postoperatively. *Cleve Clin Q* 1982;49:1–11.

22. Leung JM, Goehner P, O'Kelly BF, et al. Isoflurane anesthesia and myocardial ischemia: Comparative risk versus sufentanil anesthesia in patients undergoing coronary artery bypass graft surgery. The SPI (Study of Perioperative Ischemia) Research Group. *Anesthesiology* 1991;74:838–847.

23. Baron JF, Bertrand M, Barre E, et al. Combined epidural and general anesthesia versus general anesthesia for abdominal aortic surgery. *Anesthesiology* 1991;75:611–618.

24. Christopherson R, Beattie C, Frank SM, et al. Perioperative morbidity in patients randomized to epidural or general anesthesia for lower extremity vascular surgery: Perioperative Ischemia Randomized Anesthesia Trial Study Group. *Anesthesiology* 1993;79:422–434.

25. Slogoff S, Eeats AS. Randomized trial of primary anesthetic agents on outcome of coronary artery bypass operations. *Anesthesiology* 1989;70:179–188.

26. Tuman KJ, McCarthy RJ, Spiess BD. Epidural anaesthesia and analgesia decreases postoperative hypercoagulability in high-risk vascular patients. *Anesth Analg* 1990;70:S414.

27. Gianrossi R, Detrano R, Mulvihill D, et al. Exercise-induced ST depression in the diagnosis of coronary artery disease: A meta-analysis. *Circulation* 1989;80:87–98.

28. Detrano R, Gianrossi R, Mulvihill D, et al. Exercise-induced ST segment depression in the diagnosis of multivessel coronary disease: A meta-analysis. *J Am Coll Cardiol* 1989;14:1501–1508.

29. Weiner DA, Ryan TJ, McCabe CH, et al. Prognostic importance of a clinical profile and exercise test in medically treated patients with coronary artery disease. *J Am Coll Cardiol* 1984;3:772–779.

30. McCabe CJ, Reidy NC, Abbott WM, et al. The value of electrocardiogram monitoring during treadmill testing for peripheral vascular disease. *Surgery* 1981;89:183–186.

31. Cutler BS, Wheeler HB, Paraskos JA, et al. Applicability and interpretation of electrocardiographic stress testing in patients with peripheral vascular disease. *Am J Surg* 1981;141:501–506.

32. Arous EJ, Baum PL, Cutler BS, et al. The ischemic exercise test in patients with peripheral vascular disease: Implications for management. *Arch Surg* 1984;119:780–783.

33. Gardine RL, McBride K, Greenberg H, et al. The value of cardiac monitoring during peripheral arterial stress testing in the surgical management of peripheral vascular disease. *J Cardiovasc Surg (Torino)* 1985;26:258–261.

34. von Knorring J, Lepantalo M. Prediction of perioperative cardiac complications by electrocardiographic monitoring during treadmill exercise testing before peripheral vascular surgery. *Surgery* 1986;99:610–613.

35. Leppo J, Plaja J, Gionet M, et al. Noninvasive evaluation of cardiac risk before elective vascular surgery. *J Am Coll Cardiol* 1987;9:269–276.

36. Hanson P, Pease M, Berkoff H, et al. Arm exercise testing for coronary artery disease in patients with peripheral vascular disease. *Clin Cardiol* 1988;11:70–74.

37. McPhail N, Calvin JE, Shariatmadar A, et al. The use of preoperative exercise testing to predict cardiac complications after arterial reconstruction. *J Vasc Surg* 1988;7:60–68.

38. Carliner NH, Fisher ML, Plotnick GD, et al. Routine preoperative exercise testing in patients undergoing major noncardiac surgery. *Am J Cardiol* 1985;56:51–58.

39. Kopecky SL, Gibbons RJ, Hollier LH. Preoperative supine exercise radionuclide angiogram predicts perioperative cardiovascular events in vascular surgery. *J Am Coll Cardiol* 1986;7:226A.

40. Urbinati S, Di Pasquale G, Andreoli A, et al. Preoperative noninvasive coronary risk stratification in candidates for carotid endarterectomy. *Stroke* 1994;25:2022–2027.

41. Boucher CA, Brewster DC, Darling RC, et al. Determination of cardiac risk by dipyridamole-thallium imaging before peripheral vascular surgery. *N Engl J Med* 1985;312:389–394.

42. Cutler BS, Leppo JA. Dipyridamole thallium 201 scintigraphy to detect coronary artery disease before abdominal aortic surgery. *J Vasc Surg* 1987;5:91–100.

43. Fletcher JP, Antico VF, Gruenewald S, et al. Dipyridamole-thallium scan for screening of coronary artery disease prior to vascular surgery. *J Cardiovasc Surg (Torino)* 1988;29:666–669.

44. Sachs RN, Tellier P, Larmignat P, et al. Assessment by dipyridamole-thallium-201 myocardial scintigraphy of coronary risk before peripheral vascular surgery. *Surgery* 1988;103:584–587.

45. McEnroe CS, O'Donnell RF Jr, Yeager A, et al. Comparison of ejection fraction and Goldman risk factor analysis of dipyridamole-thallium-201 studies in the evaluation of cardiac morbidity after aortic aneurysm surgery. *J Vasc Surg* 1990;11:497–504.

46. Younis LT, Aguirre F, Byers S, et al. Perioperative and long-term prognostic value of intravenous dipyridamole thallium scintigraphy in patients with peripheral vascular disease. *Am Heart J* 1990;119:1287–1292.

47. Mangano DT, London MJ, Tubau JF, et al. Dipyridamole thallium-201 scintigraphy as a preoperative screening test: A reexamination of its predictive potential. Study of Perioperative Ischemia Research Group. *Circulation* 1991;84:493–502.

48. Strawn DJ, Guernsey JM. Dipyridamole thallium scanning in the evaluation of coronary artery disease in elective abdominal aortic surgery. *Arch Surg* 1991;126:880–884.

49. Watters TA, Botvinick EH, Dae MW, et al. Comparison of the findings on preoperative dipyridamole perfusion scintigraphy and intraoperative transesophageal echocardiography: Implications regarding the identification of myocardium at ischemic risk. *J Am Coll Cardiol* 1991;18:93–100.

50. Hendel RC, Whitfield SS, Villegas BJ, et al. Prediction of late cardiac events by dipyridamole thallium imaging in patients undergoing elective vascular surgery. *Am J Cardiol* 1992;70:1243–1249.

51. Lette J, Waters D, Cerino M, et al. Preoperative coronary artery disease risk stratification based on dipyridamole imaging and a simple three-step, three-segment model for patients undergoing noncardiac vascular surgery or major general surgery. *Am J Cardiol* 1992;69:1553–1558.

52. Madsen PV, Vissing M, Munck O, et al. A comparison of dipyridamole thallium 201 scintigraphy and clinical examination: I. The determination of cardiac risk before arterial reconstruction. *Angiology* 1992;43:306–311.

53. Brown KA, Rowen M. Extent of jeopardized viable myocardium determined by myocardial perfusion imaging best predicts perioperative cardiac events in patients undergoing noncardiac surgery. *J Am Coll Cardiol* 1993;21:325–330.

54. Kresowik TF, Bower TR, Garner SA, et al. Dipyridamole thallium imaging in patients being considered for vascular procedures. *Arch Surg* 1993;128:299–302.

55. Baron JF, Mundler O, Bertrand M, et al. Dipyridamole-thallium scintigraphy and gated radionuclide angiography to assess cardiac risk before abdominal aortic surgery. *N Engl J Med* 1994;330:663–669.

56. Bry JD, Belkin M, O'Donnell TF Jr, et al. An assessment of the positive predictive value and cost-effectiveness of dipyridamole myocardial scintigraphy in patients undergoing vascular surgery. *J Vasc Surg* 1994;19:112–121.

57. Camp AD, Garvin PJ, Hoff J, et al. Prognostic value of intravenous dipyridamole thallium imaging in patients with diabetes mellitus considered for renal transplantation. *Am J Cardiol* 1990;65:1459–1463.

58. Iqbal A, Gibbons RJ, McGoon MD, et al. Noninvasive assessment of cardiac risk in insulin dependent diabetic patients being evaluated for pancreatic transplantation using thallium-201 myocardial perfusion scintigraphy. *Transplant Proc* 1991;23(part 2):1690–1691.

59. Coley CM, Field TS, Abraham SA, et al. Usefulness of dipyridamole-thallium scanning for preoperative evaluation of cardiac risk for nonvascular surgery. *Am J Cardiol* 1992;69:1280–1285.

60. Shaw L, Miller DD, Kong BA, et al. Determination of perioperative cardiac risk by adenosine thallium-201 myocardial imaging. *Am Heart J* 1992;124:861–869.

61. Takase B, Younis LT, Byers SL, et al. Comparative prognostic value of clinical risk indexes, resting two-dimensional echocardiography, and dipyridamole stress thallium-201 myocardial imaging for perioperative cardiac events in major nonvascular surgery patients. *Am Heart J* 1993;126:1099–1106.

62. Younis L, Stratmann H, Takase B, et al. Preoperative clinical assessment and dipyridamole thallium-201 scintigraphy for prediction and prevention of cardiac events in patients having major noncardiovascular surgery and known or suspected coronary artery disease. *Am J Cardiol* 1994;47:311–317.

63. Stratmann H, Tamesis B, Wittry M, et al. Dipyridamole sestamibi tomography optimizes perioperative outcome and defines late prognosis in vascular surgery patients. *Circulation* 1993;88:I–440.

64. Ritchie JL, Bateman TM, Bonow RO, et al. Guidelines for clinical use of cardiac radionuclide imaging: A report of the American College of Cardiology/American Heart Association Task Force on Assessment of Diagnostic and Therapeutic Cardiovascular Procedures (Committee on Radionuclide Imaging), developed in collaboration with the American Society of Nuclear Cardiology. *J Am Coll Cardiol* 1995;25:521–547.

65. Berthe C, Pierard LA, Hiernaux M. Predicting the extent and location of coronary artery disease in acute myocardial infarction by echocardiography during dobutamine infusion. *Am J Cardiol* 1986;58:1167–1172.

66. Cohen JL, Green TO, Ottenweller J, et al. Dobutamine digital echocardiography for detecting coronary artery disease. *Am J Cardiol* 1991;67:1311–1318.

67. Sawada SG, Segar DS, Ryan T, et al. Echocardiographic detection of coronary artery disease during dobutamine infusion. *Circulation* 1991;83:1605–1614.

68. Martin TW, Seaworth JF, Johns JP, et al. Comparison of adenosine, dipyridamole, and dobutamine in stress echocardiography. *Ann Intern Med* 1992;116:190–196.

69. Marwick T, Willemart B, D'Hondt AM, et al. Selection of the optimal nonexercise stress for the evaluation of ischemic regional myocardial dysfunction and malperfusion: Comparison of dobutamine and adenosine using echocardiography and 99mTc-MIBI single photon emission computed tomography. *Circulation* 1993;87:345–354.

70. Lane RT, Sawada SG, Segar DS, et al. Dobutamine stress echocardiography for assessment of cardiac risk before noncardiac surgery. *Am J Cardiol* 1991;68:976–977.

71. Lalka SG, Sawada SG, Dalsing MC, et al. Dobutamine stress echocardiography as a predictor of cardiac events associated with aortic surgery. *J Vasc Surg* 1992;15:831–840.

72. Poldermans D, Fioretti PM, Forster T, et al. Dobutamine stress echocardiography for assessment of perioperative cardiac risk in patients undergoing major vascular surgery. *Circulation* 1993;87:1506–1512.

73. Eichelberger JP, Schwarz KQ, Black ER, et al. Predictive value of dobutamine echocardiography just before noncardiac vascular surgery. *Am J Cardiol* 1993;72:602–607.

74. Langan EM III, Youkey JR, Franklin DP, et al. Dobutamine stress echocardiography for cardiac risk assessment before aortic surgery. *J Vasc Surg* 1993;18:905–911.

75. Davila-Roman VG, Waggoner AD, Sicard GA, et al. Dobutamine stress echocardiography predicts surgical outcome in patients with an aortic aneurysm and peripheral vascular disease. *J Am Coll Cardiol* 1993;21:957–963.

76. Shaw LJ, Eagle KA, Gersh BJ, et al. Meta-analysis of intravenous dipyridamole-thallium-201 imaging (1985 to 1994) and dobutamine echocardiography (1991 to 1994) for risk stratification before vascular surgery. *J Am Coll Cardiol* 1996;27:787–798.

77. Cambria RP, Brewster DC, Abbott WM, et al. The impact of selective use of dipyridamole-thallium scans and surgical factors on the current morbidity of aortic surgery. *J Vasc Surg* 1992;15:43–51.

78. Froehlich JB, Karavite D, Russman PL, et al. American College of Cardiology/American Heart Association preoperative assessment guidelines reduce resource utilization before aortic surgery. *J Vasc Surg* 2002;36:758–763.

79. Diehl JT, Cali RF, Hertzer NR, et al. Complications of abdominal aortic reconstruction: An analysis of perioperative risk factors in 557 patients. *Ann Surg* 1983;197:49–56.

80. Crawford ES, Morris GC Jr, Howell JF, et al. Operative risk in patients with previous coronary artery bypass. *Ann Thorac Surg* 1978;26:215–221.

81. Reul GJ Jr, Cooley DA, Duncan JM, et al. The effect of coronary bypass on the outcome of peripheral vascular operations in 1093 patients. *J Vasc Surg* 1986;3:788–798.

82. Nielsen JL, Page CP, Mann C, et al. Risk of major elective operation after myocardial revascularization. *Am J Surg* 1992;164:423–426.

83. Huber KC, Evans MA, Bresnahan JF, et al. Outcome of noncardiac operations in patients with severe coronary artery disease successfully treated preoperatively with coronary angioplasty. *Mayo Clin Proc* 1992;67:15–21.

84. Elmore JR, Hallett JW Jr, Gibbons RJ, et al. Myocardial revascularization before abdominal aortic aneurysmorrhaphy: Effect of coronary angioplasty. *Mayo Clin Proc* 1993;68:637–641.

85. Allen JR, Helling TS, Hartzler GO. Operative procedures not involving the heart after percutaneous transluminal coronary angioplasty. *Surg Gynecol Obstet* 1991;173:285–288.

86. Hassan SA, Hlatky M, Boothroyd D, et al. Impact of prior coronary bypass surgery and angioplasty on perioperative cardiac outcomes in patients undergoing noncardiac surgery: Data from Bypass Angioplasty Revascularization Investigation (BARI) study [abstr]. *Circulation* 1999;100(suppl I):I-529.

87. Kaluza GL, Joseph J, Lee JR, et al. Catastrophic outcomes of noncardiac surgery soon after coronary stenting. *J Am Coll Cardiol* 2000;35:1288–1294.

88. Coriat P, Daloz M, Bousseau D, et al. Prevention of intraoperative myocardial ischemia during noncardiac surgery with intravenous nitroglycerin. *Anesthesiology* 1984;61:193–196.

89. Thomson IR, Mutch WA, Culligan JD. Failure of intravenous fentanyl-pancuronium anesthesia. *Anesthesiology* 1984;61:385–393.

90. Gallagher JD, Moore RA, Jose AB, et al. Prophylactic nitroglycerin infusions during coronary artery bypass surgery. *Anesthesiology* 1986;64:785–789.

91. Godet G, Coriat P, Baron JF, et al. Prevention of intraoperative myocardial ischemia during noncardiac surgery with intravenous diltiazem: A randomized trial versus placebo. *Anesthesiology* 1987;66:241–245.

92. Pasternack PF, Imparato AM, Baumann FG, et al. The hemodynamics of beta-blockade in patients undergoing abdominal aortic aneurysm repair. *Circulation* 1987;76(suppl 3, pt 2):III-1–III-7.

93. Stone JG, Foex P, Sear JW, et al. Myocardial ischemia in untreated hypertensive patients: Effect of a single small oral dose of a beta-adrenergic blocking agent. *Anesthesiology* 1988;68:495–500.

94. Pasternack PF, Grossi EA, Baumann FG, et al. Beta blockade to decrease silent myocardial ischemia during peripheral vascular surgery. *Am J Surg* 1989;158:113–116.

95. Dodds TM, Stone JG, Coromilas J, et al. Prophylactic nitroglycerin infusion during noncardiac surgery does not reduce perioperative ischemia. *Anesth Analg* 1993;76:705–713.

96. Poldermans D, Boersma E, Bax JJ, et al. The effect of bisoprolol on perioperative mortality and myocardial infarction in high-risk patients undergoing vascular surgery. *N Engl J Med* 1999;341:1789–1794.

97. Mangano DT, Hollenberg M, Fegert G, et al. Perioperative myocardial ischemia in patients undergoing noncardiac surgery: I. Incidence and severity during the 4 day perioperative period. *J Am Coll Cardiol* 1991;17:843–850.

98. Mangano DT, Layug EL, Wallace A, Tateo I. Effect of atenolol on mortality and cardiovascular morbidity after noncardiac surgery. Multicenter Study of Perioperative Ischemia Research Group. *N Engl J Med* 1996;335:1713–1720.

99. Wallace A, Layug B, Tateo I, et al. Prophylactic atenolol reduces postoperative myocardial ischemia. McSPI Research Group. *Anesthesiology* 1998;88(1):7–17.

100. Poldermans D, Boersma E, Bax JJ, et al. The effect of bisoprolol on perioperative mortality and myocardial infarction in high-risk patients undergoing vascular surgery. Dutch Echocardiographic Cardiac Risk Evaluation Applying Stress Echocardiography Study Group. *N Engl J Med* 1999;341(24):1789–1794.

101. Urban MK, Markowitz SM, Gordon MA, Urquhart BL, Kligfield P. Postoperative prophylactic administration of beta-adrenergic blockers in patients at risk for myocardial ischemia. *Anesth Analg* 2000;90(6):1257–1261.

102. Stone JG, Foex P, Sear JW, et al. Risk of myocardial ischaemia during anesthesia in treated and untreated hypertensive patients. *Br J Anaesth* 1988;61:675–679.

103. Prys-Roberts C, Meloche R, Foex P. Studies of anaesthesia in relation to hypertension: I. cardiovascular responses of treated and untreated patients. *Br J Anaesth* 1971;43:122–137.

104. Cucchiara RF, Benefiel DJ, Matteo RS, et al. Evaluation of esmolol in controlling increases in heart rate and blood pressure during endotracheal intubation in patients undergoing carotid endarterectomy. *Anesthesiology* 1986;65:528–531.

105. Magnusson J, Thulin T, Werner O, et al. Haemodynamic effects of pretreatment with metoprolol in hypertensive patients undergoing surgery. *Br J Anaesth* 1986;58:251–260.

106. Goldman L, Caldera DL. Risks of general anesthesia and elective operation in the hypertensive patient. *Anesthesiology* 1979;50:285–292.

107. Bedford RF, Feinstein B. Hospital admission blood pressure: A predictor for hypertension following endotracheal intubation. *Anesth Analg* 1980;59:367–370.

108. Slogoff S, Keats AS. Does perioperative myocardial ischemia lead to postoperative myocardial infarction? *Anesthesiology* 1985;62:107–114.

109. Gerson MC, Hurst JM, Hertzberg VS, et al. Cardiac prognosis in noncardiac geriatric surgery. *Ann Intern Med* 1985;103:832–837.

110. Dajani AS, Bisno AL, Chung KJ, et al. Prevention of bacterial endocarditis: Recommendations by the American Heart Association. *JAMA* 1990;264:2919–2922.

111. Bernard Y, Etievent J, Mourand JL, et al. Long-term percutaneous aortic valvuloplasty compared with aortic valve replacement in patients more than 75 years old. *J Am Coll Cardiol* 1992;20:796–801.

112. Logeais Y, Langanay T, Roussin R, et al. Surgery for aortic stenosis in elderly patients: A study of surgical risk and predictive factors. *Circulation* 1994;90:2891–2898.

113. Lieberman EB, Bashore TM, Hermiller JB, et al. Balloon aortic valvuloplasty in adults: Failure of procedure to improve long-term survival. *J Am Coll Cardiol* 1995;26:1522–1528.

114. Reyes VP, Raju BS, Wynne J. Percutaneous balloon valvuloplasty compared with open surgical commissurotomy for mitral stenosis. *N Engl J Med* 1994;331:961–967.

115. Grayburn, PA. Vasodilator therapy for chronic aortic and mitral regurgitation. *Am J Med Sci* 2000;320:202–208.

116. Scognamiglio R, Rahimtoola SH, Fasoli G, et al. Nifedipine in asymptomatic patients with severe aortic regurgitation and normal left ventricular function. *N Engl J Med* 1994;331:689–694.

117. Stein PD, Alpert JS, Copeland J, et al. Antithrombotic therapy in patients with mechanical and biologic prosthetic heart valves. *Chest* 1992;102(suppl):445S–455S.

118. Black IW, Fatkin D, Sagar KB, et al. Exclusion of atrial thrombus by transesophageal echocardiography does not preclude embolism after cardioversion of atrial fibrillation: A multicenter study. *Circulation* 1994;89:2509–2513.

119. Fatkin D, Kuchar DL, Thorburn CW, et al. Transesophageal echocardiography before and during direct current cardioversion of atrial fibrillation: Evidence for "atrial stunning" as a mechanism of thromboembolic complications. *J Am Coll Cardiol* 1994;23:307–316.

ANESTHESIA AND THE PATIENT WITH CARDIOVASCULAR DISEASE

David L. Reich / Alexander Mittnacht / Joel A. Kaplan

Providing anesthesia for patients with cardiovascular disease is one of the most difficult challenges facing the anesthesiologist. The constellation of anesthetic drug effects, the physiologic stresses of surgery, and underlying cardiovascular diseases complicate and limit the choice of anesthetic techniques for any particular procedure. Generally speaking, the anesthesiologist's approach to the patient with cardiovascular disease is to select agents and techniques that would optimize the patient's cardiopulmonary function. The perioperative management of a patient with cardiovascular disease requires close cooperation between the cardiologist/internist and the anesthesiologist. Each specialist has a unique knowledge base, which complements that of the other. The approach should emphasize a continuum of care from the preoperative evaluation through the extended postoperative period.

PREOPERATIVE EVALUATION

The assessment of cardiac risk and optimization of the patient's cardiovascular status are the traditional goals of the preoperative evaluation of patients with cardiovascular disease. In 1977, Goldman et al. introduced the Cardiac Risk Index Score (CRIS) to guide more quantitatively the assignment of cardiac risk in patients undergoing noncardiac surgery.[1] This study had a major impact because clinicians concluded that improvements in factors such as congestive heart failure symptomatology and general medical condition would decrease cardiac risk. While the predictive value of the CRIS remains controversial,[2] the emphasis on preoperative optimization continues and is reviewed in Chap. 82. The American College of Cardiology/American Heart Association Task Force on Practice Guidelines has published "Guidelines for Perioperative Cardiovascular Evaluation for Noncardiac Surgery," which were updated in 2002.[3] The algorithmic approach to preoperative evaluation described in these guidelines and that advocated by Mangano and Goldman[4] are valuable in that more consistent clinical approaches have emerged.

The information derived from the cardiac evaluation that is of particular value to the anesthesiologist can be summarized by answers to the following questions:

1. Are further diagnostic studies required prior to elective surgery?
2. Will the patient derive benefit from delaying surgery in order to optimize preoperative medical therapy?
3. Will the patient derive benefit from preoperative myocardial revascularization via percutaneous or surgical methods?
4. Should there be perioperative antithrombotic therapy?
5. What is the regimen of preoperative cardiovascular medications that should be continued through the perioperative period?

A cogent, clear summary of the pertinent clinical, laboratory, radiologic, echocardiographic, radionuclide, and cardiac catheterization data constitutes the ideal "medical clearance" consultation for the anesthesiologist. With the benefit of this information, the cardiologist/internist and the anesthesiologist can make intelligent decisions regarding the patient's preoperative therapy and the optimal timing of surgery.[5]

PERIOPERATIVE MONITORING

The American Society of Anesthesiologists established standards for basic intraoperative monitoring in 1986.[6] The intraoperative monitoring that is required based upon these guidelines includes (1) heart rate, (2) electrocardiogram (ECG), (3) blood pressure, (4) pulse oximetry, (5) body temperature and (6) capnometry. The indications for the use of more invasive monitors, such as intraarterial and central venous monitoring, vary by institution and practitioner. (Tables 83-1 and 83-2). The indications for pulmonary arterial catheters (PACs) are especially controversial. There are data from the intensive care setting suggesting that the PAC is harmful,[7] while other data indicate that it may provide prognostic information in the perioperative period.[8] The American Society of Anesthesiologists has published practice parameters to guide practitioners in the appropriate use of this technology.[9] A recent randomized prospective trial of PAC use in the perioperative setting demonstrated no outcome benefit.[10] Table 83-3 details specific indications for the PAC that many practitioners accept.

Various forms of proprietary electroencephalographic analysis technology have been developed that correlate with increasing sedation and loss of consciousness.[11] While incomplete amnesia is rare with current anesthetic techniques, this technology has been demonstrated to result in decreased propofol doses and faster recovery from propofol anesthesia.[12]

Transesophageal echocardiography is minimally invasive and has acquired a much larger role in intraoperative management in recent

TABLE 83-1 Indications for Intraarterial Monitoring

Major surgical procedures involving large fluid shifts and/or blood loss
Surgery requiring cardiopulmonary bypass
Surgery of the aorta
Patients with pulmonary disease requiring frequent arterial blood gases
Patients with recent myocardial infarctions, unstable angina, or severe coronary artery disease
Patients with decreased left ventricular function (congestive heart failure) or significant valvular heart disease
Patients in hypovolemic, cardiogenic, or septic shock or with multiple organ failure
Procedures involving the use of deliberate hypotension or deliberate hypothermia
Massive trauma
Patients with right heart failure, chronic obstructive pulmonary disease, pulmonary hypertension, or pulmonary embolism
Patients requiring inotropes or intraaortic balloon counterpulsation
Patients undergoing surgery of the aorta requiring cross-clamping
Patients with massive ascites
Patients with electrolyte or metabolic disturbances requiring frequent blood samples
Inability to measure arterial pressure noninvasively (e.g., morbid obesity)

TABLE 83-3 Indications for Pulmonary Artery Catheter Monitoring

Major procedures involving large fluid shifts and/or blood loss in patients with impaired left ventricular function
Patients with severely unstable angina
Patients with significant mitral or aortic valvular pathology
Patients with pericardial tamponade
Patients in hypovolemic, cardiogenic, or septic shock, or with multiple organ failure
Massive trauma
Patients with right heart failure, chronic obstructive pulmonary disease, pulmonary hypertension, or pulmonary embolism
Patients requiring high levels of positive end-expiratory pressure
Hemodynamically unstable patients requiring inotropes or intraaortic balloon counterpulsation
Patients undergoing surgery of the aorta requiring cross-clamping
Patients undergoing liver transplantation
Patients with massive ascites

ing guidelines[15] have been published, and a certifying examination is administered by the National Board of Echocardiography. A list of indications for perioperative transesophageal echocardiography is presented in Table 83-4.

years. The availability of high-frequency transducers and color-flow Doppler mapping has enhanced the ability of anesthesiologists, cardiologists, and surgeons to make intraoperative diagnoses, evaluate hemodynamic aberrations, and assess the quality of cardiac surgical interventions. The American Society of Anesthesiologists has published practice guidelines for intraoperative transesophageal echocardiography.[13] Standardized intraoperative examination guidelines for multiplane transesophageal echocardiography[14] and training guidelines have been published.

CHOICE OF ANESTHETIC TECHNIQUE

The choice of anesthetic technique is inherently a difficult one because multiple factors must be considered. These include the desires of the patient, the requirements of the surgical procedure, and the patient's underlying medical condition. While a specific anesthetic technique is occasionally desirable for a particular procedure (e.g., spinal anesthesia for transurethral resection of the prostate), it is extremely difficult to find scientific evidence that any particular anesthetic approach is superior to reasonable alternatives or that anesthetic technique per se influences patient outcome.[16,17]

There is controversy regarding the effects of regional anesthesia (with postoperative epidural analgesia) on cardiovascular morbidity/mortality in "high risk" patients. Two studies reported reduced cardiac morbidity with epidural anesthesia[18,19] and three studies found no difference.[20–22] *While some studies suggest that regional anesthesia and epidural analgesia have salutary effects in vascular surgical patients, the issue is unresolved due to the limited and conflicting clinical evidence. Additionally, there are no studies that clearly determine whether or not local anesthesia with intravenous sedation (monitored anesthesia care) is advantageous compared with general or major regional anesthetic techniques.*

Regional anesthetics and monitored anesthesia care are not infrequently converted to general anesthetics intraoperatively due to unexpectedly long surgery, patient discomfort, or changes in the surgical plan. No anesthesiologist can be certain that a particular technique will be adequate for the surgical procedure; given the unpredictability of the situation, and the anesthesiologist must have flexibility to alter the technique as needed. Therefore it is essential that the cardiologist/internist does not specifically exclude any anesthetic technique during a preoperative consultation.

TABLE 83-2 Indications for Central Venous Line Placement

Major operative procedures involving large fluid shifts and/or blood loss in patients with good left ventricular function
Intravascular volume assessment when urine output is not reliable or unavailable (renal failure or major urologic surgery)
Patients with tricuspid stenosis
Major trauma
Surgical procedures with a high risk of air embolism, such as sitting position craniotomies
Frequent blood sampling in patients who will not require an intraarterial line
Venous access for vasoactive or irritating drugs
Chronic drug administration
Inadequate peripheral IV access
Rapid infusion of IV fluids (using large cannulas)

TABLE 83-4 Practice Guidelines for Perioperative Transesophageal Echocardiography

Category I indications: supported by the strongest evidence or expert opinion
  Intraoperative evaluation of acute, persistent, and life-threatening hemodynamic disturbances in which ventricular function and its determinants are uncertain and have not responded to treatment
  Intraoperative use in valve repair
  Intraoperative use in congenital heart surgery for most lesions requiring cardiopulmonary bypass
  Intraoperative use in repair of hypertrophic obstructive cardiomyopathy
  Intraoperative use for endocarditis when preoperative testing was inadequate or extension of infection to perivalvular tissue is suspected
  Preoperative use in unstable patients with suspected thoracic aortic aneurysms, dissection, or disruption who need to be evaluated quickly
  Intraoperative assessment of aortic valve function in repair of aortic dissections with possible aortic valve involvement
  Intraoperative evaluation of pericardial window procedures
  Use in intensive care unit for unstable patients with unexplained hemodynamic disturbances, suspected valve disease, or thromboembolic problems
Category II indications: supported by weaker evidence and expert consensus
  Perioperative use in patients with increased risk of myocardial ischemia or infarction
  Perioperative use in patients with increased risk of hemodynamic disturbances
  Intraoperative assessment of valve replacement
  Intraoperative assessment of repair of cardiac aneurysms
  Intraoperative evaluation of removal of cardiac tumors
  Intraoperative detection of foreign bodies
  Intraoperative detection of air emboli during cardiotomy, heart transplant operations, and upright neurosurgical procedures
  Intraoperative use during intracardiac thrombectomy
  Intraoperative use during pulmonary embolectomy
  Intraoperative use for suspected cardiac trauma
  Preoperative assessment of patients with suspected acute thoracic aortic dissections, aneurysms, or disruption
  Intraoperative use during repair of thoracic aortic dissections without suspected aortic valve involvement
  Intraoperative detection of aortic atheromatous disease or other sources or aortic emboli
  Intraoperative evaluation of pericardiectomy, pericardial effusions, or evaluation of pericardial surgery
  Intraoperative evaluation of anastomotic sites during heart and/or lung transplantation
  Monitoring placement and function of assist devices
Category III indications: little current scientific or expert support
  Intraoperative evaluation of myocardial perfusion, coronary artery anatomy, or graft patency
  Intraoperative use during repair of cardiomyopathies other than hypertrophic obstructive cardiomyopathy
  Intraoperative use for uncomplicated endocarditis during noncardiac surgery
  Intraoperative monitoring for emboli during orthopedic procedures
  Intraoperative assessment of repair of thoracic aortic injuries
  Intraoperative use for uncomplicated pericarditis
  Intraoperative evaluation of pleuropulmonary disease
  Monitoring placement of intraaortic balloon pumps, automatic implantable cardiac defibrillators, or pulmonary artery catheters
  Intraoperative monitoring of cardioplegia administration

SOURCE: Modified from the American Society of Anesthesiologists,[13] with permission.

Regional Anesthesia

Cushing coined the term *regional anesthesia* for operations where local anesthetics were used to operate on localized areas of the body without loss of consciousness. The advantages of regional anesthesia include simplicity, low cost, and minimal equipment requirements. Many of the adverse effects of general anesthesia are avoided, such as myocardial and respiratory depression. The potential disadvantages include patients' reluctance to be awake in the operating room, local anesthetic agents of insufficient or excessive duration, local anesthetic toxicity, and the risk of neuraxial hematoma in anticoagulated patients.

The cardiovascular side effects of regional anesthesia vary depending on the technique chosen; they are described below. Regional anesthesia may also be combined with general anesthesia in adults and children in order to decrease the requirements for the general anesthetic agents and for postoperative analgesia. The institution of analgesia prior to surgical stimulation (preemptive analgesia) may have salutary effects on postoperative pain control.

REGIONAL ANESTHESIA AND ANTICOAGULATION THERAPY

Intraoperative central neuraxial anesthesia (e.g., spinal and epidural) and postoperative neuraxial analgesia are contraindicated in patients receiving significant anticoagulation or antiplatelet therapy. The increasing use of anticoagulation and antiplatelet therapy in the management of cardiovascular disease and perioperative thromboembolic prophylaxis has complicated the application of neuraxial techniques, and appropriate patient selection is essential. Very rare but potentially catastrophic hematomas within the neuraxial space

TABLE 83-5 Anticoagulation and Antiplatelet Therapy: Recommendations for Neuraxial Anesthesia (NA)

Drug	Clinical Tests	Recommendations
Unfractionated heparin (UH)	Activated partial thromboplastin time	1. NA should be avoided in fully anticoagulated patients. 2. Standard subcutaneous UH: no increased risk unless used for prolonged periods. 3. IV heparin infusion safe if started >1 h after needle placement; catheter removal 1h before subsequent dose and >2–4 hr following last heparin dose.
Low-molecular-weight heparins and heparinoids	Not useful	1. Increased risk for NA, especially when used in conjunction with antiplatelet therapy 2. >12-h interval between last dose and NA 3. Catheter removal 10–12 h after last LMWH dose; next dose 2 h after catheter removed. 4. If blood appears during placement of NA, surgery does not need to be postponed, but next dose of LMWH should be delayed for another 24 h.
Fondaparinux	Anti–factor Xa assay with fondaparinux controls	No recommendations available at present.
Warfarin	Prothrombin time	1. Warfarin should be discontinued 4–5 days prior to the planned procedure and normal PT/INR measured before administration of regional anesthesia (chronic oral anticoagulation). 2. PT and INR should be checked prior to neuraxial anesthesia if first dose was given >24 h before surgery or a second dose had been administered. 3. Neuraxial catheters should be removed when the INR is <1.5.
Lepirudin Hirudin Bivalirudin	Ecarin clotting time	No recommendations available at present.
Aspirin	Not useful	Very low risk unless used in conjunction with a second drug that affects the coagulation system.
Other NSAIDs	Not useful	No indication for increased risk unless used in conjunction with a second drug that affects the coagulation system.
Clopidogrel Ticlopidine	Not useful	1. At present, insufficient clinical data about safe time interval between drug administration and NA. 2. Recommend discontinuing clopidogrel 7 days prior to NA. 3. Recommend discontinuing ticlopidine 10–14 days prior to NA.
Tirofiban	Not useful	Recommend 8-h interval between drug administration and safe NA.
Abciximab	Not useful	Recommend 48-h interval between drug administration and safe NA.
Eptifibatide	Not useful	Recommend 8-h interval between drug administration and safe NA.

have been associated with perioperative anticoagulation.[23–25] A careful drug history and bleeding diathesis history is more effective than laboratory investigation, because low molecular weight heparins and antiplatelet drugs confer higher risk (especially in combination), but will not be detected by standard preoperative coagulation tests.[26–28]

The establishment of guidelines for the use of neuraxial anesthesia and analgesia in patients who have received or will receive anticoagulants is an evolving process. The American Society of Regional Anesthesia publishes a current set of suggested guidelines on its website. Table 83-5 summarizes these guidelines[29] and the current literature.[30–34] For patient safety, it is crucial to monitor neurologic status carefully after administration of spinal or epidural anesthesia; rapid diagnosis and treatment of neuraxial hematoma probably improves outcome.[35]

LOCAL ANESTHESIC AGENTS
The local anesthetics are classified on the basis of their chemical structure as esters or amides. The esters are hydrolyzed by esterases in the plasma, and the amides are metabolized in the liver. The duration of action of local anesthetic agents is affected by the protein-binding characteristics of the molecule and the addition of vasoconstrictors to the local anesthetic solution.[36] Toxic reactions to local anesthetics are generally characterized by central nervous system excitation (seizures), which may be followed by central nervous system depression and cardiovascular collapse.

Cocaine is the original ester local anesthetic. Its clinical use today, is mainly restricted to topical anesthesia of the nose and airway. Its major side effects result from blockade of catecholamine reuptake at sympathetic nerve terminals. Cocaine toxicity has resulted in deaths from central nervous system toxicity and arrhythmias.[37] Cocaine can also elicit myocardial ischemia, and the tachycardia associated with cocaine contraindicates its use in patients with coronary artery disease, mitral stenosis, or obstructive cardiomyopathy. *Tetracaine* is a long-acting ester local anesthetic used in spinal anesthesia. It is also used for topical anesthesia of the eye and airway but may be toxic in the larger doses required for airway topical anesthesia.

Chloroprocaine is a short-acting ester local anesthetic that is used in epidural anesthesia. This agent is very rapidly metabolized by serum cholinesterase, leading to a low incidence of toxic reactions.

Compared to the esters, the amide local anesthetics are less rapidly metabolized (in the liver) and the potential for toxic reactions is somewhat greater. Some amide compounds (e.g., lidocaine) also have antiarrhythmic actions. *Lidocaine* and *mepivacaine* are agents of intermediate duration of action that are commonly used in many types of regional blocks. *Etidocaine* and *bupivacaine* are agents of higher potency and longer duration of action that also exhibit more toxicity. Bupivacaine is particularly associated with cardiovascular collapse and arrhythmias on inadvertent intravascular injection. Ropivacaine and levobupivacaine (an enantiomer of bupivacaine) are new local anesthetics with promising profiles. They are similar in potency and duration to bupivacaine, but appear to have less cardiovascular toxicity and to cause less motor block; their use has recently been reviewed.[38–40]

Epinephrine and phenylephrine may be added in very small doses to local anesthetic solutions to prolong their duration of action by local vasoconstriction. The systemic absorption of epinephrine occurs very slowly, and the beta-adrenergic effects predominate. This results in slight tachycardia and diastolic hypotension, which is undesirable in patients with certain cardiovascular diseases.

SPINAL ANESTHESIA

The injection of a relatively small dose of local anesthetic into the subarachnoid space, producing profound motor and sensory blockade, is known as spinal anesthesia. Spinal anesthesia also produces blockade of preganglionic sympathetic fibers, resulting in a sympathetic blockade that is generally two dermatomal segments higher than the sensory dermatomal level. A high level of sympathetic blockade results in hypotension through profound arterial and venous vasodilatation, which can be prevented or treated by intravenous hydration with crystalloid solutions. If the dermatomal level of sympathetic blockade reaches T1, the patient is effectively sympathectomized. The loss of cardiac accelerator fiber function may lead to bradycardia. Complete sympathectomy always occurs with a "total spinal," which also produces respiratory insufficiency due to intercostal and phrenic nerve root blockade.

Spinal anesthesia must be undertaken cautiously, and with more intensive monitoring in patients whose cardiovascular stability depends on the maintenance of a high preload and afterload. Patients with any significant cardiac valvular disease, hypertrophic obstructive cardiomyopathy, or tetralogy of Fallot are prone to hemodynamic decompensation during spinal anesthesia. Patients with coronary artery disease (CAD) usually tolerate spinal anesthesia well as long as diastolic arterial pressure is maintained at an appropriate level to preserve coronary perfusion pressure.

EPIDURAL ANESTHESIA

The epidural space, which is filled with loose areolar tissue and a venous plexus, lies immediately external to the dura mater. An indwelling catheter is usually placed percutaneously for intermittent bolus injections or continuous infusions of local anesthetic and/or opioids. The epidural space may be entered by thoracic, lumbar, or caudal approaches.

The hemodynamic effects of epidural anesthesia are essentially similar to those of spinal anesthesia, except that the onset of sympathetic blockade is more gradual. Thus, with appropriate monitoring, cautious administration of epidural anesthetics has been safely done in patients with mitral valvular disease, aortic stenosis, or hypertrophic obstructive cardiomyopathy. It should be emphasized, though, that intraarterial and pulmonary artery catheters (PACs) may be required to monitor and treat the changes in preload and afterload that occur with epidural anesthesia in patients with severe cardiovascular disease.

By comparison with spinal anesthesia, epidural anesthesia requires higher doses of local anesthetic, which increases the potential for complications and side effects. These include inadvertent intravascular or intrathecal injections of a high dose of local anesthetic, which potentially can cause cardiovascular complications, seizures, or a "total spinal" (see above). The hemodynamic consequences of inadvertent intravenous injections of epinephrine-containing solutions may be significant for patients who cannot tolerate tachycardia. Epidural infusions of opioids for postoperative analgesia may be complicated by pruritus, nausea, urinary retention, somnolence, and respiratory depression. Thus, appropriate monitoring and nursing care are required.

COMBINED SPINAL-EPIDURAL ANESTHESIA

The injection of intrathecal anesthetic agents via a fine-bore needle placed through the epidural-introducing large-bore needle, followed by epidural catheter placement, constitutes combined spinal-epidural anesthesia. The spinal anesthetic provides a rapid onset of anesthesia, while the epidural catheter permits the administration of agents for continued intraoperative anesthesia and postoperative analgesia.[41]

NERVE BLOCKS AND INFILTRATION OF LOCAL ANESTHETIC

Nerve blocks and local anesthetic infiltration may be performed to facilitate surgery of localized areas of the body. The brachial plexus may be blocked by various approaches. The lower extremity may be anesthetized by blocking the femoral, obturator, and sciatic nerves. Local anesthetic infiltration ("field block") is performed in defined regions, such as the inguinal area to facilitate herniorrhaphies. These blocks, when properly performed, have minimal cardiovascular effects. They do, however, require large volumes of local anesthetic solution, which cause toxic reactions if inadvertent intravascular injection occurs. Intercostal blocks are associated with high blood concentrations even without intravascular injection because the neurovascular bundle enhances absorption of the local anesthetic and multiple blocks are required for clinical efficacy.

General Anesthesia

General anesthesia is a reversible state consisting of amnesia, analgesia, immobility, and the prevention of undesirable reflexes. The general anesthetics include many drugs, almost all of which have cardiovascular side effects. Intravenous agents are nearly always used for the induction of anesthesia in adults. Anesthesia is maintained using inhalational agents, intravenous agents, or a combination of the two.

Neuromuscular blocking drugs (muscle relaxants) are commonly used to facilitate tracheal intubation, lower the requirements for anesthetic agents, and prevent involuntary muscular activity in surgical cases where complete paralysis is mandatory. In children, the induction of anesthesia is highly individualized according to patient needs, practitioner, and institution. With the exception of brief operations, most general anesthesia includes tracheal intubation and mechanical ventilation. As an alternative to tracheal intubation, devices such as the laryngeal mask airway may be used to secure a patient's airway. The loss of consciousness is usually accompanied by a decrease in sympathetic tone. This, as well as the effects of positive-pressure ventilation and the cardiac depressant properties of inhalational and most intravenous anesthetic agents, causes a moderate decrease in cardiac output.

The patient with cardiovascular disease presents major concerns for the anesthesiologist. General anesthesia masks many of the symptoms of cardiovascular decompensation, such as angina, dyspnea, dizziness, and palpitations. Other signs of cardiovascular disease, such as tachycardia, are nonspecific and may be misinterpreted as hypovolemia or light anesthesia. Fluid shifts, obstructed venous return, and varying levels of noxious stimulation are other variables related to surgery that are unpredictable. It is for these reasons that appropriate monitoring and selection of anesthetic agents is vital to the intraoperative management of the patient with cardiovascular disease.

INTRAVENOUS ANESTHETICS

Intravenous anesthetic induction drugs are composed of lipophilic molecules that have an affinity for neuronal tissue or specific receptors. Their action is generally terminated by redistribution from the vessel-rich tissues (brain, heart, liver, and kidneys) to other tissues (muscle, fat, and skin). Elimination occurs via hepatic metabolism and takes place over several hours. Patients with cardiovascular disease are prone to adverse reactions to intravenous induction drugs.

Barbiturates Thiopental, an ultra-short-acting thiobarbiturate, is the prototype for agents of its class. Its cardiovascular effects are marked by dose-dependent myocardial depression and dilation of venous capacitance vessels. The decrease in cardiac output is usually compensated for by arterial vasoconstriction, so that blood pressure is minimally decreased. Standard doses of barbiturate for anesthetic induction are contraindicated in patients with preload-dependent cardiac lesions and/or severely impaired ventricular contractility. This includes patients with pericardial tamponade, mitral regurgitation, aortic regurgitation, mitral stenosis, and dilated cardiomyopathy. Reduced doses and slower injection of the drug will markedly decrease the cardiovascular effects.

Benzodiazepines Benzodiazepines may be used as premedication, to induce anesthesia, or as adjuncts to regional or general anesthesia. Their most useful therapeutic effects include sedation and amnesia. When used as sole agents, the benzodiazepines have minimal cardiovascular effects. When used in combination with other drugs, such as opioids and potent volatile anesthetics, benzodiazepines produce hypotension, which may be due to myocardial depression or decreased systemic vascular resistance.

Opioids Synthetic opioids have assumed a major role in the anesthetic care of patients with cardiovascular disease. They can be used as premedication, as supplements to regional or inhalational anesthesia, as one of the main components of "nitrous-narcotic" anesthesia, or as the primary anesthetic agent (high-dose opioid anesthesia). They are often used as supplements during anesthesia induction to block the hemodynamic response to laryngoscopy and tracheal intubation. Ventilatory support is frequently continued postoperatively following high doses of opioids because the elimination half-lives of synthetic opioids are relatively long (1.5 to 4 h). The exception is remifentanil, a new synthetic opioid that is extremely short-acting due to ester hydrolysis.[42]

High-dose synthetic (phenylpiperidine) opioid anesthesia does not depress myocardial contractility and is devoid of histamine release. It is therefore associated with markedly stable hemodynamics during anesthetic induction and maintenance in the majority of patients with cardiovascular disease. There is a recent trend toward

reducing the doses of opioids administered in cardiac anesthesia in order to facilitate more rapid tracheal extubation and discharge from the intensive care unit.[43]

Anesthesiologists only rarely administer naloxone or other opioid antagonists to reverse the effects of a systemic opioid in patients with cardiovascular disease. In surgical patients, complete reversal of the opioid effect results in the sudden onset of pain and surges in catecholamine levels. Naloxone administration has been complicated by pulmonary edema,[44,45] arrhythmias,[46] and cardiac arrest.[47] Low doses of intravenous naloxone have been safely used to reverse the pruritus and respiratory depression associated with epidural and intrathecal opioids without reversing the analgesia.

Etomidate Etomidate is an imidazole anesthetic agent that enhances gamma-aminobutyric acid (GABA)–ergic transmission. It is associated with marked hemodynamic stability during bolus administration for anesthetic induction but does not blunt the hemodynamic response to laryngoscopy and tracheal intubation. This is one of the preferred agents for anesthetic induction in patients with valvular or ventricular dysfunction, hypovolemia, or pericardial effusion.

Propofol Propofol is a substituted phenol (diisopropylphenol) that may be used for anesthetic induction and maintenance. It is mildly irritating on injection. Its main advantage is the rapid emergence and psychomotor recovery following termination of the drug infusion. Propofol may also be associated with reduced postoperative nausea and vomiting.[48] Propofol causes dose-dependent hypotension that appears to be due to a combination of myocardial depression and vasodilation. It is prudent to use reduced doses of propofol in patients with aortic or mitral valvular stenosis and cardiomyopathies. Propofol is being used increasingly for sedation in intensive care units and to facilitate "fast-track" extubation following cardiac surgery.

Ketamine Ketamine is a cyclohexanone that has indirect sympathomimetic effects and is associated with emergence delirium. Its sympathomimetic effects are advantageous, however, in certain groups of patients who are critically dependent on high resting sympathetic tone to maintain an adequate perfusion pressure: those with pericardial tamponade, hypovolemia, and systemic-to-pulmonary arterial shunts. Ketamine is relatively contraindicated in patients who cannot tolerate tachycardia, such as those with CAD or mitral stenosis.[49]

Alpha$_2$-Adrenergic Agonists Clonidine and dexmedetomidine are alpha$_2$-adrenergic agonists that are sympatholytic, sedative-anxiolytic, antiarrhythmic, analgesic, and reversible.[50,51] Clonidine has also been demonstrated to reduce anesthetic requirements and improve hemodynamic stability during the intraoperative period. Dexmedetomidine is used for sedation in the perioperative period.

INHALATIONAL ANESTHETICS

Inhalational anesthetics include nitrous oxide and the potent volatile agents. The study of the uptake and distribution of inhaled drugs with cerebral and cardiovascular effects is practically unique to anesthesiology, and cardiac output is a major determinant of uptake and distribution. The alveolar concentration of a drug is generally equal to the brain concentration. Thus, anything that hastens increases in the alveolar concentration of the drug will speed the onset of anesthesia. Two factors that speed the onset of anesthesia are a diminished cardiac output and an anesthetic agent with low solubility in the blood. Thus, patients with low cardiac output secondary to cardiovascular disease will have a more rapid onset of anesthesia when inhalational agents are used. Intracardiac right-to-left shunting will decrease the onset of anesthesia, whereas left-to-right shunting has negligible effects.

Nitrous Oxide Nitrous oxide is an excellent analgesic but not a very potent anesthetic. Concentrations up to 75% may be given safely (so as to maintain an adequate FIO_2), but incomplete amnesia and movement in response to painful stimuli are likely. Thus, nitrous oxide is nearly always administered with other anesthetic agents, such as opioids or potent volatile agents and neuromuscular blockers. It is also chosen because its relatively low solubility in the blood enhances the rapid onset and termination of its effects.

Nitrous oxide is a weak myocardial depressant, which mildly stimulates the sympathetic nervous system. It does not exacerbate pulmonary hypertension in anesthetized patients with mitral valvular disease[52] but is nevertheless avoided by most practitioners in patients with severe right ventricular dysfunction. As a sole agent, its cardiovascular effects are minimal, but cardiac output is lowered in the presence of opioids. It also accentuates the negative inotropic effects of potent volatile agents.[53]

Nitrous oxide diffuses very rapidly into closed airspaces within the body due to its low blood solubility, high lipid solubility, and the high concentrations required. Examples of closed airspaces include bowel gas, pneumothoraces, and air emboli. For this reason, nitrous oxide must be discontinued if a pneumothorax or air embolism is suspected. It is often avoided in cardiothoracic procedures, particularly in children prone to paradoxical embolization or after cardiopulmonary bypass.

Potent Volatile Agents The use of inhalational anesthesia with potent volatile agents is the most common anesthetic technique because of its relatively low cost, reliable amnesia, and bronchodilation as well as the low blood solubility and overall safety record of these agents. All are myocardial depressants and vasodilators and produce some degree of hypotension.

The effect of these agents is rapidly changed when the inspiratory concentration is adjusted. By comparison with intravenous drugs, the ability to titrate inhalational anesthesia is an advantage because the duration of surgical procedures and the degree of surgical stimulation are often unpredictable. For this reason, low doses of volatile anesthetics may be added as supplements to nitrous oxide– or intravenous-based anesthetic techniques for the control of hypertension and the prevention of awareness (incomplete amnesia).

The frequent production of nodal (junctional) rhythm is also common to these agents. The loss of atrial systole may be poorly tolerated, particularly in patients with aortic stenosis, hypertrophic cardiomyopathies, or mitral stenosis. All potent volatile agents have the potential for interactions with calcium channel blockers and beta-adrenergic blockers. Negative inotropic and conduction effects of these drugs may be augmented by the volatile anesthetic agents; however, all cardiac drugs should be continued until the time of surgery.

HALOTHANE The use of halothane in today's anesthesia practice is restricted due to its cardiovascular effects and the small incidence of hepatotoxicity. Halothane depresses the myocardium and the sinoatrial node but is not a potent vasodilator. Thus, cardiac output and heart rate are depressed in a dose-dependent fashion. This hemodynamic profile is beneficial in situations where myocardial contractility (and oxygen consumption) should be kept low and perfusion pressure high. Examples include ischemic heart disease, hypertrophic obstructive cardiomyopathy, and especially tetralogy of Fallot.

ENFLURANE Enflurane is almost equal to halothane in its negative inotropic effect, but it is more vasodilating and less of a negative chronotrope. Thus, cardiac output is better maintained, but blood pressure is lower than with equipotent dosages of halothane.

ISOFLURANE Isoflurane is somewhat less negatively inotropic than enflurane or halothane and is a potent arteriolar vasodilator, which tends to maintain cardiac output. Tachycardia frequently occurs at clinical dosages because the baroreceptor reflexes are not impaired. On the basis of its hemodynamic effects, isoflurane would be beneficial in patients with mitral or aortic regurgitation with good ventricular function. It is relatively contraindicated (as a sole agent) in patients with mitral or aortic stenosis, dilated and hypertrophic cardiomyopathies, and pericardial tamponade. Isoflurane is frequently used in patients with CAD, when it is often combined with opioids or beta-adrenergic blockers to prevent tachycardia and the dose is limited to preserve coronary perfusion pressure.

The use of isoflurane remains controversial in patients with coronary artery anatomy that predisposes to coronary "steal." Isoflurane has been shown to induce myocardial ischemia with collateral-dependent myocardial blood flow in canine models[54] and in humans.[55] The tachycardia and hypotension associated with isoflurane, as well as evidence of maldistributed myocardial blood flow, might suggest that it should not be used. Nevertheless, a prospective clinical study in patients with "steal-prone anatomy"[56] did not find intraoperative myocardial ischemia or poorer outcome with isoflurane anesthesia. A reasonable conclusion would be that isoflurane should be used with caution and appropriate monitoring in patients suspected of having "steal-prone" coronary artery anatomy.[57]

DESFLURANE Desflurane is a volatile anesthetic that was introduced into clinical practice in 1992. It is much less soluble in blood than the volatile agents described above. Its blood:gas solubility coefficient is similar to that of nitrous oxide. Thus, more rapid induction and emergence would be expected. This is particularly advantageous in ambulatory procedures. Desflurane has a unique sympathomimetic effect that is seen with rapid increases in end-tidal concentration in the absence of preanesthetic medication. The sympathomimetic action of desflurane can be blocked by fentanyl, esmolol, and clonidine.[58]

SEVOFLURANE The relatively low solubility and minimal airway irritation of sevoflurane make it a very useful anesthetic for the inhalation induction of anesthesia.[59] Its low solubility allows rapid alterations in alveolar concentration during the maintenance period of the anesthetic, thereby improving control of the depth of anesthesia.

The cardiovascular effects of sevoflurane are similar to those of isoflurane and desflurane except that sevoflurane is not associated with increases in heart rate. Sevoflurane progressively decreases blood pressure in a manner similar to the other volatile anesthetics. In animals, sevoflurane appears to be a slightly less potent coronary vasodilator than isoflurane, and it has not been associated with coronary steal.[60]

Neuromuscular Blockade

BENZYLISOQUINOLINIUM COMPOUNDS

The benzylisoquinolinium series of nondepolarizing neuromuscular blockers are all derivatives of the curare molecule. Most of these compounds have histamine-releasing properties that are dependent on the dose and rate of administration. d-Tubocurarine, metocurine, atracurium, and mivacurium are associated with clinically important histamine release following the administration of bolus doses to facilitate tracheal intubation. Cisatracurium is not associated with histamine release with large doses. While agents such as *d*-tubocurarine and metocurine are mainly dependent on renal elimination, atracurium and cisatracurium undergo a unique form of spontaneous degradation that is organ-independent (Hofmann elimination). Mivacurium undergoes enzyme-dependent ester hydrolysis.

AMINOSTEROID COMPOUNDS

Pancuronium is the classic aminosteroid nondepolarizing neuromuscular blocking drug. The atropine-like molecular structure contains two quaternary nitrogen groups. The tachycardia and hypertension associated with pancuronium have been linked to myocardial ischemia during coronary artery bypass surgery.[61] The anticholinergic effects of pancuronium, however, can be useful (e.g., in patients with mitral regurgitation) for preventing the increase in vagal tone that occurs with high-dose opioid anesthetic inductions. Vecuronium and pipecuronium have minimal cardiovascular effects at usual clinical dosages. Rocuronium has a more rapid onset of action due to its lower potency and has minimal cardiovascular side effects. While pancuronium elimination is almost entirely renal, the newer compounds are degraded by the liver.

SUCCINYLCHOLINE

Succinylcholine is a depolarizing short-acting neuromuscular blocker that is still used because of its low cost, rapid onset, and short duration of action. Its cardiovascular effects depend on whether nicotinic or muscarinic receptor effects predominate in a given patient. Thus, tachycardia and hypertension or bradycardia and hypotension may occur. Vagal effects tend to predominate with repeated doses or in children. In patients with various disorders (including neuromuscular diseases, recent burns, and massive trauma), hyperkalemic cardiac arrest may occur with succinylcholine administration because of exaggerated release of intracellular potassium from myocytes.

THE POSTOPERATIVE PERIOD AND CARDIAC COMPLICATIONS

Emergence from anesthesia is frequently accompanied by hypertension and tachycardia, which are most often due to incomplete analgesia but may also be related to withdrawal from antihypertensive drugs, hypoxemia, delirium, or bladder distention. If an underlying modifiable cause is not identified, then intravenous drugs—such as nitroglycerin, labetalol, or esmolol—are frequently used to control hemodynamics in patients with cardiovascular disease. Shivering is another phenomenon that may occur due to hypothermia or emergence from volatile anesthetics. Shivering results in severe increases in oxygen consumption, which may be poorly tolerated by patients with cardiovascular disease. Although the mechanism is unknown, low doses of meperidine decrease or eliminate shivering.[62]

In patients with risk factors, there is a high incidence of postoperative complications, such as myocardial infarction (MI), pulmonary edema, malignant ventricular arrhythmia, and cardiac death. Pain, high catecholamine levels, hypercoagulability, hypovolemia, anemia, intravascular volume shifts, drug effects, and a lower level of monitoring all probably contribute to this phenomenon. Recent prospective trials suggest that prevention of hypothermia[63] and beta-adrenergic blockade during surgery and the postoperative hospitalization[64] may decrease the incidence of these complications in high-risk patients.

Traditionally, the anesthesiologist has not played a major role in postoperative management following discharge from the postanesthesia care unit. This situation has changed with the development of multidisciplinary pain services that administer epidural analgesia and patient-controlled analgesia. As noted above, it remains controversial whether regional anesthesia and intensive postoperative analgesia are capable of reducing morbidity and mortality. It is conceivable that more effective postoperative analgesia decreases the deleterious effects of the stress response. Future efforts to reduce perioperative risk likely will concentrate on assessing the effects of more intensive perioperative hemodynamic, analgesic, and anticoagulation management.

CONCLUSIONS

The optimal perioperative care of patients with cardiovascular disease is the joint responsibility of anesthesiologists, surgeons, and cardiologists/internists. Any anesthetic agent or technique has the potential for producing adverse effects, and the margin of safety is reduced in patients with cardiovascular disease. It is the anesthesiologist's role to acquire accurate and relevant information from the preoperative evaluation, to apply appropriate monitoring technology, to select an anesthetic technique that is suited to the planned procedure and the condition of the patient, and to manage hemodynamic alterations and analgesic requirements in the perioperative period. As cardiovascular disease continues to become more prevalent in the surgical population and preoperative testing and intraoperative monitoring become more sophisticated, effective communication between the specialties of cardiology and anesthesiology will become even more important.

References

1. Goldman L, Caldera DL, Nussbaum SR, et al. Multifactorial index of cardiac risk in noncardiac surgical procedures. *N Engl J Med* 1977;297: 845–850.

2. Gilbert K, Larocque BJ, Patrick LT. Prospective evaluation of cardiac risk indices for patients undergoing noncardiac surgery. *Ann Intern Med* 2000;133(5):356–359.

3. ACC/AHA guideline update for perioperative cardiovascular evaluation for noncardiac surgery—Executive summary: A report of the American College of Cardiology/American Heart Association Task Force on Practice Guidelines (Committee to Update the 1996 Guidelines on Perioperative Cardiovascular Evaluation for Noncardiac Surgery). *Circulation* 2002;105(10):1257–1267.

4. Mangano DT, Goldman L. Preoperative assessment of patients with known or suspected coronary disease. *N Engl J Med* 1995;333: 1750–1756.

5. Katz RI, Barnhart JM, Ho G, et al. A survey on the intended purposes and perceived utility of preoperative cardiology consultations. *Anesth Analg* 1998;87(4):830–836.

6. American Society of Anesthesiologists. Standards for Basic Intraoperative Monitoring (Approved by House of Delegates on October 21, 1986 and last amended on October 21, 1998). Park Ridge, IL. <http://www.asahq.org/publicationsAndServices/standards/02.html>

7. Connors AF, Speroff T, Dawson NV, et al. The effectiveness of right heart catheterization in the initial care of critically ill patients. *JAMA* 1996;276:889–897.

8. Reich DL, Bodian CA, Krol M, et al. Intraoperative hemodynamic predictors of mortality, stroke and myocardial infarction following coronary artery bypass surgery. *Anesth Analg* 1999;88:814–822.

9. American Society of Anesthesiologists. Practice Guidelines For Pulmonary Artery Catheterization (Approved by House of Delegates on October 21, 1992, and last amended October 16, 2002). American Soci-

ety of Anesthesiologists, Park Ridge, IL. <http://www.asahq.org/publicationsAndServices/pulm_artery.pdf>

10. Sandham JD, Hull RD, Brant RF, et al. Canadian Critical Care Clinical Trials Group. A randomized, controlled trial of the use of pulmonary-artery catheters in high-risk surgical patients. *N Engl J Med* 2003; 348:5–14.

11. Glass PS, Bloom M, Kearse L, et al. Bispectral analysis measures sedation and memory effects of propofol, midazolam, isoflurane, and alfentanil in healthy volunteers. *Anesthesiology* 1997;86:836–847.

12. Gan TJ, Glass PS, Windsor A, et al. Bispectral index monitoring allows faster emergence and improved recovery from propofol, alfentanil, and nitrous oxide anesthesia. BIS Utility Study Group. *Anesthesiology* 1997;87:808–815.

13. American Society of Anesthesiologists. Practice guidelines for perioperative transesophageal echocardiography. *Anesthesiology* 1996;84:986–1006.

14. Shanewise JS, Cheung AT, Aronson S, et al. ASE/SCA guidelines for performing a comprehensive intraoperative multiplane transesophageal echocardiography examination: Recommendations of the American Society of Echocardiography Council for Intraoperative Echocardiography and the Society of Cardiovascular Anesthesiologists Task Force for Certification in Perioperative Transesophageal Echocardiography. *Anesth Analg* 1999;89:870–884.

15. Cahalan MK, Abel M, Goldman M, et al. American Society of Echocardiography and Society of Cardiovascular Anesthesiologists task force guidelines for training in perioperative echocardiography. *Anesth Analg* 2002;94:1384–1388.

16. Slogoff S, Keats AS. Randomized trial of primary anesthetic agents on outcome of coronary artery bypass operations. *Anesthesiology* 1989;70:179–188.

17. Tuman KJ, McCarthy RJ, Spiess BD, et al. Does choice of anesthetic agent significantly affect outcome after coronary artery surgery? *Anesthesiology* 1989;70:189–198.

18. Yeager MP, Glass DD, Neff RK, et al. Epidural anesthesia and analgesia in high-risk surgical procedures. *Anesthesiology* 1987;66:729–736.

19. Tuman KJ, McCarthy RJ, March RJ, et al. Effects of epidural anesthesia and analgesia on coagulation and outcome after major vascular surgery. *Anesth Analg* 1991;73:696–704.

20. Baron JF, Bertrand M, Barre E, et al. Combined epidural and general anesthesia versus general anesthesia for abdominal aortic surgery. *Anesthesiology* 1991;75:611–618.

21. Bode RH Jr, Lewis KP, Zarich SW, et al. Cardiac outcome after peripheral vascular surgery: Comparison of general and regional anesthesia. *Anesthesiology* 1996;84.3–13.

22. Christopherson R, Beattie C, Frank SM, et al. Perioperative morbidity in patients randomized to epidural or general anesthesia for lower extremity vascular surgery. *Anesthesiology* 1993;79:422–434.

23. Usubiaga J. Neurological complications following epidural anesthesia. *Int Anesthesiol Clin* 1975;13:39–45.

24. Vandermeulen E, Van Aken H, Vermylen J. Anticoagulants and spinal-epidural anesthesia. *Anesth Analg* 1994;79:1165–1177.

25. Fox J. Spinal and epidural anesthesia and anticoagulation. *Int Anesthesiol Clin* 2001;39:51–61.

26. Wu CL. Regional anesthesia and anticoagulation. *J Clin Anesth* 2001; 13:49–58.

27. Horlocker T, Wedel D. Neuraxial block and low molecular weight heparin: Balancing perioperative analgesia and thrombophylaxis. *Reg Anesth Pain Med* 1998;23:164–177.

28. Lumpkin MM. FDA public health advisory. *Anesthesiology* 1998;88:27A–28A.

29. American Society of Regional Anesthesia: Recommendations for neuraxial anesthesia and anticoagulation. Available at: <http://www.asra.com/items_of_interest/consensus_statements/>

30. Liu S, Mulroy M. Neuraxial anesthesia and analgesia in the presence of standard heparin. *Reg Anesth Pain Med* 1998;23:157–163.

31. Horlocker T, Wedel D. Neuraxial block and low-molecular weight heparin: Balancing perioperative analgesia and thrombophylaxis. *Reg Anesth Pain Med* 1998;23:164–177.

32. Kayser Enneking F, Benzon H. Oral anticoagulants and regional anesthesia: A perspective. *Reg Anesth Pain Med* 1998;23:140–145.

33. Urmey W, Rowlingson L. Do antiplatelet agents contribute to the development of perioperative spinal hematoma? *Reg Anesth Pain Med* 1998; 23:146–151.

34. Rosenquist R, Brown D. Neuraxial bleeding: Fibrinolytics/thrombolytics. *Reg Anesth Pain Med* 1998;23:152–156.

35. Lawton MT, Porter RW, Heiserman JE, et al. Surgical management of spinal epidural hematoma: Relationship between surgical timing and neurological outcome. *J Neurosurg* 1995;83:1–7.

36. Covino BG. Pharmacology of local anaesthetic agents. *Br J Anaesth* 1986;58:701–716.

37. Fleming JA, Byck R, Barash PG. Pharmacology and therapeutic applications of cocaine. *Anesthesiology* 1990;73:518–531.

38. McClure JH. Ropivacaine. *Br J Anaesth* 1996;76:300–307.

39. Foster RH, Markham A. Levobupivacaine: A review of its pharmacology and use as a local anaesthetic. *Drugs* 2000;59:551–579.

40. Gristwood RW. Cardiac and CNS toxicity of levobupivacaine: Strengths of evidence for advantage over bupivacaine. *Drug Saf* 2002;25:153–163.

41. Felsby S, Juelsgaard P. Combined spinal and epidural anesthesia. *Anesth Analg* 1995;80:821–826.

42. Dershwitz M, Randel GI, Rosow CE, et al. Initial clinical experience with remifentanil, a new opioid metabolized by esterases. *Anesth Analg* 1995;81:619–623.

43. Cheng DCH. Fast track cardiac surgery pathways: Early extubation, process of care, and cost containment. *Anesthesiology* 1998;88:1429–1433.

44. Prough DS, Roy R, Bumgarner J, et al. Acute pulmonary edema in healthy teenagers following conservative doses of intravenous naloxone. *Anesthesiology* 1984;60:485–486.

45. Johnson C, Mayer P, Grosz D. Pulmonary edema following naloxone administration in a healthy orthopedic patient. *J Clin Anesth* 1995;7:356–357.

46. Azar I, Turndorf H. Severe hypertension and multiple atrial premature contractions following naloxone administration. *Anesth Analg* 1979;58:524–525.

47. Andree RA. Sudden death following naloxone administration. *Anesth Analg* 1980;59:782–784.

48. Ewalenko P, Janny S, Dejonckheere M, et al. Antiemetic effect of subhypnotic doses of propofol after thyroidectomy. *Br J Anaesth* 1996; 77:463–467.

49. Reich DL, Silvay G. Ketamine: An update on the first 25 years of clinical experience. *Can J Anaesth* 1989;36:186–197.

50. Flacke JW. Alpha₂-adrenergic agonists in cardiovascular anesthesia. *J Cardiothorac Vasc Anesth* 1992;6:344–359.

51. Maze M, Tranquilli W. Alpha₂-agonists: Defining the role in clinical anesthesia. *Anesthesiology* 1991;74:581–605.

52. Konstadt SN, Reich DL, Thys DM. Nitrous oxide does not exacerbate pulmonary hypertension or ventricular dysfunction in patients with mitral valvular disease. *Can J Anaesth* 1990;37:613–617.

53. Stowe DF, Monroe SM, Marijic J, et al. Comparison of halothane, enflurane, and isoflurane with nitrous oxide on contractility and oxygen supply and demand in isolated hearts. *Anesthesiology* 1991;75:1062–1074.

54. Buffington CW, Romson JL, Levine A, et al. Isoflurane induces coronary steal in a canine model of chronic coronary occlusion. *Anesthesiology* 1987;66:280–292.

55. Reiz S, Balfors E, Sorensen MB, et al. Isoflurane: A powerful coronary vasodilator in patients with coronary artery disease. *Anesthesiology* 1983;59:91–97.

56. Pulley DD, Kirvassilis GV, Kelermenos N, et al. Regional and global myocardial circulatory and metabolic effects of isoflurane and halothane in patients with steal-prone coronary anatomy. *Anesthesiology* 1991;75:756–766.

57. Priebe HJ. Isoflurane and coronary hemodynamics. *Anesthesiology* 1989;71:960–976.

58. Weiskopf RB, Eger EI II, Noorani M, et al. Fentanyl, esmolol, and clonidine blunt the transient cardiovascular stimulation induced by desflurane in humans. *Anesthesiology* 1994;81:1350–1355.

59. Epstein RH, Stein AL, Marr AT, et al. High concentration versus incremental induction of anesthesia with sevoflurane in children: A comparison of induction times, vital signs, and complications. *J Clin Anesth* 1998;10:41–45.

60. Ebert TJ, Harkin CP, Muzi M. Cardiovascular responses to sevoflurane: A review. *Anesth Analg* 1995;81(6 suppl):S11–S22.

61. Thomson IR, Putnins CL. Adverse effects of pancuronium during high-dose fentanyl anesthesia for coronary artery bypass grafting. *Anesthesiology* 1985;62:708–713.

62. De Witte J, Sessler DI. Perioperative shivering: Physiology and pharmacology. *Anesthesiology* 2002;96:467–484.

63. Frank SM, Fleisher LA, Breslow MJ, et al. Perioperative maintenance of normothermia reduces the incidence of morbid cardiac events. A randomized clinical trial. *JAMA* 1997;277:1127–1134.

64. Mangano DT, Layug EL, Wallace A, et al. Effect of atenolol on mortality and cardiovascular morbidity after noncardiac surgery. Multicenter Study of Perioperative Ischemia Research Group. *N Engl J Med* 1996; 335:1713–1720.

PART FOURTEEN

MISCELLANEOUS CONDITIONS AND CARDIOVASCULAR DISEASE

THE CONNECTIVE TISSUE DISEASES AND THE CARDIOVASCULAR SYSTEM

William C. Roberts / Robert A. O'Rourke / Jose F. Roldan

The designation of *connective tissue disease* applies to both a group of heritable conditions and a group of nonheritable acquired disorders. The heritable disorders of connective tissue associated with cardiovascular disease include the Marfan syndrome (MS), Ehlers-Danlos syndrome (EDS), pseudoxanthoma elasticum (PXE), osteogenesis imperfecta (OI), annuloaortic ectasia, and familial aneurysms.[1] The nonheritable disorders of connective tissue that may have major cardiovascular involvement include systemic lupus erythematosus (SLE), polyarteritis nodosa (PN), rheumatoid arthritis (RA), ankylosing spondylitis, systemic sclerosis (SS), polymyositis and dermatomyositis, giant-cell arteritis, Churg-Strauss syndrome, antiphospholipid syndrome, and possibly syphilis.

HERITABLE CONNFCTIVE TISSUE DISEASES

Marfan Syndrome

EPIDEMIOLOGY

The prevalence of classic MS is about 5 per 100,000, without gender, racial, or ethnic predilection. Because of the great heterogeneity of the syndrome, the actual prevalence may be considerably greater, probably about 1 per 10,000.[2] MS has an autosomal dominant inheritance with high penetrance. In about 25 to 30 percent of patients, the disorder occurs without a positive family history and appears to be due to a new mutation.

MOLECULAR GENETICS

MS is associated with defects in the fibrillin-1 gene (FBN1) on chromosome 15, where 125 reported and unreported mutations (of several types) have been described[3–5] (see Chap. 72). Nearly every genotyped family has a unique mutation in the fibrillin genes, with the most common single mutation identified in just four unrelated pedigrees. This intragenic heterogenicity and the large size of the gene have precluded the routine screening of mutations to establish the diagnosis of the MS.

CLINICAL FEATURES

There is considerable variation in the clinical manifestations of MS, even within the same family. The ocular, skeletal, and cardiovascular systems are characteristically involved. The four major manifestations include a positive family history, ectopia lentis, aortic root dilatation or dissection, and dural ectasia. Many of the other, relatively mild features of MS occur with a relatively high prevalence in the general population. These features include mitral valve prolapse (MVP), early myopia, scoliosis, and joint hypermobility. Other manifestations of MS include anterior chest deformity, especially asymmetric pectus excavatum or carinatum; long, thin extremities (dolichostenomelia) with arachnodactyly; tall stature with increased lower body height (Fig. 12-7); high, narrowly arched palate; myopia; fusiform ascending aortic aneurysm (*anuloaortic ectasia*) with aortic regurgitation (AR; Fig. 84-1); and/or aortic dissection. Mitral regurgitation is due to a variety of causes, including MVP, dilatation of the mitral annulus, mitral annular calcium, rupture of mitral chordae tendineae, papillary muscle dysfunction, or infective endocarditis.[1,2]

In the absence of an unequivocally affected first-degree relative, requirements for the diagnosis include at least one major manifestation with involvement of the skeleton and at least two other systems.[5,6] In the presence of at least one unequivocally affected first-degree relative, there should be involvement of at least two systems; the presence of a major manifestation is still preferred, but this can vary depending on the family's phenotype.[5]

By echocardiogram, MVP occurs in nearly 60 percent of adults and aortic root enlargement in about 70 percent of adults with the MS.[7–9] It has been suggested that the MS and MVP are part of a phenotypic continuum.[9]

GENERAL EVALUATION

In addition to carefully recording the personal and family history and physical examination, the patient's height, arm span, and floor-to-pelvis distance should be measured. A slit-lamp ophthalmic examination and an electrocardiogram should be obtained. Patients with

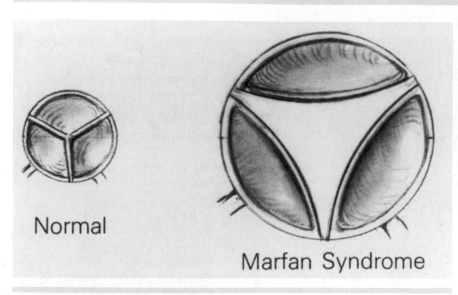

Normal

Marfan Syndrome

FIGURE 84-1 Mechanism of AR in the Marfan syndrome.

MS should be seen at least yearly, and a transthoracic echocardiogram (TTE) should be obtained annually. Consideration should be given to obtaining a transesophageal echocardiogram (TEE) or magnetic resonance imaging (MRI).[10] If the diagnosis is definite or probable, consideration should be given to screening first-degree relatives by TTE. Genetic counseling should be offered to all patients. Psychiatric counseling also is often useful. If a patient develops suggestive widening of the proximal aorta, repeat TTE or, in some instances, TEE should be performed more frequently. Patients with possible or definite MS and evidence of mitral valve abnormality should receive standard antibiotic prophylaxis prior to any surgical procedure (see Chap. 81).

MANAGEMENT

Patients with MS should avoid isometric, abrupt, or strenuous exertion; contact sports; scuba diving; and trauma. Patients with aortic dilatation and AR or MR should avoid competitive sports.[11,12] Patients without aortic dilatation and AR or MR should be allowed to perform low-to-moderate intensity static and low-intensity dynamic sports, including bowling, golf, and archery. Beta-adrenergic blockade therapy should be used in all patients including children with MS to retard the rate of dilatation of the aortic root.[13,14] Although the optimal dose has not been established, some have suggested giving the largest dose that is clinically tolerated. Selective beta$_1$-adrenergic blocking agents are preferred, although no randomized studies have been performed. Atenolol, which should be administered twice daily, appears to be the most widely used beta-adrenergic blocker in this condition.

In asymptomatic patients, repair of aortic aneurysms has been recommended at different degrees of enlargement. Thus, some have advocated repair when the aortic diameter is 55 mm or greater, when it is 60 mm or greater,[15] or when the aortic diameter increases to twice that of the uninvolved distal aorta. Some patients develop aortic dissection with aortic root dimensions less than 50 to 55 mm.[16] Surgical repair is generally recommended when the diameter reaches 55 to 60 mm.

The asymmetry of the aortic root recognized by MRI might be of clinical importance in the diagnosis of unexpected aortic root dissection.[17]

Factors resulting in earlier surgical intervention include a positive family history for aortic dissection or rupture, severe AR or MR, progressive dilatation of the aortic root on serial echocardiograms, need

for other major abdominal aortic or spinal surgical procedures, and planning for a pregnancy. In most patients, the ascending aorta and aortic valve are replaced, and the portion of the aorta containing the coronary ostia is reimplanted,[18] but there are exceptions.[19] Coronary ostial aneurysms have been in 43 percent of 40 patients with MS after coronary artery implantation.[20] Postoperatively annual assessment of the entire aorta by MRI may be useful.

In patients who require a mitral valve procedure, valve repair is usually preferred to replacement, although repair may not always be possible because of a large number of ruptured chordae tendineae, extensive annular calcium, or greatly dilated annuli.[11]

PROGNOSIS

While earlier studies indicated that the average patient's lifetime is decreased by about 35 percent,[2,12] beta-blocker therapy, antibiotic prophylaxis (against infective endocarditis), and aortic and valvular surgery have probably improved longevity. The most common causes of death of adolescents or adults with MS are rupture of a fusiform aneurysm of the ascending aorta without longitudinal dissection (Fig. 84-2), ascending aortic dissection with rupture, or congestive heart failure from AR and/or MR[16] (Fig. 84-3). The major histologic feature in the media of the wall of an aortic aneurysm is a massive loss of elastic fibers[16] (Fig. 84-4). Factors that can predispose to either aortic aneurysm or aortic dissection include systemic arterial hypertension, coarctation of the aorta, pregnancy, and trauma. In children with MS, the most common cause of death is severe MR (Fig. 84-5).

PREGNANCY

Women with MS should be counseled regarding the approximately 50 percent risk of genetic transmission of the condition. If the woman has moderate or severe AR or an aortic root diameter exceeding 40 mm, she should be advised that pregnancy greatly increases her risk of premature death. Women with an aortic root diameter of less than 40 mm usually tolerate pregnancy well, but nevertheless the chance of aortic dissection is increased by pregnancy. Beta-adrenergic blockers should be administered at least from the midtrimester onward. There may be an advantage in the use of a selective beta$_1$-adrenergic blocker.

During pregnancy, TTE should be performed every 6 to 10 weeks, depending on the initial findings. Using epidural anesthesia, vaginal delivery in the lateral decubitus position is preferred, and forceps or vacuum delivery is recommended to shorten the second stage of labor. The increases in systemic blood pressure during uterine contractions should be prevented with beta-blocking agents. Postpartum hemorrhage should be anticipated. If fetal maturity can be confirmed in a patient who requires aortic surgery during pregnancy, a Cesarean section can be done before or concomitantly with thoracic surgery.

Ehlers-Danlos Syndrome

EDS is a heterogeneous group of several disorders of connective tissue that are characterized primarily by skin fragility, easy bruising, "cigarette paper" scars, skin hyperextensibility, multiple ecchy-

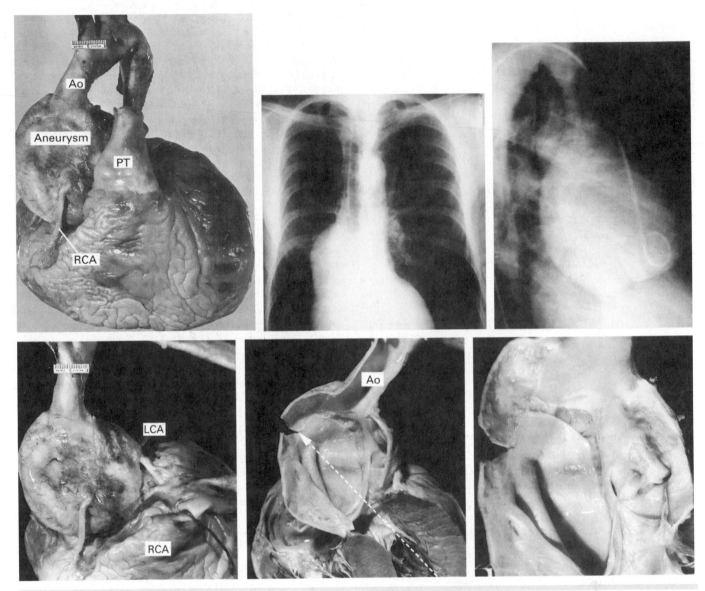

FIGURE 84-2 Heart and aorta of a 38-year-old man who was asymptomatic until exertional dyspnea appeared 5 months before death. Top left: Exterior view. Ao, ascending aorta; RCA, right coronary artery; PT, pulmonary trunk. Bottom left: Closer view of the massive aortic aneurysm after retracting the pulmonary trunk. LCA, left main coronary artery. The aneurysm does not involve the distal portion of the ascending aorta. Bottom middle: View of heart and aorta after removing their anterior half. Death resulted from rupture of the right lateral wall of the aorta at a point where blood ejected from left ventricular contacts with the aortic wall (arrow). The aneurysmal bulge is mainly to the right. Bottom right: Close-up of the multiple healed tears in the ascending aorta. One of the previously incomplete tears ruptured through and through. Posteroanterior chest roentgenogram (top middle) and lateral aortogram (top right) show massive dilatation of the ascending aorta. (From Roberts and Honig.[16] Reproduced with permission of the publisher and authors.)

moses, and joint hypermobility[1] (Fig. 12-5). Because of the complexity of previous classifications, in 1997 a new simplified classification divided EDS in 6 clinical types:[21] (1) classical, (2) hypermobility, (3) vascular, (4) kyphoscoliosis, (5) arthrochalasia, and (6) dermatosparaxis.

The numerous types of the EDS have different clinical manifestations, modes of inheritance, and natural history (see Chap. 72). In vascular type III EDS, the heart, heart valves, great vessels, and larger conduit arteries may be involved. Cardiovascular abnormalities in the EDS include: spontaneous rupture of the aorta or large arteries, coronary or intracranial aneurysms, arteriovenous fistulae, mitral and tricuspid valve prolapse, dilatation of the aortic root, ectasia of the sinuses of Valsalva, AR, renal artery aneurysms, systemic arterial hypertension, and myocardial infarction.[21,22,22a,23]

Pseudoxanthoma Elasticum

PXE is a rare heritable disorder that is characterized by the progressive accumulation of mineral precipitants within elastic fibers, particularly those of the skin, Bruch's membrane, and blood vessels. It is transmitted either as an autosomal recessive or as an autosomal dominant trait.[1,24] The estimated prevalence is 1 in 160,000 (see Chap. 72).

The elastic fiber changes cause skin, eye, gastrointestinal, and cardiovascular manifestations. The skin lesions have been described as resembling a "plucked chicken." Typically, there are yellow macules or papules that produce a rough, cobblestone texture and are maximal in the flexures of the lateral neck, axillae, antecubital fossae, groins, and popliteal spaces. They may form redundant folds

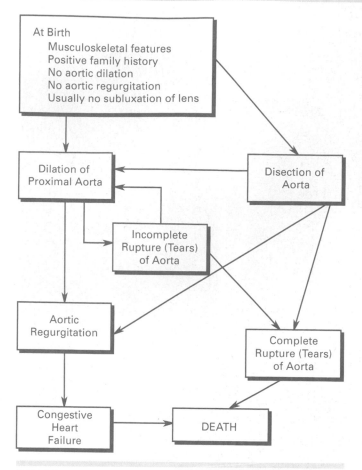

FIGURE 84-3 Scheme of development of cardiovascular complications in the Marfan syndrome. (From Roberts and Honig.[16] Reproduced with permission of the publisher and authors.)

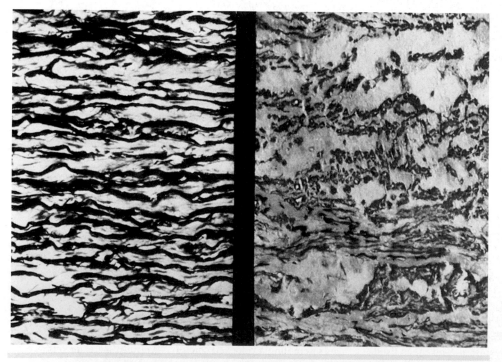

FIGURE 84-4 Left: Photomicrograph of the wall of the ascending aorta from a normal subject. Right: A similar histologic study (Movat stains) of the wall of an ascending aortic aneurysm in a 35-year-old woman with the Marfan syndrome. Note the virtual absence of elastic fibers. (From Roberts and Honig.[16] Reproduced with permission of the publisher and authors.)

of skin[1] (Fig. 12-6). The retinal changes include mottled *peau d'orange* hyperpigmentation, angioid streaks, and an increased incidence of retinal hemorrhage and disk drusen. Angioid streaks, which are breaks in Bruch's membrane behind the retina and present in 85 percent of patients with PXE, usually develop after the second decade of life. They can be found in numerous other conditions, including MS, EDS, Paget's disease, and sickle cell anemia, although PXE is most common.

It is now recognized that a mutation in the gene ABCC6 (R1141X) is associated with an increased incidence of coronary artery disease (CAD) in patients with PXE. In an study of 441 patients the odds ratio for a coronary event was 4.23 [confidence interval (CI): 1.76 to 10.20, $p = 0.001$].[24]

There may be calcific deposits in the media of medium-sized arteries. Both vascular deposits similar to Mönckeberg's arteriosclerosis and intimal plaques similar to typical atherosclerotic plaques occur in the coronary, cerebral, gastrointestinal, renal, and peripheral arteries. Angina pectoris and myocardial infarction may occur.[25]

Infrequent but fairly specific lesions in PXE are calcific deposits in the mural endocardium of the cardiac ventricles, atria, and atrioventricular valves. Both mitral stenosis and MVP also have been described in PXE. Surgery to remove mural endocardial calcific deposits has been performed with fair results.[26] Bleeding may occur in the gastrointestinal system, uterus, joints, and urinary bladder. Some bleeding complications may be prevented by avoiding aspirin, and coronary artery bypass surgery arterial grafts should not be used because of possible calcification of the internal elastic laminae.

Osteogenesis Imperfecta

OI, also known as *brittle bone disease* because of the susceptibility of affected individuals to sustain fractures from mild trauma, is a rare heritable disorder of connective tissue. The gene prevalence of OI is calculated as 4 to 5 per 100,000 persons; it is inherited in an autosomal dominant fashion with variable penetrance. More than 80 different mutations have been identified in the genes for either of the two chains that form type I collagen, which is the major structural protein of the extracellular matrix of bone, skin, and tendon. There is a wide variation in the clinical severity of OI, from some forms that are lethal in the perinatal period to other forms that may not be detected.[27] Most manifestations of OI are bony, ocular, otologic, cutaneous, and dental. The bony changes manifest themselves in a variety of ways, including short stature, in utero fractures, severe osteoporosis, and severe bone fragility, with repeated fractures and bowing of long bones. The ocular and otologic changes include blue sclerae, angioid streaks in the retina, and hearing loss. Cutaneous and dental changes result in easy bruising and occasional dentinogenesis imperfecta. An increased risk of bleeding may also be present. A major advance in the treatment of bone manifestations of OI is the use of cyclic administration of biphosphonates.[28]

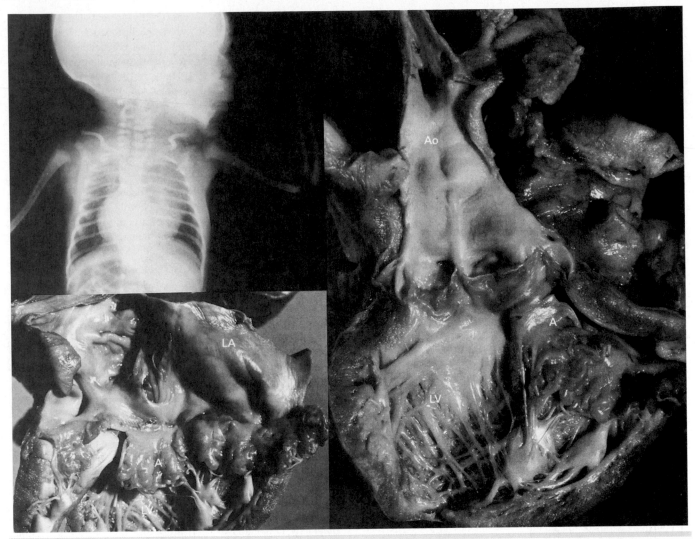

FIGURE 84-5 Congenital floppy mitral valve and floppy tricuspid valve in a 2-day-old boy who had long toes and fingers, a high-arched palate, and a grade 3/6 precordial systolic murmur typical of MR. The heart was enlarged (top left), and he died of congestive cardiac failure. At necropsy, the intima of the ascending aorta (Ao) was wrinkled (right), suggesting that the underlying media was abnormal at this early stage. Shown here are the opened aorta, aortic valve, and left ventricle (LV). A, anterior mitral leaflet. Bottom left: Opened left atrium (LA), mitral valve, and LV (LV). The mitral leaflets are considerably elongated in both longitudinal and transverse dimensions. The left atrium is dilated. (From Roberts and Honig.[16] Reproduced with permission of the publisher and author.)

The cardiovascular manifestations include AR,[27] aortic root dilatation,[27] aortic dissection,[29] and MR.[30] Mitral valve repair and reconstruction are occasionally feasible for patients with severe MR, although most patients require valve replacement. Mitral valve replacement is difficult because of weakness and friability of the tissues and poor wound healing. In addition, some patients have increased bleeding despite normal preoperative coagulation tests and bleeding times.[27,31]

Annuloaortic Ectasia

Annuloaortic ectasia, a pear-shaped enlargement of the sinus and the proximal tubular portions of the ascending aorta, is often part of MS, where it usually results in AR, partial or complete ascending aortic tears, or both. In some patients, annuloaortic ectasia is familial and no other stigmata of MS are present.[32] The genetic and molecular changes in these patients are not established. Microscopically, there is severe loss of elastic fibers in the media of the ascending aorta.

Familial Aneurysms

Various types of familial aneurysms involving cardiovascular structures have been reported, including familial aortic dissection,[33] familial aneurysms of the ventricular septum,[34] familial aneurysms of the carotid arteries,[35] and familial intracranial aneurysms.[36] At this time, it is not established that these are heritable disorders of connective tissue.

Homocystinuria

See Chap. 72.

NONHERITABLE CONNECTIVE TISSUE DISEASES

The acquired or nonheritable autoimmune or connective tissue diseases represent a subset of the arthritides and rheumatic disorders. These disorders are systemic in nature, are commonly linked by a

TABLE 84-1 Primary Cardiac Manifestations of the Nonhereditary Connective Tissue Diseases

Disease	Pericardium	Myocardium	Endocardium (Valves)	Coronary Arteries
Systemic lupus erythematosus	++	+	++	+/−
Systemic sclerosis	+	++	0	++
Polyarteritis nodosa	+/−	+	0	++
Ankylosing spondylitis	0	+/−	++	0
Rheumatoid arthritis	++	+	+	0
Polymyositis/dermatomyositis	++	++	+/−	+/−

NOTE: ++, major site of involvement; +, may be involved, but less frequently; +/−, rarely involved; 0, not involved.

diffuse abnormality of vasculature, and are characterized by inflammatory lesions in skin, joints, muscles, and connective tissue linings such as pleura and pericardium. Involvement of the kidneys, brain, and heart is usually responsible for the fatal and most serious consequences. Specific acquired connective tissue diseases that may have major cardiac involvement include SLE, PN, giant-cell arteritis, RA, ankylosing spondylitis, polymyositis and dermatomyositis, SS, and, possibly, syphilis (Table 84-1). Although certain immunogenetic factors have been identified, their etiology remains uncertain.[37]

Systemic Lupus Erythematosus

SLE, which is one of the more common autoimmune diseases, is found worldwide and affects all races, is more common among blacks and females of childbearing age, and is usually more severe in blacks than it is in whites. SLE is much more frequent among females and in patients less than 40 years of age. The female–male ratio is about 8:1. In the United States, the annual incidence of SLE is about 8 per 100,000 and the prevalence is approximately 1 per 2000.[38] The following genes of the human major histocompatibility locus antigens are associated with an increased risk for SLE: HLA-B8, HLA-DR2, HLA-DR3, HLA-DR5, HLA-DR7, HLA-DQ, and null alleles at the C2 and/or C4 loci. Genetic deficiencies of the complement system—i.e., deficiencies of C1q, C2, C4, and C8—predispose individuals to SLE and SLE-like disorders (see Chap. 72).

The inflammatory process of SLE involves multiple organ systems, including skin, joints, kidneys, brain, heart, and virtually all serous membranes. Its clinical presentation is varied and depends on the organ systems involved. Fever, arthritis and arthralgias, skin rashes (Fig. 12-21), and pleuritis are common early signs of SLE.

The immunologic abnormalities of SLE have been well characterized and enable it to be diagnosed despite the diversity of clinical presentations. Typical serologic abnormalities include the presence of antinuclear antibodies (ANAs), positive serum anti-DNA antibodies, positive anti-Smith antibodies, positive anti-ribonucleoprotein (anti-RNP) antibodies, and hypocomplementemia, i.e., low serum C3 and C4 (see Chap. 72). Less specific but frequently identified antibodies include anticytoplasmic antibodies, anticardiolipin (IgGaCL) antibodies, antiphospholipid (aPL) antibodies, and rheumatoid factor. Serum complement is decreased in most patients with SLE, and, insofar as serum complement is usually normal or elevated in other connective tissue disorders (such as RA, PN, SS, and disseminated infections), this serologic test may be useful in the diagnosis of SLE.[38] Certain patients with SLE are more likely to have elevated levels of aPL antibody, particularly those with recurrent venous thrombosis, thrombocytopenia, recurrent fetal loss, hemolytic

anemia, livedo reticularis, leg ulcers, arterial occlusions, transverse myelitis, or pulmonary hypertension.[39] Cardiac abnormalities may occur more frequently in patients with increased aPL or anticardiolipin antibody titers.[37]

Although it may have an acute, fulminating course, SLE most often is characterized by a chronic course marked with exacerbations and remissions; the 10-year survival rate exceeds 80 percent. Nephritis and seizures decrease survival approximately twofold.[40] When patients die of SLE, it is most often in the setting of acute renal failure, central nervous system disease, associated infection, infective endocarditis, or coronary artery disease (see later).

CARDIAC INVOLVEMENT

Probably about 25 percent of patients with SLE have cardiac involvement.[41] In addition to the valvular thickening or verrucae and MR or AR (or occasional stenosis), there may be pericardial thickening and/or effusion, left ventricular regional or global systolic or diastolic dysfunction, or evidence of pulmonary hypertension.[41] Either valvular regurgitation or stenosis due to SLE can require valve replacement.[41] It is unclear whether cardiac abnormalities are significantly more frequent in patients with elevated titers of aPL antibodies.[42–45] In general, valve disease in SLE is frequent but apparently independent of the presence or absence of aPL antibodies.

PERICARDITIS

SLE may cause a pancarditis with abnormalities of pericardium, endocardium, myocardium, and coronary arteries. Pericardial involvement is the most frequent, as observed clinically, by echocardiography, or at autopsy.[41] Pericardial effusions occur at some point in over one half of the patients with active SLE. Signs of active or acute pericardial disease may precede (about 5 percent) the other clinical signs of SLE.[41] In most SLE patients, the pericardial involvement is clinically silent and, when present, runs a benign course. Pericardial tamponade may occur and should be considered in patients with unexplained signs of venous congestion.[41] On rare occasions, SLE pericardial disease may lead to pericardial constriction or to acute cardiac tamponade.[41,46] Although the size of the pericardial effusion usually is not sufficiently large to allow aspiration, serologic studies of the pericardial fluid can be useful in diagnosing pericardial effusions due to SLE.

The most common type of pericardial disease in SLE is the presence of diffuse or focal adhesions or fibrinous deposits.[41] The pericardial fluid usually contains mononuclear leukocytes and occasionally lupus erythematosus (LE) cells. In patients with long-standing SLE treated with anti-inflammatory agents, pericardial abnormalities appear to occur with the same frequency as in patients not receiving these agents, but at autopsy the involvement is less extensive and more likely to be fibrous rather than fibrinous. SLE patients with fibrinous pericardial disease, particularly those with severe debilitation or renal failure, are at increased risk for purulent pericarditis, which is usually fatal.[41]

ENDOCARDITIS AND VALVE DISEASE

The cardiovascular lesion of SLE that has received the most attention is the *atypical verrucous endocarditis* first described by Libman and

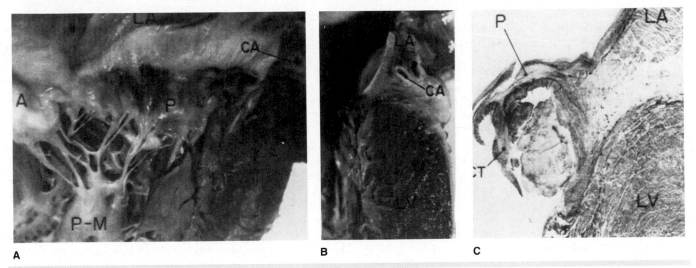

FIGURE 84-6 An example of Libman-Sacks endocarditis in systemic lupus erythematosus. *A* and *B*. The left atrium (LA) and left ventricle (LV) are open. *B* and *C*. Fibrofibrinous verrucae, present on the undersurface of the posterior leaflet (P) of the mitral valve, are often clinically silent. A, anterior leaflet of mitral valve; CA, left circumflex coronary artery; P-M, posteromedial papillary muscle; CT, chorda tendineae. H&E, ×8. (From Bulkley and Roberts.[44] Reproduced with permission from the publisher and author.)

Sacks in 1924,[47] long before SLE was recognized as a systemic disease. The lesions, as they were first described and subsequently attributed to SLE,[48] consist almost entirely of fibrin, and although they may occur on both surfaces of any of the four cardiac valves, they are now most frequently found on the left-sided valves, particularly the ventricular surface of the posterior mitral leaflet (Fig. 84-6). These *verrucae* are similar histologically to those of nonbacterial thrombotic noninfective endocarditis, the valve lesion that occurs most frequently in patients with debilitating illnesses or cancer, except that occasionally hematoxylin bodies, considered the histologic counterpart of LE cells, may be found within Libman-Sacks lesions. While valvular verrucae in SLE (Libman-Sacks lesions) are usually clinically silent, they can be dislodged and embolize and can also become infected, producing infective endocarditis.[41,45] It is prudent to recommend antibiotic prophylaxis against infective endocarditis when patients with SLE undergo procedures that may be associated with bacteremia (see Chap. 81).

Echocardiographically, SLE has a characteristic appearance, with leaflet thickening and valve masses[41,45] (see Chap. 15). The end-stage or healed form of the verrucous endocarditis of SLE is a fibrous plaque. In some instances, if the thrombotic lesions are extensive enough, their healing may be accompanied by focal scarring and deformity of the underlying valve tissue. This healed form of SLE "endocarditis" may cause valvular dysfunction, particularly MR and/or AR.[41]

MYOCARDITIS

It is unclear whether infiltration of the myocardial interstitium with acute and/or chronic inflammatory cells and focal myocardial necrosis (i.e., myocarditis) occurs as a natural part of SLE, unassociated with anti-inflammatory drug therapy (glucocorticoid treatment).[41] Several reports have described clinical features consistent with myocarditis, but actual visualization of interstitial myocardial inflammatory cells with associated myofiber necrosis has not been demonstrated histologically. Hemodynamic and echocardiographic studies, however, have shown abnormalities in both systolic and diastolic ventricular function in some SLE patients.[41] Whether these abnormalities result from an *autoimmune attack* on the myocardium or from the effects of systemic arterial hypertension, coronary artery disease, or coexisting pericardial disease is unclear (see later).

CORONARY ARTERY DISEASE

Both fatal and nonfatal acute myocardial infarction and sudden coronary death (without demonstrable infarction) from CAD may occur early in the course of SLE, particularly among young women. Studies of hearts in patients with fatal SLE have demonstrated a high incidence of CAD in patients who received treatment with glucocorticoids for more than 2 years.[41,49,50] Accelerated CAD is increasingly recognized as a leading cause of morbidity and mortality among young women patients with SLE who receive long-term glucocorticoid administration.[41,49] Although the causes of this premature CAD are uncertain, glucocorticoid treatment as well as aPL antibodies have been incriminated. It has been speculated that SLE itself may induce an underlying vasculopathy or arteritis that may facilitate premature atherogenesis from long-term glucocorticoid treatment. Coronary disease in SLE was not described before glucocorticoid therapy was introduced.[41] In one study, the presence of elevated aPL antibodies in patients with SLE correlated with left ventricular (global or segmental) dysfunction, verrucous valvular (aortic or mitral) thickening, and global valvular (mitral or aortic) thickening and dysfunction, as well as MR and AR. Coronary thrombi may occur in patients with active lupus. Acute myocardial infarction may occur in the presence of angiographically normal coronary arteries.[51] SLE also may cause coronary aneurysm;[52] aPL antibodies are known to promote platelet aggregation and to be associated with the presence of a clotting tendency, the so-called lupus anticoagulant syndrome.[42]

Inflammation (arteritis) of the wall of the sinus node artery in association with scarring of both sinus and atrioventricular nodes may account for some of the rhythm and conduction disturbances seen in these patients.[53]

PREGNANCY AND THE NEONATAL LUPUS SYNDROME

Neonatal LE is a rare disorder that arises when the so-called anti-Ro, or Sjögren's (SSA) autoantibodies—mostly immunoglobulin G (IgG)—are formed and circulate in pregnant patients, cross the placenta, and cause a lupus-like syndrome in newborns with the appearance of a skin rash and transient cytopenias from passively acquired maternal autoantibodies. Since the half-life of IgG antibodies is approximately 21 to 25 days, the neonatal lupus syndrome in newborn babies is self-limiting; it usually resolves in 3 to 6 months when all of the IgG-containing anti-Ro maternal autoantibodies have been cleared from the neonate's circulation.[53a] An unfortunate exception is complete congenital heart block, which may require the implantation of a pacemaker. Once complete heart block occurs, it is usually irreversible. One neonate has been described with first-degree heart block at birth that resolved 6 months later. Antibodies to the Ro (SSA) ribonucleoprotein complexes are present in over 85 percent of sera from mothers of infants with complete congenital heart block. In many patients, antibodies reactive to the La (SSB) antigen as well as the U1RNP protein particle are found in association with anti-Ro (SSA) antibodies.

In most cases, the neonatal lupus syndrome is a benign disorder, and most babies of mothers with anti-Ro (SSA), anti-La (SSB), or anti-U1RNP antibodies do not develop neonatal lupus. *A pregnant woman with SLE with positive anti-Ro, anti-La, or anti-RNP antibodies has a less than 3 percent risk of having a child with neonatal lupus and congenital heart block. The risk that this patient might have an infant with neonatal lupus syndrome but without congenital heart block may be as high as 1 in 3.* The neonatal lupus syndrome mediated by the presence of maternal anti-Ro antibodies can occur in babies of mothers who do not have overt SLE, who may or may not meet criteria for a diagnosis of SLE, and who may or may not have a positive test for antinuclear antibodies.[53a]

Neonatal lupus syndrome with congenital heart block can be diagnosed by the appearance of fetal bradycardia around week 23 of gestation.[51–53] The cardiac damage with conduction abnormalities in a neonate may result from binding of the passively transferred pathogenic anti-Ro antibodies to Ro (SSA)/La (SSB) antigens present in the fetal heart. It is not known whether these IgG anti-Ro antibodies represent *clinical markers* only or whether they are pathogenic. All mothers of neonates with complete congenital heart block have been HLA-DR3 positive. If a mother is HLA-DR3 positive and has circulating IgG anti-Ro antibodies, her neonate is at risk regardless of the neonate's HLA-DR status.

Other cardiac abnormalities reported in neonatal lupus syndrome include right bundle branch block, second-degree atrioventricular block, 2:1 atrioventricular block, patent ductus arteriosus, patent foramen ovale, coarctation of the aorta, tetralogy of Fallot, atrial septal defect, hypoplastic right ventricle, ventricular septal defect, dysplastic pulmonic valve, mitral and tricuspid regurgitation, pericarditis, and myocarditis. Most of these patients eventually have a pacemaker inserted.

Pregnant women with SLE should have a serum anti-Ro (SSA) antibody determination as early in pregnancy as possible. Prenatal treatment of established congenital heart block has consisted of the administration of prednisone or dexamethasone and plasmapheresis from week 23 on, although heart block has persisted in most cases.[53a] It is unclear whether aggressive anti-inflammatory therapy in an effort to diminish the generalized fetal insult and to lower the titers of circulating anti-Ro (SSA) antibodies makes a difference in fetal cardiac outcome. Fetal echocardiography is useful in following the progression of the disease and also in helping to identify decreased left ventricular contractility, increased cardiac size, tricuspid regurgitation, and pericardial effusion.

Neither dexamethasone nor plasmapheresis has had much success in reversing intrauterine third-degree heart block. Glucocorticoids, however, may be helpful in suppressing an associated inflammatory response producing pleuropericardial effusions or ascites in the fetus.

Close monitoring of the clinical course in the prospective mother is also essential because of the risk of exacerbation of the SLE. If fetal bradycardia is present, an *intrauterine therapeutic approach* for as long as possible is recommended to allow for fetal maturation to occur. Ultrasound images can be useful for assessing the degree of cardiac dysfunction present. Following delivery, the neonatologist should be prepared to have a cardiac pacemaker implanted. Otherwise, all of the other clinical and laboratory features of the neonatal lupus syndrome (with the exception of complete heart block and/or similar severe cardiac fetal disease) should slowly and gradually disappear over the first few months of the baby's life. In one study, one-third of the children with autoantibody-associated congenital heart block died in the early neonatal period[54]; most survivors required a pacemaker.

Women with SLE who are anti-Ro positive should be closely monitored during pregnancy, as should mothers of previous babies born with congenital complete heart block. Pregnant patients who are anti-Ro positive and whose babies have not had fetal bradycardia throughout most of the pregnancy should be reminded that congenital complete heart block is rare and that the neonatal cutaneous lupus syndrome is benign and transient. The long-term prognosis of mothers of children born with congenital heart block is generally fairly good.[55] In these mothers, the risk of congenital heart block in children of subsequent pregnancies is low.[54] Newborns of mothers with SLE who have a normal pulse rate are unlikely to have significant abnormalities in atrioventricular conduction.[56]

A higher incidence of clinical evidence of myocarditis and conduction defects is found in adult anti-Ro-positive patients with SLE than it is in patients who are anti-Ro negative or in healthy controls.[57] The role of the anti-Ro antibody in inducing heart blocks in adult patients with SLE is unclear.

SECONDARY EFFECTS ON THE HEART

Most of the clinically significant cardiac problems occurring in patients with SLE are secondary. Systemic arterial hypertension is common in patients with SLE, particularly those with renal disease and long-standing glucocorticoid therapy, in whom it is a major cause of cardiac enlargement and heart failure.[41] Pulmonary hypertension is also common, approaching 50 percent in a 5-year follow-up study.[58] Uremic pericarditis may occur, of course, in patients with severe renal failure. Premature or accelerated atherosclerosis has been increasingly recognized in young women with SLE receiving long-term glucocorticoid treatment.[41]

THERAPY

Therapy of cardiovascular SLE is the treatment of the underlying disease and includes nonsteroidal anti-inflammatory drugs (NSAIDs), glucocorticoids, and, in severe cases, cytotoxic agents such as azathioprine and cyclophosphamide. Systemic arterial hypertension, congestive heart failure, and arrhythmias should be treated with standard therapeutic measures. SLE-induced valve disease can require valve replacement.[41,59,60] Pericardial tamponade may require either high-dose steroids, pericardiocentesis, or placement of a pericardial window, but recurrent effusions or pericardial thickening may develop. Premature cardiovascular events from accelerated atherosclerosis may result in sudden death or myocardial infarction.[41] The antimalarial agent hydroxychloroquine lowers serum cholesterol levels in patients with SLE[61] and may decrease myocardial ischemic damage.[62] An antimalarial such as hydroxychloroquine may be beneficial as a prophylactic agent to prevent premature or accelerated atherosclerosis in young women with SLE receiving long-term treatment with glucocorticoids. Although there are no studies documenting benefit, low-dose aspirin and hydroxychloroquine are often utilized in SLE patients receiving long-term glucocorticoid therapy.

Rheumatoid Arthritis

RA, the most common of the connective tissue diseases, is characterized by its deforming erosions of the joints; these erosions result from chronic synovial inflammation and proliferation. Joint symptoms dominate its course, and symmetric involvement of the hands and wrists is most common. Other joints of the upper and lower extremities and the temporomandibular and sternoclavicular joints also may be affected. The most common systemic or extraarticular manifestations of RA include subcutaneous rheumatoid nodules, weight loss, anemia of chronic disease, and pleuritis. Less frequently, pneumonitis and a necrotizing vasculitis occur in patients with severe long-standing disease. Contrary to prior epidemiologic studies, new data support increased mortality in RA.[63]

A prospective cohort study comparing the incidence of myocardial infarction and cerebrovascular events between RA patients and non-RA patients with known CAD found that the RA patients had a greater incidence of vascular events and mortality.[64] Atherosclerosis also appears to occur at an accelerated rate in RA. There is a strong correlation between the presence of inflammatory biochemical markers and carotid atherosclerotic plaques.[65]

PERICARDIAL INVOLVEMENT

Cardiac involvement is uncommon in RA but exists in a variety of forms. A diffuse, nonspecific fibrofibrinous pericarditis occurs in about 50 percent of patients with RA; it is usually clinically silent and is overshadowed by pleuritis or joint pain.[66,67] The pericardial disease tends to be benign, but sizable effusions can occur and require pericardiocentesis, and pericardial constriction can rarely necessitate pericardiectomy. Constrictive pericarditis occurred in 4 of 47 patients with RA whose cases were followed over a 10-year period.[68] The histopathologic findings after pericardiectomy were consistent with chronic fibrosing pericardial disease. In another report, RA patients with constrictive pericarditis had a longer disease course, more severe disease, worse functional class, and more extraarticular features when compared with RA patients without cardiac constriction.[69] The presenting clinical features of cardiac constriction included dyspnea, edema, chest pain, and pulsus paradoxus. Chronic, symptomatic pericarditis may require glucocorticoid therapy. RA pericardial disease may shorten survival, especially in older patients[70] and be associated with the presence of other cardiac disease, a greater number of extraarticular manifestations, jugular venous distension, and a lower mean systemic blood pressure. Lymphocytic infiltrates of the CD8-positive type may occur in the pericardium of patients with rheumatoid pericardial disease, suggesting that these cells may play a role in the development of the pericardial disease[71] (see Chap. 80).

MYOCARDIAL AND ENDOCARDIAL INVOLVEMENT

Rarely, rheumatoid nodules focally infiltrate the heart, including the myocardium and the four cardiac valves (Fig. 84-7).[66] These nodules may produce no symptoms, but, if extensive enough or strategically located, they can compromise cardiac function. A rheumatoid nodule may extend from the mural endocardium into a chamber to present as an intracavitary mass.[72] Rheumatoid nodules developing within the valve leaflets may result in mild valvular regurgitation; if the nodule becomes necrotic, perforation of the leaflet can occur and lead to severe valvular regurgitation. The incidence of such valvular infiltration has been estimated at 1 to 2 percent in autopsy studies of patients with RA. Although distinctly uncommon, arrhythmias and conduction

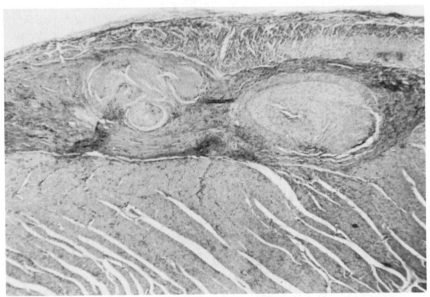

A

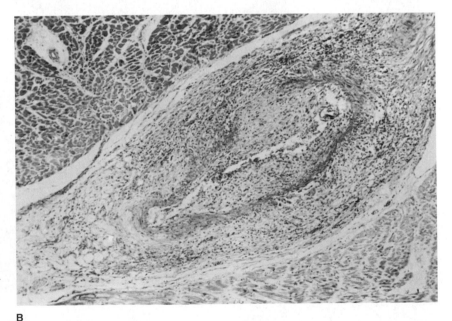

B

FIGURE 84-7 Polyarteritis nodosa. Examples of the necrotizing vasculitis affecting the extramural and intramural coronary arteries in polyarteritis. *A.* Extramural coronary arteries. *B.* Intramural coronary arteries. The intramural artery shows a necrotizing arteritis with inflammation involving the full thickness of the vessel. H&E, top, ×7; bottom, ×22.

disturbances, including complete heart block,[66] and congestive heart failure can also result from RA involvement of the heart. One echocardiographic study of 39 patients with RA detected left ventricular abnormalities in 25 percent of the patients.[73] Acute myocardial infarction may be associated with RA.[74]

THERAPY

Since most of the cardiac lesions of RA are clinically silent, it is not certain that the specific therapies used in RA, including NSAIDs, methotrexate, leflunomide, glucocorticoids and new medications, such as tumor necrosis factor alpha bocker (TNF-alpha) and tumor necrosis alpha antibodies, affect the cardiac involvement. The treatment of cardiac constriction from rheumatoid pericardial disease may include a trial of a high-dose intravenous glucocorticoid (e.g., methylprednisolone) and/or surgical therapy. Pericardiocentesis should be performed only as a lifesaving procedure.[69]

Ankylosing Spondylitis

Ankylosing spondylitis is the prototypical example within the group of the seronegative spondyloarthropathies. It is characterized by a progressive inflammatory lesion of the spine, leading to chronic back pain, deforming dorsal kyphosis (Fig. 12-24), and, in its advanced stage, fusion of the costovertebral and sacroiliac joints with immobilization of the spine. This condition is much more frequent in men than it is in women (9:1), generally first occurring early in life but with a chronic progressive course of 20 to 30 years. The HLA-B27 histocompatibility antigen is found in 90 percent of whites and in 50 percent of black patients with ankylosing spondylitis. HLA-B27 is also associated with other seronegative arthritides such as reactive arthritis (formerly called Reiter's syndrome), Crohn's disease, ulcerative colitis, and psoriatic arthritis.

CARDIAC INVOLVEMENT

Cardiovascular disease in ankylosing spondylitis, seen typically in patients with severe peripheral joint involvement and long-standing disease, takes the form of a sclerosing inflammatory lesion that is generally limited to the aortic root area. The inflammatory process, which extends immediately above and below the aortic valve, typically causes AR[74,75] (Fig. 84-8). As the inflammatory process extends below the aortic valve, it can infiltrate the basal portion of the mitral valve (which is contiguous with the aortic valve) and cause MR.[75] Extension of the inflammatory lesion into the cephalad portion of the ventricular septum, immediately caudal to the aortic valve, accounts for the associated conduction disturbances. Ventricular diastolic dysfunction may also occur.[76]

The major clinical manifestation of ankylosing spondylitis is AR, which occurs in about 5 percent of patients with this condition. Among patients with signs of spondylitis for 10 years, only 2 percent have clinical evidence of AR; by 30 years, that number increases fivefold.[74] Ankylosing spondylitis may be associated with aortic root inflammatory lesions, as may other seronegative spondyloarthropathies such as Reiter's syndrome and psoriatic arthropathy.[74]

THERAPY

Drug therapy for ankylosing spondylitis used to be directed primarily at relief of the back pain and discomfort. The treatment with TNF-alpha has been known to be effective. Patients with long-standing disease tend to be less responsive. It is unknown at this point if the natural history of the disease could be changed with the early introduction of TNF-alpha therapy.[77]

NSAIDs, methotrexate, and sulfasalazine in addition to physical therapy remain the first line of therapy. Glucocorticoids are rarely used in this condition except for treatment of uveitis. The inflammatory lesion of the heart generally runs a clinically silent course until AR develops. Not infrequently, however, the AR of ankylosing spondylitis may become severe enough to warrant aortic valve replacement[74,75] (see Chap. 56).

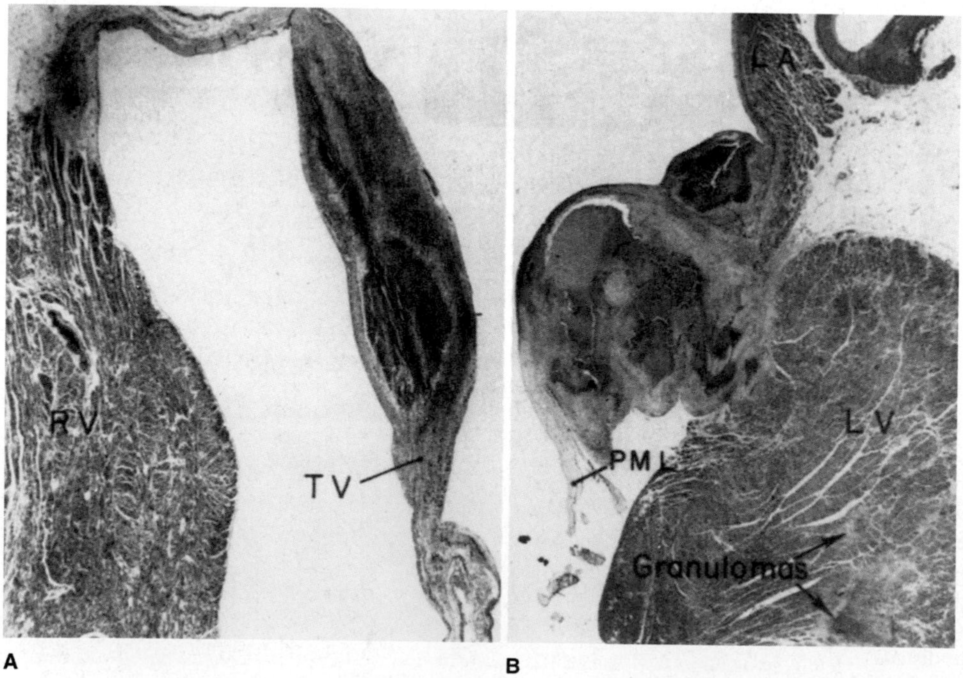

Cardiovascular Syphilis

Although this condition has traditionally not been considered to be a connective tissue disorder, cardiovascular syphilis has histologic features nearly identical to those of ankylosing spondylitis, and spirochetes have never been identified in the aorta of a patient with cardiovascular syphilis.

The distribution of the lesions, however, is distinctly different in these two conditions.[66] In cardiovascular syphilis, the process is usually limited to the tubular portion of the ascending aorta (i.e., that portion up to the origin of the innominate artery). Because the process as a rule does not extend into the wall of aorta behind the sinuses of Valsalva, AR is infrequent in syphilis. Exactly what percentage of patients with cardiovascular syphilis develop AR is unclear, but it is probably no more than about 15 percent and only those patients in whom the process

FIGURE 84-8 Rheumatoid arthritis. *A.* A tricuspid valve (TV) infiltrated by rheumatoid nodules. *B.* A mitral valve infiltrated by rheumatoid nodules. In addition, granulomas are present within the left ventricular (LV) wall. LA, left atrium; PML, posterior mitral leaflet; RV, right ventricle. H&E, A, ×12; B, ×65. (From Roberts WC, Dangel JC, Bulkley BH. Nonrheumatic valvular cardiac disease: A clinicopathologic survey of 27 different conditions causing valvular dysfunction. *Cardiovasc Clin.* Copyright 1973 by F.A. Davis Company; used by permission of F.A. Davis Company.)

extends into the wall of aorta behind the sinuses of Valsalva. In syphilis, the process *never* involves the aortic valve cusps and never extends below (caudal to) the aortic valve. In contrast, in ankylosing spondylitis, the process *always* involves basal portions of the aortic valve cusps and always extends into the membranous ventricular septum, the basal portion of the anterior mitral leaflet, or both. Thus, because the process in syphilis never extends below the aortic valve, bundle branch or complete heart block and MR never develop in cardiovascular syphilis or, if they do, they are the result of a process other than syphilis. Cardiovascular syphilis characteristically involves the entire tubular portion of the aorta, which may become either diffusely or focally dilated. In contrast, in ankylosing spondylitis, the process involves only the proximal 1 cm of the tubular portion of the ascending aorta and then usually in the areas of the aortic valve commissures. Accordingly, aneurysms of the tubular portion of the ascending aorta do not occur in ankylosing spondylitis. Syphilitic aneurysms can become so large that they burrow into the sternum or compress adjacent structures such as the right atrium, superior vena cava, or pulmonary trunk. Rupture into the adjacent structures or into the pericardial sac may also occur.

Histologically, the aortic lesions in both cardiovascular syphilis and ankylosing spondylitis are similar. Both are characterized by extensive thickening by fibrous tissue of the adventitia, with collections of plasma cells and some lymphocytes within these tissues. The vasa vasora are larger than normal, their walls are thickened, and their lumens may be severely narrowed. The inflammatory infiltrates are located primarily in the perivascular locations. The media is thinner than normal and contains scars that are generally located transversely to the long axis of the aorta. Within the scars, elastic fibers may be absent. The overlying intima is thickened, and the intimal process has the "tree bark" appearance of typical atherosclerotic plaques. Patients with cardiovascular syphilis, with or without associated AR, usually live into their 70s or 80s. In contrast to the excellent response to penicillin or ceftriazone in meningovascular syphilis, the response to antibiotic therapy in cardiovascular syphilis is less dramatic.

Systemic Sclerosis (Scleroderma)

SS, which was first identified over two centuries ago, is characterized by its striking skin manifestations; hence the name *scleroderma*. The systemic nature of this disease, and in particular its ability to affect the heart, became apparent in 1943, when Weiss and coworkers[78] described a pattern in the cardiac dysfunction of 9 patients with scleroderma and correlated these changes with abnormalities in the heart at autopsy in two patients. Moreover, they recognized that the cardiac disease was a manifestation of an underlying primary vascular disorder.

SS is characterized by fibrous thickening of the skin (Fig. 12-19) and fibrous and degenerative alterations of the fingers and of certain target organs, particularly the esophagus, small and large bowels, kidneys, lung, and heart. Central to this degenerative process are diffuse vascular lesions. Functionally, the vascular disorder is characterized by Raynaud's phenomenon, which is a prominent feature of SS. Raynaud's disease of the digits is present in almost all patients with SS and is the first clinical symptom in most. Structurally, the vascular lesions show intimal and adventitial thickening of small- and medium-sized vessels, including arterioles. The underlying pathophysiology of scleroderma that links structure and function is a Raynaud's-type phenomenon of visceral vasculature that leads to focal vascular lesions and parenchymal necrosis and fibrosis. This concept is supported by findings in the heart as well as in the lungs and kidneys. The underlying cause of the vascular disease in SS and

the role of the immune system in its pathophysiology remain unclear. SS may be related to increased activity of endothelial cells, mast cells, and fibroblasts, perhaps under the influence of immigrant cells, such as T cells, macrophages, or platelets.[77]

Like most connective tissue diseases, SS may have a variable clinical expression. Some patients may have skin involvement predominantly; others have minimal skin abnormalities but severe visceral disease that may therefore evade diagnosis.[79] Limited scleroderma (formerly called CREST syndrome) is most of the time a more benign form of scleroderma that presents with relatively mild skin changes limited to the face and fingers, *c*alcinosis, *R*aynaud's phenomenon, *e*sophageal dysmotility, *s*clerodactyly, and *t*elangiectasia. Patients with limited scleroderma have a high incidence of pulmonary hypertension. *Overlap syndromes* are seen when a patient with typical features of SS also has features of SLE, polymyositis, or RA. Although SS may run a long and benign course, the involvement of inner organs such as kidney, lung, and cardiovascular system is associated with increased morbidity and mortality.

THE CARDIOVASCULAR SYSTEM

Cardiovascular disease in patients with SS can be due to either a primary involvement of the heart by the sclerosing disease or a secondary involvement from disease of the kidney or lungs.

Primary Systemic Sclerosis of the Heart

Myocardial involvement is a major determinant of survival in SS. When the heart is involved directly by scleroderma, a myocardial fibrosis occurs that bears no direct relation to large- or small-vessel occlusions or other anatomic abnormalities. Fibrosis tends to be patchy, involving all levels of the myocardium unpredictably and the right ventricle as often as the left. Focal patchy myocardial cell necrosis may also be evident, and at autopsy over three-quarters of patients with myocardial SS have foci of necrosis. The type of necrosis is myofibrillar degeneration, or contraction-band necrosis (Fig. 84-9). This lesion is characteristic of myocardium that is subjected to transient occlusion followed by reperfusion. This could occur with vascular spasm and also may be induced experimentally by exposing myocardium to high concentrations of catecholamine. Thus, the morphologic characteristics of the myocardial lesions of primary cardiac SS are very similar to the ones seen in Raynaud's phenomenon. There is increased incidence of scleroderma renal crisis during cold weather months. Thus, it is likely that the major visceral manifestations of SS in the heart, lungs, and kidneys are related to the vascular spasm that is evident and readily detectable in the digits. Changes that are comparable to the necrosis and scarring of the fingertips can also develop in the viscera.

Present evidence suggests that the vascular system and particularly the smaller arteries and arterioles are the primary target organ of SS and that the cardiac sclerosis of scleroderma may be a consequence of focal, intermittent, and progressive ischemic injury.

Several functional studies have also suggested that microvascular spasm occurs in patients with cardiac scleroderma. Transient perfusion defects identified by thallium-201 radionuclide imaging in the setting of patent coronary arteries have also been identified in patients with SS and symptomatic cardiac disease.[80]

CLINICAL MANIFESTATIONS

The clinical features of myocardial SS include biventricular congestive heart failure, atrial and ventricular arrhythmias, myocardial infarction, angina pectoris, and sudden cardiac death.[81] These clinical manifestations reflect the underlying conditions of myocardial

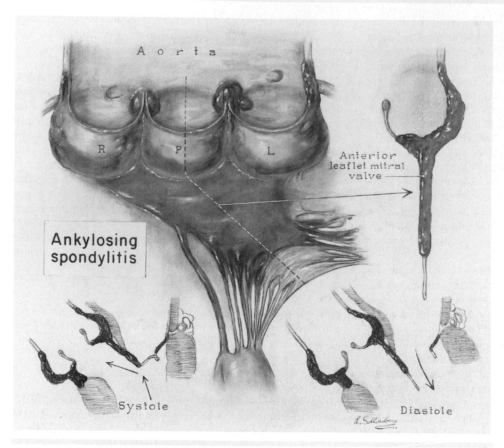

FIGURE 84-9 Diagram showing the characteristic features of ankylosing spondylitis of the heart. The aorta and aortic valve are opened, showing the thickening of the aorta in the vicinity of the aortic valve commissures and the thickening of the anterior mitral leaflet. The small diagrams at the bottom of the figure show the thickening in the wall of the aorta behind the sinuses extending below the aortic valve into the membranous ventricular septum and anterior mitral leaflet. In the patient whose heart was portrayed by this diagram, there was also some thickening in the posterior mitral leaflet.

necrosis and fibrosis and may at times mimic ischemic heart disease due to CAD. If the myocardial injury is extensive enough, hypodynamic ventricles, a syndrome resembling idiopathic dilated cardiomyopathy (see Chap. 76) may be simulated.

Patients with SS may have cardiac involvement but no cardiac symptoms.[81] One study[82] examined 18 SS patients by electrocardiography, ambulatory electrocardiography, radionuclide ventriculography, myocardial scintigraphy, and echocardiography and found a high rate of cardiac abnormalities, including ventricular tachyarrhythmias, supraventricular tachycardias, depressed left ventricular or right ventricular function, and reversible myocardial perfusion abnormalities. In other studies of patients with limited scleroderma, noninvasive cardiac techniques such as Doppler echocardiography and thallium-201 perfusion scintigraphy after a cold-stress test or radionuclide ventriculography[83] have found a number of cardiovascular abnormalities, such as mild MR, thickening of papillary muscles, abnormal left and right ventricular diastolic function, and systolic pulmonary arterial hypertension.

Skeletal muscle myositis can complicate SS, and such patients may have an increased likelihood of developing myocarditis, heart failure, and symptomatic arrhythmias, and often die suddenly.[84] Accordingly, it has been suggested that serum creatine kinase with MB fractionation and studies of left ventricular function be undertaken in patients with SS who have skeletal myositis. Autopsy studies have suggested that up to 50 percent of patients with SS have increased myocardial scar tissue and that up 30 percent of patients have exten-

sive disease.[85] Some clinical evidence of cardiac abnormalities may occur in about 40 percent of patients with SS. The cardiac disorder in about one-half of these patients has been attributed by some investigators to a myocardial scleroderma.

PERICARDIAL AND ENDOCARDIAL DISEASE

Pericardial involvement may occur in about 20 percent of patients with SS. Although the pericardial involvement is due to renal failure in as many as two-thirds of patients, some develop a fibrofibrinous or fibrous pericarditis for which no other cause is evident. Exudative pericardial effusions may accompany scleroderma pericardial disease and can be massive.[86] Most cases of pericardial effusion in scleroderma have a benign course. Rarely, pericardial tamponade may occur and may precede cutaneous thickening.[87] Rarely, constrictive pericardial disease may result from the pericardial sclerosis. MR is common in patients with SS.[88] Tricuspid regurgitation occurs in patients with very dilated right ventricular cavities.

SECONDARY CARDIOVASCULAR DISEASE

Ventricular hypertrophy and congestive heart failure may be associated with long-standing systemic arterial hypertension and renal disease. Uremic pericarditis may occur. Pulmonary hypertension with marked right ventricular hypertrophy and right-sided heart failure may result from long-standing severe pulmonary scleroderma. Mortality due to scleroderma renal crisis and malignant hypertension has dramatically decreased with the use of angiotensin-converting enzyme (ACE) inhibitors.

PULMONARY HYPERTENSIVE DISEASE

Although the pulmonary fibrosis of scleroderma had been known for years, the recognition of a pulmonary hypertensive lesion independent of parenchymal disease evolved later. Such patients tend to develop rapidly progressive dyspnea and right-sided heart failure in the setting of clear lungs. Morphologically, the pulmonary arterial lesions show the range of advanced alterations (medial and intimal thickening and plexiform lesions) as seen in the Eisenmenger syndrome and primary pulmonary hypertension. Arterial vasospasm is believed to be a major component of SS pulmonary hypertension, and the association is supported by angiographic studies. That Raynaud's phenomenon of the digits accompanies idiopathic pulmonary hypertension in about one-third of patients suggests that vascular hyperreactivity may be a common link between this disease and scleroderma (see Chap. 62).

Pulmonary hypertension portends a poor prognosis. Sudden unexpected death occurs, and hypotension and death can occur precipitously in the setting of what would appear to be relatively benign procedures such as pericardiocentesis or cardiac catheterization.

TREATMENT

There is no uniformly effective therapy for the cardiovascular disease of SS. Treatment consists of standard therapy for congestive heart failure and arrhythmias. Malignant ventricular arrhythmias in SS have responded seemingly well to insertion of an implantable cardioverter defibrillator[89] (see Chap. 30). Captopril has been shown to improve myocardial perfusion.[89a] Unlike Raynaud's disease secondary to lupus, the response to nifedipine when it is associated with scleroderma is marginal. Prazosin and hydralazine have been used with mixed results. The role of sympathectomy for severe Raynaud's disease refractory to medical treatment is highly controversial; most patients obtain only temporary relief of their symptoms. Avoiding cool temperatures is mandatory. The use of continuous intravenous infusion of epoprostenol[90] or inhaled protacyclin analogue iloprost[91] have improved dramatically the symptoms of pulmonary hypertension (see Chap. 62). A study with the oral endothelin-receptor antagonist bosentan showed promising results.[92] The use of D-penicillamine, which until recently was standard therapy, has not been proven to be efficacious.[93]

The use of high-dose glucocorticoids should be avoided in scleroderma and doses of prednisone >30 mg daily usually cause normotensive renal failure.[94]

Polymyositis and Dermatomyositis

These idiopathic autoimmune inflammatory myopathies are rare in the United States, with an estimated annual incidence of about 5 to 10 new patients per million. The clinical features include a typical heliotrope rash in dermatomyositis (DM), with periorbital edema and proximal muscle weakness present in both polymyositis (PM) and DM. Typical laboratory findings reflect the presence of muscle breakdown from the inflammatory process. Creatine kinase, myoglobulin, and serum aldolase levels are commonly elevated during acute states. The former is more sensitive in those patients who present with normal, or mildly increased, creatine kinase levels. The so-called anti-Jo-1 antibody, directed against histydil-tRNA synthetase, is detectable in the serum of 20 percent of patients with PM/DM. Its presence has been correlated with erosive arthritis, Raynaud's phenomenon, interstitial lung disease, and excess mortality, mostly due to respiratory failure. Another marker of disease severity is the anti-signal-recognition-particle (anti-SRP) antibody. Typical electromyogram (EMG) changes include short-wave potentials, low-amplitude polyphasic units, and increased spontaneous activity with muscle fibrillation. A positive skeletal muscle biopsy of a proximal muscle such as the deltoid is often confirmatory.

In addition to skeletal muscle involvement, up to 40 percent of patients may have cardiac abnormalities. A small study of 16 autopsied patients with PM/DM suggests a poor correlation between the degree of skeletal involvement and myocarditis, however.[95]

In a study of 55 patients with PM, Behan et al.[96] reported mild diffuse myocarditis, severe inflammation, or fibrosis of the cardiac conduction system in 70 percent of the patients. Also, anti-SSA (anti-Ro) antibody, which is classically associated with an increased risk of infant cardiac conduction abnormalities in the neonatal lupus syndrome, was present in 69 percent of patients with evidence of cardiovascular involvement.[96]

The role of gadolinium-DTPA enhanced MRI appears promising in diagnosing myocarditis in polymyositis.[97] Myocarditis leading to congestive heart failure is an uncommon but severe manifestation of PM/DM.[98]

Although coronary arteritis has been reported in few case reports, there are no controlled studies showing evidence of increased incidence of CAD in PM/DM. Glucocorticoids represent the mainstay of therapy. Most patients do very well on oral prednisone therapy, whereas others fail to respond to any agents. The usual practice is to begin treatment with 40 to 80 mg/d of oral prednisone or its equivalent. Methylprednisolone boluses of 500 to 1000 mg/d for 3 days is reserved for severe and acute cases. Azathioprine (Imuran) and methotrexate are used mostly as steroid-sparing agents. Intravenous immunoglobulin given in monthly boluses is an expensive therapy that is reserved for patients with severe disease and poor response to conventional immunosuppressive therapy. Response can be seen as early as 2 weeks, but typically best effects are seen only after 3 months.[99]

Polyarteritis Nodosa

PN is an uncommon disease with an annual incidence that ranges from 4.6 to 9.0 per 100.000. PN affects predominantly males with a sex ratio of 2:1.[100]

PN is characterized by segmental necrotizing inflammation of the medium- to small-sized arteries, resulting in dysfunction of multiple organ systems. The commonly involved organs are the skin, kidneys, and gastrointestinal tract. PN rarely involves the central nervous system, eyes, testes, and heart. Lungs are usually spared. A variety of cutaneous lesions may occur: livedo reticularis, palpable purpura, ulcerations, infarcts of distal digits, and nodules. Evidence of glomerulonephritis ranges from low-grade proteinuria to malignant hypertension and acute renal failure.

There is a recognized association between PN and hepatitis B infection. Hepatitis B surface antigen has been found in 15 percent of the patients. Laboratory tests are nonspecific and reflect mainly an inflammatory state. Common findings are elevated erythrocyte sedimentation rate (ESR), normochromic anemia, thrombocytosis, low C3 and C4 complement levels, and low albumin. Typically, rheumatoid factor and ANA are not present. A subset of patients with microscopic PN have antineutrophil cytoplasmic antibodies directed against myeloperoxidase. The final clinical diagnosis of PN rests on the combination of multisystem disease and biopsy evidence of active arteritis. In PN, mesenteric vessel angiograms may show aneurysmal dilatation that mimics mycotic aneurysm in infective endocarditis.

CARDIAC INVOLVEMENT

The heart and coronary arteries are infrequent targets of PN. Most often this involvement is a vasculitis of the distal subepicardial coronary arteries just as they penetrate the myocardium (Fig. 84-10). The lesions are characterized by inflammatory infiltrates in the media and adventitia and occasionally by necrosis of the full thickness of the vessel wall, with prominent involvement of the surrounding perivascular connective tissue (see Fig. 84-10). The lumens of the involved vessels may contain thrombi, and the walls may be aneurysmal. The latter is responsible for the nodular appearance of the arteries deemed characteristic of this disorder. An even later stage of the vasculitis process is evident as the lesions heal, first showing the formation of granulation tissue and subsequently fibrous tissue replacement of the original components of the artery. In this healing phase, intimal proliferation leading to coronary artery luminal narrowing is evident.[101]

The CAD of PN may lead to myocardial infarction.[102] The myocardial necrosis and subsequent replacement fibrosis tend to be focal and patchy throughout the left ventricular wall. This is in contrast to the large areas of grossly visible, regional, subendocardial, or transmural necrosis typically seen in the myocardial infarction caused by CAD (see Chap. 44).

Conduction system abnormalities have been identified in the heart of patients with PN. The size and location of the sinoatrial node

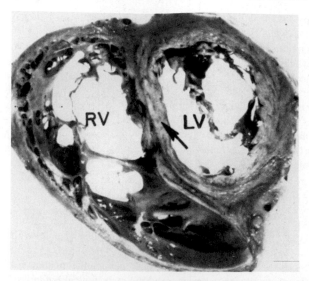

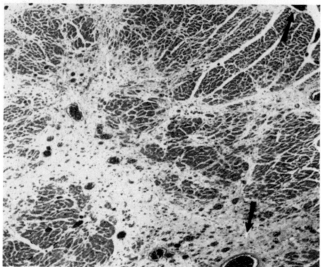

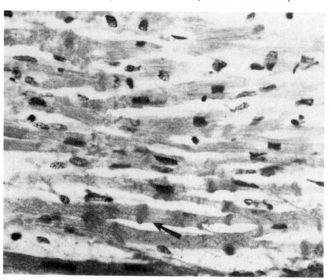

FIGURE 84-10 Systemic sclerosis (SS). Top: Cross-section through the dilated right (RV) and left (LV) ventricle of a patient with cardiac SS. Marked fibrous scarring of both ventricles is especially evident in the ventricular septum (arrow). Bottom left: Photomicrograph of myocardium showing replacement fibrosis with patent intramural coronary arteries (arrows). Bottom right: Higher-power magnification showing contraction-band necrosis of many fibers surrounding the areas of scar. H&E, ×45 and ×60. (From Bulkley BH. Progressive systemic sclerosis: Cardiac involvement. *Clin Rheum Dis* 1979; 5–131. Reproduced with permission form the publisher and author.)

and atrioventricular node arteries make them prime targets for polyarteritis.[102] Atrial and ventricular conduction disturbances may be a primary manifestation of PN, despite minimal involvement of vessels elsewhere in the heart.

Other cardiac abnormalities seen in patients with PN are those that are likely secondary to the underlying systemic arterial hypertension and renal disease. Cardiomegaly and left ventricular hypertrophy most often represent secondary cardiac manifestations of this disease. Similarly, pericardial disease may develop in a patient with PN, but this is most often due to renal insufficiency.

CLINICAL MANIFESTATIONS OF CARDIAC DISEASE

Despite the dramatic involvement of coronary arteries that may accompany PN, the most frequent cardiovascular abnormalities seen in patients with PN are unrelated to the coronary arteries per se. Systemic arterial hypertension occurs in approximately 90 percent of these patients and, in combination with chronic renal failure, is the most likely cause of congestive heart failure, which may develop in up to 60 percent of patients. Those with PN also may develop acute myocardial infarction, which poses the diagnostic question of whether the myocardial injury is due to coronary arteritis with secondary thrombosis or to atherosclerosis, in a population that is typically middle-aged, male, steroid treated, and susceptible to atherosclerotic CAD as well.[101]

THERAPY

PN has a poor prognosis. Treatment of the heart disease in PN is directed at the specific cardiac dysfunction. Glucocorticoids are still the initial mainstay of therapy. Early use of cyclophosphamide in severe disease with involvement of major organs has been associated with decreased mortality.[103]

Case reports of improvement of hepatitis-B-virus-related PN with concomitant immunosuppressive and antiviral therapy are encouraging.[104]

The use of warfarin remains controversial; low-dose aspirin, however, is usually recommended.

Giant-Cell (Cranial, Temporal, Granulomatous) Arteritis

Temporal arteritis is a systemic inflammatory vasculitis of unknown etiology that primarily involves extracranial vessels, especially branches of the external carotid artery, but can involve almost any artery in the body, as well as some veins. Giant-cell arteritis occurs almost exclusively in patients over 55 years of age. Common symptoms include headaches, scalp tenderness, jaw claudication, visual disturbances including blindness and diplopia, weight loss, anemia, and, in about 50 percent of patients, musculoskeletal symptoms attributable to polymyalgia rheumatica. Uncommon presentations of giant-cell arteritis include fever of unknown origin, chest pain from aortitis or myocardial infarction, aortic aneurysm,[105,106] peripheral gangrene, peripheral neuropathies, and large-vessel involvement with limb claudication, AR, or stroke. Typical physical findings include tenderness of the temporal or occipital arteries, nodulations of the artery, a pulseless artery, and a tender scalp.

Most giant-cell arteritis patients have a greatly elevated ESR. The only specific diagnostic test is a temporal artery biopsy that demonstrates granulomatous arterial inflammation with disruption of the internal elastica lamina. Giant cells need not be present. Unfortunately, the positive yield for giant-cell arteritis in unilateral temporal artery biopsies is no greater than 60 percent, and a contralateral biopsy may be necessary.

Since the occurrence of *skip* lesions in histologic samples is well known in giant-cell arteritis, ideally a 5-cm section of artery should be examined. Angiography is generally not helpful in diagnosis or in selecting a biopsy site. High-dose prednisone therapy is indicated to prevent blindness or to suppress inflammation in the presence of systemic involvement.

Churg-Strauss Vasculitis

Churg-Strauss syndrome, or allergic granulomatosis and angiitis, is a systemic vasculitis that develops in the setting of allergic rhinitis, asthma, and eosinophilia. Sinusitis and pulmonary infiltrates may cause confusion with Wegener's granulomatosis; the absence of cavitating pulmonary nodules or the presence of gastrointestinal involvement is often a helpful distinguishing feature. Peripheral neuropathy, cutaneous involvement, and renal disease are common clinical findings.

Pathologic studies show inflammatory lesions rich in eosinophils with intra- and extravascular granuloma formation. The major morbidity and mortality of Churg-Strauss vasculitis result from cardiac involvement. This may be associated with left ventricular dilatation and a reduced ejection fraction, as well as MR, which may require valve replacement.[105] Left ventricular systolic function may improve significantly with glucocorticoid therapy.[106]

Antiphospholipid Antibody Syndrome

The aPL antibody syndrome has been identified by the presence of aPL antibodies, usually in high titer, or the *lupus anticoagulant,* and any or all of the following clinical events:[107–116] recurrent arterial or venous thromboses, recurrent fetal losses, and thrombocytopenia. Livedo reticularis is also frequently present, and nonhealing leg ulcers and Coombs'-positive hemolytic anemia may be also. Clinically, the terms *anticardiolipin syndrome, antiphospholipid syndrome,* and *lupus anticoagulant syndrome* are usually considered to be equivalent, although some individuals may have one antibody but not the other. A false-positive Venereal Disease Research Laboratory test may also be detected in patients with aPL antibody syndrome; aPL antibodies, however, may be present in asymptomatic individuals. Often, anticardiolipin antibodies cross-react with beta$_2$-glycoprotein 1 (B2GP1) antibodies. The mechanisms whereby anticardiolipin or aPL antibodies promote intravascular thrombosis remain uncertain. These antibodies may react with lipid antigens on endothelial cells and/or platelets. The precise nature of the antigen recognized by B2GP1-dependent anticardiolipin antibodies is under active investigation. SLE is present frequently in patients with aPL antibody syndrome. The presence of anticardiolipin antibodies in patients with SLE may be associated with prolonged activated partial thromboplastin time, thrombocytopenia, and positive Coombs' test but not with the lupus anticoagulant (or the aPL) syndrome;[108] the presence of a prolonged activated partial thromboplastin time is strongly associated with venous and arterial thrombosis.

Therapy depends on the clinical setting. Patients with positive aPL antibodies but without evidence of thrombosis or recurrent fetal loss should not be treated. Patients with aPL antibody syndrome who have had thrombotic events or habitual abortions should be treated. Anticoagulation and antithrombotic therapy in these patients has included heparin, warfarin, low-dose aspirin, and the antimalarial agent hydroxychloroquine.[108] Although there is no convincing evidence of benefit, some advocate low-dose aspirin or heparin, with or without low-dose prednisone, alone or in combination, to prevent fetal loss. An increased incidence of AR or MR in association with the primary aPL antibody syndrome has been reported as well in patients with SLE who have aPL antibodies. Heart valve involvement, although frequent, appears unrelated to the presence or absence of aPL antibodies. The aPL antibody syndrome is frequently manifest by spontaneous small- and large-vessel arterial thrombosis in the cerebral and ocular circulations.[117] In healthy men, positive anticardiolipin antibody levels are a risk factor for deep venous thrombosis or pulmonary embolus, but not for ischemic stroke.[117]

Although there are no controlled trials of therapy to prevent arterial occlusion, low-dose aspirin is often used. Therapy has often included aspirin and warfarin or heparin, as well as low-dose glucocorticoids.[118]

References

1. Beighton P, ed. *McKusick's Heritable Disorders of Connective Tissue,* 5th ed. St Louis: Mosby-Year Book, 1993.
2. Pyeritz PE, McKusick VA. The Marfan syndrome: Diagnosis and management. *N Engl J Med* 1979;300:772–777.
3. Dietz HC, Curring GR, Pyeritz RE, et al. Marfan syndrome caused by a de novo missense mutation in the fibrillin gene. *Nature* 1991;352:337–339.
4. Ramirez F. Fibrillin mutations in Marfan syndrome and related phenotypes. *Curr Opin Genet Dev* 1996;6:309–315.
5. Burn J, Camm J, Davies MJ, et al. The phenotype/genotype relation and the current status of genetic screening in hypertrophic cardiomyopathy, Marfan syndrome, and the long QT syndrome. *Heart* 1997;78:110–116.
6. De Paepe A, Devereus RB, Dietz HC, et al. Revised diagnostic criteria for the Marfan syndrome. *Am J Med Genet* 1996;62:417–426.
7. Come PC, Fortuin NJ, White RI Jr, McKusick VA. Echocardiographic assessment of cardiovascular abnormalities in the Marfan syndrome: Comparison with clinical findings and with roentgenographic estimation of aortic root size. *Am J Med* 1983;74:465–474.
8. Roman MJ, Devereus RB, Kramer-Fox R, Spitzer MC. Comparison of cardiovascular and skeletal features of primary valve prolapse and Marfan syndrome. *J Cardiol* 1989;63:317–321.
9. Glesby MJ, Pyeritz RE. Association of mitral valve prolapse and systemic abnormalities of connective tissue: A phenotypic continuum. *JAMA* 1989;262:523–518.
10. Wexler L, Higgins CB. The use of magnetic resonance imaging in adult congenital heart disease. *Am J Cardiac Imaging* 1995;9:15–28.
11. David TE. Current practice in Marfan's aortic root surgery: Reconstruction with aortic valve preservation or replacement? What to do with the mitral valve. *J Cardiovasc Surg* 1997;12(suppl 2):147–150.
12. Murdoch JL, Walker BA, Halpern BL, et al. Life expectancy and causes of death in the Marfan syndrome. *N Engl J Med* 1972;286:804–808.
13. Maron BJ. Heart disease and other causes of sudden death in young athletes. *Curr Probl Cardiol* 1998;23:477–529.
14. Shores J, Berger KR, Murphy EA, Pyeritz RE. Progression of aortic dilation and the benefit of long-term beta-adrenergic blockade in Marfan's syndrome. *N Engl J Med* 1994;30:1335–1341.

15. Salim MA, Alpert BS, Ward JC, Pyeritz RE. Effect of beta-adrenergic blockade on aortic root rate of dilation in the Marfan syndrome. *Am J Cardiol* 1994;74:629–633.

16. Roberts WC, Honig HS. The spectrum of cardiovascular disease in the Marfan syndrome: A clinico-morphologic study of 18 necropsy patients and comparison to 151 previously reported necropsy patients. *Am Heart J* 1982;104:115–135.

17. Meijboom LJ, Groenink M, van der Wall EE, et al. Aortic root asymmetry in marfan patients; evaluation by magnetic resonance imaging and comparison with standard echocardiography. *Intern J Cardiac Imaging* 2000 16(3):161–168.

18. Hayashi J, Moro H, Namura O, et al. Surgical implication of aortic dissection on long-term outcome in Marfan patients. *Surg Today* 1996;26:980–984.

19. LeMaire SA, Coselli JS. Aortic root surgery in Marfan syndrome: Current practice and evolving techniques. *J Cardiovasc Surg* 1997;12(suppl 2):137–141.

20. Meijboom LJ, Nollen GJ, Merchant N, et al. Frequency of coronary ostial aneurysms after aortic root surgery in patients with the Marfan syndrome. *Am J Cardiol* 2002;1;89(9):1135–1138.

21. Beighton P, De Paepe, Steinmann B, Tsipouras P, et al. Ehlers-Danlos syndromes: revised nosology, Villefranche, 1997. Ehlers-Danlos National Foundation (USA) and Ehlers-Danlos Support Group (UK). *Am J Med Genet* 1998;77(1):31–37.

22. Slade AKB, John RM, Swanton RH. Pseudoxanthoma elasticum presenting as myocardial infarction. *Br Heart J* 1990;63:372–373.

22a. Walker DEL. Overview of inherited metabolic disorders causing cardiovascular disease. *J Inherit Metab Dis* 2003;26:245–257.

23. Takahashi T, Koide T, Yamaguchi H, et al. Ehlers-Danlos syndrome. *Ann Thorac Surg* 1994;58:1180–1182.

24. Trip MD, Smulders YM, et al: Frequent mutation in the ABCC6 gene (R1141X) is associated with a strong increase in the prevalence of coronary artery disease. *Circulation* 2002;13;106(7):773–775.

25. Kevorkian JP, Masquet C, Kural-Menasche S, et al. New report of severe coronary artery disease in an eighteen-year-old girl with pseudoxanthoma elasticum. *Angiology* 1997;48:735–741.

26. Challenor VF, Conway N, Monro JL. The surgical treatment of restrictive cardiomyopathy in pseudoxanthoma elasticum. *Br Heart J* 1988;59:266–269.

27. Wong RS, Follis FM, Shively BK, Wenly JA. Osteogenesis imperfecta and cardiovascular diseases. *Ann Thorac Surg* 1995;60:1439–1443.

28. Gloriex FH, Bishop NJ, Plotkin H, et al: Cyclic administration of pamidronate in children with severe osteogenesis imperfecta. *N Engl J Med* 1998;339:947.

29. Moriyama Y, Nishida T, Toyohira H, et al. Acute aortic dissection in a patient with osteogenesis imperfecta. *Ann Thorac Surg* 1995;60:1397–1399.

30. Fowler NO, Van der Bel-Kahn JM. Indications for surgical replacement of the mitral valve with particular reference to common and uncommon causes of mitral regurgitation. *Am J Cardiol* 1979;44:148–156.

31. Hortop J, Tsipouras P, Hanley JA, et al. Cardiovascular involvement in osteogenesis imperfecta *Circulation* 1986;73:54–61.

32. Roman MJ, Devereus RB. Heritable aortic disease. In: Lindsay J, ed. *Diseases of the Aorta*. Philadelphia: Lea & Febiger; 1994:5.

33. Pascal N, Bloor C, Godfrey M, et al. Familial aortic dissecting aneurysm. *J Am Coll Cardiol* 1989;13:811–819.

34. Chen M, Rigby ML, Redington AN. Familial aneurysms of the interventricular septum. *Br Heart J* 1991;65:104–106.

35. Jaksche VH. Familiäre Aneurysmen: Vier Karotisaneurysmen aus einer zehnköpfigen Familie. *Zentralbl Neurochir* 1986;47:351–353.

36. Elshunnar KS, Whittle IR. Familial intracranial aneurysms: Report of five families. *Br J Neurosurg* 1990;4:181–186.

37. Boumpas DT, Fessler BJ, Austin HA III, et al. Systemic lupus erythematosus: Emerging concepts. Part 2: Dermatologic and joint disease, the antiphospholipid antibody syndrome, pregnancy and hormonal therapy, morbidity and mortality, and pathogenesis. *Ann Intern Med* 1995;123:42–53.

38. Wallace DJ, Hahn BH, eds. *Dubois' Lupus Erythematosus*, 4th ed. Philadelphia: Lea & Febiger; 1993.

39. Moder KG, Miller TD, Tazelaar HD. Cardiac involvement in systemic lupus erythematosus. *Mayo Clin Proc* 1999;74:275–284.

40. Ward MM, Pyun E, Studenski S. Mortality risks associated with specific clinical manifestations of systemic lupus erythematosus. *Arch Intern Med* 1996;156:1337–1344.

41. Roberts WC, High ST. The heart in systemic lupus erythematosus. *Curr Probl Cardiol* 1999;24:1–56.

42. Nihoyannopoulous P, Gomez PM, Joshi J, et al. Cardiac abnormalities in systemic lupus erythematosus. *Circulation* 1990;82:369–375.

43. O'Rourke RA. Antiphospholipid antibodies: A marker of lupus carditis? *Circulation* 1990;82:636–638.

44. Bulkley BH, Roberts WC. The heart in systemic lupus erythematosus and the changes induced in it by corticosteroid therapy: A study of 36 necropsy patients. *Am J Med* 1975;58:243–264.

45. Roldan CA, Shively BK, Crawford MH. An echocardiographic study of valvular heart disease associated with systemic lupus erythematosus. *N Engl J Med* 1996;335:1424–1430.

46. Kahl LE. The spectrum of pericardial tamponade in systemic lupus erythematosus: Report of ten patients. *Arthritis Rheum* 1992;35:1343–1349.

47. Libman E, Sacks B. A hitherto undescribed form of valvular and mural endocarditis. *Arch Intern Med* 1924;33:701–737.

48. Gross L. The cardiac lesion in Libman-Sacks disease with a consideration of its relationship to acute diffuse lupus erythematosus. *Am J Pathol* 1940;16:375–407.

49. Sturfelt G, Eskilsson J, Nived O, et al. Cardiovascular disease in systemic disease in systemic lupus erythematosus: A study from a defined population. *Medicine (Baltimore)* 1992;71:216–223.

50. Petri M, Spence D, Bone LR, Hochberg MC. Coronary risk factors in the Johns Hopkins lupus cohort: Prevalence by patients, and preventive practices. *Medicine (Baltimore)* 1992;71:291–302.

51. Kutom AH, Gibbs HR. Myocardial infarction due to thrombi without significant coronary artery disease in systemic erythematosus. *Chest* 1991;100:571–572.

52. Sumino H, Kanda T, Saski T, et al. Myocardial infarction secondary to coronary aneurysm in systemic lupus erythematosus: An autopsy case. *Angiology* 1995;46:527–530.

53. James TN, Rupe CE, Monto RW. Pathology of the cardiac conduction system in systemic lupus erythematosus. *Ann Intern Med* 1965;63:402–410.

53a. Cimaz R, Spence DL, Hornberger L, et al. Incidence of neonatal lupus erythematosus: A prospective study of infants born to mothers with anti-Ro antibodies. *J Pediatrics* 2003;142:678–683.

54. Waltuck J, Buyon JP. Autoantibody-associated congenital heart block: Outcome in mothers and children. *Ann Intern Med* 1994;120:544–551.

55. Press J, Uziel Y, Laxer RM, et al. Long-term outcome of mothers of children with complete congenital heart block. *Am J Med* 1996;100:328–332.

56. Gobel MM, Dick M II, McCune WJ, et al. Atrioventricular conduction in children of women with systemic lupus erythematosus. *Am J Cardiol* 1993;71:94–98.

57. Logar D, Kveder T, Rozman B, Pobovisek J. Possible association between anti-Ro antibodies and myocarditis or cardiac conduction defects in adults with systemic lupus erythematosus. *Ann Rheum Dis* 1990;49:627–629.

58. Winslow TM, Ossipov MA, Fazio GP, et al. Five-year follow up study of the prevalence and progression of pulmonary hypertension in systemic lupus erythematosus. *Am Heart J* 1995;129:510–515.

59. Kalangos A, Panos A, Sezerman O. Mitral valve repair in lupus valvulitis: Report of a case and review of the literature. *J Heart Valve Dis* 1995;4:202–207.

60. Morin AM, Boyer JC, Nataf P, Gandjbakhch I. Mitral insufficiency caused by systemic lupus erythematosus requiring valve replacement: Three case reports and a review of the literature. *Thorac Cardiovasc Surg* 1996;44:313–316.

61. Petri M, Lakatta C, Madger L, Goldman D. Effect of prednisone and hydroxychloroquine on coronary artery disease risk factors in systemic lupus erythematosus: A longitudinal data analysis. *Am J Med* 1994;96: 254–259.

62. Chiariello M, Ambrosio G, Capelli-Bigazzi M, et al. Reduction in infarct size by the phospholipase inhibitor quinacrine in dogs with coronary artery occlusion. *Am Heart J* 1990;120:801–807.

63. Navarro-Cano G, Del Rincon I, Pogosian S, et al. Association of mortality with disease severity in rheumatoid arthritis, independent of comorbidity. *Arthritis Rheum* 2003;48:2425–2433.

64. Del Rincon ID, Williams K, Stern MP, et al. High incidence of cardiovascular events in a rheumatoid arthritis cohort not explained by traditional cardiac risk factors. *Arthritis Rheum* 2001;44(12):2737–2745.

65. Park YB, Ahn CW, Choi HK, et al. Atherosclerosis in rheumatoid arthritis: Morphologic evidence obtained by carotid ultrasound. *Arthritis Rheum* 2002;46(7):1714–1719.

66. Roberts WC, Dangel JC, Bulkley BH. Nonrheumatic valvular cardiac disease: A clinicopathologic survey of 27 different conditions causing valvular dysfunction. *Cardiovasc Clin* 1973;4:333–446.

67. Bacon PA, Gibson DG. Cardiac involvement in rheumatoid arthritis: An echocardiographic study. *Ann Rheum Dis* 1974;33:20–24.

68. Hakala M, Pettersson T, Tarkka M, et al. Rheumatoid arthritis as a cause of cardiac compression: Favourable long-term outcome of pericardiectomy. *Clin Rheumatol* 1993;12:199–203.

69. Escalante A, Kaufman RL, Quismorio RP Jr, Beardmore TD. Cardiac compression in rheumatoid pericarditis. *Semin Arthritis Rheum* 1990;20:148–163.

70. Hara KS, Ballard DJ, Illstrup DM, et al. Rheumatoid pericarditis: Clinical features and survival. *Medicine (Baltimore)* 1990;69: 81–91.

71. Travaglio-Encinoza A, Anaya JM, Dupuy D, et al. Rheumatoid pericarditis: New immunopathological aspects. *Clin Exp Rheumatol* 1994; 12:313–316.

72. Suriani RJ, Lansman S, Konstadt S. Intracardiac rheumatoid nodule presenting as a left atrial mass. *Am Heart J* 1994;127:463–465.

73. Maione S, Valentini G, Giunta A, et al. Cardiac involvement in rheumatoid arthritis: An echocardiographic study. *Cardiology* 1993; 83:234–239.

74. Bulkley BH, Roberts WC. Ankylosing spondylitis and aortic regurgitation: Description of the characteristic cardiovascular lesion from study of eight necropsy patients. *Circulation* 1973;48:1014–1027.

75. Roberts WC, Hollingsworth JR, Bulkley BH, et al. Combined mitral and aortic regurgitation in ankylosing spondylitis: Angiographic and anatomic features. *Am J Med* 1974;56:237–243.

76. Gould BA, Turner J, Keeling DH, et al. Myocardial dysfunction in ankylosing spondylitis. *Ann Rheum Dis* 1992;51:227 232.]

77. Gorman JD, Sack KE, Davis JC Jr. Treatment of ankylosing spondylitis by inhibition of tumor necrosis factor alpha. *N Engl J Med* 2002; 346(18):1349–1356.

78. Weiss S, Stead EA, Warren JV, Bailey OT. Scleroderma heart disease: With a consideration of certain other visceral manifestations of scleroderma. *Arch Intern Med* 1943;71:749–776.

79. Bulkley BH, Klacsmann PG, Hutchins GM. Angina pectoris, myocardial infarction and sudden death with normal coronary arteries: A clinicopathologic study of 9 patients with progressive systemic sclerosis. *Am Heart J* 1978;95:563–569.

80. Follansbee WP, Curtiss EI, Medsger TA Jr, et al. Physiologic abnormalities of cardiac function in progressive systemic sclerosis with diffuse scleroderma. *N Engl J Med* 1984;310:142–148.

81. Clements PJ, Furst DE. Heart involvement in systemic sclerosis. *Clin Dermatol* 1994;12:267–275.

82. Anvari A, Graninger W, Schneider B, et al. Cardiac involvement in systemic sclerosis. *Arthritis Rheum* 1992;35:1356–1361.

83. Candell-Riera J, Armandans-Gil L, Simeon CP, et al. Comprehensive noninvasive assessment of cardiac involvement in limited systemic sclerosis. *Arthritis Rheum* 1996;39:1138–1145.

84. Follansbee WP, Zerbe TR, Medsger TA Jr. Cardiac and skeletal muscle disease in systemic sclerosis (scleroderma): A high-risk association. *Am Heart J* 1993;125:194–203.

85. D' Angelo WA, Fries JR, Masi AT, Shulman LE. Pathologic observations in systemic sclerosis (scleroderma): A study of fifty-eight autopsy cases and fifty-eight matched controls. *Am J Med* 1969;46: 428–440.

86. Satoh M, Tokuhira M, Hama N, et al. Massive pericardial effusion in scleroderma: A review of five cases. *Br J Rheumatol* 1995;34: 564–567.

87. Perez-Bocanegra C, Fonollosa V, Simeon CP, et al. Pericardial tamponade preceding cutaneous involvement in systemic sclerosis. *Ann Rheum Dis* 1995;54:687–688.

88. Kazzam E, Caidahl K, Hallgren R, et al. Mitral regurgitation and diastolic flow profile in systemic sclerosis. *Int J Cardiol* 1990;29:357–363.

89. Martinez-Taboada V, Olalla J, Blanco R, et al. Malignant ventricular arrhythmia in systemic sclerosis controlled with an implantable cardioverter defibrillator. *J Rheumatol* 1994;21:2166–2167.

89a. Kazzam E, Caidahl K, Hallgren R, et al. Noninvasive evaluation of long-term effects of Captopril in systemic sclerosis. *J Intern Med* 1991;230:203–212.

90. Badesch DB, Tapson VF, McGoon MD, et al. Continuous intravenous epoprostenol for pulmonary hypertension due to the scleroderma spectrum of disease: A randomized, controlled trial. *Ann Intern Med* 2000; 132:425–434.

91. Hoeper MM, Schwarze M, Ehlerding S, et al. Long-term treatment of primary pulmonary hypertension with aerosolized iloprost, a prostacyclin analogue. *N Engl J Med* 2000;342:1866–1870.

92. Rubin L, Badesch DB, et al: The Bosentan Randomized Trial of Endothelin Antagonist Therapy. *N Engl J Med* 2002;346:896–903.

93. Clemens PJ, Furst DE, Wong W-K, et al: High-dose vs low-dose D-penicillamine in early diffuse systemic sclerosis. *Arthritis Rheum* 1999;42:1194.

94. Helfrich DJ, Banner B, Steen VD, et al: Normotensive renal failure in systemic sclerosis. *Arthritis Rheum* 1989;32:1128.

95. Haupt HM, Hutchins GM. The heart and cardiac conduction system in polymyositis-dermatomyositis: A clinicopathologic study of 16 autopsied patients. *Am J Cardiol* 1982;50(5):998–1006.

96. Behan WM, Behan PO, Gairns J. Cardiac damage in polymyositis associated with antibodies to tissue ribonucleoproteins. *Br Heart J* 1987; 57(2):176–180.

97. Ohata S, Shimada T, Shimizu H, et al. Myocarditis associated with polymyositis diagnosed by gadolinium-DTPA enhanced magnetic resonance imaging. *J Rheumatol* 2002;29(4):861–862.

98. Dalakas M, Illa I, Dambrosia JM, et al. A controlled trial of high-dose intravenous immune globulin as treatment for dermatomyositis. *N Engl J Med* 1993;329:1993–2000.

99. Michet CJ. Epidemiology of vasculitis. In: Conn DL, ed. *Rheumatic Disease Clinics of North America*. Philadelphia: WB Saunders; 1990: 261–268.

100. Schrader ML, Hochman JS, Bulkley BH. The heart in polyarteritis nodosa: A clinicopathologic study. *Am Heart J* 1985;109:1353–1359.

101. Chu KH, Menapace FU, Blankenship JC, et al. Polyarteritis nodosa presenting as acute myocardial infarction with coronary dissection. *Catheter Cardiovasc Diagn* 1998;44:320–324.

102. Gayraud M, Guillevin L, et al. Followup of polyarteritis nodosa, microscopic polyangiitis, and Churg-Strauss syndrome: Analysis of four prospective trials including 278 patients. French Vasculitis Study Group. *Arthritis Rheum* 2001;44(3):666–675.

103. Thiene G, Valente M, Rossi L. Involvement of the cardiac conducting system in panarteritis nodosa. *Am Heart J* 1978; 95:716–724.

104. Erhardt A, Sagir A, Guillevin L, et al. Successful treatment of hepatitis B virus associated polyarteritis nodosa with a combination of prednisolone, alpha-interferon and lamivudine. *J Hepatol* 2000;33(4): 677–683.

105. Gonzalez-Lopez L, Gamez-Nava JI, Sanchez L, et al: Cardiac manifestations in dermato-polymyositis. *Clin TXP Rheumatol* 1996; 14:373.

106. Gonzales EB, Varner WT, Lisse JR, et al. Giant-cell arteritis in the southern United States: An 11-year retrospective study from the Texas Gulf coast. *Arch Intern Med* 1989;149:1561–1565.

107. Hasley PB, Follansbee WP, Coulehan JL. Cardiac manifestations of Churg-Strauss syndrome: Report of a case and review of the literature. *Am Heart J* 1990;120:996–999.

108. Abu-Shakra M, Gladman DD, Urowitz MB, Farewell V. Anticardiolipin antibodies in systemic lupus erythematosus: Clinical and laboratory correlations. *Am J Med* 1995;99:624–628.

109. Khamashta MA, Cudrado MJ, Mujic F, et al. The management of thrombosis in the antiphospholipid-antibody syndrome. *N Engl J Med* 1995;332:993–997.

110. Beynon HLC, Walport MJ. Antiphospholipid antibodies and cardiovascular disease. *Br Heart J* 1992;67:281–284.

111. Cervera R, Asherson RA, Lie JT. Clinicopathologic correlations of the antiphospholipid syndrome. *Semin Arthritis Rheum* 1995;24:262–277.

112. Violi F, Ferro D, Quintarelli C. Antiphospholipid antibodies, hypercoagulability and thrombosis. *Haematologica* 1995;80(suppl 2):131–135.

113. Hojnik M, George J, Ziporen L, Shoenfeld Y. Heart valve involvement (Libman-Sacks endocarditis) in the antiphospholipid syndrome. *Circulation* 1996;93:1579–1987.

114. Nesher G, Ilany J, Rosenmann D, Abraham AS. Valvular dysfunction in antiphospholipid syndrome: Prevalence, clinical features, and treatment. *Semin Arthritis Rheum* 1997;27:27–35.

115. Specker C, Perniok A, Brauckmann U, et al. Detection of cerebral microemboli in APS: Introducing a novel investigation method and implications of analogies with carotid artery disease. *Lupus* 1998;7(suppl 2):S75–S80.

116. Asherson RA, Cervera R, Piette JC, et al. Catastrophic antiphospholipid syndrome: Clinical and laboratory features of 50 patients. *Medicine (Baltimore)* 1998;77:195–207.

117. Matsuura E, Kobayashi K, Yasuda T, Koike T. Antiphospholipid antibodies and atherosclerosis. *Lupus* 1998;7(suppl 2):S135–S139.

118. Ginsburg KS, Liang MH, Newcomer L, et al. Anticardiolipin antibodies and the risk for ischemic stroke and venous thrombosis. *Ann Intern Med* 1992;117:997–1002.

NEOPLASTIC HEART DISEASE*

Robert J. Hall / Denton A. Cooley / Hugh A. McAllister, Jr. / O. Howard Frazier / Robert A. O'Rourke

Benign and malignant tumors of the heart are very uncommon and present in protean ways that have challenged the acumen of physicians since the seventeenth century.[1] Intracardiac myxoma was first diagnosed, with the aid of angiography, in 1952, with a subsequent attempt to remove the tumor surgically. The first such successful removal with the use of cardiopulmonary bypass was performed in 1954; the patient, then a 40-year-old woman, was still alive 38 years later.[2] Subsequently, increased clinical awareness coupled with angiographic and noninvasive diagnostic techniques especially echocardiography led to more frequent correct diagnoses (Chap. 15).[3]

Treatment of cardiac tumors was greatly influenced by two events: the utilization of cardiopulmonary bypass by Dr. John Gibbons, which allowed a safe and reproducible approach to the cardiac chambers, and the development of clinical echocardiography, which introduced safe, noninvasive imaging and diagnosis of intracardiac masses. Operations are performed safely on cardiac tumors, with atrial myxoma having the lowest surgical mortality. The introduction of transesophageal echocardiography (TEE) further improved definition of the cardiac anatomy with visualization of the left atrial (LA) appendage and ascending aorta and increased ability to image the left atrial (LA) appendage, previously undetectable on routine transthoracic echocardiography (TTE) (Chap. 15).

The heart may be the site of a primary tumor or may be invaded secondarily by malignancies that arise in adjacent or remote organs. Whether the tumors are primary or secondary, neoplastic heart disease can be expressed in only limited ways (Table 85-1). In the presence of neoplastic disease, pericardial pain, effusion, tamponade, constriction, rapid increase in heart size, new heart murmurs, electrocardiographic (ECG) changes, atrial or ventricular arrhythmias, atrioventricular (AV) block, and unexplained heart failure are suggestive of secondary invasion of the heart. The *triad* of obstruction, embolization, and constitutional manifestations characterizes intracavitary tumors, especially myxomas.

PRIMARY TUMORS OF THE HEART

Primary tumors of the heart are extremely rare, with an incidence in autopsy series reported to be between 0.001 and 0.03 percent. These tumors usually present as intracavitary lesions, and more than 75 percent are benign.[4] Current surgical techniques permit removal and potential "cure" in many patients with primary heart tumors, thus necessitating an awareness of their clinical and hemodynamic presentation.

Myxomas constitute nearly 50 percent of all histologically benign tumors of the heart. The frequency of occurrence and classification of 533 primary tumors and cysts of the heart and pericardium collected by the Armed Forces Institute of Pathology are presented in Table 85-2.[5]

Cardiac Myxomas

Intracardiac myxoma is the most frequent benign tumor of the heart. While most (75 percent) are located in the left atrium (LA), myxomas are also found in the right atrium (RA) (18 percent), right ventricle (RV) (4 percent), and left ventricle (LV) (3 percent).[5-8] Cardiac myxomas usually originate from the region of the fossa ovalis but may arise from a variety of locations within the atria.[5] Approximately 75 percent occur in the LA. The deoxyribonucleic acid (DNA) genotype of sporadic myxomas is normal in 80 percent of patients. Tumors are likely to be associated with other abnormal conditions and have a low recurrence rate. About 5 percent of myxoma patients show a familial pattern of tumor development based on autosomal dominant inheritance; 20 percent of those with sporadic myxoma have an abnormal DNA genotype chromosomal pattern.[9-14] Most true myxomas arise only from the mural endocardium despite isolated reports that they arise from the cardiac valves, pulmonary vessels, and vena cava.[15]

PATHOLOGY

Attached to the endocardium by a broad base, myxomas are usually pedunculated, polypoid, and friable, although some may have a smooth surface and are rounded.[8,9] A myxoma appears as a soft,

*Modified and updated with permission from O. H. Frazier for the authors of Chap. 77 in the 10th edition of *Hurst's The Heart.*

TABLE 85-1 General Manifestations of Neoplastic Heart Disease

Pericardial involvement
  Pericarditis and pain
  Pericardial effusion
  Radiographic enlargement
  Arrhythmia, predominantly atrial
  Tamponade
  Constriction
Myocardial involvement
  Arrhythmias, ventricular and atrial
  Electrocardiographic changes
  Radiographic enlargement
    Generalized
    Localized
  Conduction disturbances and heart block
  Congestive heart failure
  Coronary involvement
    Angina, infarction
Intracavitary tumor
  Cavity obliteration
  Valve obstruction and valve damage
  Embolic phenomena: systemic, neurologic, and coronary
  Constitutional manifestations

TABLE 85-2 Tumors and Cysts of the Heart and Pericardium

Type	Number	Percentage
BENIGN		
Myxoma	130	24.4
Lipoma	45	8.4
Papillary fibroelastoma	42	7.9
Rhabdomyoma	36	6.8
Fibroma	17	3.2
Hemangioma	15	2.8
Teratoma	14	2.6
Mesothelioma of the AV node	12	2.3
Granular cell tumor	3	
Neurofibroma	3	
Lymphangioma	2	
Subtotal	319	59.8
Pericardial cyst	82	15.4
Bronchogenic cyst	7	1.3
Subtotal	89	16.7
MALIGNANT		
Angiosarcoma	39	7.3
Rhabdomyosarcoma	26	4.9
Mesothelioma	19	3.6
Fibrosarcoma	14	2.6
Malignant lymphoma	7	1.3
Extraskeletal osteosarcoma	5	
Neurogenic sarcoma	4	
Malignant teratoma	4	
Thymoma	4	
Leiomyosarcoma	1	
Liposarcoma	1	
Synovial sarcoma	1	
Subtotal	125	23.5
Total	533	100.0

SOURCE: McAllister and Fenoglio,[5] with permission.

gelatinous, mucoid, usually gray-white mass, often with areas of hemorrhage or thrombosis.[10–19] Myxomas vary from 1 to 15 cm in diameter, with most measuring 5 to 6 cm (Fig. 85-1A, B, and C).

On microscopic examination, the myxoma consists of an acid mucopolysaccharide myxoid matrix in which polygonal cells and occasional blood vessels are embedded. Channels, often containing red blood cells, communicate from the surface to deep within the tumor and are lined by endothelial-like cells resembling multipurpose mesenchymal cells, from which the tumor is purported to arise. Similar endothelial cells line the surface of the tumor; however, fibrin, erythrocytes, and organized thrombi also may be present on the surface. Cystic areas; focal or gross hemorrhage; calcification; glandular elements; rarely, bone formation; and even hematopoietic tissue constitute the multiple, less common, variations.[6]

A neoplastic origin of myxomas is supported by the ultrastructural characteristics of the tumor,[6] the results of biochemical analyses,[11] the cultural properties of the tumor cell,[5] and DNA analysis of the tumor.[6] Although myxomas can recur because of their incomplete removal[12] and distant growth of embolic myxomatous material has been observed,[12] the existence of a true malignant cardiac myxoma remains doubtful.[4] The occurrence of multiple tumors within the LA, bilaterally in each atrium[13] or simultaneously in the atrium and ventricle,[14] raises the likelihood of a multicentric origin rather than metastasis of the tumor.

AGE, GENDER, AND FAMILIAL OCCURRENCE

Most patients with myxomas are 30 to 60 years of age,[3] although myxomas have been discovered in children, infants, neonates,[15] and the elderly.[18] Children have a higher incidence of ventricular myxomas than do adults. A higher prevalence in females has characterized most series. Familial occurrence has been reported,[19–20] more frequently in males. Tumors are divided equally on both sides of the heart, and opposite atria are usually involved in afflicted members. Familial cases are associated with a younger age at presentation and a higher recurrence rate.[19–20]

GENERAL OR CONSTITUTIONAL MANIFESTATIONS

While asymptomatic patients with myxoma (Fig. 85-1C) have been reported, most present with one or more effects of a *triad* of constitutional, embolic, and obstructive manifestations.[3] Cardiac myxomas provoke systemic manifestations in 90 percent of the patients, characterized by weight loss, fatigue, fever, anemia (often hemolytic), elevated sedimentation rate, and elevated serum immunoglobulin concentration formed in response to tumor embolization, degenerative changes within the tumor, or overproduction of interleukin-6 by the tumor.[21] The globulin fraction most frequently elevated is immunoglobulin G (IgG); immunoglobulin A is involved only rarely.[3] Cases involving coexisting cardiac myxoma and IgG multiple myeloma,[22] and systemic AL (immunocyte-derived) amyloidosis have been reported.[23] Less common findings are leukocytosis, thrombocytopenia, clubbing, Raynaud's phenomenon, and breast fibroadenomas.[3] Polycythemia may result from tumor production of erythropoietin. Patients with hemolytic anemia have features of intravascular mechanical destruction. Hemolytic anemia is more likely to occur in patients with calcified myxomas, which are found more commonly in the RA. The protracted multisystemic symptoms pro-

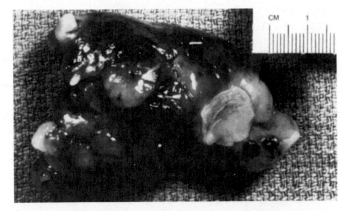

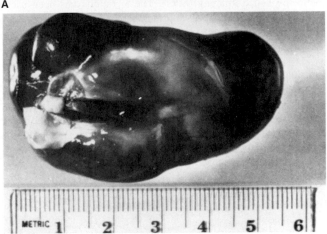

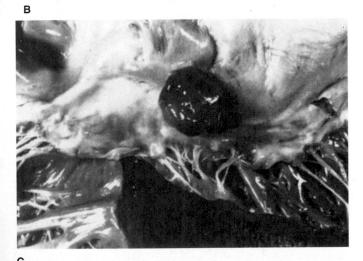

FIGURE 85-1 Left atrial myxomas. *A.* More polypoid and irregular. *B.* Smooth-surfaced and rounded. Attachment to a portion of the atrial septum is seen on each tumor. *C.* An asymptomatic sessile myxoma attached above the posterior leaflet of the mitral valve was found coincidentally at necropsy.

duced by myxomas may mimic connective tissue disease and polyarteritis nodosa.[24]

"Syndrome myxoma," or Carney's complex, characterizes a subset of patients with cardiac myxoma associated with spotty skin pigmentation and peripheral and endocrine neoplasms. These patients, in contrast to those with "sporadic myxoma," are usually younger, have a high frequency of familial myxoma, and more frequently have multiple and recurrent tumors.[25–27]

Infected Myxoma Rarely, an intracavitary myxoma becomes infected, and blood cultures have demonstrated a variety of organisms.[28] Most patients with infected myxomas experience major neurologic embolic events. Thus, surgical resection should be carried out promptly before complications occur.

Embolization Systemic tumor embolization, more commonly from myxomas with irregular, papillary, frond-like surfaces,[8,9] occurs in 40 to 50 percent of patients with LA myxoma,[2] with tumor fragments or surface clots embolizing to arteries in the brain, kidneys, and extremities.[29,30] Rarely, a complete LA myxoma becomes detached and lodges in the aortic bifurcation or the iliac arteries.[31] The size and consistency of such an embolus may require direct exploration of the aortic bifurcation. Histologic examination of emboli recovered at operation from a peripheral artery can aid in diagnosing an otherwise unsuspected intracardiac myxoma.[4] Systemic embolization, especially in a young patient with sinus rhythm, should arouse suspicion of a myxoma once bacterial endocarditis has been ruled out.

Tumor embolization of the central nervous system constitutes about 50 percent of embolic events caused by LA myxomas, may represent the first symptomatic manifestation, is more common in the left hemisphere, and may be multiple and massive.[32,32a] Embolization may be to the extracranial or intracranial cerebral vessels, with the former being amenable to surgical removal. Onset of the neurologic deficit may be gradual or sudden.

Intracranial arterial aneurysms secondary to myxomatous emboli have been demonstrated angiographically. Late rupture with intracranial hemorrhage has been reported. Care must be taken to avoid embolization during surgical removal of an intracardiac myxoma. The patient who has sustained cerebral emboli is not necessarily "cured" after the primary tumor is surgically removed because viable metastatic foci may cause symptoms years later.[33]

Retinal artery embolism can occur with transient or permanent visual impairment, confirmed by ophthalmoscopic and histopathologic evidence of particulate embolic matter in the retinal artery.[34] Only rarely has occlusion of the retinal artery occurred in the absence of multifocal neurologic manifestations.

Coronary artery embolism associated with myxoma has been documented by both angiography in living patients and histology at postmortem study.[4] Myocardial infarction occasionally is the first manifestation of a myxoma.[35]

General Features Constitutional manifestations and embolic potential are relatively common in patients with myxoma in any intracavitary location. The cardiac manifestations, symptoms, and physical findings are the consequence of the intracavitary mass and the particular location of the tumor. Myxomas of the LA may obstruct either the mitral or pulmonary venous orifices and produce pulmonary venous hypertension, secondary pulmonary hypertension, and right-sided heart failure. The clinical symptoms include dyspnea on exertion, orthopnea, paroxysmal nocturnal dyspnea, acute pulmonary edema, cough, and hemoptysis, along with palpitations, chest pain, fatigue, and peripheral edema. Episodes of syncope or dizziness are frequent, and sudden death may occur. A marked change in the severity of any symptom caused by a change in position of the patient, especially if recumbency relieves dyspnea,[3] is suggestive of myxoma.

Physical Examination On physical examination, the S_1 is loud and frequently split, with the second component corresponding to the tumor's expulsion from the mitral orifice (Chap. 12). P_2 is accentuated, and an early diastolic sound, the "tumor plop," is usually heard 80 to

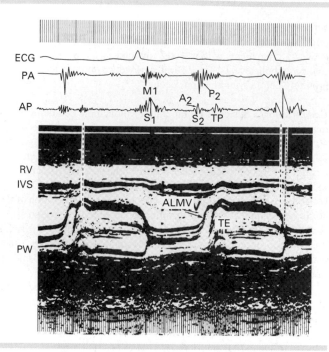

FIGURE 85-2 Recordings of a patient with a cystic left atrial myxoma, including (*top*) the electrocardiogram, (*middle*) phonocardiograms from the pulmonary area (PA) at high frequency and from the apex (AP) at medium frequency, and (*bottom*) the M-mode echocardiogram at the level of the mitral valve. Time lines equal 0.01-s intervals. The right ventricle (RV), interventricular septum (IVS), and posterior wall (PW) of the left ventricle are identified. The loud component of the first sound (M_1) is delayed (Q to M_1 = 0.09 s). The pulmonic second sound (P_2) is accentuated. Multiple linear tumor echoes (TE) are seen behind the anterior leaflet to the mitral valve (ALMV), first appearing at the mitral level 0.04 s after onset of mitral opening and completing the forward movement 0.09 s after onset of mitral opening, at which point the "tumor plop" (TP) is recorded. The A_2–TP interval measures 0.010 s.

120 ms after the A_2,[3] resembling an opening snap. The tumor plop (TP) may be confused with either an opening snap or a third heart sound and follows A_2 at an intermediate interval between these events (Fig. 85-2).

An apical diastolic or systolic murmur or both are present in many patients. The auscultatory findings may vary with the patient's change in position.[3] Features of pulmonary hypertension are frequent and may result in a murmur of tricuspid regurgitation (Chap. 12).

Electrocardiogram and Chest X-ray Results of ECG recordings are nonspecific, reflecting hemodynamic alterations similar to those of mitral valvular disease; however, sinus rhythm is generally the rule. The chest roentgenogram reveals LA enlargement and the characteristic changes of pulmonary venous congestion and pulmonary hypertension. The absence of mitral valve calcification and the presence of a LA smaller than might be expected with presumed rheumatic mitral disease are helpful differentiating clues. Calcification may be evident in the tumor even on routine chest film,[36,37] but this is better visualized and motion is better appreciated on fluoroscopy. The "wrecking ball" effect of a calcified mobile myxoma may cause destruction of the mitral valve or rupture of the chordae tendineae, resulting in severe mitral regurgitation (MR).

Echocardiography The value of TTE in the noninvasive diagnosis of intracavitary tumors has been well documented.[3,9] M-mode recordings in patients with a prolapsing LA myxoma typically demonstrate a diminished EF slope of the anterior leaflet of the mitral

valve, behind which a dense array of wavy tumor echoes is seen (Chap. 15). The TP coincides with the completion of this anterior movement of tumor echoes (Fig. 85-2). A similar array of tumor echoes may be seen in the LA during ventricular systole. TTE and TEE identify the size, shape, point of attachment, and motion characteristics of LA atrial myxomas.[38] TEE permits superior imaging of the posterior cardiac structures and LA myxomas, especially their point of attachment (Fig. 85-3) (Chap. 15). Visualization of all four chambers permits recognition of multiple tumors or tumors in less common locations. Doppler assessment of the flow patterns of the mitral valve and pulmonary vein provides further information regarding the hemodynamic consequences of LA myxomas.

Other Imaging Techniques High resolution is achieved by magnetic resonance imaging (MRI). The technique has been used to achieve excellent visualization of intracavitary atrial myxomas, providing information about the size, shape, attachment, and mobility of these tumors.[39–41]

Cardiac Catheterization Catheterization of the cardiac chambers is currently infrequently performed, since the information provided is readily obtained by echocardiographic studies. Catheterization of the right heart chambers invariably demonstrates significant pulmonary capillary wedge and pulmonary arterial hypertension.[3] A large *v* wave, even in the absence of significant MR, reflects the space-occupying effect of the tumor within the LA.

Cardiac Angiography Although angiography characterizes the size, location, and mobility of the tumor,[2] the efficacy of TTE, TEE, and other imaging techniques has largely supplanted hemodynamic studies and contrast angiography and usually permits immediate operative intervention.

Coronary Angiography Coronary angiography may demonstrate a vascular blush in the tumor from branches of both the right and/or left coronary arteries; both left and RA myxomas and ventricular myxomas have been demonstrated in this manner.[6] Neovascularization of a LA thrombus accompanying mitral stenosis may produce an appearance similar to a tumor blush. Aneurysms and occlusion of the coronary artery caused by tumor emboli have also been demonstrated by coronary angiography. Myocardial infarction in myxoma patients with normal coronary arteries has been ascribed to cytokine secretion by the tumor.[42] Cardiac catheterization and coronary angiography are indicated primarily for patients with additional heart disease and to rule out concomitant coronary artery disease.

Differential Diagnosis LA myxomas most often present as mitral valvular disease and must be differentiated from it.[1] At our institution, intracavitary myxomas were discovered in a ratio of approximately 1 per 100 patients presenting for mitral valve surgery.[3] Characteristically, the clinical course is relatively recent in origin; however, it may occasionally span many years. Fever, constitutional symptoms, and embolic phenomena mimic infective endocarditis[1]; on rare occasions the myxoma itself may be infected. Muscle pain, skin rash, and Raynaud's phenomenon may simulate peripheral vasculitis.[43] Multiple systemic arterial aneurysms secondary to myxomatous embolization have mimicked polyarteritis nodosa. Similarly, coronary artery aneurysmal dilatation and myocardial infarction have been attributed to coronary myxoma embolization. The correct diagnosis will be suspected if the physician maintains a high index of clinical suspicion in patients with diverse and protean features. TTE has greatly facilitated the recognition of intracavitary tumors and results in detection in some patients who are asymptomatic.[14] Intracavitary thrombi may at times mimic intracardiac tumor masses (Fig. 85-4).

RIGHT ATRIAL MYXOMA

Myxomas in the RA cavity constitute about one-fifth of all myxomas and tend to be more solid, have a wider attachment, and involve a greater amount of the atrial wall or septum than those in the LA. They originate from a variety of locations within the RA, including the inferior margin of the foramen ovale, the tricuspid valve, and the eustachian valve[6,44,45] and characteristically produce tricuspid valve or vena cava obstruction. A myxoma arising from the inferior vena cava has been reported, as has a myoma producing a superior vena cava syndrome.[46]

Clinical Manifestations   Clinically, symptoms of low cardiac output and manifestations of systemic venous hypertension are present, with a prominent jugular venous *a* wave, hepatomegaly, ascites, edema, and cyanosis,[6] which may be episodic and vary with the position of the patient. Persistence of sinus rhythm is common. Intermittent episodes of syncope and abrupt onset of dyspnea, features never seen with rheumatic tricuspid stenosis, are reported in one-third of these patients.[6] The pendular action of a prolapsing RA myxoma (wrecking-ball effect),[47] especially when it is calcified, may damage or destroy the tricuspid valve and produce severe tricuspid regurgitation.

Pulmonary Emboli   While embolic tumor phenomena occur less frequently with RA than with LA myxomas, pulmonary emboli have been reported[6]; at times they may be extensive and produce irreversible pulmonary hypertension.[48,49] RA myxoma has been incorrectly diagnosed as recurrent pulmonary thromboembolism.[49]

Wide dissemination of myxomatous embolization to the pulmonary arteries may occur, with active infiltration of the media and formation of aneurysms.[6] Paradoxical embolization may occur if an interatrial communication exists.

Systemic Manifestations   Constitutional symptoms are less frequent in patients with a RA myxoma.[3] Anemia, polycythemia, and cyanosis have been

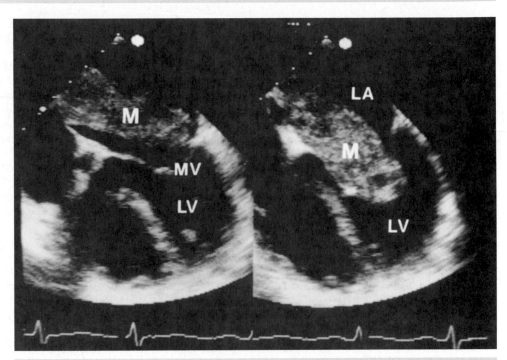

FIGURE 85-3   Transesophageal echocardiogram in the four-chamber view from a 50-year-old man who presented with exertional dyspnea and syncope. A large left atrial myxoma (M) attached to the interatrial septum is seen prolapsing across the mitral valve (MV) into the left ventricle (LV) in diastole (*right panel*). (Courtesy of Susan Wilansky, M.D., Medical Director, Noninvasive Imaging, St. Luke's Episcopal Hospital, Houston, Texas.)

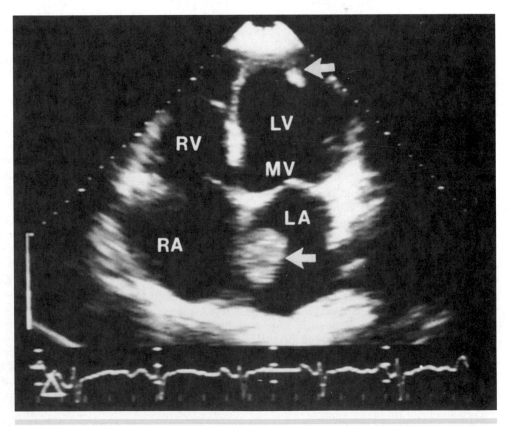

FIGURE 85-4   Two-dimensional echocardiogram, apical four-chamber view, from a patient with advanced congestive cardiomyopathy. Intracavitary masses (*arrows*), proved at autopsy to be thrombi, are present in the left atrium attached to the atrial septum (AS) and in the apex of the left ventricle. The latter masses are both sessile and pedunculated. MV = mitral valve. (Courtesy of Carlos de Castro, M.D., Department of Cardiology, St. Luke's Episcopal Hospital, Houston, Texas.)

reported. Polycythemia and cyanosis may be caused by either right-to-left shunting through a patent foramen ovale or atrial septal defect, low cardiac output and hypoxemic stimulation of the bone marrow, intravascular hemoconcentration, or erythropoietin production by the tumor. Mesenteric vasculitis of a nonembolic, probably autoimmune origin has been reported.[50]

Auscultation A loud early systolic sound may be heard. This sound occurs as late as 80 ms after the mitral component of the first sound and results from expulsion of the tumor from the right ventricle. A palpable tumor shock may coincide with this loud sound.[51] A crescendo murmur with inspiratory augmentation preceding this loud tumor expulsion sound is probably caused by early systolic tricuspid regurgitation (Chap. 12). There may be a long diastolic murmur or, more commonly, only a late diastolic rumble, augmented by inspiration, accompanying atrial systole. If major injury to the tricuspid valve occurs, the murmur of TR will be present, and large *v* waves will be seen in the jugular venous pulse (JVP) (Chap. 12). An early diastolic sound jugular venous pulse may be heard but is less constant than the TP due to a LA myxoma. The changing quality of the sound and murmurs may mimic a pericardial rub. Such sounds have been called endocardial friction rubs (Chap. 12).

Electrocardiogram and Chest X-ray The ECG is often normal, although RA enlargement frequently is suggested.[6] Low-voltage right-axis deviation and varying degrees of right bundle branch block have been reported.[6] The chest roentgenogram may reveal some prominence or enlargement of the RA shadow and, occasionally, of the RV. An important radiologic feature is the mild or moderate degree of cardiomegaly considering the severe clinical state of the patients. Calcification in the tumor is more common in patients with myxomas in the right atrium.[3]

Echocardiography TTE and TEE provide excellent images of the RA.[52] TEE provides more detail of the tumor and defines the site of attachment with greater clarity (Chap. 15). A large prolapsing atrial septal aneurysm may mimic a RA tumor.[53] With current noninvasive imaging techniques, catheterization and angiography of the right-sided heart chambers are rarely necessary.

Differential Diagnosis The clinical features of RA myxoma resemble those of rheumatic tricuspid valvular disease, although the latter is always accompanied by significant mitral and, often, aortic valve disease. There are many similarities to constrictive pericarditis and Ebstein's anomaly of the tricuspid valve. Episodic dyspnea, sudden syncope, and variability of symptoms and findings with the position of the patient are useful clues. Changing murmurs, along with fever and anemia, may suggest infective endocarditis. Tricuspid stenosis and regurgitation are prominent in patients with carcinoid syndrome, but involvement of the pulmonary valve and other features of a carcinoid tumor (discussed later) will usually distinguish it from a RA myxoma. Obstruction of the right ventricular (RV) outflow tract may resemble a RA tumor.

BILATERAL ATRIAL MYXOMA

An atrial myxoma may pass through the foramen ovale and be present in both atria.[54] The tumor is usually shaped like a dumbbell, with the common stalk attached to the margin of the fossa ovalis. Surgery has been successful most often when the correct diagnosis was made preoperatively, emphasizing the importance of echocardiographic exploration of all chambers.[13] Similar echocardiographic findings have been reported in patients with discrete tumors in each atrium.

Multichambered cardiac myxomas occasionally involve chambers other than the usual biatrial combination and are more often familial.[6]

LEFT VENTRICULAR MYXOMA

A myxoma originates from the LV in 2.5 to 4 percent of reported myxomas.[4] Most patients are under 30 years of age. Women are affected three times more often than are men, and a short duration of symptoms is also characteristic. Systemic emboli, mostly cerebral,[55] occur in two-thirds of the patients, and constitutional symptoms are usually absent. Attacks of syncope occur in nearly half of the reviewed cases. Symptoms and physical findings are suggestive of aortic or subaortic obstruction. The location and movement of the tumor mass are demonstrated particularly well by TTE and by TEE (Chap. 15).[6] Echoes from an intracavitary LV myxoma must be differentiated from LV thrombi and from ventricular septal rhabdomyomas. LV and RV myxomas have been identified by MRI (Chap. 21).[56] Planning for surgical excision can be based upon noninvasive imaging without resorting to cardiac catheterization and angiography unless coexistent cardiac or coronary disease is possible.[56,57] The tumor can be removed through a LA approach with mobilization of the anterior leaflet of the mitral valve.[58]

RIGHT VENTRICULAR MYXOMA

Myxomas of the RV are as infrequent as those of the LV. The patient will have symptoms and manifestations of right-sided heart failure, syncope, unexplained fever, and a murmur consistent with pulmonic stenosis. Pulmonary emboli may occur. An "ejection sound" has been reported, as well as delayed closure of the pulmonic valve. A right-sided TP may be heard in diastole.[6] Calcium in the tumor may be recognized on the roentgenogram. Echocardiographic imaging, both TTE and TEE, will detect most RV myxomas.[59] A RV myxoma has been diagnosed in a neonate and has been successfully removed surgically. Other tumors, producing similar outflow tract obstruction, rarely occur within the RV.[6]

SURGERY FOR INTRACAVITARY MYXOMA

Surgical resection of a myxoma is the only acceptable therapy and, in view of the dangers of embolization and sudden death, should be performed promptly.[60] For complete removal of LA myxoma, the authors use a biatrial approach, excising a full thickness of interatrial septum if the tumor is attached to the region of the fossa ovalis.[61] RA myxomas are commonly attached to the fossa ovalis, and, with right-sided tumors, a full thickness of atrial septum should also be resected. If a large portion of the septum is removed, a patch of knitted Dacron cloth should be used for repair to avoid distortion, arrhythmias, or possible atrial septal defect. Ventricular standstill with cardioplegia solution is induced before manipulating the heart, so as to reduce the possibility of fragmentation of the gelatinous tumor. LA myxomas have been removed successfully during pregnancy, utilizing cardiopulmonary bypass, with subsequent uncomplicated completion of a full-term pregnancy. Surgical removal of a RV myxoma in a neonate has been reported.[62]

By its movement within the heart, a myxoma, especially when calcified, may traumatize AV valve, which may require replacement or repair by annuloplasty.[2] Recurrences of atrial myxomas are rare and usually occur within a 48-month period.[6]

Other Benign Primary Cardiac Tumors

RHABDOMYOMA

The most frequent cardiac tumor in infants and children is a rhabdomyoma, which is probably a hamartoma rather than a true neoplasm.[63] These tumors are usually multiple, usually involve the ventricular myocardium, and project into the cavity or move freely as a pedunculated mass.[64] Associated tuberous sclerosis is present in one-third of the patients.[65,66,66a] Presenting manifestations may be caused by cardiac obstructive phenomena or by arrhythmias, AV block, pericardial effusion, ventricular preexcitation,[67] and even sudden death. These tumors can mimic pulmonary stenosis and produce hypoxic spells like those seen with tetralogy of Fallot. Ventricular outlet gradients, angiographic abnormalities, echocardiography (Chap. 15), and MRI[68] can lead to demonstration of the tumor and successful surgical resection or heart transplantation.[69] Pedunculated rhabdomyomas that arise from the LA and cause mitral stenosis have been reported. Discrete and multiple myocardial hamartomas and rhabdomyomas have caused incessant ventricular tachycardia in infants and have been successfully removed surgically.[70] Rhabdomyomas are the tumors most frequently found at fetal echocardiography, constituting 17 of 19 fetal tumors found in 14,000 fetal echocardiograms.[71]

FIBROMA

Fibromas are usually ventricular and intramural. Although reported cases have occurred in the age range from newborn to 65 years, most occur in infants and children.[76–80] Calcification is common. Sudden death, occurring in nearly one-third of the patients, likely is due to involvement of the conduction system, production of arrhythmias, or obstruction of the LV outflow tract.[74] TTE accurately delineates intramural ventricular tumors (Chap. 15). Left-axis deviation may occur as an interesting ECG feature. Total or partial resection of the tumor to relieve obstruction has been reported, with excellent probability of long-term survival.[73] Cardiac transplantation has been used in the management of a young adult with a nonresectable (1030-g) LV fibroma.[75]

PAPILLARY FIBROELASTOMA

Also referred to as papillomas or papillary fibromas, papillary fibroelastomas arise from the cardiac valves[76–80] or occasionally from the ventricular endocardium, are most commonly seen in patients over age 50, and until recently have been a coincidental finding at surgery or postmortem examination. Grossly, these tumors resemble a sea anemone, with multiple papillary fronds attached to the endothelium by a short pedicle. There is a predilection for involvement of the aortic valve,[77] where angina, infarction, or sudden death may result from coronary embolization or ostial occlusion caused by the villous tumor.[3,79] Cerebral and ocular emboli from these lesions are being reported with increasing frequency. Origin on right-sided cardiac valves is rare.[81–83] Obstruction of the RV outflow tract has been reported in a patient with a papillary tumor of the tricuspid valve. The tumor is histologically different from Lambl's excrescences, which are degenerative in origin and usually situated on the ventricular aspect of the semilunar valve along the line of closure.[4] Papillary fibroelastomas are being discovered with increasing frequency by echocardiographic (TTE and TEE) imaging of the heart; because of their potential for cerebral and coronary embolization, surgical excision is recommended for even small papillary fibroelastomas.[84]

LIPOMA

Lipomas may occur throughout the heart,[85] including the pericardium. They may be massive. Intrapericardial lipomas may cause pericardial effusion, be mistaken for a pericardial cyst, or present as asymptomatic cardiac or mediastinal enlargement. Intramyocardial lipomas are encapsulated and usually are small.[4] Occasionally, a lipoma arising from the mitral or tricuspid valve may resemble an

atrial myxoma on echocardiographic examination[86] and must also be differentiated from a cyst or lymphangioma of the mitral valve.[87] Surgical excision of lipomas yields excellent long-term results. Tissue characterization by MRI permits preoperative identification of these fatty tumors (Chap. 21).

Lipomatous hypertrophy of the atrial septum is a nonencapsulated hyperplasia of adipose tissue and may not represent a true tumor. Varying in size from 2 to 8 cm, the tumescence may bulge into the atrial cavity or superior vena cava orifice and become a consideration in the differential diagnosis of intracavitary masses.[88] Although often found coincidentally at postmortem study, lipomatous hypertrophy of the atrial septum can be associated with unexplained supraventricular rhythm and conduction disturbances, recurrent pericardial effusion, and sudden death.[4,6] Features of both TTE and TEE are distinctive and include atrial septal thickening with a bilobed appearance due to sparing of the area of the fossa ovalis. Computed tomographic (CT) scanning and MRI provide noninvasive tissue characterization of lipomas that echocardiography does not provide.[89,90] The diagnosis may be confirmed by percutaneous transvenous biopsy.

CYSTIC TUMORS OF THE ATRIOVENTRICULAR NODE

Cystic tumors of the AV node likely originate from either mesothelial or endodermal rests and are always benign.[6] Patients with these tumors tend to have partial or complete AV block, usually of long duration, and often die of complete heart block or ventricular fibrillation. These tumors are the smallest ones capable of causing sudden death.[6] Reported ages in patients have ranged from the newborn period to the ninth decade of life, with a strong female preponderance. These cystic tumors have also been referred to as mesotheliomas, lymphangioepitheliomas, and congenital polycystic tumors of the AV node.[6] Aside from chance intraoperative finding of this tumor,[91] in vivo recognition has not been reported, although the cystic structure may exceed 3 cm in size. The tumor is usually large enough to be recognized grossly at postmortem examination and should be suspected in all cases of sudden death without apparent cause, especially in children and young adults.[6] Most patients with these cystic tumors of the AV node have demonstrated complete AV block and have recurrent attacks of syncope. Even with complete AV block, a narrow QRS complex is common, and these patients may pursue a stable course for years. Electrophysiologic study discloses a block proximal to the His bundle.[6] Electronic pacing should aid in maintaining an adequate cardiac rate, but examples of electrical instability and sudden death reflect a special hazard in these patients, even during diagnostic electrophysiologic studies and after initiation of effective ventricular pacing.[92]

VASOFORMATIVE TUMORS

Hemangiomas[93] are rare cardiac tumors usually discovered at postmortem study. Coronary angiography yields a characteristic tumor blush.[6] Spontaneous resolution without treatment of a large cavernous hemangioma of the RV has been reported. Lymphangiomas and vascular hamartomas are rare primary tumors of the heart that usually present as diffuse proliferations rather than as distinct tumors. Therefore, total excision is often not practical.[94] Cardiac transplantation may be considered as an alternative in these cases.

INTRAPERICARDIAL PARAGANGLIOMA

Paragangliomas (pheochromocytomas and chemodectomas) may rarely be localized within the pericardium (Chap. 80). Although these tumors may be found overlying or within any cardiac chamber, they most commonly occur over the base of the heart in the major region of vagus nerve distribution.[95] Improved detection and localization to the mediastinum have been provided by iodine-131 metaiodobenzylguanidine nuclear scanning. MRI can further localize cardiac paragangliomas and provide detailed information for guidance of surgical excision.[96] Since these tumors are highly vascular, adherent, and difficult to resect, management with cardiac transplantation may be necessary.[97] Human cardiac explantation and autotransplantation has also been applied to a patient with a large cardiac pheochromocytoma.[98]

MISCELLANEOUS BENIGN TUMORS

The right side of the ventricular septum is rarely the site of a congenital benign thyroid rest. Enlargement results in right ventricular outflow obstruction. Complete resection is indicated, and the condition is curable. Rarely, benign teratomas occur in the ventricular myocardium and may result in sudden death.[99]

Malignant Primary Tumors of the Heart

ANGIOSARCOMA (HEMANGIOSARCOMA)

Almost all primary malignant cardiac tumors are sarcomas,[100] most frequently angiosarcomas, and they usually originate in the RA or pericardium.[101] Intense vascularity may produce a continuous murmur. One-fourth of all angiosarcomas are partially intracavitary, with valvular or vena caval[102] obstruction, and characteristically manifest right-sided heart failure and pericardial tamponade with hemorrhagic fluid. Cardiac rupture due to a RA angiosarcoma has been reported.[6] Atrial angiosarcomas exhibit highly variable histologic patterns, which may overlap those of Kaposi's sarcoma. Echocardiography, angiography, CT, or MRI are helpful in the diagnosis (Fig. 85-5A).[103] Coronary angiography may demonstrate angiomatous vessels in the tumor area. The course is rapid, and widespread metastases often make surgery impractical, although tumor excision, radiation, and chemotherapy may offer some relief of symptoms and palliation.[4] An iatrogenic hemangiopericytoma of the right ventricle has been reported following intense radiotherapy to the cardiac area.[104]

RHABDOMYOSARCOMA

Rhabdomyosarcoma is the second most frequent primary sarcoma of the heart and, like angiosarcoma, is prevalent in males. There is no single chamber predilection; multiple sites are common, and significant obstruction of at least one valve is present in half of the patients.[105] Excision of the main tumor mass combined with radiation and chemotherapy has been advocated as the treatment for patients with primary malignant tumor of the heart, but in general the prognosis is poor and survival is short.[4]

OTHER MALIGNANT PRIMARY TUMORS

Fibrosarcoma,[106] liposarcoma,[107] primary malignant lymphoma,[108] and occasionally sarcomas of other basic cell types constitute the remaining but infrequent primary malignant cardiac tumors.[4] The fibrous histiocytoma has a predilection for the LA and rarely involves right-sided cardiac chambers.[109]

Malignant primary cardiac tumors may obstruct cardiac chambers or valves[6] or result in peripheral embolic phenomena.

Surgery for Primary Cardiac Tumors

Effective palliation and local control of the disease can be achieved with extensive resection of malignant primary tumors.[110,111] Echocar-

diography (Chap. 15), MRI (Chap. 21), and computed tomography (CT) (Chap. 20) are all helpful in planning operative resection of cardiac tumors because these tests provide three-dimensional information (Fig. 85-5B and C).[112] Intraoperative echocardiography may be useful in guiding surgical resection.[113] Adjuvant chemotherapy and radiation therapy are necessary to improve long-term prognosis,[114] and the response to therapy can be assessed by MRI.[6] Cardiac transplantation has been utilized to completely resect an "inoperable" benign tumor and an unresectable malignant primary cardiac neoplasm.[115] Cardiac explantation and autotransplantation may facilitate resection of some cardiac tumors (Chap. 26).[116–118]

Tumors of the Pericardium

PERICARDIAL CYSTS

Pericardial, or mesothelial, cysts are the most frequent benign "tumors" of the pericardium (Chap. 80). They are usually found coincidentally on a routine roentgenogram. However, 25 to 30 percent of the patients will have chest pain, dyspnea, cough, or paroxysmal tachycardia. Pericardial cysts occur most frequently in the third or fourth decade of life and equally among men and women. The right costophrenic location is the most common, although they may present in the upper mediastinum.[119] Only rarely does the cyst connect with the pericardial cavity. Clinically and radiographically, they resemble other tumors of the pericardium. Hemodynamically significant compression of the cardiac chamber rarely results.[120] Echocardiography, CT, and MRI are most helpful in the differential diagnosis. Surgical excision completely relieves symptoms and confirms the diagnosis[4,64]; however, percutaneous aspiration of the cystic contents is an attractive alternative to surgical resection.

TERATOMA

Most teratomas are extracardiac yet intrapericardial[121] receive their blood supply from the aortic root or pulmonary artery through the vasa vasorum. Most are found in infants and children, with a strong female preponderance.[4] Diagnosis has been established in utero by fetal echocardiography. Recurrent, nonbloody pericardial effusion is common in children with this tumor, and intrapericardial teratoma is the most likely diagnosis in this setting.[6,122] Depressed cardiac function results from expansion of the tumor to considerable proportions, at times up to 15 cm in diameter. Surgical excision is the only effective therapy and is curative. It is rare for a teratoma to be intracardiac and arise from the interventricular septum, but this type of tumor can be successfully excised.[6]

MESOTHELIOMA

Mesothelioma ranks third in frequency among malignant tumors of the heart and pericardium.[5] The clinical manifestations resemble those of pericarditis, constrictive pericardial disease, and vena cava obstruction. Aspiration and histologic examination of the usually bloody pericardial fluid may be diagnostic. Males outnumber females by a ratio of 2:1, with the peak incidence in the third to fifth decades. Surgical excision is usually impossible, and treatment with radiation and chemotherapy generally produces only temporary improvement. Rarely, the pericardium is the site of a primary sarcoma.[117]

Primary Tumors of the Aorta

Primary tumors of the aorta are rare and are usually malignant sarcomas.[6,123] Presentation may mimic aortic dissection, coarctation,

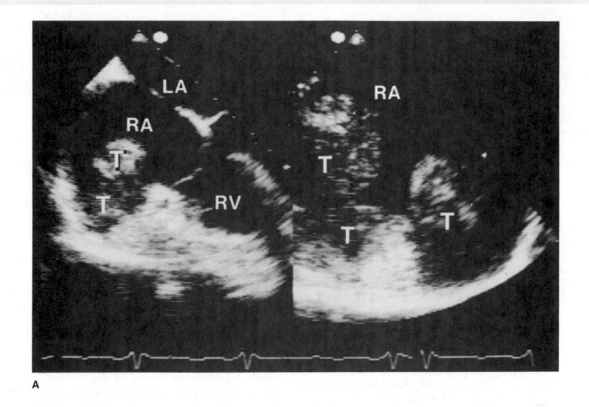

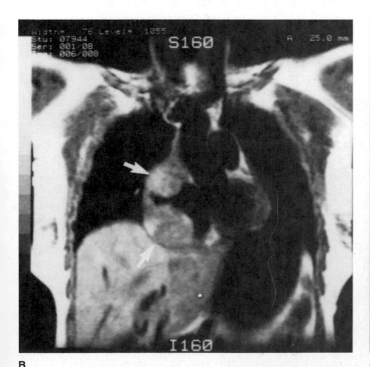

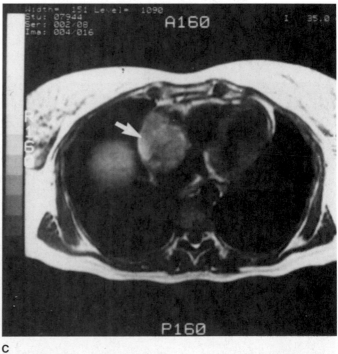

FIGURE 85-5 *A.* Biplane transesophageal echocardiogram from a 35-year-old woman who presented with shock of unknown cause. The horizontal plane (*left*) shows a tumor (T) in the right atrium (RA). The vertical plane (*right*) shows a large, bilobular tumor (T) adherent to the RA wall. Histologic examination proved this to be an angiosarcoma. (Courtesy of Susan Wilansky, M.D., Medical Director, Noninvasive Imaging, St. Luke's Episcopal Hospital, Houston, Texas.) *B* and *C.* Magnetic resonance images. Arrowheads (*B* and *C*) denote a dumbbell-shaped RA tumor of intermediate signal intensity, which is shown to abut the aorta in the coronal T1-weighted view and the tricuspid valve in the axial T1-weighted view. Note the loss of the usual high-signal-intensity margin (fat) along the right lateral aspect of the aorta in the coronal plane. This raises concern for malignant invasion of the aortic wall. (Courtesy of Clark L. Carrol, M.D., St. Luke's Episcopal Hospital, Texas Children's Hospital, and Texas Heart Institute, Houston, Texas.)

atherosclerotic occlusive disease, and malignancies in other organs. All portions of the aorta may be involved, and distal metastases are common. Surgical extirpation will relieve the obstructive phenomena, but distant metastases usually lead to disease progression.

SECONDARY TUMORS OF THE HEART

General Considerations

Metastatic tumors involve the heart, the pericardium, or both from a primary origin in some other organ 20 to 40 times more frequently than do primary tumors.[6] These secondary tumors are more frequently carcinomas than sarcomas. Cardiac metastases occur most often in people older than 50 years of age; the incidence is equal in both sexes. The development of otherwise unexplained cardiac symptoms or manifestations, cardiac enlargement, tachycardia, arrhythmias, or heart failure in the presence of neoplastic disease is suggestive of cardiac metastases.

Frequency and Origin of Secondary Tumors

In a report by the Harvard Cancer Commission of 4375 autopsies of patients who died of cancer, myocardial metastases were present in 146 patients (3.4 percent).[124] In a series of 2547 autopsies performed at Walter Reed General Hospital, 980 cases of malignant disease were observed. The heart was the site of metastatic tumor in 5.7 percent of the cases and the heart, including the pericardium, in 13.9 percent.[125] In other series, cardiac metastases have been present in patients with malignant tumors in a range as wide as 1.5 to 21 percent. A recent increased prevalence of secondary cardiac neoplasms may be related to more vigorous surgical and radiation treatment of patients with primary neoplasms. The relative infrequency of cardiac metastases has been attributed to the strong kneading action of the heart, the metabolic peculiarities of striated muscle, rapid coronary blood flow, and lymphatic connections that drain afferently from the heart.[124]

Cardiac metastases occur with all types of primary tumors. No malignant tumor tends particularly to metastasize to the heart with the possible exception of malignant melanoma, which involves the myocardium in more than 50 percent of cases.[126] Cardiac metastases are most frequent, with bronchogenic carcinoma and carcinoma of the breast occurring in one-third of the cases.[6] Cardiac infiltration, often macroscopic, is seen in one-half of cases of leukemia and in one-sixth of cases of lymphoma.

Cardiac metastases are encountered with widespread systemic tumor dissemination; only rarely is metastatic tumor limited to the heart or pericardium. Carcinomatous metastases are generally grossly visible, multiple, discrete, small, white, firm nodules; microscopically, they resemble the primary tumor and the metastases in other organs. Diffuse infiltration is characteristic of sarcomatous metastases.[127]

Metastatic tumors are classically thought to reach the heart by embolic hematogenous spread, lymphatic spread, or direct invasion, in descending order of frequency. Lymphatic spread of tumors is particularly frequent with carcinoma of the bronchus and the breast; the proximity of the heart to major mediastinal lymphatic channels seems to explain the high incidence of cardiac metastases from mediastinal tumors.

Manifestations

Secondary tumor involvement of the heart is more often symptomatic, and on rare occasions it may be the first or only expression of a remote primary tumor. At times, as with rapidly developing tamponade, recognition and appropriate therapy must be undertaken promptly. Secondary tumors of the heart may involve the pericardium, myocardium, endocardium, valves, and coronary arteries. Direct invasion of the heart through the venae cavae[128] or pulmonary veins[129] or through an expanding myocardial implant can produce an intracavitary tumor mass and result in obstruction to flow or cause valvular obstruction (Fig. 85-6). Depending on the character and location of the cardiac lesion, a variety of manifestations may serve to identify cardiac involvement.

PERICARDIAL INVOLVEMENT Pericardial involvement is often first manifest by chest pain, aggravated by inspiration, and a pericardial friction rub. Accumulation of fluid within the

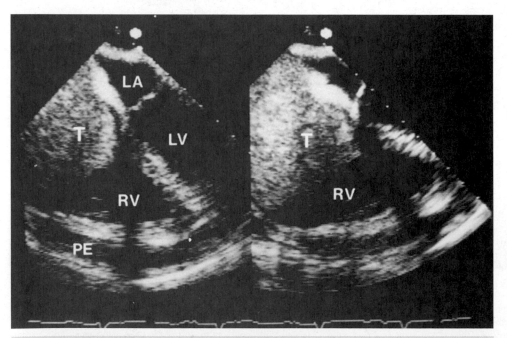

FIGURE 85-6 Transesophageal echocardiogram from a 55-year-old woman who presented with adenocarcinoma of the lung and obstructed superior vena caval syndrome. A large tumor (T) is seen in the right ventricle (RV) in systole (*left panel*) and diastole (*right panel*). Subsequent images revealed that it originated from an obstructed superior vena cava. The echo-free space anterior to the RV represented pericardial effusion (PE). (Courtesy of Susan Wilansky, M.D., Medical Director, Noninvasive Imaging, St. Luke's Episcopal Hospital, Houston, Texas.)

pericardium, often but not always bloody, may result in progressive cardiac enlargement on roentgenogram, with symptoms and signs of cardiac tamponade, and may be the first manifestation of a cardiac malignancy (Chap. 80). Clinically, the jugular venous pressure is increased, the arterial pressure is reduced, and "pulsus paradoxus" may be present (Chap. 80). Reduced electrocardiographic QRS voltage can be expected. Electrical alternation, which is generally seen in patients with large effusions and serious tamponade, may indicate the need for prompt pericardiocentesis. The echocardiogram demonstrates pericardial fluid and may demonstrate features of hemodynamic tamponade, diastolic collapse of the RA and RV,[130] inferior vena caval plethora with a blunted inspiratory response, and altered inspiratory intracardiac Doppler flow velocities (Chap. 80). Pericardial effusion and tamponade may be the first manifestations of cardiac involvement by a malignancy. The association of large quantities of pericardial fluid with tumor encasing the heart frequently results in persistent cardiac constriction, even after pericardiocentesis. Echocardiography and CT imaging are both useful for detecting pericardial metastases. Pericardioscopy performed during surgical drainage procedures has enabled visual diagnoses and guided biopsies of suspicious areas.[131]

MYOCARDIAL INVOLVEMENT

Atrial flutter and fibrillation are frequent, and a patient with either one may be unusually resistant to conventional therapy. Ventricular extrasystoles and serious ventricular arrhythmias[132] may accompany invasion of a tumor into the myocardium. Conduction disturbances and complete AV block also occur. Widespread muscle involvement by tumor invasion or obstruction of the cardiac lymphatic drainage system may cause congestive failure. Myocardial damage and heart failure may also result from some of the chemotherapeutic agents used in the treatment of patients with neoplastic diseases, and combined radiotherapy and chemotherapy may synergistically increase cardiac damage (Chap. 89). The most frequent ECG abnormalities seen in patients with neoplastic heart disease are nonspecific changes of the ST segment and the T wave due to myocardial or pericardial involvement by the tumor. Pronounced and prolonged ST-segment elevation in the absence of myocardial infarction may occur with tumor invasion of the heart.[6]

CORONARY ARTERY INVOLVEMENT

In patients with malignant tumor, angina or myocardial infarction may result from concomitant atherosclerosis, coronary occlusion by tumor embolization, or external coronary compression by the tumor as well as from coronary fibrosis or accelerated atherogenesis in patients who have received radiation to the mediastinum.[6,133] The ECG pattern of myocardial infarction can also result from massive invasion of the myocardium by a tumor or from a large pericardial effusion.

INTRACAVITARY TUMOR

Extensions of tumors such as renal cell carcinoma,[134] hepatocellular carcinoma,[135] and uterine leiomyomatosis[136] along the inferior vena cava and into the RA can present as an intracavitary obstructive mass. Leiomyosarcoma may be primary in the vena cava, most often the inferior, and extend directly into the heart. Intracavitary metastases or an expanding myocardial tumor may progressively obliterate a cardiac chamber or result in a valvular obstruction and, rarely, produce fever of unknown origin. Successful surgical resection has been reported.[137] RA and tricuspid obstruction by an intracavitary mass

can mimic pericardial constriction from tumor invasion or from previous intensive radiotherapy to the mediastinum. Systemic or pulmonary emboli, so common with primary tumors of the heart, are uncommon with secondary tumors. Right-sided intracavitary thrombi may mimic primary or secondary tumors on echographic imaging of the heart.[6]

Diagnostic Studies

Echocardiography, TTE and TEE, CT scanning, and, more recently, ultrafast CT facilitate identification of pericardial effusion and intracavitary and pericardial masses (Fig. 85-6)[6] (Chaps. 15, 20, and 21). MRI provides a global view of cardiac anatomy and plays an important role in the diagnosis and evaluation of both primary and secondary tumors of the heart, providing information about the location, extent, and attachment of the tumor. Pericardiocentesis may afford prompt symptomatic relief from pericardial tamponade and often provides a definitive cytologic diagnosis.[138] Ultrasound and fluoroscopic guidance aid in safe pericardial catheter placement. The results of endomyocardial biopsy may contribute to the diagnosis in some cases. Bone formation in metastatic osteogenic sarcoma may occasionally be visible radiographically.

Treatment

Malignant pericardial effusion usually recurs rapidly after pericardiocentesis. Depending on the cytologic type and radiosensitivity of the tumor, radiation to the cardiac area with or without systemic chemotherapy is the treatment of choice[6] (Chap. 80). The heart can tolerate 20 to 40 Gy, beyond which the risk of radiation-induced pericardial, myocardial, and valvular[139] damage is increased. Patients with malignant pericardial effusions have responded to systemic chemotherapy and to intrapericardial administration of fluorouracil, radioactive gold (nitrogen mustard), and tetracycline.[140,141] Persistent reaccumulation of fluid may require surgical creation of a pericardial "window."[142] A pericardial-pleural window has also been produced with a percutaneous balloon catheter without surgery.[143] Patients with myocardial infiltration by tumor also respond to radiation therapy and systemic chemotherapy. Recurrent ventricular tachycardia has responded to administration of amiodarone.[144] Heart block is treated with temporary or permanent electronic pacing. Surgical removal of intracavitary, obstructing secondary tumors may ameliorate symptoms and prolong survival,[145] as may chemotherapy occasionally. Documentation of tumor regression is possible with echocardiographic imaging. MRI plays an important role in characterizing the three-dimensional extent and attachment of cardiac tumors. This information is of particular importance in planning a surgical approach aimed at either complete removal or palliative debulking of a tumor mass.[146] A new biology is being developed in laboratories around the world working in these areas, and this is supported by the knowledge that is being obtained from the concerted Human Genome Project and the subsequent development of proteomics (Chap. 5). It is incumbent on the thoracic surgeon involved in the care of patients with cardiac tumors to have some degree of familiarity with the terms and promise of these advances because significant additional improvement in survival of many of these patients is unlikely to result from further advances in surgical technique. Interestingly, many sarcomas demonstrate reproducible translocations that allow for the production of novel chimeric genes, which may code for a variety of fusion proteins.

Special Considerations

LEUKEMIA

Leukemic infiltration of the heart is usually found at postmortem study.[147] Cardiac infiltrates are found in most postmortem studies of patients with acute leukemia, with most having pericardial involvement. Cardiac symptoms are unusual. Chronic lymphocytic leukemia reportedly has caused myocardial infiltration in some patients, as well as mitral valve dysfunction and congestive heart failure.[6] Myocardial rupture has been reported as an early manifestation of acute myeloblastic leukemia.[148] Massive pericardial effusion, often hemorrhagic, and pericardial tamponade have been reported, but overt pericardial effusion is rare.[6] Management consists of pericardiocentesis and chemotherapy (Chap. 80); occasionally, surgical decompression of the pericardium is necessitated by recurrent tamponade. Infective endocarditis, commonly fungal, may complicate acute leukemia. Because of advances in treatment and improved long-term remission in patients with acute lymphoblastic leukemia, complicating endocarditis has been managed by valve replacement.

MALIGNANT LYMPHOMA

Involvement of the heart in patients with malignant lymphoma is common, although it is infrequently detected before death. Cardiac or pericardial metastases occur with both Hodgkin's and non-Hodgkin's lymphoma and result from lymphatic and hematogenous spread as well as direct extension from other intrathoracic masses, resulting in predominantly epicardial and pericardial involvement. Cardiac involvement may occasionally be the direct cause of death, but antemortem detection is infrequent.

ACQUIRED IMMUNODEFICIENCY SYNDROME AND HEART NEOPLASMS

Two varieties of malignancies involving the heart have been described in patients with acquired immunodeficiency syndrome (AIDS): Kaposi's sarcoma and, less commonly, malignant lymphoma.[149] Involvement of the heart by Kaposi's sarcoma may be primary or part of a widely disseminated process. The epicardium is a common location, with involvement of the underlying myocardium. Clinical cardiac dysfunction is minimal, although fatal pericardial tamponade has been reported (Chap. 80).

Lymphomas, usually of high-grade malignant characteristics, occur with increased frequency in patients with AIDS and other immunosuppressed states (Chap. 80). Both primary and, more commonly, secondary lymphomas involve the heart either as a diffuse infiltrative process or as focal nodules in any layer of the heart. Clinical features may be absent in approximately 50 percent of patients. When present, they include cardiomegaly, pericardial effusion and tamponade, congestive failure, atrial arrhythmias, and progressive heart block.[150–153] Echocardiography is useful and demonstrates pericardial effusion, mass lesions, and wall motion abnormalities. Transvenous biopsy can be useful in making the diagnosis. There is limited experience with heart surgery in this group of patients.

CARCINOID HEART DISEASE

While carcinoid tumors are never primary in the heart and only rarely metastasize to the heart and pericardium, products of the tumor produce a distinctive endocardial and valvular pathologic pattern.[154–158,158a] Tumors producing the carcinoid syndrome most commonly arise in the gastrointestinal tract, but they may also arise in the bronchus, biliary tract, pancreas, and testis.[6,159] Appendiceal carcinoids rarely metastasize or produce the carcinoid syndrome. Ileal carcinoids, containing cytoplasmic granules that take up and reduce silver salts, frequently metastasize to the liver and produce the carcinoid syndrome. These carcinoids contain a high concentration of 5-hydroxytryptamine (5-HT), which is excreted mainly as 5-hydroxyindoleacetic acid (5-HIAA) in the urine. Bronchial, pancreatic, and gastric carcinoid tumors differ morphologically and histochemically, have a worse prognosis, and metastasize more widely than do ileal tumors. They also produce 5-HT and excrete 5-HIAA in the urine; however, the clinical picture may be atypical. Although they bear no morphologic or histochemical relation to the more typical carcinoid tumor, carcinomas of the bronchus, pancreas, or thyroid may occasionally secrete humoral substances that produce the carcinoid syndrome. In gastrointestinal carcinoid disease, the syndrome is produced by secretion of tumor products into the systemic circulation, and its recognition is delayed until after liver metastases. The carcinoid syndrome, which results from the systemic effect of circulating vasoactive amines, consists of cutaneous flushing, intestinal hypermobility, bronchial constriction, edema, and cardiac lesions. Among patients with carcinoid, those with carcinoid heart disease demonstrate strikingly higher plasma serotonin and 5-HIAA levels.[162–170]

Cardiac lesions are more commonly found in the right side of the heart than in the left (Fig. 85-6). Left-sided involvement occurs with bronchial tumors, in the presence of an intraatrial communication, or, in the absence of such a communication, when there is extensive right-sided heart involvement. Grossly glistening, white-yellow deposits are found on the pulmonary and tricuspid valves and, to varying degrees, on the RA and RV endocardium (Chap. 69). Contraction of these deposits leads to tricuspid and pulmonary valve regurgitation and stenosis and may occasionally produce a restrictive type of myopathy.[156] Mitral valve involvement may result in both stenosis and regurgitation. On microscopic examination, the endocardial lesions consist of superficial deposits of fibrous tissue beneath a normal endothelium.[154] Metastatic lesions may be found in the myocardium. Serotonin, 5-HT, and bradykinin have been implicated in the pathogenesis of the cardiac lesions. Transforming growth factor beta (TGF-β) has been shown to be produced by the fibroblasts in the carcinoid plaque and may play a critical role in progressive deposition of matrix proteins. The application of antibodies against TGF-β may potentially suppress the plaque progress.

Carcinoid heart disease cannot be recognized clinically until cardiac murmurs and signs of right-sided heart failure develop, especially elevated jugular venous pressure with inspiratory augmentation of the v wave, which is characteristic of tricuspid regurgitation (TR). A harsh, holosystolic, lower sternal border murmur with inspiratory accentuation is common, frequently followed by an early diastolic filling sound and diastolic rumble (Chap. 69). A left upper sternal midsystolic murmur of pulmonic stenosis (PS) may or may not be identified separately. Murmurs of concomitant left-sided heart valvular involvement are rarely identified. There may be a parasternal heave and systolic pulsation of the liver, although enlargement and multinodular irregularity of the liver, ascites, and edema may be features of hepatic metastases without cardiac involvement (Fig. 85-7).

Roentgenographic examination of the chest will show the lung fields to be clear and the pulmonary trunk to be normal in size; the heart may be normal in size or show evidence of RV and RA enlargement. The electrocardiogram may show evidence of RA enlargement, but RV hypertrophy is rare.

Echocardiographic imaging reveals RV volume overload and abnormal right-sided valves. The tricuspid valve is typically thickened, retracted, and fixed in a semiopen position. Doming of the tricuspid valve may be present when the valve is predominantly stenotic.

Color-flow Doppler will identify moderate to severe TR in the majority of patients. Pulmonary valve abnormalities are present in one-half of the patients, with pulmonic regurgitation more frequent than PS. With left-sided valvular involvement (7 percent of total cases), the mitral valve is affected more often than the aortic.

Diagnosis of carcinoid heart disease depends on clinical recognition of the characteristic right-sided heart findings in the setting of systemic features of the carcinoid syndrome (Chap. 89). The diagnosis is sometimes made only after the tricuspid valve has been replaced. In cases of ileal carcinoid disease, clinical recognition of multinodular deformity, along with radionuclide or CT imaging of the enlarged liver, serves to identify the prerequisite metastases to this organ. Carcinoid tumors that originate in a location that can release metabolic products outside the portal circulation do not share the latter characteristics. Urinary excretion of 5-HIAA is markedly elevated, and heavy diversion of tryptophan to this metabolic pathway may result in profound hypoproteinemia and nicotinamide deficiency (pellagra).

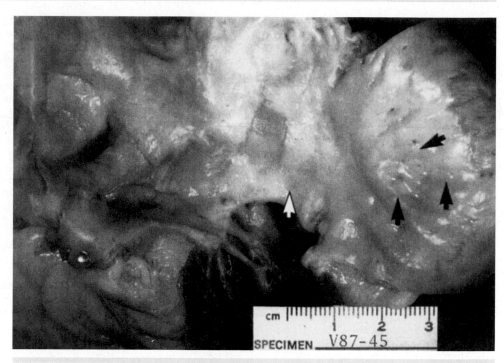

FIGURE 85-7 Carcinoid heart disease. The right atrium (RA) of a patient with carcinoid heart disease and combined tricuspid regurgitation and tricuspid stenosis. Note raised white plaques (*black arrow*) on the endocardial surface of the dilated RA and tricuspid valve (*white arrow*). Carcinoid heart disease occurs in 19 to 55 percent of patients with carcinoid.

Current chemotherapeutic programs are at least partially effective in some patients with extensive liver metastases. When hepatic metastases are present, removing the primary ileal lesion is indicated only if it is large and is producing mechanical obstruction. Occasionally, large hepatic metastases are few in number, and resection may afford symptomatic relief. Catheter embolization may permit segmental hepatic ablation in selected patients. In contrast, removal of an extraportal primary tumor can result in rapid resolution of cardiac failure. Some of the manifestations of the carcinoid syndrome may be blocked by alpha-adrenergic blockers, serotonin antagonists, and somatostatin analogues.[155]

Because heart failure is a frequent cause of disability and death when carcinoid heart disease complicates the carcinoid syndrome, tricuspid valve replacement and pulmonary valvotomy, with outflow tract enlargement if necessary, have been recommended when hemodynamically indicated. Implantation of a bioprosthetic valve[156,157] has generally been discouraged, although a review of reported cases of tricuspid valve replacement showed no significant difference in survival between patients with a bioprosthesis and those with a mechanical valve. Carcinoid plaque extending onto bioprosthetic valves early after surgery has been reported. Surgical mortality rates have been reported from 30 to 60 percent,[158–160] and only a small number of patients have undergone valve surgery. With proper care and planning, general anesthesia can be conducted with minimal risk.[161,162] Balloon valvuloplasty for tricuspid and pulmonary stenoses caused by carcinoid heart disease has been reported.[166]

References

1. Hall RJ, Cooley DA, McAllister HA Jr, et al. Neoplastic heart disease. In: Fuster V, Alexander RW, O'Rourke RA, et al, eds. *Hurst's The Heart,* 10th ed. New York: McGraw-Hill; 2001:2179–2197.

2. Chitwood WR Jr. Clarence Crafoord and the first successful resection of a cardiac myxoma. *Ann Thorac Surg* 1992;54:997–998.

3. Peters MN, Hall RJ, Cooley DA, et al. The clinical syndrome of atrial myxoma. *JAMA* 1974;230:695–701.

4. McAllister HA Jr. Primary tumors and cysts of the heart and pericardium. *Curr Probl Cardiol* 1979;4:1–51.

5. McAllister HA, Fenoglio JJ. *Tumors of the Cardiovascular System.* Washington, DC: Armed Forces Institute of Pathology; 1978.

6. McAllister H, Hall R, Cooley D. Tumors of the heart and pericardium. *Curr Probl Cardiol* 1999;24:57–116.

7. Burke A, Virmani R. Tumors of the heart and great vessels. In: Rosai J, Sobin LH, eds. *Atlas of Tumor Pathology.* Vol 3d ser, fascicle 16. Washington, DC: Armed Forces Institute of Pathology; 1996:231.

8. Burke AP, Virmani R. Cardiac myxoma: A clinicopathologic study. *Am J Clin Pathol* 1993;100:671–680.

9. Ha JW, Kang WC, Chung N, et al. Echocardiographic and morphologic characteristics of left atrial myxoma and their relation to systemic embolism. *Am J Cardiol* 1999;83(suppl A8):1579–1582.

10. Wold LE, Lie JT. Scanning electron microscopy of intracardiac myxoma. *Mayo Clin Proc* 1981;56:198–200.

11. Bashey RI, Nochumson S: Cardiac myxoma. Biochemical analyses and evidence for its neoplastic nature. *NY State J Med* 1979;79:29–32.

12. Read RC, White HJ, Murphy ML, et al. The malignant potentiality of left atrial myxoma. *J Thorac Cardiovasc Surg* 1974;68:857–868.

13. Dashkoff N, Boersma RB, Nanda NC, et al. Bilateral atrial myxomas: Echocardiographic considerations. *Am J Med* 1978;65:361–366.

14. Morgan DL, Palazola J, Reed W, et al. Left heart myxomas. *Am J Cardiol* 1977;40: 611–614.

15. Gowda, RM, Khan IA, Mehta NJ, et al. Cardiac papillary fibroelastoma originating from pulmonary vein: A case report. *Angiology* 2002; 53(6):745–748.

16. Balsara RK, Pelias AJ. Myxoma of right ventricle presenting as pulmonic stenosis in a neonate. *Chest* 1983;83:145–146.

17. Erdil N, Ates S, Cetin L, Demirkilic U, et al. Frequency of left atrial myxoma with concomitant coronary artery disease. *Surg Today* 2003;33:328–331.

18. Davison ET, Mumford D, Zaman Q, et al. Left atrial myxoma in the elderly: Report of four patients over the age of 70 and review of the literature. *J Am Geriatr Soc* 1986;34:229–233.

19. van Gelder HM, O'Brien DJ, Staples ED, et al. Familial cardiac myxoma. *Ann Thorac Surg* 1992;53:419–424.

20. Farah MG. Familial cardiac myxoma: A study of relatives of patients with myxoma. *Chest* 1994;105:65–68.

21. Mochizuki Y, Okamura Y, Iida H, et al. Interleukin-6 and "complex" cardiac myxoma. *Ann Thorac Surg* 1998;66:931–933.

22. Graham SL, Sellers AL. Atrial myxoma with multiple myeloma. *Arch Intern Med* 1979;139:116–117.

23. Molstad P, Smith G, Aukrust P. Left atrial myxoma and systemic AL-amyloidosis. *Eur Heart J* 1992;13:143–144.

24. Boussen K, Moalla M, Blondeau P, et al. Embolization of cardiac myxomas masquerading as polyarteritis nodosa. *J Rheumatol* 1991;18: 283–285.

25. Carney JA. Carney complex: The complex of myxomas, spotty pigmentation, endocrine overactivity, and schwannomas. *Semin Dermatol* 1995;14:90–98.

26. Casey M, Mah C, Merliss AD, et al. Identification of a novel genetic locus for familial cardiac myxomas and Carney complex. *Circulation* 1998;98:2560–2566.

27. Gurijala DNB, Abraham KA. Familial cardiac myxoma: Carney's complex. *Tex Heart Inst J* 2003;30(1):80–82.

28. Revankar SG, Clark RA. Infected cardiac myxoma: Case report and literature review. *Medicine (Baltimore)* 1998;77:337–344.

29. Diflo T, Cantelmo NL, Haudenschild CC, et al. Atrial myxoma with remote metastasis: Case report and review of the literature. *Surgery* 1992;111:352–356.

30. Misago N, Tanaka T, Hoshii T, et al. Erythematous papules in a patient with cardiac myxoma: A case report and review of the literature. *J Dermatol* 1995;22:600–605.

31. McMullin GM, Lane R. A rare cause of acute aortic occlusion. *Aust N Z J Surg* 1993;63:65–68.

32. Browne WT, Wijdicks EF, Parisi JE, et al. Fulminant brain necrosis from atrial myxoma showers. *Stroke* 1993;24:1090–1102.

32a. O'Rourke F, Dean N, Mouradian MS, et al. Atrial myxoma as a cause of stroke: Case report and discussion. *CMAJ* 2003;169:1049–1051.

33. Furuya K, Sasaki T, Yoshimoto Y, et al. Histologically verified cerebral aneurysm formation secondary to embolism from cardiac myxoma: Case report. *J Neurosurg* 1995;83:170–173.

34. Rafuse PE, Nicolle DA, Hutnick CM, et al. Left atrial myxoma causing ophthalmic artery occlusion. *Eye* 1997;11:25–29.

35. Cheitlin MD, McAllister HA, de Castro CM. Myocardial infarction without atherosclerosis. *JAMA* 1975;231:951–959.

36. Sharratt GP, Grover ML, Monro JL. Calcified left atrial myxoma with floppy mitral valve. *Br Heart J* 1979;42:608–610.

37. Chachques JC, Argyriadis PG, Latremouilli C, et al. Cardiomyoplasty: Ventricular reconstruction after tumor resection. *J Thorac Cardiovasc Surg* 2002;123(5):889–894.

38. Tighe DA, Rousou JA, Kenia S, et al. Transesophageal echocardiography in the management of mitral valve myxoma. *Am Heart J* 1995; 130:627–629.

39. Matsuoka H, Hamada M, Honda T, et al. Morphologic and histologic characterization of cardiac myxomas by magnetic resonance imaging. *Angiology* 1996;47:693–698.

40. Kamata J, Yoshioka K, Nasu M, et al. Myxoma of the mitral valve detected by echocardiography and magnetic resonance imaging. *Eur Heart J* 1995;16:1435–1438.

41. Rittoo D, Cotter L. Detection of a small left atrial myxoma: Value and limitations of four imaging modalities. *J Am Soc Echocardiogr* 1997;10:874–876.

42. Isobe N, Kanda T, Sakamoto H, et al. Myocardial infarction in myxoma patients with normal coronary arteries: Case reports. *Angiology* 1996;47:819–823.

43. Huston KA, Combs JJ Jr, Lie JT, et al. Left atrial myxoma simulating peripheral vasculitis. *Mayo Clin Proc* 1978;53:752–756.

44. Kuroda H, Nitta K, Ashida Y, et al. Right atrial myxoma originating from the tricuspid valve. *J Thorac Cardiovasc Surg* 1995;109: 1249–1250.

45. Teoh KH, Mulji A, Tomlinson CW, et al. Right atrial myxoma originating from the eustachian valve. *Can J Cardiol* 1993;9:441–443.

46. Price CE, Arouni AJ, LaMadid L, et al. Atrial myxoma as a cause of superior vena cava syndrome. *Chest* 2001;120(4 suppl):362S.

47. Hickie JB, Gibson H, Windsor HM. "The wrecking ball": Right atrial myxoma. *Med J Aust* 1970;2:82–86.

48. Heck HA Jr, Gross CM, Houghton JL. Long-term severe pulmonary hypertension associated with right atrial myxoma. *Chest* 1992;102: 301–303.

49. Jardine DL, Lamont DL. Right atrial myxoma mistaken for recurrent pulmonary thromboembolism. *Heart* 1997;78:512–514.

50. Park JM, Garcia RR, Patrick JK, et al. Right atrial myxoma with a nonembolic intestinal manifestation. *Pediatr Cardiol* 1990;11: 164–166.

51. Massumi R. Bedside diagnosis of right heart myxomas through detection of palpable tumor shocks and audible plops. *Am Heart J* 1983; 105:303–310.

52. Lyons SV, McCord J, Smith S. Asymptomatic giant right atrial myxoma: Role of transesophageal echocardiography in management. *Am Heart J* 1991;121:1555–1558.

53. Angelini P, Wilansky S, Gaos C, et al. Prolapsing large aneurysm of the atrial septum simulating a right atrial mass. *Catheter Cardiovasc Diagn* 1992;26:122–126.

54. Peachell JL, Mullen JC, Bentley MJ, et al. Biatrial myxoma: A rare cardiac tumor. *Ann Thorac Surg* 1998;65:1768–1769.

55. Abo-Auda WS, Chidambaram BS, Baker K, et al. Ventricular myxoma presenting as acute visual loss. *Tenn Med* 1998;91:391–392.

56. Camesas AM, Lichtstein E, Kramer J, et al. Complementary use of two-dimensional echocardiography and magnetic resonance imaging in the diagnosis of ventricular myxoma. *Am Heart J* 1987;114:440–442.

57. Gulbins H, Reichenspurner H, Wintersperger BJ, et al. Minimally invasive extirpation of a left-ventricular myxoma. *Thorac Cardiovasc Surg* 1999;47:129–130.

58. Talwalkar NG, Livesay JJ, Treistman B, et al. Mobilization of the anterior mitral leaflet for excision of a left ventricular myxoma. *Ann Thorac Surg* 1999;67:1476–1478.

59. Nass PC, Niemeyer MG, Brutal de la Riviere A, et al. Left atrial and right ventricular cardiac myxoma: A case report. *Eur J Cardiothorac Surg* 1989;3:468–470.

60. Jones DR, Warden HE, Murray GF, Hill RC, et al. Biatrial approach to cardiac myxomas: A 30-year clinical experience (comments). *Ann Thorac Surg* 1995;59:851–856.

61. Massetti M, Babatasi G, Le Page O, et al. Modified biatrial approach for the extensive resection of left atrial myxomas. *Ann Thorac Surg* 1998;66:275–276.

62. Abushaban L, Denham B, Duff D. 10 year review of cardiac tumours in childhood (comments). *Br Heart J* 1993;70:166–169.

63. Fenoglio JJ Jr, McAllister HA, Ferrans VJ. Cardiac rhabdomyoma: A clinicopathologic and electron microscopic study. *Am J Cardiol* 1976; 38:241–251.

64. Howanitz EP, Teske DW, Qualman SJ, et al. Pedunculated left ventricular rhabdomyoma. *Ann Thorac Surg* 1977;41:443–445.

65. Korf BR. Clinical and molecular genetics of tuberous sclerosis. *Pediatr Dermatol* 1999;16(1):78–79.

66. Hyman MH, Whittemore VH. National Institutes of Health Consensus Conference: Tuberous sclerosis complex. *Arch Neurol* 2002;57(5): 662–665.

66a. Lonergan GJ, Smirniotopoulos JG. Case 64: Tuberous sclerosis. *Radiology* 2003;229:385–388.

67. Mehta AV. Rhabdomyoma and ventricular preexcitation syndrome: A report of two cases and review of literature. *Am J Dis Child* 1993;147: 669–671.

68. Boxer RA, La Corte MA, Singh S, et al. Diagnosis of cardiac tumors in infants by magnetic resonance imaging. *Am J Cardiol* 1985;56: 831–832.

69. Demkow M, Sorensen K, Whitehead BF, et al. Heart transplantation in an infant with rhabdomyoma. *Pediatr Cardiol* 1995;16:204–206.

70. Garson A Jr, Smith RI Jr, Moak JP, et al. Incessant ventricular tachycardia in infants: Myocardial hamartomas and surgical cure. *J Am Coll Cardiol* 1987;10:619–626.

71. Holley DG, Martin GR, Brenner JI, et al. Diagnosis and management of fetal cardiac tumors: A multicenter experience and review of published reports (comments). *J Am Coll Cardiol* 1995;26:516–520.

72. Busch U, Kampmann C, Meyer R, et al. Removal of a giant cardiac fibroma from a 4-year-old child. *Tex Heart Inst J* 1995;22:261–264.

73. Williams DB, Danielson GK, McGoon DC, et al. Cardiac fibroma: Long-term survival after excision. *J Thorac Cardiovasc Surg* 1982;84:230–236.

74. Biancaniello TM, Meyer RA, Gaum WE, et al. Primary benign intramural ventricular tumors in children: Pre- and postoperative electrocardiographic, echocardiographic, and angiocardiographic evaluation. *Am Heart J* 1982;103:852–857.

75. Jamieson SW, Gaudiani VA, Reitz BA, et al. Operative treatment of an unresectable tumor of the left ventricle. *J Thorac Cardiovasc Surg* 1981;81:797–799.

76. Ryan PE Jr, Obeid AI, Parker FB Jr. Primary cardiac valve tumors. *J Heart Valve Dis* 1995;4:222–226.

77. al-Mohammad A, Pambakian H, Young C. Fibroelastoma: Case report and review of the literature. *Heart* 1998;79:301–304.

78. Grote J, Mugge A, Schafers HJ, et al. Multiplane transoesophageal echocardiography detection of a papillary fibroelastoma of the aortic valve causing myocardial infarction. *Eur Heart J* 1995;16: 426–429.

79. Eckstein FS, Schafers HJ, Grote J, et al. Papillary fibroelastoma of the aortic valve presenting with myocardial infarction. *Ann Thorac Surg* 1995;60:206–208.

80. Prahlow JA, Barnard JJ. Sudden death due to obstruction of coronary artery ostium by aortic valve papillary fibroelastoma. *Am J Forensic Med Pathol* 1998;19:162–165.

81. Lee CC, Celik C, Lajos TZ. Excision of papillary fibroelastoma arising from the septal leaflet of the tricuspid valve. *J Card Surg* 1995;10: 589–591.

82. Paelinck B, Vermeersch P, Kockx M. Calcified papillary fibroelastoma of the tricuspid valve. *Acta Cardiol* 1998;53:165–167.

83. Brown RD Jr, Khandheria BK, Edwards WD. Cardiac papillary fibroelastoma: A treatable cause of transient ischemic attack and ischemic stroke detected by transesophageal echocardiography. *Mayo Clin Proc* 1995;70:773–778.

84. Grinda JM, Couetil JP, Chauvaud S, et al. Cardiac valve papillary fibroelastoma: Surgical excision for revealed or potential embolization. *J Thorac Cardiovasc Surg* 1999;117:106–110.

85. Sankar NM, Thiruchelvam T, Thirunavukkaarasu K, et al. Symptomatic lipoma in the right atrial free wall: A case report. *Tex Heart Inst J* 1998;25:152–154.

86. Barberger-Gateau P, Paquet M, Desaulniers D, et al. Fibrolipoma of the mitral valve in a child: Clinical and echocardiographic features. *Circulation* 1978;58:955–958.

87. Leatherman L, Leachman RD, Hallman GL, et al. Cyst of the mitral valve. *Am J Cardiol* 1968;21:428–430.

88. Basu S, Folliguet T, Anselmo M, et al. Lipomatous hypertrophy of the interatrial septum. *Cardiovasc Surg* 1994;2:229–231.

89. Mortele KJ, Mergo PJ, Williams WF. Lipomatous hypertrophy of the atrial septum: Diagnosis with fat suppressed MR imaging. *J Magn Reson Imaging* 1998;8:1172–1174.

90. Meaney JF, Kazerooni EA, Jamadar DA, et al. CT appearance of lipomatous hypertrophy of the interatrial septum. *AJR* 1997;168: 1081–1084.

91. Balasundaram S, Halees SA, Duran C. Mesothelioma of the atrioventricular node: First successful follow-up after excision. *Eur Heart J* 1992;13:718–719.

92. Bharati S, Bauernfeind R, Josephson M. Intermittent preexcitation and mesothelioma of the atrioventricular node: A hitherto undescribed entity. *J Cardiovasc Electrophysiol* 1995;6:823–831.

93. Pigato JB, Subramanian VA, McCaba JC. Cardiac hemangioma: A case report and discussion. *Tex Heart Inst J* 1998;25:83–85.

94. Trout HHD, McAllister HA Jr, Giordano JM, et al. Vascular malformations. *Surgery* 1985;97:36–41.

95. Dresler C, Cremer J, Logemann F, et al. Intrapericardial pheochromocytoma. *Thorac Cardiovasc Surg* 1998;46:100–102.

96. Hamilton BH, Francis IR, Gross BH, et al. Intrapericardial paragangliomas (pheochromocytomas): Imaging features. *AJR* 1997;168: 109–113.

97. Jeevanandam V, Oz MC, Shapiro B, et al. Surgical management of cardiac pheochromocytoma: Resection versus transplantation. *Ann Surg* 1995;221:415–419.

98. Cooley DA, Frazier OH, Angelini P. Human cardiac explantation and autotransplantation: Application in a patient with a large cardiac pheochromocytoma. *Tex Heart Inst J* 1985;12:171–176.

99. Swalwell CI. Benign intracardiac teratoma: A case of sudden death. *Arch Pathol Lab Med* 1993;117:739–742.

100. Raaf HN, Raaf JH. Sarcomas related to the heart and vasculature. *Semin Surg Oncol* 1994;10:374–382.

101. Adachi K, Tanaka H, Toshima H, et al. Right atrial angiosarcoma diagnosed by cardiac biopsy. *Am Heart J* 1988;115: 482–485.

102. Uchita S, Hata T, Sushima Y, et al. Primary cardiac angiosarcoma with superior vena caval syndrome: Review of surgical resection and interventional management of venous inflow obstruction. *Can J Cardiol* 1998;14:1283–1285.

103. Herrmann MA, Shankerman RA, Edwards WD, et al. Primary cardiac angiosarcoma: A clinicopathologic study of six cases. *J Thorac Cardiovasc Surg* 1992;103:655–664.

104. Schmid KW, Thurner J Jr, Gruenewald K. Hemangiopericytoma of the heart following treatment of Hodgkin's disease: A case report. *Virchows Arch A Pathol Anat Histopathol* 1987;411:485–488.

105. Schmaltz AA, and Apitz J. Primary rhabdomyosarcoma of the heart. *Pediatr Cardiol* 1982;2:73–75.

106. Knobel B, Rosman P, Kishon Y, et al. Intracardiac primary fibrosarcoma: Case report and literature review. *Thorac Cardiovasc Surg* 1992;40:227–230.

107. Cafferty LL, Epstein JI. Primary liposarcoma of the right atrium. *Hum Pathol* 1987;18:408–410.

108. Cairns P, Butany J, Fulop J, et al. Cardiac presentation of non-Hodgkin's lymphoma. *Arch Pathol Lab Med* 1987;111:80–83.

109. Teramoto N, Hayashi K, Miyatani K, et al. Malignant fibrous histiocytoma of the right ventricle of the heart. *Pathol Int* 1995;45: 315–319.

110. Putnam JB Jr, Sweeney MS, Colon R, et al. Primary cardiac sarcomas. *Ann Thorac Surg* 1991;51:906–910.

111. Turner A, Batrick N. Primary cardiac sarcomas: A report of three cases and a review of the current literature. *Int J Cardiol* 1993;40:115–119.

112. Rienmuller R, Tiling R. MR and CT for detection of cardiac tumors. *J Thorac Cardiovasc Surg* 1990;38 (suppl 2):168–172.

113. Mora F, Mindich BP, Guarino T, et al. Improved surgical approach to cardiac tumors with intraoperative two-dimensional echocardiography. *Chest* 1987;91:142–144.

114. Burke AP, Cowan D, Virmani R. Primary sarcomas of the heart. *Cancer* 1992;69:387–395.

115. Goldstein DJ, Oz MC, Rose EA, et al. Experience with heart transplantation for cardiac tumors. *J Heart Lung Transplant* 1995;14:382–386.

116. Harlamert HA, Moulton JS, Lewis W. Images in cardiovascular medicine: Primary malignant fibrous histiocytoma of the heart treated with orthotopic heart transplantation. *Circulation* 1998;97:703–704.

117. Reardon MJ, DeFelice CA, Sheinbaum R, et al. Cardiac autotransplant for surgical treatment of a malignant neoplasm. *Ann Thorac Surg* 1999;67:1793–1795.

118. Wagner S, Hutchisson B, Baird MG. Cardiac explantation and autotransplantation. *AORN J* 1999;70:99–100, 102, 104–112.

119. Stoller JK, Shaw C, Matthay RA. Enlarging, atypically located pericardial cyst: Recent experience and literature review. *Chest* 1977;89: 402–406.

120. Ng AF, Olak J. Pericardial cyst causing right ventricular outflow tract obstruction (comments). *Ann Thorac Surg* 1997;63:1147–1148.

121. MacDonald S, Fay JE, Lynn RB. Intrapericardial teratoma: A continuing challenge. *Can J Surg* 1983;26:81–82.

122. Lazoglu AH, DaSilva MM, Iwahara M, et al. Primary pericardial sarcoma. *Am Heart J* 1994;127:453–458.

123. Neri E, Miracco C, Luzi P, et al. Intimal-type primary sarcoma of the thoracic aorta presenting as a saccular false aneurysm: Report of a case with evidence of rhabdomyosarcomatous differentiation. *J Thorac Cardiovasc Surg* 1999;118:371–372.

124. Prichard RW. Tumors of the heart: Review of the subject and report of one hundred and fifty cases. *Arch Pathol* 1951;51:98–128.

125. DeLoach JF, Haynes JW. Secondary tumors of the heart and pericardium: Review of the subject and report of one hundred thirty-seven cases. *Arch Int Med* 1953;91:224–249.

126. Emmot WW, Vacek JL, Agee K, et al. Metastatic malignant melanoma presenting clinically as obstruction of the right ventricular inflow and outflow tracts: Characterization by magnetic resonance imaging. *Chest* 1987;92:362–364.

127. Blocklage T, Leslie K, Yousem S, et al. Extracutaneous angiosarcomas metastatic to the lungs: Clinical and pathologic features of twenty-one cases. *Mod Pathol* 2001;14(12):1216–1225.

128. Hayashi J, Ohzeki H, Tsuchida S, et al. Surgery for cavoatrial extension of malignant tumors. *Thorac Cardiovasc Surg* 1995;43:161–164.

129. Hussain R, Neligan MC. Metastatic malignant schwannoma in the heart. *Ann Thorac Surg* 1993;56:374–375.

130. Levine MJ, Lorell BH, Diver DJ, et al. Implications of echocardiographically assisted diagnosis of pericardial tamponade in contemporary medical patients: Detection before hemodynamic embarrassment. *J Am Coll Cardiol* 1991;17:59–65.

131. Millaire A, Wurtz A, de Groote P, et al. Malignant pericardial effusions: Usefulness of pericardioscopy. *Am Heart J* 1992;124:1030–1034.

132. Sheldon R, Isaac D. Metastatic melanoma to the heart presenting with ventricular tachycardia. *Chest* 1991;99:1296–1298.

133. Virmani R, Khedekar RR, Robinowitz M, et al. Tumor embolization in coronary artery causing myocardial infarction. *Arch Pathol Lab Med* 1983;107:243–245.

134. Chatterjee T, Muller MF, Carrel T, et al. Images in cardiovascular medicine: Renal cell carcinoma with tumor thrombus extending through the inferior vena cava into the right cardiac cavities. *Circulation* 1997;96:2729–2730.

135. Fujisaki M, Kurihara E, Kikuchi K, et al. Hepatocellular carcinoma with tumor thrombus extending into the right atrium: Report of a successful resection with the use of cardiopulmonary bypass. *Surgery* 1991;109:214–219.

136. Nakayama Y, Kitamura S, Kawachi K, et al. Intravenous leiomyomatosis extending into the right atrium. *Cardiovasc Surg* 1994;2:642–645.

137. Peh WC, Cheung DL, Ngan H. Smooth muscle tumors of the inferior vena cava and right heart. *Clin Imaging* 1993;17:117–123.

138. Luck SR, DeLeon S, Shkolnik A, et al. Intracardiac Wilms' tumor: Diagnosis and management. *J Pediatr Surg* 1982;17:551–554.

139. Salcedo EE, Cohen GI, White RD, et al. Cardiac tumors: Diagnosis and management. *Curr Probl Cardiol* 1992;17:73–137.

140. McAllister HA, Hall RJ. Iatrogenic heart disease. In: Cheng TO, ed. *The International Textbook of Cardiology.* New York: Pergamon Press; 1977:871.

141. Primrose WR, Clee MD, Johnston RN. Malignant pericardial effusion managed with vinblastine. *Clin Oncol* 1983;9:67–70.

142. Chan A, Rischin D, Clarke CP, et al. Subxiphoid partial pericardiectomy with or without sclerosant instillation in the treatment of symptomatic pericardial effusions in patients with malignancy. *Cancer* 1991;68:1021–1025.

143. Palacios IF, Tuzcu EM, Ziskind AA, et al. Percutaneous balloon pericardial window for patients with malignant pericardial effusion and tamponade (comments). *Catheter Cardiovasc Diagn* 1991;22:244–249.

144. Leak D. Amiodarone for control of recurrent ventricular tachycardia secondary to cardiac metastasis. *Tex Heart Inst J* 1998;25:198–200.

145. Chen RH, Gaos CM, Frazier OH. Complete resection of a right atrial intracavitary metastatic melanoma (comments). *Ann Thorac Surg* 1996;61:1255–1257.

146. Lynch M, Balk MA, Lee RB, et al. Role of transesophageal echocardiography in the management of patients with bronchogenic carcinoma invading the left atrium. *Am J Cardiol* 1995;76:1101–1102.

147. Terry LN Jr, Kligerman MM. Pericardial and myocardial involvement by lymphomas and leukemias: The role of radiotherapy. *Cancer* 1970; 25:1003–1008.

148. Bjorkholm M, Ost A, Biberfeld P. Myocardial rupture with cardiac tamponade as a lethal early manifestation of acute myeloblastic leukemia. *Cancer* 1982;50:1777–1779.

149. Lewis W. AIDS: Cardiac findings from 115 autopsies. *Prog Cardiovasc Dis* 1989;32:207–215.

150. Aboulafia DM, Bush R, Picozzi VJ. Cardiac tamponade due to primary pericardial lymphoma in a patient with AIDS. *Chest* 1994;106: 1295–1299.

151. Chyu KY, Birnbaum Y, Naqvi T, et al. Echocardiographic detection of Kaposi's sarcoma causing cardiac tamponade in a patient with acquired immunodeficiency syndrome. *Clin Cardiol* 1998;21:131–133.

152. Azrak EC, Kern MJ, Bach RG. Hemodynamics of cardiac tamponade in a patient with AIDS-related non-Hodgkin's lymphoma. *Catheter Cardiovasc Diagn* 1998;45:287–291.

153. Estok L, Wallach F. Cardiac tamponade in a patient with AIDS: A review of pericardial disease in patients with HIV infection. *Mt Sinai J Med* 1998;65:33–39.

154. Schiller VI, Fishbein MC, Siegel RJ. Unusual cardiac involvement in carcinoid syndrome. *Am Heart J* 1986;112:1322–1323.

155. Le Metayer P, Constans J, Bernard N, et al. Carcinoid heart disease: Two cases of left heart involvement diagnosed by transthoracic and transoesophageal echocardiography. *Eur Heart J* 1993;14:1721–1723.

156. Pelikka PA, Tajik AJ, Khandheria BK, et al. Carcinoid heart disease: Clinical and echocardiographic spectrum in 74 patients. *Circulation* 1993;87:1188–1196.

157. Strickman NE, Hall RJ. Carcinoid heart disease. In: Kapoor AS, Reynolds RD, eds. *Cancer and the Heart.* New York: Springer-Verlag; 1986:135.

158. Koch CA, Azumi N, Furlong MA, et al. Carcinoid syndrome caused by an atypical carcinoid of the uterine cervix. *J Clin Endocrinol Metab* 1999;84:4209–4213.

158a. Wee JO, Sepic JD, Mihaljevic T, Cohn LH. Metastatic carcinoid tumor of the heart. *Ann Thorac Surg* 2003;76:1721–1722.

159. Robiolio PA, Rigolin VH, Wilson JS, et al. Carcinoid heart disease: Correlation of high serotonin levels with valvular abnormalities detected by cardiac catheterization and echocardiography. *Circulation* 1995;92:790–795.

160. Johnston SD, Johnston PW, O'Rourke D. Carcinoid constrictive pericarditis. *Heart* 1999;82:641–643.

161. McAllister HA Jr. Endocrine diseases and the cardiovascular system. In: Silver MD, ed. *Cardiovascular Pathology,* 2d ed. New York: Churchill Livingstone; 1991:1181.

162. Oates JA. The carcinoid syndrome. *N Engl J Med* 1986;315:702–704.

163. Ridker PM, Chertow GM, Karlson EW, et al. Bioprosthetic tricuspid valve stenosis associated with extensive plaque deposition in carcinoid heart disease. *Am Heart J* 1991;121:1835–1838.

164. Ohri SK, Schofield JB, Hodgson H, et al. Carcinoid heart disease: Early failure of an allograft valve replacement. *Ann Thorac Surg* 1994; 58:1161–1163.

165. Knott-Craig CJ, Schaff HV, Mullany CJ, et al. Carcinoid disease of the heart: Surgical management of ten patients. *J Thorac Cardiovasc Surg* 1992;104:475–481.

166. Robiolio PA, Rigolin VH, Harrison JK, et al. Predictors of outcome of tricuspid valve replacement in carcinoid heart disease. *Am J Cardiol* 1995;75:485–488.

167. Connolly HM, Nishimura RA, Smith HC, et al. Outcome of cardiac surgery for carcinoid heart disease. *J Am Coll Cardiol* 1995;25:410–416.

168. Propst JW, Siegel LC, Stover EP. Anesthetic considerations for valve replacement surgery in a patient with carcinoid syndrome. *J Cardiothorac Vasc Anesth* 1994;8:209–212.

169. Neustein SM, Cohen E. Anesthesia for aortic and mitral valve replacement in a patient with carcinoid heart disease. *Anesthesiology* 1995;82: 1067–1070.

170. Onate A, Alcibar J, Inguanzo R, et al. Balloon dilation of tricuspid and pulmonary valves in carcinoid heart disease. *Tex Heart Inst J* 1993; 20:115–119.

DIABETES AND CARDIOVASCULAR DISEASE

Michael E. Farkouh / Elliot J. Rayfield / Valentin Fuster

Globally, diabetes mellitus has become a major threat to human health. An increase in the prevalence of diabetes has been observed, which in part can be attributed to the aging of the population as well as an increase in the rate of obesity and sedentary lifestyle in the United States. Diabetes mellitus, whether type 1 or type 2, is a very strong risk factor for the development of coronary artery disease (CAD) and stroke[1,2] (Table 86-1). Eighty percent of all deaths among diabetic patients are due to atherosclerosis, compared with about 30 percent among nondiabetic persons. A large National Institutes of Health (NIH) cohort study revealed that heart disease mortality in the general U.S. population is declining at a much greater rate than it is

in diabetic subjects. In fact, diabetic women suffered an increase in heart disease mortality over that period.[3] Among all hospitalizations for diabetic complications, more than 75 percent are due to atherosclerosis. An increase in the prevalence of diabetes has been noted, which in part can be attributed to the aging of the population and an increase in the rate of obesity and the sedentary lifestyle in the United States.

Diabetes accelerates the natural course of atherosclerosis in all groups of patients and involves a greater number of coronary vessels with more diffuse atherosclerotic lesions[4–7] (Fig. 86-1). Cardiac catheterizations in diabetic patients have shown significantly more

TABLE 86-1 Clinical Evaluation of Risk Factors for the Development of Cardiovascular Disease in Diabetic Patients

Cigarette smoking
  Assess pack-years
Blood pressure
  Duration (if known), current and previous medications, assess presence of orthostatic hypertension
Serum lipids and lipoproteins
  Dietary habits, alcohol intake, amount of exercise and whether aerobic
  Family history of dyslipidemia, eruptive xanthoma, lipemia, retinalis, xanthelasma, thyroid function tests
  LDL, HDL, cholesterol, fasting triglycerides
Spot albumin/creatinine ratio (in micro- and macroalbuminuria)
  Serum creatinine
  Do not rely on dipstick protein, since negative results may reflect lack of sensitivity of test
Glycemic status
  Duration of diabetes; family history of diabetes; vascular, renal, and retinal complications
  Laboratory: FPG, hemoglobin A_1c q 3 months: Dx FPG > 126 × 2: impaired fasting glucose 110–126 × 2; when in doubt, have patient undergo 2-h oral glucose tolerance test

ABBREVIATIONS: FPG = fasting blood glucose; HDL = high density lipoprotein; LDL = low-density lipoprotein.

severe proximal and distal CAD.[8–11] In addition, plaque ulceration and thrombosis have been found to be significantly higher in diabetic patients.[12,13] Cardiovascular complications include CAD, peripheral

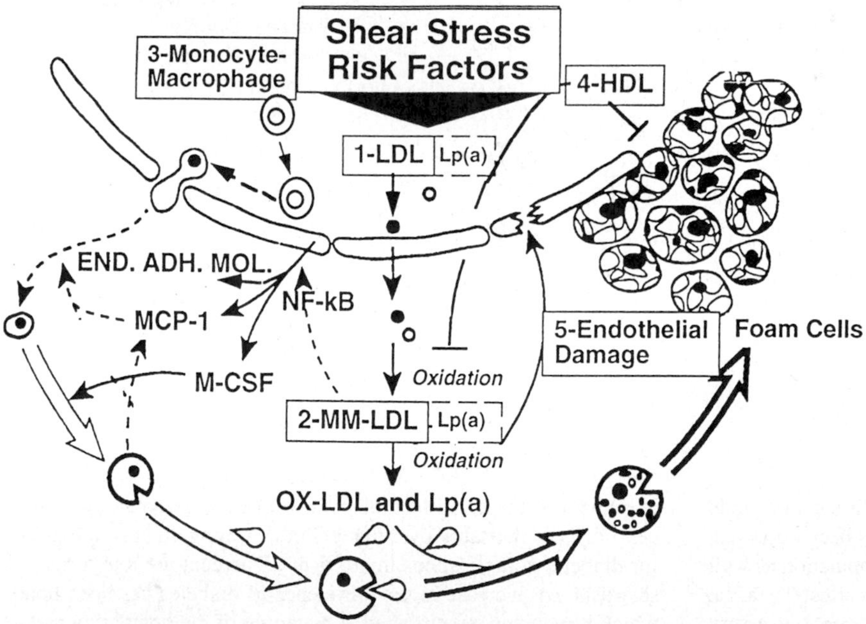

FIGURE 86-1 Schematic of staging (phases and lesion morphology of the progression of coronary atherosclerosis according to the gross pathologic and clinical findings). LDL = low-density lipoprotein; OX-LDL = oxidized low-density lipoprotein; MM-LDL = minimally modified low-density lipoprotein; HDL = high-density lipoprotein; Lp (a) = lipoprotein a; END.ADH.Mol. = endothelial adhesion molecule; MCP-1 = monocyte chemoattractant protein; NF-kB = nuclear factor kappa B; M-CSF = macrophage colony-stimulating factor; Numbers 1-->5 = stages of progression of coronary atherosclerosis. (See text for more details.)

artery disease, nephropathy, retinopathy, cardiomyopathy, and possible neuropathy (involvement of vasa vasorum). These observations underscore the heightened risks of a diabetic patient to develop vascular disease and compel the physician to correct all the metabolic abnormalities. By understanding the mechanisms underlying all these risks, physicians will be poised to prevent them.

CLINICAL PRESENTATIONS OF DIABETES MELLITUS

The risk factors for the development of diabetes are well established (Table 86-2). About 80 percent of all diabetic patients have type 2 diabetes mellitus, which characteristically occurs after age 40 years. The metabolic mechanisms of type 2 diabetes are the combination of insulin resistance and a genetically programmed defect in the pancreatic beta-cell secretion of insulin. Insulin resistance precedes the onset of type 2 diabetes by about 8 to 10 years and is associated with other cardiovascular risk factors: dyslipidemia, hypertension, and a procoagulant state.[14,15] The combination of these risk factors has been called syndrome X, the metabolic syndrome, and the cardiovascular dysmetabolic syndrome. Many patients with the metabolic syndrome exhibit either impaired fasting glucose (IFG) or impaired glucose tolerance (IGT) for many years before they develop frank diabetes.[16,17]

There are new criteria for the diagnosis of diabetes.[16] The cutoff for the diagnosis of diabetes has been lowered from 140 mg/dL to 126 mg/dL. The upper threshold for normoglycemia has been lowered from 115 mg/dL to 110 mg/dL. A fasting plasma glucose of 110 to 125 mg/dL is now referred to as IFG. These changes eliminate the need for oral glucose tolerance testing for the diagnosis of diabetes, which now rests on an elevation of the fasting plasma glucose level.

In contrast to type 2 diabetes, type 1 diabetes (10 percent of the diabetic population) usually is induced by immunologic destruction of pancreatic beta cells.[18] Type 1 diabetes classically has two peaks (at 4 years and 13 years of age) but can occur at any age. It typically produces microvascular disease (nephropathy, retinopathy) but also results in CAD.

Stroke

Compared to nondiabetic subjects, the mortality from stroke in diabetic patients is almost threefold higher.[19] The small paramedial penetrating arteries are the most common sites of cerebrovascular disease. In addition, diabetes increases the likelihood of severe carotid atherosclerosis.[20,21] Diabetic patients are likely to suffer increased brain damage with carotid emboli that would result in a transient ischemic attack in a nondiabetic individual.

Renal Disease

Nephropathy occurs in 40 percent of patients with type 1 and type 2 diabetes. Risk factors include poor glycemic control, hypertension, and ethnicity (blacks, Mexicans, Pima Indians).[22] Table 86-3 summarizes the key points for the assessment of renal status in a diabetic patient. The earliest

TABLE 86-2 Assessment of Predisposing Risk Factors in Diabetic Patients

Body weight and fat distribution
  History
    Age of onset of overweight, family history of obesity
  Physical examination
    Measure body weight (kg), height (m); calculate body mass index (BMI, kg/m^2), BMI of 25–29.9 = overweight, >30.0 = obese, BMI >27 in a diabetic patient should be treated as high risk; measure waist circumference (abdominal obesity is >40 in. in men and >36 in. in women)
  Physical Activity
    History: job, activity in sports, walking, aerobics; in women, child care, housework
    Physical examination: assess level of cardiovascular fitness in cardiac rehabilitation facility
  Family history
    History of heart disease, sudden death, elevated cholesterol level, cigarette smoking; hypertension; diabetes, especially in first-degree relatives
  Laboratory
    Measure fasting glucose and lipids in first-degree relatives

ABBREVIATION: BMI = body mass index.

TABLE 86-3 Evaluation of Renal Status

Urine albumin and protein
  Yearly screen for microalbumin in type 1 and type 2 diabetes; microalbumin/creatinine ratio collected in a spot urine, ideally first morning urine specimen (normal <30 mg/g creatinine); must rule out other diseases that cause proteinuria.
  If urine albumin/creatinine is >300 mg/g in first morning specimen, macroalbuminuria is present and is usually not reversible with ACE inhibitors; nephrology consult.
  Nephrotic syndrome: urine protein >3 g/day; nephrology consult.
  Other reasons to consult nephrologists are diabetic patients with increasing creatinine from 1.4 to over 2.0, elevated creatinine and symptoms of uremia, microalbuminuria not responding to ACE inhibitor.
Urinalysis
  Red cells, pyuria, casts require nephrology consult.
Blood pressure evaluation
  If hypertension is present, exclude secondary causes, including with advancing renal insufficiency.
  Treatment with an ACE inhibitor is preferred first choice even in African-Americans (except if precluded by hyperkalemia or other complications).
Blood urea nitrogen, serum creatinine, and glomerular filtration rate
  Yearly creatinine clearance should be obtained with 24-h urine collection and serum creatinine; most accurate way to estimate kidney function without using a radioisotope.

ABBREVIATION: ACE = angiotensin-converting enzyme.

clinical finding of diabetic kidney disease is microalbuminuria, which may occur at a time when renal histology is essentially normal.[23,24] The Diabetes Control and Complications Trial (DCCT) and the United Kingdom Prospective Diabetes Study group trial (UKPDS) showed that the development and progression of microalbuminuria can be prevented through strict glycemic control. Even once dipstick-positive proteinuria has developed, preliminary data from pancreatic transplant patients show improvement in glomerular pathology at 10 years.[25]

The UKPDS in type 2 diabetics and studies in patients with type 1 diabetes[26] using captopril have shown that control of hypertension slows the progression of nephropathy. The blood pressure should be maintained at <130/85, and angiotensin-converting enzyme (ACE) inhibitors are the preferred antihypertensive agents.[27,28] The UKPDS trial, however, showed no difference in blood pressure control with captopril versus atenolol. The benefit of antihypertensive therapy with an ACE inhibitor in type 1 diabetes can be shown early in the course of disease, when microalbuminuria is the only abnormality.[29–31]

There is insufficient evidence to recommend ACE inhibitors in normotensive patients without microalbuminuria.[32] Although screening for microalbuminuria is not as useful in type 2 diabetes patients in predicting the progression to overt nephropathy as it is in type 1 diabetes patients, once microalbuminuria develops, the rate of loss of the glomerular filtration rate (GFR) is equivalent to that in type 1 diabetes.[33,34] Nonetheless, physicians should still recommend screening on at least a yearly basis, since the risk/benefit ratio of diagnosing microalbuminuria justifies treatment with an ACE inhibitor, if not for renal disease alone,[35,36] then for reducing the incidence of myocardial infarction.[37,38]

Patients on ACE inhibitors should be monitored for potassium, since they may develop hyperkalemia in the presence of a type 4 renal tubular acidosis.[27] Sodium restriction reduces hypertension and therefore is advised. Dietary protein should be adjusted to 0.8 g/kg per day to decrease intraglomerular pressure.

More recently, clinical trials evaluating angiotensin receptor blockers (ARBs), including losartan and irbesartan, have demonstrated a significant renal protective effect in the diabetic patient with nephropathy. There were no differences between the ARB and usual care groups with regard to cardiovascular outcomes.[39,40,41]

An optimal approach toward diabetic nephropathy combines control of hypertension, preferably with an ACE inhibitor or ARB; glycemic control; sodium restriction; and adjustment of protein intake.

PROGRESSIVE RENAL INSUFFICIENCY IN DIABETES[42]

If increasing macroalbuminuria occurs or if renal insufficiency is progressive despite these measures, the patient should be referred to a nephrologist. It is strongly recommended that renal arteriography be avoided. Dietary protein restriction in patients who have progressive renal insufficiency will reduce accumulation of nitrogen-containing waste products and can have a beneficial influence on progression of renal insufficiency.

Type 2 Diabetes and Coronary Artery Disease

CAD is strongly associated with type 2 diabetes mellitus and is the leading cause of death regardless of the duration of disease. There is a twofold to fourfold increase in the relative risk ratio of cardiovascular disease in type 2 diabetes patients compared to the general population.[2,43–47] This increase is particularly disproportionate in diabetic women when compared with diabetic men.[43,45,48] The protection that premenopausal women have against CAD is not seen if they suffer from diabetes.[49,50] The degree and duration of hyperglycemia are a strong risk factor for the development of microvascular complications,[51] but, in type 2 diabetes, macrovascular complications have not been documented to be associated with the length or severity of a patient's diabetes.[5,44,47,52] Even impaired glucose tolerance increases cardiovascular risk although there is minimal hyperglycemia.[45,51–54]

The first detectable sign of a problem in people genetically prone to develop type 2 diabetes is insulin resistance, which can be seen as long as 15 to 25 years before the onset of diabetes. Several atherogenic factors are associated with insulin resistance,[55–62] which can start the atherosclerotic process years before clinical hyperglycemia ensues.[63,64] It is unclear whether the compensatory hyperinsulinemia plays a role in atherosclerosis generation in insulin-resistant patients. A number of prospective studies have shown an association between fasting or postprandial hyperinsulinemia and the future development of CAD.[62–64] However, this association has been demonstrated in middle-aged white men[65–67] but not in women[68] or in other ethnic groups.[69,70]

Hyperglycemia itself plays an important role in enhancing the progression of atherosclerosis in type 2 diabetes. The threshold above which hyperglycemia becomes atherogenic is not known but may be in the range defined as impaired glucose tolerance (i.e., fasting plasma glucose level <126 mg/dL with 30-, 60-, or 90-min plasma glucose concentrations >200 mg/L and a 2-h plasma glucose level of 140 to 200 mg/dL during an oral glucose tolerance test).[71]

Despite the role played by all these factors, population-based studies show that the degree of hyperglycemia increases the risk for CAD and cardiovascular events.[72–74]

Type 1 Diabetes and Coronary Artery Disease

In contrast to type 2 diabetes, cardiovascular risk factors can be examined in relation to hyperglycemia in type 1 diabetes patients. Long-term follow-up of these patients has shown that the incidence of cardiovascular mortality rises after age 30.[75] There is evidence that diabetes accelerates the process of early atherosclerosis that occurs at a young age in the general population. The coronary mortality rate in type 1 diabetes is markedly accelerated, and one-third of these

patients will die of CAD by age 55.[75] The protective effect of the premenopausal state is lost for females with type 1 diabetes.

It has been demonstrated that diabetic nephropathy dramatically increases the prevalence of CAD. *Diabetic nephropathy* is defined by proteinuria, a reduced GFR, and hypertension. Patients with proteinuria can be divided into two groups: those with macroalbuminuria (greater than 300 mg/d) and those with microalbuminuria (30 to 300 mg/d). The presence of overt proteinuria increases the risk of cardiovascular mortality almost tenfold compared with the risk in patients without proteinuria.[76] In another cohort, the risk of developing CAD was almost 15 times greater in patients with proteinuria than it was in those without diabetic nephropathy.[75] Since this risk of developing CAD morbidity and mortality has been demonstrated for both macro- and microalbuminuria patients, both must be considered vital in the cardiovascular evaluation of a diabetic patient (Fig. 86-2).

LIPID DISORDERS

Lipid disorders constitute one of the cornerstones in the cardiovascular management of diabetic patients. Many factors influence the lipid profile in these patients, including glycemic control, whether the diabetes is type 1 or type 2, and the presence of diabetic nephropathy.

TYPE OF DIABETES

In type 1 diabetes mellitus, the major determinant of the lipid profile is the level of glycemic control. Low-density lipoprotein (LDL) is moderately increased, triglycerides are markedly increased, and high-density lipoprotein (HDL) is decreased when the level of glycemic control is impaired. For patients with type 2 diabetes, lipid abnormalities are related not only to hyperglycemia but also to the interplay of the insulin-resistant state. Patients with type 2 diabetes may have normal LDL levels but elevated levels of the very-low-density lipoprotein (VLDL) triglycerides moiety and reduced HDL levels. The expected elevation in VLDL triglyceride is usually no more than 100 percent.

LOW-DENSITY LIPOPROTEIN CHOLESTEROL

Although LDL levels in patients with controlled type 1 or type 2 diabetes are normal, the atherogenic properties of LDL are increased. There is glycosylation of both apoprotein B[77] and the phospholipid component of LDL,[78] which changes LDL clearance and susceptibility to oxidative modifications. Glycosylation of apoprotein B occurs mainly in the LDL receptor–binding area[77] and is directly related to glucose levels. As a result, there is impairment in the LDL receptor–mediated uptake and therefore clearance of LDL.[79,80] Glycosylation also makes LDL more susceptible to oxidative modification. The product generated by the combined glycosylation and oxidation of

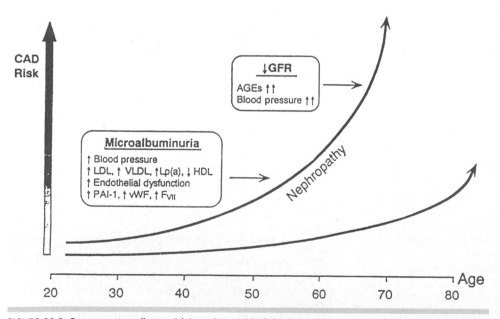

FIGURE 86-2 Coronary artery disease risk in patients with diabetes mellitus. A subset of genetically predisposed patients develops diabetic nephropathy. In these patients, the risk for CAD increases dramatically. (From Aronson and Rayfield,[142] with permission.)

LDL is more atherogenic than is either glycosylated or oxidized LDL alone.[78,81] Such LDL molecules are taken up more easily by the aortic intimal cells and macrophages, resulting in the formation of foam cells.[82–84]

Type 2 diabetic patients with insulin resistance have LDL particles that are small and rich with triglycerides but have little cholesterol in them (small, dense LDL).[85,86] These LDL particles increase the risk of CAD independent of the total LDL level, probably because of their increased susceptibility to oxidative modification. Therefore, even though LDL levels may be normal in these patients, high levels of small, dense LDL may contribute to the increased risk of CAD in such patients.[87]

VERY-LOW-DENSITY LIPOPROTEIN CHOLESTEROL

Diabetic patients have elevated levels of VLDL as a result of increased free fatty acid mobilization and high glucose levels. There is an increase in triglyceride production by the liver, which results in large, triglyceride-rich VLDL particles.[88] The size of these VLDL particles, which is dependent primarily on the amount of triglycerides available, is an important factor in determining their eventual fate. The conversion of large VLDL particles to LDL is not efficient[89]; therefore, they are cleared from circulation by other pathways. Since the removal of VLDL by lipoprotein lipase also is affected, the level of VLDL triglyceride rises. Furthermore, the abundance of large triglyceride-rich VLDL is associated with an increase in small, dense, atherogenic LDL particles.[90] Numerous studies have shown that elevated triglyceride levels are associated with increased risk for CAD in diabetic patients.[48,91–93] In contrast, elevated triglycerides are not associated with CAD risk in nondiabetic patients.

HIGH-DENSITY LIPOPROTEIN CHOLESTEROL

Low HDL level is a strong risk factor for the development of CAD in both diabetic and nondiabetic patients. There is decreased production and increased catabolism of HDL in diabetes. The decreased HDL production is a result of decreased lipoprotein lipase (LPL) activity. The failure of LPL to efficiently catabolize VLDL results in reduced availability of surface components for HDL production. By contrast, increased catabolism of HDL results from the hypertriglyceridemia of diabetes, producing triglyceride-rich HDL$_2$ that is prone to catabolism by liver enzymes.[94,95]

MANAGEMENT OF LIPID DISORDERS

Consistent with the National Cholesterol Education Program, the American Diabetes Association has published its consensus document concerning the management of lipid disorders.[96] For the most part, the cornerstone of therapy in diabetes revolves around dietary modifications, weight loss, physical exercise, and maximization of glycemic control. The Adult Treatment Panel III of the National Cholesterol Education Program (NCEP) reported their executive summary on the treatment of hyperlipidemia.[97]

One of the most striking modifications was the raising of patients with diabetes without coronary heart disease (CHD) to the same risk level as someone with CHD. The goal for LDL cholesterol, therefore, is <100 mg/dL for all those with diabetes regardless of CHD.

TYPE OF DIABETES

As was previously mentioned, the management of lipid disorders in type 1 diabetes is closely coupled to glycemic control. For type 1 patients, the front-line strategy begins with glycemic control.

In type 1 diabetes, glycemic control can lead to marked reductions in triglyceride levels, but with little or no impact on HDL levels. In type 2, pharmacotherapy is often required sooner than later, given the modest impact of nonpharmacologic strategies.[96]

Medical therapy for hyperlipidemia is similar in diabetic and nondiabetic patients, but diabetic patients require certain considerations.

The hypertriglyceridemia of diabetes can be treated effectively with fibric acid derivatives[98,99] without an adverse effect on glucose metabolism. Type 2 diabetic patients experience a reduction in the cardiovascular event rate when treated with gemfibrozil.[100] These drugs cause a 5- to 15-percent drop in LDL levels in patients with normal triglyceride levels, but in patients with hypertriglyceridemia, LDL levels go up. This elevation probably is due to the catabolism of the atherogenic LDL particle, resulting in less atherogenic LDL.[101]

Although nicotinic acid lowers both cholesterol and triglyceride levels while raising HDL levels, it generally is not indicated in diabetes. It has an adverse effect on glycemic control,[102] which results from the induction of insulin resistance.

Hydroxymethylglutaryl coenzyme A (HMG-CoA) reductase inhibitors are another group of drugs that are useful in lowering cholesterol levels in type 2 diabetes patients without having an adverse effect on glycemic control.[103] In a study assessing the effectiveness of a cholesterol-lowering drug for secondary prevention of morbidity and mortality in patients with angina or prior myocardial infarction, simvastatin was found to be more efficacious in diabetic patients than it was in the overall group.[104]

Bile acid resins can decrease the levels of LDL in diabetic patients,[105] but they can cause a significant rise in triglyceride levels, especially if VLDL levels are already high or if the diabetes is poorly controlled. In patients with high levels of both LDL and VLDL, bile acid resins can be used in low doses in combination with fibric acid derivatives.

Thrombosis

Diabetes mellitus is widely recognized as being perhaps the most significant risk factor for the development of acute coronary syndromes. The relation between diabetes and acute coronary thrombosis is multifactorial, with the interaction of plaque disruption and the interplay of local and systemic thrombogenic factors playing the primary roles.

Plaque Disruption

The inciting role of acute plaque disruption in the development of acute coronary thrombosis is well described. Although the lipid-rich core in plaque is felt to be causative in this process, more aggressive medical management of diabetes can have a favorable impact by decreasing plaque rupture and improving the clinical outcome.[106]

It is well described that not all disruptions of atherosclerotic plaques lead to clinical events. The complex interaction of local and systemic thrombogenic factors is an important determinant of whether clinically significant thrombus formation will occur.

Prothrombosis

Patients with diabetes demonstrate enhanced platelet aggregation[107,108] that correlates with increased cardiovascular events.[109]

Diabetic patients have been shown to have platelets that are hypersensitive to agonists of aggregation.[110,111] The major mechanism is felt to be increased thromboxane production.[112,113] An increased incidence of cardiovascular events in diabetic patients has been shown to be correlated with platelet hyperaggregation.

Diabetic patients have elevated levels of von Willebrand factor that correlate with vascular complications.[114,115] In addition, a relation has been shown between the insulin resistance syndrome and elevated plasma von Willebrand levels.[116] Similarly, diabetic patients often demonstrate elevated fibrinogen levels, which are also predictive of cardiovascular complications.[117–119] Fibrinogen levels mirror glycemic control.

Factor V, VII, X, XI, and XII levels also are elevated in diabetic patients.[120–122] Factor VII levels correlate directly with fasting plasma glucose levels.[122] Evidence exists linking activation of the coagulation cascade with hyperglycemia. Since antithrombin III activity is decreased with hyperglycemia, glycemic control may play a pivotal role in limiting thrombosis and thrombosis-related complications in diabetic patients.[123]

The insulin resistance syndrome is marked by increased plasminogen-activator inhibitor-1 (PAI-1) levels. Impaired plasma fibrinolytic activity therefore can increase the risk for myocardial infarction.[124] Fasting plasma insulin levels have been shown to be directly correlated to the concentration of PAI-1. Glucose has a direct effect on PAI-1-producing tissues, leading to another explanation for the presence of impaired fibrinolysis in diabetic patients. Even when insulin resistance is adjusted for, serum triglyceride levels have been closely linked to impaired fibrinolysis.[125–127]

Endothelial Dysfunction

Hyperglycemia induces the expression of adhesion molecules such as VCAM-1, ICAM-1, and E-selectin[128] (Fig. 86-3). The binding of advanced glycosylation end products (AGEs) to their receptor results in oxidative stress and the transcription factor NF-KB[129,130] and VCAM-1.[131] These early stages in diabetic atherosclerosis may be the consequence of increased adhesive interactions of monocytes and the endothelial cell surface. Hyperglycemia-induced endothelial dysfunction is believed to result primarily from increased generation of oxygen-free radicals that inactivate endothelium-derived relaxing factor (EDRF).[132,133] Enhanced levels of free radicals in the setting of sustained hyperglycemia result in the autooxidation of glucose,[134] the oxidation of lipids,[135] and the metabolism of AGEs.[136] AGEs rapidly inactivate nitric oxide and result in a reduction of endothelium-dependent vasodilatation.[137] Endothelial dysfunction is measured clinically by the vasodilatory response of forearm resistance vessels to endothelium-dependent agents such as acetylcholine. It has been determined that in vivo endothelial dysfunction occurs in subjects whose fasting plasma glucose concentrations fall in the range of 110 to 126 mg.[138]

Advanced Glycosylation End Products

AGEs are formed by nonenzymatic glucose-protein and lipoprotein interactions, with subsequent cross-linking on vascular tissues.[139,140] In the setting of aging and diabetes, AGEs form at a rate determined by the glucose concentration and the length of exposure.[141] AGEs accelerate atherogenesis by multiple mechanisms that can be classified as receptor-mediated or non-receptor-mediated.[142] AGE deposits have been demonstrated in atherosclerotic plaques and myocardium by immunohistochemistry in patients with diabetes and atherosclerosis.[143] In addition, serum levels of AGEs are significantly increased in type 2 diabetes patients with CAD in contrast to those without CAD.[144] Serum levels of AGEs correlate positively with isovolumetric relaxation time (IVRT) and left ventricular diameter during diastole in type 1 diabetic patients.[145] The systolic parameters did not correlate with serum levels of AGEs.[145]

AGEs can be prevented from forming by pharmacologic means. Aminoguanidines prevent the earlier nonenzymatic Amadori products from progressing to AGEs,[146] and cross-link breakers can break up AGEs in vascular tissues that are already formed.[147]

The cellular interactions for AGE are via a specific receptor for AGE determinants on the cell membrane.[144] Indeed, AGE receptors are present on all cells participating in atherogenesis, such as the monocyte-derived macrophages, endothelial cells, and smooth muscle cells (SMCs)[148,149] (Table 86-4). When AGE binds to its receptor, monocytes undergo chemotaxis,[150] followed by mononuclear infiltration through an intact endothelial monolayer.[151,152] Pathologic studies of human atherosclerotic plaques showed infiltration of cells with AGE receptors in a thickened intima.[149] Monocyte-macrophage interactions with AGEs promote several mediators, including interleukin-1 (IL-1), tumor necrosis factor-alpha (TNF-α), platelet-derived growth factor (PDGF), and IGF-1.[151,153,154]

There is increased cellular proliferation in smooth muscle cells, in the binding of AGE-modified proteins to

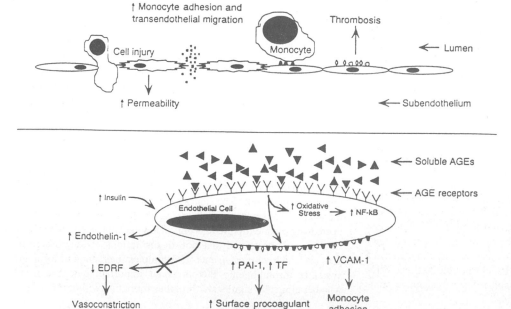

FIGURE 86-3 Generation of a dysfunctional endothelium caused by diabetes. PAI-1 = plasminogen-activator inhibitor-1; TF = tissue factor. (See text for further details.) (From Aronson and Rayfield,[142] with permission.)

TABLE 86-4 Atherosclerosis-Promoting Effects of Advanced Glycosylation End Products

Promoting inflammation
  *Secretion of cytokines (TNFα, IL-1)[146]
  *Chemotactic stimulus for monocytes-macrophages[147,148]
Induction of cellular proliferation
  *Stimulation of PDGF[147] and IGF-1[149] secretion from monocyte and (?) SMCs
Endothelial cells
  *Increased permeability of EC monolayers[150,151]
  *Increased procoagulant activity
  *Increased expression of adhesion molecules
  *Increased intracellular oxidative stress
Extracellular matrix
  Collagen cross-linking
  Enhanced synthesis of extracellular matrix components[156]
  Trapping of LDL in subendothelium
  Glycosylated subendothelium matrix quenches NO
Lipoprotein modifications
  Glycosylated LDL
  Reduced LDL recognition by cellular LDL receptors[79,80]
  Increased susceptibility of LDL to oxidative modification[78,81]

NOTE: Asterisks indicate receptor-mediated events, whereas lack of an asterisk signifies non-receptor-mediated processes. EC: endothelial cells; IGF-1: insulin-like growth factor-1; IL-1: interleukin 1; PDGF: platelet-derived growth factor; LDL: low-density lipoproteins; NO: nitric oxide; SMC: smooth muscle cells; TNFα: tumor necrosis factor-alpha.

the AGE receptor by cultured rat SMCs.[155] One can speculate that the response is induced by cytokines or growth factors. In summary, enhanced AGE formation involves receptor-mediated interaction of AGE protein with vascular wall cells, with subsequent migration of

inflammatory cells into the lesion and the elaboration of growth factors and cytokines.

Non-Receptor-Mediated Mechanisms

Glycosylated modification of proteins and lipoproteins can interfere with their normal function (Table 86-4). Glycosylation of matrix components such as type IV collagen, laminen, and vitronectin decreases the binding of anionic heparin sulfate (HS), promoting a greater turnover of HS. The absence of HS may induce a compensatory overproduction of other matrix components by means of altered partitioning of growth factors between matrix-bound proteoglycans and cells.[156] Modification of the cell-binding domain of type IV collagen results in decreased endothelial cell adhesion.[156]

CLINICAL IMPLICATIONS

Lipid Disorders

The Adult Treatment Panel III of the National Cholesterol Education Program (NCEP) reported their executive summary on the treatment of hyperlipidemia.[157] One of the most striking modifications was the raising of patients with diabetes without CHD to the same risk level as someone with CHD. As stated previously, the goal for LDL cholesterol, therefore, is <100 mg/dL for all those with diabetes regardless of CHD. Patients with a metabolic syndrome were also targeted for aggressive lifestyle modification in this document.

The management of diabetic patients with lipid abnormalities is a unique challenge to the cardiologist. Important evidence from large randomized trials of lipid-lowering therapies is based on subgroup analyses in which diabetic patients represented less than 10 percent of all the patients enrolled (Table 86-5). The 4S study enrolled 202 diabetic patients with a prior history of CAD.[158] Although this number was too small, the comparison of simvastatin with a placebo showed almost a 50 percent reduction in coronary events in favor of simvastatin (45 vs 23 percent, p = not significant). Similar trends

TABLE 86-5 Hyperlipidemia

Trial	Treatment	Outcome	Events Control Group	Events Treatment Group	Relative Risk Reduction, %	Number Needed to Treat	p
4S[158] (secondary prevention) n = 4444; 202 DM	Simvastatin	Death, nonfatal MI, revascularization	44/97 (45%)	24/105 (23%)	49	5	<.05
HPS[a] (primary and secondary prevention) n = 5963 DM	Simvastatin	Coronary death, nonfatal MI	748/n (25.1%)	601/n (20.2%)	20	20	p < 0.0001
CARE[159] (primary prevention) n = 4159; 586 DM	Pravastatin	Death, nonfatal MI, revascularization	112/304 (37%)	81/282 (29%)	21	12	.05
Helsinki Heart Study[b] (primary prevention) n = 4081 135 DM	Gemfibrozil	Death, nonfatal MI, revascularization	8/76 (10.5%)	2/59 (3.4%)	67	14	<.02

n = total number of patients. [a]Heart Protection Study Collaborative Group. MRC/BHF Heart Protection Study of cholesterol-lowering with simvastatin in 5963 people with diabetes: A randomized placebo-controlled trial. *Lancet* 2003;361:2003–2016. [b]Koskinen P, Manttari M, Manninen V, et al. Coronary heart disease incidence in NIDDM patients in the Helsinki Heart Study. *Diabetes Care* 1992;15:820–825.
ABBREVIATIONS: CARE = cholesterol and current events trial; DM = diabetes mellitus patients; MI = myocordial infarction.

were observed in the Cholesterol and Current Events (CARE) Trial, which compared pravastatin with a placebo in secondary prevention.[159] In the CARE trial, the baseline mean LDL concentration in diabetic patients was 136 mg/dL. LDL was reduced 27 percent in the group receiving pravastatin, which translated into a 25 percent reduction in coronary events over 5 years compared with that of the control group.[160] Table 86-5 demonstrates the relatively low number needed to treat (NNT) to prevent a major cardiovascular complication in three of the main lipid-lowering trials. These therapies are the cornerstone of diabetic management in the current era.

In the trials of statin therapy with hyperlipidemia, the relative benefit appears similar between diabetic patients and nondiabetic patients. The concern for the clinician is that larger trials focusing on the diabetic population have to be carried out before the magnitude of the benefit of lipid-lowering therapy in reducing cardiovascular events can be determined.

Glycemic Control

The pathophysiology of type 2 diabetes is a consequence of peripheral resistance to insulin action (in muscle and fat cells), increased hepatic glucose production, and decreased secretion of insulin by pancreatic beta cells. About 80 percent of people with type 2 diabetes are obese.[156]

POSTPRANDIAL HYPERGLYCEMIA AND CARDIOVASCULAR RISK

Postprandial glycemia may be an important factor in predicting future cardiovascular risk in epidemiologic studies.

The DECODE study showed that an elevated 2-h postprandial glucose level was independently associated with an increased mortality (Fig. 86-4).[161,162]

Diet and exercise remain the cornerstone in the management of type 2 diabetes. Pharmacologic agents available to treat type 2 diabetes are insulin, insulin secretagogues (sulfonylureas, repaglinide), alpha glucosidase inhibitors (acarbose, miglitol), and insulin sensitizers (biguanides, thiazolidinediones). Each of these agents targets a different mechanism responsible for the hyperglycemia. Figure 86-5 shows each of these agents and the target organs involved in its mode of action.

The standards of care in patients with diabetes (American Diabetes Association) are preprandial glucose levels of 80 to 120, bedtime glucose levels of 100 to 140, and hemoglobin A_{1c} (Hb A_{1c}) below 7 percent.[163]

Plasma Hb A_{1c} reflects the average glucose level of the previous 8 weeks and allows a uniform measure for achieving a target as well as comparing the efficacies of different therapies.

PHARMACOLOGIC MANAGEMENT

Sulfonylureas

Sulfonylureas are the typical therapy for lean patients with type 2 diabetes and are used in combinations with other agents in obese type 2 patients. Sulfonylureas bind to a receptor on the beta cells and inhibit the sodium-adenosine triphosphate (Na-ATP) channel; an increase in intracellular calcium results in insulin exocytosis.

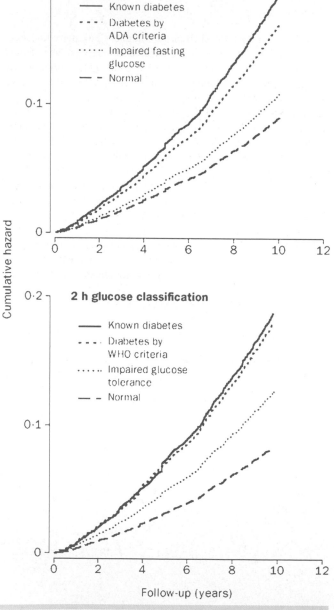

FIGURE 86-4 Cumulative hazard curves for American Diabetes Association fasting glucose criteria and the World Health Organization 2-h glucose criteria adjusted by age, sex, and study center. (From the DECODE study group,[162] with permission.)

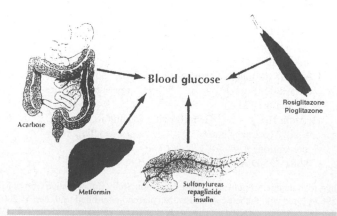

FIGURE 86-5 Mechanism of action of hypoglycemic agents.

Some experts point to a possible risk of increased myocardial damage in patients with known CAD who use sulfonylureas at the time of an ischemic event.[164] Prevention of protective ischemic preconditioning of the heart by inhibition of the potassium (K)-ATP channel is the putative mechanism.[165] The UKPDS data do not support this concern. The authors agree and use sulfonylureas in appropriate patients with CAD.

Repaglinide

This newer insulin secretagogue binds to a different receptor site than do the sulfonylureas on the K-ATP channel.[166] The half-life of this agent is 3.7 h, which makes it effective for postprandial rather than preprandial hyperglycemia, for use in the elderly and for diabetic patients with chronic renal failure.[166]

Metformin

Metformin is a biguanide drug that has been in use in Europe for over 30 years and was approved in the United States in 1995.[167] The main mode of action of metformin is decreasing hepatic glucose output primarily by inhibiting gluconeogenesis,[168] typically without hypoglycemia.[167]

Metformin is effective alone[169] or in combination with insulin,[170] sulfonylureas,[171] and thiazolidinediones.[172] The drug usually results in weight loss as a result of decreased appetite for up to 1 year after the initiation of therapy.

Significant decreases in LDL cholesterol and triglycerides occur.[171,173] The incidence of lactic acidosis with metformin is 9 per 100,000 person-years.[174] Contraindications to its use include an elevated creatinine level (>1.4 in women, >1.5 in men), congestive heart failure, severe pulmonary disease, or any hypoxic state.[175]

Thiazolidinediones

Thiazolidinediones promote insulin-stimulated glucose transport in muscles and adipocytes through a mechanism of action involving actuating peroxisome proliferator activated receptor-gamma (PPAR-γ) ligands (Fig. 86-6). Binding to the nuclear receptor promotes differentiation of adipocytes and increased expression of glucose transporter.[176] Thiazolidinediones also may act by antagonizing the effects of cytokines such as TNF-α.[177] Troglitazone has been shown to be effective both as monotherapy and in combination with insulin,[178,179] sulfonylureas,[180] and metformin.[172]

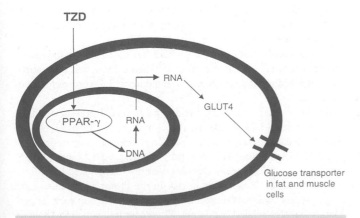

FIGURE 86-6 Mechanism of action of thiazolidinediones.

Endogenous C peptide is necessary for all the thiazolidinediones to be effective when used in combination with insulin. These agents can result in a reduction from two injections of insulin a day to one. Triglyceride levels can be lowered with troglitazone.[181,182] There is a small increase in the plasma LDL concentration, along with a favorable increase in the ratio of the buoyant LDL to the more atherogenic small dense LDL.[183] The thiazolidinediones are associated with weight gain partly resulting from improvement in glycemic control. With troglitazone, monitoring of liver function should be done monthly for the first year and quarterly thereafter.

Troglitazone has resulted in fulminant hepatic failure in about 1 in 60,000 patients on the medication; this is felt to be an idiosyncratic reaction. Patients with a history of liver disease, possibly including hepatitis C (depending on severity), and those who ingest more than a moderate amount of alcohol should not be started on this agent. Because of the potential for liver disease, troglitazone has been removed from use by the FDA.

Two other drugs in this class were approved by the U.S. Food and Drug Administration (FDA) in mid-1999, and the data to date support equal efficacy with less hepatotoxicity. No head-to-head studies of these agents are available. Monitoring of liver function tests with rosiglitazone and pioglitazone is recommended every 2 months for the first year and periodically thereafter, since it has not been determined that serious liver events with troglitazone are a class effect of the thiazolidinediones or are specific to troglitazone.

Rosiglitazone monotherapy results in a decrease of Hb A_{1c} of 0.8 to 1.5 percent greater than that seen with placebo, with the greatest reduction seen when it was given in two divided doses.[184,185] Combination studies of rosiglitazone with metformin for 26 weeks resulted in a 1.0-to 1.2-percent placebo-adjusted decrease in Hb A_{1c}.[186] Although rosiglitazone is currently approved for use as monotherapy and in combination therapy with metformin, it also is expected to be efficacious with sulfonylureas or insulin. Rosiglitazone has been reported to result in an increase in LDL and HDL cholesterol concentrations between 12 and 19 percent, with changes in serum triglycerides similar to those seen with placebo.[187]

Pioglitazone, the newest thiazolidinedione, has been approved for use as monotherapy and in combination with metformins, sulfonylureas, and insulin. In three randomized, double-blind placebo-controlled trials of 16 to 26 weeks' duration, changes in Hb A_{1c} were 1.0 to 1.4 percent.[188] Increases in alanine aminotransferase (ALT) occurred in 0.26 percent of treated patients, a result that was not different from that with placebo.[188] Patients treated with pioglitazone showed a decrease in serum triglyceride (9.3 to 9.6 percent), increases in HDL (12.2 to 19.1 percent), and increases in LDL (5.2 to 6.0 percent) with the 30- to 45-mg doses, respectively.[188]

Alpha-Glucosidase Inhibitors

Acarbose and miglitol work in the intestine to reversibly inhibit brush border alpha-glucosidases, resulting in a delay in carbohydrate absorption. Only about 1 percent of the drug is absorbed from the gastrointestinal tract. These drugs cause a 30 percent decrease in postprandial glucose in contrast to a 10 percent decrease in fasting glucose levels. They are adjuncts to other oral agents and rarely are potent enough to be used as monotherapy.

Insulin

The natural history of type 2 diabetes is one of progressive beta-cell failure. Therefore, after approximately 10 years of the use of oral hypoglycemic agents, insulin will be required either in combination

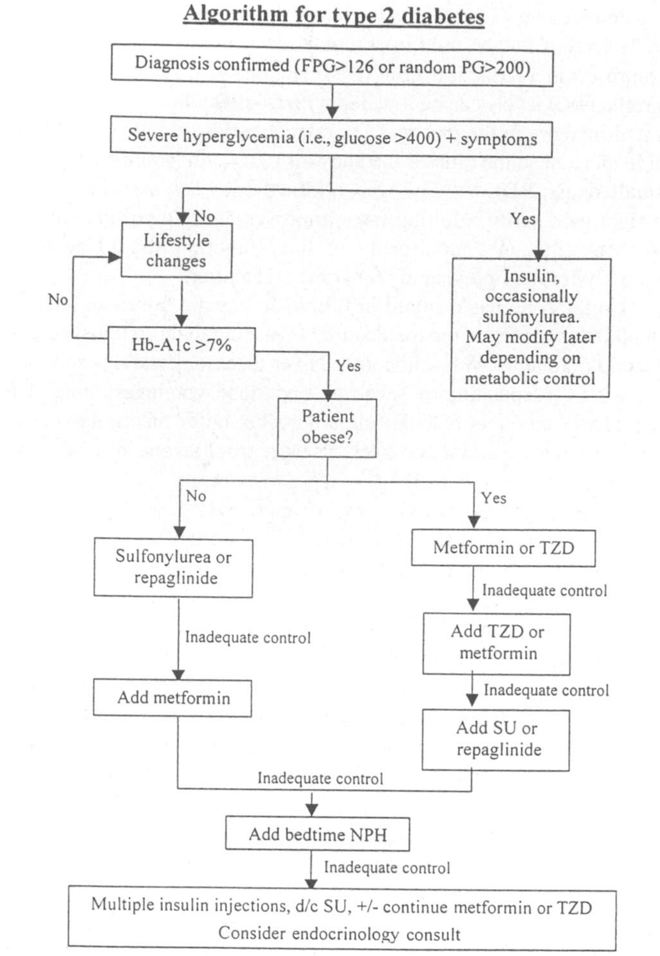

Algorithm for type 2 diabetes

FIGURE 86-7 Algorithm for type 2 diabetes. Note: Acarbose or miglitol can be added anywhere along the treatment pathway. SU, sulfonylurea; TZD, thiazolidinedione.

with oral agents or as the sole therapy. Although endogenous hyper-insulinemia is clearly associated with atherogenesis, there is no compelling evidence of increased risk of cardiovascular disease or increased mortality from exogenous insulin therapy.

Diabetes clinics nationwide have strived to optimize the glycemic control of patients with a view to minimizing the development of coronary and other vascular disease. Figure 86-7 shows an algorithm that is reasonable to use in the management of patients with type 2 diabetes. Table 86-6 shows the clinical trial evidence supporting intensive glycemic control.

NEW ADVANCES IN DIABETIC TREATMENT

A landmark study from Canada was reported addressing the promising islet cell transplantation initiative in type 1 diabetic patients.[189] Seven patients with a history of metabolic instability and severe hypoglycemia underwent islet cell transplantation with a glucocorticoid-free immunosuppressive regimen. Almost immediately after the procedure all patients attained an insulin-free status with relatively good tolerance for the antirejection therapy. Larger series are planned in the United States to verify these findings. Furthermore, the impact of this procedure on cardiovascular outcomes will also need to be addressed.

Type 2 Diabetes: United Kingdom Prospective Diabetes Study Group Trial

A number of important trials have evaluated the effects of glycemic control in cardiac patients with type 2 diabetes. Before the publication of the United Kingdom Prospective Diabetes Study Group Trial (UKPDS), there was a great deal of controversy about the benefit of intensive glycemic control in type 2 patients. Both the University Group Diabetes Program study and other reports have questioned whether sulfonylureas adversely affect the heart by blocking the ATP-dependent potassium channels.[190,191] Two small, randomized trials suggested that intensive glycemic control with insulin for type 2 diabetic patients is effective in reducing cardiovascular events. The UKPDS trial is the largest and best conducted study of glycemic control in type 2 diabetic patients. It addresses the issue of the influence of tight glycemic control in reducing micro- and macroangiopathy in newly diagnosed patients with type 2 diabetes mellitus.[192,193] In this multicenter randomized controlled trial, 5102 patients in 23 centers in the United Kingdom were studied between 1977 and 1991. A hypertension study was included to assess whether treating high blood pressure in patients with type 2 diabetes could reduce the risk of diabetic complications.[194]

The first study compared the effects of intensive blood glucose control with either sulfonylurea or insulin and conventional treatment on the risk of micro- and macrovascular complications in type 2 diabetes patients. *Intensive glycemic control* was defined as a fasting plasma glucose (FPG) level of <108 mg/dL. Over a 10-year period, Hb A_{1c} was 7.0 percent in the intensive group compared with 7.9 percent in the conventional group. There was a 25 percent risk reduction in microvascular endpoints in the intensively treated group. No difference existed between the three agents used for intensive glycemic control (chlorpropamide, glibenclimide, and insulin). Patients in the intensive group had more hypoglycemic episodes than did those in the conventional group ($p < .0001$). Finally, none of the individual agents had an adverse effect on cardiovascular outcomes.

UKPDS 34, the second arm of the study, assessed whether intensive glucose control with metformin had any specific advantage or disadvantage.[193] Mean Hb A_{1c} was 7.4 percent in the metformin group compared with 8.0 percent in the conventional group. Given that intensive glycemic control with metformin appears to decrease the risk of diabetes-related endpoints in overweight diabetes patients and is associated with less weight gain and fewer hypoglycemic attacks than insulin or sulfonylureas, the authors suggested that metformin may be the first-line pharmacologic therapy of choice in these patients. It should be noted that the UKPDS was conducted before the clinical availability of the thiazolidinediones as well as the statins (although the study did not address the issue of cholesterol reduction in diabetic patients).

A noteworthy finding in the UKPDS was a decrease in the risk of myocardial infarction of 16 percent.[192] The decrease was not statistically significant but demonstrated a trend toward fewer macrovascular events.

UKPDS determined whether intensive blood pressure control prevents micro- and macrovascular complications in patients with type 2 diabetes. *Tight blood pressure control* was defined as <150/85. The angiotensin-converting enzyme (ACE) inhibitor captopril and the beta blocker atenolol were the drugs used to achieve the tight control. Reductions in risk in the group assigned to tight blood pressure control compared with the control group were 24 percent in diabetes-related endpoints, 32 percent in death from diabetic complications, 44 percent in strokes, and 37 percent in microvascular

TABLE 86-6 Glycemic Control

Trial	Treatment	Outcome	Events Control Group	Events Treatment Group	Relative Risk Reduction, %	Number Needed to Treat	p
Type 1 DM DCCT[197] *n* = 1441 patients[a] free of cardiac disease, HTN, and dyslipidemia	Intensive glycemic control versus conventional therapy	Macrovascular events	40/730 (5.5%)	23/711 (3.2%)	42	43	.08
Type 2 DM UKPDS[192–195] In newly diagnosed diabetes mellitus *n* = 3867	Sulfonylurea or insulin versus conventional therapy	Diabetes-related outcomes	438/1138 (38.4%)	963/2729 (35.2%)	8.3	31	.029
Steno-2[136] *n* = 160	Intensive comprehensive (includes HTN, dyslipidemia, and glycemic control) therapy versus standard therapy	Macrovascular events Death MI Stroke Vascular ischemia	42/78 (53.8%)	26/77 (33.7%)	37.3	5	.03

[a]*n* = total number of patients.

ABBREVIATIONS: DCCT = the diabetes control and complications trial research group; DM = diabetes mellitus; HTN = hypertension; MI = myocordial infarction. Steno-2 = a trial of type 2 diabetic patients comparing the macrovascular complications of an intensive multifactorial risk factor modification intervention with conventional therapy; UKPDS = United Kingdom Prospective Diabetes Study.

disease (almost all of which were statistically significant). There was a nonsignificant reduction in all-cause mortality.[194]

UKPDS 39 investigated whether tight blood pressure control with either a beta blocker (atenolol) or an ACE inhibitor (captopril) has a specific advantage in terms of preventing the macro- and microvascular complications of type 2 diabetes. This study involving 1148 hypertensive patients showed that each agent was equally efficacious in reducing blood pressure, the risk of macrovascular endpoints, and deterioration of retinopathy.[195] Using these two classes of antihypertensive agents, the investigators showed that the blood pressure reduction per se was more important than was the treatment used.

The current strategy for type 2 diabetes mellitus is to optimize Hb A_{1c} levels with sulfonylureas, insulin-sensitizing agents, or insulin when necessary (see the previous discussion).

Type 1 Diabetes: Diabetes Control and Complications Trial

Intensive diabetes control versus standard therapy was evaluated in the Diabetes Control and Complications Trial (DCCT).[196,197] The primary outcome was the development and progression of microvascular disease, but patients were followed for over 6 years so that cardiac events did ensue. There was almost a doubling of the cardiac event rate in patients treated in a conventional manner (40 versus 23 events), but this did not reach statistical significance. Since the patients in this study were between ages 13 and 39 and did not have diabetes for a long enough period, a nearly significant reduction in cardiovascular events is not surprising. Diabetic renal disease is a strong predictor of subsequent cardiovascular events, and therefore, the promising result of reduced proteinuria with intensive therapy in DCCT may translate into a cardioprotective effect in the long term. The current strategy for type 1 diabetes is to optimize glycemic control with multiple injections of insulin or with an insulin pump. Such patients should have a concomitant consultation with an endocrinologist.

PREVENTION OF TYPE II DIABETES MELLITUS

Increasing evidence suggests that an atherogenic prediabetic state exists prior to the development of diabetes. In the San Antonio Heart Study, patients converting to overt diabetes had significantly higher blood pressure, body mass index, waist circumference, and triglyceride levels and lower HDL cholesterol levels at baseline compared to nonconvertors.[198]

Investigators from Finland conducted a randomized trial of 522 middle-aged overweight subjects with impaired glucose tolerance (350 women, mean age 55 years).[199] Patients were randomized to a control group or an intervention group that consisted of individualized counseling aimed at reducing weight, total intake of fat, and intake of saturated fat and increasing intake of fiber and physical activity. Over 4 years of follow-up, the cumulative incidence of diabetes was 11 percent in the intervention group and 23 percent in the control group (58 percent reduction, $p < 0.001$; Fig. 86-8). The authors concluded that indeed type-2 diabetes could be prevented with an intensive lifestyle modification program (Table 86-7).

Another trial, the Diabetes Prevention Program, evaluated over 3000 nondiabetic subjects with impaired fasting and postglucose loading plasma glucose levels showed that when compared to placebo, a lifestyle intervention reduced the incidence of developing diabetes by 58 percent (95 percent confidence interval, 48 to 66 percent and NNT of 7) whereas metformin reduced the incidence by 31 percent (95 percent confidence interval, 17 to 43 percent and NNT of 14).[200] When compared head to head the intervention group fared better than did the metformin group.[192]

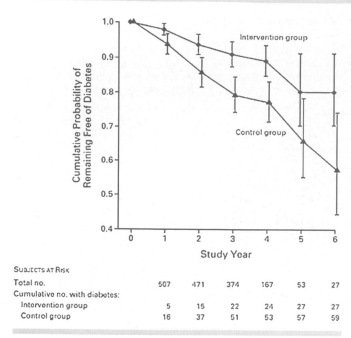

Subjects at Risk

Total no.	507	471	374	167	53	27
Cumulative no. with diabetes:						
Intervention group	5	15	22	24	27	27
Control group	16	37	51	53	57	59

FIGURE 86-8 Finnish Trial of Lifestyle Modification in Preventing Diabetes. Proportion of subjects without diabetes during the trial. (From Tuomilehto et al.,[199] with permission.)

Pharmacologic Therapies Prevent Progression to Diabetes

Evidence from large clinical trials has emerged to suggest that treatments that modify cardiovascular risk may also reduce the incidence of developing type 2 diabetes.

The WOSCOPS investigators reported on 5974 patients who were not diabetic or glucose intolerant on entry into the pravastatin primary prevention study. Therapy with pravastatin as compared with placebo was associated with a 30 percent relative reduction risk for developing overt type diabetes.[201]

Treatment with ramipril in nondiabetic patients with known vascular disease in the Heart Outcomes Prevention Evaluation Study (HOPE) trial was associated with a 34 percent reduction in the development of type 2 diabetes.[202,203] This effect may be mediated by a potential anti-inflammatory effect as well as by improved insulin sensitivity.

Early Detection of Diabetes

Because of the significant increase in major microvascular complications and the risk of premature death, it is important to begin to screen for diabetes at a younger age than 45 years, the current recommendation.[204,205] Selecting populations at the highest risk for developing diabetes for aggressive screening strategies probably will occur in the next 10 years.

Current measures of cardiovascular surveillance for CAD in asymptomatic diabetic patients focus on routine stress testing in accordance with the American College of Cardiology/American Heart Association (ACC/AHA) guidelines[206] (Table 86-8). Exercise testing in diabetic patients is more likely to be accurate when combined with echocardiography or radionuclide imaging. Diabetic patients are less likely to have an appropriate blood pressure and heart rate response to exercise and less likely to experience any pain corresponding to ST-segment changes caused in part by autonomic dysfunction. The AHA recommends that the finding of subclinical CAD should prompt clinicians to initiate more aggressive preventative measures[207] (see Table 86-8).

AHA Prevention VI: Risk Stratification[42]

For patients with diabetes, office-based assessment of risk factors is useful to define targets for intervention to reduce cardiovascular risk; additional noninvasive testing is not recommended on a routine basis at this time because it would not change management or lead to improvement in outcomes.

ANKLE-BRACHIAL BLOOD PRESSURE INDEX[42]

The ankle-brachial blood pressure index (ABI) is performed by measuring blood pressure in both arms and the posterior tibial and dorsalis pedis arteries and computing an ankle-average arm blood pressure ratio. An ABI <0.90 constitutes a diagnosis of peripheral arterial disease.

Hypertension and Nephropathy

To date, there have been no randomized trials primarily evaluating the role of hypertension treatment with nephropathy as the endpoint in type 1 diabetic patients without microalbuminuria. Hypertensive diabetic patients are treated primarily with ACE inhibitors or ARBs.

Compared with nondiabetic subjects, diabetic patients in the SHEP (Systolic Hypertension in the Elderly Program cooperative research group) study experienced a more pronounced benefit from treatment with clorthalidone. The 5-year rates of major cardiovascular events are illustrated in Fig. 86-9.[208]

The UKPDS demonstrated no advantage of captopril over atenolol in reducing macrovascular complications.[197] Clearly, this illustrates the significant role lowering of blood pressure plays in reducing adverse events independent of the agent used. The role of further blood pressure re-

TABLE 86-7 Success in Achieving the Goals of the Intervention by 1 Year, According to Treatment Group*

Group	Intervention Group (%)	Control Group (%)	P Value[†]
Weight reduction .5%	43	13	0.001
Fat intake <30% of energy intake	47	26	0.001
Saturated-fat intake <10% of energy intake	26	11	0.001
Final intake >15 g/1000 kcal	25	12	0.001
Exercise >4 h/week[‡]	86	71	0.001

*Nutrient intakes were calculated from 3-day food records.
[†]P values were determined by the chi-square test for the difference between the groups.
[‡]Exercise frequency was reported by the subjects who chose one of the four categories. The goal identified here was a frequency category 2 or higher.

TABLE 86-8 Detection of Clinical and Subclinical Cardiovascular Disease in Diabetic Patients

A. Stress testing for coronary heart disease
  Consult AHA guidelines for exercise treadmill testing
  Considerations for testing in diabetic patients
    Blunting of heart rate and blood pressure responses
    Painless ST-segment depression common in diabetic patients (autonomic neuropathy)
    Diagnostic specificity of ST-segment depression may be reduced (previous silent myocardial infarction, etc.)
    Exercise or pharmacologic testing (^{99m}Tc) perfusion scintography favorable for exercise testing in diabetic patients
    Ambulatory ECG monitoring may be helpful in special instances in diabetic patients to diagnose silent ischemia, but not
      routinely
B. Noninvasive evaluation of cardiac function
  Echocardiography (Doppler) and radionuclide ventriculography issues in diabetic patients
    Diastolic dysfunction commonly and often precedes systolic dysfunction
    Left ventricular wall motion abnormalities suggest diabetic cardiomyopathy
C. Evaluation of autonomic dysfunction
  In bedside evaluation two or more of these tests are abnormal
    Resting heart rate (supine), 100
    Excess diastolic blood pressure response to handgrip exercise
    Abnormal expiratory/inspiratory RR-interval ratio
    Postural hypotension
  Significance of autonomic dysfunction in diabetic patients
    50% 5-year mortality
    Sudden death common; consider electrophysiologic study
    Greater complications after elective surgery
    Increased danger with general anesthesia
D. Diagnosis of subclinical cardiovascular disease
  History: symptoms of claudication, angina, dyspnea on exertion, cerebrovascular disease
  Physical examination: routine checkup with evaluation of carotid and femoral bruits, peripheral arterial pulses, ratio of
    ankle to brachial artery systolic blood pressure (marker of subclinical peripheral vascular disease)
  Laboratory: urinary creatinine/albumin ratio (Table 86-1)
  ECG: left ventricular hypertrophy a strong predictor of CAD morbidity and mortality
  Electron beam CT: coronary calcium score highly correlated with total coronary atherosclerosis burden
  Carotid ultrasound: detects subclinical carotid atherosclerosis.

ABBREVIATIONS: AHA = American Heart Association; CAD = coronary heart disease; CT = computed tomography; ECG = electrocardiogram.

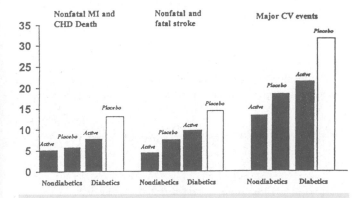

FIGURE 86-9 Five-year rates of nonfatal myocardial infarction (MI) and coronary heart disease (CHD) death, stroke, and major cardiovascular (CV) events by diabetes status and treatment (chlorthalidone vs placebo) in the Systolic Hypertension in the Elderly Program. (Data from Curb et al.[208] and from Furberg CD. Hypertension and diabetes: Current issues. *Am Heart J* 1999; 138:5401, with permission.)

duction even when high-risk patients such as diabetic patients are in the normal range needs to be delineated further. The Hypertension Optimal Treatment (HOT) study showed that the risk of major cardiovascular events in diabetic patients was halved if they had a target diastolic pressure ≤80 mmHg compared with those with a diastolic pressure ≤90 mmHg (*p* for trend = .005).[209] There was a lower but still significant decrease in the risk of silent myocardial infarction and about a 30 percent risk reduction in the rate of stroke in the ≤80 mmHg group compared with the ≤90 mmHg group.

The Captopril Prevention Projects (CAPPP) trial showed significant lowering of cardiovascular events in hypertensive patients treated with captopril instead of standard therapy with beta-blockers or diuretics (Table 86-9).[210] Approximately 5 percent of the patients had diabetes in this trial, and in these patients, similar trends in favor of captopril were observed. The Appropriate Blood pressure Control in Diabetics (ABCD) study also observed a benefit of ACE inhibitors when compared with conventional therapy in the treatment of hypertension in diabetic patients.[211]

TABLE 86-9 Hypertension

Trial	Treatment	Outcome	Control Group	Treatment Group	Relative Risk Reduction, %	p
CAPPP[210] n = 10985 572 DM[a]	Captopril versus conventional therapy	Cardiac death, nonfatal MI, stroke	263	309	33	.03

[a]n = total number of patients.

ABBREVIATIONS: captopril prevention projects; DM = diabetes mellitus patients; MI = myocardial infarction.

The use of nondihydropyridine calcium channel blockers is acceptable but not frontline therapy.

The HOPE trial evaluated over 9000 high-risk patients with evidence of vascular disease or diabetes in a randomized trial comparing ramipril with placebo over a 5-year period.[202] A total of 3578 of these patients had diabetes. This study demonstrated a 22 percent reduction in primary cardiovascular endpoints of death, myocardial infarction, and stroke in favor of ramipril. The beneficial effect of ramipril was observed over all predefined subgroups. Interestingly, there was a 30 percent reduction in the diagnosis of new diabetic patients in the ramipril-treated arm. This result also was observed in the CAPPP study. Ramipril lowered systolic blood pressure by a mean of only 6 mmHg. This would account for only approximately 40 percent of the reduction in the rate of stroke and about a 25 percent reduction in the rate of myocardial infarction. Therefore, there is some benefit of ramipril independent of the blood pressure-lowering effect that accounts for the impressive cardiovascular protective effect. HOPE provides level 1 evidence supporting the front-line use of ACE inhibitors in the treatment of diabetic patients at risk for cardiovascular events regardless of whether they are hypertensive. In the diabetic subgroup there was even a greater relative risk reduction in primary cardiovascular events (25 percent; Table 86-10).

STENO-2

Steno 2 demonstrated that a comprehensive multifactorial strategy (including lifestyle and pharmacologic interventions) to reduce cardiovascular risk in type 2 diabetic patients with microalbuminuria was highly effective (hazard ratio, 0.47; 95 percent confidence interval, 0.24 to 0.73) when compared to usual care after a mean time of 7.8 years (Fig. 86-10).[212]

The number needed to treat was only 5 patients in order to prevent a major cardiovascular event. The approach included targets of Hb A_{1C} less than 6.5 percent, blood pressure less than 130/80, total cholesterol less than 175 mg/dL and triglycerides below 150 mg/dL. Patients were prescribed aspirin and an ACE inhibitor or ARB.

This study validates the multidisciplinary approach to the cardiovascular care of the diabetic patient.

ACUTE CORONARY SYNDROMES

Diabetic patients represent a high-risk group for developing and surviving acute myocardial infarction.[213] In particular, patients with type 1 diabetes have a worse outcome than do patients with type 2 disease, and diabetic women have almost twice the risk of mortality compared with diabetic men.[8,214–216]

Reperfusion therapy is the cornerstone of the management of acute myocardial infarction. In a meta-analysis of all major thrombolytic trials, diabetic patients had a nonsignificant trend toward increased reductions in 35-day mortality rates compared with nondiabetic patients.[217] The potential advantage of angioplasty over thrombolytic therapy has not been addressed in the diabetic population.

New treatment strategies are emerging. The utilization of insulin and glucose infusion for at least 24 h after admission followed by intensive long-term insulin was compared with usual care in the DIGAMI trial (Fig. 86-11 and Table 86-11). A total of 620 diabetic patients were randomized, and the trial demonstrated a 30 percent reduction in mortality at 12 months for the group treated under the intensive program.[218]

Aspirin remains the mainstay of ongoing therapy. Beta blockers are generally underutilized in diabetic patients despite convincing evidence dating back to the prethrombolytic era that demonstated both an early- and late-survival benefit that was more impressive than that observed in the nondiabetic cohort. The standard contraindications to beta-blockers still apply, namely, atrioventricular conduction disturbances and bronchospasm.

CHRONIC CORONARY ARTERY DISEASE

The association between CAD and diabetes is strong and has led to screening strategies in diabetic patients even before they are sympto-

TABLE 86-10 Prevention Study

Trial	Treatment	Outcome	Events Control Group	Events Treatment Group	Relative Risk Reduction, %	Number Needed to Treat	p
HOPE[202] 3578 DM n = 9297[a]	Ramipril (10 mg qd)	Cardiac death, nonfatal MI, stroke	351/1769 (19.8%)	277/1808 (15.3%)	25	22	.0004

[a]n = total number of patients;

ABBREVIATIONS: DM = diabetes mellitus patients; HOPE = heart outcomes prevention evaluation study; MI = myocardial infarction.

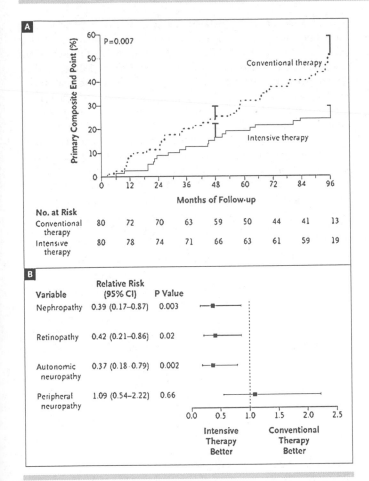

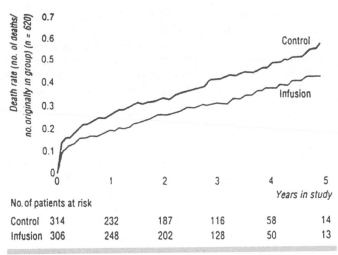

FIGURE 86-11 Actuarial mortality curves during long-term follow-up in patients receiving insulin-glucose infusion and in the control group among total DIGAMI cohort. Absolute reduction in risk was 11 percent; relative risk was 0.72 (0.55 to 0.92); p = .011. (From Malmberg, for the DIGAMI Study group,[218] with permission.)

FIGURE 86-10 Kaplan–Meier estimates of the composite endpoint of death from cardiovascular causes, nonfatal myocardial infarction, coronary-artery bypass grafting, percutaneous coronary intervention, nonfatal stroke, amputation, or surgery for peripheral atherosclerotic artery disease in the Conventional-Therapy Group and the Intensive-Therapy Group (Panel A) and the relative risk of the development or progression of nephropathy, retinopathy, and autonomic and peripheral neuropathy during the average follow-up of 7.8 years in the Intensive-Therapy Group, as compared with the Conventional-Therapy Group (Panel B). (From Gæde et al.,[212] with permission.)

matic. In addition, diabetic patients often are unaware of myocardial ischemic pain, and so silent myocardial infarction and ischemia are markedly increased in this population.[219] There is a heightened concern for the development of sudden cardiac death in those with diabetes. Therapeutic modalities in diabetic patients with CAD revolve

around standard therapy with aspirin, beta blockers, calcium channel blockers, and nitrates.

Epidemiologic evidence from the Bezafibrate Infarction Prevention Study registry shows almost a 50 percent reduction in mortality for type 2 patients with chronic CAD who were treated with beta blockers compared with controls.[220] Other randomized trial evidence has demonstrated that diabetes is a strong predictor of death and that diabetic patients may benefit more from beta blocker therapy than do non-diabetics.[221] In general, beta blockers are extremely well tolerated, and masking or prolonging of hypoglycemic symptoms appears to be highly infrequent, particularly with cardioselective beta blockers.

CORONARY REVASCULARIZATION

Diabetes mellitus accelerates the natural course of atherosclerosis in all groups of patients and involves a greater number of coronary vessels with more diffuse atherosclerotic lesions.[222–225] Cardiac catheterizations in diabetic patients have shown significantly more severe proximal and distal CAD.[226–229] In addition, rates of plaque ulceration and thrombosis have been found to be significantly higher in diabetic patients.[230,231]

TABLE 86-11 Myocardial Infarction

Trial	Treatment	Outcome	Events Control Group	Events Treatment Group	Relative Risk Reduction, %	Number Needed to Treat	p
DIGAMI[218] After MI n = 620[a]	Standard therapy with glucose-insulin infusion versus standard therapy	Long-term (3.4 years) all cause mortality	138/314 (43.9%)	102/306 (33.3%)	24	9	.011

[a]n = total number of patients; DIGAMI, MI = myocardial infarction.

The management of diabetic patients with CAD entails both pharmacologic and revascularization strategies.[232] Over the past several years, there have been many advances in the medical management of the diabetic patient with CAD. Aspirin, beta-blockers, statins, and ACE inhibitors are routinely administered. These agents may provide clinical benefit not only by treating ischemia but also by stabilizing atherosclerotic plaque and inhibiting endovascular thrombosis, thereby preventing acute coronary events.[233]

Coronary revascularization procedures have become a mainstay of therapy for CAD patients, providing both symptomatic relief and mortality reduction in certain anatomic subsets. Several studies have attempted to rationalize the use of different revascularization techniques by comparing them to medical therapy and to each other in various clinical settings.[234,235] Evidence from well-designed, prospective, randomized clinical trials suggests that surgical revascularization provides a survival advantage compared to medical therapy alone in patients with obstructive left main CAD and in patients with multivessel CAD with decreased left ventricular ejection fraction (LVEF). In addition, surgical revascularization provides symptomatic improvement compared to medical therapy in patients with multivessel CAD and normal left ventricular systolic function. Although none of the preceding studies was specifically conducted in diabetic patients, subgroup analyses of these studies indicated that diabetic patients (1) are at greater risk for cardiac death and ischemic complications than nondiabetic patients[236] and (2) despite a greater surgical risk, diabetic patients may indeed derive a greater long-term benefit from revascularization than do nondiabetic patients.

Options for Revascularization in Diabetic Patients: Coronary Artery Bypass Graft Surgery versus Balloon Angioplasty

In the Bypass Angioplasty Revascularization Investigation (BARI) randomized trial ($n = 1829$ patients in total), diabetic patients taking an oral agent or insulin ($n = 347$) undergoing coronary artery bypass graft (CABG) had a 5-year survival rate of 80.6 percent compared with 65.5 percent in the balloon angioplasty arm.[237,238] In-hospital mortality was similar in the two subgroups (0.6 percent with angioplasty, 1.2 percent with CABG, $p = 1.0$; Fig. 86-12). In addition, the CABG group had fewer repeat revascularization procedures and less angina. Although this was not a prespecified subgroup analysis according to the BARI protocol, these striking results lead to a warning issued by the NIH that recommended CABG as the revascularization strategy of choice in diabetic patients with multivessel CAD.[239]

In comparison, the BARI Registry (comprising patients eligible for but not enrolled in the BARI trial for any reason in the same medical centers) evaluating the outcome of physician-guided (i.e., nonrandomized) assignment of therapy resulted in no difference in overall long-term survival between CABG and angioplasty patients.[240] Even though the majority of patients underwent angioplasty (65 percent) rather than CABG in the BARI Registry, the 7-year mortality rate was identical in both groups: 14 percent for all patients and 26 percent for treated diabetic patients. Patients treated with balloon angioplasty, however, were less likely to have triple vessel disease, or left ventricular systolic dysfunction, and had fewer significantly obstructive lesions than those referred for CABG.

Following these conflicting findings (BARI Randomized Trial versus BARI Registry), there remains a controversy regarding the most appropriate revascularization method in diabetic patients with multivessel CAD. Significantly, the BARI Randomized Trial analysis on diabetic patients was a secondary subgroup analysis not specified by the initial protocol, and bears all the relevant methodological (statistical) limitations of this type of analysis (Fig. 86-13).[237,238,241]

The Northern New England Registry of 2766 consecutive coronary interventions among diabetic patients demonstrated a significant mortality benefit in favor of CABG.[242] Using Cox proportional hazards methods, the hazards ratio was 1.49 ($p = 0.04$) for percutaneous coronary intervention (PCI) versus CABG after adjusting for differences in baseline characteristics. Patients with three-vessel disease had the greatest benefit from CABG. The consistent message derived from this Registry and the BARI Randomized Trial is that patients (especially diabetics) with the greatest burden of disease benefit more from CABG than they do from conventional PCI treatment.

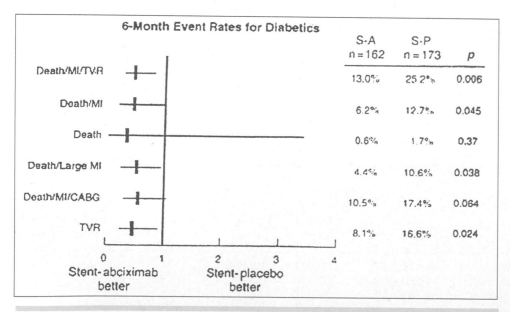

FIGURE 86-12 Absolute percentage of events, 95 percent confidence limits, and point estimates of listed endpoints for diabetic patients randomized to stenting-abciximab (S-A) or stenting-placebo (S-P). (From Marso et al.[274] with permission.)

Theoretical Explanation for the Advantage of Coronary Artery Bypass Graft over Balloon Angioplasty in Patients with Treated Diabetes

When compared with balloon angioplasty, CABG provides a greater likelihood of "complete revascularization"; can treat total chronic occlusions, left main stem stenosis, complex bifurcation disease; and diffuse disease. In diabetic patients, balloon angioplasty is associated with high rates of reocclusion and restenosis, which may provide the mechanistic basis for the BARI Randomized Trial results.[238] Kip et al. reported more repeat procedures after initial angioplasty strategy with intended incomplete revascularization, which may be an important technical limitation of the percutaneous interventional approach.[243] Van Belle et al. reported that in diabetic patients this

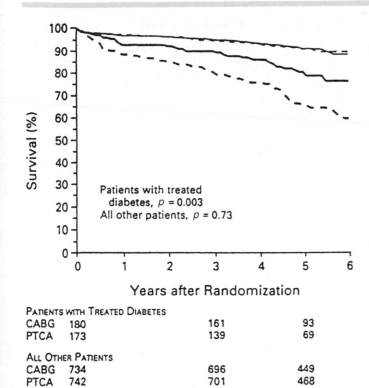

FIGURE 86-13 Survival among patients who were being treated for diabetes at baseline (heavy lines) and all other patients (light lines). Patients assigned to coronary artery bypass graft (CABG) are indicated by solid lines, and those assigned to percutaneous transluminal coronary angioplasty (PTCA) by dashed lines. The numbers of patients at risk are shown below the graph at baseline, 3 years, and 5 years. [From the Bypass Angioplasty Revascularization Investigation (BARI) Investigators,[237] with permission.]

higher reocclusion and restenosis rate after balloon angioplasty was associated with higher mortality.[244] In addition, balloon angioplasty strategies may be associated with a higher rate of progression of native coronary atherosclerosis in treated (or nontreated) vessels, or with less protection from ischemic events when new atherosclerotic lesions appear or rupture, both of which may be important factors in long-term morbidity and mortality associated with CAD and diabetes mellitus.[245] In contrast, CABG surgery also has limitations, in particular, higher perioperative morbidity and mortality in diabetic patients than it has in nondiabetic patients. CABG surgery is more invasive by nature than angioplasty, with general involvement of multiple organs. Therefore, excessive comorbidity may be prohibitive for CABG in certain patient cohorts. Finally, CABG surgery is associated with prolonged rehabilitation and may significantly degrade neuropsychiatric function, either transiently or permanently.[246]

Modern Percutaneous Coronary Intervention Techniques (Before Drug-Eluting Stents)

Before the use of stents and IIb/IIIa antagonists, the rate of restenosis after angioplasty in diabetic patients was shown to be as high as 47 to 71 percent.[247–255] The mechanism of restenosis is believed to be related to neointimal hyperplasia, which is tightly linked to the interplay between platelet-thrombus deposition, various growth factors present after injury, and endothelial dysfunction.[256,257]

Many of the technical limitations of balloon angioplasty have been overcome by coronary stent implantation during PCI.[258] Stenting is more predictable, giving a more reliable angiographic result in a wide variety of lesion types and is associated with lower restenosis in many lesion subsets. In the STRESS Trial, patients with relatively simple de novo lesions randomized to stent implantation had a 31.6 percent rate of restenosis compared to 42.1 percent in the balloon angioplasty group ($p < 0.05$).[259] Similarly, in the BENESTENT Trial, patients with relatively simple de novo native lesions randomized to stent implantation had a 22 percent rate of restenosis, compared to 32 percent in the angioplasty group ($p = 0.02$).[260] This initial clinical benefit shown in the BENESTENT trial has been sustained for 5 years during follow-up assessments.[261] Sustained patency of the target vessel is associated with superior clinical results, including less angina and improved regional left ventricular wall motion, compared to vessels with recurrent restenosis or reocclusion.[262,263] The advantage of stent implantation versus percutaneous transluminal coronary angioplasty (PTCA) alone with respect to angiographic restenosis and the need for repeat revascularization procedures has also been applicable to diabetic patients. This was evident from subgroup analyses from the stent versus angioplasty trials, since none of the studies was specifically conducted exclusively in diabetic patients.[259,260] What is clear is that diabetic patients are at significantly higher risk for restenosis after either balloon angioplasty or stent implantation compared to nondiabetic patients, as shown in all previous clinical studies on restenosis.[264–269]

A large body of evidence from prospective, randomized, double-blinded clinical trials supports the use of platelet glycoprotein IIb/IIIa inhibitors during PCI; derived mainly from the abciximab clinical trials.[270-273] A prespecified analysis of clinical outcomes in diabetic patients was included in the EPISTENT trial (20 percent of total cohort or 491 patients with diabetes).[274] Patients were assigned to a strategy of stent-implantation plus placebo, stent-implantation plus abciximab, or angioplasty plus abciximab. For diabetic patients receiving stent and abciximab, compared to stent alone, there was a >50 percent reduction in death, nonfatal myocardial infarction, or urgent revascularization rate at 6-month follow-up. In addition, diabetic patients were less likely to require repeat target-vessel revascularization, if they were treated with stent plus abciximab (8.1 percent), compared with either stent plus placebo (16.6 percent, $p = 0.02$) or angioplasty plus abciximab (18.4 percent, $p = 0.008$). Thus, it appears that the benefit of abciximab is additive to the benefit of stent implantation in diabetic patients. One-year mortality was also marginally lower with stent plus abciximab versus stent plus placebo (1.2 vs 4.1 percent, $p = 0.11$). (See Table 86-12.)

Clinical studies have demonstrated that intravascular treatment with catheter-based ionizing radiation (intravascular brachytherapy) is efficacious in reducing in-stent restenosis, but does not prevent restenosis as an adjunct to stent implantation in de novo lesions.[266,275]

Multivessel Stenting versus Coronary Artery Bypass Graft in Patients with Treated Diabetes Mellitus

The introduction and generalized application of stenting gave promise that by reducing restenosis and preventing repeat revascularizations, diabetic patients may further benefit from a PCI approach, thus achieving parity with CABG as a revascularization strategy.[276,277] The Arterial Revascularization Trial Study (ARTS) randomized trial compared the clinical outcomes of aggressive stenting versus CABG surgery in 1205 patients with multivessel coronary disease[278] and demonstrated no important differences in death, myocardial infarction, or stroke at 1 year. However, there was still a 14 percent difference, favoring CABG, in 1-year repeat revascularization rates. The diabetes subset from the ARTS revealed that multivessel stenting had a poorer 1-year major adverse cardiac event rate than did CABG (63.4 vs 84.4 percent, $p < 0.001$); the results were mainly driven by

TABLE 86-12 Coronary Revascularization

Trial	Treatment	Outcome	Events Control Group	Events Treatement Group	Relative Risk Reduction, %	Number Needed to Treat	p
BARI[237] Multivessel CAD $n = 1829^a$	CABG vs. PTCA	Mortality from all cause	PTCA 131/915 (14.3%)	CABG 111/914 (12.1%)	15.3	45	.19
Diabetics $n = 353$ CABG 180 PTCA 173	Same	Same	34.5%	19.4%	43.7	7	.003
EPISTENT[273] $n = 2399$ Diabetics[274] $n = 335$	Stent + abciximab versus Stent + placebo	Death and nonfatal MI at 6 months	Stent + placebo 22/173 (12.7%)	Stent + abciximab 10/162 (6.2%)	51.2	15	.041
$n = 318$	Stent + abciximab versus PTCA + abciximab	Same	PTCA + abciximab 12/156 (7.8%)	Stent + abciximab 10/162 (6.2%)	20.5	62	.13

^{a}n = total number of patients.
ABBREVIATIONS: CABG, coronary artery bypass graft; CAD = coronary artery disease; MI = myocardial infarction; PTCA = percutaneous transluminal coronary angioplasty.

the higher incidence of repeat revascularization after stenting than after CABG (8 percent repeat of CABG and 14.3 percent repeat of PCI, vs no repeat CABG and 3.1 percent repeat PCI, respectively).[279]

ARTS and other studies (the SOS trial),[280] which have indicated a benefit of CABG surgery versus PCI with stenting, have been limited by (1) the absence of an effective antirestenosis agent in conjunction with stent implantation, and (2) the absence of routine use of platelet glycoprotein IIb/IIIa inhibitors, which have been shown to reduce ischemic complications after angioplasty and stent procedures and to potentially reduce mortality after intracoronary stent implantation procedures in diabetic patients.

Restenosis Prevention

Treatments directed at reducing neointimal proliferation and/or geometric arterial remodeling after PCI procedures[281–285] should reduce the incidence of restenosis after balloon angioplasty and the need for repeat revascularization procedures. Since stent implantation eliminates the remodeling process,[286–288] the single target to prevent in-stent restenosis is prevention of neointimal hyperplasia.[289,290] After arterial injury, multiple mitogenic and proliferative factors have been identified as triggers leading to vascular smooth muscle cell (VSMC) activation.[291,292] The neointimal proliferation process is markedly exaggerated specifically in diabetic patients, as assessed by serial intravascular ultrasound imaging,[281,282,293] and diabetes mellitus has been identified as an independent predictor of recurrent in-stent restenosis.[264] In the past, pharmacologic therapies for the prevention of restenosis have been generally unsuccessful. While numerous animal studies have identified agents that can reduce intimal hyperplasia associated with balloon angioplasty or after stent implantation, clinical results using systemic agents or after local catheter administration have been disappointing.[291,292,294,295] A possible reason for the repeated failure is that agents given systemically or via local catheters cannot reach sufficient therapeutic levels at the injured site

within the artery to inhibit significantly the localized restenotic process without producing serious systemic side effects.

POTENTIAL USE OF DRUG-ELUTING STENTS

Sustained local delivery of an antiproliferative therapeutic agent will provide higher tissue concentrations than will systemic administration. The combination of mechanical scaffolding provided by stent implantation (to reverse arterial remodeling) with the sustained high-dose local drug delivery (via the stent) of an agent that effectively inhibits neointimal hyperplasia could provide a unique method to improve target lesion patency after PCI. This delicate balance incorporating a highly deliverable stent platform, a drug carrier vehicle (such as a nonreactive encapsulating polymer), and an effective antiproliferative agent has been achieved with the very effective clinical application of the Sirolimus drug-eluting stent.[296,297]

Multiple other drug-eluting stents have entered experimental animal or early clinical evaluations. Therapeutic agents currently undergoing assessment include paclitaxel and other taxane derivatives, actinomycin D, battimastat, tacrolimus, dexamethasone, and c-myc antisense. Drug delivery from the stent can be accomplished by a variety of means, including direct application, using either nonerodable or erodable polymers (which encapsulate the stent), phosphoryl-choline coatings, and ceramic coatings. Thus far, paclitaxel, delivered via direct application or eluted from a copolymer matrix, on three different stent platforms, has shown improved clinical outcomes and reduced restenosis in phase I or dose-ranging clinical studies.

Bypass Outcomes

CABG with use of an internal mammary artery (IMA) as a bypass conduit has been shown to be more advantageous to CABG with saphenous vein bypass conduits because of greater long-term durability of the arterial conduit.[298,299] The internal mammary artery has been shown to be significantly stenosed or occluded in approximately 8 percent of patients early after CABG surgery,[300] but has 90 to 95 percent long-term patency; sustained patency of the IMA conduit has also been shown to be associated with prolonged patient survival.[301,302] Bypass conduits attrition rates are higher in diabetic patients than they are in nondiabetic patients.[298] Bilateral IMA grafting has been shown to provide even further survival advantage than left IMA plus saphenous vein grafts; these data have led to an increased application of CABG with total arterial revascularization.[299,303] Nonetheless, the use of bilateral IMA grafting in diabetic patients remains controversial due to the potentially increased risk for sternal wound infection.[304,305,306]

Clinical Sirolimus Drug-Eluting Stent Studies: First In Man Experience

The First in Man (FIM) experience evaluated patients with stable or unstable angina undergoing single lesion treatment with the Sirolimus-eluting BX Velocity stent (Cordis, Inc., conducted in Brazil). The first 15 patients were treated with the fast-release formulation and the subsequent 30 patients were treated with the slow-release formulation Sirolimus-eluting stents. The combination of aspirin plus clopidogrel was given for 60 days after stent implantation.[296,297]

Quantitative coronary angiography evaluations at 4 to 6 months after stenting indicated no restenosis (>50 percent diameter stenosis at follow-up) and no evidence of intimal hyperplasia (0-mm late loss and 0 loss index). Intravascular ultrasound studies revealed an average percent lumen volume obstruction <3 percent for both fast- and slow-release formulations at 4 to 6 months follow-up. Extended follow-up at 2 years postprocedure is in progress. To date, there was no angiographic or intravascular ultrasound evidence of edge restenosis, late restenosis within the stent, aneurysm formation, or other abnormal pathologic findings. There were no episodes of target lesion revascularization in any of the FIM clinical cases. Importantly, rigorous assessment of patient safety revealed the following: (1) no

episodes of early- or late-stent thrombosis; (2) one patient with in-hospital intracranial hemorrhage and death (due to concomitant glycoprotein IIb/IIIa inhibitor therapy); (3) one patient with myocardial infarction 14 months after the stent procedure, due to disease progression in an area near the stent edge, as demonstrated by serial intravascular ultrasound imaging; and (4) one patient with late disease progression (left main segment) distant from the stent site detected at routine 2-year follow-up.

Intravascular ultrasound study results of the FIM experience were compared to the intravascular ultrasound study results of an earlier clinical trial using standard (bare) stainless steel, tubular slotted stents, indicating a tenfold reduction of in-stent and in-lesion neointimal tissue volume at follow-up with the use of a Sirolimus drug-eluting stent.[297,307]

Clinical Sirolimus-Eluting Stent Studies: First Double-Blind, Randomized Clinical Trial

The First Double-Blind, Randomized Clinical Trial (RAVEL) multicenter, prospective, double-blinded, randomized trial ($n = 238$ patients), performed in Europe and South America, involved single-lesion treatment with either bare stents or Sirolimus-eluting stents.[308] Six-month angiographic follow-up indicated no angiographic restenosis in the Sirolimus-eluting Bx Velocity arm versus 26 percent in the "bare" stent arm ($p < 0.0001$). Importantly, no acute, subacute or late stent thrombosis or edge restenosis events were reported. Major adverse cardiac events (MACE) at 7 months were also significantly reduced with use of the Sirolimus-eluting stents (Table 86-13). Importantly, subgroup analysis of the diabetic patients ($n = 42$) indicated no 6-month restenosis with the Sirolimus-eluting stent versus 42 percent with the bare stent ($p < 0.0001$), and similarly reduced 7-month MACE rates. Late lumen loss, an angiographic measure of neointimal hyperplasia, with the Sirolimus-eluting stent was <0.1 mm in both diabetic and nondiabetic patients (see Table 86-13).

Results from RAVEL clearly indicate that the Sirolimus-eluting stent (during single-vessel intervention) manifests striking angiographic efficacy in reducing restenosis and late lumen loss, with no important clinical safety concerns.

TABLE 86-13 The RAVEL Trial Results

	DIABETIC SUBSET		ALL PATIENTS	
	Sirolimus	Control	Sirolimus	Control
	$n = 19$	$n = 25$	$n = 120$	$n = 118$
Lesion length (mm)	9.74	9.42	9.56	9.61
Reference vessel diameter (mm)	2.52	2.55	2.60	2.64
Minimal lumen diameter, pre (mm)	0.99	0.93	0.94	0.95
Minimal lumen diameter, post (mm)	2.37	2.36	2.43	2.41
Minimal lumen diameter, follow-up (mm)	2.31*	1.56	2.42*	1.64
Late lumen loss (mm)	0.08*	0.82	−0.01 6 ± 0.33*	0.80 ± 0.53
Late loss index (late loss/acute gain)	0.05*	0.57	−0.02	0.57
Diameter stenosis at follow-up (%)	16*	38	15*	37
Binary restenosis rate at 6 months (%)	0*	42	0*	26
Major adverse cardiac events at 7 months (%)	0*	48	3.3*	27.1

Values are means or percentages;
* indicates $p < 0.0001$ versus control.
ABBREVIATIONS: RAVEL, first, double-blind, randomized clinical trial.

TABLE 86-14 SIRIUS Trial Results

	DIABETIC SUBGROUP* (N = 279)			ALL PATIENTS (N = 1078)		
	Sirolimus	Control	P Value	Sirolimus	Control	P Value
	(n = 131)	(n = 148)		(n = 553)	(n = 525)	
Mean late loss (mm) in-stent	0.29	1.20	< 0.001	0.17	1.00	< 0.001
In-stent restenosis	8.3%	48.5%	< 0.001	3.2%	35.4%	< 0.001
TLR	7.2%	22.3%	< 0.001	4.1%	16.6%	< 0.001
MACE	9.2%	25.0%	< 0.001	7.1%	18.9%	< 0.001

Lesion length = 14.5 mm and reference vessel size = 2.75 mm.
ABBREVIATIONS: TLR = target lesion revascularization; MACE = major adverse cardiac events; SIRIUS, Pivotal USA Randomized Clinical Trial.

Clinical Sirolimus Drug-Eluting Stent Studies: Pivotal USA Randomized Clinical Trial

The Pivotal USA Randomized Clinical Trial (SIRIUS) study compared the Sirolimus-eluting Bx Velocity stent versus the bare Bx Velocity stent in patients with stable or unstable angina involving lesions 15 to 30 mm in length and in vessels 2.5 to 3.5 mm in diameter.[309] The Sirolimus-eluting stents had the same Sirolimus dose and release formulation (slow-release) as used in RAVEL. Patients were treated with the combination of Aspirin plus Clopidogrel for 3 months after stent treatment. The primary endpoint is "target vessel failure" at 9 months (procedural success and the absence of MACE), and there are extensive angiographic and intravascular ultrasound study follow-up substudies to examine critically comparative late anatomic responses. Patient demographics in SIRIUS include 27 percent diabetic patients.

Significantly, although SIRIUS still includes only single-vessel treatment, the lesion morphology favors more diffuse disease in smaller vessels necessitating treatment with longer or multiple stents, a commonly observed anatomic subset in diabetic patients.

Table 86-14 summarizes the impressive findings in the diabetic subgroup, which were presented at the TCT 2002 Annual Meeting.

CONGESTIVE HEART FAILURE

Diabetic cardiomyopathy is a term used by clinicians that encompasses the multifactorial etiologies of diabetes-related left ventricular failure characterized by both systolic and diastolic function. The Framingham Heart Study showed that men with diabetes who have congestive heart failure were twice as common as their nondiabetic counterpart and that females with diabetes had a fivefold increase in the rate of congestive heart failure.[310] The spectrum of heart failure ranges from asymptomatic to overt systolic failure. Diabetes complicated by hypertension represents a particularly high-risk group for the development of congestive heart failure.[311,312] Diastolic dysfunction is exceedingly common (>50 percent prevalence in some studies) and may be linked to diabetes without the presence of concomitant hypertension.[313–316]

The etiology of impaired left ventricular function may involve any of the following mechanisms: (1) coronary atherosclerotic disease, (2) hypertension, (3) left ventricular hypertrophy, (4) obesity, (5) endothelial dysfunction, (6) coronary microvasculature disease, (7) autonomic dysfunction, and (8) metabolic abnormalities.

The diabetes and cardiovascular communities have embraced the concept of diabetic cardiomyopathy as a distinct entity independent of ischemic heart disease and hypertension. This was first described in the early 1970s when autopy specimens of diabetic patients with nephropathy demonstrated a myopathic process in the absence of epicardial CAD.[317]

Echocardiographic studies have confirmed that diastolic abnormalities occur in young diabetic patients who have no known diabetic complications. Diabetic patients who are hypertensive have increased left ventricular mass when compared to their nondiabetic counterparts and left ventricular function may in fact be hyperdynamic.[318] An Australian group has now confirmed that diabetic patients demonstrate early findings of systolic dysfunction preceding any change in the left ventricular ejection fraction.[319] The management of heart failure with preserved left ventricular systolic function usually includes beta blockers and ACE inhibitors, but evidence for this is sparse.

Once CAD develops in the diabetic patient, the left ventricular systolic dysfunction that ensues responds to all the same therapies as in the nondiabetic population. The findings of the HOPE trial suggest that early initiation of ACE inhibition retards the progression to overt CHF.

FUTURE DIRECTIONS

On the clinical front, there are still many challenges in the prevention and management of diabetic cardiovascular complications. Given the findings of the HOPE trial, the potential for an expanded role for ACE inhibitors in the prevention of cardiovascular and renal disease in all diabetic patients needs to be explored. Glycemic control appears to be the mainstay of long-term diabetes management (Table 86-15). Thus, development of better therapies and devices (e.g., closed-loop pumps, islet and pancreatic transplants) for achieving and maintaining Hb A_{1c} at not only <7 percent but in the normal range of <6 percent will be a primary goal in the next decade. Clarification of the best glycemic control strategy in preventing CHD is required in order to validate the hypothesis that an insulin sensitization strategy may be more cardioprotective. The advent of drug-eluting-stents during coronary percutaneous revascularization has led to a reevaluation of the need for coronary bypass surgery in multivessel disease. Confirmation of the results of small trials demonstrating a benefit of intravenous glucose-insulin infusion during acute myocardial infarction is needed before this therapy can be adopted. Finally, the role of gene therapy in the management of diabetic atherosclerotic vascular disease needs to be addressed within the context of all other advances.

TABLE 86-15 Guide to Comprehensive Risk Reduction for Patients with Coronary and Other Vascular Disease Who Have Diabetes

Risk intervention	Recommendations
Smoking Goal: complete cessation	Urge smoking cessation Try nicoderm patches or xyban; enroll in smoking cessation program
Blood pressure control Goal: <135/85 mmHg	Initiate lifestyle modification; weight reduction, increased physical activity; alcohol moderation; sodium restriction in all patients with blood pressure >135/85 Add BP medication if BP not below above goal
Lipid management Primary goal: LDL ≤100 mg/dL	Start AHA Step II Diet in all patients: ≤30% fat, <7% saturated fat, <200 mg/dL cholesterol Assess fasting lipid profile. Immediately start cholesterol-lowering drugs when baseline LDL > 130 mg/gL

Secondary goals: HDL>35 mg/DL TG<200 mg/dL	LDL<100 mg/dL No drug therapy	LDL 100–129 mg/dL Consider adding drug therapy to diet as follows		LDL≥130 mg/dL Add drug therapy as follows	HDL<35 mg/dL Weight management, physical activity, and smoking cessation
		↘ Suggested drug therapy ↙			
		TG<200 mg/dL	TG 200–400 mg/dL	TG>400 mg/dL	
		Statin or resin	Statin or fibrate	Consider combined drug therapy (statin + fibrate)	

Risk intervention	Recommendations
Glucose control Goal: nearly normal fasting glucose Goal: Hb-A 1c ≤1% above normal	First-step therapy: lifestyle modifications Second-step therapy: oral hypoglycemic agents (see algorithm) Third-step therapy: insulin therapy (see algorithm)
Physical activity Goal: minimum 30 minutes, 3–4 times a week	Assess risk, preferably with exercise test, to guide prescription Encourage minimum of 30–60 min of moderate-intensity activity 3–4 times weekly (walking, jogging, cycling, etc.) supplemented by an increase in daily lifestyle activities (e.g., walking breaks at work, using stairs, household work) Maximum benefit 5 to 6 h a week Advise medically supervised programs for moderate- to high-risk patients
Weight management	Start intensive dietary therapy and appropriate physical activity, as outlined above, in patients whose BMI is ≥25 kg/m^2 Particularly emphasize need for weight loss in patients with hypertension, elevated triglycerides, or elevated glucose levels
Antiplatelet agents/ anticoagulants	Start aspirin 325 mg/day if not contraindicated Manage warfarin to INR of 2–3.5 for post-MI patients not able to take aspirin
ACE inhibitors in post-MI patients	Start early post-MI in stable high-risk patients [anterior MI, previous MI, Killip class II (S$_3$ gallop, rales, radiographic congestive heart failure)] Continue indefinitely for all with LV dysfunction (ejection fraction ≤40%) or symptoms of failure Use as needed to manage blood pressure or symptoms in all other patients
Beta blockers	Start in high-risk post-MI patients (arrhythmia, LV dysfunction, inducible ischemia) at 5 to 28 days; continue 6 months minimum; observe usual contraindications; appropriate use of beta-blockers not contraindicated in patients with diabetes; use as needed to manage angina, rhythm, or blood pressure in all other patients
Estrogen	Observational studies (but not clinical trials) suggest benefit in regard to osteoporosis but not CAD, individualize recommendation consistent with other health risks

ABBREVIATIONS: AHA = American Heart Association; BP = blood pressure; CAD = coronary heart disease; HDL = high-density lipoproteins; INR = international normalized ratio; LDL = low-density lipoprotein; LV = left-ventricle; MI = myocardial infarction; TG = triglycerides.

References

1. Schwartz CJ, Valente AJ, Sprague EA, et al. Pathogenesis of the ather-osclerotic lesion: Implications for diabetes mellitus. *Diabetes Care* 1992;15:1156–1167.

2. Stamler J, Vaccaro O, Neaton JD, Wentworth D. Diabetes, other risk factors and 12-year cardiovascular mortality for men screened in the multiple risk factor intervention trial. *Diabetes Care* 1993;16: 434–444.

3. Gu K, Cowie CC, Harris MI. Diabetes and decline in heart disease mortality in US adults. *JAMA* 1999;281:1291–1297.

4. Kawate R, Yamakido M, Nishimoto Y, et al. Diabetes mellitus and its vascular complications in Japanese migrants on the island of Hawaii. *Diabetes Care* 1979;2:161–170.

5. Head J, Fuller JH. International variations in mortality among diabetic patients: The WHO Multinational Study of Vascular Disease in Diabetics. *Diabetologia* 1990;33:447–481.

6. Vigorita VJ, Morre GW, Hutchens GM. Absence of correlation between coronary arterial atherosclerosis and severity or duration of diabetes mellitus of adult onset. *Am J Cardiol* 1980;46:535–542.

7. Waller BF, Palumbo PJ, Lie JT, Roberts WC. Status of the coronary arteries at necropsy in diabetes mellitus after age 30 years: Analysis of 229 diabetic patients with and without evidence of coronary heart disease and comparison to 183 control subjects. *Am J Med* 1980;69: 498–506.

8. Granger CB, Califf RM, Young S, et al. Outcome of patients with diabetes mellitus and acute myocardial infarction treated with thrombolytic agents: The Thrombolysis and Angioplasty in Myocardial Infarction (TAMI) Study Group. *J Am Coll Cardiol* 1993;21:920–925.

9. Mueller HS, Cohen LS, Braunwald E, et al., for the TIMI investigators. Predictors of early mortality and morbidity after thrombolytic therapy of acute myocardial infarction. *Circulation* 1992;85:1254–1264.

10. Stein B, Weintraub WS, Gebhart SSP, et al. Influence of diabetes mellitus on early and late outcome after percutaneous transluminal coronary angioplasty. *Circulation* 1995;91:979–989.

11. Barzilay JI, Kronmal RA, Bittner V, et al. Coronary artery disease and coronary artery bypass grafting in diabetic patients aged >65 years (Report from the coronary artery surgery study [CASS] registry). *Am J Cardiol* 1994;74:334–339.

12. Davis M, Bland J, Hangartner J, et al. Factors influencing the presence or absence of acute coronary artery thrombi in sudden ischemic death. *Eur Heart J* 1989;10:203–208.

13. Silva JA, Escobar A, Collins TJ, et al. Unstable angina: A comparison between diabetic and non-diabetic patients. *Circulation* 1995;92: 1731–1736.

14. Hopkins PN, Hunt SC, Wu LL, et al. Hypertension, dyslipidemia, and insulin resistance: Links in a chain or spokes on a wheel? *Curr Opin Lipidol* 1996;7:241–253.

15. Gray RS, Fabsitz RR, Cowan LD, et al. Risk factor clustering in the insulin resistance syndrome: The Strong Heart Study. *Am J Epidemiol* 1998;148:869–878.

16. The Expert Committee on the Diagnosis and Classification of Diabetes Mellitus. Report of the Expert Committee on the Diagnosis and Classification of Diabetes Mellitus. *Diabetes Care* 1997;20:1183–1202.

17. Haffner SM, Stern MP, Hazuda HP, et al. Cardiovascular risk factors in confirmed prediabetic individuals: Does the clock for coronary heart disease start ticking before the onset of clinical diabetes? *JAMA* 1990;263:2893–2898.

18. Unger RH, Foster DW. Diabetes mellitus. In: Wilson JD, Foster DW, Kronenberg HM, Larsen PR, eds. *Williams Textbook of Endocrinology.* Philadelphia: Saunders;1998:973.

19. Stamler J, Vaccaro O, Neaton JD, Wentworth D. Diabetes, other risk factors, and 12-year cardiovascular mortality for men screened in the Multiple Risk Factor Intervention Trial (MRFIT). *Diabetes Care* 1993;16:434–444.

20. Folsom AR, Eckfeldt JH, Weitzman S, et al. Atherosclerosis Risk in Communities Study Investigators. Relation of carotid artery wall thickness in diabetes mellitus, fasting glucose and insulin, body size and physical activity. *Stroke* 1994;25:66–73.

21. O'Leary DH, Polak JF, Kronmal RA, et al. Distribution and correlates of sonographically detected carotid artery disease in the Cardiovascular Health Study. *Stroke* 1992;23:1752–1760.

22. Cooper ME. Pathogenesis, prevention, and treatment of diabetic nephropathy. *Lancet* 1998;352:213–219.

23. Chavers BM, Bilous RW, Ellis EN, et al. Glomerular lesions and urinary albumin excretion in type I diabetes without overt proteinuria. *N Engl J Med* 1989;320:966–970.

24. Ismail N, Becker B, Strzelczyk P, Ritz E. Renal disease and hypertension in non-insulin-dependent diabetes mellitus. *Kidney Int* 1999;55:1–28.

25. Lebovitz HE, Wiegmann TB, Cnaan A, et al. Renal protective effects of enalapril in hypertensive NIDDM: Role of baseline albuminuria. *Kidney Int* 1994;45:S150–S155.

26. Lewis EJ, Hunsicker LG, Bain RP, Rohde RD. The effect of angiotensin-converting-enzyme inhibition on diabetic nephropathy: The Collaborative Study Group. *N Engl J Med* 1993;329:1456–1462.

27. Grundy SM, Benjamin IJ, Burke GL, et al. Diabetes and cardiovascular disease: A statement for healthcare professionals from the American Heart Association. *Circulation* 1999;100:1134–1146.

28. Rose BD. Treatment of diabetic nephropathy. Up to Date Computer CD, Feb. 24, 1999.

29. Viberti G, Mogensen CE, Groop LC, Pauls JF. Effect of captopril on progression to clinical proteinuria in patients with insulin-dependent diabetes mellitus and microalbuminuria: European Microalbuminuria Captopril Study Group. *JAMA* 1994;271:275–279.

30. The Microalbuminuria Captopril Study Group. Captopril reduces the risk of nephropathy in IDDM patients with microalbuminuria. *Diabetologia* 1996;39:587–593.

31. Ravid M, Savin H, Jutrin I, et al. Long-term stabilizing effect of angiotensin-converting enzyme inhibition on plasma creatinine and on proteinuria in normotensive type II diabetic patients. *Ann Intern Med* 1993;118:577–581.

32. Golan L, Birkmeyer JD, Welch HG. The cost-effectiveness of treating all patients with type 2 diabetes with angiotensin-converting enzyme inhibitors. *Ann Intern Med* 1999;131:660–667.

33. Gaber L, Walton C, Brown S, Bakris G. Effects of different antihypertensive treatments on morphologic progression of diabetic nephropathy in uninephrectomized dogs. *Kidney Int* 1994;46:161–169.

34. Ritz E, Stefanski A. Diabetic nephropathy in type II diabetes. *Am J Kidney Dis* 1996;27:167–194.

35. Berkman J, Rifkin H. Unilateral nodular diabetic glomerulosclerosis (Kimmelstiel-Wilson): Report of a case. *Metabolism* 1973;22:715–722.

36. Austin SM, Lieberman JS, Newton LD, et al. Slope of serial glomerular filtration rate and the progression of diabetic glomerular disease. *J Am Soc Nephrol* 1993;3:1358–1370.

37. Bohlen L, de Courten M, Weidmann P. Comparative study of the effect of ACE-inhibitors and other antihypertensive agents on proteinuria in diabetic patients. *Am J Hypertens* 1994;7:84S–92S.

38. Tatti P, Pahor M, Byington RP, et al. Outcome results of the Fosinopril versus Amlodipine Cardiovascular Events Randomized Trial (FACET) in patients with hypertension and NIDDM. *Diabetes Care* 1998;21: 597–603.

39. Brenner BM, Cooper ME, de Zeeuw D, et al. Effects of losartan on renal and cardiovascular outcomes in patients with type 2 diabetes and nephropathy. *N Engl J Med* 2001;345:861–869.

40. Lewis EJ, Hunsicker LG, Clarke WR, et al. Renoprotective effect of the angiotensin-receptor antagonist irbesartan in patients with nephropathy due to type 2 diabetes. *N Engl J Med* 2001;345: 870–878.

41. Feit F, Brooks MM, Sopko G, et al. Long-term clinical outcome in the Bypass Angioplasty Revascularization Investigation Registry: Comparison with the randomized trial. BARI Investigators. *Circulation* 2000;101:2795-2802.

42. Grundy SM, Howard B, Smith S Jr, et al. Prevention conference VI: diabetes and cardiovascular disease executive summary. *Circulation* 2002;105: 2231–2239.

43. Kannel W, McGee D. Diabetes and glucose tolerance as risk factors for cardiovascular disease: The Framingham Study. *Diabetes Care* 1979;2:120–126.

44. Jarrett RJ, Shipley MJ. Type 2 (non-insulin dependent) diabetes mellitus and cardiovascular disease μ putative association via common antecedents: Further evidence from the Whitehall Study. *Diabetologia* 1988;31:737–740.

45. Jarrett RJ, McCarthney P, Keen H. The Bedford Study: Ten-year mortality rates in newly diagnosed diabetics, borderline diabetics and normoglycemic controls and the risk indices for coronary heart disease in borderline diabetics. *Diabetologia* 1982;22:79–84.

46. Fontbonne A, Eschwege E, Cambien F, et al. Hypertriglyceridemia as a risk factor for coronary heart disease mortality in subjects with impaired glucose tolerance or diabetes: Results from the 11-year follow-up of the Paris Prospective Study. *Diabetologia* 1989;32:300–304.

47. Donahue RP, Orchard TG. Diabetes mellitus and macrovascular complications: An epidemiological perspective. *Diabetes Care* 1992; 15:1141–1155.

48. Barrett-Connor E, Cohn B, Wingard D, Edelstein SL. Why is diabetes mellitus a stronger risk factor for fatal ischemic heart disease in women than in men? The Rancho Bernardo Study. *JAMA* 1991;256: 627–631.

49. Barrett-Connor E, Wingard DL. Sex differential in ischemic heart disease mortality in diabetics: A prospective population-based study. *Am J Epidemiol* 1983;118:489–496.

50. Nathan DM. Long-term complications of diabetes mellitus. *N Engl J Med* 1993;328:1676–1685.

51. Fuller JH, Shipley MJ, Rose G, et al. Coronary heart disease and impaired glucose tolerance: The Whitehall Study. *Lancet* 1980;1: 1373–1376.

52. American Diabetes Association. Consensus statement: Role of cardiovascular risk factors in prevention and treatment of macrovascular disease in diabetes. *Diabetes Care* 1993;16:72–78.

53. Yamasaki Y, Kawamori R, Matsushima H, et al. Asymptomatic hyperglycemia is associated with increased intimal plus medial thickness of the carotid artery. *Diabetologia* 1995;38:585–591.

54. Crub JD, Rodriguez BL, Burchfiel CM, et al. Sudden death, impaired glucose tolerance and diabetes in Japanese American men. *Circulation* 1995;91:2591–2595.

55. Kahn CR. Insulin action, diabetogenes and the cause of type II diabetes. *Diabetes* 1994;43:1066–1084.

56. Ferrannini E, Buzzigoli G, Bonadonna R, et al. Insulin resistance in essential hypertension. *N Engl J Med* 1987;317:350–357.

57. Zavaroni I, Bonora E, Pagliara M, et al. Risk factors for coronary artery disease in healthy persons with hyperinsulinemia and normal glucose tolerance. *N Engl J Med* 1989;320:702–706.

58. Larsson B, Savardsudd K, Welin L, et al. Abdominal adipose tissue distribution, obesity and risk of cardiovascular disease and death: 13-year follow-up of participants in the study of men born in 1913. *Br Med J* 1984;288:1401–1404.

59. Peiris AN, Sothmann MS, Hoffman RG, et al. Adiposity, fat distribution and cardiovascular risk. *Ann Intern Med* 1989;110:867–872.

60. Laakso M, Barrett-Connor E. Asymptomatic hyperglycemia is associated with lipid and lipoprotein changes favoring atherosclerosis. *Atherosclerosis* 1989;9:665–672.

61. Modan M, Halkin H, Luskyn A, et al. Hyperinsulinemia is characterized by jointly disturbed plasma VLDL, LDL, and HDL levels. *Arteriosclerosis* 1988;8:227–236.

62. Laws A, King AC, Haskell WL, Reaven GM. Relation of fasting plasma insulin concentrations to high-density lipoprotein cholesterol and triglyceride concentration in men. *Arterioscler Thromb* 1991;11: 1636–1642.

63. Reaven GM. Role of insulin resistance in human disease (syndrome X): An expanded definition. *Annu Rev Med* 1993;44:121–131.

64. Reaven GM, Laws A. Insulin resistance, compensatory hyperinsulinemia and coronary heart disease. *Diabetologia* 1994;37:948–952.

65. Fontbonne A, Charles MA, Thibult N, et al. Hyperinsulinemia as a predictor of coronary heart disease mortality in a healthy population: The Paris Prospective Study, 15-year follow-up. *Diabetologia* 1991; 34:356–361.

66. Pyorala K, Savolainen E, Kaukola S, Haapakoski J. Plasma insulin as coronary heart disease risk factor: Relationship to other risk factors and predictive value over 9.5 year follow-up of the Helsinki Policeman Study population. *Acta Med Scand* 1985;701(suppl):38–52.

67. Despres J-P, Lamarche B, Mauriege P, et al. Hyperinsulinemia is an independent risk factor for ischemic heart disease. *N Engl J Med* 1996; 334:952–957.

68. Modan M, Or J, Karasik A, et al. Hyperinsulinemia, sex and risk of atherosclerotic cardiovascular disease. *Circulation* 1991;84:1165–1175.

69. Liu QZ, Knowler WC, Nelson RG, et al. Insulin treatment, endogenous insulin concentration and ECG abnormalities in diabetic Pima Indians: Cross sectional and prospective analysis. *Diabetes* 1992;41:1141–1150.

70. Ferrara A, Barrett-Connor E, Edelstein SL. Hyperinsulinemia does not increase the risk of fatal cardiovascular disease in elderly men and women without diabetes: The Rancho Bernardo Study, 1984 to 1991. *Am J Epidemiol* 1994;140:857–869.

71. Gerstein HC, Yusuf S. Dysglycemia and risk of cardiovascular disease. *Lancet* 1996;347:949–950.

72. Singer DE, Nathan DM, Anderson KM, et al. Association of HbA1c with prevalent cardiovascular disease in the original cohort of the Framingham Heart Study. *Diabetes* 1992;41:202–208.

73. Kuusisto J, Makkanen L, Pyorala K, Laakso M. NIDDM and its metabolic control predicts coronary heart disease in elderly subjects. *Diabetes* 1994;43:960–967.

74. Uusitupa MI, Niskanen LK, Siitonen O, et al. Ten-year cardiovascular mortality in relation to risk factors and abnormalities in lipoprotein composition in type 2 (non-insulin-dependent) diabetic and nondiabetic subjects. *Diabetologia* 1993;36:1175–1184.

75. Krolewski AS, Kosinki EJ, Warram JH, et al. Magnitude and determinants of coronary artery disease in juvenile-onset, insulin-dependent diabetes mellitus. *Am J Cardiol* 1987;59:750–755.

76. Borch-Johnsen K, Kreiner S. Proteinuria: Value as predictor of cardiovascular mortality in insulin-dependent diabetes mellitus. *Br Med J* 1987;294:1651–1654.

77. Bucala R, Mitchell R, Arnold K, et al. Identification of the major site of apolipoprotein B modification by advanced glycosylation end products blocking uptake by the low density lipoprotein receptor. *J Biol Chem* 1995;270:10828–10832.

78. Bucala R, Makita Z, Koschinsky T, et al. Lipid advanced glycosylation: Pathway for lipid oxidation in vivo. *Proc Natl Acad Sci USA* 1993;90:6434–6438.

79. Bucala R, Makita Z, Vega G, et al. Modification of low-density lipoprotein by advanced glycosylation end products contributes to the dyslipidemia of diabetes and renal insufficiency. *Proc Natl Acad Sci USA* 1994;91:9441–9445.

80. Steinbrecher UP, Witztum JL. Glycosylation of low density lipoproteins to an extent comparable to that seen in diabetics slows their catabolism. *Diabetes* 1984;33:130–134.

81. Lyons TJ. Glycation and oxidation: A role in the pathogenesis of atherosclerosis. *Am J Cardiol* 1993;71:26B–31B.

82. Sobenin IA, Tertov VV, Koschinsky T, et al. Modified low-density lipoprotein from diabetic patients causes cholesterol accumulation in human intimal aortic cells. *Atherosclerosis* 1993;100:41–54.

83. Lyons TJ, Klein R, Baynes JW, et al. Stimulation of cholesterol-ester synthesis in human monocyte-derived macrophages by low-density lipoproteins from type I (insulin-dependent) diabetic patients: The influence of nonenzymatic glycosylation of low-density lipoprotein. *Diabetologia* 1987;30:916–923.

84. Klein RL, Laimins M, Lopes-Varella MF. Isolation, characterization and metabolism of the glycated and nonglycated subfractions of low-density lipoproteins isolated from type I diabetic patients and nondiabetic subjects. *Diabetes* 1995;44:1093–1098.

85. Fiengold KR, Grunfeld C, Pang M, et al. LDL subclass phenotype and triglyceride metabolism in non-insulin-dependent diabetes. *Arterioscler Throm* 1992;12:1496–1502.

86. Stewart MW, Laker MF, Dyer RG, et al. Lipoprotein compositional abnormalities and insulin resistance in type II diabetic patients with mild hyperlipidemia. *Arterioscler Throm* 1993;13:1046–1052.

87. Austin MA, Mykkanen L, Kuusisto J, et al. Prospective study of small LDLs as a risk factor for non-insulin-dependent diabetes mellitus in elderly men and women. *Circulation* 1995;92:1770–1778.

88. Howard BV, Abbott WF, Beltz WF, et al. The effect of non-insulin-dependent diabetes on very low density lipoprotein and low density lipoprotein metabolism in men. *Metabolism* 1987;36:870–877.

89. Packard CJ, Munro A, Lorimer AR, et al. Metabolism of apolipoprotein B in large triglyceride-rich very low density lipoproteins of normal and hypertriglyceridemic subjects. *J Clin Invest* 1984;84:2178–2192.

90. Austin MA, King MC, Vranizan KM, Krauss RM. Atherogenic lipoprotein phenotype: A proposed genetic marker for coronary heart disease risk. *Circulation* 1990;82:495–506.

91. West KM, Ahuja MMS, Bennett PH, et al. The role of circulation glucose and triglyceride concentration and their interaction with other "risk factors" as determinants of arterial disease in nine diabetic population samples from the WHO multinational study. *Diabetes Care* 1983;6:361–369.

92. Goldschmid MG, Barrett-Connor E, Edelstein SL, et al. Dyslipidemia and ischemic heart disease mortality among men and women with diabetes. *Circulation* 1994;89:991–997.

93. Laasko M, Lehto S, Penttila I, Pyorala K. Lipids and lipoproteins predicting coronary heart disease mortality and morbidity in patients with non-insulin-dependent diabetes. *Circulation* 1993;88:1421–1430.

94. Ginsberg HN. Diabetic dyslipidemia: Basic mechanisms underlying the common hypertriglyceridemia and low HDL cholesterol levels. *Diabetes* 1996;45(suppl):27S–30S.

95. Patsch JR, Prasad S, Gotto AM, et al. High density lipoprotein 2: Relationship of the plasma levels of this lipoprotein species to its composition, to the magnitude of postprandial lipemia, and to the activities of lipoprotein lipase and hepatic lipase. *J Clin Invest* 1984;80:341–347.

96. American Diabetes Association. Consensus statement: Detection and management of lipid disorders in diabetes. *Diabetes Care* 1993;16:828–839.

97. Expert Panel on Detection, Evaluation and Treatment of High Blood Cholesterol in Adults. Executive Summary of the Third Report of the National Cholesterol Education Program (NCEP) Expert Panel on Detection, Evaluation, and Treatment of High Blood Cholesterol in Adults (Adult Treatment Panel III) *JAMA* 2001 285: 2486-2497.

98. Vinik AI, Colwell JA. Effects of gemfibrozil on triglyceride levels in patients with NIDDM. *Diabetes Care* 1993;16:37–44.

99. Vega GL, Grundy SM. Gemfibrozil therapy in primary hypertriglyceridemia associated with coronary heart disease: Effect on metabolism of low-density lipoproteins. *JAMA* 1985;253:2398–2403.

100. Koskinen P, Manttrai M, Manninen V, et al. Coronary heart disease incidence in NIDDM patients in the Helsinki Heart Study. *Diabetes Care* 1992;15:820–825.

101. Lahdenpera S, Tilly-Kiesi M, Vuorinen-Markkola H, et al. Effects of gemfibrozil on low-density lipoprotein size, density distribution and composition in patients with type II diabetes. *Diabetes Care* 1993;16:584–592.

102. Garg A, Grundy SM. Nicotinic acid as therapy for dyslipidemia in non-insulin-dependent diabetes mellitus. *JAMA* 1990;264:723–726.

103. Garg A, Grundy SM. Lovastatin for lowering cholesterol levels in non-insulin dependent diabetes mellitus. *N Engl J Med* 1988;318:81–86.

104. Scandinavian Simvastatin Survival Study Group. Randomized trial of cholesterol lowering in 4444 patients with coronary heart disease: Scandinavian Simvastatin Survival Study (4S). *Lancet* 1994;344:1383–1389.

105. Garg A, Grundy SM. Cholestyramine therapy for dyslipidemia in non-insulin-dependent diabetes mellitus. *Ann Intern Med* 1994;121:416–422.

106. Hope investigators. Effects of an angiotensin converting enzyme inhibitor, ramipril, on cardiovascular events in high-risk patients. *N Engl J Med* 2000;342:145–153.

107. Winocour PD. Platelet abnormalities in diabetes mellitus. *Diabetes* 1992;41(suppl 2):26–31.

108. Tschoepe D, Rosen P, Schwippert B, Gries FA. Platelets in diabetes: The role of the hemostatic regulation in atherosclerosis. *Semin Thromb Hemost* 1993;19:122–128.

109. Breddin H, Krzywanek H, Althoff P, et al. Platelet aggregation as a risk factor in diabetes. *Horm Metab Res Suppl* 1985;15:63–68.

110. Winocour PD. Platelet abnormalities in diabetes mellitus. *Diabetes* 1992;41(suppl 2):26–31.

111. Winocour PD. Platelet turnover in advanced diabetes. *Eur J Clin Invest* 1994;24(suppl 1):34–37.

112. Janero DR. Malondialdehyde and thiobarbituric acid-reactivity as diagnostic indices of lipid peroxidation and peroxidative tissue injury. *Free Radic Biol Med* 1990;9:515–540.

113. Davi G, Catalano I, Averna M, et al. Thromboxane biosynthesis and platelet function in type II diabetes mellitus. *N Engl J Med* 1990;322:1769–1774.

114. Stehouwer CDA, Nauta JJP, Zeldenrust GC, et al. Urinary albumin excretion, cardiovascular disease and endothelial dysfunction in non-insulin-dependent diabetes mellitus. *Lancet* 1992;340:319–323.

115. Stehouwer CDA, Donker AJM. Urinary albumin excretion and cardiovascular disease in diabetes mellitus: Is endothelial dysfunction the missing link? *J Nephrol* 1993;6:72–92.

116. Conlan MG, Folsom AR, Finch A, et al. Associations of factor VII and von-Willebrand factor with age, race, sex and risk factors for atherosclerosis: The atherosclerosis in communities (ARIC) study. *Thromb Haemost* 1993;70:380–385.

117. Ganda OP, Arkin CF. Hyperfibrinogenemia: An important risk factor for vascular complications in diabetes. *Diabetes Care* 1992;15:1245–1250.

118. Kannel WB, D'Agostino RB, Wilson RB, et al. Diabetes, fibrinogen and risk of cardiovascular disease: The Framingham experience. *Am Heart J* 1990;120:672–676.

119. De Feo P, Gaisano GM, Haymond MW. Differential effects of insulin deficiency on albumin and fibrinogen synthesis in humans. *J Clin Invest* 1991;88:833–840.

120. Garcia Frade LJ, de la Calle H, Alava I, et al. Diabetes mellitus as a hypercoagulable state: Its relationship with fibrin fragments and vascular damage. *Thromb Res* 1987;47:533–540.

121. Landgraf-Leurs MM, Ladik T, Smolka B, et al. Increased thromboplastic potential in diabetes: A multifactorial phenomenon. *Klin Wochenschr* 1987;65:600–606.

122. Ceriello A. Coagulation activation in diabetes mellitus: The role of hyperglycaemia and therapeutic prospects. *Diabetologia* 1993;36:1119–1125.

123. Husted SE, Nielsen HK, Bak JF, Beck-Nielsen H. Antithrombin III activity, von Willebrand factor antigen and platelet function in young diabetic patients treated with multiple insulin injections versus insulin pump treatment. *Eur J Clin Invest* 1989;19:90–94.

124. Hamsten A, de Faire U, Walldius G, et al. Plasminogen activator inhibitor in plasma: Risk factor for recurrent myocardial infarction. *Lancet* 1987;2:3–9.

125. Mussoni L, Mannucci L, Sirtori M, et al. Hypertriglyceridemia and regulation of fibrinolytic activity. *Arterioscler Thromb* 1992;12:19–27.

126. Mehta J, Mehta P, Lawson D, Saldeen T. Plasma tissue plasminogen activator inhibitor levels in coronary artery disease: Correlation with age and serum triglyceride concentrations. *J Am Coll Cardiol* 1987;9:263–268.

127. Grant PJ, Kruithof EK, Felley CP, et al. Short-term infusions of insulin, triacylglycerol and glucose do not cause acute increases in plasminogen activator inhibitor-1 concentrations in man. *Clin Sci* 1990;79:513–516.

128. Richardson M, Hadcock SJ, DeReske M, Cybulsky MI. Increased expression in vivo of VCAM-1 and E-selectin by the aortic endothelium of normolipemic and hyperlipemic diabetic rabbits. *Arterioscler Thromb* 1994;14:760–769.

129. Yan SD, Schmidt AM, Anderson GM, et al. Enhanced cellular oxidant stress by the interaction of advanced glycation end products with their receptors/binding proteins. *J Biol Chem* 1994;269:9889–9897.

130. Wautier JL, Wautier MP, Schmidt AM, et al. Advanced glycation end products (AGEs) on the surface of diabetic erythrocytes bind to the vessel wall via a specific receptor inducing oxidant stress in the vasculature: A link between surface-associated AGEs and diabetic complications. *Proc Natl Acad Sci USA* 1994;91:7742–7746.

131. Schmidt AM, Hori O, Chen JX, et al. Advanced glycation end products interacting with their endothelial receptor induce expression of vascu-

lar cell adhesion molecule-1 (VCAM-1) in cultured human endothelial cells and in mice. A potential mechanism for the accelerated vasculopathy of diabetes. *J Clin Invest* 1995;96:1395–1403.

132. Keegan A, Walbank H, Cotter MA, Cameron NE. Chronic vitamin E treatment prevents defective endothelium-dependent relaxation in diabetic rat aorta. *Diabetologia* 1995;38:1475–1478.

133. Ting HH, Timimi FK, Boles KS, et al. Vitamin C improves endothelium-dependent vasodilation in patients with non-insulin-dependent diabetes mellitus. *J Clin Invest* 1996;97:22–28.

134. Hunt JV, Dean RT, Wolff SP. Hydroxyl radical production and autoxidative glycosylation: Glucose autoxidation as the cause of protein damage in the experimental glycation model of diabetes mellitus and ageing. *Biochem J* 1988;256:205–212.

135. Hunt JV, Smith CC, Wolff SP. Autoxidative glycosylation and possible involvement of peroxides and free radicals in LDL modification by glucose. *Diabetes* 1990;39:1420–1424.

136. Mullarkey CJ, Edelstein D, Brownlee M. Free radical generation by early glycation products: A mechanism for accelerated atherogenesis in diabetes. *Biochem Biophys Res Commun* 1990;173:932–939.

137. Bucala R, Tracey KJ, Cerami A. Advanced glycosylation products quench nitric oxide and mediate defective endothelium-dependent vasodilation in experimental diabetes. *J Clin Invest* 1991;87:432–438.

138. Vehkavaara S, Seppala-Lindroos A, Westerbacka J, et al. In vivo endothelial dysfunction characterizes patients with impaired fasting glucose. *Diabetes Care* 1999;22:2055–2060.

139. Vlassara H. Advanced glycation end-products and atherosclerosis. *Ann Med* 1996;28:419–426.

140. Stitt AW, Bucala R, Vlassara H. Atherogenesis and advanced glycation: Promotion, progression and prevention. *Ann NY Acad Sci* 1997; 811:115–129.

141. Brownlee M, Cerami A, Vlassara H. Advanced glycation end-products in tissue and the biochemical basis of diabetic complications. *N Engl J Med* 1988;318:1315–1321.

142. Aronson D, Rayfield EJ. Diabetes. In: Topol E, ed. *Textbook of Cardiovascular Medicine*. Philadelphia: Lippincott-Raven;1998:171.

143. Nakamura Y, Horii Y, Nishino T, et al. Immunohistochemical localization of advanced glycosylation end products in coronary atheroma and cardiac tissue in diabetes mellitus. *Am J Pathol* 1993;143:1649–1656.

144. Kilhovd BK, Berg TJ, Birkeland KI, et al. Serum levels of advanced glycation end products are increased in patients with type 2 diabetes and coronary heart disease. *Diabetes Care* 1999;22:1543–1548.

145. Berg TJ, Snorgaard O, Faber J, et al. Serum levels of advanced glycation end products are associated with left ventricular diastolic function in patients with type-1 diabetes. *Diabetes Care* 1999;22:1186–1190.

146. Brownlee M, Vlassara H, Kooney A, et al. Aminoguanidine prevents diabetes-induced arterial wall protein cross-linking. *Science* 1986;232:1629–1632.

147. Vasan S, Zhang X, Zhang X, et al. An agent cleaving glucose-derived protein crosslinks in vitro and in vivo. *Nature* 1996;382:275–278.

148. Schmidt AM, Hori O, Brett J, et al. Cellular receptors for advanced glycation end-products: Implications for induction of oxidant stress and cellular dysfunction in the pathogenesis of vascular lesions. *Arterioscler Thromb* 1994;14:1521–1528.

149. Brett J, Schmidt AM, Yan SD, et al. Survey of the distribution of a newly characterized receptor for advanced glycation end-products in tissues. *Am J Pathol* 1993;143:1699–1712.

150. Schmidt AM, Yan SD, Brett J, et al. Regulation of human mononuclear phagocyte migration by cell surface-binding proteins for advanced glycation end-products. *J Clin Invest* 1993;91:2155–2168.

151. Kirstein M, Brett J, Radoff S, et al. Advanced protein glycosylation induces selective transendothelial human monocyte chemotaxis and secretion of PDGF: Role in vascular diseases of diabetes and aging. *Proc Natl Acad Sci USA* 1990;87:9010–9014.

152. Vlassara H, Fuh H, Makita Z, et al. Exogenous advanced glycosylation end products induce complex vascular dysfunction in normal animal: A model for diabetic and aging complications. *Proc Natl Acad Sci USA* 1992;89:12043–12047.

153. Vlassara H, Brownlee M, Manogue KR, et al. Cachetin/TNF and IL-1 induced by glucose modified proteins: Role in normal tissue remodelling. *Science* 1988;240:1546–1548.

154. Kirstein M, Aston C, Hintz R, Vlassara H. Receptor-specific induction of IGF-1 in human monocytes by advanced glycosylation end product-modified proteins. *J Clin Invest* 1992;90:439–446.

155. Vlassara H, Bucala R, Striker L. Pathogenic effects of advanced glycosylation: Biochemical, biologic, and clinical implications for diabetes and aging. *Lab Invest* 1994;70:138–151.

156. Brownlee M. Glycation and diabetic complications. *Diabetes* 1994;43:836–841.

157. Expert Panel ATP III. Executive summary of the NCEP expert panel on the detection, evaluation, and treatment of high blood cholesterol in adults (ATP III). *JAMA* 2001;285:2486–2497.

158. Pyorala K, Pedersen DR, Kjekshus J, et al. Cholesterol lowering with simvastatin improves prognosis of diabetic patients with coronary heart disease. *Diabetes Care* 1997;20:614–620.

159. Sacks FM, Pfeffer MA, Moye LA, et al. The effect of pravastatin on coronary events after myocardial infarction in patients with average cholesterol levels. *N Engl J Med* 1996;335:1001–1009.

160. CARE Circulation: Goldberg RB, Mellies MJ, Sacks FM, et al. Cardiovascular events and their reduction with pravastatin in diabetic and glucose-intolerant myocardial infarction survivors with average cholesterol levels: Subgroup analyses in the cholesterol and recurrent events (CARE) trial: The Care investigators. *Circulation* 1998;98:2513–2519.

161. The DECODE study group. Glucose tolerance and mortality: comparison of WHO and American Diabetes Association diagnostic criteria. *Lancet* 1999;354:617–621.

162. The DECODE study group. Glucose tolerance and mortality: comparison of WHO and American Diabetes Association diagnostic criteria. *Lancet* 1999;354:617–621.

163. American Diabetes Association. Standard of medical care for patients with diabetes mellitus. *Diabetes Care* 2000;23(suppl 1):S532–S542.

164. Muhlhauser I, Sawicki PT, Berger M. Possible risk of sulfonylureas in the treatment of non-insulin-dependent diabetes mellitus and coronary artery disease. *Diabetologia* 1997;40:1492–1496.

165. Cleveland JC, Meldrum DR, Cain BS, et al. Oral sulfonylurea hypoglycemic agents prevent ischemic preconditioning in human myocardium. *Circulation* 1997;96(1):29–32.

166. Owens DR. Repaglinide μ prandial glucose regulator: A new class of oral antidiabetic drugs. *Diabetes Med* 1998;15(suppl 4):S28–S36.

167. Metformin for non-insulin-dependent diabetes mellitus. *Med Lett Drugs Ther* 1995;37(948):41–42.

168. Stumvoll M, Nurjhan N, Perriello G, et al. Metabolic effects of metformin in non-insulin-dependent diabetes mellitus. *N Engl J Med* 1995;333(9):550–554.

169. Garber AJ, Duncan TG, Goodman AM, et al. Efficacy of metformin in type II diabetes: Results of a double-blind, placebo-controlled, dose-response trial. *Am J Med* 1997;102:491–497.

170. Giugliano D, Quatraro A, Consoli G, et al. Metformin for obese, insulin-treated, diabetic patients: Improvement in glycemic control and reduction of metabolic risk factors. *Eur J Clin Pharmacol* 1993;44:107–112.

171. DeFronzo RA, Goodman AM, and the Multicenter Metformin Study Group. Efficacy of metformin in patients with non-insulin-dependent diabetes mellitus. *N Engl J Med* 1995;333:541–549.

172. Inzucchi SE, Maggs DG, Spollett GR, et al. Efficacy and metabolic effects of metformin and troglitazone in type II diabetes mellitus. *N Engl J Med* 1998;338:867–872.

173. Robinson AC, Burke J, Robinson S, et al. The effects of metformin on glycemic control and serum lipids in insulin-treated NIDDM patients with suboptimal metabolic control. *Diabetes Care* 1998;21(5):701–705.

174. Stang MR, Wysowski DK, Butler-Jones D. Incidence of lactic acidosis in metformin users. *Diabetes Care* 1999;22:925–927.

175. *Physicians' Desk Reference*, 52nd ed. Montvale, NJ: Medical Economics. 1998:795–800.

176. Tafuri SR. Troglitazone enhances differentiation, basal-glucose uptake and Glut 1 protein levels in 3T3-L1 adipocytes. *Endocrinology* 1996; 137:4706–4712.

177. Miles PDG, Romeo OM, Higo K, et al. TNF-α-induced insulin resistance in vivo and its prevention by troglitazone. *Diabetes* 1997;46: 1678–1683.

178. Schwartz S, Raskin P, Fonseca V, Graveline JF, for the Troglitazone and Exogenous Insulin Study Group. Effect of troglitazone in insulin-treated patients with type II diabetes mellitus. *N Engl J Med* 1998;338: 861–866.

179. Buse JB, Gumbiner B, Mathias NP, et al. The Troglitazone Insulin Study Group: Troglitazone use in insulin-treated type II diabetic patients. *Diabetes Care* 1998;21:1455–1461.

180. Horton ES, Whitehouse F, Ghazzi MN, et al. The Troglitazone Study Group: Troglitazone in combination with sulfonylurea restores glycemic control in patients with type II diabetes. *Diabetes Care* 1998;21: 1462–1469.

181. Ghazzi MN, Perez JE, Antonucci TK, et al. The Triglitazone Study Group, Whitcomb RW. Cardiac and glycemic benefits of troglitazone treatment in NIDDM. *Diabetes* 1997;46:433–439.

182. Maggs DG, Buchanan TA, Burant CF, et al. Metabolic effects of troglitazone monotherapy in type 2 diabetes mellitus. *Ann Intern Med* 1998;128:176–185.

183. Tack CJJ, Smits P, Demacker PNM, Stalenhoff AFH. Troglitazone decreases the proportion of small, dense LDL and increases the resistance of LDL to oxidation in obese subjects. *Diabetes Care* 1998;21:796–797.

184. Patel J, Miller E, Patwardhan R, the Rosiglitazone Study Group. Rosiglitazone improves glycemic control when used as monotherapy in type 2 diabetic patients. *Diabetic Med* 1998;15(suppl 2):S38.

185. Grunberger G, Weston WM, Patwardhan R, Rappaport EB. Rosiglitazone once or twice daily improves the glycemic control in patients with type 2 diabetes. *Diabetes* 1998;48(suppl 1):A102.

186. Fonesca V, Biswas N, Salzman A. Once-daily rosiglitazone in combination with metformin effectively reduces hyperglycemia in patients with type 2 diabetes. *Diabetes* 1999;48(suppl 1):A100.

187. Package insert. Philadelphia: SmithKline Beecham Pharmaceuticals.

188. Package insert. Lincolnshire, IL: Takeda Pharmaceuticals.

189. Shapiro AMJ, Lakey JRT, Ryan EA, et al. Islet transplantation in seven patients with type I diabetes mellitus using a glucocorticoid-free immunosuppressive regimen. *N Engl J Med*, 2000;348:230–238.

190. University Group Diabetes Program. A study of the effects of hypoglycemic agents on vascular complications in patients with adult onset diabetes. *Diabetes* 1976;25:1129–1153.

191. Garratt KN, Hassinger N, Grill DE, et al. Sulfonylurea drug use is associated with increased early mortality during direct coronary angioplasty for acute myocardial infarction among diabetic patients. *J Am Coll Cardiol* 1997;29:493A (Abstr).

192. UK Prospective Diabetes Study Group. Intensive blood glucose control with sulfonylureas or insulin compared with conventional treatment and risk of complications in patients with type-2 diabetes. UKPDS 33. *Lancet* 1998;352:837–853.

193. UK Prospective Diabetes Study Group. Effect of intensive blood glucose control with metformin on complications in overweight patients with type-2 diabetes. UKPDS 34. *Lancet* 1998;352:854–865.

194. UK Prospective Diabetes Study Group. Tight blood pressure control and risk of macrovascular and microvascular complications in type-2 diabetes. UKPDS 38. *BMJ* 1998;317:703–713.

195. UK Prospective Diabetes Study Group. Efficacy of atenolol and captopril in reducing risk of macrovascular and microvascular complications in type 2 diabetes. UKPDS 39. *BMJ* 1998;317:713–720.

196. The Diabetes Control and Complications Trial Research Group. The effect of intensive treatment of diabetes on the development and progression of long-term complications in insulin-dependent diabetes mellitus. *N Engl J Med* 1993;329:977–986.

197. The Diabetes Control and Complications Trial Research Group. Effect of intensive diabetes management on macrovascular events and risk factors in the Diabetes Control and Complications Trial. *Am J Cardiol* 1995;75:894–903.

198. Haffner SM, Mykanen L, Festa A, et al. Insulin-resistant pre-diabetic subjects have more atherogenic risk factors than insulin-sensitive prediabetic subjects: Implications for preventing coronary heart disease during the pre-diastolic state. *Circulation* 2000;101:975–980.

199. Tuomilehto J, Lindstrom J, Eriksson JG, et al. Prevention of type 2 diabetes melllitus by changes in lifestyle among subjects with impaired glucose tolerance. *N Engl J Med* 2001;344:1343-1350.

200. Diabetes Prevention Program Research Group. Reduction in the incidence of type 2 diabetes with lifestyle modification or metformin. *N Engl J Med* 2002;346:393-403.

201. Freeman DJ, Norrie J, Sattar N, et al. Pravastatin and the development of diabetes mellitus: Evidence for a protective treatment effect in the West of Scotland Coronary Prevention Study. *Circulation* 2001;103: 357-362.

202. Heart Outcomes Prevention Evaluation Study Investigators. Effects of ramipril on cardiovascular and microvascular outcomes in people with diabetes mellitus: Results of the HOPE study and MICRO-HOPE substudy. *Lancet* 2000;355:253–259.

203. Heart Outcomes Prevention Evaluation Study Investigators. Effects of ramipril on cardiovascular and microvascular outcomes in people with diabetes mellitus: Results of the HOPE study and MICRO-HOPE substudy. *Lancet* 2000;355:253–259.

204. The cost-effectiveness of screening for type 2 diabetes. CDC Diabetes Cost-Effectiveness Study Group, Centers for Disease Control and Prevention. *JAMA* 1998;280:1757–1763.

205. The cost-effectiveness of screening for type 2 diabetes. CDC Diabetes Cost-Effectiveness Study Group, Centers for Disease Control and Prevention. *JAMA* 1998;280:1757–1763.

206. Gibbons RJ, Balady GJ, Beasley JW, et al. ACC/AHA guidelines for exercise testing: Executive summary: A report of the American College of Cardiology/American Heart Association Task Force on Practice Guidelines (Committee on Exercise Testing). *Circulation* 1997; 96:345–354.

207. Grundy SM, Benjamin IJ, Burke GL, et al. Diabetes and cardiovascular disease: A statement for healthcare professionals from the American Heart Association. *Circulation* 1999;100:1134–1146.

208. Curb JD, Pressel SL, Cutler JA, et al. Effect of diuretic-based antihypertensive treatment on cardiovascular disease risk in older diabetic patients with isolated systolic hypertension: Systolic Hypertension in the Elderly Program Cooperative Research Group. *JAMA* 1996;276: 1886–1892.

209. Hansson L, Zanchetti A, Carruthers SG, et al., for the HOT Study Group. Effects of intensive blood-pressure lowering and low-dose aspirin in patients with hypertension: Principal results of Hypertension Optimal Treatment (HOT) randomized trial. *Lancet* 1998;351: 1755–1762.

210. Hansson L, Lindholm LH, Niskanen L, et al., for the Captopril Prevention Projects (CAPPP) study group. Effect of angiotensin-converting-enzyme inhibition compared with conventional therapy on cardiovascular morbidity and mortality in hypertension: The Captopril Prevention Project (CAPPP) randomised trial. *Lancet* 1999;353:611–616.

211. Estacio RO, Jeffers BW, Hiatt WR, et al. The effect of nisoldipine as compared with enalapril on cardiovascular outcomes in patients with non-insulin-dependent diabetes and hypertension. *N Engl J Med* 1998; 338:645–652.

212. Gæde P, Vedel P, Larsen N, et al. Multifactorial intervention and cardiovascular disease in patients with type 2 diabetes. *N Engl J Med* 2003;348:383-393.

213. Woodfield SL, Lundergan CF, Reiner JS, et al. Angiographic findings and outcome in diabetic patients treated with thrombolytic therapy for acute myocardial infarction: The GUSTO-1 experience. *J Am Coll Cardiol* 1996;28:1661–1669.

214. Jaffe AS, Spadaro JJ, Schechtman K, et al. Increased congestive heart failure after myocardial infarction of modest extent in patients with diabetes mellitus. *Am Heart J* 1984;108:31–37.

215. Savage MP, Krolewski AS, Kenien GG, et al. Acute myocardial infarction in diabetes mellitus and significance of congestive heart failure as a prognostic factor. *Am J Cardiol* 1988;62:665–669.

216. Stone PH, Muller JE, Hartwell T, et al., for the MILIS Study Group. The effect of diabetes mellitus on prognosis and serial left ventricular function after acute myocardial infarction: Contribution of both coronary disease and left ventricular dysfunction to the adverse prognosis. *J Am Coll Cardiol* 1989;14:49–57.

217. Fibrinolytic Therapy Trialists (FTT) Collaborative Group. Indications for fibrinolytic therapy in suspected acute myocardial infarction: Collaborative overview of early mortality and major morbidity results from all randomized trials of more than 1000 patients. *Lancet* 1994;343:311–322.

218. Malmberg K, for the DIGAMI Study Group. Prospective randomised study of intensive insulin treatment on long-term survival after acute myocardial infarction in patients with diabetes mellitus. *BMJ* 1997; 314:1512–1515.

219. Zarich S, Waxman S, Freeman RT, et al. Effect of autonomic nervous system dysfunction on the circadian pattern of myocardial ischaemia in diabetes mellitus. *J Am Coll Cardiol* 1994;24:956–962.

220. Jonas M, Reicher-Reiss H, Boyko V, et al. Usefulness of beta-blocker therapy in patients with non-insulin-dependent diabetes mellitus and coronary heart disease. *Am J Cardiol* 1996;77:1273–1277.

221. Kendall MJ, Lynch KP, Hjalmarson A, Kjekshus J. Beta-blockers and sudden cardiac death. *Ann Intern Med* 1995;123:358–367.

222. Kawate R, Yamakido M, Nishimoto Y, et al. Diabetes mellitus and its vascular complications in Japanese migrants on the Island of Hawaii. *Diabetes Care* 1979;2: 161-70.

223. Vigorita VJ, Moore GW, Hutchins GM. Absence of correlation between coronary arterial atherosclerosis and severity or duration of diabetes mellitus of adult onset. *Am J Cardiol* 1980;46:535–542.

224. Waller BF, Palumbo PJ, Lie JT, Roberts WC. Status of the coronary arteries at necropsy in diabetes mellitus with onset after age 30 years. Analysis of 229 diabetic patients with and without clinical evidence of coronary heart disease and comparison to 183 control subjects. *Am J Med* 1980;69:498–506.

225. Head J, Fuller JH. International variations in mortality among diabetic patients: The WHO Multinational Study of Vascular Disease in Diabetics. *Diabetologia* 1990;33:477–81.

226. Granger CB, Califf RM, Young S, et al. Outcome of patients with diabetes mellitus and acute myocardial infarction treated with thrombolytic agents. The Thrombolysis and Angioplasty in Myocardial Infarction (TAMI) Study Group. *J Am Coll Cardiol* 1993;21:920–925.

227. Mueller HS, Cohen LS, Braunwald E, et al. Predictors of early morbidity and mortality after thrombolytic therapy of acute myocardial infarction. Analyses of patient subgroups in the Thrombolysis in Myocardial Infarction (TIMI) trial, phase II. *Circulation* 1992;85:1254–1264.

228. Stein B, Weintraub WS, Gebhart SP, et al. Influence of diabetes mellitus on early and late outcome after percutaneous transluminal coronary angioplasty. *Circulation* 1995;91:979–989.

229. Barzilay JI, Kronmal RA, Bittner V, et al. Coronary artery disease and coronary artery bypass grafting in diabetic patients aged > or = 65 years (report from the Coronary Artery Surgery Study [CASS] Registry). *Am J Cardiol* 1994;74:334–339.

230. Davies MJ, Bland JM, Hangartner JR, et al. Factors influencing the presence or absence of acute coronary artery thrombi in sudden ischaemic death. *Eur Heart J* 1989;10:203–208.

231. Silva JA, Escobar A, Collins TJ, et al. Unstable angina. A comparison of angioscopic findings between diabetic and nondiabetic patients. *Circulation* 1995;92:1731–1736.

232. Detre KM, Guo P, Holubkov R, et al. Coronary revascularization in diabetic patients: A comparison of the randomized and observational components of the Aypass Angioplasty Revascularization Investigation (BARI). *Circulation* 1999;99:633–640.

233. Rauch U, Osende JI, Fuster V, et al. Thrombus formation on atherosclerotic plaques: Pathogenesis and clinical consequences. *Ann Intern Med* 2001;134:224-238.

234. Yusuf S, Zucker D, Chalmers TC. Ten-year results of the randomized control trials of coronary artery bypass graft surgery: Tabular data compiled by the collaborative effort of the original trial investigators, Part 1. *J Curr Clin Trials* 1994;145.

235. Yusuf S, Zucker D, Chalmers TC. Ten-year results of the randomized control trials of coronary artery bypass graft surgery: tabular data compiled by the collaborative effort of the original trial investigators, Part 2. *J Curr Clin Trials* [serial online] 1994;144.

236. Barsness GW, Peterson ED, Ohman EM, et al. Relationship between diabetes mellitus and long-term survival after coronary bypass and angioplasty. *Circulation* 1997;96:2551–2556.

237. *BARI* Investigators. Comparison of coronary bypass surgery with angioplasty in patients with multivessel disease. The Bypass Angioplasty Revascularization Investigation (BARI) Investigators. *N Engl J Med* 1996;335:217–225.

238. *BARI* Investigators. Influence of diabetes on 5-year mortality and morbidity in a randomized trial comparing CABG and PTCA in patients with multivessel disease: The Bypass Angioplasty Revascularization Investigation (BARI). *Circulation* 1997;96:1761–1769.

239. Ferguson JJ. NHLI BARI clinical alert on diabetics treated with angioplasty. *Circulation* 1995;92:3371.

240. Feit F, Brooks MM, Sopko G, et al. Long-term clinical outcome in the Bypass Angioplasty Revascularization Investigation Registry: Comparison with the randomized trial. BARI Investigators. *Circulation* 2000;101:2795-2802.

241. BARI Investigators. Protocol for the Bypass Angioplasty Revascularization Investigation. *Circulation* 1991;84:V-1-v-27.

242. Niles NW, McGrath PD, Malenka D, et al. Survival of patients with diabetes and multivessel coronary artery disease after surgical or percutaneous coronary revascularization: Results of a large regional prospective study. Northern New England Cardiovascular Disease Study Group. *J Am Coll Cardiol* 2001;37:1008–1015.

243. Kip KE, Bourassa MG, Jacobs AK, et al. Influence of pre-PTCA strategy and initial PTCA result in patients with multivessel disease: The Bypass Angioplasty Revascularization Investigation (BARI). *Circulation* 1999;100:910-917.

244. Van Belle E, Ketelers R, Bauters C, et al. Patency of percutaneous transluminal coronary angioplasty sites at 6- month angiographic follow-up: A key determinant of survival in diabetics after coronary balloon angioplasty. *Circulation* 2001;103:1218–1224.

245. Kuntz RE. Importance of considering atherosclerosis progression when choosing a coronary revascularization strategy: The diabetes-percutaneous transluminal coronary angioplasty dilemma. *Circulation* 1999;99:847-51.

246. Newman MF, Kirchner JL, Phillips-Bute B, et al. Longitudinal assessment of neurocognitive function after coronary- artery bypass surgery. *N Engl J Med* 2001;344:395–402.

247. Holmes DR Jr, Vlietstra RE, Smith HC, et al. Restenosis after percutaneous transluminal coronary angioplasty (PTCA): A report from the PTCA Registry of the National Heart, Lung and Blood Institute. *Am J Cardiol* 1984;53:77C–81C.

248. Weintraub WS, Kosinski AS, Brown CL, King SB. Can restenosis after coronary angioplasty be predicted from clinical variables? *J Am Coll Cardiol* 1993;21:6–14.

249. Vandormael MG, Deligonul U, Kern MJ, et al. Multilesion coronary angioplasty: Clinical and angiographic outcome. *J Am Coll Cardiol* 1987;10:246–252.

250. Quigley PJ, Hlatky MA, Hinohara T, et al. Repeat percutaneous transluminal coronary angioplasty and predictors of recurrent restenosis. *Am J Cardiol* 1989;63:409–413.

251. Lambert M, Bonan R, Cote G, et al. Multiple coronary angioplasty: A model to discriminate systemic and procedural factors related to restenosis. *J Am Coll Cardiol* 1988;12:310–314.

252. Galan KM, Hollman JL. Recurrence of stenosis after coronary angioplasty. *Heart Lung* 1986;15:585–587.

253. Rensing BJ, Hermans RM, Vos J, et al. Luminal narrowing after percutaneous transluminal coronary angioplasty. *Circulation* 1993;88: 975–985.

254. Wong SC, Baim DS, Schatz RA, et al. Immediate results and late outcomes after stent implantation in saphenous vein graft lesions: The multicenter US Palmaz-Schatz stane experience: The Palmaz-Schatz Stent Study Group. *J Am Coll Cardiol* 1995;26:704–712.

255. Bach R, Jung F, Kohsiek I, et al. Factors affecting the restenosis rate after percutaneous transluminal coronary angioplasty. *Thromb Haemost* 1994;74(suppl 1):55S–77S.

256. Kornowski R, Mintz GS, Kent KM, et al. Increased restenosis in diabetes mellitus after coronary interventions is due to exaggerated intimal hyperplasia. *Circulation* 1997;95:1366–1369.

257. Aronson D, Bloomgarden Z, Rayfield EJ. Potential mechanisms promoting restenosis in diabetes mellitus. *J Am Coll Cardiol* 1996;27:528–535.

258. Leon MB, Popma JJ, Mintz GS, et al. An overview of US coronary stent trials. *Semin Interv Cardiol* 1996;1:247–254.

259. Fischman DL, Leon MB, Baim DS, et al. A randomized comparison of coronary-stent placement and balloon angioplasty in the treatment of coronary artery disease. Stent Restenosis Study Investigators. *N Engl J Med* 1994;331:496–501.

260. Serruys PW, de Jaegere P, Kiemeneij F, et al. A comparison of balloon-expandable-stent implantation with balloon angioplasty in patients with coronary artery disease. Benestent Study Group. *N Engl J Med* 1994;331:489–495.

261. Kiemeneij F, Serruys PW, Macaya C, et al. Continued benefit of coronary stenting versus balloon angioplasty: five-year clinical follow-up of Benestent-I trial. *J Am Coll Cardiol* 2001;37:1598–1603.

262. Ruygrok PN, Webster MW, de Valk V, et al. Clinical and angiographic factors associated with asymptomatic restenosis after percutaneous coronary intervention. *Circulation* 2001;104:2289–2294.

263. Ruygrok PN, Melkert R, Morel MA, et al. Does angiography six months after coronary intervention influence management and outcome? Benestent II Investigators. *J Am Coll Cardiol* 1999;34:1507–1511.

264. Mehran R, Dangas G, Abizaid AS, et al. Angiographic patterns of in-stent restenosis: Classification and implications for long-term outcome. *Circulation* 1999;100:1872–1878.

265. Kuntz RE, Gibson CM, Nobuyoshi M, Baim DS. Generalized model of restenosis after conventional balloon angioplasty, stenting and directional atherectomy. *J Am Coll Cardiol* 1993;21:15–25.

266. Kuntz RE, Baim DS. Prevention of coronary restenosis: the evolving evidence base for radiation therapy. *Circulation* 2000;101:2130–2133.

267. El-Omar MM, Dangas G, Iakovou I, Mehran R. Update on Instent Restenosis. *Curr Interv Cardiol Rep* 2001;3:296-305.

268. Ahmed JM, Hong MK, Mehran R, et al. Influence of diabetes mellitus on early and late clinical outcomes in saphenous vein graft stenting. *J Am Coll Cardiol* 2000;36:1186–1193.

269. Abizaid A, Kornowski R, Mintz GS, et al. The influence of diabetes mellitus on acute and late clinical outcomes following coronary stent implantation. *J Am Coll Cardiol* 1998;32:584–589.

270. EPIC Investigators. Use of a monoclonal antibody directed against the platelet glycoprotein IIb/IIIa receptor in high-risk coronary angioplasty. *N Engl J Med* 1994;330:956–961.

271. The EPILOG Investigators. Platelet glycoprotein IIb/IIIa receptor blockade and low-dose heparin during percutaneous coronary revascularization. *N Engl J Med* 1997;336:1689–1696.

272. Randomised placebo-controlled trial of abciximab before and during coronary intervention in refractory unstable angina: The CAPTURE Study. *Lancet* 1997;349:1429–1435.

273. Lincoff AM, Califf RM, Moliterno DJ, et al. for the Evaluation of Platelet IIb/IIIa Inhibition in Stenting Investigators. Complementary clinical benefits of coronary-artery stenting and blockade of platelet glycoprotein IIb/IIIa receptors. *N Engl J Med* 1999;341:319–327.

274. Marso SP, Lincoff AM, Ellis SG, et al. Optimizing the percutaneous interventional outcomes for patients with diabetes mellitus: Results of the EPISTENT (Evaluation of Platelet IIb/IIIa Inhibitor for Stenting Trial) diabetic substudy. *Circulation* 1999;100:2477–2484.

275. Teirstein PS, Massullo V, Jani S, et al. Catheter-based radiotherapy to inhibit restenosis after coronary stenting. *N Engl J Med* 1997;336:1697–1703.

276. Serruys PW, Unger F, Sousa JE, et al. Comparison of coronary-artery bypass surgery and stenting for the treatment of multivessel disease. *N Engl J Med* 2001;344:1117–1124.

277. Bakhai A, Stables RH, Prasad S, Sigwart U. Trials comparing coronary artery bypass grafting with percutaneous transluminal coronary angioplasty and primary stent implantation in patients with multivessel coronary artery disease. *Curr Opin Cardiol* 2000;15:388–394.

278. The Diabetes Control and Complication Trial Research Group. The effect of intensive treatment of diabetes on the development and progression of long-term complications in insulin-dependent diabetes mellitus. *N Engl J Med* 1993;329:977–986.

279. Abizaid A, Costa MA, Centemero M, et al. Clinical and economic impact of diabetes mellitus on percutaneous and surgical treatment of multivessel coronary disease patients: Insights from the Arterial Revascularization Therapy Study (ARTS) trial. *Circulation* 2001;104:533–538.

280. The SOS Investigators. Coronary artery bypass surgery versus percutaneous coronary intervention with stent implantation in patients with multivessel coronary artery disease (the Stent or Surgery trial): A randomized controlled trial. *Lancet* 2002;360:965–970.

281. Mintz GS, Popma JJ, Pichard AD, et al. Intravascular ultrasound predictors of restenosis after percutaneous transcatheter coronary revascularization. *J Am Coll Cardiol* 1996;27:1678–1687.

282. Mintz GS, Popma JJ, Pichard AD, et al. Arterial remodeling after coronary angioplasty: A serial intravascular ultrasound study. *Circulation* 1996;94:35–43.

283. Mintz GS, Popma JJ, Hong MK, et al. Intravascular ultrasound to discern device-specific effects and mechanisms of restenosis. *Am J Cardiol* 1996;78:18–22.

284. Mintz GS, Kent KM, Pichard AD, et al. Intravascular ultrasound insights into mechanisms of stenosis formation and restenosis. *Cardiol Clin* 1997;15:17–29.

285. Kimura T, Kaburagi S, Tamura T, et al. Remodeling of human coronary arteries undergoing coronary angioplasty or atherectomy. *Circulation* 1997;96:475–483.

286. Lansky AJ, Mintz GS, Mehran R, et al. Insights into the mechanism of restenosis after PTCA and stenting. *Indian Heart J* 1998;50(suppl 1):104–108.

287. Painter JA, Mintz GS, Wong SC, et al. Serial intravascular ultrasound studies fail to show evidence of chronic Palmaz-Schatz stent recoil. *Am J Cardiol* 1995;75:398–400.

288. Popma JJ, Lansky AJ, Ito S, et al. Contemporary stent designs: Technical considerations, complications, role of intravascular ultrasound, and anticoagulation therapy. *Prog Cardiovasc Dis* 1996;39:111–128.

289. Hoffmann R, Mintz GS, Dussaillant GR, et al. Patterns and mechanisms of instent restenosis. A serial intravascular ultrasound study. *Circulation* 1996;94:1247–1254.

290. Dussaillant GR, Mintz GS, Pichard AD, et al. Small stent size and intimal hyperplasia contribute to restenosis: A volumetric intravascular ultrasound analysis. *J Am Coll Cardiol* 1995;26:720–724.

291. Dangas G, Fuster V. Management of restenosis after coronary intervention. *Am Heart J* 1996;132:428-436.

292. Sigwart U. Prevention of restenosis after stenting. *Lancet* 1999;354:269–270.

293. Kornowski R, Mintz GS, Kent KM, et al. Increased restenosis in diabetes mellitus after coronary interventions is due to exaggerated intimal hyperplasia. A serial intravascular ultrasound study. *Circulation* 1997;95:1366–1369.

294. Bittl JA. Advances in coronary angioplasty. *N Engl J Med* 1996;335:1290–1302.

295. Hong MK, Mehran R, Mintz GS, Leon MB. Restenosis after coronary angioplasty. *Curr Probl Cardiol* 1997;22:1–36.

296. Sousa JE, Costa MA, Abizaid A, et al. Lack of Neointimal Proliferation After Implantation of Sirolimus-Coated Stents in Human Coronary Arteries: A Quantitative Coronary Angiography and Three-Dimensional Intravascular Ultrasound Study. *Circulation* 2001;103:192–195.

297. Sousa JE, Costa MA, Abizaid AC, et al. Sustained suppression of neointimal proliferation by sirolimus-eluting stents: One-year angiographic and intravascular ultrasound follow-up. *Circulation* 2001;104:2007–2011.

298. Mack MJ, Osborne JA, Shennib H. Arterial graft patency in coronary artery bypass grafting: what do we really know? *Ann Thorac Surg* 1998;66:1055–1059.

299. Lytle BW, Blackstone EH, Loop FD, et al. Two internal thoracic artery grafts are better than one. *J Thorac Cardiovasc Surg* 1999;117:855–872.

300. Berger PB, Alderman EL, Nadel A, Schaff HV. Frequency of early occlusion and stenosis in a left internal mammary artery to left anterior descending artery bypass graft after surgery through a median sternotomy on conventional bypass: Benchmark for minimally invasive direct coronary artery bypass. Circulation 1999;100:2353.

301. Leavitt BJ, O'Connor GT, Olmstead EM, et al. Use of the internal mammary artery graft and in-hospital mortality and other adverse outcomes associated with coronary artery bypass surgery. *Circulation* 2001;103:507–512.

302. Loop FD, Lytle BW, Cosgrove DM, et al. Influence of the internal-mammary-artery graft on 10-year survival and other cardiac events. *N Engl J Med* 1986;314:1–6.

303. Tatoulis J, Buxton BF, Fuller JA, Royse AG. Total arterial coronary revascularization: Techniques and results in 3,220 patients. *Ann Thorac Surg* 1999;68:2093–2099.

304. Lytle BW, Cosgrove DM, Loop FD, et al. Perioperative risk of bilateral internal mammary artery grafting: analysis of 500 cases from 1971 to 1984. *Circulation* 1986;74:III37–IIII41.

305. Uva MS, Braunberger E, Fisher M, et al. Does bilateral internal thoracic artery grafting increase surgical risk in diabetic patients? *Ann Thorac Surg* 1998;66:2051–2055.

306. Borger MA, Cohen G, Buth KJ, et al. Multiple arterial grafts. Radial versus right internal thoracic arteries. *Circulation* 1998;98:II7-II13;discussion II13-II14.

307. Morice MD, Serruys PW, Sousa JE, et al. A random comparison of a sirolimus-eluting stent with a standard stent for coronary revascularization. *N Engl J Med* 2002;346:1773–1780.

308. Moses JW, Leon MB, Popma JJ, et al. Sirolimus-eluting stents versus standard stents in patients with stenosis in a native coronary artery. *N Engl J Med* 2003;349:1315–1323.

309. SIRIUS Investigators. SIRIUS Trial. Presented at the TCT Annual Meeting 2002.

310. Kannel WB, Hjortland M, Castelli WP. Role of diabetes in congestive heart failure: The Framingham Study. *Am J Cardiol* 1974;34:29–34.

311. Van Hoeven KH, Factor SM. A comparison of the pathological spectrum of hypertensive, diabetic, and hypertensive-diabetic heart disease. *Circulation* 1990;82:848–855.

312. Jain A, Avendaro G, Dharamsey S, et al. Left ventricular diastolic dysfunction in hypertension and role of plasma glucose and insulin: Comparison with diabetic heart. *Circulation* 1996;93:1396–1402.

313. Zarich SW, Arbuckle BE, Cohen LR, et al. Diastolic abnormalities in young asymptomatic diabetic patients assessed by pulse Doppler echocardiography. *J Am Coll Cardiol* 1988;12:114–120.

314. Raev DC. Which left ventricular function is impaired earlier in the evolution of diabetic cardiomyopathy? An echocardiographic study of young type I diabetic patients. *Diabetes Care* 1994;17:633–639.

315. Paillole C, Dahan M, Payche F, et al. Prevalence and significance of left ventricular filling abnormalities determined by Doppler echocardiography in young type I (insulin-dependent) diabetic patients. *Am J Cardiol* 1990;64:1010–1016.

316. Mildenerger RR, Bar-Shlomo B, Druck MN, et al. Clinically unrecognized ventricular dysfunction in young diabetic patients. *J Am Coll Cardiol* 1984;4:234–238.

317. Rubler S, Dlugash J, Yuceoglu YZ, et al. New type of cardiomyopathy associated with diabetic glomerulosclerosis. *Am J Cardiol* 1972;30:595–602.

318. Palmieri V, Bella JN, Arnett DK, et al. Effect of type 2 diabetes mellitus on left ventricular geometry and systolic function in hypertensive subjects. *Circulation* 2001;103:102–107.

319. Fang ZY, Yuda S, Anderson V, et al. Echocardiographic detection of early diabetic myocardial disease. *J Am Coll Cardiol* 2003;41:611–617.

THE METABOLIC SYNDROME, OBESITY, AND DIET

H. Robert Superko

The cardiovascular importance of the metabolic syndrome, obesity, and diet relates to the 110-year-old observation by Sir William Osler, that "A man is only as old as his arteries," and the modern physiologic and social factors that contribute to premature arterial aging.[1] Among the most important modern contributors to prematurely aged arteries are the metabolic syndrome and obesity. Excess body fat has gradually but consistently increased among people in the United States over the past 20 years. According to the National Health and Nutrition Examination Survey (NHANES), in 1980, 14.5 percent of the U.S. population were defined as obese.[2] In 1994, 22.5 percent were defined as obese, which is a 55 percent increase in the number of people suffering from obesity.[3] The combined prevalence of an overweight status and obesity [or a body mass index (BMI) $\geq$ 25 kg/ m²] in the United States is 63 percent in men and 55 percent in women.[4] The burden of obesity is disproportionately high in black and Hispanic women as well as Asian and Pacific Islanders, Native Americans, Native Alaskans, and Native Hawaiians. The increase in obesity is not uniform across age groups; it appears to be greatest in younger groups. Between 1991 and 1998 the growth in obesity in 18- to 29-year-olds was 70 percent; 30- to 39-year-olds, 50 percent; 40- to 49-year-olds, 34 percent; 50- to 59-year-olds, 48 percent; 60- to 69-year-olds, 45 percent; and > 70-year-olds, 29 percent.[5] This increase in younger age groups is of particular concern, since overweight children and adolescents suffer from increased mortality as adults. The degree of obesity is related to years of life lost compared to nonobese individuals and is most obvious in the younger age groups. Although there are ethnic and gender differences, in general, 20- to 30-year-olds with a BMI of 30 to 35 have 5 years of life lost and those with a BMI of 35 to 40 have 7 years of life lost.[6]

One way of discussing excess body fat is by using the body mass index (BMI), which is weight in kilograms divided by height in meters squared (kg/m²). From the standpoint of cardiovascular health, excess body fat can be defined as a BMI > 25 to 30, which reflects a moderately increased risk, and > 30, which reflects a greatly increased risk.[7] The rapid and widespread increase in obesity meets the definition of an epidemic, attacking many people in a region at the same time, which is widely diffused and rapidly spreading.

The relationship between overweight status and risk for coronary artery disease (CAD) is directly influenced by an atherogenic stew of metabolic disorders that substantially contribute to increased CAD risk even in the setting of "normal" blood cholesterol values. These include aspects of normal metabolism that, under the stress of the "western" lifestyle, create an atherogenic milieu that would not exist in a lifestyle more closely representative of the environment in which, for hundreds of thousands of years, homo sapiens lived, survived, and thrived. This view of metabolic disorders linked to CAD and lifestyle can be exemplified by the "thrifty gene" concept. With a great degree of prescience, Neel in 1962 hypothesized that a gene or gene cluster must exist that helps humans survive in a primitive environment represented by brief periods of caloric excess separated by periods of caloric deficiency and the need for endurance physical activity, such as chasing animals on the hunt.[8] Such a gene would allow humans to efficiently store excess calories in the form of body fat, which would be used at a later time when calories were not readily available in the diet. This genetic trait would allow maintenance of the body fat needed for women to menstruate and become pregnant and to help everyone in the tribe survive.

While such a genetic proclivity would be of great survival benefit in a primitive society, these survival genes may become deadly genes in a society represented by an abundance of calories and relative lack of physical activity. Further, if these high-risk CAD genes have a survival benefit, they must be relatively common compared to other genes that contribute to fatal medical problems. The hallmark of this disorder is the presence of multiple metabolic issues, which, under the pressure of the modern western lifestyle, lead to an increased risk of CAD. This chapter reviews the constellation of metabolic disorders that has recently been given the name "metabolic syndrome" but which has been part of the medical establishment for decades. Included in this discussion are the roles of excess body fat, diet, exercise, and some pharmacologic interventions.

METABOLIC SYNDROME

Definition

The metabolic syndrome, as defined by the Adult Treatment Panel III (ATP-III) of the National Cholesterol Education Program, includes three or more of the following: a dyslipidemia defined as fasting triglycerides > 150 mg/dL, high-density lipoprotein cholesterol (HDL-C) < 40 mg/dL in men and < 50 mg/dL in women, abdominal obesity as defined by a waist circumference > 40 in. in a man and > 35 in. in a woman, hypertension (≥130/≥85 mmHg), and insulin resistance as defined by fasting blood sugar (FBS) ≥ 110 mg/dL.[7] Since the metabolic syndrome and overweight status are so closely linked, it is of no surprise that approximately 20 to 25 percent of the U.S. population have the metabolic syndrome; in some groups, this figure approaches 50 percent.[9] The 2003 American Heart Association/American College of Cardiology (AHA/ACC) update for the management of chronic stable angina points to accumulating evidence that the risk for future CAD events can be reduced beyond that achieved by therapy to lower low-density lipoprotein cholesterol (LDL-C). It suggests that this can be done by modifying a specific secondary target of therapy, the metabolic syndrome, and recommends weight reduction and increased physical activity in persons with the metabolic syndrome or obesity.[10]

A second definition of the metabolic syndrome has been put forth by the World Health Organization (WHO), based on the European Group for the Study of Insulin Resistance; it includes hyperinsulinemia or elevated fasting glycemia and two or more of the following: abdominal obesity, dyslipidemia, or hypertension.[11] This alternative definition is useful, since the ATP-III definition is less consistently predictive of cardiovascular disease (CVD) and all-cause mortality.[12] The reason for this difference appears to be the use of a set waist circumference cutoff by the ATP-III definition compared to a waist-to-hip ratio in the WHO definition (Table 87-1). In the Kuopio Ischaemic Heart Disease Risk Factor Study, conducted in men free of CVD or diabetes, individuals with the metabolic syndrome as defined by the WHO or ATP-III were 2.9 to 4.2 times more likely to die of CAD after adjustment for conventional CV risk factors.[12]

The metabolic syndrome is characterized by physiologic complexity and strong statistical intercorrelation among its variables. The central role of insulin in the metabolic syndrome and syndrome X is generally accepted. Factor analysis (a multivariate correlation technique) of clustering of characteristics of syndrome X indicate that the syndrome is characterized by the linking of hyperinsulinemia, dyslipidemia, obesity, and hypertension which is independent of gender and age in both black and white populations.[13,14] However, factor analysis of the Framingham Offspring Study indicates that more than one independent physiologic process underlies the variability in clustering of the features of the metabolic syndrome.[15] It is important to appreciate that individuals can be insulin-resistant without meeting the ATP-III criteria for the metabolic syndrome. While hyperinsulinemia is a key component of the metabolic syndrome, it alone does not appear to underlie all features of the insulin-resistance syndrome.

History

The metabolic syndrome has a long history. The dyslipidemia associated with it is not a new discovery but dates back at least 50 years to Gofman's description in 1966 of a dyslipidemia, associated with elevated CAD risk characterized by an abundance of small, dense LDL and triglyceride-rich IDL and very low density lipoprotein (VLDL). This description was based on blood samples from the Berkekely–Lawrence Livermore and Framingham studies and recently linked to Reaven's description of the insulin-resistance syndrome as "syndrome X" in 1993.[16,17] However, as early as 1966, the potentially adverse effects of high-carbohydrate diets on triglycerides, in what later was to be termed the metabolic syndrome, was described by Farquhar and colleagues.[18,19] Additional credit must be given to Modan and colleagues, who, in 1985, described the relationship between hyperinsulinemia and insulin resistance and proposed the link between obesity, insulin resistance, hypertension, and glucose intolerance.[20]

Clinical Cardiovascular Impact

Dr. Gofman's analysis in 1966 of the Berkeley and Framingham samples resulted in an "atherogenic index" that predicted CAD risk and included aspects of the dylipidemia associated with the metabolic syndrome. Part of the atherogenic index was an abnormal abundance of LDL particles that were particularly small and dense; this was later termed the atherogenic lipoprotein profile (ALP) or LDL pattern B.[21] Over the years, many clinical trials have documented that the presence of an abundance of small LDL particles increases CAD risk threefold and is independent of most CV risk factors including LDL-C.[22] The presence of the metabolic syndrome is a strong predictor of CV risk and is particularly powerful in a population without elevated LDL-C. In the Turkish Adult Risk Factor Study, the metabolic syndrome was the major determinant of CAD risk and imposed an overall excess risk of approximately 70 percent.[23] In patients with established CAD, the presence of an abundance of small LDL particles portends a twofold greater rate of arteriographic progression but greater arteriographic benefit from treatment.[24] Change in LDL-C density or reduction in small LDL subclasses has been associated with arteriographic benefit.[25,26] The clinical importance of this knowledge lies in the fact that while the ATP-III criteria for a dyslipidemia (triglycerides > 150 mg/dL and HDL-C < 40 mg/dL in men and < 50 mg/dL in women) helps to identify individuals with this dys-

TABLE 87-1 ATP-III and WHO Criteria for the Definition of the Metabolic Syndrome*

ATP-III	Modified WHO
≥ 3 of the following:	Hyperinsulinemia (upper
Fasting glucose > 110 mg/dL	quartile of nondiabetic
Abdominal obesity:	population or FBS ≥ 110 mg/dL)
waist girth men > 40 in.	AND ≥ 2 of the following:
waist girth women > 35 in.	abdominal obesity:
Triglycerides ≥ 150 mg/dL	waist-hip >0.90 or BMI ≥ 30
HDL-C men < 40 mg/dL	Triglycerides ≥ 150 mg/dL
HDL-C women < 50 mg/dL	or HDL-C < 35 mg/dL
Blood pressure ≥ 130/85	Blood pressure ≥ 140/90
Prothrombotic and proinflammatory states	

*This table has been modified from Reference 12.

lipidemia, 34 percent of CAD patients with triglycerides between 100 and 150 mg/dL and HDL-C > 40 mg/dL still have an abundance of small LDL particles.[27]

Further clinical impact of the metabolic syndrome can be appreciated by the CV risk associated with other components of the metabolic syndrome, a 50 to 70 percent increased risk associated with obesity, and further increased risk associated with hypertension, insulin resistance, and disorders of the thrombotic system.[28] While each metabolic abnormality increases CAD risk by itself, the combination of disorders exponentially increases risk. This can be illustrated by the findings of the Quebec Cardiovascular Study, in which the presence of small LDL particles as the only metabolic abnormality increased CV risk threefold, while the combination of small LDL and elevated apolipoprotein B (apo B) increased CV risk sixfold, and the combined presence of small LDL and elevated apo B plus elevated fasting insulin levels increased CV risk 20-fold.[29]

OBESITY

Definition

Obesity has been defined as a BMI > 30.[7] (See Table 87-2.) However, reliance on a cut point for the definition of overweight status as it relates to CAD risk can be misleading. CAD risk increases even with a mild increase in BMI. In middle-aged women, a BMI > 23 but < 25 means a 50 percent increase in risk for nonfatal or fatal CAD; in middle-aged men, a BMI > 25 but < 29 means a 72 percent increase in risk.[30,31] Likewise, the use of waist circumference to define overweight status, as in ATP-III, can be misleading due to size and anthropomorphic characteristics of the individual subjects. Obesity is an individual excess amount of body fat that contributes to metabolic disturbances which, in turn, contribute to the risk of atherosclerosis.

Assessment of Body Fat

Many techniques are used to assess the degree of obesity as a percent of the total body mass represented by fat weight. Each technique has strengths and weaknesses. Hydrostatic weighing is the method historically used to assess percent body fat and is the "gold standard." However, limitations include the lack of information regarding anatomic fat location, the equipment necessary to accurately conduct an analysis involving not only an underwater weighing tank but also that needed to determine pulmonary residual volume by nitrogen dilution. In order to obtain an accurate measurement, subjects must hold their breath for 10 to 15 s on multiple runs. The test-retest variability is approximately +2.5 percent and varies significantly based on subject cooperation and technician discipline and/or experience. BMI is used frequently in the medical literature, in part because it is simple to determine. However, no indication of actual leanness or fatness can be determined, so there is a wide range of individual "fatness" within any one BMI range. BMI does not give an indication of where on the body the fat is carried. Skin fold measurements rely on multiple caliper determined skin fold thicknesses and a mathematical formula that approximates the calculated number to a percent body fat compared to hydrostatic weighing. One method requires the determination of seven sites: chest, triceps, subscapular area, axilla, suprailiac area, abdomen, and thigh. The validity of this method compared to hydrostatic weighing is approximately +6 percent. Girth measurements are easy to use and rely on the assumption that body fat is distributed at various sites on the body. Various girths are determined and used to calculate body fat. Accuracy is ±5 percent compared to hydrostatic weighing. One measure of the waist-to-hip ratio (WHR) is the circumference of the waist divided by the circumference of the hips, which takes into account abdominal obesity and may be a better predictor of the sequelae associated with adult obesity than BMI. A WHR > 1.0 in men and > 0.8 in women predicts the complications from obesity independent of BMI.[32] Bioelectrical impedance has been used since 1880 to measure conductivity in the body. Lean body tissue is more conductive due to its higher water content compared to fat tissue. The more lean tissue there is, the greater the conductive potential measured in ohms. This method uses linear regression formulas to predict body fat, which appears to be valid for a "normal" population but underpredicts body fat for obese subjects and overpredicts body fat for lean subjects. The accuracy is approximately ±5-6 percent. Perhaps the most clinically useful tool is the well established "pinch an inch" concept, where overweight status is determined if there is more than 1 in. of fat when the layer of skin near the umbilicus is pinched.

Clinical Cardiovascular Impact

Obesity has long been linked to increase CAD risk. As noted above, one population group that has a 60 to 70 percent increase in obesity over the course of 7 years comprises relatively young individuals aged 18 to 29 years.[5] This is of concern, since the Pathobiological Determinants of Atherosclerosis in Youth (PDAY) study has reported that in approximately 3000 individuals aged 15 to 34 years who died of causes other than CVD, autopsy evidence of raised lesions in the right coronary artery (RCA) and stenosis in the left anterior descending artery (LAD), was greatest in male subjects with a BMI > 30 kg/m² and those with increased panniculus thickness.[33] This relationship was not seen in women. The increase in obesity in the young is of particular concern, since weight gain during childhood, rather than absolute childhood weight, is a determinant of adult CV risk.[34] This rate of weight gain and increase in body mass and CV risk factors is particularly powerful for fasting insulin values in young adulthood and significantly associated with the rate of change of BMI ($r = 0.29, p < 0.0001$).

PATHOPHYSIOLOGY AND CARDIOVASCULAR-RELATED ISSUES

Pathophysiology

Underlying the metabolic syndrome is the condition of insulin resistance. An understanding the role of the adipocyte in the metabolic syndrome and insulin resistance is key to understanding the impact of overweight and obesity on CVD. Body fat stores can be divided into two main endocrine organs for purposes of discussing the

TABLE 87-2 BMI Definitions of Overweight and Obesity[146]

	BMI
Normal weight	18.5–24.9 kg/m²
Overweight	5–29
Obesity	> 30.0
Obesity class I	30.0–34.9
Obesity class II	35.9–39.9
Obesity class III	>50

metabolic syndrome: central and visceral adiposity. The most metabolically harmful adipose stores appear to be visceral, which contribute more to insulin resistance than does subcutaneous obesity.[35] This observation is what has led to the lay concept that individuals with an "apple-shaped" body morphology are at higher CAD risk than those with the "pear-shaped" body morphology. However, this concept is open to wide interpretation.

Adipose tissue functions primarily as an energy storage unit. In the physiologically nonoverweight condition, this function results in few or no adverse metabolic issues. However, when excess free fatty acid (FFA) turnover is present, as in obesity, multiple metabolic disruptions occur that contribute to CAD risk. Increased FFA flux inhibits lipolysis by insulin, and the increased FFA availability can result in lipotoxicity, increased inflammatory markers, increased angiotensin II, enhanced prothrombotic state, and lipoprotein disorders. High levels of FFA increases oxidative stress and reduces NO synthesis.[36] The term *lipotoxicity* describes the toxic effects of an abundance of triglycerides and FFA on normal cell health. Excess FFA contributes to cardiac myocyte apoptosis, which can be evident in the myocardium and conduction system.[37] Advanced glycation end products (AGEs) play a major role in the atherosclerosis associated with diabetes and the metabolic syndrome.[38] AGEs can crosslink macromolecules and promote vessel wall stiffness. They can also form part of the trapped matrix that forms the atherogenic plaque, and they can trigger a local inflammatory response. AGEs can be produced as part of normal physiologic function. However, the presence of sugars or phospholipids, as characterized by the metabolic syndrome, accelerates glycoxidation reactions and may become a chronic condition that promotes atherosclerosis.

This is of relevance to the cardiologist, since the process that eventually results in a fatty streak, mature atherosclerosis, and an unstable plaque involves a multi-factorial process that provides multiple treatment opportunities. In a healthy state, the endothelial cell layer acts to separate circulating compounds from the arterial intima and media wall. When circulating factors, such as those comprising the metabolic syndrome, are present for prolonged periods of time, the endothelial border loses its protective nature. Factors that contribute to the loss of endothelial border integrity include modified lipoproteins that are susceptible to oxidative damage; after crossing the endothelial border, these lipoproteins bind to matrix molecules such as collagen and proteoglycans.[39,40] The ALP, which is characteristic of the metabolic syndrome, is particularly damaging in this regard, since the small LDL particle allows endothelial penetration 50 percent faster than large LDLs, is more susceptible to oxidative damage, and binds more avidly to proteoglycan than large LDL particles.[41] In addition, reverse cholesterol transport is adversely affected by abnormalities of HDL composition and function.[42] This process leads to increased production of procoagulants, adhesion molecules, chemotatic factors, and cytokines, promoting monocyte infiltration into the artery wall, with resultant differentiation into macrophages. The scavenger receptor on the macrophage consumes modified lipoproteins at a rapid rate and eventually develops into a fatty streak and then a mature atherosclerotic lesion; thereafter, with the development of a necrotic lipid core and thin fibrous cap, plaque rupture and an often fatal CV event can ensue.

The Small-LDL Trait

A major sequel of the overweight status is a dyslipidemia characterized by low HDL-C, elevated triglycerides, and an abundance of small, dense LDLs; together, these constitute the ALP.[21] ALP contributes to increased atherosclerosis risk through a variety of associations, all or only a few of which may be present at any one time in an individual. These associations include increased throboxane synthesis, increased postprandial lipemia, increased proteoglycan binding, increased insulin resistance, reduced HDL2b, reduced phospholipase A2, increased oxidative susceptibility, and increased LDL uptake into the artery wall.[43–50] ALP is associated with insulin resistance and may be particularly relevant since the presence of the small LDL trait has been reported to be a predictor for the development of type 2 diabetes mellitus.[51] The excess FFA flux results in increased VLDL–apo B secretion, which, in the presence of obesity-related hepatic lipase activity, results in an abundance of the atherogenic small LDLs and reduced levels of HDL2b, reflecting impaired reverse cholesterol transport.

Early studies reported a relation between fasting triglycerides, HDL-C, and LDL peak particle diameter.[52] While this statistical relationship is valid, attention to correlation coefficients alone can be clinically misleading. Figure 87-1 illustrates the relationship between fasting triglycerides and LDL peak particle diameter in 544 patients with fasting triglycerides < 500 mg/dL, as seen at the Cardiology of Georgia medical practice. While

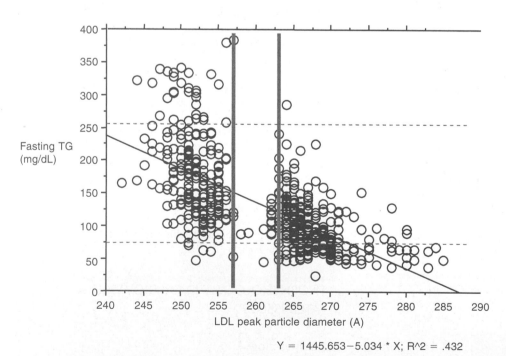

$$Y = 1445.653 - 5.034 * X; R^2 = .432$$

FIGURE 87-1 Fasting triglycerides and the relationship to LDL peak particle diameter (angstroms) in 525 patients with established CAD. Large LDL diameter is > 263 Å and small LDL diameter < 257 Å. Mean (±SD) fasting triglycerides in large LDL pattern Å subjects = 92 ± 35 mg/dL and in small LDL pattern B subjects = 187 ± 67 mg/dL. While the mathematical relationship between fasting triglycerides and LDL peak particle diameter is valid, there is significant overlap within the triglyceride range of 75 to 250 mg/dL, which renders the use of fasting triglycerides as a surrogate marker of LDL peak particle diameter problematic for accurate individual patient management.

most subjects with fasting triglycerides greater than 250 mg/dL express small LDL particles and most subjects with fasting triglycerides less than 75 mg/dL express large LDL particles, patients with fasting triglycerides between 75 and 250 mg/dL (73 percent of the patients) have a wide overlap between triglyceride level and LDL peak particle diameter, which makes the use of fasting triglycerides within this fasting triglyceride range unreliable as clinical marker of small LDL in individual patient management. A similar relationship holds for HDL-C in that, in general, values < 35 mg/dL are often associated with small LDL particles and values > 65 mg/dL are often associated with large LDL particles, but patients with HDL-C in the range of 35 to 65 mg/dL have a wide range of LDL particle size. The unreliability of triglycerides and HDL-C to predict LDL size and the fact that 40 percent of subjects have an LDL profile with at least one second LDL peak that is more than half the height of the primary peak has led to the use of percent distribution in seven LDL subclasses as a reflection of the extent of small-LDL expression. LDL I is the largest, followed by progressively smaller LDLs IIa and IIb. Small LDLs start with IIIa, followed by progressively smaller IIIb, IVa, and IVb.[53]

The assessment of these specific subclasses has become clinically important, since they have been reported to be independently associated with impaired vasoreactivity, and carotid intima-media thickness and progression (Fig. 87-2).[54,55] Several large clinical trials—and including the Boston Heart Study, the Stanford Five City Project, the Harvard Physician's Health Study, and the Quebec Cardiovascular Study— have indicated that LDL peak particle diameter is a significant predictor of CAD events in healthy populations.[56–59] LDL peak particle diameter is an independent marker of threefold increased CV risk.[60]

Arteriographic studies have also reported that the presence of small LDL identifies CAD patients with rapid arteriographic progression; with proper treatment, however, this group exhibits the most arteriographic benefit.[61–64] Most recently, two arteriographic investigations, the Stanford Coronary Risk Intervention Project and the Emory Angioplasty versus Surgery Trial, have reported that small LDL particles independently predict arteriographic progression and new lesion formation. It has therefore been recommended that these measurements be incorporated into clinical practice.[65,66]

Syndrome X

In 1988, prior to the 2001 ATP-III description of the metabolic syndrome, the constellation of abnormalities likely to appear as manifestations of a defect in insulin action was designated as syndrome X.[67] A defect in insulin action, as a component of ALP, was reported in 1993.[46] Individuals with an abundance of small LDL particles have significantly higher insulin values after a glucose load than those with predominantly large LDL particles. Thus, the term *metabolic syndrome X* has been used to describe a major component of the ATP-III–defined metabolic syndrome. However, syndrome X, insulin resistance, and the metabolic syndrome are not synonymous, and the term *syndrome X* has given way to the term *insulin resistance*.

Insulin Resistance

The term *insulin resistance* describes a metabolic state in which insulin's action in the peripheral tissues is less efficient than normal, which results in increased insulin secretion in order to maintain normal blood glucose levels. Insulin resistance, a major component of the metabolic syndrome, is of particular interest to cardiologists because of a link to restenosis following angioplasty and stent placement.

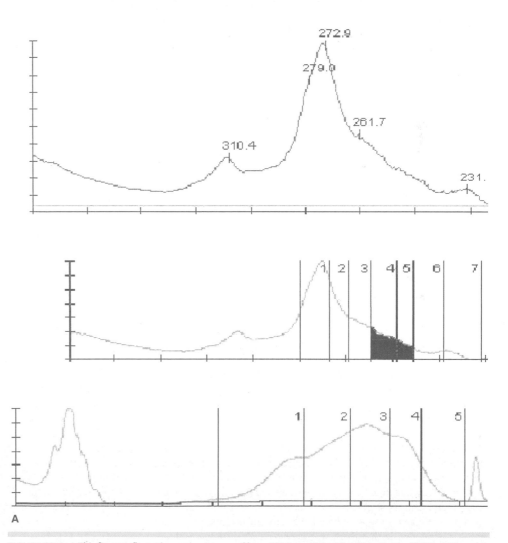

A

FIGURE 87-2 *A.* This figure reflects the predominance of large LDL in an LDL pattern A patient with Trig 100 mg/dL, LDL-C 148 mg/dL, HDL 51 mg/dL. The distribution of all LDLs are distributed within the 7 columns. 1, 2, and 3 are large LDL regions, while 4, 5, 6, 7 are small LDL regions. The peak LDL particle diameter is 272.9 angstroms and only 12.3 percent of the LDL is in the small LDL region IIIa (region 4) and IIIb (region 5) (blackened). HDL subclass distribution is represented on the bottom tracing, and column 1 represents HDL2b. In this case 14 percent of the HDLs are in the HDL2b region. *B.* This figure reflects the predominance of small LDL in an LDL pattern B patient with Trig 173 mg/dL, LDL-C 116 mg/dL, HDL-C 41 mg/dL. The peak LDL particle diameter is 247.9 angstroms with a secondary peak in the large region at 264.1 angstroms and 43.4 percent of the LDL in the small LDL region IIIa (region 4) and IIIb (region 5) (blackened); 10 percent of the HDLs are in the HDL2b region.

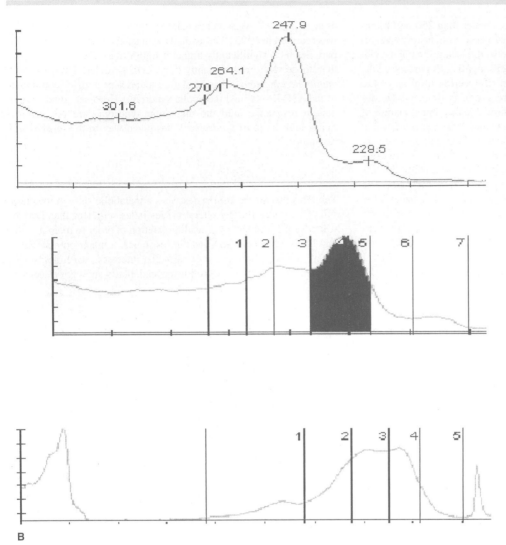

B

FIGURE 87-2 (Continued)

It is established that insulin promotes smooth muscle replication in cell culture and animal models.[68] Its important role in humans has recently been elucidated by reports that levels of insulin after a glucose load are significantly higher in patients who have undergone percutaneous coronary angioplasty (PTCA) and experienced stent restenosis compared with those who do not exhibit restenosis.[69,70] In those who, on 3.5-month repeat angiography, showed a > 50 percent loss of diameter gain, the integration of insulin concentrations (μU/mL), over the period of a 3-h oral glucose tolerance test was significantly higher in the restenosis group compared to the no restenosis group ($p = 0.01$).[69] Following Palmaz-Schatz stent placement, those with a significantly greater level of neointimal formation 6 months later had significantly higher fasting (7.7 vs. 4.7 μU/mL) insulin and 2-h post-glucose-load insulin level (98.3 vs. 44.1 μU/mL) compared to those with a lower level of neointimal formation.[70] Of interest is that there was no difference in fasting blood sugar (98 vs. 97 mg/dL) between the groups, which indicates that a test of the fasting blood sugar is not adequate to detect this condition of high restenosis risk. Of additional interest is the elevated postglucose insulin response observed in the patients having the "B" pattern of small LDL compared with similarly elevated postglucose insulin levels in PTCA or stent patients who exhibited restenosis.[17] Following a standard glucose load, individuals with the large LDL "A" pat-

tern trait had a 1-h post-glucose-load insulin level of approximately 59 μU/mL, compared to approximately 115 μU/mL in the individuals having the "B" pattern of small LDL. This can be compared to the 1-h level of approximately 65 μU/mL in those free of restenosis, compared to approximately 110 μU/mL in patients who had undergone PTCA. Thus, elevated post-glucose-load insulin values not only mark the insulin-resistant condition but are also linked to the atherogenic small-LDL trait and restenosis risk.

The statistical relationship between the ATP-III criteria for the metabolic syndrome and insulin resistance can be misinterpreted.[71] While obesity is related to insulin resistance, the European Group for the Study of Insulin Resistance has concluded, based on insulin-mediated glucose disposal in 1100 subjects, that only about 25 percent of obese individuals can be classified as insulin-resistant. Thus, not all overweight individuals are insulin-resistant and not all insulin-resistant individuals are overweight, as illustrated in Fig. 87-3.

Insulin resistance is determined in the research laboratory with the euglycemic insulin clamp technique. This involves continuous intravenous administration of insulin and glucose over a 3 h period, after which insulin sensitivity is calculated by measuring the amount of glucose required to maintain normal glucose levels. This method is not practical for clinical purposes. Although fasting plasma insulin concentrations are less accurate than the values obtained from the euglycemic clamp technique, the former provide a reasonable clinical alternative. Values < 15 mU/L are considered normal, 15 to 20 mU/L borderline high, and > 20 mU/L high.[72] Laboratory insulin methods are not standardized on a national level, as is total cholesterol, and laboratory methodology and standardization must be considered in the interpretation of individual patient values. Fasting glucose between 110 and 126 mg/dL is predictive of insulin resistance, but it is not a sensitive marker and most subjects with insulin resistance have a fasting glucose < 110 mg/dL. While hypertension is statistically associated with insulin resistance, it also has poor sensitivity. Although not absolute, the most sensitive clinical marker appears to be the triglyceride/HDL-C ratio.

Type 2 Diabetes

The development of overt type 2 diabetes mellitus is the eventual outcome for many patients with the metabolic syndrome. The increased CAD risk associated with type 2 diabetes is now well established. Multiple large clinical studies—including the Framingham Study, the Israeli Ischemic Heart Study, the Whitehall Study, the Paris Prospective Study, the Finnish Social Insurance Institute Study, the Gothenburg Population Study, and the Multiple Risk Intervention Trial—have consistently reported an increased CAD risk of 1.5 to 3.0 in diabetic patients. Autopsy studies in type 2 diabetics without clinical CAD have revealed that 79 percent of men and 70 percent of women have a high-grade coronary lesion.[73] The ATP-III has classified type 2 diabetes as a CAD equivalent, which affords it treatment implications similar to those of CAD.

The presence of type 2 diabetes has major implications for CV procedures. Repeat revascularization following stent placement is significantly higher in diabetic versus nondiabetic patients. The National Heart, Lung, and Blood Institute (NHLBI) dynamic registry has reported that repeat revascularization was needed in 17.2 percent of diabetic patients requiring stent placement, compared to 10.1 percent for nondiabetics (RR 1.77, 95 percent CI 1.38 to 2.26).[74]

A major metabolic characteristic of type 2 diabetes is a dyslipidemia that is often identical to the metabolic syndrome and the ALP trait.[75] This is of interest because small LDL has been shown to be a significant predictor of the development of type 2 diabetes.[51] The relevance of this lies in the finding that the arteriographic severity in type 2 diabetics is significantly ($p < 0.01$) related to the presence of intermediate-density and triglyceride-rich lipoproteins (Sf12-60), which are a characteristic of ALP.[76]

Since type 2 diabetes is considered a CAD equivalent, prevention or delay in the onset of type 2 diabetes may be considered a productive step in the prevention or delay of CAD. It is recommended that individuals over the age of 45 years with a BMI > 25 kg/m^2 be screened to detect prediabetes.[77] Four well-designed randomized trials justify an approach to detecting high-risk individuals and provide intervention, because this can facilitate a significant reduction in the development of type 2 diabetes.[77] In the Finnish study, 3.2 years of intensive individualized instruction on weight reduction, diet, and exercise in obese subjects with impaired glucose tolerance resulted in a 58 percent reduction in the incidence of diabetes.[78] In the Diabetes Prevention Program (DPP), 2.8 years of treatment with either intensive diet and exercise or metformin in obese glucose-intolerant subjects resulted in a 58 percent relative reduction in diabetes in the lifestyle intervention group and a 31 percent reduction in the metformin group.[79] The Troglitazone in Prevention of Diabetes (TRIPOD) study treated Hispanic women

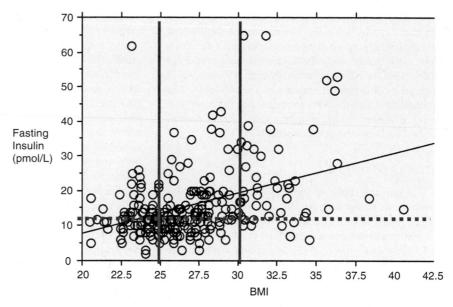

$$Y = -15.228 + 1.156 * X; R^2 = .164$$

A

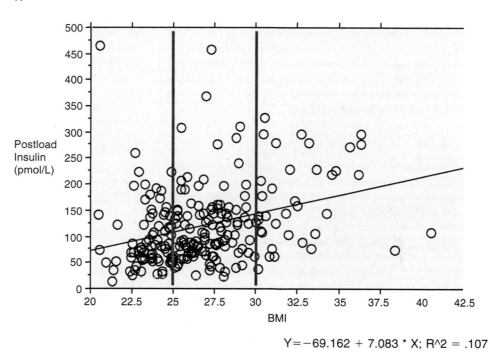

$$Y = -69.162 + 7.083 * X; R^2 = .107$$

B

FIGURE 87-3 The relationship between BMI and fasting insulin levels (A) and post-glucose-load insulin levels (B) in 246 subjects in the Stanford Coronary Risk Intervention Project. Defining overweight status as a BMI > 25 but < 30 (solid line), and obesity as > 30 (solid line), the relationship between insulin levels and BMI can be appreciated. Mean ($\pm$SD) fasting insulin = 16.1 $\pm$ 10.3 pmol/L and postglucose load = 120.6 $\pm$ 75.8 pmol/L. Fasting insulin > 12 pmol/L has been associated with increased CAD risk (dotted line). While a valid statistical relationship between insulin and BMI exists, for the majority of individual patients, in the middle range, the relationship is too scattered to be of clinical use.

with previous gestational diabetes with troglitazone for 30 months, and a 56 percent relative reduction in diabetes was reported.[80] The STOP-NIDDM study treated obese subjects with impaired glucose tolerance with the α-glucosidase inhibitor acabose for 3.3 years and reported a 25 percent reduction in realtive risk for progression to diabetes.[81] Thus, with either intensive lifestyle or pharmacologic intervention, significant reductions (25 to 58 percent) in the appearance of type 2 diabetes in high risk individuals can be achieved. The number needed to treat (NNT) in order to prevent one case of progression to type 2 diabetes is surprisingly low. In the Finnish study, the NNT to prevent one case in 5 years was 5; in the DPP, the NNT to prevent one case in 3 years was 7; with metformin, the NNT to prevent one case in 3 years was 14. This compares quite favorably with the NNT to prevent one CV event with LDL-C–lowering treatment, which is approximately 26 in patients without established CAD and 7 in post-MI patients.[82,83]

Left Ventricular Dysfunction

Heart failure is a growing cause of significant CV morbidity and mortality. Components of the metabolic syndrome are associated with LV changes linked to heart failure and predict long-term development of ventricular dysfunction. A link exists between aspects of heart failure and aspects of the metabolic syndrome. In hypertensive patients, LV wall thickness is related to blood pressure ($r = 0.4$, $p < 0.004$) and independently related to insulin sensitivity ($r = -0.59$, $p < 0.0001$), indicating that LV hypertrophy and diastolic dysfunction are associated with the insulin-resistance metabolic syndrome.[84] In a 20-year follow-up of middle-aged men, factors associated with insulin resistance were found to precede LV systolic dysfunction independently of CAD and hypertension.[85] In young individuals, fasting insulin is an independent predictor ($p < 0.02$) of LV mass, indexed by height, and indicates that an excessive load on the heart relatively early in life is associated with the metabolic syndrome even after accounting for the effects of race, gender, and blood pressure.[86] For this reason it has been suggested that LV dysfunction is a part of the insulin resistance syndrome.

Hypertension

Elevations in blood pressure have long been noted to be associated with an overweight status, but the link between the metabolic syndrome and hypertension is less well understood than the dyslipidemia and prothrombotic aspects. The link between hypertension and the metabolic syndrome is tightly linked to the central adiposity component of the syndrome. The Olivetti Heart Study has reported that waist circumference was the strongest independent predictor of blood pressure ($p < 0.001$) and its association with increased blood pressure was independent of BMI and insulin resistance.[87]

Leptin

Leptin, a hormone secreted from adipocytes, has an action on the central hypothalamic nuclei that affects the consumption of calories and expenditure of body energy. A rich field of research exists in mouse models, but the exact role that leptin plays in human obesity and CV risk remains unclear. Much like insulin resistance, the concept of leptin resistance has been discussed. Leptin resistance implies that elevated levels of circulating leptin are often found in obese individuals and that the resistance may be tissue- and individual-specific.[88] One important insight from leptin research that helps clarify the mechanism of obesity-associated thrombosis risk is the finding that leptin increases platelet aggregation and arterial thrombosis.[89]

Inflammation

Various components of the inflammatory response play important roles in the development and progression of atherosclerosis. Adipose tissue is a source of inflammatory mediators such as cytokines, tumor necrosis factor alpha (TNF-α), and interleukin-6.[90] This proinflammatory state is characterized by elevated high-sensitivity C-reactive protein (hs-CRP), which, in 7 prospective investigations, was found to contribute to clinical CV events.[91] It remains unclear if the association of elevated CRP and atherosclerosis is an epiphenomenon or if CRP itself is involved in the initiation and progression of atherosclerosis. Several studies have described a relation between plasma CRP and fasting insulin concentrations in both type 2 diabetic patients and in nondiabetic, insulin-resistant patients, indicating that elevated levels of inflammatory markers such as CRP, fibrinogen, and plasminogen activator-1 are components of the insulin-resistant or metabolic syndrome.[92] Further, the Insulin Resistance Athersclerosis Study (IRAS) has shown that in insulin-resistant subjects, there is a linear relationship between CRP level and the number of components of the metabolic syndrome present, which include dyslipidemia, upper-body adiposity, insulin resistance, and hypertension.[92] The greater the number of components, the higher the CRP.

The link between overweight status, insulin resistance, and elevated CRP is not consistent or direct. In individuals who are obese but classified as either insulin-resistant (IR) or insulin-sensitive by a modification of the insulin suppression test before and after weight loss, CRP was found to correlate with insulin resistance but not BMI or waist circumference.[93] Weight loss was achieved in both the IR and non-IR group but was associated with a significant reduction in CRP only in the IR group. Thus, the association of elevated CRP is found primarily in IR obese subjects and the benefit of weight loss in regard to CRP reduction was noted primarily in IR obese subjects who lost weight but not in obese subjects who were not IR and lost weight. Four possible explanations for the association of markers of inflammation with the insulin-resistance syndrome have been proposed.[92] First, the association may reflect an inflammatory trigger to insulin resistance and type 2 diabetes; second, elevated CRP could be the result of the atherosclerotic process; third, decreased insulin sensitivity could enhance CRP expression; and fourth, adipose tissue derived cytokines could be the trigger for this process.

Thrombotic Issues

An important component of the metabolic syndrome is dysfunction within the atherorthrombosis system. This dysfunction includes aspects of both fibrinolysis and thrombosis. Contributing to the atherosclerotic process are disorders of the fibrinolytic system. Fibrinolysis can be suppressed due to elevated plasminogen activator inhibitor (PAI)-1 concentrations, increased factor VII, fibrinogen, and von Willebrand factor, all of which have been linked to the development of myocardial infarction.[94,95] Increased PAI-1 is associated with the insulin-resistance syndrome and atherosclerosis and atherothrombotic risk.[96] Increased PAI-1 overexpression is a direct effect of insulin, and pharmacologic reduction in insulin levels has been reported to reduce PAI-1 levels and improve carotid wall intimal medial thickness.[97,98] A causative link between atherothrombosis and inflammation exists in the observation CRP induces PAI-1 expression and activity in human aortic endothelial cells.[99]

Enhanced thrombosis risk has been linked to fibrinogen, factor VII, factor VIII, and von Willebrand factor in the setting of components of the metabolic syndrome. Elevated fibrinogen levels are linked to increased CAD risk. The Atherosclerosis Risk in Communities (ARIC) study has presented evidence that fibrinogen levels are linked to attributes of the metabolic syndrome, including body size, fasting insulin, diabetes, and inversely with HDL-C.[100] In the Framingham Study, an increase in plasma fibrinogen was found to increase CV risk substantially; for each 56 mg/dL increase in fibrinogen level, CV risk increases approximately 20 percent.[101]

Elevation in factor VII levels are often noted in association with features of the insulin-resistance syndrome and increases in proportion to postprandial hyperlipidemia.[102,103] Subjects with the dyslipidemia identified with the metabolic syndrome have enhanced postprandial lipemia, which creates the setting for chronic elevations in factor VII during the postprandial state, which comprises approximately 70 percent of the day.[44] The ARIC study has revealed that factor VIII and von Willebrand factor are associated with attributes of the metabolic syndrome, including BMI, waist-to-hip ratio, serum insulin, and triglycerides.[104] Similar findings were reported from the Framingham Offspring Study, which found that von Willebrand factor, factor VII, PAI-1, and tissue plasminogen activator were increased across fasting insulin quintiles in subjects with normal glucose tolerance.[105]

Insulin resistance adversely affects platelet function. Insulin receptors are located on platelets and play a role in normal platelet function. Insulin appears to inhibit platelet aggregation in healthy nonobese individuals.[106] Obese and nonobese individuals have a different insulin/platelet interaction. In nonobese individuals, insulin inhibits platelet deposition on collagen, but it does not have this effect in obese individuals and does not increase platelet cyclic guanosine monophosphate, as it does in nonobese individuals.[107]

Advanced glycosylation end-products (AGEs) play an important role in the atherothrombotic process and are clinically relevant in the type 2 diabetes and the insulin-resistance metabolic milieu. Glucose can react with an amino group of a protein to produce AGEs, of which hemoglobin A1c is the best known. AGEs act as molecular binding agents that promote atherosclerosis by contributing to an inflammatory response, smooth muscle cell hypertrophy, vessel wall stiffness, cell adhesion, and eventually platelet activation.[108]

Endothelial Dysfunction

Endothelial dysfunction can be defined as an impaired response to endothelium-dependent vasodilators and has been reported to be present in patients with type 2 diabetes, insulin resistance, and obesity.[109] Insulin promotes production of nitrous oxide (NO) within the endothelium, but this response is blunted in subjects with diabetes or insulin resistance.[110] Atherogenic components of the metabolic syndrome have been linked to endothelial dysfunction. Assessment of forearm blood flow in healthy subjects has revealed that individuals with small LDL exhibit a significantly impaired blood flow response to acetylcholine infusion and that the association is independent of triglycerides, LDL-C, and HDL-C.[111]

Nonalcoholic Steatohepatitis

Nonalcoholic steatohepatitis (NASH) comprises a spectrum of conditions characterized by macrovesicular fatty change in the liver associated with an absence of alcohol consumption, which would be considered detrimental to the liver. It is associated with increasing fibrosis, which may proceed to cirrhosis.[112] It is now considered that insulin resistance is the fundamental operative mechanism as the first step in the development of NASH and that oxidative stress is the second.[113] Clinical characteristics associated with NASH include obesity, hyperlipidemia, diabetes mellitus, and hypertension, all of which have been associated with impaired insulin signaling and elevated insulin levels.[114] NASH is the second most common chronic liver disease in the United States, with a prevalence of approximately 3 percent. Liver biopsy is often required to make the diagnosis. Treatment is not well established but includes gradual reduction of excess body fat, control of hyperlipidemia, improvement of insulin sensitivity, and antioxidants.[115] Polyunsaturated fatty acids (PUFA) may play an important role in this process, as they increase fatty acid oxidation by acting as ligand activators of PPAR-α and induce the transcription of genes affiliated with fatty acid oxidation.[116]

TREATMENT

The treatment of the metabolic syndrome should not focus on a single variable but entail a multifactorial approach that includes lifestyle modification directed to the individual disorder and, if necessary, pharmacologic intervention. It must be stressed that the effectiveness of pharmacologic intervention is greatly enhanced by even modest lifestyle improvements. The clinical relevance of multifactorial intervention has been highlighted by the significant 50 percent reduction in CV and microvascular events in type 2 diabetic patients with microalbuminuria who were treated with multifactorial intervention as opposed to conventional therapy.[117]

Weight Loss and Exercise

Energy balance is the foundation for management of the metabolic syndrome and obesity. This involves the amount and type of dietary calories consumed each day balanced against the energy expenditure through physical activity. Mathematical models exist to assist in the approximation of calories necessary to sustain human life under various levels of activity. An individual's metabolic rate is the resting metabolic rate plus the number of calories consumed by daily activities, which can vary widely from person to person. One equation to determine the resting metabolic rate (RMR) in kilocalories is the Harris-Benedict equation:

$$\text{Men: RMR} = 66.473 + 13.751 \times \text{BW} + 5.0033 \times \text{HT} - 6.755 \times \text{age}$$

$$\text{Women: RMR} = 655.0955 + 9.463 \times \text{BW} + 1.8496 \times \text{HT} - 4.6756 \times \text{age}$$

where BW = body weight in kilograms, HT = height in centimeters, and age is given in years. To determine the total daily metabolic rate, the number of calories spent in physical activity must be added and can be approximated by adding an additional 15 percent for men and women who are sedentary; an additional 40 and 35 percent for men and women, respectively, doing light activity; an additional 50 and 45 percent, respectively, for men and women doing moderate activity; an additional 85 and 70 percent, respectively, for men and women who are very active (such as full-time athletes or forestry and mine workers); and 110 and 100 percent, respectively, for men and women who are exceptionally active, such as lumberjacks.

Loss of excess body fat is the foundation of treatment of the metabolic syndrome. The beneficial metabolic effects of fat weight loss is different in insulin-resistant and insulin-sensitive patients. Obese women characterized as insulin-resistant by the insulin suppression test who loose weight significantly reduce their fasting triglyceride concentrations and day-long concentrations of plasma glucose and insulin, while obese women who are not insulin-resistant yet achieve the same weight loss, do not.[93] Direct identification of the metabolic insulin-resistant state allows identification of subjects who have the best metabolic response to weight reduction. The amount of weight loss that can result in significant health benefit is surprisingly low.

Long-term studies have shown that a sustained, moderate weight reduction of approximately 10 percent improves glycemic control by improving insulin resistance and is associated with better control of hypertension, increased HDL-C, decreased LDL-C, and decreased triglycerides.[118] These metabolic benefits are most marked in obese subjects and those with visceral fat accumulation. In the Finnish study and the Diabetes Prevention Program, weight reduction of 5 to 7 percent was typical, and 74 percent of subjects maintained at least 150 min/week of moderate physical activity. This amount of lifestyle modification significantly reduced the onset of type 2 diabetes over a period of approximately 3 years.[78,79] Side effects from lifestyle modification are minimal.

One possible therapy for weight reduction and improvement in the metabolic syndrome is gastric surgery. Gastric surgery, such as the Swedish adjustable gastric banding method, has been suggested as a possible therapy for the metabolic syndrome in obese subjects. This procedure has been reported to reduce BMI from a mean ($\pm$SD) of 43.3 ± 6.9 to 34.5 ± 7.4 ($p < 0.001$) 1 year after surgery and was associated with a significant ($p < 0.001$) reduction in insulin resistance and the prevalence of the metabolic syndrome (58.8 percent decreasing to 21.6 percent).[119] The beneficial effect of gastric surgery on CV outcomes in patients with established CAD is well documented by the Program On the Surgical Control of the Hyperlipidemias (POSCH), trial in which the distal 200 cm of the small intestine was bypassed, with restoration of bowel continuity by an end-to-side ileocecostomy in patients who had experienced a previous myocardial infarction.[120] LDL-C was reduced approximately 38 percent and lipoprotein A1 and HDL-C increased significantly.[121] After 5 years, CV endpoints were reduced significantly; at 18 years of follow-up, significant ($p < 0.05$ to 0.001) reductions in overall mortality, coronary atherosclerosis mortality, nonfatal myocardial infarction, and the need for coronary artery bypass grafting were observed.

Diet

In addition to physical activity, proper diet modification and reduction of excess dietary calories is the second foundation for treatment of the metabolic syndrome. Diet composition can affect insulin secretion and the probability of expressing hyperinsulinemia. The Coronary Artery Risk Development in Young Adults (CADIA) study examined 2909 individuals 18 to 30 years old and found a powerful link between dietary fiber, blood pressure, plasma triglycerides, HDL-C, LDL-C, and fibrinogen. However, compared to dietary fat, carbohydrates, and protein, fiber had a more powerful association with these metabolic disorders linked to CAD risk.[122] Fiber consumption predicted (inversely) insulin levels, weight gain, and other CVD risk factors more strongly than did total or saturated fat consumption. Fat-substitute products for dietary consumption reduce total blood cholesterol a minor amount and have the potential to reduce excess body fat. However, a report from the AHA Nutrition Committee concludes that factors affecting energy balance, specifically portion size control and physical activity, are likely to have a greater impact on weight than does the use of fat-modified products. That is, substitution of low-fat for full-fat products may not be effective in lowering body weight if other strategies for weight control are not implemented.[123] The increase in overweight and the metabolic syndrome may be linked to the finding that in 1995, some 150 lb of sugar were consumed each year per adult in the United States, compared to 120 lb per year in 1970. In 1995, simple sugars averaged 25 percent of the average American's diet calories.[124]

Some debate has arisen regarding the CV benefit of very low carbohydrate and high-protein diets. This debate is often clouded by the short-term weight loss associated with high-protein diets compared to the high amounts of carbohydrates often seen with low-fat diets. A focus on reduced-fat diets often results in diets higher in carbohydrates as a source of calories, and when these are simple carbohydrates, there is an adverse effect on CV risk. For this reason, the AHA has recommended that a high intake of sugar be avoided.[124] Even with no change in daily calories or physical activity level, consumption of a diet with a greater percentage of calories derived from carbohydrates results in an increase in triglycerides, a reduction in HDL-C, and an increased expression of the small-LDL trait.[125] Diet carbohydrates vary considerably in their effect on increasing blood sugar. They have been classified based on a glycemic index (GI) based on the rise in blood sugar compared with glucose or white bread with a standard carbohydrate content of 50 g.[126] Consumption of meals with lower GI scores can result in improved blood sugar control and lipid profiles.

Dietary fats can be simply classified into saturated, monounsaturated, and polyunsaturated. Consumption of diets rich in saturated fats increases LDL-C but also increases HDL-C and reduces triglycerides. Consumption of diets rich in mono- or polyunsaturated fats results in a modest decrease in LDL-C, a slightly lower increase in HDL-C, and a reduction in triglycerides compared to saturated fats.[127] Some polyunsaturated fats in the diets appear to have adverse CV health consequences. Trans fatty acids (often found in stick margarine and bakery goods) increase LDL-C and Lp(a).[128] Four clinical studies indicate that consumption of trans fatty acids in the diet is associated with a significant increase in CV risk.[127] The consumption of omega-3 fatty acids has been associated with reduced CV risk in 16 studies.[127] This may be particularly important in patients with established CAD. The Diet and Reinfarction Trial, the GISSI-Prevention trial, the India fish and mustard oil study, and the Lyon Diet Heart Study all strongly suggest that diets enriched in omega-3 fatty acids are associated with improved coronary outcomes.[129–132] Garlic supplementation appears to have no significant effect on lipoprotein metabolism that could benefit CAD risk.[133]

Moderate alcohol consumption in general has been associated with reduced CV risk in epidemiologic studies even in patients with type 2 diabetes.[134] The Insulin Resistance and Atherosclerosis Study (IRAS) has reported that a U-shaped relationship exists between alcohol consumption and measures of insulin resistance, so that the greatest degree of insulin sensitivity was found in subjects whose self-reported drinking consisted of approximately 18.6 g/day or ~1.5 drinks per day.[135] This was associated with the lowest BMI and smallest waist circumference, so that the improved insulin sensitivity associated with alcohol consumption may be a function of BMI and central adiposity more favorable to higher insulin sensitivity. Although some recent observational studies have suggested that alcohol consumption may help protect against heart disease, there are adverse effects of alcohol consumption that may be particularly disadvantages in patients with the metabolic syndrome. As early as 1974, it was reported that moderate alcohol consumption is associated with a significant increase in triglycerides, and further work indicated that individuals with the small-LDL pattern B trait had significantly greater postprandial triglyceride increases with isocoloric test meals with and without alcohol compared to LDL pattern A subjects.[136,137] Thus, while alcohol consumption may be associated with reduced CV risk in some subjects, individuals in whom it has an adverse effect on lipid metabolism are those with the atherogenic lipoprotein profile and excessive body fat.

Drugs

FIBRIC ACID DERIVATIVES

The fibric acid derivatives clofibrate, gemfibrozil, and fenofibrate are well-established medications that are effective in reducing triglycerides, increasing HDL-C, and reducing small LDL.[138] They work as PPAR-α agonists to upregulate gene expression of lipoprotein lipase (LPL) and apo A1.[139] The clinical effectiveness of this class of drugs in patients with elevated plasma insulin levels was established by the VA-HIT subgroup analysis.[140] In this investigation, the presence of diabetes was associated with an increased risk for CV events. In subjects without diabetes but a fasting plasma insulin > 39 μU/mL, a 31 percent increase in CV events was reported ($p = 0.03$). Gemfibrozil treatment was most effective in those with established diabetes, reducing CV events by 41 percent, and in those with elevated insulin levels, reducing CV events by 35 percent ($p = 0.04$). The combination of a fibric acid derivative and a statin can have significantly better lipid effects in type 2 diabetic patients with combined hyperlipidemia than can either agent alone.[141] The combination of fenofibrate and atorvastatin has been reported to achieve a 46 percent reduction in LDL-C, 50 percent reduction in triglycerides, 22 percent increase in HDL-C, and a 19 percent reduction in fibrinogen, with no change in Hb A1c or significant adverse side effects for 6 months. The interaction of the gemfibrozil-statin combination appears to increase the risk of myopathy, but this has not been reported to the U.S. Food and Drug Administration (FDA) with a fenofibrate-statin combination.[142] Gemfibrozil, but not fenofibrate, appears to inhibit the glucuronidation-mediated lactonization of simvastatin and the glucuronidation of a beta-oxidation product that contributes to the myositis risk when some statins and gemfibrozil are used in combination.[143]

NICOTINIC ACID

Nicotinic acid is a well-established drug that has substantial effects on reducing triglycerides, small LDL, and Lp(a) and in increasing HDL-C, HDL-2b and apo A1. Its role in the treatment of type 2 diabetes and insulin resistance has been questioned based on an early study in 13 type 2 diabetics that used 4500 mg of niacin per day and reported a 16 percent increase in fasting blood sugar and a 21 percent increase in Hgb A1c.[144] The potential adverse effect of niacin on glucose and insulin has been clarified by more recent and larger investigations. The Arterial Disease Multiple Intervention Trial (ADMIT) treated 125 type 2 diabetic patients with either 3000 mg/day of immediate-release niacin or placebo; significant ($p < 0.001$) reductions in triglycerides and increases in HDL-C were reported.[145] Mean Hgb A1c was unchanged and fasting glucose increased 8.1 percent ($p < 0.04$), while fasting insulin increased 13 percent in the group with type 2 diabetes as compared to 4 percent in the placebo group ($p = 0.09$). In an investigation of extended-release niacin in stable type 2 diabetic patients, 1000 mg/day niacin had no significant effect on glycosylated hemoglobin levels; in the group receiving 1500 mg/day, glycosylated hemoglobin levels rose from a mean of 7.2 percent at baseline to 7.5 percent ($p = 0.05$).[146] While nicotinic acid has the potential to increase glucose and insulin levels in doses ranging from 1500 to 2500 mg/day, this effect is minimal and must be weighed against the substantial lipid and LDL and HDL subclass benefits, which have been linked to clinical benefit.[147] Incidence of myopathy with niacin-statin combination are significantly lower than with gemfibrozil-statin. Of the 871 adverse event reports (AERs) of the FDA on statin-induced rhabdomyolysis, 4 (all outside the United States) were associated with niacin, compared to 80 cases with fibrates. No cases of myopathy have been reported with extended-release niacin in the AERs to the FDA or clinical trials in a total of 1700 patients.

HMG-CoA REDUCTASE INHIBITORS

Standard lipid therapy to reduce LDL-C affects the clinical outcome of type 2 diabetics positively. After 5 years of treatment with simvastatin, the Heart Protection Study reported a 19.7 percent reduction in major CV events in patients with type 2 diabetes who did and did not have a previous CV event.[148] The Scandinavian Simvastatin Survival Study reported a significant reduction in coronary events and death rates in patients with type 2 diabetes receiving simvastatin treatment, and the Cholesterol and Recurrent Events study revealed a reduction in CAD events with pravastatin treatment in both type 2 diabetes and patients with impaired fasting glucose (110 to 125 mg/dL).[149,150] The combination of a statin and nicotinic acid is more effective than either agent alone in correcting the dyslipidemia associated with the insulin-resistant condition.[151]

AGENTS THAT INCREASE TISSUE SENSITIVITY TO INSULIN

The thiazolidinedione class of medications are peroxisome proliferator–activated receptor gamma (PPAR-g) agonists that bind to nuclear receptors and regulate gene expression that impacts insulin action and lipid metabolism.[152] Troglitazone 400 mg/day has a statistically significant ($p < 0.01$) but relatively minor effect on increasing LDL peak particle diameter as assessed by gradient gel electrophoresis.[153] These agents may improve factors associated with the metabolic syndrome by improving insulin sensitivity, attenuating the migration of monocytes, and reducing intimal hyperplasia.[154]

Metformin is a biguanide that enhances tissue insulin sensitivity by inhibiting hepatic glucose production. It is frequently associated with some degree of weight loss and triglyceride reduction. In the Diabetes Prevention Program, 2.8 years of treatment with metformin in obese glucose-intolerant subjects resulted in a 31 percent relative reduction in diabetes.[79]

ACARBOSE

Acarbose is an α-glucosidase inhibitor. α-Glucosidase is an enzyme that breaks polymeric sugar chains into individual monosaccharide units and inhibits intestinal absorption of the sugars. It was used in the STOP-NIDDM trial and reduced type 2 diabetes risk by 32 percent.[81]

CONCLUSION

The metabolic syndrome is a complex interaction of physiologic pathways that may have had a survival benefit in a "primitive hunter-gather" lifestyle. However, because of the excessive consumption of calories and sedentary nature of modern "western" lifestyles, these otherwise normal pathways now contribute to greatly enhanced CAD risk. The foundation of this risk is the role of the adipocyte and greatly enhanced FFA flux in the overweight state. The number of people classified as overweight or obese has increased 55 percent in the past decade; currently, 63 percent of American men and 55 percent of American women can be classified as overweight or obese. The increase in obesity is greatest in younger age groups.

Insulin resistance is a major physiologic characteristic of the metabolic syndrome, which also includes central obesity, dyslipidemia, hypertension, enhanced thrombosis, LV dysfunction, proinflammatory states, endothelial dysfunction, and NASH. Single or multiple components of the metabolic syndrome may be present in any one individual. Risk increases with the increasing number of metabolic syndrome components.

Key to treatment is appropriate physical activity, weight management, and proper nutrition. Medications such as thiozolodinediones and metformin may directly improve insulin resistance, and lipid-lowering drugs such as fibrates, nicotinic acid, and statins can improve dyslipidemia.

Without adequate control of the epidemic of metabolic syndrome and overweight, the incidence of CAD will increase in the next decades as the current cohort of overweight young adults reach middle age. With adequate control of the metabolic syndrome, substantial progress in the prevention of CAD can be made.

References

1. Osler W. *The Principles and Practice of Medicine.* New York: Appleton; 1892:664.
2. National Center for Health Statistics. Prevalence of overweight and obesity among adults: United States, 1999 (initial results from the 1999 National Health and Nutrition Examination Survey). Hyattsville, MD: Centers for Disease Control; 2000. Available at http://www.cdc.gov/nchs/products/pubs/pubd/hestats/obese/obe\se99.htm.
3. Flegal KM, Carroll MD, Kuczmarski RT, et al. NHANES. *Int J Obes Rel Metab Disord* 1998;22:39–47.
4. Must A, Spandano J, Coakley EH, et al. The disease burden associated with overweight and obesity. *JAMA* 1999;282:1523–1559.
5. Mokdad AH, Serdula MK, Dietz WH, et al. The spread of the obesity epidemic in the United States, 1991–1998. *JAMA* 1999;282:1519–1522.
6. Fontaine KR, Redden DT, Wang C, et al. Years of life lost due to obesity. *JAMA* 2003;289:187–193.
7. NCEP ATP-III. Expert Panel on Detection, Evaluation, and Treatment of High Blood Cholesterol in Adults. Executive Summary of the Third Report of the National Cholesterol Education Program (NCEP) Expert Panel on Detection, Evaluation, and Treatment of High Blood Cholesterol in Adults (Adult Treatment Panel III). *JAMA* 2001;285:2486–2497.
8. Neel JV. Diabetes mellitus: A thrifty genotype rendered detrimental by progress. *Am J Hum Genet* 1962;14:353–362.
9. Ford ES, Giles WH, Dietz WH. Prevalence of the metabolic syndrome among US adults. *JAMA* 2002;287:356–359.
10. Gibbons RJ, Alpert JS, Antman EM, et al. ACC/AHA 2002 guideline update for the management of patients with chronic stable angina—Summary article. *Circulation* 2003;107:149–158.
11. Balkau B, Charles MA. Comment on the provisional report from the WHO consultation: European Group for the Study of Insulin Resistance (EGIR). *Diabet Med* 1999;16:44–443.
12. Lakka HM, Laaksonen DE, Niskanen LK, et al. The metabolic syndrome and total and cardiovascular disease mortality in middle-aged men. *JAMA* 2002;288:2709–2716.
13. Chen W, Srinivasan SR, Elkasabany A, Berenson GS. Cardiovascular risk factors clustering features of insulin resistance syndrome (syndrome X) in a biracial (black-white) population of children, adolescents, and young adults: The Bogalusa Heart Study. *Am J Epidemiol* 1999;150:667–674.
14. Hanley AJ, Karter AJ, Festa A, et al. The Insulin Resistance Atherosclerosis Study. Factor analysis of metabolic syndrome using directly measured insulin sensitivity: The Insulin Resistance Atherosclerosis Study. *Diabetes* 2002;51:2642–2647.
15. Meigs JB, D'Agostino RB, Wilson PW, et al. Risk variable clustering in the insulin resistance syndrome. The Framingham Offspring Study. *Diabetes* 1997;46:1594–1600.
16. Gofman JW, Young W, Tandy R. Ischemic heart disease, atherosclerosis and longevity. *Circulation* 1966;34:679–697.
17. Reaven GM, Ida Chen YD, Jeppesen J, et al. Insulin resistance and hyperinsulinemia in individuals with small, dense low density lipoprotein particles. *J Clin Invest* 1993;92:141–146.
18. Farquhar JW, Frank A, Gross RC, Reaven GM. Glucose, insulin, and triglyceride responses to high and low carbohydrate diets in man. *J Clin Invest* 1966;45(10):1648–1656
19. Reaven GM. Role of insulin resistance in human disease (syndrome X): An expanded definition. *Annu Rev Med* 1993;44:121–131
20. Modan M, Halkin H, Almog S, et al. hyperinsulinemia: A link between hyertension, obesity, and glucose intolerance. *J Clin Invest* 1985;75:809–817.
21. Krauss RM. Heterogeneity of plasma low-density lipoproteins and atherosclerosis risk. *Curr Opin Lipidol* 1994;5:339–349.
22. Austin MA. Triglyceride, small, dense low-density lipoprotein, and the atherogenic lipoprotein phenotype. *Curr Atheroscler Rep* 2000;2(3):200–207.
23. Onat A, Ceyhan K, Basar O, et al. Metabolic syndrome: Major impact on coronary risk in a population with low cholesterol levels—A prospective and cross-sectional evaluation. *Atherosclerosis* 2002;165;285–292.
24. Miller BD, Alderman EL, Haskell WL, et al. Predominance of dense low-density lipoprotein particles predicts angiographic benefit or therapy in the Stanford Coronary Risk Intervention project. *Circulation* 1996;94: 2146–2153
25. Zambon A, Hokanson JE, Brown BG, Brunzell JD. Evidence for a new pathophysiological mechanism for coronary artery disease regression. *Circulation* 1999;99:1959–1964
26. Williams PT, Superko HR, Alderman EA. Small low density lipoprotein III but not low density lipoprotein cholesterol is related to arteriographic progression. *Circulation* 2000;102:II-848.
27. Brown C, Garrett B, Superko HR. Small LDL and hs-CRP as New CAD Risk Factors. *J Med Assoc Georgia* 2001;90:11–18.
28. Eckel RH, Wassef M, Chait A, et al. Diabetes and cardiovascular disease writing group II: Pathogenesis of atherosclerosis in diabetes. *Circulation* 2002;105:e138–e143.
29. Lamarche B, Tchernof A, Mauriege P, et al. Fasting insulin and apolipoprotein B levels and low-density lipoprotein particle size as risk factors for ischemic heart disease. *JAMA* 1998;279:1955–1961.
30. Manson JE, Willett WC, Stanpfer MJ, et al. Body weight and mortality among women. *N Engl J Med* 1995;333:677–685.
31. Rimm EB, Stampfer MJ, Giovannucci E, et al. Body size and fat distribution as predictors of coronary heart disease among middle-aged and older US men. *Am J Epidemiol* 1995;141:1117–1127.
32. Bjorntorp P. Regional patterns of fat distribution. *Ann Intern Med* 1985;103:994–995.
33. McGill HC, McMahan A, Herderick EE, et al. Obesity accelerates the progression of coronary atherosclerosis in young men. *Circulation* 2002;105:2712–2718.
34. Sinaiko AR, Donahue RP, Jacobs DR, Prineas RJ. Relation of weight and rate of increase in weight during childhood and adolescence to body size, blood pressure, fasting insulin, and lipids in young adults. *Circulation* 1999;99:1471–1476.
35. Guo Z, Hensrud DD, Johnson CM, Jensen MD. Regional post-prandial fatty acid metabolism in different obesity phenotypes. *Diabetes* 1999;48:1586–1592.
36. Egan BM, Lu G, Greene EL. Vascular effects of non-esterified fatty acids: Implications for the cardiovascular risk factor cluster. *Prostaglandins Leukot Essent Fatty Acids* 1999;60:411–420.
37. Alpert MA. Obesity cardiomyopathy: Pathophysiology and evolution of the clinical syndrome. *Am J Med Sci* 2001;321:225–236.
38. Bierhaus A, Hofmann MA, Ziegler R, et al. AGEs and their interaction with AGE-receptors in vascular disease and diabetes mellitus. I: The AGE concept. *Cardiovasc Res* 1998;37:586–600.
39. Eckel RH, Wassef M, Chait A, et al. Diabetes and cardiovascular disease writing group II: Pathogenesis of atherosclerosis in diabetes. *Circulation* 2002;105:e138–e143.
40. Ross. R. Atherosclerosis—An inflammatory disease. *N Engl J Med* 1999;340:115–126.

41. Krauss RM. The tangled web of coronary risk factors. *Am J Med* 1991;90:36S–41S.

42. Quintao EC, Medina WL, Passarelli M. Reverse cholesterol transport in diabetes mellitus. *Diabetes Metab Res Rev* 2000;16:237–250.

43. Weisser B, Locher R, de Graaf J, et al. Low density lipoprotein subfractions increase thromboxane formation in endothelial cells. *Biochem Biophys Res Commun* 1993;192(3):1245–1250.

44. Superko HR, Krauss RM. Garlic powder: Effect on plasma lipids, post prandial lipemia, LDL particle size, HDL subclass distribution, and Lp(a). *J Am Coll Cardiol* 2000;35:321–326.

45. La Belle M, Krauss RM. Differences in carbohydrate content of low density lipoproteins associated with low density lipoprotein subclass patterns. *J Lipid Res* 1990;31:1577–1588.

46. Reaven GM, Ida Chen YD, et al. Insulin resistance and hyperinsulinemia in individuals with small, dense low density lipoprotein particles. *J Clin Invest* 1993;92:141–146.

47. Williams PT, Vranizan KM, Austin MA, Krauss RM. Familial correlations of HDL subclasses based on gradient gel electrophoresis. *Arterioscler Thromb* 1992;12:1467–1474.

48. Tselepis AD, Dentan C, Karabina SAP, et al. PAF-degrading acetyl-hydrolase is preferentially associated with dense LDL and VHDL-1 in human plasma. *Arterioscler Thromb Vasc Biol* 1995;15:1764–1773.

49. Tribble DL, van den Berg JJM, Motchnik PA, et al. Oxidative susceptibility of low density lipoprotein subfractions is related to their Ubiquinol-10 and alpha-tocopherol content. *Proc Natl Acad Sci USA* 1994;91:1183–1187.

50. Nordestgaard BG, Wootton R, Lewis B. Selective retention of VLDL, IDL, and LDL in the arterial intima of genetically hyperlipidemic rabbits in vivo. Molecular size as a determinant of fractional loss from the intima-inner media. *Arterioscler Thromb Vasc Biol* 1995;15:534–542.

51. Austin MA, Mykkanen L, Kuusisto J, et al. Prospective study of small LDLs as a risk factor for non-insulin-dependent diabetes mellitus in elderly men and women. *Circulation* 1995;92:1770–1778.

52. Austin MA, King MC, Vranizan KM, Krauss RM. Atherogenic lipoprotein phenotype. A proposed genetic marker for coronary heart disease risk. *Circulation* 1990;82:495–506.

53. Krauss RM, Blanche PJ. Detection and quantitation of LDL subfractions. *Curr Opin Lipidol* 1992;3:377–383.

54. Vakkilainen J, Makimattila S, Seppala-Lindroos A, et al. Endothelial dysfunction in men with small LDL particles. *Circulation* 2000;102:716–721.

55. Skoglund-Anderson C, Tang R, Bond MG, et al. LDL particle size distribution is associated with carotid intima-media thickness in healthy 50-year-old men. *Arterioscler Thromb Vasc Biol* 1999;19:2422–2430.

56. Austin MA, Breslow JL, Hennekens CH, et al. Low density lipoprotein subclass patterns and risk of myocardial infarction. *JAMA* 1988;260:1917–1921.

57. Lamarche B, Tchernof A, Mauriege P, et al. Fasting insulin and apolipoprotein B levels and low-density lipoprotein particle size as risk factors for ischemic heart disease. *JAMA* 1998;279:1955–1961.

58. Stampfer MJ, Krauss RM, Blanche PJ, et al. A prospective study of triglyceride level, low density lipoprotein particle diameter, and risk of myocardial infarction. *JAMA* 1996;276:882–888.

59. Gardner CD, Fortmann SP, Krauss RM. Association of small low-density lipoprotein particles with the incidence of coronary artery disease in men and women. *JAMA* 1996;276:875–881.

60. Austin MA, Kamigaki A, Hokanson JE. Low-density lipoprotein particle size is a risk factor for coronary heart disease independent of triglyceride and HDL cholesterol: A meta-analysis of three prospective studies in men (abstr). *Circulation* 1999;99:1124.

61. Krauss RM, Lindgren FT, Williams PT, et al. Intermedicate-density lipoproteins and progression of coronary artery disease in hypercholesterolaemic men. *Lancet* 1987;2:62–65.

62. Watts GF, Lewis B, Brunt JNH, et al. Effects on coronary artery disease of lipid-lowering diet, or diet plus cholestyramine, in the St Thomas' Atherosclerosis Regression Study (STARS). *Lancet* 1992;339:563–569.

63. Zambon A, Hokanson JE, Brown BG, Brunzell JD. Evidence for a new pathophysiological mechanism for coronary artery disease regression. *Circulation* 1999;99:1959–1964.

64. Miller BD, Alderman EL, Haskell WL, et al. Predominance of dense low-density lipoprotein particles predicts angiographic benefit or therapy in the Stanford Coronary Risk Intervention project. *Circulation* 1996;94:2146–2153.

65. Williams PT, Superko HR, Alderman EA. Small low density lipoprotein III but not low density lipoprotein cholesterol is related to arteriographic progression. *Circulation* 2000;102:II-848.

66. Zhao XQ, Kosinski AJS, Malinow MR, et al. Association of LDL heterogeneity and native coronary disease progression at 3 years following PTCA or CABG in EAST. *Circulation* 2000;102:II-698.

67. Reaven GM, Ida Chen YD, Jeppesen J, et al. Insulin resistance and hyperinsulinemia in individuals with small, dense low density lipoprotein particles. *J Clin Invest* 1993;92:141–146.

68. Weisser B, Locher R, Lehmann E, et al. Proliferative effects of low-density lipoprotein subfractions on vascular smooth muscle cells: Potentiation by insulin. *J Hypertens Suppl* 1993;11(suppl 5):S126–S127.

69. Nishimoto Y, Miyazaki Y, Toki Y, et al. Enhanced secretion of insulin plays a role in the development of atherosclerosis and restensosis of coronary arteries: Elective percutaneous transluminal coronary angioplasty in patients with effort angina. *J Am Coll Cardiol* 1998;32:1624–1629.

70. Takagi T, Yoshida K, Akasaka T, et al. Hyperinsulinemia during oral glucose tolerance test is associated with increased neointimal tissue proliferation after coronary stent implantation in nondiabetic patients. *J Am Coll Cardiol* 2000;36:731–738.

71. Reaven G. Metabolic Syndrome. *Circulation* 2002;106:286–288.

72. Williams CL, Hayman LL, Daniels SR, et al. Cardiovascular health in childhood. *Circulation* 2002:106:143–160.

73. Goraya TY, Leibson CL, Palumbo PJ, et al. Coronary atherosclerosis in diabetes mellitus. *J Am Coll Cardiol* 2002;40:946–953.

74. Laskey W, Selzer F, Vlachos HA, et al. Comparison of in-hospital and one-year outcomes in patients with and without diabetes mellitus undergoing percutaneous catheter intervention. *Am J Cardiol* 2002;90:1062–1067.

75. Superko HR. Current and future trends in therapy for dyslipidemias. *Endocr Pract* 1997;3:255:263.

76. Tkac I, Kimball BP, Lewis G, et al. The severity of coronary atherosclerosis in type 2 diabetes mellitus is related to the number of circulating triglyceride-rich lipoprotein particles. *Arterioscler Thromb Vasc Biol* 1997;17(12):3633–3638.

77. Sherwin RS, Anderson RM, Buse JB, et al. The prevention of delay of type 2 diabetes. *Diabetes Care* 2003;26:S62–S69.

78. Tuomilehto J, Lindstrom J, Eriksson JG, et al. Prevention of type 2 diabetes mellitus by changes in lifestyle among subjects with impaired glucose tolerance. *N Engl J Med* 2001;344:1343–1350.

79. Diabetes Prevention Research Group: Reduction in the evidence of type 2 diabetes with life-style intervention or metformin. *N Engl J Med* 2002;346:393–403.

80. Buchanan TA, Xiang AH, Peters RK, et al. Preservation of pancreatic beta-cell function and prevention of type 2 diabetes by pharmacological treatment of insulin resistance in high-risk Hispanic women. *Diabetes* 2002;51(9):2796–2803.

81. Chiasson JL, Josse RG, Gomis R, et al. Acarbose for prevention of type 2 diabetes mellitus: The STOP-NIDDM randomised trial. *Lancet* 2002;359(9323):2072–2077.

82. Robinson JG, Boland LL, McGovern PG, Folsom AR. A comparison of NCEP and absolute risk stratification methods for lipid-lowering therapy in middle aged adults: The ARIC study. *Prev Cardiol* 2001;4:148–157.

83. Sacks FM, Pfeffer MA, Moye LA, et al. The effect of pravastatin on coronary events after myocardial infarction in patients with average cholesterol levels. *N Engl J Med* 1996;335:1001–1009.

84. Lind L, Andersson PE, Andren B, et al. Left ventricular hypertrophy in hypertension is associated with the insulin resistance metabolic syndrome. *J Hypertens* 1995;13:433–438.

85. Arnlov J, Lind L, Zethelius B, et al. Several factors associated with the insulin resistance syndrome are predictors of left ventricular systolic dysfunction in a male population after 20 years of follow-up. *Am Heart J* 2001;142:720–724.

86. Davis CL, Kapuku G, Snieder H, et al. Insulin resistance syndrome and left ventricular mass in healthy young people. *Am J Med Sci* 2002;324:72–75.

87. Siani A, Cuppuccio FP, Barba G, et al. The relationship of waist circumference to blood pressure: The Olivetti Heart Study. *Am J Hypertens* 2002;15:780–786.

88. Frederich RC, Hamann A, Anderson S, et al. Leptin levels reflect body lipid content in mice: Evidence for diet-induced resistance to leptin action. *Nat Med* 1995;1:1311–1314.

89. Konstantinides S, Schafer K, Koschnick S, et al. Leptin-dependent platelet aggregation and arterial thrombosis suggests a mechanism for atherothrombotic disease in obesity. *J Clin Invest* 2001;108:1533–1540.

90. Rader DJ. Inflammatory markers of coronary risk. *N Engl J Med* 2000;343:1179–1182.

91. Lemieux I, Pascot A, Prud'Homme D, et al. Elevated C-reactive protein, another component of the atherothrombotic profile of abdominal obesity. *Arterioscler Thromb Vasc Biol* 2001;21:961–967.

92. Festa A, D'Agostino R Jr, Howard G, et al. Chronic subclinical inflammation as part of the insulin resistance syndrome: The Insulin Resistance Atherosclerosis Study (IRAS). *Circulation* 2000;10:42–47.

93. McLaughlin T, Abbasi F, Lamendola C, et al. Differentiation between obesity and insulin resistance in the association with C-reactive protein. *Circulation* 2002;106:2908–2912.

94. Heinrich J, Balleisen L, Schulte H, et al. Fibrinogen and factor VII in the prediction of coronary risk. Results from the PROCAM study in healthy men. *Arterioscler Thromb Vasc Biol* 1994;14:54–59.

95. Hamsten A, de Faire U, Walldius G, et al. Plasminogen activator inhibitor in plasma: Risk for recurrent myocardial infarction. *Lancet* 1987/II:3–9.

96. Juhan-Vague I, Alessi M, Vague P. Increased plasma PAI-1 levels. A possible link between insulin resistance and atherothrombosis. *Diabetologia* 1991;34:457–462.

97. Sobel BE. Increased plasminogen activator inhibitor-1 and vasculopathy: A reconcilable paradox. *Circulation* 1999;99: 2496–2498.

98. Minamikawa J, Yamauchi M, Inoue D, et al. Another potential use of troglitazone in non-insulin-dependent diabetes mellitus. *J Clin Endocrinol Metab* 1998;83:1041–1042.

99. Devaraj S, Xu DY, Jialal I. C-reactive protein increases plasminogen activator inhibitor-1 expression and activity in human aortic endothelial cells: Implications for the metabolic syndrome and atherothrombosis. *Circulation* 2003;107:398–404.

100. Folsom AR, Wu KK, Davies CE, et al. Population correlates of plasma fibrinogen and factor VII: Putative cardiovascular risk factors. *Atherosclerosis* 1991;91:191–205.

101. Kannel WB, D'Agostino RB, Belanger AJ. Long-term influence of fibrinogen on initial vs recurrent cardiovascular events: The Framingham Study. *J Am Coll Cardiol* 1996:27:25A

102. Mansfield MW, Heywood DM, Grant PJ. Circulating levels of factor VII, fibrinogen, and von Willlebrand factor and features of insulin resistance in first-degree relatives of patients with NIDDM. *Circulation* 1996;94:2171–2176.

103. Miller GJ. Lipoprotein and thrombosis: Effects of lipid lowering. *Curr Opin Lipidol* 1995;6:38–42.

104. Conlan MG, Folsom AR, Finch A, et al. Association of factor VIII and von Willebrand factor with age, race, and risk factors for atherosclerosis. The Atherosclerosis Risk in Communities (ARIC) study. *Thromb Haemost* 1993;70:380–385.

105. Meigs JB, Mittleman MA, Nathan DM, et al. Hyperinsulinemia, hyperglycemia, and impaired hemostasis: The Framingham Offspring Study. *JAMA* 2000;283:221–228.

106. Trovati M, Anfossi G, Cavalot F, et al. Insulin directly reduces platelet sensitivity to aggregating agents: Studies in vitro and in vivo. *Diabetes* 1988;37:780–786.

107. Westerbacka J, Yki-Jarvinen H, Turpeinen A, et al. Inhibition of platelet-collagen interaction. An in vivo action of insulin abolished by insulin resistance in obesity. *Arterioscler Thromb Vasc Biol* 2002;22:167–172.

108. Kohler HP. Insulin resistance syndrome: Interaction with coagulation and fibrinolysis. *Swiss Med Wkly* 2002;132:241–252.

109. Calles-Escandon J, Cipolla M. Diabetes and endothelial dysfunction: A clinical perspective. *Endocr Rev* 2001;22:36–52.

110. Tack CJ, Ong MK, Lutterman JA, et al. Insulin-induced vasodilation and endothelial function in obesity/insulin resistance: Effects of troglitazone. *Diabetologia* 1998;41:569–576.

111. Vakkilainen J, Makimattila S, Seppala-Lindroos A, et al. Endothelial dysfunction in men with small LDL particles. *Circulation* 2000;102:716–721.

112. Contos MJ, Sanyal AJ. The clinicopathologic spectrum and management of nonalcoholic fatty liver disease. *Adv Anat Pathol* 2002;9:37–51.

113. Chitturi S, George J. Interaction of iron, insulin resistance, and nonalcoholic steatohepatitis. *Curr Gastroenterol Rep* 2003;5:18–25.

114. Harrison SA, Kadakia S, Lang KA, Schenker S. Nonalcoholic steatohepatitis: What we know in the new millennium. *Am J Gastroenterol* 2002;97:2714–2724.

115. Mehta K, Van Thiel DH, Shah N, Mobarhan S. Nonalcoholic fatty liver disease: Pathogenesis and the role of antioxidants. *Nutr Rev* 2002;60:289–293.

116. Clarke SD. Nonalcoholic steatosis and steatohepatitis. I. Molecular mechanism for polyunsaturated fatty acid regulation of gene transcription. *Am J Physiol Gastrointest Liver Physiol* 2001;281:G865–G869.

117. Gaede P, Vedel P, Larsen N, Jensen GVH, et al. Multifactorial intervention and cardiovascular disease in patients with type 2 diabetes. *N Engl J Med* 2003;348:383–393.

118. Pasanisi R, Contaldo F, de Simone G, Mancini M. Benefits of sustained moderate weight loss in obesity. *Nutr Metab Cardiovasc Dis* 2001;11:401–406.

119. Gazzaruso C, Giordanette S, La Manna A, et al. Weight loss after Swedish adjustable gastric banding: Relationships to insulin resistance and metabolic syndrome. *Obes Surg* 2002;12:841–845.

120. Buchwald H, Varco RL, Boen JR, et al. Effective lipid modification by partial ileal bypass reduced long-term coronary heart disease mortality and morbidity: Five-year posttrial follow-up report from the POSCH. *Arch Intern Med* 1998;158:1253–1261.

121. Campos CT, Matts JP, Fitch LL, et al. Lipoprotein modification achieved by partial ileal bypass: Five year results for the program on the surgical control of the hyperlipidemias. *Surgery* 1987;102:424–432.

122. Ludwig DS, Pereira MA, Kroenke CH, et al. dietary fiber, weight gain, and cardiovascular disease risk factors in young adults. *JAMA* 1999;282:1539–1546.

123. Wylie-Rosett J. Fat Substitutes and Health. *Circulation* 2002;105:2800–2804.

124. Howard B, Wylie-Rosett J. Sugar and cardiovascular disease: A statement for healthcare professionals from the Committee on Nutrition of the Council on Nutrition, Physical Activity, and Metabolism of the American Heart Association. *Circulation* 2002; 106(4):523–527.

125. Dreon DM, Fernstrom H, Miller B, Krauss RM. Low density lipoprotein subclass patterns and lipoprotein response to a reduced-fat diet in men. *FASEB J* 1994;8:121–126.

126. Jenkins DJ, Wolever TM, Taylor RH, et al. Glycemic index of foods: A physiological basis for carbohydrate exchange. *Am J Clin Nutr* 1981;34:362–366.

127. Hu FB, Willett WC. Optimal diets for prevention of coronary heart disease. *JAMA* 2002;288:2569–2578.

128. Nestel P, Noakes M, Belling BE. Plasma lipoprotein and Lp(a) changes with substitution of elaidic acid for oleic acid in the diet. *J Lipid Res* 1992;33:1029–1036.

129. Burr ML, Fehily AM, Gilbert JF, et al. Effects of changes in fat, fish, and fibre intakes on death and myocardial reinfarction: Diet and Reinfarction Trial (DART). *Lancet* 1989;2:757–761.

130. GISSI-Prevenzione Investigators. Dietary supplementation with n-3 polyunsaturated fatty acids and vitamin E after myocardial infarction: Results from the GISSI-Prevenzione trial. *Lancet* 1999;354:447–455.

131. Singh RB, Niaz MA, Sharma JP, et al. Randomized, double-blind, placebo controlled trial of fish oil and mustard oil in patients with suspected acute myocardial infarction: The Indian Experiment of Infarct Survival 4. *Cardiovasc Drugs Ther* 1997;11:485–491.

132. De Lorgeril M, Renaud S, Mamelle N, et al. Mediterranean alpha-linolenic acid–rich diet in secondary prevention of coronary heart disease. *Lancet* 1994;343:1454–1459.

133. Superko HR, Krauss RM. Garlic powder: Effect on plasma lipids, post prandial lipemia, LDL particle size, HDL subclass distribution, and Lp(a). *J Am Coll Cardiol* 2000:35:321–326.

134. Ajani UA, Gaziano JM, Lotufo PA, et al. Alcohol consumption and risk of coronary heart disease by diabetes status. *Circulation* 2000;102(5):500–505.

135. Bell R, D'Agostino RB, Mayer-Davis EJ, et al. Associations between alcohol consumption and insulin sensitivity and cardiovascular disease risk factors. *Diabetes Care* 2000;23:1630–1636.

136. Ginsberg H, Olefsky J, Farquhar J, Reaven GM. Moderate ethanol ingestion and plasma triglyceride levels. A study in normal and hyper-triglyceridemic persons. *Ann Intern Med* 1974;80:143–149.

137. Superko HR. Effects of acute and chronic alcohol consumption on postprandial lipemia in healthy normotriglyceridemic men. *Am J Cardiol* 1992;69:701–704.

138. Feher MD, Caslake M, Foxton J, et al. Atherogenic lipoprotein phenotype in type 2 diabetes: Reversal with micronised fenofibrate. *Diabetes/Metab Res Rev* 1999;395–399.

139. Staels B, Auwerx J. Regulation of apo A-I gene expression by fibrates. *Atherosclerosis* 1998;137(suppl):S19–S23.

140. Rubins HB, Robins SJ, Nelson DB, et al and the VA-HIT Study Group. Diabetes, plasma insulin, and cardiovascular disease. *Arch Intern Med* 2002;162:2597–2604.

141. Athyros VG, Papageorgiou AA, Athyrou VV, et al. Atorvastatin and micronized fenofibrate alone and in combination in type 2 diabetes with combined hyperlipidemia. *Diabetes Care* 2002;25:1198–1202.

142. Thompson PD, Clarkson P, Karas RH. et al. Statin-associated myopathy. *JAMA* 2003;289(13):1681–1690.

143. Prueksaritanont T, Tang C, Qiu Y, et al. Effects of fibrates on metabolism of statins in human hepatocytes. *Drug Metab Dispos* 2002;30:1280–1287.

144. Garg A, Grundy SM. Nicotinic acid as therapy for dyslipidemia in non insulin dependent diabetes mellitus. *JAMA* 1990;264:723–726.

145. Elam MB, Hunninghake DB, Davis KB, et al for the ADMIT Investigators. Effect of niacin on lipid and lipoprotein levels and glycemic control in patients with diabetes and peripheral arterial disease. *JAMA* 2000;284:1263–1270

146. Grundy SM, Pasternak R, Greenland P, et al. Assessment of cardiovascular risk by use of multiple-risk-factor assessment equations. *Circulation* 1999;100:1481–1492

147. Superko HR. Hypercholesterolemia and dyslipidemia. *Curr Treat Options Cardiovasc Med* 2000;2:173–187.

148. Heart Protection Study Collaborative Group. MRC/BHF heart protection study of cholesterol lowering with simvastatin in 20,536 high-risk individuals: A randomized placebo-controlled trial. *Lancet* 2002;360:7–22.

149. Pyorala K, Pedersen TR, Kjekshus J, et al. Cholesterol lowering with simvastatin improves prognosis of diabetic patients with coronary heart disease. *Diabetes Care* 1997;20:614–620.

150. Goldberg RB, Mellies MJ, Sacks FM, et al. Cardiovascular events and their reduction with pravastatin in diabetic and glucose intolerant myocardial infarction survivors with average cholesterol levels: Subgroup analyses in the Cholesterol and Recurrent Events (CARE) trial. *Circulation* 1998;98:2513–2559.

151. Tsalamandris C, Panagiotopoulos S, Sinha A, et al. Complementary effects of pravastatin and nicotinic acid in the treatment of combined hyperlipidaemia in diabetic and non-diabetic patients. *J Cardiovasc Risk* 1994;1:231–239.

152. Lebovitz HE, Banerji MA. Insulin resistance and its treatment by thiazolidinediones. *Recent Prog Horm Res* 2001;56:265–294.

153. Sunayama S, Watanabe Y, Ohmura H, et al. Effects of troglitazone on atherogenic lipoprotein phenotype in coronary patients with insulin resistance. *Atherosclerosis* 1999;146(1):187–193.

154. Hsueh WA. PPAR-gamma effects on the vasculature. *J Invest Med* 2001;49:127–129.

AIDS AND THE CARDIOVASCULAR SYSTEM

Melvin D. Cheitlin

The pandemic of acquired immunodeficiency syndrome (AIDS) continues to take a tragic toll on lives in the United States and is resulting in a catastrophe in Africa and Southeast Asia. Russia, China, and India are recognizing the growing epidemic in their countries. AIDS is now the fourth largest cause of death worldwide.[1] By the end of 2002, 42 million people worldwide were infected with the human immunodeficiency virus (HIV), 95 percent occurring in developing countries. Worldwide, 50 percent of adults living with HIV or AIDS are women.[1a] The disease is increasingly seen in women with the proportion of women increasing in the United States from 7 percent in 1985 to 23 percent in 1998.[1,2] In the United States, over 1 million people are HIV positive, and about 2 million have been diagnosed with AIDS.[2,3] In the 9 countries in Africa with the highest prevalence of AIDS, life expectancy by 2010 to 2015 will fall on average by 16 years, according to the United Nations Population Division.[3]

AIDS is caused by infection with a virus of the family Retroviridae. This group of retroviruses comprises enveloped ribonucleic acid (RNA) viruses possessing an RNA-dependent deoxyribonucleic acid (DNA) polymerase (reverse transcriptase). There are two classes of AIDS viruses: HIV-1 and HIV-2.

The most specific definition of infection by HIV is by identification of the HIV organism in the host's tissues. Isolation of the virus is not easily done and, therefore, lacks sensitivity. Thus, a patient with repeated positive screening test results for antibodies to HIV, as with an enzyme-linked immunosorbent assay (ELISA) and confirmed by a supplemental test such as the Western blot immunofluorescence assay, should be considered to be infected by HIV.

The following classification system for the different stages of HIV infection as proposed by the United States Centers for Disease Control and Prevention (CDC) is helpful[4]:

Group I: Acute infection
Group II: Asymptomatic infection
Group III: Persistent generalized lymphadenopathy (PGL)
Group IV: Chronic disease: AIDS with constitutional disease (such as unexplained diarrhea, weight loss, or fever for more than 1 month), neurologic disease, secondary infectious diseases, secondary cancers (Kaposi's sarcoma, non-Hodgkin's lymphoma, and primary lymphoma of the brain)

In January 1993, the CDC, together with other state and territorial health departments, broadened the surveillance definition for AIDS adding a measure of immunosuppression (a CD4+ T-lymphocyte count <200/μL or a CD4+ percentage <14), as well as three additional clinical conditions: pulmonary tuberculosis, recurrent pneumonia (two or more episodes within 1 year), or invasive cervical cancer.[5]

Patients with HIV infection have also been divided into three clinical categories. Category A includes asymptomatic patients, those with acute HIV infection or progressive lymphadenopathy. Category B includes symptomatic patients without AIDS-defining conditions. Category C includes patients with 25 AIDS-defining conditions, including opportunistic infections, tumors, central nervous system abnormalities, wasting syndrome, pulmonary tuberculosis, invasive cervical carcinoma, and recurrent pneumonia.[5]

The HIV infection, a zoonosis in chimpanzees, was first recognized in humans in 1981. In the last 2 decades AIDS has become pandemic, with many aspects of epidemics of the past, such as those of poliomyelitis and the black plague. This infection is due to a retrovirus that invades the nucleus of certain cells containing a specific receptor on their cell membranes and incorporates the DNA copy of HIV in the host's genetic material or genome. After an asymptomatic latent period from infection of 2 to 6 weeks, most patients experience a primary HIV-1 infection that is a self-limited viral syndrome not unlike infectious mononucleosis, characterized by fever, fatigue, pharangitis, lymphadenopathy, and maculopapular rash.[6] Over 95 percent of the patients seroconvert to a positive HIV serology within 6 months, most within 6 to 12 weeks.[7] After an apparent incubation (dormant) period of a mean of 8 to 10 years, the virus can eventually express itself by releasing into the cytoplasm double-stranded DNA copies of the virus, thus killing the cell and invading other immune cells, usually T-helper lymphocytes, to the point that the host's immune defense mechanisms are compromised.[8] Studies have demonstrated a high rate of viral replication in the lymph nodes during this quiescent period, indicating active progression of the disease, despite the low levels of infectious HIV in the plasma of some patients.[9]

A long-term prospective study showed the actuarial rate of progression from the time of infection to the appearance of AIDS to be 53 percent at 10 years and 68 percent at 14 years after infection, with an increasing progression after 5 years of infection.[10] About 30 percent of patients with PGL will progress to AIDS in 5 years.[11] A minority of patients have an accelerated course and develop full-blown AIDS in 1 or 2 years.[12] Small groups of patients have also been described who have had HIV infection for over 10 years without any symptoms.[13] At some point, there is a breakdown of the body's immunologic defense with the development of opportunistic infections, gastrointestinal disease, non-Hodgkin's lymphoma, and Kaposi's sarcoma. These complications lead inevitably, at least in a very high percentage of cases, to death.

The average length of life after infection in the absence of treatment is approximately 10 years.[10] With the introduction of highly active antiretroviral therapy (HAART) including nucleoside reverse-transcriptase inhibitors and especially the protease-inhibitor drugs, elimination of the virus from the peripheral blood and prolongation of life have been demonstrated.[14] The impact of the new treatment with multiple drugs is seen in a fall in the rate of AIDS deaths by 12 percent in the United States in 1996 and by 47 percent in 1997.[15]

At the beginning of the epidemic in the United States, the HIV organism struck mainly at the male homosexual population. Later it was found to be transmitted not only through sexual intercourse but also through blood-borne contamination, soon affecting the population using intravenous drugs and those receiving blood products, such as those with hemophilia. The disease is also transmitted perinatally, so that an increasing number of pediatric patients with AIDS are being seen. Although in the United States, male-to-male sexual activity and intravenous drug users account for 75 percent of cases, in the developing world heterosexual transmission accounts for the majority of cases.[16]

From work with HIV-1, it has been found that the usual way in which the virus attacks cells is through interaction with a receptor on the surface membrane of the cell, the so-called CD4 receptor. This is present in T-helper lymphocytes. Macrophages, microglia, and Langerhans' cells may have specific receptors for HIV other than CD4. Other cells seem to lack an HIV receptor and therefore are much less often found to be sites of infection; the myocardial cell is one such cell.

From the beginning of the epidemic, it was recognized that the heart could be involved but that significant clinical involvement of the heart was unusual. Originally it was believed, through autopsy studies, that the heart was involved mainly because of pericarditis or metastatic Kaposi's sarcoma.[17] On further review of autopsy series and clinical series and especially with the study of patients with AIDS who had echocardiography, it was apparent that abnormalities of the heart were seen frequently, even though clinical manifestations of heart disease still remained unusual.

AUTOPSY FINDINGS

The incidence of cardiac involvement at autopsy varies, depending on the definition of cardiac disease. In 15 autopsy series, the incidence of cardiac involvement varies from none to 70 percent of the hearts, depending on whether lymphocytic infiltration with or without myocardial necrosis is included.[17–22] The presence of autopsy-proven cardiac involvement in patients who, during life, had clinically significant cardiac involvement is less impressive, especially if one includes the patients with localized, isolated collections of myocardial lymphocytes.

In large series of consecutive autopsies of AIDS patients, between 5 and 20 percent appear to have had cardiac lesions of potential clinical importance. These include patients with myocarditis with clinical manifestations, mainly with known pathogens such as toxoplasmosis, clinically evident pericarditis, or nonbacterial endocarditis, which can cause systemic emboli.

The largest most recent autopsy series is by Barbero et al., with 440 AIDS patients. Cardiac involvement was documented in 18.6 percent and dilated cardiomyopathy in 2.7 percent.[23]

More important are the relatively few patients in whom cardiac abnormality was listed as the cause of death. The most common cause of death is respiratory failure and infection.[20,24,24a] Neoplasm, lymphoma, and encephalopathy are also frequent causes of death.[25] Of 858 autopsied patients with AIDS from 15 series in the literature, only 9 (1 percent) had the cause of death listed as cardiac. If the cases with a recognized etiology for heart disease are removed, only 0.5 percent of deaths were possibly due to HIV "myocarditis."

Right ventricular hypertrophy and/or dilatation was reported in 12 of 71 patients (16.9 percent)[21] and in 18 of 115 patients (15.7 percent).[20] Pericarditis varied in frequency from 3 of 41 (7.3 percent)[18] to 3 of 101 (3 percent).[19]

ECHOCARDIOGRAPHIC FINDINGS

Echocardiography in patients with either AIDS or PGL has been reported in a number of studies.[26–31] The prevalence of echocardiographic abnormalities varies from 15 to 60 percent. The prevalence of left ventricular hypokinesis also varies from 12.5 to 41 percent in three large series.[26–28] In one series,[26] 4 of the 8 patients had congestive heart failure; 1 died and at autopsy had a dilated cardiomyopathy without evidence of inflammatory myocarditis or cardiac opportunistic infections. In this study only clinical congestive heart failure was mentioned.[26] Dilated cardiomyopathy was seen only in the hospitalized patients. In a large prospective echocardiographic study of 296 HIV-infected adults that was conducted over 4 years, Currie and colleagues found 13 (4 percent) with dilated cardiomyopathy.[29]

Cecchi and colleagues[30] selected 127 patients (9 percent) from 1398 admitted for HIV infection with a clinical suspicion of cardiac disease. Echocardiograms showed 92 (72 percent) had evidence of cardiac involvement, 6.5 percent of total HIV patients; 38 (2.7 percent) had pericardial effusion, and 20 (1.4 percent) had dilated cardiomyopathy.[30]

The finding of pericardial effusion was common, varying from 20 to 40 percent.[27,28,30] The incidence of tamponade varies: In one series[27] of 18 patients with pericardial effusion, 5 (28 percent) had tamponade. In this report of 300 patients with AIDS, 16 (5 percent) had clinically apparent heart disease, due in most cases to opportunistic infection or tumor.[27]

Steffen and colleagues[31] reported the prospectively collected results of echocardiography in 151 HIV-seropositive patients, 92 percent of whom were men with a median age of 37 years. Of these, 13 percent were intravenous drug users, of whom 74 percent were in Walter Reed stages IV to VI, a classification using counts of T4 helper cells and clinical data.[32] A total of 107 patients (71 percent) had normal echocardiograms. Echocardiographic abnormalities attributed to HIV infection were present in 31 patients (21 percent). There was an association of abnormal echocardiographic findings with advanced clinical stages of the disease. The mortality during follow-up was the same for those with normal echocardiograms (35 of 102) as it was for those with abnormal echocardiograms (12 of 29; $p = .48$). Even in those with the most advanced clinical disease, there was no independent prognostic significance of the echocardiographic cardiac involvement, with 44 percent of both echo-normal and echo-abnormal patients dying. This study shows a remarkably low incidence of HIV-associated echocardiographic abnormalities, most often asymptomatic pericardial effusion.

These studies suggest that the prevalence of echocardiographic abnormalities in HIV-positive patients depends on the stage of their clinical illness, with the sickest patients having the most abnormalities. Katz and Sadaniantz have recently published a review of echocardiography in HIV cardiac disease.[32a]

PERICARDIAL INVOLVEMENT

In general, pericardial effusion and pericarditis constitute the most commonly recognized cardiac involvement in AIDS. At autopsy, Kaposi's sarcoma involvement and lymphoma may be clinically silent, accompanied by asymptomatic pericardial effusion, or they may be clinically important because of pericardial tamponade.[33] Pericarditis due to specific organisms has frequently been reported. These organisms are most commonly *Mycobacterium tuberculosis*[27,34,35] or *Mycobacterium avium–intracellulare*.[34,36] One study[27] reported pericardial tamponade in 5 patients and large pericardial effusions in 6. Of the patients with clinical heart disease in this study, 22 percent had echocardiographic evidence of tamponade, and another 33 percent had large pericardial effusions.

In a review of 15 autopsy and echocardiographic studies involving 1139 patients with HIV disease, the incidence of pericardial disease was 21 percent. Most cases were asymptomatic without an identifiable etiology. In those that were symptomatic, about two-thirds were caused by infection or neoplasm and one-third were of undetermined etiology. In the 66 published cases of pericardial tamponade, 26 percent were caused by *M. tuberculosis*.[34]

In a prospective echocardiographic study among 231 patients recruited over a 5-year period, the prevalence of pericardial effusion for AIDS patients entering into the study was 5 percent. Over the follow-up time, the incidence of pericardial effusion increased as the stage of the HIV progressed from 0 percent per year in asymptomatic HIV-infected patients to 11 percent per year in patients with AIDS; 80 percent of these effusions were small and asymptomatic.[35] The survival of the AIDS patients who developed pericardial effusion was significantly shorter than the survival of those who did not, 36 percent versus 93 percent at 6 months. This shortened survival period remained significant even after adjustment for lead-time bias and was independent of CD4+ T-cell count.[35] Since death was not due directly to pericardial effusion, the development of pericardial effusion in the setting of HIV infection probably suggests end-stage HIV disease.

Flum and colleagues[36] also reported that AIDS-associated pericardial effusion was a grave prognostic sign. They reported 29 patients who had surgical windows for large effusions; only in 2 patients did this result in a change in clinical management. The mortality was 69 percent at 8 weeks after the pericardial window.[36] They concluded that pericardial biopsy for diagnosis provided little practical therapeutic information and that surgical windows were justified only to relieve tamponade.

The etiology of pericardial effusion or pericarditis is not obvious; it may be HIV infection or other opportunistic viral infections with coxsackievirus, cytomegalovirus, or neoplasm.[37] Tuberculous pericarditis is particularly common in Africa.[38] Occasionally, pericarditis has been reported to be caused by common organisms such as *Staphylococcus*,[39] *Cryptococcus neoformans*,[40] or herpes simplex virus.[41]

MYOCARDIAL INVOLVEMENT

For a number of years, involvement of the pericardium and myocardium with both common and unusual opportunistic infections and neoplasms, such as Kaposi's sarcoma and lymphoma, has been recognized. At times, this involvement appears to be incidental and associated with the presence of organisms in many tissues, including the heart. Often, this involvement is not accompanied by signs of cell necrosis or even inflammation. At other times, the infection is accompanied by an intense myocarditis. Opportunistic infection has included viruses (herpes simplex, cytomegalovirus, and coxsackievirus), bacteria, protozoa (*Toxoplasma gondii*), and fungi (*Candida albicans, C. neoformans,* and *Aspergillus fumigatus*).[40,42,43] These specific infections have been diagnosed at autopsy but also during life with myocardial biopsy. The importance of identifying a specific organism as the cause of the myocarditis rests in the potential for treatment[34,44]; for instance, amphotericin B and flucytosine may be used to treat cryptococcosis. Albrecht and colleagues[45] reported a case of *T. gondii* myocarditis in a 45-year-old man with AIDS who was treated successfully with appropriate antiprotozoal therapy.

The most common neoplasms are Kaposi's sarcoma and lymphoma of the non-Hodgkin's type.[17,20,46] With Kaposi's sarcoma, the tumor involvement of the myocardium or pericardium is most frequently an incidental finding. On occasion, myocardial involvement by lymphoma is diagnosed by needle biopsy of the myocardium.

One study reported a collection of 21 cases of lymphoma in AIDS patients, 3 with Hodgkin's and 18 with non-Hodgkin's lymphoma of various histologic types, almost all of which were in the high-grade categories.[47] Unfortunately, these tend to be histologically aggressive tumors involving many organs, and they respond poorly to treatment. At times, the patient presents with pericardial tamponade or even superior vena cava syndrome.[48] Echocardiography revealing infiltration into the myocardium and/or myocardial or pericardial masses is most helpful in establishing a diagnosis.

CARDIOMYOPATHY

In 1986, Cohen and colleagues reported 3 patients with AIDS who had clinical, echocardiographic, and morphologic findings of dilated cardiomyopathy.[49] A subsequent report described 58 consecutively autopsied patients.[50] Seven (12 percent) had major clinical cardiovascular abnormalities, including 4 with congestive heart failure and others with ventricular tachycardia. All were late in the course of their disease. All patients with these major clinical cardiac abnormalities had focal myocarditis at autopsy. The etiology in these cases was not obvious but was believed to be viral myocarditis.

In another study of 71 patients with AIDS, 8 had left ventricular dilatation and decreased contractility and 4 had congestive heart failure.[26] In a similar echocardiographic study, none of 102 AIDS patients had congestive heart failure, although 41 percent had left ventricular hypokinesia.[28]

In autopsy studies reported in the literature, cardiac causes of death have been rare; clinically, the incidence of congestive heart failure has been extremely small, although microscopic focal myocarditis is frequently described. In 14 studies in the literature, 1009 patients with AIDS were reported. A total of 8 died of cardiac involvement. One had cryptococcal myocarditis, and 1 had toxoplasmic myocarditis; 5 came from one institution.[26]

Symptomatic cardiomyopathy in association with HIV-1 infection is uncommon; however, echocardiographic evidence of left ventricular dysfunction is more common, especially in patients with advanced HIV disease. Individual reports of 1 to 5 cases of patients with either dilated left ventricle, hypokinetic left ventricle, or both have been frequent enough to require explanation.[51] Furthermore, the occurrence of cardiomyopathy in children, in whom a disease unrelated to HIV infection would be rare, further suggests a relationship between HIV disease and cardiomyopathy.[52] In a study by Langston and colleagues[52] in infants and children dying with HIV infection, the frequency of cardiac disease as the cause of death increased with age, 0 percent by age 1 year and 25 percent after age 10 years.

Lipshultz and colleagues[53] did a prospective study on 196 HIV-infected children, median age 2.1 years. Only 2 had congestive heart failure at enrollment. An echocardiogram done every 4 months revealed a 2-year accumulative incidence of cardiomyopathy of 4.7 percent (95 percent confidence interval, 1.5 to 7.9 percent).[53]

Prospective echocardiographic studies have been reported that show a high prevalence of myocardial dysfunction. DeCastro and colleagues[54] did serial echocardiograms prospectively on 136 HIV-positive patients over a mean follow-up time of 415 ± 220 days. Seven AIDS patients developed clinical and echocardiographic findings of global left ventricular dysfunction. Of the 6 who died, 5 were autopsied: 3 had acute lymphocytic myocarditis, 1 had cryptococcal myocarditis, and 1 had myocardial fibrosis.[54]

Blanchard and colleagues[55] did serial echocardiograms on 70 HIV-positive outpatients. Of the 50 patients with AIDS, 7 (14 percent) had echocardiographic evidence of left ventricular dysfunction. On a repeat echocardiogram, 3 of the 7 had improved left ventricular function, implying a transient problem that caused a transient decrease in left ventricular function.[55]

At San Francisco General Hospital, the cases of 74 AIDS outpatients were prospectively followed using serial quantitative Doppler echocardiography every 4 months. Control populations included HIV-positive patients without disease, HIV-positive patients with AIDS-related complex, and HIV-negative gay men. Over the follow-up period of 16.5 ± 12 months, no differences in left ventricular systolic or diastolic function were detected between the groups and no differences were found in the mean values from the first to the last echocardiogram.[56]

The prospective study by Barbaro and colleagues[57] reported 952 asymptomatic HIV-positive patients whose cases were followed clinically and by echocardiography for 60 ± 5.3 months. With the echocardiogram, dilated cardiomyopathy was diagnosed in 76 (8 percent) of patients, an incidence of 1.6 cases per 100 patients per year. A myocardial biopsy was done on all patients with cardiomyopathy, and a histologic diagnosis of myocarditis made in 83 percent. By in situ hybridization HIV nucleic acid sequences were found in 58 patients but only 36 (62 percent) had active myocarditis. Of these 36 patients, 25 percent had other cardiotropic virus infections with Coxsackie B virus in 6 (17 percent), cytomegalovirus in 2 (6 percent), and Epstein-Barr virus in 1 (3 percent). The authors concluded that dilated cardiomyopathy might be related either to direct HIV infection or to an autoimmune process induced by HIV, possibly in association with other cardiotropic viruses. Heart failure appearing rapidly is a bad prognostic sign, with about half the patients dying within 6 months to one year.[53,57]

Possible Reasons for Cardiomyopathy

There are many theories on the etiology of the echocardiographic reduction in left ventricular function with or without left ventricular dilatation in patients with AIDS who may or may not have heart failure.[32a] The most frequently mentioned etiology is that of myocarditis or postmyocarditis cardiomyopathy. There are occasional reports of a virus grown from cardiac muscle. In 1987, Calabrese and colleagues[58] were the first to report the culturing of HIV from a right ventricular myocardial biopsy of a patient with a hypokinetic right ventricle and a normal left ventricle.

There is some evidence that HIV itself invades the myocardial cell. The myocyte has no CD4+ receptors, which are the major way by which the virus enters the cell. Although there are other ways and possibly other receptors by which the virus could invade the cell, no one has convincingly shown the virus or a portion of the viral DNA or RNA within the genome of the myocardial cell.[59,60] One study reported detecting HIV nucleic acid sequences by in situ hybridization in cardiac tissue sections from 6 of 22 patients examined who had died of AIDS.[61] The hybridization target was thought to be myocytes, but this could not be proved by this technique. Furthermore, the myocardial cells showing the positive hybridization signal were sparse, comprising only one or a few cells per section; the myocardium was normal by light microscopy; and none of the patients had clinical evidence of cardiac disease. Still, the most compelling evidence for the ability of HIV virus to enter the myocardial cell comes from the previously mentioned study by Barbaro and colleagues.[57]

Other Theories for the Development of Cardiomyopathy

OPPORTUNISTIC INFECTIONS

Patients with AIDS are exposed to and susceptible to multiple bacterial, viral, mycotic, and protozoal infections. Epstein-Barr virus and cytomegalovirus are both known to cause myocarditis in AIDS patients.[57,58] *Cryptococcus neoformans* and *T. Gondii* myocarditis have been well described.[24,44,62] Myocarditis due to *M. avium--intracellulare* has been reported.[18] *Aspergillus* endocarditis and myocarditis have been reported.[63]

DILATED CARDIOMYOPATHY AS A POSTVIRAL DISORDER

The study of patients with myocarditis without AIDS has shown that myocarditis can be precipitated by viral infection and that the inflammatory reaction can progress when the virus is no longer recoverable from either the heart or even the patient. The viral infection precipitates an immune reaction either to viral antigen that cross-reacts with a myocardial protein or to altered myocardial protein, which acts as a foreign antigen, thus precipitating the immune reactions that continue the myocardial necrosis and inflammatory cell infiltration[64] (see also Chap. 76).

The evidence that congestive cardiomyopathy is precipitated by a previous viral myocarditis includes the biopsy finding of inflammatory infiltrate in some patients with dilated cardiomyopathy[65] and detection of increased elevated viral antibody titers and viral-specific RNA sequences in myocardial biopsies.[66] Thus, cardiomyopathy can result from a previous infection with a number of organisms that are no longer recoverable from the myocardium.

Herskowitz and colleagues[67] reported the histologic and immunopathologic results of 37 endomyocardial biopsy samples from patients infected with HIV-1 who developed unexplained global left ventricular dysfunction. Twenty-eight patients had New York Heart

Association (NYHA) class III and IV congestive heart failure. Four patients had myocarditis secondary to known etiologies. Of the remaining 33 patients, 17 (52 percent) had histologic evidence of idiopathic active or borderline myocarditis. Specific hybridization within myocytes was abnormal in 5 patients with HIV-1 antisense riboprobe and in 16 of the 33 with cytomegalovirus immediate early (IE-2) antisense riboprobe. This study is compatible with the possibility that cardiotropic virus infection and myocarditis may be important in the pathogenesis of HIV-associated cardiomyopathy.[67]

IMPAIRMENT OF THE IMMUNE MECHANISM LEADING TO CARDIOMYOPATHY

Humorally mediated autoimmune reactions involving antimyosin antibodies may also be implicated in the development of cardiomyopathy.[68] Circulating cardiac autoantibodies have been identified in AIDS patients with cardiomyopathy and in none of the HIV-positive patients without cardiomyopathy. In situ hybridization with genomic probes failed to show evidence of HIV or any other viruses within the heart muscle. Results of ELISA showed a high titer of immunoglobulin G antibody to myosin and to cardiac mitochondrial adenine nucleotide transporter. In this study, it was concluded that the cardiomyopathy might be related not to HIV infection of the heart but rather to autoimmunity. Currie and colleagues reported an increased frequency of cardiac-specific autoantibodies in HIV-infected patients (15 percent) vs. in control patients (3.5 percent). Those with left ventricular dysfunction had the highest prevalence of cardiac autoantibodies (43 percent).[68a] Apparent improvement of left ventricular function in children with AIDS by using intravenously administered immunoglobulin is also suggestive of an immunologic etiology for the left ventricular dysfunction.[69]

ROLE OF CYTOKINES IN MYOCARDITIS

Ho and colleagues[70] proposed a primary role for neuroglial cell damage from the cytolytic effect of release of substances termed cytokines from HIV-infected monocytes, the "innocent bystander" destruction mechanism. Cytokines are biologically active mediators and are soluble proteins released by immune cells. Reversible myocardial depression is well documented in human and canine septic shock.[71] This was subsequently demonstrated to be due to a "myocardial depressant factor." The exact nature of this myocardial depressant factor is not agreed upon, but it could be related to a variety of mediators of sepsis such as endotoxin, cytokine tumor necrosis factor (TNF), and interleukin-2.[72]

Other studies showed that the administration of endotoxin-released TNF caused depression of left ventricular function independent of left ventricular volume or loading conditions,[73] and elevated circulating levels of TNF have been noted in patients with severe chronic heart failure.[74] Increased circulating levels of TNF have been noted in patients with advanced HIV-1 infection.[75] This is consistent with a finding of increased production of the cytokine TNF by peripheral monocytes of patients with AIDS.[76]

Barbaro and colleagues[77] investigated the myocardial expression of TNF-α and inducible nitric oxide synthase (INOS) in endomyocardial biopsies in patients with HIV dilated cardiomyopathy and compared them with myocardium from patients with idiopathic dilated cardiomyopathy. The mean intensity of both TNF-α and INOS immunostaining was greater in the patients with HIV than it was in the patients with idiopathic cardiomyopathy. The staining intensity of both TNF-α and INOS was inversely correlated with the CD4 count.

Liu and colleagues[78] demonstrated by immunostaining in the hearts of patients with AIDS that macrophages in the heart from those with cardiomyopathy were positive for cyclooxygenase-2 (COX-2) and INOS and were not in those without cardiomyopathy. This suggests that COX-2 activated HIV infected monocytes, macrophages, and T cells play a crucial role in the progression of HIV-1 myocarditis to cardiomyopathy.[78] Shannon[79] studied a Simian Immunodeficiency Viral (SIV) infection in nonhuman primates and reported that the SIV is localized to CD4-bearing inflammatory cells and not to cardiac myocytes, suggesting that the heart is an innocent bystander in AIDS cardiomyopathy.

The increased levels of cytokines including TNF, interleukins-1 and -2, and alpha-interferon might lead to myocardial dysfunction, either acting locally in a paracrine fashion on adjacent myocardium, or systemically causing a decrease in myocardial function.[77,80]

Twu and colleagues, using immunocytochemistry and computerized image analysis, demonstrated that patients with HIV cardiomyopathy had significant cardiomyocyte apoptosis related to the expression by inflammatory cells of gp120 and TNF-α. In HIV cardiomyopathic hearts, active caspase 9, a component of the mitochondrion-controlled apoptotic pathway, and elements of the death receptor-mediated pathway, TNF-α and Fas ligand were strongly expressed on macrophages and weakly on cardiomyocytes. There was greater macrophage infiltration on the cardiomyopathic hearts than in those without cardiomyopathy. They concluded that the cardiomyocytes die through both the mitochondrion- and death receptor-controlled apoptotic pathways.[80a]

CACHEXIA

Many patients with AIDS have marked weight loss and cachexia. In patients with anorexia nervosa, wall motion as assessed by two-dimensional echo Doppler was found to be abnormal in 8 of 14 patients but not in control subjects; also, lower stroke volume was found in patients compared with controls, possibly because of decreased heart size.[81] Starvation and refeeding studies in animals have demonstrated myofibrillar atrophy and cardiac interstitial edema, which are accompanied by a decrease in left ventricular compliance and decreased peak systolic force.[82] These changes are thought to be due to protein-calorie malnutrition. Congestive heart failure may occur, especially during refeeding and recovery.[83]

VITAMIN- AND SELENIUM-DEFICIENCY STATES

Cachectic people can have vitamin-deficiency states; it is doubtful that many patients with cardiomyopathy have this as a prime etiology. Selenium deficiency has been described, together with reduced cardiac selenium levels in AIDS, similar to Keshan's disease seen in Chinese people with selenium deficiency. In one study, 10 patients with AIDS who had decreased left ventricular fractional shortening on echocardiography received sodium selenite for 23 days.[84] Of 8 patients, 6 showed a return toward normal of left ventricular fractional shortening within 21 days. Selenium deficiency has been reported to be common in malnourished pediatric patients with AIDS.[85]

DRUG-INDUCED CARDIOMYOPATHY

The effect of drugs, both recreational and therapeutic, on myocardial function is not well delineated in patients with AIDS. In most patients with AIDS and cardiomyopathy, however, drugs do not seem to be the cause[61, 86]; nevertheless, in patients with AIDS, drugs such as doxorubicin, alpha$_2$-interferon, and interleukin-2 have been shown to produce cardiomyopathy that is sometimes reversible. One report described 3 cases of reversible cardiac dysfunction associated with alpha$_2$-interferon therapy in AIDS patients with Kaposi's sarcoma.[87]

Cocaine use has been associated with myocarditis and dilated cardiomyopathy, which occasionally has been reported to be reversible.[88] Cocaethylene, an active cocaine metabolite, coadministered with alcohol results in a marked alteration of host immunity and to increased susceptibility to infection with coxsackievirus B3, cytomegalovirus, and murine AIDS.[89] Alcohol consumption during murine-acquired immunodeficiency syndrome has been shown to accentuate cardiac pathology due to coxsackievirus.[90] Pentamidine has been reported to cause ventricular tachycardia.[91] Zidovudine (AZT), a nucleoside analogue, is a drug that inhibits replication of HIV in vitro, probably by inhibiting the reverse-transcriptase enzyme, which is essential to the replication of the retrovirus. No adverse cardiac effects have been reported in phase 1 clinical trials, and one study failed to show cardiotoxicity[92]; however, a toxic mitochondrial myopathy caused by long-term AZT after 12.8 months of therapy has been reported.[93] This myopathy is characterized by abnormal mitochondria with paracrystalloid inclusions. AZT-induced cardiomyopathy in rats has been shown to be related to oxidative damage and activated ADP-ribosylation reactions damaging mitochondrial energy production.[94] An extensive review of the subject has recently been reported by Lewis.[94a] In AIDS mice, a combination of zidovudine, lamivudine, and indinavir was given for 35 days. Left ventricular mass increased 160 percent by echocardiography, and the markers for cardiomyopathy; atrial natriuretic factor mRNA increased 250 percent, and sarcoplasmic calcium ATPase (SERCA 2) decreased 57 percent. Microscopically, damaged mitochondria were seen.[95] Whether this can occur in cardiac muscle in some patients is not clear. Foscarnet therapy for the treatment of cytomegalovirus infection has also been reported to produce a reversible cardiomyopathy.[96]

Conclusions

Clinical heart muscle disease and heart failure in AIDS are unusual. When this condition occurs, there may be explanations other than direct infection with HIV. The exact incidence of heart muscle disease in AIDS is as yet unknown but must be small, and the mechanisms that can cause failure are probably multiple. With prolonged survival with HAART, cardiomyopathy may become more frequent.

METABOLIC CARDIOVASCULAR COMPLICATIONS OF ANTIVIRAL DRUGS

With the introduction of protease inhibitors, a class of drugs that suppresses HIV replication, to the treatment of patients with HIV infection, metabolic abnormalities have been seen that have potential for development of cardiovascular disease. The metabolic abnormalities seen consist of hypertriglyceridemia, lowered HDL, hyperglycemia, and insulin resistance.[97] Insulin resistance is common and is found in about half the patients on protease inhibitors compared to about one-fourth of patients on nucleoside therapy.[97a] New-onset hyperglycemia similar to type II diabetes mellitus has been described, as well as worsening of preexisting diabetes in 1 to 6 percent of patients. This problem has been described with all of the protease inhibitors.[98] The cause of the hyperglycemia is not known, but it does respond to sulfonylureas, suggesting that the drug causes increased resistance to the peripheral effects of insulin, although it is not possible to rule out a reduction in insulin secretion.[99] The treatment of hyperglycemia is similar to that of type 2 diabetes: diet and oral hypoglycemic drugs.

Lipid metabolic abnormalities have also been seen in patients taking protease inhibitors with extremely high triglyceride levels over 1000 mg/dL,[100] which can occur within 2 weeks of starting therapy. In a study of ritonavir plus saquinavir, 11 percent of patients developed triglycerides above 1500 mg/dL. There were no instances of pancreatitis. There are also elevations in serum cholesterol.[101]

A lipodystrophy syndrome has been described consisting of wasting of adipose tissues in the face, arms, and upper chest with central fat distribution, and, although seen before protease inhibitors were introduced, has been more prominently recognized since the introduction of HAART.[97,101a] There is a loss of subcutaneous fat from the face and limbs (partial lipodystrophy), and the development of fat deposits in the abdomen ("protease pouch") and dorsocervical fat pad ("buffalo hump").[102] The abdominal fat may be either in the subcutaneous tissue or in the intraabdominal visceral fat.[103] The abnormal fat distribution appears to be associated with the use of ritonavir–saquinavir combinations rather than with indinavir and does not respond to dietary restriction or exercise. In patients with a buffalo hump, hypercortisolism has been ruled out as a cause, and half the patients with a buffalo hump had never been on protease inhibitors.[102] The relation of these abnormalities to protease inhibitors is still not clear.[101a]

Although the mechanism by which this drug induces hyperlipidemia is unknown, there is a 60 percent homology of the catalytic region of the HIV-1 protease to which the drugs bind to two proteins regulating lipid metabolism: cytoplasmic retinoic acid-binding protein type I (CRABP-I) and low-density lipoprotein-receptor-related protein (LRP). Binding of the protease inhibitors to LRP would impair hepatic chylomicron uptake and triglyceride clearance.[99] The elevated triglycerides respond to gemfibrozil. Patients with lipodystrophy syndrome have been shown to have accelerated lipolysis, explaining the lipoatrophy seen in the limbs, and increased hepatic reesterification promoting the observed hypertriglyceridemia.[104] Insulin resistance and hyperglycemia have been shown to be related to impaired glucose transport and phosphorylation causing reduced insulin-mediated glucose uptake by skeletal muscle.[105]

The treatment of dyslipidemia associated with protease inhibitors begins with switching the patient to a protease inhibitor less likely to cause dyslipidemia. This is especially effective if the patient is taking ritonavir.[105a] In some studies, substituting nonnucleoside reverse-transcriptase inhibitors for protease inhibitors has had a beneficial effect.[105b] Dietary and drug treatment of dyslipidemia associated with HIV treatment follows the recommendations of the National Cholesterol Education Program (NCEP) Adult Treatment Panel III (ATPIII).[105c]

In 45 HIV-infected patients taking protease inhibitors who had abnormally elevated lipids, the National Cholesterol Education Program Guidelines were followed without disrupting the HIV therapy. Mean serum cholesterol rose from 170 mg/dL before to 289 mg/dL after starting the protease inhibitor, and the triglycerides were 879 mg/dL. On diet, gemfibrozil alone, or with atorvastatin, the cholesterol fell to 201 mg/dL ($p = .01$) over a 10-month period.[106] Bezafibrate has also been shown to effectively reduce triglycerides by 35 percent over 6 months in lipodystrophy patients with diet-resistant hyperlipidemia.[107]

Since the protease inhibitors are such important drugs in the management of patients with HIV infection, every attempt must be made to control their metabolic side effects without stopping the drug. Diet and oral hypoglycemic drugs can control the hyperglycemia. Fibrates and HMG-CoA reductase inhibitors decrease the elevated triglycerides, cholesterol, and low-density lipoproteins, as noted. A potential problem is that protease inhibitors are metabolized by the hepatic cytochrome P450 CYP4-A system, and these drugs can both induce and/or inhibit the system. Therefore, other drugs metabolized by the cytochrome P450 system can have their plasma levels either decreased or increased when used together with the protease inhibitors, resulting in an extensive list of drug interactions and possibly drug toxicity. Pravastatin is the only 3-hydroxy-3-methylglutaryl coenzyme A (HMG CoA) reductase drug that is not metabolized by other statin drugs will be markedly elevated.[108] The importance of treating the metabolic abnormalities, however, is seen in the increasing number of reports of premature, extensive coronary artery disease in patients taking protease inhibitors.[108]

RISK OF INCREASED ATHEROSCLEROSIS AND CORONARY ARTERY DISEASE

With increasing advances in therapy and especially with the protease inhibitors and combination therapy (HAART), there has been a decrease in morbidity and mortality in HIV infected patients.[1] In 1255 patients with advanced AIDS with a CD4+ count of <100/mm³, the mortality decreased from 29.4/100 patient-years in 1995 to 8.8/100 patient-years in 1997. There was also a decrease in AIDS-related opportunistic infections.[15,109] With the introduction of protease inhibitors there have been increasing reports of premature myocardial infarctions raising the possibility of an increase in atherosclerosis, including coronary artery disease as a result of the metabolic changes seen with protease inhibitors.

Studies investigating the possible relation between antiretroviral therapy and subclinical atherosclerosis have yielded mixed results. Using ultrasound, Maggi and colleagues[110] showed carotid intimal-medial thickening in 52.7 percent of AIDS patients on protease inhibitors, 14.9 percent of AIDS patients not on protease inhibitors, and only 6.7 percent of healthy controls. Mercie and colleagues[111] studied 423 HIV-infected patients with carotid ultrasound and found with multivariant analysis that the effect of HAART disappeared after adjustment for the conventional atherosclerotic risk factors.

An increasing incidence of patients with presumably premature coronary artery disease has also been described.[112] In 5672 outpatients with HIV-1 infection seen between 1993 and 2000 the frequency of myocardial infarction increased after introduction of protease inhibitors in 1996. Myocardial infarction occurred in 19 of 3247 patients taking protease inhibitors and in only 2 of 2425 patients not on protease inhibitors, an odds ratio of 7.1.[113] Not all the evidence favors an increased risk of coronary disease in patients treated with protease inhibitors. Klein and associates reported a study of Kaiser Permanente patients from Northern California before and after protease inhibitors use and before and after antiretroviral therapy. Coronary heart disease and myocardial infarction hospitalization rates were not significantly different before versus after protease inhibitors (6.2 vs 6.7 event/1000 person years) or before or after antiretroviral therapy (5.7 vs 6.8 event/1000 person years). However, comparing HIV positive and negative patients, the coronary heart disease hospitalization rate was significantly higher (6.5 vs 3.8 event/1000 person years $p = 0.003$) and the difference in the myocardial infarction rate was also higher (4.3 vs 2.9 event/1000 person years $p = .07$).[113a] With greater longevity and increased use of highly effective antiretroviral agents, increasing morbidity and mortality due to coronary artery disease will be seen.

PULMONARY HYPERTENSION

Right ventricular hypertrophy and dilatation due to pulmonary hypertension is seen in patients with HIV-1 infection.[114,114a] Mesa and colleagues[115] in 88 reported cases of pulmonary hypertension in AIDS patients from the literature found no correlation with CD4 counts or history of pulmonary infection. The 1-year survival was 51 percent for patients with pulmonary hypertension. In 33 patients where tissue was examined microscopically, 28 (85 percent) had the plexogenic variant of pulmonary arterial hypertension. The cause of the pulmonary hypertension is unknown but cytokine-related stimu-

lation and proliferation of endothelium is postulated.[116] Another possibility is that hyperplasia of the smooth muscle cells in the pulmonary arterioles is stimulated by receptor-mediated action of viral proteins. The HIV envelope protein gp120 has been shown to be a potent mitogen for vascular smooth muscle cells.[117]

INFECTIVE ENDOCARDITIS

Infective endocarditis in patients with HIV infection is almost exclusively seen in intravenous drug users. Cicalini and colleagues[118] reported 108 episodes of infective endocarditis in 105 HIV-infected patients of whom 94.3 percent were intravenous drug users. As with infective endocarditis in non-AIDS intravenous drug users, the most common valve involved was the tricuspid valve (52 percent) and the most frequent organism, S. aureus. Left-sided valves were involved in 46 percent of patients.

CLINICAL WORKUP AND THERAPY

The workup of patients with AIDS and suspected cardiac involvement begins with the history and physical examination for symptoms and signs of cardiac disease. Since there is no therapeutic advantage to finding subclinical cardiovascular involvement, there is no justification for screening electrocardiograms or echocardiograms. If there are signs or symptoms suggesting cardiovascular disease such as shortness of breath, a friction rub, an S_3 gallop, or other evidence of congestive heart failure, an echocardiogram is useful in identifying pericardial effusion and in evaluating right and left ventricular size and function. Invasive diagnostic studies are rarely necessary.

If left ventricular dilatation and hypokinesis are found with or without clinical evidence of heart failure, consideration should be given to stopping all drugs that are not absolutely essential.[119] If, in a 2-week follow-up, echocardiography reveals improvement, the suspected drug should be eliminated.

The question of whether a myocardial biopsy is helpful is controversial. The finding of a treatable cause of biopsy-proved myocarditis is rare. Furthermore, there is no evidence that treating biopsy-proved focal myocarditis with steroids or antimetabolites is effective.[120] Therefore, by available evidence, myocardial biopsy is of little value. There is no specific treatment for pulmonary hypertension without obvious secondary cause. Calcium channel blocking drugs, prostacyclin (intravenous epoprostenol or oral bosentan) or phosphodiesterase-5 inhibitors (sildenafil) can be tried in an attempt to lower the pulmonary vascular resistance.[121]

The potential cardiotoxic roles of drugs for opportunistic infection,[122] as well as other known etiologies such as hypertension, hypertrophic cardiomyopathy, and coronary artery disease, should be considered. The treatment of congestive heart failure is similar to that of the treatment of heart failure from other etiologies (e.g., diuretics, digoxin, and angiotensin-converting enzyme inhibitors (see Chap. 21).

CARDIOVASCULAR SURGERY IN AIDS PATIENTS

There has been an increased interest in whether AIDS health care workers can become infected, or, if infected, can infect patients and accelerate the disease through surgery. The problem is illustrated by the following questions:

1. Are we performing an expensive procedure that will cause prolonged hospitalization and probably not affect the outcome in AIDS patients?
2. What is the risk of accelerating the disease by surgery?

3. What is the risk of HIV infection to health care workers?
4. What is the risk of getting HIV infection during open-heart surgery?

In general, it is not wise to perform expensive procedures with some degree of morbidity and mortality that result in prolonged hospitalization of patients with a limited life span due to their underlying disease. For this reason, patients with AIDS should not be subjected to surgery that will most probably not significantly affect their survival. Before protease inhibitors were available, probably 70 percent of patients found to have AIDS would die within 3 to 4 years of the diagnosis.[123] Now, with newer drugs, life has been markedly prolonged.[15] Therefore, if patients with AIDS have medically uncontrollable symptoms, invasive procedures that can ameliorate these symptoms are indicated.

With infective endocarditis, the vast majority of HIV-infected patients are intravenous drug users, and the most common valve involved is the tricuspid valve, which almost always can be treated medically. The most frequent problem in which the question of cardiovascular surgery arises in a relatively young subgroup involves the intravenous drug user with infective endocarditis on the aortic and/or mitral valve and congestive heart failure. The presence of HIV disease in these patients, who overall have a high mortality and poor results from surgery, would suggest that they be treated medically for as long as possible.[124] If failure persists, valvular replacement should be done.

HIV-positive patients and patients with PGL who have not had an opportunistic infection or cancer can have a prolonged course over many years and, in general, should be treated like patients without HIV disease. In fact, life span might be prolonged after HIV infection by using combinations of drugs, including reverse-transcriptase inhibitors and the new protease inhibitors. In this subgroup, cardiovascular surgery should be considered for the usual indications.

The question of whether progression of the HIV disease is accelerated by the immunologic challenge that occurs from cardiopulmonary bypass is largely unanswered. Instances of HIV-positive patients who developed AIDS shortly after open heart surgery have been reported. It is known that cardiopulmonary bypass temporarily depresses phagocytic function and immune globulin production.[125] Cardiopulmonary bypass per se in HIV-negative patients causes prolonged abnormalities in the CD4+/CD8+ T-cell ratio up to 6 days postoperatively.[126] There is, therefore, a basis for concern that cardiopulmonary bypass surgery could accelerate the progression of HIV disease, and this must be taken into consideration.

Whether all patients undergoing cardiovascular surgery or other invasive procedures should have HIV testing is a matter of heated debate. Although the risk to health care personnel is small, HIV infection is usually tantamount to a chronic and eventually fatal infection; fear is great among both health care workers and the public. In contrast, AIDS is an emotional subject, and patients who are known to be HIV positive may be subjected to prejudice and discrimination. At present, HIV testing of both health care workers and patients is voluntary; however, there are proposed recommendations requiring disclosure to patients that a health care worker is HIV positive and informed consent from patients before any invasive procedure is done. This matter is still under considerable debate. Knowledge of the patient's HIV status or awareness of the patient's high-risk status for such infection did not appear to influence the rate of exposure, suggesting that preoperative testing for HIV infection would not decrease the frequency of accidental exposure to blood.

In combined data from 20 prospective studies of the risk of HIV-1 transmission to health care workers, there were 6498 parenteral exposures among 1948 subjects.[127] The chance of seroconversion was 0.32 percent per exposure (95 percent confidence interval, 0.18 to 0.46 percent); in 2885 mucous membrane exposures, there was 1 seroconversion (0.03 percent per exposure). The risk of a health care worker developing HIV seroconversion from work-related activities was very low: approximately 1 infection in 300 documented exposures to HIV-positive blood.[127a]

Still, because of the risk, some cardiovascular surgeons and cardiologists are refusing to operate on or catheterize an HIV-positive person or a patient who will not allow an HIV test to be done. In 1989, a survey was done of the attitudes of cardiac surgeons in the United States concerning operating on HIV-positive patients.[128] More than half responded, and two-thirds of these were reportedly willing to perform open heart surgery on HIV-positive patients no matter how the patients had acquired their HIV infection. One-quarter of the surgeons would not operate no matter how the HIV infection was acquired, and the rest were uncertain. Once the patient has gone from the HIV-carrier state to AIDS, two-thirds of the cardiac surgeons would not operate. Of those responding, 90 percent want to be able to test all their patients for HIV status. In 1992 a national survey of surgeons showed that only 8 percent knew the risk of acquiring HIV infection if they sustained percutaneous injury with contaminated blood and only 61 percent were familiar with the CDC guidelines on universal precautions.[129] A physician's fear of becoming infected with HIV is understandable, but as in the case of other professions that involved personal dangers, the profession of the physician requires performance. Both the American College of Physicians and the American Medical Association currently have standards stating that physicians may not ethically refuse to treat patients solely because the patients are HIV positive.

References

1. Fauci AS. The AIDS epidemic. N Engl J Med 1999;341:1046–1050.
1a. www.cdc.gov/hiv/stats.htm exposure 2/15/03
2. Centers for Disease Control: HIV/AIDS Surveillance Report, vol. 10, no. 2. Atlanta: Centers for Disease Control and Prevention 1998:1–43.
3. Department of Economic and Social Affairs of the United Nations Secretariat. The Demographic Impact of HIV/AIDS. New York: United Nations, 1999.
4. Centers for Disease Control. Classification system for human T-lymphotropic virus type III/lymphadenopathy-associated virus infections. MMWR Morb Mortal Wkly Rep 1986;35:334–339.
5. Centers for Disease Control. 1993 Revised classification system for HIV infection and expanded surveillance case definition for AIDS among adolescents and adults. MMWR 1992;41(RR-17):1–19.
6. Schacker T, Collier AC, Hughes J, et al. Clinical and epidemiologic features of primary HIV infection. Ann Intern Med 1996;125:257–264.
7. Horsburgh CR Jr, Ou CY, Jason J, et al. Duration of human immunodeficiency virus infection before detection of antibody. Lancet 1989;2:637–640.
8. Bacchetti P, Moss AR. Incubation period of AIDS in San Francisco [letter]. Nature 1989;338:251–253.
9. Feinberg MB, Greene WC. Molecular insights into human immunodeficiency virus type 1 pathogenesis. Curr Opin Immunol 1992;4:466–474.
10. Rutherford GW, Lifson AR, Hessol NA, et al. Course of HIV-1 infection in a cohort of homosexual and bisexual men: An 11 year follow-up study. BMJ 1990;301:1183–1188.
11. Osmond D. Progression to AIDS in persons testing seropositive for antibody to HIV. In: Cohen PT, Sande MA, Volberding PA, eds. The

AIDS Knowledge Base. Waltham, MA: Medical Publishing Group; 1990:1.1.6.

12. Piatak M Jr, Saag MS, Yang LC, et al. High levels of HIV-1 in plasma during all stages of infection determined by competitive PCR. *Science* 1993;259:1749–1754.

13. Pantaleo G, Menzo S, Vaccarezza M, et al. Studies in subjects with long-term nonprogressive human immunodeficiency virus infection. *N Engl J Med* 1995;332:209–216.

14. Balfour HH Jr. Antiviral drugs. *N Engl J Med* 1999;340:1255–1268.

15. Palella FJ, Delaney KM, Moorman AC, et al. Declining morbidity and mortality among patients with advanced human immunodeficiency virus infection. The HIV outpatient study investigators. *N Engl J Med* 1998;338:853–860.

16. Mann J, Ching , Piot P, et al. The international epidemiology of AIDS. *Sci Am* 1988;259:82–89.

17. Silver MA, Macher AM, Reichert CM, et al. Cardiac involvement by Kaposi's sarcoma in acquired immune deficiency syndrome (AIDS). *Am J Cardiol* 1984;53:983–985.

18. Cammarosano C, Lewis W. Cardiac lesions in acquired immune deficiency syndrome (AIDS). *J Am Coll Cardiol* 1985;5:703–706.

19. Wilkes MS, Fortin AH, Felix JC, et al. Value of necropsy in acquired immunodeficiency syndrome. *Lancet* 1988;2:85–88.

20. Lewis W. AIDS: Cardiac findings from 115 autopsies. *Prog Cardiovasc Dis* 1989;32:207–215.

21. Anderson DW, Virmani R, Reilly JM, et al. Prevalent myocarditis at necropsy in the acquired immunodeficiency syndrome. *J Am Coll Cardiol* 1988;11:792–799.

22. Segal BH, Factor SM. Myocardial risk factors other than human immunodeficiency virus infection may contribute to histologic cardiomyopathic changes in acquired immune deficiency syndrome. *Mod Pathol* 1993;6:560–564.

23. Barbaro G, DiLorenzo G, Grisorio B, et al. Cardiac involvement in the acquired immunodeficiency syndrome: A multicenter clinical and pathological study. Gruppo Italiano par lo studio cardiologico dei pazienti affetti da AIDS Investigators. *AIDS Res Hum Retroviruses* 1998; 14:1071–1077.

24. Masliah E, DeTeresa RM, Mallory ME, et al. Changes in pathological findings at autopsy in AIDS cases for the last 15 years. *AIDS* 2000;14:69–74.

24a. Selik RM, Byers RH Jr, Dworkin MS. Trends in diseases reported in U.S. Death Certificates that mention HIV infection 1987–1999. *J Acquir Immune Defic Syndr* 2002;29:378–387.

25. Murray JF, Garay SM, Hopewell PC, et al. Pulmonary complications of the acquired immunodeficiency syndrome. An update. Report of the second National Heart, Lung and Blood Institute workshop. *Am Rev Respir Dis* 1987;135:504–509.

26. Himelman RB, Chung WS, Chernoff DN, et al. Cardiac manifestations of human immunodeficiency virus infection: A two-dimensional echocardiographic study. *J Am Coll Cardiol* 1989;13:1030–1036.

27. Monsuez JJ, Kinney EL, Vittecoq D, et al. Comparison among acquired immune deficiency syndrome patients with and without clinical evidence of cardiac disease. *Am J Cardiol* 1988;62:1311–1313.

28. Corallo S, Mutinelli MR, Moroni M, et al. Echocardiography detects myocardial damage in AIDS: Prospective study in 102 patients. *Eur Heart J* 1988;9:887–892.

29. Currie PF, Jacob AJ, Foreman AR, et al. Heart muscle disease related to HIV infection: Prognostic implications. *BMJ* 1994;309:1605–1607.

30. Cecchi E, Parrini I, Chinaglia A, et al. Cardiac complications in HIV infections. *G Ital Cardiol* 1997;27:917–924.

31. Steffen HM, Muller R, Schrappe-Bächer M, et al. Prevalence of echocardiographic abnormalities in human immunodeficiency virus 1 infection. *Am J Noninvasive Cardiol* 1991;5:280–284.

32. Redfield RR, Wright DC, Tramont EC. The Walter Reed staging classification for HTLV-III/LAV infection: Special report. *N Engl J Med* 1986;314:131–132.

32a. Katz AS, Sadaniantz A. Echocardiography in HIV cardiac disease. *Prog Cardiovasc Dis* 2003; 45:285–292.

33. Chyu KY, Birnbaum Y, Naqvi T, et al. Echocardiographic detection of Kaposi's sarcoma causing cardiac tamponade in a patient with acquired immunodeficiency syndrome. *Clin Cardiol* 1998;21:131–133.

34. Estok L, Wallach F. Cardiac tamponade in a patient with AIDS: A review of pericardial disease in patients with HIV infection. *Mt Sinai J Med* 1998;65:33–39.

35. Heidenreich PA, Eisenberg MJ, Kee LL, et al. Pericardial effusion in AIDS: Incidence and survival. *Circulation* 1995;92:3229–3234.

36. Flum DR, McGinn JT Jr, Tyras DH. The role of the "pericardial window" in AIDS. *Chest* 1995;107:1522–1525.

37. Azrak EC, Kern MJ, Bach RG. Hemodynamics of cardiac tamponade in a patient with AIDS-related non-Hodgkin's lymphoma. *Catheter Cardiovasc Design* 1998;45:287–291.

38. Hakim JG, Ternouth I, Mushangi E, et al. Double blind randomised placebo controlled trial of adjunctive prednisolone in the treatment of effusive tuberculous pericarditis in HIV seropositive patients. *Heart* 2000;84(2):183–188.

39. Decker CF, Tuazon CU. *Staphylococcus aureus* pericarditis in HIV-infected patients. *Chest* 1994;105:615–616.

40. Zuger A, Louie E, Holzman RS, et al. Cryptococcal disease in patients with acquired immunodeficiency syndrome: Diagnostic features and outcome of treatment. *Ann Intern Med* 1986;104:234–240.

41. Freedberg RS, Gindea AJ, Dieterich DT, et al. Herpes simplex pericarditis in AIDS. *NY State J Med* 1987;87:304–306.

42. Francis CK. Cardiac involvement in AIDS. *Curr Probl Cardiol* 1990; 15:571–639.

43. Hofman P, Drici MD, Gibelin P, et al. Prevalence of toxoplasma myocarditis in patients with the acquired immunodeficiency syndrome. *Br Heart J* 1993;70:376–381.

44. Kinney EL, Monsuez JJ, Kitzis M, et al. Treatment of AIDS-associated heart disease. *Angiology* 1989;40:970–976.

45. Albrecht H, Stellbrink HJ, Fenske S, et al. Successful treatment of *Toxoplasma gondii* myocarditis in an AIDS patient. *Eur J Clin Microbiol Infect Dis* 1994;13:500–504.

46. Little RF, Gutierrez M, Jaffe ES, et al. HIV-associated non-Hodgkin lymphoma: Incidence, presentation, and prognosis. *JAMA* 2001;285:1880–1885.

47. Ioachim HL, Cooper MC, Hellman GC. Lymphomas in men at high risk for acquired immune deficiency syndrome (AIDS): A study of 21 cases. *Cancer* 1985;56:2831–2842.

48. Levitt LJ, Ault KA, Pinkus GS, et al. Pericarditis and early cardiac tamponade as a primary manifestation of lymphoscarcoma cell leukemia. *Am J Med* 1979;67:719–723.

49. Cohen IS, Anderson DW, Virmani R, et al. Congestive cardiomyopathy in association with the acquired immunodeficiency syndrome. *N Engl J Med* 1986;315:628–630.

50. Reilly JM, Cunnion RE, Anderson DW, et al. Frequency of myocarditis, left ventricular dysfunction and ventricular tachycardia in the acquired immune deficiency syndrome. *Am J Cardiol* 1988;62:789–793.

51. Lipshultz SE, Orav EJ, Sanders SP, et al. Cardiac structure and function in children with human immunodeficiency virus infection treated with zidovudine. *N Engl J Med* 1992;327:1260–1265.

52. Langston C, Cooper ER, Goldfarb J, et al. Human immunodeficiency virus-related mortality in infants and children: Data from the pediatric pulmonary and cardiovascular complications of vertically transmitted HIV (P(2)C(2)) Study. *Pediatrics* 2001;107:328–338.

53. Lipshultz SE, Easley KA, Orav EJ, et al. Left ventricle structure and function in children with human immunodeficiency virus: The prospective P2 C2 HIV Multicenter Study. Pediatric Pulmonary and Cardiac Complications of Vertically Transmitted HIV Infection (P2 C2 HIV) Study Group. *Circulation* 1998;97:1246–1256.

54. DeCastro S, d'Amati G, Gallo P, et al. Frequency of development of acute global left ventricular dysfunction in human immunodeficiency virus infection. *J Am Coll Cardiol* 1994;24:1018–1024.

55. Blanchard DG, Hagenhoff C, Chow LC, et al. Reversibility of cardiac abnormalities in human immunodeficiency virus (HIV)-infected individuals: A serial echocardiographic study. *J Am Coll Cardiol* 1991;17:1270–1276.

56. Cheitlin MD. Cardiovascular complications of HIV infection. In: Sande MA, Volberding PA, eds. *The Medical Management of AIDS,* 4th ed. Philadelphia: Saunders; 1995:332.

57. Barbaro G, Di Lorenzo G, Grisorio B, et al. Incidence of dilated cardiomyopathy and detection of HIV in myocardial cells of HIV-positive patients. Gruppo Italiano per lo Studio Cardilogico dei Pazianti Affetti, da AIDS. *N Engl J Med* 1998;339:1093–1099.

58. Calabrese LH, Proffitt MR, Yen-Lieberman B, et al. Congestive cardiomyopathy and illness related to the acquired immunodeficiency syndrome (AIDS) associated with isolation of retrovirus from myocardium. *Ann Intern Med* 1987;107:691–692.

59. Okano M, Gross TG. A review of Epstein-Barr virus infection in patients with immunodeficiency disorders. *Am J Med Sci* 2000;319: 392–396.

60. Grody WW, Cheng L, Lewis W. Infection of the heart by the human immunodeficiency virus. *Am J Cardiol* 1990;66:203–206.

61. Kaminski HJ, Katzman M, Wiest PM, et al. Cardiomyopathy associated with the acquired immune deficiency syndrome. *J AIDS* 1988;1: 105–110.

62. Acierno LJ. Cardiac complications in acquired immunodeficiency syndrome (AIDS): A review. *J Am Coll Cardiol* 1989;13: 1144–1154.

63. Cox JN, Di Dio F, Pizzolato GP, et al. *Aspergillus* endocarditis and myocarditis in a patient with the acquired immunodeficiency syndrome (AIDS): A review of the literature: Case report. *Virchows Arch* [A] 1990;417:255–259.

64. Lowry PJ, Thompson RA, Littler WA. Cellular immunity in congestive cardiomyopathy: The normal cellular immune response. *Br Heart J* 1985;53:394–399.

65. Parrillo JE, Aretz HT, Palacios I, et al. The results of transvenous endomyocardial biopsy can frequently be used to diagnose myocardial disease in patients with idiopathic heart failure: Endomyocardial biopsy in 100 consecutive patients revealed a substantial incidence of myocarditis. *Circulation* 1984;69:93–101.

66. Bowles NE, Richardson PJ, Olsen EGJ, et al. Detection of Coxsackie-B-virus-specific RNA sequences in myocardial biopsy samples from patients with myocarditis and dilated cardiomyopathy. *Lancet* 1984;1:1120–1123.

67. Herskowitz A, WU T-C, Willoughby SB, et al. Myocarditis and cardiotrophic viral infection associated with severe left ventricular dysfunction in late-stage infection with human immunodeficiency virus. *J Am Coll Cardiol* 1994;24:1025–1032.

68. Herskowitz A, Ansari AA, Neumann DA, et al. Cardiomyopathy in acquired immunodeficiency syndrome: Evidence for autoimmunity [abstr]. *Circulation* 1989;80(suppl II):II–322.

68a. Currie PF, Goldman JH, Caforio AL, et al. Cardiac autoimmunity in HIV-related heart muscle disease. *Heart* 1998;79:599:604.

69. Lipshultz SE, Orav J, Sanders SP, et al. Immunoglobulins and left ventricular structure and function in pediatric HIV infection. *Circulation* 1995;92:2220–2225.

70. Ho DD, Pomerantz RJ, Kaplan JC. Pathogenesis of infection with human immunodeficiency virus. *N Engl J Med* 1987;317:278–286.

71. Natanson C, Fink MP, Ballantyne HK, et al. Gram-negative bacteremia produces both severe systolic and diastolic cardiac dysfunction in a canine model that simulates human septic shock. *J Clin Invest* 1986;78:259–270.

72. Cunnion RE, Parrillo JE. Myocardial dysfunction in sepsis: Recent insights [editorial]. *Chest* 1989;95:941–945.

73. Suffredini AF, Fromm RE, Parker MM, et al. The cardiovascular response of normal humans to the administration of endotoxin. *N Engl J Med* 1989;321:280–287.

74. Levine B, Kalman J, Mayer L, et al. Elevated circulating levels of tumor necrosis factor in severe chronic heart failure. *N Engl J Med* 1990; 323:236–241.

75. Lähdevirta J, Maury CPJ, Teppo AM, et al. Elevated levels of circulating cachectin/tumor necrosis factor in patients with acquired immunodeficiency syndrome. *Am J Med* 1988;85:289–291.

76. Wright SC, Jewett A, Mitsuyasu R, et al. Spontaneous cytotoxicity and tumor necrosis factor production by peripheral blood monocytes from AIDS patients. *J Immunol* 1988;141:99–104.

77. Barbaro G, Di Lorenzo G, Soldini M, et al. Intensity of myocardial expression of inducible nitric oxide synthase influences the clinical course of human immunodeficiency virus-associated cardiomyopathy. Gruppo Italiano per lo Studio Cardiologico dei pazienti affetti dei AIDS (GISCA). *Circulation* 1999;100:933–939.

78. Liu QN, Reddy S, Sayre JW, et al. Essential role of HIV type 1-infected and cyclooxygenase 2-activated macrophages and T cells in HIV type 1 myocarditis. *AIDS Res Hum Retroviruses* 2001;17: 142–133.

79. Shannon RP. SIV cardiomyopathy in nonhuman primaes. *Trends Cardiovasc Med* 2001;11:242–246.

80. Yamamoto N. The role of cytokines in the acquired immunodeficiency syndrome. *Int J Clin Lab Res* 1995;25:29–34.

80a. Twu C, Liu NQ, Popik W, et al. Cardiomyocytes undergo apoptosis in human immunodeficiency virus cardiomyopathy through mitochondrion- and death receptor-controlled pathways. *PNAS* 2002;99: 14386–14391.

81. Goldberg SJ, Comerci GD, Feldman L. Cardiac output and regional myocardial contraction in anorexia nervosa. *J Adolesc Health Care* 1988;9:15–21.

82. Abel RM, Grimes JB, Alonso D, et al. Adverse hemodynamic and ultrastructural changes in dog hearts subjected to protein-calorie malnutrition. *Am Heart J* 1979;97:733–744.

83. Schocken DD, Holloway JD, Powers PS. Weight loss and the heart: Effects of anorexia nervosa and starvation. *Arch Intern Med* 1989;149:877–881.

84. Dworkin BM, Antonecchia PP, Smith F, et al. Reduced cardiac selenium content in the acquired immunodeficiency syndrome. *J Parenter Enteral Nutr* 1989;13:644–647.

85. Kavanaugh-McHugh AL, Ruff A, Perlman E, et al. Selenium deficiency and cardiomyopathy in acquired immunodeficiency syndrome. *J Parenter Enteral Nutr* 1991;15:347–349.

86. Kaul S, Fishbein MC, Siegel RJ. Cardiac manifestations of acquired immune deficiency syndrome: A 1991 update. *Am Heart J* 1991;122: 535–544.

87. Deyton LR, Walker RF, Kovacs JA, et al. Reversible cardiac dysfunction associated with interferon alpha therapy in AIDS patients with Kaposi's sarcoma. *N Engl J Med* 1989;321:1246–1249.

88. Chokshi SK, Moore R, Pandian NG, et al. Reversible cardiomyopathy associated with cocaine intoxication. *Ann Intern Med* 1989;111: 1039–1040.

89. Liu Y, Montes S, Zhang D, et al. Cocaethylene and heart disease during murine AIDS. *Int Immunopharmacol* 2002;2:139–150.

90. Sepulveda RT, Jiang S, Besselsen DG, et al. Alcohol consumption during murine acquired immunodeficiency syndrome accentuates heart pathology due to coxsackievirus. *Alcohol Alcohol* 2002;37: 157–163.

91. Wharton JM, Demopulos PA, Goldschlager N. Torsade de pointes during administration of pentamidine isothionate. *Am J Med* 1987;83: 571–576.

92. Richman DD, Fischl MA, Grieco MH, et al. The toxicity of azidothymidine (AZT) in the treatment of patients with AIDS and AIDS-related complex: A double-blind, placebo-controlled trial. *N Engl J Med* 1987;317:192–197.

93. Dalakas MC, Illa I, Pezeshkpour GH, et al. Mitochondrial myopathy caused by long-term zidovudine therapy. *N Engl J Med* 1990;322: 1098–1105.

94. Szabados E, Fischer GM, Toth K, et al. Role of reactive oxygen species and poly-ADP-ribose polymerase in the development of AZT-induced cardiomyopathy in rats. *Free Radic Biol Med* 1999;26: 302–317.

94a. Lewis W. Mitochondrial DNA replication, nucleoside reverse-transcriptase inhibitors, and AIDS cardiomyopathy. *Prog Cardiovasc Dis* 2003;45:305–318.

95. Lewis W, Haase CP, Raidel SM, et al. Combined antiretroviral therapy causes cardiomyopathy and elevates plasma lactate in transgenic AIDS mice. *Lab Invest* 2001;81:1527–1536.

96. Brown DL, Sather S, Cheitlin MD. Reversible cardiac dysfunction associated with foscarnet therapy for cytomegalovirus esophagitis in an AIDS patient. *Am Heart J* 1993;125:1439–1441.

97. Krishnaswamy G, Chi DS, Kelley JL, et al. The cardiovascular and metabolic complications of HIV infection. *Cardiol Rev* 2000;8:260–268.

97a. Van der Valk M, Bisschop PH, Rumijn JA, et al. Lipodystrophy in HIV-1-positive patients is associated with insulin resistance in multiple metabolic pathways. *AIDS* 2001;15:2093–2100.

98. Eastone JA, Decker CF. New onset diabetes mellitus associated with the use of protease inhibitors. *Ann Intern Med* 1997;127:948.

99. Carr A, Samaras K, Chisholm DJ, et al. Pathogenesis of HIV-1 protease inhibitor-associated peripheral lipodystrophy, hyperlipidemia, and insulin resistance. *Lancet* 1998;351:1881–1883.

100. Danner SA, Carr A, Leondard J, et al. Safety, pharmacokinetics and preliminary efficacy of ritonavir, an inhibitor of HIV-1 protease. *N Engl J Med* 1995;333:1528–1533

101. Cameron DW, Japour AJ, Xu Y, et al. Ritonavir and saquinavir combination therapy for the treatment of HIV infection. *AIDS* 1999;13:213–224.

101a. Kotler DP. HIV infection and lipodystrophy. *Prog Cardiovasc Dis* 2003;45:269–284.

102. Lo JC, Mullighan K, Tai VW, et al. Buffalo hump in men with HIV-1 infection. *Lancet* 1998;351:867–870.

103. Miller KD, Jones E, Janovsk JA, et al. Visceral abdominal fat accumulation associated with use of indinavir. *Lancet* 1998;351:871–875.

104. Sekhar RV, Jahoor F, White AC, et al. Metabolic basis of HIV-lipodystrophy syndrome. *Am J Physiol Endocrinol Metab* 2002;283:E332–E337.

105. Behrens GM, Boerner AR, Weber K, et al. Impaired glucose phosphorylation and transport in skeletal muscle cause insulin resistance in HIV-1-infected patients with lipodystrophy. *J Clin Invest* 2002;110:1319–1327.

105a. Stein JH. Dyslipidemia in the era of HIV protease inhibitors. *Prog Cardiovasc Dis* 2003;45:293–304.

105b. Dube MP, Sprecher D, Henry WK, et al. Preliminary guidelines for the evaluation and management of dyslipidemia in adults infected with human immunodeficiency virus and receiving antiretroviral therapy: Recommendations of the Adult AIDS Clinical Trial Group Cardiovascular Disease Focus Group. *Clin Infect Dis* 2000;31:1216–1224.

105c. Executive Summary of the Third Report of the National Cholesterol Education Program (NCEP) Expert Panel on Detection, Evaluation, and Treatment of High Blood Cholesterol in Adults (Adult Treatment Panel III) (ATPIII). *JAMA* 2001;285:2486–2497.

106. Melroe NH, Kopaczewski J, Henry K, et al. Intervention for hyperlipidemia associated with protease inhibitors. *J Assoc Nurses AIDS Care* 1999;10:55–69.

107. Periard D, Telenti A, Sudre P, et al. Atherogenic dyslipidemia in HIV-infected individuals treated with protease inhibitors. The Swiss HIV Cohort Study. *Circulation* 1999;100:700–705.

108. Currier JS. Cardiovascular risk associated with HIV therapy. *J Acquir Immune Defic Syndr* 2002;31 Suppl 1:S16–2.

109. Louie JK, Hsu LC, Osmond DH, et al. Trends in causes of death among persons with acquired immunodeficiency syndrome in the era of highly active antiretroviral therapy, San Francisco, 1994–1998. *J Infect Dis* 2002;186:1023–1027.

110. Maggi P, Serio G, Epifani G, et al. Premature lesions of the carotid vessels in HIV-1-infected patients treated with protease inhibitors. *AIDS* 2000;14:F123–F128.

111. Mercie P, Thiebaut R, Lavignolle V, et al. Evaluation of cardiovascular risk factors in HIV-1 infected patients using carotid intima-media thickness measurement. *Ann Med* 2002;34:55–63.

112. Tabib A, Leroux C, Mornex JF, et al. Accelerated coronary atherosclerosis and arteriosclerosis in young human-immunodeficiency-virus-positive patients. *Coron Artery Dis* 2000;11:41–46.

113. Holmberg SD, Moorman AC, Williamson JM, et al. Protease inhibitors and cardiovascular outcomes in patients with HIV-1. *Lancet* 2002;360:1747–1748.

113a. Klein D, Hurley LB, Quesenberry CP Jr, et al. Do protease inhibitors increase the risk for coronary heart disease in patients with HIV-1 infection? *J Acquir Immune Defic Syndr* 2002;30:471–477.

114. Himelman RB, Dohrmann M, Goodman P, et al: Severe pulmonary hypertension and cor pulmonale in the acquired immunodeficiency syndrome. *Am J Cardiol* 1989;64:1396–1399.

114a. Mehta NJ. Khan IA, Mehta RN, et al. HIV-related pulmonary hypertension: Analytic review of 131 cases. *Chest* 2000;118:1133–1141.

115. Mesa RA, Edell ES, Dunn WF, et al. Human immunodeficiency virus infection and pulmonary hypertension: Two new cases and a review of 86 reported cases. *Mayo Clin Proc* 1998;73:37–45.

116. Pellicelli AM, Palmieri F, Cicalini S, et al. Pathogenesis of HIV-related pulmonary hypertension. *Ann N Y Acad Sci* 2001;946:82–94.

117. Kim J, Ruff M, Karwatowska-Prokopczuk E, et al. HIV envelope protein gp120 induces neuropeptide Y receptor-mediated proliferation of vascular smooth muscle cells: Relevance to AIDS cardiovascular pathogenesis. *Regul Pept* 1998;25;75–76:201–205.

118. Cicalini S, Forcina G, De Rosa FG. Infective endocarditis in patients with human immunodeficiency virus infection. *J Infect* 2001;42:267–271.

119. Herskowitz A, Willouby SB, Baughman KL, et al. Cardiomyopathy associated with antiretroviral therapy in patients with HIV infection: A report of six cases. *Ann Intern Med* 1992;116:311–313.

120. Mason JW, O'Connell JB, Herskowitz A, et al. A clinical trial of immunosuppressive therapy for myocarditis: The Myocarditis Treatment Trial Investigators. *N Engl J Med* 1995;333:269–275.

121. Maloney JP. Advances in the treatment of secondary pulmonary hypertension. *Curr Opin Pulm Med* 2003;9:139–143.

122. Piscitelli SC, Gallicano KD. Interactions among drugs for HIV and opportunistic infections. *N Engl J Med* 2001;344:984–996.

123. Centers for Disease Control. Acquired immunodeficiency syndrome: United States Update. *MMWR* 1986;35:17–21.

124. Ribera E, Miro JM, Cortes E, et al. Influence of human immunodeficiency virus 1 and degree of immunosuppression in the clinical characteristics and outcome of infective endocarditis in intravenous drug users. *Arch Intern Med* 1998;158:2043–2050.

125. Utley JR. Pathophysiology of cardiopulmonary bypass: Current issues. *J Card Surg* 1990;5:177–189.

126. Pollock R, Ames F, Rubio P, et al. Protracted severe immune dysregulation induced by cardiopulmonary bypass: A predisposing etiologic factor in blood transfusion-related AIDS? *J Clin Lab Immunol* 1987;22:1–5.

127. Gerberding JL. Management of occupational exposures to bloodborne viruses. *N Engl J Med* 1995;332:444–451.

127a. Gerberding JL. Occupational exposure to HIV in health care settings. *N Engl J Med* 2003;348:826–833.

128. Condit D, Frater RWM. Human immunodeficiency virus and the cardiac surgeon: A survey of attitudes. *Ann Thorac Surg* 1989;47:182–186.

129. Shelley GA, Howard RJ. A national survey of surgeons' attitudes about patients with human immunodeficiency virus infections and acquired immunodeficiency syndrome. *Arch Surg* 1992;127:206–211.

EFFECT OF NONCARDIAC DRUGS, ELECTRICITY, POISONS, AND RADIATION ON THE HEART

Andrew L. Smith / Wendy M. Book

This chapter deals with a number of deleterious side effects of treatments and environmental agents on the heart. Toxic effects may occur acutely and require emergent intervention or may be chronic and not be manifest until days or years after exposure.

NONCARDIAC DRUGS

Chemotherapeutic Agents

Chemotherapeutic agents may result in acute or chronic cardiovascular toxicity. The heart, composed of nonproliferating myocytes, was traditionally thought to be protected from the effects of drugs on rapidly dividing cells. A number of these agents are now recognized to cause cardiovascular complications including cardiomyopathy, myocarditis, pericarditis, myocardial ischemia, arrhythmias, and peripheral hypotension or vasospasm (Table 89-1).[1]

Cardiovascular alterations in the patient receiving chemotherapy may be the result of a specific drug or combination of drugs or be related to tumor-associated factors such as hypercoagulability or release of myocardial depressant factors. Correlating a specific therapy with a particular adverse event may be difficult; however, knowledge of side effects of each agent should be considered when prescribing therapy.

ANTHRACYCLINES

The anthracycline antineoplastics—doxorubicin, daunorubicin, and epirubicin—are the leading cause of chemotherapy-related heart disease. These agents may cause cardiac problems during therapy, weeks after completion of therapy, or, unexpectedly, years later.[2] During acute therapy, electrocardiogram (ECG) changes occur in ap-

proximately 30 percent of patients and usually regress within weeks. Findings include ST-T changes, decreased QRS voltage, prolongation of the QT interval, and atrial and ventricular ectopy. Sustained atrial or ventricular arrhythmias are rare. The occurrence of early ECG abnormalities does not predict cardiomyopathy and is not an indication to discontinue therapy.[1] The development of persistent sinus tachycardia in an otherwise stable oncology patient (although nonspecific), however, may raise the suspicion of ventricular dysfunction and impending congestive heart failure.

Congestive heart failure is related to the cumulative dose of the anthracycline administered. The incidences of heart failure at specific doses of doxorubicin include 0.4 percent at 400 mg/m^2 of body surface area, 7 percent at 550 mg/m^2, and 18 percent at 700 mg/m^2 (Fig. 89-1).[3] Traditionally, the cardiac limiting dose has been described as 550 mg/m^2 because of the acute rise in heart failure seen above this dose. There is great individual variability, however, with reports of heart failure occurring with doses less than 100 mg/m^2 and, conversely, with some patients tolerating greater than 1000 mg/m^2 without cardiac compromise.[3,4] Risk factors for anthracycline-induced cardiomyopathy are debated but include prior chest radiation, young age (0-12), age greater than 70, and preexisting heart disease.[3–5] Young females may be at particularly increased risk for late cardiac dysfunction.[5] Rapid infusion schedules associated with higher peak drug concentration appear to result in greater cardiotoxicity. Combination therapy with cyclophosphamide is an additional risk factor,[1] with cardiotoxicity noted at doses of 300 mg/m.[2]

The pathogenesis of anthracycline-induced cardiotoxicity is not known. Theories generally implicate free radical damage. One proposal is that enzymatic reduction of the anthracycline quinone ring results in lipid peroxidation and cell membrane damage. Another theory involves the formation of an anthracycline–iron complex, which

TABLE 89-1 Chemotherapeutic Agents Commonly Associated with Cardiovascular Toxicity

Drug	Associated Toxicity
Anthracyclines	
Doxorubicin	Cardiomyopathy
Daunorubicin	
Epirubicin	
Idarubicin	
Mitoxantrone	
Alkylating agents	
Cyclophosphamide	Reversible systolic dysfunction, hemorrhagic myocarditis
Cisplatin	Raynaud's phenomenon
Antimetabolites	
5-Fluorouracil	Coronary vasospasm
Other	
Amsacrine	Arrhythmias
Paclitaxel	Arrhythmias
Trastuzumab	Cardiomyopathy
Interleukin 2	Hypotension, myocarditis
Interferon alpha	Hypotension, cardiomyopathy

undergoes "redox cycling" that results in oxygen radicals and degradation of microsomal, mitochondrial, and membrane lipids. Disturbances of calcium exchange have also been noted.[6]

The average time to clinical development of heart failure symptoms is 1 month from the end of anthracycline therapy but may occur anytime within 1 year. Patient presentation is similar to that for other dilated cardiomyopathies (see Chap. 76).

Biventricular systolic dysfunction occurs, and restrictive hemodynamics have been described.[7] The clinical course varies from fulminant heart failure to gradually progressive deterioration. Some patients have reversibility of systolic dysfunction. Therapy, in addition to withholding further anthracycline dosing or other myocardial toxins, is generally considered the same as recommended for patients with heart failure from dilated cardiomyopathy (see Chap. 25).

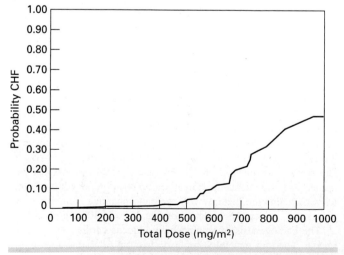

FIGURE 89-1 The development of doxorubicin-induced heart failure is related to cumulative dose. Toxicity may occur at any dose, but at 550 mg/m² the probability increases significantly. (From Von Hoff et al.[3])

Noninvasive assessment of left ventricular function has been utilized to guide anthracycline dosing and prevent cardiac toxicity. Serial echocardiography and/or radionuclide angiography (see Chaps. 15 and 19) are most commonly used.[8–10] Improved echocardiographic technologies have increased the use of this modality. The most commonly used parameter is resting left ventricular ejection fraction. Recognition that resting left ventricular ejection fraction is relatively insensitive for detecting early cardiotoxicity[2] has resulted in the investigation of other variables (exercise or dobutamine echocardiography,[9] Doppler velocities, and systolic time intervals) in assessing this problem. These methods have generally been evaluated in small-sized studies and have not gained widespread acceptance in current therapy guidelines. Adult guidelines for serial assessment have been developed.[21] A drop in left ventricular ejection fraction greater than 10 percent (EF units) and to below a normal value of 50 percent is an indication to discontinue therapy. A baseline left ventricular ejection fraction less than 30 percent has generally been considered a contraindication to initiating anthracycline therapy.[10]

Compared to the noninvasive methods, endomyocardial biopsy is considered more specific and provides earlier sensitivity in detection of anthracycline cardiotoxicity. The Billingham score, which quantifies cytoplasmic changes and the percent of myocytes damaged has been utilized to assess the risk of congestive heart failure.[11] Clinical utility has been limited because of the invasive nature of this procedure and the special expertise required in obtaining and reading the specimens. Additionally, variability of histologic changes and the potential for sampling error have been noted.[12]

There is growing recognition of the occurrence of cardiac dysfunction years after completion of anthracycline therapy. This is particularly of concern in children. One study reported a 23 percent incidence of late cardiac abnormalities (decreased systolic function by noninvasive testing) in survivors of pediatric malignancies treated with anthracycline therapy.[13] The incidence of abnormalities was higher in the patients with the longer elapsed times since therapy, with a 38 percent incidence in patients with a follow-up period greater than 10 years. This study, as well as others,[14] suggests that subclinical myocardial damage may not become clinically evident until years after therapy. Although fewer than 5 percent of these patients had developed clinical heart failure, the potentially progressive nature of systolic dysfunction raises the issue of need for long-term clinical follow-up. There are presently no accepted guidelines, however, in either the pediatric or adult population for chronic monitoring. Early treatment of systolic dysfunction with angiotensin-converting enzyme inhibitors may be warranted in asymptomatic patients.[2] Additionally, patients presenting late after anthracycline therapy with exertional fatigue and normal resting ejection fractions have been noted to have abnormalities on dobutamine echocardiography. This observation suggests abnormalities in cardiac reserve that may lead to symptoms.

Clinical strategies for preventing anthracycline cardiotoxicity have had to balance the need for antineoplastic efficacy. Lower clinical toxicity in adults has been noted with prolonged infusions of doxorubicin over 48 to 96 h in order to avoid high-peak concentrations.[15] In contrast, continuous infusion schedules in children do not offer a cardioprotective advantage.[16] Several antioxidants have been evaluated but with inconclusive results.[6,16] *Dexrazoxane,* an iron-chelating agent, reduces free-radical generation by anthracyclines and is currently recommended for consideration for patients with metastatic breast cancer who have received more than 300 mg/m² of doxorubicin.[17] Studies demonstrate a decrease in cardiotoxicity and most, but not all, trials have suggested preserved efficacy of antitumor activity. Epirubicine, an anthracycline, may have a lower risk of cardiotoxicity. Unfortunately, at cumulative doses above 1000 mg/m² the incidence of cardiotoxicity is reported to be 16 to 35 percent.[17]

OTHER CHEMOTHERAPEUTIC AGENTS

Mitoxantrone, an anthracendione lacking the amino sugar of anthracyclines, causes cardiotoxicity with features similar to anthracycline-induced cardiomyopathy.[1] This drug appears to have less cardiotoxicity than doxorubicin at equal myelotoxic doses. Cumulative doses above 160 mg/m² are associated with an increasing incidence of congestive heart failure. There has been increasing concern that mitoxantrone in high doses and particularly when combined with other chemotherapeutic agents may result in a high incidence of delayed myocardial toxicity.[18] High-dose *cyclophosphamide* (120 to 240 mg/kg over several days) used in bone marrow transplantation may cause acute cardiac toxicity.[1,19] Symptomatic systolic dysfunction, usually reversible with drug discontinuation, is associated with decreased QRS voltage on the ECG. Pericardial effusions have been noted, and a hemorrhagic myocarditis may result in death. Necropsy data demonstrate endothelial injury with resultant interstitial fibrin deposition and capillary microthrombosis. The cardiotoxicity of cyclophosphamide is likely due to damage from its biologically active metabolites. Rapid metabolizers of cyclophosphamide appear to be prone to cardiotoxicity. The metabolites cause toxic endothelial damage leading to muscle damage.[19] Cyclophosphamide may also potentiate the cardiotoxic effects of the anthracyclines.[1,18]

5-Fluorouracil may occasionally cause angina, electrocardiographic changes, and rarely myocardial infarction.[1,20] The majority of episodes occur during the first cycle of therapy and resolve spontaneously after discontinuation. Arrhythmias and systolic dysfunction have been observed. The understanding of 5-fluorouracil toxicity is complicated because combination chemotherapy is generally utilized, patients may be systemically ill, and many receiving this medication have preexisting coronary artery disease.[20] The incidence of cardiac toxicity is uncertain but ranges from 1 to 8 percent.[21] Patients with known coronary artery disease are at higher risk for serious cardiotoxicity. The mechanism of toxicity remains unclear, although coronary vasospasm has been suspected. Coronary catheterization has generally failed to demonstrate vasomotor hyperreactivity with 5-fluorouracil or ergonovine challenge.

Amsacrine (AMSA P-D) has been associated with prolongation of the QT interval. Malignant ventricular arrhythmias may occur in <1 percent of patients and are exacerbated by hypokalemia.[22]

Paclitaxel (Taxol) is being used with increased frequency for breast and ovarian cancer. The most common cardiovascular effect is the development of transient asymptomatic bradycardia, occurring in up to 30 percent of patients. Bradycardia with adverse consequences occurs in only 0.1 percent of patients. Paclitaxel alters anthracycline pharmacokinetics and is known to increase doxorubicin cardiotoxicity.[23]

Trastuzumab (recombinant humanized anti-HER2 antibody) is a relatively new treatment for breast cancer that has had favorable antitumor effects when added to standard chemotherapy in selected patients. A retrospective review described a 27 percent incidence of cardiotoxicity when this agent was given with an anthracycline and cyclophosphamide, a 13 percent incidence in combination with paclitaxel, and a 3 to 7 percent incidence given alone. The majority of these patients had received prior anthracycline therapy.[24] The pathophysiology and true incidence trastuzumab cardiotoxicity is uncertain. Clinically symptoms occur more acutely than anthracycline toxicity and the majority of patients experience improvement with standard heart failure treatment.[25]

Immunomodulating Agents

The biologic response modifiers, *interleukin (IL) 2* and *interferon alpha*, have been associated with cardiovascular toxicity predominantly secondary to peripheral vasodilatation. IL-2 causes tachycardia and hypotension, as well as capillary leak syndrome. Myocarditis has been reported in patients who died soon after initiation of therapy. IL-2 therapy requires pretreatment assessment of cardiovascular risks and close monitoring during drug administration.

Interferon alpha may cause supraventricular tachyarrhythmias. A reversible cardiomyopathy has been described.[1,19,26,27]

Psychotropic Agents

Psychiatric illness, particularly depression, is common in patients with cardiovascular disease (see Chap. 91). Morbidity and mortality following cardiac events are increased in patients with depression, particularly if untreated.[28,29] A variety of psychotropic agents have conduction or vascular effects. A thorough understanding of these therapeutic, but potentially toxic, agents is necessary in the treatment of patients with preexisting cardiac disease. Intentional overdose with these drugs may result in serious cardiac manifestations.

TRICYCLIC ANTIDEPRESSANTS

The tricyclic antidepressants, including the tertiary (amitryptyline, clomipramine, doxepin, imipramine, trimipramine) and secondary (desipramine, nortriptyline, protriptyline) amines, have potentially serious cardiovascular effects. These effects include increased heart rate, orthostatic hypotension, ECG changes, and possible depression of ventricular function. These drugs have electrophysiologic properties similar to the type IA antiarrhythmics. There is the potential for late proarrhythmia in patients with structural heart disease who are taking these agents.[30]

The tricyclic antidepressants have several properties that account for the majority of cardiovascular effects. These drugs inhibit uptake of both norepinephrine and serotonin, resulting in greater toxicity compared to the selective serotonin reuptake inhibitors (SSRIs). A hyperadrenergic state may result in tachycardia. Alpha blockade occurs at higher drug levels and may cause marked hypotension in the setting of overdose. The anticholinergic effects result in tachycardia, dry mouth, and constipation, and in overdose they may delay gastrointestinal absorption of the drug. Sodium channel blockade, typical of the type IA antiarrhythmic compounds, results in conduction abnormalities and the potential to suppress ventricular function.[31]

The most frequent side effect of tricyclic antidepressant treatment, orthostatic hypotension, is common in older patients and does not generally improve with reducing doses to lower levels that will still maintain antidepressant effects. Orthostasis, mediated predominantly by alpha₁ blockade, may occur with all of these drugs but is less likely with nortriptyline.[30–32]

The most common electrocardiographic changes include nonspecific ST-T changes and prolongation of the QT interval, PR interval, and QRS duration. PR prolongation is due to prolonged infranodal conduction. Patients with preexisting conduction disease, particularly bundle branch block, are at increased risk of toxicity.[33] The tricyclic antidepressants have type IA antiarrhythmic properties and may potentially suppress ventricular ectopy. The results of antiarrhythmic studies, however, including those with type I agents, suggest the potential for a proarrhythmic effect for these drugs at therapeutic doses in patients with serious structural heart disease.[30,34] Tricyclic antidepressants are generally contraindicated in the recovery phase following myocardial infarction. Although tricyclic antidepressant therapy may be indicated in the treatment of severely depressed patients, the threshold for use should rise as the severity of heart disease increases or when there is QT prolongation.[30] These issues are discussed in detail in Chap. 91.

Tricyclic antidepressants may impair left ventricular function in patients with severe systolic dysfunction; however, decreases in left ventricular ejection fraction have generally not been noted in patients with moderately impaired function.

Tricyclic antidepressant overdose carries a mortality of 2 to 3 percent, which is generally related to cardiac complications. Clinical status at initial presentation and serum drug levels are not predictive of prognosis. QRS prolongation is a sign of toxicity but may be absent in the patient with serious cardiac complications. Rightward deviation of the terminal 40 ms of the frontal plane QRS axis is a more sensitive marker. This finding, manifested by a terminal R wave in lead aVR, has an 83 percent sensitivity and 63 percent specificity for toxicity.[35]

Aggressive support measures in tricyclic antidepressant overdose should be initiated immediately and include airway maintenance, gastric lavage, and repeated dosing of activated charcoal. Alkalinization with intravenous sodium bicarbonate decreases unbound drug and reverses cardiac and central nervous system conduction defects. Alkalinization is indicated in cardiac arrest, hypotension, arrhythmias, acidosis, and QRS prolongation. Hypotension refractory to volume loading and bicarbonate therapy should be treated with vasopressors, including norepinephrine or phenylephrine, and with vasopressor doses of dopamine. Type I antiarrhythmics (quinidine, procainamide, disopyramide) should not be used. Sodium bicarbonate is the initial therapy for ventricular dysrhythmias.[36]

The duration of monitoring after tricyclic overdose is controversial. Signs of major toxicity generally occur within 6 h of presentation in the emergency department. If clinical or ECG evidence of toxicity is absent and two doses of activated charcoal have been given, patients may not require admission for medical monitoring. Fluoxetine increases tricyclic antidepressant serum levels, and additional monitoring is recommended in patients receiving this medication. Patients with cardiac disease or other serious medical problems may require a longer period of observation.[35]

OTHER ANTIDEPRESSANTS

SSRIs have not been studied extensively in patients with cardiac disease. Case reports of cardiac toxicity are rare, despite the increasing popularity of these agents in the treatment of depression. These agents have rarely been associated with orthostatic hypotension and with bradycardia. Cardiac function does not appear to be depressed by these agents.[37] The SSRIs may affect the cytochrome P$_{450}$ system and may therefore alter the metabolism of a variety of drugs, including agents used in cardiovascular disease such as antiarrhythmic medications, beta blockers, calcium channel blockers, and warfarin.[37–40]

The monoamine oxidase (MAO) inhibitors have little effect on cardiac conduction or myocardial contractility. Orthostatic hypotension is common, particularly in elderly patients. The major concern with these agents is interaction with other drugs or tyramine-containing substances, resulting in hypertensive crisis. Lithium, used commonly in the treatment of bipolar disorder, is generally well tolerated in patients with cardiac disease. Suppression of sinus node automaticity, resulting in bradycardias, is the most common complication.[41] In patients free of known heart disease, clinically significant sinus node dysfunction occurs in fewer than 1 percent and is reversible with discontinuation of lithium therapy. Preexisting sinus node disease or concomitant therapy with drugs altering sinus node function, however, may result in sinus bradycardia. Lithium-induced

hypothyroidism may be a contributing factor.[42] Pacemaker therapy may be required to allow continuation of lithium therapy.

Lithium therapy has been associated with electrocardiographic changes simulating hypokalemia. T-wave inversion, prominent U waves, and QT prolongation may occur. PR prolongation, bundle branch block, and complete heart block are rare.[41] Overdose with lithium may result in severe bradycardias requiring temporary pacemaker therapy. A low anion gap may suggest the presence of lithium toxicity.[43]

ANTIPSYCHOTIC AGENTS

The phenothiazine antipsychotic agents have potential cardiac toxicity similar to that of the tricyclic antidepressants. These drugs may cause sinus tachycardia, PR and QT prolongation, and disturbances of intraventricular conduction. Chlorpromazine and thioridazine[44] are the most commonly implicated phenothiazines as causes of torsades de pointes. The butyrophenone, haloperidol, is also associated with torsades de pointes at high doses given intravenously.[45]

Noncardiac Drugs and Toxic Antidepressants Causing Torsades de Pointes

As discussed earlier, tricyclic, phenothiazine, and other psychotropic agents may prolong the QT interval and induce torsades de pointes. A variety of antiarrhythmic agents, particularly the type I agents, are most strongly associated with this potentially fatal arrhythmia. Other toxic causes of torsades de pointes[46] are listed in Table 89-2.

The antibiotics erythromycin and trimethoprim-sulfamethoxazole[47,48] have only rarely been associated with torsades de pointes, the exception being the effect of erythromycin on the metabolism of terfenadine and astemizole. Liquid protein diets and starvation[49] may cause marked electrolyte and chemical disturbances, triggering QT prolongation. Probucol,[50] may prolong the QT interval, resulting in torsades de pointes.

The QT prolongation and torsades de pointes reported with the antihistamines terfenadine and astemizole and with cisapride have been associated with high drug levels from excessive dosing or altered metabolism.[51,52] Terfenadine-, astemizole-, and cisapride-induced prolongation of the QT interval is due to the electrophysiologic activity of blocking HERG, the ion channel that is responsible for the rapid component of the delayed rectifier current for potassium (I_{kr}).[52] These drugs are metabolized by cytochrome P$_{450}$ 3A.[53] A variety of agents inhibit this isoenzyme including antifungals (ketoconazole, fluconazole, itraconazole), erythromycin or clarithromycin (not azithromycin), SSRIs (fluvoxamine, nefazodone, fluoxetine, sertraline), quinine, and grapefruit juice. Serious cardiac arrhythmias have been reported in patients taking terfenadine, astemizole, or cis-

TABLE 89-2 Noncardiac Drugs and Toxins Known to Cause Torsades de Pointes

Psychotropic agents	Antihistamines
Tricyclic antidepressants	Terfenadine
Tetracyclic antidepressants	Astemizole
Phenothiazines	Other
Haloperidol	Cisapride
Chloral hydrate	Pentamidine
Antibiotics	Probucol
Erythromycin	Arsenic
Trimethoprim-sulfa-	Organophosphates
methoxazole	Liquid protein diets

TABLE 89-3 Drug-Related Valvular Disease

Agents
    Methysergide
    Ergotamine
    Dexfenfluramine
    Fenfluramine
    Pergolide
Pathology
    Fibroendocardial plaque formation on normal valvular
        architecture
Echocardiographic findings
    Valve thickening and retraction
    Valvular regurgitation

apride with drugs that inhibit cytochrome P_{450} 3A isoenzyme. Patients with a history of prolonged QT interval or those with serious underlying cardiac disease are at higher risk for this problem. Some women appear to have slow metabolism of these drugs, and thus female gender is a risk factor for drug-induced arrhythmia.[52]

Drug-Related Valvular Heart Disease

Valvular heart disease, resembling that seen with carcinoid syndrome has been associated with antimigraine drugs methysergide and ergotamine, the weight loss medications dexfenfluramine and fenfluramine, and in several instances to pergolide mesylate used to treat Parkinson's disease and restless leg syndrome (Table 89-3).[54–62]

The incidence of valvular abnormalities is more common with methysergide compared to ergotamine and appears to be greater with the chronic use of dexfenfluramine and the combination of fenfluramine and phentermine. Dexfenfluramine and fenfluramine were withdrawn from the market in 1997 when up to 30 percent of users were reported to develop asymptomatic valve regurgitation.[57] Later reports suggested a lower incidence of problems including reports of valvular regurgitation in approximately 7 percent of dexfenfluramine treated patients versus 2 to 5 percent of controls.[58] The true incidence of valvular problems is uncertain and differences in reported cases may be secondary to differences in length of therapy, time from therapy to cardiac evaluation, and methods used to determine abnormalities. Mild aortic regurgitation is the most common finding. Abnormalities often improve with cessation of therapy.[59,60]

Antimigraine Drugs

In addition to ergotamine and methysergide, sumatriptan is used to treat migraines. Sumatriptan, a selective serotonin type I agonist, may cause coronary artery vasospasm. Sumatriptan should not be taken within 24 hours of treatment with ergotamine-like medications because of the risk of prolonged vasoconstriction.[63]

Ergotamine, methysergide, and sumatriptan are generally contraindicated in patients with obstructive coronary artery disease because of vasoconstrictor effects and the possibility of precipitating angina.[64]

Chloroquine

The antimalarial agent, chloroquine, is commonly used to treat collagen vascular and dermatologic disorders. Irreversible retinal damage is the primary concern with long-term or high-dose therapy. Skeletal myopathy and less commonly cardiomyopathy may occur. With cardiac involvement, features of restrictive cardiomyopathy are most common. Myocardial biopsy with analysis by electron microscopy showing curvilinear and myeloid bodies is diagnostic. These findings may be seen on skeletal muscle biopsy. The ECG may demonstrate T-wave changes and conduction abnormalities. Acute chloroquine poisoning results in hypotension, tachycardia, and prolongation of the QRS and is often fatal.[65,66]

Anabolic Steroids

Illicit use of androgens has been identified as a problem in competitive athletes and body builders. It is estimated that 300,000 persons in the United States have had recent steroid use and over 1 million have had prior use.[67–69] Anabolic steroids, including testosterone, stanozolol, and nandrolone, are frequently used in combination and at high doses for intermittent periods of several weeks to months. Doses commonly exceed 100 times the doses used for medical purposes.[67] Animal data indicate that these agents can cause abnormal lipids left ventricular hypertrophy, increased blood volume, and hypertension. Data on human toxicity are limited but suggest similar toxicity.[70] Stanozolol and nandrolone reduce total high-density lipoprotein levels by over 50 percent and increase low-density lipoprotein levels by over 30 percent.[71] Isolated reports of young men (< age 35) developing severe coronary atherosclerosis, myocardial infarctions, or stroke exist in the literature.[67,72] Because of the secrecy surrounding the use of these agents, the full clinical significance of abuse is not known.

Cocaine

Cocaine is a common drug of abuse and has potentially lethal cardiac toxicity. It is estimated that over 30 million Americans have used cocaine at least once and that 5 million use it regularly.[73] Cocaine may be swallowed, inhaled nasally, smoked, or injected intravenously. Cardiovascular toxicity is broad, ranging from sudden death to chronic cardiomyopathy.[74] A summary of the cardiovascular syndromes associated with illicit cocaine use is shown in Table 89-4. Use of cocaine with other drugs such as ethanol[75] or tobacco[76] may

TABLE 89-4 Cardiovascular Complications of Cocaine

Sudden death
Acute myocardial infarction
Chest pain without myocardial infarction
Accelerated coronary atherosclerosis
Intimal hyperplasia of coronary vessels
Electrocardiographic abnormalities
    Sinus tachycardia
    Premature ventricular complexes
    Ventricular tachycardia
    Torsades de pointes
    Ventricular fibrillation
    Prolongation of QT interval
    Early repolarization (ST-segment change)
Acute reversible myocarditis
Dilated cardiomyopathy
Acute severe hypertension
Acute aortic dissection, rupture
Pneumopericardium
Stroke
Subarachnoid hemorrhage
Endocarditis (intravenous use)

have combined detrimental effects. Cardiovascular susceptibility in an individual is difficult to predict due to the lack of dose-response relationship and the high degree of variability in the individual response to cocaine.[77]

Cocaine has a generalized sympathomimetic effect and has local anesthetic properties. Cocaine blocks the reuptake of norepinephrine and dopamine on preganglionic sympathetic nerve terminals. This produces sympathetic stimulation both centrally and peripherally. These catecholamine effects acutely result in tachycardia, hypertension, increased myocardial contractility, and vascular constriction. The local anesthetic effect, occurring through blockade of the fast sodium channel, results in slowed conduction in myocardial tissues. This may result in electrocardiographic abnormalities including prolongation of the PR, QRS, and QT intervals similar to that seen with toxicity from type I antiarrhythmic agents. These effects increase the vulnerability to reentrant ventricular arrhythmias.[73,74,78]

Cocaine may result in increased thrombogenicity.[74,76] Platelet aggregation is enhanced and endothelial function is altered, resulting in the potential for development of coronary thrombosis in the absence of coronary atherosclerosis. Chronic use of cocaine is associated with premature coronary atherosclerosis.[74,79] Cocaine indirectly causes constriction of both diseased and nondiseased coronary artery segments, but its effect is more marked in diseased vessels. Ethanol use and tobacco smoking may worsen the potential for vasospasm.[75,76] Up to one-third of reported cases of patients with cocaine-induced myocardial infarctions have normal coronary arteries.[74] The combined cardiac effects, including early coronary atherosclerosis, coronary vasospasm, increased thrombogenicity, increased myocardial oxygen demands, and proarrhythmic effects, make this drug a lethal threat to users of all ages.

Cocaine may have direct or indirect myocardial toxicity. Animal studies suggest a direct negative inotropic effect on the heart, possibly related to its local anesthetic properties. Chronic dosing has demonstrated myocardial contraction bands, myofibrillar disorganization, interstitial edema, and mitochondrial swelling. Mononuclear infiltrates have been noted. Myocardial changes may mimic those seen with catecholamine excess as in pheochromocytoma. Clinical case reports have described transient toxic cardiomyopathy, acute myocarditis, and permanently dilated cardiomyopathy.[74]

Chest pain is the most common reason for cocaine users to seek medical attention. Over 64,000 patients are evaluated annually for cocaine-related chest pain, of whom over half are admitted to the hospital. The evaluation of cocaine-related chest pain is difficult.[80,81] Prospective studies demonstrate that approximately 6 percent of patients presenting to the emergency room with cocaine-related chest pain have myocardial infarction. These patients are often young men without other risk factors for coronary artery disease except for tobacco smoking. The duration and quality of discomfort does not readily distinguish those eventually noted to have enzyme documentation of infarction. Many young patients have early repolarization patterns, with ST elevation in leads V_1 to V_3, a normal variant that may be confused with acute infarction. Infarction has been noted in patients with normal or nonspecific ECGs. Because of the difficulty in excluding myocardial infarctions, patients are often monitored for a period of at least 12 h until enzymes have excluded infarction.[80]

Treatment strategies for cocaine-induced myocardial ischemia have been developed based on the known cardiac and nervous system toxicity of the drug.[73,78] Randomized prospective trials of therapy do not exist. Patients presenting with anxiety, tachycardia, or hypertension may respond well to benzodiazepines. Nitroglycerin may reverse coronary vasoconstriction induced by cocaine. Aspirin may prevent thrombus formation. Patients not responding to these

measures may benefit from the alpha-adrenergic antagonist phentolamine or from calcium channel blocker therapy with verapamil.[73] Beta-adrenergic antagonists have been avoided because of the potential of enhanced coronary vasoconstriction and for unopposed alpha-mediated hypertensive crisis. Combined alpha and beta blockade with labetalol has been utilized to treat tachyarrhythmias but is not an accepted therapy for myocardial ischemia.[73] However, the bias against beta blockade is undergoing clinical reevaluation with recognition that beta blockers may block the hyperadrenergic effects that result in thrombosis and vasospasm.[82]

In documented myocardial infarction, thrombolytic therapy is highly effective; however, over 40 percent of patients without infarction will meet accepted electrocardiographic criteria for use of lytic therapy.[83] The early repolarization pattern common in young men makes diagnosis difficult, particularly when a prior ECG is not available. Thrombolytic therapy carries increased risk of hemorrhagic stroke in patients with recently uncontrolled hypertension. Therefore, emergent coronary angiography may be necessary to document coronary occlusion and direct strategies such as primary angioplasty or thrombolysis (see Chap. 56).

Management of supraventricular or ventricular tachyarrhythmias may be facilitated by administration of benzodiazepines. Rhythm disturbances may be exacerbated by acidosis or electrolyte disorders. Intravenous sodium bicarbonate and magnesium may be beneficial. Lidocaine should be used cautiously because of concerns of lowered seizure threshold and potential proarrhythmic effects following recent cocaine use.[78]

Patients with cocaine-associated chest pain not related to myocardial infarction have a favorable 1-year prognosis, particularly if cocaine use is discontinued. Urgent diagnostic cardiac evaluation is not generally recommended. Unfortunately, recurrent cocaine use after cocaine-associated chest pain occurs in over 60 percent of cases.[73]

Methamphetamines

The biologic effects of methamphetamines are similar to that of cocaine, but vasoconstriction is less.[84] Cardiovascular toxicity is common and includes tachycardia, hypertension, and arrhythmias. Chest pain and myocardial infarction are less common than with cocaine.[85] Chronic use may result in a catecholamine-mediated dilated cardiomyopathy.[86]

Ethanol

See Chap. 76.

ELECTRICITY INJURY

Environmental Accidents

Accidental contact with electricity may occur in the home, where young children are particularly vulnerable.[87] Job-related electrical injuries are most common in construction and electrical workers but also on any job in which electrical equipment is used, including the health care setting. Approximately 1200 deaths related to domestic electrical injury occur each year in the United States.[88] There are two to three times as many serious injuries, including burns and neurologic complications.[88,89] Lightning kills at least 100 people per year in the United States, representing a 30 percent mortality rate in reported cases. Lightning injuries generally occur between May and

September in the late afternoon hours and affect predominantly young people involved in outdoor recreational activities.[90] Death following electrical shock is usually secondary to immediate cardiac rhythm disturbances, although later cardiac complications secondary to internal injury may occur.

Pathophysiology

The degree of total body injury from electricity is determined by the amount of current delivered, tissue resistance, and duration of contact.[89] Specific organs or tissues injured are in part determined by the path of the current. Electrical injuries are classified as high voltage (> 1000 V) or low voltage (< 1000 V). High-voltage electrical wires and household current (120 or 220 V) are alternating currents (AC) that may result in prolonged exposure due to tetatanic muscle contractions and inability of the victim to "let go." The frequencies of domestically generated AC (50 to 60 cycles per second) result in an increased risk for ventricular fibrillation even at household voltages.[88] Sources of domestic direct current (DC) are usually low voltage (3 to 24 V), including batteries, appliance transformers, and portable emergency generators and are less likely to cause injury. Lightning is an extremely high-voltage, direct current of brief duration.

Heat injury tissue necrosis is more severe with high-voltage AC. These burns are often internal and may mimic crush injuries.[91] Tissue resistance to current flow is least in nervous and vascular tissues, and therefore the heart and neurovascular bundles may serve as conduits for electrical current through the thorax.[92] Arm-to-arm pathway of current is associated with greater risk for cardiac injury, followed by arm-to-leg pathways determined by entry and exit sites. A stride potential, leg-to-leg, is infrequently associated with cardiac effects.[88]

Cardiovascular Effects

Cardiac damage in electrical injury may occur as a result of contusion injury or myocardial necrosis or may be in part related to massive release of catecholamines. Typical symptoms or signs of myocardial damage may be absent.[93] Lightning injuries result from brief, high-voltage direct current. Immediate death may be secondary to asystole or ventricular fibrillation or result from apnea secondary to injury of the central respiratory centers. Lightning strikes may occur by a direct hit, side splash, or ground strike. Direct hits cause mechanical trauma to organs secondary to dissipated energy.[89] Strikes to the chest can result in severe, often reversible global myocardial dysfunction or localized myocardial contusion. Electrocardiographic abnormalities, including QT prolongation and ST-T abnormalities, may be the result of cardiac or neurologic injury. ST elevation has been noted with direct strikes. Conduction abnormalities, including right bundle branch block and complete heart block, have been noted.[90] Pericardial effusions may develop following direct strikes. Elevated levels of creatine kinase-MB (CK-MB) are generally noted.[89,90] Splash strikes in which a tree or other object is hit prior to the victim being hit are associated with CK-MB release in less than two-thirds of patients. Severe myocardial injury is unlikely unless there is a short distance between the directly hit object and the victim. Ground strikes generally do not cause a significant cardiac injury but may be associated with nonspecific ST-T abnormalities.[90]

Domestic AC accidents may cause myocardial necrosis and conduction abnormalities. An injury pattern mimicking infarction may be seen on the ECG but is generally related to direct myocardial injury and not from coronary thrombosis.[88] Household voltages (120 to 220 V) may cause sudden death, particularly when they involve arm-to-arm pathways or low skin resistance in a wet victim. Serious myocardial damage is rare.[87]

Treatment for cardiac arrest should be initiated immediately after the patient is disconnected from the current source. Resuscitation efforts should be continued for a prolonged period. In lightning strikes involving multiple victims, attention should be directed first to those who are "apparently dead."[92] This is because there is a higher resuscitation rate for these individuals compared to those with medical cardiac arrest. Of note, lightning victims with vital signs generally survive without immediate medical attention.

Patients surviving high-voltage injuries generally require hospital admission, usually for attention to neurologic complications and internal or external burn injuries and less commonly for cardiac monitoring. An initially normal ECG carries a favorable cardiac prognosis leading some clinicians to question the need for 24-h electrocardiographic monitoring. Patients with arm-to-arm or arm-to-leg passage of current may be at risk for postadmission rhythm disturbances, and a higher index of suspicion is required in such patients.[94]

Adults and children presenting to the emergency department following low-voltage shocks of less than 240 V have a low incidence of myocardial injury, and most do not require further monitoring.[87]

Electroconvulsive Therapy

Electroconvulsive therapy (ECT) is accepted therapy for a variety of psychiatric illnesses including depression resistant to pharmacologic therapy, severe suicidal ideation with vegetative signs, acute mania, and depression with intolerance to medication side effects secondary to cardiac problems.[95] ECT is performed with a brief unilateral or bilateral electrical stimulus to the brain while the patient is under short-acting anesthesia with a hypnotic drug and a muscle depolarizing agent.[96] ECT produces brief, intense stimulation of the central nervous system. Cardiovascular complications may result from this stimulation or from the drugs used to modify the response.

Initially, the ECT stimulus activates the vagus nerve and may produce bradycardia, hypotension, and rarely asystole.[97,98] Sympathetic discharge occurs, which is amplified by a 15-fold rise in epinephrine and threefold rise in norepinephrine levels, resulting in tachycardia and hypertension.[97] Transient atrial and ventricular tachyarrhythmias may occur in approximately 10 percent of patients with known or suspected cardiovascular disease.[99] Transient electrocardiographic alterations, including ST-T-wave changes, QRS changes, QT prolongation, and peaked T waves, may occur.

The mortality rate of ECT is less than 3 in 10,000, and the complication rate is approximately 0.3 percent. Patients with severe heart disease may successfully undergo ECT with acceptable risk. Prior to ECT, electrolyte abnormalities should be corrected and systemic hypertension should be controlled. Patients with pulmonary disease require special evaluation because hypoxia and respiratory acidosis may precipitate cardiovascular events.[95,100]

Following ECT, hypertension and tachycardia may be controlled with adrenergic blockade with intravenous labetolol or esmolol.[101] Other antihypertensive agents such as clonidine or calcium channel blockers may be utilized. Sustained ventricular arrhythmias are treated with lidocaine, but pretreatment with lidocaine is not indicated. Patients with cardiac pacemakers can safely undergo ECT.[102] Currently used pacemakers are not likely to be affected by ECT current. Although these newer devices have not been systematically studied, the 50 to 100 W delivered to the scalp during ECT are probably inadequate to reprogram current pacemakers.

TABLE 89-5 Common Naturoceutical Agents for Cardiovascular Conditions or with Cardiac Effects

Naturoceutical	Popular Use	Reported/Possible Side Effects	Reported/Possible Medication Interactions
Aconite	Hypertension, mental health	Ventricular arrhythmias, death	
Belladonna	Anxiety, muscle spasm	Anticholinergic, CNS depressant	Tricyclic antidepressants, quinidine, amantadine
Birch leaf	Edema	Electrolyte abnormalities	Diuretics
Capsaicin	Claudication, muscle pain, neuropathy	Hypertension, flushing, headache	
Coenzyme Q 10	Heart failure, hypertension, coronary artery disease, arrhythmias	Abnormal liver function tests	
Danshen	Angina, poor circulation	Decreased platelet aggregation, hypotension, (+) inotrope, (−) chronotrope	Anticoagulants, vasoactive medications
Feverfew	Migraine	Prostaglandin inhibition, mouth ulcers	
Garlic	Hyperlipidemia, hypertension	Decreased platelet aggregation and thromboxanes, increased fibrinolysis, hypoglycemia	Anticoagulants, hypoglycemic agents
Ginger	Nausea, energy booster	Increased bleeding time, antiplatelet effects	Anticoagulants
Ginseng	Libido, energy booster	Hypertension, palpitations	Digitalis potentiation, diuretic resistance
Ginkgo biloba	Memory aid, circulation, vascular disease	Antiplatelet, headache, gastrointestinal effects	Anticoagulants
Guarana	Energy booster	High caffeine content, hypertension, decreased platelet aggregation	Stimulants, methylxanthines
Grapeseed extract	Hyperlipidemia, coronary artery disease	Antioxidant, gastrointestinal effects	
Hawthorn	Heart failure, angina, arrhythmias	Hypotension, bradycardia, (+) inotrope	Digitalis potentiation, vasodilator potentiation
Horse chestnut	Edema, venous insufficiency	Palpitations, renal, hepatic, gastrointestinal effects; "pseudolupus;" death	
Indian snakeroot	Hypertension, anxiety	Reserpine source, depression, fatigue	Vasoactive medications, digitalis, barbiturates, levodopa
Ma Huang (ephedra)	Weight loss, energy, asthma	Hypertension, palpitations, stroke, myocardial infarction, death	Stimulants, α, β agonists, halothane, monoamine oxidase inhibitors

(Continued)

TABLE 89-5 Common Naturoceutical Agents for Cardiovascular Conditions or with Cardiac Effects (*Continued*)

Naturoceutical	Popular Use	Reported/Possible Side Effects	Reported/Possible Medication Interactions
Motherwort	Heart aid, thyroid	Contains cardiac glycosides and alkaloids	Digitalis
Nettle	Prostate	Hepatitis, contains glycosides	Digitalis
Plantain	Various	Contains digitalis lanata	Digoxin toxicity
Saw palmetto	Prostate	Edema	
Squill	Edema, cardiac, renal	Diuretic effects, electrolyte abnormalities, cardiac glycosides, arrhythmias	Diuretics, digitalis, quinidine, glucocorticoids, calcium
Stephnia tetranda	Hypertension	Calcium channel blocking effects, decreases aldosterone, nephrotoxicity	Potentiation of calcium channel blockers
St. John's wort	Depression	"Serotonin" syndrome	Serotonin reuptake inhibitors, cyclosporine, tacrolimus, digoxin
Uva ursi	Edema, diet aid	Diuretic effects, electrolyte abnormalities	Diuretics
Valerian	Sleep aid, angina	Gastrointestinal effects, abnormal liver function tests	
Vitamin E	Supplement	Bleeding	Anticoagulants, cyclosporine
White willow	Arthritis	Contains salicin	Anticoagulants
Yohimbine	Impotence	Hypertension, hypotension, tachycardia	Vasoactive medication

SOURCE: Modified with permission from Hermann DD. Naturoceutical agents and cardiovascular medicine: The hope, the hype and the harm, *ACC Curr J Rev 1999;8:56.*

Lithotripsy

Extracorporeal shock wave lithotripsy used to treat renal stones and gallstones has the potential to cause cardiac arrhythmias. Rhythm disturbances may be related to electrical stimulus from the shock wave or from enhanced vagal tone associated with the procedure. Electrocardiographic monitoring is recommended for patients with cardiac disease. Gating of the shock waves to the QRS cycle may be necessary in high-risk patients, although ungated lithotripsy with newer devices is reportedly safe in most patients.[103,104]

POISONS

Complementary and Alternative Medicines

Many people now use complementary and alternative therapies including herbal medicines, acupuncture and meditation (see Chap. 108). Most physicians are unaware that their patients are using these therapies in conjunction with orthodox medicine. Few physicians are knowledgeable about potential side effects and drug interactions of

botanical medication. In addition, since these products are considered dietary supplements, they are not subject to government regulations mandating safety and efficacy. Therefore, quality and purity of these products cannot be assured.[105] Commonly used alternative therapies are listed in Table 89-5 with their purported use, possible side effects and potential medication interactions (see also Chap. 108).[106]

Concerns have been raised regarding the safety of ephedra, a dietary supplement utilized for weight loss and enhancement of athletic performance. Ephedra and ephedrine-alkaloid containing products have been associated with palpitations, cerebrovascular accidents, myocardial infarction, and death.[107]

The National Heart, Lung, and Blood Institute and the National Center for Alternative and Complementary Medicine are pursuing scientific evaluation of botanicals, chelation therapy, meditation, and acupuncture.[105] Calcium chelation with ethylenediamine tetraacetic acid (EDTA) is proposed to benefit patients with vascular disease; however, no clinical trials have been performed. Similarly, exochelin is a chelator that may arrest the growth of smooth muscle cells and may potentially have a role in cardiovascular disease and angioplasty restenosis. Acupuncture has been shown to lower blood pressure but persistent antihypertensive effects have yet to be proven. Meditation may reduce blood pressure and lower levels of stress-related hormones such as cortisol.[105] Few side effects are associated with meditation and acupuncture.

HERBAL–MEDICATION INTERACTIONS

St. John's wort is commonly used by patients to treat mild depression. Hypericin and hyperforin, two components of St. John's wort are responsible for its antidepressant effects. Hyperforin acts as an inducer of the cytochrome P_{450} CYP3A4 and therefore may lower serum levels of medications metabolized by this pathway.[108] St. John's wort has been shown to decrease plasma cyclosporine levels, protease inhibitors such as indinavir, and decrease the effectiveness of oral contraceptives.[108,109] St. John's wort may also decrease the effectiveness of warfarin.[109] Other herbal therapies that interact with the cytochrome P_{450} system and thus may interfere with metabolism of medication through these pathways include milk thistle (Silymarin), ginseng, garlic, danshen, and licorice.[108] Specific interactions are shown in Table 89-5.

PURPORTED BENEFITS IN CARDIOVASCULAR DISEASE

Many adults use alternative medicines to treat cardiovascular diseases despite proven lack of benefit and potential harm. The more commonly used alternative treatments for cardiovascular disease include antioxidants, L-arginine, fish oils, coenzyme Q, and soy protein. Antioxidants theoretically may benefit patients with cardiovascular disease. The efficacy of antioxidant supplements such as vitamin E, however, has yet to be proven.[110] Similarly, coenzyme Q has not been shown to affect outcomes or symptoms in patients with congestive heart failure.[110] Soy protein may help reduce cholesterol, and current recommendations are for 25 g/d of soy protein.[110] Routine use of dietary supplements to treat cardiovascular disease is not supported by the existing literature.

VENOMS AND TOXINS

Snakebites are a rare cause of death in the United States but account for over 40,000 deaths worldwide. The majority of these fatal bites occur in Asia, South America, and Africa. Scorpion stings are a common problem in India, Southeast Asia, Mexico, Israel, and the Southwestern United States. The cardiovascular effects of some snake venom, scorpion venom, arthropod stings, and marine toxins are shown in Table 89-6.[111–115]

HALOGENATED HYDROCARBONS

Halogenated hydrocarbons are used in fire extinguishers, solvents, and refrigerants and in the manufacture of pesticides and plastics. Heavy acute exposure to these compounds may result in cardiac arrhythmias and sudden death.[116] Direct cardiac effects include depression of myocardial contractility[117] and sensitization to the arrhythmogenic effects of catecholamines. Indirect cardiotoxicity may result from hypoxia or central nervous system toxicity.

ORGANOPHOSPHATES

Organophosphates, used commercially in pesticides, are powerful inhibitors of acetylcholinesterase, and this inhibition can result in parasympathetic overstimulation. Suicide attempts account for the majority of fatalities associated with ingestion of large doses of organophosphates. Signs and symptoms of ingestion include respiratory depression, bronchospasm and secretion, and pulmonary edema. Deaths are generally related to respiratory failure. Cardiac toxicity is generally associated with QT prolongation. Torsades de pointes, atrioventricular conduction disturbances, and ST-T abnormalities have been noted. Cardiac arrhythmias have been noted up to 15 days after exposure. Direct myocardial toxicity has been postulated, in addition to cholinergic hyperactivity.[118] Treatment includes continued atropine administration at doses sufficient to dry mucous membranes and increase heart rate to 100 beats per minute. Obidoxime therapy has also been studied in severe overdoses.[119]

CARBON MONOXIDE

Toxicity from carbon monoxide is related to tissue hypoxia. Carbon monoxide has a much higher affinity for hemoglobin than does oxygen, preventing adequate oxygen exchange. Carbon monoxide exposure worsens angina pectoris and increases the risk of myocardial infarction.[120] Carbon monoxide poisoning results in electrocardiographic abnormalities, including sinus tachycardia, atrial fibrillation, atrioventricular block, and ST-T abnormalities. Cardiac enzyme elevation may occur. Severe exposure can result in myocardial necrosis and cardiomyopathy. Transient evidence of cardiac toxicity, however, is not necessarily associated with long-term sequelae.[121]

TABLE 89-6 Cardiovascular Effects of Reptile, Arthropod, and Marine Toxins

Toxins	Effects
Snakes and Scorpions[111,112]	
Cobra venom	Augments myocardial contraction at low doses, asystole at high doses
Rattlesnake venom	Depresses myocardial contractility
Cobra, mamba, coral snake, taipan[118]	Neuromuscular toxicity, pulmonary hypertension
Scorpion stings—*Buthidae* venom	Tachycardia, hypertension, arrhythmias, myocardial depression from massive catecholamine release, myocarditis, congestive heart failure, cardiac arrest
Arthropods[113]	
Bee, hornet, wasp	Anaphylaxis
Bee venom	Direct cardiac effects, ischemia
Black widow (*Lactrodectus*)	Rare cardiac manifestations, hypertension, tachycardia may occur
Marine Organisms[114,115]	
Stingray venom	Phosphodiesterase may cause arrhythmias
Sea cucumber	Holothurin may cause cardiac glycoside toxicity
Pufferfish	Tetrodotoxin may cause bradycardia and vascular collapse
Lionfish (*Pterois volitans*)	Negative inotropic and chronotropic effects

RADIATION

Mediastinal radiation—commonly used to treat Hodgkin's disease, lung cancer, breast cancer, and seminoma—may result in acute or late cardiac sequelae. Prior to the 1960s, the heart was thought to be resistant to the effects of clinical radiation. It is now known that radiation can lead to acute or chronic pericarditis, coronary artery disease, systolic and diastolic ventricular dysfunction, conduction defects, and valvular dysfunction.[122] Many cancer patients now have improved long-term survivals, and thus are more prone to late complications of mediastinal irradiation (Table 89-7). Risk factors for the development of radiation-induced heart disease include total radiation dose > 35 Gy, high fractionated dose (> 2.0 Gy/d), volume of heart irradiated, young age at exposure, long time from exposure, mediastinal tumor, traditional cardiovascular risk factors, and concomitant anthracycline administration.[122]

Pericardial Disease

Acute pericarditis, constrictive pericarditis and effusive-constrictive pericarditis may follow radiation therapy. While up to 40 percent of patients treated with older techniques developed pericarditis, the incidence with modern techniques (total dose < 30 Gy, subcarinal blocking and daily fraction size < 2 Gy) is approximately 2.5 percent.[123] Clinically apparent pericarditis may occur 4 to 12 months after radiation therapy. Acute pericarditis, asymptomatic pericardial effusion, or pericardial tamponade may occur. Other etiologies of pericarditis should be considered particularly malignant involvement of the pericardium. Pericarditis occurring during treatment of a mediastinal mass contiguous to the heart is generally secondary to tumor effect and does not correlate with late pericardial complications.[124,125]

Radiation may cause an exudative pericarditis followed by pericardial fibrosis due to fibroblast proliferation and collagen deposition. Although the majority of patients with pericardial effusion recover spontaneously, up to 20 percent may develop chronic and/or constrictive pericarditis 5 to 10 years after therapy.[122]

Treatment for acute pericarditis is based on relief of symptoms including antipyretics, anti-inflammatory agents, and pericardiocentesis when indicated. Surgical mortality in patients with constrictive pericarditis may be as high as 40 percent.[126] Extensive mediastinal and pericardial fibrosis make pericardiectomy technically challenging. Radiation-induced constriction is often associated with coronary artery disease, valvular heart disease, and/or myocardial dysfunction. Candidates for pericardiectomy should be carefully selected.

Myocardial Dysfunction

Radiation causes diffuse interstitial fibrosis, which more commonly leads to diastolic dysfunction. Systolic dysfunction is rare and is usually associated with prior anthracycline treatment. Asymptomatic patients may have varying degrees of myocardial fibrosis that may be patchy or diffuse. Microcirculatory damage leading to ischemia may also contribute myocardial cell death and fibrosis.[122]

Coronary Artery Disease

Premature coronary artery disease may result from prior radiation therapy. The coronary ostia and left main coronary artery are frequently involved in radiation-induced coronary artery disease. Microscopically, these lesions demonstrate intimal proliferation and fibrosis.[122] In one study, 23 percent of patients undergoing cardiac surgery for radiation-related valvular disease also had left main disease.[126] Mediastinal and pericardial fibrosis make surgical revascularization more difficult. In addition, the left internal mammary artery, which is often used as a graft, is often included in the radiation field. The long-term patency of the internal mammary graft in radiation-related coronary artery disease is not known, but early occlusion has been reported.[127] Routine assessment of cardiovascular risk factors is indicated in all patients, regardless of age, who have received radiation therapy to the chest. Annual measurement of lipid profiles, high sensitive C-reactive protein, and thyroid function are recommended. Modifications of traditional risk factors including smoking cessation, blood pressure control, weight maintenance, and treatment of diabetes are important. Exercise electrocardiography or stress perfusion testing should be considered in high-risk individuals who may not develop anginal chest pain even in the presence of significant coronary stenosis.[122]

Conduction Disturbances and Arrhythmias

Radiation may result in fibrosis of the nodal and infranodal pathways causing all levels of atrioventricular block. Right bundle branch block is more common than left. Sick sinus syndrome has been reported as well. Persistent tachycardia may also occur, similar to the denervated heart, and may be related to autonomic nervous system dysfunction. Radiation-related conduction abnormalities are associated with total dose > 40 Gy, a delay of 10 years or more since therapy, interval abnormal ECG (bundle branch block), and prior pericardial involvement.[122]

Valvular Disease

Clinically significant valvular heart disease secondary to radiation is rare, but when present, usually involves the aortic or mitral valves. Coexisting pericardial disease is the rule. At autopsy fibrous thickening of the valves is seen. This most commonly leads to asymptomatic aortic and mitral regurgitation. Stenotic lesions are rare. Echocardiographic studies have demonstrated characteristic thickening and fibrotic changes of the aortic-mitral curtain, distinct from the appearance of rheumatic valvular disease.[128] Successful surgical replacement of symptomatic regurgitant valves depends on the absence of concomitant constrictive pericarditis. Conduction abnormalities requiring pacemaker placement are also common in the perioperative period.[128]

TABLE 89-7   Radiation-Induced Cardiac Disease

Pericardial
   Acute pericarditis
   Chronic pericarditis
   Constrictive pericarditis
Myocardial
   Restrictive cardiomyopathy
   Dilated cardiomyopathy (concomitant anthracyclines)
Coronary artery disease
Conduction abnormalities
   Atrioventricular block
   Right bundle branch block
   Left bundle branch block
Valvular disease

References

1. Frishman WH, Sung HM, Yee HCM, et al. Cardiovascular toxicity with cancer chemotherapy. *Curr Probl Cardiol* 1996;21:225–288.

2. Shan K, Lincoff AM, Young JB. Anthracycline-induced cardiomyopathy. *Ann Intern Med* 1996;125:47–58.

3. Von Hoff DD, Layard MW, Basa P, et al. Risk factors for doxorubicin-induced congestive heart failure. *Ann Intern Med* 1979;91:710–717.

4. Bristow MR, Mason JW, Billingham ME, Daniels JR. Doxorubicin cardiomyopathy: Evaluation of phonocardiography, endomyocardial biopsy, and cardiac catheterization. *Ann Intern Med* 1978;88:168–175.

5. Lipschultz SE, Lipsitz SR, Mone SM, et al. Female sex and higher drug dose as risk factors for late cardiotoxic effects of doxorubicin therapy for childhood cancer. *N Engl J Med* 1995;332:1738–1743.

6. Singal PK, Iliskovic N. Doxorubicin-induced cardiomyopathy. *N Engl J Med* 1998;339:900–905.

7. Moreg JS, Oglon DJ. Outcomes of clinical congestive heart failure induced by anthracycline chemotherapy. *Cancer* 1992;70:2637–2641.

8. Steinherz J, Graham T, Hurwitz R, et al. Guidelines for cardiac monitoring of children during and after anthracycline therapy: Report of the Cardiology Committee of the Children's Cancer Study Group. *Pediatrics* 1992;89:942–949.

9. Weegner KM, Bledsoe M, Chauvenet A, Wofford M. Exercise echocardiography in the detection of anthracycline cardiotoxicity. *Cancer* 1991;68:435–438.

10. Schwartz RG, McKenzie WB, Alexander J, et al. Congestive heart failure and left ventricular dysfunction complicating doxorubicin therapy: Seven-year experience using radionuclide angiocardiography. *Am J Med* 1987;82:1109–1118.

11. McKillop JH, Bristow MR, Goris ML, et al. Sensitivity and specificity of radionuclide ejection fraction in doxorubicin cardiotoxicity. *Am Heart J* 1983;106:1048–1056.

12. Isner JM, Ferrans VJ, Cohen SR, et al. Clinical and morphologic cardiac findings after anthracycline chemotherapy: Analysis of 64 patients studied at necropsy. *Am J Cardiol* 1983;51:1167–1174.

13. Steinherz LJ, Steinherz PG, Tan CTC, et al. Cardiac toxicity 4 to 20 years after completing anthracycline therapy. *JAMA* 1991;266:1672–1677.

14. Kramer LC, Van Dalen EC, Offringam, et al. Anthracycline-induced clinical heart failure and a cohort of 607 children: Long-term followup study. *J Clin Oncol* 2001;19:191–196

15. Legha SS, Benjamin RS, MacKay B, et al. Reduction of doxorubicin cardiotoxicity by prolonged continuous intravenous infusion. *Ann Intern Med* 1982;89:133–139.

16. Lipshultz SE, Giantris, AL, Lipsitz SR, et al. Doxorubicin administration by continous infusion is not cardioprotective: Dana-Farber 91-01 Acute Lymphoblastic Leukemia protocol. *J Clin Oncol* 2002;20:1677–1682.

17. Schuchter LM, Hensley ML, Meropol NJ, et al. 2002 Update of recommendations for the use of chemotherapy and radiotherapy protectants: Clinical practice Guidelines of the American Society of Clinical Oncology. *J Clin Oncol* 2002;20:2895–2903.

18. Gralow JR, Livingston RB. University of Washington high dose cyclophosphamide, mitoxantrone, etoposide experience in metastatic breast cancer: unexpected cardiac toxicity. *J Clin Oncol* 2001;19:3903–3904.

19. Feenstra J, Grobbee DE, Remme WJ, Stricker BH. Drug induced heart failure. *J Am Coll Cardiol* 1999;33:1152–1162.

20. Robben NC, Pippas AW, Moore JO. The syndrome of 5-fluorouracil cardiotoxicity: An elusive cardiopathy. *Cancer* 1993;71:493–509.

21. Akhtar SS, Salim KP, Bano ZA. Symptomatic cardiotoxicity with high dose 5-fluorouracil infusion: A prospective study. *Oncology* 1993;50:441–445.

22. Weiss RB, Grillo-Lopez AJ, Marsoni S, et al. Amsacrine-associated cardiotoxicity: An analysis of 82 cases. *J Clin Oncol* 1986;4:918–928.

23. Salminen E, Syvanen K, Korpela J, et al. Docetaxel with epirubicin–Investigations on cardiac safety. *Anti-cancer* 2003;14:73–77.

24. Sideman A, Hudis C, Pierri N. Cardiac dysfunction in the trastuzumab *J Clin Oncol* 2002;20:1215–1221.

25. Spire J. Cardiac dysfunction in the trastuzumab clinical experience. *J Clin Oncol* 2002;20:1156–1157.

26. DuBois JS, Udelson JE, Atkins B. Severe reversible, global and regional ventricular dysfunction associated with high-dose interleukin-2 immunotherapy. *J Immunother* 1995;18:119–123.

27. Kuwatu A, Ohashi M, Sugiyama M, et al. A case of reversible dilated cardiomyopathy after α interferon therapy in a patient with renal cell carcinoma. *Am J Med Sci* 2002;324:331–334.

28. Roose SP, Dalak GW. Treating the depressed patient with cardiovascular problems. *J Clin Psychiatry* 1992;53(9, suppl):25–31.

29. Fraser-Smith N, Lesperance F, Talajic M. Depression following myocardial infarction: Impact on 6-month survival. *JAMA* 1993;270:1819–1825.

30. Glassman AH, Roose SP, Bigger JT. The safety of tricyclic antidepressants in cardiac patients—risk benefit reconsidered. *JAMA* 1993;269:2673–2675.

31. Franco-Bronson K. The management of treatment-resistant depression in the medically ill. *Psychiatr Clin North Am* 1996;19:329–348.

32. Glassman AH, Preud'home XA. Review of the cardiovascular effects of heterocyclic antidepressants. *J Clin Psychiatry* 1983;54(2, suppl):16–22.

33. Roose SP, Glassman AH, Gardina EGV, et al. Tricyclic antidepressants in depressed patients with cardiac conduction disease. *Arch Gen Psychiatry* 1987;44:273–275.

34. The Cardiac Arrhythmia Suppression Trial II Investigators. Effect of the antiarrhythmic agent moricizine on survival after myocardial infarction. *N Engl J Med* 1992;327:227–233.

35. Wolfe TR, Caravati EM, Rollin DE. Terminal 40-ms frontal plane QRS axis as a marker for tricyclic antidepressant overdose. *Ann Emerg Med* 1989;18:348–351.

36. Shanon M. Toxicology reviews: Targeted management strategies for cardiovascular toxicity from tricyclic antidepressant overdose: The pivotal role for alkalinization and sodium loading. *Pediatr Emerg Care* 1998;14:293–298.

37. Ciraulo DA, Shader RI. Fluoxetine drug-drug interactions: I. Antidepressants and antipsychotics. *J Clin Psychopharmacol* 1990;48:1990.

38. Sheline YI, Freedland KE, Carney RM. How safe are serotonin reuptake inhibitors for depression in patients with coronary heart disease? *Am J Med* 1997;102:54–59.

39. Strik JJMH, Honig A, Lousberg R, et al. Cardiac side-effects to two selective serotonin reuptake inhibitors in middle-aged and elderly depressed patients. *Internat Clin Psychopharm* 1998;13:263–267.

40. Rudorfer MV, Manji HK, Potter WZ. Comparative tolerability profiles of the newer versus older antidepressants. *Drug Safety* 1994;10:18–46.

41. Rosenqvist M, Bergfeldt L, Aili H, Mathe AA. Sinus node dysfunction during long-term lithium treatment. *Br Heart J* 1993;70:371–375.

42. Numata T, Abe H, Terao T, Nakashima Y. Possible involvement of hypothyroidism as a cause of lithium-induced sinus node dysfunction. *PACE* 1999;22:954–957.

43. Simard M, Gumbiner B, Lee A, et al. Lithium carbonate intoxication: A case report and review of the literature. *Arch Intern Med* 1989;149:36–46.

44. Kemper AJ, Dunlap R, Pietro DA. Thioridazine-induced torsade de pointes. Successful therapy with isoproterenol. *JAMA* 1983;249:2931–2934.

45. Di Salvo TG, O'Gara PT. Torsades de pointes caused by high-dose intravenous haloperidol in cardiac patients. *Clin Cardiol* 1995;18:285–290.

46. Haverkamp W, Shenasa M, Borggrefe M, Breithardt G. Torsades de pointes. In: Zipes DP, Jalife J, eds. *Cardiac Electrophysiology: From Cell to Bedside,* 2nd ed. Philadelphia: Saunders;1995:885–899.

47. Orban Z, MacDonald LL, Peters MA, Guslits B. Erythromycin-induced cardiac toxicity. *Am J Cardiol* 1995;75:859–861.

48. Lopez JA, Harold JG, Rosenthal ML, et al. QT prolongation and torsades de pointes after administration of trimethoprim-sulfamethoxazole. *Am J Cardiol* 1987;59:376–377.

49. Pringle TH, Scorbie IN, Murray RG, et al. Prolongation of the QT interval during therapeutic starvation: A substrate for malignant arrhythmias. *Int J Obes* 1983;7:253–261.

50. Reinoehl J, Frankovich D, Machado C, et al. Probucol-associated tachyarrhythmic events and QT prolongation: Importance of gender. *Am Heart J* 1996;131:1184–1191.

51. Vitola J, Vukanovic J, Roden D. Cisapride-induced torsades de pointes. *J Cardiovasc Electrophysiol* 1998;9:1109–1113.

52. Priori SG. Exploring the hidden danger of noncardiac drugs. *J Cardiovasc Electrophysiol* 1998;9:1114–1116.

53. Nemeroff CB, DeVane CL, Pollack BG. Newer antidepressants and the cytochrome P450 system. *Am J Psychiatry* 1996;153:311–320.

54. Redfield MM, Nicholson WJ, Edwards WD, Tajik AJ. Valve disease associated with ergot alkaloid: Echocardiographic and pathologic correlations. *Ann Intern Med* 1992;117:50–52.

55. Mason JW, Billingham ME, Friedman JP. Methysergide-induced heart disease: A case of multivalvular and myocardial fibrosis. *Circulation* 1977;56:889–890.

56. Connolly HM, Crary JL, McGoon MD, et al. Valvular heart disease associated with fenfluramine-phentermine [published correction appears in *N Engl J Med* 1997;337:1783]. *N Engl J Med* 1997;337:581–588.

57. Cardiac valvulopathy associated with exposure to fenfluramine or dexfenfluramine: US Department of Health and Human Services interim public health recommendations, Nov 1997. *MMWR Morb Mortal Wkly Rep* 1997;46:1061–1066.

58. Weissman NJ, Tighe JF Jr, Gottdiener JS, Gwynne JT. Sustained-Release Dexfenfluramine Study Group. An assessment of heart valve abnormalities in obese patients taking dexfenfluramine, sustained-release dexfenfluramine, or placebo. *N Engl J Med* 1998;339:725–732.

59. Hensrud DD, Connolly HM, Grogan M, et al. Echocardiographic improvement over time after cessation of use of fenfluramine and phentermine. *Mayo Clin Proc* 1999;74:1191–1197.

60. Shively BK, Roldan CA, Gill EA, et al. Prevalence and determinants of valvulopathy in patients treated with dexfenfluramine. *Circulation* 1999;100:2161–2167.

61. Pritchett AM, Morrison JF, Edwards WD. Valvular heart disease in patients taking pergolide. *Mayo Clin Pro* 2002;77:1280–1286.

62. Rahimtoola MB. Drug-related valvular heart disease: here we go again: Will we do better this time? *Mayo Clin Pro* 2002;77:1275–1277.

63. Liston H, Bennett L, Usher B, Nappi J. The association of the combination of sumtriptan and methysergide in myocardial infarction in a premenopausal woman. *Arch Intern Med* Mar 1999;159:511–513.

64. VanDenBrink AM, Reekers M, Bax W, et al. Coronary side-effect potential of current and prospective antimigraine drugs. *Circulation* 1998;98:25–30.

65. Cubero GI, Reguero JJ, Ortega JM. Restrictive cardiomyopathy caused by chloroquine. *Br Heart J* 1993;69:451–452.

66. Ratliff NB, Estes ML, Myles JL et al. Diagnosis of chloroquine cardiomyopathy by endomyocardial biopsy. *N Engl J Med* 1987;316:191–193.

67. Bagatell CJ, Bremner WJ. Androgens in men—uses and abuses: *New Engl J Med* 1996;334:707–714.

68. Yesalis CE, Kennedy NK, Kopstein AN, Bahrke MS. Anabolic-adrogenic steroid use in the United States. *JAMA* 1993;270:1217–1221.

69. Nieminen MS, Ramo MP, Viitasalo M, Heikkila P, et al. Serious cardiovascular side effects of large doses of anabolic steroids in weight lifters. *Eur Heart J* 1996;17:1576–1583.

70. Blue JG, Lombardo JA. Steroids and steroid-like compounds. *Clinics in Sports Med* 1999;18:667–689.

71. Glazer G. Atherogenic effects of anabolic steroids on serum lipid levels: A literature review. *Arch Intern Med* 1991;151:1925–1933.

72. Mewis C, Spyridopulous I, Kuhlkamp V, Seipel L. Manifestation of severe coronary heart disease after anabolic drug abuse. *Clin Cardiol* 1996;19:153–155.

73. Hollander JE. The management of cocaine-associated myocardial ischemia. *N Engl J Med* 1995;333:1267–1272.

74. Kloner RA, Hale S, Alker Rezkalla S. The effects of acute and chronic cocaine use on the heart. *Circulation* 1992;85:407–419.

75. Pirwitz MJ, Willard JE, Landau C, et al. Influence of cocaine, ethanol, or their combination epicardial coronary arterial dimensions in humans. *Arch Intern Med* 1995;155:1186–1191.

76. Moliterno DJ, Willard JE, Lange RA, et al. Coronary-artery vasoconstriction induced by cocaine, cigarette smoking, or both. *N Engl J Med* 1994;330:454–459.

77. Knuepfer MM, Mueller PJ. Review of evidence for a novel model of cocaine-induced cardiovascular toxicity. *Pharmacol Biochem and Behavior* 1999;63:489–500.

78. Om A, Ellahham S, Disciascio G. Management of cocaine-induced cardiovascular complications. *Am Heart J* 1993;125:469–475.

79. Hollander JE, Hoffman RS, Burstein JL, et al. Cocaine-associated myocardial infarction: Mortality and complications. *Arch Intern Med* 1995;155:1081–1086.

80. Weber JE, Shofer FS, Larkin GL, et al. Validation of a brief observation period for patients with cocaine-associated chest pain. *N Engl J Med* 2003;348:510–517.

81. Kloner RA, Rezkalla SH. Cocaine and the heart. *N Engl J Med* 2003;348:487–488.

82. Leikin JB. Cocaine and B-adrenergic blockers: A remarriage after a decade-long divorce? *Crit Care Med* 1999;27:688–689.

83. Gitter MJ, Goldsmith SR, Dunbar DN, Sharkey SW. Cocaine and chest pain: Clinical features and outcome of patients hospitalized to rule out myocardial infarction. *Ann Intern Med* 1991;115:277–282.

84. Pitts DK, Marwah J. Cocaine and central monoaminergic neurotransmission: A review of electrophysiologic studies and comparison to amphetamine and antidepressants. *Life Sci* 1988;42:949–968.

85. Derlet RW, Rice P, Horowitz BZ, Lord RV. Amphetamine toxicity: Experiences with 127 cases. *J Emerg Med* 1989;7:157–161.

86. Hong R, Matsuyama E, Nur K. Cardiomyopathy associated with the smoking of crystal amphetamine. *JAMA* 1991;265:1152–1154.

87. Bailey B, Gaudreauh HP, Thivierge RL, Turgeon JP. Cardiac monitoring of children with household electrical injuries. *Ann Emerg Med* 1995;25:612–617.

88. Carleton SC. Cardiac problems associated with electrical injury. *Cardiol Clin* 1995;13:263–277.

89. Browne BJ, Gaasch WR. Electrical injuries and lightning. *Emerg Med Clin North Am* 1992;10:211–229.

90. Lichtenberg R, Dries D, Ward K, et al. Cardiovascular effects of lightning strikes. *J Am Coll Cardiol* 1993;21:531–536.

91. Artz CP. Electrical injury simulates crush injury. *Surg Gynecol Obstet* 1967;125:1316.

92. Robinson NMK, Chamberlain DA. Electrical injury to the heart may cause long-term damage to conducting tissue: A hypothesis and review of the literature. *Int J Cardiol* 1966;53:273–277.

93. Jain S, Bandi V. Electrical and lightning injuries. *Critical Care Clinics* 1999;15:319–331.

94. Jenson PJ, Thomsen PEB, Bagger JP, et al. Electrical injury causing ventricular arrhythmias. *Br Heart J* 1987;57:279–283.

95. Banazak DA. Electroconvulsive therapy: A guide for family physicians. *Am Fam Physician* 1996;53:273–278.

96. Sackeim HA, Devanand DP, Prudie J. Stimulus intensity, seizure threshold, and seizure duration: Impact on the efficacy and safety of electroconvulsive therapy. *Psychiatr Clin North Am* 1991;14:803–843.

97. Gerring JP, Shields HM. The identification and management of patients with a high risk for cardiac arrhythmias during modified ECT. *J Clin Psychiatry* 1982;43:140–143.

98. Graybar G, Goethe J, Levy T, et al. Transient large upright T-wave on the electrocardiogram during multiple monitored electroconvulsive therapy. *Anesthesiology* 1983;59:467–469.

99. Gould L, Copalaswamy C, Chandy F, Kim B. Electroconvulsive therapy induced ECG changes simulating a myocardial infarction. *Arch Intern Med* 1983;143:1786–1787.

100. Banazak DA. Electroconvulsive therapy: A guide for family physicians. *Am Fam Physician* 1996;53:273–278.

101. Leslie JB, Kalayjiam RW, Sirgo MA, et al. Intravenous labetolol for the treatment of postoperative hypertension. *Anesthesiology* 1987;67:413–421.

102. Abiusa P, Dunkelman R, Proper M. Electroconvulsive therapy in patients with pacemakers. *JAMA* 1978;240:2459–2462.

103. Greenstein A, Kaver I, Lechtman V, et al. Cardiac arrhythmias during nonsynchronized extracorporeal shock wave lithotripsy. *J Urol* 1995;154:1321–1322.

104. Zeng ZR, Lindstedt E, Roijer A, Olsson SB. Arrhythmia during extracorporeal shock wave lithotripsy. *Br J Urol* 1993;71:10–16.

105. Lin MC, Gershwin ME, Linghurst JC, Wu KK. State of complementary and alternative medicine in cardiovascular, lung, and blood research. *Circulation* 2001;103:2038.

106. Hermann DD. Naturoceutical agents and cardiovascular medicine: the hope, the hype and the harm. *ACC Current Journal Review* 1999;Sept/Oct:53–57.

107. Shekelle PG, Hardy ML, Morton SC, et al. Efficacy and safety of ephedra and ephedrine for weight loss and athletic performance: a meta-analysis. *JAMA* 2003;289:1537–1545.

108. Ioannides C. Pharmacokinetic interactions between herbal remedies and medicinal drugs. *Xenobiotica* 2002;32(6):451–478.

109. DeSmet PAGM. Herbal Remedies. *NEJM* 2002;347(25):2046–2056.

110. Chagan L, Ioselovich A, Asherova L, Cheng JW. Use of alternative pharmacotherapy in management of cardiovascular diseases. *Am J Manag Care* 2002;8:270–285.

111. Karalliedde L. Animal toxins. *Br J Anaesth* 1995;75:319–327.

112. Meki AAM, El-Deen ZMM, El-Deen HMM. Myocardial injury in scorpion envenomed children: significance of assessment of serum troponin I and Interleukin-8. *Neuroendocrinology Letters* 2002;23:133–140.

113. Gueron M, Ilia R, Margulis G. Arthropod poisons and the cardiovascular system. *Am J Emerg Med* 2000;18:708–714.

114. Church JE, Hodgson WC. Adrenergic and cholinergic activity contributes to the cardiovascular effects of lionfish *(Pterois volitans)*. *Toxicon* 2001;40:787–796.

115. Brown CK, Shepherd SM. Marine trauma, envenomations and intoxications. *Emerg Med Clin North Am* 1992;10:385–408.

116. Weill H. Cardiorespiratory effects of inhalant occupational exposures. *Circulation* 1981;63:250A–252A.

117. Zakhari S, Aviado DM. Cardiovascular toxicology of aerosol propellants, refrigerants, and related solvents. In: Van Stee EW, ed. *Cardiovascular Toxicology*. New York: Raven; 1982:281–314.

118. Roth A, Zellinger I, Arad M, Atsmon J. Organophosphates and the heart. *Chest* 1993;103:576–578.

119. Thiermann H, Mast U, Klimmek R, et al. Obidoxime therapy in OP poisoned patients. Cholinesterase status, pharmacokinetics and laboratory findings during obidoxime therapy in organophosphate poisoned patients. *Hum Exp Toxicol* 1997;16:473–480.

120. Marius-Nunez AL. Myocardial infarction with normal coronary arteries after acute exposure to carbon monoxide. *Chest* 1990;97:491–494.

121. Roberts JR, Bain M, Klachko MN, et al. Successful heart transplantation from a victim of carbon monoxide poisoning. *Ann Emerg Med* 1995;26:652–655.

122. Adams MJ, Hardenbergh PH, Constine LS, Lipshultz SE. Radiation-associated cardiovascular disease. *Crit Rev Onol Hematol* 2003;45:55–75.

123. Arsenian MA. Cardiovascular sequlae of therapeutic thoracic radiation. *Pro Cardiovasc Dis* 1991;33:299–311.

124. Ni Y, Von Segesser LK, Turina M. Futility of pericardiectomy for postirradiation constrictive pericarditis. *Ann Thorac Surg* 1990;49:445–448.

125. Shapiro CL, Hardenbergh PH, Gelman R, et al. Cardiac effects of adjuvant doxorubicin and radiation therapy in breast cancer patients. *J Clin Oncol* 1998;16:3493–3501.

126. Handa N, McGregor CGA, Danielson GK, et al. Valvular heart operation in patients with previous mediastinal radiation therapy. *Ann Thorac Surg* 2001;71:1880–1884.

127. Khan MH, Ettinger SM. Post mediastinal radiation coronary artery disease and its effects on arterial conduits. *Catheter Cardiovasc Interv* 2001;52:242–248.

128. Brand MD, Abadi CA, Aurigemma GP, et al. Radiation-associated valvular heart disease in Hodgkin's disease is associated with characteristic thickening and fibrosis of the aortic-mitral curtain. *J Heart Valve Dis* 2001;10:681–685.

ADVERSE CARDIOVASCULAR DRUG INTERACTIONS AND COMPLICATIONS

William H. Frishman / Lionel H. Opie / Domenic A. Sica

Toxicities from drug interactions have been shown to be a cause of morbidity and death in patients,[1] and these interactions are often associated with the loss of individual drug efficacy.[2] Recent technologies have resulted in an explosion of information concerning the cytochrome P450 isoenzyme system involved in the metabolism of cardiovascular (CVR) drugs.[3–10] In addition to the isoenzyme inhibition and induction by various drugs, microsomal drug metabolism is affected by genetic polymorphisms,[9] age, nutrition, gender,[6] and hepatic diseases.[3,4,7] P-glycoprotein, which mediates the transcellular transport of many drugs, may also play an important role in clinically significant drug–drug interactions.[5]

Today, a knowledge of CVR drug interactions is regarded as basic to our understanding of the pharmacologic properties of CVR drugs. Such interfaces can be either pharmacokinetic, whereby one agent interferes with the metabolism of another, or pharmacodynamic, whereby the hemodynamic properties of one agent are added or subtracted from those of another (Fig. 90-1). An example of a pharma-cokinetic interaction is the decreased rate of hepatic metabolism of lidocaine during cimetidine therapy, wherein the risk of lidocaine toxicity increases. An example of a pharmacodynamic interaction arises when nifedipine is added to beta-adrenergic blockade in the therapy of severe angina pectoris, sometimes with excess hypotension as a potential side effect of treatment.

This chapter includes discussions of the drug interactions of the major classes of CVR drugs, following an established sequence of these drugs.[11,12]

BETA-ADRENERGIC–BLOCKING DRUGS

Beta-adrenergic blockers demonstrate relatively few serious drug interactions (Table 90-1). An example of a pharmacokinetic interaction is that with cimetidine,[13] which reduces hepatic metabolism and therefore increases blood levels of carvedilol, propranolol, labetalol,

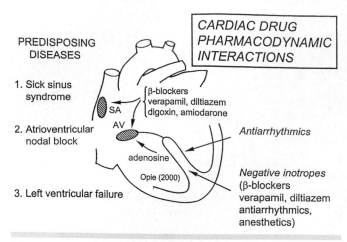

FIGURE 90-1 Cardiac drug pharmacodynamic interactions at the levels of the SA node, AV node, conduction system, and myocardium. The predisposing disease conditions are shown on the left. (Figure Copyrighted by LH Opie.)

and metoprolol, which are metabolized in the liver by the cytochrome oxidase system (Fig. 90-2). However, there is no interaction of cimetidine with beta blockers such as atenolol, sotalol, and nadolol, which are not metabolized in the liver. Another pharmacokinetic interaction occurs when verapamil raises blood levels of metoprolol through a hepatic interaction[14]; presumably, other beta blockers metabolized by the liver may be subject to a similar interaction.

Now used with increasing frequency in the acute phase of myocardial infarction, beta blockers may depress hepatic blood flow, thereby decreasing the hepatic inactivation of lidocaine.[15] Thus, beta blockade increases lidocaine blood levels, with an enhanced risk of toxicity. An example of a pharmacodynamic interaction with beta blockers is that seen with nonsteroidal anti-inflammatory drugs (NSAIDs), including indomethacin, which may attenuate the antihypertensive effects of beta blockers, possibly by decreasing the formation of vasodilatory prostaglandins.[16]

NITRATES

The chief drug interactions of nitrates are pharmacodynamic (Table 90-2). For example, during triple therapy of angina pectoris (nitrates, beta blockers, and calcium channel blockers (CCBs)), the overall efficacy of the combination may be lessened because each drug can predispose patients to excess hypotension.[17] Even two components of triple therapy, such as diltiazem and nitrates, may interact adversely to cause moderate hypotension.[18] Nonetheless, high doses of diltiazem can improve persistent effort angina when added to maximum doses of propranolol and isosorbide dinitrate without any report of significant hypotension.[19] Therefore individual patients vary greatly in their susceptibility to triple therapy–related hypotension. A dangerous drug–drug interaction is that of nitrates with sildenafil (Viagra) or vardenafil (Levitra), drugs for the treatment of erectile dysfunction that can intensify the hypotensive effects of nitrates.[20] Sildenafil should not be used within 24 h of nitrate use. There is a reported beneficial interaction between nitrates and hydralazine whereby the latter drug appears to lessen nitrate tolerance.[21]

High doses of nitroglycerin may induce heparin resistance by altering the activity of antithrombin III.[22] Nitroglycerin can also lessen the therapeutic effects of the tissue plasminogen activator (t-PA) alteplase.

CALCIUM ANTAGONISTS

Many of the interactions of CCBs are pharmacodynamic (Table 90-2),[23,24] such as added effects on the atrioventricular (AV) or sinus nodes (verapamil or diltiazem plus beta blockers, excess digitalis, or amiodarone) or on systemic vascular resistance (e.g., nifedipine plus beta blockers causing excess hypotension). However, it is now increasingly recognized that verapamil and diltiazem (but probably not nifedipine) inhibit the hepatic oxidation of some drugs, the blood levels of which consequently increase. Such agents include cyclosporine (diltiazem), the antiepileptic carbamazepine (verapamil), prazosin (verapamil), lovastatin, atorvastatin and simvastatin (diltiazem), theophylline (verapamil), some human immunodeficiency virus (HIV) protease inhibitors (diltiazem), and quinidine (verapamil). In addition, nifedipine and verapamil increase hepatic blood flow, potentially enhancing first-pass metabolism of agents such as propranolol, resulting in decreased beta-blocker blood levels.[7] The effects of some dihydropyridine CCBs (e.g., felodipine and nifedipine) are potentiated by the ingestion of grapefruit juice.[25] The potential for toxic drug–drug interactions with bepridil is so great that it is viewed as a last-resort therapy.[26,27]

Verapamil and Beta Blockers

Intravenous verapamil added to beta-adrenergic blockade carries the risk of added hypotension or nodal inhibition.[28,29] In patients with angina pectoris already receiving beta blockers, verapamil given either intravenously[30] or orally[31] can reduce myocardial contractility,[31] increase heart size,[32] and cause sinus bradycardia.[33] Verapamil also interacts pharmacokinetically with hepatically metabolized beta blockers to raise blood levels.[7,34] Despite such pharmacokinetic interactions (e.g., verapamil with propranolol) in normal subjects, pharmacodynamic changes remain more important.[35] The combination of verapamil and beta blockade in the therapy of angina pectoris must be used with extreme care when myocardial failure is clinically apparent and/or sinoatrial (SA) or AV-nodal suppression is present. The combination of verapamil and beta blockade, more so than either agent alone, improves myocardial function during exercise.[36] Verapamil plus a beta blocker may prove additive in the treatment of hypertension, though this combination carries a small risk of inhibition of sinus rate, AV conduction, and left ventricular function.[37]

Verapamil and Digoxin

Verapamil can increase blood digoxin levels by over 50 percent[38]; thus dosage reduction of a similar magnitude is warranted.

In digitalis toxicity, rapid intravenous administration of verapamil is absolutely contraindicated because the additive AV-nodal inhibitory effects of these two agents can prove fatal. Experimentally, verapamil can inhibit the Ca^{2+}-dependent delayed afterdepolarizations, which drive the ventricular automaticity found in digitalis toxicity. Oral verapamil and digitalis can, however, be combined in the absence of digitalis toxicity or AV block because their pharmacologic sites of action differ; nevertheless, digoxin levels need careful monitoring. The combination is often used in the management of supraventricular tachycardias.

TABLE 90-1 Drug Interactions of Beta-Adrenergic-Blocking Agents

Cardiac Drug	Interacting Drugs	Mechanism	Consequences	Prophylaxis
HEMODYNAMIC INTERACTIONS				
All beta blockers	Calcium antagonists, especially nifedipine	Added hypotension	Risk of myocardial ischemia	Blood pressure control, adjust doses
	Verapamil or diltiazem	Added negative inotropic effect	Risk of myocardial failure	Check for CHF, adjust doses
	Flecainide		Hypotension	Check LV function flecainide levels
	Sympathomimetics (S)	Opposing effects	Loss of clinical benefit	Avoid S
ELECTROPHYSIOLOGIC INTERACTIONS				
All beta blockers	Verapamil	Added inhibition of SA, AV nodes	Bradycardia, asystole, complete heart block	Exclude "sick-sinus" syndrome, AV nodal disease; adjust dose, exclude predrug LV failure
	Diltiazem	Added negative inotropic effect	Excess hypotension	
HEPATIC INTERACTIONS				
Propranolol (P)	Cimetidine (C)	C decreases P metabolism	Excess propranolol effects	Reduce both drug doses
	Lidocaine	Low hepatic blood flow	Excess lidocaine effects	Reduce lidocaine dose
Metoprolol (M)	Verapamil (V)	V decreases M metabolism	Excess M effects	Reduce M dose
	Cimetidine (C)	C decreases M metabolism	Excess M effects	Reduce both drug doses
Labetalol (L)	Cimetidine (C)	C decreases L metabolism	Excess L and C effects	Reduce both drug doses
Carvedilol (CV)	Cimetidine (C)	C decreases CV metabolism	Excess CV effects	Reduce both drug doses
ANTIHYPERTENSIVE INTERACTIONS				
Beta blockers	Indomethacin (I), NSAIDs	I inhibits vasodilatory prostaglandins	Decreased antihypertensive effect	Omit indomethacin; use alternative drugs
IMMUNE-INTERACTING DRUGS				
Acebutolol	Other drugs altering immune status: procainamide, hydralazine, captopril	Theoretical risk of additive immune effects	Theoretical risk of lupus or neutropenia	Check antinuclear factors and neutrophils; low doses during cotherapy

ABBREVIATIONS: AV = atrioventricular; CHF = congestive heart failure; LV = left ventricular; SA = sinoatrial.

Verapamil and Prazosin

The combination of verapamil with prazosin for hypertension is additive.[39] A hepatic pharmacokinetic interaction with enhanced bioavailability of prazosin may explain this effect.[40,41]

Verapamil and Quinidine

Verapamil and quinidine may interact to cause excess hypotension,[42] either by combined inhibition of peripheral alpha receptors or by an increase in quinidine levels[43] owing to a hepatic interaction.

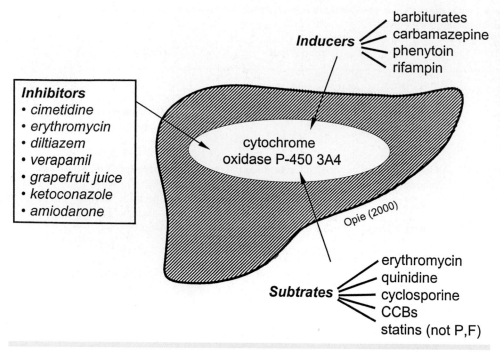

FIGURE 90-2 Potential hepatic pharmacokinetic interactions at the level of cytochrome oxidase P450 and potential pharmacodynamic interactions due to altered hepatic blood flow. (Figure copyrighted by LH Opie.)

Verapamil and Disopyramide

Both verapamil and disopyramide are powerful negative inotropes. Thus, the combination should be reserved for situations where left ventricular function is normal and can be closely monitored after initiation of therapy.

Verapamil and Theophylline

Verapamil may inhibit the hepatic metabolism of theophylline and thereby increase blood theophylline levels.[44]

Verapamil and Protease Inhibitors

Verapamil may decrease the hepatic metabolism of several HIV protease inhibitors and increase exposure to active drug. The significance of this interaction is unclear at this time.[24]

Nifedipine

The combination of nifedipine with beta blockade is generally well tolerated except for the risk of hypotension.[11] Nifedipine and propranolol may have a pharmacokinetic interaction whereby blood levels of propranolol increase; it is thought that nifedipine increases hepatic blood flow so that the hepatic breakdown of propranolol increases.[45] A pharmacokinetic and pharmacodynamic interaction exists with the combination of diltiazem and nifedipine, with diltiazem potentially raising nifedipine blood levels, leading to an increased risk of hypotension.[46] Although nifedipine is an afterload reducer, it also has a direct negative inotropic effect. Hence, its combination with beta blockers, disopyramide, or any other negative inotropic agent should occur with caution. Nifedipine in combination with prazosin hydrochloride may cause excess hypotension[47]; thus low initial additive doses are recommended.

Diltiazem

Diltiazem, like verapamil, may modestly (some studies report no change) increase blood digoxin levels. Diltiazem in combination with long-acting nitrates[18] or nifedipine[48] occasionally causes excess hypotension. The combination of high-dose diltiazem with beta blockade may cause bradycardia or hypotension.[49] Intravenous diltiazem can be expected to produce a spectrum of drug interactions comparable to those of intravenous verapamil. As diltiazem is metabolized by CYP3A4, it interacts with other similarly metabolized compounds (e.g., cyclosporine and cilostazol), increasing the blood levels of both drugs.[50,51] Blood levels of some statins increase with diltiazem (Table 90-2).

ANTIARRHYTHMIC AGENTS

During antiarrhythmic therapy, numerous and sometimes serious drug interactions are possible (Table 90-3).[52,53] Patients with serious ventricular arrhythmias often have underlying angina pectoris (potentially necessitating treatment with CCBs or beta blockers) or congestive heart failure (CHF) (requiring digitalis and diuretics). Gastroesophageal reflux, a common symptom in patients with chronic cardiac conditions, may require cimetidine, a drug with the potential for numerous hepatic interactions (Table 90-3). The most frequent antiarrhythmic drug interactions occur with digoxin (the levels of which increase with quinidine and verapamil), with diuretics (there is a risk of QT prolongation with antiarrhythmics, such as quinidine, disopyramide, amiodarone, and sotalol, which prolong duration of the action potential), and at the level of hepatic enzyme induction (cimetidine decreases hepatic metabolism of quinidine[54]; phenytoin and barbiturates have an opposite effect). There is also the risk of antiarrhythmic drug–drug interactions. Thus, amiodarone, when added to quinidine, enhances the risk of QT prolongation while quinidine levels increase, so that quinidine toxicity is also more likely.[53] The combination of antiarrhythmic drugs that depress SA node function, such as amiodarone, beta blockers or CCBs, can also lead to life-threatening bradycardia. Type I antiarrhythmic drugs should not be used with certain macrolide antibiotics (erythromycin) because both drugs can prolong the QT interval, precipitating torsades de pointes, especially in women.[55–57] Other drugs that prolong the QT interval are shown in Fig. 90-2.

Quinidine

Because quinidine increases blood digoxin levels, the dose of quinidine must be decreased and blood digoxin levels checked when these drugs are coadministered.[58] Quinidine may enhance the effects of other hypotensive agents, including verapamil,[42] or of agents inhibiting the sinus node (beta blockers, verapamil, diltiazem, and alpha methyldopa). Quinidine increases the effects of coumarin anticoagulants by a hepatic interaction.[59] When hepatic enzymes are induced

TABLE 90-2 Drug Interactions of Nitrates and Calcium Channel Blocking Agents

Cardiac Drug	Interacting Drugs	Mechanism	Consequences	Prophylaxis
HEMODYNAMIC INTERACTIONS				
All nitrates	Calcium antagonists	Excess vasodilation	Syncope, dizziness	Monitor blood pressure
	Prazosin (PZ)	Excess vasodilation	Syncope, dizziness	Check blood pressure, use low doses initially
	Sildenafil (S) (Viagra)[a]	Excess hypotension	Syncope, dizziness, myocardial infarction	Before giving nitrates for acute coronary syndrome, question for use of sildenafil in the preceding 24 h
	Alteplase (t-PA)	Decrease t-PA effect	Thrombolytic benefit less	Avoid or reduce nitrate dose, policy not clear
CALCIUM ANTAGONIST DRUGS				
Verapamil (V)	Beta blockers	SA and AV nodal inhibition; myocardial failure	Added nodal and negative inotropic effects	Careful observation, check ECG, blood pressure, and pulse rate
	Cimetidine	Hepatic metabolic interaction	Blood V increases	Adjust dose
	Digoxin (D)	Decreased D clearance	Risk of D toxicity	Reduce D dose by 50%; check D blood level
	Digitalis poisoning	Added SA and AV nodal inhibition	Asystole; complete heart block after IV D	Avoid IV D in digitalis poisoning
	Disopyramide	Pharmacodynamic	Hypotension, constipation	Check blood pressure, LV function, and gut
	Flecainide (F)	Added negative inotropic effect	Hypotension	Check left ventricular function and F levels
	Prazosin and other alpha blockers	Hepatic interaction	Hypotension	Check blood pressure during combined therapy
	Quinidine (Q)	Added alpha-receptor inhibition; V decreases Q clearance	Hypotension; increased Q levels	Check Q levels and blood pressure
	Theophylline (T)	Inhibition of hepatic metabolism	Increased T blood levels	Reduce T dose and check levels
Nifedipine (N)	Beta blockers	Additive negative inotropism	Hypotension	Check blood pressure and use a low initial dose
	Cimetidine	Hepatic metabolic interaction	Blood N levels increase	Reduce N dose by about 50%
	Digoxin (D)	Minor to modest changes in D	Increased D levels	Check D blood level
	Prazosin and other alpha blockers	Prazosin blocks alpha reflex to N	Postural hypotension	Low initial dose of prazosin of N
	Propranolol (P)	N and P have opposing effects on liver blood flow	N decreases P levels; increases N levels	Adjust P and N doses as needed
	Quinidine (Q)	N improves LV function; Q is cleared more rapidly	Decreased Q effect	Check Q levels
	Diltiazem	Hepatic metabolism of N inhibited	Hypotension	Adjust doses of N and diltiazem

(Continued)

TABLE 90-2 Drug Interactions of Nitrates and Calcium Channel Blocking Agents (*Continued*)

Cardiac Drug	Interacting Drugs	Mechanism	Consequences	Prophylaxis
Diltiazem	Beta blockers	Added SA nodal inhibition; negative inotropism	Bradycardia, hypotension	Monitor ECG and LV function
	Cimetidine	Hepatic metabolism interaction	Increased levels of diltiazem	Monitor ECG and LV function
	Cyclosporine (C)	Hepatic metabolism of C inhibited	Increased blood levels of C	Adjust C doses
	Digoxin (D)	Fall in D clearance	Relevant only in renal failure	Monitor D levels
	Flecainide (F)	Additive negative inotropic effect	Hypotension	Check LV function and monitor F levels
	Ciliostazol (Ci)	Hepatic metabolism of Ci inhibited	Increased Ci levels	Empirically decrease Ci dose
	Simvastain, lovastatin, and atorvastatin	Hepatic metabolism inhibited (less common with atorvastatin)	Increased levels	Decrease doses of respective statin
Nicardipine (see nifedipine)	Cyclosporine (C)	Hepatic metabolism of C inhibited	Increased blood C levels	Adjust C doses
	Digoxin (D)	Decreased D clearance	Doubling of D level	Decrease D dose and monitor levels

*a*Sildenafil is metabolized by the 3A4 isoform, so that inhibitors predispose to excess levels of the drug and to nitrate interaction.
ABBREVIATIONS: ECG = electrocardiogram; IV = intravenous; LV = left ventricular; T-PA = tissue plasminogen activator.

by drugs such as phenytoin, phenobarbital, and rifampin (rifampicin), the hepatic metabolism of quinidine may markedly increase, with a decrease in the steady-state concentrations of quinidine.[60,61] Conversely, cimetidine can inhibit hepatic enzymes and decrease the metabolism of quinidine with opposite effects. Ranitidine does not have similar effects.[62] Verapamil may increase quinidine levels. Conversely, nifedipine may lower plasma quinidine levels, probably by improving left ventricular systolic function.[63,64]

Hypokalemia decreases the antiarrhythmic effect of quinidine and predisposes to QT prolongation by quinidine. When quinidine is combined with other drugs that also prolong the QT interval, such as amiodarone, sotalol, or thiazide diuretics, careful monitoring of the QT interval is mandated.[65]

Quinidine is a vagolytic drug and lessens the effects of procedures that enhance vagal activity, such as carotid sinus massage. Quinidine also inhibits muscarinic receptors and reduces the effects of anticholinesterases in myasthenia gravis.

Procainamide

Procainamide (PA) and n-acetylprocainamide (NAPA) are organic cations extensively secreted by the renal organic cation secretory pathway. Cimetidine competes for their secretion and therefore decreases the renal clearance of PA. The ensuing increase in blood levels necessitates a reduction in the dose of PA.[66]

Disopyramide

Since disopyramide is a negative inotrope, there is the potential for its reducing cardiac output in patients already receiving other nega-

tive inotropes, such as the CCB verapamil,[67] beta blockers, or flecainide and in patients with preexisting systolic dysfunction. It is also potentially dangerous to combine disopyramide with drugs likely to depress nodal or conduction tissues, such as quinidine, digoxin, beta blockers, and alpha-methyldopa. Disopyramide is ineffective in digitalis toxicity and should be avoided. There is no interaction with disopyramide and lidocaine. The concomitant use of disopyramide with other type I antiarrhythmic agents or beta blockers should be reserved for life-threatening arrhythmias because of the increased risk of bradycardia and hypotension. The risk of QT prolongation requires that disopyramide not be combined with other drugs prolonging the QT interval, such as tricyclic antidepressants and antiarrhythmic agents such as amiodarone or sotalol. Hepatic enzyme inducers, such as phenytoin and rifampin, may lower plasma levels of disopyramide.[68] Pyridostigmine bromide may interact favorably with disopyramide by inhibiting cholinesterase activity, reducing its anticholinergic side effects.[69]

Lidocaine/Tocainide

In patients receiving cimetidine[70] or halothane,[71] the hepatic clearance of lidocaine is reduced and toxicity may occur more readily. Lidocaine may cause SA-nodal arrest, especially with coadministration of other agents that depress nodal function,[72] including beta blockers. There are no currently recognized drug interactions for tocainide.

Dofetilide and Ibutilide

Dofetilide is eliminated by both glomerular filtration and active secretion via the cation transport system. Amiloride and metformin

TABLE 90-3 Drug Interactions of Antiarrhythmic Drugs

Cardiac Drug	Interacting Drugs	Mechanism	Consequences	Prophylaxis
		CLASS 1 A		
Quinidine (Q)	Amiodarone	Added QT effects; blood Q levels rise	Torsades de pointes	Check QT intervals and K$^+$
	Antibiotics (some)	Quinidine inhibits muscarinic receptors	Increased antibiotic-induced muscular weakness	Clinical care, drug levels
	Anticholinesterases (AChE)	Quinidine inhibits muscarinic receptors	Decreased AChE efficacy in myasthenia gravis	Avoid Q if possible
	Antihypertensive agents Beta blockers	Added hypotensive and SA nodal effects	Hypotension, excess bradycardia	Check BP and ECG
	Cimetidine (C)	C inhibits oxidative metabolism of Q	Increased Q levels, risk of toxicity	Q levels, consider switch to ranitidine
	Warfarin, other coumarin anticoagulants	Hepatic interaction with Q	Bleeding	Check INR
	Digoxin (D)	Decrease D clearance; inhibition of P-glycoprotein	Risk of D toxicity	Check D levels
	Diltiazem	Added inhibition of SA node	Excess bradycardia	Check ECG, heart rate
	Disopyramide	Added QT prolongation	Torsades de pointes	Check QT intervals and K$^+$ levels
	K$^+$ losing diuretics	Hypokalemia and QT prolongation	Torsades de pointes	Check QT intervals and K$^+$ levels
	Hepatic enzyme inducers (phenytoin, barbiturates, rifampin)	Increased Q hepatic metabolism by CYP3A4	Decreased Q levels	Q levels, dose alteration
	Nifedipine	Increased Q clearance	Decreased Q levels	Q levels, doses
	Class III agents: sotalol, amiodarone, dofetilide, ibutilide	Added QT prolongation	Torsades de pointes	Check QT intervals and K$^+$ levels
	Verapamil	Decreased Q clearance	Excess bradycardia	Check ECG, Q levels
	Warfarin	Hepatic interaction with Q	Bleeding	Check INR
Procainamide (P)	Cimetidine	Decreased renal P clearance	Prolonged P half-life, excess P effect	Reduce P dose; consider ranitidine
Disopyramide (Dis)	Agents prolonging APD (quinidine, amiodarone, sotalol)	Added QT prolongation, especially if hypokalemia is present	Torsades de pointes	Check QT intervals and K$^+$ levels
	Beta blockers	Combined negative inotropism	Hypotension	Reduce doses
	Cimetidine	Hepatic Dis metabolism falls	Increased blood Dis levels	Reduce doses
	Digitalis toxicity	Added SA, AV nodal depression	SA, AV block	Avoid Dis in digitalis toxicity
	Hepatic enzyme inducers (phenytoin, rifampin, barbiturates)	Enhanced Dis hepatic metabolism	Blood Dis levels fall; readjust Dis dose	Readjust Dis dose
	Drugs inhibiting SA or AV nodes/conduction system (quinidine, beta blockers, methyldopa, digoxin)	Pharmacodynamic additive effects	SA, AV block; conduction block	Check ECG; decrease doses

(Continued)

TABLE 90-3 TABLE 90-3 Drug Interactions of Antiarrhythmic Drugs (*Continued*)

Cardiac Drug	Interacting Drugs	Mechanism	Consequences	Prophylaxis
	Pyridostigmine (Py)	Inhibition of cholinesterase activity	Beneficial effect of Py on Dis; harmful effect of Dis on P	In myasthenia gravis, avoid Dis
		CLASS 1B		
Lidocaine (L)	Verapamil, Diltiazem	Combined negative inotropism	Hypotension	Avoid IV diltiazem or verapamil cotherapy
	Cimetidine	Decreased hepatic metabolism	Increased L levels	Decrease L infusion rate
	Halothane	Decreased hepatic blood flow	Increased L levels	Decreased L infusion rate
	Propranolol	Decreased hepatic blood flow	Increased L levels	Decrease L infusion rate
	Other beta blockers	Decreased hepatic blood flow	Increased L levels	Decrease L infusion rate
Mexiletine (M)	Hepatic enzyme inducers (phenytoin, barbiturates, rifampin)	Increased hepatic metabolism	Decreased plasma M levels	Increase M dose
		CLASS 1C		
Flecainide (F)	Amiodarone	Unknown	Blood F rises, added effect on nodes, myocardium	Decrease F dose
	Digoxin (D)	Decreased D clearance	Blood D rises slightly	Check D level
	Drugs inhibiting SA or AV nodes, IV conduction or myocardial function	Pharmacodynamic additive effects	SA, AV block; conduction block, cardiogenic shock	Avoid combinations, decrease doses
	Cimetidine	Decreased hepatic metabolism	Blood F rises	Check F dose
Propafenone	Digoxin (D)	Pharmacokinetic, inhibition of P-glycoprotein	Increased D level	Decrease D dose
Moricizine (Mo)	Cimetidine	Decreased Mo metabolism	Blood Mo rises	Decrease Mo dose
		CLASS III		
Amiodarone (A)	Drugs prolonging QT interval (quinidine, disopyramide, phenothiazines, tricyclic antidepressants, thiazide diuretics, sotalol)	Additive effects on repolarization and QT interval	Torsades de pointes	Avoid low K$^+$; avoid combinations
	Quinidine (Q)	CYP2D6 inhibition	Blood Q rises	Check Q levels
	Procainamide (P)	Pharmacokinetic	Blood P rises	Check P dose
Sotalol, dofetilide, ibutilide	Procainamide	Hypokalemia plus class III action, as for amiodarone	Torsades de pointes	Avoid low K$^+$ situations; consider K$^+$ sparing diuretic
		CLASS IV		
Adenosine (Ad)	Disopyramide (Dis)	Dis inhibits breakdown of Ad	Excess nodal inhibition	Reduce Ad down to 25% or less
	Theophylline (T)	T blocks Ad receptor	Decrease Ad effect	Carefully adjust Ad dose upward

ABBREVIATIONS: APD = action potential duration; AV = atrioventricular; BP = blood pressure; ECG = electrocardiogram; INR = international normalized ratio; IV = intravenous; SA = sinoatrial.

also undergo renal cationic secretion. These drugs may compete with dofetilide for tubular secretion and should be used together cautiously. In addition, drugs known to directly prolong the QT interval and induce torsades de pointes (e.g., tricyclic antidepressants, antiarrhythmics, cisapride, erythromycin, and haloperidol) should be used carefully if at all when dofetilide or ibutilide are being given.[73]

Mexiletine

Narcotics delay the gastrointestinal absorption of mexiletine. Rifampin, barbiturates, and phenytoin all induce hepatic enzymes, reducing the plasma levels of mexiletine. The renal clearance of mexiletine decreases significantly with urinary alkalinization. Cimetidine inhibits the CYP2D6 hepatic isoform that breaks down mexiletine. It should, but does not, increase plasma levels of mexiletine.[74] Rather, cimetidine decreases the gastrointestinal symptoms associated with mexiletine. Disopyramide and mexiletine given together may predispose to a negative inotropic effect.[75] Mexiletine may, however, be combined with quinidine,[76–77] beta-adrenergic blockers,[78] and amiodarone[79] provided that the appropriate contraindications for each drug are observed and the patient is closely monitored for CHF.

Flecainide

Since flecainide inhibits sinus and AV-nodal function, its combination with beta blockers, verapamil, diltiazem, and digitalis can cause bradycardia and these combinations should be given carefully. Flecainide also has additive negative inotropic effects that may exaggerate those of beta blockers,[80] verapamil, or disopyramide. Combined inhibitory effects on His-Purkinje conduction may arise during cotherapy with quinidine or procainamide and to a lesser extent with disopyrarmide. Flecainide blood levels are increased by amiodarone; its dose should be decreased by about one-third when these drugs are used together.[81] Studies of healthy volunteers suggest that cimetidine delays the clearance of flecainide[82] and that flecainide increases blood digoxin levels by about 25 percent.[80]

Propafenone

Propafenone is a class IC antiarrhythmic drug; therefore it may interact adversely with other drugs, depressing nodal function, intraventricular conduction, or the inotropic state. Nonetheless, propafenone can be combined with quinidine or procainamide at reduced doses of both drugs.[74] Propafenone substantially increases serum digoxin levels likely related to a decrease in its nonrenal clearance.[83]

Amiodarone

The most serious interaction with amiodarone[65] is the potential for accentuating the proarrhythmic effect of other drugs that prolong the QT interval, such as class IA antiarrhythmic agents, sotalol, phenothiazines, tricyclic antidepressants, and thiazide diuretics. Amiodarone ordinarily does not depress the SA node, but it may do so when combined with beta blockers or CCBs such as verapamil or diltiazem.[23] In patients receiving warfarin, amiodarone further prolongs the INR; therefore close monitoring is required.[84] Amiodarone also significantly increases digoxin levels (Table 90-3).

Sotalol

Treatment with any agents that may cause hypokalemia (e.g., diuretics) or drugs that prolong the action potential duration (e.g., quinidine,

disopyramide, amiodarone, tricyclic antidepressants, or probucol) may precipitate torsades de pointes.[85]

Adenosine

Adenosine has an indirect cardiac effect, similar to that of the CCB antagonist verapamil by enhancing the flow of the current $I_{k(ACh)}$. Aminophylline or theophylline, by competing with adenosine for the receptor sites, completely inhibits the adenosine-induced effect on AV conduction. Dipyridamole, on the other hand, inhibits the breakdown of adenosine and/or its uptake into the tissues, so that the amount of adenosine available for the antiarrhythmic effect is increased.[12] Effective doses of adenosine in patients receiving prolonged dipyridamole therapy may only be one-quarter to one-eighth normal doses.

POSITIVE INOTROPIC AGENTS

Drug interactions of digitalis and other positive inotropic agents are shown in Table 90-4.

Digoxin

The quinidine–digoxin interaction is best described (Fig. 90-3). Quinidine approximately doubles blood digoxin levels by decreasing both renal and extrarenal clearance.[38,86–88] The prior dose of digoxin should generally be halved and the plasma digoxin rechecked. Quinine, the diastereomer of quinidine given for muscle cramps, acts in a similar fashion. Recent evidence indicates that quinidine inhibits digoxin transport across epithelial cell membranes (especially in the kidney) owing to its high affinity for p-glycoprotein on the ATP-dependent efflux pump encoded by the *mdrla* gene.[88,89]

The verapamil–digoxin interaction is equally significant; digoxin levels increase by 60 to 90 percent with this combination.[38] The other CCBs, nifedipine and diltiazem, increase digoxin levels much less than verapamil.[87,90,91] Adjustment of the digoxin dose with these latter agents is usually unnecessary. Nicardipine causes only a modest rise of digoxin levels.[92] Nitrendipine, however, resembles verapamil in that it approximately doubles the digoxin levels.[93] There are no simple rules that explain CCB effect on digoxin levels; thus careful clinical monitoring is indicated whenever a CCB is added to digoxin.

Among other vasodilators, prazosin increases digoxin levels in canine experimental studies by reducing its plasma and tissue binding.[94] Among antiarrhythmics other than quinidine or verapamil, amiodarone and propafenone[83] also elevate serum digoxin levels. Other antiarrhythmics, including procainamide and mexiletine, have no interaction with digoxin. There is a relatively small rise in digoxin levels with coadministration of flecainide.[80] When co-administered medications elevate digoxin levels, the features of digitalis toxicity may be agent-specific. With quinidine and digoxin, tachyarrhythmias become more likely; amiodarone and verapamil seem to suppress the ventricular arrhythmias of digitalis toxicity, making bradycardia and AV block more likely.[95]

Diuretics may indirectly precipitate digitalis toxicity by causing hypokalemia, which, when particularly severe (plasma $K^+ < 3$ meq/L), may reduce the tubular secretion of digoxin. K^+-sparing diuretics (amiloride, triamterene, and spironolactone)[96,97] as well as captopril decrease digoxin clearance by about 20 to 30 percent and may also elevate serum K^+ levels. However, spironolactone and its metabolite canrenone may decrease digitalis toxicity[97] as a result of an increase in K^+ levels derived from inhibition of aldosterone tubular

TABLE 90-4 Drug Interactions of Digitalis and Other Positive Inotropic Agents

Cardiac Drug	Interacting Drugs	Mechanism	Consequences	Prophylaxis
		POSITIVE INOTOROPIC AGENTS		
Digitoxin	Verapamil	Nonrenal clearance of digitoxin falls	Digitoxin levels up by one-third	Check and adjust digitoxin levels
	Other drugs interacting with digoxin	Altered digitoxin clearance (?)	Digitoxin levels increase (?)	Check and adjust digitoxin levels
Digoxin (D)	Amiodarone	Reduced renal clearance of D via inhibition of p-glycoprotein transport	D level may double	Check D level; reduce dose by 50%
	Captopril	Reduced D clearance	Blood D increases	Check and adjust D dose
	Diltiazem	Variable decrease of D clearance	Variable increase in blood D; bradycardia or heart block	Check and adjust D level
	Diuretics; potassium-sparing amiloride, triamterene,	Reduced extrarenal D clearance	D levels up by 20%	Check and adjust D level
	spironolactone (S)	S reduces renal D clearance and S may falsely elevate D levels by assay interference	D levels may increase	Complex effects; check and adjust D levels but do so monitoring for D toxicity symptoms
	Nifedipine	Variable fall of D clearance	Variable rise in D levels	Check and adjust D level
	Nitrendipine	Reduced D clearance	Blood D doubles	Check D level; reduce dose by 50%
	Prazosin (PZ)	PZ displaces D from binding sites; mechanism not clear in humans	Blood D rises	Check D level; reduce dose empirically based on level
	Propafenone	Not defined	D level increases	Check and adjust D level
	Quinidine, quinine	Reduced D clearance	Blood D doubles	Check D level; reduce dose by 50%
	Verapamil	Reduced D clearance	Blood D doubles or more; bradycardia or heart block	Check D level; reduce dose by 50%
		SYMPATHOMIMETIC INOTROPES		
Dobutamine, Inamrinone, Milrinone	Thiazide or loop diuretics	Additive hypokalemic effects	Increased risk of arrhythmias	Monitor blood potassium values
Dopamine	MAO inhibitors	Decreased metabolism of dopamine	Increase in the vasopressor effect of dopamine	Reduce dopamine dose by 90%
	Ergot derivatives	Additive vasoconstrictor effect	Limb ischemia	Avoid combination use

effect. Nonetheless, the combination of digoxin-quinidine-spironolactone has been reported to markedly elevate digoxin levels.[98]

The gastrointestinal absorption of digoxin may be decreased by cholestyramine, probably because of adsorption of digoxin to the resin; digoxin should therefore be given several hours before the resin,

or else digoxin capsules may be used (Lanoxicaps; 0.2 mg = 0.25 mg of digoxin). Digoxin capsules also decrease the interaction with kaolin pectate and acarbose,[99] which reduce digoxin absorption, and with erythromycin and tetracycline, which suppress gastrointestinal flora that otherwise inactivate digoxin and thereby increase digoxin blood levels. Cancer chemotherapeutic agents may damage intestinal mucosa and depress digoxin absorption. NSAIDs decrease the renal clearance of digoxin, thereby increasing plasma digoxin levels. Rifampin and phenobarbital, through hepatic enzyme induction and/or an increase in intestinal p-glycoprotein, can reduce plasma digoxin levels.[90]

SYMPATHOMIMETIC AGENTS

Dopamine

Dopamine is metabolized by monoamine oxidase (MAO), and dopamine effects will be prolonged in patients receiving MAO inhibitors. The interaction can result in severe hypertension and/or cardiac arrhythmias. No more than one-tenth of the usual dose of dopamine should be given to patients receiving MAO inhibitors. Dopamine and ergot derivatives should not be coadministered, as this leads to the more frequent occurrence of peripheral ischemia and gangrene of hands and feet. Dopamine is also contraindicated during the use of cyclopropane or halogenated hydrocarbon anesthetics (enhanced risk of arrhythmias). The glomerular filtration rate (GFR) may increase when dopamine corrects systemic hypotension, which may be associated with an increased clearance of renally cleared drugs.

Dobutamine

Dobutamine decreases plasma potassium (K^+) levels, which in part relates to its effecting a transcellular shift of K^+. It should be used cautiously with diuretics if significant diuretic-related hypokalemia is expected.

PHOSPHODIESTERASE INHIBITORS

Inamrinone and Milrinone

Inamrinone and milrinone are phosphodiesterase inhibitors that can provoke arrhythmias. During diuretic therapy, plasma K^+ should be monitored. Although the digoxin level does not increase when these drugs are combined with digitalis, digoxin toxicity is possible in the context of the proarrhythmic effects of these compounds. Dosage adjustments with inamrinone and milrinone may become necessary for patients with renal failure in that these compounds undergo significant renal clearance.

DIURETICS

Drug interactions with diuretics are summarized in Table 90-5.

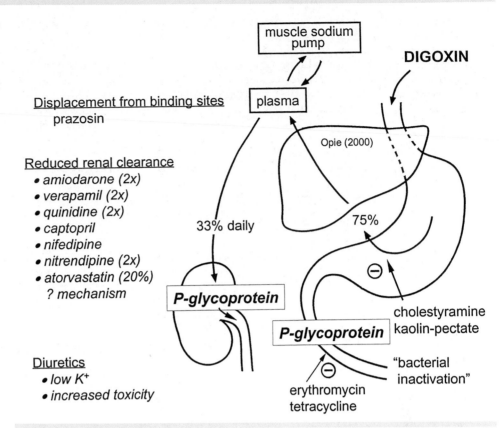

Displacement from binding sites
prazosin

Reduced renal clearance
- *amiodarone (2x)*
- *verapamil (2x)*
- *quinidine (2x)*
- *captopril*
- *nifedipine*
- *nitrendipine (2x)*
- *atorvastatin (20%)*
  ? mechanism

Diuretics
- *low K^+*
- *increased toxicity*

FIGURE 90-3 Potential site of digoxin interactions. Note the importance of reduced renal clearance; 2× means that an approximate doubling of digoxin blood levels has been reported. (Figure copyrighted by LH Opie.)

Loop Diuretics

Hypokalemia and/or hypomagnesemia, which can occur when loop diuretics are given, may precipitate digitalis toxicity. Finally, NSAIDs attenuate the diuretic effect of loop diuretics and therefore may increase the likelihood of exacerbating CHF.[100,101]

An interesting and complex set of interactions between furosemide and captopril has emerged. On the one hand, captopril decreases the tubular delivery of furosemide, which is a prerequisite for furosemide's effect. This may explain why captopril reduces furosemide-induced natriuresis to less than half.[102] This effect of captopril in altering furosemide excretion seems not to be shared by other angiotensin-converting enzyme (ACE) inhibitors.[103] There is also an important pharmacodynamic interaction between captopril and furosemide. When captopril is given in a standard dose of 25 mg, furosemide has little or no diuretic effect, whereas a 1 mg dose of captopril enhances the diuretic effect of furosemide.[104] The proposed mechanism is that the very low dose of captopril does not completely suppress the production of angiotensin II. This allows sufficient circulating angiotensin II to maintain some efferent arteriolar tone and thereby to preserve GFR, which is a necessary element for diuretic effect. Both of these interactions, therefore, argue for captopril to be given in low doses with furosemide if a volume endpoint is the therapeutic goal.

In patients with hyponatremic CHF, which is an indirect indicator of a high-renin state, ACE inhibitor monotherapy is often therapeutically ineffective in correcting the hyponatremia; however, the addition of a loop diuretic will produce a hypotonic diuresis and correct the sodium abnormality.[105] Quite apart from the complex interactions described above, it is generally regarded as a wise precaution to

TABLE 90-5 Drug Interactions of Diuretics

Cardiac Drug	Interacting Drugs	Mechanism	Consequences	Treatment
Loop and thiazide diuretics	Indomethacin and other NSAIDs and likely COXIBs	Pharmacodynamic	Decreased antihypertensive and diuretic effect	Increase the diuretic dose or change the timing of its administration to be more distant from that of the NSAID or COXIB
	Probenecid	Decreased tubular delivery of diuretic	Decreased diuretic effect	Increase diuretic dose or dose frequency
	ACE inhibitors	Excess diuresis, renin axis activation	Excess hypotension; prerenal azotemia	Temper diuresis, liberalize sodium intake, reduce the ACE inhibitor dose or temporarily discontinue its use
Furosemide (F)	Captopril	Possible interference with tubular secretion of F; potential for added efferent arteriolar vasodilatation	Loss of diuretic efficacy of F; decreased glomerular filtration rate	Reduce dose of captopril or consider a renally and hepatically cleared ACE inhibitor or increase furosemide dose
K^+-retaining diuretics	ACE inhibitors and ARBs	Additive K^+ retention	Hyperkalemia	Monitor K^+ levels

ABBREVIATIONS: ACE = angiotensin-converting enzyme; ARBs = angiotensin-receptor blockers; AII = angiotensin II; COXIB = cyclooxygenase inhibitor; NSAID = nonsteroidal anti-inflammatory drug.

reduce the diuretic dose of patients with CHF before addition of an ACE inhibitor. The aim of this procedure is to lessen excessive first-dose hypotension, which is commonly observed in the CHF patient who has been overdiuresed.[106]

Thiazide Diuretics

NSAIDs may attenuate the antihypertensive effect of thiazide-type diuretics.[107] Diuretic-induced hypokalemia or hypomagnesemia may predispose to ventricular arrhythmias, including torsades de pointes; when that happens, an antiarrhythmic agent—such as a class III agent (including sotalol, dofetilide, ibutilide, and probably to a lesser extent amiodarone) as well as a class Ia agent, (such as quinidine or disopyramide)—is usually administered.[11] This phenomenon is more frequent in females.[108]

Diuretics may reduce the renal clearance of lithium, particularly if the patient so treated becomes volume-contracted (and experiences a fall in GFR); therein lies the increased risk of lithium toxicity in diuretic-treated patients.[109] Diuretic-related hyponatremia is more common with thiazide diuretics, particularly in elderly women.[110]

Spironolactone and Other Potassium-Sparing Diuretics

Several medications can precipitate hyperkalemia when administered to patients with underlying renal insufficiency or other disturbances in K^+ homeostasis, such as congestive heart failure. ACE inhibitors and angiotensin receptor blockers (ARB)s are two such medications that promote K^+ retention, particularly if combined with K^+-sparing diuretics, as was often the case in the Randomized Aldactone Evaluation Study (RALES) study and the Eplerenone Post-Acute Myocardial Infarction Heart Failure Efficacy and Survival Study (EPHESUS).[111,112] In RALES, serious hyperkalemia ($K^+ > 6.0$ meq/L) occurred in 14 (2 percent) of patients treated with spironolactone (dose range 25 to 50 mg/day) and in 10 subjects

(1 percent) treated with placebo. This trial excluded patients with serum creatinine values of > 2.5 mg/dL and serum K^+ values of 5.0 meq/L.[111] The same exclusion criteria were applied in the recently completed EPHESUS study, where serious hyperkalemia ($K^+ > 6.0$ meq/L) occurred in 5.5 and 3.9 percent of eplerenone and placebo-treated patients respectively.[112] Other compounds that may increase the chance of developing hyperkalemia in ACE- or ARB-treated patients include trimethoprim and heparin (decreased renal excretion of K^+) or beta blockers (decreased cellular entry).[113]

VASODILATORS

Drug interactions with vasodilators, ACE inhibitors, and ARBs are listed in Table 90-6.

Nitroprusside and Hydralazine

Nitroprusside and hydralazine may increase the renal elimination of digoxin in CHF and thereby decrease digoxin levels as the result of improved left ventricular function and an increase in effective renal plasma flow.[114] By creating hepatic shunts, hydralazine may also increase the oral bioavailability and thereby the blood levels of hepatically cleared beta blockers such as propranolol, oxprenolol, and metoprolol.[115] This occurs more frequently in a fasting state and does not occur with sustained-release beta blockers. In patients with systolic CHF, the use of oral hydralazine together with nitrates prevents early development of nitrate tolerance and results in a persistent nitrate-mediated hemodynamic effect on systemic, pulmonary artery, and left ventricular filling pressures.[21]

Prazosin, Doxazosin, and Terazosin

There is an interaction between prazosin and the calcium antagonists verapamil and nifedipine resulting in excessive hypotension. In the

TABLE 90-6 Drug Interactions of Vasodilators, Angiotensin-Converting Enzyme Inhibitors, and Angiotensin II Receptor Blockers

Cardiac Drug	Interacting Drugs	Mechanism	Consequences	Prophylaxis
		VASODILATORS		
Hydralazine	Beta blockers (BB) hepatically metabolized	Hepatic shunting	BB metabolism ↓ Blood levels ↑	Propranolol, metoprolol dose ↓
Hydralazine	Nitrates (N)	Renal blood flow ↑, added vasodilation; free radicals scavenged	Less N tolerance; risk of excessive hypotension	Possibility of serious interaction with Viagra
Hydralazine/ nitroprusside	Digoxin (D)	Increased renal D excretion	Decreased D levels	Check D levels
Prazosin (P) and other α-blockers	Nifedipine (Nif)	Pharmacodynamic	Excess hypotension	Start with low dose of the α-blocker or dihydropyridine CCB
	Nitrates	Pharmacodynamic	Syncope, hypotension	Decrease P dose
	Verapamil	Hepatic metabolism	Synergistic antihypertensive effect	Adjust doses
Cilostazol (C)	Inhibitors of CYP450 3A4: diltiazem, verapamil, cyclosporine	↓ hepatic metabolism	Increased C levels, risk of increased mortality in heart failure	Reduce the dose of C or avoid entirely
		ANGIOTENSIN-CONVERTING ENZYME (ACE) INHIBITORS		
ACE inhibitor (class effect)	Diuretics	High renin levels in overdiuresed patients	"First dose" hypotension; risk of renal failure	Reduce diuretic dose; correct volume depletion
ACE inhibitor (class effect)	Potassium-sparing diuretics	Additional potassium retention	Hyperkalemia	Avoid combination or combine with care
ACE inhibitor (class effect)	Indomethacin	Less vasodilation	Less BP ↓; less antifailure effects	Avoid if possible
ACE inhibitor (class effect?)	Aspirin	Less vasodilation	Less antifailure effects	Low-dose aspirin
Captopril	Loop diuretic	Possible interference with tubular secretion	Lessened diuretic effect of furosemide	Consider alternate ACE inhibitor
Captopril	Immunosuppressive drugs, procainamide, hydralazine, possibly acebutolol	Added immune effects	Increased risk of neutropenia	Avoid combination; check neutrophil count
	Probenecid (P)	P inhibits tubular secretion of captopril	Small rise in captopril levels	Decrease dose of captopril according to blood pressure response
		ANGIOTENSIN II RECEPTOR BLOCKERS (ARBs)		
ARBs (class effect)	Diuretics	High renin levels in overdiuresed patients	First-dose hypotension, risk of renal failure	Reduce diuretic dose; correct volume depletion
	Potassium-sparing diuretics	Additional potassium retention	Hyperkalemia	Avoid combination or combine with care

case of verapamil, part of the effect may be explained by verapamil, a known inhibitor of cytochrome P450, increasing the bloods levels of prazosin when it is coadministered. In beta blocker–treated patients, the first dose hypotensive response to an alpha$_1$-adrenergic blocking drug may be exaggerated, particularly with prazosin. Both nitrates and prazosin may cause syncope, and these agents should be combined with care. Experimentally, prazosin may increase the plasma digoxin level. Similar interactions may hold for the other agents in this group.

ANGIOTENSIN-CONVERTING ENZYME INHIBITORS

Several class-specific drug interactions occur with drugs in this class (Table 90-6). For example, the concurrent administration of lithium with an ACE inhibitor is associated with a greater likelihood of lithium toxicity.[116] K$^+$ supplements or K$^+$-sparing diuretics when given with an ACE inhibitor increase the probability of developing hyperkalemia. NSAIDs such as indomethacin reduce the antihypertensive effect of ACE inhibitors.[117] NSAIDs also attenuate the natriuretic response seen with ACE inhibitors. Finally, both ACE inhibitors and NSAIDs can lead to functional renal insufficiency, particularly in those taking diuretics. This combination of drugs should be administered with extreme care to highly vulnerable patients, such as the elderly.[118]

The issue of whether aspirin attenuates the effects of an ACE inhibitor in hypertension and/or CHF has been a matter of some controversy.[119] To whatever extent the improvement in symptoms and survival rendered by treatment with ACE inhibitors is attributable to their effects on the circulation and the kidneys, this benefit can be rescinded by concomitant administration of aspirin.[120] There is a wealth of data suggesting an important interaction between aspirin and ACE inhibitors in patients with chronic stable CVR disease. An interaction is biologically plausible because there is considerable evidence that ACE inhibitors exert important effects through increasing the production of vasodilator prostaglandins, whereas aspirin blocks their production through the inhibition of cyclooxygenase, even at low doses. There is some evidence that low-dose aspirin may also increase systolic and diastolic blood pressure. There is also considerable evidence that aspirin may entirely neutralize the clinical benefits of ACE in patients with CHF, possibly by blocking endogenous vasodilator prostaglandin production and/or by enhancing the vasoconstrictor potential of endothelin. In patients requiring treatment for CHF, aspirin should be avoided if possible and the integrity of prostaglandin metabolism respected; the more severe the CHF, the more compelling the argument. As an alternative in these patients, antiplatelet therapy should be considered with agents that do not block the cyclooxygenase system.[121]

Finally, combining an ACE inhibitor with allopurinol is associated with a higher risk of hypersensitivity reactions, with several reports of the Stevens-Johnson syndrome due to the combination of captopril and allopurinol having been described.[122] Quinapril reduces the absorption of tetracycline by ≈ 35 percent, which may be due to the high magnesium content of quinapril tablets.

ANGIOTENSIN II RECEPTOR BLOCKERS

Losartan (CYP2C9 and CYP3A4) and irbesartan (CYP2C9) are metabolized by the P450 system. To date, a clinical relevant drug–drug interaction has not been observed with either compound when given with inhibitors or suppressors of the P450 system.[123] Blood pressure may fall precipitously when these drugs are given to individuals having been excessively diuresed or with high-renin hypertension. Hyperkalemia can occur with ARB therapy—particularly in patients with renal failure and/or diabetes—though this occurs less commonly than is the case with ACE inhibitors.[124] There is a 49 percent increase in digoxin peak plasma concentration and a 20 percent increase in trough digoxin concentration when digoxin is coadministered with telmisartan. The mechanism is unknown; however, it is not thought to be related to the CYP450 system (Table 90-6).[125]

ANTITHROMBOTIC AND THROMBOLYTIC AGENTS

Table 90-7 summarizes the drug interactions of antithrombotic agents.

Aspirin

Since blood levels of uric acid may be increased by both aspirin and thiazide diuretics, special care is required with their use in patients with a history of gout.[126] Conversely, aspirin may decrease the uricosuric effect of sulfinpyrazone and probenecid. Aspirin is not dissimilar to NSAIDs in that each can reduce vasodilator prostaglandin production (Fig. 90-4). Thus, aspirin can diminish the natriuretic effect of spironolactone (and other diuretics) as well as reduce the efficacy (and possibly the mortality benefits) of ACE inhibitors in CHF. Aspirin-induced gastrointestinal bleeding may be a greater hazard in patients receiving other NSAIDs and/or corticosteroid therapy. Antacids, by altering the pH of the stomach, may decrease the efficacy of enteric-coated aspirin preparations and, by alkalinizing the urine, increase the renal excretion of aspirin. CYP450 inducers (e.g., barbiturates, phenytoin, and rifampin) increase aspirin breakdown. Aspirin can cause hypoglycemia in patients receiving oral hypoglycemics and/or insulin. Aspirin, especially in high doses, may make evident a bleeding tendency and worsen anticoagulant-induced bleeding.[127] In bypass surgery patients, the dipyridamole-warfarin combination causes less bleeding than the aspirin-warfarin combination.[128] All aspirin-related drug interactions should be less intense if the doses are kept low, as is the current trend.

Sulfinpyrazone

Sulfinpyrazone increases the effects of warfarin primarily by inhibiting the cytochrome P450-mediated oxidation of (S)-warfarin, the biologically more potent enantiomer. The increased clearance of (R)-warfarin with sulfinpyrazone results not from induction but from its selective displacement from plasma protein binding sites. Like aspirin, sulfinpyrazone may increase the likelihood of hypoglycemia in patients given sulfonylureas. In addition, the use of sulfinpyrazone has been demonstrated to decrease the renal excretion of aspirin.

Dipyridamole

Dipyridamole is a potent vasodilator. Thus, care is required when it is used in combination with other vasodilators. Caffeine reduces the CVR responses to intravenous dipyridamole in a dose-dependent fashion. Dipyridamole use can be accompanied by bronchospasm, bradycardia, and occasionally asystole. Note the interaction with adenosine, as discussed above.

TABLE 90-7 Drug Interactions of Antithrombotic Agents

Cardiac Drug	Interacting Drugs	Mechanism	Consequences	Prophylaxis
Aspirin (A)	ACE inhibitors	Vasodilation ↓	Less antifailure effect	Low A dose
	Hepatic enzyme inducers (barbiturates, phenytoin, rifampin)	Increased A metabolism	Decreased A effect	Adjust A dose; check A side effects
	Sulfinpyrazone (S), Probenecid (P)	A decreases urate excretion at low doses (< 3 g/day)	Decreased uricosuric effect of S or P	Increase dose of S or P or switch to alternative therapy such as allopurinol
	Thiazide diuretics	A decreases urate excretion by competition for urate secretion	Hyperuricemia	Check blood urate values; no specific treatment for values < 12 mg/dL
	Warfarin (W)	A is antithrombotic	Excess bleeding	Check INR periodically
Sulfinpyrazone (S)	Warfarin	S displaces W from plasma proteins	Excess bleeding	Check INR periodically
POTENTIATING DRUGS				
Warfarin (W)	Allopurinol	Mechanism unknown	Excess bleeding	Check INR periodically
	Amiodarone	Mechanism unknown	Sensitizes to W for months	Avoid combination when possible
	Aspirin	Added bleeding tendency	Excess bleeding	Check INR intermittently
	Cimetidine	Decreased W degradation	Excess bleeding	Check INR intermittently
	Quinidine	Hepatic interaction	Excess bleeding	Check INR intermittently
	Statins	Hepatic interaction?	Excess bleeding	Check INR
	Sulfinpyrazone	Displaces W from plasma proteins	Excess bleeding	Check INR or prothrombin
INHIBITORY DRUGS				
	Cholestyramine, colestipol	Decrease absorption of W	Decreased W effect	Check INR or prothrombin
Alteplase, t-PA	Nitrates	Decreased t-PA effect	Less thrombolytic benefit	Avoid or reduce nitrate dose;? Increase t-PA dose

ABBREVIATIONS: INR = international normalized ratio; t-PA = tissue plasminogen activator.

Ticlopidine

Ticlopidine is an antiplatelet agent that interferes with ATP-induced platelet aggregation and, unlike aspirin, does not appear to interfere with the vasodilating activity of ACE inhibitors.[119] Ticlopidine is a potent inhibitor of CYP2D6 and CYP2C19 and can be associated with toxicity when coadministered with phenytoin—a compound metabolized by CYP2C19. Ticlopidine has been associated with the development of aplastic anemia and thrombotic thrombocytopenic purpura. Ticlopidine should be discontinued if the absolute neutrophil count falls below 1200/mm^3 or if the platelet count falls below 80,000/mm^3. Clopidogrel, an antiplatelet drug, is activated by hepatic cytochrome P450 (CYP) 3A4 and is responsible for variable platelet inhibitor when given with other substances that promote CYP3A4.[119a]

Warfarin

Warfarin may be subject to many (up to 80) drug interactions.[12] Furthermore, there is a *diet-drug* interaction for warfarin. Warfarin's effects are lessened by a diet rich in vitamin K, as found in dark green vegetables and certain plant oils. A good rule with warfarin therapy is to maintain a constant diet to minimize fluctuations in the international normalized ratio (INR). The safest rule is to tell patients receiving oral anticoagulation not to use any new or over-the-counter drugs without consultation and for the physician to carefully check out any added compounds. More frequent measurements of the INR time and dose adjustments are required when potentially interfering drugs, including herbal agents, are added.

The major known sites of interaction are, first, the plasma proteins to which warfarin is bound and second the cytochrome P450 CYP2C9 isozyme, which is responsible for warfarin breakdown. *Interfering* drugs include those that reduce absorption of vitamin K or warfarin, such as cholestyramine.[12] Sulfinpyrazone increases warfarin levels by displacing it from plasma proteins. Other interfering drugs are those that induce hepatic enzymes, which then increase the rate of warfarin metabolism. Yet other *potentiating* drugs decrease the hepatic degradation of warfarin to increase the anticoagulant effect, including antibiotics such as metronidazole (Flagyl) and cotrimoxazole (Bactrim). Cimetidine likewise inhibits hepatic degradation; ranitidine does not. Other potentiating cardiovascular agents are allopurinol, clofibrate, quinidine, statins, and amiodarone.[12,129]

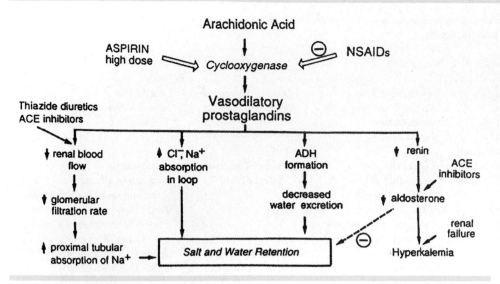

FIGURE 90-4 Possible mechanism whereby nonsteroidal anti-inflammatory drugs (NSAIDs), including aspirin, block the cyclooxygenase pathway and thereby inhibit the formation of vasodilatory prostaglandins. The resultant salt and water retention may decrease the effects of almost all antihypertensives, including angiotensin-converting enzyme inhibitors. In addition, NSAIDs decrease renin and aldosterone through an entirely different mechanism, which would tend to lessen salt and water retention. (Adapted from Houston MC. Nonsteroidal anti-inflammatory drugs and antihypertensives. *Am J Med* 1991;90(suppl 5A):42S–47S. Reproduced with permission from the publisher and authors.)

Amiodarone is especially dangerous because of its excessively long half-life, such that the interaction can occur even upon discontinuation of this compound. Grapefruit juice, which works on CYP3A4 (and not CYP2C9), does not potentiate the action of warfarin. Heparin or aspirin may potentiate bleeding with warfarin, although there are large interindividual variations.[130] Very high doses of aspirin can impair the synthesis of clotting factors. It must be reemphasized that sulfinpyrazone has a powerful effect in displacing warfarin from blood proteins; thus the required dose of warfarin may be as low as 1 mg.

Heparins

Physically, heparin (including the low-molecular-weight heparins) is incompatible with certain substances in an aqueous solution, including antibiotics, antihistamines, phenothiazines, hydrocortisone, and reteplase. Direct pharmacokinetic or pharmacodynamic drug interactions have not been described for heparins except for a controversial interaction with nitrates.[131]

Tissue-Type Plasminogen Activator

Concurrent use of intravenous nitroglycerin diminishes the efficacy of recombinant tissue-type plasminogen activator (t-PA, or alteplase); possibly because of increased hepatic blood flow and an enhanced catabolism of t-PA as well as enhanced in vitro degradation.[132,133]

LIPID-LOWERING AGENTS

Interactions with Warfarin

A number of lipid-lowering agents may interact with warfarin, either by decreasing absorption (cholestyramine) or by interference with metabolism (clofibrate, benzafibrate, fenofibrate, or gemfibrozil). No interactions occur with niacin, colesevalem, or ezitimibe.

The package inserts for gemfibrozil and fenofibrate both give prominent warnings that the warfarin dose should be reduced and the prothrombin time determined more frequently when these drugs are coadministered.[134] In general, there appear to be less potential for interaction between statins and warfarin than is the case for fibrates and warfarin.

Other Interactions

There are few serious interactions with lipid-lowering agents (Table 90-8). As a group, these drugs are well tolerated apart from two uncommon but potentially serious adverse effects: elevation of liver enzymes and skeletal muscle abnormalities, which range from benign myalgias to life-threatening rhabdomyolysis. Adverse effects with statins are frequently associated with drug interactions; the recent withdrawal of cerivastatin as a result of numerous deaths from rhabdomyolysis illustrates the clinical importance of such interactions.[135]

Drug interactions involving the statins may have either a pharmacodynamic or pharmacokinetic basis or both. The CYP450 enzyme system plays an important part in the metabolism of the statins, leading to clinically relevant interactions with other agents, particularly cyclosporine, erythromycin, itraconazole, ketoconazole, and HIV protease inhibitors, which are also metabolized by this system. The CYP3A family metabolizes lovastatin, simvastatin, atorvastatin, and rosuvastatin, whereas CYP2C9 metabolizes fluvastatin. Pravastatin is not significantly metabolized by the CYP450 system.[135] In addition, the statins are substrates for P-glycoprotein, a drug transporter present in the small intestine that may influence their oral bioavailability. In clinical practice, the risk of a serious interaction causing myopathy is enhanced when statin metabolism is markedly inhibited. Thus, rhabdomyolysis has occurred following the coadministration of cyclosporine, a potent CYP3A4 and P-glycoprotein inhibitor, and lovastatin. Verapamil and itraconazole have been shown to increase the exposure to simvastatin.[136] Pharmacodynamically, there is an increased risk of myopathy when statins are coprescribed with fibrates or nicotinic acid.[137] This occurs relatively infrequently, but is particularly associated with the combination of cerivastatin and gemfibrozil.[135,138] In clinical practice, the advantage of better lipid control with combined therapy seems to outweigh these risks. Serum creatine kinase levels should be checked periodically, especially after increasing doses or after starting combination therapy.

ANTIHYPERTENSIVE DRUGS

Interactions for diuretics, beta-adrenergic blockers, CCBs, ACE inhibitors, ARBs, and alpha₁-adrenergic blockers have already been considered. In general, NSAIDs (aspirin is not prone to cause the same interaction) and COXIBs reduce the blood pressure–lowering effect of most antihypertensives with the possible exception of CCBs.[139–142] When CCBs are employed as antihypertensives, part of their effect derives from natriuresis; thus, when a diuretic is added to a CCB, the ensuing reduction in blood pressure is more modest.[143]

TABLE 90-8 Drug Interactions of Lipid-Lowering Agents

Cardiac Drug	Interacting Drugs	Mechanism	Consequence	Prophylaxis
Fibric acids (gemfibrozil, clofibrate, benzafibrate, fenofibrate)	Warfarin; statins (see below)	Hepatic interference	Risk of bleeding	Check prothrombin time
Bile acid sequestrants (cholestyramine, colestipol)	Warfarin (W); many other drugs	Decreased absorption	Decreased W effect	Check prothrombin time; space doses
HMG-CoA reductase inhibitors (statins) (lovastatin, simvastatin, pravastatin), atorvastatin, fluvastatin)	Fibrates, inhibitors of CYP3A4 (erythromycin, antifungal azoles and others) nicotinic acid, niacin, cyclosporine	Increased likelihood of muscle damage and myositis	Rhabdomyolysis and risk of renal failure; increased cyclosporine levels	Check creatinine phosphokinase levels; avoid whenever possible
Statins	Warfarin	Hepatic interaction	Increased risk of bleeding	Check INR or prothrombin time
Pravastatin	Cyclosporine	Hepatic interaction; cyclosporine hepatotoxicity	Rhabdomyolysis and risk of renal failure; increased cyclosporine levels	Check creatine phosphokinase levels; avoid if possible

HERBAL MEDICINES

Herbal supplements are commonly used by patients for various cardiac conditions and are often taken without the treating physician's knowledge.[144,145] Many herbs are cardiotoxic or can interact unfavorably with known cardiac drugs, although the true risks of these interactions and effects are difficult to characterize owing to the limited number and nature of existing reports. Moreover, an herb that may be safe in small doses may become dangerous at higher doses. The risk of overdose is higher with herbal preparations than with conventional medications because of the variability in the content of these products.

Chamomile has antispasmodic actions and warfarin-like effects. Feverfew, garlic, *Gingko,* ginger, and ginseng may alter bleeding time and can pose safety risks in patients taking warfarin. *Gingko* and ginseng should be avoided in patients receiving warfarin and heparin. Dong quai contains coumarin and thereby increases the risk of bleeding.[146] Gossypol and licorice are associated with renal loss of K^+ and should not be used with thiazides/loop diuretics or digoxin. Plantain, kyushin, licorice, uzara root, ginseng, and hawthorn berries can mimic digitalis or potentiate digitalis toxicity.

Kelp can interfere with the antiarrhythmic effects of amiodarone. St. John's wort can lower serum digoxin levels by reducing digoxin absorption, possibly by inducing p-glycoprotein in the gut.[5,147] St. John's wort induces a variety of P450 isozymes (CYP3A4, CYP2C9, and CYP1A2) and thereby also increases metabolism of compounds such as warfarin, cyclosporine, and oral contraceptives.[148] The degree of induction is unpredictable due to factors such as the variable quality and quantity of constituent(s) in St. John's wort preparations.

References

1. Doucet J, Chassagne P, Trivalle C, et al. Drug-drug interactions related to hospital admissions in older adults: A prospective study of 1000 patients. *J Am Geriatr Soc* 1996;44:944–948.
2. Lacombe PS, Garcia Vicente JA, Costa Pagès J, Morselli PL. Causes and problems of nonresponse or poor response to drugs. *Drugs* 1996; 51:552–570.
3. Michalets EL. Update: Clinically significant cytochrome P-450 drug interactions. *Pharmacotherapy* 1998;18:84–112.
4. Cheng JWM. Cytochrome P450 mediated cardiovascular drug interactions. *Heart Dis* 2000;2:254–258.
5. Yu DK. The contribution of p-glycoprotein to pharmacokinetic drug-drug interactions. *J Clin Pharmacol* 1999;39:1203–1211.
6. Tran C, Knowles SR, Liu BA, Shear NH. Gender differences in adverse drug reactions. *J Clin Pharmacol* 1998;38:1003–1009.
7. Sokol SI, Cheng-Lai A, Frishman WH, Kaza CS. Cardiovascular drug therapy in patients with hepatic diseases and patients with congestive heart failure. *J Clin Pharmacol* 2000;40:11–30.
8. Be alert for interactions between prescription and OTC drugs. *Drugs Ther Perspect* 1996;7:12–14.
9. Huang J-D, Chuang S-K, Cheng C-L, Lai M-L. Pharmacokinetics of metoprolol enantiomers in Chinese subjects of major CYP2D6 genotypes. *Clin Pharmacol Ther* 1999;65:402–407.
10. Strayhorn VA, Baciewicz AM, Self TH. Update on rifampin drug interactions: III. *Arch Intern Med* 1997;157:2453–2458.
11. Opie LH. Adverse cardiovascular drug reactions. *Curr Prob Cardiol* 2000;25:621–676.
12. Opie LH. Cardiovascular drug interactions. In: Frishman WH, Sonnenblick EH, Sica DA, eds. *Cardiovascular Pharmacotherapeutics.* 2d ed. New York: McGraw Hill; 2003:875.
13. Kirch W, Spahn H, Kohler H, Mutschler E. Influence of β-receptor antagonists on pharmacokinetics of cimetidine. *Drugs* 1983;25 (suppl 2):127–130.

14. McLean AJ, Knight R, Harrison PM, Harper RW. Clearance-based oral drug interaction between verapamil and metoprolol and comparison with atenolol. *Am J Cardiol* 1985;5:1628–1629.

15. Ochs HR, Carstens G, Greenblatt DJ. Reduction in lidocaine clearance during continuous infusion and by coadministration of propranolol. *N Engl J Med* 1980;303:373–377.

16. Webster J. Interactions of NSAIDs with diuretics and β-blockers: Mechanism and clinical implications. *Drugs* 1985;30:32–41.

17. Tolins M, Weir K, Chesler E, Pierpont GL. "Maximal" drug therapy is not necessarily optimal in chronic angina pectoris. *J Am Coll Cardiol* 1984;3:1051–1057.

18. Bruce RA, Hossack KF, Kusumi F, et al. Excessive reduction in peripheral resistance during exercise and risk of orthostatic symptoms with sustained-release nitroglycerin and diltiazem treatment of angina. *Am Heart J* 1985;109:1020–1026.

19. Boden WE, Bough EW, Reichman MJ, et al. Beneficial effects of high-dose diltiazem in patients with persistent effort angina on β-blockers and nitrates: A randomized, double-blind, placebo-controlled, crossover study. *Circulation* 1985;71:1197–1205.

20. Cheitlin MD, Hutter AM Jr, Brindis RG, et al. ACC/AHA Expert Consensus Document: Use of sildenafil (Viagra) in patients with cardiovascular disease. *J Am Coll Cardiol* 1999;33:273–282.

21. Gogia H, Mehra A, Parikh S, et al. Prevention of tolerance to hemodynamic effects of nitrates with concomitant use of hydralazine in patients with chronic heart failure. *J Am Cardiol* 1995;26:1575–1580.

22. Becker RC, Corrao JM, Bovill EG, et al. Intravenous nitroglycerin-induced heparin resistance: A qualitative antithrombin III abnormality. *Am Heart J* 1990;119:1254–1261.

23. Reicher-Reiss H, Neufeld HN, Ebner FX. Calcium antagonists: Adverse drug interactions. *Cardiovasc Drug Ther* 1987;1:403–409.

24. Abernethy DR, Schwartz JB. Calcium antagonist drugs. *N Engl J Med* 1999;341:1447–1457.

25. Abernethy DR. Grapefruits and drugs: When is statistically significant clinically significant? *J Clin Invest* 1997;10:2297–2298.

26. Frishman WH. Comparative efficacy and concomitant use of bepridil and beta blockers in the management of angina pectoris. *Am J Cardiol* 1992;69(suppl):50D–60D.

27. Mullins ME, Horowitz Z, Linden DHJ, et al. Life-threatening interaction of mibefradil and β-blockers with dihydropyridine calcium channel blockers. *JAMA* 1998;280:157–158.

28. Yeh R, Gulamhusein SS, Klcin GJ. Combined verapamil and propranolol for supraventricular tachycardia. *Am J Cardiol* 1984;53:757–763.

29. Ellrodt AG, Ault MJ, Riedinger MS, Murati GH. Efficacy and safety of sublingual nifedipine in hypertensive emergencies. *Am J Med* 1985; 79(suppl 4A):19–25.

30. Kieval J, Kirsten EB, Kessler KM, et al. The effects of intravenous verapamil on hemodynamic status of patients with coronary artery disease receiving propranolol. *Circulation* 1982;65:653–659.

31. Packer M, Meller J, Medina N, et al. Hemodynamic consequences of combined beta-adrenergic and slow calcium channel blockade in man. *Circulation* 1982;65:660–668.

32. Johnston DL, Lesoway R, Humen DP, Kostuk WJ. Clinical and hemodynamic evaluation of propranolol in combination with verapamil, nifedipine and diltiazem in exertional angina pectoris: A placebo-controlled, double-blind, randomized, cross-over study. *Am J Cardiol* 1985;55:680–687.

33. Winniford MD, Fulton KL, Corbett JR, et al. Propranolol-verapamil versus propranolol-nifedipine in severe angina pectoris of effort: A randomized, double-blind, cross-over study, *Am J Cardiol* 1985;55: 281–285.

34. Hamann SR, Kaltenborn KE, Vore M, et al. Cardiovascular pharmacokinetic consequences of combined administration of verapamil and propranolol in dogs. *Am J Cardiol* 1985;56:147–156.

35. Murdoch DL, Thomson GD, Thompson GG, et al. Evaluation of potential pharmacodynamic and pharmacokinetic interactions between verapamil and propranolol in normal subjects. *Br J Clin Pharmacol* 1991;31:323–332.

36. Johnston DL, Gebhardt VA, Donald A, Kostuk WJ. Comparative effects of propranolol and verapamil alone and in combination on left ventricular function in patients with chronic exertional angina: A double-blind, placebo-controlled, randomized, cross-over study with radionuclide ventriculography. *Circulation* 1983;68:1280–1289.

37. McInnes GT, Findlay IN, Murray G, et al. Cardiovascular responses to verapamil and propranolol in hypertensive patients. *J Hypertens* 1985; 3(suppl 3):S219–S221.

38. Pedersen KE. Digoxin interactions: The influence of quinidine and verapamil on the pharmacokinetics and receptor binding of digitalis glycosides. *Acta Med Scand* 1985;697(suppl):12–40.

39. Elliott HL, Pasanisi F, Meredith PA, Reid JL. Acute hypotensive response to nifedipine added to prazosin. *BMJ* 1984;288:238.

40. Pasanisi F, Elliott HL, Meredith PA, et al. Combined alpha-adrenoceptor antagonism and calcium channel blockade in normal subjects. *Clin Pharmacol Ther* 1984;36:716–723.

41. Reid JL, Meredith PA, Pasanisi F. Clinical pharmacological aspects of calcium antagonists and their therapeutic role in hypertension. *J Cardiovasc Pharmacol* 1985;7(suppl 4):S18–S20.

42. Maisel AS, Motulsky HJ, Insel PA. Hypotension after quinidine plus verapamil: Possible additive competition at alpha-adrenergic receptors. *N Engl J Med* 1985;312:167–171.

43. Trohman RG, Estes DM, Castellanos A, et al. Increased quinidine plasma concentrations during administration of verapamil: A new quinidine-verapamil interaction. *Am J Cardiol* 1986;57:706–707.

44. Hansten PD, Horn JR. Calcium channel blocker-induced drug interactions: Evidence for metabolic inhibition. *Drug Interact Newsl* 1986; 6:35–40.

45. Kleinbloesem CH, van Brummelen P, Sandberg TH, et al. Kinetic and haemodynamic interactions between nifedipine and propranolol in healthy subjects utilizing controlled rates of drug input. In: Kleinbloesem CH, ed. *Nifedipine: Clinical Pharmacokinetics and Haemodynamic Effects.* The Hague: Drukkerij JH Pasmans BV; 1985:151.

46. Goldberger J, Frishman WH. Clinical utility of nifedipine and diltiazem plasma levels in patients with angina pectoris receiving monotherapy and combination treatment. *J Clin Pharmacol* 1989; 29(7):628–634.

47. Kiss I, Farsang C. Nifedipine-prazosin interaction in patients with essential hypertension. *Cardiovasc Drugs Ther* 1989;3:413–415.

48. Frishman WH, Charlap S, Kimmel B, et al. Diltiazem compared to nifedipine and combination treatment with stable angina: Effects on angina, exercise tolerance and the ambulatory ECG. *Circulation* 1988; 77:774–786.

49. Hung J, Lamb IH, Connolly SJ, et al. The effect of diltiazem and propranolol, alone and in combination, on exercise performance and left ventricular function in patients with stable effort angina: A double-blind, randomized, and placebo-controlled study. *Circulation* 1983;68: 560–567.

50. Jones TE, Morris RG, Mathew TH: Diltiazem-cyclosporin pharmacokinetic interaction-dose-response relationship. *Br J Clin Pharmacol* 1997;44:499–504.

51. Cheng JWM. Cilostazol. *Heart Dis* 1999;1:182–186.

52. Bigger JT, Giardina EG. Drug interactions in antiarrhythmic therapy. *Ann NY Acad Sci* 1984;427:140–161.

53. Jaillon P. Antiarrhythmic drug interactions: Are they important? *Eur Heart J* 1987;8(suppl A):127–132.

54. Hardy BG, Zador IT, Golden L, et al. Effects of cimetidine on the pharmacokinetics of quinidine. *Am J Cardiol* 1983;52:172–175.

55. Drici M-D, Knollman BC, Wang W-X, Woosley RL. Cardiac actions of erythromycin: Influence of female sex. *JAMA* 1998;280:1774–1776.

56. Mishra A, Friedman HS, Sinha AK. The effects of erythromycin on the electrocardiogram. *Chest* 1999;115:983–986.

57. Lee KL, Jim M-H, Tang SC, Tai Y-T. QT prolongation and Torsades de pointes associated with clarithromycin. *Am J Med* 1998;104:395–396.

58. Hager WD, Fenster P, Mayersohn M, et al. Digoxin-quinidine interaction: Pharmacokinetic evaluation. *N Engl J Med* 1979;300: 1238–1241.

59. Koch-Weser J. Quinidine-induced hypoprothrombinemic hemorrhage in patients on chronic warfarin therapy. *Ann Intern Med* 1968;68:511–517.

60. Dada JL, Wilkinson GR, Nies AJ. Interaction of quinidine with anticonvulsant drugs. *N Engl J Med* 1976;294:699–702.

61. Twum-Barima Y, Carruthers SG. Quinidine-rifampicin. *N Engl J Med* 1981;304:1466–1469.

62. Farringer JA, McWay-Hess K, Clementi WA. Cimetidine-quinidine interaction. *Clin Pharmacol* 1984;3:81–83.

63. Green JA, Clementi WA, Porter C, Stigelman W. Nifedipine-quinidine interaction. *Clin Pharmacol* 1983;2:461–465.

64. Van Lith RM, Appleby DH. Quinidine-nifedipine interaction. *Drug Intell Clin Pharm* 1985;19:829–830.

65. Marcus FI. Drug interactions with amiodarone. *Am Heart J* 1983;106:924–930.

66. Christian CO, Meredith CG, Speeg KV. Cimetidine inhibits procainamide clearance. *Clin Pharmacol Ther* 1984;36:221–227.

67. Lee JT, Davy JM, Kates RE. Evaluation of combined administration of verapamil and disopyramide in dogs. *J Cardiovasc Pharmacol* 1985;7:501–507.

68. Kapil RP, Axelson JE, Mansfield IL, et al. Disopyramide pharmacokinetics and metabolism: Effect of inducers. *Br J Clin Pharmacol* 1987;24:781–791.

69. Teichman SL, Fisher JD, Matos JA, Kim SG. Disopyramide-pyridostigmine: Report of a beneficial drug interaction. *J Cardiovasc Pharmacol* 1985;7:108–113.

70. Feely J, Wilkinson GR, McAllister CB, Wood AJ. Increased toxicity and reduced clearance of lidocaine by cimetidine. *Ann Intern Med* 1982;96:592–594.

71. Boyce JR, Cervenko FW, Wright FJ. Effects of halothane on the pharmacokinetics of lidocaine in digitalis-toxic dogs. *Can Anaesth Soc J* 1978;25:323–328.

72. Jeresaty RM, Kahn AH, Landry AB. Sinoatrial arrest due to lidocaine in a patient receiving quinidine. *Chest* 1972;61:683–685.

73. Frishman WH, Cheng-Lai A, Chen J, eds. Antiarrhythmic agents. In: *Current Cardiovascular Drugs,* 3d ed. Philadelphia: Current Medicine; 2000:54.

74. Klein AL, Sami MH: Usefulness and safety of cimetidine in patients receiving mexiletine for ventricular arrhythmia. *Am Heart J* 1985;109:1281–1286.

75. Breithardt G, Selpel L, Abendroth RR. Comparative cross-over study of the effects of disopyramide and mexiletine on stimulus-induced ventricular tachycardia (abstr). *Circulation* 1980;62(suppl 3):153.

76. Duff HJ, Roden D, Primm RK, et al. Mexiletine in the treatment of resistant ventricular arrhythmias: Enhancement of efficacy and reduction of dose-related side-effects by combination with quinidine. *Circulation* 1983;67:1124–1128.

77. Greenspan AM, Spielman SR, Webb CR, et al. Efficacy of combination therapy with mexiletine and a type 1A agent for inducible ventricular tachyarrhythmias secondary to coronary artery disease. *Am J Cardiol* 1985;56:277–284.

78. Leahey EB, Heissenbuttel RH, Giardina EG, Bigger JT. Combined mexiletine and propranolol treatment of refractory ventricular tachycardia. *BMJ* 1980;2:357–358.

79. Waleffe A, Mary-Rabine L, Legrand V, et al. Combined mexiletine and amiodarone treatment of refractory recurrent ventricular tachycardia. *Am Heart J* 1980;100:788–793.

80. Lewis GP, Holtzman JL. Interaction of flecainide with digoxin and propranolol. *Am J Cardiol* 1984;53:52B–57B.

81. Shea P, Lal R, Kim SS, et al. Flecainide and amiodarone interaction. *J Am Coll Cardiol* 1986;7:1127–1130.

82. Tjandra Maga TB, van Hecken A, van Melle P, et al: Altered pharmacokinetics of oral flecainide by cimetidine. *Br J Clin Pharmacol* 1986;22:108–110.

83. Calvo MV, Martin-Suarez A, Martin Luengo C, et al. Interaction between digoxin and propafenone. *Ther Drug Monit* 1989;11:10–15.

84. Martinowitz U, Rabinovich J, Goldfarb D, et al. Interaction between warfarin sodium and amiodarone. *N Engl J Med* 1981;304:671–672.

85. Cavusoglu E, Frishman WH. Sotalol: A new β-adrenergic blocker for ventricular arrhythmias. *Prog Cardiovasc Dis* 1995;37:423–440.

86. Vincent JL, Dufaye P, Berre J, Kahn RJ. Bretylium in severe ventricular arrhythmias associated with digitalis intoxication. *Am J Emerg Med* 1984;2:504–506.

87. Peipho RW, Culbertson VL, Rhodes RS. Drug interactions with the calcium-entry blockers. *Circulation* 1987;75:181–194.

88. Hauptman PJ, Kelley RA. Digitalis. *Circulation* 1999;99:1265–1270.

89. Greiner B, Eichelbaum M, Fritz P, et al. The role of intestinal p-glycoprotein in the interaction of digoxin and rifampin. *J Clin Invest* 1999;104:147–153.

90. Kirch W, Hutt HJ, Dylewicz P, Ohnhaus EE. Dose-dependence of the nifedipine-digoxin interaction. *Clin Pharmacol Ther* 1986;39:35–39.

91. Lessem JN. Interaction between Ca^{2+} antagonists and digitalis. *Cardiovasc Drugs Ther* 1988;1:441–446.

92. Lessem J, Bellinetto A. Interaction between digoxin and the calcium antagonists nicardipine and tiapamil. *Clin Ther* 1983;5:595–602.

93. Kirch W, Hutt HJ, Heidemann H, et al. Drug interactions with nitrendipine. *J Cardiovasc Pharmacol* 1984;6:S982–S985.

94. Plunkett LM, Gokhale RD, Vallner JJ, Tackett RL. Prazosin alters free and total plasma digoxin levels in dogs. *Am Heart J* 1985;109:847–851.

95. Marcus FI. Pharmacokinetic interactions between digoxin and other drugs. *J Am Coll Cardiol* 1985;5(suppl A):82A–90A.

96. Waldorff S, Andersen JD, Heeboil-Nielsen N, et al. Spironolactone-induced changes in digoxin kinetics. *Clin Pharmacol Ther* 1978;24:162–167.

97. Waldorff S, Hansen PB, Egeblad H, et al. Interactions between digoxin and potassium-sparing diuretics. *Clin Pharmacol Ther* 1983;33:418–423.

98. Fenster PE, Hager WD, Goodman MM. Digoxin-quinidine-spironolactone interaction. *Clin Pharmacol Ther* 1984;36:70–73.

99. Miura T, Ueno K, Tanaka K, et al. Impairment of absorption of digoxin by acarbose. *J Clin Pharmacol* 1998;38:654–657.

100. Dzau VJ, Packer M, Lilly LS, et al. Prostaglandins in severe congestive heart failure: Relation to activation of the renin-angiotensin system and hyponatremia. *N Engl J Med* 1984;310:347–352.

101. Feenstra J, Heerdink ER, Grobbee DE, Stricker BH. Association of nonsteroidal anti-inflammatory drugs with first occurrence of heart failure and with relapsing heart failure: The Rotterdam Study. *Arch Intern Med* 2002;162:265–270.

102. McLay JS, McMurray JJ, Bridges AB, et al. Acute effects of captopril on the renal actions of furosemide in patients with chronic heart failure. *Am Heart J* 1993;126:879–886.

103. Van Hecken AM, Verbresselt R, Buntinx A, et al. Absence of a pharmacokinetic interaction between enalapril and furosemide. *Br J Clin Pharmacol* 1987;23:84–87.

104. Motwani JG, Fenwick MK, Morton JJ, Struthers AD: Furosemide-induced natriuresis is augmented by ultra-low-dose captopril but not by standard dose of captopril in chronic heart failure. *Circulation* 1992;86:439–445.

105. Dzau VJ, Hollenberg NK. Renal response to captopril in severe heart failure: Role of furosemide in natriuresis and reversal of hyponatremia. *Ann Intern Med* 1984;100:777–782.

106. Sica DA. Dosage considerations with perindopril for systemic hypertension. *Am J Cardiol* 2001;88(7 suppl):13i–18i.

107. Gurwitz JH, Everitt DE, Monane M, et al. The impact of ibuprofen on the efficacy of antihypertensive treatment with hydrochlorothiazide in elderly persons. *J Gerontol A Biol Sci Med Sci* 1996;51:M74–79.

108. Wolbrette DL. Risk of proarrhythmia with class III antiarrhythmic agents: Sex-based differences and other issues. *Am J Cardiol* 2003;91:39D–44D.

109. Crabtree BL, Mack JE, Johnson CD, Amyx BC. Comparison of the effects of hydro-chlorothiazide and furosemide on lithium disposition. *Am J Psychiatry* 1991;148:1060–1063.

110. Sharabi Y, Illan R, Kamari Y, et al. Diuretic induced hyponatraemia in elderly hypertensive women. *J Hum Hypertens* 2002;16:631–635.

111. Pitt B, Zannad F, Remme WJ, et al. The effect of spironolactone on morbidity and mortality in patients with severe heart failure. *N Engl J Med* 1999;341:709–717.

112. Pitt B, Remme W, Zannad F, et al. Eplerenone, a selective aldosterone blocker, in patients with left ventricular dysfunction after myocardial infarction. *N Engl J Med* 2003;348:1309–1321.

113. Perazella MA. Drug-induced hyperkalemia: Old culprits and new offenders. *Am J Med* 2000;109:307–314.

114. Cogan JJ, Humphreys MH, Carlson CJ, et al. Acute vasodilator therapy increases renal clearance of digoxin in patients with congestive heart failure. *Circulation* 1981;64:973–976.

115. Schneck DW, Vary JE. Mechanism by which hydralazine increases propranolol bioavailability. *Clin Pharmacol Ther* 1948;35:447–453.

116. Correa FJ, Eiser AR. Angiotensin-converting enzyme inhibitors and lithium toxicity. *Am J Med* 1992;93:108–109.

117. Conlin PR, Moore TJ, Swartz SL, et al. Effect of indomethacin on blood pressure lowering by captopril and losartan in hypertensive patients. *Hypertension* 2000;36:461–465.

118. Adhiyaman V, Asghar M, Oke A, et al. Nephrotoxicity in the elderly due to co-prescription of angiotensin converting enzyme inhibitors and nonsteroidal anti-inflammatory drugs. *J R Soc Med* 2001;94:512–514.

119. Cleland JG, John J, Houghton T. Does aspirin attenuate the effect of angiotensin-converting enzyme inhibitors in hypertension or heart failure? *Curr Opin Nephrol Hypertens* 2001;10:625–631.

119a. Lau WC, Gurbel PA, Watkins PB, et al. Contribution of hepatic cytochrome P450 3A4 metabolic activity to the phenomenon of clopidogrel resistance. *Circulation* 2004;109:166–171.

120. Hall D. Controversies in heart failure. Are beneficial effects of angiotensin-converting enzyme inhibitors attenuated by aspirin in patients with heart failure? *Cardiol Clin* 2001;19:597–603.

121. Spaulding C, Charbonnier B, Cohen-Solal A, et al. Acute hemodynamic interaction of aspirin and ticlopidine with enalapril: Results of a double-blind, randomized comparative trial. *Circulation* 1998;98:757–765.

122. Samanta A, Burden AC. Fever, myalgia, and arthralgia in a patient on captopril and allopurinol. *Lancet* 1984;1:679.

123. Sica DA. Newer antihypertensive agents: Angiotensin-receptor antagonists. In: Hollenberg N, ed. *Atlas of Hypertension*, 4th ed. Philadelphia: Current Medicine; 2003:301–324.

124. Bakris GL, Siomos M, Richardson D, et al. ACE inhibition or angiotensin receptor blockade: Impact on potassium in renal failure. VAL-K Study Group. *Kidney Int* 2000;58:2084–2092.

125. Stangier J, Su CA, Hendriks MG, et al. The effect of telmisartan on the steady-state pharmacokinetics of digoxin in healthy male volunteers. *J Clin Pharmacol* 2000;40:1373–1379.

126. Grayzel AI, Liddle L, Seegmiller JE. Diagnostic significance of hyperuricemia in arthritis. *N Engl J Med* 1961;265:763–768.

127. Moroz L. Increased blood fibrinolytic activity after aspirin ingestion. *N Engl J Med* 1977;296:525–529.

128. Chesebro JH, Fuster V, Elveback LR, et al. Trial of combined warfarin plus dipyridamole or aspirin therapy in prosthetic heart valve replacement: Danger of aspirin compared with dipyridamole. *Am J Cardiol* 1983;51:1537–1541.

129. Lin JC, Ito MK, Stolley SN, et al. The effect of converting from pravastatin to simvastatin on the pharmacodynamics of warfarin. *J Clin Pharmacol* 1999;39:86–90.

130. O'Reilly RA, Sahud MA, Aggeler PM. Impact of aspirin and chlorthalidone on the pharmacodynamics of oral anticoagulant drugs in man. *Ann NY Acad Sci* 1971;179:173–186.

131. Koh KK, Park GS, Song JH, Moon TH. Interaction of intravenous heparin and organic nitrates in acute ischemic syndromes. *Am J Cardiol* 1995;76:706–709.

132. Romeo F, Rosano GM, Martuscelli E, De Luca F. Concurrent nitroglycerin administration reduces the efficacy of recombinant tissue-type plasminogen activator in patients with acute anterior wall myocardial infarction. *Am Heart J* 1995;130:692–697.

133. White CM, Fan C, Chen BP, et al. Assessment of the drug interaction between alteplase and nitroglycerin: An in vitro study. *Pharmacotherapy* 2000;20:380–382.

134. Rindone JP, Keng HC. Gemfibrozil-warfarin drug interaction resulting in profound hypoprothrombinemia. *Chest* 1998;114:641–642.

135. Sica DA, Gehr TW. 3-Hydroxy-3-methylglutaryl coenzyme A reductase inhibitors and rhabdomyolysis: Considerations in the renal failure patient. *Curr Opin Nephrol Hypertens* 2002;11:123–133.

136. Lees RS, Lees AM. Rhabdomyolysis from the coadministration of lovastatin and the antifungal agent intraconazole. *N Engl J Med* 1995;333:664–665.

137. Ballantyne CM, Corsini A, Davidson MH, et al. Risk for myopathy with statin therapy in high-risk patients. *Arch Intern Med* 2003;163:553–564.

138. Williams D, Feely J. Pharmacokinetic-pharmacodynamic drug interactions with HMG-CoA reductase inhibitors. *Clin Pharmacokinet* 2002;41:343–370.

139. Houston MC. Nonsteroidal anti-inflammatory drugs and antihypertensives. *Am J Med* 1991;90(suppl 5A):42S–47S.

140. NSAIDs and hypertension: Is it clinically important? *Drugs Ther Perspect* 1998;11:14–16.

141. Salvetti A, Magagna A, Abdel-Haq B, et al. Nifedipine interactions in hypertensive patients. *Cardiovasc Drugs Ther* 1990;4:963–968.

142. Johnson DL, Hisel TM, Phillips BB. Effect of cyclooxygenase-2 inhibitors on blood pressure. *Ann Pharmacother* 2003;37:442–446.

143. Weinberger MH. The relationship of sodium balance and concomitant diuretic therapy to blood pressure response with calcium channel entry blockers. *Am J Med* 1991;90(suppl 5A):15S–20S.

144. Sinatra ST, Frishman WH, Peterson SJ, Lin G. Use of alternative/complementary medicine in treating cardiovascular disease. In: Frishman WH, Sonnenblick EH, Sica DA, eds. *Cardiovascular Pharmacotherapeutics*, 2d ed. New York: McGraw-Hill; 2003:857.

145. Sinatra St, Frishman WH, Peterson SJ. Use of alternative medicines in treating cardiovascular disease. In: Frishman WH, Sonnenblick EH, Sica DA, eds. *Cardiovascular Pharmacotherapeutic Manual*, 2d ed. New York: McGraw-Hill; 2004:485.

146. Fugh-Berman A. Herb-drug interactions. *Lancet* 2000;355:134–138.

147. Johne A, Brockmöller Bauer S, Maurer A, et al. Pharmacokinetic interaction of digoxin with an herbal extract from St. John's wort (*Hypericum perforatum*). *Clin Pharmacol Ther* 1999;66:338–345.

148. Henderson L, Yue QY, Bergquist C, et al. St. John's wort (*Hypericum perforatum*): Drug interactions and clinical outcomes. *Br J Clin Pharmacol* 2002;54:349–356.

EFFECTS OF MOOD AND ANXIETY DISORDERS ON THE CARDIOVASCULAR SYSTEM

Dominique L. Musselman / Bruce Rudisch / William M. McDonald / Charles B. Nemeroff

And now here's my secret, a very simple secret: It is only with the heart that one can see rightly; what is essential is invisible to the eye.

Antoine de Saint-Exupery, The Little Prince, *1943*

DEPRESSION AND COMORBID MEDICAL ILLNESS

The interactions of personality traits, psychiatric symptoms and syndromes, and environmental stressors with the cardiovascular system have long intrigued investigators interested in the factors that contribute to the development and progression of atherosclerotic heart disease. Differences in rates of ischemic heart disease (IHD) remain substantially unexplained even after surveillance of the well-established risk factors. Although the type A personality pattern has been studied intensely as a risk factor for coronary artery disease (CAD),[1] lack of a consistent association between type A behavior and the subsequent development of IHD has stimulated questions about the contributions of the psychological concept of hostility,[2] as well as the syndrome of major depression. Increasing evidence is accumulating that suggests that major depression (Table 91-1),[3]—a mood disorder—is associated with drastically elevated morbidity and mortality after an index myocardial infarction (MI) and also acts as an independent risk factor in the development of atherosclerotic heart disease.

Depressive syndromes and major depression are exceedingly common. The most recent comprehensive study done in the United States, the National Comorbidity Study, reported lifetime prevalence rates of major depression (13 percent) and dysthymia (5 percent).[4] Point prevalence rates of major depression in primary care outpatients range from 2 to 16 percent and 9 to 20 percent for all depressive disorders[4–6] and are even higher among medical inpatients: 8 percent for major depression and 15 to 36 percent for all depressive disorders.[7,8]

Minor depressive disorder (depressive symptoms subthreshold in severity compared with major depression and dysthymia) is also common in the community[9] and in primary care clinics.[10] The Epidemiologic Catchment Area Study of over 18,500 individuals reported the lifetime prevalence rate of subthreshold depressive symptoms to be 23 percent in comparison to 6 percent, the sum of the prevalence rates of major depression and dysthymia.[9] Recognition and treatment of major depression is crucial, especially for patients after an MI. Not only do depressed patients experience great difficulties in problem solving and coping with challenges, depression adversely affects compliance with medical therapy[11] and rehabilitation[12] and quality of medical care received.[13] Minor depressive disorder also is associated with significant functional impairment and substantial increases in health care utilization.[9,14] Since the 1960s, multiple cross-sectional and longitudinal studies have scrutinized the association of cardiovascular disease (CVD), especially CAD and congestive heart failure (CHF), with depressive symptoms as well as major depression.

EPIDEMIOLOGY

Depression and Cardiovascular Disease: Clinical Samples

Relatively consistent point prevalence rates of depression have been documented in patients with CAD, ranging from 15 to 23 percent, despite the potential methodologic weaknesses of some of the studies (such as the use of unmodified psychiatric diagnostic instruments

TABLE 91-1 DSM-IV Diagnostic Criteria for Depressive Disorders[3]

Major Depressive Disorder
- Five (or more) of the following symptoms have been present during the same 2-week period and represent a change from previous functioning; at least one of the symptoms is either (1) depressed mood or (2) loss of interest or pleasure.
  (1) Depressed mood
  (2) Markedly diminished interest or pleasure
  (3) Significant weight loss or weight gain, or decrease or increase in appetite
  (4) Insomnia or hypersomnia
  (5) Psychomotor agitation or retardation (observable by others)
  (6) Fatigue or loss of energy nearly every day
  (7) Feelings of worthlessness or excessive or inappropriate guilt
  (8) Diminished concentration or indecisiveness
  (9) Recurrent thoughts of death (not just fear of dying) or suicide
- The symptoms cause clinically significant distress or impairment in social, occupational, or other important areas of functioning.
- The symptoms are not due to the direct physiological effects of a substance or a general medical condition.
- The symptoms are not better accounted for by bereavement.

Dysthymic Disorder
A. Depressed mood for most of the day, for more days than not, for at least 2 years
B. Presence, while depressed, of two (or more) of the following:
  (1) Poor appetite or overeating
  (2) Insomnia or hypersomnia
  (3) Low energy or fatigue
  (4) Low self-esteem
  (5) Poor concentration or difficulty making decisions
  (6) Feelings of hopelessness
C. The disturbance is not better accounted for by chronic major depressive disorder.

Reprinted with permission from the *Diagnostic and Statistical Manual of Mental Disorders*, 4th ed. Copyright 1994, American Psychiatric Association.

to determine the prevalence of depression, excluding patients because of CVD severity, and measuring depressive symptoms at different times after hospital admission) and methodologic differences (dissimilar patient populations, diagnostic instruments, etc.).[15–24]

Although the prevalence of depressive symptoms in patients after coronary artery bypass graft (CABG) surgery,[25] or those hospitalized for CHF,[22,26] has not been as well studied, preliminary evidence indicates that these patients have equally as elevated, or even greater, rates of major depression.

The presence of depression in patients with preexisting cardiovascular disease is a risk factor for future cardiovascular events and death. The seminal studies of Frasure-Smith and colleagues[20,27] demonstrated that post-MI depression was a significant predictor of mortality ($p < .001$) in 222 patients both 6 and 18 months after an MI. Depression remained a significant predictor of mortality ($p = .01$) even after multivariate statistical methodology was used to factor out the effects of left ventricular dysfunction and previous MI. Multiple logistic regression analyses revealed that depression was significantly related to 18-month cardiac mortality even after controlling for other significant multivariate predictors of mortality [previous MI, Killip class, frequency of premature ventricular contractions (PVCs) ($p = .003$)]. More recent studies have been consistent with these results.[28,29] Indeed, in a cohort of 870 post-MI patients recruited between 1991 and 1994, the greater the severity of depressive symptoms during the index hospital admission, the more

severely diminished the long-term (5-year) cardiac mortality, independent of established prognostic factors. Depression severity had as great an impact upon survival as left ventricular dysfunction or diabetes.[30] Other investigators have subsequently extended the finding of depression's negative impact on prognosis to patients with CHF[31,32] and patients who are post-CABG.[25]

Despite these findings, however, other investigators have been critical of the association between post-MI depression and mortality given the possible confounding effect of severity of CVD.[33] Although many positive studies have taken the confounding effects of disease severity into account through multivariate analysis, including the seminal studies of Frasure-Smith et al., or by making adjustments for surrogate markers of disease severity such as fatigue and dyspnea,[34] Carroll and Lane have urged caution when using these multivariate techniques, given the possibility of underadjustment for confounding risk factors.[33]

Depression as a Risk Factor for Ischemic Heart Disease in Community Samples

The notion that having a psychiatric illness such as major depression increases one's risk for developing IHD remains controversial and often has been "explained" intuitively by the hypothesis that persons with psychiatric disorders generally have other risk factors for the development of CAD.[1] Nevertheless, studies using the most rigorous methods (prospective in design; using structured clinical interviews or diagnostic instruments; inclusion of other risk factors for CVD in the analysis such as hypertension, hypercholesterolemia, nicotine, other substance abuse, and physical inactivity; and controlling for demographic factors such as age, sex, and socioeconomic status) have consistently, though not unanimously, demonstrated that depression does indeed serve as an independent risk factor for the development and expression of CVD.[35–55] Such large epidemiologic studies may use self-report instruments rather than clinical interviews to evaluate the importance of psychological factors in predicting CVD. Assessments of this type typically are added to large, multiple-risk-factor studies in which population-based samples are followed up prospectively.[1] The advantage of using "dimensional" measures of depression (rather than a categorical diagnosis of major depression) lies in the increased statistical power that allows these studies to detect smaller "effects." Indeed, the use of dimensional measures of depression has allowed for the demonstration of a dose-response relation, with several studies demonstrating graded relative risks for cardiac events for increasing depression severity,[39,44,45,48,51,54,55] providing further evidence for a causal role of depression in the development of CVD.

A number of these studies of antecedent depression and cardiovascular risk were subjected to a recent metanalysis.[56] Taken as a group, the relative risk of developing heart disease in patients who were initially depression-free was 1.64 (95 percent confidence interval 1.29–2.08 $p < 0.001$), implicating depression *as an independent risk factor* in the pathophysiologic progression of CVD, rather than merely as a secondary emotional response to cardiovascular illness.

PATHOPHYSIOLOGY

Hypothalamic-Pituitary-Adrenocortical and Sympathomedullary Hyperactivity

Advances in biological psychiatry have included the discovery of numerous neurochemical, neuroendocrine, and neuroanatomic alterations in unipolar depression. Often proposed as important adjuncts in the diagnosis of depressed subjects, some of these biological markers may reflect important pathophysiologic alterations that con-

tribute to the increased vulnerability of depressed patients to CVD. These markers include hypothalamic-pituitary-adrenocortical (HPA) and sympathoadrenal hyperactivity, diminished heart rate variability (HRV), alterations in platelet receptors and/or reactivity, increased secretion of proinflammatory cytokines, and ventricular instability and myocardial ischemia in reaction to mental stress (Fig. 91-1, Plate 108).

Two primary components that are central to the "fight or flight" stress response observed by Cannon in 1911[57] and the "general adaptation syndrome" described by Selye in 1956[58] are the HPA axis and the sympathoadrenal system. In response to stress, hypothalamic neurons containing corticotropin-releasing factor (CRF) increase the synthesis and release of corticotropin (ACTH), β-endorphin, and other pro-opiomelanocortin (POMC) products from the anterior pituitary gland. Many studies have documented evidence of HPA axis hyperactivity in medication-free patients with major depression (i.e., elevated CRF concentrations in cerebrospinal fluid),[59–61] blunting of the ACTH response to CRF administration, nonsuppression of cortisol secretion after dexamethasone administration, hypercortisolemia,

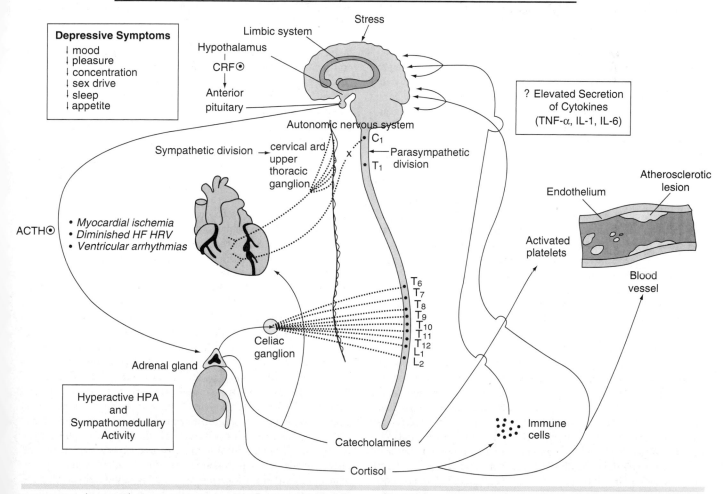

The Relationship Between Major Depression and Cardiovascular Disease

FIGURE 91-1 (Plate 108) Hypothetical schema of pathophysiologic findings associated with depression that probably contributes to increased susceptibility to cardiovascular disease. Autonomic nervous system innervation of the heart via the parasympathetic vagus (X) nerve and sympathetic (postganglionic efferents from the cervical and upper thoracic paravertebral ganglia) nerves is shown. ACTH = corticotropin; CRF = corticotropin-releasing factor; HRV = heart rate variability; HPA = hypothalamic-pituitary-adrenocortical axis; IL-1 = interleukin-1; IL-6 = interleukin-6; TNF-α = tumor necrosis factor-α. (From *Arch Gen Psychiatry*, July 1998;55: p 583. Copyright (1998), American Medical Association.)

and pituitary and adrenal gland enlargement, as well as direct evidence of increased numbers of hypothalamic CRF neurons in postmortem brain tissue from depressed patients compared with controls.[62] Administered corticosteroids have long been known to induce hypercholesterolemia, hypertriglyceridemia, and hypertension. Other atherosclerosis-inducing actions of steroids include injury to vascular endothelial cells[63] and intima[64] and the inhibition of normal healing.[65] Indeed, elevated morning plasma cortisol concentrations have been significantly correlated with moderate-to-severe coronary atherosclerosis in young and middle-aged men.[66]

Many patients with major depression also exhibit dysregulation of the sympathoadrenal system. The adrenal medulla and sympathetic nervous system (SNS) together constitute the sympathoadrenal system. Although central nervous system (CNS) regulation of the sympathoadrenal system has been only partially characterized, hypothalamic CRF-containing neurons provide stimulatory input to several autonomic centers that are involved in regulating sympathetic activity.[67] Nerve impulses from regulatory centers in the CNS control catecholamine release from the sympathoadrenal system. Physiologic and pathologic conditions causing sympathoadrenal activation include physical activity, coronary artery ischemia, heart failure, and mental stress. Epinephrine in plasma is derived from the adrenal medulla, whereas plasma norepinephrine (NE) concentrations reflect the secretion of NE largely from sympathetic nerve terminals, with the remaining NE provided by the adrenal medulla and extraadrenal chromaffin cells. Peripheral plasma NE concentrations are determined not only by the rate of release from sympathetic nervous system nerve terminals but also by reuptake into presynaptic terminals, local metabolic degradation, and redistribution into multiple physiologic compartments. Hypersecretion of NE in unipolar depression has been documented by elevated plasma NE and NE metabolite concentrations[68] and elevated urinary concentrations of NE and its metabolites, though discordant reports exist.[69] Not only do depressed patients exhibit higher basal plasma concentrations of NE, those with melancholia exhibit even greater elevations in plasma NE concentrations when subjected to orthostatic challenge than do normal control subjects and depressed patients *without* melancholia.[70] Furthermore, depressed patients who are dexamethasone (DST) nonsuppressors exhibit significantly higher basal and cold-stimulated plasma concentrations of NE than do depressed patients who are DST suppressors.[70] After treatment with tricyclic antidepressants (TCAs), urinary excretion of NE and its metabolites diminish together with plasma NE concentrations,[71,72] although Veith and colleagues[68] reported that chronic treatment with desipramine increased plasma concentrations of NE. Thus, sympathoadrenal hyperactivity seems to represent a state rather than a trait marker of depression, possibly reflecting increased CRF release within the CNS.

Sympathoadrenal hyperactivity contributes to the development of CVD through effects of catecholamines on the heart, blood vessels, and platelets. Sympathoadrenal activation modifies the function of circulating platelets through direct effects on platelets, catecholamine-induced changes in hemodynamic factors (increased shear stress), circulating lipids, and inhibition of vascular eicosanoid synthesis.[73] Arachidonic acid metabolites such as prostaglandins and leukotrienes contribute to diverse circulatory and hemostatic functions, including inhibition of platelet aggregation, and vascular contractility and permeability.[74] Elevations of plasma NE levels are found most frequently in young hypertensive patients[75] and in subjects with high-cardiac-output borderline hypertension who later proceed to established high-resistance hypertension.[76] Even normotensive depressed patients have been found to exhibit greater heart rates at rest, after orthostasis, and after exercise in comparison with normal controls. These depressed patients also exhibited increased plasma concentrations of NE and serotonin (5-HT) at rest.[77] Thus, the sympathoadrenal hyperactivity observed in many patients with major depression may contribute to the development of CVD through the effects of catecholamines on cardiac function and platelets.

Diminished Heart Rate Variability

Alterations in autonomic nervous system activity, as demonstrated by exaggerated responses in heart rate to orthostatic challenge[69] or reduction in HRV, represent yet another mechanism that potentially contributes to the diminished survival of depressed patients with CVD. The beat-to-beat fluctuations in hemodynamic parameters are thought to reflect the dynamic response of cardiovascular control systems to a myriad of naturally occurring physiologic perturbations, such as fluctuations in heart rate associated with respiration. Therefore, HRV may provide a sensitive measure of the functioning of the rapidly reacting sympathetic, parasympathetic, and renin-angiotensin systems. Cardiovascular homeostasis is maintained by the parasympathetic and sympathetic nervous systems through afferent pressor receptors and chemoreceptors and efferents that alter heart rate, atrioventricular conduction, and contractility and impinge on the peripheral vasculature, altering arterial and venous vasomotor tone.[78] HRV is the standard deviation of successive R-R intervals in sinus rhythm and reflects the interplay and balance between sympathetic and parasympathetic input on the cardiac pacemaker. Peripheral control of HRV occurs mainly through the parasympathetic cholinergic vagus nerve.[79] Central generation and control of heart rate are regulated by the hypothalamus, the limbic system, and the brainstem. Numerous CNS neurotransmitters are involved in modulating HRV, including acetylcholine, NE, 5-HT, and dopamine.[80]

A high degree of HRV is observed in normal hearts with good cardiac function, whereas HRV can be decreased significantly in patients with severe CAD or heart failure.[81] Moreover, the relative risk of sudden death after an acute MI is significantly higher in patients with decreased HRV.[82–84] Heart rate variability is one of many prognostic factors after an infarction [e.g., age, left ventricular ejection fraction (LVEF), and frequency of arrythmias]. Its positive predictive power, like that of other factors after an MI, is relatively modest when considered in isolation. Although positive predictive accuracy is not high when HRV is considered alone, in combination with other prognostic factors, clinically useful levels of negative predictive accuracy can be achieved.[85] Among the many arrhythmogenic factors, autonomic tone is the most difficult to measure,[86] and, therefore, interest in HRV continues. Power spectral analysis measurements of HRV often are used because certain frequency bands of the heart period power spectrum have been associated with autonomic nervous system control of the sinus node.[87] The low-frequency power of the heart period power spectrum reflects modulation of sympathetic and vagal tone by baroreflex activity,[88] while high-frequency power reflects modulation of vagal tone, primarily by respiratory frequency and depth (i.e., respiratory sinus arrhythmia).[89] The physiologic mechanisms that contribute to ultralow-frequency and very low frequency power of the heart period spectrum (which account for more than 90 percent of the total power in a 24-h period) remain obscure. In a study of 715 patients after MI, certain frequency bands (total, ultralow, and very low frequencies) of the heart period power spectrum were strongly associated with mortality during 4 years of follow-up, even after adjustment for other major risk factors. Indeed, very-low-frequency power was most strongly associated with death secondary to arrhythmia.[90]

Reduced high-frequency HRV has been observed in depressed patients in comparison with nondepressed groups,[91] although discrepant reports exist.[92] In patients with angiographically confirmed CAD, diminished HRV during 24-h Holter monitoring was significantly more common in depressed patients than in matched nondepressed patients.[93] Diminished high-frequency HRV is thought to reflect decreased parasympathetic tone, possibly predisposing patients to ventricular arrhythmias and perhaps to the excessive cardiovascular mortality found in CVD patients with a comorbid major depressive disorder.[94] Diminished HRV in patients with major depression also may be contributed to by a deficiency of omega-3 fatty acids[95] in this patient population. Not only have multiple studies documented a deficiency of omega-3 fatty acids in patients with major depression,[96–98] these polyunsaturated lipids possess antiarrhythmic properties and reduce the risk of ventricular arrhythmias.[99,100]

Few studies have documented improvement of reduced HRV after effective depression treatment, either antidepressant[101] or cognitive behavioral psychotherapy.[102] Nevertheless, the complexity and chaos of HRV of depressed patients is increasingly characterized using nonlinear techniques, though the physiologic significance of such nontraditional methods requires further examination.[103] Nevertheless, the prognostic importance of improvement in diminished HRV in depressed patients remains an intriguing area of research. Subsequent investigations will also seek to determine the processes that underlie ultralow and very-low-frequency bands of the heart power spectrum; whether these bands are altered in depressed patients (with or without CVD) remains obscure.

Alterations in Platelet Receptors and/or Reactivity

The adverse effects of depression on cardiovascular disease also may be mediated by platelet mechanisms. Markovitz and Matthews[104] first proposed that enhanced platelet responses to psychologic stress may trigger adverse coronary artery ischemic events. This association between platelet activation and vascular disease is supported indirectly by studies linking cerebrovascular disease and depression. The Established Populations for Epidemiologic Studies of the Elderly prospectively studied 10,294 persons age 65 and older for 6 years and determined that rates of stroke (adjusted for age, physical disability, and other medical disorders) were 2.3 to 2.7 times higher in persons designated with "high" versus "low" levels of depressive symptoms.[42] In another prospective study, 103 consecutive stroke patients[105] were assessed for major depression or dysthymia approximately 2 weeks after a stroke. Patients with major depression or dysthymia were 3.4 times more likely to have died during the 10-year follow-up period than were nondepressed patients ($p = .007$), even after controlling for confounding variables (age, medical comorbidity, type of stroke, and lesion location; $p = .03$).

Platelets play a central role in hemostasis, thrombosis, the development of atherosclerosis, and acute coronary syndromes[106] through their interactions with both subendothelial components of damaged vessel walls and plasma coagulation factors, primarily thrombin. Human platelets contain adrenergic, serotonergic, and dopaminergic receptors. Through activation of platelet alpha$_2$ adrenoceptors, increases in circulating catecholamines (>4 nmol/L) potentiate the effects of other agonists and, at higher concentrations, initiate platelet thrombotic responses, including secretion, aggregation, and activation of the arachidonate pathway. After injury to vessel endothelium, platelets and circulating leukocytes attach to the newly exposed subendothelial layer. Platelet adhesion to exposed collagen (and other components of the subendothelial matrix) and to thrombin stimulates platelet activation. Activation converts platelet membrane GPIIb/IIIa complexes into functional receptors for fibrinogen. Activation also is accompanied by extrusion or secretion of platelet storage granule contents into the extracellular environment. Platelets activated at the site of an injury to the vessel wall accelerate the local formation of thrombin and release a variety of products from their storage granules, including chemotactic and mitogenic factors, inducing leukocyte migration from the bloodstream and vascular cell proliferation. These secreted platelet products [e.g., platelet factor 4, β-thromboglobulin (β-TG), and 5-HT] stimulate and recruit other platelets and cause irreversible platelet–platelet aggregation, ultimately leading to the formation of a fused platelet thrombus. Platelets also contribute to vascular damage by stimulating lipoprotein uptake by macrophages and mediating vasoconstriction through the production and/or release of substances such as thromboxane A$_2$, platelet-activating factor, and 5-HT.[73] Clinical trials have confirmed the importance of platelets in vascular damage; antiaggregating medications are useful in secondary prevention,[107,108] delay the progression of atherosclerotic lesions,[109] and improve post-MI outcomes.[110,111]

The authors sought to determine whether heightened susceptibility to platelet activation might be a mechanism by which depression in physically healthy young volunteers acts as a significant risk factor for cardiovascular and cerebrovascular disease and/or increased mortality after MI. Utilizing fluorescence-activated flow cytometric analysis, we discovered that in comparison to normal controls, relatively, young, medically healthy, depressed patients without any other risk factors for CAD exhibited enhanced baseline platelet activation as well as increased platelet responsiveness.[112] Moreover, in another study, in comparison to normal controls, depressed patients *with* one or more traditional risk factors for CAD exhibited, under *basal* conditions, increased circulating platelets that had proceeded to irreversible degranulation.[113]

Indeed patients suffering from comorbid CVD and major depression also exhibit increased platelet activation as measured by markedly elevated plasma concentrations of the platelet secretion products PF4 and β-TG compared with *non*depressed, age-matched patients with CVD.[114] Interestingly, increased platelet activation has also been documented in CVD patients with the negative emotion, hostility, in comparison to healthy controls.[115] Although the mechanism or mechanisms responsible remain unknown, heightened susceptibility to platelet activation and secretion may contribute, at least in part, to the increased vulnerability of depressed patients to CVD and/or mortality after an MI.

Serotonin secreted by platelets induces both platelet aggregation and coronary vasoconstriction, both of which are mediated by 5-HT$_2$ receptors. Vasoconstriction occurs especially when normal endothelial cell counterregulatory mechanisms of vascular relaxation are defective, as often occurs in patients with CAD.[116] Indeed, essential hypertension, elevated plasma cholesterol levels, older age, and smoking, which are well-known predisposing factors for the development of CVD, all contribute to 5-HT-mediated platelet activation. Moreover, alterations in platelet 5-HT-mediated activation also have been described in affective disorders, most notably major depression. Considerable evidence has accrued in the last two decades that supports the hypothesis that alterations in CNS and platelet serotonergic function occur in depressed patients.[117]

Serotonin-mediated platelet activation can contribute to the development of atherosclerosis, thrombosis, and vasoconstriction. Even though 5-HT is a weak platelet agonist, it markedly amplifies platelet reactions to a variety of other agonists such as adenosine diphosphate (ADP), thromboxane A$_2$, catecholamines, and thrombin. Through an action on 5-HT$_2$ receptors, serotonin enhances platelet aggregation and the release of intragranular products and arachidonic acid metabolites in response to otherwise ineffective agonist concentrations.[118] This 5-HT-induced platelet amplification occurs at the low concentrations attained when 5-HT is released from seeping platelets subjected to shear stresses[119] and from platelet activation by contact with an arterial wall lesion.[120] Interestingly, several investigators have reported *increases* in platelet 5-HT$_2$ binding density in depressed patients.[121–122] Moreover, the changes appear to be state-dependent in that 5-HT$_2$-binding-site density returned to control values only in patients who showed clinical improvement. Depressed patients have been found to exhibit significant *reductions* in the number of platelet and brain 5-HT transporter sites as detected by [^{3}H] imipramine binding[123] as well as by the more selective ligand [^{3}H] paroxetine.[124] The increased 5-HT$_2$-receptor-binding density and decreased 5-HT-transporter sites suggest that depressed patients may be particularly susceptible to 5-HT-mediated platelet activation and coronary artery vasoconstriction. Decreased numbers of platelet 5-HT transporters would potentially hinder the uptake and storage of periplatelet serotonin, exposing the increased numbers of 5-HT$_2$ receptors to 5-HT.[125]

Platelets from depressed patients also exhibit significantly increased elevations of intracellular free calcium concentration, [Ca^{2+}]i, after 5-HT-induced stimulation in comparison to controls.[126] Even functionally trivial increases in intraplatelet calcium "prime" the platelet secretion and aggregation response to stimulation by even a "weak" agonist such as 5-HT[127] or in response to increased blood flow. Thus, platelets with elevated [Ca^{2+}]i, as are observed in depressed patients, probably would exhibit increased activation in comparison with normal comparison subjects under basal conditions or in response to shear-induced aggregation (e.g., after an orthostatic challenge). More recently, antidepressants that inhibit the reuptake of serotonin into neurons (and platelets) have been shown to normalize the abnormally heightened platelet activation and secretion observed in patients with depression, without[113] and with CVD.[128]

Increased Secretion of Proinflammatory Cytokines

Inflammation and associated secretion of proinflammatory cytokines may mediate the association of depression and atherosclerotic progression.[129] During inflammation, infection, and other conditions,[130] intercellular signaling polypeptides known as cytokines are secreted by activated cells such as endothelial cells, fibroblasts, macrophages, and monocytes. Though cytokines exert a variety of effects in the acute-phase response, the proinflammatory cytokines, interleukin (IL)-1, IL-6, and tumor necrosis factor-α (TNF-α), stimulate production of hepatic-derived acute-phase proteins, such as C-reactive protein and fibrinogen, and also induce "sickness" behavior. Sickness behavior, a constellation of nonspecific signs and symptoms that accompanies the physiologic response to infection and inflammation, includes fatigue, anorexia, anhedonia, decreased psychomotor activity, and disappearance of body-care activities,[131] which overlap with the symptoms of major depression. Perhaps not surprisingly, IL-6 is elevated in many patients with major depression,[132–134] along with elevations of acute phase reactants,[135] including fibrinogen.[132] Given reports linking increased secretion of proinflammatory cytyokines to symptoms of exhaustion in clinical samples,[136] and elevations of fibrinogen in depressed individuals in large-scale, prospective, community-based, epidemiologic studies,[137,138] future studies will ascertain whether inflammatory markers mediate the increased incidence of CVD and cardiac-related mortality in patients with depressive syndromes.

Myocardial Ischemia and Ventricular Instability in Reaction to Mental Stress

The combination of a vulnerable myocardium after MI, acute ischemia, and negative emotional arousal has long been thought to trigger fatal ventricular arrythmias.[139] Indeed, Jiang and colleagues[140] longitudinally assessed 126 patients with CAD over a 5-year period. Mental stress-induced myocardial ischemia at baseline in CAD patients was associated with significantly higher rates of subsequent fatal and nonfatal cardiac events independently of age, baseline LVEF, and previous MI. This study proposed that the relation between psychological stress and adverse cardiac events is mediated by myocardial ischemia. Although myocardial ischemia probably is the most significant factor in predisposition to ventricular instability, other factors also contribute. CNS control mechanisms can significantly decrease the threshold for ventricular fibrillation.[141] Ventricular fibrillation is believed to be the mechanism underlying sudden cardiac death, the most common cause of fatality among patients with CAD.[142] Indeed, psychological stress predisposes to abnormal ventricular activity by lowering the ventricular vulnerable-period threshold even to the point of fibrillation. The vagus nerve, however, exerts antiarrthymic activity through a direct action on the ventricular myocardium and interference with sympathetic activity.[143] Increased parasympathetic activity has a protective effect on myocardium electrically destabilized by increased adrenergic tone.[142]

Psychological and physical events can elicit a stress response, which usually is defined as the reaction of an organism to deleterious forces that disturb physiologic homeostasis.[144] Psychological stress in humans with CAD increases ventricular ectopic activity and increases the risk of ventricular fibrillation.[145] There are several similarities between the stress response and major depression: both can be characterized by increased blood pressure and heart rate as well as increased arousal and increased mobilization of energy stores.[146] Particularly relevant to both the stress response and depression are the critical brain structures—the locus coeruleus and the central nucleus of the amygdala—which both are innervated by CRF-containing nerve terminals.[147] The stress response and major depression differ in some respects, however. In depression, some aspects of the normal stress response seem to escalate to a pathologic state[148] that fails to respond appropriately to usual counterregulatory responses, resulting in a sustained version of a usually transient phenomenon (i.e., hyperactivity of the HPA axis or the sympathoadrenal system). Although many studies have linked stressful life events to the onset of major depression,[149,150] some depressions are clearly "endogenous" (i.e., they have no obvious environmental precipitant).

Frasure-Smith and colleagues[27] proposed that depression worsens the prognosis after an MI through another mechanism: PVCs. The risk of sudden cardiac death associated with significant depressive symptoms (Beck Depression Inventory score $\geq$ 10) was greatest among patients with 10 or more PVCs per hour (60 percent of these patients died within 18 months), suggesting arrythymia as the link between depression and sudden cardiac death.[27] Depressed patients with CAD are not more likely to have arrhythmias than are nondepressed patients with CAD, but the risk associated with depression is confined largely to patients with PVCs. Patients who were *not* depressed experienced little increase in risk associated with PVCs even in the presence of a low LVEF.[27] Thus, the prognostic impact of PVCs may be related more to depression than to PVCs per se. In the Cardiac Arrhythmia Suppression Trial (CAST),[151] suppression of PVC frequency in post-MI patients did not reduce but actually increased mortality even though PVCs are associated with increased mortality after an MI. Thus, treatment of depression may be necessary to improve survival in depressed patients with PVCs.[152]

ANXIETY DISORDERS AND CARDIOVASCULAR DISEASE

Epidemiology

Anxiety disorders are the most prevalent psychiatric disorders in the United States (Table 91-2), with simple phobias being the most common (9 percent) and social phobia (8 percent) being the most often observed (Tables 91-3 and 91-4). A survey of adult primary care patients ($n = 637$) enrolled in a health maintenance organization revealed that 10 percent had untreated anxiety disorders.[153]

Unfortunately, anxiety disorders, though common, remain largely undiagnosed and undertreated.[154] Stereotyped as the "worried well," patients with anxiety disorders such as phobias, panic disorder, and generalized anxiety disorder have substantially higher rates of health service utilization, increased social and role disability, diminished quality of life, and poor health outcomes.[153,155] Moreover, the comorbidity of anxiety and affective disorders is substantial. Nearly 60 percent of patients with major depression in the National Comorbidity Survey suffered from a comorbid anxiety disorder.[4] Indeed, patients with mixed anxiety and depressive symptoms (or comorbid anxiety and depressive syndromes) suffer increased emotional disability as well as poorer social and role function in comparison to patients with either condition alone.[153] After elective catheterization, the physical disability of patients with CAD at 1 year of follow-up was associated with the severity of these patients' anxiety and depressive symptoms at catheterization, *not* with the number of main coronary vessels stenosed.[154]

The prevalence of anxiety disorders in patients with CVD has been largely understudied, with most studies focusing on patients with mitral valve prolapse or individuals referred for evaluation of chest pain. Substantial numbers of patients each year who undergo coronary angiography because of symptoms of chest pain (yet have normal coronary arteries) are thought to have anxiety disorders such as panic disorder. Subsequently categorized as having "atypical chest pain," these patients may suffer chest pain in response to anxiety and/or hyperventilation.[156,157]

However, a large, multicity survey of 875 primary care outpatients revealed that patients with CHF or MI exhibited a point prevalence rate of at least one anxiety disorder (panic disorder, phobia, or generalized anxiety disorder) of 18 percent[155] (Table 91-5). Whether the prevalence of anxiety disorders is elevated in patients who are hospitalized for CAD (e.g., elective coronary catheterization, post MI, or unstable angina) remains to be determined.

TABLE 91-2 12-Month Prevalence of DSM-III-R Disorders in the National Comorbidity Survey (NCS)[4]

Disorder	%
Any anxiety disorder	19.3
Any addictive disorder	11.3
Any mood disorder	11.3
Nonaffective psychosis	0.3
Any NCS disorder	30.9

TABLE 91-3 12-Month Prevalence of Diagnosed Anxiety Disorders in the National Comorbidity Survey[4]

Disorder	%
Simple phobia	8.8
Social phobia	7.9
Posttraumatic stress disorder	3.9
Generalized anxiety disorder	3.1
Agoraphobia	2.8
Panic disorder	2.3
Obsessive-compulsive disorder	<1.0
Any anxiety disorder	19.3

A small number of prospective epidemiologic studies (which control for many of the commonly accepted risk factors for IHD) indicate an increased relative risk of nonfatal and fatal CVD events in patients with anxiety symptoms, even among individuals who have "simple" phobias (e.g., claustrophobia and fear of illness, heights, crowds, or going out alone).[158-163] A dose-response relationship has been demonstrated in these studies, with minimal symptoms of anxiety sufficient to elevate risk, suggesting that nonclinical, or "normal" levels of anxiety may play some role in the development of IHD.[164] Moreover, an ancillary study of 348 CAST and CAST II participants who had asymptomatic ventricular arrhythmias after MI and were treated with placebo revealed that stressful life events during the initial 4 months of participation in CAST trial and higher anxiety were predictive of mortality independently of the effects of physiologic variables such as diabetes and ejection fraction.[152]

PATHOPHYSIOLOGY OF ANXIETY

The neurocircuitry of anxiety has been postulated to arise from the amygdala, the brain area that registers the emotional significance of environmental stimuli and stores emotional memories. The efferent pathways from the central nucleus of the amygdala travel to a multiplicity of critical brain structures, including the parabrachial nucleus (resulting in dyspnea and hyperventilation), the dorsomedial nucleus of the vagus nerve and nucleus ambiguous (activating the parasympathetic nervous system), and the lateral hypothalamus (resulting in SNS activation).[165] Through reciprocal neuronal pathways connecting the amygdala to the medial prefrontal cortex, cognitive experience of the specific anxiety disorder differs, although fear symptoms may overlap. During panic attacks the fear is of imminent death; in social phobia, the fear is of embarassment; in posttraumatic stress disorder, the traumatic memory is remembered or reexperienced; in obsessive-compulsive disorder, obsessional ideas recur and intrude; and in generalized anxiety disorder, anxiety is "free-floating" (i.e., not conditioned to specific situations or triggers).[166]

Described in the past with terms such as *cardiac neurosis, irritable heart syndrome, battle fatigue,* and *soldier's heart,* panic disorder is the anxiety disorder most often associated with cardiovascular symptoms of chest pain, tachycardia, and dyspnea. Discrete panic attacks can be induced in the laboratory setting, especially in patients with panic disorder, by a variety of stimuli: sodium lactate, caffeine, isoproterenol, serotonin receptor agonist m-chlorophenylpiperazine (m-CPP), cholecystokinin tetrapeptide (CCK_4), inhalation of CO_2-enriched air, and voluntary acute hyperventilation of room air. The common element among these disparate inducers may be their ability

TABLE 91-4 Diagnostic Criteria of the Most Common DSM-IV Anxiety Disorders[3]

DSM-IV Criteria of Simple Phobia

Marked and persistent fear that is excessive or unreasonable, cued by the presence or anticipation of a specific object or situation (e.g., flying, heights, animals, receiving an injection, seeing blood).

Exposure to the phobic stimulus almost invariably provokes an immediate anxiety response, which may take the form of a situationally bound or situationally predisposed panic attack.

The person (adults only) recognizes that the feature is excessive or unreasonable.

The phobic situation is avoided or else is endured with intense anxiety or distress.

The avoidance, anxious anticipation, or distress in the feared situations interferes significantly with the person's normal routine, occupational (or academic) functioning, or social activities or relationships.

Or there is marked distress about having the phobia.

DSM-IV Diagnostic Criteria of Social Phobia

Marked fear of being focus of attention; avoidance of meeting unfamiliar people and close scrutiny by others.

Fear of behaving in embarassing or humiliating way.

Extreme anticipatory anxiety, which may manifest itself as a panic attack.

DSM-IV Diagnostic Criteria of Posttraumatic Stress Disorder

Experience of a traumatic event.

Reexperienced by intrusive and distressing recollection, dreams, flashbacks, distress in similar situations.

Persistent avoidance of stimuli associated with trauma.

Persistent symptoms of increased arousal.

Duration of disturbance of at least 1 month.

DSM-IV Diagnostic Criteria of Panic Disorder

Recurrent and unexpected panic attacks.

Plus one or more of the following:

- Persistent concern about having additional attacks (anticipatory anxiety) or
- Worry about the consequences of the attacks or
- A significant change in behavior related to the attacks (phobic avoidance)

Not due to a substance, medical condition, or mental illness.

At least 2 unexpected panic attacks for diagnosis.

Definition of Panic Attack

A period of intense fear or discomfort in which at least 4 of the following symptoms develop suddenly:

- Palpitations or increased heart rate
- Sweating
- Trembling or shaking
- Sensations of shortness of breath or smothering
- Feeling of choking
- Nausea or abdominal distress
- Chest pain or discomfort
- Dizziness, light-headedness, or faintness
- Derealization or depersonalization
- Fear of losing control or going crazy
- Chills or hot flashes
- Paresthesia (numbness or tingling)
- Fear of dying

DSM-IV Criteria of Generalized Anxiety Disorder

Excessive anxiety and worry for more days than not for past 6 months.

Difficulty controlling worry.

Functional impairment and/or distress.

Symptoms not attributable to other causes.

Physical symptoms	Psychological symptoms
• Restlessness or feeling keyed up/on edge • Fatigue • Muscle tension	• Excessive anxiety or worry • Difficulty controlling worry • Irritability • Difficulty concentrating or mind going blank • Sleep disturbance

Reprinted with permission from the *Diagnostic and Statistical Manual of Mental Disorders,* 4th ed. Copyright 1994, American Psychiatric Association.

to stimulate the respiratory rate with the induction of an accompanying subjective sense of breathlessness.[167] Although some researchers have proposed that patients with panic disorder have only a heightened sensitivity to and develop a learned intolerance of tachypnea,[168] the higher concordance rate of panic disorder observed in monozygotic as compared with dizygotic twins[169] and evidence of altered respiratory rhythym during sleep[170] provide proof of a genetic diathesis and a biological abnormality, respectively, underlying the phenotype of panic disorder.[170]

A Focus on the Cardiovascular System

Although the neurobiology of specific anxiety disorders has not been explored as fully as that of unipolar depression, potential neurochemical, neuroendocrine, and neuroanatomic alterations have not only been identified but have been increasingly scrutinized. Patients with major depression or anxiety disorders may experience common symptoms (e.g., alterations in psychomotor activity, impairment of sleep, increased appetite, and reduced concentration). Moreover, there are several shared neurobiological findings between patients with certain common syndromal anxiety disorders and those with depression, although differences also exist. The neurobiology of patients with certain anxiety disorders is subsequently reviewed, with attention to mechanisms that contribute to the development of cardiovascular disease and/or cardiac-related mortality: HPA axis activity, sympathomedullary activity, diminished HRV, and alterations in platelet receptor number or function.

While limited and inconsistent evidence suggests that alterations of HPA axis activity occur across the anxiety disorder spectrum,[171,172] altered HPA axis activity has been most consistently documented in individuals with posttraumatic stress disorder (PTSD). In nearly all controlled studies of PTSD patients, alterations of HPA axis hyperactivity have been documented, including elevations of cerebrospinal fluid (CSF) CRF concentrations[173] and blunting of the ACTH response to CRF stimulation.[174] In comparison to control subjects, however, PTSD

TABLE 91-5 Prevalence of Comorbid Anxiety Disorders in Primary Care Outpatients*

	Major Depression (%)	Hypertension (%)	Diabetes (%)	Heart Disease (%)
Panic disorder	9.4	0.9†	1.1†	1.2†
Phobia	22.7	5.5†	4.8†	9.2†
Generalized anxiety disorder	54.1	10.4†	11.9†	12.4†
Any anxiety disorder	66.3	14.6†	15.5†	17.8†

*Diagnosis of congestive heart failure or myocardial infarction within the previous year, adjusted for patient age, sex, race, education, marital status, income, study site, and each of the other medical or psychiatric conditions.
†Value significantly different from that of patients with current depression ($p \leq .05$), based on regression coefficients.
SOURCE: Sherbourne et al.[155]

patients generally exhibit reduced plasma cortisol concentrations, diminished 24-h urinary cortisol concentrations, and a greater suppression of plasma cortisol concentrations in response to low doses (e.g., 0.5 mg) of dexamethasone.[175,176] However the two studies that measured CSF CRF concentrations in PTSD[177,173] found results identical to those repeatedly reported in depression: elevated CSF CRF concentrations. Whether patients with PTSD experience an increased (or decreased) relative risk of CVD is not known. Potential confounds in those studies include the very high rate of comorbid substance abuse and alcoholism as well as tobacco abuse in PTSD patients. Patients with panic disorder do not appear to exhibit alterations in HPA axis function consistently; scrutiny continues of patients with social phobia, generalized anxiety disorder, and obsessive-compulsive disorder.

Sympathomedullary function has been investigated intensively in patients with panic disorder. As was discussed previously, plasma concentrations of catecholamines are determined by the rate of release, local metabolic degradation, synaptic reuptake, and redistribution into other extravascular spaces.[178] To examine systemic as well as regional sympathomedullary kinetics, investigators infuse intravenous trace amounts of radiolabeled NE and epinephrine (EPI). Arterial or "arterialized venous" samples of endogenous catecholamines are then obtained, and a "compartmental analysis" is performed to mathematically fit the data into a two-compartment ("whole-body" versus "cardiac" or "extravascular" versus "vascular"/plasma compartments) model. Whole-body NE "spillover" (the rate of NE appearance in plasma), a sensitive measure of systemic SNS activity, is similar under basal conditions in panic patients and control subjects[179] and increases to a similar degree in both groups under laboratory mental stress.[179] Panic patients do, however, exhibit significantly higher cardiac spillover rates of coronary sinus (cardiac-derived) EPI under basal conditions, increased whole-body EPI secretion during laboratory mental stress, and surges of EPI whole-body spillover during panic attacks. Such increases in EPI in panic patients presumably are due to "loading" of sympathetic neuronal stores by uptake from plasma during surges of EPI secretion during panic attacks.[179] Further investigation of cardiac and/or systemic sympathomedullary activation during spontaneous or pharmacologically provoked panic attacks is needed to confirm these findings, along with prospective investigations of the cardiac-related risk of patients with panic disorder.[180,181] However, multiple prospective cohort studies (which control for other accepted risk factors for IHD) report that increasing severity of anxiety is associated with an increased risk for developing elevated systolic blood pressure[181] or hypertension.[182,183] However, given the comorbidity between anxiety and depressive symptoms and syndromes, further studies are required to determine whether the evidence of increased risk for the development of CAD (or hypertension) in anxiety disorder patients is independent of the contribution of depression.[164]

Another area awaiting investigation in patients with anxiety disorders is platelet receptor function, particularly the receptors most integral to thrombovascular repair and disease. Psychobiological studies of patients with panic disorder, in contrast to reports of patients with major depression, have not detected alterations of platelet 5-HT transporters and platelet 5-HT$_2$ receptors. In comparison to control subjects, however, patients with panic attacks have been reported, like those with depression, to exhibit increased plasma concentrations of PF4 and β-TG, providing evidence of increased platelet secretion. Moreover, after treatment of panic patients with alprazolam, plasma concentrations of these alpha granule-specific proteins were reduced significantly.[184] The presence of anxiety disorders has been hypothesized to trigger coronary events through atherosclerotic plaque rupture, coronary vasospasm, ventricular arrhythmias, or atrial arrhthymias.[164] Panic-induced hyperventilation is a well-known precipitant of coronary spasm,[185] which in turn may induce ventricular arrhythmias and MI.[161]

Emergency room physicians and cardiologists are well acquainted with the challenges of evaluating patients with an acute onset of chest discomfort, combined with painful and overwhelming anxiety symptoms, which may or may not be associated with clinically significant cardiovascular disease (Table 91-6). The most compelling evidence regarding the association of anxiety disorders and cardiovascular dysfunction comes from reports of abnormal cardiac autonomic control.[164] Examination of HRV in patients with anxiety

TABLE 91-6 Medical Conditions Associated with Anxiety Symptoms

- Cardiovascular disorders: mitral valve prolapse, coronary artery disease, paroxysmal tachycardia, hypertension, hypotension
- Endocrinopathies: hyperthyroidism, hypothyroidism, diabetes, hypoglycemia, hypocalcemia, porphyria, endocrine tumors
- Neurologic disorders: migraine headaches, transient ischemic attacks, temporal lobe seizures
- Pulmonary disease: asthma, chronic obstructive pulmonary disease, pulmonary embolus
- Vestibular dysfunction: Meniere's disease
- Infectious diseases: tuberculosis, brucellosis, human immunodeficiency virus or acquired immunodeficiency syndrome
- Drug effects: cocaine abuse, alcohol or sedative withdrawal, sympathomimetics, caffeine, monosodium glutamate, akathisia

disorders has revealed that patients with panic disorder[186,187] and patients with generalized anxiety disorder[188] exhibit reductions in high-frequency HRV.[189] As was noted earlier, diminished HRV increases the risk of arrhythmias and sudden cardiac death. Indeed, patients with panic disorder or agoraphobia exhibit a higher density of PVCs in comparison to patients with other anxiety disorders[190] and normal comparison subjects.[191] Whether patients with panic disorder (or other anxiety disorders) exhibit increased rates of sudden cardiac death remains to be determined.

Although so-called mental disorders may produce effects on cardiovascular function, perhaps less well understood are the cardiovascular contributions to certain anxiety disorders. Whether cardiovascular abnormalities or dysfunction reliably produce symptoms of anxiety is an intriguing area of investigation (e.g., is worsening of CHF associated with an increased incidence of panic attacks?). In comparison to gender- and age-matched controls, individuals with cardiac arrhythmias exhibited significantly higher self-reported anxiety scores.[192] Whether a causal biological mechanism exists between PVCs and anxiety symptoms or disorders or there is merely an association remains to be determined.[193]

Certainly, the impact of anxiety disorders on the development of and worsening of CVD should be more completely discriminated from the contributions of depressive symptoms or syndromes.[164] Such knowledge carries the promise of anxiety symptom reduction and improved quality of life and the potential for new treatment modalities to enhance cardiovascular function in patients with CVD who have comorbid anxiety disorders.

Treatment of Major Depression and Anxiety Disorders in Patients with Cardiovascular Disease

As with other medical disorders, effective treatment of major psychiatric illnesses such as major depression and panic disorder, respectively, require patient access to informed health care practioners, accurate diagnosis, affordable treatment, and safe, effective treatment modalities. Factors hampering well-conducted psychiatric (psychotherapeutic or psychopharmacologic and somatic) treatment include patient reluctance, social stigma regarding psychiatric treatment, managed care restrictions, and a dearth of psychiatrists and psychologists, particularly in rural areas. However, the evidence of the adverse impact of affective and anxiety disorders on relatively young and physically healthy individuals as well as medically ill patients heralds an opportunity and an accompanying incentive to prevent or limit the personal suffering, economic cost, and social disability associated with mental disorders. Although the safety and efficacy of anxiolytic and antidepressant treatment in patients with cardiovascular disease remain to be extensively established in randomized clinical trials, these agents, particularly the newly introduced ones, are prescribed routinely to patients with heart disease. This seems appropriate given the drastic reduction in psychosocial function associated with anxiety or depressive disorders and the extant literature demonstrating the safety and efficacy of these psychotropic agents in generally healthy populations, existing data from psychopharmacologic treatment of medically ill patients, and the paucity of psychiatric practitioners available to patients with severe CVD.

Many heart patients believe that their persistent "worry," "lack of enjoyment of life," or "loss of interest" constitutes an understandable (and untreatable) condition. However, given the prevalence of major depression in patients with heart disease, the astute clinician's index of suspicion should always be heightened. Third-party information (particularly from a spouse or other caregiver) is often more reveal-

ing of the true extent of a patient's symptoms (e.g., irritability, social isolation, or listlessness), including attempts to "self-medicate" through abuse of alcohol, prescription medication, or illicit substances. A thorough evaluation of anxiety, panic attacks (if any), and depressive symptoms should be performed, including queries regarding feelings of pessimism, hopelessness, and the wish not to continue living. While the preferences of cardiac patients, as with any medical disorder, should be respected, cardiac patients and their families should always be gently apprised of the risks of untreated depression (CVD-related morbidity and mortality) versus the options of psychotherapeutic and/or psychopharmacologic treatment. Consultation with a knowledgeable mental health provider can assist in the discrimination of depressive disorders from complicated or pathologic grief, delirium, ascertainment of coexisting anxiety disorders (such as generalized anxiety disorder or social phobia), detection of intoxication or withdrawal syndromes, and appropriate emotional reactions.

The efficacy (and safety) of psychotherapeutic and psychopharmacologic treatment of post-MI patients with comorbid major depression or any of the anxiety disorders is an area undergoing intense investigation. In two large-scale, randomized, multicenter studies, the Montreal Heart Attack Readjustment Trial (M-HART) ($n = 1376$)[194] and the Enhancing Recovering in Coronary Heart Disease (ENRICHD) Patients Study ($n = 2481$), sponsored by the National Heart, Lung, and Blood Institute,[195] the psychosocial interventions were not superior to routine care in reducing cardiac events or prolonging survival. Whereas the individual and group cognitive behavior psychotherapy of ENRICHD was effective in reducing depressive symptoms (57 percent reduction in depression in the treatment arm versus 47 percent reduction in the control group) and improving social support (27 percent improvement in social support in the treatment group compared with an 18 percent improvement in the usual care group), the home-based telephone monitoring and psychosocial nursing intervention of M-HART appeared detrimental to women with depression or lack of social support.[194] Older, smaller studies have reported successful psychological interventions with post-MI patients[196,197] targeted primarily to diminish "psychological distress"[198] or alter type A personality traits.[199]

With the introduction of fluoxetine (Prozac) in the United States and citalopram (Celexa) in Europe in 1989, over a decade of clinical information has been gleaned regarding the selective serotonin reuptake inhibitor (SSRI) class of antidepressants. Furthermore, during the 1990s, the SSRIs and more recently the 5-HT and NE reuptake inhibitor (SSNRI) venlafaxine superseded the benzodiazepines as the first-line treatment of choice for anxiety disorders.[205] These newer antidepressants provide significant reduction of anxiety symptoms in approximately 60 percent of medically healthy patients without having a potential for addiction. SSRIs and SSNRIs have been approved by U.S. Food and Drug Agency for the treatment of panic disorder (paroxetine, Paxil, and sertraline, Zoloft), social anxiety disorder (social phobia, paroxetine), obsessive-compulsive disorder (paroxetine, sertraline, fluoxetine and fluvoxamine, Luvox), and generalized anxiety disorder (paroxetine, venlafaxine, Effexor) (Table 91-7). It is important to note that the SSRIs, although they all are potent 5-HT reuptake inhibitors, also exert unique effects on other neurotransmitter systems. Thus, paroxetine is a very potent inhibitor of NE reuptake, whereas sertraline is a potent inhibitor of dopamine (DA) reuptake. The clinical sequelae of these pharmacologic properties remain obscure.

During the time (often 6 to 8 weeks) before the onset of an antidepressant's anxiolytic effect, benzodiazepines such as lorazepam, alprazolam, and clonazepam may be utilized. These agents are rap-

TABLE 91-7 Cardiac-Related Side Effects of Psychotropic Agents Commonly Utilized for Treatment of Anxiety or Depression

Class	Cardiovascular Side Effects	Likely Mechanism of Side Effect	Other Effects and Benefits
Tricyclic and related cyclic antidepressants	Orthostatic hypotension	Postsynaptic alpha$_1$-receptor blockade	
Nortriptyline (Pamelor) Imipramine (Tofranil) Amitriptyline (Elavil)			Nortriptyline with lowest incidence of orthostatic hypotension[200–201]
Desipramine (Norpramin) Clomipramine (Anafranil)	Tachycardia	Secondary to hypotension	
Doxepin (Sinequan)	Decreased heart rate variability	Postsynaptic cholinergic receptor blockade	Urinary retention, dry mouth, constipation, confusion, exacerbation of narrow-angle glaucoma
Trimipramine (Surmontil) Protriptyline (Vivactil)	Slowing of intraventricular conduction	Quinidine-like effects	Avoid in patients with bifascicular block, left bundle branch block, QTc > 44 ms, or QRS > 11 ms
Monoamine oxidase inhibitors Phenelzine (Nardil) Tranylcypromine (Parnate) Isocarboxazid (Marplan)	Orthostatic hypotension Hypertensive crisis	Inhibition of metabolism of serotonin and catecholamines	Fatal in overdose Requires adherence to tyramine-free diet, and avoidance of other antidepressants, and sympathomimetics
Selective serotonin reuptake inhibitors (SSRIs)		Postsynaptic serotonin receptor blockade	Fatal in overdose Typical SSRI side effects: nausea, insomnia, sexual dysfunction, nervousness
Fluoxetine (Prozac)	Sinus bradycadia[202]	Unknown	Requires 8 weeks for complete washout Inhibitor of CYP$_{450}$ IID6 and CYP$_{450}$ IIIA4 enzymes Also FDA-approved for treatment of adult and pediatric obsessive compulsive disorder (OCD), bulimia, pediatric depression
Paroxetine (Paxil)	Clinically insignificant decreases in heart rate[203]	Unknown	Inhibitor of CYP$_{450}$ IID6 enzyme Also FDA-approved for treatment of social phobia, panic disorder, OCD, generalized anxiety disorder (GAD)
Sertraline (Zoloft)	None known		In high doses, inhibitor of CYP$_{450}$ IID6 enzyme Also FDA-approved for treatment of panic disorder, adult and pediatric OCD, post-traumatic stress disorder (PTSD)
Fluvoxamine (Luvox)	None known		Potent inhibitor of multiple CYP$_{450}$ enzymes Also FDA-approved for treatment of adult and pediatric OCD

(continued)

TABLE 91-7 Cardiac-Related Side Effects of Psychotropic Agents Commonly Utilized for Treatment of Anxiety or Depression (*Continued*)

Class	Cardiovascular Side Effects	Likely Mechanism of Side Effect	Other Effects and Benefits
Citalopram (Celexa)	None known		
Escitalopram (Lexapro)	None known		SSRI with most selective binding to serotonin transporter
Venlafaxine (Effexor)	Arrhythmia or cardiac block in overdose[204]	Unknown	No significant inhibition of CYP_{450} enzymes
			Also FDA-approved for treatment of GAD
	Increased diastolic blood pressure in doses > 300 mg/d[205]	Presynaptic inhibition of norepinephrine reuptake	Side-effect profile similar to SSRIs
Presynaptic alpha$_2$-receptor antagonist			
Mirtazapine (Remeron)	None known	Postsynaptic histamine$_1$-receptor blockade	Very sedating in low doses
			Weight gain
			Minimal sexual side effects
			No significant inhibition of CYP_{450} enzymes
Dopamine and norepinephrine reuptake inhibitor			
Bupropion (Wellbutrin; Zyban)	Significant increases in blood pressure in patients with preexisting hypertension[200]	Presynaptic inhibition of norepinephrine reuptake	No significant inhibition of CYP_{450} enzymes
			Minimal sexual side effects
			Not proven effective in the treatment of anxiety disorders
			FDA-approved for treatment of nicotine dependence
Atypical serotonergic agents			
Trazodone (Desyrel)	Orthostatic hypotension	Postsynaptic alpha$_1$-receptor blockade	Sedation, confusion, dizziness
	Cardiac arrhythmias rare[206]	unknown	Rare cases of priapism
Nefazodone (Serzone)	Sinus bradycardia[207]	unknown	Similar side-effect profile as trazodone (except without priapism)
			Minimal sexual side effects
			Potent inhibitor of multiple CYP_{450} enzymes
			Liver failure rare
Psychostimulants			
Dextroamphetamine (Dexedrine)	Rarely increases blood pressure or induces tachycardia in therapeutic doses	Release of dopamine and catecholamines	Avoid in patients with hyperthyroidism, severe hypertension, severe angina, tachyarrhythmias
Methylphenidate (Ritalin)			
Benzodiazepines		Allosteric alteration of GABA$_A$ receptors	Rapid relief of anxiety symptoms
Alprazolam (Xanax)			
Clonazepam (Klonopin)			
Lorazepam (Ativan)	Hypotension	Muscle relaxation via GABA$_A$ spinal cord receptors	Can cause fatigue, ataxia, drowsiness, amnesia, and behavioral dyscontrol
Oxazepam (Serax)			Relatively safe in overdose
			Physiologic and psychologic dependence and withdrawal symptoms if dosage not gradually tapered

(continued)

TABLE 91-7   Cardiac-Related Side Effects of Psychotropic Agents Commonly Utilized for Treatment of Anxiety or Depression (*Continued*)

Class	Cardiovascular Side Effects	Likely Mechanism of Side Effect	Other Effects and Benefits
Partial 5-HT$_{1A}$-receptor agonist Buspirone (BuSpar)	None known		FDA-approved for treatment of GAD Nonaddictive
Omega$_1$-receptor agonist Zolpidem (Ambien)	None known	Potentiation of GABA$_A$ receptor	Sedating Nonaddictive
Zaleplon (Sonata)	None known		
Lithium	Sinus node dysfunction Sinoatrial block T-wave inversion or flattening, Particularly in patients >60 years of age Arrhythmias and sudden death in patients with cardiac disease	Unknown	Narrow therapeutic index (.6-1.2 mmol/L) Many medications alter lithium plasma levels* Fatal in overdose Mood stabilizer for patients with bipolar disorder Yearly ECG in patients over 50

*Medications that increase lithium levels: nonsteroidal anti-inflammatory drugs, diuretics (thiazides, ethacrynic acid, spironolactone, triamterene), angiotensin-converting enzyme inhibitors, metronidazole, tetracycline. Medications that decrease lithium levels: acetazolamide, theophylline, aminophylline, caffeine, osmotic diuretics.[204]

ABBREVIATION: GABA = gamma-aminobutyric acid.

idly effective but should be used only for short-term treatment (6- to 8-week duration) of disabling anxiety symptoms. Benzodiazepines are sedating, produce gait instability, impair memory, may induce behavioral disinhibition, are ineffective in the treatment of coexisting depressive syndromes, and place patients at risk of physiologic (and psychologic) dependence.

The use of tricyclic and structurally related antidepressants should be limited in patients with CVD because of the myriad of side effects of these drugs on the cardiovascular system, including orthostatic hypotension, tachycardia, reduction in HRV, and slowing of intraventricular conduction (as a result of quinidine-like effects; see Table 91-7). These antidepressants should never be prescribed for patients with bifascicular and left fascicular block.[208] As might be expected, examination of prescription databases has revealed an increased risk of MI with administration of TCAs in comparison to SSRIs and atypical antidepressants.[209,210] Monoamine oxidase inhibitors and trazodone are generally free of effects on cardiac conduction but, like the TCAs, may cause postural hypotension.[211] Because of their fewer potential adverse effects on the cardiovascular system and the lack of lethality from an overdose, pharmacotherapeutic treatment with SSRIs, the SSNRI venlafaxine, or other "atypical" antidepressants (such as bupropion, nefazodone, and mirtazapine) may offer significant advantages in depressed or anxious patients with CVD.

The only known cardiac effect of SSRIs is severe sinus node slowing, which to date has been reported in only a few cases.[212,213] 5-HT has been implicated in both platelet aggregation and coronary artery vasoconstriction; the SSRIs, which are widely used to treat major depression, produce effects on platelet function. The case reports of altered hemostasis[214,215] with SSRI treatment, combined with findings of in vivo clinical studies indicate that SSRIs reduce platelet activation in patients with major depression, without[113,216] and with,[128] CAD. Though potentially advantageous in patients with heightened platelet activation (e.g., smokers[217]), retrospective examinations of large-scale medication databases have revealed no such

cardioprotective effective[218] or even an increased risk of upper gastrointestinal bleeding with SSRI antidepressants,[219] especially when coprescribed with nonsteroidal anti-inflammatory drugs.[220] Conversely, other investigators have not documented an increased risk of upper gastrointestinal bleeding in SSRI-treated patients,[221] or a propensity for intracranial hemorrage.[222]

Because of inhibition of some cytochrome P$_{450}$ isoenzymes, certain SSRIs may alter the metabolism of medications often used in patients with heart disease. The SSRIs that inhibit the P$_{450}$ 2D6 isoenzyme (fluoxetine, paroxetine, fluvoxamine, and higher doses of sertraline) should be used with caution in patients receiving medications metabolized by the P$_{450}$ 2D6 (e.g., lipophilic beta blockers and type 1C antiarrhythmics: flecainide, mexiletine, propafenone). SSRIs that inhibit the P$_{450}$ 3A4 isoenzyme (fluoxetine, fluvoxamine, nefazodone) may increase the plasma concentrations of calcium channel blockers and warfarin.[223] Although the antidepressants venlafaxine, bupropion, citalopram, and mirtazapine exhibit minimal hepatic P$_{450}$ enzyme inhibition, their safety remains to be established in patients with CVD who have comorbid depression or anxiety disorders.

After short-term treatment with buproprion,[224] fluoxetine,[225] paroxetine, fluvoxamine,[92] or paroxetine,[203] depressed patients exhibit no changes in HRV. A randomized, double-blind, multicenter study compared the efficacy of nortriptyline and paroxetine in depressed patients with IHD.[203] Both antidepressants were effective in the treatment of depression, but not surprisingly, there were more dropouts because of side effects and more cardiac-related effects with the TCA. The SADHART study, a randomized, multicenter, double-blind trial of sertraline ($n = 186$) versus placebo ($n = 183$) attempted to determine the safety and efficacy of this SSRI in the treatment of patients hospitalized for unstable angina or index MI. Sertraline exerted no significant effect upon LVEF, in comparison to placebo, or did it exact increases in ventricular premature complex runs or QTc interval, or other cardiac parameters. Moreover, in comparison to placebo-treated patients, depressed individuals with at least one prior episode of depression exhibited a significant improvement in depressive symptoms (72 vs 51 percent; $p = .003$), especially those who exhibited depressive symptoms of moderate or greater severity (78 vs 45 percent; $p = .001$). The SADHART sertraline efficacy data are generally congruent with efficacy of other oral antidepressants in "medically healthy" patients with major depression. That is, any of the available oral antidepressants will usually produce a therapeutic response (an improvement in depressive symptoms by 50 percent or more, in comparison to pretreatment severity of depressive symptoms) in 60 to 70 percent of depressed patients, provided that the antidepressant is administered in sufficient dosage over a treatment duration of 5 to 6 weeks.[226] While there is limited, case-control evidence suggesting a role for SSRIs in decreasing the likelihood of MI in smokers,[217] there are as yet no prospective, randomized, controlled trials demonstrating that treatment with SSRIs diminishes future cardiac morbidity or mortality.

Another somatic treatment modality, electroconvulsive therapy (ECT), is effective in up to 80 percent of patients with either unipolar or bipolar depression.[227,228] ECT has several advantages over medication management of depression. The time to response for ECT is 1 to 3 weeks compared to the 4 to 8 weeks needed for antidepressants, and ECT is clearly the most effective treatment for depression. The most recent trial of ECT in middle-aged and older adults with severe treatment-resistant depression found that more than 80 percent had complete remission of their depressive symptoms.[229] A comparable group of patients treated with antidepressants would be expected to have a remission rate of no better than 30 to 40 percent.

ECT is the treatment of choice in depressed patients who are severely ill (e.g., at nutritional risk from severe calorie loss or dehydration) and require a rapid clinical response. ECT also should be considered for patients who have experienced a previous positive response to ECT, do not respond to oral antidepressants, or cannot tolerate the associated side effects of antidepressants. Patient variables associated with a positive response include increasing age[229] and the presence of psychotic (e.g., hallucinations and delusions) and catatonic symptoms.[227]

The morbidity and mortality associated with ECT have decreased dramatically over the past 60 years. The introduction of curare and, later succinylcholine, decreased the incidence of orthopedic complications from almost 20 percent of cases to being a rare complication. In fact, patients recovering from such orthopedic surgery as that involving the hip can safely be given ECT. Complications related to cognitive dysfunction, such as delirium and amnesia, also have been decreased through the use of brief pulse (versus sine wave) and unilateral (versus bilateral) ECT.

ECT produces a seizure by providing a brief pulse (approximately 1 to 2 s in duration) of electrical charge over the scalp in the area of the right parietal lobe (right unilateral ECT) or over both temples (bilateral ECT). This pulse elicits a generalized convulsive seizure that lasts approximately 30 to 60 s. The patient is anesthetized during the procedure with a short-acting barbiturate (e.g., methohexital), propofol, or etomidate and paralyzed with a muscle relaxant such as succinylcholine. Respirations are controlled by masked ventilation, and intubation is not required unless there have been recurrent episodes of aspiration.

Structural brain studies using magnetic resonance images have shown no evidence of brain damage secondary to ECT.[230] Moreover, most studies of memory problems associated with ECT have reported that patients have transient amnesia. Memory loss is increased with the use of bilateral rather than unilateral ECT and is directly correlated with the number of treatments administered and higher stimulus intensity.[228] Evidence for amnesia should be monitored carefully during ECT as some patients may experience permanent retrograde memory loss.[231] However, more commonly, anterograde and retrograde memory problems occur in a temporal gradient around the time of ECT and clear completely within 6 months of the ECT treatment period.

ECT-related delirium is relatively rare, however; the risk for delirium increases in patients who are older, have comorbid neurologic disorders with associated brain pathology (e.g., Alzheimer's disease, Parkinson's disease, or periventricular white matter changes on magnetic resonance imaging) and/or are receiving more than 8 to 10 treatments. The delirium usually clears within 24 h and can be minimized by changing the treatment parameters (e.g., using unilateral rather than bilateral electrode placement) and treating 2 rather than 3 times a week.

Until recently, the cardiac complications from ECT resulted in the most serious adverse events. As recently as the 1980s, deaths from ECT were estimated to be approximately 1 per 10,000 treatments (most patients receive 6 to 10 treatments per ECT trial), primarily as a result of cardiac complications. Two major cardiac complications occur in relation to the ECT stimulus: an initial asystole secondary to vagal nerve stimulation followed closely by the release of EPI with tachycardia and hypertension. Although the patient is paralyzed, the ECT electrode that conducts up to 100 Joules of energy to stimulate the seizure also produces a direct stimulus of the masseter muscles (a bite block is kept in place during the treatments) and the vagus nerve. The stimulation of the vagus nerve can subsequently cause asystole. Within seconds of vagal stimulation, an adrenergic discharge related to the onset of a generalized seizure causes the release of EPI with tachycardia, hypertension, and the potential for myocardial ischemia or arrhythmias. The tachycardia is relatively brief (1 to 2 min).

Certain clinical situations increase the risk of complications from a course of ECT (i.e., diseases that affect the CNS and/or the cardio-thrombovascular system): a cerebral vascular accident (CVA) during the previous 6 months, any illness that increases intracranial pressure (e.g., brain tumor), medical disorders that disrupt the blood-brain barrier (e.g., meningitis), a cerebral or aortic aneurysm, MI, severe valvular heart disease, a high-grade atrioventricular block, symptomatic ventricular arrhythmias, supraventricular arrhythmias with uncontrolled ventricular rate, and coagulation or bleeding disorders.[232] Implanted cardiac pacemakers and defibrillators are usually not problematic during ECT.[233] Some practitioners choose to convert a demand pacemaker to a fixed mode, and an electrophysiologist should be consulted to determine whether the defibrillator's function should be inhibited during each ECT treatment. Electroconvulsive therapy also is tolerated by cardiac transplant patients who have normal cardiac function.[234]

Electroconvulsive therapy can be conceptualized as a cardiac stress test with peak heart rates of 120 to 140 BPM; however, because of the general anesthesia, the patient cannot report symptoms such as chest pain, and the seizure stimulating the tachycardia cannot be terminated abruptly. Therefore, the pre-ECT workup should include a complete review of systems and a screen for exercise intolerance, angina, evidence of congestive heart failure (patients will receive approximately 1 L of fluid per ECT treatment) or diabetes, extent of smoking history, cholesterol level, and other cardiac risk factors. The basic pre-ECT screening includes measurement of serum electrolytes (with particular attention to hydration status and potassium) and hemoglobin and the obtaining of an electrocardiogram (ECG). Chest x-rays are obtained in case of evidence of CHF or pulmonary disease. Patients with a history of back pain are evaluated with spine films; neuroimaging is used to determine whether there has been a recent CVA or increased intracranial pressure in patients with neurologic dysfunction. Although "beta blockers" are used during ECT treatment (see later), cardiovascular screening should determine whether the patient can tolerate transient tachycardia and hypertension. Patients with evidence for CAD can be screened with a relatively inexpensive treadmill test establishing a peak heart rate of at least 120. ECT patients with severe depression, however, are typically sedentary, elderly, and often unable to tolerate even minimal physical activity. Many would be unable to complete a treadmill test, and more expensive tests such as a persantine thallium stress test can be substituted when appropriate.

Modern ECT suites are equipped with continuous ECG and blood pressure and heart rate monitors as well as pulse oximetry and an electroencephalograph to record seizure activity. Patients should continue their pulmonary (except theophylline) and cardiac (except lidocaine) medications during a course of ECT treatment. Theophylline and lidocaine are discontinued because of prolongation and reduction of seizure duration, respectively. As a result of the increase in intraocular pressure during an ECT-induced seizure, glaucoma medications generally are continued, except for acetylcholinesterases. Hypoglycemic agents should not be administered the morning of ECT to prevent hypoglycemia in diabetic patients. Patients must not ingest food or fluids before ECT treatments but may receive intravenous fluids as tolerated. In addition to usual ECT medications (methohexital 1 mg/kg and succinylcholine 0.75 to 1.50 mg/kg), patients with hypertension, CAD, valvular heart disease, and CHF routinely receive prophylactic medication to prevent cardiac complications from the transient hypertension and tachycardia induced by ECT.[235] Such a "cardiac-modified" ECT protocol[236] should be utilized for elderly patients and those with cardiac disease. Usually either of two beta blockers, labetalol or esmolol, is utilized to reduce maximal heart rate, mean arterial pressure, and arrhythmia frequency during ECT. Labetalol, a selective alpha$_1$- and nonselective beta-adrenergic receptor blocker, with an elimination half-life of 5 to 8 h, may induce significant hypotension.[237] Esmolol (beta$_1$ selective at the usual doses, rapid onset, and an elimination half-life of 9 min) may replace labetalol if labetalol induces prolonged bradycardia and hypotension. Esmolol, however, has been associated with shortened seizure duration during ECT. If elderly patients pretreated with a beta blocker continue to exhibit transient increases in blood pressure, a calcium channel blocker may be added. Nicardipine has replaced nifedipine as the calcium channel blocker of choice because nicardepine may be administered intravenously and has a shorter duration of action. The ECT protocol also involves adequate hydration before ECT, discontinuation of psychotropic medication whenever possible, and provision of anticholinergic medication (0.4 to 0.8 mg intravenous atropine or 0.2 mg of glycopyrrolate) to decrease oropharyngeal secretions and prevent bradycardias whenever beta blockers are used.[238] Caffeine sodium benzoate (usual dose = 120 to 140 mg) may be administered intravenously prior to ECT to maintain adequate seizure duration[239] and does not appear to significantly affect peak pulse rates during ECT. Continuous blood pressure monitoring and ECG monitoring should be performed during all treatments, along with monitoring for shortness of breath or chest pain.

The third most common cardiac complication is orthostatic hypotension, which usually occurs in the recovery room, particularly in elderly debilitated patients and patients with medical conditions associated with autonomic dysfunction (e.g., Parkinson's disease). As was noted earlier, consideration should be given to the utilization of shorter-acting beta blockers that have less alpha-adrenoreceptor blockade (esmolol for labetalol) and/or shorter-acting calcium channel blockers (nicardepine for nifedipine). After each ECT treatment, patients recover for over an hour in a setting similar to an outpatient surgical suite. Patients remain on a cardiac monitor with intravenous fluids and supplemental oxygen provided until they are oriented and exhibit no orthostatic hypotension (approximately 20 to 30 min). They are then dressed and asked to be seated upright in a chair until they are fully alert and able to ingest fluids orally (approximately 20 to 30 min in duration).

In summary, the magnitude of the risks associated with ECT are approximately equivalent to those of general anesthesia. The incidence of delirium during ECT can be reduced to less than 5 percent in elderly patients through the administration of twice-weekly ECT treatments and the use of unilateral electrode placement on the right temporal area in patients at risk (patients with structural brain changes, concomitant medical illness, Alzheimer's disease, Parkinson's disease, advanced age, and concomitant administration of psychotropic medications).[238] Cardiac complications are not uncommon with ECT but are reduced significantly with a cardiac ECT protocol. Although generally a safe and effective treatment, ECT in elderly patients with cardiovascular disease requires a multispecialty coordinated effort among a specially trained ECT-nursing service, psychiatrist, anesthesiologist, and cardiologist.

FUTURE DIRECTIONS FOR RESEARCH

Usually underdiagnosed and undertreated, major depression and anxiety disorders are encountered commonly in patients with CAD and patients referred for evaluation of chest pain. However, a burgeoning literature on the importance of major depression and anxiety disorders in patients with heart disease has accumulated over the past two decades. Several studies have shown depression and its associated symptoms to be a major risk factor in both the development of CVD and death after an index MI. Further evidence is accumulating regarding the increased risk of patients with anxiety disorders or anxiety symptoms for the development of IHD, although currently there is a dearth of information about the prevalence of anxiety disorders in patients with CAD or CHF. An intriguing area of investigation involves the possible effects of anxiety disorders on the thrombovascular system and the "reciprocal" cardiovascular contributions to anxiety symptoms or anxiety syndromes, such as panic disorder. Although treatment of depression in many patients with CVD improves their dysphoria and other signs and symptoms of depression, are these agents safe and effective in the treatment of anxiety disorders as well? One of many important questions to be answered is whether aggressive and consistent treatment of anxiety and depressive syndromes in patients with CVD not only improves their quality of life but diminishes cardiovascular-related morbidity and improves survival. Which treatment modalities (psychotherapeutic versus psychopharmacologic or a combination) will be most effective in patients with recurrent or more severe depression remains to be determined. Treatment studies also may assess the relation between depression and subsequent compliance with medication and modification of risk factors for CVD.[27] Future studies undoubtedly should continue to scrutinize whether there are gender-specific psychiatric and psychobiological differences in susceptibility to CVD,[240] symptom presentation,[241] vulnerability to adverse outcomes after treatment for CVD (e.g., CABG),[25] and response to depression treatment.[242,243] Although women are more vulnerable to depression and CVD is the leading cause of death among adult women in the United States, the question of whether the impact of depression and anxiety on CVD differs by gender has been understudied, with the results to date conflicting.[48,244,245]

The associations between diseases of the CNS (anxiety and depressive disorders) and disorders of peripheral "end organs" such as the heart raise intriguing questions regarding what is "cardiovascular" or "psychiatric." Molecular biological techniques may provide further opportunity for the elucidation of the relation between cardiovascular and psychiatric diseases, given the possibility that clinically distinct disorders, such as depression and IHD, may share several genetic susceptibility loci.[246] Illumination of the interplay between anxiety disorders, depressive syndromes, and the thrombovascular system, particularly in patients with CVD, undoubtedly will lead to the development of new treatment modalities that not only will improve patients' quality of life but potentially will decrease their morbidity and improve long-term survival rates.

ACKNOWLEDGMENTS

This research was supported by grants MH-01399, NIMH 156617-03, MH-42088, MH-49523, and RR-00039 from the National Institutes of Health, Bethesda, MD, an Established Investigator Award from the National Alliance for Research on Schizophrenia and Depression (CB Nemeroff), and a Research Award from the Dana Foundation (DL Musselman). We are also grateful for the assistance of Mr. Angelo Brown.

References

1. Hayward C. Psychiatric illness and cardiovascular disease risk. *Epidemiol Rev* 1995;17:129–138.

2. Williams R, Schneiderman N. Resolved: Psychosocial interventions can improve clinical outcomes in organic disease. *Psychosom Med* 2002;64:552–557.

3. American Psychiatric Association. *Diagnostic and Statistical Manual of Mental Disorders,* 4th ed. Washington, DC: American Psychiatric Association, 1994.

4. Kessler RC, McGonagle KA, Zhao S, et al. Lifetime and 12-month prevalence of DSM-III-R psychiatric disorders in the United States. *Arch Gen Psychiatry* 1994;51:8–19.

5. Von Korff M, Shapiro S, Burke JD, et al. Anxiety and depression in a primary care clinic: Comparison of Diagnostic Interview Schedule, General Health Questionnaire, and practitioner assessments. *Arch Gen Psychiatry* 1987;44:152–156.

6. Cohen-Cole SA, Kaufman KG. Major depression in physical illness: Diagnosis, prevalence, and antidepressant treatment (a ten year review: 1982–1992). *Depression* 1993;1:181–204.

7. Magni G, Schifano F, DeLeo D. Assessment of depression in an elderly medical population. *J Affective Disord* 1986;11:121–124.

8. Feldman E, Mayou R, Hawton K, et al. Psychiatric disorder in medical inpatients. *Q J Med* 1987;63:405–412.

9. Johnson J, Weissman MM, Klerman GL. Service utilization and social morbidity associated with depressive symptoms in the community. *JAMA* 1992;267:1478–1483.

10. Ormel J, Koeter MWJ, van den Brink W, et al. Recognition, management, and course of anxiety and depression in general practice. *Arch Gen Psychiatry* 1991;48:700–706.

11. DiMatteo MR, Lepper HS, Croghan TW. Depression is a risk factor for noncompliance with medical treatment: Meta-analysis of the effects of anxiety and depression on patient adherence. *Arch Int Med* 2000;160:2101–2107.

12. Mayou R, Foster A, Williamson B. Medical care after myocardial infarction. *J Psychosom Res* 1979;23:23–26.

13. Druss BG, Bradford D, Rosenheck RA, et al. Quality of medical care and excess mortality in older patients with mental disorders. *Arch Gen Psychiatry* 2001;58:565–572.

14. Wells KB, Stewart A, Hayes RD, et al. The functioning and well-being of depressed patients. Results of the Medical Outcomes Study. *JAMA* 1989;262:914–919.

15. Carney RM, Rich MW, Freedland KE, et al. Major depressive disorder predicts cardiac events in patients with coronary artery disease. *Psychosom Med* 1988;50:627–633.

16. Robins LN, Helzer JE, Croughnan J, et al. *NIMH Diagnostic Interview Schedule: Version III-R.* Rockville, MD: National Institutes of Mental Health, 1987.

17. Schleifer SJ, Macarini-Hinson MM, Coyle DA, et al. The nature and course of depression following myocardial infarction. *Arch Intern Med* 1989;149:1785–1789.

18. Endicott J, Spitzer RL. A diagnostic interview: The Schedule for Affective Disorders and Schizophrenia. *Arch Gen Psychiatry* 1978;35:837–844.

19. Freedland KE, Carney RM, Rich MW, et al. Depression in elderly patients with heart failure. *J Geriatr Psychiatry* 1991;24:59–71.

20. Frasure-Smith N, Lesperance F, Talajic M. Depression following myocardial infarction: Impact on 6-month survival. *JAMA* 1993;270:1819–1861.

21. Gonzalez MB, Snyderman TB, Colket JT, et al. Depression in patients with coronary artery disease. *Depression* 1996;4:57–62.

22. Koenig HG. Depression in hospitalized older patients with congestive heart failure. *Gen Hosp Psychiatry* 1998;20:29–43.

23. Kaufmann PG, McMahon RP, Becker LC, et al. The psychophysiological investigations of myocardial ischemia (PIMI) study: Objective, methods, and variability of measures. *Psychosom Med* 1999;60:56–63.

24. Lesperance F, Frasure-Smith N, Juneau M, et al. Depression and 1-year prognosis in unstable angina. *Arch Intern Med.* 2000;160:1354–1360.

25. Connerney I, Shapiro PA, McLaughlin JS, et al. Relation between depression after coronary artery bypass surgery and 12 month outcome: A prospective study. *Lancet* 2001;358:1766–1771.

26. Freedland KE, Rich MW, Skala JA, et al. Prevalence of depression in hospitalized patients with congestive heart failure. *Psychosom Med* 2003;65:119–128.

27. Frasure-Smith N, Lesperance F, Talajic M. Depression and 18-month prognosis after myocardial infarction. *Circulation* 1995;91:999–1005.

28. Bush D, Ziegelstein R, Tayback M, et al. Even minimal symptoms of depression increase mortality risk after acute myocardial infarction. *Am J Cardiol* 2001;88:337–341.

29. Frasure-Smith N, Lesperance F, Juneau M, et al. Gender, depression, and one-year prognosis after myocardial infarction. *Psychosom Med* 1999;61:26–37.

30. Lesperance F, Frasure-Smith N, Talajic M, et al. Five-year risk of cardiac mortality in relation to initial severity and one-year changes in depression symptoms after myocardial infarction. *Circulation* 2002;105:1049–1053.

31. Jiang W, Hasselblad V, Krishnan RR, et al. Patients with CHF and depression have greater risk of mortality and morbidity than patients without depression.[comment]. *J Am Coll Cardiol* 2002;39:919–921.

32. Vaccarino V, Kasl SV, Abramsom J, et al. Depressive symptoms and risk of functional decline and death in patients with heart failure. *J Am Coll Cardiol* 2001;38:199–205.

33. Carroll D, Lane D. Depression and mortality following myocardial infarction: The issue of disease severity. *Epidmiol Psych Soc* 2002;11:65–68.

34. Irvine J, Basinski A, Baker B, et al. Depression and risk of sudden cardiac death after myocardial infarction: Testing for the confounding effects of fatigue. *Psychosom Med* 1999;61:729–737.

35. Ostfeld AM, Lebovits BZ, Shekelle RB, et al. A prospective study of the relationship between personality and coronary heart disease. *J Chronic Dis* 1964;17:265–276.

36. Brozek J, Keyes A, Blackburn H. Personality differences between potential coronary and noncoronary subjects. *Ann NY Acad Sci* 1966;134:1057–1064.

37. Goldberg EL, Comstock GW, Hornstra RK. Depressed mood and subsequent physical illness. *Am J Psychiatry* 1979;136:530–534.

38. Murphy JM, Monson RR, Olivier DC, et al. Affective disorders and mortality. *Arch Gen Psychiatry* 1987;44:473–480.

39. Anda R, Williamson D, Jones D, et al. Depressed affect, hopelessness, and the risk of ischemic heart disease in a cohort of U.S. adults. *Epidemiology* 1993;4:285–294.

40. Aromaa A, Raitasalo R, Reunanen A, et al. Depression and cardiovascular diseases. *Acta Psychiatria Scandinavia* 1994;377:77–82.

41. Vogt T, Pope C, Mullooly J, et al. Mental health status as a predictor of morbidity and mortality: A 15-year follow-up of members of a health maintenance organization. *Am J Public Health* 1994;84:227–231.

42. Simonsick EM, Wallace RB, Blazer DG, et al. Depressive symptomatology and hypertension-associated morbidity and mortality in older adults. *Psychosom Med* 1995;57:427–435.

43. Everson SA, Goldberg DE, Kaplan GA, et al. Hopelessness and risk of mortality and incidence of myocardial infarction and cancer. *Psychosom Med* 1996;58:113–121.

44. Barefoot JC, Schroll M. Symptoms of depression, acute myocardial infarction, and total mortality in a community sample. *Circulation* 1996;93:1976–1980.

45. Pratt LA, Ford DE, Crum RM, et al. Depression, psychotropic medication, and risk of myocardial infarction: Prospective data from the Baltimore ECA follow-up. *Circulation* 1996;94:3123–3129.

46. Wassertheil-Smoller S, Applegate WB, Berge K, et al. Change in depression as a precursor of cardiovascular events. *Arch Intern Med* 1996;156:553–561.

47. Callahan CM, Wolinsky FD, Stump TE, et al. Mortality, symptoms, and functional impairment in late-life depression. *J Gen Intern Med* 1998;13:746–752.

48. Mendes de Leon CF, Krumholz HM, Seeman TS, et al. Depression and risk of coronary heart disease in elderly men and women: New Haven EPESE, 1982–1991. *Arch Intern Med* 1998;158:2341–2348.

49. Ford DE, Mead LA, Chang PP, et al. Depression is a risk factor for coronary artery disease in men: The Precursors Study. *Arch Intern Med* 1998;158:1422–1426.

50. Schwartz SW, Cornoni-Huntley J, Cole SR, et al. Are sleep complaints an independent risk factor for myocardial infarction? *AEP* 1998;8: 384–392.

51. Sesso H, Kawachi I, Vokonas PS, et al. Depression and the risk of coronary heart disease in the Normative Aging Study. *Am J Cardiol* 1998;82:851–856.

52. Whooley MA, Browner WS. Association between depressive symptoms and mortality in older women. Study of Osteoporotic Fractures Research Group. *Arch Intern Med* 1998;158:2129–2135.

53. Ariyo AA. Depression and coronary mortality in the elderly. *Circulation* 2000;102:1773–1779.

54. Ferketich AK, Schwartzbaum JA, Frid DJ, et al. Depression as an antecedent to heart disease among women and men in the NHANES I study. *Arch Intern Med* 2000;160:1261–1268.

55. Pennix BWJH, Beekman ATF, Honig A, et al. Depression and cardiac morbidity: Results from a community-based longitudinal study. *Arch Gen Psychiatry* 2001;58:221–227.

56. Rugulies R. Depression as a predictor for coronary heart disease. A review and meta-analysis. *Am J Prev Med* 2002;23:51–61.

57. Vingerhoets A. *Psychosocial Stress: An Experimental Approach.* Groningen, The Netherlands: Swets & Zeitlinger, 1985.

58. Selye H. *The Stress of Life.* New York: McGraw Hill, 1956.

59. Nemeroff CB, Widerlov E, Bissette G, et al. Elevated concentrations of CSF corticotropin-releasing factor-like immunoreactivity in depressed patients. *Science* 1984;226:1342–1344.

60. Banki CM, Karmasci L, Bissette G, et al. CSF corticotropin-releasing and somatostatin in major depression: Response to antidepressant treatment and relapse. *Eur Neuropsychopharmacol* 1992;2:107–113.

61. Risch SC, Lewine RJ, Kalin NH, et al. Limbic-hypothalamic-pituitary-adrenal axis activity and ventricular-to-brain ratio studies in affective illness and schizophrenia. *Neuropsychopharmacology* 1992;6:95–100.

62. Raadsheer FC, van Heerikhuize JJ, Lucassen PJ, et al. Corticotropin-releasing hormone mRNA levels in the paraventricular nucleus of patients with Alzheimer's disease and depression. *Am J Psychiatry* 1995;152:1372–1376.

63. Bjorkerud S, ed. Effect of Adrenocortical Hormones on the Integrity of Rat Aortic Endothelium. Berlin: Springer-Verlag, 1973.

64. Valigorsky JM. Metaplastic transformation of aortic smooth muscle cells in cortisone-induced dissecting aneurysms in hamsters. *Fed Proc* 1969;28:802.

65. Ross R, Harker L. Hyperlipidemia and atherosclerosis. *Science* 1976;193:1094–1100.

66. Troxler RG, Sprague EA, Albanese RA, et al. The association of elevated plasma cortisol and early atherosclerosis as demonstrated by coronary angiography. *Atherosclerosis* 1977;26:151–162.

67. Swanson LW, Sawchenko PE, Rivier J, et al. Organization of ovine corticotropin-releasing factor immunoreactive cells and fibers in the rat brain: An immunohistochemical study. *Neuroendocrinology* 1983;36:165–186.

68. Veith RC, Lewis L, Linares OA, et al. Sympathetic nervous system activity in major depression: Basal and desipramine-induced alterations in plasma NE kinetics. *Arch Gen Psychiatry* 1994;51:411–422.

69. Carney RM, Freedland KE, Veith RC, et al. Major depression, heart rate, and plasma norepinephrine in patients with coronary heart disease. *Biological Psychiatry* 1999;45:458–463.

70. Roy A, Guthrie S, Pickar D, et al. Plasma NE responses to cold challenge in depressed patients and normal controls. *Psychiatry Res* 1987;21:161–168.

71. Golden RN, Markey SP, Risby ED, et al. Antidepressants reduce whole-body norepinephrine turnover while enhancing 6-hydroxymelatonin output. *Arch Gen Psychiatry* 1988;45:150–154.

72. Linnoila M, Guthrie S, Lane EA, et al. Clinical studies on NE metabolism: How to interpret the numbers. *Psychiatry Res* 1986;17:229–239.

73. Anfossi G, Trovati M. Role of catecholamines in platelet function: Pathophysiological and clinical significance. *Eur J Clin Invest* 1996;26:353–370.

74. Gerritsen ME. Physiological and pathophysiological roles of eicosanoids in the microcirculation. *Cardiovasc Res* 1996;32:720–732.

75. Goldstein DS. Plasma catecholamines and essential hypertension: An analytical review. *Hypertension* 1983;5:86–99.

76. Lund-Johansen P. *Hemodynamic Alterations in Early Essential Hypertension: Recent Advances.* New York: Raven Press, 1983.

77. Lechin F, van der Dijs B, Orozco B, et al. Plasma neurotransmitters, blood pressure, and heart rate during supine-resting, orthostasis, and moderate exercise conditions in major depressed patients. *Biological Psychiatry* 1995;38:166–173.

78. Akselrod S, Gordon D, Ubel FA, et al. Power spectrum analysis of heart rate fluctuation: A quantitative probe of beat-to-beat cardiovascular control. *Science* 1981;213:220–222.

79. Low PA. Autonomic nervous system function. *J Clin Neurophysiol* 1993;10:14–27.

80. Shields RW. Functional anatomy of the autonomic nervous system. *J Clin Neurophysiol* 1993;10:2–13.

81. Dalack GW, Roose SP. Perspectives on the relationship between cardiovascular disease and affective disorder. *J Clin Psychiatry* 1990; 51(7 suppl):4–9, discussion 10–11.

82. Bigger JT, Kleiger RE, Fleiss JL, et al. Components of HR variability measured during healing of acute myocardial infarction. *Am J Cardiol* 1988;61:208–215.

83. LaRovere MT, Specchia G, Mortana A, et al. Baroreflex sensitivity, clinical correlates, and cardiovascular mortality among patients with a first myocardial infarction: A prospective study. *Circulation* 1988;78: 816–824.

84. Cripps T, Malik M, Farrell T, et al. Prognostic value of reduced heart rate variability after myocardial infarction: Clinical evaluation of a new analysis method. *Brit Heart J* 1991;65:14–19.

85. Viskin S, Belhassen B. Noninvasive and invasive strategies for the prevention of sudden death after myocardial infarction. Value, limitations and implications for therapy. *Drugs* 1992;44:336–355.

86. Campbell RWF. *Can Analysis of Heart Rate Variability Predict Arrhythmias and Antiarrhythmic Effects?* Dordrecht, Netherlands: Kluwer Academic Publishers, 1996.

87. Pagani M, Lombardi F, Guzzetti S, et al. Power spectral analysis of heart rate and arterial pressure variabilities as a marker of sympathovagal interaction in man and conscious dog. *Circ Res* 1986;59:178–193.

88. Koizumi K, Terui N, Kollai M. Effect of cardiac vagal and sympathetic nerve activity on heart rate in rhythmic fluctuations. *J Auton Nerv Syst* 1985;12:251–259.

89. Fouad FM, Tarazzi RC, Gerrario CM, et al. Assessment of parasympathetic control of heart rate by a noninvasive method. *Am J Physiol* 1984;246:H838–H842.

90. Bigger TJJ, Fleiss JL, Steinman RC, et al. Frequency domain measures of heart period variability and mortality after myocardial infarction. *Circulation* 1992;85:164–171.

91. Stein PK, Carney RM, Freedland KE, et al. Severe depression is associated with markedly reduced heart rate variability in patients with stable coronary artery disease. *J Psychosom Res* 2000;48:493–500.

92. Rechlin T, Weis M, Claus D. Heart rate variability in depressed patients and differential effects of paroxetine and amitriptyline on cardiovascular autonomic functions. *Pharmacopsychiatry* 1994;27:124–128.

93. Carney RM, Saunders RD, Freedland KE, et al. Association of depression with reduced heart rate variability in coronary artery disease. *Am J Cardiol* 1995;76:562–564.

94. Roose SP, Glassman AH, Dalack GW. Depression, heart disease, and tricyclic antidepressants. *J Clin Psychiatry* 1989;50 (suppl 7):12–16.

95. Severus WE, Ahrens B, Stoll AL. Omega-3 fatty acids—the missing link? (letter). *Arch Gen Psychiatry* 1999;56:380–381.

96. Adams PB, Lawson S, Sanigorski A, et al. Arachidonic acid to eicosapentaenoic acid ratio in blood correlates positively with clinical symptoms of depression. *Lipids* 1996;31:S157–S161.

97. Maes M, Smith R, Christophe A, et al. Fatty acid composition in major depression: Decreased omega 3 fractions in cholesteryl esters and increased C20:4 omega-6/C20:5 omega-3 ratio in cholesteryl esters and phospholipids. *J Affective Disord* 1996;38:35–46.

98. Edwards R, Peet M, Shay J, et al. Omega-3 polyunsaturated fatty acid levels in the diet and in red blood cell membranes of depressed patients. *J Affective Disord* 1998;48:149–155.

99. Christensen JH, Korup E, Aaroe J, et al. Fish consumption, n-3 fatty acids in cell membranes, and heart rate variability in survivors of myocardial infarction with left ventricular dysfunction. *Am J Cardiol* 1997;79:1670–1673.

100. Albert CM, Hennekens CH, O'Donnell CJ, et al. Fish consumption and risk of sudden cardiac death. *JAMA* 1998;279:23–28.

101. Balogh S, Fitzpatrick DF, Hendricks SE, et al. Increases in heart rate variability with successful treatment in patients with major depressive disorder. *Psychopharmacol Bull* 1993;29:201–206.

102. Carney RM, Freedland KE, Stein PK, et al. Change in heart rate and heart rate variability during treatment for depression in patients with coronary heart disease. *Psychosom Med* 2000;62:639–647.

103. Selz KA, Mandell AJ. Style as mechanism: From man to a map of the interval and back. *Chaos Med Biol: SPIE Proc* 1994;2036:174–182.

104. Markovitz JH, Matthews KA. Platelets and coronary heart disease: Potential psychophysiologic mechanism. *Psychosom Med* 1991;53:643–668.

105. Morris PLP, Robsin RG, Andrzejewski P, et al. Association of depression with 10-year poststroke mortality. *Am J Psychiatry* 1993;150:124–129.

106. Lefkovits J, Plow EF, Topol EJ. Platelet glycoprotein IIb/IIIa receptors in cardiovascular medicine. *N Engl J Med* 1995;332:1553–1559.

107. Antiplatelet Trialists' Collaboration: Secondary prevention of vascular disease by prolonged antiplatelet treatment. *BMJ (Clin Res ed)* 1988;296:320–331.

108. Verstraete M. Risk factors, interventions and therapeutic agents in the prevention of atherosclerosis-related ischaemic diseases. *Drugs* 1991;42 (suppl 5):22–38.

109. Ridker PM, Manson JE, Buring JE, et al. The effect of chronic platelet inhibition with low-dose aspirin on atherosclerotic progression and acute thrombosis: Clinical evidence from the Physicians' Health Study. *Am Heart J* 1991;122:1588–1592.

110. Second IToISCG. Randomized trial of intravenous streptokinase, oral aspirin, both, or neither among 17,187 cases of suspected acute myocardial infarction: ISIS-2. *Lancet* 1988;2:349–360.

111. Antiplatelet Trialists' Collaboration. Collaborative overview of randomized trials of antiplatelet therapy, I: Prevention of death, myocardial infarction, and stroke by prolonged antiplatelet therapy in various categories of patients. *BMJ* 1994;308:81–106.

112. Musselman DL, Tomer A, Manatunga AK, et al. Exaggerated platelet reactivity in major depression. *Am J Psychiatry* 1996;153:1313–1317.

113. Musselman DL, Marzec UM, Manatunga A, et al. Platelet reactivity in depressed patients treated with paroxetine: Preliminary findings. *Arch Gen Psychiatry* 2000;57:875–882.

114. Kuijpers PMJC, Hamulyak K, Strik JJMH, et al. Beta-thromboglobulin and platelet factor 4 levels in post-myocardial infarction patients with major depression. *Psychiatry Res* 2002;109:207–210.

115. Markovitz JH, Matthews KA, Kiss J, et al. Effects of hostility on platelet reactivity to psychological stress in coronary heart disease patients and healthy controls. *Psychosom Med* 1996;58:143–149.

116. Laghrissi-Thode F, Wagner WR, Pollock BG, et al. Elevated platelet factor 4 and β-thromboglobulin plasma levels in depressed patients with ischemic heart disease. *Biol Psychiatry* 1997;42:290–295.

117. Owens MJ, Nemeroff CB. Role of serotonin in the pathophysiology of depression: Focus on the serotonin transporter. *Clin Chem* 1994;40:288–295.

118. DeClerck F. Effects of serotonin on platelets and blood vessels. *J Cardiovasc Pharmacol* 1991;17 (suppl 5):S1–S5.

119. Osim EE, Wyllie JH. Evidence for loss of 5-hydroxytryptamine from circulating platelets. *J Physiol (London)* 1982;326:25P–26P.

120. Ashton JH, Ogletree ML, Michel IM, et al. Cooperative mediation by serotonin S2 and thromboxane S2/prostaglandin H2 receptor activation of cyclic flow variation in dogs with severe coronary artery stenosis. *Circulation* 1987;76:952–959.

121. Biegon A, Essar N, Israeli M, et al. Serotonin 5-HT2 receptor binding on blood platelets as a state dependent marker in major affective disorder. *Psychopharmacology* 1990;102:73–75.

122. Pandey GN, Pandey SC, Janicak PG. Platelet serotonin-2 binding sites in depression and suicide. *Biol Psychiatry* 1990;28:215–222.

123. France RD, Urban B, Krishnan KRR, et al. CSF corticotropin-releasing factor-like immunoreactivity in chronic pain patients with and without major depression. *Biolog Psychiatry* 1988;23:86–88.

124. Nemeroff CB, Knight DL, Franks J, et al. Further studies on platelet transporter binding in depression. *Am J Psychiatry* 1994;151:1623–1625.

125. Cerrito F, Lazzaro MP, Gaudio E, et al. 5HT2-receptors and serotonin release: Their role in human platelet aggregation. *Life Sci* 1993;53:209–215.

126. Plein H, Berk M, Eppel S, et al. Augmented platelet calcium uptake in response to serotonin stimulation in patients with major depression measured using Mn^{2+} influx and $^{45}Ca^{2+}$ uptake. *Life Sci* 1999;66:425–431.

127. Ware JA, Smith M, Salzman EW. Synergism of platelet aggregating agents. Role of elevation of cytoplasmic calcium. *J Clin Invest* 1987;80:267–271.

128. Pollock BG, Laghrissi-Thode F, Wagner WR. Evaluation of platelet activation in depressed patients with ischemic heart disease after paroxetine or nortriptyline treatment. *J Clin Psychopharmacol* 2000;20:137–140.

129. Ross R. Atherosclerosis: An inflammatory disease. *N Engl J Med* 1999;340:115–126.

130. Gabay C, Kushner I. Acute-phase proteins and other systemic responses to inflammation. *N Engl J Med* 1999;340:448–454.

131. Yirmiya R. Endotoxin produces a depressive-like episode in rats. *Brain Res* 1996;711:163–174.

132. Maes M, Delange J, Ranjan R, et al. Acute phase proteins in schizophrenia, mania and major depression: Modulation by psychotropic drugs. *Psychiatry Res* 1996;66:1–11.

133. Musselman DL, Miller AH, Porter MR, et al. Higher than normal plasma interleukin-6 concentrations in cancer patients with depression. *Am J Psychiatry* 2001;158:1252–1257.

134. Miller GE, Stetler CA, Carney RM, et al. Clinical depression and inflamatory risk markers for coronary heart disease. *Am J Cardiol* 2002;90:1279–1283.

135. Gumnick JF, Pearce BD, Miller AH. The impact of depression on the immune system and immune-related disorders. In Thakore J, ed. *Physical Consequences of Depression.* England, Wrightson Biomedical; 2001:153–180.

136. Wirz PH, von Kanel R, Fischer JE. Glucocorticoid sensitivity of monocyte interleukin-6 production is reduced in vitally exhausted men. Paper presented at the Annual Scientific Meeting of the American Psychosomatic Society. 2003:A-11; Phoenix, Arizona.

137. Everson SA, Kaplan GA. Hopelessness is a determinant of fibrinogen levels in middle-aged men. *Am J Epidemiol* 2001;153:S66.

138. Castilla-Puentes R, Zhang Y, Bromberger JT, et al. Depressed women have elevated coagulation factors in midlife. Paper presented at the Annual Scientific Meeting of the American Psychosomatic Society. 2003:A-23; Phoenix, Arizona.

139. Verrier RL. *Behavioral stress, myocardial ischemia, and arrhthmias.* Toronto: Saunders, 1990.

140. Jiang W, Babyak M, Krantz DS, et al. Mental stress-induced myocardial ischemia and cardiac events. *JAMA* 1996;21:1651–1656.

141. Lown B, DeSilva RA, Reich P, et al. Psychophysiologic factors in sudden cardiac death. *Am J Psychiatry* 1980;137:1325–1335.

142. Lown B, Verrier RL. Neural activity and ventricular fibrillation. *N Engl J Med* 1976;294:1165–1170.

143. Zaza A, Schwartz PJ. Role of the autonomic nervous system in the genesis of early ischemic arrhythmias. *J Cardiovasc Pharmacol* 1985; 7(5 suppl):S8–S12.

144. Heit S, Owens MJ, Plotsky PM, et al. Corticotropin-releasing factor, stress, and depression. *Neuroscientists* 1997;3:186–194.

145. Follick MJ, Gorkin L, Capone RJ, et al. Psychological distress as a predictor of ventricular arrhythmias in a post-myocardial infarct population. *Am Heart J* 1988;116:32–36.

146. Gold PW, Goodwin FK, Chrousos GP. Clinical and biochemical manifestations of depression. Relation to the neurobiology of stress. *N Engl J Med* 1988;319:413–420.

147. Curtis AL, Pavcovich LA, Grigoriadis DE, et al. Previous stress alters corticotropin-releasing factor neurotransmission in the locus coeruleus. *Neuroscience* 1995;65:541–550.

148. Chrousos GP, Gold PW. The concepts of stress and stress system disorders. Overview of physical and behavioral homeostasis. *JAMA* 1992;267:1244–1252.

149. Paykel E. Causal relationships between clinical depression and life events. In: Barrett JE, ed. *Stress and Mental Disorder.* New York: Raven Press, 1979.

150. Kendler KS, Kessler RC, Neale MC, et al. The prediction of major depression in women: Toward an integrated etiologic model. *Am J Psychiatry* 1993;150:1139–1148.

151. Echt DS, Liebson PR, Mitchell LB, et al. Mortality and morbidity in patients receiving ecainide, flecenaide or placebo: The Cardiac Arrythmia Suppression Trial. *N Engl J Med* 1991;324:781–788.

152. Thomas SA, Friedmann E, Wimbush F, et al. Psychosocial factors and survival in the Cardiac Arrhythmia Suppression Trial (CAST): A reexamination. *Am J Crit Care* 1997;6:116–126.

153. Fifer SK, Mathias SD, Patrick DL, et al. Untreated anxiety among adult primary care patients in a health maintenance organization. *Arch Gen Psychiatry* 1994;51:740–750.

154. Sullivan MD, LaCroix AZ, Baum C, et al. Functional status in coronary artery disease: A one-year prospective study of the role of anxiety and depression. *Am J Med* 1997;103:348–356.

155. Sherbourne CD, Jackson CA, Meredith LS, et al. Prevalence of comorbid anxiety disorders in primary care outpatients. *Arch Fam Med* 1996;5:27–34.

156. Beck JG, Berisford MA, Taegtmeyer H. The effects of voluntary hyperventilation on patients with chest pain without coronary artery disease. *Behav Res Ther* 1991;29:611–621.

157. Lynch P, Bakal DA, Whitelaw W, et al. Chest muscle activity and panic anxiety: A preliminary investigation. *Psychosom Med* 1991;53:80–89.

158. Haines AP, Imeson JD, Meade TW. Phobic anxiety and ischaemic heart disease. *BMJ (Clin Res ed)* 1987;295:297–299.

159. Eaker ED, Pinsky J, Castelli WP. Myocardial infarction and coronary death among women: Psychosocial predictors from a 20-year follow-up of women in the Framingham Study. *Am J Epidemiol* 1992;135:854–864.

160. Kawachi I, Colitz GA, Ascherio A. Prospective study of phobic anxiety and risk of coronary heart disease in men. *Circulation* 1994; 89:1992–1997.

161. Kawachi I, Sparrow D, Vokonas PS, et al. Symptoms of anxiety and risk of coronary heart disease. The Normative Aging Study. *Circulation* 1994;90:2225.

162. Kubzansky LD, Kawachi I, Spiro A III, et al. Is worrying bad for your heart? A prospective study of worry and coronary heart disease in the Normative Aging Study. *Circulation* 1997;95:818–824.

163. Herrmann C, Brand-Driehorst S, Buss U, et al. Effects of anxiety and depression on 5-year mortality in 5057 patients referred for exercise testing. *J Psychosom Res* 2000;48:455–462.

164. Kubzansky LD, Kawachi I, Weiss ST, et al. Anxiety and coronary heart disease: A synthesis of epidemiological, psychological, and experimental evidence. *Ann Behav Med* 1998;20:47–58.

165. Davis M. The role of the amygdala in fear-potentiated startle: Implications for animal models of anxiety. *Trends Pharmacol Sci* 1992;13:35–41.

166. Ninan PT. The functional anatomy, neurochemistry, and pharmacology of anxiety. *J Clin Psychiatry* 1999;60(suppl 22):12–17.

167. Stein MB, Uhde TW. Biology of anxiety disorders. In: Schatzberg AF, Nemeroff CB, eds. *The American Psychiatric Association Textbook of Psychopharmacology,* 2d ed. Washington, DC: American Psychiatric Association, 1998:609–628.

168. McNally RJ, Eke M. Anxiety sensitivity, suffocation fear, and breath-holding duration as predictors of response to carbon dioxide challenge. *J Abnormal Psychol* 1996;105:146–149.

169. Torgersen S, ed. *Twin Studies in Panic Disorder.* New York: Alan R. Liss, 1990.

170. Stein MB, Millar TW, Larsen DK, et al. Irregular breathing during sleep in patients with panic disorder. *Am J Psychiatry* 1995;152:1168–1173.

171. Condren RM, O'Neill A, Ryan MC, et al. HPA axis response to a psychological stressor in generalised social phobia. *Psychoneuroendocrinology* 2002;27:693–703.

172. Marshall RD, Blanco C, Printz D, et al. A pilot study of noradrenergic and HPA axis functioning in PTSD vs. panic disorder. *Psychiatry Res* 2002;110:219–230.

173. Baker DG, West SA, Nicholson WE, et al. Serial CSF corticotropin-releasing hormone levels and adrenocortical activity in combat veterans with posttraumatic stress disorder. *Am J Psychiatry* 1999;156:585–588.

174. Smith MA, Davidson J, Ritchie JC, et al. The corticotropin-releasing hormone test in patients with posttraumatic stress disorder. *Biol Psychiatry* 1989;26:349–355.

175. Yehuda R, Boisoneau D, Lowy MT, et al. Dose-response changes in plasma cortisol and lymphocyte glucocorticoid receptors following dexamethasone administration in combat veterans with and without posttraumatic stress disorder. *Arch Gen Psychiatry* 1995;52:583–593.

176. Stein MB, Yehuda R, Koverola C, et al. Enhanced dexamethasone suppression of plasma cortisol in adult women traumatized by childhood sexual abuse. *Biolog Psychiatry* 1997;42:680–686.

177. Bremner JD, Randall P, Vermetten E, et al. Magnetic resonance imaging-based measurement of hippocampal volume in posttraumatic stress disorder related to childhood physical and sexual abuse—A preliminary report. *Biol Psychiatry* 1997;41:23–32.

178. Linares OA, Zech LA, Jacquez JA, et al. Effect of sodium-restricted diet and posture on norepinephrine kinetics in humans. *Am J Physiol* 1988;254:E222–E230.

179. Wilkinson DJC, Thompson JM, Lambert GW, et al. Sympathetic activity in patients with panic disorder at rest, under laboratory mental stress, and during panic attacks. *Arch Gen Psychiatry* 1998;55:511–520.

180. Weissman MM, Markowitz JS, Quellette R, et al. Panic disorder and cardiovascular/cerebrovascular problems: Results from a community survey. *Am J Psychiatry* 1990;147:1504–1508.

181. Coryell W, Noyes R, Clancy J. Excess mortality in panic disorder: A comparison with primary unipolar depression. *Arch Gen Psychiatry* 1982;39:701–703.

182. Jonas BS, Franks P, Ingram DD. Are symptoms of anxiety and depression risk factors for hypertension? Longitudinal evidence from

the national Health and Nutrition Examination Survey I Epidemiologic Follow-Up Study. *Arch Fam Med* 1997;6:43–49.

183. Rutledge T, Hogan BE. A quantitative review of prospective evidence linking psychological factors with hypertension development. *Psychosom Med* 2002;64:758–766.

184. Sheehan DV, Coleman JH, Greenblatt DJ, et al. Some biochemical correlates of panic attacks with agoraphobia and their response to a new treatment. *J Clin Psychopharmacol* 1984;4:66–75.

185. Freeman IJ, Nixon PGF. Are coronary artery spasm and progressive damage to the heart associated with the hyperventilation syndrome? *BMJ* 1985;291:851–852.

186. Yeragani VK, Pohl R, Berger R, et al. Decreased heart rate variability in panic disorder patients: A study of power-spectral analysis of heart rate. *Psychiatry Res* 1993;46:89–103.

187. Sloan EP, Natarajan M, Baker B, et al. Nocturnal and daytime panic attacks—Comparison of sleep architecture, heart rate variability, and response to sodium lactate challenge. *Biol Psychiatry* 1999;45:1313–1320.

188. Lyonsfield JD. *An Examination of Image and Thought Processes in Generalized Anxiety.* New York, NY: Association for the Advancement of Behavior Therapy. 1991.

189. Thayer JF, Friedman BH, Borkovec TD. Autonomic characteristics of generalized anxiety disorder and worry. *Biol Psychiatry* 1996;39:255–266.

190. Shear MK, Kligfield P, Harshfield G, et al. Cardiac rate and rhythm in panic patients. *Am J Psychiatry* 1987;144:633–637.

191. Chignon J-M, Lepine J-P, Ades J. Panic disorder in cardiac outpatients. *Am J Psychiatry* 1993;150:780–785.

192. Katz C, Martin RD, Landa B, et al. Relationship of psychologic factors to frequent symptomatic ventricular arrhythmia. *Am J Med* 1985;78:589–594.

193. Follick MJ, Ahern DK, Gorkin L, et al. Relation of psychosocial and stress reactivity variables to ventricular arrhythmias in the Cardiac Arrhythmia Pilot Study (CAPS). *Am J Cardiol* 1990;66:63–67.

194. Frasure-Smith N, Lesperance F, Prince RH, et al. Randomised trial of home-based psychosocial nursing intervention for patients recovering from myocardial infarction. *Lancet* 1997;350:473–470.

195. Kandzari DE, Kay J, O'Shea JC, et al. Highlights from the American Heart Association annual scientific sessions 2001: November 11 to 14, 2001. *Am Heart J* 2002;143:217–228.

196. Frasure-Smith N, Lesperance F, Juneau M. Differential long-term impact of in-hospital symptoms of psychological stress after non-Q-wave and Q-wave myocardial infarction. *Am J Cardiol* 1992;69:1128–1134.

197. Jones DA, West RR. Psychological rehabilitation after myocardial infarction: Multicentre randomised controlled trial. *BMJ* 1996;313:1517–1521.

198. Frasure-Smith N. In-hospital symptoms of psychological stress as predictors of long-term outcome after acute myocardial infarction in men. *Am J Cardiol* 1991;67:121–127.

199. Friedman M, Thoresen CE, Gill JJ, et al. Alteration of type A behavior and its effect on cardiac recurrences in post myocardial infarction patients: Summary results of the recurrent coronary prevention project. *Am Heart J* 1986;112:653–665.

200. Roose SP, Glassman AH, Siris SG, et al. Comparison of imipramine- and nortriptyline-induced orthostatic hypotension: A meaningful difference. *J Clin Psychopharmacol* 1981;1:316–319.

201. Thayssen P, Bjerre M, Kragh-Sorensen P. Cardiovascular effects of imipramine and nortriptyline in elderly patients. *Psychopharmacology* 1981;74:360–364.

202. Feder R. Bradycardia and syncope induced by fluoxetine [letter]. *J Clin Psychiatry* 1991;52:139.

203. Roose SP, Laghriss-Thode F, Kennedy JS, et al. Comparison of paroxetine and nortriptyline in depressed patients with ischemic heart disease. *JAMA* 1998;279:287–291.

204. Franco-Bronson K. The management of treatment-resistant depression in the medically ill. *Psych Clin North Am* 1996;19:329–350.

205. Feighner JP. Cardiovascular safety in depressed patients: Focus on venlafaxine. *J Clin Psychiatry* 1995;56:574–579.

206. Hyman SE, Arana GW, Rosenbaum JF. *Handbook of Psychiatric Drug Therapy.* Boston: Little, Brown, 1995.

207. Robinson DS, Roberts DL, Smith JM, et al. The safety profile of nefazodone. *J Clin Psychiatry* 1996;57(suppl 2):31–38.

208. Roose SP, Dalack GW. Treating the depressed patient with cardio-vascular problems. *J Clin Psychiatry* 1992;53:25–31.

209. Cohen HW, Gibson G, Alderman MH. Excess risk of myocardial infarction in patients treated with antidepressant medications: Association with use of tricyclic agents. *Am J Med* 2000;108:2–8.

210. Hippisley-Cox J, Pringle M, Hammersley V, et al. Antidepressants as risk factor for ischaemic heart disease: Case-control study in primary care. *BMJ* 2001;323:666–669.

211. Arana GW, Hyman SE. *Handbook of Psychiatric Drug Therapy,* 2nd ed. Boston: Little, Brown, 1995.

212. Ellison JM, Milofsky JE, Ely E. Fluoxetine-induced bradycardia and syncope in two patients. *J Clin Psychiatry* 1990;51:385–386.

213. Enemark B. The importance of ECG monitoring in antidepressant treatment. *Nordic J Psychiatry* 1993;47(suppl 30):57–65.

214. Yaryura-Tobias JA, Kirschen H, Ninan P, et al. Fluoxetine and bleeding in obsessive-compulsive disorder [letter]. *Am J Psychiatry* 1991;148:949.

215. Alderman CP, Moritz CK, Ben-Tovim DI. Abnormal platelet aggregation associated with fluoxetine therapy. *Ann Pharmacother* 1992;26:1517–1519.

216. Markovitz JH, Shuster JL, Chitwood WS, et al. Platelet activation in depression and effects of sertraline treatment: An open-label study. *Am J Psychiatry* 2000;157:1006–1008.

217. Sauer WH, Berlin J, Kimmel SE. Selective serotonin reuptake inhibitors and myocardial infarction. *Circulation* 2001;104:1894–1898.

218. Meier CR, Schlienger RG, Jick H. Use of selective serotonin reuptake inhibitors and risk of developing first-time acute myocardial infarction. *Br J Clin Pharmacol* 2001;52:179–184.

219. van Walraven C, Mamdani MM, Wells PS, et al. Inhibition of serotonin reuptake by antidepressants and upper gastrointestinal bleeding in elderly patients: Retrospective cohort study. *BMJ* 2001;323:655–661.

220. Dalton SO, Johansen C, Mellemkjaer L, et al. Use of selective serotonin reuptake inhibitors and risk of upper gastrointestinal tract bleeding. *Arch Intern Med* 2003;163:59–64.

221. Layton D, Clark DW, Pearce GL, et al. Is there an association between SSRIs and risk of abnormal bleeding? Results from a cohort study based on prescription monitoring in England. *Eur J Clin Pharmacol* 2001;57:167–176.

222. Bak S, Tsiropoulos I, Kjaersgaard JO, et al. Selective serotonin reuptake inhibitors and the risk of stroke: A population-based case-control study. *Stroke* 2002;33:1465–1473.

223. Callahan AM, Marangell LB, Ketter TA. Evaluating the clinical significance of drug interactions: A systematic approach. *Harvard Rev Psychiatry* 1996;4:153–158.

224. Roose SP, Dalack GW, Glassman AH, et al. Cardiovascular effects of buproprion in depressed patients with heart disease. *Am J Psychiatry* 1991;148:512–516.

225. Roose SP, Glassman AH, Attia E, et al. Cardiovascular effects of fluoxetine in depressed patients with heart disease. *Am J Psychiatry* 1998;155:660–665.

226. Glassman AH, O'Connor CM, Califf RM, et al. Sertraline treatment of major depression in patients with acute MI or unstable angina. *JAMA* 2002;288:701–709.

227. Petrides G, Fink M, Husain MM, et al. ECT remission rates in psychotic versus nonpsychotic depressed patients: A report from CORE. *J ECT* 2001;17:244–253.

228. American PATFoET. The practice of electroconvulsive therapy: Recommendations for treatment, training, and privileging. Washington, DC: *Am Psychiatr Assoc Press,* 2001.

229. O'Connor MK, Knapp R, Husain M, et al. The influence of age on the response of major depression to electroconvulsive therapy: A report from C.O.R.E. *J ECT* 2001;17.

230. Weiner RD. Does electroconvulsive therapy cause brain damage? *Behav Brain Sci* 1984;7:1–53.

231. Sackheim HA. Memory and ECT: From polarization to reconciliation [editorial; comment]. *J ECT* 2000;16:87–96.

232. Applegate RJ. Diagnosis and management of ischemic heart disease in the patient scheduled to undergo electroconvulsive therapy. *Convulsive Ther* 1997;13:128–144.

233. Pornnoppadol C, Isenberg K. ECT and the implantable converter defibrillator. *JECT* 1998;14:124–126.

234. Block M, Admon D, Bonne O, et al. Electroconvulsive therapy in depressed cardiac transplant patients. *Convulsive Ther* 1992;8:290–293.

235. Maneksha FR. Hypertension and tachycardia during electroconvulsive therapy: To treat or not to treat. *Convulsive Ther* 1991;70:28–35.

236. Figiel GD, McDonald L, LaPlante R. Cardiac modified ECT in the elderly [letter]. *Am J Psychiatry* 1994;151:790–791.

237. Stoudemire A, Knos G, Gladson M, et al. Labetalol in the control of cardiovascular responses to electroconvulsive therapy in high-risk depressed medical patients. *J Clin Psychiatry* 1990;51:508–512.

238. Figiel G, McDonald WM, McCall WV, et al. Electroconvulsive therapy. In: Schatzberg AF, Nemeroff CB, eds. *American Psychiatric Association Textbook of Psychopharmacology*. 2nd ed. Washington, DC: American Psychiatric Association, 1998:523–545.

239. Coffey CE, Weiner RD, Hinkle PE, et al. Augmentation of ECT seizures with caffeine [erratum appears in *Biol Psychiatry*]. *Biol Psychiatry* 1987;22:637–649.

240. Knopp RH. Risk factors for coronary artery disease in women. *Am J Cardiol* 2002;89:28E–34E.

241. Sheps DS, Kaufmann PG, Sheffield D, et al. Sex differences in chest pain in patients with documented coronary artery disease and exercise-induced ischemia: Results from the PIMI study. *Am Heart J* 2001;142:864–871.

242. Lesperance F, Frasure-Smith N, Talajic M. Major depression before and after myocardial infarction: Its nature and consequences. *Psychosom Med* 1996;58:99–110.

243. Kon Koh K, Mincemoyer R, Bui MN, et al. Effects of hormone-replacement therapy on fibrinolysis in postmenopausal women. *N Engl J Med* 1997;336:683–690.

244. Hippisley-Cox J, Fielding K, Pringle M. Depression is risk factor for ischemic heart disease in men: A population based study. *BMJ* 1998;316:1714–1719.

245. Pennix BWJH, Guralnik JM, Mendes de Leon C, et al. Cardiovascular events and mortality in newly and chronically depressed persons > 70 years of age. *Am J Cardiol* 1998;81:988–994.

246. Kendell R, Jablensky A. Distinguishing between the validity and utility of psychiatric diagnoses. *Am J Psychiatry* 2003;160:4–12.

HEART DISEASE AND PREGNANCY

John H. McAnulty / James Metcalfe / Kent Ueland

Pregnancy alters the cardiovascular system and the heart; also, congenital and acquired heart disease affects pregnancy. An understanding of the cardiovascular changes during a normal pregnancy is important for optimal care. Failure to recognize and treat heart disease, when it exists, may adversely affect both the mother and the child.

HEART DISEASE ISSUES UNIQUE TO PREGNANCY

In the case of a woman with heart disease during pregnancy, some issues are always important. These are outlined below.

Health Priorities

Concerning the mother and child, the health of one importantly influences that of the other. The well-being of the fetus is always considered, but the safety of the mother is always the highest priority. Ideally, treatment of the mother with drugs, diagnostic studies, or surgery should be avoided. If required for maternal safety, however, they should be used.

Maternal Fragility

Despite advances in the recognition and management of heart disease, pregnancy puts the mother at risk. The normal hemodynamic changes of pregnancy may result in disability or death. The risk is so great with some cardiovascular abnormalities[1,2] that a recommendation of avoidance or interruption of pregnancy is well supported

(Table 92-1). Emotional stability is also threatened by pregnancy in the woman with heart disease. Misconceptions and apprehension are common; it is important to keep a pregnant woman and her family informed and comfortable.

Fetal Vulnerability

The fetus depends on its mother for a continuous supply of oxygen and nutrients. The mother must also remove the products of fetal metabolism, including heat. The maternal commitment to the fetus is exceptional, but if the mother requires a redistribution of volume for her own safety, blood is preferentially diverted away from the uterus. In the woman with no cardiac disease, blood flow to the fetus is adequate, even during periods of physical and emotional stress. In the woman with heart disease, however, where uterine blood flow may already be compromised, the possibility of inadequate uterine perfusion increases. Treatment of maternal heart disease may also jeopardize the fetus. Diagnostic studies, drugs, or surgery may increase fetal loss, result in teratogenicity, or alter fetal growth.

Newborn Infant Vulnerability

The health of a newborn infant is a concern when the mother has heart disease. This fragility may be due to a marginal uterine blood flow during pregnancy or to lingering effects of the medications used to treat the mother. Additionally, there will be an increased incidence of congenital heart disease among the live-born infants of parents with congenital heart disease. Early infant nourishment may be jeopardized if maternal heart disease is severe enough to interfere with breast-feeding. Even if the mother is capable of breast-feeding,

TABLE 92-1 Cardiovascular Abnormalities Placing a Mother and Infant at Extremely High Risk

Advise *avoidance* or *interruption of pregnancy*
  Pulmonary hypertension
  Dilated cardiomyopathy with congestive failure
  Marfan's syndrome with dilated aortic root
  Cyanotic congenital heart disease
Pregnancy counseling and close clinical follow-up required
  Prosthetic valve
  Coarctation of the aorta
  Marfan's syndrome
  Dilated cardiomyopathy in asymptomatic women
  Obstructive lesions

SOURCE: Modified from McAnulty JH, Morton MJ, Ueland K. The heart and pregnancy. *Curr Probl Cardiol* 1988; 13:589–665. Reproduced with permission from the publisher and authors.

cardiovascular medications may be transmitted to the infant in breast milk. Finally, the infant is at risk of losing a parent, since life expectancy with many forms of heart disease is significantly reduced.

Maternal Heart Disease May Not Be "Typical"

Many women with heart disease who become pregnant have a form of heart disease that is relatively new, having existed for less than 50 years. They have "mechanically altered" heart disease. Although new information has been acquired about hearts that have been altered by surgery (or a catheter), there is still much that remains unknown. It is best not to consider a previous lesion to have been mechanically "corrected," because there is always some residual disease.

CARDIOVASCULAR ADJUSTMENTS DURING A NORMAL PREGNANCY

Maternal adaptation to pregnancy includes remarkable cardiovascular changes. These explain in part why some cardiac abnormalities are poorly tolerated during pregnancy, resulting in symptoms and signs even in a normal pregnancy. These may be difficult to distinguish from those symptoms and signs that occur with heart disease.

Hemodynamic Changes at Rest

Resting cardiac output (CO) increases by over 40 percent during pregnancy. The increase begins early, with the cardiac output reaching its highest levels by the 20th week. In the last half of pregnancy, CO is significantly affected by body position (Fig. 92-1), as the enlarged uterus reduces venous return from the lower extremities.[3–8] Compared with measurements made near term, when the woman is in the left lateral position, CO is lower by an average of 0.6 L/min when a woman is supine and by 1.2 L/min when she assumes the upright position.[7] In general, this results in few or no symptoms; but in some women, maintenance of the supine position may result in symptomatic hypotension, possibly in those whose collateral vessels are not well developed.[9] Symptoms of this "supine hypotensive syndrome of pregnancy" can be corrected by having the woman turn onto her side.

The hemodynamic changes associated with or causing the variation in CO also change dramatically (Fig. 92-2). CO is the product of heart rate times stroke volume. Its early rise is due mainly to an increase in stroke volume.[3,6] By the 20th week, stroke volume gradually begins to fall because of obstruction of the vena cava by the enlarged uterus and increased dilation of the venous bed. The heart rate increases gradually throughout pregnancy, reaching a level that is approximately 25 percent above the nonpregnant levels by the time of delivery.

CO is also related directly to the mean blood pressure (BP) and inversely to the systemic vascular resistance. There is a fall in BP early in pregnancy, with a gradual return to nonpregnant levels by term. The fall in systemic vascular resistance is more marked, decreasing to two-thirds of resting nonpregnant values at about the 20th week of pregnancy and then gradually rising through the remainder of pregnancy, although not achieving nonpregnant levels until a few weeks after delivery.[3,6]

Finally, the CO is equal to the oxygen consumption divided by the systemic arteriovenous oxygen difference. The mother's oxygen consumption (which includes that of her fetus) increases by 20 percent within the first 20 weeks of pregnancy and increases steadily to a level that is approximately 30 percent above the nonpregnant levels by the time of delivery.[6] This increase is due both to the metabolic needs of the fetus and the increased metabolic needs of the mother. The increase in CO occurs earlier than the rise in oxygen

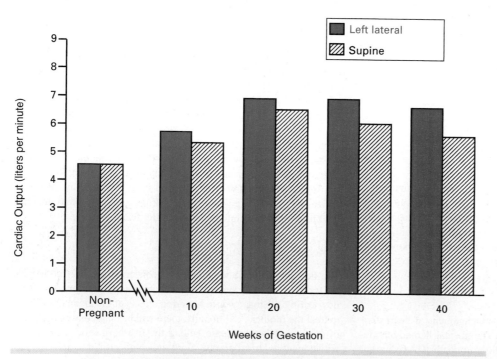

FIGURE 92-1 Cardiac output values during normal pregnancy when measured in the supine and left lateral positions. The values are derived from measurements made in many studies.[3–7]

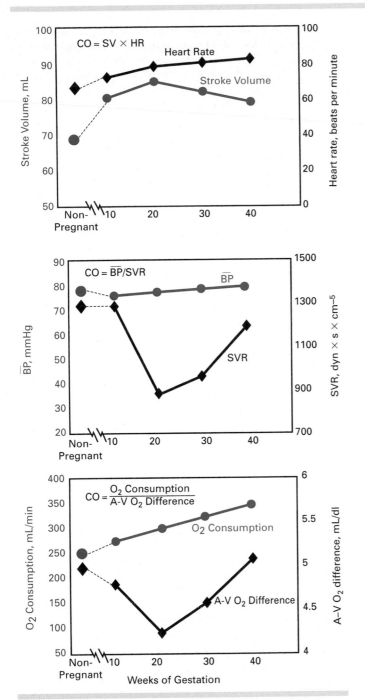

FIGURE 92-2 The cardiac output(CO) can be determined from other parameters in at least three ways: CO = heart rate (HR) × stroke volume (SV); CO = mean arterial pressure (BP) minus the RA pressure/systemic vascular resistance (SVR); CO = oxygen (O₂) consumption/arteriovenous (AV) O₂ difference. The expected values for these parameters measured in the supine position during pregnancy are based on information acquired from many studies.[3–7]

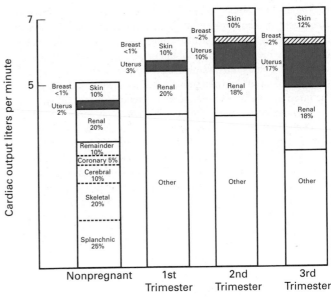

FIGURE 92-3 The changes in cardiac output and its distribution at rest in nonpregnant women. Data used in this graph are fragmentary, especially early in pregnancy.

the use of general anesthesia reduces it still further. Following delivery, the CO briefly approaches 10 L/min[10] (7 to 8 L/min with cesarean section)[11]; it then falls rapidly to near-normal, nonpregnant values within a few weeks after delivery. A slight elevation in CO can persist for as long as a year.[12] The increase in maternal CO in women with twins or triplets is slightly greater than that in women with single pregnancies.[13]

The distribution of blood flow is affected by changes in local vascular resistance (Fig. 92-3). Resistance changes are still not fully understood. Hopefully, new imaging modalities will allow us to know if the estimate of organ flow described in the past are accurate.[14] Renal blood flow increases by approximately 30 percent in the first trimester and remains at that level or declines slightly throughout the pregnancy. Nonpregnant mammary blood flow is usually less than 1 percent of the CO but can be approximately 2 percent of the CO at term. Blood flow to the skin increases by 40 to 50 percent—a mechanism for heat dissipation.

In the nonpregnant woman, uterine blood flow is approximately 100 mL/min (2 percent of the CO); it increases to approximately 1200 mL/min at term, a value approaching the mother's blood flow to her own kidneys.[15,16] During pregnancy, uterine blood vessels are maximally dilated; flow can increase, but this must result from increased maternal arterial pressure and flow. Excitement, heat, anxiety,[17] exercise, and decrease in venous return all decrease uterine blood flow. Vasoconstriction caused by endogenous catecholamines, vasoconstrictive drugs, maternal mechanical pulmonary ventilation, and some anesthetics as well as that associated with preeclampsia and eclampsia can decrease perfusion of the uterus. Although uterine blood flow can potentially be limited even in a healthy woman, the concern about diversion of flow from the uterus is greater in the mother with heart disease.

Hemodynamic Changes with Exercise

Pregnancy changes the hemodynamic response to exercise.[8] For any given level of exercise in the sitting position, the CO is greater than

consumption; thus the arteriovenous oxygen difference narrows early in pregnancy with a gradual increase in oxygen extraction throughout pregnancy, so that by term, the systemic arteriovenous oxygen difference exceeds nonpregnant values.

At the beginning of labor, CO measured in the supine position increases to over 7 L/min. This rises to over 9 L/min with each uterine contraction due to extrusion of approximately 500 mL of blood into the central venous system and to an increase in heart rate. Administration of epidural anesthesia reduces this CO to about 8 L/min, and in nonpregnant women, and maximum CO is reached at lower exercise levels. In a nonpregnant woman, training or conditioning results in a greater increase in stroke volume and a smaller increment in heart rate with exercise than would occur in an untrained individual. During pregnancy, this training effect is not seen, possibly because the increase in stroke volume is limited as a result of compression of the inferior vena cava or the increased venous distensibility.[18]

Exercise during pregnancy is not clearly any more dangerous or beneficial to the mother with heart disease than when she is not pregnant. It does affect the fetus. In animal models, maternal exercise has been associated with a fall in uterine blood flow. In humans, it is known that the type of exercise affects maternal hemodynamics and uterine perfusion.[19,20] As an example, maximal exercise by swimming causes less fetal bradycardia (a marker of uterine blood flow) than the same level of cycling.[21] Additionally, regular aerobic endurance exercise during pregnancy has been associated with a reduction in birth weight. Since most of the reduction is due to a decrease in neonatal fat mass, it is not clear if it is detrimental.[22,23]

Infants born to mothers who work in a standing position may be abnormally small at birth.[23] Although the long-term effects of this are not clear, the implications in relation to exercise and work in the upright position are likely greater for women with heart disease.[24–26] This question, relating to exercise and the effect on the fetus, has become more important with an increasing enthusiasm for recreational exercise in the United States. Although there are insufficient data to suggest that the healthy pregnant woman should avoid recreational exercise, an argument can be made for advising the woman with heart disease to keep the exercise level below that which causes symptoms.[27]

Mechanisms for Hemodynamic Changes

The mechanisms evoking the hemodynamic adaptation to pregnancy are not fully understood. They may in part be due to volume changes. Total body water increases steadily throughout pregnancy by 6 to 8 L (most is extracellular).[28] Sodium retention results in an excess accumulation of 500 to 900 meq by the time of delivery. As early as 6 weeks after conception, plasma volume increases, approaching its maximum of $1\frac{1}{2}$ to 2 times normal by the second trimester, where it stays throughout the pregnancy.[29] The red blood cell mass also increases, but not to the same degree as the increase in plasma volume. As a result, the hematocrit falls, though rarely to less than 30 percent. Peak hemodilution occurs at 24 to 26 weeks; then the hematocrit gradually increases.

Vascular alterations also contribute to the hemodynamic changes of pregnancy. Arterial compliance is increased.[30,31] Venous capacitance increases as well, although there is an increase in venous vascular tone.[31,32] These changes are advantageous in maintaining the hemodynamics of a normal pregnancy. There may be disadvantages as well; vascular accidents, when they occur in women, frequently do so during pregnancy.[33–36] Additionally, the venous changes may explain in part the increase in thromboemboli during pregnancy.[37]

Intrinsic cardiac changes can also explain some of the hemodynamic changes.[38,39] The stroke volume increases by approximately 25 percent. The ejection fraction does not change; thus the heart has to enlarge (since the ejection fraction is the stroke volume divided by the end-diastolic volume). Since the increases in left ventricular (LV) end-diastolic and systolic volumes are small and not adequate to explain the constant ejection fraction, the heart must become reconfigured as well. If so, this occurs with only a 10 to 15 percent increase in myocardial mass during pregnancy and an alteration in LV compliance.[40]

The ultimate cause of these recognized changes is uncertain. Complex interactions of the renin-angiotension-aldosterone system, the reproductive hormones, prostaglandins, nitric oxide, and atrial natriuretic factor contribute to the fluid and sodium changes. Currently, the effects of the increased level of circulating steroid hormones seem to explain the vascular and myocardial changes satisfactorily.

DIAGNOSIS OF HEART DISEASE

Clinical Evaluation

The recognition and definition of heart disease are often difficult during pregnancy. Symptoms suggesting heart disease—including fatigue, dyspnea, orthopnea, pedal edema, and chest discomfort—occur commonly in pregnant women with normal hearts. Although they should alert a caregiver to the possibility of heart disease, the concern should increase if the dyspnea or orthopnea is progressive and limiting or if a woman develops hemoptysis, syncope with exertion, or chest pain clearly related to effort. Common examination features of a normal pregnancy include pedal edema, basilar pulmonary rales, a third heart sound, a systolic murmur, and prominent neck vein pulsations (Chap. 12). However, cyanosis or clubbing, a loud systolic murmur (grade 3 or louder), cardiomegaly, a "fixed split" second heart sound, or a left parasternal lift and loud P_2 do not occur as part of a normal pregnancy. A diastolic murmur is unusual enough during pregnancy, and it generally indicates heart disease if care is taken to exclude the venous hum or internal mammary flow sounds (the mammary souffle), which have diastolic components and are normal (Chap. 12).

Diagnostic Studies

It is preferable to evaluate the cardiovascular status during pregnancy with the history and physical examination alone. On occasion, additional diagnostic studies are required. They should be chosen with a consideration of the risks to the mother and to the fetus and performed by medical personnel experienced with the changes of pregnancy so as to avoid a mistake in diagnosis, with consequent anxiety, apprehension, and unnecessary expense.

ECHOCARDIOGRAPHY WITH DOPPLER FLOW STUDIES
Echocardiography with evaluation of flow by Doppler is so safe (no known risk to the mother or fetus) and is so diagnostically useful that overuse, expense, and potential misinterpretation are the only significant concerns (Chap. 15).

RADIOGRAPHIC PROCEDURES
All x-ray procedures should generally be avoided, particularly early in pregnancy. They increase the risk of abnormal fetal organogenesis or of a subsequent malignancy in the child, particularly leukemia. If a study is required, it should be delayed to as late in pregnancy as possible, the radiation dose should be kept to a minimum, and shielding of the fetus should be optimal (Chap. 14).[41] Every woman of childbearing age should be questioned about the possibility of pregnancy before any x-ray procedure. The exposure to a fetus is small (estimated to be 10 to 1400 μGy) and has not been associated with any recognizable increase in congenital malformations or malignancies. This information can be given to worried parents if a chest x-ray was performed.

ELECTROCARDIOGRAPHY

Electrocardiography is safe. Pregnancy makes interpretation of ST-T wave variations even more difficult than usual; inferior ST-segment depression is common enough to possibly be the result of a normal pregnancy. There is a leftward shift of the QRS axis during pregnancy, but true axis deviation (−30 degrees) implies heart disease (Chap. 13.)

RADIONUCLIDE STUDIES

Although many radionuclides should attach to albumin and thus not reach the fetus, separation can occur and fetal exposure is possible. It is preferable to avoid these studies. On occasion, a pulmonary ventilation/perfusion scan or even a thallium myocardial perfusion scan is required during pregnancy. Estimated exposure to the fetus is low (400 μGy) (Chap. 19).[37]

MAGNETIC RESONANCE IMAGING

No adverse fetal effects have been reported with the use of this procedure during pregnancy. It should be avoided in women with implanted pacemakers or defibrillators (Chap. 21).

CARDIOVASCULAR DRUGS AND PREGNANCY

Nearly all cardiac drugs cross the placenta and are secreted in breast milk. Since information about the use of any drug is incomplete, it is best to avoid their use but, if required for maternal safety, they should not be withheld.[42,43]

Diuretics

Diuretics can and should be used for treatment of congestive heart failure that is uncontrolled by sodium restriction, and they are first-line therapy for the treatment of hypertension.[43–45] No one agent is clearly contraindicated; experience is greatest with the thiazide diuretics and with furosemide.[43,44] Diuretics should not be used for prophylaxis against toxemia or for treatment of pedal edema.

Inotropic Agents

The indications for the use of digitalis are not changed by pregnancy. Fetal serum levels approximate those in the mother. The same dose of digoxin in general will yield lower maternal serum levels during pregnancy than in the nonpregnant state.[43] Digitalis may shorten the duration of gestation and labor due to an effect on the myometrium similar to the inotropic effect on the myocardium.

When intravenous inotropic or vasopressor agents are required, the standard agents (dopamine, dobutamine, and norepinephrine) may be used, but the fetus is jeopardized because all such agents increase resistance to uterine blood flow and may stimulate uterine contractions. Ephedrine is an appropriate initial vasopressor drug since, at least in animal models, it does not adversely affect uterine blood flow.

There is no available information about the efficacy or safety of the phosphodiesterase inhibitors (amrinone, milrinone).

Adrenergic-Receptor-Blocking Agents

Observations that beta blockers may decrease umbilical blood flow, initiate premature labor, and result in a small and infarcted placenta with the potential for low-birth-weight infants have led to concerns about their use. However, beta-blocking drugs have been used in a large number of pregnant women without adverse effects. Their use for the usual clinical indications is reasonable.[46,47] All the available beta-blocking agents cross the placenta, are present in human breast milk, and can reach significant levels in the fetus or newborn. Recent concerns about low birth weights from maternal use of atenolol early in pregnancy[48] make use of alternative beta$_1$-selective agents preferable. If these agents are used during pregnancy, it is appropriate to monitor fetal heart rate as well as, immediately after delivery, the newborn infant's heart rate, blood sugar, and respiratory status.

Experience with the alpha-blocking agents phenoxybenzamine and phentolamine is sparse. Clonidine, prazosin, and labetalol, with their mixed alpha- and beta-blocking effects, have been used for the treatment of hypertension during pregnancy without clear detrimental effects.[49]

Calcium Channel Blocking Drugs

The dihydiopyridine agents (nifedipine, nicardipine, isradipine, felopidine) are effective antihypertensive and afterload-reducing agents that have been used without any adverse effect on the fetus or newborn infant.[43,50] If a nondihydropyridine agent is desired, verapamil is the drug of choice. The calcium channel blockers also cause relaxation of the uterus; nifedipine has been used for this purpose.

Antiarrhythmic Agents

Atrioventricular (AV) node blockade is occasionally required during pregnancy. This can be achieved with digoxin, beta blockers, and calcium blockers. Early reports suggest that adenosine can also be safely used as an AV node–blocking agent.[51] As a general rule, it is preferable to avoid the standard antiarrhythmic drugs in any patient. This is true during pregnancy as well. When such drugs are essential for the treatment of recurrent arrhythmias or for maternal safety, they should be used. However, there is insufficient accumulated information as to whether these drugs increase the risk to the fetus or child.[43,52,53] If intravenous drug therapy is required, lidocaine or procainamide provide reasonable first-line therapy; there is *no reported* experience with intravenous *amiodarone*.

If oral antiarrhythmic therapy is necessary, it may still be appropriate to begin with quinidine, since—given its long-term availability—it is the drug that has been most frequently used without clear adverse fetal effects.[43,52,53] Information about procainamide, disopyramide, mexiletine, and dofetilide is sparse. Flecainide and sotalol are the drugs most often given to the mother to treat fetal arrhythmias; this and clinical experience makes them seem reasonable choices for the treatment of arrhythmias in the mother.[53,54] The early available information concerning amiodarone indicates a 10 percent chance of fetal thyroid abnormalities and an increased likelihood of fetal loss and deformity.[55,56] Thus it should be avoided unless its use is essential for maternal or fetal safety.

Vasodilator Agents

When needed for a hypertensive crisis or emergency afterload and preload reduction, nitroprusside is the vasodilator drug of choice. Despite a paucity of information about its use during pregnancy, this controversial recommendation is made because the drug is highly effective, works instantly, and is easily titrated; its effects dissipate immediately when the drug is stopped. The concern about the use of this drug is that its metabolite, cyanide, can be detected in the fetus. This has not been demonstrated to be a significant problem in humans.[57,58] The appearance of this metabolite is a reason to limit the duration of use of this drug whenever possible. Intravenous hydralazine, nitroglycerin, or labetalol are alternative options for parenteral therapy.

Chronic afterload reduction to treat hypertension, aortic or mitral regurgitation, or ventricular dysfunction during pregnancy has been achieved with the calcium blocking drugs hydralazine and methyldopa.[49,59] Adverse fetal effects have not been reported.

The angiotensin-converting enzyme (ACE) inhibitors increase the risk of abnormalities in fetal renal development and are *contraindicated in pregnancy*.[49,60] A series of case reports of similar problems with the angiotensin II receptor blockers suggest that their use should be avoided until more data are available.[61,62]

Antithrombotic Agents

The chronic use of warfarin is associated with a 1 to 5 percent chance per year of significant bleeding. Warfarin crosses the placenta, and fetal exposure during the first 3 months (particularly weeks 7 to 12) is associated with a 5 to 25 percent incidence of malformations that comprise the "warfarin embryopathy syndrome" (facial abnormalities, optic atrophy, digital abnormalities, epithelial changes, and mental impairment).[63–65] The syndrome may be dose-related, with one study suggesting that it occurs only with doses greater than 5 mg/day.[66] The use of warfarin at any time during pregnancy increases the risk of fetal bleeding or maternal uterine hemorrhage.

Self-administered subcutaneous high-dose unfractionated heparin (16,000 to 24,000 U/day) is a feasible alternative.[67,68] This drug does not cross the placenta. Accumulating data suggest that low-molecular-weight heparin, while currently more expensive, is effective, easier to use (once or twice daily without the need to follow serial blood tests), and as safe as standard heparin.[68a] Although evaluated for the prophylaxis of venous thrombosis, its value in preventing thromboemboli in patients with mechanical prostheses has not yet been proven.[64,65,69a] (Chap. 71).

When anticoagulation is required, unfractionated heparin and, more recently, low-molecular heparin[69a] has been advocated for the first trimester and warfarin for the next 5 months, with a return to heparin therapy prior to labor and delivery. Although successful pregnancies have been achieved with this approach, the authors favor avoidance of warfarin during pregnancy; especially when the pregnant woman or her family are capable of heparin administration at home.

Antiplatelet agents increase the chance of maternal bleeding, and they cross the placenta. Aspirin has been associated with an increased incidence of abortion and fetal growth retardation. Its inhibition of prostaglandin synthesis may result in closure of the ductus arteriosus during fetal life.[70] Still, it has frequently been used and even recommended by some for specific indications and as prophylaxis against preeclampsia.[71] These trade-offs are difficult to evaluate; thus aspirin should be avoided unless it is necessary. There are no data available on the effects of dipyridimole, clopidogrel, or the IIb, IIIa glycoprotein platelet receptor inhibitors during pregnancy.

Anesthetic Agents

Anesthesia for surgery during pregnancy and at the time of labor and delivery can adversely affect a woman with heart disease. In most cases, lumbar epidural anesthesia with a pudendal nerve block to minimize pain is effective and least likely to result in hemodynamic compromise.[72]

MANAGEMENT OF CARDIOVASCULAR SYNDROMES

Cardiovascular complications can occur with any form of heart disease. The management of each patient must be individualized, but some recommendations are applicable in most cases.

Low-Cardiac-Output Syndrome

A low CO is ominous in any patient, and this is particularly true in pregnancy. Although potentially treatable causes such as tamponade or severe valvular stenosis should be considered, low CO is most often due to intravascular volume depletion. This should be prevented when possible and corrected when recognized. Although it is a concern in any pregnant woman, volume depletion is particularly dangerous in those with lesions that limit blood flow, such as pulmonary hypertension, aortic or pulmonic valve stenosis, hypertrophic cardiomyopathy, or mitral stenosis. Measures to prevent or treat a fall in central blood volume are outlined in Table 92-2.

Congestive Heart Failure

The management of congestive heart failure during pregnancy should not differ greatly from that at other times *except* that the ACE inhibitors and angiotensin II receptor blockers should not be used. Congestive heart failure is one situation where maintaining a woman in the supine position may be beneficial by causing preload reduction with obstruction of return of blood from the inferior vena cava to the heart.

Thromboembolic Complications

The risk of venous thromboemboli increases fivefold during and immediately after pregnancy,[37,73,74] and there is arguably an increase in arterial emboli as well.[75] Both may be the result of a woman's hypercoagulable status during pregnancy, and the likelihood of venous thrombosis is increased by venous stasis. Prevention is optimal. Prophylactic full-dose heparin or low-molecular-weight heparin[76] is indicated in those at high risk for a thromboembolic complication including women with thromboemboli during a previous pregnancy (percent risk of thrombus/embolus is 4 to 15 percent), antithrombin

TABLE 92-2 Measures to Protect Against a Fall in Central Blood Volume

Position
    45–60° left lateral
    10° Trendelenburg
Full-leg stockings
Volume preloading for surgery and delivery 1500 mL of
    glucose-free normal saline
Drugs
    Avoid vasodilator drugs
    Ephedrine for hypotension unresponsive to fluid
      replacement
Anesthetics (if required)
    Regional: serial small boluses
    General: emphasis on benzodiazepines and narcotics,
      low-dose inhalation agents

III deficiency (70 percent), protein C deficiency (33 percent), protein S deficiency (17 percent), and the anticardiolipin antibody syndrome.[37] Prothrombin gene mutations and factor V mutation resulting in the resistance to activated protein C (found in 3 to 5 percent of the population) may eventually be shown to be a reason for prophylaxis as well.[77–78]

If a thrombus or embolus is identified, 5 to 10 days of intravenous heparin therapy followed by full-dose subcutaneous heparin is recommended.[37] If a thromboembolus is life-threatening (e.g., a massive pulmonary embolus or a thrombosed prosthetic valve), thrombolytic therapy can be used[79,80] (Chaps. 54 and 63).

Hypertension

Hypertension can be present before pregnancy (in 1 to 5 percent) and persist throughout pregnancy, or it can develop with pregnancy.[49,80] When normotensive women become pregnant, 5 to 7 percent will develop hypertension. Because of the marked early fall in systemic vascular resistance, hypertension often does not occur until the second half of pregnancy. It has been identified as *pregnancy-induced* or *gestational hypertension* or *toxemia*. When associated with proteinuria, pedal edema, central nervous system (CNS) irritability, elevation of liver enzymes, and coagulation disturbances, the hypertension syndrome is called *preeclampsia*. If convulsions occur, the diagnosis is *eclampsia*. It is not clear that hypertension alone puts the mother or fetus at risk during pregnancy, but preeclampsia increases maternal risk (1 to 2 percent chance of CNS bleed, convulsions, or other severe systemic illness) and may cause fetal growth retardation (10 to 15 percent). Maternal and fetal morbidity and mortality increase still further with eclampsia.

Guidelines for the level of BP control are not well established. Until more is known, an argument can be made for keeping the systolic BP below 160 mmHg and the diastolic BP below 100 mmHg. This may provide a margin of safety against severe hypertensive episodes and possibly will improve fetal survival. Unless the patient has previously demonstrated salt-sensitive hypertension, sodium restriction is generally inadvisable, since pregnant women with hypertension have lower plasma volumes than normotensive women. Despite this, if drug treatment is required, a thiazide drug is optimal firsts-line therapy. If an additional drug is needed, experience is greatest with methyldopa.[49,81–84] This otherwise infrequently used antihypertensive agent has been used with normal development of the fetus and neonate. Beta$_1$-selective blockers and calcium channel blockers have been proven to be effective. Again, ACE inhibitors *should not be used,* and the safety of angiotension II blocking agents has been questioned.[61,62]

Pulmonary Hypertension

Whether pulmonary hypertension (PH) (Chap. 62) is primary or secondary to prolonged left-to-right shunting (Eisenmenger's syndrome), drug abuse, a primary vascular disease syndrome, or recurrent pulmonary emboli, maternal mortality ranges from 30 to 70 percent.[85,86] Even with maternal survival, fetal loss exceeds 40 percent. Maternal death can occur at any time during pregnancy, but the mother is most vulnerable during the time of labor and delivery and in the first postpartum week. If PH is recognized early in pregnancy, interruption of the pregnancy is advised. If this is declined or if the PH is recognized late in pregnancy, close follow-up is required. Intravascular volume depletion puts these patients at greatest risk. Systemic vascular resistance and pressure must be maintained in patients with PH who have a right-to-left shunt, and meticulous attention to

intravenous catheters is essential to avoid systemic emboli. At the time of labor and delivery, a central venous line allows adequate fluid administration, and a radial artery catheter makes determinations of BP and oxygen saturation easier. These lines should be used for 48 to 72 h postdelivery.

Arrhythmias

In the woman with dizziness, palpitations, and light-headedness, pregnancy offers many other explanations, but arrhythmias should be considered as a possible cause. The rules for treatment should be the same as in the nonpregnant patient with the possible exception that a rhythm causing hemodynamic instability should be treated somewhat more rapidly because of concern about diversion of blood flow away from the uterus. As always, if a potentially reversible cause can be identified, it should be corrected.

Tachyarrhythmias are as frequent during pregnancy. The presence of *atrial* or *ventricular premature beats* or of *sinus tachycardia* is a reason to identify and correct the cause but not a reason to institute specific treatment for arrhythmias.

Paroxysmal supraventricular tachycardia is the most common sustained abnormal rhythm occurring with pregnancy.[53,87,88] Initial treatment with vagal maneuvers is as appropriate as at other times. If medical treatment is required, intravenous adenosine or verapamil is effective. Cardioversion can be used if required.[59] If recurrent episodes necessitate a daily drug, verapamil or a beta blocker is often effective. Digoxin is less effective and should be avoided if the patient has preexcitation.

Management of *atrial fibrillation* and *flutter* should be as in the nonpregnant woman. If these rhythms occur in a woman with mitral stenosis, severe left ventricular dysfunction, or a previous thromboembolic event, antithrombotic therapy with heparin is indicated (Chaps. 28 and 29).

If necessary for refractory arrhythmias, radiofrequency catheter ablation can be performed, optimally later in pregnancy and with radiation shielding.[41]

Ventricular tachycardia may occur during pregnancy.[52,53,90] If it is suggestive of a right ventricular outflow tract tachycardia (a left bundle branch block with vertical axis morphology), beta-blocker therapy may be effective (Chap. 31). Emergency management of rapid ventricular tachycardia or ventricular fibrillation should be as recommended for the nonpregnant woman.[91,92] If possible, during acute management, the pelvis should be rolled to the left to enhance blood return from the lower extremities. If pregnancy has proceeded beyond 24 weeks and maternal survival is in question, emergency cesarean section should be considered. Pregnancies have been successful in women with implanted cardioverter/defibrillators; treatment shocks have no demonstrated adverse effects on the baby.

Abnormalities that predispose young adults to ventricular fibrillation are not well characterized during pregnancy. Most is known about the prolonged QT-interval syndrome.[93,94] If this is recognized (usually from transient arrhythmia symptoms) and it is an acquired form, the presumed cause (usually a drug) should be eliminated. If the syndrome is congenital, beta-blocker therapy during pregnancy is warranted (Chap. 28). Implantable defibrillators have been used with recurrent ventricular arrhythmias, but their value remains unproven in this syndrome even when it is unrelated to pregnancy. In patients with a congenital syndrome, transmission with autosomal dominance can affect the child.

Bradyarrhythmias may also occur during pregnancy (Chap. 32). Although they are a reason to look for a reversible cause, treatment is generally not required unless the patient has clear hemodynamic compromise. Complete heart block, which in this age group is most likely to be congenital in origin, is consistent with a successful pregnancy.[95] If required, a permanent pacemaker can be inserted.

Loss-of-Consciousness Spells

Pregnancy makes an assessment of a loss-of-consciousness spell even more difficult than usual. If a seizure disorder cannot be excluded as a cause, appropriate evaluation with electroencephalography is indicated. If a seizure is unlikely or excluded, the syndrome of syncope should include a consideration of the usual causes, most of which are due to an imbalance of vascular volume and tone or to cardiac abnormalities (Chap. 40).

Endocarditis

Infective endocarditis can occur during pregnancy in women without a recognized heart abnormality, but structural abnormalities place individuals at much greater risk (Chap. 81). The clinical presentation of endocarditis is the same during pregnancy as at other times.[96,97] *Streptococcus* is the most common cause. Intravenous drug abusers are more likely to have staphylococcal infections, and women with genitourinary tract infections are more likely to have gram-negative infections, most commonly due to *Escherichia coli*. Optimal management includes prevention. Although it is not the recommendation of the American Heart Association committee addressing this issue,[97] most physicians caring for women with heart disease recommend antibiotic prophylaxis at the time of dental or surgical procedures or at labor and delivery. If endocarditis does occur, it should be treated aggressively with medical therapy, and the usual indications for surgery are appropriate during pregnancy. If open-heart surgery is required late in pregnancy, simultaneous cesarean section should be considered.

Surgery

Although surgery is not exactly a complication of pregnancy, pregnant women with heart disease have the same 0.5 to 2.0 percent chance of requiring surgery as those who are not pregnant. If surgery is required, maintenance of central volume can be enhanced utilizing the measures outlined in Table 92-2. Fetal monitoring should be performed. If it is essential to perform heart surgery during pregnancy, the risks are greater than in the nonpregnant woman and fetal risk is high.[98,99]

SPECIFIC FORMS OF HEART DISEASE

Other sections of this book discuss specific cardiovascular abnormalities in detail. The remainder of this chapter relates these to pregnancy. In assessing each, it is appropriate to consider antibiotic prophylaxis against endocarditis with dental or surgical procedures. Though of unproven value, it is as appropriate during pregnancy as at other times[97] and is recommended at labor and delivery.

Rheumatic Heart Disease

Rheumatic fever remains a common and virulent disease worldwide but is uncommon in the United States. The resultant valve and myocardial disease are probably the most common cardiac abnormalities affecting pregnancy.[100] In the United States, clinically recognized rheumatic fever is uncommon but does occur. In a woman

presenting with myocarditis, rheumatic fever as a cause should be considered, particularly if it is associated with fever, joint discomfort, subcutaneous nodules, erythema marginatum, or chorea and if there is evidence of a group A streptococcal infection.[101] Rheumatic fever is the cause of almost all mitral stenosis; of some isolated mitral, aortic, or tricuspid regurgitation; and of some double- and triple-valve disease. Definition of valve morphology by echocardiography can help to clarify the etiology. Recognition of rheumatic fever as the cause of heart disease is important because it identifies those who need antibiotic prophylaxis to prevent recurrence of the disease.[102]

Valve Disease

MITRAL STENOSIS

The increased CO, tachycardia, and fluid retention of pregnancy may double the resting pressure gradient across a stenotic mitral valve.[68a,103] Symptoms attributable to an increase in left atrial pressure occur in up to 25 percent of patients with mitral stenosis (MS) during pregnancy.[1,104,105] They usually become apparent by the 20th week and may be aggravated still further at the time of labor and delivery. Maternal death is rare when there is careful attention to the management of congestive heart failure.[1] Although potentially at risk from the elevated left atrial pressure, the patient with MS also depends on this pressure to fill the LV. Because the pregnant woman is especially liable to sudden shifts in the distribution of blood volume, preservation of an adequate intravascular volume is essential to prevent a dramatic fall in CO.

If a woman contemplating pregnancy has symptomatic MS, balloon dilation or valve surgery is appropriate before conception. If MS is first recognized during pregnancy and symptoms develop, standard medical therapy is appropriate. If this does not control symptoms, balloon valvuloplasty can be performed (with appropriate radiation shielding of the fetus).[106,107] Mitral valve surgical commissurotomy or valve replacement has been performed, but fetal loss exceeds 30 percent.[99] Atrial fibrillation is of particular concern during pregnancy. The usual rapid ventricular response further compromises diastolic flow time and can result in pulmonary edema. Emergency treatment should include intravenous verapamil or cardioversion (Chap. 67).

MITRAL REGURGITATION

Mitral regurgitation (MR) may be due to rheumatic fever, but unlike MS, the majority of cases are due to other causes (Chap. 67). In general MR is well tolerated during pregnancy.[1,68a,105] If it is severe, symptomatic, or associated with LV dysfunction, valve repair before pregnancy is recommended. Afterload reduction is an important component of therapy, remembering that ACE inhibitors and angiotensin II receptor blockers should not be used. One cause of mitral regurgitation is *mitral valve prolapse* (Chap. 68). The volume and pressure changes of pregnancy may alter examination findings in a woman with mitral valve prolapse (Chap. 68). Associated arrhythmias, endocarditis, cerebral emboli, and hemodynamically significant regurgitation may be rare complications and are no more likely to occur during pregnancy than at other times.[108,109]

AORTIC STENOSIS

The diagnostic criteria for aortic valve stenosis (AS) are the same during pregnancy as at other times. Pregnancy in the presence of AS can be successful, but if stenosis is severe, maternal deaths have occurred and congestive heart failure is common.[1,68a,105,110] The offspring can have as high as a 20 percent incidence of congenital heart disease, a value that interestingly can potentially be halved by correcting the outflow tract obstruction prior to pregnancy.[111]

If severe AS is recognized before pregnancy, balloon valvotomy or a surgical commissurotomy is recommended prior to conception. If pregnancy does occur in the presence of severe aortic stenosis, measures to avoid hypovolemia are particularly important. If congestive heart failure develops, it can be treated as previously described. If severe symptoms persist, a balloon valvuloplasty or aortic valve surgery can be performed during pregnancy,[112-114] the latter being associated with increased fetal loss (Chap. 66).

AORTIC REGURGITATION

Like AS, aortic regurgitation (AR) may be congenital, but other causes include rheumatic fever, endocarditis, dilation of the aortic root, or, more ominously, aortic dissection. A dilated root or dissection should raise the consideration of Marfan's syndrome. Aortic regurgitation is generally well tolerated during pregnancy; however, if it is severe, symptomatic, or associated with LV dysfunction, valve surgery should be considered before pregnancy.[1,2,105,112] If congestive heart failure occurs with pregnancy, treatment should include afterload reduction. *ACE inhibitors and angiotensin-receptor blockers should be avoided.* If endocarditis should occur and the infection is not rapidly controlled, mortality with medical therapy is high and surgical therapy is indicated. If this occurs late in pregnancy, consideration of associated cesarean section is appropriate.

PULMONIC VALVE DISEASE

Many women with pulmonic valve disease will have had previous valve comissurotomy or balloon valvuloplasty for valve stenosis or as part of the correction of tetralogy of Fallot. The residual stenosis and invariable regurgitation are potential concerns but in general do not adversely affect the outcome of pregnancy. The occasional patient with significant pulmonic valve stenosis who has not been treated appears to tolerate pregnancy well. Intravascular volume depletion should be avoided. If severe symptoms (recurrent syncope, uncontrolled dyspnea, and chest pain) occur, balloon valvuloplasty can be performed.

TRICUSPID VALVE DISEASE

Significant tricuspid valve disease is also uncommon during pregnancy. The incidence of regurgitation has increased because of intravenous drug use, with its resultant right-sided endocarditis. This regurgitation requires no specific therapy during pregnancy. Tricuspid stenosis is rare. If it is encountered, avoidance of intravascular volume depletion would seem to be important.

PROSTHETIC VALVE DISEASE

An artificial valve can perhaps be considered the ultimate form of valve disease (Chap. 70). Although many have benefited from these valves, all are left with "prosthetic heart valve disease." One or more of its major associated complications—thromboemboli, bleeding (from anticoagulation), endocarditis, valve dysfunction, reoperation, or death—affects patients at a rate of greater than 5 percent per year throughout their lives.[115,116] Pregnancy increases the risk of each of these complications, and the prosthetic valve and its treatment can adversely affect the fetus.[65,68,117,118] All these are reasons that a prosthetic valve is a relative contraindication to pregnancy. Still, women with prosthetic valves often become pregnant. Anticoagulation is required in those with a *mechanical* prosthesis. Full-dose subcutaneous heparin is the therapy of choice, maintaining anticoagulation at the "high therapeutic level" by following factor Xa levels; partial thromboplastin levels are unreliable during pregnancy. Low-

molecular-weight heparin is a reasonable alternative but has not been evaluated in patients with prosthetic valves[69,69a] (Chap. 70). There is insufficient data to reliably predict or compare clinical outcomes or to confirm the safety of enoxaparin, unfractionated heparin, or warfarin with mechanical heart valves. A *heterograft* or *homograft* prosthesis is an alternative to a mechanical prosthesis. Because of the inherently lower thromboembolic rates associated with these tissue prostheses, anticoagulation is not needed. However, they do not completely eliminate the concern about thromboemboli, and the rate of heterograft degeneration is high in young women, resulting in the need for early valve replacement[119] (see Chap. 70). On balance, when choosing a prosthetic valve for a woman of childbearing age, we recommend a mechanical prosthesis for those capable of heparin management. If the safe use of anticoagulation is questionable, a bioprosthesis may be preferable.

Congenital Heart Disease

Congenital heart disease is now the most common heart disease encountered in women of childbearing age in the United States. In most, it has been altered by surgery. Each abnormality is unique, but some issues apply to all. First, some abnormalities significantly increase the risk of maternal morbidity and mortality during pregnancy. Second, there is an increased risk of fetal death,[2] which increases with the severity of the maternal lesions. Third, the presence of a congenital cardiac abnormality in either parent or in a sibling increases the risk of cardiac and other congenital abnormalities in the fetus. Congenital heart disease is recognized in 0.8 percent of all live births in the United States.[120,121] Its presence in a parent increases this risk to 2 to 15 percent.[120] Although some have shown that the risk is two to three times greater if it is the mother rather than the father who has congenital heart disease,[121,124] this finding has not been universal.[123] Actually, the risk that a child will have heart disease can reach 50 percent when the abnormality is transmitted as an autosomal dominant trait, as in the case of Marfan's syndrome, the congenital long-QT syndrome, or hypertrophic cardiomyopathy. When recognized, maternal congenital heart disease should be corrected prior to surgery. In some cases, this will make the pregnancy safer for the mother and may provide a better intrauterine environment for fetal development. Fourth, the implications of residual or inoperable lesions must be clearly understood before pregnancy is undertaken. Finally, as with valve disease, antibiotic prophylaxis against endocarditis is as appropriate during pregnancy as at other times.

LEFT-TO-RIGHT SHUNTS

Some women with left-to-right shunts reach adulthood and become pregnant often without previous recognition of their disease. Although left-to-right shunting increases the chances of PH, right ventricular (RV) failure, arrhythmias, and emboli, it is not clear that these complications are made more likely by a pregnancy. The degree of shunting is generally not affected by pregnancy since the resistances of the systemic and pulmonary vascular circuits fall to a similar degree.[125] The RV volume overload associated with the shunts is generally well tolerated during pregnancy.

Atrial septal defects are the most common cause of left to right shunts with *ventricular septal defects* or a *patent ductus arteriosus* occasionally presenting at the time of pregnancy. In each case, pregnancy is generally well tolerated. There is a 15 to 20 percent fetal loss rate and the offspring have a 5 to 15 percent chance of having a congenital heart abnormality (an incidence not affected by previous corrective procedures).[126] Correction, if anything, makes pregnancy even safer.

RIGHT-TO-LEFT SHUNT ("CYANOTIC" HEART DISEASE)

Right-to-left shunting can occur through septal defects when pulmonary vascular resistance exceeds systemic vascular resistance or when there is an obstruction to RV outflow and pulmonary vascular resistance is normal. All are forms of "cyanotic" heart disease. The presence of cyanosis, especially when sufficient to result in elevated hemoglobin levels, is associated with high fetal loss, prematurity, and reduced infant birth weights.[1,2,112,127,128] The situation of elevated pulmonary vascular resistance, or Eisenmenger's syndrome, has been discussed earlier under "Pulmonary Hypertension." With this problem, it is advisable to avoid or interrupt pregnancy. When the cyanosis is not due to Eisenmenger's syndrome, maternal mortality is less, but women are at increased risk of heart failure (approximately 15 percent) from thromboemboli, arrhythmias, and endocarditis (4.5 percent).[127]

Tetralogy of Fallot This is the most common form of right-to-left shunting resulting from obstruction to pulmonary flow when pulmonary vascular resistance is normal. If it is uncorrected, successful pregnancy can be achieved, but maternal mortality is high and fetal loss can exceed 50 percent. After surgical correction of the defect, maternal mortality does not clearly exceed that of a woman without heart disease[128]; the offspring have a 5 to 10 percent chance of having congenital heart disease.

OBSTRUCTIVE LESIONS

Two recommendations apply in women with obstructive cardiac lesions. First, volume depletion should be avoided, since it can result in a significant fall in CO whether the obstruction is on the left or right side of the heart. Second, surgical or catheter treatment for a left- or right-sided obstructive lesion is recommended prior to pregnancy, not only to increase maternal safety but also to decrease the chance of congenital heart disease in the offspring.[111]

Two LV obstructive disease processes warrant further discussion: coarctation of the aorta and hypertrophic obstructive cardiomyopathy.

Coarctation of the Aorta More common in men, coarctation may occur in women who reach childbearing age and conceive (Chap. 74). Maternal mortality rates range from 3 to 8 percent.[1] Surgical correction prior to pregnancy reduces the risk of aortic dissection or rupture.[129] If pregnancy occurs in a woman with a coarctation, BP control is appropriate. Antibiotic prophylaxis is recommended because of the associated bicuspic aortic valve. The effects of catheter dilation of a coarctation on subsequent pregnancies are uncertain, but they are as likely to decrease the risks associated with pregnancy as the surgical procedure. It is not clear whether mechanical treatment decreases the rate of rupture of associated intracranial aneurysms.

Hypertrophic Cardiomyopathy *Hypertrophic cardiomyopathy* (HCM) is inherited as an autosomal dominant trait with variable penetrance; thus offspring have a 50 percent chance of having the abnormality, although phenotypes may vary (Chap. 77). It may occur with or without an LV outflow tract obstruction at rest or with stress. The fall in peripheral vascular resistance and peripheral pooling of blood can cause hypotension, and the intermittent high catecholamine state of pregnancy can increase LV outflow tract obstruction. An increase in the symptoms of dyspnea, chest discomfort, and palpitations has been noted during pregnancy.[130,130a] It is not clear that pregnancy increases the approximately 1 to 3 percent chance per year of sudden death, but deaths with pregnancy may exceed 1 percent.[131] This is another obstructive lesion where it is important to avoid hypovolemia. Beta-blocker therapy has been recommended at the time of labor and delivery.

COMPLEX CONGENITAL LESIONS

Predicting the outcome of pregnancy becomes more difficult as maternal abnormalities become more complex. In general, maternal and fetal morbidity and mortality are high, particularly when the abnormality results in maternal cyanosis or marked functional limitation. Still, surgery has made pregnancy a consideration, even in women with the most severe disease, such as a functional single-ventricle or tricuspid atresia.[132]

Transposition of the Great Vessels Women with d-transposition of the great arteries (some with single ventricles) may become pregnant. The little available information available indicates a very poor maternal and fetal outcome.[2,133] Partial or complete surgical correction of the lesion prior to pregnancy improves the outcome for the mother as well as the fetus.[133,134] If l-transposition ("corrected" transposition) is not complicated by cyanosis, ventricular dysfunction, or heart block, pregnancy should be well tolerated.[135]

Ebstein's Anomaly of the Tricuspid Valve This condition may be mild and unrecognized during pregnancy. Increasing problems of RV dysfunction, obstruction to right-sided heart flow, and right-to-left shunting resulting in cyanosis increase the risk to the woman during pregnancy. Maternal morbidity and mortality are low if the patient does not have severe disease, and fetal loss is approximately 25 percent: significant right-to-left shunting is a reason to avoid pregnancy.[137]

Marfan's Syndrome It may be difficult, but it is important to diagnose Marfan's Syndrome in young women (Chap. 84). First, anecdotally, the risk of death from aortic rupture or dissection during pregnancy is high in women with Marfan's syndrome, particularly if the aortic root is enlarged (greater than 40 mm by echocardiography).[35,137,138] Second, the expected life span of the woman with Marfan's syndrome is reduced to about half of normal, implying that her years of motherhood will be limited. Third, half of the offspring will be affected with the syndrome. These are reasons that women with Marfan's syndrome should be advised to avoid pregnancy. The risks are sufficient to recommend interruption if pregnancy has occurred. Should the parents elect to continue the pregnancy, activity should be restricted and hypertension prevented. While unproven, prophylactic of beta blockers during pregnancy seems reasonable. This is the one cardiovascular syndrome where cesarean delivery is recommended in order to avoid the hemodynamic stresses of labor.

MYOCARDIAL DISEASE

Hypertrophic Cardiomyopathy

HCM has been discussed as an obstructive or nonobstructive lesion. A concentric hypertrophic cardiomyopathy may be the result of aortic stenosis or hypertension[130a] (Chap. 77).

DILATED CARDIOMYOPATHY

The cause of a dilated cardiomyopathy is often unclear (Chap. 71), but up to 30 to 50 percent of these cases are familial.[139,140] Its occurrence is a reason to suggest that pregnancy should be avoided. This strong recommendation is not supported by data from prospective trials but is given because myocardial dysfunction is the feature associated with increased maternal and fetal mortality in many forms of heart disease. It also comes from the observations of those who develop this problem in the third trimester or first 6 weeks postpartum.

This *peripartum cardiomyopathy* may simply be a dilated cardiomyopathy occurring in pregnancy, but given the timing of onset, it may be a unique entity.[141–143] Case reports have suggested that myocarditis may be a part of this disease, but it is not clearly more common than other forms of cardiomyopathy.[144] Small studies have suggested a possible role for treatment with immune globulin.[145] In the woman with a dilated cardiomyopathy during pregnancy, standard treatment for heart failure, thromboemboli, and arrhythmias is appropriate (Chap. 76).

If ventricular function does not return to normal after pregnancy, subsequent pregnancies have been associated with maternal mortality rates of 19 to 50 percent.[146] Even in those whose LV function returns to normal, deaths have been reported with subsequent pregnancies.

Coronary Artery Disease

Chest discomfort is common during a normal pregnancy and for the most part is due to abdominal distension or gastroesophageal reflux. Coronary artery disease (CAD) is an uncommon but possible cause, and both angina and myocardial infarctions have been reported during pregnancy. CAD in pregnancy can result from atherosclerosis, particularly in those with familial hyperlipidemia, diabetes, hypertension, or a smoking history.[147] Other explanations have been dissection of the coronary artery, spasm, emboli, or vasculitis. If CAD is a consideration, an electrocardiogram and exercise stress test may help with the diagnosis. If essential, thallium imaging or angiography can be performed. When it is suspected or demonstrated, CAD should be treated with standard medical therapy. If symptoms are not relieved, angioplasty or bypass surgery can be performed.[148,149]

Pregnancy following Cardiac Transplantation

Many cardiac transplant recipients are women of childbearing age (Chap. 26). Successful pregnancies after transplantation have been reported,[150] but the potential hazards to the mother and fetus—which include maternal heart failure, immunosuppressive therapy, maternal infections, and serial diagnostic studies—have already been recognized as causing problems in the fetus and in newborns. The potential for a shortened maternal life span must also be considered when a patient is counseled about the advisability of pregnancy.

References

1. Siu SC, Sermer M, Coleman JM, et al. Prospective multicenter study of pregnancy outcomes in women with heart disease. *Circulation* 2001;104(5):515–521.
2. Siu SC, Colman JM, Sorensen S, et al. Adverse neonatal and cardiac outcomes are more common in pregnant women with cardiac disease. *Circulation* 2002;105(18):2179–2184.
2a. Reimold SC, Rutherford JD. Valvular heart disease in pregnancy. *N Engl J Med* 2003;349:52–59.
3. Ueland K, Novy MJ, Peterson EN, Metcalfe J. Maternal cardiovascular dynamics: IV. The influence of gestational age on the maternal cardiovascular response to posture and exercise. *Am J Obstet Gynecol* 1969;104:856–864.
4. Capeless EL, Clapp JF. Cardiovascular changes in early phase of pregnancy. *Am J Obstet Gynecol* 1989;161:1449–1453.
5. Easterling TR, Benedetti TJ, Schmucher BC, Millard SP. Maternal hemodynamics in normal and preeclamptic pregnancies: A longitudinal study. *Obstet Gynecol* 1990;76:1061–1069.
6. Robson SC, Hunter S, Boys RJ, Dunlop W. Serial study of factors influencing changes in cardiac output during human pregnancy. *Am J Physiol* 1989;256:H1060–H1065.
7. Clark SL, Cotton DB, Pivarnik JM, et al. Position change and central hemodynamic profile during normal third-trimester pregnancy and postpartum. *Am J Obstet Gynecol* 1991;164:883–887.
8. Sady MA, Haydon BB, Sady SP, et al. Cardiovascular response to maximal cycle exercise during pregnancy and at two and seven months postpartum. *Am J Obstet Gynecol* 1990;162:1181–1185.
9. Kinsella SM, Lohmann G. Supine hypotensive syndrome (review). *Obstet Gynecol* 1994;83:774–788.
10. Robson S, Dunop W, Boys R, Hunter S. Cardiac output during labor. *BMJ* 1987;295:1169–1172.
11. James C, Banner T, Caton D. Cardiac output in women undergoing cesarean section with epidural or general anesthesia. *Am J Obstet Gynecol* 1989;160:1178–1183.
12. Clapp JF III, Capeless E. Cardiovascular function before, during, and after the first and subsequent pregnancies. *Am J Cardiol* 1997;80:1469–1473.
13. Rovinsky JJ, Jaffin H. Cardiovascular hemodynamics in pregnancy: II. Cardiac output and left ventricular work in multiple pregnancy. *Am J Obstet Gynecol* 1966;95:781–784.
14. Metcalfe J, McAnulty JH, Ueland K. *Heart Disease in Pregnancy: Physiology and Management.* Boston: Little, Brown; 1986:1–54.
15. Thoresen M, Wesche J. Doppler measurements of changes in human mammary and uterine blood flow during pregnancy and lactation. *Acta Obstet Gynecol Scand* 1988;67:741–745.
16. Thaler I, Manor D, Itskovitz J, et al. Changes in uterine blood flow during human pregnancy. *Am J Obstet Gynecol* 1990;162:121–125.
17. Teixerira JM, Fisk NM, Glover V. Association between maternal anxiety in pregnancy and increased uterine artery resistance index: Cohort based study. *BMJ* 1999;318:1288–1289.
18. Morton MJ, Paul MS, Campos GR, et al. Exercise dynamics in late gestation: Effects of physical training. *Am J Obstet Gynecol* 1985;152:91–97.
19. Veille JC, Hellerstein HK, Bacevice AE. Maternal left ventricular performance during bicycle exercise. *Am J Cardiol* 1992;69:1506–1508.
20. Rauramo I, Forss M. Effect of exercise on maternal hemodynamics and placental blood flow in healthy women. *Acta Obstet Gynecol Scand* 1988;67:21–25.
21. Watson WJ, Katz VL, Hackney AC, et al. Fetal responses to maximal swimming and cycling exercise during pregnancy. *Obstet Gynecol* 1991;77:382–386.
22. Clapp JF III, Capeless EL. Neonatal morphometrics after endurance exercise during pregnancy. *Am J Obstet Gynecol* 1990;163:1805–1811.
23. Naeye RL, Peters EC. Working during pregnancy: Effects on the fetus. *Pediatrics* 1982;69:724–727.
24. Clapp JF III. Pregnancy outcome: Physical activities inside versus outside the workplace. *Semin Perinatol* 1996;20(1):70–76.
25. Sternfeld B. Physical activity and pregnancy outcome: Review and recommendations. *Sports Med* 1997;23(1):33–47.
26. Campbell MK, Mottola MF. Recreational exercise and occupational activity during pregnancy and birth weight: A case-control study. *Am J Obstet Gynecol* 2001;184(3):403–408.
27. Practice ACO. ACOG Committee opinion. Number 267, January 2002: Exercise during pregnancy and the postpartum period. *Obstet Gynecol* 2002;99(1):171–173.
28. Lindheimer MC, Katz AL. Sodium and diuretics in pregnancy. *N Engl J Med* 1973;299:891–894.
29. Chesley LC. Plasma and red cell volumes during pregnancy. *Am J Obstet Gynecol* 1972;112:440–450.
30. Hart MV, Morton MJ, Hosenpud JD, Metcalfe J. Aortic function during normal human pregnancy. *Am J Obstet Gynecol* 1986;154:887–891.
31. Poppas A, Shroff SG, Korcarz CE, et al. Serial assessment of the cardiovascular system in normal pregnancy: Role of arterial compliance and pulsatile arterial load. *Circulation* 1997;95:2407–2415.
32. Edouard DA, Pannier BM, London GM, et al. Venous and arterial behavior during normal pregnancy. *Am Physiol* 1998;274:H1605–612.

33. Anderson RA, Fineron PW. Aortic dissection in pregnancy: Importance of pregnancy-induced changes in the vessel wall and bicuspid aortic valve in pathogenesis. *Br J Obstet Gynaecol* 1994;101:1085–1088.

34. Nolte JE, Rutherford RB, Nawaz S, et al. Arterial dissections associated with pregnancy (review). *J Vasc Surg* 1995;21:515–520.

35. Elkayam U, Ostrzega E, Shotan A, Mehra A. Cardiovascular problems in pregnant women with the Marfan syndrome (review). *Ann Intern Med* 1995;123:117–122.

36. Lipscomb KJ, Smith JC, Clarke B, et al. Outcome of pregnancy in women with Marfan's syndrome. *Br J Obstet Gynecol* 1997;104(2):201–206.

37. Toglia MR, Weg JH. Venous thromboembolism during pregnancy. *N Engl J Med* 1996;335:108–113.

38. Katz R, Karliner JS, Resnik R. Effects of a natural volume overload state (pregnancy) on left ventricular performance in normal human subjects. *Circulation* 1978;58:434–441.

39. Sadaniantz A, Kocheril AG, Emans SP, et al. Cardiovascular changes in pregnancy evaluated by two-dimensional and Doppler echocardiography. *J Am Soc Echo* 1992;5:253–258.

40. Veille JC, Kitzman DW, et al. Left ventricular diastolic filling response to stationary bicycle exercise during pregnancy and the postpartum period. *American Journal of Obstetrics & Gynecology* 2001;185(4);822–827.

41. Damilakis J, Theocharopoulos N, Perisinakis K, et al. Conceptus radiation dose and risk from cardiac catheter ablation procedures. *Circulation* 2001;104(8):893–897.

42. Committee on Drugs, American Academy of Pediatrics. The transfer of drugs and other chemicals into human breast milk. *Pediatrics* 1994;93:137.

43. Cox JL, Gardner MJ. Cardiovascular drugs in pregnancy and lactation. In: Gleicher N, Gall SA, Sibai BM, et al, eds. *Principles and Practice of Medical Therapy in Pregnancy,* 3d ed. Norwalk, CT: Appleton & Lange; 1998:911–926.

44. Collins R, Yusuf S, Peto R. Overview of randomized trials of diuretics in pregnancy. *BMJ* 1985;290:17–23.

45. ALLHAT Collaborative Research Group. Major outcomes in high-risk hypertensive patients randomized to angiotensin-converting enzyme inhibitor or calcium channel blocker vs diuretic. *JAMA* 2002;2888:2981–2997.

46. Frishman WH, Chesner M. Beta-andrenergic blockers in pregnancy. *Am Heart J* 1988;115:147–152.

47. Magee LA, Elran E, Bull SB, et al. Risks and benefits of beta-receptor blockers for pregnancy hypertension: Overview of the randomized trials. *Eur J Obstet Gynecol Reprod Biol* 2000;88(1):15–26.

48. Lydakis C, Lip GY, Beevers M, Beevers DG. Atenolol and fetal growth in pregnancies complicated by hypertension. *Am J Hypertens* 1999;12:541–547.

49. Sibai BM. Treatment of hypertension in pregnant women (review). *N Engl J Med* 1996;335:257–265.

50. Wide-Swensson DH, Ingemarsson I, Lunell NO, et al. Calcium channel blockade (isradipine) in treatment of hypertension in pregnancy: A randomized placebo-controlled study. *Am J Obstet Gynecol* 1995;173:872–878.

51. Elkayam U, Goodwin TM. Adenosine therapy for supraventricular tachycardia during pregnancy. *Am J Cardiol* 1995;75:521–523.

52. Page RL. Treatment of arrhythmias during pregnancy (review). *Am Heart J* 1995;130:871–876.

53. Tan HL, Lie KI. Treatment of tachyarrhythmias during pregnancy and lactation. *Eur Heart J* 2001;22(6):458–464.

54. Oudijk MA, Michon MM, Kleinman CS, et al. Sotalol in the treatment of fetal dysrhythmias. *Circulation* 2000;101(23):2721–2726.

55. Ovadin M, Brito M, Hoyer GL, Marcus FI. Human experience with amiodarone in the embryonic period. *Am J Cardiol* 1994;73:316–317.

56. Magee LA, Downar E, Sermer M, et al. Pregnancy outcome after gestational exposure to amiodarone in Canada. *Am J Obstet Gynecol* 1995;172:1307–1311.

57. Stempel JE, O'Grady JP, Morton MJ, Johnson KA. Use of sodium nitroprusside in complications of gestational hypertension. *Obstet Gynecol* 1982;60:533–538.

58. Shoemaker CT, Meyers M. Sodium nitroprusside for control of severe hypertensive disease of pregnancy: A case report and discussion of potential toxicity. *Am J Obstet Gynecol* 1984;149:171–173.

59. Cunningham FG, Lindheimer MD. Hypertension in pregnancy. *N Engl J Med* 1992;326:927–932.

60. Hanssens M, Keirse MJ, Vankelecom F, et al. Fetal and neonatal effects of treatment with angiotensin converting enzyme inhibitors in pregnancy. *Obstet Gynecol* 1991;78:128–135.

61. Saji H, Yamanaka M, Hagiwara A, et al. Losartan and fetal toxic effects (comment). *Lancet* 2001;357(9253):363.

62. Lambot MA, Vermeylen D, Noel JC. Angiotensin-II-receptor inhibitors in pregnancy. *Lancet* 2001;357(9268):1619–1620.

63. Hall JT, Pauli RM, Wilson KM. Maternal and fetal sequelae of anticoagulation during pregnancy. *Am J Med* 1980;68:122.

64. Iturbe-Alessio I, Fonseca MC, Mutchinik O, et al. Risks of anticoagulant therapy in pregnant women with artificial heart valves. *N Engl J Med* 1986;315:1390–1393.

65. Hung L, Rahimtoola SH. Prosthetic heart valves and pregnancy. *Circulation* 2003;107:1240–1246.

66. Vitale N, De Feo M, De Santo LS, et al. Dose-dependent fetal complications of warfarin in pregnant women with mechanical heart valves. *J Am Coll Cardiol* 1999;33:1637–1641.

67. Ginsberg JS, Kowalchuk G, Hirsh J, et al. Heparin therapy during pregnancy. *Arch Intern Med* 1989;149:2233–2236.

68. Elkayam U. Anticoagulation in pregnant women with prosthetic heart valves: A double jeopardy (editorial). *J Am Coll Cardiol* 1996;27:1704–1706.

68a. Reimold SC, Rutherford JD. Valvular heart disease in pregnancy. *N Engl J Med* 2003;349:52–59.

69. Topol EJ, Casele H, Elkayam U, et al. for the Anticoagulation in Prosthetic Valves and Pregnancy Consensus Report (APPCR) Panel and Scientific Roundtable. Anticoagulation and enoxaparin use in patients with prosthetic heart valves and/or pregnancy. *Clin Cardiol Consensus Rep* 2002;3(9):1–20.

69a. Ginsberg JS, Chan WS, Bates SM, et al. Anticoagulation of pregnant women with mechanical heart valves. *Arch Intern Med* 2003;163:694–698.

70. Werler MM, Mitchell AA, Shapiro S. The relation of aspirin use during the first trimester of pregnancy to congenital cardiac defects. *N Engl J Med* 1989;321:1639–1642.

71. DuBard MB, Cutter GR. Low-dose aspirin therapy to prevent preeclampsia. *Am J Obstet Gynecol* 1993;168:1083–1091.

72. McAnulty JH. Anesthesia during pregnancy in the patient with heart disease. In: Bonica JJ, McDonald JS, eds. *Principles and Practice of Obstetric Analgesia and Anesthesia.* Philadelphia: Lea & Febiger; 1994:1013–1039.

73. Haemostatis and Thrombosis Task Force. Guidelines on the prevention, investigation and management of thrombosis associated with pregnancy: Maternal and neonatal haemostasis working papers of the Haemostasis and Thrombosis Task Force. *J Clin Pathol* 1993;46:489–496.

74. Greer IA. Thrombosis in pregnancy: Maternal and fetal issues. *Lancet* 1999;353:1258–1265.

75. Kittner SJ, Stern BJ, Feeser BR, et al. Pregnancy and the risk of stroke. *N Engl J Med* 1996;335:768–774.

76. Sturridge F, de Swiet M, Letsky E. The use of low molecular weight heparin for thrombophylaxis in pregnancy. *Br J Obstet Gynaecol* 1994;101:69–71.

77. Hellgren M, Svensson PJ, Dahlback B. Resistance to activated protein C as a basis for venous thromboembolism associated with pregnancy and oral contraceptives. *Am J Obstet Gynecol* 1995;173:210–213.

78. Gerhart A, Scharf RE, Beckmann MW, et al. Prothrombin and factor V mutations in women with a history of thrombosis during pregnancy and the puerperium. *N Engl J Med* 2000;342:374–380.

79. Turrentine MA, Braems G, Ramirez MM. Use of thrombolytics for the treatment of thromboembolic disease during pregnancy (review). *Obstet Gynecol Surv* 1995;50:534–541.

80. Lengyel M, Fuster V, Keltai M, et al. Guidelines for management of left-sided prosthetic valve thrombosis: A role for thrombolytic therapy. *J Am Coll Cardiol* 1997;30:1521–1526.

81. Rey E, LeLorier J, Burgess E, et al. Report of the Canadian Hypertension Society Consensus Conference: 3. Pharmacologic treatment of hypertensive disorders in pregnancy. *Can Med Assoc J* 1997;157: 1245–1254.

82. Witlin AG, Sibai BM. Hypertension. *Clin Obstet Gynecol* 1998;41: 533–544.

83. Churchill D. The new American guidelines on the hypertensive disorders of pregnancy. *J Hum Hypertens* 2001;15:583–585.

84. Phillips RA, Greenblatt J, Krakoff LR. Hypertensive emergencies: Diagnosis and management. *Prog Cardiovasc Dis* 2002;45:33–48.

85. Avila S, Grinberg M, Snitcowsky R, et al. Maternal and fetal outcome in pregnant women with Eisenmenger's syndrome. *Eur Heart J* 1995; 16:460–464.

86. Weiss BM, Hess OM. Pulmonary vascular disease and pregnancy: Current controversies, management strategies, and perspectives. *Eur Heart J* 2000;21:104–115.

87. Widerhorn J, Widerhorn AL, Rahimtoola SH, Elkayam U. WPW syndrome during pregnancy: Increased incidence of supraventricular arrhythmias. *Am Heart J* 1992;123:796–798.

88. Lee SH, Chan SA, Wu TJ, et al. Effects of pregnancy on first onset and symptoms of paroxysmal supraventricular tachycardia. *Am J Cardiol* 1995;76:675–678.

89. Rosemond RL. Cardioversion during pregnancy. *JAMA* 1993;269: 3167.

90. Brodsky M, Doria R, Allen V, Sato D. New onset ventricular tachycardia during pregnancy. *Am Heart J* 1992;123:933–941.

91. Dildy GA, Clark SL. Cardiac arrest during pregnancy. *Obstet Gynecol Clin North Am* 1995;22:303–314.

92. Kloeck W, Cummins RO, Chamberlain D, et al. Special resuscitation situations: An advisory statement from the International Liaison Committee on Resuscitation. *Circulation* 97(8):2196–2210.

93. McCurdy CM, Rutherford SE, Coddington CC. Syncope and sudden arrhythmic death complicating pregnancy: A case report of Ramano-Ward syndrome. *J Reprod Med* 1993;38:233–234.

94. Rashba EJ, Zareba W, Moss AJ, et al. Influence of pregnancy on the risk for cardiac events in patients with hereditary long QT syndrome. LQTS Investigators. *Circulation* 1998;97:451–456.

95. Dalvi BV, Chaudhuri A, Kulkarni HL, Kale PA. Therapeutic guidelines for congenital complete heart block presenting in pregnancy. *Obstet Gynecol* 1994; 79:802–804.

96. Ebrahimi R, Leung CY, Elkayam U, Reid CL. Infective endocarditis. In: Gleicher N, ed. *Principles and Practice of Medical Therapy in Pregnancy,* 2d ed. Norwalk, CT: Appleton & Lange; 1992:795–801.

97. Dajani AS, Taubert KA, Wilson W, et al. Prevention of bacterial endocarditis: Recommendations by the American Heart Association. *JAMA* 1997;277:1794–1801.

98. Chambers CE, Clark SL. Cardiac surgery during pregnancy (review). *Clin Obstet Gynecol* 1994;37:316–323.

99. Sullivan HJ. Valvular heart surgery during pregnancy (review). *Surg Clin North Am* 1995;75:59–75.

100. McAnulty JH. Rheumatic heart disease. In: Gleicher N, Gall SA, Sibai BM, et al, eds. *Principles and Practice of Medical Therapy in Pregnancy,* 2d ed. Norwalk, CT: Appleton & Lange; 1992: 783–788.

101. Special Writing Group of the Committee on Rheumatic Fever, Endocarditis, and Kawasaki Disease of the Council on Cardiovascular Disease in the Young of the American Heart Association. Guidelines for the diagnosis of rheumatic fever: Jones criteria, 1992 update. *JAMA* 1992;268:2069–2073.

102. Dajani AS, Bisno AL, Chung KJ, et al. Prevention of rheumatic fever. *Circulation* 1988;78:1082–1086.

103. Bryg RJ, Gordon PR, Kudesia VS, Bhatia RK. Effect of pregnancy on pressure gradient in mitral stenosis. *Am J Cardiol* 1989;63:384–386.

104. Desai DK, Adanlawo M, Naidoo DP, et al. Mitral stenosis in pregnancy: A four-year experience at King Edward VIII Hospital, Durban, South Africa. *Br J Obstet Gynaecol* 2000;107(8):953–958.

105. Hameed A, Karaalp IS, et al. The effect of valvular heart disease on maternal and fetal outcome of pregnancy. *J Am Coll Cardiol* 2001; 37(3):893–899.

106. Gupta A, Lokhandwala YY, Satoskar PR, Salvi VS. Balloon mitral valvotomy in pregnancy: Maternal and fetal outcomes. *J Am Coll Surg* 1998;187:409–415.

107. Mangione JA, Lourenco RM, dos Santos ES, et al. Long-term follow-up of pregnant women after percutaneous mitral valvuloplasty. (comment). *Catheter Cardiovasc Interv* 2000;50(4):413–417.

108. Cowles T, Gonik B. Mitral valve prolapse in pregnancy. *Semin Perinatol* 1990;14:34–41.

109. Nishimura RA, McGoon MD. Perspectives on mitral-valve prolapse. *N Engl J Med* 1999;341(1):48–59.

110. Lao TT, Sermer M, McGee L, et al. Congenital aortic stenosis and pregnancy—A reappraisal (review). *Am J Obstet Gynecol* 1993;169: 540–545.

111. Whittemore R, Hobbins JC, Engle MA. Pregnancy and its outcome in women with and without surgical treatment of congenital heart disease. *Am J Cardiol* 1982;50:641–651.

112. American College of Cardiology/American Heart Association Task Force on Practice Guidelines (Committee on Management of Patients with Valvular Heart Disease). ACC/AHA Guidelines for the management of patients with valvular heart disease. *J Am Coll Cardiol* 1998; 32:1486–1588.

113. Banning AP, Pearson JF, Hall RJ. Role of balloon dilatation of the aortic valve in pregnant patients with severe aortic stenosis. *Br Heart J* 1993;70:544–545.

114. Lao TT, Adelman AG, Sermer M, Colman JM. Balloon valvuloplasty for congenital aortic stenosis in pregnancy. *Br J Obstet Gynaecol* 1993;100:1141–1142.

115. Bloomfield P, Wheatley DJ, Prescott RJ, Miller HC. Twelve-year comparison of a Bjork-Shirley mechanical heart valve with porcine bioprostheses. *N Engl J Med* 1991;324:573–579.

116. Rahimtoola SH. Choice of prosthetic heart valve for adult patients. *J Am Coll Cardiol* 2003;41:893–904.

117. North RA, Sadler L, Stewart AW, et al. Long-term survival and valve-related complications in young women with cardiac valve replacements. *Circulation* 1999;99:2669–2676.

118. Elkayam U. Pregnancy through a prosthetic valve. *J Am Coll Cardiol* 1999;33:1643–1645.

119. Jamieson WR, Miller DC, Akins CW, et al. Pregnancy and bioprostheses: Influence on structural valve deterioration. *Ann Thorac Surg* 1995;60:S282–S286.

120. Mitchell SC, Korones SB, Berendes HW. Congenital heart disease in 56,109 births: Incidence and natural history. *Circulation* 1971;43: 323–332.

121. Nora JJ, Nora AH. The evolution of specific genetic and environmental counseling in congenital heart disease. *Circulation* 1978;57:205–213.

122. Morris CD, Menashe VD. Evidence for maternal transmission of congenital heart defects. *Circulation* 1993;88(suppl):1–98.

123. Whittemore R, Wells JA, Castellsagne X. A second-generation study of 427 probands with congenital heart defects and their 837 children. *J Am Coll Cardiol* 1994;23:1459–1467.

124. Nora J. From generational studies to a multilevel genetic-environmental interaction (editorial). *J Am Coll Cardiol* 1994;23:1468–1471.

125. Metcalfe J, Ueland K. Maternal cardiovascular adjustments to pregnancy. *Prog Cardiovasc Dis* 1974;16:363–374.

126. Morris CD, Manashe VD. 25-year mortality after surgical repair of congenital heart defect in childhood: A population-based cohort study. *JAMA* 1991;266:3447–3452.

127. Neill CA, Swanson S. Outcome of pregnancy in congenital heart disease. *Circulation* 1961;24:1003–1011.

128. Presbytero P, Sommerville J, Stone S, et al. Pregnancy and cyanotic congenital heart disease, outcome of mother and fetus. *Circulation* 1994;89:2673–2676.

129. Beauchesne LM, Connolly HM, Ammash NM, et al. Coarctation of the aorta: Outcome of pregnancy. *J Am Coll Cardiol* 2001:38(6):1728–1733.

130. Piacenza JM, Kirkorian G, Audra PH, Mellier G. Hypertrophic cardiomyopathy and pregnancy. *Eur J Obstet Gynecol Reprod Biol* 1998;80(1):17–23.

130a. Autore C, Conte MR, Piccininno M, et al. Risk associated with pregnancy in hypertrophic cardiomyopathy. *J Am Coll Cardiol* 2002;40:1864–1869.

131. Autore C, Conte MR, Piccininno M, et al. Risk associated with pregnancy in hypertrophic cardiomyopathy. *J Am Coll Cardiol* 2002;40(10):1864–1869.

132. Conobbio MM, Mair DD, Velde M, Koos BJ. Pregnancy outcomes after the Fontan repair. *J Am Coll Cardiol* 1996;28:763–767.

133. Patton DE, Lee W, Cotton DB, et al. Cyanotic maternal heart disease in pregnancy. *Obstet Gynecol Surv* 1990;45:594–600.

134. Clarkson PM, Wilson NJ, Neutze JM, et al. Outcome of pregnancy after the Mustard operation for transposition of the great arteries with intact ventricular septum. *J Am Coll Cardiol* 1994;24:190–193.

135. Connolly H, Grogan M, Warnes CA. Pregnancy among women with congenitally corrected transposition of great arteries. *J Am Coll Cardiol* 1999;33:1692–1695.

136. Connolly HM, Warnes CA. Ebstein's anomaly: Outcome of pregnancy. *J Am Coll Cardiol* 1994;23:1194–1198.

137. Mor-Yosef S, Younis J, Granat M, et al. Marfan's syndrome in pregnancy. *Obstet Gynecol Surv* 1988;43:382–385.

138. Pyeritz RE. Maternal and fetal complications of pregnancy in the Marfan syndrome. *Am J Med* 1981;71:784–790.

139. Grunig E, Tasman JA, Kucherer H, et al. Frequency and phenotypes of familial dilated cardiomyopathy. *J Am Coll Cardiol* 1998;31:86–94.

140. Olson TM, Michels VV, Thibodeau SN, et al. Actin mutations in dilated cardiomyopathy, a heritable form of heart failure. *Science* 1998;280:750–752.

141. Damakil JG, Rahimtoola SH, Sutton GC, et al. Natural course of peripartum cardiomyopathy. *Circulation* 1971;44:1053–1061.

142. O'Connell JB, Costanzo-Mordin MR, Surbranian R, et al. Peripartum cardiomyopathy: Clinical, hemodynamic, histologic and prognostic characteristics. *J Am Coll Cardiol* 1986;8:52–56.

143. Heider AL, Kuller JA, Strauss RA, Wells SR. Peripartum cardiomyopathy: A review of the literature. *Obstet Gynecol Surv* 1999;54:526–531.

144. Rizeq MN, Rickenbacher PR, Fowler MB, Billingham ME. Incidence of myocarditis in peripartum cardiomyopathy. *Am J Cardiol* 1994;74:474–477.

145. Sutton MS, Cole P, Plappert M, et al. Effects of subsequent pregnancy on left ventricular function in peripartum cardiomyopathy. *Am Heart J* 1991;121:1776–1778.

146. Elkayam U, Tummala PP, Rao K, et al. Maternal and fetal outcomes of subsequent pregnancies in women with peripartum cardiomyopathy. (comment) [erratum appears in *N Engl J Med* 2001 Aug 16;345(7):552]. *N Engl J Med* 2001;344(21):1567–1571.

147. Roth A, Elkayam U. Acute myocardial infarction associated with pregnancy. *Ann Intern Med* 1996;125:751–762.

148. Cowan NC, de Belder MA, Rothman MT. Coronary angioplasty in pregnancy. *Br Heart J* 1988;59:588–592.

149. Garry D, Leikin E, Fleisher AG, Tejani N. Acute myocardial infarction in pregnancy with subsequent medical and surgical management. *Obstet Gynecol* 1996;87(5 pt 2):802–804.

150. Morini A, Spina V, Aleandri V, et al. Pregnancy after heart transplant: Update and case report. *Hum Reprod* 1998;13:749–757.

151. Ishikawa A, Matsura S. Occlusive thromboaortopathy (Takayasu's disease) and pregnancy. *Am J Cardiol* 1982;50:1293–1300.

152. Railton A, Allen DG. Takayasu's arteritis in pregnancy: A report of 4 cases. *S Afr Med J* 1988;73:123–127.

TRAUMATIC HEART DISEASE

Panagiotis N. Symbas

Accidental or intentional trauma is the leading cause of death, hospitalization, and loss of working days in American society, particularly among young people.[1-3] Cardiac and great vessel injuries are a major contributor to this mortality and morbidity.[4]

The heart and/or great vessels are usually injured from penetrating and nonpenetrating trauma. Other causes of cardiac injuries include iatrogenic trauma caused by the various diagnostic, therapeutic, and resuscitative procedures[5-7,7a]; and ionizing radiation[8] and electric currents.[9]

Many nonpenetrating injuries and an occasional penetrating injury of the heart are well tolerated. In addition, frequently these cardiac injuries are overshadowed by the more overt manifestations of cerebral, abdominal, or musculoskeletal trauma. As a result, they may be overlooked unless a high index of suspicion is maintained and specific studies are obtained.

PENETRATING INJURIES

Penetrating injuries usually are observed with wounds of the precordium but also may be associated with wounds elsewhere in the chest, neck, or upper abdomen. They usually are due to missile or knife wounds but occasionally are caused by a missile embolus reaching the heart through the venous system.

Penetrating Cardiac Trauma

Although penetrating cardiac trauma frequently involves only the free cardiac wall, injury to cardiac valves, chordae tendineae, papillary muscles, atrial or ventricular septum, coronary arteries, and the conduction system may occur. The multiplicity of heart and great vessel lesions that may be produced by penetrating wounds is indicated in Table 93-1.

The relative frequency of a single penetrating wound of the free cardiac wall is due to its area of exposure on the anterior chest wall. In decreasing order of frequency, the structures affected are the right ventricle, left ventricle, right atrium, and left atrium.[10] Cardiac wounds may be single or multiple; the latter more commonly are caused by missiles.[11-13]

The pathophysiologic consequences and clinical manifestations of penetrating injuries to the heart depend on the size and site of the wound, the mode of injury, and especially the state of the pericardial wound. When the pericardial wound remains open and bleeding occurs freely into the pleural space, there are signs and symptoms of hemothorax and loss of circulating blood volume. When there is in-trapericardial hemorrhage with a sealed pericardial wound, cardiac tamponade (see Chap. 80) is the presenting clinical picture. The diagnosis of cardiac injury should be suspected in a patient with chest, lower neck, epigastric, or especially precordial penetrating wounds and with symptoms and signs of cardiac tamponade and/or hemothorax and loss of circulating blood volume. The management of penetrating wounds of the heart consists of immediate thoracotomy and cardiorrhaphy.[10,12,14] When this cannot be done or while appropriate arrangements are made for thoracotomy, the patient's blood volume should be expanded; pericardiocentesis is performed only to provide time for a safe operation.

Although the management of symptomatic patients with a suspected penetrating cardiac wound is clearly defined, the management of the asymptomatic patients with a penetrating precordial wound presented a considerable dilemma in the past, when the options were either exploratory surgery or observation. Currently, the immediate use of echocardiography makes the treatment of these patients safer by avoiding unnecessary surgery or observation, with its accompanying risk of sudden deterioration and even death.[15]

Residual or Delayed Sequelae of Penetrating Cardiac Trauma

Patients with penetrating cardiac wounds should be observed closely immediately postoperatively and after discharge for the clinical manifestations of residual or delayed sequelae. Such sequelae may include (1) ventricular or atrial septal defect; (2) injury of the valve cups, leaflets, or chordae tendineae; (3) aortocardiac or aortopulmonary communication, or communication from the coronary artery to the coronary vein or the cardiac chamber; (4) ventricular aneurysms; (5) posttraumatic or postoperative pericarditis; and (6) electrocardiographic abnormalities.[16,17] When symptoms and signs of a structural defect are detected, echocardiography and/or cardiac catheterization should be performed to define the lesion and its hemodynamic significance and determine the proper mode of therapy.

Posttraumatic pericarditis, which is similar to the postcardiotomy syndrome seen after cardiac surgery, occurs in approximately 20 percent of all cases of penetrating heart wounds. Symptomatic management is the treatment of choice for this syndrome unless cardiac tamponade or other sequelae, such as purulent or constrictive pericarditis, require surgical intervention.

Missile wounds also may result in the presence of a projectile within the heart after either a direct injury to the heart or an injury to a systemic vein with subsequent migration of the missile to the heart.

TABLE 93-1 Penetrating Wounds of the Heart

I. Pericardial damage
   A. Laceration or perforation
   B. Hemopericardium with or without cardiac tamponade
   C. Serofibrinous or suppurative pericarditis
   D. Pneumopericardium
   E. Constrictive pericarditis
II. Myocardial damage
   A. Laceration
   B. Penetration or perforation
   C. Retained foreign body
   D. Structural defects
      1. Aneurysm formation
      2. Septal defects
      3. Aorticocardiac fistula
III. Valvular injury
   A. Leaflet or cusp injury
   B. Papillary muscle or chordae tendineae laceration
IV. Coronary artery injury
   A. Laceration or thrombosis with or without myocardial infarction
   B. Arteriovenous fistula
   C. Aneurysm
V. Embolism
   A. Foreign body
   B. Thrombus (septic or sterile)
VI. Infective endocarditis
VII. Rhythm or conduction disturbances

SOURCE: Prepared by Loren F. Parmley, MD, and Thomas W. Mattingly, and modified with permission.

The missile or the thrombus associated with it may embolize into the systemic or pulmonary arteries.[18–20] Bacterial endocarditis also may occur if the projectile is not completely embedded in the myocardium.[21] Rarely, a patient with a projectile in the heart may develop cardiac neurosis.[22] In many patients, however, the retained missile in the heart results in no ill effects over a long period of observation.[23,24] Therefore, treatment for missiles in the heart should be individualized according to the patient's clinical course and the location, size, and shape of the missile.[23,24] Missiles that cause symptoms should be removed. Similarly, missiles that are free or partially protruding into a left cardiac chamber should be removed, because their embolization to the systemic arterial system may have serious consequences.[23,24] Missiles in the right side of the heart may be removed or left to embolize to the pulmonary vascular bed, from which they can be retrieved easily.[19] Intramyocardial and intrapericardial bullets and pellets are generally well tolerated and may be left in place.

A missile that has embolized to the systemic arterial bed should be removed without delay unless it has resulted in a significant neurologic deficit.[20] Projectiles adjacent to or embedded within the wall of one of the great or coronary arteries should be extracted to prevent subsequent erosion and bleeding.

Coronary Artery Penetrating Trauma

Coronary artery injuries can result in cardiac tamponade and varying degrees of myocardial ischemia or myocardial infarction. The management of these wounds is dependent on the amount of myocardium at risk. Wounds of major branches of the coronary arterial system are repaired or bypassed, whereas small terminal vessels are ligated. Coronary artery aneurysms and arteriovenous fistulas are rare sequelae of injury, and their treatment should be individualized.[25]

Penetrating Trauma of the Aorta and Great Vessels

The pathophysiology of penetrating wounds to the great vessels is quite similar to that of penetrating wounds to the heart and depends on whether the site of the wound is intra- or extrapericardial.[26,27] In addition to the obvious results of immediate or delayed hemorrhage, a penetrating wound of a great vessel may result in the formation of a false aneurysm, with possible subsequent rupture, or an arteriovenous fistula, producing immediate or latent signs and symptoms of congestive heart failure.[28] Traumatic arteriovenous fistulas occasionally are complicated by the development of bacterial endarteritis and endocarditis.[29] These traumatic vascular lesions should be detected and repaired as soon as possible.

NONPENETRATING INJURIES

The vast majority of blunt injuries to the heart are due to automobile accidents, although other forms of blunt trauma also may result in this type of injury. The cardiac injury usually is caused by direct compressing or decelerating forces delivered to the chest or rarely by an indirect force delivered to the abdomen that results in a marked increase in intravascular pressures. A wide variety of injuries are produced by nonpenetrating trauma (Table 93-2).

Cardiac Contusion

Contusion of the heart usually refers to blunt injury that causes identifiable histopathologic changes within the myocardium. The patho-

TABLE 93-2 Nonpenetrating Trauma of the Heart

1. Pericardial injury
   a. Hemopericardium
   b. Rupture or laceration
   c. Serofibrinous pericarditis
   d. Constrictive pericarditis
2. Myocardial injury
   a. Contusion
   b. Rupture of free cardiac wall, early or delayed
   c. Rupture of septum
   d. Aneurysm
   e. Laceration
3. Disturbances of rhythm or conduction
4. Valve injury
   a. Rupture of valve leaflets, cusp, or chordae tendineae
   b. Contusion of papillary muscle
5. Coronary artery injury
   a. Thrombosis with or without myocardial infarction
   b. Arteriovenous fistula
   c. Laceration with or without myocardial infarction
6. Great vessel injury
   a. Rupture
   b. Aneurysm formation
   c. Aorta-cardiac chamber fistula
   d. Thrombotic occlusion

logic lesions of myocardial contusion vary considerably, ranging from small areas of petechiae or ecchymosis to contusion of the full thickness of the myocardial wall with or without rupture of the heart.[1]

The forces that produce nonpenetrating lesions of the heart are such that external evidence of chest injury may be meager or undetectable. This lack of evidence of chest wall injury and the frequent absence of symptoms from the cardiac injury, along with the common presence of other, more obvious injuries to the body, may impede the early diagnosis of cardiac contusion.

Patients with contusions of the heart are commonly asymptomatic, but they may occasionally complain of pain that is identical to myocardial ischemia and/or myocardial infarction.[30] The pain is usually transient unless there is concomitant coronary artery injury or occult atherosclerotic coronary heart disease.[31] Coronary thrombosis can result from nonpenetrating trauma, but this is rare and usually is associated with existing atherosclerotic coronary artery disease.[32] Dyspnea and hypotension rarely may be presenting symptoms. In mild or moderate myocardial contusion, these signs may be transient and are usually absent. Cardiac failure is relatively rare; when it is present, the possibility of an associated cardiac injury, such as rupture of the ventricular septum or of one of the cardiac valves, is high. The diagnosis of cardiac contusion should be suspected in all patients with significant blunt trauma, particularly to the precordium. Unfortunately, none of the currently available diagnostic tests for myocardial contusion can conclusively establish the diagnosis in all patients. The appropriate use and interpretation of the available tests, however, can assist in the diagnosis of myocardial contusion with reasonable accuracy.

Electrocardiography has been the most widely used test for the diagnosis of contusion of the heart. Various electrocardiographic abnormalities have been considered suggestive of cardiac contusion, such as nonspecific ST-T or Q-wave changes, supraventricular tachyarrhythmias, and ventricular arrhythmias, including fibrillation, which is usually the cause of death at the time of the traumatic impact.[33,34] However, a variety of other clinical conditions[35–37] that are frequently present in traumatized patients (i.e., pain, anxiety, hemorrhage, hypoxia, hypokalemia, head trauma, or alcohol or cocaine toxicity) may cause many of these abnormalities. Therefore, the presence of these other causes must be excluded before the electrocardiographic abnormalities are attributed to contusion of the heart.[38,39]

Elevation of the serum level of the MB fraction of creatinine kinase (CK) has been extrapolated from its use in acute myocardial infarction as a diagnostic aid in patients with cardiac contusion. Other clinical conditions that cause elevation in the level of this enzyme [i.e., tachyarrhythmias and skeletal muscle diseases, including trauma (see Chap. 52)] must be excluded before an abnormal level is ascribed to contusion of the heart.[38,39]

Two-dimensional transthoracic and transesophageal echocardiography (TTE and TEE) are useful in the diagnosis of cardiac contusion, particularly of the structural lesions associated with cardiac contusion.[40,41] The sensitivity and specificity of these tests for diagnosing contusion of the heart, however, have not been clearly defined (see Chap. 15).

Circulating cardiac troponin I was measured in a limited number of blunt trauma victims. It was concluded that this test is accurate for diagnosing cardiac contusion.[42] Additional studies are needed, however, to determine its absolute accuracy.

The treatment of myocardial contusion is symptomatic. Prevention and early treatment of arrhythmias are the most important therapeutic measures. Appropriate antiarrhythmic agents (see Chap. 35) should be used to control ectopic rhythms, and congestive heart fail-

ure should be treated with angiotensin-converting enzyme (ACE) inhibitors. If the myocardial contusion is severe, support with inotropic drugs (see Chap. 25) may be necessary. When all these measures fail, balloon counterpulsation[43] or even a left ventricular assist device[44] may be utilized.

Cardiac Rupture

Although minor, insignificant myocardial contusion of the right ventricle is the most common blunt cardiac injury; the most fatal lesion is rupture of the heart. The rupture may occur in the free cardiac wall or the ventricular septum. Rupture of the free cardiac wall is extremely difficult to diagnose and treat in a timely manner because of the frequently rapid demise of the patient and because traumatic cardiac rupture is often only one of many severe bodily injuries. As a result, rupture of the heart frequently has not been amenable to therapy. The currently immediately available echocardiography in emergency rooms, however, may increase the number of successfully treated patients.[45]

Residual or Delayed Sequelae of Blunt Injury to the Heart

Contusion of the heart usually heals with little or no obvious scarring or impairment of cardiac function. Large contusions, however, may cause a decrease in cardiac output, and extensive necrosis may lead to rupture or, rarely, congestive heart failure and the formation of a true or false aneurysm.[46] Cardiac aneurysms may cause arrhythmias, congestive heart failure, rupture, and mural thrombosis with embolism. Because of these complications, surgical repair of a traumatic aneurysm is advisable. Localized areas of necrosis and hemorrhage involving the cardiac conduction system may produce various conduction defects.

The most commonly injured valve in surviving patients is the aortic valve, with aortic regurgitation characteristically causing the rapid development of congestive heart failure. Injury of the atrioventricular valves is an uncommon result of nonpenetrating cardiac injury and usually occurs in the presence of severe cardiac trauma, resulting in death. Rupture of the mitral valve leaflet can have hemodynamic consequences somewhat similar to those of aortic valve injury but rarely is encountered clinically. In contrast, tricuspid valve injury may be tolerated for years before surgical correction is required.

Rupture of the papillary muscle or chordae tendineae occurs more frequently than does rupture of valve leaflets. Cardiac contusion also may cause papillary muscle dysfunction with secondary mitral or tricuspid regurgitation.[47] The clinical outcome depends on whether the structures involved are on the right side of the heart, where the lesion may be well tolerated, or the left side, where the high-pressure system can lead to more serious hemodynamic sequelae. The murmurs produced by these lesions are generally typical of valvular regurgitation, but unusual high-pitched systolic and diastolic murmurs of variable loudness also may result (see Chap. 12). Tricuspid regurgitation may be present despite the absence of a detectable murmur.[48] Prompt and correct diagnosis by echocardiographic, hemodynamic, and angiographic studies is important. Patients with hemodynamically significant valvular injury should undergo valvuloplasty or valve replacement.

Pericardial lesions often are overlooked and frequently heal without incident. Hemopericardium may occur but usually is due to the coexisting myocardial injury. Posttraumatic pericarditis develops less frequently with blunt than with penetrating cardiac injuries. The symptoms and signs of posttraumatic pericarditis are similar to those of pericarditis produced by a wide variety of causes (see Chap. 80). When hemopericardium or hydropericardium is suspected, echocardiography can confirm the diagnosis. Pericardial laceration usually is well tolerated, but herniation of the heart may occur, leading to more serious consequences and death.[49]

Aortic Rupture

Rupture of the aorta is the most common blunt injury of the great vessels. Rupture or avulsion of the innominate, carotid, or left subclavian arteries or the venae cavae also has been observed. Because of the variety of mechanical forces produced by blunt trauma (Fig. 93-1), combined with anatomic factors, the most common sites of rupture of the aorta from blunt injury are the descending aorta just distal to the origin of the left subclavian artery (aortic isthmus) and the ascending aorta commonly just above the aortic valve.[50–52] Because of the high incidence of severe cardiac injury in patients with rupture of the ascending aorta, most of the patients who survive aortic rupture long enough to receive definitive surgical correction are those who have sustained rupture of the aortic isthmus. About 20 percent of patients with aortic rupture survive the original injury. A false aneurysm is formed in these patients at the site of rupture, the wall of which consists of adventitia and/or parietal pleura and other mediastinal structures. The intactness of these structures maintains continuity of the circulation.

The common manifestations of traumatic rupture of the aorta are chest and/or midscapular pain, a new murmur, increased pulse am-

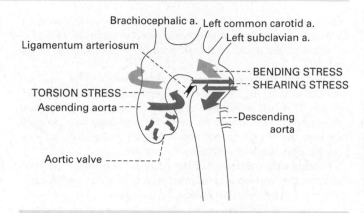

FIGURE 93-1 Diagrammatic illustration of the forces acting on the aortic wall during rupture of the aorta from blunt trauma. (From Symbas PN. *Traumatic Injuries of the Heart and Great Vessels.* Springfield, IL: Charles C Thomas; 1971:153. Courtesy of Charles C Thomas, Publisher, Springfield, Illinois.)

plitude, and hypertension of the upper extremities. Some patients, however, are surprisingly free of any major symptoms or signs from the aortic rupture. Although there are occasionally no obvious signs of external injury, patients with rupture of the aorta usually have associated injuries of the skeleton, abdominal viscera, or central nervous system that can mask the signs of aortic rupture. For this reason, *any patient who has sustained severe blunt trauma or has been exposed to major deceleration forces should be suspected of having*

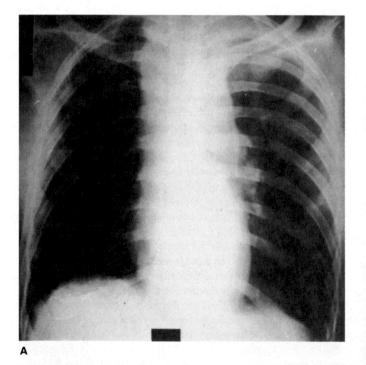

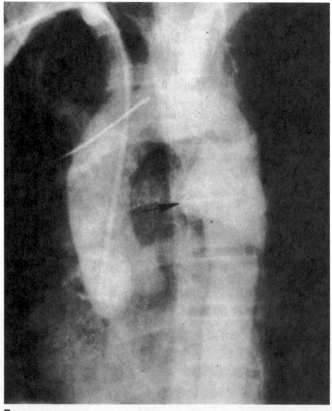

FIGURE 93-2 *A.* Chest roentgenogram of a young man who shortly before admission was involved in an automobile accident. Note the mediastinal widening. *B.* Aortogram the same day showing a false aneurysm distal to the origin of the left subclavian artery and two filling defects, one proximal and one distal to the aneurysm.

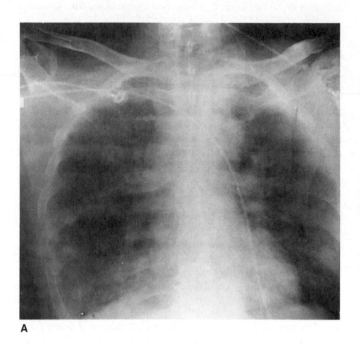

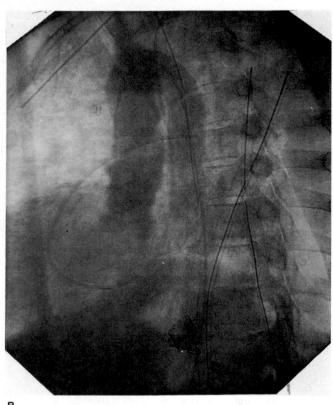

FIGURE 93-3 *A.* Chest roentgenogram of a young man shortly after a vehicular accident. *B.* Aortogram showing rupture of the ascending aorta.

aortic rupture if there is an increased pulse pressure, upper extremity hypertension, and especially widening of the upper mediastinal silhouette.

Chest roentgenography is of great diagnostic value in patients with aortic rupture. Widening of the superior mediastinal shadow, depression of the left main bronchus, displacement of the trachea and esophagus to the right, and especially obliteration of the aortic knob shadow are common roentgenographic abnormalities associated with injury at the aortic isthmus (Fig. 93-2). Widening of the mediastinum also has been observed in all cases with rupture of the aortic arch and in about 79 percent with rupture of the ascending aorta (Fig. 93-3).[52] The most definitive procedure to establish the diagnosis of aortic rupture is aortography, which should be performed immediately in all patients whose history, physical examination, and, particularly, chest roentgenogram suggest the possibility of this injury. Computed tomography scanning also is used widely to evaluate patients with a widened mediastinum.[53] The approximately 55 percent sensitivity and 65 percent sensitivity of this test limit its contribution to the definitive management of these patients.[54] TEE appears to be a useful diagnostic test (see Chap. 15), but there has been no comprehensive study of its diagnostic value for aortic rupture. Until further experience is gained, caution should be exercised when it is used as the sole technique for establishing the diagnosis. Treatment should be undertaken as soon as possible.

Patients with no other organ injuries that add unacceptable risk to the surgical treatment should be operated on as soon as possible. The remaining patients, such as those with trauma to the central nervous system, contaminated wounds, respiratory insufficiency from lung contusion or other causes, body surface burns, blunt cardiac injury, tears of solid organs that will undergo nonoperative management, retroperitoneal hematoma, and medical comorbidities should be treated medically to maintain the mean systemic blood pressure below 70 mmHg and control the aortic wall tension until the other injuries or complications cease to add unacceptable risk to the surgical treatment.[55]

References

1. Symbas PN. *Cardiothoracic Trauma.* Philadelphia: Saunders; 1989.
2. James S. Injury mortality. In: *National Summary of Injury Mortality Data, 1987–1993.* Washington, DC: U.S. Department of Health and Human Services, Public Health Service, Centers for Disease Control and Prevention; June 1996.
3. Price PR, Mackenzie EJ. Cost of injury—United States: A report to Congress. *JAMA* 1989;262:2803–2804.
4. Kemmerer WT, Eckert WG, Gathwright JB, et al. Patterns of thoracic injuries in fatal traffic accidents. *J Trauma* 1961;1:595–599.
5. Bredlau CE, Roubin GS, Leimgruber PP, et al. In-hospital morbidity and mortality in patients undergoing elective coronary angioplasty. *Circulation* 1985;72:1044–1052.
6. Gaul G, Hollman J, Simpendorfer C, Franco I. Acute occlusion in multiple lesion coronary angioplasty: Frequency and management. *J Am Coll Cardiol* 1989;13:283–228.
7. Nobuyoshi M, Hamasaki N, Kimura T, et al. Indications, complications and short-term clinical outcome of percutaneous transvenous mitral commissurotomy. *Circulation* 1989;80:782–792.
7a. Salehian O, Teoh K, Mulji A Blunt and penetrating cardiac trauma: A review. *Can J Cardiol* 2003;19:1054–1059.
8. Cohn KE, Stewart JR, Fajardo LF, Hancock EW. Heart disease following radiation. *Medicine (Baltimore)* 1967;46:281–298.

9. Jackson SH, Parry DJ. Lightning and the heart. *Br Heart J* 1980;43: 454–527.

10. Symbas PN, Harlaftis N, Waldo WJ. Penetrating wounds: A comparison of different therapeutic methods. *Ann Surg* 1976;183:377–381.

11. Symbas PN. *Cardiothoracic Trauma: Current Problems in Surgery.* St. Louis: Mosby Year Book; 1991:742.

12. Thourani VH, Filiciano DV, Cooper WA, et al. Penetrating cardiac trauma at an urban trauma center: A 22-year experience. *Am Surg* 1999; 65: 811–818.

13. Trinkle JK, Toon RS, Franz JL, et al. Affairs of the wounded heart: Penetrating cardiac wounds. *J Trauma* 1979;19:467–472.

14. Mitchell ME, Muakkassa FF, Poole GV, et al. Surgical approach of choice for penetrating cardiac wounds. *J Trauma* 1993;34:17–20.

15. Rozycki GS, Feliciano DV, Schmidt JA, et al. The role of surgeon-performed ultrasound in patients with possible cardiac wounds. *Ann Surg* 1996;224:1–8.

16. Symbas PN, DiOrio DA, Tyras DH, et al. Penetrating cardiac wounds: Significant residual and delayed sequelae. *J Thorac Cardiovasc Surg* 1973;6:526–532.

17. Symbas PN. *Traumatic Heart Disease: Current Problems in Cardiology.* St Louis: Mosby Year Book; 1991:539.

18. Bland EF, Beebe GW. Missles in the heart: A 20-year follow-up report of world war cases. *N Engl J Med* 1966;274:1039–1046.

19. Symbas PN, Hatcher CR Jr, Mansour KA. Projectile embolus of the lung. *J Thorac Cardiovasc Surg* 1968;56:97–103.

20. Symbas PN, Harlaftis N. Bullet emboli in the pulmonary and systemic arteries. *Ann Surg* 1977;185:318–320.

21. Decker HR. Foreign bodies in the heart and pericardium: Should they be removed? *J Thorac Surg* 1939;9:62.

22. Turner GG. Bullets in the heart for 23 years. *Surgery* 1942;9:832–852.

23. Symbas PN, Picone AL, Hatcher CR Jr, Vlasis SE. Cardiac missiles: A review of the literature and personal experience. *Ann Surg* 1990;211: 639–648.

24. Symbas PN, Vlasis SE, Picone AL, Hatcher CR Jr. Missiles in the heart. *Ann Thorac Surg* 1989;48:192–194.

25. Konecke LL, Spitzer S, Mason D, et al. Traumatic aneurysm of the left coronary artery. *Am J Cardiol* 1971;27:221–223.

26. Symbas PN, Schdava JS. Penetrating wounds of the thoracic aorta. *Ann Surg* 1970;171:441–450.

27. Symbas PN, Kourias E, Tyras DH, Hatcher CR Jr. Penetrating wounds of the great vessels. *Ann Surg* 1974;179:757–762.

28. Symbas PN, Schlant RC, Logan WD Jr, et al. Traumatic aorticopulmonary fistula complicated by postoperative low cardiac output treated with dopamine. *Ann Surg* 1967;165:614–619.

29. Parmley LF Jr, Orbison JA, Hughes CW, Mattingly TW. Acquired arteriovenous fistulas complicated by endarteritis and endocarditis lenta due to *Streptococcus faecalis. N Engl J Med* 1954;250:305–309.

30. Kissane RW. Traumatic heart diseases, especially myocardial contusion. *Postgrad Med* 1954;15:114–119.

31. Stern T, Wolf RY, Reichart B, et al. Coronary artery occlusion resulting from blunt trauma. *JAMA* 1974;230:1308–1309.

32. Levy H. Traumatic coronary thrombosis with myocardial infarction: Postmortem study. *Arch Intern Med* 1949;84:261–276.

33. Louhimo I. Heart injury after blunt thoracic trauma: An experimental study on rabbits. *Acta Chir Scand Suppl* 1968;380:1–60.

34. Dolara A, Morando P, Pampaloni M. Electrocardiographic findings in 98 consecutive nonpenetrating chest injuries. *Dis Chest* 1967;52:50–56.

35. Potkin RT, Werner JA, Trobaugh GB, et al. Evaluation of noninvasive tests of cardiac damage in suspected cardiac contusion. *Circulation* 1982;66:627–631.

36. Marriott HJ, Nizet PM. Physiologic stimuli simulating ischemic heart disease. *JAMA* 1967;200:715.

37. Tindall GT, Iwata K, McGraw CP, Vanderveer RW. Cardiorespiratory changes associated with intracranial pressure waves: Evaluation of these changes in 27 patients with head injuries. *South Med J* 1975;68: 407–412.

38. Manor A, Alpan G. Specificity of creatine kinase MB isoenzyme for myocardial injury. *Clin Chem* 1978;24:2206.

39. Snow N, Richardson JD, Flynt LM Jr. Myocardial contusion: Implication for patients with multiple traumatic injuries. *Surgery* 1982;92: 744–750.

40. Miller FA Jr, Seward JB, Gersh BJ, et al. Two-dimensional echocardiographic findings in cardiac trauma. *Am J Cardiol* 1982;50:1022–1027.

41. Shapiro NG, Yanofsky SD, Trapp I, et al. Cardiovascular evaluation in thoracic blunt trauma using transesophageal echocardiography (TEE). *J Trauma* 1991;131:835–839.

42. Adams JE III, Davila-Roman VG, Bessey PQ, et al. Improved detection of cardiac contusion with cardiac troponin I. *Am Heart J* 1996;131: 308–312.

43. Snow N, Luca AE, Richardson JD. Intra-aortic balloon counterpulsation for cardiogenic shock from cardiac contusion. *J Trauma* 1982;22: 426–429.

44. Chavanon O, Dutheil V, Hacini R, et al. Treatment of severe cardiac contusion with a left ventricular assist device in a patient with multiple trauma. *J Thorac Cardiovasc Surg* 1999;118:189–190.

45. Symbas NP, Bongiorno PF, Symbas PN. Blunt cardiac rupture: The utility of emergency department ultrasound. *Ann Thorac Surg* 1999;67: 1274–1276.

46. Singh R, Nolan SP, Schrank JP. Traumatic left ventricular aneurysm: Two cases with normal coronary angiograms. *JAMA* 1975;234: 412–414.

47. Schroeder JS, Stinson EB, Bieber CP, et al. Papillary muscle dysfunction due to nonpenetrating chest trauma, recognition in a potential cardiac donor. *Br Heart J* 1972;34:645–647.

48. Marvin RF, Schrank JP, Nolan SP. Traumatic tricuspid insufficiency. *Am J Cardiol* 1973;32:723–726.

49. Anderson M, Fredens M, Olesson KH. Traumatic rupture of the pericardium. *Am J Cardiol* 1971;27:566–569.

50. Feczko JD, Lynch L, Pless JE, et al. An autopsy case review of 142 nonpenetrating (blunt) injuries of the aorta. *J Trauma* 1992; 33:846–849.

51. Symbas PN, Tyras DH, Ware RE, DiOrio DA. Traumatic rupture of the aorta. *Ann Surg* 1973;178:6–12.

52. Symbas PJ, Horsley SW, Symbas PN. Rupture of the ascending aorta caused by blunt trauma. *Ann Thorac Surg* 1998;66:113–117.

53. Fenner MN, Fisher KS, Sergel NL, et al. Evaluation of possible traumatic thoracic aortic injury using aortography and CT. *Am Surg* 1990; 56:497–499.

54. Miller FB, Richardson JD, Thomas HA, et al. Role of CT in diagnosis of major arterial injury after blunt thoracic trauma. *Surgery* 1989;106: 596–603.

55. Symbas PN, Sherman AS, Silver JM, et al. Traumatic rupture of the aorta immediate or delayed repair? *Ann Surg* 2002;235:796–802.

THE HEART AND KIDNEY DISEASE

Tahsin Masud / William E. Mitch

Cardiovascular disease is the number one cause of death in patients with end-stage renal disease (ESRD) undergoing dialysis.[1] Almost half of the deaths of dialysis patients in the United States are caused by cardiovascular disease; acute myocardial infarction causes 20.8 deaths per 1000 patient-years.[2] The cardiovascular mortality rate in ESRD patients on dialysis is approximately 10 to 20 times higher than in the general population (Fig. 94-1).[3] In several prospective studies,[4,5] chronic renal insufficiency (CRI) has been independently associated with incident cardiovascular events and cardiovascular mortality. Cardiovascular atherosclerosis begins long before ESRD. The incidence of major cardiovascular events was increased by 40 percent even when serum creatinine just exceeded the normal upper level of 1.4 mg/dL.[6]

The higher prevalence of cardiovascular disease in patients with renal disease may be the consequence of the high prevalence of hypertension, diabetes, aging, and hyperlipidemia. There are, however, other specific risk factors for coronary artery disease (CAD) and cardiovascular morbidity in dialysis patients, such as a high prevalence of left ventricular hypertrophy,[7] anemia,[8] and hypotension during hemodialysis (HD),[9] and abnormal calcium and phosphate metabolism[10] leading to hyperparathyroidism and vascular calcification. Beside coronary disease, CRI is associated with an increased risk of pericardial disease, infective endocarditis, and fluid and electrolyte disturbances that contribute significantly to cardiac dysfunction.

CARDIOVASCULAR RISK FACTORS IN CHRONICALLY UREMIC PATIENTS

Systemic Arterial Hypertension

Almost 80 percent of CRI patients have systemic hypertension before beginning dialysis therapy.[1] Hypertension in dialysis or ESRD patients, as in normal subjects, is associated with an increased risk for left ventricular hypertrophy, CAD, congestive heart failure, and cerebrovascular complications, as well as mortality.[11] The pathogenesis of hypertension includes both an expanded extracellular fluid volume (ECV)[12,13] and vasoconstriction, mediated by overactivity of the sympathetic nervous system and the renin–angiotensin axis.[14–16] Hypertension caused or aggravated by sodium retention leading to ECV expansion is associated with an increase in cardiac output plus an increase in total peripheral vascular resistance.[17] These findings contrast with the normal value of cardiac output and high peripheral resistance found in hypertensive subjects with normal renal function. The increase in cardiac output found in CRI patients may be related to anemia from lack of erythropoietin. Finally, there is the possibility that some unidentified factor in uremia changes cardiac muscle metabolism. For example, Lin et al.[18] reported that even normotensive HD patients have an increased left ventricular mass despite the absence of hypertension or ECV expansion.

Direct evidence that ECV expansion plays a principal role in the hypertension of chronic renal failure is found in reports indicating that hypertension rapidly resolves when the ECV is reduced by diuretics or vigorous dialysis.[12,13] In comparison, many ESRD patients also have a high peripheral vascular resistance in addition to ECV expansion. As an extreme example, there appears to be a small group (~10 percent) of ESRD patients who exhibit dialysis-resistant hypertension and high levels of plasma renin activity. Drugs inhibiting the renin–angiotensin axis can control hypertension in this group, implicating a role for this axis in the pathogenesis of dialysis-resistant hypertension.

The mechanisms causing arterial vasoconstriction in CRI patients may be more complicated than activation of the renin–angiotensin system alone. It has been proposed that circulating inhibitors of Na^+-K^+-ATPase increase peripheral vascular resistance by causing an increase in intracellular sodium, resulting in an increase in intracellular calcium and, hence, contraction of vascular smooth muscle cells.[19,20] Second, overactivity of the sympathetic nervous system has been observed in CRI patients. This abnormality is reversed by nephrectomy,[21] suggesting it is mediated by an afferent signal from

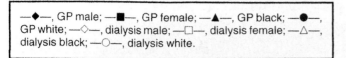

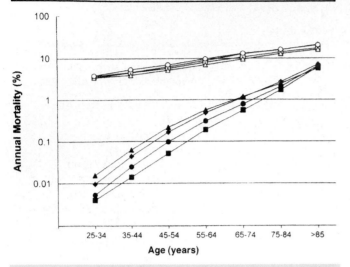

FIGURE 94-1 Cardiovascular mortality defined as death due to arrhythmias, cardiomyopathy, cardiac arrest, myocardial infarction, atherosclerotic heart disease, or pulmonary edema in the general population (GP) is compared to ESRD patients treated by dialysis. Data are stratified by age, race, and gender. [Reproduced with permission from the *American Journal of Kidney Diseases* 1998;32(5, suppl 3):S115, Fig. 1; Copyright 1998 by the National Kidney Foundation.]

the kidneys. Other proposed mechanisms causing hypertension in CRI patients include impaired endothelium-dependant vasodilatation because of impaired nitric oxide production due to high plasma levels of asymmetric dimethylarginine and/or hyperhomocysteinemia.[22] Finally, it has been suggested that secondary hyperparathyroidism causes hypertension by facilitating calcium entry into smooth muscle cells of the arterial wall. This hypothesis has been questioned, however, because of conflicting reports about the response of hypertension to parathyroidectomy and is a topic that needs further research.[23–24]

Another possible mechanism for hypertension involves responses to recombinant human erythropoietin (rHuEPO), since administration of rHuEPO worsens hypertension in approximately 20 to 30 percent of dialysis patients.[22] In this case, the proposed mechanisms of hypertension are an increase in peripheral vascular resistance from a higher hemoglobin or rHuEPO-induced stimulation of the release of vasoconstricting endothelin.[25] Other suggested mechanisms are related to an increase in blood viscosity, an increase in vascular resistance associated with correction of hypoxemic-mediated vasodilatation, a direct vasopressor effect of rHuEPO and inhibition of nitric oxide synthesis.[22]

One hypothesis links the presence of a high serum uric acid to the development of hypertension and possibly vascular disease.[26] The basis for this hypothesis is that humans have higher serum uric acid levels than do nonprimates because of a mutation that interferes with uricase activity. When the serum uric acid level in rats was raised, the investigators found that vascular disease and hypertension related to salt sensitivity developed. The vascular disease involved preglomerular and other vessels and is related to smooth muscle cell proliferation. It is tempting to attribute the almost universal presence of hypertension in patients with kidney disease to such a mechanism

because salt-sensitive hypertension is invariably present as is higher serum uric acid. The increase in uric acid in CRI patients is due to decreased excretion but the increase is somewhat lower than predicted from the decrease in clearance because the uric acid that is produced is degraded to metabolic products, presumably by gastrointestinal bacteria.[27]

In patients with kidney disease and hypertension, ECV expansion is the most common mechanism; most patients with so-called *dialysis-resistant* hypertension can be effectively treated by vigorous removal of ECV. For this reason the cornerstone of correcting hypertension in dialysis patients must be to reduce ECV (i.e., to lower the patient's "dry weight" assignment). The dry weight of a dialysis patient is defined as that weight at which there is no ECV expansion (e.g., edema or effusions), and blood pressure is normal. Unfortunately, achieving a dry weight is difficult because patients can become symptomatically hypotensive or develop leg cramps and these symptoms make it difficult to establish a "true" dry weight. The effectiveness of a vigorous dialysis strategy is that daily dialysis corrects hypertension and these patients generally do not require vasodilating drugs.[28]

In patients who have persistent hypertension despite attempts to reduce ECV, antihypertensive medications that inhibit the renin–angiotensin axis [angiotensin receptor inhibitors, angiotensin converting enzyme (ACE) inhibitors, or beta blockers] are the logical choice. These drugs also have "cardioprotective" properties.[6] If they are ineffective, calcium channel blockers, clonidine or minoxidil, can be used, but again the "best medicine" is to reduce the ECV. The dosage of antihypertensive drugs (like other medicines) must be adjusted for the degree of renal failure. Antihypertensive drugs are generally withheld on HD treatment days so that more ECV can be removed without causing hypotension. Bilateral nephrectomy has rarely been used to treat malignant or treatment-resistant hypertension.[29]

Diabetes Mellitus

The number of patients starting maintenance dialysis with the diagnosis of diabetic nephropathy has been consistently rising over the last 10 years. In the year 2000, approximately 44 percent of all CRI patients who began maintenance dialysis had diabetes and it is predicted that this percentage will continue to increase.[1] Diabetic dialysis patients have more cardiovascular morbidity and mortality and all-cause mortality compared to dialysis patients without diabetes.[1] The presumed reason for this risk pattern is the accelerated development of diabetic and hypertensive vascular damage.

Hyperlipidemia

Hyperlipidemia is more common in patients with CRI than it is in the general population, but the types of abnormalities differ.[30] In nephrotic patients and those treated with chronic peritoneal dialysis (CPD) or patients with a renal transplant, an elevated plasma level of low-density lipoprotein (LDL) is common. The degree of LDL elevation is correlated with the tendency for cardiovascular disease. In patients with CRI before or after beginning dialysis treatments, hypertriglyceridemia is the most common plasma lipid abnormality, and often it occurs in association with a low HDL although it may occur without a high LDL or total cholesterol level.[30] Lipoprotein(a) [Lp(a)] serum levels are elevated in patients with uremia. The plasma concentration of Lp(a) generally correlates with the severity of proteinuria, and it rises more when there is activation of the acute-phase response.[31] Elevated Lp(a) is considered to be an independent risk factor of death from CAD in HD patients.[32]

Impaired activity of lipoprotein lipase with impaired degradation of very low-density lipoprotein appears to be the major mechanism causing hypertriglyceridemia.[33] In CPD patients, the high concentration of glucose in the dialysate contributes to the development of hypertriglyceridemia.[34] As in other subjects, diuretics and beta blockers can contribute to hyperlipidemia in CRI patients before or after beginning dialysis therapy.

Strategies for lowering triglycerides and LDL cholesterol include restricting dietary fat, participating in regular exercise, giving fish-oil supplements, and avoiding alcohol or drugs known to cause an abnormal lipid profile. The 3-hydroxy-3-methylglutaryl coenzyme A (HMG-CoA) reductase inhibitors ("statins") are the preferred drugs for treating high plasma triglycerides and LDL-cholesterol levels. They appear to be safe in ESRD patients, but the dose may need to be adjusted. In contrast, the dose of a statin must be reduced for patients taking cyclosporine or tacrolimus after renal transplantation. Clofibrate or gemfibrozil are rarely used because they have been associated with an increased incidence of myositis or hepatotoxicity in dialysis patients. In a reported study of a prospective cohort,[35] statins were associated with a reduction in both cardiovascular-specific death and total mortality in dialysis patients. This has led to ongoing prospective, randomized, placebo-controlled studies: the 4D-trial[36] (Die Deutsche Diabetes Dialysis), the CHORUS study[37] (Cerivastatin in Heart Outcomes in Renal Disease: Understanding Survival), and the ALERT[38] study (Assessment of Lescol in Renal Transplantation). Until data from these investigations are available, the National Cholesterol Education Program Adult Treatment Panel guidelines are recommended for classifying and treating lipid abnormalities in patients with chronic renal disease.[39]

Homocysteine

Plasma levels of homocysteine are often elevated in patients with renal failure. The exact mechanism is unknown, although reduced clearance by the damaged kidneys appears to play a role.[40] Results from small prospective, case-control studies have led to the conclusion that there is an association between an elevated homocysteine level and adverse cardiovascular events in dialysis[41] and renal transplant[42] patients. Rather than assign a cause effect relation to this finding, it should be remembered that hyperhomocysteinemia could simply be due to reduced renal function in patients with other risk factors for atherosclerotic disease. Regarding treatment, predialysis and dialysis patients who were given 1 to 5 mg of folic acid daily had plasma homocysteine levels reduced by 25 to 30 percent; a folate intake of >10 mg/d by HD patients did not lower plasma homocysteine levels further.[43] Whether lowering plasma homocysteine will be associated with a decreased risk of cardiovascular complications in ESRD patients is unknown. In a randomized, placebo-controlled trial, sponsored by the National Institutes of Health, the effect of homocysteine-lowering therapy on cardiovascular events is being examined in 4000 stable renal transplant recipients.[44]

Hemodialysis-Associated Hypotension

Clinically significant hypotension occurs in approximately 10 to 30 percent of HD treatments.[45] Usually the consequences are minor, but cerebrovascular insufficiency and/or cardiovascular instability (myocardial ischemia and arrhythmias) can occur. These complications of hypotension may account at least in part for the "U-shaped" relation between systolic blood pressure and cardiovascular mortality in

HD patients.[9] The relative death rate for patients with postdialysis systolic blood pressures below 110 mmHg was double that of the reference group (those with a postdialysis blood pressure of 140 to 149 mmHg).[9] Theoretically, hypotension contributed to the increased relative risk of death in ESRD patients by several mechanisms including the acute coronary syndrome, autoregulation dysfunction, ischemia, and development of arrhythmias.

As noted earlier, the major factor that causes intradialytic hypotension is the removal of a large amount of ECV over a short period. Cardiovascular compensatory mechanisms that should be activated to maintain blood pressure will be blunted. Rapid lowering of plasma osmolality due to removal of urea or other molecules shifts fluid from the extracellular to the intracellular compartment. The mechanism involves the fact that osmotically active molecules do not move out of cells as rapidly as dialysis removes them from blood.[46] Another mechanism relates to the use of an acetate-based dialysate as acetate can cause arterial vasodilatation and interfere with the vasoconstrictor response that should occur when ECV is reduced. Other factors favoring hypotension during HD include the following: (1) systolic and/or diastolic cardiac dysfunction; (2) a rapid reduction in serum potassium and calcium leading to depressed cardiac contractility; (3) autonomic neuropathy (particularly in diabetic patients); (4) sepsis; (5) occult hemorrhage (e.g., retroperitoneal hemorrhage after percutaneous vein catheterization to place a dialysis access catheter or gastrointestinal bleeding); (6) eating prior to or during dialysis resulting in splanchnic vasodilation; (7) interference of compensatory responses to hypotension because antihypertensive medications were taken on the day of dialysis; or (8) rarely, profound hypotension can develop because of a paradoxical decrease in or withdrawal of sympathetic nervous system activity. This should be suspected in patients with slowing of heart rate and low systemic vascular resistance.[47] Finally, there may be unsuspected pericardial effusion producing the physiology of cardiac tamponade when ECV is reduced during dialysis.

Methods that reduce the incidence of hypotension include the use of a high-sodium dialysate with a bicarbonate buffer (rather than an acetate buffer). The high sodium content tends to counteract the shift of fluid from the extracellular to the intracellular space while the bicarbonate buffer does not cause vasodilatation. Other strategies for preventing hypotension are to remove ECV at a slower rate and extent. This approach absolutely requires the help of a dietitian to assist the patient in not drinking too much fluid while avoiding foods that contain excess salt. Finally, antihypertensive medications should be withheld on HD days and the temperature of dialysate can be lowered as this leads to a vasoconstrictive response.[48]

Hyperphosphatemia, Vitamin D, and Coronary Artery Calcification

Hyperphosphatemia is common in CRI patients, especially those treated by dialysis. It occurs because the intake of phosphates exceeds the ability to excrete them or remove them by dialysis. A high serum phosphorus is the major cause of progressively severe secondary hyperparathyroidism and the concomitant calcification of blood vessels and visceral organs. Note that phosphorus in the body is in various phosphate salts, but the laboratory measures these ions collectively as serum phosphorus concentration. In ESRD patients, the histologic and radiologic evidence of coronary arterial calcification is much more striking than it is in the general population and this is frequent even among young patients [7 to 30 years, mean (S/D) 19 ± 7].[49] There are strong relations among cardiac death in HD patients and high serum phosphorus, high serum calcium $\times$ phosphorus concentration product, or high serum parathyroid hormone (PTH) levels.[10] This association is especially pertinent to deaths due to coronary artery disease and sudden death syndrome. An important risk factor for vascular or soft tissue calcification is a high calcium $\times$ phosphorus level (>60 mg^2/dL^2),[50,51] but the deposition of calcium and phosphates in soft tissues is even more closely linked to a high serum phosphorus level. For example, the presence of a high phosphate level in the incubation medium directly enhances calcification of human aortic smooth muscle cells via a sodium-dependent, phosphate transporter-sensitive mechanism.[52]

A second factor controlling parathyroid status involves vitamin D and the control of bone and blood calcium and phosphorus levels. The kidney is the organ that converts vitamin D to its most active fragment—1,25dihydroxycholecalciferol, or calcitriol. With the loss of kidney function, plasma calcitriol decreases. This abnormality can be corrected by administering cacitriol to dialysis patients with hyperparathyroidism. Calcitriol, however, increases intestinal absorption of both calcium and phosphates and, hence, when serum phosphorus is high, cacitriol administration can aggravate vascular calcification. An echocardiography evaluation of dialysis patients revealed that 90 percent of patients with valvular calcification were receiving vitamin D therapy compared to only 10 percent of patients without calcification.[53] Vitamin D not only inhibits vascular smooth muscle cell proliferation but also induces these cells to assume an osteoblastic phenotype.[53] Another important, but often overlooked complication of cacitriol administration is overzealous suppression of PTH secretion leading to "low-turnover" bone disease. Besides vitamin D and its analogues, warfarin may play a role in vascular calcification by interfering with the function of matrix Gla protein, a vitamin-K-dependent molecule that inhibits vascular calcification and is secreted by vascular smooth muscle.[54]

The amount of calcium in the coronary arteries has been examined using electron beam computed tomography. The values in dialysis patients are high and are thought to reflect the total amount of calcium in the atherosclerotic plaque.[55] The clinical significance of coronary artery calcification detected by this methodology is still being investigated. Regardless, patients with CRI before or after beginning dialysis treatment are considered to represent a high-risk group for the presence of CAD, so that aggressive risk-factor modification should be undertaken independently of the findings of coronary artery calcification.[56]

The principal strategy for preventing or treating secondary hyperparathyroidism must be based on correcting hyperphosphatemia. This can be accomplished only if patients adhere to a diet containing less than 1 g of phosphorus per day. Even with dietary compliance, many patients will need to take phosphate binders after meals. For patients with high calcium $\times$ phosphorus concentration product, a noncalcium-containing phosphate binder, such as sevelamer hydrochloride (Renagel) should be selected to reduce the amount of ingested calcium. In contrast, if the serum calcium is low, calcium carbonate or calcium acetate should be used but only as long as the serum calcium is not high. If hypocalcemia persists and serum phosphorus is normal (especially if there is evidence of secondary hyperparathyroidism), vitamin D therapy can be useful. If the serum phosphorus is above 6 mg/dL, administering vitamin D could enhance calcium and phosphorus absorption and, ultimately, soft tissue calcification. In considering specific therapies for hyperparathyroidism, calcitriol has a special property; it increases the sensitivity of parathyroid cells to the inhibitory effects of an increase in calcium on parathyroid hormone secretion. In dialysis patients, a rise in serum calcium suppresses parathyroid hormone levels and this response occurs at a lower level of serum calcium following calcitriol administration. In summary, careful monitoring of serum calcium, phosphorus, and parathyroid hormone levels are necessary to avoid hypercalcemia and soft tissue calcification. There is an additional problem related to oversuppression of parathyroid hormone with the development of distinctly abnormal bone morphology. As this brief description emphasizes, the management of calcium, phosphate, and parathyroid hormone metabolism is complicated.

Inflammation and Serum Albumin

Much has been made of a low serum albumin level as an index of malnutrition, yet there are several other causes for a patient being treated by dialysis to have a low serum albumin level and loss of protein stores.[57] The presence of a low serum albumin level is important because it is the strongest independent predictor of total and cardiovascular mortality in ESRD patients.[58,59] A serum albumin level below 3.5 g/dL is found in 44 percent of CPD patients and in 20 percent of those on HD.[60] The serum albumin concentration is influenced by age, fluid overload, capillary leakage, and evidence of inflammation, as well as dietary protein stores.[57] Reports have proposed that inflammation per se plays a key role in the development of atherosclerosis and, hence, the increased risk of cardiovascular death in the general population.[61,62] The evidence for inflammation in these reports is the finding of a high C-reactive protein (CRP). Similar associations between a high CRP and increased mortality have been reported from cross-sectional evaluations of both HD[63] and CPD[64] patients. For example, Stenvinkle et al.[65] concluded that there is a strong association between the presence of atherosclerosis, a low serum albumin level and a high CRP in CRI patients who were not treated by dialysis. Such patients frequently also have high plasma levels of Lp(a) and fibrinogen, two acute-phase reactants considered to be independent atherogenic factors.[66] Elevated plasma levels of the proinflammatory cytokines, interleukin-1, interleukin-6, and tumor necrosis factor are also associated with increased mortality.[67] These findings suggest that inflammation, mediated by proinflammatory cytokines, cause the serum albumin to be low and cause the loss of lean body mass and the development of cardiovascular disease in patients with kidney disease. In this case, the decline in protein stores should be linked to increased protein breakdown initiated by responses to inflammation rather than to an abnormal diet (as would be the case in malnutrition).[57,68] The reason for emphasizing this distinction is that there is persuasive evidence indicating that serum albumin levels increase when dietary protein is restricted for patients with renal insufficiency who are not dialysed.[69,70] What is needed is a method of blocking inflammation and then observing changes in serum albumin concentration.

The mechanisms causing inflammatory responses in ESRD patients remain unclear and proposed mechanisms are summarized in Table 94-1. Specific therapies directed at controlling the degree of inflammation, such as blocking cytokines or their effects will have to be tested for safety and efficacy in CRI patients.

ISCHEMIC HEART DISEASE

Ischemic coronary artery disease (CAD) is the major cause of morbidity and mortality in ESRD patients.[1] Compared with the general population, ESRD patients not only have an increased risk of an acute coronary event but they also have poor survival after a myocardial infarction; the 2-year mortality is 73 percent.[71] Specifically, the prevalence of angiographically confirmed CAD in a 45 year-old patient starting HD varies from 73 percent in symptomatic patients to 54 percent in asymptomatic patients.[72] The risk of myocardial in-

TABLE 94-1 Potential Causes of Inflammation in Renal Disease Patients

Comorbid conditions
Congestive heart failure
Ischemic heart disease

Reduced renal function
Reduced clearance of cytokines
Accumulation of advanced glycation end-products

Infections
Dialysis catheter related
Graft and fistula
Peritonitis

Dialysis-related stimuli
Bioincompatibility of dialysis membrane and
  peritoneal dialysate solutions
Exposure to endotoxins and cytokines-inducing substances
  from contaminated dialysate

farction is understandably related to the high prevalence of hypertension, ECV overload, anemia, hypotension and hypoxia during HD, and increased blood flow through the arteriovenous fistula.[73] Angina pectoris is frequent in the dialysis patient but it is also notable that 25 to 30 percent of these patients will have electrocardiogram (ECG) or perfusion scans indicating CAD even in the absence of significant narrowing of a major coronary artery.[74] Angina in such patients, could be due to an imbalance between oxygen supply to, and demand from, the myocardium. Decreased oxygen supply would be related to anemia, reduced vasodilator reserve, abnormal endothelial vasomotor function, and intramyocardial vessel disease. The latter could be a consequence of left ventricular hypertrophy and/or impaired cellular energy utilization. In addition, asymptomatic severe CAD is quite common because of uremic or diabetic autonomic neuropathy and a sedentary lifestyle.[75]

Regarding the ECG, dialysis per se changes the amplitude of the QRS complex related to removal of extracellular water,[76] especially in patients with left ventricular hypertrophy. The classical ECG changes of acute myocardial ischemia or infarction are similar to those seen in patients without renal disease. Exercise stress tests, however, are limited by the presence of an abnormal resting ECG, blunted or absent tachycardia (autonomic neuropathy) during the test, or a markedly reduced exercise capacity. Finally, changes in serum potassium or ionized calcium levels during dialysis or between treatments may complicate interpretation of the ECG. Serial measures of biochemical markers of myocardial ischemia such as creatine kinase MB isoenzyme and/or lactic dehydrogenase are reliable in diagnosing acute myocardial infarction in dialysis patients, but they have poor specificity.[77] In dialysis patients, the serum troponin-T level is related to left ventricular mass and is an independent predictor of all-cause and cardiovascular mortality.[78] For these patients, the serum troponin-I is considered the most accurate biochemical marker for detecting acute myocardial injury.[79] When serum troponin-I levels are above 0.8 ng/mL, the sensitivity and specificity for the diagnosis of acute myocardial injury is reported to be 83 and 91 percent, respectively.[80] Consequently, a minimal increase in serum troponin-I should be interpreted with caution in dialysis patients.

Nuclear scintigraphic screening techniques for CAD include dipyridamole–thallium testing, but this test is considered to be of limited value in screening for CAD because of a sensitivity of 37 to 86 percent, a specificity near 75 percent, and a positive predictive value of approximately 70 percent.[81] Better results were found with the unusual strategy of stressing patients with both dipyridamole infusion and exercise, and performing thallium imaging This group was then observed for the development of any major coronary event. The sensitivity, specificity, positive and negative predictive values, and overall accuracy of this approach to detect CAD were 92, 89, 71, 98, and 90 percent, respectively.[82] Dobutamine stress echocardiography reportedly has a sensitivity in the range of 69 to 95 percent in patients with chronic renal disease and a specificity of approximately 95 percent, making this another good choice for detecting CAD in patients with suspicious symptoms or those awaiting a kidney transplant.[81]

The American Society of Transplant Physicians[81] recommends that all patients evaluated for a kidney transplant receive screening for CAD unless their risk is low (i.e., no history of CAD or congestive heart failure (CHF), did not have diabetes, and were <50 years old). Patients at highest risk (those with symptoms of angina and a history of CAD or asymptomatic individuals with diabetes and >50 years old) are recommended to have coronary arteriography to detect CAD. For others, coronary arteriography is reserved unless there is a positive result from noninvasive testing. Similar screening guidelines are applicable for dialysis patients who require other types of major surgical procedures.

At present, coronary angiography is considered the gold standard for defining the presence and extent of CAD in CRI patients but, as in other patients, this invasive procedure should be reserved for those in whom an intervention (i.e., coronary bypass grafting or percutaneous coronary angioplasty) is contemplated. The dose of contrast dye used in patients should be minimized in order to avoid loss of residual renal function. Special consideration is required for patients with diabetes or proteinuria. With dialysis patients, there is no need to send patients for dialysis after the procedure unless there is concern about the consequences of hyperosmolar contrast solution precipitating heart failure or hyperkalemia.

The management of angina pectoris in patients with uremia is similar to that used for patients with no kidney disease except that the drug dosages should be adjusted appropriately (Table 94-2). Nitrates, beta blockers, angiotensin-converting enzyme (ACE) inhibitors, angiotensin II receptor blockers (ARBs), and calcium channel blockers are well tolerated by kidney patients (these drugs are usually withheld before dialysis to avoid hypotension). The usefulness of antiplatelet therapy and anticoagulation for patients with uremia and CAD is uncertain. The overwhelming evidence for a beneficial effect of low-dose aspirin in preventing myocardial infarction in the general population outweighs the theoretical concerns about impairing platelet function and increasing the risk of bleeding of dialysis patients, but it must not be forgotten that these patients undergo systemic heparinization 3 times each week.[83] Fractionated low-molecular-weight heparin exerts an unpredictable activity in ESRD patients because they accumulate small peptides. For this reason, this therapy is not recommended for patients with renal failure. Supportive therapy for CAD includes erythropoietin to correct anemia to a hemoglobin of 10 to 11 g/dL as this level reduces exercise-induced cardiac ischemia in dialysis patients.[84] Raising hemoglobin to normal values does not benefit the survival of ESRD patients with congestive heart failure or ischemic heart disease.[85]

Treatment of angina pectoris occurring during a dialysis treatment includes (1) stopping ultrafiltration to avoid more ECV depletion; (2) reducing blood flow through the dialyzer to limit cardiac oxygen demand; and (3) administering oxygen. If there is hypotension, the patient should be placed in Trendelenburg's position while

TABLE 94-2 Dosing of Selected Cardiovascular Drugs in Renal Failure

Drug	Method of Modification	GFR >50	GFR 10–50	GFR <10	Supplemental Dose after Hemodialysis
ADRENERGIC AGENTS					
Clonidine	D	100%	100%	100%	No
Doxazosin	D	100%	100%	100%	No
Methyldopa	I	q8h	q8–q12h	q12–q24h	250 mg
Prazosin	D	100%	100%	100%	No
Terazosin	D	100%	100%	100%	?
ANGIOTENSIN-CONVERTING ENZYME INHIBITORS					
Benazepril	D	100%	75–100%	50%	No
Captopril	D	100%	75%	50%	25–30%
Cilazapril	D	75%	50%	10–25%	No
	I	q24h	q24–48h	q72h	
Enalapril	D	100%	75–100%	50%	20–25%
Fosinopril	D	100%	100%	75%	No
Lisinopril	D	100%	50–75%	25–50%	20%
Pentopril	D	100%	50–75%	50%	?
Perindopril	D	100%	75%	50%	25–50%
Quinapril	D	100%	75–100%	50%	25%
Ramapril	D	100%	50–75%	25–50%	20%
ANGIOTENSIN-II-RECEPTOR ANTAGONISTS					
Losartan	D	100%	100%	100%	?
Valsartan	D	100%	100%	50%	?
ANTIARRHYTHMICS					
Amiodarone	D	100%	100%	100%	No
Bretylium	D	100%	25–50%	25%	No
Disopyramide	I	q8h	q12–24h	q24–48h	No
Flecainide	D	100%	100%	50–75%	No
Lidocaine	D	100%	100%	100%	No
Mexiletine	D	100%	100%	50–75%	No
N-Acetyl-procainamide	D	100%	50%	25%	No
	I	q6–8h	q8–q12h	q12–q18h	
Procainamide	I	q4h	q6–12h	q8–24h	200 mg
Propafenone	D	100%	100%	100%	No
Quinidine	D	100%	100%	75%	100–200 mg
Tocainide	D	100%	100%	50%	200 mg
BETA BLOCKERS					
Acebutolol	D	100%	50%	30–50%	No
Atenolol	D	100%	50%	30–50%	25–50 mg
	I	q24h	q48h	q96h	
Betaxolol	D	100%	100%	50%	No
Bisoprolol	D	100%	75%	50%	?
Carvedilol	D	100%	100%	100%	No
Labetalol	D	100%	100%	100%	No
Metoprolol	D	100%	100%	100%	50 mg
Nadolol	D	100%	50%	25%	40 mg
Pindolol	D	100%	100%	100%	No
Propranolol	D	100%	100%	100%	No
Sotalol	D	100%	30%	15–30%	80 mg
Timolol	D	100%	100%	100%	No

(Continued)

TABLE 94-2 Dosing of Selected Cardiovascular Drugs in Renal Failure (*Continued*)

Drug	Method of Modification	GFR >50	GFR 10–50	GFR <10	Supplemental Dose after Hemodialysis
CALCIUM CHANNEL BLOCKERS—NO ADJUSTMENT NECESSARY					
CARDIAC GLYCOSIDES					
Digitoxin	D	100%	100%	50–75%	No
Digoxin	D	100%	25–75%	10–25%	No
	I	q24h	q36h	q48h	
IONOTROPIC AGENTS					
Amrinone	D	100%	100%	50–75%	?
Dobutamine	D	100%	100%	100%	?
Milrinone	D	100%	100%	50–75%	?
VASODILATORS					
Hydralazine	I	q8h	q8h	q16h	No
Fenoldopam	D	100%	100%	100%	No
Minoxidil	D	100%	100%	50–75%	No
Nitroprusside	D	100%	100%	50–75%	No

ABBREVIATIONS: GFR = glomerular filtration rate; D = Dose; I = interval; ? = unknown.
SOURCE: Adapted from Aronoff GR, Berns JS, Brier ME, et al. *Drug Prescribing in Renal Failure: Dosing Guidelines for Adults,* 4th ed. Philadelphia: American College of Physicians; 1999:24–37.

saline is infused. The blood pressure should be raised before administering sublingual nitroglycerin, which can cause hypotension. If there is no hypotension, nitroglycerin can be administered immediately but the blood pressure must be monitored.

Acute and long-term management strategies for myocardial infarction in ESRD patients are similar to those used for patients who do not have uremia. Controlling the degree of changes in ECV is important, and to accomplish this goal, salt and fluid intake must be restricted to avoid excess accumulation of ECV and body weight. Hypertension and anemia are managed as outlined earlier. The usual concentration of potassium in the dialysate is 2 meq/L, but it can be raised to 3 to 3.5 meq/L to prevent arrhythmias in patients with CAD (or those receiving digoxin). Again, control of dietary potassium is critical and as a general rule, must be restricted in all dialysis patients and potassium supplements or infusions should be avoided. There is a serious risk of developing life-threatening hyperkalemia, and the means of removing potassium could take hours and require an unnecessary dialysis treatment with additional cardiovascular stress. The use of antiarrhythmic drugs should be guided by serum levels.

There are scarce results of trials comparing medical therapy versus coronary intervention in treating CAD in patients with uremia. The same is true for prospective randomized trials comparing the outcomes of percutaneous transluminal coronary angioplasty (PTCA) versus coronary artery bypass grafting (CABG) in patients with uremia. There was a small randomized study of diabetic renal transplant candidates that revealed decreased mortality and cardiac events following revascularization (CABG or PTCA) when compared to medical therapy (calcium channel blocker plus aspirin).[86] There also are some retrospective studies suggesting more favorable results in ESRD patients after CABG surgery compared to PTCA.[87,88] This is relevant because CABG carries a mortality rate of approximately 12 percent in dialysis patients.[87,89] Perioperative mortality is reported to be greater in this population as are the lengths of

hospital and intensive care stays, and ventilator care time.[83] These data emphasize that the physician recommending this operation should be convinced there will be an improved quality of life after CABG.

Dialysis should be performed the day before cardiac surgery to optimize ECV status and to control serum potassium and acidosis. The initial success rate of PTCA in patients with ESRD is roughly the same as in general population in terms of dilatation of the lesion (76 to 96 percent), but relief of angina is less successful and ranges from 57 to 92 percent.[83] Moreover, the restenosis rate following PTCA seems to be much higher in ESRD patients (41 to 80 percent), compared to roughly 33 percent in patients who do not have diabetes or uremia.[75] Coronary stenting in dialysis patients appears to result in long-term patency with a restenosis rate that is not different from that of nondialysis patients (30 vs 25 percent).[90] Unfortunately, however, the mortality rate at 2-years after stenting was higher in the dialysis group (15 vs 5 percent) than it was in the reference group. In summary, CABG appears to be the treatment of choice when coronary revascularization is indicated in stable ESRD patient. But the predicted quality of life must be better before surgery is recommended. PTCA with stenting should be reserved for dialysis patients with single vessel disease or those who are not CABG candidates.

CONGESTIVE HEART FAILURE

CHF is present in 36 percent of dialysis patients[91] and when present upon starting dialysis, is associated with a 93 percent increase in mortality, independently of age or presence of diabetes or ischemic heart disease[92] (Fig. 94-2). Echocardiograms in ESRD patients reveal a high prevalence of "hypertrophic cardiomyopathy" characterized by left ventricular hypertrophy, asymmetric septal hypertrophy, and/or impaired contractility, as well as dilated cardiomyopathy.[93]

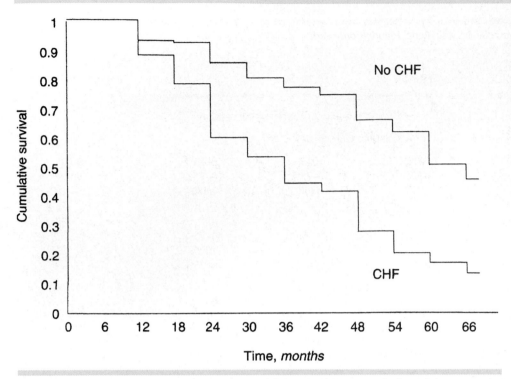

FIGURE 94-2 The cumulative percent survival in patients with and without congestive heart failure on starting ESRD therapy. (Reproduced with permission from *Kidney International* 1996;49:1428.)

Concentric left ventricular hypertrophy occurs in patients with current or previous hypertension. Risk factors for developing CHF include hypertension, diabetes, persistent ECV expansion, anemia, arteriovenous fistula, ischemic heart disease, metabolic acidosis, electrolyte disturbances, hypercalcemia, hyperphosphatemia,[91] and possibly the uremic state per se.[94] Successful HD can improve cardiac function dramatically,[95] by suggested mechanisms that include controlling hypertension, correcting volume overload, removing uremic toxins, and normalizing blood pH and electrolyte levels (particularly, ionized calcium and potassium).[96] The prevention of CHF in dialysis patients requires strict control of ECV and hypertension. Consequently, dietary restriction of salt and fluid are critical so that the patient's weight can be kept as close as possible to the estimated dry weight (see earlier). Note that a dry weight may be erroneously assigned when there is a loss of muscle mass that is unrecognized while ECV increases and maintains a constant body weight. Finally, the adverse influence of an arteriovenous fistula can be tested by occluding it and determining whether or not the heart rate slows (Branham's sign).[97] If the heart rate slows, revision of the fistula can decrease excessive blood shunting and the consequent increase in oxygen demands of the heart.

Management of CHF in predialysis patients requires bed rest, loop diuretics to remove excess ECV, and the use of ACE inhibitors or ARBs. In patients with type 2 diabetes with nephropathy, the frequency of hospitalization is reduced by treatment with ARBs.[98] This benefit occurred in patients with well-defined kidney damage (serum creatinine level 1.9 mg/dL) and proteinuria. The benefit was virtually independent of the treatment of hypertension suggesting a special effect of the drug to benefit the cardiovascular system. For some CHF patients with renal insufficiency, it may be necessary to add metolazone to furosemide to improve the loss of ECV. In such cases, serum potassium levels must be monitored. The major factor increasing potassium excretion in patients treated with loop diuretics is hyperaldosteronism.[99] If digitalis is also prescribed, an adjustment of dosage

and frequent monitoring of plasma levels are necessary. Treatment of CHF in dialysis patients includes bed rest and oxygen therapy plus fluid removal by dialysis and screening for other problems such as myocardial infarction, arrhythmias, pericarditis, or infective endocarditis.

Therapy of CHF using ACE inhibitors in patients with no renal insufficiency improves survival.[100–102] The role of ACE inhibitors in treating CHF in patients with moderate or severe renal failure is not so well studied. However, dialysis patients who were treated with ACE inhibitors for 3 years had a decrease in left ventricular mass, in comparison with patients who had the same degree of blood pressure control, hemoglobin concentration, and adequacy of dialysis.[103] A retrospective analysis of dialysis patients with diabetes revealed better survival when patients were treated with ACE inhibitors.[104] Despite these positive reports, ACE inhibitor treatment requires vigilance as patients undergoing dialyses with synthetic AN69 membranes can develop an anaphylactoid reaction when treated with ACE inhibitors.[105] The reaction results from accumulation of bradykinin, because this type of dialysis membrane stimulates bradykinin release and ACE inhibitors block bradykinin degradation. Another problem is that ACE inhibitor therapy of patients with renal insufficiency can precipitate an acute decrease in glomerular filtration rate (see later). Often the decrease in kidney function is short-lived but, in certain patients, the decrease in kidney function persists. The patients at risk for this complication are those with a serum sodium level <130 mmol/L, a systolic blood pressure below 100 mmHg, with severe chronic obstructive lung disease and cor pulmonale.[106] To manage the abrupt decline in kidney function, it is important to measure serum creatinine and serum potassium a week after starting ACE inhibitors in patients with any of these problems. Patients who are unable to tolerate ACE inhibitors can benefit from hydralazine plus nitrates to achieve "afterload reduction." ARBs have not been extensively evaluated in the treatment of CHF in CRI patients, but they do have other benefits relative to ACE inhibitor therapy such as a lower incidence of hyperkalemia,[107] cough,[108] angioedema,[109] and hypersensitivity reactions with synthetic AN69 dialysis membranes.[110] It also is unknown whether spironolactone will be tolerated or will prove to be beneficial in treating CHF in CRI patients.[111] There are also very limited data about the use of beta blockers in patients with CHF and renal disease. Given the clear benefit of beta blockers in nonrenal patients with mild to moderate CHF, it seems likely these agents will also prove to be beneficial for kidney disease patients.

PERICARDIAL DISEASE

Before dialysis was widely available, pericarditis was regarded as a preterminal event in uremic patients. At present, the incidence of clinically apparent pericarditis has decreased from 50 to 5 to 20 percent.[112] The cause of uremic pericarditis is unknown but most likely is related to accumulation of uremic toxins, since vigorous dialysis is generally associated with its resolution. Moreover, pericarditis is diagnosed most often in patients who receive inadequate dialysis. Other factors that have been associated with pericarditis include infections with hepatitis or cytomegalovirus viruses or with tuberculosis, or the presence of systemic lupus erythematosus, hypercalemia, and/or hyperparathyroidism.[112] Pericarditis appears to occur less frequently in CPD patients than it does in HD patients, possibly because CPD has a higher clearance of "middle molecules."[113] The identity of these middle molecules or toxins is unknown.

The primary treatment for dialysis-associated pericarditis is intensive dialysis (e.g., daily HD for 1 to 2 weeks); heparin is eliminated to avoid hemorrhage into the pericardial space. The efficacy of indomethacin in treating pericarditis is questionable; results from a prospective, double-blind study led to the conclusion that the principal benefit of indomethacin is to reduce fever and clinical resolution of the disorder was not shortened.[114]

Pericardial effusion is even more frequent in dialysis patients because it is linked to ECV expansion. Although an effusion often complicates pericarditis, cardiac tamponade is rare. *An important clue to the presence of impending cardiac tamponade is the occurrence of repeated and/or severe hypotension during dialysis.* Treatment of a large pericardial effusion with or without pericarditis is tricky. Intensification of dialysis may result in improvement but aggressive fluid removal can cause serious hypotension. If there is no improvement or if hemodynamic compromise occurs with dialysis, surgical drainage[115,116] of the pericardium is the preferred procedure. Constrictive pericarditis is rare in dialysis patients, even those with pericarditis.[117] It should be suspected when there is intractable right-sided heart failure in patients with a normal-sized or small heart. Cardiac catheterization will verify the diagnosis, and pericardiectomy is the definitive treatment (see Chap. 80).

INFECTIVE ENDOCARDITIS

Bacteremia occurs in approximately 10 to 20 percent of HD patients.[118,119] The most frequent organism is *Staphylococcus aureus* and the incidence of bacteremia by this organism is about 1.2 episodes per 100 patient-months.[119] Besides *S. aureus*, organisms frequently causing endocarditis are *S. epidermidis*, *Streptococcus viridans*, enterococci, and gram-negative organisms.[118,120] As expected, infective endocarditis is most common when there has been percutaneous placement of permanent or temporary dialysis catheters (59 percent); arteriovenous grafts (38 percent) and arteriovenous fistulas (3 percent) also are associated with this problem.[120] Other factors associated with infective endocarditis are aortic valve calcifications (28 to 55 percent) and mitral valve calcifications (10 to 40 percent).[121,122] When calcified valves are the nidus for infection, the aortic valve is involved in over 80 percent of cases.[118]

When endocarditis is suspected, repeated blood cultures, physical examinations, and an echocardiographic assessment are mandatory. Transesophageal echocardiography is the procedure of choice for the diagnosis of endocarditis in a patient with bacteremia (sensitivity of 100 percent compared to 33 percent with transthoracic echocardiography).[123] Treatment of infective endocarditis consists of 4 to 6 weeks of parenteral antibiotics (see Chap. 81). Survival of HD patients undergoing valve replacement for endocarditis is poor.[124]

CARDIAC ARRHYTHMIAS

Risk factors for cardiac arrhythmias in dialysis patients include ischemic heart disease, calcification of the conduction system from secondary hyperparathyroidism, pericarditis, dialysis-associated hy-

potension, dialysis-induced acid-base and electrolyte disturbances (hyper- and hypokalemia, hyper- and hypocalcemia, and hypermagnesemia), and hypoxemia. Fortunately, serious arrhythmias are uncommon except in patients with underlying heart disease, those receiving digitalis, or those with severe hypokalemia.[125,126] The risk for atrial and ventricular arrhythmias in dialysis patients receiving digitalis increases sharply during dialysis because of rapid shifts of potassium. Therefore, digitalis should be prescribed with the lowest therapeutic dosage. Notably, the potassium concentration in the dialysate can be raised to decrease the risk of digitalis-toxic arrhythmias but, in such patients, dietary potassium must be rigidly restricted to prevent hyperkalemia.

RENAL FUNCTION IN HEART FAILURE

In heart failure, enhanced sympathetic activity and activation of the renin–angiotensin–aldosterone axis enhance salt reabsorption by the kidney. These responses expand the ECV and plasma volume leading to edema and increased end-diastolic volume.[127] CHF can also cause vasopressin release leading to excessive water reabsorption. These responses coupled with increased water intake (possibly related to angiotensin-II-stimulated central thirst receptors) cause hyponatremia, an important indicator of a poor prognosis.[128]

Renal vasoconstriction in CHF patients can cause a blood urea nitrogen (BUN) to serum creatinine ratio above 10:1. Although this may arise from decreased perfusion of the kidney (prerenal azotemia), a high ratio is also a signal to search for gastrointestinal bleeding. When salt and water reabsorption are stimulated (e.g., with heart failure), urine flow and sodium excretion fall, leading to a high urine specific gravity and osmolality. To diagnose prerenal azotemia, the urinalysis and stool guaiac tests are critical. With prerenal azotemia, both tests should be normal; there should be no proteinuria or cellular or granular casts as the latter signifies kidney damage. Diuretic therapy may mask these characteristics by reducing the urine specific gravity and osmolality and diluting cellular or granular casts so they are less easily identified compared to findings in a concentrated urine sample.

Factors that can precipitate or exacerbate renal insufficiency include excessive diuresis, use of ACE inhibitors or nonsteroidal anti-inflammatory drugs (NSAIDs), and worsening cardiac function. The basis for renal insufficiency in each of these cases is a decrease in kidney blood flow. The glomerular filtration rate becomes dependent on angiotensin-II-induced constriction of the efferent glomerular arteriole and blocking this response with ACE inhibitors or ARBs can markedly decrease the glomerular filtration rate.[129] NSAIDs reduce the glomerular filtration rate by blocking the release of prostaglandins so that the prostaglandin-induced stimulation of the renin–angiotensin system is absent.[130] Finally, antihypertensive agents (e.g., hydralazine) can reduce glomerular filtration by causing systemic hypotension and reducing renal perfusion pressure.

The management of renal insufficiency in CHF patients is aimed primarily at improving cardiac function (see Chap. 25). NSAIDs should be avoided, and diuretics should be used judiciously because excessive diuresis can predispose the patient to a further decrease in clearance. Careful attention to changes in the blood urea nitrogen (BUN) concentration relative to serum creatinine concentration and to serum potassium level is mandatory to avoid these problems. The reduced renal clearance (i.e., a sharp rise in serum creatinine) associated with ACE inhibitor therapy of CHF is usually a transient physiologic response. But, if the serum creatinine level does not return to pretreatment levels, the drug should be withdrawn and a diagnosis of renal artery stenosis considered.

RENAL FAILURE FOLLOWING CARDIAC CATHETERIZATION

Contrast Nephropathy

The risk of renal damage following radiocontrast dye is high in patients with diabetes mellitus, multiple myeloma, preexisting renal failure, and, especially, proteinuria, volume depletion, heart failure, and large amounts of contrast dye.[131] Renal failure after contrast dye is typically brief (approximately 5 to 7 days) unless there is preexisting renal damage.

Contrast agents reduce renal function by altering renal hemodynamics and by exerting toxic effects through generation of oxygen-free radicals.[132] In high-risk patients, contrast dye studies should be avoided but if required, the amount of contrast dye should be minimized. Studies examining the role of acetylcysteine compared to hydration with 0.5 normal saline alone in the prevention of contrast-agent-induced nephrotoxicity have shown conflicting results.[133,134] The benefit was apparent when acetylcysteine was administered in divided doses at least 24 h before the angiography procedure and serum creatinine level was above 1.5 mg/dL.[135–137]

Atheroembolic Nephropathy

This complication usually occurs in elderly patients with erosive aortic atherosclerosis. Kidney damage is due to cholesterol emboli to the kidneys and is most commonly detected after invasive vascular procedure, such as manipulation of the aorta during angiography or vascular surgery or after anticoagulant and fibrinolytic therapy.[138] The reported incidence of atheroembolic renal failure following coronary angiography is less than 2 percent.[139] In atheroembolic nephropathy, the serum creatinine level rises and usually does not return to basal levels. Instead, renal insufficiency progressively declines. Atheroembolization to other organs such as the eyes (cholesterol plaques seen by funduscopy), pancreas (pancreatitis), and skin (livedo reticularis or gangrene) may be present.[138] Urinalysis is important because it typically does not contain cellular or granular casts (the signs of acute tubular damage). The disease can activate inflammation yielding an "active" urinary sediment with hematuria and cellular casts, hypocomplementemia, eosinophilia, and a high sedimentation rate.[138,140] Biopsy of an affected organ (e.g., skin or kidney) would help establish the diagnosis, but the absence of atheroemboli in a kidney biopsy does not exclude the diagnosis since the affected vessels may be missed. There is no specific treatment for this condition.

CARDIAC DRUGS IN RENAL FAILURE

Many drugs used to treat cardiovascular diseases are eliminated (i.e., cleared) by the kidneys. To avoid toxic side effects, the doses of these drugs must be modified depending on the level of the patient's glomerular filtration rate. Dosing guidelines for commonly prescribed cardiovascular drugs in patients with diminished renal function are listed in Table 94-2.

Digoxin

The volume of distribution of digoxin is reduced 30 to 50 percent in ESRD patients and, hence, the loading dose of digoxin should be reduced. The digitalis maintenance dosage should also be decreased because its primary route of elimination is by glomerular filtration.

Because of individual variations in digoxin pharmacokinetics, only general guidelines for maintenance dosages are available: 0.0625 to 0.125 mg every other day may result in a therapeutic plasma level but the serum level must be measured and the dose adjusted based on this value. If a loading dose is not administered or if adjustments are made in the maintenance dose, the time required to attain a new steady state can be prolonged to approximately 3 weeks (the half-life of digoxin in renal failure is 4.4 days versus 1.6 days in normal subjects).[141] Concomitant administration of quinidine or verapamil can increase plasma digoxin levels and produce clinical toxicity.

Beta Blockers

Since atenolol (Tenormin) and nadolol (Corgard) are eliminated primarily by the kidneys, a dose reduction of 50 to 70 percent is necessary for patients with chronic renal failure.[142] These drugs should be withheld on the day of a HD treatment because a significant fraction is removed by the dialysis procedure. The usual dose is then given after dialysis (see Table 94-2).

Sodium Nitroprusside

In dialysis or predialysis patients, infusion of nitroprusside leads to accumulation of thiocyanate.[143] Thiocyanate can cause neurologic toxicities such as confusion, hyperreflexia, and seizures. Therefore, the dose of nitroprusside should be minimized for CRI patients and the drug given for as short a period as possible. Both the cyanide and thiocyanate levels in plasma should be monitored to avoid toxicity.

Fenoldopam, a dopamine$_1$ receptor agonist, increases renal blood flow and glomerular filtration rate; this agent may be a good alternative to nitroprusside for the treatment of severe hypertension in patients with renal disease.[144]

Angiotensin-Converting Enzyme Inhibitors

The doses of the ACE inhibitors (except fosinopril) should be reduced by approximately 50 percent for patients with moderate to advanced CRI because the drug itself or its metabolites are excreted by the kidney.[145] Accumulation of converting enzyme inhibitors can cause hematologic toxicity manifested as low granulocyte count to aplastic anemia. ACE inhibitors and ARBs can exert two other types of toxic effects in predialysis patients. First, they can cause hyperkalemia by blocking angiotensin-stimulated aldosterone release leading to reduced potassium excretion. Second, they can cause rapid loss of renal function in patients with renal artery stenosis or other conditions associated with activation of the renin–angiotensin system, including CHF.[129] The mechanism for the decrease in glomerular filtration rate is inhibition of angiotensin-induced constriction of the efferent glomerular arterioles. The resulting dilation leads to a decrease in the hydrostatic pressure across the glomerular capillary wall. These drugs, like other antihypertensive agents, should be withheld on the morning of a HD treatment to avoid hypotension.

Cyclosporine and Tacrolimus

The use of cyclosporine A and tacrolimus in heart transplant recipients is often associated with an acute reduction in renal function and this response can progress to chronic renal failure.[146] These agents constrict both afferent and efferent glomerular arterioles, resulting in reduced kidney blood flow and glomerular filtration. There is also proximal tubular injury (vacuolar changes, inclusion bodies, and giant mitochondria). Hyperkalemia and renal tubular acidosis also may occur with acute administration but these are usually reversible when the dose is reduced. With chronic injury, irreversible nephrotoxicity develops related to the presence of tubulointerstitial fibrosis, tubular atrophy, hyaline arteriolar degeneration, and glomerular sclerosis. Although these changes may remain stable, approximately 7 percent of heart transplant patients treated chronically with cyclosporine A progress to ESRD.[147] The hemolytic uremic syndrome, presumably due to endothelial cell damage, has also been described with these agents but this is uncommon.[148] The mechanism causing this problem is unknown.

References

1. U.S. Renal Data System, USRDS 2002 Annual Data Report: Atlas of End-Stage Renal Disease in the United States, National Institutes of Health, National Institute of Diabetes and Digestive and Kidney Diseases, Bethesda, MD, 2002.

2. Causes of Death. United States Renal Data System 1999 Annual Report. *Am J Kidney Dis* 1999;34(suppl 1):S87–S94.

3. Foley RN, Parfrey PS, Sarnak MJ. Clinical epidemiology of cardiovascular disease in chronic renal disease. *Am J Kidney Dis* 1998; 32(suppl 3): S112–S119.

4. Ruilope LM, Salvetti A, Jamersom K, et al. Renal function and intensive lowering of blood pressure in hypertensive participants of the hypertension optimal treatment (HOT) study. *J Am Soc Nephrol* 2001; 12:218–225.

5. Shilpak MG, Fried LF, Crump C, et al. Cardiovascular disease risk status in elderly persons with renal insufficiency. *Kidney Int* 2002, 62:997–1004.

6. Mann JF, Gerstein HC, Pogue J, et al. Renal insufficiency as a predictor of cardiovascular outcomes and the impact of Ramipril: The HOPE randomized trial. *Ann Intern Med* 2001,134:629–636.

7. Stack AG, Saran R. Clinical correlates and mortality impact of left ventricular hypertrophy among new ESRD patients in the United States. *Am J Kidney Dis* 2002;40:1202–1210.

8. Ma J, Ebben J, Xia H, Collins A. Hematocrit level and associated mortality in hemodialysis patients. *J Am Soc Nephrol* 1999;10: 610–619.

9. Zager PG, Nikolic J, Brown RH, et al. "U-shaped" curve association of blood pressure and mortality in hemodialysis patients. *Kidney Int* 1998;54:561–569.

10. Ganesh SK, Stack AG, Levin NW, et al. Association of elevated serum PO_4, $CA \times PO_4$ product, and parathyroid hormone with cardiac mortality risk in chronic hemodialysis patients. *J Am Soc Nephrol* 2001;12:2131–2138.

11. Mailloux LU, Haley WE. Hypertension in the ESRD patient: pathophysiology, therapy, outcomes, and future directions. *Am J Kidney Dis* 1998;32:705–719.

12. Ritz E, Charra B, Leunissen KML, et al. How important is volume excess in the etiology of hypertension in dialysis patients? *Semin Dial* 1999;12:296–299.

13. Vertes V, Cangiano JL, Berman LB, Gould A. Hypertension in end-stage renal disease. *N Engl J Med* 1969;280:978–981.

14. Ligtenberg G, Blankestijn PJ, Oey PL, et al. Reduction of sympathetic hyperactivity by enalapril in patients with chronic renal failure. *N Engl J of Med* 1999;340:1321–1328.

15. Kim KE, Onesti G, Schwartz AB, et al. Hemodynamics of hypertension in chronic end-stage renal disease. *Circulation* 1972;46:452–464.

16. Acosta JH. Hypertension in chronic renal disease. *Kidney Int* 1982; 22:702–712.

17. Kim KE, Onesti G, DelGuercio ET, et al. Sequential hemodynamic changes in end-stage renal disease and the anephric state during volume expansion. *Hypertension* 1991;2:102–110.

18. Lin Y, Chen C, Yu W, et al. Left ventricular mass and hemodynamic overload in normotensive hemodialysis patients. *Kidney Int* 2002; 62:1828–1838.

19. Kelly RA, O'Hara DS, MitchWE, et al. Endogenous digitalis-like factors in hypertension and chronic renal insufficiency. *Kidney Int* 1986;30:723–729.

20. Glatter KA, Graves SW, Hollenberg NK, et al. Sustained volume expansion and (Na-K) ATPase inhibition in chronic renal failure. *Am J Hypertens* 1994; 7:1016–1025.

21. Converse RL Jr, Jacobsen TN, Toto RD, et al. Sympathetic overactivity in patients with chronic renal failure. *N Engl J Med* 1992;327: 1912–1918.

22. Hörl MP, Hörl WH. Hemodialysis-associated hypertension: Pathophysiology and therapy. *Am J Kidney Dis* 2002;39:227–244.

23. Goldsmith DJA, Covic AA, Venning MC, et al. Blood pressure reduction after parathyroidectomy for secondary hyperparathyroidism: Further evidence implicating calcium homeostasis in blood pressure regulation. *Am J Kidney Dis* 1996;27:819–825.

24. Ifudu O, Matthew JJ, Macey LJ, et al. Parathyroidectomy does not correct hypertension in patients on maintenance hemodialysis. *Am J Nephrol* 1998;18:28–34.

25. Stefanidis I, Mertens PR, Wurth P, et al. Influence of recombinant human erythropoietin therapy on plasma endothelin-1 levels during hemodialysis. *Int J Artif Organs* 2001;24:367–373.

26. Wantanabe S, Kang D, Feng L, et al. Uric acid, hominoid evolution, and the pathogenesis of salt-sensitivity. *Hypertension* 2002;40:355–360.

27. Kelly RA, Mitch WE. Creatinine, uric acid and other nitrogenous waste products: Clinical implication of the imbalance between production and elimination in uremia. *Semin Nephrol* 1983;3:286–294.

28. Charra B, Schulman G, Breyer JA, et al. Survival as an index of adequacy of dialysis. *Kidney Int* 1992;41:1286–1291.

29. Zazgornik J, Biesenbach G, Janko O, et al. Bilateral nephrectomy: The best, but often overlooked, treatment for refractory hypertension in hemodialysis patients. *Am J Hypertension* 1998;11:1364–1370.

30. Kaski BL. Hyperlipidemia in patients with chronic renal disease. *Am J Kidney Dis* 1998;32(suppl 3):S142–S156.

31. Quaschning T, Krane V, Metzer T, et al. Abnormalities in uremic lipoprotein metabolism and its impact on cardiovascular disease. *Am J Kidney Dis* 2001;38(suppl 1):S14–S19.

32. Koda Y, Nishi S, Suzuki M, et al. Lipoprotein(a) is a predictor of cardiovascular mortality of hemodialysis patients. *Kidney Int* 1999, 56(suppl 71):S251–S253.

33. Chan MK, Persaud J, Varghese Z, et al. Pathogenic roles of post-heparin lipases in lipid abnormalities in hemodialysis patients. *Kidney Int* 1984;25:812–818.

34. Lindholm B, Norbeck HE. Serum lipids and lipoproteins during continuous ambulatory peritoneal dialysis. *Acta Med Scand* 1986; 220:143–151.

35. Seliger SL, Weiss NS, Gillen DL, et al. HMG-COA reductase inhibitors are associated with reduced mortality in ESRD patients. *Kidney Int* 2002, 61:297–304.

36. Wanner C, Krane V, Ruf G, et al. Rationale and design of a trial improving outcome of type 2 diabetics on hemodialysis. *Kidney Int* 1999,56(suppl 71):S222–S226.

37. Keane WF, Brenner BM, Mazzu A, et al. The CHORUS (Cerivastatin in Heart Outcomes in Renal disease: Understanding Survival) protocol: A double-blind, placebo-controlled trail in patients with ESRD. *Am J Kidney Dis* 2001;37(suppl 2):S48–S53.

38. Holdaas H, Fellstrom B, Holme I, et al. Effects of fluvastatin on cardiac events in renal transplant patients: ALERT (Assessment of Lescol in Renal Transplantation) study design and baseline data. *J Cardiovasc Risk* 2001;8:63–71.

39. Talbert RL. New therapeutic options in the National Cholesterol Education Program Adult Treatment Panel III. *Am J Manag Care* 2002;8(12, suppl):S301–S307.

40. Kitiyakara C, Gonin J, Massy Z, et al. Non-traditional cardiovascular disease risk factors in end-stage renal disease: oxidate stress and hyperhomocysteinemia. *Curr Opin Nephrol Hypertens* 2000;9: 477–487.

41. Moustapha A, Naso A, Nahlawi M, et al. Prospective study of hyperhomocysteinemia as an adverse cardiovascular risk factor in

end-stage renal disease [published erratum appears in *Circulation* 1998; 97:711]. *Circulation* 1998;97:138–141.

42. Ducloux D, Motte G, Challier B, et al. Serum total homocysteine and cardiovascular disease occurrence in chronic stable renal transplant recipients: a prospective study. *J Am Soc Nephrol* 2000;11:134–137.

43. Masud T. Trace elements and vitamins. In: Mitch WE, Klahr S, eds. *Handbook of Nutrition and the Kidney*, 4th ed. Philadelphia: Lippincott Williams and Wilkins, 2002:233–252.

44. De Vries AS, Verbeke F, Schrijvers BF, et al. Is folate a promising agent in the prevention and treatment of cardiovascular disease in patients with renal failure? *Kidney Int* 2002;61:1199–1209.

45. Perazella MA. Pharmacological options available to treat symptomatic intradialytic hypotension. *Am J Kidney Dis* 2001; 38(suppl4): S26–S36.

46. Keshaviah P, Shapiro F. A critical examination of dialysis-induced hypotension. *Am J Kidney Dis* 1982;2:290–301.

47. Converse RL Jr, Jacobsen TN, Jost CMT, et al. Paradoxical withdrawal of reflex vasoconstriction as a cause of hemodialysis-induced hypotension. *J Clin Invest* 1992;90:1657–1665.

48. Deehnan S, Henrich WL. Preventing dialysis hypotension: A comparison of usual protective maneuvers. *Kidney Int* 2001;59:1175–1181.

49. Goodman WG, Goldin J, Kuizon BD, et al. Coronary-artery calcification in young adults with end-stage renal disease who are undergoing dialysis. *N Engl J Med* 2000;342:1478–1483.

50. McGonigle RJS, Fowler MB, Timmis AB, et al. Uremic cardiomyopathy: Potential role of vitamin D and parathyroid hormone. *Nephron* 1984;36:94–100.

51. Moe SM, O'Neill KD, Duan D, Ahmed S, et al. Medial artery calcification in ESRD patients is associated with deposition of bone matrix protein. *Kidney Int* 2002;61:638–647.

52. Giachelli CM, Jono S, Shioi JS, et al. Vascular calcification and inorganic phosphate. *Am J Kidney Dis* 2001;38[suppl 1]:S34.

53. Qunibi WY, Nolan CA, Ayus JC. Cardiovascular calcification in patients with end-stage renal disease: A century-old phenomenon. *Kidney Int* 2002;62[suppl 82]:S73–S80.

54. Price PA, Faus SA, Williamson MK. Warfarin-induced artery calcification is accelerated by growth and vitamin D. *Aterioscler Thromb Vasc Biol* 2000;20:317–327.

55. Schwarz U, Buzello M, Ritz E, et al. Morphology of coronary atherosclerotic lesions in patients with end-stage-renal disese. *Nephrol Dial Transplant* 2000:15:218–213.

56. Fatica RA, Dennis VW. Cardiovascular mortality in chronic renal failure: Hyperphophatemia, coronary calcification, and role of phosphate binders. *Cleve Clin J Med* 2002;69[suppl 3]:S21–S27.

57. Mitch WE. Malnutrition: a frequent misdiagnosis for hemodialysis patients. *J Clin Invest* 2002;110:437–439.

58. Lowrie EG, Lew NL. Death risk in hemodialysis patients: the predictive value of commonly measured variables and evaluation of death rate differences between facilities. *Am J Kidney Dis* 1990; 15:458–482.

59. Avram MM, Goldwasser P, Errora M, et al. Predictors of survival in continuous ambulatory peritoneal dialysis patients: The importance of prealbumin and other nutritional and metabolic parameters. *Am J Kidney Dis* 1994;23:91–98.

60. Health Care Financing Administration. 2000 Annual report: ESRD clinical performances measures project. *Am J Kidney Dis* 2001; 37(suppl 3):S35–S52.

61. Ross R. Atherosclerosis-An inflammatory disease. *N Engl J Med* 1999; 340:115–126.

62. Ridker PM, Cushman M, Stampfer MJ, et al. Inflammation, aspirin, and risk of cardiovascular disease in apparently healthy men. *N Engl J Med* 1997;336:973–979.

63. Zimmermann J, Herrlinger S, Pruy A, et al. Inflammation enhances cardiovascular risk and mortality in hemodialysis patients. *Kidney Int* 1999;55:648–658.

64. Haubitz M, Brunkhorst R. C-reactive protein and chronic chlamydia pneumonia infection-long term predictors of cardiovascular disease survival in patients on peritoneal dialysis. *Nephrol Dial Transplant* 2001;16:809–815.

65. Stenvinkle P, Heimburger O, Paultre F, et al. Strong association between malnutrition, inflammation, and atherosclerosis in chronic renal failure. *Kidney Int* 1999;55:1899–1911.

66. Haijar KA, Nachman RL. The role of lipoprotein (a) in atherogenesis and thrombosis. *Ann Rev Med* 1996;47:423–442.

67. Bergstrom J, Lindholm B. What are the causes and consequences of the chronic inflammatory state in chronic dialysis patients? *Semin Dial* 2000;13:163–175.

68. Kaysen GA, Dubin JA, Muller HG, et al. Levels of alpha1 acid glycoprotein and ceruloplasmin predict future albumin levels in hemodialysis patients. *Kidney Int* 2001;60:2360–2366.

69. Walser M, Hill S. Can renal replacement be deferred by a supplemented very low protein diet? *J Am Soc Nephrol* 1999;10: 110–116.

70. Aparicio M, Chauveau P, De Precigout V, et al. Nutrition and outcome on renal replacement therapy of patients with chronic renal failure treated by a supplemented very low protein diet. *J Am Soc Nephrol* 2000;11:708–716.

71. Herzog CA, Ma JZ, Collins AJ. Poor long-term survival after myocardial infarction among patients on long-term dialysis. *N Engl J Med* 1998;339:799–805.

72. Joki N, Hase H, Nakamura R, et al. Onset of coronary artery disease prior to initiation of hemodialysis in patients with end-stage renal disease. *Nephrol Dial Transplant* 1997;12:718–723.

73. Ori Y, Korzets A, Katz M, et al. Hemodialysis arteriovenous access -a prospective hemodynamic evaluation. *Nephrol Dial Transplant* 1996; 11:94–97.

74. Rostand SG. Coronary heart disease in chronic renal insufficiency: Some management considerations. *J Am Soc Nephrol* 2000;11: 1948–1956.

75. Goldsmith D, Covic A. Coronary artery disease in uremia: Etiology, diagnosis, and therapy. *Kidney Int* 2001;60:2059–2078.

76. Ojanen S, Koobi T, Korhonen P, et al. QRS amplitude and volume changes during hemodialysis. *Am J Nephrol* 1999;19:423–427.

77. George SK, Singh AK. Current markers of myocardial ischemia and their validity in end-stage renal disease. *Curr Opin Nephrol Hypertens* 1999;8:719–722.

78. Mallamaci F, Zoccali C, Parlongo S, et al. Troponin is related to left ventricular mass and predicts all-cause and cardiovascular mortality in hemodialysis patients. *Am J Kidney Dis* 2002;40:68–75.

79. Martin GS, Becker BN, Schulman G. Cardiac troponin-I accurately predicts myocardial injury in renal failure. *Nephrol Dial Transplant* 1998;13:1709–1712.

80. Ikeda J, Zenimoto M, Kita M, et al. Usefulness of cardiac troponin I in patients with acute myocardial infarction. *Rinsho Byori. (Japanese)* 2002;50:982–986.

81. Murphy SW, Foley RN, Parfrey PS. Screening and treatment for cardiovascular disease in patients with chronic renal disease. *Am J Kidney Dis* 1998;32(suppl 3):S184–S189.

82. Dahan M, Viron BM, Faraggi M, et al. Diagnostic accuracy and prognostic value of combined dipyridamole-exercise thallium imaging in hemodialysis patients. *Kidney Int* 1998;54:255–262.

83. Rabelink TJ, Truin G, Jaegere P. Treatment of coronary artery disease in patients with renal failure. *Nephrol Dial Transplant* 2001;15(suppl 5):117–121.

84. Macdougall IC, Lewis NP, Sanders MJ, et al. Long-term cardio-respiratory effects of amelioration of renal anemia by erythropoietin. *Lancet* 1990;335:489–493.

85. Sunder-Plassmann G, Horl WH. Effect of erythropoietin on cardio-vascular diseases. *Am J Kidney Dis* 2001;38:(suppl 1):S20–S25.

86. Manske CL, Wang Y, Rector T, et al. Coronary revascularization in insulin-dependant diabetic patients with chronic renal failure. *Lancet* 1992;340:998–1002.

87. Herzog CA, Ma Z, Collins AJ. Long-term outcome of dialysis patients in the United States with coronary vascularization procedures. *Kidney Int* 1999;56:324–332.

88. Herzog CA, Ma Z, Collins AJ. Comparative survival of dialysis patients in the United States after coronary angioplasty, coronary

artery stenting, and coronary artery bypass surgery and impact of diabetes. *Circulation* 2002;106:2207–2211.

89. Hillis LD. Coronary artery bypass surgery: Risks and benefits, realistic and unrealistic expectations. *J Invest Med* 1995;43:17–27.

90. Le Feuvre C, Dambrin G, Helft G, et al. Comparison of clinical outcome following coronary stenting or ballon angioplsty in dialysis versus non-dialysis patients. *Am J Cardiol* 2000;85:1365–1368.

91. Stack AG, Bloembergen WE. A cross-sectional study of the prevalence and clinical correlates of congestive heart failure among incident US dialysis patients. *Am J Kidney Dis* 2001;38:992–1000.

92. Harnett JD, Foley RN, Kent GM, et al. Congestive heart failure in dialysis patients: Prevalence, incidence, prognosis and risk factors. *Kidney Int* 1995;47:884–890.

93. Pafrey PS, Foley RN, Harnett JD et al. The outcome and risk factors for left ventricular disorders in chronic uremia. *Nephrol Dial Transplant* 1996;11:1277–1285.

94. Al-Ahmad A, Sarnak MJ, Salem DN et al. Cause and management of heart failure in patients with chronic renal disease. *Semin Nephrol* 2001;21:3–12.

95. Hung J, Harris PJ, Uren RF, et al. Uremic cardiomyopathy-effect of hemodialysis on left ventricular function in end-stage renal failure. *N Engl J Med* 1980;230:547–551.

96. Van der Sande FM, Cheriex EC, van Kuijk WH, et al. Effect of dialysate calcium concentration on intradialytic blood pressure course in cardiac-compromised patients. *Am J Kidney Dis* 1998;32: 125–131.

97. Young PR Jr, Rohr MS, Marterre WF Jr. High output cardiac failure secondary to brachiocephalic arteriovenous hemodialysis fistula: Two cases. *Am Surg* 1998;64:239–241.

98. Brenner BM, Cooper ME, de Zeeuw D, et al. Effects of losartan on renal and cardiovascular outcomes in patients with type 2 diabetes and nephropathy. *N Engl J Med* 2001;345:861–869.

99. Wilcox CS, Mitch WE, Kelly RA, et al. Factors affecting potassium balance during furosemide administration. *Clin Sci (London)* 1984; 67:195–203.

100. The SOLVD investigators: Effect of enalapril on survival in patients with reduced left ventricular ejection fractions and congestive heart failure. *N Eng J Med* 1991;325:293–302.

101. The CONSENSUS trial study group. Effects of enalapril on mortality in severe congestive heart failure: Results of the Cooperative North Scandanavian Enalapril Study (CONSENSUS). *N Engl J Med* 1987; 316:1429–1435.

102. Carson P, Johnson G, Fletcher R, et al. Mild systolic dysfunction in heart failure (left ventricular ejection fraction >35%): Baseline characteristics, prognosis and response to therapy in the Vasodilator in Heart Failure Trials (V-HeFT). *J Am Coll Cardiol* 1996;27:642–649.

103. Paoletti E, Cassottana P, Bellino D, et al. Left ventricular geometry and adverse cardiovascular events in chronic hemodialysis patients on prolonged therapy with ACE inhibitors. *Am J Kidney Dis* 2002;40: 728–736.

104. Stoves J, Baczkowski AJ, Turney JH. Factors influencing survival of diabetic patients after initiation of renal replacement therapy. *Nephrology* 2001;6:79–82.

105. Brunet P, Jaber K, Berland Y, et al. Anaphylactoid reactions during hemodialysis and hemofiltration: role of associating AN69 membrane and angiotensin I-converting enzyme inhibitors. *Am J Kidney Dis* 1992;19:444–447.

106. Davies MK, Gibbs CR, Lip GH. ABC of heart failure. Management: Diuretics, ACE inhibitors, and nitrates. *BMJ* 2000;320:428–431.

107. Bakris GL, Siomos M, Richardson D, et al. ACE inhibition or angiotensin receptor blockade: impact on potassium in renal failure. VAL-K Study Group. *Kidney Int* 2000;58:2084–2092.

108. Benz J, Oshrain C, Henry D. Valsartan, a new angiotensin II receptor antagonist: a double-blind study comparing the incidence of cough with lisinopril and hydrochlorothiazide. *J Clin Pharmacol* 1997;37: 101–107.

109. Sica DA, Black HR. Angioedema in heart failure: Occurrence with ACE inhibitors and safety of angiotensin receptor blocker therapy. *Congest Heart Fail* 2002;8:334–341.

110. Tepel M, van der Giet M, Zidek W. Efficacy and tolerability of angiotensin II type 1 receptor antagonists in dialysis patients using AN69 dialysis membranes. *Kidney Blood Press Res* 2001;24:71–74.

111. Barbour MM, McKindley DS. Pharmacology and pharmacotherapy of cardiovascular drugs in patients with chronic renal disease. *Semin Nephrol* 2001;21:66–78.

112. Ganukula SR, Spodick DH. Pericardial disease in renal patients. *Semin Nephrol* 2001;21:52–56.

113. Silverberg S, Oreopoulos DG, Wise DJ, et al. Pericarditis in patients undergoing long-term hemodialysis and peritoneal dialysis. *Am J Med* 1977;63:874–879.

114. Spector D, Alfred H, Siedlecki M, et al. A controlled study of the effect of indomethacin in uremic pericarditis. *Kidney Int* 1983;24:663–669.

115. Luft FC, Kleit SA, Smith RN, et al. Management of uremic pericarditis with tamponade. *Arch Intern Med* 1974;134:488–490.

116. Daugirdas JT, Leehey DJ, Popli S, et al. Subxiphoid pericardiostomy for hemodialysis-associated pericardial effusion. *Arch Intern Med* 1986;146:1113–1115.

117. Moraski RE, Bousvaros G. Constrictive pericarditis due to chronic uremia. *N Engl J Med* 1969;281:542–543.

118. Robinson DL, Fowler VG, Sexton DJ, et al. Bacterial endocarditis in hemodialysis patients. *Am J Kidney Dis* 1997;30:521–524.

119. Marr KA, Kong L, Fowler VG, et al. Incidence and outcome of *Staphylococcus aureus* bacteremia in hemodialysis patients. *Kidney Int* 1998;54:1684–1689.

120. Maraj S, Jacobs LE, Kung SC, et al. Epidemiology and outcome of infective endocarditis in hemodialysis patients. *Am J Med Sci* 2002; 324:254–260.

121. Ribeiro S, Ramos A, Brandao A, et al. Cardiac valve calcification in haemodialysis patients: Role of calcium phosphate metabolism. *Nephrol Dial Transplant* 1998;13:2037–2040.

122. Straumann E, Meyer B, Misteli M, et al. Aortic and mitral valve disease in patients with end-stage renal failure on hemodialysis. *Br Heart J* 1992;67:236–239.

123. Fowler VG, Li J, Corey GR, et al. Role of echocardiography in evaluation of patients with staphylococcus aureus bacteremia: experience in 103 patients. *J Am Coll Cardiol* 1997;30:1072–1078.

124. Baglin A, Hanslik T, Vaillant JN, et al. Severe valvular heart disease in patients on chronic dialysis: A five-year multicenter French survey. *Ann Med Interne (Paris)* 1997;148:521–526.

125. Kyriakidis M, Voudiclaris S, Kremastinos D, et al. Cardiac arrhythmias in chronic renal failure. *Nephron* 1984;38:26–29.

126. Weber H, Schwarzer C, Stummvoll HK, et al. Chronic hemodialysis: High risk patients for arrhythmias? *Nephron* 1984;37:180–185.

127. Schrier RW, Abraham WT. Hormones and hemodynamics in heart failure. *N Engl J Med* 1999;341:577–585.

128. Lee WH, Packer M. Prognostic importance of serum sodium concentration and its modification by converting-enzyme inhibition in patients with severe chronic heart failure. *Circulation* 1986;73:257–267.

129. Suki WN. Renal hemodynamic consequences of angiotensin-converting enzyme inhibition in congestive heart failure. *Arch Intern Med* 1989; 149:669–673.

130. Dzau VJ, Packer M, Lilly LS, et al. Prostaglandins in severe congestive heart failure. *N Engl J Med* 1984;310:347–352.

131. Solomon R. Contrast-medium-induced acute renal failure. *Kidney Int* 1998;53:230–242.

132. Andrews NP, Prasad A, Quyyumi AA. *N*-acetylcysteine improves coronary and peripheral vascular function. *J Am Coll Cardiol* 2001; 37:117–123.

133. Tepel M, van der Giet M, Schwarzfeld C, et al. Prevention of radiographic contrast agent-induced reductions in renal function by acetylcysteine. *N Engl J Med* 2000;343:180–184.

134. Durham JD, Caputo C, Dokko J, et al. A randomized controlled trial of N-acetylcysteine to prevent contrast nephropathy in cardiac angiography. *Kidney Int* 2002;62:2202–2207.

135. Briguori C, Manganelli F, Scarpato P, et al. Acetylcysteine and contrast agent-associated nephrotoxicity. *J Am Coll Cardiol* 2002;40: 298–303.

136. Kou-G S, Cheng JJ, Kuan P, et al. Acetylcysteine protects against acute renal failure in patients with abnormal renal function undergoing a coronary procedure. *J Am Coll Cardiol* 2002;40:1383–1388.

137. Diaz-Sandoval LJ, Kosowsky BD, Losord DW, et al. Acetylcysteine to prevent angiography-related renal tissue injury (the APART trial). *Am J Cardiol.* 2002;89:356–358.

138. Scolari F, Tardanico R, Zani R, et al. Cholestrol crystal embolism: A recognizable cause of renal disease. *Am J Kidney Dis* 2000;36: 1089–1109.

139. Saklayen MG, Gupta S, Suryaprasad A, et al. Incidence of atheroembolic renal failure after coronary angiography. A prospective study. *Angiology* 1997;48:609–613.

140. Rudnick MR. Nephrotoxic risks of renal angiography: Contrast media-associated nephrotoxicity and atheroembolism-A critical review. *Am J Kidney Dis* 1994;24:713–727.

141. Jelliffe RW. An improved method of digoxin therapy. *Ann Intern Med* 1968;69:703–717.

142. Kirch W, Gorg KG. Clinical pharmacokinetics of atenolol–A review. *Eur J Drug Metab Pharmacokinet* 1982;7:81–91.

143. Cohn JN, Burke LP. Nitroprusside. *Ann Intern Med* 1979;91:752–757.

144. Murphy MB, Murray C, Shorten GD. Fenoldopam: A selective peripheral dopamine-receptor agonist for the treatment of severe hypertension. *N Engl J Med* 2001; 345:1548–1557.

145. White CM. Pharmacologic, pharmacokinetic, and therapeutic differences among ACE inhibitors. *Pharmacotherapy* 1998;18:588–599.

146. Ader JL, Rostaing L. Cyclosporin nephrotoxicity: Pathophysiology and comparison with FK-506. *Curr Opin Nephrol Hypertension* 1998; 7:539–545.

147. Goldstein DJ, Zuech N, Sehgal V, et al. Cyclosporin-associated end-stage nephropathy after cardiac transplantation. *Transplantation* 1997; 63:664–668.

148. De Mattos AM, Olyaei AJ, Bennett WM. Pharmacology of immuno-suppressive medications used in renal diseases and transplantation. *Am J Kidney Dis* 1996;28:631–667.

EXERCISE AND THE CARDIOVASCULAR SYSTEM

Gerald F. Fletcher / Thomas R. Flipse / Keith R. Oken

Exercise benefits healthy individuals and those at high risk for cardiovascular disease, as well as those with manifest cardiovascular disease. This chapter addresses the hemodynamics and health benefits of exercise, conditioning programs, the athlete's heart, and exercise-induced sudden death.

ACUTE HEMODYNAMICS

During physical activity, energy expenditure increases. The compensatory cardiovascular response represents an integration of neural, biochemical, and physiologic factors.

The cardiovascular "control center" is believed to reside in the ventrolateral medulla of the brain and responds to both central and peripheral input. Central impulses arise from somatomotor centers of the brain. Peripheral impulses are generated by mechanorceptors, found in muscles, joints, and the vascular system; chemoreceptors, found in the muscles and the vascular system; and baroreceptors, found in the vascular system. These impulses transit autonomic afferent fibers. The control center regulates cardiac output (CO) and its distribution to organs and tissues according to metabolic demand.

The "feed-forward" command system, located in the motor cortex provides a coordinated and rapid cardiovascular response to optimize tissue perfusion and maintain central blood pressure. This central command provides the greatest control over heart rate (HR) during exercise[1] and is also involved in the preexercise anticipatory response.[2] Stimulation of the central control center by the higher command centers leads to alteration of autonomic tone. This may explain the influence of "emotions" on the cardiovascular response.

The cardiovascular control center also receives input from peripheral receptors. Stretch and tension of muscular and articular mechanoreceptors trigger afferent impulses that are important in the regulation of the circulatory response to dynamic exercise.[3] Muscle chemoreceptors stimulated by products of metabolism influence the control center as well. This reflex neural input, termed the *exercise pressor reflex,* provides rapid feedback modifying the autonomic outflow in response to physical activity.[4]

Vascular baroreceptors are located in the aortic arch and carotid sinuses. They respond to changes in arterial blood pressure and regulate HR by eliciting reciprocal changes in sympathetic and parasympathetic activity. The arterial baroreceptors protect the cardiovascular system from relatively short-term changes in blood pressure, as seen during physical exercise. Tonically active cardiopulmonary mechanoreceptors in the atria, ventricles, and pulmonary vessels help regulate the circulatory response. An increase in blood pressure elicits reflex slowing of the heart. The converse applies during hypotension. During physical activity, this feedback mechanism is altered so that blood pressure is permitted to rise. The aortic and carotid bodies contain chemoreceptors sensitive to arterial oxygen, carbon dioxide, and hydrogen ion concentrations. Decreased arterial oxygen levels trigger an increase in arterial pressure, while changes in carbon dioxide and hydrogen ion concentration have a relatively small effect.

Circulatory Adjustments with Exercise

The circulatory response to exercise involves a complex series of adjustments resulting in an increase in CO proportional to metabolic demands. These changes ensure that the metabolic needs of exercising muscles are met, that hyperthermia does not occur, and that blood flow to essential organs is protected. Adequate blood flow is delivered to exercising muscles through increased CO and redistribution of blood flow away from the viscera. CO is defined as the product of stroke volume (SV) and HR. The average CO at rest is about 5 L/min for both trained and untrained men. In women the value is approximately 25 percent lower.

Resting CO increases immediately before the onset of physical exercise as a result of "anticipatory changes" in the autonomic nervous system resulting in tachycardia and increased venous return. After the onset of exercise, CO increases rapidly until steady-rate exercise is reached. CO then rises gradually until a plateau is achieved. The magnitude of the hemodynamic response during physical activity depends on the intensity and the muscle mass involved. In sedentary individuals, CO during maximal exercise increases approximately 4 times, to an average of 20 to 22 L/min. In elite-class athletes the CO may rise eightfold, to values of 35 to 40 L/min.

HEART RATE RESPONSE TO EXERCISE

From rest to strenuous exercise, HR increases rapidly to levels of 160 to 180 beats per minute. During short periods of maximal exercise, rates of 240 beats per min have been recorded. The initial rapid increase is likely the result of central command influences or a rapid reflex from muscle mechanoreceptors. The instant acceleration in heart rate is largely due to vagal withdrawal. Later increases result from reflex activation of the pulmonary stretch receptors, which trigger increased sympathetic tone and more parasympathetic withdrawal. Increased circulating catecholamines play a role as well. During exercise, changes in HR account for a greater percent of the increase in CO than does SV. SV plateaus when the CO has increased to only one-half of its maximum. Further increases in CO occur by increases in the HR.

STROKE VOLUME CHANGES WITH EXERCISE

Two physiologic mechanisms influence SV. Increased venous return elicits enhanced diastolic filling and more forceful systolic contraction. Neurohormonal influences also enhance contractility through direct effects.

ENHANCED DIASTOLIC FILLING

Diastolic ventricular filling (preload) is enhanced by slower HR or increased venous return. Increased end-diastolic volume stretches myocardial fibers enhancing overlap of sarcomeral myofilaments and improving ventricular compliance. This in turn results in enhanced contractility and greater SV. It is believed that this mechanism is responsible for increased SV during transition from rest to exercise or from the upright to the supine position. Resting CO and SV are highest in the supine position. Supine SV is nearly maximal at rest and increases only slightly during exercise. In the normal supine individual, increased CO with exercise results predominantly from an increase in HR, with little increase in SV. Venous return to the heart is lower in the upright position resulting in a lower resting SV and CO. During upright exercise, however, SV can approach maximum SV observed in the recumbent position, usually without an increase in ventricular diastolic dimensions.[5]

IMPROVED SYSTOLIC EMPTYING

Increases in SV during upright exercise most likely occur through the combined effect of enhanced diastolic filling and more complete emptying during systole. Exercise-induced increases in circulating catecholamines enhance myocardial contractility. In the early phase of upright exercise, CO rises due to a simultaneous increase in SV and HR. In the later phases of exercise, increases in HR are primarily responsible for further increases in CO.

DISTRIBUTION OF CARDIAC OUTPUT DURING EXERCISE

Blood flow to tissues is generally proportional to metabolic activity. At rest, about 20 percent of CO is distributed to the skeletal muscle. During physical activity, the majority (up to 85 percent) of the increased CO is diverted to the working muscles. This represents an increase from 4 to 7 to 50 to 75 mL blood every minute per 100 g of muscle. Even within active muscle, the increased blood flow is highly regulated. The greatest amount of blood is delivered to the oxidative portions of the muscle at the expense of the tissue with high glycolytic capacity.

Local metabolic conditions as well as neural and hormonal regulation of vasomotor tone control the shunting of blood to active muscles. The local response is due primarily to the buildup of vasodilatory metabolites in exercising muscle.

During exertion, parasympathetic activity is withdrawn and sympathetic discharge is maximal. This results in increased release of norepinephrine from sympathetic postganglionic nerve endings. Plasma epinephrine levels are also increased. As a result, most vascular beds constrict, except those in exercising muscles, influenced by vasodilating metabolites. Blood flow to the skin increases during light and moderate exercise, favoring body cooling. Further increases in workload cause a progressive decrease in skin flow as the rising cutaneous sympathetic vascular tone overcomes the thermoregulatory vasodilatory response.[2] The kidneys and splanchnic tissues extract only 10 to 25 percent of the oxygen available in their blood supply. Consequently, considerable reductions in blood flow to these tissues can be tolerated via increased oxygen extraction.[6] Some tissues cannot accommodate such reductions in blood supply. At rest, the heart extracts about 75 percent of the oxygen in the coronary blood flow. Because of limited margin of reserve and increased myocardial demands, coronary blood flow increases fourfold during exercise. Cerebral blood flow also increases during exercise by approximately 25 to 30 percent.[7] During maximal exercise, however, cerebral flow may decrease due to hyperventilation and respiratory alkalosis.

On cessation of exercise, there is an abrupt decrease in HR and CO secondary to withdrawal of sympathetic tone and reactivation of vagal activity. In contrast, systemic vascular resistance remains lower for some time due to persistent vasodilation in the muscles. As a result, arterial pressure falls, often below preexercise levels, for periods up to 12 h into recovery.[8] Blood pressure is then stabilized at normal levels by baroreceptor reflexes.

Exercise Type and Cardiovascular Response

Different types of exercise impose different loads on the cardiovascular system. Isotonic (dynamic) exercise is defined as muscular contraction of large muscle groups resulting in movement. It primarily induces a volume load to the heart. Isometric (static) exercise is defined as a constant muscular contraction of a smaller muscle group without movement. It provokes more pressure than volume load to the heart. Significant increases in both CO and oxygen consumption (VO_2) and a fall in systemic vascular resistance characterize the acute load posed by isotonic exercise. In contrast, isometric exercise increases systemic vascular resistance while producing only minimal changes in CO and VO_2.[9] A third type of exercise is resistance exercise. This is a combination of isometric and isotonic exercise evoked by using muscular contraction with movement, as in free-weight lifting. Most activities, such as sports or employment-related activities, combine all three types of exercise (Table 95-1).

ISOTONIC (DYNAMIC) EXERCISE

The response to isotonic exercise is mediated through central and peripheral adaptations that increase oxygen delivery to exercising muscles. In normal sedentary individuals, VO_2 typically increases tenfold from rest to maximal exertion,[10] while in world-

TABLE 95-1 Types of Exercise

	Isotonic	Isometric	Resistance
Alternative terminology	Dynamic	Static	Resistive
Example	Running	Static hand grip	Weight lifting
Oxygen uptake	Greatest	Least	Intermediate
CO	Greatest	Least	Intermediate
Peripheral resistance	Greatest decrease	Least decrease	Intermediate
Blood pressure	Decreases	Increases	Increases

ABBREVIATIONS: CO = cardiac output.

class athletes the increase is significantly greater. Maximal VO_2 is considered an indicator of the level or degree of conditioning.[11]

During acute isotonic exercise, such as running, peripheral vascular resistance falls. Marked vasodilation of vessels in exercising muscles overcomes vasoconstriction of the splanchnic and renal vessels. In active muscles, local autoregulation in response to hypoxia, falling pH, and increased local temperature results in vasodilation.

During prolonged dynamic exercise, skeletal muscle metabolism is primarily aerobic and requires a significant increase in oxygen supply to meet the increased demand for adenosine triphosphate. The increased oxygen requirements are met by an augmentation of the local blood flow and improved oxygen extraction.

ISOMETRIC (STATIC) EXERCISE

The acute cardiovascular response to isometric exercise is different. The oxygen requirements needed to sustain the contraction of smaller muscle groups are lower. With isometric exercise, the necessary VO_2 is maintained with a smaller increase in CO. Increases in regional blood flow are limited by mechanical compression of blood vessels during sustained muscular contraction.[12] Regional blood flow may actually decrease. In order to maintain regional perfusion, a pressor response is evoked, which is mediated, at least in part, by reflexes originating in the contracting muscles.[13] The increase in blood pressure is proportional both to the relative muscle tension and the mass of the muscle groups involved.

Stroke volume usually declines as a result of increased blood pressure and the absence of augmented venous return. In its "pure state," static exercise represents a pressure, or systolic, load. In order to maintain the higher CO, the HR must increase, often out of proportion to the metabolic needs of the active muscle groups.

RESISTANCE (RESISTIVE) EXERCISE

Resistance exercises are activities that use repetitive movements against a resistance, generating a low-to-moderate rise in muscle tension. The response to resistance exercise is determined by the extent of both the isotonic and isometric components.

Weight lifting is considered the prototype resistance exercise and is thought to have a high isometric component. Blood pressure and HR responses during weight lifting are proportional to the relative intensity of muscle contraction, the mass of the muscle groups involved, and the duration of the contraction.[14] Weight-training exercises have been shown to cause an acute increase in blood pressure.[15] This is thought to be the result of restricted muscle perfusion and a centrally mediated pressor response caused by enhanced muscle tension. The HR response during maximal upper body resistance exercise is lower than that seen during maximal isotonic exercise.[16] This contributes to a lower heart rate–blood pressure product during maximal resistance exercise compared to maximal dynamic exercise.

Previous concerns regarding the safety of resistance training have been rebutted by several reports that reveal that moderate resistance training programs are safe even in subjects with cardiac disease.[17,18] At this time, it is believed that resistance training (done on a regular schedule) is useful for promoting muscle strength, flexibility, and functionality but probably contributes less significantly than does isotonic exercise to overall cardiovascular health and longevity.

CONDITIONING TRAINING

Physical conditioning affects the cardiovascular and musculoskeletal systems in a variety of ways that improve work performance and exercise capacity. Maximal VO_2 may increase two- to threefold through conditioning induced by repetitive periods of dynamic exercise. In-

creased CO and peripheral adaptations that improve oxygen extraction contribute equally.[19] Conditioning alters cardiac structure and function, enhancing exercise-induced increases in stroke volume.

At rest, CO is similar for both trained and untrained individuals. Endurance training induces an increase in resting parasympathetic tone and reduces resting sympathetic activity. Heart rates below 30 beats per minute have been recorded for some healthy athletes. Cardiac output is maintained in such individuals by increased SV. Training-induced increase in blood volume and intrinsic myocardial factors have been cited as the source of this enhanced resting and exercise SV (Table 95-2). During exercise, trained individuals achieve a larger maximal CO than do sedentary persons. In the untrained person, there is only a small increase in SV during the transition from rest to exercise, while the major augmentation in CO is induced by tachycardia. The improved cardiac performance after conditioning is secondary to both the Frank-Starling mechanism and augmented myocardial contraction and relaxation.

In previously sedentary individuals, 8 weeks of aerobic training increases SV. This change is associated with increased left ventricular end-diastolic dimension with preservation or even reduction of the end-systolic size.[20] The enhanced end-diastolic dimensions are, however, much lower than those of well-trained athletes.[21] It is not known whether this discrepancy results from prolonged training, genetic factors, or a combination of both. After cessation of training, changes largely regress within 3 weeks.

Several factors contribute to the cardiac adaptations of exercise training. Parasympathetically mediated bradycardia prolongs diastolic filling time. Expanded plasma volume also increases preload.[22] These changes enhance contractility through Frank-Starling mechanisms. Some studies have shown that endurance training results in increased compliance of the left ventricle.[23] This is probably due to enhanced early diastolic filling and increased peak myocardial lengthening during exercise.[24,25] (See Table 95-2.)

These physiologic changes are accompanied by biochemical and ultrastructural alterations of the myocardial fibers, which have been demonstrated in the hearts of physically conditioned animals. There is an increase in lactic dehydrogenase and pyruvate kinase activity, which enhances the respiratory capacity of the cardiac myocytes. Myocytes enlarge and manifest more mitochondria and myofibrils. Observed ultrastructural changes in the sarcolemma and sarcoplasmic reticulum probably influence intracellular calcium homeostasis and may explain the improved diastolic function of the conditioned heart.

The cross-sectional area of the epicardial coronary arteries increases in response to exercise. Alterations in the coronary microcirculation have also been identified. Animal studies reveal increased capillary density and capillary-to-fiber ratio. Decreased diffusion distance between the capillaries and myocytes has also been observed.[26] Some data suggest that training can promote coronary collateral formation in ischemic vascular beds.[27] These adaptations may

TABLE 95-2 Clinical Effects of Exercise Training

Increase in oxygen consumption
Increase in cardiac stroke volume
Increase in maximal exercise CO
Increase in resting parasympathetic tone
Decrease in resting sympathetic tone
Decrease in resting heart rate

ABBREVIATIONS: CO = cardiac output.

enable the heart to better tolerate transient ischemia and to function at a lower percentage of its total oxidative capacity during exercise.[28] Thus, training-induced myocardial adaptations appear to protect against myocardial ischemia.

Skeletal muscle also adapts to long-term training with changes that enhance oxygen extraction. Capillary density and capillary-to-fiber ratio increase.[29] The number of mitochondria increases, as do mitochondrial concentrations of oxidative enzymes. Other cellular adaptations include increases in myoglobin levels, increased concentrations of enzymes involved in lipid metabolism, and enhanced ATPase activity.[30]

Gender Differences

Available data suggest qualitatively similar responses to dynamic and static exercise in both women and men. Some quantitative differences have been demonstrated in teenage girls who manifest a 5 to 10 percent greater CO than boys at any level of submaximal oxygen uptake.[31] This is likely related to a 10 percent lower hemoglobin concentration in women. In order to deliver the same amount of oxygen, there is a proportionate increase in CO. The gross maximal aerobic capacity in women is approximately 50 percent lower than it is in men.[32] When adjusted to lean body mass, the difference is 10 to 15 percent, a more accurate reflection of gender-related differences. The absolute number of skeletal muscle fibers and the fiber-type distribution are similar in women and men.[33] For reasons that are unclear, muscle fibers in men are hypertrophied, resulting in greater cross-sectional muscle mass. Although strength adjusted to cross-sectional muscle area is similar in men and women, men's increased muscle mass yields generally greater isometric strength.[34]

Exercise-induced increases in SV also differ between the sexes. Men manifest a progressive increase in ejection fraction with little or no increase in end-diastolic volume. In contrast, women tend to increase end-diastolic volume without a significant increase in ejection fraction.[35] This results in a plateau of the ejection fraction during exercise compared to a progressive increase in men.

Aging Differences

Special considerations must be addressed when prescribing exercise for the elderly. In these subjects, maximal end-diastolic volume increases, whereas maximal HR, left ventricular ejection fraction, and CO are all lower than they are in the young individuals. Coronary disease is common in the elderly and may affect the cardiac response to exercise. In addition, the increased potential for exercise-related myocardial ischemia and arrhythmias may increase the risk of adverse events. A critical factor in an elderly (>65 years) person's ability to function independently is mobility.[36–42] The overall focus for exercise training should be to enhance health-related fitness, reduce the risk of various chronic diseases, and improve overall quality of life. Considerable evidence demonstrates that physical activity, both endurance and resistance-type exercise, can significantly improve these indices and facilitate functional independence and overall well-being.

Elderly persons should ideally undergo a medical evaluation before initiating an exercise program. This assessment should include not only a "focused" physical examination but should identify any psychosocial limitations to participation, which are prevalent in this age group.[42–47] For older, apparently healthy persons desiring to participate in a low-to-moderate intensity activity such as walking, an exercise test may not be required. However, for more vigorous activities and for all cardiac patients, an exercise test is appropriate. In addition, a search for any dietary inadequacies that may be compounded by increases in caloric expenditure should be done. A review of the individual's medication regimen for possible interactions with activity programs should be performed.[48]

As with young persons, the combination of endurance and resistance exercise is best for achieving the health and fitness goals of the elderly.[49–52] However, some specific comments regarding intensity, frequency, duration, and mode of exercise for the elderly are required. The exercise capacity of the elderly, both before and after exercise training, is usually lower.[37,53] Furthermore, because many in this age group have been sedentary for years, specific muscle groups are often markedly deconditioned. In addition, musculoskeletal limitations, particularly arthritis, can be severely limiting. Thus it is important to prescribe an exercise program with low-level energy expenditure, particularly during the first few weeks, with gradual increases thereafter. In these instances, however, participants are encouraged to increase the frequency of exercise (with shorter duration), even to perhaps 3 or 4 times per day. Higher intensity training must be recommended with caution in this age group because of the potential for musculoskeletal injury.

Those whose exercise duration is limited (<15 min per session) because of physical or psychosocial limitations should also attempt to exercise more frequently. Conversely, for those not limited, increasing the duration of activity to as much as 45 to 60 min per session is valuable for increasing caloric expenditure and improvement of risk factors, including obesity, lipid abnormalities, hypertension, and elevated blood glucose.

Many elderly persons have symptomatic concomitant medical and physical limitations (orthopedic, neurologic, and vascular) that may be exacerbated by weight-bearing exercise, especially higher impact activities such as jogging. Even walking may be difficult for the elderly person. Thus, even seemingly innocent activities should be carefully considered for potential adverse effects in this age group, especially when the activity requires individuals to bear their entire weight.

Implementation of Exercise Training

The type of activity, frequency, duration, intensity, and progression determine the effect of physical activity. Epidemiologic studies suggest that moderate-intensity activities, such as brisk walking, performed on a regular basis confer cardioprotection to both men and women.[54–58] More vigorous activity may confer greater cardioprotection, but the majority of the benefit is accrued with moderate levels of exertion.[57–59] Moreover, fitness appears to be a powerful, independent predictor of cardiovascular risk.[60,61] High-intensity exercise programs are often associated with poor compliance rates and more musculoskeletal injuries. Thus, a highly structured program of vigorous exercise, especially in the elderly, is not generally recommended.

Current guidelines recommend that persons of all ages perform exercise of moderate intensity for 30 to 60 min, 4 to 6 times weekly or at least 30 min of moderate-intensity physical activity on a daily basis.[62–65] At the present, only 10 to 20 percent of the population meets this recommendation.[63,66] Since only a small percentage of the population is employed in a physically demanding occupation, most need to perform this activity in their leisure time. Examples of recommended activities include brisk walking, cycling, swimming, and active yard work. The duration of any period of activity should be at least 10 min, and the accumulated daily duration should be at least

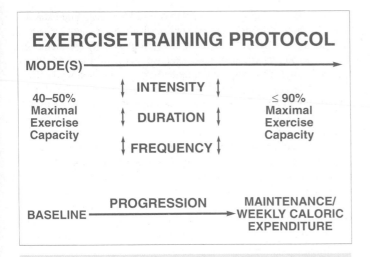

FIGURE 95-1 Exercise training model protocol. *Mode* refers to the type of exercise, such as jogging, swimming, or biking. *Maximal exercise capacity* refers to that achieved at peak exercise testing and can be expressed in terms of oxygen consumption, metabolic units, caloric expenditure, or perceived exertion. Intensity, duration, and frequency are each increased or decreased appropriately to ultimately achieve a maintenance level of total weekly caloric expenditure.

30 min. Those who are sedentary should be encouraged to initially perform a duration of activity that is "comfortable" and to gradually increase to 30 to 60 min of daily activity. People who meet these daily standards and who wish to increase their activity further should be encouraged to do so. Figure 95-1 displays an exercise training protocol for an effective training program. Resistance exercises should be added to the activity program to increase muscle strength. Resistance training using 8 to 10 different exercise sets with 10 to 15 repetitions each (arms, shoulders, chest, trunk, back, hips, and legs) performed at a moderate to high intensity (e.g., 10 to 15 lbs of free weight) for a minimum of 2 days per week is recommended.

Physicians and other health professionals should encourage the general public and their patients to follow these guidelines. Incorporating preventive services into medical practice is challenging due to time and financial constraints. To address these issues, the Centers for Disease Control and Prevention developed the Physician-Based Assessment and Counseling for Exercise (PACE) project.[67] This system includes a simple discussion of physical activity counseling and illustrates how a clinician can efficiently incorporate physical activity counseling into a busy clinical practice through the use of paramedical personnel.

THE ATHLETE'S HEART

The hearts of apparently healthy, highly trained athletes differ structurally from the rest of the population. Regardless of age, intensive exercise training induces an increase in left ventricular mass. This cardiac hypertrophy is considered a physiologic response to an increased workload.

The duration of training and the type of activity influence the magnitude of change in cardiac size and structure. Short-term training is not associated with changes in cardiac dimensions, although there is an improvement in maximal VO$_2$ and submaximal HR.[68,69] Prolonged endurance training elicits left ventricular enlargement, which regresses to pretraining levels after cessation of training. This

involution is not associated with any apparent deleterious effects.[70] Although specific training demands determine the structural changes in an athlete's heart, the response to training varies widely among individuals.[71,71a,71b]

Isotonically trained athletes develop eccentric hypertrophy with a slight increase in wall thickness as well as an increase in end-diastolic volume. The ratio of left ventricular volume to wall thickness remains normal. These athletes have a higher prevalence of multivalvular regurgitation, perhaps due to increased annular dimensions of the atrioventricular valves.[72] In contrast, athletes involved in isometric training show a concentric hypertrophy defined by symmetrically thickened myocardium and little difference in end-diastolic volume compared to the sedentary. Concentric hypertrophy of isometric training is not associated with changes in ventricular compliance.[73] Contrarily, diastolic filling indices of isometrically trained athletes who used anabolic steroids are abnormal.[73,74] These studies suggest that anabolic steroids may alter normal physiologic hypertrophy, leading to increased myocardial "stiffness."

The effect of structural cardiac adaptation to exercise on myocardial blood flow and long-term cardiovascular health is unknown. The functional hypertrophy that occurs in response to exercise training is different from pathologic hypertrophy. During exercise training, the myocardial overload is only temporary, allowing for a "recuperative period" between exercise sessions. The cardiac hypertrophy associated with training is not accompanied by progressive "weakening" of the left ventricle. Even though the hearts of elite athletes are larger than those of sedentary control subjects, the size is usually at the upper limits of normal when indexed to body size. Nonetheless, nearly 15 percent manifest dimensions compatible with dilated cardiomyopathy. This dilatation is without systolic dysfunction and appears to be an extreme physiologic adaptation, the long-term consequences of which are unknown. There is no compelling evidence that exercise training can "harm" a normal heart. To the contrary, the functional capacity of the athlete's heart is much greater, as measured by SV and maximal CO.

The cardiovascular examination of an athlete is characterized by resting bradycardia, and an exaggerated respiratory variation in HR. The bradycardia is due to increased vagal tone. Although HRs of 30 to 40 beats per minute are frequently seen, no specific intervention is necessary if the athlete is asymptomatic. The apical impulse may be slightly displaced due to left ventricular enlargement, but wide displacements suggest cardiac pathology. Both third and fourth heart sounds are often heard in athletes, especially in the supine position. These are considered normal in this population. Systolic murmurs are also relatively common, reflecting a larger SV or functional regurgitation due to annular dilatation of the atrioventricular valves.

Electrocardiographic abnormalities are often seen in highly trained athletes (Table 95-3). These include sinus bradycardia with

TABLE 95-3 Electrocardiographic Changes Seen in Highly Trained Athletes

Sinus bradycardia and sinus pauses
Atrioventricular block
   First degree
   Type I second degree
Morphologic P-wave changes
QRS voltage of left ventricular hypertrophy
T-wave changes

sinus arrhythmia, sinus pauses with junctional escape beats, first-degree atrioventricular block, and periods of Möbitz type I second-degree atrioventricular block.[75] These are likely vagally mediated and resolve with exercise or atropine administration. P-wave changes are frequently noted as a result of atrial enlargement. QRS voltage suggesting ventricular hypertrophy is often seen associated with T-wave inversion in the inferior leads. Juvenile T-wave pattern (T-wave inversions in the anterior leads) and elevated early "takeoff" of the T-wave is often seen. "Strain" patterns, with downsloping ST-T changes indicating abnormal repolarization, are uncommon but can be seen in athletes who perform isometric exercise.[76] Chest roentgenograms may reveal cardiomegaly with a cardiothoracic ratio between 0.5 and 0.6. Such findings are not considered pathologic.

Echocardiography is the best tool for assessing cardiac hypertrophy associated with physical conditioning and is useful in differentiating functional hypertrophy from hypertrophic cardiomyopathy. At times, left ventricular wall thickness exceeding 13 mm or asymmetric septal hypertrophy pose diagnostic challenges. The distinction is important because hypertrophic cardiomyopathy may confer a risk of sudden death during exercise (see also Chap. 77). In these cases, screening of relatives and/or attempts to induce regression through a period of deconditioning may be warranted. The clinician's role is to distinguish physiologic adaptations to exercise from pathologic conditions, which occur in athletes with similar frequency to the general population.

SUDDEN DEATH

Sudden death in the athlete occurs rarely but invariably captures public attention, especially when the victim is young, vigorous, and apparently healthy. Through the efforts of the American Heart Association (AHA) and other organizations, regular exercise has been encouraged as part of a healthy lifestyle. Consequently, physicians and other health care workers may be asked to defend their recommendations in the presence of media attention and may find themselves addressing the anxieties of athletes, parents, and coaches when sudden death occurs. Fortunately, sudden death with exercise is a rare phenomenon; accidents, homicides, and illicit drug use pose a much greater risk (see also Chap. 41).[77]

One of the earliest reports of sudden death during exercise dates back to 490 B.C. when Phidippides died after running 26 miles from Marathon to Athens to report the defeat of the Persian army. More recently, the incidence of sudden death during exercise is small. Each year there are approximately 4 million competitive high school athletes, 500,000 collegiate athletes, and 5000 professional athletes participating in sports.[78] One review reported 134 deaths in young competitive athletes over a 10-year period.[79] While underreporting is likely, sudden death in young athletes remains a rare event. It is estimated that 1:200,000 to 300,000 high school and college athletes suffer sudden cardiovascular death each academic year, and 1:70,000 will succumb over a 3-year high school career.[77]

The incidence of sudden death during exercise in older athletes (>35 years of age) is higher. In one review in Seattle, 11 percent of 316 consecutive victims of sudden death died during or immediately after exercise; and, in Miami, 17 percent of 150 patients had exertion-related sudden death.[80] The majority of these victims had coronary artery disease. Nationally, the frequency of sudden death in apparently healthy men is 1:15,000 joggers, and 1:50,000 marathoners.[78] There appears to be a causal relation between exertion and sudden death. Data from Rhode Island revealed 1 death per 396,000 h of jogging, while the death rate for nonvigorous activity was 1 death per 3 million person-hours.[80,81]

There may be an association between sudden death and exercise intensity. In Seattle, the incidence of exercise-related sudden death is estimated at 5.4 per 100,000. During vigorous activity the incidence is 5 times higher for men who exercise frequently and 56 times higher for men who exercise infrequently.[82] Among men who participate regularly in high-intensity exercise, the increase in risk during athletic training and competition is outweighed by a decrease in risk of sudden cardiac death at other times; therefore, their overall risk of sudden death was lower.[83]

Gender influences the incidence of exercise-related sudden death. Approximately 10 percent of these events occur in women. Historically, women have been less likely to participate in high school and college sports and have been subjected to less intensive training demands, although these trends are changing. Women participate less frequently in sports associated with the greatest risk for sudden cardiac death, and they less commonly manifest hypertrophic cardiomyopathy (HCM).[77] Racial difference in rates of exercise-related sudden death also exist. This may relate, in part, to differences in access to health care and underreporting of high-risk conditions, such as hypertrophic cardiomyopathy (see also Chap. 77).[77] In Maron's series of 134 athletes with sudden death, 52 percent were white, and 44 percent were African-American. The majority of events occurred during high school years, with a median age of 17 years. Basketball, football, and track were the most common sports associated with sudden death, and 63 percent occurred between 3 P.M. and 9 P.M., coinciding with the peak participation time for these sports.[79] Ninety percent of victims collapse during or immediately after a training session. A prodromal complaint, such as chest pain, shortness of breath, or light-headedness, was present in 90 percent of victims immediately prior to the event, and 18 percent had symptoms in the 3 years before their death.[79]

Sudden cardiac death may be due to mechanical abnormalities, but the majority is due to dysrhythmias (i.e., ventricular fibrillation). The healthy heart does not appear to be vulnerable to exercise-induced ventricular arrhythmias, except in cases of significant electrolyte abnormalities, drug use, heat stroke, or blunt trauma to the chest wall.[84] Structural abnormality provides the requisite substrate for arrhythmia. Although an ill-timed ventricular ectopic beat is usually the trigger, exercise may facilitate the development of ventricular fibrillation in susceptible individuals. This may be due to transient myocardial ischemia, caused by hypoxia and increased myocardial oxygen demand in the setting of reduced coronary perfusion time. Alterations in autonomic tone, enhanced coagulability, and release of coronary vasoconstrictor substances, including thromboxane A_2, may also play a role. Acidosis, electrolyte derangements, rise in body temperature, and elevated concentrations of circulating free fatty acids may also contribute.[84]

The most frequent cardiac pathology associated with sudden death in athletes >35 is coronary disease. The majority have no evidence of acute intracoronary thrombi at necropsy, suggesting transient myocardial ischemia (due to fixed obstruction or coronary vasospasm) may be arrhythmogenic during increased myocardial oxygen demand.[84] Coronary artery thrombi are seen in only 25 percent of exercise-induced sudden death victims with coronary disease.[85] Plaque rupture may occur due to twisting of epicardial arteries during exaggerated changes in systolic and diastolic dimensions during exercise. Alternatively, the rise in systolic blood pressure may cause an increase in shear forces. Catecholamine-induced platelet aggregation may also play a role.[82] The majority of exercise-related sudden death due to coronary disease occurs in victims with risk factors for this condition or with prodromal symptoms such as chest pain.[81,85,86] This suggests that efforts directed at screening and counseling patients on symptoms may be effective at preventing sudden death in this population.

For young athletes (<35 years of age), coronary disease is a rare cause of exercise-induced sudden death. It is usually attributable to congenital cardiac anomalies, with HCM the most common. HCM is present in 0.2 percent of the general population but is associated with 36 percent of cases of sudden death in young athletes.[77,79] A subset of individuals with HCM have a propensity for malignant ventricular arrhythmias, and exercise-induced alterations in circulating cate-cholamines, blood volume, and electrolytes enhance this risk.[77] Sudden cardiac death with exercise may be more likely if there is a family history of sudden death, personal history of syncope, marked left ventricular hypertrophy, or ventricular or atrial arrhythmias.[84] Genetic characteristics such as abnormalities in the gene coding for troponin, charge-altering mutations in β-myosin heavy chain gene, and certain ACE gene polymorphism may also define subsets at in-creased risk.[87–89] The heterogeneity of this disorder precludes accu-rate stratification of the risk of sudden death.[77] The 26th Bethesda Conference report recommended that athletes with a diagnosis of HCM avoid intense athletic training and competition.[90] Observa-tional data suggest that prophylactic automatic defibrillation implan-tation is effective in preventing sudden death in patients with HCM deemed to be at increased risk.[91] There is no data, however, regard-ing their use to facilitate continued participation in competitive ath-letics.[92] The 26th Bethesda Conference, explicitly advises against "all moderate and high-intensity sports" for those athletes with im-plantable defibrillators.[90] (For a list of conditions associated with sudden cardiac death, see Table 95-4.)

There are inherent limits to large-scale screening of young athletes for sudden death because events are rare and very few par-ticipants are at risk. Cardiac abnormalities conferring a predisposi-tion toward sudden death are rare in the young,[78] and large-scale screening strategies must be designed with this in mind. Italy boasts the world's most aggressive screening program. The Italian govern-ment mandates that all persons between 12 to 35 years of age partic-ipating in sports have annual medical clearance. In addition to a history and physical examination, an electrocardiogram (ECG), an exercise test, and a pulmonary function test are required. Echocar-diograms are also required in selected Italian professional sports.[77]

In the United States, there are no accepted standards for screening high school and college athletes. Five states do not require an exam-ination, and 11 do not have a standard medical form.[78] In addition to nurses and physician assistants, some states allow chiropractors and "naturopathic" clinicians to perform preparticipation examina-tions.[78] The AHA has recommended a national standard for prepar-ticipation evaluations and that they be performed by a physician or, in select instances, a registered nurse or physician assistant. In any case, the individual performing the evaluation should have the train-ing and skills to perform the history and physical examination and to recognize potential cardiovascular disease.[78]

The AHA has also recommended a screening history and physical examination for everyone before participating in high school and col-legiate sports. In high school, screening should be repeated every 2 years, including an interim history. For collegiate athletes, an in-terim history and blood pressure measurement should be obtained in the third or fourth year, but repeated screening is not necessary.[78,93] The cardiovascular history should inquire about chest pain, syncope, unexplained shortness of breath, or diminished exercise tolerance. A history of heart murmur or hypertension and any family history of premature death or significant cardiovascular conditions should be documented. At minimum, the cardiovascular examination should include brachial blood pressure in the sitting position, assessment of femoral pulses to exclude coarctation of the aorta, evaluation for physical stigmata of Marfan's syndrome, and precordial auscu-ltation in supine and standing positions to identify a murmur associated with dynamic left ventricular outflow obstruction.[78] If a cardiovascular abnormality is suspected, the athlete should be referred to a cardiologist for evaluation.

The routine use of diagnostic tests as part of preparticipation screening evaluations is limited by low specificity, low disease preva-lence, and cost. The ECG is abnormal in 95 percent of individuals with HCM. It proved useful in identifying HCM in a large series from Italy.[94] It is often abnormal in those with coronary anomalies and may identify the long-QT syndrome. Analysis of ECG screening in high school athletes suggests such screening can be helpful (see Table 95-3).[95] (Echocardiography is accurate in the detection of hypertrophic cardiomyopathy, valvular heart disease, aortic root dilation, and left ventricular systolic dysfunction, but cost currently restricts its use to carefully selected individuals.)

The routine use of exercise testing to detect coronary disease in older athletes is not justified because of its low-positive predictive value. However, for an athlete with an intermediate pretest probabil-ity of coronary disease (e.g. diabetics), exercise testing is useful. Con-sensus guidelines also favor preparticipation stress testing in patients with congenital complete heart block and chronic aortic regurgita-tion.[96] The potential for false-positive test results, unnecessary dis-qualification from athletic participation, and heightened anxiety also contribute to contemporary resistance to add routine diagnostic test-ing to preparticipation screening programs. This position is supported by the low yield of screening programs.

A retrospective study suggests that screening history and physical examinations reveal suspected cardiovascular abnormalities in only 3 percent of athletes who died suddenly.[77] Even with the addition of noninvasive testing, it would not be possible to identify many ath-letes at risk, and cost prohibits routine aggressive testing. However, a uniform screening process such as the one outlined by the AHA is expected to identify more cardiovascular abnormalities in athletes and, by disqualifying such individuals from intense athletic activity, may decrease the incidence of sudden death.[77]

TABLE 95-4 Cardiovascular Abnormalities Associated with Sudden Death

Aortic stenosis
Arrhythmogenic right ventricular dysplasia
Coarctation of the aorta
Commotio cordis
Congenital malformations of the coronary arteries
Coronary artery disease
Drug-related morphologic changes
Hypertrophic cardiomyopathy
Idiopathic dilated cardiomyopathy
Idiopathic left ventricular hypertrophy
Idiopathic ventricular tachycardia
Kawasaki's disease
Long-QT syndrome
Marfan's syndrome
Mitral valve prolapse
Myocardial bridging of coronary arteries
Myocarditis
Sarcoidosis
Wolff-Parkinson-White syndrome

References

1. Williamson JW, Nobrega AC, Garcia JA, et al. Cardiovascular responses at the onset of static exercise in patients with dual-chamber pacemakers. *J Appl Physiol* 1995;79:1668–1672.

2. Rowell LB. *Human Cardiovascular Control*. New York: Oxford University Press, 1993:xv, 500.

3. Strange S, Secher NH, Pawelczyk JA, et al. Neural control of cardiovascular responses and of ventilation during dynamic exercise in man. *J Physiol (London)* 1993;470:693–704.

4. Rowell LB, O'Leary DS. Reflex control of the circulation during exercise: Chemoreflexes and mechanoreflexes. *J Appl Physiol* 1990;69:407–418.

5. Bevegard S, Holmgren A, Jonsson B. Circulatory studies in well-trained athletes at rest and during heavy exercise, with special reference to stroke volume and the influence of body position. *Acta Physiol Scand* 1963;57:26.

6. Musch TI, Haidet GC, Ordway GA, et al. Training effects on regional blood flow response to maximal exercise in foxhounds. *J Appl Physiol* 1987;62:1724–1732.

7. Thomas SN, Schroeder T, Secher NH, et al. Cerebral blood flow during submaximal and maximal dynamic exercise in humans. *J Appl Physiol* 1989;67:744–748.

8. Pescatello LS, Fargo AE, Leach CN, Jr., et al. Short-term effect of dynamic exercise on arterial blood pressure. *Circulation* 1991;83:1557–1561.

9. Bechuza GR, Lenser MC, Hanson PG, et al. Comparison of hemodynamic responses to static and dynamic exercise. *J Appl Physiol* 1982;53:1589–1593.

10. Bruce RA, Kusumi F, Hosmer D. Maximal oxygen intake and normographic assessment of functional aerobic impairment in cardiovascular disease. *Am Heart J* 1973;85:546–562.

11. Saltin B, Astrand PO. Maximal oxygen uptake in athletes. *J Appl Physiol* 1967;23:353–358.

12. Asmussen E. Similarities and dissimilarities between static and dynamic exercise. *Circ Res* 1981;48:I3–10.

13. Hanson P, Nagle F. Isometric exercise: Cardiovascular responses in normal and cardiac populations. In: Hanson P, ed. *Exercise and the Heart, Cardiology Clinics*. Philadelphia: Saunders; 1987:157–170.

14. Seals DR, Washburn RA, Hanson PG, et al. Increased cardiovascular response to static contraction of large muscle groups. *J Appl Physiol* 1983;54:434–437.

15. Wescott W, Howeff B. Blood pressure response during weight training exercises. *NSCA J* 1983;5:67–71.

16. DeBusk RF, Valdez R, Houston N, et al. Cardiovascular responses to dynamic and static effort soon after myocardial infarction. Application to occupational work assessment. *Circulation* 1978;58:368–375.

17. Ghilarducci LE, Holly RG, Amsterdam EA. Effects of high resistance training in coronary artery disease. *Am J Cardiol* 1989;64:866–870.

18. Sparling PB, Cantwell JD, Dolan CM, et al. Strength training in a cardiac rehabilitation program: A six-month follow-up. *Arch Phys Med Rehabil* 1990;71:148–152.

19. Rowell LB. Human cardiovascular adjustments to exercise and thermal stress. *Physiol Rev* 1974;54:75–159.

20. Ehsani AA, Hagberg JM, Hickson RC. Rapid changes in ventricular dimensions and mass in response to physical conditioning and deconditioning. *Am J Cardiol* 1972;42:52–56.

21. Saltin B: Physiologic effects on physical conditioning. *Med Sci Sports* 1969;1:50–56.

22. Convertino VA. Blood volume: Its adaptation to endurance training. *Med Sci Sports Exerc* 1991;23:1338–1348.

23. Levy WC, Cerqueira MD, Abrass IB, et al. Endurance exercise training augments diastolic filling at rest and during exercise in healthy young and older men. *Circulation* 1993;88:116–126.

24. Matsuda M, Sugishita Y, Koseki S, et al. Effect of exercise on left ventricular diastolic filling in athletes and nonathletes. *J Appl Physiol* 1983;55:323–328.

25. Granger CB, Karimeddini MK, Smith VE, et al. Rapid ventricular filling in left ventricular hypertrophy: I. Physiologic hypertrophy. *J Am Coll Cardiol* 1985;5:862–868.

26. Anversa P, Levicky V, Beghi C, et al. Morphometry of exercise-induced right ventricular hypertrophy in the rat. *Circ Res* 1983;52:57–64.

27. Froelicher V, Jensen D, Atwood JE, et al. Cardiac rehabilitation: Evidence for improvement in myocardial perfusion and function. *Arch Phys Med Rehabil* 1980;61:517–522.

28. Starnes JW, Bowles DK: Role of exercise in the cause and prevention of cardiac dysfunction. *Exerc Sport Sci Rev* 1995;23:349–373.

29. Hermansen L, Wachtlova M. Capillary density of skeletal muscle in well-trained and untrained men. *J Appl Physiol* 1971;30:860–863.

30. Holloszy JO, Booth FW. Biochemical adaptations to endurance exercise in muscle. *Annu Rev Physiol* 1976;38:273–291.

31. Bar-Or O, Shephard RJ, Allen CL. Cardiac output of 10- to 13-year-old boys and girls during submaximal exercise. *J Appl Physiol* 1971;30:219–223.

32. Drinkwater BL. Women and exercise: Physiological aspects. *Exerc Sport Sci Rev* 1984;12:21–51.

33. Costill DL, Daniels J, Evans W, et al. Skeletal muscle enzymes and fiber composition in male and female track athletes. *J Appl Physiol* 1976;40:149–154.

34. Astrand PO, Rodahl K. *Textbook of Work, Physiology, Physiological Basis of Exercise*. New York: McGraw-Hill; 1986:756.

35. Higginbotham MB, Morris KG, Coleman RE, et al. Sex-related differences in the normal cardiac response to upright exercise. *Circulation* 1984;70:357–366.

36. King AC, Haskell WL, Young DR, et al. Long-term effects of varying intensities and formats of physical activity on participation rates, fitness, and lipoproteins in men and women aged 50 to 65 years. *Circulation* 1995;91:2596–2604.

37. Elia EA. Exercise and the elderly. *Clin Sports Med* 1991;10:141–155.

38. Brown M, Holloszy JO. Effects of a low intensity exercise program on selected physical performance characteristics of 60- to 71-year olds. *Aging (Milano)* 1991;3:129–139.

39. King AC, Haskell WL, Taylor CB, et al. Group- vs home-based exercise training in healthy older men and women. A community-based clinical trial. *JAMA* 1991;266:1535–1542.

40. Shephard RJ: Exercise and aging: Extending independence in older adults. *Geriatrics* 1993;48:61–64.

41. Stewart AL, King AC, Haskell WL: Endurance exercise and health-related quality of life in 50-65 year-old adults. *Gerontologist* 1993;33:782–789.

42. Emery CF, Hauck ER, Blumenthal JA. Exercise adherence or maintenance among older adults: 1-year follow-up study. *Psychol Aging* 1992;7:466–470.

43. Hassmen P, Ceci R, Backman L. Exercise for older women: A training method and its influences on physical and cognitive performance. *Eur J Appl Physiol* 1992;64:460–466.

44. King AC, Taylor CB, Haskell WL. Effects of differing intensities and formats of 12 months of exercise training on psychological outcomes in older adults. *Health Psychol* 1993;12:292–300.

45. Marcus BH, Simkin LR. The stages of exercise behavior. *J Sports Med Phys Fitness* 1993;33:83–88.

46. Barry HC, Eathorne SW. Exercise and aging. Issues for the practitioner. *Med Clin North Am* 1994;78:357–376.

47. Courneya KS. Understanding readiness for regular physical activity in older individuals: An application of the theory of planned behavior. *Health Psychol* 1995;14:80–87.

48. Rich MW, Palmeri S, McCluskey ER, et al. Calcium channel blockers for hypertension in older patients. *Cardiovasc Rev Rep* 1991;12:11–14.

49. Brown M, Holloszy JO. Effects of walking, jogging and cycling on strength, flexibility, speed and balance in 60- to 72-year olds. *Aging (Milano)* 1993;5:427–434.

50. McAuley E. Self-efficacy and the maintenance of exercise participation in older adults. *J Behav Med* 1993;16:103–113.

51. Rogers MA, Evans WJ. Changes in skeletal muscle with aging: Effects of exercise training. *Exerc Sport Sci Rev* 1993;21:365–379.

52. Franklin BA, Whaley MH, Howley ET. A*CSM's Guidelines for Exercise; Testing and Prescription*. Philadelphia: Lippincott Williams & Wilkins; 2000.

53. Williams MA, Maresh CM, Esterbrooks DJ, et al. Early exercise training in patients older than age 65 years compared with that in younger patients after acute myocardial infarction or coronary artery bypass grafting. *Am J Cardiol* 1985;55:263–266.

54. Powell KE, Thompson PD, Caspersen CJ, et al. Physical activity and the incidence of coronary heart disease. *Annu Rev Public Health* 1987; 8:253–287.

55. Berlin JA, Colditz GA. A meta-analysis of physical activity in the prevention of coronary heart disease. *Am J Epidemiol* 1990;132: 612–628.

56. O'Connor GT, Buring JE, Yusuf S, et al. An overview of randomized trials of rehabilitation with exercise after myocardial infarction. *Circulation* 1989;80:234–244.

57. Manson JE, Greenland P, LaCroix AZ, et al. Walking compared with vigorous exercise for the prevention of cardiovascular events in women. *N Engl J Med* 2002;347:716–725.

58. Lee IM, Rexrode KM, Cook NR, et al. Physical activity and coronary heart disease in women: Is "no pain, no gain" passe? *JAMA* 2001;285: 1447–1454.

59. Lee IM, Hsieh CC, Paffenbarger RS, Jr. Exercise intensity and longevity in men. The Harvard Alumni Health Study. *JAMA* 1995;273: 1179–1184.

60. Myers J, Prakash M, Froelicher V, et al. Exercise capacity and mortality among men referred for exercise testing. *N Engl J Med* 2002;346: 793–801.

61. Laukkanen JA, Lakka TA, Rauramaa R, et al. Cardiovascular fitness as a predictor of mortality in men. *Arch Intern Med* 2001;161:825–831.

62. Fletcher GF, Balady GJ, Amsterdam EA, et al. Exercise standards for testing and training: A statement for healthcare professionals from the American Heart Association. *Circulation* 2001;104:1694–1740.

63. U. S. Department of Health and Human Services. *Physical Activity and Health: A Report of the Surgeon General.* CoDCaP US Department of Health and Human Services, National Center for Chronic Disease Prevention and Health Promotion, ed. Pittsburgh: President's Council on Physical Fitness and Sports, 1996:278.

64. Pate RR, Pratt M, Blair SN, et al. Physical activity and public health. A recommendation from the Centers for Disease Control and Prevention and the American College of Sports Medicine. *JAMA* 1995;273: 402–407.

65. NIH Consensus Development Panel. Physical activity and cardiovascular health. *JAMA* 1996;276:241–246.

66. Caspersen CJ, Christenson GM, Pollard RA. Status of the 1990 physical fitness and exercise objectives—Evidence from NHIS 1985. *Public Health Rep* 1986;101:587–592.

67. Patrick K, Calfas KJ, Sallis JF, et al. Basic principles of physical activity counseling: Project PACE. In: Thomas R, ed. *The Heart and Exercise.* New York: Igaku-Shoin; 1996:33–50.

68. Ricci G, Lajoie D, Petitclerc R, et al. Left ventricular size following endurance, sprint, and strength training. *Med Sci Sports Exerc* 1982;14: 344–347.

69. Thompson PD, Lewis S, Varady A, et al. Cardiac dimensions and performance after either arm or leg endurance training. *Med Sci Sports Exerc* 1981;13:303–309.

70. Dickhuth HH, Horstmann T, Staiger J, et al. The long-term involution of physiological cardiomegaly and cardiac hypertrophy. *Med Sci Sports Exerc* 1989;21:244–249.

71. Maron BJ. Structural features of the athlete heart as defined by echocardiography. *J Am Coll Cardiol* 1986;7:190–203.

71a. Fagard R. Athlete's heart. *Heart* 2003;89:1455–1461.

71b. Sharma S. Athlete's heart: Effect of age, sex, ethnicity and sporting discipline. *Exp Physiol* 2003;88:665–669.

72. Douglas PS, Berman GO, O'Toole ML, et al. Prevalence of multivalvular regurgitation in athletes. *Am J Cardiol* 1989; 64:209–212.

73. Pearson AC, Schiff M, Mrosek D, et al. Left ventricular diastolic function in weight lifters. *Am J Cardiol* 1986;58:1254–1259.

74. Urhausen A, Holpes R, Kindermann W. One- and two-dimensional echocardiography in bodybuilders using anabolic steroids. *Eur J Appl Physiol* 1989;58:633–640.

75. Zehender M, Meinertz T, Keul J, et al. ECG variants and cardiac arrhythmias in athletes: Clinical relevance and prognostic importance. *Am Heart J* 1990;119:1378–1391.

76. Buttrick PM, Scheuer J. Exercise and the heart: Acute hemodynamics, conditioning training, the athlete's heart, and sudden death. In: Schlant RC, Alexander RW, eds. *Hurst's The Heart*, 8th ed. New York: McGraw-Hill; 1994:2057–2066.

77. Maron BJ. Cardiovascular risks to young persons on the athletic field. *Ann Intern Med* 1998;129:379–386.

78. Maron BJ, Thompson PD, Puffer JC, et al. Cardiovascular preparticipation screening of competitive athletes. A statement for health professionals from the Sudden Death Committee (clinical cardiology) and Congenital Cardiac Defects Committee (cardiovascular disease in the young), American Heart Association. *Circulation* 1996;94:850–856.

79. Maron BJ, Shirani J, Poliac LC, et al. Sudden death in young competitive athletes. Clinical, demographic, and pathological profiles. *JAMA* 276:1996;199–204.

80. Cobb LA, Weaver WD. Exercise: A risk for sudden death in patients with coronary heart disease. *J Am Coll Cardiol* 1986;7:215–219.

81. Thompson PD, Funk EJ, Carleton RA, et al. Incidence of death during jogging in Rhode Island from 1975 through 1980. *JAMA* 1982;247: 2535–2538.

82. Thompson PD. The cardiovascular complications of vigorous physical activity. *Arch Intern Med* 1996;156:2297–2302.

83. Siscovick DS, Weiss NS, Fletcher RH, et al. The incidence of primary cardiac arrest during vigorous exercise. *N Engl J Med* 1984;311:874–877.

84. Franklin BA, Fletcher GF, Gordon NF, et al. Cardiovascular evaluation of the athlete. Issues regarding performance, screening and sudden cardiac death. *Sports Med* 1997;24:97–119.

85. Virmani R, Burke AP, Farb A, et al. Causes of sudden death in young and middle-aged competitive athletes. *Cardiol Clin* 1997;15:439–466.

86. Northcote RJ, Ballantyne D. Sudden cardiac death in sport. *BMJ (Clin Res Ed)* 1983;287:1357–1359.

87. Watkins H, McKenna WJ, Thierfelder L, et al. Mutations in the genes for cardiac troponin T and alpha-tropomyosin in hypertrophic cardiomyopathy. *N Engl J Med* 1995;332:1058–1064.

88. Anan R, Greve G, Thierfelder L, et al. Prognostic implications of novel beta cardiac myosin heavy chain gene mutations that cause familial hypertrophic cardiomyopathy. *J Clin Invest* 1994;93:280–285.

89. Marian AJ, Yu QT, Workman R, et al. Angiotensin-converting enzyme polymorphism in hypertrophic cardiomyopathy and sudden cardiac death. *Lancet* 1993;342:1085–1086.

90. Maron BJ, Mitchell JH. 26th Bethesda Conference: recommendations for determining eligibility for competition in athletes with cardiovascular abnormalities. *J Am Coll Cardiol* 1994;24:845–99.

91. Maron BJ, Shen WK, Link MS, et al. Efficacy of implantable cardioverter-defibrillators for the prevention of sudden death in patients with hypertrophic cardiomyopathy. *N Engl J Med* 2000;342:365–373.

92. Maron BJ, Mitten MJ, Quandt EF, et al. Competitive athletes with cardiovascular disease—The case of Nicholas Knapp. *N Engl J Med* 1998;339:1632–1635.

93. Maron BJ, Thompson PD, Puffer JC, et al. Cardiovascular preparticipation screening of competitive athletes: addendum: an addendum to a statement for health professionals from the Sudden Death Committee (Council on Clinical Cardiology) and the Congenital Cardiac Defects Committee (Council on Cardiovascular Disease in the Young), American Heart Association. *Circulation* 1998;97:2294.

94. Corrado D, Basso C, Schiavon M, et al. Screening for hypertrophic cardiomyopathy in young athletes. *N Engl J Med* 1998;339:364–369.

95. Fuller CM. Cost effectiveness analysis of screening of high school athletes for risk of sudden cardiac death. *Med Sci Sports Exerc* 2000;32: 887–890.

96. Gibbons RJ, Balady GJ, Bricker JT, et al. ACC/AHA 2002 guideline update for exercise testing: A report of the American College of Cardiology/American Heart Association Task Force on Practice Guidelines (Committee on Exercise Testing) 2002. American College of Cardiology Web site. Available at: www.acc.org/clinical/guidelines/exercise/dirindex.htm.

CARDIOVASCULAR AGING IN THE ABSENCE OF CLINICAL DISEASE AND THERAPEUTIC CONSIDERATIONS FOR OLDER PATIENTS WITH CLINICAL CARDIOVASCULAR DISEASES

Edward G. Lakatta / Steven P. Schulman / Gary Gerstenblith

As persons age, cardiovascular structure and function change and alter the substrate upon which specific pathophysiologic disease mechanisms become superimposed. While epidemiologic studies have discovered that lipid levels, diabetes, sedentary lifestyle, and genetic factors are risks for coronary disease, hypertension, and stroke—the quintessential cardiovascular (CV) diseases within our society—advancing age unequivocally confers the major risk.

The percentage of older persons in the population is increasing worldwide. It is estimated that, by the year 2035, nearly one in four individuals will be 65 years of age or older. The incidence and prevalence of clinically manifest major CV diseases increase steeply with advancing age (Fig. 96-1). Moreover, in a substantial percentage of older, community-dwelling, otherwise healthy volunteers, subclinical or occult disease—such as silent coronary atherosclerosis (Fig. 96-2)—increases with age as well. Left ventricular hypertrophy, heart failure, and atrial fibrillation also increase dramatically with age (Fig. 96-1D to G).

The enhanced likelihood of older persons to develop, for a given time at risk, diseases depicted in Figs. 96-1 and 96-2 points to interactions between mechanisms that underlie aging and those that underlie diseases. In other words, age-associated changes in CV structure and function become "partners" with pathophysiologic disease mechanisms in determining the threshold, severity, and prognosis of CV disease occurrence in older persons. The nature of age-disease interactions is complex and involves mechanisms of aging per se, multiple defined disease risk factors, and as yet undefined risk factors—e.g., those that may have a genetic basis. The role of specific age-associated changes in CV structure and function in such age-disease interactions has formerly been, and largely continues to be, unrecognized by those who shape medical policy. Thus, specific aspects of CV aging have remained largely outside the bailiwick of clinical cardiology and, until recently, have not been considered in most epidemiologic studies of CV disease.

Quantitative information on age-associated alterations in CV structure and function in health is essential to define and target the specific characteristics of CV aging that render it such a major risk factor for CV diseases. Such information is also required to differentiate between the limitations of an elderly person that relate to disease and those that are within expected normal limits. During the past two decades, a sustained effort has been applied to characterize the

Prevalence of Hypertension in US Adult Population

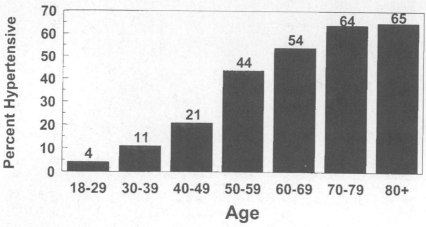

Based on NHANES III survey: 1988-1991
HTN defined by BP >140/90 or treated

A

Incidence of Atherothrombotic Stroke by Age in Framingham

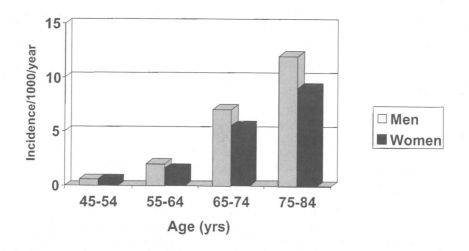

B

FIGURE 96-1 *A.* Prevalence of hypertension, defined as systolic blood pressure $> = 140$ or diastolic blood pressure $> = 90$ or current use of medication for purposes of treating high blood pressure. Data are based on National Health and Nutrition Examination Survey III (1988–1991). *B.* Incidence of atherothrombotic stroke (per 1000 subjects per year) by age in men (*light bars*) and women (*dark bars*) from the Framingham Heart Study. *C.* Incidence of coronary heart disease by age in men (*light bars*) and women (*dark bars*) from the Framingham Heart Study. (*A, B,* and *C* from Lakatta EG, Levy D. Arterial and cardiac aging: Major shareholders in cardiovascular disease enterprises. Part I. Aging arteries: A "set-up" for vascular disease. *Circulation* 2003;107:129–146. With permission.) *D.* Prevalence of echocardiographic left ventricular hypertrophy in women according to baseline age and systolic blood pressure. *E.* Prevalence of echocardiographic left ventricular hypertrophy in men according to baseline age and systolic blood pressure. *F.* Prevalence of heart failure by age in Framingham Heart Study men (*light bars*) and women (*dark bars*). *G.* Prevalence of atrial fibrillation by age in subjects from the Framingham Heart Study. (*D, E, F,* and *G* from Lakatta EG, Levy D. Arterial and cardiac aging: Major shareholders in cardiovascular disease enterprises. Part II: The aging heart in health: Links to heart disease. *Circulation* 2003;107:346–354. With permission.)

Incidence of CHD by Age and Sex

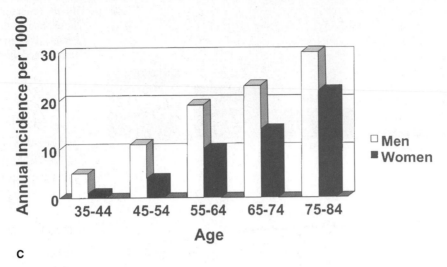

C

Age-Adjusted Prevalence of LVH

Women

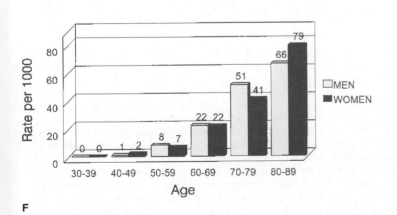

D

Age-Adjusted Prevalence of LVH

Men

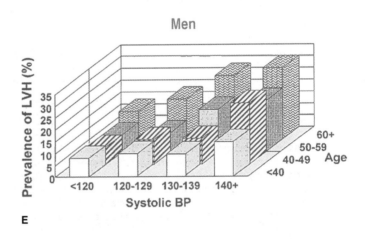

E

Prevalence of Heart Failure by Age in Framingham

F

Prevalence of AF by Age in Framingham

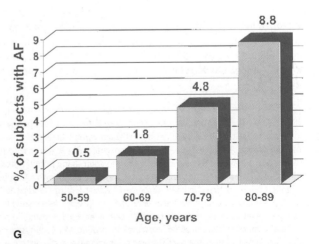

G

FIGURE 96-1 (Continued)

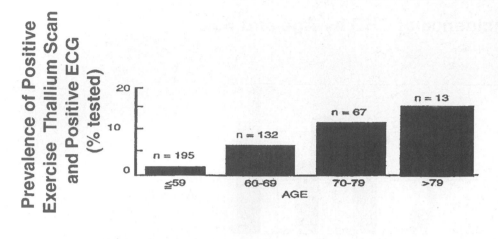

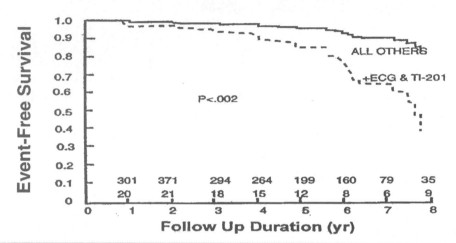

are characterized with respect to lifestyle (e.g., exercise habits) in an attempt to clarify the interactions of these factors and those changes that result from aging per se. Perspectives gleaned from these studies are emphasized throughout this chapter.

AGE-ASSOCIATED CHANGES IN CENTRAL ARTERIAL STRUCTURE AND FUNCTION IN PERSONS WITHOUT A VASCULAR DISEASE DIAGNOSIS

Arterial Thickening and Stiffening

Cross-sectional studies in humans have found that wall thickening and dilatation are prominent structural changes that occur within large elastic arteries during aging (see Ref. 1 for review). While the carotid wall intimal media (IM) thickness increases two- to threefold between 20 and 90 years of age in BLSA subjects rigorously screened to exclude carotid or coronary arterial stenosis (Fig. 96-3A), marked heterogeneity in IM thickness is observed among individuals, particularly at older ages. There is currently no detailed information regarding the factors involved in progressive IM thickening with aging in humans.

Postmortem studies indicate that aortic wall thickening that occurs with aging consists mainly of intimal thickening, even in populations with a low incidence of atherosclerosis[2]; changes in endothelial cell properties with aging are likely involved in this remodeling.[3]

IM thickening is accompanied by both luminal dilatation (Fig. 96-3B) and a reduction in compliance or distensibility (Fig. 96-3C), i.e., an increase in vessel stiffness. Pulse wave velocity (PWV), a relatively convenient, noninvasive index of vascular stiffening, increases with age both in men and women (Fig. 96-3D). Increased PWV has tradi-

FIGURE 96-2 *Top.* The prevalance of silent ischemia in apparently healthy asymptomatic volunteer subjects from the Baltimore Longitudinal Study on Aging (BLSA). Silent ischemia is defined as both a positive thallium-201 (Tl-201) scan and a positive electrocardiogram (ECG) during maximal exercise. *N* = number of test performed. *Bottom.* The event-free survival in those with a double-positive (ECG + Tl-201) test is markedly reduced compared to all other volunteers tested. Within 5 years, 50 percent of those with a double-positive test for silent ischemia developed their initial clinical manifestation of coronary artery disease. Numbers in the lower part of the figure represent the number of subjects monitored during the follow-up period; lower numbers = all double-positive test; top number = all others. (From Lakatta EG, Levy D. Arterial and cardiac aging: Major shareholders in cardiovascular disease enterprises. Part II: The aging heart in health: Links to heart disease. *Circulation* 2003;107:346–354. With permission.)

effects of aging in health on multiple aspects of CV structure and function in a single study population, the Baltimore Longitudinal Study on Aging (BLSA). These community-dwelling volunteers are rigorously screened to detect both clinical and occult CV disease and

reduction in compliance or distensibility (Fig. 96-3C), i.e., an increase in vessel stiffness. Pulse wave velocity (PWV), a relatively convenient, noninvasive index of vascular stiffening, increases with age both in men and women (Fig. 96-3D). Increased PWV has tradi-

FIGURE 96-3 *A.* The common carotid intimal medial thickness in healthy volunteers from the Baltimore Longitudinal Study on Aging (BLSA) as a function of age. (From Nagai Y, Metter EJ, Earley CJ, et al. Increased carotid artery intimal-medial thickness in asymptomatic older subjects with exercise-induced myocardial ischemia. *Circulation* 1998;98:1504–1509. With permission.) *B.* Aortic root diameter measured via M-mode echocardiography. (From Gerstenblith G, Frederiksen J, Yin FC. Echocardiographic assessment of a normal adult aging population. *Circulation* 1977;56:273–278. With permission.) *C.* The stroke volume index/pulse pressure, an index of total systemic vascular compliance, increases with aging. (From Fleg JL, O'Connor FC, Gerstenblith G. Impact of age on the cardiovascular response to dynamic upright exercise in healthy men and women. *J Appl Physiol* 1995;78:890–900. With permission.) *D.* Aortic pulse-wave velocity as a function of age in healthy BLSA volunteer subjects. Pulse-wave pressure (PWV) determined in part by the intrinsic stress/strain relationship (stiffness) of the vascular wall and in part by the mean arterial pressure. *E.* Increased pulse-wave velocity results in reflected pulse waves arriving back to the base of aorta at an earlier time within the cardiac cycle (i.e., prior to closure of the aortic valve), producing a late-systolic augmentation of the central pressure pulse contour. Early reflected pulse waves in conjunction with a resetting of the baroflex lead to an increase in the resting systolic pressure with aging, which, by definition in normotensives, occurs within the clinically normal range. (*D* and *E* from Vaitkevicius PV, Fleg JL, Engel JH, et al. Effects of age and aerobic capacity on arterial stiffness in healthy adults. *Circulation* 1993;88:1456–1462. With permission.). *F.* Pulse pressure in healthy BLSA individuals. (From Pearson JD, Morrell CH, Brant LJ, et al. Age-associated changes in blood pressure in a longitudinal study of healthy men and women. *J Gerontol Med Sci* 1997;52:M177–M183. With permission.)

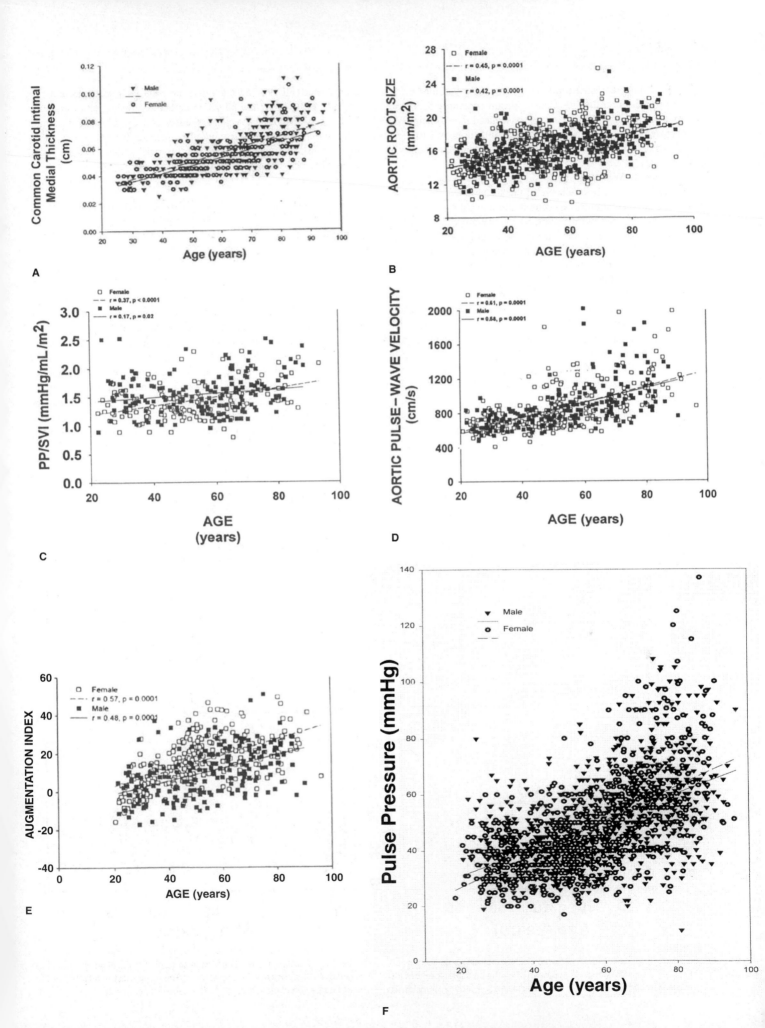

tionally been linked to structural alterations in the vascular media, including increased collagen, reduced elastin content, elastin fractures, and calcification. Prominent age-associated increases in PWV have been demonstrated in populations with little or no atherosclerosis, indicating that vascular stiffening can occur independently of atherosclerosis.[4]

An increased PWV causes reflected pulse waves to reach the base of aorta earlier (i.e., prior to closure of the aortic value), producing a late systolic augmentation of the central pressure pulse contour (Fig. 96-3E). Early reflected pulse waves, in conjunction with a resetting of the baroflex, lead to an increase in the resting systolic pressure with aging within the clinically "normal" range. On average, the diastolic pressure does not increase after middle age and, in many older persons, becomes reduced due to the reduced conduit artery compliance and early reflected pulse waves occurring centrally in late systole rather than in diastole. Peripheral vascular resistance calculated from the resting mean arterial pressure and cardiac output increases modestly or does not appreciably change at rest with aging in otherwise healthy, normotensive persons. The net result is a dramatic increase in pulse pressure (PP) with increasing age (Fig. 96-3F). Pulse pressure is thus a useful but not perfect hemodynamic indicator of conduit artery vascular stiffness.

Endothelial function (Fig. 96-4A) becomes measureably altered in about the sixth decade of life, a time when total systemic arterial

compliance (Fig. 96-3C) and pulse pressure begin to appreciably elevate (Fig. 96-3F). Thus, altered endothelial function with aging may be a mechanism that not only increases aortic stiffness and permits arterial pulse pressure to rise but also underlies the importance of increased stiffness and pulse pressure as risk factors for CV events, even when accounting for systolic pressure (see below).

SPECIFIC LINKS OF ARTERIAL AGING TO ARTERIAL DISEASE

Intimal Medial Thickening

It has been argued that the age-associated increase in IM thickness with aging in humans represents an early stage of atherosclerosis. Indeed, excessive IM thickening at a given age predicts the coexistence of *silent* coronary artery disease (CAD).[5] Since silent CAD often progresses to overt clinical CAD, it is not surprising that increased IM thickness predicts future clinical CV disease events. A plethora of other epidemiologic studies of individuals, not initially screened to exclude the presence of occult CV disease, have indicated that increased IM thickness is an independent predictor of future CV events. The risk gradation among quintiles of IM thickening is non-

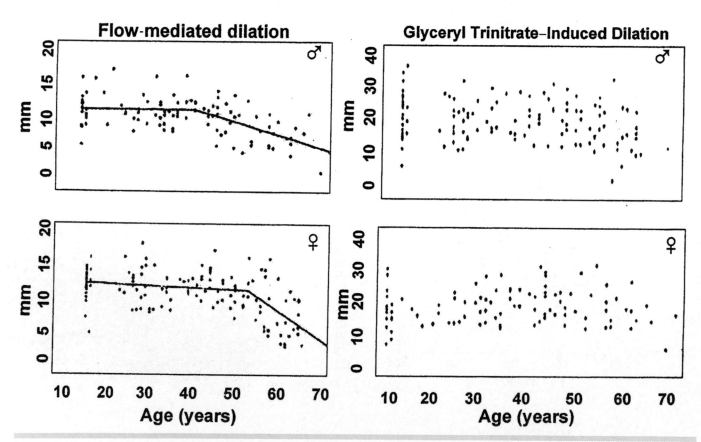

FIGURE 96-4 Endothelial (flow)-mediated and nonendothelial (glyceryl trinitrate)-induced arterial dilatation in apparently healthy persons. Note that the marked age associated decline occurs about a decade later in females vs. males. (From Lakatta EG, Levy D. Arterial and cardiac aging: Major shareholders in cardiovascular disease enterprises. Part II: The aging heart in health: Links to heart disease. *Circulation* 2003;107:346–354. With permission.)

linear, with the greatest risk occurring in the upper quintile.[6] Thus, those older persons in the upper quintile of IM thickness may be considered to have aged "unsuccessfully" or to have "subclinical" vascular disease. The potency of IM thickness as a risk factor in other individuals equals or exceeds that of most other more "traditional" risk factors.[6] However, the difference between those older and younger persons without evidence of coronary disease far exceeds the difference between older persons free of coronary disease and those with disease.

Molecular and Cellular Links between Intimal Thickening and Atherosclerosis

Findings from the rodent and nonhuman primate models of arterial aging[7,8] clearly indicate that central arterial intimal/medial thickening is an age-associated process that is separate from atherosclerosis, since both of these animal models are devoid of atherosclerosis. The age-associated cellular, enzymatic, and molecular mechanisms that underlie the phenotypic appearance of intimal/medial thickening— including the migration of activated vascular smooth muscle cell (SMC) into the intima and the elevated levels or activity of molecules—such as matrix metalloproteinase 2 (MMP-2), membrane type 1 matrix metalloproteinase (MT1-MMP), angiotensin II (Ang II), transforming growth factor-beta (TGF-β), and interstitial cell adhesion molecule-1 (ICAM-1)—create a metabolically active environment that induces, contributes to, or is a result of endothelial dysfunction and its attendant endothelial permeability. These same metabolic, enzymatic, cellular, and endothelial alterations are increasingly recognized as playing a critical role in the genesis of atherosclerosis and in promoting oxidant stress, vascular inflammation, and vascular remodeling.[9] In other words, many of the same factors that underlie the age-associated structural and functional intimal alterations are also implicated in the pathogenesis of clinical CV diseases. These culprits could thus represent the missing links that explain the "risky" component of arterial aging in humans.

The blurring of the boundaries between the aging and the atherosclerotic processes may have been fueled and aggravated in part by a poor selection of terminology. The age-associated intimal/medial thickening that is observed in humans is often ascribed to "subclinical" atherosclerosis.[10,11] This concept has become so pervasive that intimal/medial thickening is now widely seen by epidemiologists and clinicians as a valid surrogate measure of atherosclerosis. Intimal/medial thickening, per se, however, is only weakly associated with the extent and severity of coronary artery disease.[12] Indeed, referring to age-associated intimal/medial thickening as "subclinical atherosclerosis" gives the false impression that the atherosclerotic process is already present in the arterial wall, whereas, as noted above, intimal/medial thickening and endothelial dysfunction clearly occur in the absence of atherosclerosis. In other words, excessive age-associated arterial changes—i.e., intimal/medial thickening—in humans is *not* necessarily synonymous with "early" or "subclinical" atherosclerosis.[13] Rather, as the arterial wall becomes remodeled during aging, it becomes supersensitive to risk factors (e.g., high-fat diets, etc.) not usually encountered by animals. In the absence of these and other risk factors, diffuse intimal thickening is not likely to evolve into atherosclerosis. Hence, referring to diffuse intimal/-medial thickening per se as subclinical atherosclerosis is misleading.

Rather, vascular aging and vascular disease are partners; each contributes specific components to what is currently referred to as *vascular disease*. Thus, what clinical medicine and epidemiology now refer to as vascular disease might be regarded as the *vascular*

aging–vascular disease interaction. The heart and aging blood vessels provide the milieu in which CV diseases can flourish.

Arterial Stiffening

Recent studies have demonstrated that increased vascular stiffness is a risk factor for CV events, even when accounting for the effect of blood pressure. Data emerging from epidemiologic studies indicate that increased central arterial stiffening occurs in the context of atherosclerosis and diabetes.[14,15] Abnormalities of the endothelium have been identified to occur early on in the pathophysiology of atherosclerosis, diabetes, and hypertension.[16] The link between endothelial dysfunction and stiffness may be that stiffness is governed not only by the structural changes within the matrix, as noted above, but also by endothelial regulation of vascular smooth muscle tone and other aspects of vascular wall structure/function. There are compensatory mechanisms to normalize blood pressure that fail with advancing age. Increased large arterial stiffening precedes the development of hypertension.[17] The risk of increased vascular stiffness has been overshadowed by the idea that an increase in mean arterial pressure or peripheral resistance is the predominant cause of increased large artery stiffness. In other words, while a "secondary" increase in large artery stiffness is attributable to an increase in mean pressure that occurs in hypertension, evidence now exists that a "primary" increase in large artery stiffness—i.e., that which accompanies aging—precedes an elevation of arterial pressure. Normotensive individuals who fall within the upper quartiles for measures of arterial stiffness are more likely to develop hypertension. Observations such as this give rise to the notion that hypertension is in part a disease of the arterial wall.

Increased Arterial Pressure

As our definition of "disease" continues to evolve, we may find that many subjects who were formerly thought to be healthy are not. For example, systolic pressure above 140 mmHg is now considered to be hypertension—i.e., disease. Larger studies have shown that individuals who manifest modest elevations in systolic and pulse pressures are more likely to develop clinical disease or to die from it. Owing to the decline in diastolic pressure in older men and women in whom systolic pressure is increasing, "isolated systolic hypertension" emerges as the most common form of hypertension above age 50; even when mild in severity (stage 1), it is associated with an appreciable increase in CV disease risk.[18,19] But based on long-term follow-up of middle-aged and older subjects, Framingham researchers have found pulse pressure to be a better predictor of coronary disease risk than the systolic or diastolic pressure.[20] In older subjects, diastolic blood pressure, when considered jointly with the systolic pressure, is inversely related to coronary risk. Consideration of the systolic and diastolic pressures jointly may be preferable to consideration of either value alone.[18,19,21]

AGE-ASSOCIATED CHANGES IN CARDIAC STRUCTURE AND FUNCTION IN PERSONS WITHOUT A HEART DISEASE DIAGNOSIS

There is a continuum of expression of cardiac structural and functional alterations with age in healthy humans, and these age-associated cardiac changes appear to have relevance to the steep increases in left ventricular hypertrophy (LVH), chronic heart failure, and atrial fibrillation (Fig. 96-1) with increasing age.

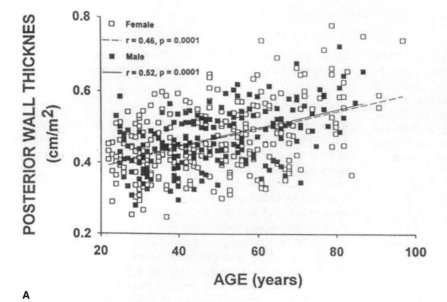

A

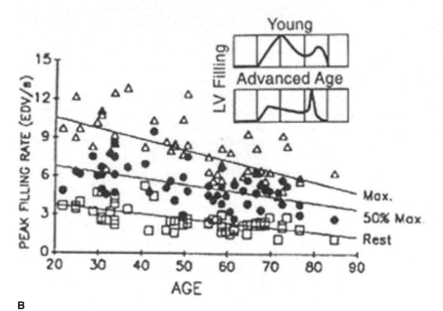

B

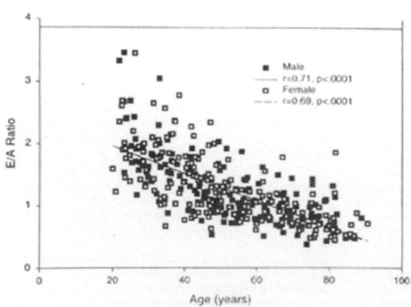

C

Cross-sectional studies of sedentary BLSA volunteer subjects without CV disease indicate that the left ventricular (LV) wall thickness, measured via M-mode (one-dimensional) echocardiography, increases progressively with age in both sexes (Fig. 96-5A).[22] This is mostly due to an increase in average myocyte size. In older, hospitalized patients without apparent CV disease, autopsy studies indicate that overall LV mass decreased with age, and cardiac myocyte enlargement was observed concurrently with an estimated decrease in myocyte number.[23] The observed frequency of apoptotic myocytes is higher in older male than female hearts.[24] An increase in the amount and a change in the physical properties of collagen (purportedly due to nonenzymatic cross-linking) also occur within the myocardium with aging. However, the cardiac myocyte-to-collagen ratio in the older heart either remains constant or increases.

Left Ventricular Filling and Preload

The early diastolic filling rate progressively slows after the age of 20 years, so that by 80 years the rate is reduced up to 50 percent (Fig. 96-5B). This reduction in filling rate is likely attributable either to structural (fibrous) changes within the LV myocardium or to residual myofilament Ca^{2+} activation from the preceding systole.

Despite the slowing of LV filling early in diastole, more filling occurs in late diastole, due in part to a more vigorous atrial contraction. Hence the ratio of early to late LV filling decreases with age (Fig. 96-5C). The augmented atrial contraction is accompanied by atrial enlargement and is manifested on auscultation as a fourth heart sound (atrial gallop). Despite the age-associated changes in the diastolic filling pattern in older men, their LV end-dias-

FIGURE 96-5 *A*. Left ventricular posterior wall thickness, measured by M-mode echocardiography, increases with age in healthy BLSA men and women. Note that the marked age-associated increase in LVWT in these healthy BLSA participants is within what is considered to be the clinically "normal" range. (From Gerstenblith G, Frederiksen J, Yin FC. Echocardiographic assessment of a normal adult aging population. *Circulation* 1977;56:273–278. With permission.) *B*. Maximum left ventricular filling rate at rest and during vigorous cycle exercise assessed via equilibrium gated blood-pool scans in healthy volunteers from the Baltimore Longitudinal Study on Aging. (From Schulman SP, Lakatta EG, Fleg JL, et al. Age-related decline in left ventricular filling at rest and exercise. *Am J Physiol* 1992;263:H1932–H1938. With permission.) EDV = end-diastolic volume. *C*. The ratio of early LV diastolic filling rate (E) to the atrial filling component (A) declines with aging, and the extent of this E/A decline with aging in healthy BLSA volunteers is identical to that in participants of the Framingham Study (From Benjamin EJ, Levy D, Anderson KM et al. Determinants of Doppler indexes of left ventricular diastolic function in normal subjects (the Framingham Heart Study). *Am J Cardiol* 1992;70:508–515, and Schulman SP, Lakatta EG, Fleg JL, et al. Age-related decline in left ventricular filling at rest and exercise. *Am J Physiol* 1992;263:H1932–H1938. With permission.)

tolic volume index (EDVI),—i.e., normalized for body surface area in the supine position at rest—does not substantially differ from that in their younger counterparts (Fig. 96-5A).

The acute reserve capacity of specific functions (e.g., EDV) that determine cardiac performance can be conveniently illustrated by depicting these over a wide range of demand for blood flow and pressure regulation—e.g., assumption of the sitting posture and during submaximal and exhaustive (maximal) upright exercise (Figs. 96-5B and 96-6). Assumption of the sitting position reduces EDVI in younger but not in older individuals (Fig. 96-6A); the age-associated decline in the maximum LV filling rate observed at rest persists. During submaximal cycle-seated exercise, EDVI increases equivalently at all ages; but during exhaustive exercise, EDVI drops to the seated rest level in young men but remains elevated in older men (Fig. 96-6A). Thus, for EDVI, the average, acute, dynamic EDV reserve range during the postural change and during graded upright exercise is moderately greater at 85 than at 20 years. This does not support the widely held concept that the dynamic range of filling volumes is compromised in older hearts despite a reduction in LV early diastolic filling rate (Fig. 96-5B). In fact, during vigorous (maximal) exercise, the LV at end-diastole becomes acutely dilated in healthy, older but not younger persons.

The interindividual variation of EDVI within the age-associated patterns depicted during exhaustive exercise (maximal) by the regression line for men in Fig. 96-6 is illustrated for both men and women in Fig. 96-7. Whether the capacity for further acute dilation of the LV of older persons beyond that observed in Figs. 96-6 and 96-7 is compromised cannot readily be determined. In older BLSA persons with occult silent coronary disease, however, as evident by both electrocardiographic (ECG) evidence and thallium scan perfusion deficits during exhaustive exercise but not at rest, the LVEDVI at maximum exercise is greater than that in healthy age-matched subjects [as is the increase in LV end-systolic volume index (ESVI) and reduction in ejection fraction[25]]. Thus, at least in older patients with silent ischemia, the capacity exists for acute EDVI dilation during exercise beyond that observed in healthy individuals.

Left Ventricular Ejection

Figure 96-6B illustrates a remarkable age-associated reduction in the range of reserve in the ESVI: in younger men, the ESVI becomes progressively reduced with increasing demands for CV perfusion from supine rest to maximum upright exercise, but the range of acute ESV reserve at age 85 is only about one-fifth of that at age 20. The age-associated failure in ESV regulation across the various levels of demand depicted in Fig. 96-6B causes a similar age-associated loss of ejection fraction regulation (Fig. 96-6C). See Fig. 96-7B and C for interindividual variations in ESVI and ejection fraction at maximal exercise in both men and women.

The net result of the age-associated changes in EDVI and ESVI regulation depicted in Fig. 96-6A and B is that the stroke volume index (SVI) in older persons is preserved at the level achieved by younger persons over a wide range of performance (Fig. 96-6D). Specifically, the Frank-Starling mechanism is utilized in older men with the assumption of an upright, seated posture at rest (Fig. 96-6A) to produce a modest age-associated increase in SVI (Fig. 96-6D). During progressive exhaustive exercise, however, the failure of older men to reduce ESVI (Fig. 96-6B) impairs the ejection fraction (Fig. 96-6C), and SVI is not augmented in older compared with younger men, as would be anticipated on the basis of their augmented EDVI. In other words, while healthy older persons utilize the Frank-Starling mechanism during vigorous exercise, this mechanism is impaired

due to impaired LV ejection. See Fig. 96-7D for interindividual variation of SVI in both men and women at maximum effort.

Heart Rate

In the supine position at rest, the heart rate in healthy BLSA men is not age-related (Fig. 96-6E). In other populations, a reduction in the spontaneous and respiratory variations in resting heart rate is observed and reflects altered autonomic modulation with aging (see below). With assumption of the seated resting position, heart rate increases slightly less in older than in younger men (Fig. 96-6E). The magnitude of this age-associated reduction increases progressively during exercise. The net result is that maximum acute dynamic reserve range of heart rate is reduced by about one-third between 20 and 85 years of age. See Fig. 96-7E for individual variation in heart rate in both men and women at maximum effort.

Cardiac Output

The cardiac index, as expected from the behavior of the SVI and heart rate functions in Fig. 96-6D and E, does not vary with age in either posture at rest (Fig. 96-6E) but is reduced at maximal exercise in older men. This reduction is entirely due to a reduction in heart rate reserve, as SVI at maximal exercise is preserved in healthy men rigorously screened to exclude occult coronary disease at older age. The loss of acute cardiac output reserve from seated rest to exhaustive, seated cycle exercise averages about 30 percent in healthy, community-dwelling BLSA volunteer men. Alternatively stated, subjects at the older end of the age range can augment their cardiac index 2.5-fold over seated rest, whereas those at the younger end of the spectrum can increase their cardiac index 3.5-fold. See Fig. 96-7 for interindividual variation in the maximum cardiac output in both BLSA men and women.

The same pattern of age-associated endogenous deficits depicted in BLSA subjects during graded, upright exercise in Figs. 96-6 and 96-7 is observed during prolonged exercise (> 1 h) at a fixed (70 percent of $\dot{V}O_2$max) relative submaximal workload.[26]

Aerobic Capacity

The extent to which the maximum aerobic capacity declines with aging, as well as its suspected underlying mechanisms, vary among studies (see Ref. 1 for review). Aerobic capacity estimated by either peak oxygen consumption or work capacity accompanying the hemodynamic pattern at maximal exercise (Figs. 96-6 and 96-7) declines approximately 50 percent. Thus, in this study population rigorously prescreened to exclude disease, the age-associated reduction in the cardiac component accounts for roughly half of the age-associated decline in aerobic capacity, the remainder being attributable to age-associated differences in oxygen (O_2) utilization. Such reductions in O_2 utilization during vigorous exercise result from age-associated reduction in muscle mass and from a reduction in the shunting of blood from viscera to working muscles during exercise as well as the amount of O_2 consumed per unit of working muscle mass per amount of O_2 delivered to the muscle.

The patterns of hemodynamic reserve function measured across the range of demands as illustrated in Fig. 96-6 for men are nearly identical in women. Exceptions are that, at seated rest, women do not exhibit a modest age-associated increase in EDVI because, in women, unlike men, assumption of the upright posture does not produce a greater reduction in EDVI in younger than in older subjects. Due to the absence in women of an age-associated increase in EDVI

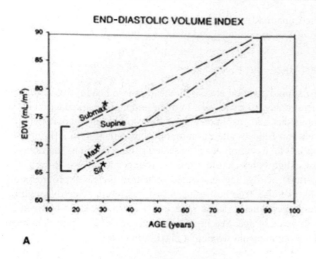

A

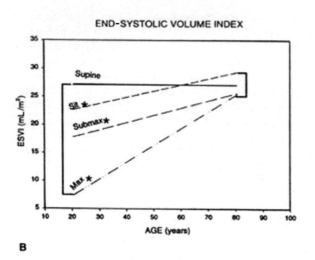

B

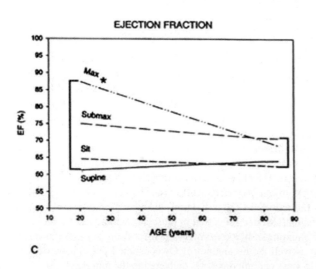

C

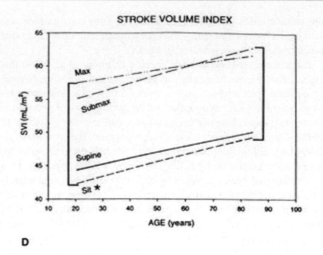

D

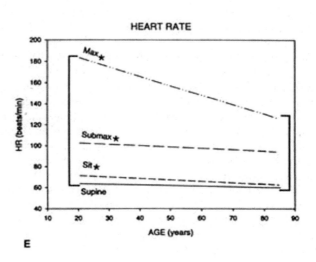

E

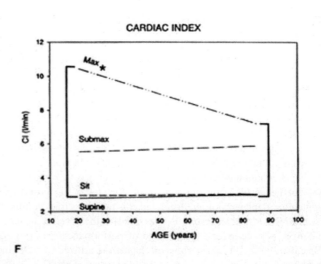

F

in the seated position, the SVI does not increase with age at seated rest, and, in contrast to men, the calculated cardiac index at seated rest decreases modestly with age in women. At maximal exercise, the age-associated increase of EDVI is of borderline statistical significance in women. However, the change in EDVI from rest to maximal exercise in a given individual (not shown in the figure) significantly increases with age and is nearly identical in both men and women.[27]

In summary, Figs. 96-6 and 96-7 illustrate that when CV function in adult volunteer community-dwelling subjects ranging in age from 20 to 85 years is compared, impaired cardioacceleration and LV ejection reserve capacity are the most dramatic changes in cardiac function with aging in health. Impaired ejection reserve, indicated by the failure of older persons to regulate ESV (Figs. 96-6B and 96-7B) as effectively as younger ones do, is accompanied by LV dilation at end-diastole (Figs. 96-6 and 96-7A and D) and an altered diastolic filling pattern (Fig. 96-5B and C).

MECHANISMS OF IMPAIRED LV EJECTION WITH AGING IN PERSONS WITHOUT CLINICAL CV DISEASE

Myocardial Contractility

Information as to how aging affects factors that regulate intrinsic myocardial contractility in humans is incomplete because the effectiveness of intrinsic myocardial contractility in the intact circulation is difficult to separate from loading and autonomic modulatory influences on contractility. A deficit in maximal intrinsic contractility of older persons might be expected on the basis of the reduced maximum heart rate (Figs. 96-6 and 96-7), as the heart rate per se is a determinant of the myocardial contractile state. Additional supporting evidence for reduced LV contractility with aging comes from studies in which the LV of older but not younger healthy BLSA men in the presence of beta-adrenergic blockade dilates at end-diastole in response to a given increase in afterload.[28]

The most reliable estimate of myocardial systolic stiffness or elastance, the slope of the ESP/ESV coordinates measured across a range of EDVs at rest, has not been estimated in a homogeneous, healthy study population across a broad age range and by convention cannot be accessed during exercise. A single point, depicting end-systolic pressure (ESP)/end-systolic volume (ESV) as a contractility index at each overall CV level of performance in Fig. 96-6, presents an age-associated pattern of myocardial contractile reserve that is nearly indentical to the age-associated change in the pattern of ejection fraction in Fig. 96-6.[27]

Left Ventricular Afterload   Cardiac afterload has two components, one generated by the heart itself and the other by the vasculature. The cardiac component of afterload during exercise can be expected to increase slightly with age because the heart's size increases in older persons throughout the cardiac cycle during exercise.[27] The vascular load on the heart has four components: conduit artery compliance characteristics, reflected pulse waves, resistance, and inertance. Inertance is determined by the mass of blood in the large arteries that requires acceleration prior to LV ejection. As the central arterial diastolic diameter increases with aging (Fig. 96-3B), the inertance component of afterload also likely increases. Thus, each of the pulsatile components of vascular load, measured at rest, increase with age. Hence, the aortic impedance, a composite function of the determinants of vascular afterload, increases with age (see Ref. 1 for review).

Increased vascular loading on the heart is a likely cause of the increase in LV wall thickness with aging (Fig 96-7A). Studies in large populations of broad age range demonstrate that arterial pressure, which varies directly with vascular loading, is a major determinant of LV mass, and that the relative impact of age and arterial pressure on LV wall thickness varies with the manner in which study subjects are screened with respect to hypertension.[29] The increase in LV wall thickness with aging reduces the expected increase in cardiac afterload due to increased LV volume in older persons during stress.[27]

Arterial/Ventricular Load Matching   Optimal and efficient ejection of blood from the heart occurs when ventricular and vascular loads are matched. (Note that in this context, *stiffness* refers to time-varying cardiac elastance throughout the cardiac cycle due to combined effects of active contractile and "passive" structural properties and to the interaction of both of these.) It has been suggested that the precise cardiac and vascular load matching that is characteristic in younger persons is preserved at older ages, at least at rest, because the increased vascular stiffness in older persons at rest is matched by increased resting ventricular stiffness.[30]

During exercise, in order for the ejection fraction to increase, the LV end-systolic elastance (E_{LV}) must increase to a greater extent than the vascular elastance, (E_A)—i.e., E_A/E_{LV} must decrease. With increasing age, however, the increase of E_{LV} fails to increase in proportion to the increase in E_A; hence the E_A/E_{LV} during exercise in older persons decreases to a lesser extent than it does in younger persons (Fig. 96-8A).[31] This altered arterial-ventricular load matching in older versus younger persons during exercise is a mechanism for the deficit in the acute LVEF reserve that accompanies advancing age in many individuals. Thus, the LVEF, often attributed by cardiologists to a measure of LV pump function, is in fact determined by both cardiac and vascular properties, and both change with age. An acute

FIGURE 96-6 Least-squares linear regression on age of left ventricular volumes, ejection fraction (EF), heart rate (HR), and cardiac index (CI) at rest and during graded cycle exercise in 149 healthy males from the Baltimore Longitudinal Study on Aging (BLSA) who exercised to at least a 100-W workload. The asterisk indicates that regression on age is statistically significant. The overall magnitude of the acute, dynamic range of reserve of a given function in younger compared with older subjects can quickly be gleaned from the length of the brackets depicted at the extremes of the regression lines. For end-diastolic volume index (EDVI), the average, acute, dynamic EDV reserve range during the postural change and during graded upright exercise is moderately greater at 85 than at 20 years. A. There is a remarkable age-associated reduction in the range of reserve in the end-systolic volume index (ESVI) (B), which causes a similar age-associated loss of EF regulation (C). The stroke volume index (SVI) is preserved in older persons over a wide range of performance (D). During progressive exhaustive exercise, however, the failure to reduce ESVI (B)

impairs the EF in older men (C). Thus, SVI is not augmented in older compared with younger men, as would be anticipated on the basis of their augmented EDVI. The maximum acute dynamic reserve range of HR is reduced by about one-third between 20 and 85 years of age (E). The loss of acute cardiac output reserve from seated rest to exhaustive, seated cycle exercise averages about 30 percent in healthy, community-dwelling BLSA volunteer men (F). This reduction is entirely due to a reduction in HR reserve, as SVI at maximal exercise is preserved. At maximal exercise, the age-associated increase in EDVI is of borderline statistical significance in women, but the change in EDVI from rest to maximal exercise in a given individual (not shown) significantly increases with age and is nearly identical in both men and women. (From Fleg JL, O'Connor FC, Gerstenblith G, et al. Impact of age on the cardiovascular response to dynamic upright exercise in healthy men and women. *J Appl Physiol* 1995;78: 890–900. With permission.)

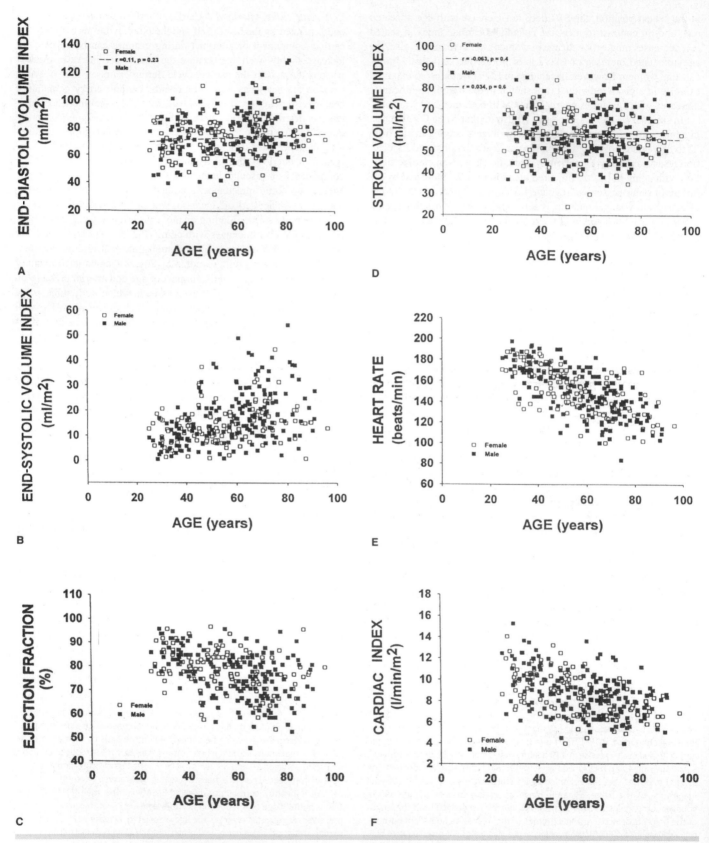

FIGURE 96-7 Scatterplots of heart rate and cardiac volumes, ejection fraction, and cardiac index in healthy sedentary men from the Baltimore Longitudinal Study on Aging (BLSA) depicted in Fig. 96-7 and for 113 BLSA women who exercised to a 75-W workload. Illustrated is the heterogeneity among individuals at a given age. In some instances (e.g., end-systolic volume index and ejection fraction), this heterogeneity increases with age. (From Fleg JL, O'Connor FC, Gerstenblith G, et al. Impact of age on the cardiovascular response to dynamic upright exercise in healthy men and women. *J Appl Physiol* 1995;78:890–900. With permission.)

Arterial-Ventricular Coupling

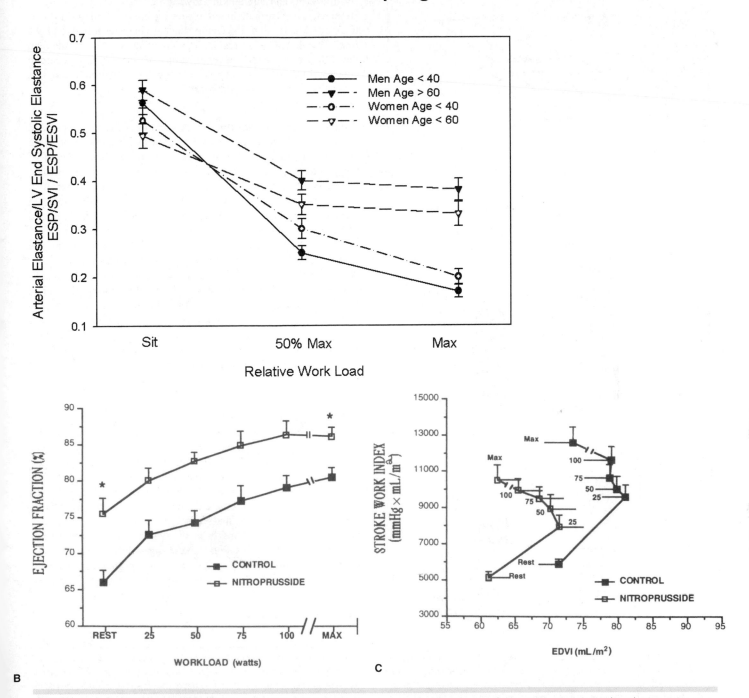

B

C

FIGURE 96-8 *A.* Load mismatch during exercise. (*A* and *B* from Nussbacher A, Gerstenblith G, O'Connor FC, et al. Hemodynamic effects of unloading the old heart. *Am J Physiol* 1999;277:H1863–H1871. With permission.) *B.* Ejection fraction at seated, at upright rest, at intermediate common submaximal workloads, and at maximum effort in healthy volunteers aged 71 ± 7 prior to and during sodium nitroprusside (SNP) infusion. At any level of effort, ejection fraction is substantially increased by SNP. *C.* Ventricular function, depicted as stroke work index versus end-diastolic volume index (EDVI) relationship at upright, at seated rest, and during exercise in the presence and absence of SNP. The relationship is shifted leftward and downward with SNP, indicating a smaller EDVI and lower stroke work index at any exercise load. (From Nussbacher A, Gerstenblith G, O'Connor FC, et al. Hemodynamic effects of unloading the old heart. *Am J Physiol* 1999;277:H1863–H1871. With permission.)

pharmacologic reduction in both cardiac and vascular components of LV afterload by sodium nitroprusside (SNP) infusions in older, healthy BLSA volunteers augments LVEF (Fig. 96-8*B*) in these subjects (at rest and exercise).[32] Because of concomitant reductions in preload and afterload during SNP infusion, the LV of older persons delivers the same SV stroke work and cardiac output while working at a smaller size (Fig. 96-8*C*).

Sympathetic Modulation The essence of sympathetic modulation of the CV system is to ensure that the heart beats faster; to ensure that it

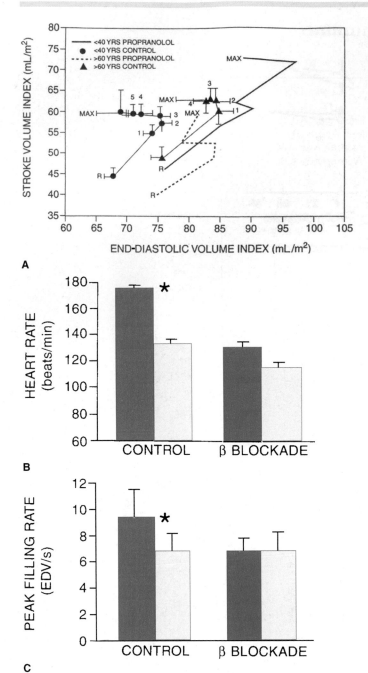

A

B

C

retains a small size by reducing the diastolic filling period, reducing LV afterload, and augmenting myocardial contractility and relaxation; and to redistribute blood to working muscles and to skin so as to dissipate heat. All of the factors that have been identified to play a role in the deficient CV regulation with aging—i.e., heart rate (and thus filling time), afterload (both cardiac and vascular), myocardial contractility, and redistribution of blood flow—exhibit a deficient sympathetic modulatory component.

Sympathetic Neurotransmitters Apparent deficits in sympathetic modulation of cardiac and arterial functions with aging occur in the presence of exaggerated neurotransmitter levels. Plasma levels of norepinephrine and epinephrine, during any perturbation from the supine basal state, increase to a greater extent in older than in younger healthy humans (see Ref. 33 for review). The age-associated increase in plasma levels of norepinephrine results from an increased spillover into the circulation and, to a lesser extent, to reduced plasma clearance. The degree of norepinephrine spillover into the circulation differs among body organs; increased spillover occurs within the heart.[34] It has been suggested that a deficient norepinephrine reuptake mechanism at nerve endings is the primary mechanism for increased spillover. During prolonged exercise, however, diminished neurotransmitter reuptake might also be associated with depletion, reduced release, and spillover.[35] Thus, depending on the duration of the stress, enhanced or deficient neurotransmitter release might be a basis for apparent impairment of sympathetic CV regulation with aging (Figs. 96-6*B*, 96-7, and 96-8).

Deficits in Cardiac Beta-Adrenergic-Receptor Signaling The age-associated increase in neurotransmitter spillover into the circulation during acute stress implies a greater heart and vascular receptor occupancy by these substances. Experimental evidence indicates that this leads to desensitization of the postsynaptic signaling components of sympathetic modulation. Indeed, multiple lines of evidence support the idea that the efficiency of postsynaptic beta-adrenergic signaling declines with aging (see Ref. 33 for review).

One line of evidence stems from the observation that acute beta-adrenergic receptor (BAR) blockade changes the exercise hemodynamic profile of younger persons to resemble that of older ones (Fig. 96-9). The reduction in heart rate during exercise in the pres-

FIGURE 96-9 *A.* Stroke volume index as a function of end-diastolic volume (EDV) index at rest (R) and during graded cycle workloads in the upright seated position in healthy men from the Baltimore Longitudinal Study on Aging (BLSA), in the presence and absence (*dashed line*) of beta-adrenergic blockade. R = seated rest; 1–4 or 5 = graded submaximal workloads on cycle ergometer; max = maximum effort. Stroke volume/end-diastolic functions with symbols are those measured in the absence of propranolol; dashed and solid line functions without symbols are the stroke volume compared with end-diastolic function measured in the presence of propranolol. Note that, in the absence of propranolol, the stroke volume versus EDV relation in older persons is shifted rightward from that in younger ones. This indicates that the left ventricle of older persons in the sitting position compared with that of younger ones operates from a greater preload both at rest and during submaximal and maximal exercise. Propranolol markedly shifts the stroke volume/EDV relationship in younger persons (*solid line without points*) rightward but does not markedly offset the curve in older persons (*dashed line without points*). Thus, with respect to this assessment of ventricular function curve, β-adrenergic blockade with propranolol makes younger men appear like older ones. The abolition of the age-associated differences in the left ventricular (LV) function curve after propranolol are ac-

companied by a reduction or abolition of the age-associated reduction in heart rate, which, at maximum, is shown in *B.* Note, however, that beta-adrenergic blockade in younger individuals in this figure causes stroke volume index to increase to a greater extent than during beta-blockade in older ones, suggesting that mechanisms other than deficient beta-adrenergic regulation compromise LV ejection. One potential mechanism is an age-associated decrease in maximum intrinsic myocardial contractility. Another likely mechanism is enhanced vascular afterload due to the structural changes in compliance arteries noted above and possibly also to impaired vasorelaxation during exercise. (From Fleg JL, Schulman S, O'Connor F, et al. Effects of acute beta-adrenergic receptor blockade on age-associated changes in cardiovascular performance during dynamic exercise. *Circulation* 1994;90: 2333–2341. With permission.) *B.* Peak exercise heart rate in the same subjects as in *A* in the presence and absence of acute beta-adrenergic blockade by propranolol. *C.* The age-associated reduction in peak LV diastolic filling rate at maximum exercise in healthy BLSA subjects is abolished during exercise in the presence of beta-adrenergic blockade with propranolol. Solid = less than 40 years; light = more than 60 years. (From Schulman SP, Lakatta EG, Fleg JL, et al. Age-related decline in left ventricular filling at rest and exercise. *Am J Physiol* 1992;73:H1932–H1938. With permission.)

ence of acute beta-adrenergic blockade is greater in younger than in older subjects (Fig. 96-9*B*), and significant beta blockade–induced LV dilatation occurs only in younger subjects (Fig. 96-9*A*). The age-associated deficits in LV early diastolic filling rate both at rest and during exercise (Fig. 96-9*C*) also are abolished by acute beta-adrenergic blockade.[36] Note, however, that beta-adrenergic blockade in younger individuals in Fig. 96-9 causes SVI to increase to a greater extent than in beta blockade in older ones, suggesting that mechanisms other than deficient beta-adrenergic regulation compromise LV ejection. One potential mechanism is an age-associated decrease in maximum intrinsic myocardial contractility. Another likely mechanism is enhanced vascular afterload due to the structural changes in compliance arteries, noted above and possibly also to impaired vasorelaxation during exercise. In this regard, it has been observed that the increase in aortic impedance during exercise in old dogs is abolished by beta-adrenergic blockade.[37]

The second type of evidence for a diminished efficacy of synaptic BAR signaling is that CV responses at rest to beta-adrenergic agonist infusions decrease with age (see Ref. 1 for review).

Physical Deconditioning

A marked reduction in physical activity accompanies advancing age in a majority of adults. Thus, it may be hypothesized that a reduction in physical conditioning status might be implicated as a factor in the reduced CV reserve of older, healthy sedentary individuals, as discussed. Alternatively, the issue arises as to whether physical conditioning via aerobic training of sedentary older persons can affect deficits in CV reserve capacity due to the aging process per se.

It has been amply documented that physical conditioning of older persons can substantially increase their maximum aerobic work capacity and peak oxygen consumption. The extent to which this conditioning effect results from enhanced central cardiac performance or from augmented peripheral circulatory and O_2 utilization mechanisms, including changes in skeletal muscle mass, varies with the characteristics of the population studied, the type and degree of conditioning achieved, gender, body position during study (see Ref. 1 for review), and likely genetic factors. A longitudinal study of older men in the upright position indicates that an enhanced physical conditioning status increases O_2 consumption and work capacity, in part by increases in the maximum cardiac output (CO) by increasing the maximum stroke volume (SV), and in part by increasing the estimated total body atrioventricular (AV) O_2 utilization.[38] The augmentation of maximum SVI is due to an augmented reduction of LVESV (Fig. 96-10*A*) and, thus, a concomitant increase in LV ejection fraction, as the effect of conditioning status to increase LVEDI exercise is minimal (recall that LVEDI during acute vigorous exercise is already moderately increased in older, sedentary, preconditioned men). This minor effect of physical conditioning on LVEDVI in older persons is in contrast to the effect of physical conditioning in younger persons, which substantially increases EDVI and SVI on the basis of the Frank-Starling mechanism, as well as via an enhanced LV ejection fraction. In contrast to the improved LV ejection, the maximal heart rate of older persons did not vary with physical conditioning status (Fig. 96-10*A*). There is no strong evidence that physical conditioning of older persons can offset the deficiency in sympathetic modulation. Rather, conditioning effects to increase LV ejection appear to relate to the reduction in vascular afterload, as reflected in a reduced pulse wave velocity,[39] and to carotid augmentation index (AGI) (Fig. 96-10*B*) in older athletes compared with sedentary controls as well as possibly to an augmentation of the maximum intrinsic myocardial contractility. In animal models, some but not all

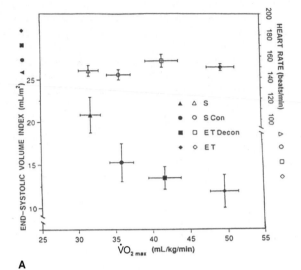

MAX EXERCISE

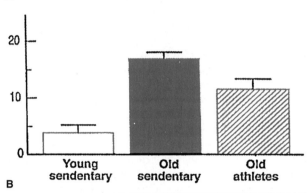

FIGURE 96-10 *A*. Heart rate and end-systolic volume during peak seated, upright exercise on a cycle ergometer across a broad range of aerobic capacity in healthy males who have been exercise-conditioned or deconditioned. S = sedentary; ET = exercise-trained; SCon = sedentary men after conditioning; ET Decon = men who had been exercise-trained but stopped their training for the study to become detrained or deconditioned (DeCon). The figure shows that the extent to which the left ventricle empties, as manifest by the end-systolic volume, varies with the level of aerobic capacity ($\dot{V}O_2$max), which was varied among the four groups by either conditioning or deconditioning protocols. In contrast, the peak heart rate achieved does not vary with aerobic capacity. (From Schulman SP, Fleg JL, Goldberg AP, et al. Continuum of cardiovascular performance across a broad range of fitness levels in healthy older men. *Circulation* 1996;94:359–367. With permission.)

studied determinants of the latter are affected by physical conditioning status (see Ref. 1 for review).

Heart Conduction and Rhythm

There is an increase in elastic and collagenous tissue in all parts of the conduction system with advancing age. Fat accumulates around the sinoatrial node, sometimes producing a partial or complete separation of the node from the atrial musculature. There may be a pronounced decrease in the number of pacemaker cells in the sinoatrial node beginning at age 60, and by age 75 the sinoatrial node cell number may become substantially reduced. A variable degree of calcification of the left side of the cardiac skeleton, which includes the aortic and mitral annuli, the central fibrous body, and the summit of the interventricular septum, also occurs with aging. Because of their proximity to these structures, the atrioventricular (AV) node, AV bundle, bifurcation, and proximal left and right bundle branches may be affected by this process.

The P-R interval increases with aging due to a prolongation of the A-H time with no change in the H-V time.[40] While the supine basal heart rate is not affected by aging, beat-to-beat fluctuation of heart rate, commonly known as heart rate variability, declines steadily with age.[41] Reduced heart rate variability is an indicator of cardiac autonomic regulation commonly found in older people and has been linked to increased risk for morbid and fatal outcomes.[41]

An increase in the prevalence and complexity of both supraventricular and ventricular arrhythmias—whether detected by resting ECG, ambulatory monitoring, or exercise testing—occurs in otherwise healthy older as opposed to younger persons. Isolated atrial premature beats (APBs) appear on the resting ECG in 5 to 10 percent of subjects above 60 years of age and are generally not associated with heart disease. Isolated APBs are detected in 6 percent of resting healthy BLSA volunteers above 60 years of age, in 39 percent during exercise testing, and in 88 percent during ambulatory 24-h monitoring.[42] Over a 10-year mean follow-up period, isolated APBs, even if frequent, are not predictive of increased cardiac risk in these individuals.[43]

Short bursts of paroxysmal supraventricular tachycardia (PSVT) are observed in 1 to 2 percent of apparently healthy individuals above 65 years of age who were rigorously screened to exclude disease. Several 24-h ambulatory monitoring studies have demonstrated short runs of this PSVT (usually three to five beats) in 13 to 50 percent of clinically healthy older subjects.[42,44] While the presence of nonsustained PSVT did not predict an increase in risk of a future coronary event in BLSA subjects, 15 percent with PSVT later developed de novo atrial fibrillation, compared with fewer than 1 percent subjects without PSVT. The incidence of PSVT during exercise, typically asymptomatic three- to five-beat salvos, increases with age, from nil in the youngest age group to about 10 percent in the ninth decade.[45] While those individuals with exercise-induced PSVT were not at a greater risk for coronary events over a multiyear follow up, 10 percent developed a spontaneous atrial tachyarrhythmia, compared with only 2 percent of the control group. Thus, PSVT at rest or induced by exercise is an early clue that some healthy individuals are at increased risk for future atrial fibrillation (AF). Another risk factor for AF may be the increase in left atrial size that accompanies advancing age in otherwise healthy persons.[46]

In older subjects without apparent heart disease, the limited data available support a marked age-associated increase in the prevalence and complexity of ventricular ectopy (VE), both at rest and during exercise, at least in men. A steep increase in the prevalence of VE with advancing age occurs both in those clinically free of heart disease and in unselected populations. In healthy BLSA volunteers with a normal ST-segment response to treadmill exercise, isolated VE occurred at rest in 8.6 percent of men over age 60 compared to only 0.5 percent in those 20 to 40 years of age. In women, interestingly, the prevalence of VE at rest was not age-related. Among 98 carefully screened asymptomatic BLSA participants above 60 years of age, 35 percent had multiform VE, 11 percent ventricular couplets, and 4 percent short runs of ventricular tachycardia on 24-h monitoring[42]; all occurred substantially more commonly in older than in healthy younger subjects. Neither the prevalence nor the complexity of resting VE was a determinant of future coronary events over a 10-year mean follow-up period.[43] Isolated VE during or after maximal treadmill exercise increased in prevalence fivefold, from 11 to 57 percent

between the third and ninth decades in apparently healthy BLSA volunteers.[47]

Many of the age-associated changes in cardiac and arterial structure or function that have been observed in humans also occur across a wide range of other species. Insights gained from cellular and molecular studies in these animal models may hold clues that will assist in directing future efforts toward developing novel therapies for age-associated arterial structural and functional remodeling in humans. The results of studies have recently been reviewed.[3,9,48]

SUMMARY

In summary, there is a growing body of evidence that increased large artery thickening and stiffness and endothelial dysfunction in apparently otherwise healthy older persons and the ensuing increase in systolic and pulse pressure, formerly thought to be part of "normal" aging, precede clinical disease and predict a higher risk for developing clinical atherosclerosis, hypertension, and stroke (Table 96-1). There is also evidence of a vicious cycle: altered mechanical properties of the vessel wall influence the development of atherosclerosis, and the latter, via endothelial cell dysfunction and other mechanisms, influences vascular stiffness. Some of the vascular changes that occur with aging in normotensive humans, including endothelial dysfunction, have been observed in hypertensives at an earlier age and are more marked than in normotensives. Such otherwise asymptomatic individuals might be considered to manifest "unsuccessful" vascular aging. When stated in this context, "unsuccessful vascular aging" becomes the risk factor for eventual clinical disease manifestations. Combinations of age associated endothelial dysfunction, intimal medial thickening, arterial stiffening, and arterial pulse pressure widening occurring to varying degrees determine the overall vascular aging profile of a given individual. Worse combinations may lead to a vessel wall with the most "unsuccessful" aging.

In western society, additional risk factors—including hypertension, smoking, dyslipidemia, diabetes, diet, and heretofore unidentified genetic factors—interact with vascular aging (as described above) to activate an atherosclerotic plaque. According to this view, the development and progression of atherosclerosis in older persons differs from that in younger persons and from that in experimental younger animals because it represents an *interaction* of atherosclerotic risk factors and their effect to produce atherosclerotic plaque at any age and intrinsic of vascular aging. Evidence in support of this view comes from studies in which an atherogenic diet resulting in the same elevation of plasma lipids caused markedly more severe atherosclerotic lesions in older than in younger rabbits and nonhuman primates.[49,50]

When CV function in healthy, adult community-dwelling volunteers, ranging in age from 20 to 85 years, is assessed, increased LV wall thickness, alterations in the diastolic filling pattern, impaired LV ejection and heart rate reserve capacity, and altered heart rhythm are the most dramatic changes in cardiac function with aging. The extents to which the end-systolic volume is reduced and the ejection fraction increased at peak exercise are reduced with aging, and these deficits probably result from deficient intrinsic myocardial performance and from an augmented afterload, both due in part to a deficiency in beta-adrenergic stimulation to enhance myocardial contractility or to reduce the pulsatile components of vascular afterload. A decrease in the maximum capacity for physical work with aging is due to both diminished cardiac (heart rate) and peripheral factors. Some of the CV deficits that accompany aging in health can be retarded by physical conditioning.

TABLE 96-1 Relationship of Cardiovascular Human Aging in Health to Cardiovascular Diseases

Age-Associated Changes	Plausible Mechanisms	Possible Relation to Human Disease
CARDIOVASCULAR STRUCTURAL REMODELING		
⇑ Vascular intimal thickness	⇑ Migration of and ⇑ matrix production by VSMC Possible derivation of intimal cells from other sources	Promotes development of atherosclerosis
⇑ Vascular stiffness	Elastin fragmentation ⇑ Elastase activity ⇑ Collagen production by VSMC and ⇑ Cross-linking of collagen Altered growth factor regulation/tissue repair mechanisms	Systolic hypertension Left ventricular wall thickening Stroke Atherosclerosis LVH ??
⇑ LV wall thickness	⇑ LV myocyte size with altered Ca^{2+} handling ⇓ Myocyte number (necrotic and apoptotic death) Altered growth-factor regulation Focal matrix collagen deposition	Retarded early diastolic cardiac filling ⇑ Cardiac filling pressure Lower threshold for dyspnea ⇑ Likelihood of heart failure with relatively normal systolic function LVH??
⇑ Left atrial size	⇑ Left atrial pressure/volume	⇑ Prevalence of atrial fibrillation and other atrial arrhythmias
CARDIOVASCULAR FUNCTIONAL CHANGES		
Altered regulation of vascular tone	⇓ NO production/effects	Vascular stiffening; hypertension Early atherosclerosis
Reduced threshold for cell Ca^{2+} overload	Changes in gene expression of proteins that regulate Ca^{2+} handling; increased $\omega6{:}\omega3$ polyunsaturated fatty acids ratio in cardiac membranes	Lower threshold for atrial and ventricular arrhythmia Increased myocyte death Increased fibrosis Reduced diastolic and systolic function
⇓ Cardiovascular reserve	⇑ Vascular load ⇓ Intrinsic myocardial contractility Ventricular-vascular load mismatch during stress ⇑ Plasma levels of catecholamines ⇓ β-adrenergic modulation of heart rate myocardial contractility and vascular tone due to postsynaptic signaling deficits	Lower threshold for heart failure and increased severity of HF
REDUCED PHYSICAL ACTIVITY		
	Learned lifestyle	Exaggerated age Δ's in some aspects of cardiovascular structure and function, e.g., arterial stiffening Negative impact on atherosclerotic vascular disease, hypertension, and heart failure

ABBREVIATIONS: LVH = left ventricular hypertrophy; VSMC = vascular smooth muscle cell; Δ = changes; $\omega6{:}\omega3$ = ratio of omega six to omega three.

Changes in cardiac properties that accompany aging alter the substrate upon which CV disease is superimposed in several ways (Table 96-1 and Fig. 96-11) and thus alter the occurrence, presentation, and manifestations of heart disease in older persons. While these age-associated cardiac changes per se do not result in clinical heart disease, they do compromise the cardiac reserve capacity. They also affect the threshold for symptoms and signs in response to any given disease-related challenge (Table 96-1). Age-associated cardiac changes also explain the increased risk for LVH, atrial fibrillation, and congestive heart failure (systolic and diagnostic), with advancing age (Fig. 96-1D to G). The three cardiac diagnoses become interrelated in older persons, in part due to this link with age-associated cardiac changes. An age-dependent increase in LV stiffness promotes an increase in end-diastolic filling pressure, which is an important contributor to diastolic heart failure in older persons. A mild degree of ischemia-induced relaxation abnormality that may not induce clinical symptoms in a younger patient may cause dyspnea in an older one, who, by virtue of age alone, has preexisting slowed and delayed early diastolic relaxation. Similarly, a progressive decline in LV compliance with age may go unnoticed for many years, (i.e., subclinical diastolic dysfunction); but with the occurrence of an acute stress, the subclinical dysfunction can become acutely manifest as overt heart failure. A classic example is the development of

AGING: THE MAJOR RISK FACTOR FOR CARDIOVASCULAR MORBIDITY AND MORTALITY

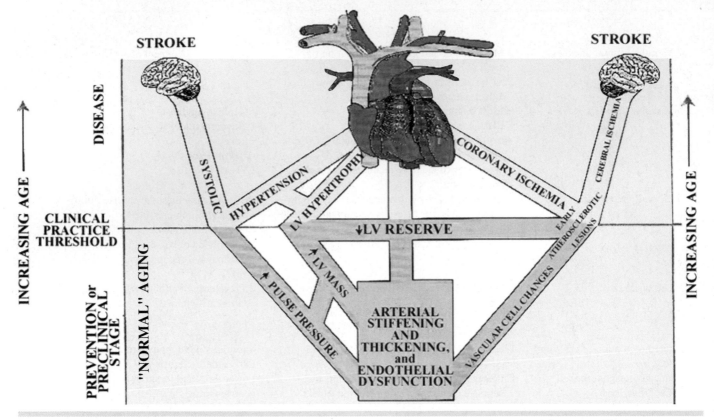

FIGURE 96-11 Changes in the vasculature and heart with aging in health. Age-related changes in vascular and cardiac structure and function are nearly ubiquitous. Central arteries stiffen with age, and this process raises systolic blood pressure and pulse pressure. Isolated systolic hypertension, the most common form of hypertension in older people, is associated with increased risk for various manifestations of cardiovascular disease (Table 96-1). In addition, the age-dependent increase in blood pressure contributes to increasing left ventricular mass, which has been identified as a risk factor for cardiovascular disease independent of the high blood pressure that may have contributed to its development. Congestive heart failure, a common and dire condition in the elderly, is often a late consequence of age-related alterations in blood pressure and cardiac and vascular structure and function. Age-associated changes in cardiovascular structure and function depicted below the "clinical threshold" line ought not to be considered to reflect "normal" or "physiologic" aging. Rather, these, in addition to other already acknowledged risk factors, might be construed as contributory factors to the diseases to which they relate. Thus, excessive age-associated changes in heart and blood vessels are risk factors for cardiovascular disease, leading to heart and brain disorders in older persons (see text for details). (From Lakatta EG. Cardiovascular regulatory mechanisms in advanced age. *Physiol Rev* 1993;73:413–465. With permission.)

atrial fibrillation with the loss of atrial contraction coupled with abbreviated diastolic filling time due to tachycardia, which can precipitate pulmonary edema in a matter of minutes when the conducive structural and functional milieu is present, as in the aging heart.

Age-associated changes may also alter the manifestations and presentation of common cardiac diseases. This usually occurs in patients with acute infarction in whom the diagnosis is delayed because of atypical symptoms resulting in increased time to onset of therapy. Age-associated changes, including those in beta-adrenergic responsiveness and in vascular stiffness, also influence the response to and therefore the selection of different therapeutic inventions in older individuals with CV disease. Thus, in one sense, those processes below the line in Fig. 96-11 ought not to be considered to reflect normal or physiologic aging. Rather, they might be construed as specific risk factors for the diseases that they relate to and thus might be targets of future interventions designed to decrease the occurrence and/or manifestations of CV disease at later ages.

Recent advances in our understanding of the age-associated alterations in vascular and cardiac structure and function, at both the cellular and molecular levels, provide valuable clues that will hopefully assist in directing future efforts to develop effective therapies to prevent, delay, or attenuate the CV changes that accompany aging. These age-associated changes are themselves increasingly recognized as risk factors for CV diseases, and future efforts to modulate them will require the close collaboration of a consortium of researchers, including molecular cardiologists, CV physiologists, and translational clinical trialists.

WHAT TO DO NOW ABOUT "UNSUCCESSFUL" AGING OF THE HEART AND BLOOD VESSELS

Extreme age-associated changes in CV structure/function that are perceived as deleterious aspects of CV aging in otherwise healthy persons ought to be interpreted to reflect "unsuccessful" CV aging. Indeed, as noted above, data emerging from epidemiologic studies indicate that specific aspects of cardiac and vascular aging in otherwise apparently healthy persons confer an increased risk for CV events.

If cardiac and vascular aging are risk factors for disease, these represent a potential target for treatment and prevention. Lifestyle intervention or pharmacotherapy, to retard the rate of progression of subclinical disease, might be considered before clinical disease becomes manifest.

With respect to lifestyle, the risk factor of lack of vigorous exercise increases dramatically with age in otherwise healthy persons.[51] It is noteworthy that the pulse pressure, pulse-wave velocity, and carotid augmentation index are lower[39,52] and baroreceptor reflex function is improved[53] in older persons who are physically conditioned than in those who are sedentary. Exercise conditioning also improves endothelial function in older persons.[54] There is also evidence to indicate that diets low in sodium are associated with reduced arterial stiffening with aging.[55] Exercise conditioning improves LV reserve function. Intriguingly, it has recently been shown in the rat model[56] as well as in elderly patients[57] that physical activity and exercise training restore the cardiac protective effects of ischemic preconditioning and preinfarction angina that are otherwise lost during aging.

With respect to pharmacotherapy, angiotensin-converting enzyme (ACE) inhibitors have been shown to retard vascular aging in rodents.[58,59] An emerging concept in the treatment of hypertension recognizes that progressive vascular damage can continue to occur even when arterial pressure is controlled. It is conceivable that drugs that retard or reverse age-associated vascular wall remodeling and increased stiffness will be preferable to those that lower pressure without affecting the vascular wall properties. In this regard, a novel drug that breaks such cross-links has been shown to reduce indices of arterial stiffness measures in rodents, dogs, and nonhuman primates as well as in humans.[60–63] Retardation or reduction in IM thickness in humans has been achieved by drug/diet intervention.[64–68] It is thus far unproved if such treatment can "prevent" unsuccessful aging of the vasculature in individuals of early middle age who exhibit excessive subclinical evidence of unsuccessful aging.

Accelerated cardiac and vascular aging in apparently healthy younger and middle-aged adults—i.e., those who exhibit measurements of heart or vascular aging that usually occur later in life—may indicate the need for interventions designed to decrease the occurrence and/or manifestations of CV disease at later ages. Similarly, exaggerated heart or vascular aging in older persons, such as those with age-associated vascular measurements in the upper tercile, may merit similar consideration. Specifically, prime targets for intervention are those persons presently perceived as "normal" individuals without a "textbook" CV disease diagnosis whose arteries and hearts are placing them at increased risk for the occurrence of CV disease. Such a strategy would thus advocate treating "unsuccessful" aging. However, additional studies of the effectiveness of treatment regimens to delay or prevent each change are required for this strategy to be put into practice.

THERAPEUTIC CONSIDERATIONS IN OLDER PATIENTS WITH CLINICAL CARDIOVASCULAR DISEASES

Ischemic Heart Disease

Increasing age is the most powerful predictor of future coronary artery disease in asymptomatic individuals (Fig. 96-1).[69] Autopsy studies demonstrate that the prevalence of obstructive coronary disease increases from approximately 10 to 20 percent in the fourth decade to 50 to 70 percent in the eighth decade.[70] Advancing age is also associated with more severe, diffuse atherosclerosis and more damage to the LV, with the prevalence of triple-vessel and left main coronary disease doubling from ages 40 to 80. Elevated end-diastolic pressure and wall motion abnormalities on left ventriculography are also more common in the elderly patient with coronary artery disease.[71] Therefore almost all clinical manifestations of ischemic heart disease have a higher mortality rate and a worse outcome in the older population. The higher prevalence and severity of disease also influence the interpretation of diagnostic testing, with a significant increase in sensitivity and modest decrease in specificity of exercise treadmill testing to detect coronary artery disease in the elderly.[72] Finally, the clinical assessment of the elderly patient with coronary artery disease is often limited by the coexistence of diseases that make interpretation of symptoms difficult.[73] Thus, in the elderly, a high clinical index of suspicion plus the use of objective parameters such as stress test results are important in assessing and diagnosing ischemic heart disease.

ACUTE CORONARY SYNDROMES

The incidence of myocardial infarction appears to have been increasing in the elderly over the last 15 years, particularly in older women.[74] Despite increased utilization of therapies shown to be effective in patients who have experienced acute myocardial infarction (AMI), 5-year survival has not changed over the last 15 years in AMI patients at least 75 years of age.[74] Older patients with AMI are more likely to be female; to have a history of angina, heart failure, hypertension, and diabetes; and to have experienced a non-Q-wave AMI.[75,76] Older patients are also more likely to present with atypical symptoms of acute myocardial ischemia and infarction, such as shortness of breath, confusion, and failure to thrive.[77] Furthermore, nearly one-half of myocardial infarctions in the elderly go unrecognized clinically (see also Chaps. 51 and 52).[77]

Age is a powerful independent predictor of short- and long-term mortality in patients with AMI.[76–79] In patients admitted with a first ST-segment elevation myocardial infarction and treated with thrombolytic therapy, in-hospital mortality increases exponentially as a function of age from 1.9 percent among patients 40 years of age or younger to 31.9 percent among patients above age 80.[78] Similarly, in the Global Utilization of Streptokinase and Tissue Plasminogen Activator for Occluded Arteries (GUSTO-1) trial, 30-day mortality following a ST-segment elevation myocardial infarction increased from 3 percent in patients under 65 years of age to 19.6 percent in patients 75 to 85 years of age and to 30.3 percent in patients over age 85.[80] Age was the most powerful predictor of in-hospital and 30-day mortality in this trial. Age is also a powerful predictor of recurrent ischemia and 30-day mortality in patients with non-ST-segment-elevation acute coronary syndromes.[81] In the Platelet glycoprotein IIb/IIIa in Unstable Angina: Receptor Suppression Using Integrilin (eptifibatide) Therapy (PURSUIT) trial of 9461 patients with unstable angina or non-ST-segment elevation, age was the most powerful predictor of 30-day mortality.[82]

Elderly acute infarct patients experience a much greater incidence of heart failure, atrial fibrillation, and cardiogenic shock in spite of the fact that indices of infarct size—such as creatinine phosphokinase levels and QRS scores—do not change with age.[76,78,80] Age is a powerful predictor of cardiogenic shock in both ST-segment and non-ST-segment elevation acute coronary syndromes.[83] The risks of heart failure and shock increase three- to fourfold in patients over 85 years of age compared to those below age 65.[80] This higher incidence of heart failure and shock may result from age-related changes in diastolic filling (Fig. 96-6) and aortic compliance (Fig. 96-3) and decreased sensitivity to catecholamine stimulation, resulting in diminished cardiac reserve and afterload mismatch following ischemic damage. Mortality in older patients with myocardial infarction as opposed to younger ones is less likely to result from ventricular fibrillation, but the former are much more likely to have electromechanical dissociation and cardiac rupture on autopsy. The risk of death following hospital discharge also increases exponentially with increasing age, by almost 6 percent per year.[78]

The high morbidity and mortality associated with acute ischemic syndromes in the elderly dictate an aggressive approach to management. Thrombolytic therapy in AMI reduces mortality, and data suggest a possible benefit in the elderly. In a metanalysis of large randomized trials of thrombolytic therapy, subset analyses of the nearly 5800 patients above 74 years of age showed a nonsignificant trend toward thrombolytic benefit, with a net saving of 1 life per 100 patients treated at 35 days after infarction. Although the relative decreases in mortality is less in older compared to younger patients treated with thrombolytics, the absolute benefit in terms of number of lives saved with treatment is similar.[84] Large registry data in the United States show that thrombolytic-eligible patients above age 75 are significantly less likely to receive reperfusion therapy than patients below age 65, with an odds ratio of 0.4.[85] Part of the reluctance of physicians to use thrombolytic agents in this age group arises from the concerns about intracranial hemorrhage. Age is an important predictor of suffering a hemorrhagic stroke with thrombolytic therapy.[80,86] This increased risk of reperfusion strategies in the elderly was confirmed in recent thrombolytic trials. Patients with ST-segment-elevation AMI were randomized to standard bolus thrombolytic therapy with unfractionated heparin or to bolus thrombolytic therapy with low-molecular-weight heparin or half-dose bolus thrombolytic therapy and full-dose platelet glycoprotein IIb/IIIa inhibitors. In patients 75 years of age and above, major bleeding rates and intracranial hemorrhage were greater in the experimental arms compared to conventional therapy.[87,88] Recent large observational studies in older patients with ST-segment-elevation myocardial infarction also raise concerns about the use of thrombolytic therapy in the elderly. These data suggest that in patients above the age of 75 years, thrombolytic therapy may increase short-term mortality compared to conservative therapy.[89,90] Given the increase hemorrhagic risk and reduced benefit of thrombolytic therapy, careful risk stratification of the patient above age 75 with an ST-segment-elevation infarction must be considered. These factors include the age and weight of the patient, the number of leads with ST-segment elevation, duration of symptoms, as well as the proximity of the hospital to a high-volume center with facilities for on-site percutaneous coronary intervention.

Primary angioplasty has been compared with thrombolytic therapy in several trials showing beneficial effects on mortality, recurrent myocardial infarction, and recurrent ischemia.[91,92] Patients treated with direct angioplasty have a lower overall stroke and hemorrhagic stroke risk compared to those treated with thrombolytics.[93] A recent randomized trial of 87 patients above age 75 with ST-segment-elevation myocardial infarction show a significant decrease in death, reinfarction, and stroke 30-days and 20 months following direct angioplasty compared to thrombolytic therapy.[94] Importantly, these studies involve operators with great expertise from high-volume angioplasty centers.

In patients with unstable angina or non-ST-segment elevation myocardial infarction, studies show that the addition of a parenteral glycoprotein IIb/IIIa inhibitor to standard anti-ischemic therapy including aspirin and heparin reduces short-term risks of death, myocardial infarction, and refractory angina.[95,96] In a recent metanaly-

sis of all major randomized clinical trials involving the glycoprotein IIb/IIIa inhibitors in which percutaneous coronary revascularization was not mandated by protocol design,[97] the mean age of the patient population (31,402 patients) was 64 years. There is a modest 9 percent relative decrease in 30-day death or nonfatal myocardial infarction with the addition of a glycoprotein IIb/IIIa inhibitor compared to placebo. There was no heterogeneity of effect across age subgroups. The greatest benefits of a glycoprotein IIb/IIIa inhibitor were in higher-risk patient subgroups, including those with positive troponin or ST-segment depression and patients proceeding to coronary revascularization. Although bleeding is more common with glycoprotein IIb/IIIa inhibitor therapy compared to placebo, it is generally mild, with no increase in stroke rate or risk of intracranial hemorrhage. Therefore age should not exclude the addition of a glycoprotein IIb/IIIa inhibitor to standard anti-ischemic therapy for unstable angina or non-ST-segment elevation myocardial infarction, particularly in higher-risk elderly patients proceeding to coronary revascularization. The theinopyridine derivative clopidogrel was evaluated in 12,562 patients with non-ST-segment elevation acute coronary syndrome patients treated with aspirin.[98] The primary endpoint of CV mortality, nonfatal myocardial infarction, or stroke was reduced 20 percent compared to placebo following a mean of 9 months of therapy. This benefit was evident in the 6208-patient subgroup above age 65. Therefore, in those elderly patients with a low bleeding risk and non-ST-segment acute coronary syndromes, clopidogrel plus aspirin reduce future CV events.

Finally, three recent trials assessed the impact of a conservative medical strategy versus an invasive approach on short-term outcomes of death, myocardial infarction, and recurrent ischemic events in patients with non-ST-segment-elevation acute coronary syndromes.[99–101] These studies show a decrease in the primary endpoint for an initial invasive compared to conservative strategy. The benefit of an invasive approach was much more evident in higher-risk patients, including those with positive troponin, ST-segment depression on ECG, and, importantly, the large subgroup of patients above age 65 in these studies. These data suggest that since older patients with acute coronary syndromes are often at increased risk for adverse outcomes, an early invasive approach should be considered for many such patients (see also Chaps. 51 and 52).

Beta-blocker therapy is greatly underprescribed in older post-myocardial infarction patients. In the Cooperative Cardiovascular Project, investigators reviewed records of approximately 200,000 Medicare beneficiaries who suffered a myocardial infarction. Only 34 percent of this elderly cohort were discharged home on a beta-blocker.[102] Paradoxically, patients leaving hospital without beta-blocker therapy have comorbidities that place them at the highest mortality risk. Confirming the older randomized trials, all subgroups of patients in this database had a large survival advantage (approximately 40 percent reduction in 2-year mortality) with beta-blocker therapy. Similarly, aspirin therapy decreases mortality and reinfarction in elderly infarct subjects.[103,104] Nevertheless, among 10,000 Medicare beneficiaries with an AMI with no contraindication to aspirin therapy, only 61 percent received it within the first 2 hospital days.[105] Aspirin therapy in this large group of elderly infarct patients was independently associated with a lower 30-day mortality. Furthermore, only 76 percent of elderly subjects without any contraindications were discharged home on aspirin following a myocardial infarction.[106] Aspirin use is independently associated with improved 6-month outcome in this group.

ACE-inhibitor therapy following AMI reduces morbidity and mortality. In the randomized, placebo-controlled clinical trials that involved high-risk patients with LV dysfunction or clinical congestive heart failure, there was a large survival benefit in older patients randomized to ACE-inhibitor therapy compared to placebo.[107–109] In the Survival and Ventricular Enlargement Trial, the angiotensin converting enzyme inhibitor captopril resulted in a 23 percent long-term mortality reduction compared to placebo in the 783 patients 65 years of age and older with a LV ejection fraction of less than 40 percent post–myocardial infarction.[107] In the Acute Infarction Ramipril Efficacy Study of ramipril compared with placebo in 2006 postinfarction patients with clinical congestive heart failure, the mean age of the population was 65 years.[108] After an average of 15 months follow-up, mortality was reduced from 23 percent in the placebo group to 17 percent in the ramipril group. Patients over 65 years of age had a larger survival advantage with the ACE inhibitor (39 percent reduction) compared to those under 65 years of age. In the 1749 postinfarct patients (mean age 67.7 years) with echocardiographic evidence of LV dysfunction who were randomized to the ACE inhibitor trandolapril versus placebo, long-term survival was significantly improved with ACE-inhibitor therapy.[109] The 1121 patients at least 65 years of age had a 38 percent reduction in mortality with trandolapril compared to placebo. Therefore older patients with large infarctions, LV dysfunction, or clinical heart failure have a large survival advantage with long-term ACE-inhibitor therapy. For lower-risk elderly patients, the benefits are clearly less and individualized treatment (i.e. risk of hypotension or renal insufficiency) must be considered in this lower risk group.

CHRONIC CORONARY DISEASE

The use of percutaneous coronary intervention has increased significantly as therapy for ischemic heart disease in the elderly, with improved outcomes likely due to increased operator experience, new tools, the introduction of coronary stents, and better antiplatelet therapies. In spite of increasing age and greater comorbidities among patients, the procedural success rate of percutaneous coronary intervention in the elderly has significantly improved with reduction in complications, less need for emergent coronary artery bypass surgery, and decreased length of hospital stay.[110–112]

Use of bypass surgery has also increased in the very elderly.[113] Thirty-day and 1 year mortality in a large cohort 80 years and older averaged 11.5 and 19.2 percent, respectively, both 2.5-fold greater than the corresponding operative mortality in the 65- to 70-year-olds. In spite of the high short-term morbidity and mortality, the 3-year mortality rate of this group was similar to that in the general octogenarian population. Independent predictors of short- and long-term mortality included increasing age, female gender, admission with AMI, congestive heart failure, cerebral or peripheral vascular disease, and chronic renal disease. Increasing age is also a significant independent predictor of stroke, which occurs in about 8 percent of the very elderly who undergo bypass surgery.[114] Recent data also suggest that older age is a powerful predictor of both short-term and 5-year cognitive decline following coronary artery bypass surgery.[115] An important addition to the treatment of the elderly patient with critical multivessel coronary artery disease may be off-pump coronary artery bypass surgery, which theoretically reduces the risk of the neurologic complications that occur with aortic cross-clamping. Although a recent randomized trial in low-risk patients (mean age 61 years) to standard versus off-pump bypass showed no difference in short-term or 1-year stroke, death, myocardial infarction, or coronary reintervention,[116] observational data suggest that older patients may particularly benefit from off-pump bypass surgery, with a decrease in stroke risk.[117] Prospective trials are needed in the elderly to

fully address the risks and benefits of off-pump bypass surgery in this important and growing group of patients.

Previous randomized trials of medical versus revascularization therapy in patients with stable coronary artery disease excluded the elderly. An important recent trial prospectively randomized patients aged 75 years and older (mean 80 years) with moderate angina despite treatment with at least two antianginal drugs to coronary angiography and revascularization versus optimal medical therapy.[118] The primary endpoint of this trial was quality-of-life score at 6 months. Seventy-four percent of patients randomized to the invasive arm had anatomy appropriate for either percutaneous intervention (54 percent) or CABG (20 percent). These data dispel the myth that older patients usually have diffuse coronary disease not amenable to revascularization. Although quality of life improved in both groups by 6 months, the group randomized to invasive therapy had a significantly better quality of life compared to medically treated patients. Secondary endpoints of 6-month death, myocardial infarction, or hospitalization for unstable angina were significantly lower in those elderly patients randomized to invasive therapy (19 percent) versus medical therapy (49 percent). Furthermore, one-third of patients in the medical arm crossed over to revascularization due to refractory symptomatology. This important study suggests that age alone is not a contraindication to an invasive approach to the treatment of moderate to severe angina. (See also Chap. 57.)

Although several trials have randomized patients with stable coronary artery disease to percutaneous coronary intervention versus coronary artery bypass surgery, the elderly were generally excluded. A recent randomized trial of 454 high-risk veterans with medically refractory angina were randomized to percutaneous coronary intervention with or without stents or coronary artery bypass surgery.[119] The high-risk group included patients > 70 years, prior bypass, LV ejection fraction < 35 percent, recent myocardial infarction, or need for intraaortic balloon pump intervention. Survival at 30 days was excellent in both groups (95 percent versus 97 percent for bypass and angioplasty, respectively). Survival up to 3 years remained similar in the two groups. These data suggest that high-risk patients with medically refractory angina, including the elderly, can undergo revascularization with angioplasty or bypass surgery with excellent survival as well as relief of angina.

Risk Factors for Coronary Artery Disease

Although elderly patients with coronary artery disease are less likely to be prescribed statin therapy, they derive the same relative reduction in morbidity and mortality as young subjects; thus the absolute benefit is far greater in the elderly (see also Chap. 43).[120] In the Cholesterol and Recurrent Events Trial evaluating either 40 mg of pravastatin or placebo over 5 years in patients with a myocardial infarction who had total cholesterol levels below 240 mg/dL and low-density-lipoprotein levels between 115 to 174 mg/dL, 1283 patients were aged 65 to 75 years of age.[121] In this group, lipid-lowering therapy reduced the primary endpoint of cardiac death or nonfatal myocardial infarction by 39 percent. The individual secondary endpoints of cardiac death, nonfatal reinfarction, stroke, and need for coronary artery bypass surgery were also reduced.

The Scandinavian Simvastatin Survival Study (4S) included 1848 patients 65 to 70 years of age with chronic coronary artery disease and an elevated baseline total cholesterol.[122] After 5.4 years of follow-up, cholesterol lowering with simvastatin resulted in significant decreases in total mortality, coronary heart disease mortality, major coronary events, and revascularization procedures. Similarly, the

Pravastatin Pooling Project demonstrated a relative risk reduction of 26 percent in patients between 65 to 75 years of age.[123] Finally, the recently reported Heart Protection Study included over 5800 subjects 70 years of age and older in addition to nearly 1300 subjects 75 to 80 years of age with stable coronary disease, peripheral vascular or carotid disease, or diabetes mellitus and randomized to simvastatin versus placebo.[124] Elderly subjects had the same degree of benefit in terms of reduction in vascular events as younger subjects on statin therapy. Therefore lipid-lowering therapy should be a treatment goal in elderly patients with established coronary disease, vascular disease, or diabetes.

HYPERTENSION

The prevalence of hypertension increases dramatically with age (Fig. 96-1) and remains in this age group a major risk factor for myocardial infarction, stroke, and heart failure.[125] Approximately 65 percent of Americans 70 years of age and older have hypertension.[126] Systolic pressure rises progressively with age, while diastolic pressure tends to plateau and even decline after age 60.[65] Therefore isolated systolic hypertension is very common in the elderly and often inadequately treated. The consequent rise in pulse pressure, due primarily to an increase in central vascular stiffness, is a strong and independent risk factor for CV events,[20] for adverse consequences following an infarction,[127] and for the development of heart failure.[128] Numerous trials demonstrate the value of antihypertensive therapy for even mild diastolic hypertension in the elderly population.[129] In isolated systolic hypertension, prospective randomized trials have demonstrated that therapy with a diuretic[130] and a long-acting dihydropyridine calcium antagonist[131] decrease the risk of stroke, congestive heart failure, and myocardial infarction or death in older patients with this entity. Although the general blood pressure goal is 140/90, lower goals are indicated in the presence of diabetes, target-organ damage, and clinical CV disease.[132]

Nonpharmacologic therapy, consisting of restricted salt intake and weight reduction, decreases blood pressure in elderly hypertensives.[133] The selection of pharmacologic therapy should be based on prospective randomized trials,[134] the presence of associated comorbidities (e.g., ischemia, renal insufficiency, congestive heart failure), and the duration of action and side-effect profile of the agent. Despite the widespread choice and effectiveness of proven therapies, the vast majority of hypertensive patients do not reach the appropriate blood pressure goal.[132] Many patients require several antihypertensive agents to achieve satisfactory blood pressure control, particularly in the presence of diabetes and/or renal insufficiency.

SMOKING

Although smoking is a more frequent risk factor in young patients with myocardial infarction,[135] it is still an important reversible risk factor in older patients with coronary artery disease. Following AMI, continued smoking poses a powerful risk for recurrent ischemic events independent of age.[136] The reduction in morbidity and mortality risk from smoking cessation in older patients with coronary disease is comparable to that in younger patients who quit.[137]

DIABETES MELLITUS

Diabetes is a powerful risk factor for the development of coronary disease and of coronary disease mortality.[138] Older diabetics with coronary disease are at particularly high risk for morbidity and mortality.[125] The prevalence of insulin resistance and diabetes mellitus increases dramatically with increasing age, such that the metabolic syndrome is found in many older patients with coronary artery disease.[139] In older patients with the metabolic syndrome, weight loss,

exercise, and blood pressure control are important additional factors to treat.[140] In the high-risk older patient with type 2 diabetes, a multifactorial intervention program with aggressive treatment designed to control blood pressure, blood glucose, and hyperlipidemia—in association with a program to encourage exercise and weight loss—results in a substantial reduction in future CV events.[141]

Congestive Heart Failure

In contrast to other CV disorders, the prevalence of chronic heart failure (CHF) is dramatically increasing (see Fig. 96-1). Approximately 5 million Americans have CHF, and each year 550,000 new cases are diagnosed.[142,143] The incidence of heart failure doubles with each decade of life, and the prevalence rises to almost 10 percent of those above 80 years of age.[144] In part this is because heart failure represents a final common pathway for most other cardiac disorders and in part because of the more successful treatments of heart failure[145] and acute ischemic disease. These successes increase the numbers surviving, albeit with heart failure or at increased risk for it.

CHF is also a highly lethal condition, with significant mortality, morbidity, and associated costs in the older population. Analyses in over 160,000 Medicare recipients with newly diagnosed CHF indicate a median survival of only 2 to 4 years.[146] More than 90 percent of CHF deaths occur in adults above 65 years of age.[147] CHF is also the leading cause of hospitalization in Medicare beneficiaries,[148] and hospitalization in these patients is itself a major risk factor for subsequent re-hospitalization, mortality, and functional decline.[149]

Age-associated biological factors themselves are unlikely to result in heart failure, but they increase the likelihood of the development of symptoms in the presence of ischemic or hypertensive disease. Increased vascular load due to increased central vascular stiffness and decreased endothelium-dependent vasodilatation (see above) increase the likelihood of progressive LV dysfunction, adverse clinical outcomes, and a more variable and complicated response to conventional therapeutic interventions in older individuals with ischemic or hypertension-induced LV damage.[128,150] In addition, the age-associated decrease in sympathetic responsiveness limits the ability of the older person to augment heart rate and cardiac function in the presence of superimposed heart disease, particularly in the setting of acute depression of LV function. Finally, the decrease in early LV filling and the presumptive increase in LV filling pressures during exercise may worsen heart failure symptoms, especially in association with diseases that also impair LV filling, such as coronary artery disease, tachyarrhythmias, and systemic arterial hypertension.

Evaluation of the older patient presenting with failure symptoms should include a noninvasive study to determine whether the primary problem is systolic dysfunction. Up to 40 percent of older individuals with heart failure have normal systolic function.[151] An evaluation for the presence of ischemic, hypertensive, and valvular disease should be performed. Diuretics are particularly useful in patients with increased vascular stiffness presenting with acute congestive symptoms, since significant reductions in pressure occur with relatively small changes in intravascular volume. In patients with systolic dysfunction and sinus rhythm, digitalis may improve signs and symptoms of heart failure.[152] However, the maintenance dose should be reduced to 0.125 mg/day because of the age-associated decreased volume of distribution and creatinine clearance. ACE inhibitors are a cornerstone of therapy in patients with systolic dysfunction, and their benefit extends to the elderly.[153] Studies indicating the value of the beta blockers[154] as well as aldosterone[155] in patients with continued symptoms despite ACE-inhibitor therapy probably extend to the older population as well. New devices may also significantly improve outcomes in patients with persistent failure despite medical therapy. The use of atrial-synchronized biventricular pacing in patients with heart failure and a QRS duration of $\geq$ 130 ms improves functional class and quality of life and decreases hospitalization.[156] The use of experimental long-term LV assist devices[157] may be particularly helpful in older patients with concomitant diseases and contraindications to transplantation, although the cost of these interventions may be prohibitive (see also Chaps. 23–25).

Although systolic dysfunction is present in at least half of the patients with CHF, the presence of a normal or elevated ejection fraction is more common in the older group, particularly women and those with diabetes and hypertension. Although the existence of this entity is sometimes questioned, these patients do experience significant limitations in exercise duration and quality of life, increases in neurohormonal activation and CHF markers such as natriuretic peptide,[158] as well as increased mortality, hospitalization rates, and health care costs when compared with the general population.[159,160] The report of a group of patients with acute pulmonary edema in the setting of a normal ejection fraction which did not change after resolution of the symptoms in the absence of known ischemic, pulmonary, and valvular disease also supports the existence of the syndrome,[161] The etiology is not clear, although, in addition to abnormalities in diastolic filling, hypertension is almost invariably present, and increased pulse pressure with exercise suggests increased central vascular stiffness.[158]

There are no controlled, randomized trials of interventions in this patient population. Increased vascular and LV chamber stiffness increase the likelihood of significant pressure shifts with relatively small changes in volume. Thus diuretics, although extremely useful in the acute setting, may be associated with symptomatic hypotension in the absence of volume overload. Careful control of blood pressure is also important. Interventions which decrease LV mass and improve diastolic filling are theoretically helpful, but clinical trials are not yet completed.[162]

The importance of the individual patient's role as a partner in his or her care and of individualizing treatment and monitoring plans cannot be overemphasized. Although patients may carry the same heart failure diagnosis, they differ markedly in terms of disease severity and complexity, associated comorbidities, social support, education, ingrained habits, access to medical personnel and knowledge, and understanding of health care information and directions. Noncompliance with medications or diet is often cited as a major factor contributing to hospitalization in heart failure patients. The most common factors contributing to possibly preventable readmissions are noncompliance, failure to seek help promptly, and poor social support. It is possible to predict which heart failure patients are at increased risk for early readmission. In these patients, a multidisciplinary team approach including simplification of the medical regimen, close monitoring, and intensive patient education can decrease hospital admission and improve quality of life.[163–165]

Arrhythmias

Supraventricular and ventricular arrhythmias increase in frequency with aging (see Fig. 96-1), probably due to age-associated changes in the impulse formation and conduction system, including loss of pacemaker and conducting cells and fibrosis as well as increased incidence of mitral annular and aortic calcification, hypertension, and ischemic disease. Other illnesses may frequently present with arrhythmias in the elderly as well, including hyperthyroidism, anemia, hypoxia, electrolyte imbalance, and infection. Age-associated changes in both passive and active state diastolic properties as well as

decreased systolic reserve (see above) may increase the likelihood that the older individual will develop hemodynamic compromise and/or ischemia during an arrhythmic episode.

Evaluation of the older patient presenting with symptomatic or asymptomatic arrhythmias, therefore, should include a search for concomitant illnesses as well as other presenting triggers such as chest pain, unusual exertion, smoking, caffeine, electrolyte abnormalities, and medicine and alcohol ingestion. Ambulatory ECG monitoring during the patient's normal activities is most likely to determine the nature and severity of the arrhythmia. Invasive electrophysiology studies can be used to not only diagnose the arrhythmia but also to determine its mechanism, obtain prognostic information, and determine the suitability of different therapeutic approaches.

Atrial fibrillation is common in the elderly. In the population based Cardiovascular Health Study of 5201 men and women aged $\geq$ 65 years, 4.8 percent of women and 6.2 percent of men had atrial fibrillation.[166] In five randomized trials of anticoagulation for the prevention of stroke in atrial fibrillation, the mean age of enrolled patients was 69 years, with 25 percent over age 75.[167] Atrial fibrillation in the elderly is associated with increasing age, heart failure, valvular heart disease, stroke, diabetes, and hypertension. Older individuals are more likely to experience hemodynamic compromise resulting from the increased ventricular rate and loss of atrial/ventricular synchrony accompanying the arrhythmia because of the age-associated changes in relaxation properties and increased dependence on atrial contribution. Because of the increased likelihood of coronary disease, the higher rate is also more likely to be associated with myocardial ischemia. Atrial fibrillation may also result in atrial remodeling, which increases the likelihood of maintenance of the arrhythmia,[168] cardiomyopathy due to the rapid rate[169] and lower output related to the irregularity of the rhythm.[170] The risk of embolic stroke in atrial fibrillation is also increased with age. The Framingham Study reported that the risk of stroke attributed to atrial fibrillation rose from 7.3 percent in those 60 to 69 years of age to 30.8 percent in those aged 80 to 89 (see also Chaps. 27 and 28).[171]

Therapeutic goals in patients with atrial fibrillation include stroke prevention, rate control, and possibly rhythm control. In randomized trials, anticoagulation has prevented embolic strokes in most patients with atrial fibrillation, including those over 75 years of age.[172] This benefit of anticoagulation is greater than that of aspirin therapy in the elderly, although there is a higher rate of intracranial hemorrhage. Careful monitoring of the international normalized ratio (INR) is important, as most embolic strokes in the elderly occur when the ratio is under 2.0 and most cerebral hemorrhages occur when the ratio is above 3.0. Although the benefits of aspirin are less significant, aspirin can be used in older patients who have a contraindication to warfarin therapy, including an inability to carefully monitor the INR. Rate control in patients without systolic dysfunction may be attempted with diltiazem, verapamil, and beta blockers; in patients with systolic dysfunction, amiodarone or digitalis may be used. A useful goal is a rate of < 80/min at rest and < 110/min on a 6-min walk test. If patients are intolerant of medical therapy or if medical therapy is ineffective, AV-nodal ablation and pacemaker insertion[173] or AV-nodal modification, which results in slowed AV conduction but not complete heart block should be considered. Cardioversion should be attempted in patients who are hemodynamically compromised, in acute atrial fibrillation, and for those who are at low likelihood of reversion to atrial fibrillation if conversion does occur. This can be attempted with electrical or pharmacologic approaches. A randomized study compared several weeks of warfarin therapy before cardioversion with more immediate cardioversion if transesophageal echocardiography revealed no atrial thrombi; it demonstrated similar rates of thromboembolism and maintenance of sinus rhythm but a lower hemorrhage rate in the transesophageal group.[174] Either approach would be reasonable, but it is important to continue warfarin for at least 1 month following cardioversion.

Two recent studies compared rate-control and rhythm-control strategies in primarily older (mean ages 70 and 68 years) patients with atrial fibrillation.[175,176] In the AFFIRM trial, 5-year estimates indicated that a higher proportion of patients were in sinus rhythm in the rhythm-control group, 63 percent, than in the rate-control group, 35 percent. In the second study, 39 percent of the rhythm-control and 10 percent of the rate-control groups were in sinus rhythm at follow-up. There were no significant differences in mortality in either study, although subgroup analysis indicated a higher mortality in the rhythm-control group for those 65 years of age and older. Ischemic stroke and thromboembolic events were nonsignificantly higher in the rhythm-control group in the first and second studies, respectively, and were associated with discontinuation of anticoagulation or subtherapeutic treatment. In the AFFIRM trial, rates of hospitalization were higher in the rhythm-control group. Thus, rate control is a reasonable strategy in older patients with atrial fibrillation that is not associated with significant symptoms or hemodynamic compromise. Anticoagulation should be maintained regardless of a rate- or rhythm-control strategy. If rhythm control is attempted, flecanide and propafenone may be used in patients without ischemic or structural heart disease. In those with ischemic disease, sotalol may be used. In patients with heart failure, dofetilide increases the likelihood of conversion to and maintenance of sinus rhythm[177] without the increase in mortality associated with some other antiarrhythmic agents in patients with heart failure. Amiodarone is useful in nearly all patient populations and in a randomized trial was more effective than sotalol or propafenone in preventing recurrences of atrial fibrillation.[178]

The recognition that rapid firing of atrial myocytes located near the pulmonary veins may be responsible for some episodes of atrial fibrillation has led to the use of catheter ablation to terminate atrial fibrillation.[179] It is possible that this approach may result in improved outcomes as compared with pharmacologic therapy and/or a rate-control strategy.

About half of all pacemakers are placed because of sinus node dysfunction with bradycardia.[180] The use of programmable pacemakers to appropriately time atrial and ventricular systole may be particularly useful in older patients, because in them diastolic filling and cardiac output are more dependent on atrial contribution. In the Medicare population, after adjustment for confounding patient characteristics, dual-chamber pacing is associated with improved 1- and 2-year survival when compared with single-chamber pacing.[180] In a randomized trial comparing the two pacing modalities in patients with sinus node dysfunction, there was no difference in stroke-free mortality, but the risk of new and chronic atrial fibrillation and signs and symptoms of heart failure were significantly reduced and quality of life was higher in patients assigned to dual-chamber pacing.[181]

Ventricular arrhythmias in the elderly are to be approached in the same fashion as in younger individuals—i.e., those that are asymptomatic and unassociated with evidence of cardiac disease can be viewed as less serious than those associated with evidence of LV dysfunction and/or ischemia. Both older and younger postmyocardial infarction patients benefit from beta-blocker therapy with a reduction in sudden death. Life-threatening ventricular arrhythmias are common in the elderly patient with severe coronary disease and LV dysfunction. As in younger subjects, aggressive management of elderly survivors of cardiac arrest and of those with hypotensive ventricular tachycardia is justified. Antiarrhythmic therapy selected with electrophysiologic testing and/or placement of an automatic implantable

cardioverter/defibrillator (AICD) are well tolerated in the elderly and lead to improved survival.[182] In the MADIT-II trial, patients with an ejection fraction of ≤ 0.30 and a prior myocardial infarction randomized to an AICD experienced improved survival as compared to those randomized to conventional therapy. For those ≥ 70 years of age, the hazard ratio of death was decreased by more than 30 percent.[183]

Valvular Heart Disease

The most frequent valvular heart disease in the elderly is calcific aortic stenosis. The development of clinically significant aortic stenosis may be very rapid in this age group, as calcification and severe scarring occur rather abruptly. In addition, animal studies demonstrate that there is less compensatory hypertrophy in response to increased impedance to LV ejection in the aged heart, which could also contribute to the development of heart failure. (see Chap. 66).[184]

There is considerable evidence that calcific aortic stenosis in the elderly is not the result of a degenerative process per se but actually involves an active inflammatory process similar to that present in atherosclerotic vascular lesions. This is supported by pathologic findings of lesions containing low-density lipoprotein (LDL), Lp(a), macrophages, and T lymphocytes[185] as well as macrophages that produce osteopontin, a protein which enhances tissue calcification.[186] The presence of calcific disease is also related to traditional atherosclerotic risk factors including cigarette use, diabetes, hypertension, and hyperlipidemia.[187] Finally, in a retrospective study of 174 patients with mild to moderate calcific aortic stenosis, those who were on a "statin" regimen (taking an HMG-CoA reductase inhibitor) had a smaller increase in peak and mean gradients and a smaller decrease in aortic valve area over a mean follow-up of 21 months.[188]

By far the most helpful study one can perform in assessing an elderly subject for significant aortic stenosis is a Doppler echocardiogram for severe aortic valve calcification with decreased mobility, a small aortic valve area, and a significant transvalvular gradient. The presence of LVH can be assessed as well as LV function. It seems that asymptomatic elderly patients with significant aortic stenosis by echocardiography can be followed carefully without surgical intervention until the first symptoms appear.[189] It should be noted, however, that if the older patient is limited by other disease—e.g., arthritis—he or she may not be able to exercise to the point where symptoms occur despite the presence of significant disease requiring surgery. In the presence of asymptomatic severe stenosis or if the assessment of symptoms is difficult because of concomitant diseases, physician-supervised exercise testing is safe in patients with moderate-to-severe asymptomatic aortic stenosis and can identify those who would benefit from surgery.[190] As in younger patients, a low calculated valve area in the presence of a low cardiac output may be due to incomplete valve opening rather than severe stenosis. Calculation of the valve area during dobutamine administration in these instances will provide a more accurate assessment of valvular stenosis.[191]

Coronary angiography should be performed in older individuals prior to aortic valve surgery to assess the need for bypass grafting. Aortic valve replacement often results in marked improvement in symptoms and LV function as well as expected survival in the older patient.[192] Predictors of surgical mortality with aortic valve replacement include low ejection fraction and congestive heart failure, atrial fibrillation, associated surgical procedures, and an emergency procedure, suggesting that aortic valve replacement for symptomatic aortic stenosis should not be delayed merely because the patient is elderly.[193] Percutaneous aortic valvuloplasty in the elderly is associated with poor outcomes, including early restenosis, aortic regurgitation, stroke, high mortality, and heart failure.[194] It is useful only for palliation and as a "bridge" to valve replacement in very ill patients[195] or to decrease risk associated with urgent noncardiac surgery.

Chronic aortic regurgitation may occur in elderly individuals secondary to aortic root dilatation. Symptoms include angina, even in patients without significant coronary disease, and congestive heart failure. It is important to recognize, however, that symptoms may not occur until significant LV dysfunction is present; therefore the onset of dysfunction is sufficient to prompt surgery, rather than awaiting the occurrence of symptoms. Vasodilator therapy may be helpful in patients with normal LV function. In a randomized trial, nifedipine was shown to reduce LV volume and mass, increase ejection fraction, and delay the occurrence of systolic dysfunction.[196] Best operative results occur in individuals with no or minimal symptoms, mild to moderate ventricular dysfunction, and a brief duration of LV dysfunction.

The most common cause of mitral stenosis in the elderly is rheumatic disease, which at times may not result in symptoms until the patient reaches old age. The diagnosis may be more difficult in the elderly because calcification of the valve may decrease the intensity of the first heart sound and the opening sound, and diminished cardiac output may decrease the intensity of the diastolic rumble. Doppler echocardiography is very useful in diagnosing the presence of significant disease. If symptoms are more than mild or if pulmonary hypertension develops, surgery or balloon mitral valvuloplasty should be considered. Atrial fibrillation often triggers functional deterioration in older individuals because the dependence of filling on atrial contribution is exaggerated in the presence of mitral stenosis. Balloon mitral valvuloplasty compares favorably with open surgical commissurotomy in appropriate candidates—i.e., those with minimal calcification, good mobility, little subvalvular disease, and only mild mitral regurgitation; it should be considered for elderly patients with symptomatic mitral stenosis.[197,198]

Mitral regurgitation in the elderly is most often related to ischemic heart disease and myxomatous degeneration of the mitral valve. As is true for aortic insufficiency, symptoms may be recognized only after significant LV dysfunction has occurred, and intervention should be considered on the basis of dysfunction rather than awaiting the onset of symptoms.[199] It should also be remembered that favorable unloading conditions will raise the ejection fraction in the presence of significant mitral regurgitation. Therefore, an ejection fraction of under 60 should be considered abnormal and is associated with a poorer postsurgical prognosis. Vasodilator therapy improves symptoms in patients with ventricular dilatation and impaired systolic function.[200] For elderly patients with mitral regurgitation, mitral valve repair is associated with a lower operative mortality and improved late outcomes; it eliminates the need for anticoagulation in patients without atrial fibrillation and results in excellent long-term results. Thus repair rather than replacement should be performed if possible. If repair is not possible, chordal preservation should be attempted.[201]

For elderly patients requiring valve replacement, the choice of a mechanical valve with the bleeding risk of lifelong anticoagulation must be balanced against a bioprosthetic valve and risk of structural deterioration. Additional factors in the choice include candidacy for anticoagulation and other requirements for anticoagulation such as atrial fibrillation, age, and valve position. In a series of elderly subjects receiving aortic or mitral mechanical valve replacements, freedom from major anticoagulant-related hemorrhage was 76 percent at 10 years.[202] A bioprosthetic valve in the mitral position deteriorates more rapidly than in the aortic position. In a large series of elderly patients receiving porcine bioprostheses, freedom from structural deterioration at 10 years for the aortic valve bioprostheses was 98 percent and for the mitral valve bioprosthesis 79 percent, with excellent long-term survival free of major morbidity.[203]

ACKNOWLEDGMENTS

The editorial assistance of Christina R. Link is appreciated in preparing this chapter.

References

1. Lakatta EG. Cardiovascular regulatory mechanisms in advanced age. *Physiol Rev* 1993;73: 413–465.
2. Virmani R, Avolio AP, Mergner WJ, et al. Effect of aging on aortic morphology in populations with high and low prevalence of hypertension and atherosclerosis. Comparison between occidental and Chinese communities. *Am J Pathol* 1991;139(5):1119–1129.
3. Lakatta EG. Cellular and molecular clues to heart and arterial aging. *Circulation* 2003;107:490–497.
4. Avolio A. Genetic and environmental factors in the function and structure of the arterial wall. *Hypertension* 1995;26:34–37.
5. Nagai Y, Metter EJ, Earley CJ, et al. Increased carotid artery intimal-medial thickness in asymptomatic older subjects with exercise-induced myocardial ischemia. *Circulation* 1998;98:1504–1509.
6. O'Leary DH, Polak JF, Kronmal RA, et al. for the Cardiovascular Health Study Collaborative Research Group. Carotid-artery intima and media thickness as a risk factor for myocardial infarction and stroke in older adults. *N Engl J Med* 1999;340:14–22.
7. Li Z, Froehlich J, Galis ZS, et al. Increased expression of matrix metalloproteinase-2 in the thickened intima of aged rats. *Hypertension* 1999;33:116–123.
8. Wang M, Lakatta EG. In situ imbalance of matrix metalloproteinase-2 activators and inhibitors in age associated aortic remodeling. *Hypertension* 2002;39:865–873.
9. Najjar SS, Lakatta EG. Vascular aging: From molecular to clinical cardiology. In: *The Textbook of Molecular Cardiology.* Totowa, NJ: Humana Press, 2002.
10. Salonen R, Nyssonen K, Porkkala-Sarataho E, et al. The Kuopio Atherosclerosis Prevention Study (KAPS): Effect of pravastatin treatment on lipids, oxidation resistance of lipoproteins, and atherosclerotic progression. *Am J Cardiol* 1995;76:34C–39C.
11. Woo KS, Chook P, Raitakari OT, et al. Westernization of Chinese adults and increased subclinical atherosclerosis. *Arterioscler Thromb Vasc Biol* 1999;19:2487–2493.
12. Adams MR, Nakagomi A, Keech A, et al. Carotid intima-media thickness is only weakly correlated with the extent and severity of coronary artery disease. *Circulation* 1995;92:2127–2134.
13. Homma S, Hirose N, Ishida H, et al. Carotid plaque and intima-media thickness assessed by B-mode ultrasonography in subjects ranging from young adults to centenarians. *Stroke* 2001;32:830–835.
14. Dart AM, Kingwell BA. Pulse pressure—A review of mechanisms and clinical relevance. *J Am Coll Cardiol* 2001;37:975–984.
15. Blacher J, Asmar R, Djane S, et al. Aortic pulse wave velocity as a marker of cardiovascular risk in hypertensive patients. *Hypertension* 1999;33:1111–1117.
16. Gimbrone MA Jr. Vascular endothelium, hemodynamic forces, and atherogenesis. *Am J Pathol* 1999;155:1–5.
17. Liao D, Arnett DK, Tyroler HA, et al. Arterial stiffness and the development of hypertension: The ARIC Study. *Hypertension* 1999;34:201–206.
18. Franklin SS, Larson MG, Khan SA, et al. Does the relation of blood pressure to coronary heart disease risk change with aging? The Framingham Heart Study. *Circulation* 2001;103:1245–1249.
19. Sesso HD, Stampfer MJ, Rosner B, et al. Systolic and diastolic blood pressure, pulse pressure, and mean arterial pressure as predictors of cardiovascular disease risk in men. *Hypertension* 2000;36:801–807.

20. Franklin SS, Khan SA, Wong ND, et al. Is pulse pressure useful in predicting risk for coronary heart disease? The Framingham Heart Study. *Circulation* 1999;100:354–360.

21. Miura K, Dyer AR, Greenland P, et al. Pulse pressure compared with other blood pressure indexes in the prediction of 25-year cardio-vascular and all-cause mortality rates: The Chicago Heart Association Detection Project in Industry Study. *Hypertension* 2001;38:232–237.

22. Lakatta EG.: Cardiovascular aging research: The next horizons (review). *J Am Geriatr Soc* 1999;47: 613–625.

23. Olivetti G, Melissari M, Capasso JM, et al. Cardiomyopathy of the aging human heart: Myocyte loss and reactive cellular hypertrophy. *Circ Res* 1991;68:1560.

24. Olivetti G, Giordano G, Corradi D, et al. Gender differences and aging: Effects in the human heart. *J Am Coll Cardiol* 1995;26:1068.

25. Fleg JL, Schulman SP, Gerstenblith G, et al. Additive effects of age and silent myocardial ischemia on the left ventricular response to upright cycle exercise. *J Appl Physiol* 1993;75:499.

26. Correia LC, Lakatta EG, O'Connor FC, et al. Attenuated cardio-vascular reserve during prolonged submaximal cycle exercise in healthy older subjects. *J Am Coll Cardiol* 2002;40:1290–1297.

27. Fleg JL, O'Connor FC, Gerstenblith G, et al. Impact of age on the cardiovascular response to dynamic upright exercise in healthy men and women. *J Appl Physiol* 1995;78:890–900.

28. Yin FCP, Raizes GS, Guarnieri T, et al. Age-associated decrease in ventricular response to haemodynamic stress during beta-adrenergic blockade. *Br Heart J* 1978;40:1349–1355.

29. Chen C-H, Ting C-T, Lin S-J, et al. Which arterial and cardiac parameters best predict left ventricular mass? *Circulation* 1998;98: 422.

30. Chen C-H, Nakayama M, Talbot M, et al. Verapamil acutely reduces ventricular-vascular stiffening and improves aerobic exercise performance in elderly individuals. *J Am Coll Cardiol* 1999;33: 1602–1609.

31. Schulman SP, Gerstenblith G, Fleg JL, et al. Relationship of age and sex on ventricular vascular coupling at rest and exercise. *Circulation* 2000(suppl);102:II-602.

32. Nussbacher A, Gerstenblith G, O'Connor F, et al: Hemodynamic effects of unloading the old heart. *Am J Physiol* 1999;277:H1863–H1871.

33. Lakatta EG. Deficient neuroendocrine regulation of the cardiovascular system with advancing age in healthy humans (point of view). *Circulation* 1993;87:631.

34. Esler MD, Turner AG, Kaye DM, et al. Aging effects on human sympathetic neuronal function. *Am J Physiol* 1995;268:R278–R285.

35. Seals DR, Dempsey JA. Aging, exercise and cardiopulmonary function. In: Lamb DR, Gisolfi CV, Nadel E, eds. *Perspectives in Exercise Science and Sports Medicine*. Vol 8. Carmel, IN: Cooper Publishing Group, 1995, pp 237–304.

36. Fleg JL, Schulman S, O'Connor F, et al. Effects of acute β-adrenergic receptor blockade on age-associated changes in cardiovascular performance during dynamic exercise. *Circulation* 1994;90:2333.

37. Yin FCP, Weisfeldt ML, Milnor WR. Role of aortic input impedance in the decreased cardiovascular response to exercise with aging in dogs. *J Clin Invest* 1981;68:28–38.

38. Schulman SP, Fleg JL, Goldberg AP, et al. Continuum of cardio-vascular performance across a broad range of fitness levels in healthy older men. *Circulation* 1996;94:359–367.

39. Tanaka H, DeSouza CA, Seals DR: Absence of age-related increase in central arterial stiffness in physically active women. *Arterioscler Thromb Vasc Biol* 1998;18:127–132.

40. Das DN, Fleg JL, Lakatta EG. Effect of age on the components of atrioventricular conduction in normal man. *Am J Cardiol* 1982;49(2): 1031.

41. Tsuji H, Larson MG, Venditti FJ, et al. Impact of reduced heart rate variability on risk for cardiac events. *Circulation* 1996;94:2850–2855.

42. Fleg JL, Kennedy HL. Cardiac arrhythmias in a healthy elderly population: Detection by 24-hour ambulatory electrocardiography. *Chest* 1982;81:302–307.

43. Fleg JL, Kennedy HL. Long-term prognosis significance of ambulatory electrocardiographic findings in apparently healthy subjects 60 years of age. *Am J Cardiol* 1992;70:748–751.

44. Manolio TA, Furberg CD, Rautaharju PM, et al. Cardiac arrhythmias on 24-hour ambulatory electrocardiography in older women and men: The Cardiovascular Health Study. *J Am Coll Cardiol* 1994;23:916–925.

45. Maurer MS, Shefrin EA, Fleg JL. Prevalence and prognostic significance of exercise-induced supraventricular tachycardia in apparently healthy volunteers. *Am J Cardiol* 1995;756:788–792.

46. Gerstenblith G, Fredricksen J, Yin FCP, et al. Echocardiographic assessment of a normal adult aging population. *Circulation* 1977;56: 273–278.

47. Busby MJ, Shefrin EA, Fleg JL. Prevalence and long-term significance of exercise-induced frequent or repetitive ventricular ectopic beats in apparently healthy volunteers. *J Am Coll Cardiol* 1989;14(7): 1659–1665.

48. Lakatta EG, Sollott SJ. The "heartbreak" of older age. *J Pharmacol Exp Ther* 2003. In press.

49. Spagnoli LG, Bonanno E, Mauriello A, et al. Multicentric inflammation in epicardial coronary arteries of patients dying of acute myocardial infarction. *J Am Coll Cardiol* 2002;40:1579–1588.

50. Clarkson TB. Nonhuman primate models of atherosclerosis. *Lab Anim Sci* 1998;48:569–572.

51. Talbot LA, Metter EJ, Fleg JL. Leisure-time physical activities and their relationship to cardiorespiratory fitness in healthy men and women 18–95 years old. *Med Sci Sports Exer* 2000;32:417–425.

52. Vaitkevicius PV, Fleg JL, Engel JH, et al. Effects of age and aerobic capacity on arterial stiffness in healthy adults. *Circulation* 1993;88: 1456–1462.

53. Hunt BE, Farquhar WB, Taylor JA. Does reduced vascular stiffening fully explain preserved cardiovagal baroreflex function in older, physically active men? *Circulation* 2001;103:2424–2427.

54. Rywik TM, Blackman R, Yataco AR, et al. Enhanced endothelial vasoreactivity in endurance trained older men. *J Appl Physiol* 1999;87: 2136–2142.

55. Avolio AP, Clyde KM, Beard TC, et al. Improved arterial distensibility in normotensive subjects on a low salt diet. *Arteriosclerosis* 1986;6: 166–169.

56. Abete P, Calabrese C, Ferrara N, et al. Exercise training restores ischemic preconditioning in the aging heart. *J Am Coll Cardiol* 2000; 36:643–650.

57. Abete P, Ferrara N, Cacciatore F, et al. High level of physical activity preserves the cardioprotective effect of preinfarction angina in elderly patients. *J Am Coll Cardiol* 2001;38:1357–1365.

58. Michel JB, Heudes D, Michel O, et al. Effect of chronic ANG I-converting enzyme inhibition on aging processes. II. Large arteries. *Am J Physiol* 1994;267:R124–R135.

59. Levy BI, Michel JB, Salzmann JL, et al. Remodeling of heart and arteries by chronic converting enzyme inhibition in spontaneously hypertensive rats. *Am J Hypertens* 1991;4:240S–245S.

60. Wolfenbuttel BHR, Boulanger CM, Crijns FRL, et al. Breakers of advanced glycation end products restore large artery properties in experimental diabetes. *Proc Natl Acad Sci USA* 1998;95:4630–4634.

61. Asif M, Egan J, Vasan S, et al. An advanced glycation endproduct cross-link breaker can reverse age-related increases in myocardial stiffness. *Proc Natl Acad Sci USA* 2000;97:2809–2813.

62. Vaitkevicius PV, Lane M, Spurgeon HA, et al. A cross-link breaker has sustained effects on arterial and ventricular properties in older rhesus monkeys. *Proc Natl Acad Sci USA* 2001;98:1171–1175.

63. Kass DA, Shapiro EP, Kawaguchi M, et al. Improved arterial compliance by a novel advanced glycation end-product crosslink breaker. *Circulation* 2001;104:1464–1470.

64. Glynn RJ, Chae CU, Guralnik JM, et al. Pulse pressure and mortality in older people. *Arch Intern Med* 2000;160:2765–2772.

65. Franklin SS, Gustin W IV, Wong ND, et al. Hemodynamic patterns of age-related changes in blood pressure. The Framingham Heart Study. *Circulation* 1997;96:308–315.

66. Benetos A, Zureik M, Morcet J, et al. A decrease in diastolic blood pressure combined with an increase in systolic blood pressure is associated with a higher cardiovascular mortality in men. *J Am Coll Cardiol* 2000;35:673–680.

67. Blacher J, Guerin AP, Pannier B, et al. Impact of aortic stiffness on survival in end-stage renal disease. *Circulation* 1999;99:2434–2439.

68. Fagard RH, Pardaens K, Staessen JA, et al. The pulse pressure-to-stroke index ratio predicts cardiovascular events and death in uncomplicated hypertension. *J Am Coll Cardiol* 2001;38:227–231.

69. Wilson PWF, D'Agostino RB, Levy D, et al. Prediction of coronary heart diseases using risk factor categories. *Circulation* 1998;97:1837–1847.

70. Elveback L, Lie JT. Continued high prevalence of coronary artery disease at autopsy in Olmstead County, Minnesota 1950 to 1979. *Circulation* 1984;70:345–349.

71. Gersh BJ, Kronmal RA, Frye RL. Coronary arteriography and coronary artery bypass surgery; morbidity and mortality in patients aged 65 years or older: A report from the Coronary Artery Surgery Study. *Circulation* 1983;67:483–491.

72. Hlatky M, Pryor DB, Harrell FE. Factors affecting sensitivity and specificity of exercise elctrocardiography: Multivariate analysis. *Am J Med* 1984;77:64–71.

73. Frishman WH, DeMaria AN, Ewy GA. Clinical assessment. *J Am Coll Cardiol* 1987;10:48A–51A.

74. Roger VL, Jacobsen SJ, Weston SA, et al. Trends in the incidence and survival of patients with hospitalized myocardial infarction, Olmstead County, Minnesota, 1979 to 1994. *Ann Intern Med* 2002;136:341–348.

75. Nicod P, Gilpin E, Dittrich H, et al. Short- and long-term clinical outcome after Q wave and non-Q wave myocardial infarction in a large population. *Circulation* 1989;79:528.

76. Goldberg RJ, Gore JM, Gurwitz JH, et al. The impact of age on the incidence and prognosis of initial acute myocardial infarction: The Worcester Heart Attack Study. *Am Heart J* 1989;117:543–549.

77. Nadelmann J, Frishman WH, Ooi WL, et al. Prevalence, incidence and prognosis of recognized and unrecognized myocardial infarction in persons aged 75 years or older: The Bronx Aging Study. *Am J Cardiol* 1990;66:533–537.

78. Maggioni AP, Maseri A, Fresco C, et al. Age-related increase in mortality among patients with first myocardial infarctions treated with thrombolysis. *N Engl J Med* 1993;329:1442–1448.

79. Keller NM, Feit F. Atherosclerotic heart disease in the elderly. *Curr Opin Cardiol* 1995;10:427–433.

80. The GUSTO Investigators. An international randomized trial comparing four thrombolytic strategies for acute myocardial infarction. *N Engl J Med* 1993;329:673–682.

81. Armstrong PW, Fu Yuling, Chang W-C, et al. for the GUSTO-IIb Investigators. Acute coronary syndromes in the GUSTO-IIb trial. *Circulation* 1998;98:1860–1868.

82. Boersma E, Pieper KS, Steyerberg EW, et al. for the PURSUIT Investigators. Predictors of outcome in patients with acute coronary syndromes without persistent ST-segment elevation. *Circulation* 2000; 10:2557–2567.

83. Hasdai D, Topol EJ, Califf RM, et al. Cardiogenic shock complicating acute coronary syndromes. *Lancet* 2000;356:749–756.

84. Fibrinolytic Therapy Trialists' Collaborative Group. Indications for fibrinolytic therapy in suspected acute myocardial infarction: Collaborative overview of early mortality and major morbidity results from all randomized trials of more than 1000 patients. *Lancet* 1994;343: 311–322.

85. Barron HV, Bowlby LJ, Breen T, et al. Use of reperfusion therapy for acute myocardial infarction in the United States: Data from the National Registry of Myocardial Infarction 2. *Circulation* 1998;97: 1150–1156.

86. Gore JM, Granger CB, Simoons ML, et al. Stroke after thrombolysis. Mortality and functional outcomes in the GUSTO-I Trial. *Circulation* 1995;92:2811–2818.

87. The Assessment of the Safety and Efficacy of a New Thrombolytic Regimen (ASSENT)-3 Investigators. Efficacy and safety of tenecteplase in combination with enoxaparin, abciximab, or unfractionated heparin: The ASSENT-3 randomised trial in acute myocardial infarction. *Lancet* 2001;358:605–613.

88. GUSTO V Investigators. Reperfusion therapy for acute myocardial infarction with fibrinolytic therapy or combination reduced fibrinolytic therapy and platelet glycoprotein IIb/IIIa inhibition: The GUSTO V randomised trial. *Lancet* 2001;357:1905–1914.

89. Soumerai SB, McLaughlin TJ, Ross-Degnan D, et al. Effectiveness of thrombolytic therapy for acute myocardial infarction in the elderly. *Arch Intern Med* 2002;161:561–568.

90. Thiemann DR, Coresh J, Schulman SP, et al. Lack of benefit of thrombolysis in patients with myocardial infarction who are older than 75 years. *Circulation* 2000;101:2239–2246.

91. Grines CL, Browne KF, Marco J, et al. A comparison of immediate angioplasty with thrombolytic therapy for acute myocardial infarction. *N Engl J Med* 1993;328:672–679.

92. Zijlstra F, Hoorntje JCA, de Boer M-J, et al. Long-term benefit of primary angioplasty as compared with thrombolytic therapy for acute myocardial infarction. *N Engl J Med* 1999;341:1413–1419.

93. Weaver WD, Simes RJ, Betriu A, et al. Comparison of primary coronary angioplasty and intravenous thrombolytic therapy for acute myocardial infarction. *JAMA* 1997;278:2093–2098.

94. de Boer M-J, Ottervanger J-P, van't Hof AWJ, et al. Reperfusion therapy in elderly patients with acute myocardial infarction. *J Am Coll Cardiol* 2002;39:1723–1728.

95. The Platelet Receptor Inhibition in Ischemic Syndrome Management in Patients Limited by Unstable Signs and Symptoms (PRISM-PLUS) Study Investigators. Inhibition of the platelet glycoprotein IIb/IIIa receptor with tirofiban in unstable angina and non-Q wave myocardial infarction. *N Engl J Med* 1998;338:1488–1497.

96. The PURSUIT Trial Investigators. Inhibition of platelet glycoprotein IIb/IIIa with eptifibatide in patients with acute coronary syndromes. *N Engl J Med* 1998;339:436–443.

97. Boersma E, Harrington RA, Moliterno DJ, et al. Platelet glycoprotein IIb/IIIa inhibitors in acute coronary syndromes: A meta-analysis of all major randomised clnical trials. *Lancet* 2002;359:189–198.

98. The Clopidogrel in Unstable Angina to Prevent Recurrent Events Trial Investigators. Effects of clopidogrel in addition to aspirin in patients with acute coronary syndromes without ST-segment elevation. *N Engl J Med* 2001;345:494–502.

99. Fox KAA, Poole-Wilson RA, Clayton TC, et al. for the Randomized Intervention Trial of unstable Angina (RITA) investigators. Interventional versus conservative treatment for patients with unstable angina or non-ST segment elevation myocardial infarction: The British Heart Foundation RITA 3 randomised trial. *Lancet* 2002;360:743–751.

100. Cannon CP, Weintraub WS, Demopoulos LA, et al for the TACTICS-Thrombolysis in Myocardial Infarction 18 Investigators. Comparison of early invasive and conservative strategies in patients with unstable coronary syndromes treated with the glycoprotein IIb/IIIa inhibitor tirofiban. *N Engl J Med* 2001;344:1879–1887.

101. Fragmin and Fast Revascularization during Instability in Coronary artery disease (FRISC II) Investigators. Invasive compared with non-invasive treatment in unstable coronary-artery disease: FRISC II prospective randomised multicentre study. *Lancet* 1999;354:708–715.

102. Gottlieb SS, McCarter RJ, Vogel RA. Effect of beta-blockade on mortality among high-risk and low-risk patients after myocardial infarction. *N Engl J Med* 1998;339:489–497.

103. ISIS-2. Randomised trial of intravenous streptokinase, oral aspirin, both or neither among 17,187 cases of suspected acute myocardial infarction. *Lancet* 1988;2:349–360.

104. Antithrombotic Trialists' Collaboration. Collaborative meta-analysis of randomised trials of antiplatelet therapy for prevention of death, myocardial infarction, and stroke in high risk patients. *BMJ* 2002; 324:71–86.

105. Krumholz HM, Radford MJ, Ellerbeck EF, et al. Aspirin in the treatment of acute myocardial infarction in elderly Medicare beneficiaries. Patterns of use and outcomes. *Circulation* 1995;92:2841–2847.

106. Krumholz HM, Radford MJ, Ellerbeck EF, et al. Aspirin for secondary prevention after acute myocardial infarction in the elderly: Prescribed use and outcomes. *Ann Intern Med* 1996;124:292–298.

107. Pfeffer MA, Braunwald E, Moye LA, et al. Effect of captopril on mortality and morbidity in patients with left ventricular dysfunction after myocardial infarction. *N Engl J Med* 1992;327:669–677.

108. The Acute Infarction Ramipril Efficacy (AIRE) Study Investigators. Effect of ramipril on mortality and morbidity of survivors of acute myocardial infarction with clinical evidence of heart failure. *Lancet* 1993;342:821–828.

109. Kober L, Torp-Pedersen C, Carlsen JE, et al for the Trandolapril Cardiac Evaluation (TRACE) Study Group. A clinical trial of the angiotensin-converting-enzyme inhibitor trandolapril in patients with left ventricular dysfunction after myocardial infarction. *N Engl J Med* 1995;333:1670–1676.

110. Weintraub WS, Manohey E, Ghazzal Z. Trends in outcome and costs of coronary intervention in the 1990's. *Am J Cardiol* 2001;88:597–503.

111. Thompson RC, Holmes DR Jr, Grill DE, et al. TIMI IIIB Investigators. Effects of tissue plasminogen activator and a comparison of early invasive and conservative strategies in unstable angina and non-Q-wave myocardial infarction: Results of the TIMI IIIB Trial. *Circulation* 1994;89:1545.

112. Abenhaim HA, Eisenberg MJ, Schechter D. Comparison of six-month outcomes of percutaneous transluminal coronary angioplasty in patients $\geq$ 75 with those < 75 years of age (The ROSETTA Registry). *Am J Cardiol* 2001;87:1392–1395.

113. Peterson ED, Cowper PA, Jollis JG, et al. Outcomes of coronary artery bypass graft surgery in 24,461 patients aged 80 years or older. *Circulation* 1995;92(suppl II):II-85–II-91.

114. Freeman WK, Schaff HV, O'Brien PC, et al. Cardiac surgery in the octogenarian: Perioperative outcome and clinical follow-up. *J Am Coll Cardiol* 1991;18:29–35.

115. Newman MF, Kirchner JL, Phillips-Bute B, et al for the Neurological Outcome Research Group and the Cardiothoracic Anesthesiology Research Endeavors Investigators. Longitudinal assessment of neurocognitive function after coronary-artery bypass surgery. *N Engl J Med* 2001;344(6):395–402.

116. Nathoe HM, van Dijk D, Jansen WEL, et al. A comparison of on-pump and off-pump coronary bypass surgery in low-risk patients. *N Engl J Med* 2003;348:394–402.

117. Cleveland JC Jr, Shroyer AL, Chen AY, et al. Off-pump coronary artery bypass grafting decreases risk-adjusted mortality and morbidity. *Ann Thorac Surg* 2001;72:1282–1288.

118. The Sixth Report of the Joint National Committee on The TIME Investigators. Trial of invasive versus medical therapy in elderly patients with chronic symptomatic coronary-artery disease (TIME): A randomised trial. *Lancet* 2001;358:951–957.

119. Morrison DA, Sethi G, Sacks J, et al. Percutaneous coronary intervention versus coronary artery bypass graft surgery for patients with medically refractory myocardial ischemia and risk factors for adverse outcomes with bypass: A multicenter, randomized trial. *J Am Coll Cardiol* 2001;38:143–149.

120. Maycock CAA, Muhlestein JB, Horne BD, et al. Statin therapy is associated with reduced mortality across all age groups of individuals with significant coronary disease, including very elderly patients. *J Am Coll Cardiol* 2002;40:1777–1785.

121. Lewis SJ, Moye LA, Sacks FM, et al for the CARE Investigators. Effect of pravastatin on cardiovascular events in older patients with myocardial infarction and cholesterol levels in the average range. *Ann Intern Med* 1998;129:681–689.

122. Miettinen TA, Pyorala K, Olsson AG, et al for the Scandinavian Simvastatin Study Group. Cholesterol-lowering therapy in women and elderly patients with myocardial infarction or angina pectoris. *Circulation* 1997;96:4211–4218.

123. Sacks FM, Tonkin AM, Shepherd J, et al. Effect of pravastatin on coronary disease events in subgroups defined by coronary risk factors: The Prospective Pravastatin Pooling Project. *Circulation* 2000;102:1893–1900.

124. Heart Protection Study Collaborative Group. MRC/BHF Heart Protection Study of cholesterol lowering with simvastatin in 20,536 high-risk individuals: A randomized placebo-controlled trial. *Lancet* 2002;360:7–22.

125. Williams MA, Fleg JL, Ades PA, et al. Secondary prevention of coronary heart disease in the elderly (with emphasis on patients $\geq$ 75 years of age). *Circulation* 2002;105:1735–1743.

126. Burt VL, Whelton P, Roccella EJ, et al. Prevalence of hypertension in the US adult population: Results from the Third National Health and Nutrition Examination Survey, 1988–1991. *Hypertension* 1995;25:305–313.

127. Mitchell GF, Moyce LA, Braunwald E, et al. Sphygmanometrically determined pulse pressure is a powerful independent predictor of recurrent events after myocardial infarction in patients with impaired left ventricular function. *Circulation* 1997;96:4254–4260.

128. Chae CU, Pfeffer MA, Glynn RJ, et al. Increased pulse pressure and risk of heart failure in the elderly. *JAMA* 1999;281:634–639.

129. Management Committee of the Australian Therapeutic Trial in Mild Hypertension. Treatment of mild hypertension in the elderly. *Med J Aust* 1981;2:398.

130. SHEP Cooperative Research Group. Prevention of stroke by antihypertensive drug treatment in older persons with isolated systolic hypertension. *JAMA* 1991;265:3255.

131. Staessen JA, Fagard R, Thijs L, et al. Randomized double-blind comparison of placebo and active treatment for older patients with isolated systolic hypertension. *Lancet* 1997;350:757–764.

132. *Sixth Report of the Joint National Committee on Prevention, Detection, Evaluation, and Treatment of High Blood Pressure*. NIH Publ 98-4080. Bethesda, MD: National Institutes of Health, National Heart, Lung, and Blood Institute, National High Blood Pressure Education Program; November 1997.

133. Whelton PK, Appel LJ, Espeland MA, et al. Sodium reduction and weight loss in the treatment of hypertension in older persons: A randomized controlled trial of nonpharmacologic interventions in the elderly. *JAMA* 1998;279:839–846.

134. The ALLHAT Officers and Coordinators for the ALLHAT Collaborative Research Group. Major outcomes in high-risk hypertensive patients randomized to angiotensin-converting enzyme inhibitor or calcium channel blocker vs diuretic. *JAMA* 2002;288:2981–2997.

135. Zimmerman FH, Cameron A, Fisher LD, et al. Myocardial infarction in young adults: Angiographic characterization, risk factors and prognosis (Coronary Artery Surgery Study Registry). *J Am Coll Cardiol* 1995;26:654–661.

136. Rea TD, Heckbert SR, Kaplan RC, et al. Smoking status and risk for recurrent coronary events after myocardial infarction. *Ann Intern Med* 2002;137:494.

137. Hermanson B, Omenn GS, Kronmal RA, et al. Beneficial six-year outcome of smoking cessation in older men and women with coronary artery disease: Results from the CASS registry. *N Engl J Med* 1988;319:1365–1369.

138. Haffner SM, Lehto S, Ronnemaa T, et al. Mortality for coronary heart disease in subjects with type 2 diabetes and in nondiabetic subjects with and without prior myocardial infarction. *N Engl J Med* 1998;339:229–234.

139. Ford ES, Giles WH, Dietz WH. Prevalence of the metabolic syndrome among US adults. Findings from the Third National Health and Nutrition Education Survey. *JAMA* 2002;287:356–359.

140. Diabetes Prevention Program Research Group. Reduction in the incidence of type 2 diabetes with lifestyle intervention or metformin. *N Engl J Med* 2002;346:393–403.

141. Gaede P, Vedel P, Larsen N, et al. Multifactorial intervention and Cardiovascular disease in patients with type 2 diabetes. *N Engl J Med* 2003;348:383–393.

142. *2002 Heart and Stroke Statistical Update*. Dallas: American Heart Association, 2001.

143. Massie BM, Shah NH. Evolving trends in the epidemiologic factors of heart failure: Rationale for preventive strategies and comprehensive disease management. *Am Heart J* 1997;133:703–712.

144. Ho KK, Pinsky JL, Kannel WB, et al. The epidemiology of heart failure: The Framingham Study. *J Am Coll Cardiol* 1993;22(suppl):6A–13A.

145. Levy D, Kenchaiah S, Larson MG, et al. Long-term trends in the incidence of and survival with heart failure. *N Engl J Med* 2002;347:1397–1402.

146. Croft JB, Giles WH, Pollard RA, et al. Heart failure survival among older adults in the United States. *Arch Intern Med* 1999;159:505–510.

147. Centers for Disease Control and Prevention. Changes in mortality from heart failure—United States, 1980–1995. *JAMA* 1998;280: 874–875.

148. Graves EJ. National Hospital Discharge Survey: Annual summary, 1988. *Vital Health Stat* 13,1991:1–55.

149. Wolinsky FD, Overhage JM, Stump TE, et al. The sequelae of hospitalization for congestive heart failure among older adults. *J Am Geriatr Soc* 1997;45:558–563.

150. Domanski MJ, Mitchell GF, Norman JE, et al. Independent prognostic information provided by sphygmomanometrically determined pulse pressure and mean arterial pressure in patients with left ventricular dysfunction. *J Am Coll Cardiol* 1999;33:951–958.

151. Wong WF, Gold S, Fukuyama O, et al. Diastolic dysfunction in elderly patients with congestive heart failure. *Am J Cardiol* 1989;63: 1526–1528.

152. The Digitalis Investigation Group. The effect of digoxin on mortality and morbidity in patients with heart failure. *N Engl J Med* 1997;336: 525–533.

153. The CONSENSUS Trial Study Group. Effects of enalapril on mortality in severe congestive heart failure. *N Engl J Med* 1987;316:1429.

154. Packer M, Coats AJS, Fowler MB, et al. Effect of carvedilol on survival in severe chronic heart failure. *N Engl J Med* 2001;344: 1651–1658.

155. Pitt B, Zannad F, Remme WJ, et al for the Randomized Aldactone Study Investigators: The effect of spironolactone on morbidity and mortality in patients with severe heart failure. *N Engl J Med* 1999;341: 709–717.

156. Abraham WT, Fisher WG, Smith AL, et al. Cardiac resynchronization in chronic heart failure. *N Engl J Med* 2002;346:1845–1853.

157. Rose EA, Gelllins AC, Moskowitz AJ, et al. Long-term use of a left ventricular assist device for end-stage heart failure. *N Engl J Med* 2001;345:1435–1443.

158. Kitzman DW, Little WC, Anderson RT, et al. Pathophysiological characterization of isolated diastolic heart failure in comparison to systolic heart failure. *JAMA* 2002;288:2144–2150.

159. Vasan RS, Larson MG, Benjamin EJ, et al. Congestive heart failure in subjects with normal versus reduced left ventricular ejection fraction: Prevalence and mortality in a population-based cohort. *J Am Coll Cardiol* 1999;33:1948–1955.

160. Dauterman KW, Massie BM, Gheorghiade M. Heart failure associated with preserved systolic function: A common and costly clinical entity. *Am Heart J* 1998;135:S310–S319.

161. Gandhi SK, Powers JC, Nomeir A-M, et al. The pathogenesis of acute pulmonary edema associated with hypertension. *N Engl J Med* 2001; 344:17–22.

162. Swedberg K, Pfeffer M, Granger C, et al. Candesartan in heart failure—Assessment of reduction in mortality and morbidity (CHARM): rationale and design. *J Card Fail* 1999;5:276–282.

163. Rich MW, Beckham V, Wittenberg C, et al. A multidisciplinary intervention to prevent the readmission of elderly patients with congestive heart failure. *N Engl J Med* 1995;333:1190–1195.

164. Stewart S, Pearson S, Horowitz JD. Effects of a home-based intervention among patients with congestive heart failure discharged from acute hospital care. *Arch Intern Med* 1998;158:1067–1072.

165. Kasper EK, Gerstenblith G, Hefter G, et al. A randomized trial of the efficacy of multi-disciplinary care in heart failure outpatients at high risk of hospital readmission. *J Am Coll Cardiol* 39:471–480, 2002.

166. Furberg CD, Psaty BM, Manolio TA, et al. Prevalence of atrial fibrillation in elderly subjects (the Cardiovascular Health Study). *Am J Cardiol* 1994;74:236–241.

167. Alberts GW. Atrial fibrillation and stroke. *Arch Intern Med* 1994;154: 1443–1448.

168. Goette A, Honeycutt C, Langberg JJ. Electrical remodeling in atrial fibrillation: time course and mechanisms. *Circulation* 1996;94: 2968–2974.

169. Zipes D. Atrial fibrillation: A tachycardia-induced atrial cardiomyopathy. *Circulation* 1997;95:562–564.

170. Daoud EG, Weiss R, Bahu M, et al. Effect of an irregular ventricular rhythm on cardiac output. *Am J Cardiol* 1996;78:1433–1436.

171. Wolf PA, Abbott RD, Kannel WB. Atrial fibrillation: A major contributor to stroke in the elderly. *Arch Intern Med* 1987;147:1561.

172. Atrial Fibrillation Investigators: Risk factors for stroke and efficacy of antithrombotic therapy in atrial fibrillation: Analysis of pooled data from five randomized trials. *Arch Intern Med* 1994;154:1449–1457.

173. Ozcan C, Zahangir A, Friedman PA, et al. Long-term survival after ablation of the atrioventricular node and implantation of a permanent pacemaker in patients with atrial fibrillation. *N Engl J Med* 2001;344: 1043–1051.

174. Klein AL, Grimm RA, Murray RD, et al. Use of transesophageal echocardiography to guide cardioversion in patients with atrial fibrillation. *N Engl J Med* 2001;344:1411–1420.

175. The Atrial Fibrillation Follow-Up Investigation of Rhythm Management (AFFIRM) Investigators: A comparison of rate control and rhythm control in patients with atrial fibrillation. *N Engl J Med* 2002; 347:1825–1833.

176. Van Gelder IC, Hagens VE, Hosker HA, et al. A comparison of rate control and rhythm control in patients with recurrent persistent atrial fibrillation. *N Engl J Med* 2002;347:1834–1840.

177. Torp-Pedersen C, Moller M, Bloch-Thomsen PE, et al. for the Danish Investigations of Arrhythmia and Mortality on Dofetilide Study Group: Dofetilide in patients with congestive heart failure and left ventricular dysfunction. *N Engl J Med* 1999;341:857–865.

178. Roy D, Talajic M, Dorian P, et al. Amiodarone to prevent recurrence of atrial fibrillation. *N Engl J Med* 2000;342:913–920.

179. Haissaguerre M, Jais P, Shah DC, et al. Electrophysiological end point for catheter ablation of atrial fibrillation initiated from multiple pulmonary venous foci. *Circulation* 2000;101:1409–1417.

180. Lamas GA, Pashos CL, Normand S, et al. Permanent pacemaker selection and subsequent survival in elderly Medicare pacemaker recipients. *Circulation* 1995;91:1063–1069.

181. Lamas GA, Lee KL, Sweeney MO, et al. Ventricular pacing or dual-chamber pacing for sinus node dysfunction. *N Engl J Med* 2002;346: 1854–1862.

182. Tresh DD, Trouop PH, Thakur RK, et al. Comparison of efficacy of automatic implantable cardioverter defibrillator in patients older and younger than 65 years of age. *Am J Med* 1991;90:717–724.

183. Moss AJ, Zareba W, Hall J, et al. Prophylactic implantation of a defibrillator in patients with myocardial infarction and reduced ejection fraction. *N Engl J Med* 2002;346:877–883.

184. Isoyama S, Wei JY, Izumo S, et al. The effect of age on the development of cardiac hypertrophy produced by aortic constriction in the rat. *Circ Res* 1987;61:337–342.

185. Olsson M, Thyberg J, Nilsson J. Presence of oxidized low density lipoprotein in nonrheumatic stenotic aortic valves. *Arterioscler Thromb Vasc Biol* 1999;19:1218–1222.

186. O'Brien KD, Kuusisto J, Reichenbach DD, et al. Osteopontin is expressed in human aortic valvular lesions. *Circulation* 1995;92: 2163–2168.

187. Stewart BF, Siscovick D, Lind BK, et al. Clinical factors associated with calcific aortic valve disease. *J Am Coll Cardiol* 1997;29:630–634.

188. Novaro GM, Tiong IY, Pearce GL, et al. Effect of hydroxymethylglutaryl coenzyme A reductase inhibitors on the progression of calcific aortic stenosis. *Circulation* 2001;104:2205–2209.

189. Pellikka PA, Nushimura RA, Bailey KR, et al. The natural history of adults with asymptomatic hemodynamically significant aortic stenosis. *J Am Coll Cardiol* 1990;15:1012–1017.

190. Carabello BA. Aortic stenosis. *N Engl J Med* 2002;346:677–682.

191. Nishimura RA, Grantham JA, Connolly HM, et al. Low-output, low-gradient aortic stenosis in patients with depressed left ventricular systolic function. *Circulation* 2002;106(7):809–813.

192. Lindblom D, Lindblom U, Qvist J, et al. Long-term relative survival rates after heart valve replacement. *J Am Coll Cardiol* 1990;15: 566–573.

193. Logeais Y, Langanay T, Roussin R, et al. Surgery for aortic stenosis in elderly patients. A study of surgical risk and predictive factors. *Circulation* 1994;90:2891–2898.

194. Bernard Y, Etievent J, Mourand JL, et al. Long-term results of percutaneous aortic valvuloplasty compared with aortic valve replacement

in patients more than 75 years old. *J Am Coll Cardiol* 1992;20: 792–801.

195. Carabello BA, Crawford FA. Medical progress: Valvular heart disease. *N Engl J Med* 1997;337:32–41.

196. Scognamiglio R, Rahimtoola SH, Fasoli G, et al. Nifedipine in asymptomatic patients with severe aortic regurgitation and normal left ventricular function. *N Engl J Med* 1994;331:689–694.

197. Reyes VP, Raju S, Wynne J, et al. Percutaneous balloon valvuloplasty compared with open surgical commissurotomy for mitral stenosis. *N Engl J Med* 1994;331:961–967.

198. Tuzcu EM, Block PC, Griffin BP, et al. Immediate and long-term outcome of percutaneous mitral valvotomy in patients 65 years and older. *Circulation* 1992;85:963–971.

199. ACC/AHA guidelines for the management of patients with valvular heart disease: A report of the American College of Cardiology/ American Heart Association Task Force on Practice Guidelines (Committee on Management of Patients with Valvular Heart Disease). *J Am Coll Cardiol* 1998;32:1486–1588.

200. Levine HF, Gaasch WH. Vasoactive drugs in chronic regurgitant lesions of the mitral and aortic valves. *J Am Coll Cardiol* 1996;28: 1083–1091.

201. Otto CM. Evaluation and management of chronic mitral regurgitation. *N Engl J Med* 2001;345:740–746.

202. Holper K, Ottke M, Lewe T, et al. Bioprosthetic and mechanical valves in the elderly: Benefits and risks. *Ann Thorac Surg* 1995;60: S443–S446.

203. Burr LH, Jamieson RE, Munro AI, et al. Porcine bioprostheses in the elderly: Clinical performance by age groups and valve positions. *Ann Thorac Surg* 1995;60:S264–S269.

WOMEN AND CORONARY ARTERY DISEASE

Pamela Charney

Cardiovascular mortality is increasing in American women while it is decreasing in men (Fig. 97-1). Yet, the importance of coronary artery disease (CAD) in women has not adequately captured public and physician attention.[1] In a national telephone survey of over 1000 American women, only 33 percent identified heart disease as a leading cause of death in women,[2] despite evidence to the contrary (Fig. 97-2).

The impact of the interaction between sex and age is clinically important. Middle-aged women have a lower CAD mortality rate than middle-aged men. In middle-aged populations around the world, there is a consistent ratio of male-to-female CAD deaths, varying from 2.5 to 4.5.[3] The etiology of excess CAD mortality in middle-aged men has not been determined, although the variable differences between countries suggest that "sex is not destiny with regard to CHD [coronary heart disease]."[3] With increasing age, the differences in mortality rates between women and men decrease. As CAD identification and risk-factor management have focused on middle-aged men, rates of CAD mortality have dropped. To affect CAD mortality in women, increased attention will have to be given to these issues for women by both physicians and patients.

PREVENTION: GENDER-SPECIFIC ISSUES

Tobacco

Tobacco exposure is the single most important coronary artery risk factor for women and men.[1,4,5] Tobacco exposure can occur through personal use of tobacco or by inhaling secondhand smoke. In epidemiologic studies, greater exposure in amount and duration is related to higher CAD events in a dose-related fashion.[6,7] More white women smoke than Hispanic or black women.[8] Cigarette smoking has been associated with an earlier age of first myocardial infarction (see also Chap. 43) and menopause.[5] Since middle-aged women experience less symptomatic CAD than middle-aged men, the increased risk of myocardial infarction and sudden death related to tobacco use is greater for women than men. There is a dose-response relationship for CAD in diabetic women who smoke, as discussed further below, in the discussion of diabetes.[6]

Over the last several decades, American women's personal use of cigarettes has not decreased as dramatically as it has among men (Fig. 97-3). The prevalence of cigarette use among women reflects both higher initiation rates and greater difficulty discontinuing cigarette use.[4] Women smokers are more likely than men to report that smoking cigarettes helps them to deal with emotional stress.

Women have more difficulty quitting cigarette use both initially and in the long term. However, successful tobacco cessation for women, as for men, dramatically decreases the risk of further coronary events.[4–6] Black smokers also have low both short- and long-term cigarette cessation rates.[4,9]

Women contemplating smoking cessation are often concerned about potential weight gain, a common consequence of efforts to stop smoking.[4,9] Weight gain with tobacco cessation is on average 7 to 10 lb, with fewer than 10 percent gaining more than 20 lb. Weight gain tends to be higher among women, blacks, and smokers who inhale more than 25 cigarettes per day. In contrast, women smokers report that they are unwilling to experience any or minimal weight increase as a result of smoking cessation.[4,9] Yet smokers trying to lose weight are still interested in discontinuing the use of tobacco.[9]

To avoid weight gain with tobacco cessation, several types of interventions have been recommended.[4] Realistic expectations may be helpful as well as exercise, careful choice of snacks, and appropriate pharmacotherapy. Increasing physical activity contributes to success in smoking cessation, as does an increased expenditure of calories, even if it does not modify weight gain.[10] Craving for sweets may occur, and having on hand sweet snacks that are low in sugar may limit caloric consumption.

Multiple pharmacologic therapies are available.[4,11,12] Nicotine replacement products about double tobacco cessation success compared with tobacco cessation groups alone. The patch has the highest compliance rate and provides smoother levels than the gum, spray, or lozenge. The use of the patch with a shorter-acting nicotine replacement product providing a rapid boost in nicotine level is safe and improves success.[11] Bupropion has been found to be effective in

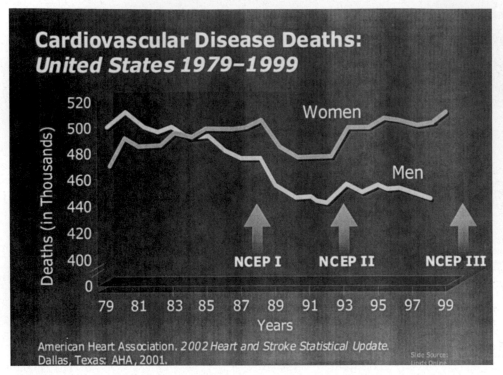

FIGURE 97-1 Graph comparing rates of coronary artery disease for women and men over the last two decades, with marks when cholesterol guidelines were released. (Developed from the American Heart Association 2002 Heart and Stroke Statistical Update data by www.lipidsonline.org. With permission.)

may have more trouble giving up tobacco than white smokers.[12–14] Physiologic addiction in black smokers may previously have been underestimated, resulting in undertreatment of nicotine addiction. In a comparison of black and white smokers consuming similar amounts of tobacco, black smokers were found to have higher blood levels of cotinine than white smokers.[13]

Many surveys reveal that physicians can have a powerful effect on smoking cessation, even with minimal effort.[4,15] Unfortunately, most programs to aid smokers with CAD have not focused on women's special issues.[15] Programs that promote activities to minimize weight gain and stress social support may be more effective for women. Additional research is needed. In the meantime, "Simple advice by one's physician to stop smoking is more effective than no advice at all, and as the physician-delivered smoking intervention becomes more intensive, the effects are greater."[15]

improving tobacco cessation rates in both white and black smokers[12] and is reported to minimize weight gain while it is used.[4,12] Although bupropion is an antidepressant, it has been effective in smokers who are not depressed. Bupropion is contraindicated in patients with a history of seizures (since it lowers the seizure threshold), head trauma, or heavy alcohol consumption. Bupropion can exacerbate symptoms related to anorexia and bulimia and should be avoided if there is a history of these disorders or recent use of a monoamine oxidase (MAO) inhibitor. It has been observed that black smokers

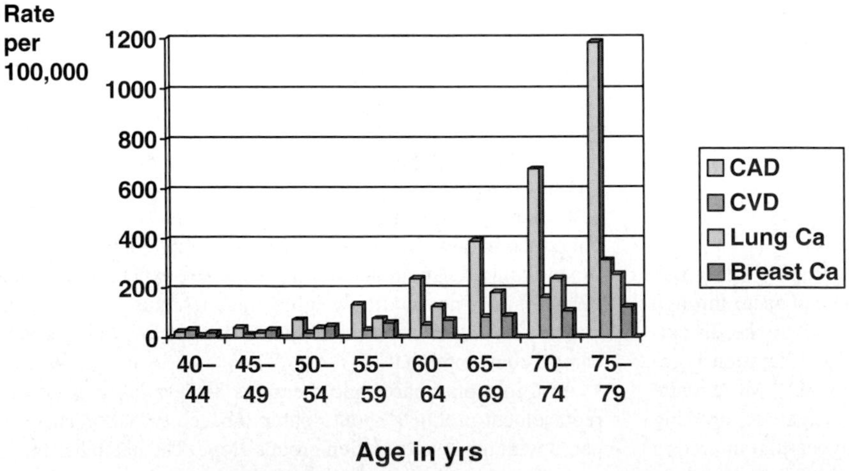

Diabetes

Diabetic individuals have higher mortality rates from coronary artery disease than nondiabetics[16–19] (see also Chap. 86). In the last decade, CHD mortality rates have increased by 23 percent in diabetic women, while they have decreased by 27 percent in nondiabetic women. This is in comparison to diabetic men, where mortality rates have declined by 13 percent, while they have decreased by 36 percent in nondiabetic men[16] (Fig. 97-4). Diabetic women have CAD rates similar to those of diabetic men, so the "female advantage" is lost.

Diabetic women also have higher in-hospital mortality after myocardial infarction (MI) and an increased incidence of congestive heart failure (CHF) than do diabetic men.[16]

In a subgroup analysis of the WHO MONICA Project (World Health Organization Multinational Monitoring of Trends and Determinants of Cardiovascular Disease), the 1-year mortality in Finland after a first hospitalization for MI was 44.2 percent in diabetic men, 32.6 percent in nondiabetic men, 36.9 percent in diabetic women, and 20.2 percent in nondiabetic women.[17] In a review of data from the National Registry of Myocardial Infarction II, women's increased mortality post-MI was not associated with glycemic control but rather with hypertension and hyperlipidemia.[20] Further research is required to determine whether these

FIGURE 97-2 Age-specific mortality for coronary artery disease (CAD), cerebrovascular disease (CVD), lung cancer, and breast cancer in women in the United States, 1997. (From Wingo PA, Calle EE, McTiernan A. *J Women's Health Gender Based Med* 2000;9(9):999–1006. With permission.)

observations reflect gender differences in risk factors or natural history, or whether less aggressive CAD prevention in diabetic women plays a role.

Diabetic women and men with hypertension have especially high rates of CAD.[20] Native Americans, Mexican Americans, and black populations have a higher prevalence of both diabetes and hypertension than American white populations.[8] Women and men generally have similar incidence rates of diabetes, although more women become hypertensive with increasing age.

Women at risk for developing diabetes include obese women and those who have experienced gestational diabetes (compared with women who have had a pregnancy without glucose intolerance).[21] Greater weight is associated with greater insulin resistance as well as a higher rate of glucose intolerance. Even a moderate increase in physical activity (such as walking 3 h per week) and avoiding weight gain decreases the risk of developing diabetes.[16]

Lipid abnormalities are common in diabetic patients. At the time of diagnosis of type II diabetes, women have substantially lower high-density lipoprotein (HDL) cholesterol than age-matched nondiabetic women.[22] Other lipid abnormalities are also present, including elevated triglycerides. Subgroup analysis of diabetic patients treated with HMG-CoA reductase inhibitors documented improved lipoprotein patterns with treatment and fewer CAD events.[16] Studies including more women diabetics are in progress.

Insulin resistance is characterized by elevated levels of circulating insulin and is associated with glucose intolerance, higher levels of free fatty acids, central obesity, and hypertension.[16] One clinical example is polycystic ovarian syndrome, where increased androgens, lower HDL, and higher triglycerides and higher rates of coronary artery disease have been noted.[23] Genetic mapping suggests that polycystic ovarian syndrome is related to inherited alterations in insulin production.[24] In women with polycystic ovarian syndrome, treatment with metformin appears to reduce systolic blood pressure and hyperinsulinemia and to aid amenorrhea.

The "metabolic syndrome" was defined in the Third Report of the National Cholesterol Education Program Expert Panel on Detection, Evaluation, and Treatment of High Blood Cholesterol[25] to include obesity, glucose intolerance, hypertension, and lipid abnormalities (see Chap. 87). The metabolic syndrome is present in 22 to 24 percent of evaluated Americans over 20 years of age, with greater rates with increasing age.[26]

For diabetic women, the dose-response hazards of tobacco use have been documented in the Nurses' Health Study with 20 years' follow-up.[6] The relative risk for a CAD event was 2.68 for current

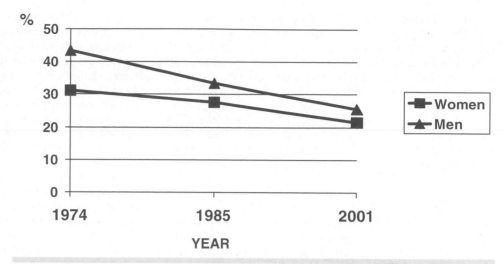

FIGURE 97-3 Prevalence of smoking among men and women in the United States. (Data from Thorndike AN, Rigotti NA, Stafford RS, Singer DE. National patterns in the treatment of smokers by physicians. *JAMA* 1998;279(8): 604–608 and U.S. Department of Health and Human Services. Centers for Disease Control and Prevention, Office of Smoking and Health. *MMWR* 2001;52:303–307. With permission.)

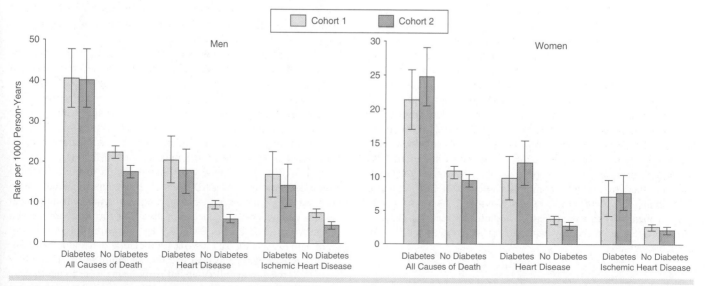

FIGURE 97-4 Change in mortality rates in women and men diabetics compared with nondiabetics. Cohort 1 was defined in 1971–1975 and followed up through 1982–1984, while cohort 2 was defined in 1982–1984 and followed through 1992–1993. (From Gu K, Cowie C, Harris M. Diabetes and decline in heart disease mortality in U.S. adults. JAMA 1999;281(14):1291–1297. With permission.)

diabetic smokers of more than 15 cigarettes daily, 1.66 for current diabetic smokers of less than 15 cigarettes daily, and 1.21 for past diabetic smokers, all compared with women who had never smoked ($p < 0.001$ for trend). Diabetic women who had not smoked for 10 years had a risk similar to that of nonsmoking diabetic women.

In summary, diabetic women should be considered at high risk for coronary artery disease events.[16-18] Aggressive management of tobacco use,[8] lipoprotein abnormalities,[16,22] and hypertension,[16] if present, is beneficial. Regular exercise can also improve glucose control[16] and insulin resistance.[16,27] There is some evidence that glucose control decreases vascular disease.[16]

Hypertension

The prevalence of hypertension also increases with advancing age, and since life expectancy is greater for women than men, there are more elderly women with hypertension.[28] At all ages, black women and men have about double the incidence of hypertension as their white counterparts. Generally, women are more likely to have controlled blood pressure (BP) than men.

Both systolic and diastolic blood pressures have been found in population, cohort, and treatment studies to predict coronary events. Framingham data revealed that with a systolic BP greater than 180, the annual incidence of coronary heart disease (angina, coronary insufficiency, myocardial infarction, or death from these diagnoses) in women over 65 years of age is greater than 30 percent, while for older men above age 65, it is about 50 percent.[29] In other epidemiologic studies, higher diastolic BP also predicts greater rates of clinical CAD.[30]

While treatment trials have also documented that lower BP decreases the incidence of a first MI and sudden death, this effect has been less dramatic than the decrease in stroke occurrence with BP control. Analysis of MI prevention in women has also been limited by the smaller number of first MIs in middle-aged women, the age group predominantly studied in early pharmacologic treatment trials.[31] Once older subjects were studied in clinical trials, the benefit of treating hypertension to prevent coronary events received greater recognition.[32,33] As Kannel states, "coronary disease is the most common and lethal sequela of hypertension, equaling in incidence all the other cardiovascular outcomes combined."[34]

Gender-specific information about pharmacologic therapy of hypertension with thiazide diuretics and angiotensin-converting enzyme (ACE) inhibitors is available. Thiazide diuretics are a preferred first choice in the treatment of hypertension in women as well as men (Chap. 61) and are also beneficial for bone health.[35] Epidemiologic studies have documented a reduction of about one-third in hip fracture with the use of thiazide diuretics. In a randomized, double-blind, placebo-controlled trial, thiazides were associated with preservation of hip and spine bone mineral density.[35] ACE inhibitors should be utilized cautiously in women of reproductive age because these drugs are potentially teratogenic, especially in the second trimester.[36] Potentially fertile women must understand the risk to the fetus before initiating therapy. Cough, a common side effect of first-generation ACE inhibitors, occurred substantially more frequently in women than in men.[36] With the advent of angiotensin receptor blockers (ARBs), alternative therapy without this side effect has become available.

Lipids

There are important gender differences in lipoprotein profiles.[37] Total cholesterol peaks in women from age 55 to 64 and in men at around age 50. HDL is usually greater in women than in men, with

HDL levels remaining similar with increasing age. Many experts consider HDL more predictive for women than any other lipoprotein component, with the strongest correlation between low HDL levels and CAD events. Low-density lipoprotein (LDL) levels increase with increasing age for both women and men and are especially predictive of events in men. Triglyceride levels may be important in women but have not been shown to be independently important in men.

Secondary prevention with pharmacologic treatment of hyperlipidemia decreases CAD events in women as well as men. Yet these agents are underprescribed after MI and target treatment levels are not reached.[38] Primary prevention trials for hyperlipidemia in women have often lacked adequate power. With the inclusion of older subjects and newer agents, such as the HMG-CoA reductase inhibitors (which simultaneously decrease LDL and increase HDL), clearer evidence of benefit for primary prevention is emerging.

With the latest cholesterol treatment guidelines, diabetic women are candidates for primary prevention with aggressive treatment of lipid abnormalities.[25] There is still controversy about the cost-benefit ratio for aggressive treatment in the woman at low risk for vascular disease.

Treatment of hyperlipidemia is discussed in detail in Chap. 43. In short-term studies, the HMG-CoA reductase inhibitors have been compared with hormone replacement therapy regimens.[39,40] Although both types of agents improve HDL, the HMG-CoA reductase inhibitors are more effective in improving LDL than is hormonal therapy. Triglyceride levels often increase with hormonal therapy and decrease with the HMG-CoA reductase inhibitors.[39,40] Further on in this chapter, the risks and potential benefits of hormonal therapy are discussed.

Obesity

The prevalence of obesity has been steadily increasing, as illustrated in comparing U.S. prevalence rates in 1990 and 2000 (Fig. 97-5A and B). Over 50 percent of black or Mexican-American women and 30 percent of white women are obese. In the recent third National Health and Nutrition Examination Survey, body mass index (BMI) was greater among black and Mexican-American women than white women (mean BMI was 29.2 kg/m^2 for black women, 28.6 kg/m^2 for Mexican-American women, and 26.3 kg/m^2 for white women).[41] Racial differences in BMI, as well as glycosylated hemoglobin, start in childhood, with black and Mexican-American girls having less favorable profiles than white girls.[8]

Obesity is linked to multiple cardiac risk factors (including insulin resistance, diabetes, hypertension, and hyperlipidemia) and independently associated with coronary artery event rates.[42] The pattern of weight distribution is also predictive of coronary events, with more events among women with the "apple" shape, with a greater central or abdominal girth, than among those with the "pear" shape, with more weight on the hips and buttocks.[43,44] A greater waist circumference increases health risk regardless of BMI.[44]

Increased physical activity or limited weight loss is associated with a decreased risk of CAD events.[43] Behavioral interventions to decrease weight have been most successful when there is a physical activity component.[43,44] One innovative trial for 40 obese women (mean weight 89.2 kg and BMI 32.9 kg) compared a 16-week program with instruction on a low-fat 1200-calorie diet and either training to increase daily physical exertion or addition of an aerobics class.[44] At the 1-year follow-up, all participants were found to have lost weight. Women who had increased their activities of daily living most successfully sustained weight reduction after a year. A study of obese twins revealed that lack of physical activity correlated with which twin was more obese.[43] While new pharmacologic treatments

Obesity Trends* Among U.S. Adults
BRFSS, 1990

(*BMI ≥ 30, or ~ 30 lbs overweight for 5′4″ woman)

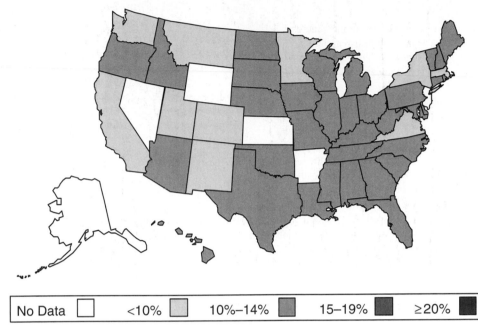

| No Data ☐ | <10% ☐ | 10%–14% ☐ | 15–19% ☐ | ≥20% ■ |

Source: Mokdad AH.

A

Obesity Trends* Among U.S. Adults
BRFSS, 2000

(*BMI ≥ 30, or ~ 30 lbs overweight for 5′4″ woman)

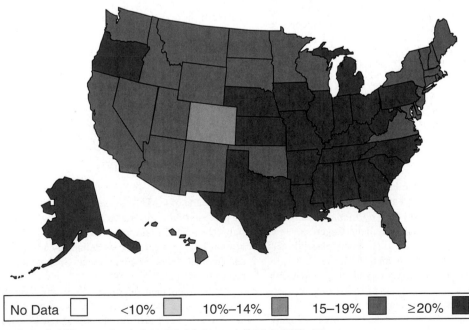

| No Data ☐ | <10% ☐ | 10%–14% ☐ | 15–19% ☐ | ≥20% ■ |

Source: Mokdad AH, et al. *J Am Med Assoc* 2001;286:10

B

FIGURE 97-5 *A* and *B*. Obesity prevalence maps of the United States in 1990 and 2000. (From the Centers for Disease Control, 2001.)

for obesity have been developed, many have been documented to be hazardous.[45]

Physical Activity and Exercise

Generally, women have smaller hearts, so cardiac output is increased by raising heart rate. Men, in comparison, accomplish an increase in cardiac output by increasing stroke volume. Therefore women's physiologic response to exercise includes a lower work capacity and oxygen uptake.[46]

Studies on women and physical activity have substantial limitations, since historically data collection has excluded housework and child care. These reports may have greatly underestimated the actual amount of energy expended daily. Yet in national surveys, sedentary lifestyles are reported by as many as 70 percent of adult women, with higher rates among black and Hispanic women and those with less education or lower income.[41] Especially for women, encouraging increased activity during activities of daily living is probably more important than counseling them on initiating an exercise program.

Physical activity is also important as secondary prevention. Both women and men benefit from referral to cardiac rehabilitation programs after MI. Currently, fewer women than men are referred for cardiac rehabilitation.[47]

Menopause and Hormonal Replacement Therapy

The importance of menopause as a risk factor for CAD in women is still being defined. Women with early menopause after gynecologic surgery have been considered at higher risk for CAD and osteoporosis on the basis of less hormonal exposure.[48] However, a 1999 analysis from the Nurses' Health Study found only women smokers with a younger age of menopause have a greater risk of CAD.[49]

Many American postmenopausal women use hormonal replacement therapy, and these medications were the second most frequently filled prescription in the United States in 2000.[50] Although population surveys have suggested that hormonal replacement therapy may decrease the risk of CAD, the women using hormones reported less tobacco exposure, greater levels of exercise, and readier access to medical care; they also tended to be healthier and wealthier.[50–52] Results of prospective randomized clinical trials indicate that the combination of estrogen and progestin after menopause increases CAD risk. Evaluation of the preventive value of estrogen alone in women without a uterus is currently ongoing. Estrogen alone is contraindicated in women with a uterus because of the associated increased risk of endometrial cancer. The Women's Health Initiative (WHI)[51] and Heart & Estrogen/Progestin Replacement Study (HERS)[53] are critical to our understanding of the impact of hormone replacement therapy on cardiovascular disease.

The Women's Health Initiative is the largest study of aging ever funded; it enrolled women age 50 to 79 years of age.[53] There are four arms of this national randomized control trial: hormonal therapy (estrogen with progestin for women with a uterus and estrogen alone for women after hysterectomy); very low fat diet versus placebo; calcium and vitamin D versus placebo, and a control arm.

The safety monitoring board prematurely halted the estrogen with progestin arm in 2002 because, with 5.2 years of follow-up, the overall health risks were greater than the benefit. The absolute additional risk was 7 more CAD events, 8 additional strokes, 8 more pulmonary emboli, and 8 additional invasive breast cancers for each 1000 women treated for 10 years. In contrast, there would be only 6 fewer colon cancers and 5 fewer hip fractures in 1000 women treated for 10 years. The risk of CAD events increased within the first year (Fig. 97-6), as did the risk of developing pulmonary emboli.

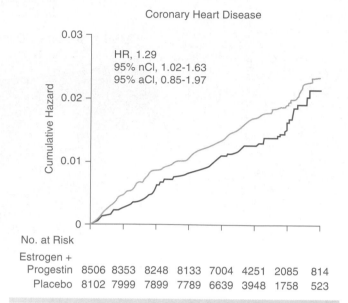

FIGURE 97-6 The effect of hormone replacement therapy over the first few years on coronary heart disease events. (From Writing Group for the Women's Health Initiative Investigators. Risks and benefits of estrogen plus progestin in healthy postmenopausal women: Principal results from the Women's Health Initiative randomized controlled trial. *JAMA* 2002;288:321–333. With permission.)

While HERS was a secondary prevention clinical trial of hormonal therapy, results also did not demonstrate cardiovascular benefit.[53] These postmenopausal women had evidence of CAD [MI, coronary artery bypass grafting (CABG), percutaneous transluminal coronary angioplasty (PTCA) for occlusion greater than 50 percent, or angiography with more than one major coronary artery]. With no overall reduction in CAD events, substantially more venous thrombotic events occurred in the group receiving hormonal therapy. Therefore hormonal replacement therapy should be avoided in the setting of acute coronary ischemia. Also remarkable in HERS was the lack of secondary prevention reported in these women with known heart disease (Fig. 97-7).

National guidelines have reflected WHI and HERS results and emphasize other modalities for the prevention of heart disease in women.[52] In counseling menopausal women, a review of cardiovascular prevention should be a focus. Hormonal therapy is generally used to control severe vasomotor symptoms.

Psychosocial Risk Factors

Both socioeconomic and psychological factors affect the prevalence and outcome of CAD[54,55] (see Chap. 91). Coronary disease morbidity and mortality are greater among those of lower socioeconomic status (SES).[54,55] Markers for SES have included years of formal education, owning a car, income defined by absolute or relative amount, and parental status.[55] More recently SES has also been defined independently of race.[8,41]

Women and men of lower SES from several United Kingdom studies were at increased risk for symptomatic CAD compared to those of a higher SES from the same area.[55–57] Lower SES has also been related to higher rates of tobacco use and higher inpatient mortality after MI.[56] Differences in event rates were greater for women than for men between different socioeconomic classes.

Depression, which is diagnosed twice as often in women as in men, affects outcomes in CAD.[54,58,59] Prospective data from the Baltimore Epidemiologic Catchment Area Study correlated a history of dysphoria or a major depressive episode with an increased risk of MI for both women and men.[58] A positive response to a single question was central: "In your lifetime, have you ever had 2 weeks or more during which you felt sad, blue, depressed, or when you lost all interest and pleasure in things that you usually cared about or enjoyed?" The positive answer was associated with a 2.07 odds ratio of self-reporting an MI infarction at 13 years follow-up, compared with those giving a negative response, independent of other coronary risk factors. Depression diagnosed with a patient interview 5 to 15 days after MI was a significant predictor of mortality at 6 months.[60] Although fewer women than men agreed to participate in this observational study, depression was more common in women than in men. As early as 1991, the question of whether a higher rate of depression in women after MI correlated with gender differences in prognosis was raised[61]; the answer is still unclear. Although an adequate pharmacologic interventional trial of depression diagnosed after MI in women has not yet been reported, the selective serotonin reuptake inhibitors have been found to be clinically safe in the presence of cardiac disease.[59]

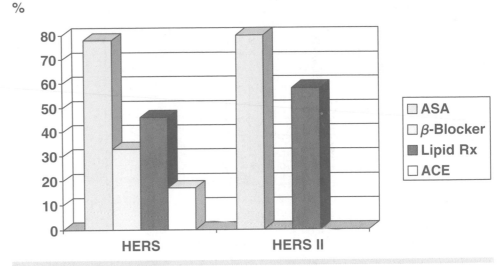

FIGURE 97-7 Bar graph showing use of preventive medications by participants in HERS at enrollment. (Adapted from Grady D, Herrington D, Bittner V, et al. Cardiovascular disease outcomes during 6.8 years of hormone therapy: Heart and Estrogen/Progestin Replacement Study Follow-Up (HERS II). *JAMA* 2002;288:49–57. With permission.)

Race, Women, and Coronary Artery Disease

Black women's CAD mortality rates are related to traditional CAD risk factors as well as racial and socioeconomic issues.[55] Combined analysis of data from the 1986 National Mortality Feedback Survey, the 1985 National Health Interview Survey, and the U.S. Bureau of the Census revealed that young black women (age <55) had more than twice the rate of CAD mortality (sudden and nonsudden) as young white Americans.[62] CAD death rates for young black women in this study exceeded rates for young men and white women. Importantly, family income, educational level, and occupational status accounted for more of this observed difference than traditional coronary risk factors.[62] In HERS, a large secondary prevention trial of estrogen/progestin, black women were at increased risk for coronary events at 6 years of follow-up [relative hazard (RH) 2.05 with confidence interval (CI) 1.52 to 2.77, $p < 0.001$].[63]

With the application of careful methodology, Mexican-American women have coronary heart disease mortality rates higher or equal to those of non-Hispanic white American women.[64] This observation is consistent with the higher rates of obesity, hypertension, and diabetes among Mexican-American women than among white women, even if tobacco use is less frequent.[41] The prevalence of the metabolic syndrome is substantially greater among Mexican Americans (32 percent) than among white and black Americans.[26] Other Hispanic populations have not been studied as extensively.

Racial differences in physiology have also begun to be considered. Differences among electrocardiographic findings among black and white healthy subjects were detailed in 1998.[66] Differences in tobacco metabolism, such as slower cotinine clearance and higher serum cotinine levels, are seen in black smokers compared with white and Hispanic smokers.[13,67]

DIAGNOSIS OF CORONARY ARTERY DISEASE IN WOMEN

Since CAD is often diagnosed clinically by a careful history, preconceived biases can affect perception of CAD risk. In one study, an actress portrayed a woman twice with the same script but with different clothes and affect. Physicians who reviewed the video in which the actress described chest pain with "exaggerated emotional presentation style" predicted less CAD than when the same script was presented with a "businesslike effect."[68] More recently, physicians were recruited to view a video of different actors (black and white women and men) accompanied by the same written information. The black woman was least likely to be referred for cardiac catheterization.[69] If the diagnosis of CAD is not considered, then evaluation and management will not occur. The clinical history typical for angina and acute coronary syndromes is reviewed at the beginning of the appropriate sections below as well as in Chap. 12.

Once CAD is considered as a diagnosis, further evaluation is required to assess disease presence and severity. Noninvasive stress testing can help assess disease control and determine which patients with an intermediate risk for CAD will benefit from further interventions.[70] More extensive discussion can be found in Chap. 16, but potential gender differences in noninvasive testing are discussed briefly here. Unfortunately, each of the noninvasive techniques has limitations in women.[71,72]

Exercise stress testing is the oldest noninvasive way to assess CAD risk. However, if a completed exercise stress test reveals ST-segment changes and depression greater than 1 mm, especially in younger women (where the prevalence of ST-segment depression is less), this may indicate significant CAD.[73] In comparison, a negative exercise stress test with adequate exertion is often helpful because it decreases the need to consider cardiac catheterization.[70,74] Gender-specific criteria have been proposed to compensate for the generally smaller ST-segment changes seen in women.[74] The discussion of angina below includes a review of the potential impact of the menstrual cycle on stress testing.

As a rule, stress imaging techniques are favored in assessing a woman for possible CAD or staging the severity of disease. Local

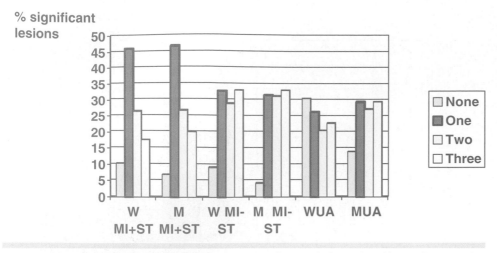

% significant
lesions

FIGURE 97-8 Comparison of clinical presentations of women and men with the number of lesions documented at catheterization. (From Weiner DA, Ryan TJ, McCabe CH, et al. Exercise stress testing: Correlations among history of angina, ST-segment response and prevalence of coronary artery disease in the Coronary Artery Surgery Study (CASS). N Engl J Med 1979; 301:230–235. With permission.)

expertise is an important consideration in deciding between nuclear medicine and echocardiography techniques. Nuclear stress perfusion testing in women can be potentially hindered by soft tissue attenuation from breast tissue with the use of thallium, so technetium may be preferred. Stress echocardiography is highly dependent on operator expertise and may be technically difficult in obese patients. Many authors prefer stress imaging tests, with their lower false-positive rates, to exercise stress tests for women.[71]

Patterns of referral for cardiac catheterization may vary by gender, with some appropriate differences.[71,74] Because cardiac catheterization is less likely to reveal CAD in women, many clinicians initially evaluate women at intermediate risk with stress imaging techniques. For example, anginal symptoms are less predictive of abnormal coronary anatomy in women than in men (Fig. 97-8). In the Coronary Artery Surgery Study (CASS), CAD was diagnosed by cardiac catheterization in 63 percent of women with definitive angina, 40 percent in women with probable angina, and 4 percent in women with nonischemic pain.[75] Direct referral to cardiac catheterization should occur with a high suspicion of significant CAD that might benefit from intervention or after an abnormal noninvasive stress test.

MANAGEMENT OF CLINICAL CORONARY ARTERY DISEASE IN WOMEN

Asymptomatic Women

Some individuals are truly asymptomatic with respect to CAD. Others may have had atypical symptoms that have not yet been diagnosed as possible CAD. When Framingham researchers interviewed patients who had developed evidence of an interim MI by electrocardiography (ECG) (25 percent of all MIs), almost 50 percent, in retrospect, reported some symptoms.[76]

For truly asymptomatic women, national guidelines for prevention have been increasingly developed.[77] Counseling of asymptomatic women about CAD should include a review of the common risk factors and symptoms of CAD as well as encouragement for implementing a healthy lifestyle.[1,78] The single most important intervention for prevention is avoiding exposure to tobacco.[1,4,78]

Prospective cohort studies have been used to develop models predicting the impact of one or more risk factors on the likelihood of

future coronary artery events.[25,41,78] When multiple individual risk factors are present, the cumulative risk of CAD is greater than the sum of its parts.[25,78] The prevalence and impact of risk factors has been explored for women in several studies including the Third National Health and Nutrition Examination Survey,[41] and the Framingham Heart Study.[78,79]

The Third National Health and Nutrition Examination Survey (NHANES III) explored the intersection between race, SES, and the prevalence of cardiovascular risk factors.[41] Among women, tobacco use, systolic BP, BMI, leisure-time activity, non–high density lipoprotein cholesterol, and the presence of non-insulin-dependent diabetes were assessed in black ($n = 1762$), Mexican-American ($n = 1481$), and white women ($n = 2023$) age 25 to 64 years old. SES status was defined by the highest educational level attained, and a poverty income ratio was derived from family income and size. Compared with prior studies in which comparisons were attempted, more low-SES white women were included.

In NHANES III, as expected, increasing age was associated with a greater prevalence of all risk factors. The importance of race, even when SES was included, in a CAD risk model was revealed. Black and Mexican-American women had a higher BMI and systolic BP and more diabetes; they also reported less leisure-time activity (as well as lower tobacco use) than white women of a similar SES. With increasing age, black and Mexican-American women had greater prevalence rates of hypertension than white women. In contrast, with greater age, smoking rates decreased for white women and were generally stable for black and Mexican-American women.

Clustering of risk factors was also an important predictor in the Framingham Offspring Study (age 30 to 74 years at enrollment), where 17 percent of all participants had three of the six risk factors [lowest-quintile high-density lipoprotein (HDL) cholesterol, highest-quintile cholesterol, BMI, systolic BP, triglycerides, and glucose].[79] With 16 years of follow-up for coronary artery events (MI or sudden death), there were 79 first coronary artery events among the 1818 women who were initially free of symptomatic CAD, compared with 229 events among the 1759 men. However, CAD events were associated with three or more risk factors for 48 percent of the CAD events in women and 20 percent of the CAD events in men.

Long-term cardiovascular outcome has also been considered among white women with a low risk-factor profile in the Chicago Heart Association Detection Project in Industry.[80] A low risk-factor profile was defined as not a current smoker, BP ≤ 120/80, total cholesterol <200, no history of diabetes or MI, and no ECG abnormalities. At entry, only 6.8 percent of the cohort age 40 to 59 years met these criteria. However, these women had substantially lower CAD mortality with a mean follow-up of 22 years (3.5 compared with 14.5 age-adjusted mortality rate per 10,000 person-years, RR 0.21, 95 percent; CI 0.05 to 0.84).

In summary, these studies indicate that risk factors are additive and women without traditional cardiovascular risk factors (tobacco, hypertension, high cholesterol, diabetes, physical inactivity, family history, and old age) or low SES are at relatively low risk for coronary events.

Angina

As described from Framingham data, the first presentation of symptomatic CAD is typically angina in women and MI in men.[81]

The clinical diagnosis of angina can be challenging. Women generally visit physicians more often than men and report more symptoms, including chest pain. To determine whether angina is the most probable diagnosis, attention to the type and duration of symptoms and the impact of activities often provides important clues. The chest pain associated with angina classically may be a heavy pressure or squeezing but may also be described as a burning, aching, or stabbing. Typically duration varies between 10 and 20 min, with MI more likely after 30 min of sustained pressure or pain. Often angina is precipitated by exertion. Women compared with men with angina more frequently report angina with emotional or mental stress.[1] Too often, older women ascribe their decreased ability to complete housework or walk to "getting old." Therefore it is essential to explore a patient's exercise tolerance and if a decrease occurs, consider CAD in the differential.

Managing angina in women is complicated by the observation that anginal symptoms in them are less predictive of abnormal coronary anatomy than in men[75] (Fig. 97-8). Data on women with unstable angina also reveal lower rates of CAD at cardiac catheterization.[76] In a 6-year follow-up of patients seen for the first time with unstable angina in the emergency department in Olmstead County, Minnesota, women were older and more often had atypical angina and a history of hypertension. Fewer noninvasive and invasive procedures were completed on women, yet after adjustment for confounders, women had fewer cardiac events with 6 years of follow-up.[76] Potential physiologic differences to explain why anatomic lesions are less common in women include differences in vascular tone and microvascular or endothelial dysfunction.[82]

The potential role of vascular spasm has been explored in several pertinent studies.[83–85] When consecutive patients with a history of chest pain without evidence of acute ischemia, cardiomyopathy, or congestive heart failure were found to have no more than slight coronary artery abnormalities on angiography, intracoronary acetylcholine infusion was completed.[83] Of the 58 men and 59 women studied, large-artery spasm ($n = 63$) occurred predominantly in men (40 men vs. 23 women), while microvascular spasm ($n = 29$) occurred more often in women (20 women vs. 9 men). Patients with microvascular spasm had less coronary artery constriction after acetylcholine infusion, although angina (93 percent) and ischemic changes on ECG (83 percent) were often noted. Lactate levels in the coronary sinus were higher after acetylcholine infusion in patients with microvascular spasm (82 percent) than in those with large-artery spasm (53 percent).

Furthermore, the relationship between the menstrual cycle and vascular spasm is beginning to receive increasing attention.[84,85] The menstrual cycle can be divided into menstrual, follicular (from menses to ovulation, high estrogen levels), and luteal (ovulation to menses, low estrogen and high progesterone levels) phases utilizing historical timing, basal body temperature, bleeding patterns, and laboratory results. An important study of 10 women with vasospastic angina throughout the menstrual cycle has added to our knowledge.[83] Participants were premenopausal women with a history of vasospastic angina (all with a normal cardiac catheterization followed by intracoronary acetylcholine infusion leading to both symptoms and typical ST-segment elevation). All cardiac medication was held for a full menstrual cycle, with every other morning estrogen and progesterone levels, ST Holter monitoring, and flow-mediated dilation measurement of the brachial artery (Doppler study of the brachial artery before and after BP cuff elevation above systolic pressure). The average number of ischemic episodes inversely correlated with flow-mediated vasodilatation of the brachial artery (Fig. 97-9). In contrast to hormonal stimuli, similar amounts of vasodilatation in

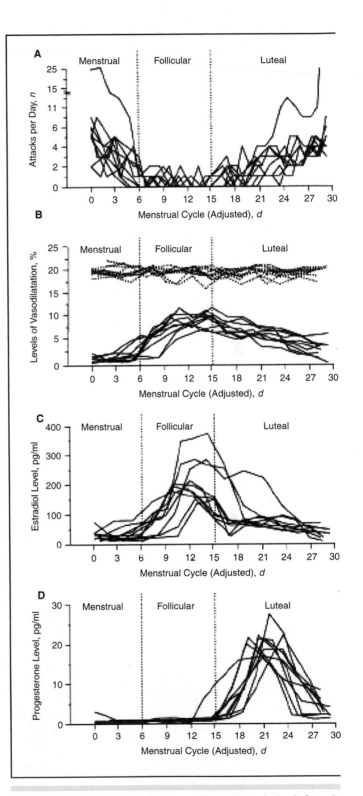

FIGURE 97-9 Comparison of the frequency of anginal attacks, level of vasodilation, and hormonal levels with the menstrual cycle in women off cardiac medication and documented to have vasospastic angina. (From Kawano H, Motoyama T, Ohgushi M, et al. Menstrual cyclic variation of myocardial ischemia in premenopausal women with variant angina. *Ann Intern Med* 2001; 135(11):977–981. With permission.)

different parts of the menstrual cycle occurred after nitroglycerin exposure. Other studies have also raised speculation about the importance of documenting when in the menstrual cycle a stress test is completed. More research is required in this area.[84,85]

Secondary prevention should be initiated with the diagnosis of angina, including control of risk factors and appropriate pharmacologic therapies (aspirin, lipid-lowering agents, but usually not hormone replacement therapy). Underuse of these agents in women is discussed in the section on MI, below. In one Swiss study, elderly women with angina had a less favorable 6-month outcome and reported a lower quality of life than men despite less frequent coronary obstruction at cardiac catheterization.[86]

Acute Coronary Ischemia Including Acute Myocardial Infarction

There are substantial gender differences in the presentation and natural history of acute coronary ischemia (including unstable angina and MI). Extensive general discussions of acute coronary ischemia syndromes can be found in other chapters. This section focuses on gender differences in presentation, prognosis, and management.

Gender differences in acute ischemia at the time of presentation and during short-term follow-up have been explored.[1,78,87–90] In the National Registry of Myocardial Infarction–I, women had a higher mortality during the index hospitalization.[87] As in earlier studies, women arrived later for evaluation after symptoms began; they also received less thrombolytic treatment as well as fewer invasive interventions (catheterization, PTCA, and CABG). Women had higher mortality rates than men, even at similar ages or after similar interventions, from cardiogenic shock, sudden death, arrhythmias, myocardial rupture, and electromechanical dissociation (in descending order). Complementary results were noted in a Spanish registry of patients less than 80 years of age experiencing a first MI.[88] As well as a later presentation for care, women had higher mortality during hospitalization and within 6 months. Women more often developed acute pulmonary edema or cardiogenic shock (25 percent of women vs. 11 percent of men) and less often developed at least one episode of ventricular fibrillation or sustained ventricular tachycardia requiring immediate medical care (15 percent of women vs. 24 percent of men).

Prospective subgroup gender analysis of patients enrolled in Global Use of Strategies to Open Occluded Coronary Arteries in Acute Coronary Syndromes (GUSTO IIb) compared initial presentations, evaluation, and 30-day mortality.[89] Although most subjects enrolled had had an acute MI (54 percent of women and 67 percent of men), substantial numbers of participants had unstable angina (Fig. 97-10). At presentation, women were more often diagnosed with unstable angina than men (46 vs. 36 percent, $p < 0.001$; odds ratio 1.51, 95 percent CI 1.34 to 1.69). Women subjects with acute coronary ischemia were older and had more comorbid conditions (diabetes, hypertension, angina, congestive heart failure) than the men, who were more likely to be smokers or to have had a prior MI, angioplasty, or CABG surgery. With MI, the initial entry ECG in women compared with men was less likely to indicate ST-segment elevation (27 vs. 37 percent, $p < 0.001$).

In GUSTO IIb, after cardiac catheterization (completed in 53 percent of women and 59 percent of men), women were about twice as likely to demonstrate no vessels with CAD compared with men. Specifically women compared to men with unstable angina (30 versus 14 percent, $p < 0.001$), after MI with ST-segment elevation (10 versus 7 percent, $p < 0.02$) or MI without ST-segment elevation (9 versus 4 percent, $p < 0.001$) had no lesions at angiography. These results are similar to those from the National Registry of Myocardial Infarction–II (MITI-II).[90]

Mortality by gender within 30 days after hospitalization for MI has been further elucidated by the GUSTO IIb and MITI-II reports.[89,90] Overall in GUSTO IIb, within 30 days, mortality for women was higher than for men (6.0 versus 4.0 percent, $p < 0.001$) despite similar reinfarction rates (6.2 percent for women, 5.6 percent for men, $p = 0.19$), with the difference explained by baseline variables such as older age and more comorbid conditions.[88] Among those with unstable angina, women had lower mortality and reinfarction rates within 30 days than did men (odds ratio 0.65, 95 percent CI 0.49 to 0.87, $p = 0.003$).

The interaction of gender and age was explored with data available from the National Registry of Myocardial Infarction–II.[90] Women with MI are often older and have more comorbid conditions than do men. Although overall there was a 14 percent early mortality in women after hospitalization for MI compared with 10 percent in men, when age was further considered, the picture became more complex. Upon analysis of the interaction of gender and age, the 30-day mortality after MI was about twice as great for women age 30 to 50 compared with men of the same age and progressively decreased with increasing age until reaching unity at age 75 (Fig. 97-11).

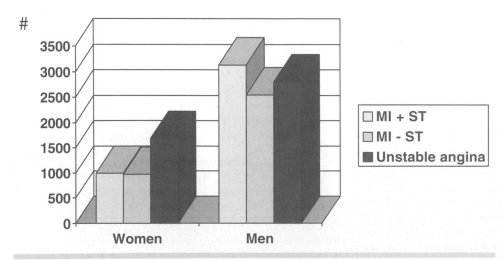

Acute Coronary Diagnosis GUSTO II b

FIGURE 97-10 Comparison of acute ischemia presentations at time of enrollment in the emergency department. (From Hochman JS, Tamis J, Thompson TD, et al. Sex, clinical presentation, and outcome in patients with acute coronary syndromes. *N Engl J Med* 1999;341:226–232. With permission.)

In long-term follow-up after MI, women have more symptoms than men, although long-term mortality is better or similar.[91] Women tend to have more angina and congestive heart failure despite better systolic left ventricular function.[90] Women as well as men most often develop congestive heart failure from ischemic heart disease.[46]

Finally, the initiation and follow-up of secondary prevention measures is essential for women as well as men. In the Third National Health and Nutrition Survey a focus on secondary prevention revealed women, blacks, and those age 46 to 65 years were more likely to have more than two poorly controlled major risk factors.[92] Pharmacologic therapies that are efficacious in women as well as men are often not prescribed (i.e., aspirin and agents to lower cholesterol.)[38,63,79,87,92] Furthermore, treatment goals have often not been met (like achieving BP or lipid control).[38,63,92] Cardiac rehabilitation is equally effective for women, although more men then women historically have participated.

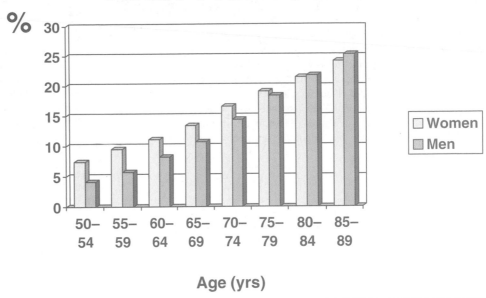

FIGURE 97-11 Mortality after myocardial infarction: Sex differences by age. (From Vaccarino V, Parsons L, Every NR, et al. Sex-based differences in early mortality after myocardial infarction. *N Engl J Med* 1999; 341:217–225. With permission.)

Interventions for Coronary Artery Disease

Gender differences in the prevalence and complications of angioplasty and CABG surgery are evolving. Both procedures are utilized less in women than in men, and there has been controversy as to whether women are undertreated or men overtreated.[1,77,93,94] Initially, angioplasty in women was associated with a higher procedure complication rate that improved with the development of smaller coronary artery catheters.[81] The higher in-hospital mortality and vascular and bleeding complication rates in women have been gradually approaching rates in men.[81]

CABG surgery is also more commonly performed in men than women. The conduit selected is less often the internal mammary artery in women than in men, although this graft is associated with the best short- and long-term results. Reasons for this might include higher rates of diabetes in women undergoing CABG and the decreased use of internal mammary artery grafting in the setting of osteoporosis.[95] Inpatient mortality is about twice higher for women than men, and most dramatic in young women.[81] Similar to PTCA, women undergoing CABG also have more vascular and bleeding complications than men.[81,95] Gender differences are less apparent with follow-up after several years.[81,94,96]

Sudden Death

Sudden death occurs 30 percent less in American women than men.[97] However, from 1989 to 1998 the rate of sudden death for women 35 to 44 years of age increased 21 percent compared with a 2.8 percent decrease in men.[97] In the Nurses' Health Study Cohort 636 women or 57.3 percent of the cohort died out of the hospital or in the emergency department. There was no prior history of heart disease in 69 percent of the women with sudden death. At least one coronary risk factor

was present in 94 percent of those who died. The strongest associations were with cigarette smoking, diabetes, and hypertension.[97] Out-of-hospital arrest survival is similar for women and men; however, men had higher rates of ventricular fibrillation.[98]

Silent MI in the Framingham Study was common, representing 25 percent of MI when diagnosed on the basis of new Q waves on the screening ECG.[55] Despite obtaining further history, almost half of the subjects had no symptoms. Silent MI was more common in women than in men (35 vs. 28 percent). At 30 years of follow-up, the first presentation of MI resulted in death among 39 percent women and 31 percent of men.[84] The prognosis of silent MI has not been adequately studied; sudden death is one possible sequela, as documented in an autopsy study where clinical history was obtained after sudden death ($n = 51$) or death after trauma ($n = 15$).[99] On autopsy, only 2 of 51 women had a documented prior MI, although 35 percent of the sample had evidence of a prior MI. The acute thrombus associated with plaque erosion (often noted in early atherosclerosis) occurred more often in younger women smokers without obesity, high cholesterol, or elevated glycohemoglobin. In comparison, plaque rupture was more often found in older women with elevated cholesterol.

Arrhythmias

Women have a higher heart rate than men and respond to increasing cardiac demand by increasing heart rate rather than increasing stroke volume. Women also have a longer QT interval and shorter sinus node recovery time.[36,100]

Gender differences in incidence and natural history have been noted. Atrioventricular node reentrant tachycardia and orthodromic supraventricular tachycardia have a female predominance, although men are more likely to have atrial and ventricular fibrillation associated with Wolff-Parkinson-White syndrome.[36,101] Paroxysmal atrial fibrillation in women may be associated with faster heart rates and longer duration.[101] After MI, women are more likely to have atrial fibrillation.[89] Overall, women have a higher risk of dying of atrial fibrillation.[102] A pacemaker registry retrospective review from Germany (with 31,913 entries) found that when pacemakers are implanted, women are more likely to receive a single-chamber pacer, while men are more likely to receive a dual-chamber pacer.[103]

It is generally known that torsades de pointes occurs more commonly in women.[36,101] Potential contributors to the development of torsades de pointes include QT duration and heart rate variability.[104] Drugs that prolong repolarization are associated with a higher prevalence of torsades de pointes in women.[36] Heart rate variability differs in adult women and men but becomes similar by the seventh decade.[104]

SUMMARY

Over the past few decades significant differences in individual patient factors that affect diagnosis and management have begun to be further defined and explored. The diagnosis of CAD must be considered in women with typical or atypical symptoms. All physicians and patients must focus on primary and secondary prevention for both women and men.

References

1. Charney P, ed. *Coronary Artery Disease in Women: Prevention, Diagnosis and Management*. Philadelphia: American College of Physicians; 1999.
2. Mosca L, Jones WK, King KB, et al. Awareness, perception, and knowledge of heart disease risk and prevention among women in the United States: American Heart Association Women's Heart Disease and Stroke Campaign Task Force. *Arch Fam Med* 2000;9:506–515.
3. Barrett-Connor E. Sex differences in coronary heart disease: Why are women so superior? The 1995 Ancel Keys Lecture. *Circulation* 1997; 95:252–264.
4. Ockene JK, Bonollo DP, Adams A. Smoking. In: Charney P, ed. *Coronary Artery Disease in Women*. Philadelphia: American College of Physicians; 1999.
5. Center for Disease Control and Prevention. Women and Smoking: a report of the Surgeon General (Executive Summary). *MMWR Morb Mortal Wkly Rep* 2002;51(No RR.12):1–13.
6. Al-Delaimy WK, Manson JE, Solomon CG, et al. Smoking and the risk of coronary heart disease among women with type 2 diabetes mellitus. *Arch Intern Med* 2002;162:273–279.
7. Willet W, Green A, Stampfer M, et al. Relative and absolute excess risks of coronary heart disease among women who smoke cigarettes. *N Engl J Med* 1987;317:1303–1309.
8. Winkleby MA, Robinson TN, Sundquist J, Kraemer HC. Ethnic variations in cardiovascular disease risk factors among children and young adults: Findings from the third National Health and Nutrition Examination Survey, 1988–1994. *JAMA* 1999;281:1006–1013.
9. Wee CC, Rigotti N, Davis RB, et al. Relationship between smoking and weight control efforts among adults in the United States. *Arch Intern Med* 2001;161:546–550.
10. Marcus BH, Albrecht AE, King TK, et al. The efficacy of exercise as an aid for smoking cessation in women: A randomized controlled trial. *Arch Intern Med* 1999;159:1229–1234.
11. Blondal T, Gudmundsson LJ, Olafsdottir I, et al. Nicotine nasal spray with nicotine patch for smoking cessation: Randomized trial with six year follow-up. *BMJ* 1999;318:285–288.
12. Ahluwalia JS, Harris KJ, Catley D, et al. Sustained-release bupropion for smoking cessation in African Americans: A randomized controlled trial. *JAMA* 2000;288:468–474.
13. Carballo RS, Giovino GA, Perchaeck TF, et al. Racial and ethnic differences in serum cotinine levels for cigarette smokers: Third National Health and Nutrition Examination Survey, 1988–1991. *JAMA* 1998; 280:135–139.
14. Thorndike AN, Rigotti NA, Stafford RS, Singer DE. National patterns in the treatment of smokers by physicians. *JAMA* 1998;279(8):604–608.
15. Fiore M, Bailey W, Cohen S, et al. *Smoking Cessation: Clinical Practice Guidelines No. 18.* Publication 96-0692. Rockville, MD: USDHHS, PHS, AHCPR; 1996.
16. Rennert NJ, Charney P. Preventing cardiovascular disease in diabetes and glucose intolerance: Evidence and implications for care. *Primary Care Clin North Am.* 2003;30:569–592.
17. Miettinen H, Lehto S, Salomaa V, et. al. for the FINMONICA Myocardial Infarction Register Study Group: Impact of diabetes on mortality after the first myocardial infarction. *Diabetes Care* 1998;21: 69–75.
18. Douglas P, ed. *Cardiovascular Health and Disease in Women,* 2d ed. Philadelphia: Saunders; 2002.
19. Gu K, Cowie C, Harris M. Diabetes and decline in heart disease mortality in U.S. adults. *JAMA* 1999;281(14):1291–1297.
20. Vaccarino V, Parsons L, Every N, et al. Impact of history of diabetes mellitus on hospital mortality in men and women with first acute myocardial infarction. *Am J Cardiol* 2000;85:1486–1489.
21. Sullivan M. Criteria for the oral glucose tolerance test in pregnancy. *Diabetes* 1964;13(13):278–285.
22. Prospective Diabetes Study Group. United Kingdom Prospective Diabetes Study 27: Plasma lipids and lipoproteins at diagnosis of NIDDM by age and sex, UK. *Diabetes Care* 1997;20(11):1683–1687.
23. Wild R. Polycystic ovary syndrome: A risk for coronary artery disease? *Am J Obstet Gynecol* 2002;186(1):35–43.
24. Waterworth DM, Bennett ST, Gharani N, et al. Linkage and association of insulin gene VNTR regulatory polymorphism with polycystic ovarian syndrome. *Lancet* 1997;349:986–990.
25. National Cholesterol Education Program (NCEP) Expert Panel on Detection, Evaluation and Treatment of High Blood Cholesterol in Adults (Adult Treatment Panel III) *JAMA* 2001;285:2486–2497.
26. Ford E, Giles W, Dietz WH. Prevalence of the metabolic syndrome among U.S. adults—Findings from the Third National Health and Nutrition Examination Survey. *JAMA* 2002;287(3):356–359.
27. Mayer-Davis EJ, D'Agostino R, Karter AJ, et al. Intensity and amount of physical activity in relation to insulin sensitivity: The Insulin Resistance Atherosclerosis Study. *JAMA* 1998;279:669–674.
28. The Women's Caucus, Working Group on Women's Health of the Society of General Internal Medicine. Hypertension in women: What is really known? *Ann Intern Med* 1991;115:287–293.
29. Sagie A. The natural history of borderline isolated systolic hypertension. *N Engl J Med* 1993;329:1912–1917.
30. Stamler J, Stamler R, Neaton JD, et al. Blood pressure, systolic and diastolic, and cardiovascular risks: U.S. population data. *Arch Intern Med* 1993;153:598–615.
31. Quan A, Kerlikowske K, Gueyffier F, et al. Efficacy of treating hypertension in women. *J Gen Intern Med* 1999;14:718–729.
32. SHEP Cooperative Research Group. Prevention of stroke by antihypertensive drug treatment in older persons with isolated systolic hypertension: Final results of the Systolic Hypertension in the Elderly Program (SHEP). *JAMA* 1991;265(24):3255–3264.
33. Dahlof B, Lindholm LH, Hansson L, et al. Morbidity and mortality in the Swedish Trial in Old Patients with Hypertension (STOP-Hypertension). *Lancet* 1991;338:1281–1285.
34. Kannel WB. Blood pressure as a cardiovascular risk factor: Prevention and treatment. *JAMA* 1996;275:1571–1576.
35. LaCroix AZ, Ott SM, Ichikawa L, et al. Low-dose hydrochlorothiazide and preservation of bone mineral density in older adults: a randomized, double-blind, placebo-controlled trial. *Ann Intern Med* 2000;133(7): 516–526.
36. Schaefer BM, Caracciolo V, Frishman WH, Charney P. Gender, ethnicity and genetics in cardiovascular disease: Part II. Implications for pharmacotherapy. *Heart Dis* 2003;5:202–214.

37. Walsh ME. Lipids: Natural history and pharmacologic management. In: Charney P, ed. *Coronary Artery Disease in Women*. Philadelphia: American College of Physicians; 1999:101–128.

38. Majumdar SR, Gurwitz JH, Soumerai SB. Undertreatment of hyperlipidemia in the secondary prevention of coronary artery disease. *J Gen Intern Med* 1999;14:711–717.

39. Davidson MH, Testolin LM, Maki KC, et al. A comparison of estrogen replacement, pravastatin, and combined treatment for the management of hypercholesterolemia in postmenopausal women. *Arch Intern Med* 1997;157:1186–1192.

40. Darling GM, Johns JA, McCloud PI, Davis SR. Estrogen and progestin compared with simvastatin for hypercholesterolemia in postmenopausal women. *N Engl J Med* 1997;337:595–601.

41. Winkleby M, Kraemer HC, Ahn DK, Varady AN. Ethnic and socioeconomic differences in cardiovascular disease risk factors: Findings for women from the Third National Health and Nutrition Examination Survey, 1988–1994. *JAMA* 1998;280:356–362.

42. Wilson PF, D'Agostino RB, Sullivan L, et al. Overweight and obesity as determinants of cardiovascular risk: The Framingham experience. *Arch Intern Med* 2002;162:1867–1872.

43. Samaras K, Kelly PJ, Chiano MN, et al. Genetic and environmental influences on total-body and central abdominal fat: The effect of physical activity in female twins. *Ann Intern Med* 1999;130:873–882.

44. Andersen RD, Wadden TA, Bartlett SJ, et al. Effects of lifestyle activity vs. structured aerobic exercise in obese women. *JAMA* 1999;381(4):335–340.

45. Yanoviski SZ, Yanoviski JA. Obesity. *N Engl J Med* 2002;346:591–602.

46. Beniaminovitz A, Mancini D. Congestive heart failure. In: Charney P, ed. *Coronary Artery Disease in Women: Prevention, Diagnosis and Management*. Philadelphia: American College of Physicians; 1999:476–495.

47. Fair JM, Berra K, King AC. Exercise as primary and secondary prevention in Charney P, ed. *Coronary Artery Disease in Women: Prevention, Diagnosis and Management*. Philadelphia: American College of Physicians; 1999:209–235.

48. Oliver MF, Boyd GS. Effect of bilateral ovariectomy on coronary artery disease and serum lipid levels. *Lancet* 1959;2:690.

49. Hu FB, Grodstein F, Hennekens CH, et al. Age at natural menopause and risk of cardiovascular disease. *Arch Intern Med* 1999;159:1061–1066.

50. Fletcher SW, Colditz GA, eds. Failure of estrogen plus progestin therapy for prevention. *JAMA* 2002;288:266–267.

51. Writing Group for the Women's Health Initiative Investigators. Risks and benefits of estrogen plus progestin in healthy postmenopausal women: Principal results from the Women's Health Initiative randomized controlled trial. *JAMA* 2002;288:321–333.

52. U.S. Preventive Task Force. Postmenopausal hormone replacement therapy for primary prevention of chronic conditions: recommendations and rationale. *Ann Intern Med* 2002;137:834–839.

53. Grady D, Herrington D, Bittner V, et al. Cardiovascular disease outcomes during 6.8 years of hormone therapy: Heart and Estrogen/Progestin Replacement Study Follow-Up (HERS II). *JAMA* 2002;288:49–57.

54. Jacobs SC, Stone PH. Psychosocial issues. In: Charney P, ed. *Coronary Artery Disease in Women*. Philadelphia: American College of Physicians; 1999:496–534.

55. Charney P. Future directions. In: Charney P, ed. *Coronary Artery Disease in Women: Prevention, Diagnosis and Management*. Philadelphia: American College of Physicians; 1999:575–593.

56. Morrison C, Woodward M, Leslie W, Turnstall-Pedoe H. Effect of socioeconomic group on incidence of, management of, and survival after myocardial infarction and coronary death: Analysis of community coronary event register. *BMJ* 1997;314:541–546.

57. Marmot MG, Bosma H, Hemingway H, et al. Contribution of job control and other risk factors to social variations in coronary heart disease incidence. *Lancet* 1997;350:235–239.

58. Pratt LA, Ford DE, Crum RM, et al. Depression, psychotropic medication, and risk of myocardial infarction: Prospective data from the Baltimore ECA follow-up. *Circulation* 1996;94:3123–3129.

59. Carney RM, Jaffe AS, ed. Treatment of depression following acute myocardial infarction. *JAMA* 2002;288:750–752.

60. Creed F. The importance of depression following myocardial infarction. *Heart* 1999;82:406–408.

61. Carney RM, Freedland KE, Smith L, et al. Relation of depression and mortality after myocardial infarction in women (letter). *Circulation* 1991;84(4):1876–1877.

62. Escobedo LG, Giles WH, Anda RF. Socioeconomic status, race, and death from coronary heart disease. *Am J Prev Med* 1997;13:123–130.

63. Vittinghoff E, Shlipak MG, Varosy PD, et al. Risk factors and secondary prevention in women with heart disease: the Heart and Estrogen/progestin Replacement Study. *Ann Intern Med* 2003:138:81–89.

64. Pandey DK, Labarthe DR, Goff DC Jr, et al. Community-wide coronary heart disease mortality in Mexican Americans equals or exceeds that in Non-Hispanic whites: The Corpus Christi Heart Project. *Am J Med* 2001;110:81–87.

65. Shaukat N, Lear J, Lowy A, et al. First myocardial infarction in patients of Indian subcontinent and European origin: Comparison of risk factors, management, and long term outcome. *BMJ* 1997;314:639–642.

66. Vitelli LL, Crow RS, Shahar E, et al. Electrocardiographic findings in a healthy biracial population. *Am J Cardiol* 1998;81:453–459.

67. Perez-Stable EJ, Herrera B, Jacob P, Benowitz NL. Nicotine metabolism and intake in black and white smokers. *JAMA* 1998;280:152–156.

68. Birdwell BG, Herbers JE, Kroenke K. Evaluating chest pain: The patient's presentation style alters the physician's diagnostic approach. *Arch Intern Med* 1993;153:1991–1995.

69. Schulman KA, Berlin JA, Harless W, et al. The effect of race and sex on physician's recommendations for cardiac catheterization. *N Engl J Med* 1999;340:618–626.

70. Roger VL, Jacobsen SJ, Weston SA, et al. Sex differences in evaluation and outcome after stress testing. *Mayo Clin Proc* 2002;77:638–645.

71. Shaw LJ, Peterson ED, Johnson LL. Noninvasive testing techniques for diagnosis and prognosis. In: Charney P, ed. *Coronary Artery Disease in Women*. Philadelphia: American College of Physicians; 1999:341–345.

72. Kwok Y, Kim C, Grady D, et al. Meta-analysis of exercise testing to detect coronary artery disease in women. *Am J Cardiol* 1999;83:660–663.

73. Okin PM, Kligfield P. Gender-specific criteria and performance of the exercise electrocardiogram. *Circulation* 1995;92(5):1209–1216.

74. Roger V, Jacobsen SJ, Weston SA, et al. Sex differences in evaluation and outcome after stress testing. *Mayo Clin Proc* 2002;77:638–645.

75. Weiner DA, Ryan TJ, McCabe CH, et al. Exercise stress testing: Correlations among history of angina, ST segment response and prevalence of coronary artery disease in the Coronary Artery Surgery Study (CASS). *N Engl J Med* 1979;301:230–235.

76. Roger VL, Farkouh ME, Weston SA, et al. Sex differences in evaluation and outcome of unstable angina. *JAMA* 2000;283:646–652.

77. Mosca L, Grundy SM, Judelson D, et al. Guide to preventive cardiology for women. *Circulation* 1999;99:2480–2484.

78. Wilson PWF, Kannel WB, Silbershatz H, D'Agostino RB. Clustering of metabolic factors and coronary heart disease. *Arch Intern Med* 1999;159:1104–1109.

79. Hubert HB, Eaker ED, Garrison R, Castelli WP. Life-style correlates of risk factor change in young adults: An eight-year study of coronary heart disease risk factors in the Framingham offspring. *Am J Epidemiol* 1987;125(5):812–831.

80. Stamler J, Stamler R, Neaton JD, et al. Low risk-factor profile and long-term cardiovascular and noncardiovascular mortality and life expectancy: Findings for 5 large cohorts of young adults and middle-aged men and women. *JAMA* 1999;282:2012–2018.

81. Lerner DS, Kannel W. Patterns of heart disease morbidity and mortality in the sexes: A 26-year follow-up of the Framingham population. *Am Heart J* 1986;111:383–390.

82. Jacobs AK. Coronary vascularization in women in 2003: Sex revisited. *Circulation* 2003;107(3):375–377.

83. Mohri M, Koyanagi M, Egashira K, et al. Angina pectoris caused by coronary microvascular spasm. *Lancet* 1998;351:1165–1169.

84. Kawano H, Motoyama T, Ohgushi M, et al. Menstrual cyclic variation of myocardial ischemia in premenopausal women with variant angina. *Ann Intern Med* 2001;135(11):977–981.

85. Charney P. Coronary artery disease in young women: The menstrual cycle and other risk factors. *Ann Intern Med* 2001;135(11):1002–1004.

86. Kuster GM, Buser P, Osswald S. Comparison of presentation, perception, and six month outcome between women and men ≥75 years of age with angina pectoris. *Am J Cardiol* 2003;91:436–439.

87. Chandra NC, Ziegelstein RC, Rogers WJ, et al. Observations of the treatment of women in the United States with myocardial infarction: A report from the National Registry of Myocardial Infarction I. *Arch Intern Med* 1998;158:981–988.

88. Marrugat JM, Sala J, Masia R, et al. Mortality differences between men and women following first myocardial infarction. *JAMA* 1998; 280:1405–1409.

89. Hochman JS, Tamis J, Thompson TD, et al. Sex, clinical presentation, and outcome in patients with acute coronary syndromes. *N Engl J Med* 1999;341:226–232.

90. Vaccarino V, Parsons L, Every NR, et al. Sex-based differences in early mortality after myocardial infarction. *N Engl J Med* 1999;341:217–225.

91. Collins LJ, Douglas PS. Acute coronary syndromes. In: Charney P, ed. *Coronary Artery Disease in Women*. Philadelphia: American College of Physicians; 1999:407–413.

92. Qureshi AI, Suri FK, Guterman LR, et al. Ineffective secondary prevention in survivors of cardiovascular events in the U.S. population: Report from the Third National Health and Nutrition Examination Survey. *Arch Intern Med* 2001;161:1621–1628.

93. Bickell NA, Pieper KS, Lee KL, et al. Referral patterns for coronary artery disease treatment: Gender bias or good clinical judgement. *Ann Intern Med* 1992;116:791–797.

94. Gahli WA, Faris PD, Galbraith D, et al. Sex differences in access to coronary revascularization after cardiac catheterization: Importance of detailed clinical data. *Ann Intern Med* 2002;136:723–732.

95. Hartz RS, Charney P. Coronary artery bypass grafting: Is it worth the risk? In: Charney P, ed. *Coronary Artery Disease in Women*. Philadelphia: American College of Physicians; 1999:438–462.

96. Haan CK, Chiong JR, Coombs LP, et al. Comparison of risk profiles and outcomes in women versus men ≥75 years of age undergoing coronary artery bypass grafting. *Am J Cardiol* 2003;91:1255–1258.

97. Albert CM, Chae CU, Grodstein F, et al. Prospective study of sudden cardiac death among women in the United States. *Circulation* 2003; 107(16):2096–2101.

98. Kim C, Fahrenbruch CE, Eisenberg MS. Out-of-hospital arrest in men and women. *Circulation* 2001:104:2699–2703.

99. Oparil S. Pathophysiology of sudden coronary death in women: Implications for prevention. *Circulation* 1998:97:2103–2104.

100. Burke JH, Ehlert FA, Kruse JT, et al. Gender-specific differences in the QT interval and the effect of autonomic tone and menstrual cycle in healthy adults. *Am J Cardiol* 1997;79:178–181.

101. Hnatkova K, Waktare JE, Murgatroyd FD, et al. Age and gender influences on rate and duration of paroxysmal atrial fibrillation. *Pacing Clin Electrophysiol* 1998;21:2455–2458.

102. Benjamin EJ, Wolf PA, D'Agostino RB, et al. Impact of atrial fibrillation on the risk of death: the Framingham Heart Study. *Circulation* 1998;98:946–952.

103. Schuppel R, Buchele G, Batz L, Koenig W. Sex differences in selection of pacemakers: Retrospective observation study. *BMJ* 1988;316: 492–495.

104. Stein PK, Kleiger RE, Rottman JN. Differing effects of age on heart rate variability in men and women. *Am J Cardiol* 1997; 80:302–305.

PART FIFTEEN

DISEASES OF THE GREAT VESSELS AND PERIPHERAL VESSELS

DISEASES OF THE AORTA

Jonathan L. Halperin / Jeffrey W. Olin

THE NORMAL AORTA

The aorta is the major conductance vessel of the body, an elastic artery with a trilaminar wall: the *tunica intima, tunica media,* and *tunica adventitia.* The innermost component of the tunica intima is the endothelium, resting on a thin basal lamina. The subendothelial tissue comprises fibroblasts, collagen fibers, elastic fibers, and mucoid ground substance. An internal elastic membrane forms the outer lining of the tunica intima. The tunica media is approximately 1 mm thick, comprising elastin, smooth muscle cells, collagen, and ground substance. It is the predominance of elastic fibers in the aortic wall and their arrangement as circumferential lamellae that distinguish this elastic artery from the smaller muscular arteries. A lamellar unit comprises two concentric elastic lamellae and the smooth muscle cells, collagen, and ground substance contained within.[1,2] The thoracic aorta incorporates 35 to 56 lamellar units and the abdominal aorta about 28 units.[3] Surrounding the tunica media is the tunica adventitia, which is composed of loose connective tissue, including fibroblasts, relatively small amounts of collagen fibers, elastin, and ground substance. Within the tunica adventitia lie the *nervi vasorum* and *vasa vasorum.* The arteries arising along the course of the aorta give rise to the vasa vasorum, which develop into a capillary network supplying the adventitia and media of the thoracic aorta. The vasa vasorum do not supply the media of the abdominal aorta.[4]

The ascending aorta is approximately 5 cm in length and 3 cm in maximum diameter, depending on age, gender, and body surface area[5]; the aortic arch is approximately 4 cm long with a diameter ranging from 2.5 to 3.5 cm. As it descends in the posterior mediastinum, the thoracic aorta tapers slightly in diameter approximately 20 cm beyond the arch from an average of 2.3 to 2 cm. The abdominal aorta begins in the median plane at the aortic hiatus of the diaphragm, descends approximately 15 cm in front of the vertebral column to the level of the fourth lumbar vertebra, and then divides into two common iliac arteries. Along this course, its diameter narrows from 2.0 to 2.6 cm above to 1.7 to 1.9 cm below, averaging 2 mm larger in males than in females (Table 98-1). Aside from gender, aortic root dimension is principally related to age, height, and weight. The influence of blood pressure is small though statistically significant. The gender difference in aortic root dimension is not consistently explained by body surface area.[6]

The force of left ventricular ejection creates a pressure wave that traverses the aorta, producing radial expansion and contraction of the arterial walls.[7] Potential energy derived from myocardial contraction and stored in the aortic wall during systole is transformed during diastolic recoil into kinetic energy, which drives blood into the peripheral vessels.[8] The pressure wave is conducted at an approximate velocity of 5 m/s, increasing in amplitude as it traverses the aorta. Forward flow in the aorta begins when the aortic valve opens, and systolic pressure rises as the pressure wave courses along the length of the aorta. The velocity of flow rises rapidly to a peak and then gradually decreases. With aortic valve closure there is a transient period of backward flow before forward flow recurs during diastole, particularly in the descending thoracic and abdominal aorta, albeit at considerably less than systolic velocity. The *incisura,* present in the proximal portion of the thoracic aorta, gradually disappears and is generally absent in the abdominal aorta.[9]

Changes with Age

Each of the four components of the aortic wall—elastic tissue, collagen fibers, smooth muscle cells, and mucoid ground substance—changes with age (Fig. 98-1). Elastic fibers fragment, collagen becomes more prominent at the expense of smooth muscle cells, and glycosaminoglycans accumulate.[10–13] As a result, the aorta becomes less distensible, reducing its capacity to absorb the forces derived from left ventricular contraction.[14] Weakening of the aortic wall leads to dilatation of the lumen as well as elongation and uncoiling of the aortic arch, collectively producing ectasia.[15,16]

The elderly aorta is characterized by dilatation and elongation. Accompanying these changes are alterations in aortic wall structure, with fragmentation of elastic fibers, loss of smooth muscle cell nuclei (*medionecrosis*),[17] accumulation of collagenous tissue, and deposition of basophilic ground substance.[12] As the aorta dilates because of disease of the medial layer, tension on the aortic wall leads to increasing shear stress. This process is accelerated by hypertension, particularly when pulsatile forces are high. Under conditions of

TABLE 98-1 Echocardiographic Measurements of Aortic Root Diameter in Relation to Age, Gender, Blood Pressure, and Body Indices in the Framingham Heart Study

Variable	Men	Women
	(n = 1849)	(n = 2152)
Age, years	48 + 14	49 + 14
Weight, kg	80 + 11	62 + 9
Height, m	1.7 + 0.1	1.6 + 0.1
BSA, m^2	1.95 + 0.15	1.64 + 0.13
MBI, kg/m^2	26 + 3.2	24 + 3.6
SBP, mmHg	126 + 16	121 + 18
DBP, mmHg	79 + 9	75 + 9
MAP, mmHg	95 + 10	90 + 11
PP, mmHg	47 + 13	46 + 14
Prior SBP, mmHg	125 + 14	118 + 15
Prior DBP, mmHg	80 + 9	75 + 9
Prior MAP, mmHg	95 + 10	90 + 10
Aortic root dimension, mm	32 + 3	28 + 3[a]
Aortic root/height	19 + 1.8	18 + 2[a]
Aortic root/weight	0.41 + 0.06	0.46 + 0.07[a]
Aortic root/BMI	1.26 + 0.16	1.20 + 0.18[a]
Aortic root/BSA	16.7 + 1.8	17.3 + 2.0[a]

[a] $p < 0.0001$ compared with men. Values are mean + SD.
ABBREVIATIONS: BSA = body surface area; BMI = body mass index; SBP = systolic blood pressure; DBP = diastolic blood pressure; MAP = mean arterial pressure; PP = pulse pressure. Prior blood pressure values were obtained from an examination 8 years earlier.
SOURCE: Adapted from the Framingham Heart Study.[6] With permission.

increased peripheral vascular resistance, a reflected wave has an impact additive to that of antegrade pulsatile flow. The combination of congenital, degenerative, mechanical, and hemodynamic factors adversely affects the medial layer of the aortic wall, leading to dilatation and setting the stage for the catastrophes of aortic dissection or rupture.

ANEURYSMAL DISEASE OF THE AORTA

The designation *aortic aneurysm* implies that the diameter of the aorta is more than $1\frac{1}{2}$ times larger than normal[18,19]; it has been suggested that the term be restricted to situations where the diameter of the aorta exceeds 3 cm.[20] The pathologic term *aneurysm*—derived from the Greek *aneurysma*, referring to dilation—is distinguished from *ectasia*, which refers to the modest generalized dilation of the aorta that occurs with aging.[16] Aneurysms may be classified according to morphology, etiology, or location. The gross morphologic classification distinguishes true aneurysms of the aorta as *fusiform* or *saccular*. A fusiform aneurysm is cylindrical and affects the entire circumference of the aorta; a saccular aneurysm is an outpouching of only a portion of the aortic wall. Frequently, a small neck provides continuity between the aortic lumen and the saccular aneurysm. Fusiform aneurysms are more common than the saccular type. The most common aneurysms associated with atherosclerosis involve the infrarenal abdominal segment and are almost exclusively fusiform. Thoracic aortic aneurysms are occasionally saccular, with a relatively narrow communication between the cavity of the aneurysm and the aortic lumen. This limited orifice may protect the thin wall of the aneurysm from the force of intraaortic pressure and reduce the risk of rupture, in contrast to fusiform aneurysms, in which the entire circumference of the dilated segment is exposed to the pulsatile distending forces of cardiac systole.

Beyond their morphology, aortic aneurysms may also be classified according to the segment involved, as thoracic, thoracoabdominal, or abdominal. This simplifies understanding because pathogenesis, clinical presentation, natural history, and treatment depend in large measure on location. Aneurysm formation is considerably more widespread along the length of the aorta than obstructive atherosclerotic disease, potentially affecting almost the entire vessel, whereas obstruction tends to involve only the abdominal portion of the aorta, when the iliac arteries are commonly affected as well. Dilatation of the aorta may occur as a consequence of atherosclerosis alone as well as of aging, infection, inflammation, trauma, congenital anomalies, and medial degeneration or in combinations of pathologic states. The pathologic changes that accompany these conditions cause the aorta to thicken, thin, bulge, tear, rupture, narrow, or dissect or to be altered by combinations of these conditions.

In distinction to the normal aorta, the striking histologic feature of aortic aneurysms is destruction of the media and elastic tissue. Excessive proteolytic enzyme activity may promote deterioration of structural matrix proteins, such as elastin and collagen, in the aortic wall.[21] Smooth muscle cells derived from patients with aortic aneurysms, compared to those from normal aortas, display invasive properties. This increased migration, which appears to be due to overproduction of the matrix metalloproteinase MMP-2, may lead to extracellular matrix remodeling and subsequent medial disruption in the aneurysmal aorta.[22] Abnormal biochemical elastolytic and active proteolytic activity also has been identified in tissue from aneurysmal aortas.[23] An abnormal presence of macrophages[24] and elevated levels of cytokines[25] in aneurysmal aortic tissue likewise indicate that an active inflammatory process may contribute to the pathogenesis of aortic aneurysms. Cultured smooth muscle cells from aneurysmal aortas, compared with cells from normal aortas, produce elevated levels of plasminogen activators.[26] This could increase the amount of plasmin available for zymogen activation of matrix metalloproteinases, which would favor proteolysis in the absence of a reciprocal rise in plasmin activator inhibitor. Matrix metalloproteinases thus may play a major role in the aortic wall degeneration that leads to aneurysm formation.

Cystic Medial Necrosis

Over the course of normal aging, degenerative changes occur throughout most of the length of the aorta, leading to a mild form of cystic medial necrosis. Although essentially physiologic, this process develops more rapidly in patients with bicuspid aortic valve, during pregnancy, and very markedly in the Marfan syndrome, in which over 11 percent of patients suffer dissections of the aorta. The mechanism by which the medial layer of the aorta is subject to this accelerated rate of degeneration is a subject of active molecular genetic investigation. *Cystic medial necrosis,* a form of vascular pathology unique to the aorta, was first described by Gsell and shortly afterward by Erdheim.[27,28] Histologic evidence of severe elastic fiber degeneration, necrosis of muscle cells, and cystic spaces filled with mucoid material is most often encountered in the ascending aorta from the region of the valve to the brachiocephalic artery, though similar changes may be seen in the remainder of the aorta as well. Because of the dilatation of the aortic root, aortic regurgitation may be a secondary feature, although the valve leaflets themselves are histologically unaffected.

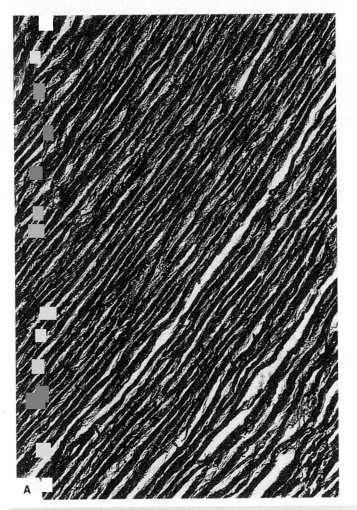

FIGURE 98-1 Histology of the normal aorta of a child (*panel A*) and an elderly adult (*panel B*). With aging, elastic fibers fragment, collagen becomes more prominent, smooth muscle cells diminish, and acid mucopolysaccharide ground substance accumulates. Weakening of the aortic wall leads to dilation of the lumen as well as elongation and uncoiling of the aortic arch. Orcein and Giesen stain, magnification × 414. (From Nichols and O'Rourke.[291] With permission.)

Cystic medial necrosis is the most common cause of ascending aortic aneurysm,[27,29] and although this type of aortic pathology is typical of patients with the Marfan syndrome, it may also occur in the absence of any clinical Marfan's stigmata. Aneurysms caused by cystic medial necrosis are usually fusiform and may involve the sinuses of Valsalva. Increasingly recognized is the association of proximal aortic dilation with congenital bicuspid aortic valve with or without hemodynamically significant valvular stenosis or regurgitation.[30] Whether this is mediated by cystic medial necrosis of the aorta in all or some cases is not yet clear, though the prognosis appears better than in aortic aneurysm associated with other features of the Marfan syndrome.

The Marfan Syndrome

This inherited disorder, described in 1896, is characterized by dolichostenomelia, ligamentous redundancy, ectopia lentis, ascending aortic dilatation, and incompetence of either the aortic or mitral valves or both.[31] The syndrome is linked to an autosomal dominant anomaly in the genes regulating synthesis of fibrillin type 1, a large lipoprotein that helps direct and orient elastin in the developing aorta.[32,33–37] The mutation in chromosome 15 is linked to the rate of aortic disease as a familial trait, but it may also occur sporadically without a family history of Marfan's syndrome or aortic disease. A mutation of chromosome 5 has also been identified in patients with Marfan's syndrome; this can also arise spontaneously, and in some cases there may be concurrent mutations in both chromosomes 5 and 15. This variability in fibrillin gene mutations accounts for the broad spectrum of aortic disease severity in patients with Marfan's syndrome and may explain the occurrence of cystic medial necrosis of the aorta in patients with congenitally bicuspid aortic valves. What is not clear is whether these mutations lead to a qualitative or quantitative defect of elastin—or both—but there is a link between the pathology of the aortic media and the identification of specific genetic mutations of these two chromosomes.[38,39]

In patients with the Marfan syndrome, the aortic root tends to enlarge in fusiform fashion in association with aortic valvular regurgitation, and about half of these patients have mitral insufficiency as well (Fig. 98-2). The aneurysms involve the sinuses of Valsalva and the tubular portion of the aorta, producing annuloaortic ectasia characterized by degeneration of elastic fibers and accumulation of mucoid material within the medial layer of the aortic wall. According to some pathologists but not others, neither cysts nor necrotic tissue characterize the histologic changes in the aorta that occur in the

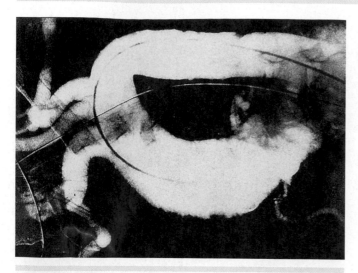

FIGURE 98-2 Aortogram of a patient with Marfan's syndrome. Aneurysms are characterized by annuloaortic ectasia, involving the sinuses of Valsalva and the tubular portion of the aorta, produced by degeneration of elastic fibers and the accumulation of mucoid material within the medial layer of the aortic wall, grossly resembling cystic medial necrosis. (From Creager et al.[292] With permission.)

Marfan syndrome, yet the gross pathology resembles that of cystic medial necrosis.[16] Abnormalities associated with the Marfan syndrome typically affect the entire length of the aorta, though dissection most often involves the thoracic portion,[40] with or without other histologic features of the syndrome or aortic valvular incompetence.

Atherosclerotic Thoracic Aortic Aneurysm

Atherosclerosis is an unusual cause of ascending aortic aneurysms; when it is the etiology, there is usually evidence of atherosclerosis elsewhere. Proximal atherosclerotic aneurysms are typically fusiform and extend into the arch. Aneurysms of the aortic arch are therefore often contiguous with aneurysms in the ascending aorta, and they occur more frequently in men than in women.[41] More frequently, atherosclerotic aneurysms affect the distal aspect of the arch and descending thoracic aorta.[42] All proximal aortic aneurysms caused by atherosclerosis are usually part of a more diffuse atherosclerotic process and must be distinguished from cystic medial necrosis as well as syphilitic and other aneurysms of infectious or inflammatory etiologies in this location.

In contrast to the ascending aorta, the majority of aneurysms of the descending thoracic aorta are associated with atherosclerosis.[43–45] These may extend to the level of the abdominal aorta, are typically fusiform, and often begin distal to the origin of the left subclavian artery.[46] Descending thoracic aneurysms may also occur in patients with aortic coarctation.[47]

Aneurysms of the thoracic aorta typically produce no symptoms, but a variety of symptom complexes may arise, related to the size of the aneurysm and its location within the thorax. Patients with aneurysms of the ascending aorta may develop congestive heart failure as a consequence of aortic valvular regurgitation. Enlargement of the sinuses of Valsalva may cause myocardial ischemia or infarction due to direct compression of the coronary arteries or coronary arterial thromboembolism.[48] Right ventricular outflow tract obstruction and tricuspid regurgitation may result from aneurysmal deformation of the noncoronary sinus.[30] Aneurysms of the sinuses of Valsalva may rupture directly into the right ventricular cavity, right atrium, or pul-

monary artery, causing heart failure associated with a continuous murmur.[49,50] Chest pain may occur when the aneurysm compresses surrounding structures or erodes into adjacent bone, such as the ribs or sternum. Compression of the superior vena cava may produce venous congestion of the head, neck, and upper extremities. Rupture may occur into the left pleural space, pericardium, pulmonary artery, or superior vena cava.[30,40,51]

Aneurysms of the aortic arch may produce symptoms by compression of contiguous structures, but most are asymptomatic. Dyspnea or cough may be caused by compression of the trachea or mainstem bronchi, dysphagia by compression of the esophagus, or hoarseness secondary to left vocal cord paralysis related to compression of the left recurrent laryngeal nerve.[52] Superior vena cava syndrome and pulmonary artery stenosis result when these vessels are compressed.[53–55] Chest pain related either to compression of adjacent structures or to erosion of ribs or vertebrae is typically positional. Physical examination may demonstrate right sternoclavicular lift or tracheal deviation. Aneurysms of the aortic arch may rupture into the mediastinum, pleural space, tracheobronchial tree (causing hemoptysis), or esophagus (causing hematemesis). Arteriovenous fistulas may result from rupture into the superior vena cava or pulmonary artery.

Symptoms of descending thoracic aortic aneurysms include chest pain from compression of surrounding soft tissues or erosion of vertebrae. Irritation of the recurrent laryngeal nerve may produce hoarseness.[45] Dyspnea may result from bronchial compression, and hemoptysis from direct erosion into the lung parenchyma.[43,56] Dysphagia and hematemesis are features of esophageal compression or erosion. Rupture may occur into the mediastinum or left pleural space.

Primary prophylactic operation is indicated in cases where the aneurysm is 6 cm in maximum diameter, or 5 cm in cases of the Marfan syndrome. As noted above, symptoms are frequently a harbinger of rupture or death in patients with thoracic aortic aneurysm, calling for a more aggressive approach.

Thoracoabdominal Aortic Aneurysm

As suggested by the nomenclature, thoracoabdominal aortic aneurysms have features of both thoracic and abdominal aortic aneurysms (Fig. 98-3). Although they constitute only about 3 percent of all aortic aneurysms, thoracoabdominal aneurysms are considered as a separate class because of the diffuse and extensive aortic involvement and special considerations for surgical repair, which may entail reimplantation of the origins of visceral arteries.[57] Among the various proposed classification schemes, Crawford and colleagues delineated four types of thoracoabdominal aortic aneurysms, according to the segment and extent of aorta involved.[58] In keeping with the notion that thoracoabdominal aortic aneurysms represent a diffusely atherosclerotic and ectatic aorta with one or more aneurysmal segments of variable length, two types that are essentially confined to the abdominal aorta are included. The principal clinical implication is that surgical repair may require reimplantation or reconstruction of the origins of major branch arteries, which entails risks of ischemic tissue injury greater than those associated with aneurysmectomy alone.

Because they occur less frequently than discrete aneurysms of the aorta, relatively little information is available regarding the natural history of thoracoabdominal aneurysms. The etiologic factors and clinical presentation are more comparable to aneurysms of the abdominal than the thoracic aorta; thus, it has been speculated that the risk of rupture is similar to that of abdominal aortic aneurysms of

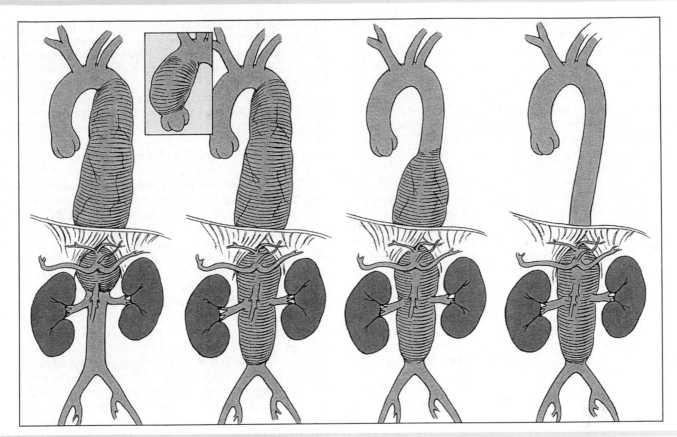

FIGURE 98-3 Classification of thoracoabdominal aortic aneurysms. Type I aneurysms involve most of the descending aorta from near the origin of the left subclavian artery to the abdominal vessels, but the renal arteries are not involved. Type II aneurysms also begin near the origin of the left subclavian artery but extend below the origins of the renal arteries in the abdomen. Type III aneurysms arise more distally and involve less of the descending thoracic aorta but often more of the abdominal aorta than type I and II aneurysms. Type IV aneurysms arise at the level of the diaphragm and typically extend to a point below the origins of the renal arteries. (From Crawford and Coselli.[293] With permission.)

equivalent diameter. In one autopsy series involving 7642 cases between 1935 and 1954, a total of 7 thoracoabdominal aneurysms were found, 4 of which had ruptured.[57] The patients manifested diffuse atherosclerosis, and mortality might have been a consequence of concomitant coronary or cerebrovascular disease.

Although most patients with thoracoabdominal aortic aneurysms are asymptomatic, discomfort occasionally develops in the epigastrium or left upper quadrant of the abdomen. Back or flank pain may occur when the patient lies in left lateral decubitus position. Erosion of the anterior surfaces of the vertebral bodies may occur, leading to radiculopathy.[59–61] Visceral artery occlusion may occur, but frank ischemia and infarction are infrequent.[61] Patients who complain of claudication may also have occlusive atherosclerotic disease of the aorta or the iliac or more distal arteries. Because mural thrombosis is so common in atherosclerotic aneurysms, they may be the source of peripheral atheroembolism, causing occlusion of distal vessels.[62,63] Rupture of the thoracic component of these aneurysms generally occurs into the left pleural space, producing a hemothorax; the abdominal component may rupture into the retroperitoneum, inferior vena cava, or duodenum.

Abdominal Aortic Aneurysm

Aneurysms of the abdominal aorta account for approximately 15,000 deaths annually in the United States.[64] The incidence of abdominal aortic aneurysms in autopsy series has ranged from 1.8 to 6.6 percent of cases, leading to an estimated occurrence rate of 15 to 37 cases per

100,000 patient-years.[65–75] The incidence increases with age, ranging from less than 2.1 per 100,000 patient-years between the ages of 40 and 49 to more than 280 per 100,000 patient-years among individuals above age 80.[73,74] Abdominal aortic aneurysms occur two to five times more frequently in men than women and more often in whites than blacks.[73,74] One autopsy series reported an incidence of 4.2 percent among white men, compared with 1.5 percent among black men.[68] The prevalence of abdominal aortic aneurysms is higher in patients with clinical evidence of atherosclerosis. In patients with coronary artery disease, for instance, the prevalence of abdominal aneurysms is approximately 5 percent, and nearly 10 percent of patients with atherosclerotic peripheral arterial obstructive disease have associated abdominal aortic aneurysms.[67,76–78]

In over 90 percent of cases, the superior margins of abdominal aortic aneurysms are below the level of the renal arteries.[79–81] Atherosclerosis has been held responsible for the majority, although some authors have suggested that atherosclerosis may be a secondary phenomenon in aneurysmal disease.[82–84] Several reports of familial clustering of abdominal aortic aneurysm have appeared, and decreased type 3 collagen and elastin content of the aortic wall as well as increased collagenase activity have been identified in some familial cases.[85–90] Whether atherosclerosis is the inciting cause of these aneurysms or a cofactor in otherwise predisposed individuals remains uncertain[91]; it has been proposed that atherosclerosis may represent a secondary response to vascular injury resulting from primary changes in elastin and collagen in patients predisposed to abdominal aortic aneurysm.[92]

Survival is limited in patients with abdominal aortic aneurysms because of the potential for aortic rupture and the prevalence of coronary artery disease. In 1950, the survival rates of 102 patients with abdominal aortic aneurysms identified on physical examination or radiography, most atherosclerotic,[93] were 67 percent at 1 year, 49 percent at 3 years, and 19 percent at 5 years. Of the fatalities, 63 percent were related to rupture. Others have subsequently reported similar statistics.[94–97] The survival rate for patients with aneurysms smaller than 6 cm in one series was 75 percent after 1 year, 68 percent after 3 years, and 48 percent after 5 years. For those with aneurysms larger than 6 cm, the first-year survival rate was 48 percent, at 3 years 12 percent, and at 5 years 6 percent. Follow-up after up to 20 years of 127 patients initially deemed medically unfit for surgery (predominantly because of severe coexisting coronary artery disease) found the mortality rate 71 percent, 28 percent of which was due to rupture.[98] In other series, rupture was reported in 20 percent of patients over a 30-year period, most with aneurysms over 5 cm in diameter,[74] and the following survival rates have been described in patients with untreated abdominal aortic aneurysms: 62 percent after 1 year, 32 percent after 3 years, and 19 percent after 5 years.[99] Thirty-eight percent of the patients died as a consequence of rupture; 55 percent of those with aneurysms larger than 6 cm died of rupture, compared with 16 percent of those with aneurysms smaller than 6 cm in diameter. In a group of patients with aneurysms initially 3 to 6 cm in diameter, the mean expansion rate was 0.4 cm per year.[100]

The pathophysiologic processes that underlie aneurysm expansion have not been clearly defined but appear to involve elastolysis and collagenolysis promoted by inflammatory changes within the aortic wall and by hypertension.[101] Despite the greater risk of rupture with large aneurysms, it has been difficult to establish a clear correlation between the rate of aneurysm expansion and the risk of rupture. The problem may be one of observational methodology, however, and there is little reason to doubt that rapid expansion is a harbinger of rupture.[102] It is widely believed but difficult to prove that symptomatic aneurysms or those that generate a local or systemic inflammatory response show an earlier propensity to rupture. The prevalence of abdominal aortic aneurysm increases with age, occurring more frequently in patients aged 60 to 70 years than in younger individuals, although affected individuals range from ages 30 to over 90.[103,104] Coronary artery disease, peripheral arterial disease, and other manifestations of systemic atherosclerosis occur frequently in patients with abdominal aortic aneurysms, and hypertension often coexists.[105] Whether hypertension correlates with the risk of rupture is controversial.[106]

A relationship between inflammatory processes and aortic aneurysmal disease is supported by an abnormal accumulation of macrophages and elevated levels of cytokines in aneurysmal aortic tissue.[24,25] In a case-control study,[107] 30 patients with inflammatory aneurysm were compared to 60 control patients who had noninflammatory aneurysms. There were no distinctions between the two groups of patients with respect to risk factors, treatment requirements, or prognosis, but inflammatory aneurysms tended to present with more symptoms, a higher erythrocyte sedimentation rate, a larger diameter, and more of a retroperitoneal inflammatory reaction than conventional aneurysms. In another series of 355 patients who underwent surgical repair, 5.6 percent of abdominal aortic aneurysms had inflammatory clinical features and 11 percent had histologic evidence of inflammation.[108] The early and late results of surgery were no different between patients with inflammatory or noninflammatory aneurysms.

An elevated baseline level of C-reactive protein, a marker of inflammation, correlates with poor prognosis in patients with symptomatic aortic aneurysms or dissection.[109]

CLINICAL MANIFESTATIONS

Most patients with abdominal aortic aneurysms are asymptomatic, yet symptoms may take the form of abdominal discomfort or back pain, and some patients become aware of abdominal pulsation.[110,111] Less frequently, pain may occur in the legs, chest, or groin; anorexia, nausea, vomiting, constipation, or dyspnea may develop. Compression of the left iliac vein may cause left leg swelling, just as compression of the left ureter may cause hydronephrosis or compression of testicular veins may cause varicocele. As the aneurysm expands and compresses vertebrae and lumbar nerve roots, pain may develop in the lower back and radiate to the posterior aspects of the legs. Flank pain radiating to the anterior left thigh or scrotum may reflect compression of the left genitofemoral nerve. Nausea and vomiting may occur as the aneurysm compresses the duodenum. Bladder compression may cause urinary frequency or urgency.

The key physical finding is a pulsatile abdominal mass. Typically, aneurysms larger than 4 cm in diameter are palpable except those occurring in obese individuals or in cases where adequate examination is inhibited by guarding. The patient should be positioned supine with the knees flexed. A pulsatile epigastric or periumbilical mass may be visible as well as palpable. To distinguish an abdominal aortic aneurysm from paraaortic masses requires that the examiner's hands address the lateral borders. An aneurysm expands laterally with each systole. This technique also permits estimation of the transverse diameter of the aneurysm.[112] Auscultation may reveal a bruit over the mass, but abdominal bruits are not specific for aneurysm formation, and only about 40 percent of such aneurysms are associated with bruits. The finding of a pulsatile mass in the groin, suggesting an iliac artery aneurysm, or in the popliteal fossa, suggesting a popliteal artery aneurysm, raises the index of suspicion that an abdominal aortic aneurysm may be present, since multiple aneurysms often coexist. Physical signs may reflect atherosclerosis of other vessels, including carotid bruits or diminished arterial pulses in the lower extremities.

The triad of chronic abdominal pain, weight loss, and an accelerated sedimentation rate in a patient with an abdominal aortic aneurysm is highly suggestive of an inflammatory aneurysm. Inflammatory aortic or iliac aneurysms were present in 4.5 percent of the 2816 patients who underwent elective abdominal aortic aneurysm repair at the Mayo Clinic from 1955 to 1985.[113] Compared to patients with noninflammatory atherosclerotic aneurysms, those with inflammatory aneurysms were more likely to have symptoms (66 vs. 20 percent, $p < 0.0001$), weight loss (21 vs. 10 percent, $p < 0.05$), a higher sedimentation rate (73 vs. 33 percent, $p < 0.0001$), and a higher operative mortality rate (7.9 vs. 2.4 percent, $p < 0.002$).

ULTRASOUND SCREENING

How best to approach the problem of screening is an important health economic conundrum, considering the prevalence of and mortality associated with abdominal aneurysmal disease. In a population-based investigation of 67,800 men aged 65 to 74 years initiated in the United Kingdom in 1997, a total of 33,839 were randomly invited to undergo abdominal ultrasound scanning and compared with 33,961 in a control group in whom scans were not performed.[114] Men with aortic aneurysms measuring at least 3 cm in diameter were followed with repeat scans for a mean of 4.1 years and surgical treatment was considered when the diameter reached 5.5 cm, when expansion occurred at a rate of over 1 cm/year, or when symptoms occurred. Over 27,000 (80 percent) of the men invited agreed to screening, and 1333 aneurysms were detected. There were 65 aneurysm-related deaths (absolute risk 0.19 percent) in this group, compared with 113 (0.33 percent) in the control group (relative risk reduction, 42 percent; 95

percent CI 22–58 percent; $p = 0.0002$), including a 53 percent reduction of risk (95 percent CI 30–64 percent) among those who actually underwent screening. The 30-day mortality rate was 6 percent (24 of 414) after elective aneurysm repair, compared to 37 percent (30 of 81) after emergency operations. Over 4 years, 47 fewer deaths related to abdominal aortic aneurysms occurred in the screened group than in the control group, but the additional costs incurred were 2.2 million British pounds (approximately US $3.5 million). After adjustment for censoring and a discount of 6 percent, the mean additional cost of screening was £63.4/$98 (95 percent CI, £53.3 to £73.5/$84 to $116) per patient. Over 4 years, the mean incremental cost-effectiveness ratio for screening was £28,400/$45,000 per life-year gained, corresponding approximately to £36,000/$57,000 per quality-adjusted life-year. After 10 years, this figure declined to approximately £8,000/$12,500 per life-year gained.[115]

ANEURYSM RUPTURE

Rupture of an abdominal aortic aneurysm usually produces the clinical picture of extreme distress as a result of abdominal catastrophe. Despite surgical advances, mortality is still the most frequent outcome because of the abrupt nature of circulatory collapse, which prevents timely intervention except in unusual cases. Patients frequently have severe abdominal or back pain, but the pattern of pain varies considerably. The aneurysm may rupture into the retroperitoneum or into the peritoneal or pleural cavities, leading to hypotension, tachycardia, pallor, diaphoresis, or deep shock, depending on the extent of rupture and associated blood loss into the extravascular space. On occasion, rupture occurs directly into the duodenum, causing an aortoduodenal fistula and acute gastrointestinal bleeding. This possibility should be considered when gastrointestinal bleeding is evident along with signs of an aneurysm on physical examination. Rupture may also occur into the inferior vena cava or iliac veins, producing an arteriovenous fistula; this is suggested by rapid development of leg swelling or high-output congestive heart failure in the presence of an abdominal aortic aneurysm.

SURGICAL AND ENDOGRAFT REPAIR

During the past decade, randomized trials comparing early intervention vs. expectant management of infrarenal abdominal aortic aneurysms measuring 4.0 to 5.4 cm in diameter have been conducted in the United Kingdom and by the Veterans Administration (VA).[116,117] By protocol, elective surgical treatment was not offered to patients allocated to the nonoperative cohort in each trial until aneurysms exceeded 5.4 cm in size on serial imaging studies. Women comprised 17 percent of the patients in the UK study but only 0.8 percent of the VA population. Thirty-day operative mortality rates (UK, 5.4 percent; VA, 2.1 percent) were competitive with those from other multicenter studies. Endografts were employed in 27 patients in the surgical limb of the UK trial (4.8 percent) but in just two patients in the VA trial.

After a mean follow-up of 4.9 years, early aneurysm repair produced no significant benefits with respect to the incidence of either aneurysm-related deaths or deaths from all causes in the VA trial. The same conclusions were originally reached at a mean follow-up of 4.6 years in the UK trial in 1998. While the UK surgical cohort had a lower overall mortality rate than the nonoperative cohort at 8 years ($p = 0.03$), this finding has been attributed in part to a higher rate of smoking cessation in the early-surgery group.[118] The annual rupture rate was negligible (0.6 percent) for observed aneurysms in the VA trial and 3.2 percent in the UK trial. Rupture in the UK trial was more likely to occur in women (odds ratio 4.0, 95 percent CI 2.0 to 7.9;

$p < 0.001$), accounting for 14 percent of all deaths in women compared to 4.6 percent of all deaths in men ($p < 0.001$). Aneurysm size at the time of randomization did not influence the risk for rupture in the UK trial or the long-term mortality rate in either trial, which may reflect the promptness with which intervention was performed when aneurysms reached a diameter ≥5.5 cm. Over 60 percent of the patients in the nonoperative limb of each of these trials have undergone aneurysm repair because of documented enlargement, including 81 percent of the patients in the VA trial whose aneurysms were 5.0 to 5.4 cm in diameter when recruited.

ENDOVASCULAR REPAIR

Parodi et al. first reported the technique of transfemoral catheter-based repair of infrarenal abdominal aortic aneurysms in 1991 as an alternative for management of patients at high risk of complications with conventional surgical treatment.[119] Over the following decade, a variety of stent grafts and delivery systems have been introduced, all of which require open exposure of the common femoral arteries for sheath insertion. In addition, extraperitoneal incisions may be necessary to establish temporary access conduits to the iliac arteries when the size or tortuosity of the external iliac arteries precludes transfemoral cannulation. By avoiding major abdominal/retroperitoneal surgery, however, endovascular repair under regional or local anesthesia has become a valuable alternative for patients in whom severe cardiopulmonary disease, advanced age, morbid obesity, or a previously instrumented abdomen present obstacles to safe, direct surgical reconstruction.

Most stent graft devices have a modular construction consisting of a metallic exoskeleton surrounding an intimal fabric graft to maintain linear stability and avoid kinking. The aortic stem and one contiguous iliac limb are inserted through one femoral artery and the other iliac limb is then positioned using a separate delivery system through the contralateral femoral artery. The conventional technique required an adequate aortic segment of relatively normal caliber below the renal arteries, but newer devices incorporate barbed hooks to secure the stent graft to the aorta above the renal arteries. To avoid obstructing the origins of the renal arteries by the fabric component of the endograft, at least a 1 to 1.5 cm relatively straight aortic segment measuring no more than 28 mm in diameter should be available below the renal arteries. This poses a particular challenge in females patients, in whom the aortoiliac arteries are generally smaller and more angulated than in men.[120–123]

Continued blood flow into the excluded sac of an aneurysm, termed an *endoleak*, represents an important complication of endograft repair.[124] *Type I* endoleaks are caused by incompetent proximal or distal attachments, produce high intrasac pressure that can lead to rupture, and should be repaired using intraluminal extension cuffs or conversion to an open procedure as soon as they are discovered. *Type II* endoleaks result from retrograde flow from branch vessels (e.g., the lumbar or inferior mesenteric arteries) and occur in as many as 40 percent of patients after endograft implantation. These may be corrected by selective arterial embolization, but over half seal spontaneously and when persistent do not appear to increase the risk for rupture over 18 to 36 months.[125–128] *Type III* endoleaks are caused by fabric defects or tears or disruption of modular graft components. These carry the same potential for delayed aneurysm rupture as type I endoleaks and should, therefore, be promptly repaired. *Type IV* endoleaks, the least common, result from high graft porosity and diffuse leakage through interstices, and usually occur within 30 days of implantation. Because of the potential for endoleaks, follow-up imaging every 6 to 12 months is recommended following endovascular stent-graft repair.[124,129]

Other complications of endovascular stent-graft repair of abdominal aortic aneurysms include occlusion of the iliac limbs of bifurcation endografts,[130,131] migration from the proximal attachment related to progressive aortic expansion,[132,133] which can be detected by serial imaging studies in 13 percent of patients at 1 year after endovascular aneurysm repair, in 21 percent at 2 years, and in 19 percent at 3 years.[134] These and other complications may become increasingly apparent as the follow-up of patients undergoing endograft repair grows longer.

CONCOMITANT CORONARY ARTERY DISEASE

Coronary artery disease is the most important risk factor for cardiac events and death in patients undergoing aneurysm surgery.[135–138] Since operative mortality is related mainly to myocardial ischemia, it has been suggested that coronary revascularization be performed in certain patients prior to abdominal aortic aneurysm resection.[139–142] No well-designed studies are available that compare the outcome of serial myocardial revascularization and abdominal aortic aneurysm repair with aneurysm surgery alone. Even so, an effort should be made to identify those patients at highest cardiac risk preoperatively using noninvasive diagnostic methods.[138,143,144] Abnormal findings indicative of extensive myocardial ischemia may prompt angiography to determine the nature of coronary artery disease and left ventricular function. Thereafter, decisions regarding coronary revascularization must be based on symptoms, angiographic findings, and other elements of risk. It is reasonable to consider coronary revascularization prior to aneurysm surgery in patients with left main coronary artery disease, stenosis greater than 70 percent in each of the three major coronary arteries in the presence of impaired left ventricular function, and in those with active angina pectoris.

ATHEROSCLEROSIS OF THE AORTA

Pathologic Anatomy

Pathologic evidence of atherosclerosis of the aorta is common in western society. The usual risk factors are tobacco smoking, diabetes mellitus, hypertension, hypercholesterolemia, obesity, and sedentary lifestyle as well as novel risk factors such as elevated plasma levels of homocysteine and C-reactive protein. The pathogenesis of atherosclerosis is discussed in Chap. 44.

Atherosclerosis most commonly develops in the infrarenal aorta and may be asymptomatic or produce intermittent claudication, critical limb ischemia, or atheromatous embolism. Atherosclerosis also commonly occurs at the origins of the brachiocephalic, carotid, and subclavian vessels as well as in the aortic arch.[145] Atherosclerosis involving the supraceliac portion of the abdominal aorta and the descending thoracic aorta is much less common.[146]

Atheromatous Embolism

Embolism of cholesterol-laden material and thrombus from the surface of the aorta occurs commonly in patients with severe aortic atherosclerosis.[147] Atheroembolism may be spontaneous, although it occurs more frequently after surgical or arteriographic manipulation, such as catheter-based coronary or peripheral interventions. In a retrospective study of 71 autopsies, the incidence of cholesterol embolism in patients who had undergone arteriography before death was 27 percent, compared to 4.3 percent in an age- and disease-matched control group who did not undergo angiography.[148] The severity of aortic atherosclerosis seems the most important factor

predictive of this complication. In a review of 4587 cardiac catheterizations, there were 7 cases of clinical cholesterol embolism (0.002 percent),[149] and in another series, there were 8 cases among 3733 cardiac catheterization, angioplasty, and intraaortic balloon pump procedures (0.002 percent). None were observed when access was obtained through the brachial artery.[150] In a study of 7621 patients undergoing cardiac catheterization, histologic evidence of atheroembolism was found in 41 (0.54 percent) patients, but none had clinically apparent ischemic complications.[151]

Whether anticoagulant and thrombolytic drugs can exacerbate atheroembolism associated with the "blue-toe syndrome" is controversial.[152,153] Few cases of this complication were reported in clinical trials of anticoagulation in high-risk patients with atrial fibrillation, despite the frequent finding of morphologically complex aortic plaque in this population.[154]

Patients with atheromatous embolism typically have a history of angina pectoris, myocardial infarction, transient ischemic attack, stroke, intermittent claudication, or peripheral gangrene. Clinical signs and symptoms are variable, depending on the amount, size, and site of origin of the atheromatous material as well as on the tissue affected. Macroembolism may present catastrophically as an acute ischemic limb, while patients with microembolism may have milder localized signs or a clinical picture suggesting systemic illness, including fever, weight loss, anorexia, myalgia, headache, nausea, vomiting, or diarrhea. Occasionally, the presentation may suggest vasculitis, infective endocarditis, or malignancy (Table 98-2).[155,156] Cutaneous manifestations are the most frequent findings[157] and include cyanotic toes, gangrenous digits, livedo reticularis, or nodules (Fig. 98-4).[158] When atheroembolism affects both lower extremities, the source is generally the aorta, but when only one extremity is involved, it may be difficult to determine whether the origin is a diseased ipsilateral iliofemoral artery or a more proximal or distal site.

Atheromatous embolism arising from the aortic arch or the carotid and vertebral arteries may cause stroke, transient ischemic attack, amaurosis fugax, blindness, headache, confusion, organic brain syndromes, dizziness or spinal cord infarction. Retinal artery

TABLE 98-2 Clinical Manifestations of Atheroembolism

Constitutional	Fever
	Weight loss
	Malaise
	Anorexia
Skin	Purple or blue toes
	Gangrenous digits
	Livedo reticularis
	Nodules
Kidney	Uncontrolled hypertension
	Renal failure
Nervous system	Transient ischemic attack
	Amaurosis fugax
	Stroke
	Hollenhorst plaque
Heart	Myocardial infarction
	Angina pectoris
Gastrointestinal	Abdominal pain
	Intestinal bleeding
	Mesenteric ischemia
	Pancreatitis

SOURCE: Adapted from Bartholomew and Olin.[155] With permission.

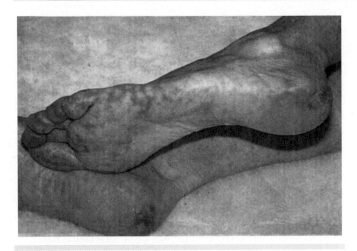

FIGURE 98-4 Typical appearance of atheromatous embolism involving the feet. There is livedo reticularis on the lateral portion of the foot, with several cyanotic toes. Note the lesions on both heels, indicating that the source of the emboli is above the aortic bifurcation. (From Bartholomew and Olin.[155] With permission.)

occlusion may be identified by Hollenhorst plaque visible on ophthalmoscopic examination as yellow, highly refractile atheromatous material at an arteriolar bifurcation. The risk of ischemic events in the central nervous system appears related to specific morphologic features of atheromatous aortic plaque defined by transesophageal echocardiography, including thickness, ulceration or the presence of mobile elements.[159,160]

Atheroembolism originating from the suprarenal aorta may involve the kidneys, producing occlusion of multiple small arteries and segmental ischemic atrophy. This small vessel occlusive disease may cause accelerated hypertension, microscopic hematuria, or renal failure. Pathologically, biconvex cholesterol crystals occlude the interlobular and afferent arterioles (150 to 200 μm in diameter). A foreign-body reaction leads to small vessel occlusion, reducing the glomerular filtration rate, activating the renin-angiotensin-aldosterone system, and accelerating hypertension. Various patterns of renal insufficiency may develop and progress over weeks or months to irreversible renal failure requiring dialysis.[155,161] The differential diagnosis includes renal artery stenosis, renal artery thrombosis, infective endocarditis, vasculitis such as polyarteritis nodosa, and other causes of acute renal failure. No single laboratory test is diagnostic, as acceleration of the erythrocyte sedimentation rate, leukocytosis with eosinophilia, and anemia are common in many systemic illnesses.[162] Blood urea nitrogen and creatinine elevations may be early manifestations of renal involvement, and the urine sediment may be abnormal. Elevated serum amylase or hepatic transaminase levels may indicate pancreatic or hepatic involvement, and creatine phosphokinase and aldolase arise from affected muscle. Renal biopsy is rarely required but may reveal pathognomonic needle-shaped cholesterol clefts within small vessels. Atheroembolic renal disease carries a poor prognosis, with a mortality rate of 81 percent (179 of 221 patients) in one series; the most common causes were cardiac, renal, or multiorgan failure.[157]

TREATMENT

Treatment seldom reverses damage, so emphasis is on prevention of subsequent ischemic events. It may be feasible to isolate or replace a discrete segment of the aorta by surgery, angioplasty, or stent-graft insertion when the source of embolism can be confirmed. Treatment should also involve symptomatic care of the affected ischemic tissue and risk-factor modification to prevent progression of atheromatous disease and promote plaque stabilization. If embolism affects the lower extremities, local care of ischemic ulcers is appropriate; when gangrene is present, amputation may be required. The role of sympathectomy is controversial, but this may be helpful when pain is intractable. In cases of renal atheroembolism, dialysis should be performed as necessary, and blood pressure controlled pharmacologically.

Optimum antithrombotic therapy (anticoagulants, platelet inhibitors, or a combination of both) has not been defined for atheromatous embolism, but these agents generally lessen the risk of cardiovascular ischemic events. Case reports of improvement with lipid-lowering therapy[163] are supported by observations in nonrandomized series[164] and evidence in coronary disease that HMG CoA-reductase inhibitor ("statin") drugs improve plaque stabilization.[165]

Surgical or endovascular therapy has been advocated to remove the source of atheroembolism, particularly when located in the aortoiliac segment. When atheromatous disease is infrarenal, as is most common, aortobi-iliac or aortobifemoral bypass is indicated. Replacement of the suprarenal aorta is generally reserved for patients with life-threatening situations because of its considerable perioperative morbidity and mortality.[166] Aortic stent grafting to overlay the atheromatous material and prevent future embolism has been described. In poor candidates for aortic replacement, ligation of the common femoral arteries along with extraanatomic bypass may prevent recurrent lower limb ischemia, but intestinal and renal ischemia is not avoided.[167] No well-designed trials have compared nonoperative with surgical therapy for patients with atheroembolism, and it is often difficult to localize the source of embolism when atherosclerosis is diffusely distributed.[168]

Atherosclerosis of the Aortic Arch

Atherosclerosis of the thoracic aorta is a strong predictor of initial and recurrent stroke, coronary events, and death.[159,169,170] The thickness and morphology (protrusion, ulceration, or mobility) of atheromatous plaque correlate with the prevalence of stroke (Table 98-3).[160,171] Whether this association has a direct atheroembolic

TABLE 98-3 Ischemic Vascular Events Related to Aortic Atheromatous Plaque

Plaque Thickness (mm)	RECURRENT BRAIN INFARCTION		ANY VASCULAR EVENT[a]	
	Follow-up (person-years)	Incidence (events per 100 person-years)	Follow-up (person-years)	Incidence (events per 100 person-years)
<1	359.3	2.8	354.0	5.9
1–3.9	312.6	3.5	308.2	9.1
≥4	92.4	11.9	88.4	26.0

[a]Includes cerebral infarction, myocardial infarction, peripheral embolism, and death from any vascular cause.
SOURCE: Adapted from the French Study of Aortic Plaques in Stroke Group.[159] With permission.

mechanism or reflects associated cerebrovascular pathology has not been conclusively determined.

Aortoiliac Occlusive Disease

Atherosclerotic occlusive disease of the infrarenal aorta and iliac arteries may occur with or without atherosclerosis of the infrainguinal vessels.[172,173] When isolated, aortoiliac atherosclerosis typically occurs in younger individuals who smoke cigarettes. Almost half the cases are women, many of whom angiographically exhibit the "hypoplastic aortic syndrome," with small-caliber aortic, iliac, and femoropopliteal arteries. The disease in these cases is usually confined to the aortic bifurcation.[174] Males are generally older and present with more diffuse disease (type II involving the aorta, common, and external iliac arteries, and type III comprising widespread disease both above and below the inguinal ligament). Disease localized to the distal aorta and common iliac arteries (type I) rarely produces limb-threatening ischemia because of extensive collateral vessels. The classic presentation is the Leriche syndrome, a clinical triad of intermittent claudication involving the low back, buttocks, hip or thigh, which is often mistaken for degenerative joint disease of the low back or hips, impotency (which occurs in 30 to 50 percent of males with aortoiliac occlusive disease) and "global atrophy" of the lower extremities, reflecting the chronicity of low-grade ischemia.[175] The femoral pulses are often weak or absent, but the ankle-brachial index may be normal at rest. A decline in ankle systolic pressure following exercise confirms hemodynamically significant stenosis.

MANAGEMENT

Treatment of patients with occlusive atherosclerosis of the aorta should include measures directed at improving symptoms (e.g., claudication or limb ischemia) and thus quality of life, as well as reduction of overall cardiovascular risk. The latter involves the same measures as management of other manifestations of systemic atherosclerosis or peripheral arterial disease (Chaps. 99–102).

Catheter-based intervention to relieve aortic obstruction should be considered in cases of critical limb ischemia or claudication that substantially compromises lifestyle. While there is controversy on this point, there is general consensus that patients with aortoiliac occlusive disease do not respond as well to exercise or medications (pentoxifylline or cilostazol) as do patients with infrainguinal peripheral arterial disease. Surgical revascularization (e.g., endarterectomy, aortoiliac or aortobifemoral bypass) has been almost entirely replaced by percutaneous catheter-based interventions under local anesthesia, which avoid abdominal incision, abbreviate hospital stay, reduce cost, accelerate recovery, and carry lower short-term morbidity and mortality.[176]

The Transatlantic Inter-societal Consensus group classified patients with aortoiliac occlusive disease into four categories. Endovascular therapy was favored for patients with type A lesions; surgery was preferred for those with type D lesions (Table 98-4).[177] Although the evidence then available was not sufficient to support firm recommendations for type B or C aortoiliac lesions, subsequent technologic advances justify an attempt at angioplasty and stenting in most cases meeting clinical criteria for revascularization unless obstructive disease extends into the common femoral artery. Surgical revascularization of aortoiliac lesions is associated with 74 to 95 percent patency rates at 5 years,[178] similar but not superior to results with catheter-based interventions.[179] A multicenter trial of primary iliac stenting in 486 patients demonstrated clinical benefit in 91 percent at 1 year, 84 percent at 2 years, and 63 percent at 43 months follow-up; angiographic patency was 92 percent.[180]

TABLE 98-4 Morphologic Stratification of Aortoiliac Atherosclerosis

Type A
- Single stenosis < 3 cm of the common iliac artery (CIA) or external iliac artery (EIA) (unilateral or bilateral)

Type B
- Single lesion 3–10 cm in length not extending into the common femoral artery (CFA)
- Total of 2 stenoses < 5 cm long in the CIA and/or EIA not extending into the CFA
- Unilateral CIA occlusion

Type C
- Bilateral 5- to 10-cm-long stenosis of the CIA and/or EIA not extending into the CFA
- Unilateral EIA occlusion not extending into the CFA
- Unilateral EIA stenosis extending into the CFA
- Bilateral CIA occlusions

Type D
- Diffuse multiple unilateral stenosis involving the CIA, EIA, and CFA (usually > 10 cm)
- Unilateral occlusion involving both the CIA and EIA
- Bilateral EIA occlusions
- Diffuse disease involving the aorta and both iliac arteries
- Iliac stenosis in a patient with an abdominal aortic aneurysm or other lesion requiring aortic or iliac surgery

SOURCE: Adapted from the Transatlantic Inter-societal Consensus (TASC).[177] With permission.

ACUTE OBSTRUCTION OF THE TERMINAL AORTA

Etiology

Sudden occlusion of the terminal aorta may result from a large "saddle" embolus,[181] trauma, dissection (see below) or in situ thrombosis superimposed on aneurysmal or atherosclerotic disease. Most emboli large enough to occlude the terminal aorta (saddle embolism) originate in the heart in patients with mitral stenosis, atrial fibrillation, acute anterior myocardial infarction or infective endocarditis, or involve paradoxical embolism through a right-to-left intracardiac shunt from a peripheral venous source. When thrombotic occlusion of the aorta develops at a point of atherosclerotic narrowing, collateral perfusion is usually sufficient to prevent acute limb ischemia. Acute aortic occlusion related to thrombosis of an abdominal aortic aneurysm is considerably less common than thrombosis of popliteal aneurysms.

CLINICAL FEATURES

Unlike gradually progressive obstruction, abrupt total or near-total interruption of flow through the terminal aorta or common iliac arteries poses an immediate threat to life and limb. Although the clinical picture varies depending on collaterals, the full-blown syndrome is characterized by abrupt onset of pain, typically severe, in the lumbar area, buttocks, perineum, abdomen, and legs. Diffuse cyanosis may be present from the umbilicus to the feet and the lower limbs may be pale and cold. Numbness, paresthesias, and paralysis dominate the picture. Pulses are absent in the lower limbs and, unless circulation is restored promptly, muscle necrosis may produce myoglobinuria, renal failure, acidosis, hyperkalemia, and death.

MANAGEMENT

In contrast to chronic aortoiliac occlusion, acute aortic occlusion calls for immediate revascularization. The optimum procedure depends on etiology and the strategy for prevention of recurrent embolism. Transfemoral catheter-based embolectomy can extract even large amounts of embolic material from the distal aorta. Even after circulation has been restored, however, mortality is high, related to the underlying disease.[182]

TABLE 98-5 Classification of Aortic Dissection

	DeBakey[287]		Stanford[288]
Type I	Ascending, transverse, descending aorta	Type A	All dissections involving the ascending aorta
Type II	Ascending aorta	Type B	Aorta distal to the origin of the left subclavian artery
Type III			
A.	Descending aorta to the diaphragm		
B.	Descending aorta to below the diaphragm		

DISSECTION OF THE AORTA

Aortic dissection may be fatal without early diagnosis and aggressive treatment. The presenting symptoms and signs are so myriad and nonspecific that dissection may be overlooked initially in up to 40 percent of cases and the diagnosis in a substantial proportion of cases is only established postmortem.[183] Few other conditions demand such prompt diagnosis and treatment, since the mortality rate of untreated dissection approaches 1 percent/hour during the first 48 h, 80 percent at 14 days, and 90 percent at 3 months.[184]

Aortic dissection is considered acute when identified within 2 weeks of onset and chronic when symptoms have been present longer. Several schemes for classification of aortic dissections have been proposed (Table 98-5), but the simplest is based on distinguishing those originating proximal or distal to the left subclavian artery. For the former, early surgical intervention is generally recommended, while the latter may be managed medically or by endovascular therapy.

PATHOGENESIS

The inciting event is usually an intimal tear that propels blood from the true lumen into the middle or outer layer of aortic media, forming a second or false lumen separated by an intimal flap.[185,186] In some cases, however, intramural hematoma precedes perforation of the intima.[187] The dissection may propagate proximally (retrograde) and/or distally (antegrade) and may narrow or occlude the origin of any branch artery arising from the aorta; the antegrade type is most common. Spiral dissection may leave some aortic branches supplied by the true lumen and others supplied by the false lumen (Fig. 98-5), or pressure from one lumen may compress portions of the other.

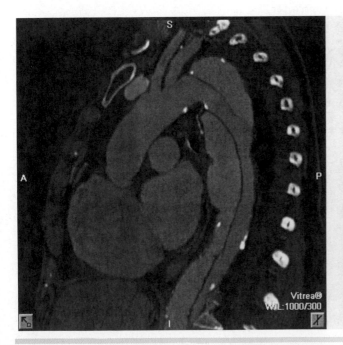 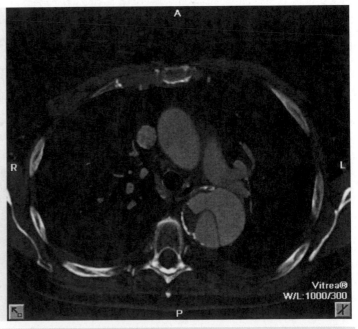

FIGURE 98-5 *A.* Magnetic resonance angiogram (MRA) in the oblique maximum-intensity projection (MIP) demonstrating dissection of the aorta beginning just distal to the origin of the left subclavian artery (type B) and spiraling along the entire descending thoracic aorta. *B.* Axial section demonstrating the true and false lumens in the proximal portion of the descending thoracic aorta.

The intimal tear originates in the ascending aorta in 65 percent of cases, transverse arch in 10 percent, upper descending aorta (just beyond the origin of the left subclavian artery) in 20 percent, and more distally in 5 percent of cases.[185] The false lumen may terminate at any point along the length of the aorta or the iliac or femoral arteries, and there are sometimes multiple flaps and levels of reentry. The false lumen can undergo retrograde dissection, thrombotic occlusion, pseudoaneurysm formation, compression, or rupture. Associated with these are obstruction of the coronary ostia, incompetence of the aortic valve, or pericardial tamponade.[188]

Left untreated, fewer than 10 percent of patients with proximal aortic dissection survive a year; most succumb within the first 3 months,[189] usually of acute aortic insufficiency, major branch vessel occlusion, or rupture into the pericardium, mediastinum, or left hemithorax. In 20 years of follow-up of 527 patients with aortic dissection, nearly 30 percent of late deaths were due to ruptured aortic aneurysm.[190]

Aortic dissection occurs more often in men than in women, with a 2-5:1 preponderance,[191] usually in the sixth and seventh decades of life. Systemic hypertension is the major predisposing risk factor. In the International Registry of Acute Aortic Dissection, 194 of 289 patients (69 percent) with proximal dissections and 132 of 175 (77 percent) with distal dissections had a history of hypertension,[192] and similar ratios were reported at the Mayo Clinic.[191] Other predisposing conditions are the Marfan syndrome, bicuspid aortic valve, Ehlers-Danlos syndrome, Turner's syndrome, Noonan's syndrome, aortic aneurysm, and annuloaortic ectasia, many of which are associated with cystic medial necrosis. The most common causes of aortic dissection in patients below 40 years of age are Marfan's syndrome and pregnancy. Iatrogenic trauma resulting from catheter manipulation is the culprit in approximately 5 percent of cases, usually involving the descending thoracic or abdominal aorta. Cocaine abuse is another predisposing factor.[193]

CLINICAL PRESENTATION

The most common symptom of aortic dissection is chest or upper back pain of sudden onset, classically described as ripping, tearing, or shearing in quality (Table 98-6).[186] In the International Registry, chest pain was present in over 95 percent of patients, 79 percent of patients with type A dissections and 63 percent of those with type B

dissections.[192] In one large series, painless dissection occurred in only 15 percent of patients.[191] Impending aortic rupture should be considered when pain subsides and later recurs.[189]

CARDIOVASCULAR MANIFESTATIONS

Aortic insufficiency occurs in 18 to 55 percent of patients with proximal aortic dissection. In the International Registry, a diastolic murmur of aortic insufficiency was identified in 44 percent of patients with proximal aortic dissection, compared with 12 percent of those with distal aortic dissection.[192] After aortic rupture, the second most common cause of death in patients with aortic dissection is acute, severe aortic insufficiency caused by dilatation of the aortic root, annulus, and valve cusps. Most patients with aortic dissection are hypertensive, but 3 to 18 percent present in shock, sometimes secondary to extension of dissection into the coronary arteries, acute myocardial infarction, left ventricular dysfunction, acute severe aortic insufficiency, cardiac tamponade or aortic rupture. Coronary perfusion may be compromised by retrograde dissection, compression by the false lumen, or hypotension.[194] Differential pulse volume and blood pressure between the right and left upper extremities was detected in 38 percent of patients with proximal aortic dissection in one series.[195] An abrupt loss of pulse can affect the carotid, subclavian, axillary, radial, ulnar, or femoral arteries and acute limb ischemia has been reported in 20 percent of patients.[196,198]

NEUROLOGIC MANIFESTATIONS

Approximately 15 to 20 percent of patients with aortic dissection develop a neurologic deficit, with transient cerebral ischemia or stroke in up to 10 percent of cases as a result of extension of dissection into the carotid or vertebral arteries.[199] In the International Registry, syncope was a presenting symptom in 13 percent of patients with proximal dissection and 4 percent of those with distal dissection.[192] Interruption of circulation to the spinal cord can lead to paraplegia.[200] Less common neurologic abnormalities include Horner's syndrome, hoarseness, and ischemic neuropathy.

DIAGNOSIS

A high index of suspicion is required to establish the diagnosis promptly, since the presentations of aortic dissection are so myriad and mimic a wide array of other diseases. Accordingly, simple diag-

TABLE 98-6 Clinical Features of Aortic Dissection

Clinical Feature (%)	PROXIMAL (TYPE I, II, A) INVESTIGATOR (REFERENCE)				DISTAL (TYPE III, B) INVESTIGATOR (REFERENCE)			
	Crawford[289] (n = 229)	Hagan[192] (n = 289)	Fradet[290] (n = 156)	Spittell[191] (n = 102)	Crawford (n = 317)	Hagan (n = 175)	Fradet (n = 103)	Spittell (n = 66)
Chest pain	66[a]							
Back pain	N/A[a]	79	51	59	79[a]	63	43	29
Abdominal pain	N/A	47	18	12	N/A	64	42	52
Cerebrovascular accident	7	22	7	8	N/A	43	14	15
Renal insufficiency	10	6	6[b]	2	3	2.3	N/A	0
Shock	N/A	N/A	N/A	N/A	12	N/A	N/A	N/A
Aortic insufficiency	55	13	18	3	N/A	1.5	3	1
Rupture	4	44	11[a]	16	N/A	12	N/A	0

[a]N/A = not available; information not provided in referenced article; information not separated into incidence in proximal vs. distal site of dissecting aneurysm.

nostic tests are employed to exclude other causes of the symptoms. An electrocardiogram should be performed to exclude acute myocardial infarction, as administration of thrombolytic drugs in patients with acute aortic dissection is associated with a high mortality rate.[201] Chest radiography was normal in 12.4 percent of 427 patients in the International Registry,[192] but it may help exclude other causes of chest pain, such as pneumothorax. The most common findings in patients with dissection include widening of the mediastinal shadow, pleural effusion, or >10 mm separation of aortic intimal calcification.[202]

The most frequently used modalities to identify dissection and define the sites of origin and termination are computed tomography (CT), transesophageal echocardiography (TEE), and magnetic resonance imaging (MRI). The primary diagnostic criterion for diagnosis of aortic dissection by CT is demonstration of two contrast-filled lumens separated by an intimal flap[203] (see also Chap. 20). The sensitivity of this method ranges from 93 to 100 percent and specificity from 87 to 100 percent.[204,206] Inaccuracy may result from inadequate contrast opacification, nonvisualization of the intimal flap, artifacts that simulate an intimal flap extending across the aortic lumen, misinterpretation of adjacent vessels or prominent sinus of Valsalva as the flap, atelectasis, and pleural thickening or thrombosis of the false lumen. Multidetector-row CT scanners offer more rapid image acquisition, variable section thickness, three-dimensional rendering, diminished helical artifacts, and smaller contrast requirements, overcoming many of these pitfalls.[207]

The sensitivity and specificity of MRI for diagnosis of aortic dissection has been reported between 95 and 100 percent.[208,210] The technique enables identification of the entry tear and the extent of dissection; defines the anatomy of the vessels arising from the aortic arch, visceral vessels, and the iliac and common femoral arteries[211–213]; and provides a measurement of blood flow velocities in both the true and false lumens.[214,215] When the false lumen is occluded by thrombus, the dissection may be missed, giving the appearance of an intact aneurysm.[203] Other shortcomings are inaccessibility of the patient for 30 to 60 min during image acquisition and unsuitability of the method for those with implanted electronic devices. On the other hand, a promising potential future application is the use of MRI to guide endovascular interventional therapeutic procedures (i.e., fenestration, stenting, and stent grafting).[216,217]

Another excellent noninvasive diagnostic test for aortic dissection, TEE, provides rapid multiplane imaging of the aorta and assessment of flow dynamics. The examination can be performed in the emergency department soon after patient presentation[218,219] with a sensitivity near 98 percent and a specificity of 63 to 96 percent.[220–223] Limitations are that the coronary arteries and the arch vessels may not be adequately visualized, extension into the visceral or iliac arteries may go undetected, there is a blind spot in the proximal aortic arch,[222] and the quality of the study is operator-dependent.

Contrast aortography, once the standard method, can accurately identify the site of intimal tear, distinguish the two lumens, define the degree of aortic valve insufficiency, and clearly delineate the branches of the aorta.[224] Comparative studies found the sensitivity of aortography to be 88 percent and the specificity 94 percent for aortic dissection.[221] Inaccuracy may arise when there is thrombosis of the false lumen or circumferential dissection. The need for injection of contrast material, the invasive nature of the examination, and delays inherent in preparing the angiography suite have made catheter aortography a secondary diagnostic modality.[183]

Intravascular ultrasonography using high-frequency transducers is a promising tool for accurate determination of the location and extent of dissection and assessment of branch vessels. This method may be particularly helpful to differentiate aortic dissection from a penetrating atherosclerotic ulcer, but it has not been widely employed.[225]

DIFFERENTIAL DIAGNOSIS

Among the conditions that may initially resemble acute or chronic aortic dissection are myocardial infarction, thoracic aortic aneurysm without dissection, musculoskeletal chest pain, mediastinal tumors, pericarditis, pleuritis, pneumothorax, pulmonary thromboembolism, cholecystitis, ureteral colic, appendicitis, mesenteric ischemia, pyelonephritis, stroke, transient ischemic attack, and limb ischemia. Given the extensive differential diagnosis, objective diagnostic testing is necessary when the diagnosis of dissection is considered. The diagnosis is most strongly suggested when migratory chest and back pain of less than 24 h duration arises in a patient with a history of hypertension.

TREATMENT

Management of patients with aortic dissection involves lowering blood pressure and the rate of rise in aortic pressure during ventricular systole (dP/dt), analgesia, and selection of patients who benefit from surgical or endovascular intervention. Both blood pressure and heart rate contribute to the shear force exerted on the aortic wall, which is the major factor responsible for progression of dissection.[226] Reduction in the velocity of ventricular contraction retards expansion of the dissection.[227] Beta-adrenergic antagonists such as intravenous esmolol, propranolol, or metoprolol are the first line of therapy and may be given concurrently with sodium nitroprusside to rapidly reduce these hemodynamic forces. Another approach is administration of the alpha- and beta-adrenergic antagonist labetalol by intravenous infusion.[228] The goal is to lower systolic blood pressure to the lowest tolerated level without compromising perfusion of vital organs, usually 90 to 110 mmHg. In patients with reactive airway disease, the calcium-channel antagonists diltiazem and verapamil represent potential alternatives to treatment with beta-blocking drugs.

Once the diagnosis is established and pain and hemodynamic forces have been controlled, surgical or endovascular intervention may be warranted. In a European cooperative study, continued medical management of patients with type B (distal) aortic dissection was associated with a survival rate no lower than management with surgical therapy.[229,230] Survival rates for patients with proximal (type A; DeBakey type I or II) aortic dissection treated medically are poor: 43, 34, and 28 percent at 2 weeks, 5 years, and 10 years, respectively.[231] A direct comparison of surgical versus medical therapy for type III aortic dissection found comparable survival rates at 1, 5, and 10 years.[230] Unless an associated illness precludes surgery, repair is indicated for patients with proximal dissection.[232] The usual procedure—replacement of the aortic segment affected by the intimal tear and aneurysmal dilatation with a tubular interposition graft[233]—is associated with a mortality rate between 5 and 32 percent.[234,235]

When insufficiency or other pathology of the aortic valve is present, emergent composite reconstruction carries an 8-year survival rate of 40 to 50 percent.[236] Perioperative complications and mortality increase when dissection extends beyond the ascending aorta into the arch, but operative techniques for reimplantation of the great vessels and coronary arteries have improved. In an international registry of 550 patients with type A aortic dissection, ascending aortic replacement was performed in 91 percent, root replacement in 32 percent, and complete arch replacement in 12.6 percent of those undergoing surgical repair.[237] The overall mortality rate was 27 percent (23 percent for patients below 70 years of age and 38 percent for those over age 70, $p = 0.003$).

The cornerstones of long-term management of survivors of aortic dissection are beta-adrenergic blockade and meticulous blood pressure control. Regardless of the initial management strategy, patients should undergo periodic surveillance imaging by MRI or CT every 6 to 12 months to monitor the diameter of the aorta, the extent of dissection, and the status of the repair, which might require additional intervention. Clinical events or significant radiographic changes in the extent of dissection or diameter of the aorta warrant consideration of surgical repair, since enlargement of the false channel and late rupture is the most common cause of death following the initial event. Leakage, rupture, arterial compromise producing tissue ischemia due to the dissection, enlargement of aortic diameter beyond 5.0 cm, extension of dissection despite therapy, persistent pain, or poorly-controlled hypertension constitute potential indications for repair.[186]

Endovascular stent-graft devices may be placed over the entry tear to control distal thoracic aortic dissection by thrombosis of the false lumen, but there is less experience with this technology in patients with type A than with type B dissections.[238] Patency of branch vessels is achieved by supplementary stenting. In one series of 23 patients, the 30-day mortality rate was 16 percent, but there were no late deaths over a follow-up period of 13 months.[239] The procedures may be combined with septal fenestration to equalize pressure in the true and false channels.[240,241] As endovascular techniques improve, their role is expected to increase.[242,243]

Penetrating Aortic Ulcer

A penetrating aortic ulcer is an ulcerated atheromatous lesion that disrupts the internal elastic lamina and erodes into the media, which in some cases may mimic or initiate aortic dissection, pseudoaneurysm formation, intramural hematoma, or rupture.[244] Among 684 aortograms in cases of suspected aortic dissection, the incidence of penetrating ulcer was 2.3 percent.[245] Penetrating ulcers typically cause sudden back or chest pain in elderly, hypertensive patients. Intramural hematoma develops without an intimal flap. The extensive atheromatous disease at the site of the ulcer is uncommon in the region of the intimal flap of a dissection (Fig. 98-6). Accurate diagnosis of this condition is critical, since medical management with blood pressure and heart rate control in patients with uncomplicated ulceration is associated with a good outcome.[246,247] Surgical intervention

is required when hemodynamic instability, pseudoaneurysm, or rupture occurs, but endovascular stent-graft repair has been successfully employed in patients.[248–250]

Intramural Hematoma

Intramural hematoma constitutes a variant of aortic dissection in which no entry point or intimal flap can be identified. Optimal therapy for this condition is not known and complications such as aortic dissection and aortic rupture occur unpredictably.[251] Whether the intramural hematoma arises from a small intimal tear or rupture of vasa vasorum within the aortic wall remains controversial.[252] On CT scan, intramural hematoma may appear as a crescent-shaped or circumferential thickening of the aortic wall with no flow in the space containing the hematoma. Up to 17 percent of patients with aortic dissection actually have intramural hematoma, but only CT or MRI imaging currently makes the distinction. The clinical course is variable: the hematoma may persist, reabsorb returning the aorta to a normal appearance, lead to aneurysm with the possibility of rupture, or convert to dissection.[253]

Among 124 patients with intramural hematoma in one series, in-hospital mortality was 7 percent for 41 patients with proximal aortic hematomas and 1 percent for 83 patients with distal hematomas,[254] substantially better than the 47 percent mortality reported with proximal intramural hematomas and 13 percent in patients with distal hematomas in another series of medically managed patients.[255] In a recent report, hematoma progressed to aortic dissection in 45 percent of 66 patients and mortality was 20 percent at 30 days. Late progression occurred in 21 percent and death in 17 percent of patients, yielding 1-, 2-, and 5-year survival rates of 76, 73, and 43 percent, respectively. Regardless of aortic diameter, type A intramural hematoma is more likely to progress, and early surgical intervention is recommended for such cases.[256] In a metanalysis of 143 patients, the mortality rate for patients with type A hematomas undergoing surgery was 14 versus 36 percent for those treated medically, a relative risk reduction of 75 percent (95 percent CI 57 to 98 percent) with surgery ($p < 0.02$). The mortality for patients with type B hematomas treated medically was 14 percent, similar to the outcome in the surgical group.[257]

AORTITIS

Inflammation of the aortic wall may occur in noninfectious diseases, such as Takayasu's disease, giant cell arteritis, the spondyloarthropathies, Behçet's syndrome, relapsing polychondritis, Cogan's syndrome, rheumatoid arthritis, systemic lupus erythematosus, sarcoidosis, idiopathic retroperitoneal fibrosis, and other disorders. Only the most common entities are discussed in detail.

Takayasu's Disease

The prototypical nonspecific aortitis, Takayasu's arteritis, was named for the Japanese ophthalmologist who first called attention to the funduscopic findings.[258] Because of its predilection for the brachiocephalic vessels, this arteritis has been labeled *pulseless disease* and *aortic arch syndrome*. The classic form occurs with the greatest frequency in Asian countries, but patients with a similar nonspecific aortitis are encountered worldwide. There are approximately 150 new cases per year in Japan, while the incidence is lower in the United States and western Europe.[259] The etiology is unknown; no infectious agent has been identified, and identification of anti-

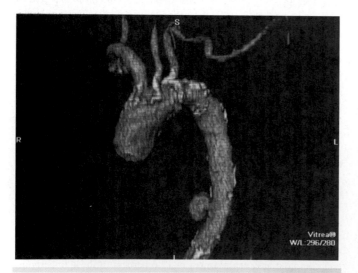

FIGURE 98-6 Magnetic resonance angiogram: surface-shaded rendering of a maximum-intensity projection demonstrating a penetrating aortic ulcer in the distal portion of the descending thoracic aorta.

endothelial antibodies in 18 of 19 patients with this disease supports an autoimmune mechanism. This finding is nonspecific; such antibodies have also been demonstrated in patients with thrombangiitis obliterans.[260,261]

HISTOPATHOLOGY

Histologic examination during active stages of the disease discloses a granulomatous arteritis similar to giant cell arteritis and to the aortitis associated with the seronegative spondyloarthropathies and Cogan's syndrome. In later stages, medial degeneration, fibrous scarring, intimal proliferation, and thrombosis result in narrowing of the vessel. Aneurysm formation is less common than stenosis, but aneurysm rupture is an important cause of death in patients with Takayasu's arteritis. Angiographically, the left subclavian artery is narrowed in about 90 percent of patients. The right subclavian artery, left carotid artery, and brachiocephalic trunk follow closely in frequency of stenosis.[262] Thoracic aortic lesions occur in two-thirds of patients, the abdominal aorta is involved in half, and aortoiliac involvement in 12 percent. Pulmonary arteritis occurs in about half the patients and may be associated with pulmonary hypertension.

CLINICAL FEATURES

In 70 to 80 percent of cases, clinical manifestations of the illness appear during the second or third decade of life, but onset in childhood and in middle life have been reported. Women are affected eight to nine times more often than men. During the early or "prepulseless" period, symptoms include fever, night sweats, malaise, nausea, vomiting, weight loss, rash, arthralgia, and Raynaud's phenomenon. Splenomegaly may occur and laboratory findings may include acceleration of the erythrocyte sedimentation rate, elevated levels of C-reactive protein, anemia, and plasma protein abnormalities.

Once arterial obstruction develops, upper extremity claudication may occur due to subclavian artery stenosis. Stroke, transient cerebral ischemia, dizziness or syncope usually indicates narrowing of the brachiocephalic arteries or subclavian steal.[263] The retinopathy that first drew the attention of Takayasu is believed to result from retinal ischemia. Hypertension, observed in over half the cases, is sometimes malignant and suggests narrowing of the aorta proximal to the renal arteries or involvement of the renal arteries themselves.[264] When arch vessel stenosis makes it difficult to measure blood pressure accurately in the upper limbs, the pressure should be measured in the lower limbs instead.

Cardiac manifestations result from severe hypertension, dilatation of the aortic root producing valvular insufficiency, or coronary artery stenosis (Fig. 98-7). Angina pectoris, myocardial infarction, and heart failure have been reported. Clinical pericarditis has been observed infrequently, but healed pericarditis is often encountered at necropsy. Involvement of the visceral arteries may result in splanchnic ischemia, and aortoiliac obstruction may produce intermittent claudication in the lower limbs. Involvement of the abdominal aorta, most common in India or South America, produces the "middle aortic syndrome," represented angiographically by long, smooth narrowing of the abdominal aorta with thick walls.[265]

Patients in whom severe aortitis is evidence at the time of diagnosis face a 25 to 30 percent risk of ischemic events or death over a period of 5 years. Those without ischemic complications at presentation tend of fare better over 5 to 10 years. Severe hypertension and cardiac involvement predict shortened life expectancy.[263]

DIAGNOSIS

The American College of Rheumatology has identified six major criteria for the diagnosis of Takayasu's arteritis.[266] Onset of illness by

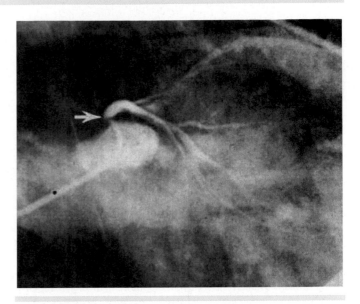

FIGURE 98-7 Typical angiographic appearance of Takayasu's arteritis, showing a tight focal ostial stenosis in the left main coronary artery. (From Jolly et al.[294] With permission.)

age 40 years avoids overlap with giant cell arteritis. Other criteria include upper extremity claudication, diminished brachial pulses, >10 mmHg difference between systolic blood pressure in the arms, subclavian or aortic bruit, and narrowing of the aorta or a major branch. The presence of three of these six criteria is associated with high diagnostic accuracy. While the erythrocyte sedimentation rate or C-reactive protein is elevated in three-quarters of patients at presentation, these indices do not accurately reflect disease activity.[259]

Arteriography typically shows long areas of smooth narrowing interspersed with areas that appear normal. Aneurysm and occlusions are also common. CT scans may show wall thickening resulting from inflammation of the media and adventitia,[267] and MRI may disclose arterial wall edema as a marker of active disease.[268-270] MR angiography of the entire aorta, arch vessels, and iliac vessels is generally recommended for all patients with suspected Takayasu's disease to define the extent of disease, identify aneurysms, and estimate the activity of disease.

MANAGEMENT

Corticosteroid therapy appears effective in suppressing inflammation during the active phase,[271,272] and favorable results have been reported with immunosuppressive and cytotoxic agents.[273] Operative treatment may be employed to relieve symptoms due to arterial obstruction, and percutaneous angioplasty has been associated with favorable results. These procedures are best reserved for patients in whom the acute inflammatory stage of the disease has been controlled.[274]

Giant Cell Arteritis

Giant cell arteritis (temporal arteritis, polymyalgia rheumatica) involves extracranial arteries, including the aorta in 10 to 13 percent of cases. A peak incidence in late life sets giant cell arteritis apart from other nonspecific arteritides. Like Takayasu's disease, giant cell arteritis may produce narrowing of the brachiocephalic arteries, aneurysms of the ascending aorta, aortic dissection, and aortic regurgitation.[275] Despite clinical, angiographic, and pathologic similarities to Takayasu's arteritis, giant cell arteritis almost always occurs in individuals over 50 years of age. While the most common presentation involves polymyalgia rheumatica with temporal arteritis, any large artery may be involved. Data from the Mayo Clinic suggest an incidence of 17.8 cases per 100,000 person-years, and this may be rising.[276]

Treatment of giant cell arteritis usually involves oral prednisone in an initial dose of 40 to 60 mg daily. In unresponsive cases (<10 percent) or in those who relapse as the dose is tapered, cytotoxic agents such as cyclosporine, azothioprine, and methotrexate may be helpful.[277] One randomized double-blind trial found a significant reduction in the rate of relapse and the cumulative mean dose of corticosteroid medication with methotrexate compared to placebo in corticosteroid-treated patients,[278] but another study did not.[279]

HLA-B27 Associated Spondyloarthropathies

Aortitis is present in a substantial proportion of patients with ankylosing spondylitis and Reiter's syndrome; more than 90 percent have the histocompatibility antigen HLA-B27. Aortic involvement is most common in those with spondylitis of long duration, peripheral joint complaints in addition to spondylitis, and iritis.[280,281] Inflammation of the aortic root and surrounding tissues manifest by aortic valve regurgitation or cardiac conduction abnormalities in patients with the HLA-B27 histocompatibility antigen may also occur without spondyloarthropathies. Histologically, the aortic lesion in this setting resembles the inflammation seen in syphilis, with focal destruction of medial elastic tissue and thickening of the intima and adventitia.

Infectious Aortitis

Primary infection of the aortic wall is a rare cause of aortic aneurysms, which are more often saccular than fusiform. Infectious or "mycotic" aneurysms may arise secondarily from an infection occurring in a preexistent aneurysm of another etiology. *Staphylococcus, Salmonella,* and *Pseudomonas* species are the most frequent pathogens causing primary aortic infections.[282] Many cases arise as complications of infective endocarditis or arterial catheterization. An intrinsically abnormal aorta, however, may become infected as a consequence of bacteremia. Such infection produces suppurative aortitis, leading to weakness of a portion of the aortic wall. In these cases aneurysms are typically saccular, yet there is a comparatively high propensity to rupture.

Syphilitic Aortitis

Chronic treponemal infection produces a chronic aortitis in about 10 percent of patients with untreated tertiary syphilis and is the primary cause of death in about the same proportion of cases, but there is evidence of the process at autopsy in about half of those patients who have had untreated syphilis for more than 10 years.[283] During the spirochetemic phase of primary syphilis, *Treponema pallidum* organisms lodge in the adventitia of the vasa vasorum and initiate an inflammatory response characterized by perivascular lymphocytic and plasma cell infiltrate. This is followed by obliterative endarteritis, resulting in patchy medial necrosis, elastic fiber fragmentation, weakening of the aortic wall and aneurysm formation. The intima of the aorta has a characteristic wrinkled appearance, frequently with superimposed atherosclerotic plaques. Because the infection is seeded through the vasa vasorum, the process is most severe in the ascending aorta and the arch, where the density of these vessels is greatest. Luetic aneurysms are typically saccular and involve the ascending

aorta whether or not the transverse and descending portions are also affected. Aortic aneurysms resulting from cardiovascular syphilis follow interruption of the elastic fibers as a result of periaortitis and mesoaortitis, which thicken but weaken the aortic wall. Rupture is the major complication, but the enlarging aneurysm may also compress or erode adjacent structures of the mediastinum. Since the inflammatory process tends to interrupt the medial layer by transverse scars, dissection is distinctly uncommon.

Aortic involvement may be asymptomatic or associated with aortic regurgitation, coronary ostial stenosis, or aortic aneurysm. Asymptomatic aortitis may sometimes be identified by linear calcification of the ascending aorta, evident on chest radiographs. Valvular regurgitation, present in 20 to 30 percent of patients with syphilitic aortitis, is mainly a consequence of aortic root dilatation. Coronary ostial stenosis, only a century ago more common than coronary atherosclerosis as a cause of angina pectoris, occurs in 25 to 30 percent of such patients, most of whom also have aortic regurgitation. While angina pectoris is common in patients with syphilitic ostial stenosis, myocardial infarction is rare. The least frequent manifestation of syphilitic aortitis is aneurysm formation, which occurs in 5 to 10 percent of affected patients. While the prognosis for patients with uncomplicated syphilitic aortitis is comparable to that of the general population, the outlook is poor when syphilitic aneurysms of the aorta are large enough to produce symptoms. The diagnosis of cardiovascular syphilis may be difficult in patients over age 50 years, when hypertensive and atherosclerotic disease often coexist. Serologically, 40 to 95 percent of patients with cardiovascular syphilis have elevated Venereal Disease Research Laboratory (VDRL) titers, and nearly all test positive on fluorescent treponemal antibody absorption (FTA-ABS).

The frequency of cardiovascular syphilis has fallen dramatically over recent decades due to early identification and treatment of the disease. Adequate antimicrobial therapy of early syphilis is the most important preventive measure, though whether such treatment retards the progression of disease once aortitis has developed has not been clearly established. Without surgical intervention, symptomatic syphilitic aortic aneurysms are associated with a high mortality rate.

Tuberculous Aortitis

Tuberculous aneurysms usually result from direct extension of infection from hilar lymph nodes and subsequent granulomatous destruction of the medial layer, leading to loss of aortic wall elasticity. The posterior or posterolateral aortic wall is usually the site of saccular aneurysm formation in these cases. Caseating granulomatous lesions affecting the medial layer of the aortic wall characterize the histology. Pseudoaneurysm formation,[284] perforation, or aortoenteric fistula may result.[285,286] Infection may occasionally invade the aortic valve ring and adjacent structures, producing a caseating perivalvular abscess.

References

1. Glagov S, Wolinsky H. New concepts of the relation of structure to function in the arterial wall. *Proc Inst Med Chicago* 1968;27:106.
2. Wolinsky H, Glagov S. Comparison of abdominal and thoracic aortic medial structure in mammals: Deviation of man from the usual pattern. *Circ Res* 1969;25:677–686.
3. Wolinsky H, Glagov S. A lamellar unit of aortic medial structure and function in mammals. *Circ Res* 1967;20:99–111.
4. Movat HZ, More RH, Haust MD. The diffuse internal thickening of the human aorta with aging. *Am J Pathol* 1958;34:1023–1031.

5. Vasan RS, Larson MG, Levy D. Determinants of echocardiographic aortic root size: The Framingham Heart Study. *Circulation* 1995;91: 734–740.

6. Vasan RS, Larson MG, Levy D. Determinants of echocardiographic aortic root size: The Framingham Heart Study. *Circulation* 1995;91: 734–740.

7. Caro CG. *The Mechanics of the Circulation.* New York: Oxford University Press; 1978.

8. Slater EE, DeSanctis RW. Diseases of the aorta. In: Braunwald E, ed. *Heart Disease.* Philadelphia: Saunders; 1984:1540–1571.

9. Kroeker EJ, Wood EH. Comparison of simultaneously recorded central and peripheral arterial pressure pulses during rest, exercise and tilted position in man. *Circ Res* 1955;3:623–632.

10. Guard HR, Bhende YM. Changes due to aging in the abdominal aorta. *Ind J Med Res* 1953;41:267–276.

11. Bunting CH, Bunting H. Acid mucopolysaccharides of the aorta. *AMA Arch Pathol* 1953;55:257–264.

12. Cornwell GG. Westermark P, Murdoch W, et al. Senile aortic amyloid: A third distinctive type of age-related cardiovascular amyloid. *Am J Pathol* 1982;108:135–139.

13. Schwartz PH et al. Amyloidosis in human and animal pathology: A comparative study. In: Wegelius O, Pasternack A, eds. *Amyloidosis.* London: Academic Press; 1976:71–102.

14. Avolio AP et al. Effects of aging on changing arterial compliance and left ventricular load in a northern Chinese urban community. *Circulation* 1983;68:50–58.

15. Virmani R, McAllister HA Jr. Pathology of the aorta and major arteries. In: Lande A, Berkmen YM, McAllister HA Jr, eds. *Aortitis: Clinical, Pathologic, and Radiographic Aspects.* New York: Raven Press; 1986:7–53.

16. Becker AE. Medionecrosis aortae. *Pathol Microbiol* 1975;43:124.

17. Schlatmann TJ, Becker AE. Histologic changes in the normal aging aorta: Implications for dissecting aortic aneurysm. *Am J Cardiol* 1977;39:13–20.

18. Crawford ES, Morris GC Jr, Myhre HO, et al. Celiac axis, superior mesenteric artery and inferior mesenteric artery occlusion: Surgical considerations. *Surgery* 1977;82:856–866.

19. Crawford ES, Hess KR. Abdominal aortic aneurysm (editorial). *N Engl J Med* 1989;321:1040–1042.

20. Weintraub AM, Gomes MN. Clinical manifestations of abdominal aortic aneurysm and thoracoabdominal aneurysm. In: Lindsay J Jr, Hurst JW, eds. *The Aorta.* New York: Grune & Stratton; 1979:131–168.

21. Davies MJ. Aortic aneurysm formation: Lessons from human studies and experimental models. *Circulation* 1998;98:193.

22. Goodall S, Porter KE, Bell PR, Thompson MM. Enhanced invasive properties exhibited by smooth muscle cells are associated with elevated production of MMP-2 in patients with aortic aneurysms. *Eur J Vasc Endovasc Surg* 2002;24:72–80.

23. Reilly JM, Brophy CM, Tilson MD. Characterization of an elastase from aneurysmal aorta which degrades intact aortic elastin. *Ann Vasc Surg* 1992;6:99.

24. Anidjar S, Dobrin PB, Eichorst M, et al. Correlation of inflammatory infiltrate with the enlargement of experimental aortic aneurysms. *J Vasc Surg* 1992;16:139.

25. Pearce WH, Koch AE. Cellular components and features of immune response in abdominal aortic aneurysms. *Ann N Y Acad Sci* 1996;800: 175.

26. Louwrens HD, Kwaan HC, Pearce WH, et al. Plasminogen activator and plasminogen activator inhibitor expression by normal and aneurysmal human aortic smooth muscle cells in culture. *Eur J Vasc Endovasc Surg* 1995;10:289–293.

27. Gsell O. Wandnekrosen der Aorta als selbstandige Erkrankung und Ihre beziehung zur Spontanruptur. *Virchows Arch Pathol Anat* 1928;270:1.

28. Erdheim J. Medionecrosis aortae idiopathica. *Virchows Arch Pathol Anat* 1929;273:454.

29. Campbell CD. Aneurysms of the ascending aorta. In: Campbell D, ed. *Aortic Aneurysms: Surgical Therapy.* Mount Kisco, NY: Futura; 1981: 19–46.

30. Hahn RT, Devereux RB. Determinants of aortic root dilatation associated with bicuspid aortic valves. *Circulation* 1990;82(suppl II).

31. Marfan AB. Un cas de deformation congenitale des quatre membres, plus prononce des extremites, caracterise par l'allongement des coeur avec un certain degre d'amincissement. *Bull Mem Soc Med Hop Paris* 1896;13:220–226.

32. Jondeau G, Delorme G, Guiti C. [Marfan syndrome]. *Rev Prat* 2002;52:1089–1093.

33. Kainulainen K, Pulkkinen L, Savolainen A, et al. Location on chromosome 15 of the gene defect causing Marfan syndrome. *N Engl J Med* 1990;323:935–939.

34. Lee B, Godfrey M, Vitale E, et al. Linkage of Marfan syndrome and a phenotypically related disorder to two different fibrillin genes. *Nature* 1991;353:330.

35. Maslen CL Corson GM, Maddox BK, et al. Partial sequencing of a candidate gene for the Marfan syndrome. *Nature* 1991;334–337.

36. Dietz HC, Pyeritz RE, Hall BD, et al. The Marfan syndrome locus: Confirmation of assignment to chromosome 15.*Genomics* 1991;9: 355–361.

37. Tsipouras P, Del Mastro R, Sarfarzi M, et al. Genetic linkage of the Marfan syndrome ectopia lentis and congenital contractural arachnodactyly to the fibrillin genes on chromosome 15 and 5. *N Engl J Med* 1992;326:905–909.

38. Francke U, Furthmayr H. Marfan's syndrome and other disorders of fibrillin. *N Engl J Med* 1994;330:1384–1385.

39. Hollister D, Goodfrey M, Sakai L, Pyeritz R. Immunohistologic abnormalities of the microfibrillar-fiber system in the Marfan syndrome. *N Engl J Med* 1990;323:152.

40. Finkbohner R, Johnston D, Crawford ES, et al. Marfan syndrome: Long-term survival and complications after aortic aneurysm repair. *Circulation* 1995;91:728–733.

41. Noon GP. Aneurysms of the aortic arch. In: Campbell AD, ed. *Aortic Aneurysms: Surgical Therapy.* Mount Kisco, NY: Futura; 1981:79–100.

42. Morse DE. Embryology, anatomy and histology of the aorta. In: Lindsay J, Hurst JW, eds. *The Aorta.* New York: Grune & Stratton; 1979:15–37.

43. Dillon ML, Young WG, Sealy WC. Aneurysms of the descending thoracic aorta. *Ann Thorac Surg* 1967;3:430–438.

44. DeBakey ME, Noon GP. Aneurysms of the thoracic aorta. *Mod Concepts Cardiovasc Dis* 1975;44:53.

45. Joyce JW, Fairbairn JF II, Kincaid OW, Juergens JL. Aneurysms of the thoracic aorta: A clinical study with special reference to prognosis. *Circulation* 1964;29:176.

46. Lindsay J Jr: Thoracic aneurysms. In: Lindsay J, Hurst JW, eds. *The Aorta.* New York: Grune & Stratton; 1979:121–130.

47. Roberts WC: The aorta: Its acquired diseases and their consequences as viewed from a morphologic perspective In: Lindsay J, Hurst JW, eds. *The Aorta.* New York: Grune & Stratton; 1979: 51–117.

48. Bulkley BH, Hutchins GM, Ross RS. Aortic sinus of Valsalva aneurysms simulating primary right sided valvular heart disease. *Circulation* 1975;52:696–699.

49. Blieden LC, Edwards JE. Anomalies of the thoracic aorta: Pathologic considerations. *Prog Cardiovasc Dis* 1973;16:25–41.

50. Davies GJ, Watt J, Muir JR. Ruptured sinus of Valsalva aneurysm with aortic-left atrial fistula. *Eur J Cardiol* 1975;3:213–218.

51. Cranley JJ, Hermann LG, Preuninger RM. Natural history of aneurysms of the aorta. *Arch Surg* 1954;69:185–197.

52. Birnholz JC, Ferrucci JT, Wyman SM. Roentgen features of dysphagia aortica. *Radiology* 1974;111:93–96.

53. Seymour J, Emanuel R, Pattinson N. Acquired pulmonary stenosis. *Br Heart J* 1968;30:776–785.

54. Drachler DH, Willis PW III. Acquired right ventricular outflow tract obstruction. *Am Heart J* 1971;82:536–540.

55. Banker VP, Maddison FE. Superior vena cava syndrome secondary to aortic disease. *Dis Chest* 1967;51:656–662.

56. Varkey B, Tristani FE. Compression of pulmonary artery and bronchus by descending thoracic aortic aneurysm. *Am J Cardiol* 1974;34: 610–614.

57. Fomon JJ, Kurzweg FT, Broadaway FK. Aneurysms of the aorta: A review. *Ann Surg* 1967;165:557–563.

58. Crawford ES, Snyder DM, Cho GC, et al. Progress in treatment of thoracoabdominal and abdominal aortic aneurysms involving celiac, superior mesenteric and renal arteries. *Ann Surg* 1978:188:404–421.

59. Creech O Jr, DeBakey ME, Morris GC Jr. Aneurysm of thoracoabdominal aorta involving the celiac, superior mesenteric and renal arteries. Report of four cases treated by resection and homograft replacement. *Ann Surg* 1956;144:549–573.

60. Etheredge SN, Yee J, Smith JV, et al. Successful resection of a large aneurysm of the upper abdominal aorta and replacement with homograft. *Surgery* 1955;38:1071–1081.

61. Hardy JD, Timmis HH, Saleh SS, et al. Thoracoabdominal aortic aneurysm: Simplified surgical management with case report. *Ann Surg* 1967;166:1008–1011.

62. Heyde MN van der Zwaveling A. Resection of an abdominal aortic aneurysm in a patient with Marfan's syndrome. *J Cardiovasc Surg* 1961;2:359–366.

63. DeBakey ME: Surgical considerations in the treatment of aneurysms of the thoracoabdominal aorta. *Ann Surg* 1965;162:650–662.

64. American Heart Association: Heart Disease and Stroke Statistics—2003 Update http://www.americanheart.org/downloadable/heart/10461207852142003HDSStats Book.pdf

65. Auerbach O, Garfinkel L. Atherosclerosis and aneurysm of the aorta in relation to smoking habits and age. *Chest* 1980;78:805–809.

66. Carlsson J, Sternby NH. Aortic aneurysms. *Acta Chir Scand* 1964;127:466–473.

67. Cole CW, Barber GG, Bouchard AG, et al. Abdominal aortic aneurysm: The consequences of a positive family history. *Can J Surg* 1989;32:117–120.

68. Allardice JT, Allwright GJ, Wafula JM, et al. High prevalence of abdominal aortic aneurysm in men with peripheral vascular disease: Screening by ultrasonography. *Br J Surg* 1988;75:240–242.

69. Darling RC, Messina CR, Brewster DC, Ottinger LW. Autopsy study of unoperated abdominal aortic aneurysms: The case for early resection. *Circulation* 1977;56(suppl 2):161.

70. Johansen K, Koepsell T. Familial tendency for abdominal aortic aneurysm. *JAMA* 1986;256:1934–1936.

71. Johnson G Jr, Avery A, McDougal EG, et al. Aneurysms of the abdominal aorta: Incidence in blacks and whites in North Carolina. *Arch Surg* 1985;120:1138–1140.

72. Leopold GR, Goldberger LE, Bernstein EF. Ultrasonic detection and evaluation of abdominal aortic aneurysms. *Surgery* 1972;72:939–945.

73. Scott RA. Ultrasound screening in the management of abdominal aortic aneurysms. *Int Angiol* 1986;5:263–267.

74. Bickerstaff LK, Hollier LH, Van Peenan HJ, et al. Abdominal aortic aneurysms: The changing natural history. *J Vasc Surg* 1984;1:6.

75. Bowers D, Cave WS. Aneurysms of the abdominal aorta: A twenty-year study. *J R Soc Med* 1985;78:812–820.

76. Cabellon S Jr, Moncrief CL, Pierre DR, et al. Incidence of abdominal aortic aneurysms in patients with atheromatous arterial disease. *Am J Surg* 1983;146:575–576.

77. Graham M, Chan A. Ultrasound screening for clinically occult abdominal aortic aneurysm. *Can Med Assoc J* 1988;138:627–629.

78. Thurmond AS, Semler HJ. Abdominal aortic aneurysm: incidence in a population at risk. *J Cardiovasc Surg* 1986;27:457–460.

79. Sommerville RL, Allen EV, Edwards JE. Bland and infected arteriosclerotic abdominal aortic aneurysms: a clinicopathologic study. *Medicine* 1959;38:207–221.

80. Friedman SA, Hufnagel CA, Conrad PW, et al. Abdominal aortic aneurysms: Clinical status and results of surgery in 100 consecutive cases. *JAMA* 1967;200:1147–1151.

81. Gliedman ML, Ayers WB, Vestal BL. Aneurysms of the abdominal aorta and its branches. *Ann Surg* 1957;146:207.

82. Schatz IJ Fairbairn JF II, Juergens JL. Abdominal aortic aneurysms: A reappraisal. *Circulation* 1962;26:200–205.

83. DeBakey ME, Crawford ES, Cooley DA, et al. Aneurysm of abdominal aorta: Analysis of graft replacement therapy 1 to 11 years after operation. *Ann Surg* 1964;160:622–639.

84. Reilly JM, Tilson MD. Incidence and etiology of abdominal aortic aneurysms. *Surg Clin North Am* 1989;69:705–711.

85. Norrgard O, Rais O, Anguist K. Familial occurrence of abdominal aortic aneurysms. *Surgery* 1984;95:650–656.

86. Tilson MD, Seashore M. Human genetics of the abdominal aortic aneurysm. *Surg Gynecol Obstet* 1984;158:129–132.

87. Tilson MD, Seashore M. Fifty families with abdominal aortic aneurysms in two or more first-order relatives. *Am J Surg* 1984;147:551–553.

88. Busuttil RW, Abou-Zamzam A, Machleder H. Collagenase activity of the human aorta: a comparison of patients with and without abdominal aortic aneurysms. *Arch Surg* 1980;115:1373–1378.

89. Menashi S, et al. Collagen in abdominal aortic aneurysm: Typing, content, and degradation. *J Vasc Surg* 1987;6:578–582.

90. Sumner D, Hokanson D, Strandness D. Stress-strain characteristics and collagen-elastin content of abdominal aortic aneurysms. *Surg Gynecol Obstet* 1970;130:459–466.

91. Kuivanieri H, Tromp G, Prockup DJ. Genetic causes of aortic aneurysms. *J Clin Invest* 1991;88:1441–1444.

92. Ernst CB. Abdominal aortic aneurysm. *N Engl J Med* 1993;328:1167.

93. Estes JE Jr. Abdominal aortic aneurysm: A study of one hundred and two cases. *Circulation* 1950;2:258.

94. Wright IS, Urdaneta E, Wright B. Reopening the case of the abdominal aortic aneurysm. *Circulation* 1956;13:754–768.

95. Blakemore AH, Voorhees AB Jr. Aneurysm of the aorta: A review of 365 cases. *Angiology* 1954;5:209–231.

96. Kampmeier RH. Aneurysm of the abdominal aorta: a study of 73 cases. *Am J Med Sci* 1936;192:97–109.

97. Szilagyi DE, Smith RF, DeRusso FJ, et al. Contribution of abdominal aortic aneurysmectomy to prolongation of life. *Ann Surg* 1966;164:678–699.

98. Szilagyi DE, Elliott JP, Smith RF. Clinical fate of the patient with asymptomatic abdominal aortic aneurysm and unfit for surgical treatment. *Arch Surg* 1972;104:600–606.

99. Foster JH et al. Comparative study of elective resection and expectant treatment of abdominal aortic aneurysm. *Surg Gynecol Obstet* 1969;129:1–9.

100. Bernstein EF, Chan EL. Abdominal aortic aneurysm in high-risk patients: Outcome of selective management based on size and expansion rate. *Ann Surg* 1984;200:255–263.

101. Anidjar S, Dobrin PB, Chejfec G, Michel JB. Experimental study of determinants of aneurysmal expansion of the abdominal aorta. *Ann Vasc Surg* 1994;8:127–136.

102. Cronenwett JL et al. Actuarial analysis of variables associated with rupture of small abdominal aortic aneurysms. *Surgery* 1985;98:472–483.

103. Gore I, Hirst AE. Arteriosclerotic aneurysms of the abdominal aorta: A review. *Prog Cardiovasc Dis* 1973;17:113–149.

104. Stokes J, Butcher HRJ. Abdominal aortic aneurysms: Factors influencing operative mortality and criteria of operability. *Arch Surg* 1973;107:297–302.

105. Hall AB et al. Surgical treatment of aortic aneurysm in the aged. *Arch Surg* 1970;100:455–460.

106. Hammond EC, Garfinkel L. Coronary heart disease, stroke, and aortic aneurysm. *Arch Environ Health* 1969;19:167–182.

107. Bonamigo TP, Bianco C, Becker M, et al. Inflammatory aneurysms of infra-renal abdominal aorta. A case-control study. *Minerva Cardioangiol* 2002;50:253–258.

108. Cavallaro A, Sapienza P, di Marzo L, et al. [Inflammatory aneurysm of the abdominal aorta. Study of 355 patients with aortic aneurysm.] *Recenti Prog Med* 2001;92:269–273.

109. Schillinger M, Domanovits H, Bayegan K, et al. C-reactive protein and mortality in patients with acute aortic disease. *Intensive Care Med* 2002;28:740–745.

110. Barrat-Boyes BG. Symptomatology and prognosis of abdominal aortic aneurysm. *Lancet* 1957;2:716–720.

111. Tallgren LG, von Bonsdorff CH. Symptomatology and prognosis of abdominal aortic aneurysm. *Acta Med Scand* 1964;175(suppl 421):287.

112. Brewster DC, et al. Assessment of abdominal aortic aneurysm size. *Circulation* 1977;56(suppl 2):164–169.

113. Pennell RC, Hollier LH, Lie JT, et al. Inflammatory abdominal aortic aneurysms: A thirty-year review. *J Vasc Surg* 1985;2:859–869.

114. Scott RA. The Multicentre Aneurysm Screening Study (MASS) into the effect of abdominal aortic aneurysm screening on mortality in men: A randomised controlled trial. *Lancet* 2002;360:1531–1539.

115. Multicentre Aneurysm Screening Study Group: Multicentre aneurysm screening study (MASS): Cost effectiveness analysis of screening for abdominal aortic aneurysms based on four year results from randomised controlled trial. *BMJ* 2002;325:1135–1142.

116. Powell JT, Greenhalgh RM, Ruckley CV, Fowkes FG. The UK Small Aneurysm Trial. *Ann N Y Acad Sci* 1996;800:249–251.

117. Lederle FA WS, Johnson GR, Reinke DB, et al. Immediate repair compared with surveillance of small abdominal aortic aneurysms. *N Engl J Med* 2002;346:1437–1444.

118. Brady A, Fowkes F, Greenhalgh R, et al. Risk factors for postoperative death following elective surgical repair of abdominal aortic aneurysm: Results from the UK Small Aneurysm Trial. *Br J Surg* 2000;87:742–749.

119. Parodi JC, Palamz JC, Barone HD. Transfemoral intraluminal graft implantation for abdominal aortic aneurysms. *Ann Vasc Surg* 1991;5:491–499.

120. Carpenter JP, Baum RA, Barker CF, et al. Impact of exclusion criteria on patient selection for endovascular abdominal aortic aneurysm repair. *J Vasc Surg* 2001;34:1050–1054.

121. Becker GJ, Kovacs M, Mathison MN, et al. Risk stratification and outcomes of transluminal endografting for abdominal aortic aneurysm: 7-year experience and long-term follow-up. *J Vasc Interv Radiol* 2001;12:1033–1046.

122. Mathison M, Becker GJ, Katzen BT, et al. The influence of female gender on the outcome of endovascular abdominal aortic aneurysm repair. *J Vasc Interv Radiol* 2001;12:1047–1051.

123. Wolf YG, Tillich M, Lee WA, et al. Impact of aortoiliac tortuosity on endovascular repair of abdominal aortic aneurysms: Evaluation of 3D computer-based assessment. *J Vasc Surg* 2001;34:594–599.

124. Veith FJ, Johnston KW. Endovascular treatment of abdominal aortic aneurysms: An innovation in evolution and under evaluation. *J Vasc Surg* 2002;35:183.

125. White RA, Donayre C, Walot I, Stewart M. Abdominal aortic aneurysm rupture following endoluminal graft deployment: Report of a predictable event. *J Endovasc Ther* 2000;7:257–262.

126. Abraham CZ, Chuter TA, Reilly LM, et al. Abdominal aortic aneurysm repair with the Zenith stent graft: Short to midterm results. *J Vasc Surg* 2002;36:217–224; discussion 24–25.

127. Zarins CK, White RA, Hodgson KJ, et al. Endoleak as a predictor of outcome after endovascular aneurysm repair: AneuRx multicenter clinical trial. *J Vasc Surg* 2000;32:90–107.

128. Zarins CK, White RA, Moll FL, et al. The AneuRx stent graft: four-year results and worldwide experience 2000. *J Vasc Surg* 2001;33:S135–S145.

129. Sapirstein W, Chandeysson P, Wentz C. The Food and Drug Administration approval of endovascular grafts for abdominal aortic aneurysm: An 18-month retrospective. *J Vasc Surg* 2001;34:180–183.

130. Stelter W, Umscheid T, Ziegler P. Three-year experience with modular stent-graft devices for endovascular AAA treatment. *J Endovasc Surg* 1997;4:362–369.

131. Amesur NB, Zajko AB, Orons PD, Makaroun MS. Endovascular treatment of iliac limb stenoses or occlusions in 31 patients treated with the ancure endograft. *J Vasc Interv Radiol* 2000;11:421–428.

132. Greenberg RK, Lawrence-Brown M, Bhandari G, et al. An update of the Zenith endovascular graft for abdominal aortic aneurysms: Initial implantation and mid-term follow-up data. *J Vasc Surg* 2001;33:S157–S164.

133. Broeders IA, Blankensteijn JD, Wever JJ, Eikelboom BC. Mid-term fixation stability of the EndoVascular Technologies endograft. EVT Investigators. *Eur J Vasc Endovasc Surg* 1999;18:300–307.

134. Makaroun MS, Deaton DH. Is proximal aortic neck dilatation after endovascular aneurysm exclusion a cause for concern? *J Vasc Surg* 2001;33:S39–S45.

135. Boucher CA, et al. Determination of cardiac risk by dipyridamole-thallium imaging before peripheral vascular surgery. *N Engl J Med* 1985;312:389–394.

136. Leppo J et al. Noninvasive evaluation of cardiac risk before elective vascular surgery. *J Am Coll Cardiol* 1987;9:269–276.

137. Raby KE et al. Correlation between preoperative ischemia and major cardiac events after peripheral vascular surgery. *N Engl J Med* 1989;321:1296–300.

138. Eagle KA et al. Combining clinical and thallium data optimizes preoperative assessment of cardiac risk before major vascular surgery. *Ann Intern Med* 1989;110:859–866.

139. Hertzer NR, et al. Coronary artery disease in peripheral vascular patients. *Ann Surg* 1984;199:223–233.

140. Jamieson WRE, et al. Influence of ischemic heart disease on early and late mortality after surgery for peripheral occlusive vascular disease. *Circulation* 1982;66:1–92.

141. Tomatis LA, Fierens EE, Verbrugge GP. Evaluation of surgical risk in peripheral vascular disease by coronary arteriography: A series of 100 cases. *Surgery* 1972;71:429–435.

142. McCollum CH, et al. Myocardial revascularization prior to subsequent major surgery in patients with coronary artery disease. *Surgery* 1977;81:302–304.

143. Fleisher LA, Rosenbaum SH, Barash PG. Preoperative silent ischemia is a predictor of postoperative cardiac events in patients undergoing elective noncardiac surgery. *Soc Cardiovasc Anesthes* 1990;12:98.

144. McCabe CJ, et al. The value of electrocardiogram monitoring during treadmill testing for peripheral vascular disease. *Surgery* 1981;89:183–186.

145. Davila-Roman VG, Murphy SF, Nickerson NJ, et al. Atherosclerosis of the ascending aorta is an independent predictor of long-term neurologic events and mortality. *J Am Coll Cardiol* 1999;33:1308–1316.

146. Khoury Z, Gottlieb S, Stern S, et al. Frequency and distribution of atherosclerotic plaques in the thoracic aorta as determined by transesophageal echocardiography in patients with coronary artery disease. *Am J Cardiol* 1997;79:23–27.

147. Khatibzadeh M, Mitusch R, Stierle U, et al. Aortic atherosclerotic plaques as a source of systemic embolism. *J Am Coll Cardiol* 1996;27:664–669.

148. Ramirez G, O'Neill WM Jr, et al. Cholesterol embolization: A complication of angiography. *Arch Intern Med* 1978;138:1430–1432.

149. Drost H, Buis B, Haan D, Hillers JA. Cholesterol embolization as a complication of left heart catheterization: Report of 7 cases. *Br Heart J* 1984;52:339.

150. Colt HG, Begg RJ, Saporito JJ. Cholesterol emboli after cardiac catheterization: Eight cases and a review of the literature. *Medicine* 1988;67:389–400.

151. Eggebrecht H, Oldenbureg O, Dirsch O, et al. Potential embolization by atherosclerotic debris dislodged from aortic wall during cardiac catheterization: Histologic and clinical findings in 7621 patients. *Catheter Cardiovasc Interv* 2000;49:389–394.

152. Hyman BT, Landas SK, Ashman RF. Warfarin-related purple toes syndrome and cholesterol microembolization. *Am J Med* 1987;82:1233–1237.

153. Bruns FJ, Segel DP, Adler S. Control of cholesterol embolization by discontinuation of anticoagulant therapy. *Am J Med Sci* 1978;275:105–108.

154. Blackshear JL, Zabalgoitia M, Pennock GD, et al for the Stroke Prevention in Atrial Fibrillation Investigators: Warfarin safety and efficacy in patients with thoracic aortic plaque and atrial fibrillation. *Am J Cardiol* 1999;83:453–435.

155. Bartholomew JR, Olin JW: Atheromatous embolization. In: Bartholomew JR, ed. *Peripheral Vascular Diseases*, 2d ed. St Louis: Mosby; 1996.

156. Olin JW. Syndromes that mimic vasculitis. *Curr Opin Cardiol* 1991;6:768–774.

157. Fine MJ, Kapoor WN, Falanga V. Cholesterol crystal embolization: A review of 221 cases in the English language. *Angiology* 1987;38:769–784.

158. Pennington M, Yeager J, Skelton J, Smith KJ. Cholesterol embolization syndrome: Cutaneous histopathological features and the variable onset of symptoms in patients with different risk factors. *Br J Dermatol* 2002;146:511–517.

159. The French Study of Aortic Plaques in Stroke Group. Atherosclerotic disease of the aortic arch as a risk factor for recurrent ischemic stroke. *N Engl J Med* 1996;334:1216–1221.

160. Cohen A AP. Atherosclerosis of the thoracic aorta: From risk stratification to treatment. *Am J Cardiol* 2002;90:1333–1335.

161. Scolari F, Tardanico R, Zani R, et al. Cholesterol crystal embolism: A recognizable cause of renal disease. *Am J Kidney Dis* 2000;36:1089–1109.

162. Kasinath BS, Lewis EJ. Eosinophilia as a clue to the diagnosis of atheroembolic renal disease. *Arch Intern Med* 1987;147:1384–1385.

163. Woolfson RG, Lachmann H. Improvement in renal cholesterol emboli syndrome after simvastatin. *Lancet* 1998;351:1331–1332.

164. Tunick PA, et al. Effect of treatment on the incidence of stroke and other emboli in 519 patients with severe thoracic aortic plaque. *Am J Cardiol* 90:1320–1325.

165. Pitt B, Waters D, Brown WV, et al. Aggressive lipid-lowering therapy compared with angioplasty in stable coronary artery disease. *N Engl J Med* 1999;341:70–76.

166. Belenfant X, Meyrier A, Jacquot C. Supportive treatment improves survival in multivessel cholesterol crystal embolization. *Am J Kidney Dis* 1999;33:840–850.

167. Keen R, McCarthy W, Shireman P, et al. Surgical management of atheroembolization. *J Vasc Surg* 1995;21:773–781.

168. Fisher DF Jr, Clagett GP, Brigham RA, et al. Dilemmas in dealing with the blue toe syndrome: Aortic versus peripheral source. *Am J Surg* 1984;148:836–839.

169. Amarenco P, Cohen A, Tzourio C, et al. Atherosclerotic disease of the aortic arch and risk of ischemic stroke. *N Engl J Med* 1994;331:1474–1479.

170. Fazio GP, Redberg RF, Winslow T, et al. Transesophageal echocardiographically detected atherosclerotic aortic plaque is a marker for coronary artery disease. *J Am Coll Cardiol* 1993;21:144–150.

171. Cohen A, Tzourio C, Bertrand B, et al. Aortic atheroma morphology and vascular events: a followup study in patients with ischemic stroke: FAPS Investigators. *Circulation* 1997;96:2828–3841.

172. Brewster DC. Clinical and anatomical considerations for surgery in aortoiliac disease and results of surgical treatment. *Circulation* 1991;83(suppl I):I-42–I-52.

173. Debakey ME, Lawrie GM, Glaeser DH. Patterns of atherosclerosis and their surgical significance. *Ann Surg* 1985;201:115–131.

174. DeLaurentis DA, Friedmann P, Wolferth CC Jr, et al. Atherosclerosis and hypoplastic aortoiliac system. *Surgery* 1978;83:37.

175. Leriche R, Morel A. The syndrome of thrombotic obliteration of the aortic bifurcation. *Ann Surg* 1948;127:193–204.

176. Diethrich EB. Endovascular treatment of abdominal aortic occlusive disease: The impact of stents and intravascular ultrasound imaging. *Eur J Vasc Surg* 1993;7:228–236.

177. Transatlantic Inter-societal Consensus (TASC). Group: Management of peripheral arterial disease. *J Vasc Surg* 2000;31(suppl):S1–S296.

178. Johnston KW. Balloon angioplasty: Predictive factors for long-term success. *Semin Vasc Surg* 1989;3:117–122.

179. Sullivan TM, Childs MB, Bacharach JM, et al. Percutaneous transluminal angioplasty and primary stenting of the iliac arteries in 288 patients. *J Vasc Surg* 1997;25:829–839.

180. Palmaz JC, Laborde JC, Rivera FJ, et al. Stenting of the iliac arteries with the Palmaz stent: experience from a multicenter trial. *Cardiovasc Intervent Radiol* 1992;15:291–297.

181. Busuttil RW, Keehn G, Milliken J, et al. Aortic saddle embolus: A twenty-year experience. *Ann Surg* 1983;197:698–706.

182. Fogarty T, Daily P, Shumway N, et al. Experience with balloon catheter technique for arterial embolectomy. *Am J Surg* 1971;122:231–237.

183. Khan IA, Nair CK. Clinical, diagnostic and management perspectives of aortic dissection. *Chest* 2002;122:311–328.

184. Hirst AE, et al. Dissecting aneurysms of the aorta: A review of 505 cases. *Medicine* 1958;37:217–279.

185. Crawford ES. The diagnosis and management of aortic dissection. *JAMA* 1990;264:2537–2541.

186. DeSanctis RW, Doroghazi RM, Austen WG, Buckley MJ. Aortic dissection. *N Engl J Med* 1990;317:1060–1067.

187. Wilson SK, Hutchins GM. Aortic dissecting aneurysms: Causative factors in 204 subjects. *Arch Pathol Lab Med* 1982;106:175–180.

188. Coplan NL, Goldman B, Mechanic G, et al. Sudden hemodynamic collapse following relief of cardiac tamponade in a patient with aortic dissection. *Am Heart J* 1986;111:405–406.

189. Meszaros I, Morocz J, Szlavi J, et al. Epidemiology and clinicopathology of aortic dissection. *Chest* 2000;117:1271–1278.

190. DeBakey ME, McCollum CH, Crawford ES, et al. Dissection and dissecting aneurysms of the aorta: Twenty-year follow up of five hundred twenty-seven patients treated surgically. *Surgery* 1982;92:1118–1134.

191. Spittell PC, Spittell JA Jr, Joyce JW, et al. Clinical features and differential diagnosis of aortic dissection: Experience with 236 cases (1980 through 1990). *Mayo Clin Proc* 1993;68:642–651.

192. Hagan PG, Nienaber CA, Isselbacher EM, et al. The International Registry of acute Aortic Dissection (IRAD). New Insights into an old disease. *JAMA* 2000;283:897–903.

193. Perron AD, Gibbs M. Thoracic aortic dissection secondary to crack cocaine ingestion. *Am J Emerg Med* 1997;12:507–509.

194. Eisenberg MJ, Rice SA, Paraschos A, et al. The clinical spectrum of patients with aneurysms of the ascending aorta. *Am Heart J* 1993;125:1380–1385.

195. von Kodolitsch Y, Schwartz AG, Nienaber CA. Clinical prediction of acute aortic dissection. *Arch Intern Med* 2000;160:2977–2982.

196. Fann JI, Sarris GE, Mitchell RS, et al. Treatment of patients with aortic dissection presenting with peripheral vascular complications. *Ann Surg* 1990;212:705–713.

197. Cambria RP, Brewster DC, Gertler J, et al. Vascular complications associated with spontaneous aortic dissection. *J Vasc Surg* 1988;7:199–209.

198. Giles J, Walters H. Aortic dissection presenting as acute leg ischemia. *Clin Radiol* 1990;42:116–117.

199. Gerber O, Heyer EJ, Vieux U. Painless dissections of the aorta presenting as acute neurologic syndromes. *Stroke* 1986;17:644–647.

200. Strouse PJ, et al. Aortic dissection presenting as spinal cord ischemia with a false negative aortogram. *Cardiovasc Intervent Radiol* 1990;13:77–82.

201. Butler J, Davies AH, Westaby S. Streptokinase in acute aortic dissection. *Br Med J* 1990;300:517–519.

202. Petasnick JP. Radiologic evaluation of aortic dissection. *Radiology* 1991;180:297–305.

203. Cigarroa JE, Isselbacher EM, DeSanctis RW, Eagle KA. Diagnostic imaging in the evaluation of suspected aortic dissection—Old standards and new directions. *N Engl J Med* 1993;128:35–43.

204. Thorsen MK, San Dretto MA, Lawson TL, et al. Dissecting aortic aneurysms: accuracy of computed tomographic diagnosis. *Radiology* 1983;148:773–777.

205. Nienaber CA, Kodolitsch Y, Nicolas V, et al. The diagnosis of thoracic aortic dissection by noninvasive imaging procedures. *N Engl J Med* 1993;328:1–9.

206. Sommer T, Fehske W, Holzknecht N, et al. Aortic dissection: A comparative study of diagnosis with spiral CT, multiplanar transesophageal echocardiography, and MR imaging. *Radiology* 1996;199:347–352.

207. Rubin GD. MDCT imaging of the aorta and peripheral vessels. *Eur J Radiol* 2003;45(suppl):S42–S49.

208. Tomiguchi S, Morishita S, Nakashima R, et al. Usefullness of turboFLASH dynamic MR imaging of dissecting aneurysms of the thoracic aorta. *Cardiovasc Intervent Radiol* 1994;17:17–21.

209. Mendelson DS, Apter S, Mitty HA, et al. Residual dissection of the thoracic aorta after repair: MRI-angiographic correlation. *Comput Med Imaging Graph* 1991;15:31–35.

210. White R, Ullyot D, Higgins CB. MR imaging of the aorta after surgery for aortic dissection. *Am J Roentgenol* 1988;150:87–92.

211. Prince MR, Narasimham DL, Stanley JC, et al: Breath-hold gadolin-ium-enhanced MR angiography of the abdominal aorta and its major branches. *Radiology* 1995;197:785–792.

212. Wolff KA, Herold CJ, Tempany CM, et al. Aortic dissection: Atypical patterns seen at MR imaging. *Radiology* 1991;181:489–495.

213. Earls JP, DeSena S, Bluemke DA. Gadolinium-enhanced three-dimensional MR angiography of the entire aorta and iliac arteries with dynamic manual table translation. *Radiology* 1998;209:844–849.

214. Chang JM, Friese K, Caputo GR, et al. MR measurement of blood flow in the true and false channel in chronic aortic dissection. *J Comput Assist Tomogr* 1991;15:418–423.

215. Mitchell L, et al. Case report: Aortic dissection: Morphology and differential flow velocity patterns demonstrated by magnetic resonance imaging. *Clin Radiol* 1988;39:458–461.

216. Adam G, Neuerburg J, Bucker A, et al. Interventional magnetic reso-nance. Initial clinical experience with a 1.5-tesla magnetic resonance system combined with c-arm fluoroscopy. *Invest Radiol* 1997;32:191–197.

217. Yang X, Bolster BD Jr, Kraitchman DL, Atalar E. Intravascular MR-monitored balloon angioplasty: An in vivo feasibility study. *J Vasc Intervent Radiol* 1998;9:953–959.

218. Omoto R, Kyo S, Matsumura M. Evaluation of biplane color Doppler transesophageal echocardiography in 200 consecutive patients. *Circu-lation* 1992;85:1237–1247.

219. Pearson AC, Castello R, Lebovitz AJ. Safety and utility of trans-esophageal echocardiography in the critically ill patient. *Am Heart J* 1990;119:1083–1089.

220. Hashimoto S, Kumada T, Osakada G, et al. Assessment of trans-esophageal Doppler echocardiography in dissecting aortic aneurysm. *J Am Coll Cardiol* 1989;14:1253–1262.

221. Erbel R, Daniel W, Visser C, et al. Echocardiography in diagnosis of aortic dissection. *Lancet* 1989;330:457–460.

222. Keren A, Kim CB, Hu BS, et al.: Accuracy of biplane and multiplane transesophageal echocardiography in diagnosis of typical acute aortic dissection and intramural hematoma. *J Am Coll Cardiol* 28:627–36, 1996

223. Balla RJ, Nanda NC, Gatewood R, et al. Usefulness of transesophageal echocardiography in assessment of aortic dissection. *Circulation* 1991; 84:1903–1914.

224. Soto B, Harman MA, Ceballos R, Barcia A. Angiographic diagnosis of dissecting aneurysm of the aorta. *Am J Roentgenol Radium Ther Nucl Med* 1972;116:146–154.

225. Weintraub AR, Erbel R, Gorge G, et al. Intravascular ultrasound imag-ing in acute aortic dissection. *J Am Coll Cardiol* 1994;24:495–503.

226. Prokop EK, Palmer RF, Wheat MW. Hydrodynamic forces in dissecting aneurysms: In-vitro studies in a tygon model and in dog aortas. *Circ Res* 1970;27:121–127.

227. Wheat MW Jr, Palmer RF. Treatment of dissecting aneurysms of the aorta without surgery. *Prog Cardiovasc Dis* 1968;11:198–210.

228. Grubb BP, Sirio C, Zelis R. Intravenous labetolol in acute aortic dissection. *JAMA* 1987;258:78–79.

229. Chirillo F, Marchiori MC, Andriolo L, et al. Outcome of 290 patients with aortic dissection: A 12-year multicentre experience. *Eur Heart J* 1990;11:311–319.

230. Glower DD, Fann JI, Speier RH, Morrison L. Comparison of medical and surgical therapy for uncomplicated descending aortic dissections. *Circulation* 1990;82(suppl IV):IV39–IV46.

231. Masuda Y, Yamada Z, Morooka N, et al. Prognosis of patients with medically treated aortic dissections. *Circulation* 1991;84(suppl III): III-7–III-13.

232. Borst HG, Laass J. Surgical treatment of thoracic aortic aneurysms. *Adv Card Surg* 1993;4:47–87.

233. Crawford ES, Svensson LG, Coselli JS, et al. Surgical treatment of aneurysm and/or dissection of the ascending aorta, transverse aortic arch and ascending aorta and transverse aortic arch. *J Thorac Cardiovasc Surg* 1989;98G 659–673.

234. Ikonomidis JS, Weisel RD, Mouradian MS, et al. Thoracic aortic surgery. *Circulation* 1991;84(suppl III):III-1–III-6.

235. Svensson LG, Crawford ES, Hess KR, et al. Dissection of the aorta and dissecting aortic aneurysm: Improving early and long-term surgical results. *Circulation* 1990;82(suppl IV):IV-24–IV-38.

236. Taniguchi K, Nakano S, Matsuda H, et al. Long-term survival and complications after composite graft replacement for ascending aortic aneurysm associated with aortic regurgitation. *Circulation* 1991; 84(suppl III):III-31–III-39.

237. Mehta RH, O'Gara PT, Bossone E, et al. Acute type A aortic dissection in the elderly: Clinical characteristics, mangament and outcomes in the current era. *J Am Coll Cardiol* 2002;40:685–692.

238. Walker PJ, Dake MD, Mitchell RS, Miller DC. The use of en-dovascular techniques for the treatment of complications of aortic dissection. *J Vasc Surg* 1993;18:1042–1051.

239. Dake MD, Kato N, Mitchell RS, et al. Endovascular stent–graft placement for the treatment of acute aortic dissection. *N Engl J Med* 1999;340:1546–1552.

240. Slonim SM, Miller DC, Mitchell RS, et al. Percutaneous balloon fenestration and stenting for life-threatening ischemic complications in patients with acute aortic dissection. *Thorac Cardiovasc Surg* 1999; 117:1118–1126.

241. Williams DM, Lee DY, Hamilton BH, et al. The dissected aorta: Percutaneous treatment of ischemic complications—principles and results. *J Vasc Intervent Radiol* 1997;8:605–625.

242. Vedantham S, Picus D, Sanchez LA, et al. Percutaneous management of ischemic complications in patients with type-B aortic dissection. *J Vasc Intervent Radiol* 2003;12:181–193.

243. Lopera J, Patino JH, Urbina C, et al. Endovascular treatment of com-plicated type-B aortic dissection with stent-grafts: Midterm results. *J Vasc Intervent Radiol* 2003;14:195–203.

244. Cooke JP, Kazmier FJ, Orszulak TA. The penetrating aortic ulcer: Pathologic manifestations, diagnosis, and management. *Mayo Clin Proc* 1988;63:718–725.

245. Stanson AW, Kazmier FJ, Hollier LH. Penetrating atherosclerotic ulcers of the thoracic aorta: Natural history and clinicopathologic correlations. *Ann Vasc Surg* 1986;1:15–23.

246. Hussain S, Glover JL, Bree R, Bendick PJ. Penetrating atherosclerotic ulcers of the thoracic aorta. *J Vasc Surg* 1989;9:710–717.

247. Movsowitz HD, Lampert C, Jacobs LE, Kotler MN. Penetrating atherosclerotic aortic ulcers. *Am Heart J* 1994;28:1210–1217.

248. Faries PL, Lang E, Ramdev P, et al. Endovascular stent-graft treat-ment of a ruptured thoracic aortic ulcer. *J Endovasc Ther* 2002;9: II-20–II-24.

249. Kos X, Bouchard L, Otal P, et al. Stent-graft treatment of penetrating thoracic aortic ulcers. *J Endovasc Ther* 2002;9:II-25–II-31.

250. Crane JS, Cowling M, Cheshire NJ. Endovascular stent grafting of a penetrating ulcer in the descending thoracic aorta. *Eur J Vasc Endovasc Surg* 2003;25:178–179.

251. Von Kodolitsch Y, Csosz SK, Koschyk DH, et al. Intramural hematoma of the aorta. Predictors of progression to dissection and rupture. *Circulation* 2003;107:1158–1163.

252. Cambria RP. Regarding "analysis of predictive factors for progression of type B aortic intramural hematoma with computed tomography. *J Vasc Surg* 2002;35:1295–1296.

253. Isselbacher EM. Intramural hematoma of the aorta: Should we let down our guard? *Am J Med* 2002;113:244–246.

254. Song JK, Kim HS, Song JM. Outcomes of medically treated patients with aortic intramural hematoma. *Am J Med* 2002;113:181–187.

255. Sawhney NS, DeMaria AN, Blanchard DG. Aortic inramural hematoma: An increasingly recognized and potentially fatal entity. *Chest* 2001;120: 1340–1346.

256. von Kodolitsch Y, Csosz SK, Koschyk DH, et al. Intramural hematoma of the aorta. Predictors of progression to dissection and rupture. *Circulation* 2003;107:1158–1163.

257. Maraj R, Rerkpattanapipat P, Jacobs LE, et al. Meta-analysis of 143 reported cases of aortic intramural hematoma. *Am J Cardiol* 2000; 86:664–648.

258. Ito I: Aortitis syndrome (Takayasu's arteritis): A review. *Jpn Heart J* 1995;36:273–281.

259. Kerr GS, Hallahan CW, Giordano J, et al. Takayasu arteritis. *Ann Intern Med* 1994;120:919–929.

260. Eichorn J, Sima D, Thiele B, et al. Anti-endothelial cell antibodies in Takayasu's arteritis. *Circulation* 1996;94:2396–2401.

261. Noris M, Daina E, Gamba S, et al. Interleukin-6 and RANTES in Takayasu's arteritis: A guide for therapeutic decisions. *Circulation* 1999;100:55–60.

262. Ishikawa K: Diagnostic approach and proposed criteria for the clinical diagnosis of Takayasu's arteriopathy. *J Am Coll Cardiol* 1998;12: 964–972.

263. Ishikawa K, Maetani S. Long-term outcome for 120 Japanese patients with Takayasu's disease. *Circulation* 1994;90:1855–1860.

264. Wolak T, Szendro G, Goleman L, Paran E. Malignant hypertension as a presenting symptom of Takayasu arteritis. *Mayo Clin Proc* 2003;78: 231–236.

265. Connolly JE, Wilson SE, Lawrence PL, Fujitani RM. Middle aortic syndrome: Distal thoracic and abdominal coarctation, a disorder with multiple etiologies. *J Am Coll Surg* 2002;194:774–781.

266. Arend WP, Michel BA, Bloch DA, et al. The American College of Rheumatology 1990 criteria for the classification of Takayasu arteritis. *Arthritis Rheum* 1990;33:1129–1134.

267. Rigby WFC, Fan CM, Mark EJ. Case records of the Massachusetts General Hospital. Weekly clinicopathological exercises. Case 39-2002—A 35-year-old man with headache, deviation of the tongue, and unusual radiographic abnormalities. *N Engl J Med* 2002; 2057–2065.

268. Flamm SD, White RD, Hoffman GS. The clinical application of "edema-weighted" magnetic resonance imaging in the assessment of Takayasu's arteritis. *Int J Cardiol* 1998;66(suppl 1):S151–S159.

269. Hoffman GS, Ahmed AE. Surrogate markers of disease activity in patients with takayasu arteritis. A preliminary report from The International Network for the Study of the Systemic Vasculitides (INSSYS). *Int J Cardiol* 66(suppl 1):1998;S191–S194.

270. Tso E, Flamm SD, White RD, et al. Takayasu's arteritis. Utility and limitations of magnetic resonance imaging in diagnosis and treatment. *Arthritis Rheum* 2002;46:1634–1642.

271. Ishikawa K. Effects of prednisolone therapy on arterial angiographic features in Takayasu's disease. *Am J Cardiol* 1991;68:410–413.

272. Fraga A, Mintz G, Valle L, et al. Takayasu's arteritis: Frequency of systemic manifestations (study of 22 patients) and favorable response to maintenance corticosteroid therapy with adrenocorticosteroids (12 patients). *Arthritis Rheum* 1972;15:617–624.

273. Hoffman GS, Leavitt RY, Kerr GS, et al. Treatment of glucocorticoid-resistant or relapsing Takayasu arteritis with methotrexate. *Arthritis Rheum* 1994;37:578–582.

274. Tyagi S, Singh B, Kaul UA, et al. Balloon angioplasty for renovascular hypertension in Takayasu's arteritis. *Am Heart J* 1993;125:1386–1393.

275. Evans JM, O'Fallon WM, Hunder GG. Increased incidence of aortic aneurysm and dissection in giant cell (temporal) arteritis. *Ann Intern Med* 1995;122:502–507.

276. Salvarani C, Gabriel S, O'Fallon WM, Hunder GG. The incidence of giant cell arteritis in Olmsted County, Minnesota: Apparent fluctuations in a cyclic pattern. *Ann Intern Med* 1995;123:192–194.

277. Nordborg E, Nordborg C. Giant cell arteritis: Epidemiological clues to its pathogenesis and an update on its treatment. *Rheumatology* 2003; 42:413–421.

278. Jover JA, Hernandez-Garcia C, Morado IC, et al. Combined treatment of giant-cell arteritis with methotrexate and prednisolone. A randomized, double-blind, placebo-controlled trial. *Ann Intern Med* 2001;134: 106–114.

279. Hoffman GS, Cid MC, Hellmann DB, et al. A multicenter randomized, double blind, placebo-controlled trial of adjuvant methotrexate treatment for giant cell arteritis. *Arthritis Rheum* 2002;46:1309–1318.

280. Bulkley BH, Roberts WC. Ankylosing spondylitis and aortic regurgitation: Description of the characteristic cardiovascular lesion from study of eight necropsy patients. *Circulation* 1973;48:1014–1027.

281. Roldan CA, Chavez J, Wiest PW, et al. Aortic root disease and valve disease associated with ankylosing spondylitis. *J Am Coll Cardiol* 1998;32:1397–1404.

282. Fiessinger JN PJ. [Inflammatory and infectious aortitis]. *Rev Prat* 2002;52:1094–1099.

283. Jackman JD, Radolf JD. Cardiovascular syphilis. *Am J Med* 1989;87: 425–433.

284. Hagino RT, Clagett GP, Valentine RJ. A case of Pott's disease of the spine eroding into the suprarenal aorta. *J Vasc Surg* 1996;24:482–486.

285. Allins AD, Wagner WH, Cossman DV, et al. Tuberculous infection of the descending thoracic and abdominal aorta: Case report and literature review. *Ann Vasc Surg* 1999;13:439–444.

286. Golzarian J, Cheng J, Giron F, et al. Tuberculous pseudoaneurysm of the descending thoracic aorta. *Texas Heart Inst J* 1999;26:232–235.

287. DeBakey ME HW, Cooley DA, et al. Surgical management of dissecting aneurysm of the aorta. *J Thorac Cardiovasc Surg* 1965;49:130.

288. Dailey PO, Trueblood HW, Stinson EB, et al. Management of acute aortic dissections. *Ann Thorac Surg* 1970;10:237–246.

289. Crawford ES, Svensson LG, Coselli JS, et al. Aortic dissection and dissecting aortic aneurysms. *Ann Surg* 1988;208:254–273.

290. Fradet G, Jamieson WR, Janusz MT, et al. Aortic dissection: current expectations and treatment. Experience with 258 patients over 20 years. *Can J Surg* 1990;33:465–469.

291. Nichols WW, O'Rourke MF. *McDonald's Blood Flow in Arteries: Theoretic, Experimental and Clinical Principles,* 3d ed. Philadelphia: Lea & Febiger; 1990.

292. Creager MA, Halperin JL, Whittemore AD. Aneurysmal disease of the aorta and its branches. In: Loscalzo JCM, Dzau VJ, eds. *Vascular Medicine: A Textbook of Vascular Biology and Diseases.* Boston: Little, Brown; 1992.

293. Crawford ES, Coselli JS. Thoracoabdominal aortic aneurysms. *Semin Thorac Cardiovasc Surg* 1991;3:302.

294. Jolly M, Bartholomew JR, Flamm S, Olin JW. Angina and coronary ostial lesions in a young woman as a presentation of Takayasu's arteritis. *J Cardiovasc Surg* 1999;7:443–446.

CEREBROVASCULAR DISEASE AND NEUROLOGIC MANIFESTATIONS OF HEART DISEASE

Megan C. Leary / Louis R. Caplan

Most vascular diseases affect both the heart and the brain. Heart diseases often lead to lesions and dysfunction within the brain, and central nervous system (CNS) diseases influence the heart and its function.

BRAIN AND CEREBROVASCULAR COMPLICATIONS OF HEART DISEASE

Cerebral complications occur when (1) the heart pumps unwanted materials into the circulation that reach the brain (embolism); (2) pump function fails and the brain is hypoperfused; and (3) drugs given to treat cardiac disease have neurologic side effects.

Direct Cardiogenic Brain Embolism

ETIOLOGY

Diagnostic criteria for cardiogenic embolism were formerly very restrictive. Embolism was diagnosed when sudden focal neurologic signs, maximal at onset, developed in patients with peripheral systemic embolism and recent myocardial infarction or rheumatic mitral stenosis.[1] Using these criteria, cardiogenic embolism was diagnosed in only 3 to 8 percent of stroke patients.[2–5] None of these criteria are secure. In various stroke registries, about 10 to 20 percent of patients diagnosed with cardioembolic strokes did not have maximal symptoms at onset.[5–8] Certain cardiac arrhythmias are now well-accepted sources of embolic stroke—atrial fibrillation. Only about 2 percent of patients with cardiogenic brain embolism have clinically recognized peripheral emboli. In necropsy studies of patients with brain embolism, however, infarcts are commonly found in the spleen and kidneys and other organs. The symptoms of peripheral embolism are often so minor and nonspecific (transient abdominal discomfort, leg cramp, etc.) that they are seldom diagnosed correctly.

Before the advent of echocardiography, 30 percent of stroke patients were deemed to most likely have cardiogenic embolism.[5,6] Subsequent studies using stricter diagnostic criteria attributed 17 percent,[7] 22 percent,[9] and 14 percent[8] of strokes to cardiogenic embolism. As more advanced diagnostic techniques have been developed, more cardiac abnormalities (and their association with stroke) are recognized. In 1991 published data from the Lausanne Stroke Registry indicated that 305 (23 percent) of 1311 patients with a first-ever stroke also had a potential cardiac source of embolism.[10,11] However, as many patients have coexisting cardiac and extracranial vascular disease,[11] criteria for the diagnosis of cardiac embolism remain controversial.

Cardiac sources of cerebral emboli can be divided into three groups[1]: (1) *cardiac wall and chamber abnormalities*—cardiomyopathies, hypokinetic and akinetic ventricular regions after myocardial infarction, atrial septal aneurysms, ventricular aneurysms, atrial myxomas, papillary fibroelastomas and other tumors, septal defects, and patent foramen ovale; (2) *valve disorders*—rheumatic mitral and aortic disease, prosthetic valves, bacterial endocarditis, fibrous and fibrinous endocardial lesions, mitral valve prolapse, and mitral annulus calcification; and (3) *arrhythmias*, especially atrial fibrillation and "sick-sinus" syndrome.

Some cardiac sources have much higher rates of initial and recurrent embolism. The Stroke Data Bank[12] divided potential sources into *strong sources* (prosthetic valves, atrial fibrillation, sick-sinus syndrome, ventricular aneurysm, akinetic segments, mural thrombi, cardiomyopathy, diffuse ventricular hypokinesia) and *weak sources* (myocardial infarct over 6 months old, aortic and mitral stenosis and regurgitation, congestive failure, mitral valve prolapse, mitral annulus calcification, hypokinetic ventricular segments).

The risk of embolism varies within individual cardiac abnormalities depending on many factors. For example, in patients with atrial fibrillation, associated heart disease, patient age, duration, chronic versus intermittent fibrillation, and atrial size all influence embolic risk. The presence of a potential cardiac source of embolism does not mean that a stroke was caused by an embolus from the heart. Coexistent occlusive cerebrovascular disease is common. In the Lausanne registry, among patients with potential cardiac embolic sources, 11 percent of patients had severe cervicocranial vascular occlusive disease (>75 percent stenosis) and 40 percent had mild-to-moderate stenosis proximal to brain infarcts.[11]

Mitral valve prolapse (MVP) is the most common form of valve disease in adults and is generally benign.[13,14] MVP as a source of embolic stroke continues to be controversial[1] (see Chap. 68). Several small clinical series have reported cerebral embolism in MVP patients who lacked other possible embolic sources.[15–18] Direct cardiac inspection in MVP patients has noted morphologic valvular lesions, such as thrombi and fibrous lesions, clearly suggestive of embolism[19–21]; fibrin-platelet depositions on the surfaces of the mitral leaflets have been noted,[18–20] as well as thrombi in the angle between the posterior mitral valve leaflet and the left atrial wall.[18,21,22] Patients with MVP also may have other disorders such as atrial fibrillation, syncope, and migraine. The rate of recurrent stroke in patients with MVP as the only known cause is very low.[17,18] Given the very high incidence of MVP, the frequency of MVP-related stroke is extremely low.[18–23] Most neurologists feel that warfarin anticoagulants are ordinarily not indicated in prophylaxis of patients with MVP, even after an initial stroke. Aspirin prophylaxis (80 to 325 mg/day) is, however, advisable. Demonstration of an intracardiac thrombus by echocardiography would change that recommendation to warfarin.

Mitral annulus calcification (MAC) is an important, often unrecognized, cause of embolism. Ulceration and extrusion of calcium through overlapping cusps have been seen at necropsy,[24] thrombi have been found on valves attached to the ulcerative process,[25] and calcific emboli have been seen in surgical embolectomies.[18,24,26] Several series show a convincing relation between MAC and brain emboli and stroke.[1,7,27–29] Bacterial endocarditis can also develop on the MAC. Obviously, there is little rationale to utilize anticoagulation to prevent calcific emboli. The decision to use antiplatelet agents versus anticoagulants should include consideration of other potential comorbid factors, such as: atrial fibrillation (which can occur 12 times more often in patients with MAC than it would in those without MAC).[14,30]

More patients may have cardiogenic embolism than are now diagnosed. Clinical features and brain investigations such as computed tomography (CT), magnetic resonance imaging (MRI), and angiography (CT, MR, and digital subtraction angiography) may suggest emboli, but often a clear source is not identified. These cases, which are termed *infarcts of unknown causes* (IUC) in the Stroke Data Bank,[6,31,32] include as many as 40 percent of patients.

Some disorders are associated with *fibrous and fibrinous lesions of the heart valves and endocardium.*[1] Similar valve lesions occur in patients with systemic lupus erythematosus (Libman-Sacks endocarditis[33]), antiphospholipid antibody syndrome,[34] and cancer and other debilitating diseases (nonbacterial thrombotic endocarditis). Mobile fibrous strands are also often found during echocardiography.[1,35–37] Fibrin-platelet aggregates may attach to these fibrous and fibrinous lesions. Warfarin anticoagulants are ineffective in prevention of embolism in these conditions.

Embolic complications are common in patients who have *infective endocarditis.*[1,38] Mycotic aneurysms can cause fatal subarachnoid bleeding. Bleeding can also result from vascular necrosis as a result of an infected embolus.[38] Embolization usually stops when infection is controlled.[35] Warfarin does not prevent embolization and is probably contraindicated unless there are other important lesions such as prosthetic valves or life-threatening pulmonary embolism (see Chaps. 63 and 71). In children and young adults with congenital heart defects, especially those with right-to-left shunts and polycythemia, brain abscess is an important complication (see Chap. 73).

Emboli often arise from sources other than the heart, such as the aorta, proximal arteries (intraarterial or so-called local embolism), leg veins (paradoxical emboli), fat in the liver or bones (fat embolism), and materials introduced by the patient or physician (drug particles or air).[1] The types of embolic material also vary (Table 99-1).[1,39] *Atheromatous plaques in the aortic arch and ascending aorta are a very important and previously neglected source of embolism to the brain* (Figs. 99-1 and 99-2). Ulcerated atheromatous plaques are often found at necropsy in patients with ischemic strokes, especially in those in whom the stroke etiology was not determined during life.[40] Transesophageal echocardiography (TEE) often shows these atheromas, but technical factors limit visualization of the entire arch.[41] The aorta can also be insonated by B-mode ultrasound probes placed in the supraclavicular fossa on each side.[42] Large (>4 mm), protruding *mobile aortic atheromas are especially likely to cause embolic strokes and are associated with a high rate of recurrent strokes.*[43] Use of oral anticoagulants rather than antiplatelet agents is recommended in these patients.[14,44,45]

CLINICAL FINDINGS

Anterior Circulation Recipient Sites Balloons placed into the circulation tend to follow the same flow patterns[46]; anterior circulation material reaches the middle cerebral arteries (MCAs) and their branches.[46] The most common sites are the main stem MCA, the upper or lower divisions of

TABLE 99-1 Embolic Materials

Cardiac	Intraarterial
1. Red fibrin-dependent thrombi	1. Red fibrin-dependent thrombi
2. White platelet-fibrin nidi	2. White platelet-fibrin nidi
3. Material from marantic endocarditis	3. Combined fibrin-platelet and fibrin-dependent clots
4. Bacteria from vegetations	4. Cholesterol crystals
5. Calcium from valves and mitral annulus calcification	5. Atheromatous plaque debris
6. Myxoma cells and debris	6. Calcium from vascular calcifications
	7. Air
	8. Mucin from tumors
	9. Talc or microcrystalline cellulose from injected drugs

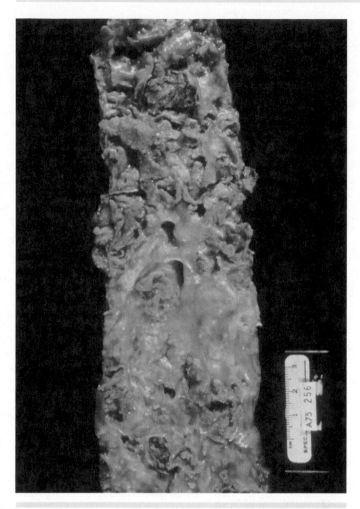

FIGURE 99-1 Descending aorta at necropsy from a patient whose transesophageal echocardiography before surgery showed severe disease of the ascending aorta and aortic arch with mobile protruding plaques. This patient died after coronary artery bypass grafting surgery having never awakened after the procedure. Submitted by Denise Barbut. (From Caplan LR. *Stroke: A Clinical Approach*, 3d ed. Boston: Butterworth-Heinemann, 2000, with permission.)

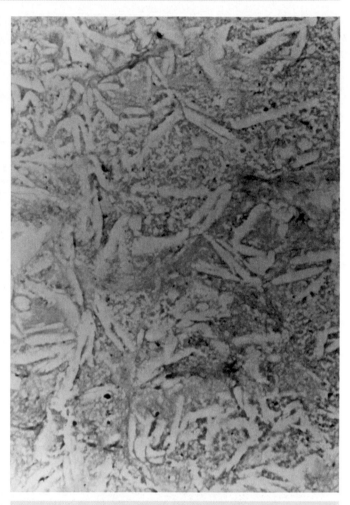

FIGURE 99-2 Cholesterol crystals and other particulate debris are caught in a filter placed in the aorta at the time that aortic clamps are removed. Submitted by Denise Barbut. (From Caplan LR. *Stroke: A Clinical Approach*, 3d ed. Boston: Butterworth-Heinemann, 2000, with permission.)

the MCA, or their branches. The upper division of the MCA supplies the frontal and parietal lobes above the sylvian fissure, and the lower division supplies the convexal temporal and inferior parietal lobes. Resultant neurologic deficits include the following:

MCA UPPER DIVISION. Contralateral hemiparesis; hemisensory loss; aphasia (left hemisphere); lack of awareness of deficit; neglect of the left visual space; and motor impersistence[47] (right hemisphere).

MCA INFERIOR DIVISION Wernicke-type fluent aphasia; agitation; right-upper-quadrantanopia (left hemisphere); agitation and hyperactivity; left neglect, poor drawing, and copying (right hemisphere).[48]

MCA MAIN STEM Findings include features of both upper and lower division infarcts.

Posterior Circulation Recipient Sites Vertebrobasilar territory symptoms are usually attributed to local disease within that circulation without consideration of possible cardiogenic embolism. In the major stroke registries,[1,5–11] however, about 20 percent of emboli of cardiac origin go to the posterior circulation. Twenty percent is expected, as about one-fifth of cerebral blood flow goes to this circulation. In the posterior circulation, certain recipient sites are favored.

POSTERIOR CEREBRAL ARTERY (PCA)[49–52] Particles and clots go to the most distal part of the system; the PCA is the terminal vessel in the vertebrobasilar circuit. The hallmark of PCA lesions is hemianopia and/or hemisensory loss contralateral to the infarct. Patients with left-PCA territory infarcts also often cannot read or name colors but retain the ability to write and spell. Amnesia is sometimes prominent and may last up to 6 months. Right-PCA territory infarction is often associated with left visual neglect.

TOP OF THE BASILAR ARTERY[50,53,54] The major clinical features are apathy and sleepiness; abnormal vertical gaze; and hallucinations, unusual reports, and other behavioral abnormalities. Bilateral PCA territory infarction causes bilateral visual field loss, amnesia, and severe agitation and delirium.

VERTEBRAL ARTERY (VA) INTRACRANIALLY AND ITS POSTERIOR INFERIOR CEREBELLAR ARTERY (PICA) BRANCH Somewhat larger emboli may occlude an intracranial VA and cause cerebellar infarction involving mostly the posterior inferior surface.[50,55] Ataxia, vomiting, and occipital headache are the most common signs.

ONSET AND COURSE

Most embolic events occur during activities of daily living but some embolic strokes have their onset during rest or sleep. Sudden coughing, sneezing, or arising at night to urinate can precipitate embolism.[1,5] Although the deficit is most often maximal at outset, 11 percent of embolic stroke patients in the Harvard Stroke Registry had a stuttering or stepwise course, whereas 10 percent had fluctuations or progressive deficits. Later progression, if it occurs, is usually within the first 48 h. Progression is usually due to distal passage of emboli. "Nonsudden" embolism is explained by an embolus moving from its initial location, as demonstrated by angiography, to a more distal branch.[1,56] Early angiography has a very high rate of showing intracranial emboli,[6,57] but angiography after 48 h shows a much lower rate of blockage.

More recently, transcranial Doppler (TCD) sonography has shown a high incidence of MCA blockage acutely in patients with sudden-onset hemispheric strokes, but later, recanalization of the MCA and normalization of the intracranial blood velocities occur.[1,58] As in all large infarcts, brain edema and swelling may develop during the 24 to 72 h after stroke, with headache, decreased alertness, and worsening of neurologic signs. The edema is often cytotoxic (inside cells) and usually does not respond to corticosteroid treatment.

DIAGNOSTIC TESTING

Emboli usually cause occlusion of distal branches and produce surface infarcts that are roughly triangular, with the apex of the triangle pointing inward. CT and MRI findings can suggest the presence of embolism by the location and shape of the lesion,[59] presence of superficial wedge-shaped infarcts in multiple different vascular territories, hemorrhagic infarction, and visualization of thrombi within arteries. Among 60 patients with cardiogenic sources of embolism studied by CT in whom occlusive atherosclerotic cerebrovascular disease had been excluded, 56 had superficial large or small cortical or subcortical infarcts and only 4 had deep infarcts.[59] Emboli can block the MCA and occasionally cause solely deep infarcts because the superficial territory has good collateral flow; these infarcts are called *striatocapsular* because they involve the internal capsule and the adjacent basal ganglia, which are supplied by lenticulostriate branches of the MCA.[1,5,60] Tiny emboli may cause small deep or superficial infarcts.

MRI, particularly with the use of MR diffusion-weighted and MR gradient-recalled echo (GRE) imaging, is more sensitive for detection of acute brain infarcts than is CT and is also superior in detecting hemorrhagic infarction by imaging hemosiderin. Hemorrhagic infarction has long been considered characteristic of embolism, especially when the artery leading to the infarct is patent.[61] The mechanism of hemorrhagic infarction is reperfusion of ischemic zones, which occurs with spontaneous passage of the embolus, after iatrogenic opening of an occluded artery (e.g., endarterectomy, fibrinolytic treatment), or after restoration of the circulation after a period of systemic hypoperfusion. Hemorrhage occurs into proximal reperfused regions of brain infarcts.[1,5,62] At times, it is also possible to image the acute embolus on CT.[1,63,64]

In unselected series of stroke patients, transthoracic echocardiography (TTE; see Chap. 15) has been variably useful in detecting sources.[1,65–67] TTE is useful in patients with known cardiac disease to clarify potential embolic sources and heart function,[5] in young patients without stroke risk factors, and in stroke patients who do not have lacunar infarction or ultrasound evidence of intrinsic atherostenosis of a major extracranial and intracranial artery. Transesophageal echocardiography (TEE) (see Chap. 15) provides much better visualization of the aorta, atria, cardiac valves, and septal regions. Reports of TEE suggest that the diagnostic yield is 2 to 10 times that of TTE.[68–71] Aortic plaques, atrial septal aneurysms, and atrial septal defects are also much better seen with TEE (Fig. 99-3). The use of an echo-enhancing agent such as agitated saline helps detect intracardiac shunts.

Echocardiography has definite limitations. Particles the size of 2 mm can block major brain arteries but are beyond the imaging resolution of current echocardiographic technology.[72] Also, thromboembolism is a dynamic process. When a clot forms in the heart and embolizes, there may be no residual evidence until a clot reforms.[1,39] Cardiac thrombi are imaged differently on sequential echocardiograms[1,73]; even large thrombi seen on one echocardiogram can disappear later.[73] Platelet scintigraphy using platelets

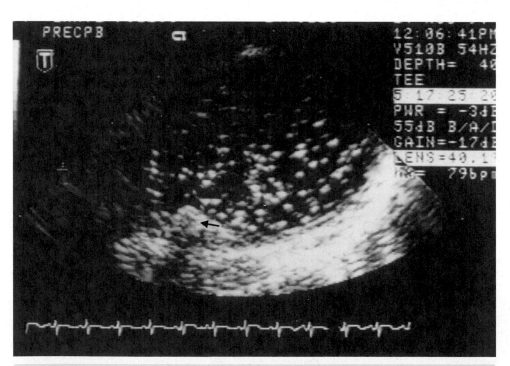

FIGURE 99-3 Transesophageal echocardiography recording during cardiac surgery from the aorta at the level of the origin of the left subclavian artery. A mobile plaque is seen protruding into the aortic lumen (small black arrow). This recording was taken after the release of aortic clamps and shows a "shower" of emboli within the aortic lumen beyond where the aorta was previously clamped. Submitted by Denise Barbut. (From Caplan LR. *Stroke: A Clinical Approach*, 3d ed. Boston: Butterworth-Heinemann, 2000, with permission.)

labeled with radionuclides may be helpful in localizing cardiac and intraarterial sources, but its sensitivity and specificity are undefined.[74]

Embolic signals are now detected by monitoring with transcranial Doppler (TCD).[1,75,76] Embolic particles passing under TCD probes produce transient, short-duration, high-intensity signals referred to as HITS (high-intensity transient signals). Examples of HITS are shown in Figs. 99-4 and 99-5. TCD monitoring of patients with atrial fibrillation,[77] cardiac surgery,[78] prosthetic valves, left ventricular assist devices,[79] carotid artery disease, and carotid endarterectomy have shown a relatively high frequency of embolic signals. In the future, monitoring of emboli with TCD will become an important diagnostic modality to guide treatment.

PREVENTION AND TREATMENT

Early studies showed that warfarin was effective in preventing brain embolism in patients with rheumatic mitral stenosis and atrial fibrillation (AF). Previously, the intensity of anticoagulation was higher than that currently used, and brain hemorrhages and other bleeding complications were common. Trials have now shown that low-dose warfarin [*international normalized ratio* (INR) 2.0 to 3.0] is also effective in preventing brain emboli in patients with nonrheumatic AF.

In the Copenhagen Atrial Fibrillation Aspirin Anticoagulation (AFASAK) study, 1007 patients (median age 74.2 years) with chronic, nonrheumatic AF were assigned to warfarin (INR 2.8 to 4.2), aspirin (75 mg/day), or placebo.[80] The study was halted prematurely when analysis of effectiveness reached a predetermined level of significance in favor of warfarin treatment. The principal outcome was the composite of ischemic or hemorrhagic stroke, transient ischemic attack (TIA), and systemic embolism. The observed reduction for warfarin compared to placebo was 64 percent, an absolute risk reduction of 3.5 percent per year. An analysis by intention to treat, which excluded TIA and minor stroke, indicated a risk reduction of

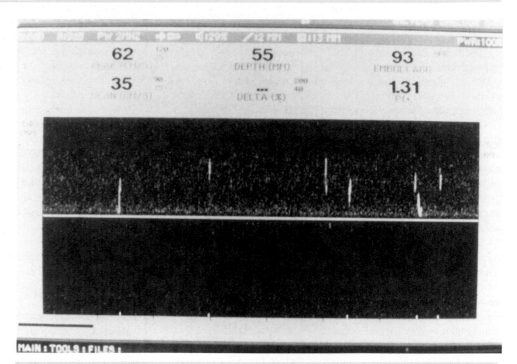

FIGURE 99-4 Transcranial Doppler recording from the middle cerebral arteries during steady state cardiac bypass surgery at a time when the aorta was being manipulated. The white streaks represent microemboli. Submitted by Denise Barbut. (From Caplan LR. *Stroke: A Clinical Approach,* 3d ed. Boston: Butterworth-Heinemann, 2000, with permission.)

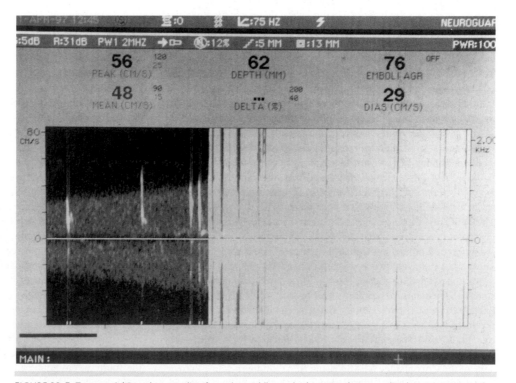

FIGURE 99-5 Transcranial Doppler recording from the middle cerebral arteries during cardiac bypass surgery. A few distinct emboli (white streaks in the left of the figure) are followed by a massive shower of emboli ("white-out") at the time of the release of aortic clamps. Submitted by Denise Barbut. (From Caplan LR. *Stroke: A Clinical Approach,* 3d ed, Boston: Butterworth-Heinemann, 2000, with permission.)

about 50 percent ($p < .05$) and an absolute reduction of about 1.5 percent per year.

The Stroke Prevention in Atrial Fibrillation (SPAF) study investigators evaluated warfarin and aspirin in patients with nonrheumatic AF.[81,82] The study evaluated two groups of patients on the basis of their eligibility for warfarin. In the first group, 627 patients judged eligible for warfarin were randomized to open label warfarin (INR 2.8 to 4.5; prothrombin time, 1.3 to 1.8 times control) or, in a double-blinded fashion, to either aspirin (325 mg daily, enteric-coated) or a matching placebo. In the second group, 703 patients ineligible for warfarin were randomized (double-blind) to aspirin (325 mg daily, enteric-coated) or placebo. The principal outcome, a composite of ischemic stroke and systemic embolism, was significantly decreased during a mean follow-up of 1.3 years. The outcome of disabling ischemic stroke or vascular death was reduced by warfarin by 54 percent ($p = .11$), an absolute reduction of 2.6 percent per year. Aspirin also decreased the principal outcome in both study groups. The risk reduction was 42 percent ($p = .02$), and the absolute reduction was 2.7 percent per year. The outcome of disabling stroke or death was reduced 22 percent by aspirin ($p = .33$) an absolute reduction of about 1 percent per year. The SPAF investigators later compared low-intensity fixed-dose warfarin (INR 1.2 to 1.5) plus aspirin (325 mg/day) with adjusted dose warfarin (INR 2.0 to 3.0) in elderly patients with one or more risk factors for embolism.[83] Ischemic stroke and systemic embolism were present in 7.9 percent of patients on fixed dose warfarin plus aspirin versus only 1.9 percent on adjusted-dose warfarin. SPAF investigators later studied the effectiveness of 325 mg aspirin in patients with low risk and found that the rate of ischemic stroke was low (2 percent per year).[84]

The SPAF study identified three risk factors for thromboembolism—recent congestive heart failure, history of hypertension, and previous thromboembolism[85,86]*—and suggested that anticoagulation with warfarin was not indicated in patients with none of the three risk factors who were at low risk for thromboembolism (2.5 percent per year).* In such patients, the dangers of anticoagulant therapy may outweigh its benefits. Aspirin (325 mg daily) is probably reasonable and safe therapy for patients with lone, nonrheumatic AF who are under 60 years of age and have none of the three identified risk factors.[85–87] In other patients with AF, long-term oral warfarin therapy (INR 2.0 to 3.0) should be used unless contraindicated.[84,87,88]

In the Boston Area Anticoagulation Trial for Atrial Fibrillation (BAATAF), 420 patients with nonrheumatic AF, mean age 68 years, were randomized unblinded to warfarin (target prothrombin time ratio, 1.2 to 1.5 x control; INR 1.5 to 2.7) or to a control group who were allowed to take aspirin.[89] The principal outcome was ischemic stroke or systemic embolism, and the mean follow-up was 2.2 years. The incidence of stroke was reduced by 86 percent in the warfarin group compared to control ($p = .002$), equivalent to an absolute risk reduction of 2.6 percent per year. There was no demonstrable benefit of aspirin, but the study was not designed to test aspirin.

In the Canadian Atrial Fibrillation Anticoagulation (CAFA) study, 187 patients were randomized to warfarin (INR target range 2.0 to 3.0) and 191 to placebo.[90] The principal outcome was the composite of nonlacunar stroke, non-CNS embolism, and fatal or intracranial hemorrhage. The relative risk reduction for warfarin was 37 percent ($p = .17$). The study was ended prematurely when the results of the Copenhagen AFASAK and SPAF studies became known.

The European Atrial Fibrillation Trial (EAFT) Study Group addressed the question of the optimal level of anticoagulation by reviewing the results of their own trial.[91] No treatment effect was found with anticoagulation responses below INRs of 2.0. The rate of thromboembolic events was lowest at INRs from 2 to 3.9; most major hemorrhages occurred at INRs of 5.0 and above. The EAFT group recommended a target of 3.0 with a range from 2 to 5.0.[91] Fixed-dose warfarin with a target of 1.3 to 1.5 was not as effective as standard adjusted-dose warfarin at an average INR of 2.4, even when aspirin 325 mg/day was added to the low fixed-dose warfarin in another study.

Warfarin is about 50 percent more effective than aspirin in preventing stroke in patients with atrial fibrillation who do not have valvular disease. The effectiveness of anticoagulation on embolism from other cardiac conditions has not been well studied. The rate of recurrence of stroke in patients with MVP is so low that warfarin is not recommended for prophylaxis except when a thrombus is seen on echocardiography (see Chap. 68). Warfarin may not be effective in preventing calcific, myxomatous, bacterial, and fibrin-platelet emboli, and warfarin has been posited to worsen cholesterol crystal embolization.[92]

The timing of the initiation of warfarin anticoagulation after embolic stroke remains controversial. Embolic brain infarcts often become hemorrhagic, and serious brain hemorrhage has occurred after anticoagulation.[93–97] Large infarcts, hypertension, large bolus doses of heparin, and excessive anticoagulation have been associated with hemorrhage. Because most hemorrhagic transformations occur within 48 h, the recommendations of the Cerebral Embolism Task Force were to avoid early anticoagulation in patients with large infarcts or hemorrhagic transformation on repeat CT.[98,99] Studies of patients with cerebral and cerebellar hemorrhagic infarction show that, in the vast majority, the cause is embolic, that hemorrhagic infarction occurs equally with and without anticoagulation, and that the development of hemorrhagic infarction is rarely accompanied by clinical worsening.[100,101] Patients with hemorrhagic transformation who were continued on anticoagulants did not worsen. The risk of reembolism must be balanced against the small but definite risk of important bleeding. If the patient has a large brain infarct, heparin should be delayed and bolus heparin infusions should be avoided. If the risk for reembolism is high, immediate heparinization is advisable, whereas if the risk seems low, it is prudent to delay anticoagulants for at least 48 h. One study showed that in patients with atrial fibrillation with embolic strokes who were treated with well-controlled heparin anticoagulation soon after stroke onset fared better than did patients treated later.[102,103]

Paradoxical Embolism

While once considered rare, emboli entering the systemic circulation through right-to-left shunting of blood are now often recognized with the advent of newer diagnostic technologies. By far the most common potential intracardiac shunt is a residual patent foramen ovale (PFO). The high frequency of PFOs in the normal adult population has made it difficult to be certain in an individual stroke patient with a PFO whether paradoxical embolism through the PFO was the cause of their stroke or whether the PFO was merely an incidental finding. Autopsy series have shown that about 30 percent of adults have a probe patent foramen ovale at necropsy.[104] Hagen et al. studied 956 patients with clinically and pathologically normal hearts and found a PFO in 27.3 percent.[104] The frequency of PFOs declined with age: 34.3 percent during the first 3 decades of life, 25.4 percent during the fourth to eighth decades, and 20.2 percent during the ninth and tenth decades. The average diameter of PFOs was 4.9 mm and the size tended to increase with age.[104] Echocardiographic studies have shown that PFOs are more common in patients with an undetermined cause of stroke than in those in whom another etiology has been defined.[105–107] Lechat et al., using transthoracic echocardiography with contrast injection during Valsalva maneuver, demonstrated right-to-left shunting through a PFO in 56 percent of patients with cryptogenic stroke, in comparison to 10 percent of the patients in the control group.[105] Webster et al., in a study of stroke patients less than 40 years of age, found a PFO in 50 percent of patients with stroke using contrast echocardiography.[108] Di Tullio et al. demonstrated the presence of a PFO in 42 percent of patients with a cryptogenic stroke, compared with 7 percent in those with a determined etiology of stroke. This was observed in the younger (47 percent compared with 4 percent) and in the older (38 percent compared with 8 percent) age subgroups.[106]

Neuroimaging studies are not conclusive with regard to the link between patent foramen ovale and embolic stroke. However, in 1998, Steiner et al. reported on a series of 95 patients with first stroke and who had PFOs.[109] Those with large PFOs demonstrated more features of embolic strokes with brain imaging than did patients with small PFOs.

Review of series of patients with paradoxical embolism[110–112] through a PFO and the authors' experience allows the derivation of five criteria that, when four or more are met, establish with a high degree of certainty the presence of paradoxical embolism.[1] The findings are (1) a situation that promotes thrombosis of leg or pelvic veins (e.g., long sitting in one position or recent surgery); (2) increased coagulability (e.g., the use of oral contraceptives, presence of Leiden factor with resistance to activated protein C or dehydration); (3) the sudden onset of stroke during sexual intercourse, straining at stool, or other activity that includes a Valsalva maneuver or that promotes right-to-left shunting of blood; (4) pulmonary embolism within a short time before or after the neurologic ischemic event, and (5) the absence of other putative causes of stroke after thorough evaluation.

Brain Hypoperfusion (Cardiac Pump Failure)

After cardiopulmonary resuscitation (CPR), the heart often recovers in individuals whose brain has been irreversibly damaged by ischemic-anoxic damage.[113] Cardiologists must be familiar with the pathology, signs, and prognosis of brain dysfunction after periods of circulatory failure.

Different brain regions have selective vulnerability to hypoxic-ischemic damage. Those regions that are most remote and that are at the edges of major vascular supply are more liable to injury. These zones have usually been referred to as "border zones" or "watersheds." The cerebral cortex is most vulnerable to injury. Damage may be diffuse or "laminar," involving layers of the cortex. The hippocampus is one of the most vulnerable areas.[114–117] In the brain, the border zone regions are between the anterior cerebral artery (ACA) and MCA and between the MCA and PCA. Damage is usually most severe in the posterior parieto-temporo-occipital region and in frontal areas most remote from the heart and thus called *distal fields*. A similar border zone exists in the cerebellum between the cerebellar arteries and in the brainstem between medial and lateral penetrating arteries. The basal ganglia and thalamus are most involved if hypoxia is severe but some circulation is preserved. This situation applies most to hanging, strangulation, drowning, and carbon monoxide exposure.[118] Cerebellar neurons, especially Purkinje cells, may also be selectively injured.[119]

When circulatory arrest is complete and abrupt, brainstem nuclei are especially vulnerable to necrosis, especially in young humans and experimental animals.[120] When hypoxia and ischemia are especially severe, the spinal cord may also be damaged.[121,122] When cortical damage is very severe and protracted, cytotoxic edema causes massive brain swelling, with cessation of blood flow and brain death.

CLINICAL FINDINGS

Very severe damage leads to mortal injury to the cortex and brainstem, irreversible coma, and brain death. When initially examined, such patients have no brainstem reflexes (pupillary, corneal, and oculovestibular and oculocephalic reflexes) and no response to stimuli except perhaps a decerebration response. These findings do not improve, and respiratory control is absent or lost.

When cerebral cortical damage is very severe but brainstem ischemic changes are reversible, brainstem reflexes are preserved but there is no meaningful response to the environment. Automatic facial movements such as blinking, tongue protrusion, and yawning usually persist. The eyes may rest slightly up and move from side to side. When this state does not improve, it is referred to as the *persistent vegetative state*[113,116,123,124] or "wakefulness without awareness." Laminar cortical necrosis causes seizures. These are often multifocal myoclonic twitches or jerks of the facial and limb muscles, which are difficult to control with anticonvulsants; oversedation should be avoided.

With severe border-zone injury, there is weakness of the arms and proximal lower extremities with preservation of face, leg, and foot movement (the "man in a barrel" syndrome). With less severe ischemia, the symptoms and signs are predominantly visual. Patients describe difficulty seeing and inability to integrate the features of large objects or scenes despite retained capacity to see small objects in some parts of their visual fields. Reading is impossible. There are features of Balint's syndrome,[113,125] including asimultagnosia (i.e., seeing things piecemeal or sequentially); optic ataxia (i.e., poor eye-hand coordination); and optic apraxia (i.e., difficulty in directing gaze). Apathy and inertia are also common and are caused by damage to the frontal lobe. Amnesia is also very common. Patients cannot make new memories and have patchy, retrograde amnesia for events during and before hospitalization. This Korsakoff-type syndrome is due to hippocampal damage and may not be fully reversible. Amnesia may be accompanied by visual abnormalities, apathy, and confusion, or may be isolated.

Action myoclonus (the Lance-Adams syndrome)[119] is thought to be due to cerebellar damage.[119] This disorder is characterized by arrhythmic fine or coarse jerking, especially on attempted movement. Reaching for an object may be accompanied by gross oscillation and tremor-like movements. Gait ataxia is also common. The findings are worsened by stress.

PROGNOSIS

Shortly after resuscitation or arrest, patients with less severe cerebral injuries show some reactivity to the environment. Eye opening and restless limb movements develop. The eyes may fixate on objects. Noise, a flashlight, or a gentle pinch arouses patients to avoid or react to stimuli. Soon patients awaken fully and may begin to speak. Cognitive and behavioral abnormalities may be detected after the patient awakens, depending on the degree of injury.

Prognostic signs and variables have been extensively studied.[113,126–129] The initial neurologic findings and their course are helpful in predicting outcome. Among patients who have meaningful responses to pain at 1 h, almost all survivors have preserved intellectual function. Patients who do not respond to pain by 24 h either die or remain in a vegetative state. Being comatose predicts a poor prognosis.[128,129] *Thus, two simple observations—the presence or absence of coma and the response to pain—predict neurologic outcome very early.*[129] Recurrent myoclonus is also a poor prognostic sign in this group of patients. Wijdicks et al. reported that in the setting of diffuse, persistent myoclonus in comatose survivors of cardiac arrest, all patients in myoclonus status died.[130]

In a study in Seattle of out-of-hospital cardiac arrests, patients who did not awaken died on average 3.5 days after arrest.[131,132] Of 459 patients, 183 never awakened (40 percent). Among those who did awaken, 91 (33 percent) had persistent neurologic deficits.[131] Prognosis could be made by analysis of pupillary light reflexes, eye movements, and motor responses.[132] Bystander initiation of CPR was not significantly related to awakening,[132] in contrast to another study that found that outcome was better if CPR were started by by-standers before the emergency team arrived.[133] Patients awake on admission were included in one study[133] but excluded in the other.[132] After in-hospital CPR, pneumonia, hypotension, renal failure, cancer, and a housebound state before hospitalization were significantly related to death in the hospital (see Chap. 42).[134]

DIAGNOSTIC TESTING

Neuroimaging and other tests have proved to be relatively unhelpful; in contrast to the neurologic examination.[113] CT is used to exclude other causes of coma such as brain hemorrhage. Electroencephalography (EEG) is helpful in studying cortical activity in unresponsive patients and in assessing brain death.

Similarly, the absence of responses to visual and somatosensory stimuli is a poor prognostic sign. TCD may be helpful in the evaluation of brain death.[135–137]

TREATMENT

Other than maintaining adequate circulation and oxygenation, treatment has not been helpful in improving outcome. Increased blood sugar correlates with poor outcome,[138] and experimental animals subjected to circulatory arrest do worse if they have been fed glucose before the arrest.[139,140] Blood calcium and the presence of free radicals and excitatory neurotoxins have all been postulated to affect neuronal cell death.[140–142] A multifaceted approach to therapy has been most successful.[143]

Neurologic Effects of Cardiac Drugs and Cardiac Encephalopathy

Drugs given to patients with cardiac disease often have neurologic side effects[144] (see Chap. 90). Digitalis can cause visual hallucinations, yellow vision, and general confusion.[145,146] Digitalis levels need not be excessively elevated; the symptoms disappear with cessation of the drug. Quinidine can cause confusion with delirium, seizures and coma, vertigo, tinnitus, and visual blurring.[147] Chronic cognitive and behavioral changes and "quinidine dementia" are less well known.[147] Similar toxicity has been seen with lithium. Patients may become acutely comatose while being treated with intravenous lidocaine. This effect has been associated with the accidental administration of very large doses; more common CNS effects of less extreme toxicity include sedation, irritability, and twitching. The latter may progress to seizures accompanied by respiratory depression. Amiodarone often causes ataxia, weakness, tremors, paresthesias, visual symptoms, and a Parkinsonian-like syndrome and occasionally causes delirium.[144]

Patients with congestive heart failure often develop an encephalopathy characterized by decreased alertness; sleepiness; decrease in all intellectual functions; asterixis; and variability of alertness and cognitive functions from minute-to-minute and hour-to-hour.[144] These patients may not have pulmonary, liver, or renal failure or electrolyte abnormalities. This cardiac encephalopathy is probably multifactoral. Posited explanations include: decreased

brain perfusion due to low cardiac output and high central venous pressure; intracranial fluid effusion similar in etiology to pericardial and pleural effusions and ascites; side effects of cardiac and other drugs.[144]

NEUROLOGIC AND CEREBROVASCULAR COMPLICATIONS OF ENDOVASCULAR CARDIAC PROCEDURES AND CARDIAC SURGERY

Patients with heart disease are diagnosed, treated, and at times even cured, with a variety of cardiac procedures. Although the implicit goal with any cardiac intervention (diagnostic or therapeutic) is to improve a patient's quality of life, these procedures often carry risk as well as the possibility of benefit.

Endovascular Cardiac Diagnostic and Therapeutic Procedures

CARDIAC CATHERIZATION

Stroke and TIA are known complications of heart catheterization. In 1977, Dawson and Fischer reported cerebrovascular complications in 10 of 1000 consecutive cardiac catheterizations. Nine out of 10 of these events were determined to be embolic.[148,149] Similarly, Mendez Dominguez et al. reported thromboembolic neurologic complications in 7 patients in a series of 2178 consecutive cardiac catheterizations. In all cases the cerebrovascular impairment occurred either during or within several minutes following the cardiac catheterization. All strokes were confirmed with CT or MRI, and the clinical profile in the majority of cases supported an embolic mechanism.[150] Central retinal artery occlusion has been reported in association with cardiac catheterization.[151] More recently, Liu et al. reported 6 ischemic strokes and 1 intracerebral hemorrhage in a series of 3648 cardiac catheterizations in children. In this study, the suspected catheterization-related stroke mechanisms included intracranial hemorrhage due to intraprocedure anticoagulation as well as cerebral embolism from local clot.[152] Other potential mechanisms for cerebrovascular events during cardiac angiography may include catheter tip thromboembolism, atherosclerotic plaque or cholesterol embolism, air emboli, arterial vasospasm, and/or hypotension.[148,153–156]

CORONARY ARTERY ANGIOPLASTY AND STENTING

The stroke rate in patients undergoing percutaneous coronary interventions for both stable as well as unstable coronary artery disease (including angioplasty for acute myocardial infarction) has been reported to be between 0 and 4 percent.[157–164] A combined analysis of data from 4 double-blind, placebo-controlled, randomized trials (EPIC, CAPTURE, EPILOG, EPISTENT) conducted between 1991 and 1997 assessed 8555 patients undergoing various percutaneous coronary interventions. Among the 8555 patients, there were 33 strokes in 31 patients (0.36 percent) within 30 days. Stroke occurred in 9 (0.29 percent) of 3079 patients receiving percutaneous coronary interventions alone: 6 were ischemic and 3 hemorrhagic. Stroke was diagnosed in 22 (0.41 percent) of 5476 patients who underwent percutaneous treatment in conjunction with abciximab treatment, of which there were 13 ischemic strokes and 9 hemorrhages.[157–162]

Galbreath et al. reported a 0.2 percent rate of focal central neurological complication in their series of 1968 percutaneous transluminal coronary angioplasties (PTCAs): 3 were ischemic strokes and 1 was a TIA. The mechanism in these cases was determined to be embolic in 3 of the cases: one patient inadvertently had air injected through the guide catheter and two had events after the ascending aorta was "scraped" with the guide catheter in search of a graft ostium. The remaining patient had an event during a period of hypotension.[163]

ELECTROPHYSIOLOGIC PROCEDURES AND ELECTRICAL CARDIOVERSION

Thromboembolic stroke can be a complication of cardiac electrophysiologic procedures, including radiofrequency catheter ablation of arrhythmia. Multicenter data are limited; however, the stroke risk appears to be less than 2 percent.[148,165–168]

Electrical cardioversion is not uncommonly used in the treatment of atrial fibrillation and atrial flutter. The risk of stroke due to direct current cardioversion has been estimated to occur in 1.3 percent of cardioverted patients.[169] Anticoagulation before and after cardioversion lowers the risk of embolism.[148,169,170]

PERCUTANEOUS VALVULOPLASTY

Percutaneous balloon mitral as well as aortic valvuloplasties have also been complicated by stroke. With regards to when the neurological events occur, Letac et al.'s 1988 series of 218 patients undergoing transcutaneous balloon aortic valvuloplasty indicates that 1 stroke occurred intraprocedure, while 3 additional strokes occurred during the postprocedure time period.[148,171–174]

INTRAAORTIC BALLOON PUMP

Intraaortic balloon pumps (IABPs) are used in patients with severe left ventricular failure or cardiogenic shock. The IABP is inserted into the patient's midthoracic aorta in order to maintain adequate perfusion. Spinal cord infarcts can occur in patients with IABPs due to local thromboembolism, aortic dissection, aortic atherosclerotic plaque rupture, or local hypoperfusion.[148,175]

Cardiovascular Surgery

Every year, an estimated 1 million patients undergo cardiac surgery throughout the world. Coronary artery bypass surgery (CABS) is the most common major cardiovascular operation performed.

It is concerning, then, that the frequency of abnormalities of intellectual function and behavior after cardiac surgery is quite high.[176,177] In general, the reported incidence of neurologic complications after cardiac surgery varies widely from 7 to 61 percent for transient complications and from 1.6 to 23 percent for permanent complications.[178,179] With regard to specific surgeries and stroke, the cerebrovascular risk may depend upon the particular procedure performed. Estimations of stroke risk for isolated CABS range from 0.8 to 1.7 percent.[180–182] There does not appear to be a significant difference in postoperative stroke rates in patients undergoing an off-pump coronary artery bypass graft (CABG) versus patients undergoing the traditional on-pump operation.[183–184] In one multicenter study, the incidence of stroke plus severe intellectual dysfunction from CABS has been reported to be 6 percent.[185] With regard to combined procedures, one multicenter investigation assessing 273 patients undergoing combined CABS and left-sided cardiac procedure (such as aortic or mitral valve replacement) estimated that 15.8 percent of patients had neurologic complications: 8.5 percent with stroke or TIA and 7.3 percent with new intellectual deterioration.[186] Clearly, this combined procedure appears to carry a higher stroke risk than CABG per-

formed in isolation. In contrast, minimally invasive cardiac surgical procedures may have a lessened stroke risk. A single center's result with direct-access, minimally invasive mitral valve surgery in 106 patients demonstrates a low rate of stroke and TIA, with a total of 0.28 percent of patients having either stroke or TIA.[187]

Overall, in prospective studies, transient complications have been noted in 61 percent of cardiac surgery patients.[188] In one series in CABS patients, 16.8 percent had stroke or encephalopathy postoperatively; the encephalopathies usually cleared, and only 2 percent of patients had severe strokes.[189] The potential mechanisms of cerebral impairment in the cardiac surgery population will be explored later.

ATHEROTHROMBOTIC, HEMODYNAMICALLY MEDIATED BRAIN INFARCTS

An estimated 12 percent of patients requiring CABG also have significant carotid artery disease.[187] One major concern regarding cardiac surgery patients has been whether the hemodynamic and circulatory stress of heart surgery will lead to underperfusion of areas supplied by already stenotic or occluded arteries, resulting in brain infarcts. This concern underlies neck auscultation for bruits, ultrasound carotid artery testing, and cerebral angiography prior to CABS. However, hemodynamically induced infarction related to preexisting atherosclerotic occlusive cervicocranial arterial disease is a rare complication of heart surgery. *Patients with carotid bruits have a very low rate of stroke after elective surgery.*[190] *In a retrospective study of CABS patients with known carotid disease, ipsilateral strokes occurred in 1.1 percent of arteries with 50 to 90 percent stenosis, in 6.2 percent of arteries with >90 percent stenosis, and in only 2 percent of vessels with carotid occlusion.*[191,192] *Intracranial flow and velocity do not show significant changes in patients with high-grade carotid stenosis during CABS.*[193]

Stroke rates vary greatly in those undergoing combined as opposed to staged procedures, taking into consideration carotid endarterectomy (CEA) and CABS.[194] Definitive management of combined cerebral and coronary artery disease awaits the outcome of clinical trials. One systematic review of 97 published studies of staged versus synchronous operations found no significant difference in outcomes between these two surgical groups. Unfortunately in this study, there were no comparable data for patients with combined carotid stenosis and cardiac disease NOT undergoing either staged or synchronous surgery.[195] It thus remains unclear whether operations aimed at minimizing the risk of hypoperfusion or watershed stroke during cardiac surgery actually decrease this stroke risk.

Most studies have relied on clinical localization of focal deficits and inference about their mechanisms. A neuroradiology study reviewed neuroimaging results from 30 patients with acute strokes in relation to CABS.[196] Only one had evidence of a hemodynamic atherostenotic mechanism, which supports the data suggesting hemodynamically induced infarction during cardiac surgery is rare. Embolism arising from cardiac and aortic sources is much more common than atherothrombotic infarcts and is of a much greater concern.[176]

BRAIN EMBOLISM

A strong point against a hemodynamic or hypoperfusion cause of many strokes is their timing. Strokes occur more frequently *after* recovery from the anesthetic. If the mechanism of stroke were hemodynamic, the major circulatory stress would be intraoperative and patients would awaken with the deficit. In two studies in which the authors record the timing of CABS-related strokes, only 16[197] and 17 percent[198] of patients had deficits noted immediately postoperatively.

The distribution of infarcts and their multiplicity on neuroimaging scans were most consistent with embolism. Embolic infarcts may involve either the anterior or the posterior circulation.[176,189,196,197] In one series of postoperative, posterior circulation strokes, the majority were embolic and followed cardiac surgery.[198]

In cardiac surgery patients, the preponderance of evidence suggests that macroemboli (greater than 200 μm in diameter) and microemboli are responsible for most neurologic complications.[178,185,189,195,199,200] Macroemboli (associated with atherosclerotic plaque disruption or rupture) are believed to precipitate focal deficits, while particulate microemboli (white blood cell and platelet aggregates, fat, or air) may be implicated in more subtle diffuse cognitive dysfunction.[185,201]

Emboli may arise from preexisting cardiac abnormalities (such as hypofunctioning ventricles, dilated atria, and aortic atheromas) or from postoperative arrhythmias.[176] *Evidence links operative and postoperative embolism to aortic ulcerative atherosclerotic lesions. Cross-clamping of the ascending aorta and aortotomy liberate cholesterol or calcific plaque debris.*[176,202] Figure 99-1 shows the aorta of a patient who died having never awakened after CABS. Figure 99-2 shows cholesterol crystals and other debris trapped within a filter placed in the aorta at the time of unclamping.

In one series in which embolic signals were monitored during CABS surgery, 34 percent of signals were detected as the aortic cross clamps were removed and another 24 percent as aortic partial occlusion clamps were removed.[202] The number of microemboli detected correlates with abnormalities of cognitive function studied after surgery.[176,203] Figure 99-3 shows microemboli within the aorta shown by TEE after release of aortic clamps. Figures 99-4 and 99-5 are TCD recordings during manipulation of the aorta and after release of aortic clamps.

Necropsy examination of patients dying after cardiac surgery has shown severe bilateral, predominantly border-zone infarcts.[204] The small arteries of the brain and other viscera (heart, kidney, spleen, pancreas) may be packed with birefringent cholesterol crystal emboli.[204] TEE makes it possible to detect protruding ulcerative plaques in the aorta preoperatively and intraoperatively.[176,205,206] In one patient with repeated peripheral emboli, a protruding atherosclerotic plaque was removed surgically.[205] Intraaortic atherosclerotic debris identified by TEE has been found to be associated with embolic events.[206] Intraoperative B-mode ultrasonography with the probe placed on the aorta has also been used to detect severe aortic atherosclerotic plaques.[207] Ultrasonic imaging showed aortic atheromas in 58 percent of patients, whereas visual examination and palpation detected plaques in only 24 percent.[207] *Atherosclerosis of the ascending aorta is a very important risk factor for post-CABS stroke.*[176,208] *In patients who are scheduled to undergo elective cardiac surgery, consideration should be given to having TEEs performed before surgery to evaluate cardiac lesions and thrombi, cardiac function, and aortic atheromas.*

Thromboembolic infarction often occurs in the days following surgery when cessation of anticoagulation is necessary. Postoperative activation of coagulation factors in cardiac surgery patients can promote hypercoagulability. Disseminated intravascular coagulation, acquired antithrombin III deficiency, and acquired protein C deficiencies are not uncommon. Activation of the coagulation-fibrinolytic system can persist for 2 months after cardiopulmonary bypass surgery.[209,210] In some patients, hypercoagulability related to surgery can precipitate occlusive thrombosis in atherostenotic arteries, and the newly formed thrombus can lead to intraarterial embolism. Cardiac, aortic, and intraarterial embolism accounts for the vast majority of cardiac-surgery-related focal neurologic deficits.

POSTOPERATIVE ENCEPHALOPATHY: MICROEMBOLI AND OTHER CAUSES

Gilman described a diffuse CNS disorder following open heart surgery (characterized by altered levels of consciousness and activity and confusion[211]) that is now referred to as *encephalopathy*. Clinical and imaging studies usually do not show important focal neurologic signs or large focal infarcts. The incidence of encephalopathy varies.[179] In one series, 57 of 1669 (3.4 percent) CABS patients had postoperative mental state changes including delirium and encephalopathy.[212] In the Cleveland Clinic prospective series, 11.6 percent were "encephalopathic" on the fourth postoperative day.[189]

Encephalopathy has multiple causes. Embolization of particulate matter was considered the leading cause, and this led to intraoperative technical improvements, including the introduction of membrane rather than bubble oxygenators and on-line filtration.[179] These technical advances have led to a decrease in the risk of macroemboli (>25 mm), but they do not protect against microemboli of air, fat, or particles.[179]

A necropsy study of patients who died after cardiopulmonary bypass or angiography has awakened interest in this subject.[179,213] Focal, small capillary and arteriolar dilatations (SCADs) were commonly found in the brain.[213] About one-half of the SCADs show birefringent crystalline material within the dilated capillaries. SCADs could, at least in part, explain the decreased cerebral blood flow found during cardiopulmonary bypass. SCADs are iatrogenically generated microemboli, but as yet their origin is unknown. Their morphology is most consistent with air or fat.[179,213]

Other causes of encephalopathy are common. Diffuse hypoxic-ischemic insults from hypotension and hypoperfusion do occur. *Drugs are a very common cause of encephalopathy in the postoperative period. Particularly important are haloperidol, narcotics, and sedatives.* Morphine is sometimes used heavily intraoperatively, and opiate withdrawal with restlessness and hyperactivity can result. Agitation and restlessness are often early signs of organic encephalopathy and may lead to the administration of haloperidol, barbiturates, phenothiazines, or benzodiazepines for calming and sedation. When these drugs wear off and the patient begins to awaken, agitation may occur and more sedatives may be given. Haloperidol causes rigidity, restlessness, agitation, hallucinations, and confusion. In experimental animals, haloperidol delays recovery from strokes by months and its use is not advised.[214,215] Phenothiazines and sedatives are also problematic; *in general, use of sedatives and narcotics should be minimized and they should be tapered as soon as possible.*

POSTOPERATIVE INTRACRANIAL HEMORRHAGE

Intracerebral or subarachnoid hemorrhages have occasionally been reported after cardiac surgery, most commonly in children who had repair of congenital heart disease[216] or in cardiac transplantation patients.[217] The postulated mechanism involves an abrupt increase in brain blood flow with rupture of small intracranial arteries unprepared for the new load. Usually, there is a prolonged period when cardiac output is low, and this output is suddenly increased by the surgery. Abrupt increases in brain blood flow or pressure in other situations have also been associated with intracerebral hemorrhage.[218]

STROKE MIMICS: POSTOPERATIVE PERIPHERAL NERVE COMPLICATIONS

Brachial plexus and peripheral nerve lesions frequently develop after cardiac surgery and can be confused with CNS complications.[219] In one series, new peripheral nervous system deficits occurred in 13 percent of patients.[219] The most common deficit is a unilateral brachial plexopathy characterized by shoulder pain and usually weakness and numbness of one hand. It is probably caused by positioning of the arm during surgery, with traction on the lower trunk of the brachial plexus. Ulnar, peroneal, and saphenous nerve injuries are also common and are also related to positioning. Diaphragmatic and vocal cord paralyses are likely related to local effects of the cardiac surgery on the recurrent laryngeal and phrenic nerves.

CARDIAC EFFECTS OF BRAIN LESIONS

Information is beginning to emerge on cardiac muscle changes (myocytolysis), arrhythmias, pulmonary edema, electrocardiogram (ECG) changes, and sudden death due to brain disease and sudden emotional stresses.[220,221]

Cardiac Lesions

The two most common lesions found in the hearts of patients dying with acute CNS lesions are patchy regions of myocardial necrosis and subendocardial hemorrhage. The abnormalities range from eosinophilic staining of cells with preserved striations to transformation of myocardial cells into dense eosinophilic contraction bands. These changes have been referred to as *myocytolysis*.[220,222] Subendocardial petechiae and frank hemorrhages are also noted. These lesions were described in the 1950s[221,223] but were considered rare.[224,225] One study found a very high incidence of myocardial abnormalities in patients dying of brain lesions that increase intracranial pressure rapidly.[226] Stress-related release of catecholamines and possibly corticosteroids may be responsible, at least in part, for the cardiac lesions found in patients with CNS lesions.[220,227–232]

Electrocardiographic and Enzyme Changes

In stroke patients, especially those with subarachnoid hemorrhage, ECGs may show a prolonged QT interval; giant, wide, roller-coaster inverted T waves; and U waves.[233] These changes are often called *cerebral T waves*. Patients with stroke who have continuous ECG monitoring have a high incidence of T-wave and ST-segment changes, various arrhythmias, and cardiac enzyme abnormalities. ECG changes may include a prolonged QT interval, depressed ST segments, flat or inverted T waves, and U waves.[220,233–236] Less often, tall, peaked T waves and elevated ST segments are noted (see Chap. 13). Myocardial enzyme release and echocardiographic wall motion abnormalities are associated with impaired left ventricular performance after subarachnoid hemorrhage. In severely affected patients, reduction of cardiac output may elevate the risk of vasospasm-induced cerebral ischemia.[237] Cardiac and skeletal muscle enzymes, including the MB isoenzyme of creatine kinase (MB-CK), are often abnormal in stroke patients.[236,238–241] During the 4 to 7 days after stroke, there is usually a slow rise and later fall in serum MB-CK levels, a pattern quite different from that found in acute myocardial infarction (see Chap. 52); the temporal pattern of cardiac isoenzyme release is more compatible with smoldering low-grade necrosis, such as patchy, focal myocytolysis.[224,238] The ST-segment and T-wave abnormalities and cardiac arrhythmias correlate significantly with raised levels of MB-CK in stroke patients.[224]

Arrhythmias

Various cardiac arrhythmias have been found in stroke patients, most frequently sinus bradycardia and tachycardia and premature ventricular contractions.[220,234–236] Some arrhythmias are manifestations of primary cardiac problems, but others are undoubtedly secondary to the brain lesions. The incidence of sinus tachycardia and bradycardia is maximal on the first day after intracerebral hemorrhage.[242] Ventricular bigeminy, atrioventricular dissociation and block, ventricular tachycardia, atrial fibrillation, and bundle branch blocks are found less often.[242] All arrhythmias are more common in patients who have primary brainstem lesions or brainstem compression.

Neurogenic Pulmonary Edema

Acute pulmonary edema may complicate strokes, especially *subarachnoid hemorrhage (SAH)* and posterior circulation ischemia and hemorrhage.[224,243] Pulmonary edema has been found in 70 percent of patients with fatal *SAH* and correlates with the severity and suddenness of development of raised intracranial pressure.[244]

Centrally mediated sympathetic discharges such as those caused by increased intracranial pressure produce intense systemic vasoconstriction.[245] Blood shifts from the high-resistance systemic circulation to the low-resistance pulmonary circulation. Increased pulmonary capillary pressure leads to pulmonary hypertension and rupture of pulmonary vessels, with lung hemorrhage. The pulmonary edema fluid has a high-protein content and can develop despite normal cardiac function.[224,245]

Sudden Death

Sudden death associated with stressful situations, including so-called "voodoo death," must involve CNS mechanisms.[232,235–249] Ventricular fibrillation, the presumed mechanism of sudden death, can be reliably elicited by stimulation of cardiac sympathetic nerves in both the normal and the ischemic heart.[250] Ischemia reduces the threshold for ventricular fibrillation.[224,248,251] Stress must cause CNS stimulation that triggers autonomic activation.[232] Sudden vagotonic stimulation can cause bradycardia and cardiac standstill. The effects of vagal stimulation on the development of ventricular arrhythmias is uncertain.[250] Patients with lateral medullary and lateral pontine infarcts affecting reticular formation structures die unexpectedly; these patients have a high incidence of various types of autonomic dysregulation, such as labile blood pressure, syncope, tachycardia, and flushing, as well as a failure of automatic respiration.[50]

COEXISTENT VASCULAR DISEASES AFFECTING BOTH HEART AND BRAIN

Atherosclerosis

The most common and important vascular disease that affects both the brain and the heart is atherosclerosis. The most frequent cause of death in stroke patients is coronary artery disease,[252] and extra- and intracranial arterial atherosclerosis[253] is common in patients with coronary artery disease.

PATHOLOGY AND PREDOMINANT SITES OF DISEASE
In white men the predominant atherosclerotic lesions involve the origins of the internal carotid artery (ICA) and the VA origins in the neck.[5,254] Fatty streaks and flat plaques first affect the posterior wall of the common carotid artery (CCA) opposite the flow divider between the ICA and the external carotid artery (ECA), a region of low sheer stress.[255,256] Atherosclerotic plaques at this site do not differ from plaques in the aorta or coronary arteries (see Chap. 44). At first, plaques expand gradually and encroach on the lumen of the ICA and

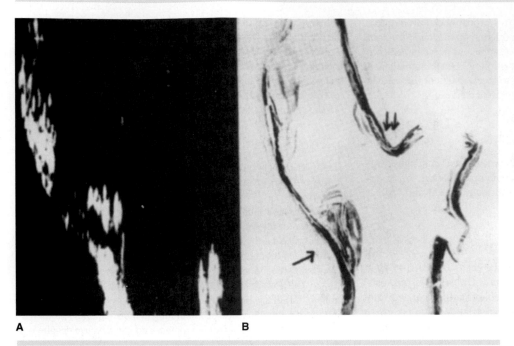

A   B

FIGURE 99-6 *A.* B-mode ultrasonic image showing plaque at internal carotid artery origin. *B.* A carotid specimen. The plaque (*single arrow*) is opposite the flow divider between the internal and external carotid arteries (*two arrows*). (From Hennerici M, Steinke W. Abbildende Ultraschallverfahren (B-scan) in duplex system. In: *Durchbluntungsstorungen des Gehirns—Neue Diagnostischen Möglichkeiten*. Gutersloh: Bertelsmann, 1987, with permission.)

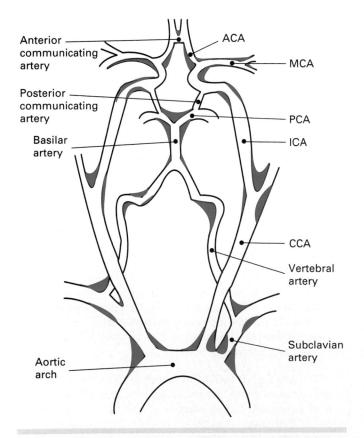

FIGURE 99-7 Sites of predilection for atherosclerotic narrowing: dark areas represent plaques. ACA, anterior cerebral artery; CCA, common carotid artery; ICA, internal carotid artery; MCA, middle cerebral arteries; PCA, posterior cerebral artery. (From Caplan LR. *Stroke: A Clinical Approach,* 3d ed. Boston: Butterworth-Heinemann, 2000, with permission.)

sometimes the CCA (Fig. 99-6). Atheromatous plaques often develop concurrently at the VA origin or spread from the parent subclavian artery to involve the VA origin.[45,257] When plaques reach a critical size, they affect turbulence, flow, and motion of the arteries, causing complications to develop within the plaques. Cracking, ulcerations, and mural thrombi develop, and the overlying endothelium is damaged with the development of occlusive thrombi.[258] Fresh thrombi loosely adherent to vascular walls rapidly propagate and embolize. Because the ICA has no nuchal branches, the clot often propagates cranially, usually extending as far as the first branch of the ophthalmic artery, which arises from the intracranial siphon portion of the ICA. In the VA, collateral channels from the ECA and thyrocervical trunk usually provide collateral channels that reconstitute the VA in the neck and limit propagation of thrombi. In the 2 to 3 weeks after the development of an occlusive thrombus, the clot gradually organizes and is much less likely to propagate or embolize. The reduction in cranial blood flow caused by severe stenosis or occlusion of the ICA or VA stimulates development of collateral circulation that usually becomes adequate.

Figure 99-7 shows diagrammatically the sites of predilection for development of atherosclerosis in the cervicocranial circulation. Note the concentration of these sites at branch points and flow dividers. There are important race and sex differences in the distribution of cerebral atherosclerosis.[259–262] White men usually develop lesions of the ICA and VA origins. Patients with ICA-origin disease have a high frequency of hypercholesterolemia, coronary artery disease, and peripheral vascular occlusive disease. With the exception of the basilar artery (BA) and the ICA siphon, intracranial occlusive disease develops only after extracranial disease is well established in this group. Blacks and individuals of Chinese, Japanese, and Thai ancestry have a much higher incidence of intracranial occlusive disease and a rather low frequency of extracranial disease.[259–263] Intracranial disease is more prevalent in women and those with diabetes. Patients with intracranial occlusive disease do not have a high incidence of coronary or peripheral vascular occlusive disease.

MECHANISMS OF ISCHEMIA

Ischemia in patients with occlusive lesions is caused by two different mechanisms—hypoperfusion and embolism.[5,50,264,265] Hypoperfusion develops only when a critical reduction in luminal diameter causes reduced distal perfusion. When flow is reduced slowly, the brain vasculature has a remarkable capacity to develop collateral circulation. Patients with severe ICA-origin occlusive disease remain asymptomatic despite marked decrease in blood flow.[266,267] Even when vascular occlusion is abrupt—as in tying neck arteries to treat brain aneurysms—surprisingly few patients develop persistent brain ischemia. In most patients, within a few days or at most 2 weeks following an arterial occlusion, collateral circulation develops maximally and stabilizes.

Intraarterial embolism is probably a much more frequent and important cause of brain infarction than hypoperfusion. However, decreased perfusion probably limits clearance (washout) of emboli.[265] In patients with anterior circulation infarcts, angiography shows a very high frequency of intraarterial intracranial emboli distal to an ICA thrombosis.[268] These emboli most often involve the MCA and its branches. If angiography is repeated or performed later than 48 h after stroke, MCA occlusion is usually not present.[5,6] Intraarterial emboli often fragment and move distally. Intraarterial embolism is also very common in the posterior circulation, where the most common donor sites are the VA origin and intracranial VA and the most frequent recipient sites for emboli are the intracranial VA, the PCA, and the distal basilar artery bifurcation.[50,269]

CLINICAL FINDINGS

Many patients with atherosclerotic occlusive disease are asymptomatic. The most frequent symptoms of hypoperfusion or embolism are headache, TIAs, and neurologic signs related to brain infarction. Headaches are due to vascular distention or brain swelling secondary to infarction. Unaccustomed headaches often precede strokes.[5,270] TIAs are caused by hypoperfusion or intraarterial emboli. Frequent, very brief stereotyped spells precipitated by postural changes suggest a hemodynamic mechanism. In contrast, emboli cause longer, less frequent attacks.[264,271] In many patients with clinical TIAs (i.e., with no lasting symptoms or signs), neuroimaging tests show brain infarcts.[272,273] Strokes may have various temporal features such as being maximal at outset, fluctuating, stepwise, or gradually progressive. The pattern is related to the adequacy of collateral circulation and the propagation and embolization of thrombi.

Neurologic symptoms and signs depend on the region of brain that is ischemic. Table 99-2 outlines the most frequent clinical patterns resulting from occlusions of the major extracranial and intracranial arteries.[5,50,254]

DIAGNOSTIC TESTING

In most patients, the nature and severity of the brain and vascular lesions causing the stroke can be defined. CT and MRI should localize brain lesions, distinguish between infarcts and hemorrhages, and determine the location, extent, and size of the processes. CT or MRI is usually the first test in patients with suspected stroke because the information allows clinicians to exclude nonvascular disease such as tumor or abscess; to differentiate hemorrhage from ischemia, and show subdural hematomas; to identify the vascular territory involved; and to define the extent of brain already damaged.

The vascular territory involved should be inferred by the nature of the neurologic symptoms and signs and the location of brain lesions on CT or MRI. Echocardiography, especially TEE, has dramatically improved the ability to detect potential cardiac sources of emboli (see Chap. 15).

Ultrasound techniques can be used to screen for obstructive lesions in the major extracranial and intracranial arteries in both anterior (carotid) and posterior (vertebrobasilar) circulation arteries. For extracranial use, the two most important are *B-mode scans* and *Doppler spectra*, both pulsed and continuous-wave (CW) Doppler. The anatomy of the carotid bifurcation (the CCA, proximal ICA, and ECA) and the proximal VAs can be imaged by high-frequency, 5- to 10-MHz, B-mode ultrasound systems, which provide images of the vessels in real time both longitudinally and in cross-section (Fig. 99-8). Plaque calcifications and clot are often difficult to image. Pulsed Doppler registers frequency shifts from moving columns of blood. Doppler analysis can show the direction and velocity of blood flow. Multigated Doppler and B-mode scanning are now used together in so-called duplex systems.[5,50,274,275] The duplex system is probably more than 90 percent effective in separating arteries that are normal or minimally narrowed from those that have moderate disease (30 to 70 percent narrowing), and from those with severe narrowing (>70 percent stenosis). B-mode scanning sometimes suggests the presence of ulceration or hemorrhage in plaques that show heterogeneous images.[275] CW Doppler uses a movable probe to measure flow velocities along the carotid and vertebral arteries; the technique is less time-consuming and less expensive than is the duplex system and, in expert hands, is very accurate in detecting high-grade stenosis.[274,276] Ultrasound techniques cannot reliably separate complete occlusion from very high degrees of stenosis. Color-flow and power Doppler can show turbulence and altered flow dynamics.

TCD ultrasound is used to analyze the presence of intracranial arterial stenoses and to provide information about the intracranial effects of extracranial occlusive lesions. The technique takes advantage

TABLE 99-2 Common Signs in Cerebrovascular Occlusive Disease at Various Sites

ICA origin	Ipsilateral transient monocular blindness; MCA and ACA signs
ICA siphon (proximal to ophthalmic artery)	Same as ICA origin
ICA siphon (distal to ophthalmic artery)	MCA and ACA signs
ACA	Contralateral weakness of the lower limb and shoulder shrug
MCA	Contralateral motor, sensory, and visual loss
	Left: Aphasia
	Right: Neglect of left space, lack of awareness of deficit, apathy, impersistence
AChA	Contralateral motor, sensory, and visual loss, usually without cognitive changes
Subclavian artery (proximal to VA)	Lack of arm stamina, cool hand, transient dizziness, veering, diplopia
VA origin	Same as subclavian, but no ipsilateral arm or hand findings
VA intracranially	Lateral medullary syndrome; staggering and veering (cerebellar infarction)
BA	Bilateral motor weakness; ophthalmoplegia and diplopia
PCA	Contralateral hemianopia and hemisensory loss
	Left: alexia with agraphia
	Right: neglect of left visual space

ABBREVIATIONS: ACA = anterior cerebral artery; AChA = anterior choroidal artery; BA = basilar artery; ICA = internal carotid artery; MCA = middle cerebral artery; PCA = posterior cerebral artery; VA = vertebral artery.

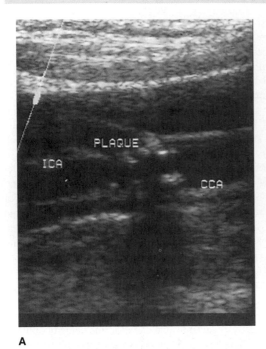

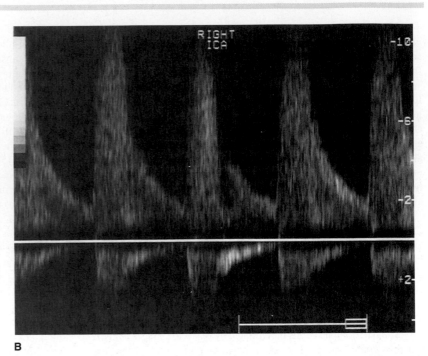

A   **B**

FIGURE 99-8 Duplex scan of carotid artery plaque. *A*. B-mode ultrasonic image showing plaque protruding into internal carotid artery (ICA) lumen. *B.* Doppler spectra at level of plaque showing high voltage related to stenosis.

of the soft spots in the temporal bones and natural foramina (the orbit and foramen magnum) that provide windows for ultrasound recording. The depth and angle of the probe recording can be varied, allowing the recording of velocities and sound spectra from all the major intracranial arteries.[5,50,135,277] Major obstructive lesions are reliably shown by both extracranial ultrasound and TCD. Continuous recording of intracranial arteries with TCD is a very sensitive and accurate method of detecting emboli passing under the probes.[176,202,278,279] Examples of microembolic signals are shown in Figs. 99-4 and 99-5.

Magnetic resonance angiography (MRA) provides an additional method of imaging both the extracranial and intracranial arteries for areas of stenosis and occlusion.[5,50,263,280] CT angiography (CTA), using a spiral (helical) CT machine and dye injected intravenously, can also image the major large craniocervical arteries.[281] Standard catheter angiography is warranted when ultrasound and CTA or MRA have not sufficiently defined the vascular lesion and treatment is clinically feasible.[5,50,263]

TREATMENT

For rational treatment, the following should be known: the location, nature, and severity of the occlusive lesion; the location, extent, and reversibility of the brain lesion; and the blood constituents and coagulability.[5,282] Treatment should *not* be guided solely by the temporal pattern of the symptoms, such as TIA, progressing stroke, or so-called completed stroke.[5,272,282,283] These time courses do not predict the cause and mechanism of ischemia, do not tell if an infarct is present, and do not identify patients who will have further or recurrent ischemia.[283]

Physicians should first decide whether or not any specific therapy is indicated. Very severe neurologic deficits, serious intercurrent illnesses (dementia, cancer, etc.), and psychosocioeconomic considerations may make patients unsuitable for specific treatments. If treatment is feasible, the next questions to be considered are what

brain tissue is at risk for further ischemia and what may be the benefit/risk ratio of specific treatments. To determine the tissue at risk, clinicians consider the cause and the deficit. For example, a man with a slight hemiplegia due to a small lacunar infarct in the anterior limb of the internal capsule may have infarcted the entire tissue supplied by an occluded small artery. In that case, treatment consists of controlling hypertension, the cause of the microvasculopathy. If, however, that same patient has a small cortical infarct in the precentral gyrus due to ICA disease, the rest of the ICA territory is at risk for further ischemia and aggressive treatment is warranted. Suppose a patient has a moderate-sized MCA infarct. If the patient were a Chinese woman with intrinsic atherosclerotic disease of that MCA, she might have little tissue at risk for further ischemia. No aggressive treatment should be given. If that same woman's infarct were due to cardiogenic embolism, the whole remainder of the brain would be at risk for further damage from another embolus. Newer MRI techniques—diffusion-weighted and perfusion MRI—along with MRA, can show, even very soon after symptoms begin, brain that is already infarcted, and brain tissue that is underperfused but not yet infarcted.[5,281,284,285]

Patients who have little tissue at risk are not candidates for specific therapy. If there is considerable residual at-risk tissue, the guidelines in Table 99-3 are used to direct treatment, which depends upon the location and severity of the causative vascular lesions. Carotid endarterectomy (CEN) has been shown to be effective in symptomatic patients with severe ICA stenosis (>70 percent).[286–289]

The Asymptomatic Carotid Artery Study (ACAS) suggested that carotid endarterectomy is slightly better than medical therapy in asymptomatic patients with severe carotid stenosis when the operation is executed by surgeons who have records of very low surgical morbidity and mortality.[290] To be effective, the operative mortality and morbidity of CEN must not be greater than 2 to 4 percent.[286–290] Surgery is also feasible on the extracranial vertebral artery in selected

TABLE 99-3 Suggested Use of Anticoagulants and Platelet Antiaggregants

HEPARIN (STANDARD DOSE)

Short term, 2–4 weeks. Usually given by intravenous infusion, keeping APTT between 60 and 100 s (1.5–2 × control APTT).
1. Immediate therapy for definite cardiac-origin cerebral embolism (large cerebral infarct, hypertension, bacterial endocarditis, or sepsis would delay or contraindicate this use).
2. Patients with severe stenosis or occlusion of the ICA origin, ICA siphon, MCA, vertebral artery, or basilar artery with less than a large clinical deficit. Subsequent treatment could consist of warfarin or surgery.

HEPARIN (SUBCUTANEOUS MINIDOSE)

For prophylaxis of deep vein occlusion in patients immobilized by stroke (unless contraindicated; see Chap. 54).

WARFARIN

Usually overlapped with heparin; keeping prothrombin time around INR of 2.0–3.0 (approximately 1.3–1.5 × control).
1. Long term (>3 months)
   a. Patients with cardiogenic cerebral embolization and rheumatic heart disease, atrial fibrillation with large atria or prior cerebral embolism, prosthetic valves, and some hypercoagulable states.
   b. Patients with severe stenosis of the ICA origin, ICA siphon, MCA stem, vertebral artery, and basilar artery. Used until studies show artery has been occluded for at least 3 weeks.
2. Short term (3–6 weeks)
   a. Patients with recent occlusion of the ICA, MCA, vertebral, or basilar arteries.

PLATELET ANTIAGGREGANTS (ASPIRIN, TICLOPIDINE, CLOPIDOGREL)

1. Patients with plaque disease of the extracranial and intracranial arteries without severe stenosis.
2. Patients with polycythemia or thrombocytosis and related ischemic attacks.

ABBREVIATIONS: APTT = activated partial thromboplastin time; ICA = internal carotid artery; INR = International Normalized Ratio; MCA = middle cerebral artery.

patients with intraarterial embolism from this site or with intractable posterior circulation hemodynamic ischemia, a rare occurrence.[50,291]

For minor and moderate degrees of stenosis in extra- and intracranial arteries, agents that alter platelet aggregation and adhesion are recommended. The most likely mechanism of ischemia in these patients is "white clot"—platelet fibrin emboli. Aspirin,[292,293] ticlopidine[294,295] clopidogrel,[296] and a tablet containing 25 mg aspirin and 200 mg of modified-release dipyridamole given 2 times a day[297] have all proven effective in randomized trials that contained large numbers of patients with TIAs and minor strokes. Many nonsteroidal anti-inflammatory drugs have antiplatelet effects, as do the omega-3 fish oils containing eicosapentanoic acid. Clopidogrel is as effective

as ticlopidine and has fewer serious hematologic complications[296] (see Chap. 54).

For patients with severe stenosis of large intracranial arteries, warfarin is recommended if there are no contraindications. The anticoagulant level should be kept at an INR of 2.0 to 3.0. Anticoagulation should be continued for at least 2 months. The state of the intracranial arteries can be monitored using TCD and/or MRA or CTA.[281] The same regimen is used for patients with severe extracranial stenosis who are not operative candidates or who refuse surgery. For patients with complete occlusions when first seen, heparin and then warfarin are prescribed for 2 to 3 months.[5]

Thrombolytic drugs, especially recombinant-tissue-type plasminogen activator (rt-PA) and streptokinase, have been given intravenously and intraarterially in patients with acute brain ischemia. In a study in which the arterial lesions were not defined, intravenous therapy with rt-PA given within 90 min and 3 h of ischemia onset, in the aggregate, provided a statistically significant benefit.[298] Unfortunately in this and other studies about 6 to 12 percent of patients treated with thrombolytic agents developed important intracranial bleeding. Uncontrolled studies show that patients with distal intracranial arterial embolic occlusions do well with intravenous thrombolytic therapy.[299–304] Patients with ICA occlusions in the neck and intracranially rarely reperfuse after intravenous thrombolytic therapy, especially if collateral circulation is poor. Intraarterially administered prourokinase thrombolysis has also been proven to be very effective in opening blocked intracranial arteries within the anterior circulation.[305] Patients with in situ thrombosis superimposed upon preexistent severe atherostenosis do less well than do patients with embolism. The dose, timing, mode of delivery, and target group for therapy remain unsettled. The authors believe vascular imaging should precede administration of thrombolytic agents. Brain and vascular imaging can guide physicians as to who should receive thrombolytics and by what route.[306]

Because all patients with atherosclerosis are at risk of developing more lesions, control of risk factors is very important and should be begun in the hospital. Risk factors include smoking, hyperlipidemia, obesity, inactivity, and hypertension (see Chap. 43). Blood pressure should not be excessively lowered during the acute ischemic period as this may decrease flow in collateral arteries. Blood pressure control can be instituted 3 to 4 weeks after the stroke. Rehabilitation must also begin early.

Management of Coexisting Coronary and Cerebrovascular Disease

In patients considered for cardiac surgery who have symptoms of brain ischemia, it is important to define the extent of cerebrovascular disease preoperatively by noninvasive means (ultrasound and/or MRA), as well as to define cardiac and coronary artery anatomy and function. Staged surgical procedures are sometimes warranted. In some patients with excessive surgical risks, anticoagulation may represent an alternative treatment. Clearly, optimal medical therapy should be instituted preoperatively and continued after surgery.

Systemic Arterial Hypertension

High blood pressure, both acute and chronic, damages deep, penetrating small intracranial arteries; accelerates the development of atherosclerosis in the extracranial and large intracranial arteries; and results in ischemic syndromes of lacunar infarction,[5,50,304,305] diffuse ischemic changes in white matter and basal gray matter structures

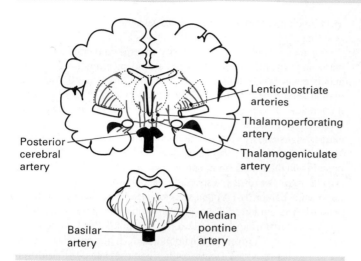

FIGURE 99-9 Deep penetrating arteries prone to the development of lipo-hyalinosis and microaneurysms (dark blue). Occlusion of these arteries causes lacunar infarcts, and rupture of these arteries causes intracerebral hemorrhage. (From Caplan LR. *Stroke: A Clinical Approach,* 3d ed. Boston: Butterworth-Heinemann, 2000, with permission.)

(Binswanger's disease[5,306]), and intracerebral hemorrhage. Hypertension is also frequent in patients with aneurysmal SAH and may contribute to enlargement and rupture of aneurysms.

Hypertension especially damages the deep arteries that penetrate perpendicularly from the major intracranial arteries (Fig. 99-9; see Chap. 61). Serial sections of these arteries in patients with hypertension show characteristic abnormalities consisting of focal microaneurysmal enlargements and small hemorrhagic extravasations through the arterial walls. Subintimal foam cells may obliterate the lumen, and pink-staining amorphous fibrinoid material is found within the walls of the small arteries. The media are often considerably thickened. In places, the vessels are often replaced by whorls, tangles, and wisps of connective tissue that completely obliterate the usual vascular layers, causing segmental arterial disorganization as a consequence of *lipohyalinosis* and *fibrinoid degeneration.*[5,50,307,308] Microaneurysms are common in patients with hypertensive intracerebral hemorrhages and in hypertensive older patients.[309–313]

The two major patterns of brain ischemia in patients with hypertension are *discrete lacunar infarcts* and a more *diffuse patchy white and gray matter degeneration with gliosis.* Both are caused by sclerotic changes in deep intracerebral arteries and arterioles. The term *lacune* (hole) refers to a small, deep infarct caused by lipohyalinosis of the penetrating artery feeding the ischemic brain tissue.[307,308,314,315] Other vascular pathologic processes such as microdissections and tiny emboli occasionally also cause lacunes.[307] Some patients are normotensive and have miniature atherosclerotic lesions (so-called microatheromas) at the orifices of the branches or within the parent arteries blocking or extending into the branches.[5,50,304] Amyloid angiopathy can also cause small, deep infarcts in normotensive and hypertensive patients. Single lacunes cause discrete clinical syndromes.[5,50,316,317] The most common syndromes are pure motor hemiparesis,[318] pure sensory stroke,[319] ataxic hemiparesis,[320] and the dysarthria–clumsy hand syndrome[321] (see Chap. 61).

Since the advent of CT and MRI, it has become widely appreciated that hypertensive patients with lacunes often have more diffuse changes in the white matter of the brain, referred to as *leukoariosis.*[306,322] The clinical picture consists of acute strokes; subacute

progression of neurologic signs; dementia, especially the frontal lobe apathetic type; slow shuffling gait disorder; and parkinsonian, pyramidal, and pseudobulbar signs.[306,323,324] The clinical signs and gross pathology are identical to those partially described by Otto Binswanger in 1894 and 1895[323] and by his students Alzheimer and Nissl.[323] The deep arteries are thickened and hyalinized and show lipohyalinosis and sometimes amyloid angiopathy in regions of white matter atrophy and gliosis. Invariably, lacunar infarcts are also found. The pathogenesis most likely is related to diffuse vascular narrowing in deep arteries and altered microvascular flow and perfusion. Some studies suggest altered hemorrheology and increased blood viscosity, and some patients have had polycythemia.[306] The diagnosis is made on the basis of the clinical findings, the CT and MRI abnormalities, and the absence of cortical infarcts, larger artery occlusive disease, or cardioembolic sources.

HYPERTENSIVE INTRACEREBRAL HEMORRHAGE

Intracerebral hemorrhage (ICH) accounts for about 10 percent of all strokes.[5,6] Head trauma, vascular malformations, bleeding diatheses, drugs (especially amphetamines and cocaine), amyloid angiopathy, and intracranial aneurysms account for some cases.[309,325] Traditionally, spontaneous ICH has usually been equated with hypertensive hemorrhage. Many of these patients, however, have no history of hypertension and no associated changes of hypertensive vasculopathy at necropsy.[218,309,326,327] Acute elevations of blood pressure and/or blood flow to the brain (Table 99-4) can cause ICH by the sudden increase in blood pressure, causing breakage of capillaries and arterioles.[218,309]

Hypertensive ICH issues from the deep penetrating arteries, so the locations parallel the distribution of these arteries. Hematomas develop in the same sites as lacunes; the most frequent locations are the putamen/internal capsule (30 to 40 percent), caudate nucleus (8 percent), lobar white matter (20 percent), thalamus (15 percent), pons (10 percent), and cerebellum (10 percent).[309] In fatal hematomas, microaneurysms and lipohyalinosis are prevalent in penetrating arteries, but the hematomas obscure findings in the middle of the lesions.[328] Along the outside, circumferentially, fibrin globules represent rupture sites.[328] Arterioles or capillaries rupture in the center of the lesion, suddenly increasing local tissue pressure and leading to pressure on adjacent capillaries, which then rupture. As the hematoma gradually grows on its periphery (Fig. 99-10), local tissue pressure and finally intracranial pressure increase until the hematoma

TABLE 99-4 Causes of Acute Changes in Blood Pressure or Blood Flow That Can Result in Intracerebral Hemorrhage

Drugs, especially cocaine and amphetamines
Recent onset of arterial hypertension
Pheochromocytoma
Cold hemorrhages (exposure to freezing ambient temperatures)
Dental chair hemorrhages
Intracranial operations on the fifth cranial nerve
Stereotactic treatment of the fifth cranial nerve for trigeminal neuralgia
Carotid endarterectomy (reflex hypertension and reperfusion)
Cardiac transplantation, especially in children
Surgical repair of congenital heart disease in children
Migraine

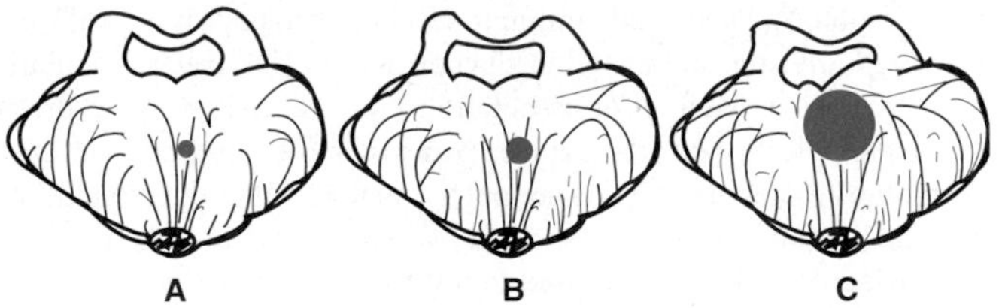

FIGURE 99-10 Gradual evolution of a hypertensive pontine intracerebral hematoma. *A.* The earliest leakage of blood from a paramedian penetrating artery. *B* and *C.* The hematoma has grown. (From Caplan LR. *Stroke: A Clinical Approach,* 3d ed. Boston: Butterworth-Heinemann, 2000, with permission.)

is contained. Alternatively, the pressure is decompressed by the lesion emptying into the ventricular system or into the subarachnoid space on the brain surface.[5,50]

Clinical Findings   Patients with ICH most often have a gradual evolution of neurologic signs; symptoms do not begin abruptly, as in SAH.[309] The first neurologic signs are related to the bleeding site (e.g., left putaminal hematoma patients might first notice right arm weakness or numbness), whereas cerebellar hematoma patients stagger and feel off balance. As the hematoma grows, focal signs worsen. When and if the hematoma increases sufficiently in size to increase intracranial pressure, headache, vomiting, and decreased levels of alertness develop.[309] In the presence of small, restricted hemorrhages, headache is absent and the patient remains alert. The course and findings mimic so-called progressing ischemic stroke. Headache is absent or not a very prominent symptom in more than half of patients with ICH. Loss of consciousness is also not invariable but is a bad prognostic sign when present. Clinical localization of the hematoma rests on an analysis of pupillary responses, eye movements, and the presence and distribution of motor signs.

Diagnosis   Noncontrast CT and MR GRE imaging both accurately show the location, size, shape, and extent of intracerebral hemorrhages. The presence of ventricular and surface drainage, surrounding edema, and pressure shifts in surrounding tissues are also demonstrated. Routine MRI (without MR susceptibility or GRE sequences) in the patient with an acute hematoma is more difficult to interpret, but old hematomas are more readily shown by imaging hemosiderin-containing cavities. Susceptibility-weighted images acquired on echo-planar machines can show even very acute intracerebral hemorrhages.[329] MRI is superior to CT in imaging arteriovenous malformations and cavernous angiomas. Lumbar puncture is seldom warranted. Atypical location, absence of hypertension, and abnormal vascular echoes on MRI are indications for angiography.

Prognosis and Treatment   Coma, increased intracranial pressure, and large hematoma size (>3 cm in one dimension on CT) all indicate a poor prognosis.[309,330] Ordinarily, severe systemic hypertension should be reduced, but not excessively. The hematoma causes increased intracranial pressure, and the spinal fluid pressure and pressure in the dural sinuses increase pari passu. Patients with ICH can die from raised intracranial pressure. In order to perfuse the brain and to maintain an arteriovenous pressure gradient, the systemic arterial pressure must rise. Overzealous reduction of systemic blood pressure can cause clinical deterioration. The patient's state of alertness and neurologic signs should be carefully monitored, together with the blood pressure.

Recent hematomas in the cerebral lobes, cerebellum, and right putamen are sometimes drained surgically without leaving a major deficit, at times using stereotactic equipment with CT guidance. The indications for drainage are increased intracranial pressure and the presence of lesions that require removal (tumor, arteriovenous malformations, aneurysm).[309] When hematomas resolve, they leave a cavity disconnecting but not destroying the overlying cortex.

Small hematomas usually resolve well without specific therapy except blood pressure control, whereas massive hematomas usually kill or maim patients before they can be treated. Medium-sized hematomas (2 to 4 cm), which increase intracranial pressure and cause worsening signs or decreased consciousness while patients are under observation, are indications for drainage if the hematoma is favorably located.

Subarachnoid Hemorrhage

SAH is not directly caused by hypertension in most cases, although an abrupt increase in blood pressure (e.g., due to cocaine or amphetamines) can sometimes lead to SAH, as can a bleeding diathesis, trauma, and amyloid angiopathy. The most frequent lesions causing SAH are abnormal vessels such as aneurysms and vascular malformations on or near the surface of the brain. SAH describes bleeding directly into the subarachnoid space with rapid dissemination into the cerebrospinal fluid (CSF) pathways. Usually blood is suddenly released under systemic arterial pressure, causing an abrupt rise in intracranial pressure and producing headache, vomiting, and interruption of conscious behavior and memory, at least temporarily.[5,331] In some patients, the jet and spread of blood cause neckache, backache, or sciatica instead of headache. Patients are usually agitated and restless or sleepy and have a stiff neck.

The most frequent cause of SAH is leakage from a berry aneurysm. Often there has been a past history of a "warning leak"— that is, a sudden-onset headache unusual for the patient that lasts days and usually prevents normal daily activities.[331,332] Aneurysms are most often located at bifurcations of major intracranial arteries. The most common sites are the ICA–posterior communicating artery junction, the ACA–anterior communicating artery junction, and the MCA bifurcation. CT can often suggest the site of rupture if blood is pooled locally near a typical site.[333] Large aneurysms are occasionally visible on contrast-enhanced CT or MRI. CTA and MRA are useful tests for screening for aneurysms.[281] Lumbar puncture is very important in the diagnosis of SAH.[334] The absence of blood in the CSF effectively excludes the diagnosis of SAH if the fluid is examined within 24 h of the onset of the headache, although bleeds that are very small in volume or older than 72 h can be missed. The CSF pressure, presence of xanthochromia, and quantification of the hemoglobin and bilirubin content of the CSF by spectrophotometry can help establish and date the bleeding and document increased intracranial pressure.[335]

The two most important complications of aneurysmal SAH are rebleeding and brain ischemia due to vasoconstriction (so-called vasospasm). Once an aneurysm has ruptured either a tiny cap of platelets and fibrin seals, the point of rupture or continued bleeding leads to death. Lysis of the fibrin cap initiates rebleeding. Surgical clipping of the aneurysmal sac or obliteration of the aneurysm by endovascular use of balloons or other devices should be attempted before rebleeding occurs.

Vasoconstriction of arteries is thought to be due to blood or blood products that bathe the adventitia of arteries.[335–338] In the presence of a large accumulation of blood, there is a much higher incidence of arterial vasoconstriction and resultant brain ischemia and infarction.

Delayed ischemia can also develop after surgery, as manipulation of vessels can precipitate or potentiate vasoconstriction. The clinical findings in patients with vasoconstriction confirmed by angiography are often those of diffuse brain swelling, such as headache, decreased alertness, and confusion. When vasoconstriction is focal or multifocal, the clinical findings are those of focal ischemia, such as hemiparesis, aphasia, hemianopia, and so on. Vasoconstriction usually has its onset 3 to 5 days after hemorrhage. The peak time for constriction is days 5 to 9; vasoconstriction usually improves after the second week unless rebleeding occurs.[339]

Vasoconstriction is detected by angiography in 30 to 70 percent of patients with SAH, depending on the timing of the study.[339,340] Severe vasoconstriction is manifested by a lumen size of <0.5 mm, delayed anterograde flow, and evidence of collateral filling distal to the vasoconstricted vessel. TCD is effective in monitoring for the presence of vasoconstriction, which increases blood flow velocities.[341] Single-photon emission computed tomography (SPECT) can also show regions of poor perfusion and document the presence of delayed ischemia.[342]

Many treatments have been tried to prevent or treat vasoconstriction after SAH.[338] These include removal of blood by lumbar puncture and at the time of early surgery; pharmacologic agents such as calcium channel blockers to minimize contraction of the arterial wall; and hypervolemia to prevent ischemia by maintaining perfusion. At present, the most popular approaches are early surgery, nimodipine (a calcium channel blocker), and hypervolemic therapy, especially after aneurysmal clipping. Hypovolemia is common after SAH, as is hyponatremia. Hypervolemia does not reverse the vasoconstriction but helps maintain brain perfusion.

Coagulopathies

Hypercoagulability and bleeding due to decreased coagulability affect most body organs, including the brain and heart. An increased tendency for clotting can be caused by abnormalities of the formed blood elements or serologic factors.[5,343–345] Increased numbers of red blood cells and platelets and qualitative abnormalities such as sickle cell disease can cause intravascular clotting, especially in the presence of dehydration and reduced plasma volume. Excessive platelet activation, or so-called sticky platelets, can also explain increased coagulability but has proved hard to measure reliably in vitro.[346,347] The level of beta-thromboglobulin is a good marker for platelet activation (see Chap. 54). Serologic abnormalities may be congenital or acquired. Decreased amounts of natural anticoagulants (antithrombin III, protein C, and protein S), resistance to activated protein C, and prothrombin gene mutations can cause hypercoagulability.[343–345,348] These proteins may be decreased in patients with hypoproteinemia, especially that due to the nephrotic syndrome and urinary protein loss. Fibrinogen levels and the levels of the various coagulation factors such as factors VIII and XI may also be high in patients with a prothrombotic state (see Chap. 54). In many of these patients—those on high-dose estrogen birth control pills, pregnant women, and patients with cancer—serologic and standard coagulation tests (in vitro) do not clarify the mechanism of the excessive clotting in vivo. Stroke patients may have serologic evidence of platelet activation and increased fibrin formation but decreased natural fibrinolytic and anticoagulant activity.[344,348]

Measurement of various serum antiphospholipid antibodies elicited considerable interest. The usually measured substances are the so-called lupus anticoagulant,[349–351] anticardiolipin antibodies, and beta$_2$-glycoprotein 1 antibodies. Increased activity of antiphospholipid antibodies (APLA) is found in patients with systemic lupus erythematosus, acquired immunodeficiency syndrome (AIDS), giant cell arteritis, and Sneddon's syndrome[351–354] (livedo reticularis and strokes), as well as in association with the use of some drugs (e.g., phenytoin, phenothiazines, procainamide, hydralazine, and quinidine). When the APLAs are not associated with other conditions and the patient has clinical evidence of excess clotting, the disorder is considered to be primary and is referred to as the *primary APLA syndrome*.[355–358] Patients with APLAs have an increased incidence of spontaneous abortions, venous occlusive disease of the legs and pulmonary embolism, brain infarcts (often multiple), thrombocytopenia, and false-positive syphilis serologic tests. Older patients with APLAs often also have important risk factors for stroke.[355–358]

Patients with systemic illnesses often have elevated erythrocyte sedimentation rates, and strokes and pulmonary emboli often follow and complicate myocardial infarction (see Chap. 52). Customarily, such brain infarcts have been attributed to cardiogenic embolism, but some undoubtedly are related to thromboses precipitated by increased levels of acute-phase reactant coagulation proteins. Cancer, especially mucinous adenocarcinoma, has been associated with multiple vascular occlusions, large and tiny brain infarcts, and venous and arterial occlusions.[359]

Deficient coagulability can lead to serious intracranial bleeding. The hemorrhage can be into the brain (ICH), CSF, SAH, or the subdural and epidural compartments. Thrombocytopenia, hemophilia, and leukemia are common conditions leading to intracranial hemorrhage. The most common iatrogenic cause of bleeding is anticoagulation with heparin or warfarin.[309,360] Brain hemorrhage has also been described after fibrinolytic treatment of patients with coronary artery disease[361,362] and after rt-PA infusion to treat cerebrovascular occlusive disease[298–303] (see Chaps. 52 and 54).

Anticoagulant-related ICH, a catastrophic complication with high morbidity and mortality, is relatively rare considering the frequency of anticoagulant use. Anticoagulant-related hemorrhages develop more insidiously and evolve more slowly and more often than do other causes of ICH.[308,360] Many are erroneously attributed to brain ischemia, especially if anticoagulants had been prescribed to treat TIAs. Any patient taking anticoagulants who develops CNS symptoms should be considered to have anticoagulant-related ICH until CT or MRI excludes the diagnosis. The hematoma grows slowly and insidiously increases intracranial pressure. Many patients require surgical drainage of their hematomas to ensure survival. Anticoagulants should be stopped immediately and their effect reversed by fresh frozen plasma or vitamin K. It is probably safe to resume anticoagulation with heparin 7 days to 2 weeks after the ICH if indicated—for prophylaxis in patients with artificial heart valves.[363] In patients treated with fibrinolytic agents, hemorrhages are most often lobar or cerebellar and may be multiple. ICH is more common when there is a past stroke, when heparin or other agents that affect coagulation are given with or after fibrinolytic agents, and when there is a hemostatic defect secondary to treatment.[362,363]

Arterial Dissection

Aortic dissections involving the innominate or carotid arteries (see Chap. 98) are a well-known cause of stroke and other manifestations of brain ischemia. Less well known are the syndromes produced by dissections of the extracranial and intracranial arteries, which are especially likely to occur in young, active individuals without risk factors for atherosclerosis or stroke but after trauma or chiropractic or other neck manipulations. They are also associated with fibromuscular dysplasia, alpha$_1$-antitrypsin deficiency, Marfan's syndrome, pseudoxanthoma elasticum, and migraine.

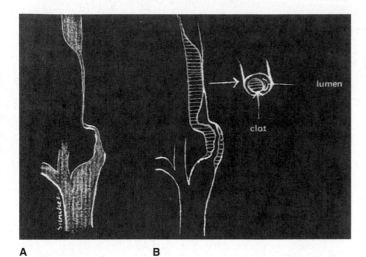

A   **B**

FIGURE 99-11 Diagrams of a carotid artery dissection. *A.* The lumen encroached upon by the intramural clot. *B.* The dissection (*cross-hatched*). (From Caplan LR. *Stroke: A Clinical Approach,* 3d ed. Boston: Butterworth-Heinemann, 2000, with permission.)

Dissections start with a tear in the media and spread longitudinally (Fig. 99-11), often disrupting adventitial fibers or even rupturing through the adventitia to produce an extravascular hematoma and a false or pseudoaneurysm within muscle and connective tissue. Intracranially, such a rupture can produce SAH. Other dissections cause arterial obstruction and secondary thrombosis of the narrowed vascular lumen. Most cerebrovascular dissections occur in the extracranial vessels, particularly the pharyngeal portion of the internal carotid artery and the nuchal vertebral arteries.[5,50,364–369]

Extracranial dissections produce sharp pain and throbbing headache; brain and retinal ischemic episodes, which may occur in rapid-fire attacks ("carotid allegro"[369]); and pressure on adjacent structures especially cranial nerves X through XII, which exit at the skull base. Strokes, usually from embolization of clots, are common but may have a benign course. Intracranial dissections have a poorer prognosis, often with vascular rupture and SAH. The diagnosis is confirmed by angiography, CT, or MRI. Ultrasound studies can be helpful in suggesting the diagnosis of dissection in the neck.[370]

Treatment consists of the use of heparin acutely, followed by warfarin. In patients in whom the dissected artery is initially occluded and remains occluded, warfarin can be stopped after 6 to 12 weeks. The authors continue warfarin in other patients until there no longer is severe luminal narrowing, monitoring the dissected arteries by noninvasive techniques (ultrasound, CTA, or MRA). Intracranial dissections with SAH have been treated surgically.[365,371,372]

References

1. Caplan LR. Brain embolism. In: Caplan LR, Hurst JW, Chimowitz MI (eds). *Clinical Neurocardiology.* New York: Marcel Dekker; 1999: 35–185.
2. Aring C., Merritt H. Differential diagnosis between cerebral hemorrhage and cerebral thrombosis. *Arch Intern Med* 1935;56:435–456.
3. Whisnant J, Fitzgibbons J, Kurland L, Sayre GP. Natural history of stroke in Rochester, Minnesota 1945–1954. *Stroke* 1971;2:11–22.
4. Matsumoto N, Whisnant J, Kurland L, Okazaki H. Natural history of stroke in Rochester, Minnesota 1955–1969. *Stroke* 1973;4:2–29.
5. Caplan LR. *Stroke: A Clinical Approach,* 3d ed. Boston: Butterworth-Heinemann, 2000.
6. Mohr J, Caplan LR, Melski J, et al. The Harvard Cooperative Stroke registry: A prospective study. *Neurology* 1978;28:754–762.
7. Caplan LR, Hier D, D'Cruz I. Cerebral embolism in the Michael Reese Stroke Registry. *Stroke* 1983;14:530–536.
8. Foulkes MA, Wolf PA, Price TR, et al. The Stroke Data Bank: Design, methods, and baseline characteristics. *Stroke* 1988;19:547–554.
9. Kunitz S, Gross C, Heyman A, et al. The Pilot Stroke Data Bank: Definition, design and data. *Stroke* 1984;15:740–746.
10. Bogousslavsky J, Van Melle G, Regli F. The Lausanne Stroke Registry: Analysis of 1000 consecutive patients with first strokes. *Stroke* 1988;19:1083–1092.
11. Bogousslavsky J, Cachin C, Regli F, et al. Cardiac sources of embolism and cerebral infarction—clinical consequences and vascular concomitants: The Lausanne Stroke Registry. *Neurology* 1991;41: 855–859.
12. Kittner SJ, Sharkness CM, Sloan M, et al. Infarcts with a cardiac source of embolism in the NINDS Stroke Data Bank: Neurologic examination. *Neurology* 1992;42:299–302.
13. Jeresaty RM. *Mitral Valve Prolapse.* New York, NY: Raven Press; 1979.
14. Salem DN, Hartnett Daudelin D, Levine HJ, et al. Antithrombotic therapy in valvular heart disease. *Chest* 2001;119:207S–219S.
15. Barnett HJM, Jones MW, Boughner DR, Kostuk WJ. Cerebral ischemic events associated with prolapsing mitral valve. *Arch Neurol* 1976;33:777–782.
16. Barnett HJM, Boughner DR, Taylor DW, et al. Further evidence relating mitral valve prolapse to cerebral ischemic events. *N Engl J Med* 1980;302:139–144.
17. Sandok BA, Giuliani ER. Cerebral ischemic events in patients with mitral valve prolapse. *Stroke* 1982;13:448–450.
18. Lauzier S, Barnett HJM. Cerebral ischemia with mitral valve prolapse and mitral annulus calcification. In: Furlan AJ (ed). *The Heart and Stroke.* London: Springer-Verlag; 1987:63–100.
19. Pomerance A. Ballooning deformity (mucoid degeneration) of atrioventricular valves. *Br Heart J* 1969;31:343–351.
20. Pomerance A, Davies MJ. Strokes: A complication of mitral leaflet prolapse. *Lancet* 1977;2:1186.
21. Kostuk WJ, Boughner DR, Barnett HJM, Silver MD. Strokes: A complication of mitral-leaflet prolapse. *Lancet* 1977;2:313–316.
22. Hanson MR, Conomy JP, Hodgman JR. Brain events associated with mitral valve prolapse. *Stroke* 1980;11:499–506.
23. Jones HR, Naggar CZ, Selyan MP, Downing ZZ. Mitral valve prolapse and cerebral ischemic events: A comparison between a neurology population with stroke and a cardiology population with mitral valve prolapse observed for 5 years. *Stroke* 1982;13:451–453.
24. Pomerance A. Pathological and clinical study of calcification in the mitral valve ring. *J Clin Pathol* 1970;23:354–361.
25. Stein JH, Soble JS. Thrombus associated with mitral valve calcification. *Stroke* 1995;26:1697–1699.
26. Fulkerson PK, Beaver BM, Auseon JC, Graven HL. Calcification of the mitral annulus—etiology, clinical associations, complications and therapy. *Am J Med* 1979;66:967–977.
27. deBono DP, Warlow CP. Mitral-annulus calcification and cerebral or retinal ischemia. *Lancet* 1979;2:383–385.
28. Korn D, DeSanctis RW, Sell S. Massive calcification of the mitral annulus. A clinicopathological study of fourteen cases. *N Engl J Med* 1962;267:900–909.
29. Benjamin EJ, Plehn JF, D'Agostino RB, et al. Mitral annular calcification and the risk of stroke in an elderly cohort. *N Engl J Med* 1992;327: 374–379.
30. Savage DD, Garrison RJ, Castelli WP, et al. Prevalence of submitral (annular) calcium and its correlations in a general population–based sample (the Framingham study). *Am J Cardiol* 1983;51: 1375–1378.
31. Sacco RL, Ellenberg JH, Mohr JP, et al. Infarcts of undetermined cause: The NINCDS Stroke Data Bank. *Ann Neurol* 1989;25:382–390.
32. Mohr JP. Infarct of unclear cause. In: Furlan AJ (ed). *The Heart and Stroke.* London: Springer-Verlag;1987:101–116.

33. Galve E, Candell-Riera J, Pigrau C, et al. Prevalence, morphology, types and evaluation of cardiac valvular disease in systemic lupus erythematosus. *N Engl J Med* 1988;319:817–823.

34. Barbut D, Borer JS, Wallerson D, et al. Anticardiolipin antibody and stroke: Possible relation of valvular heart disease and embolic events. *Cardiology* 1991;79:99–109.

35. Nighoghossian N, Derex L, Loire R, et al. Giant Lambl excrescences. An unusual source of cerebral embolism. *Arch Neurol* 1997;54:41–44.

36. Cohen A, Tzourio C, Chauvel C, et al. Mitral valve strands and the risk of ischemic stroke in elderly patients. *Stroke* 1997;28:1574–1578.

37. Caplan LR. Mitral valve strands: What are they and what is their relation to stroke? *Neurol Network Comment* 1998;2:11–14.

38. Kanter MC, Hart RG. Neurologic complications of infective endocarditis. *Neurology* 1991;41:1015–1020.

39. Caplan LR. Of birds and nests and brain emboli. *Rev Neurol (Paris)* 1991;147:265–273.

40. Amarenco P, Duyckaerts C, Tzourio C, et al. The prevalence of ulcerated plaques in the aortic arch in patients with stroke. *N Engl J Med* 1992;326:221–225.

41. Amarenco P, Cohan A, Baudrimont M, Bousser M-G. Transesophageal echocardiographic detection of aortic arch disease in patients with cerebral infarction. *Stroke* 1992;23:1056–1061.

42. Weinberger J, Azhar S, Danisi F, et al. A new noninvasive technique for imaging atherosclerotic plaque in the aortic arch of stroke patients by transcutaneous real-time B-mode ultrasonography. *Stroke* 1998;29:673–676.

43. The French Study of Aortic Plaques in Stroke Group. Atherosclerotic disease of the aortic arch as a risk factor for recurrent ischemic stroke. *N Engl J Med* 1996;334:1216–1221.

44. Dressler F, Craig W, Castello R, Labovitz AJ. Mobile aortic atheroma and systemic emboli; efficacy of anticoagulation and influence of plaques morphology on recurrent stroke. *J Am Coll Cardiol* 1998;31:134–138.

45. Ferrari E, Vidal R, Chevallier T, Baudouy M. Atherosclerosis of the thoracic aorta and systemic emboli; Efficacy of anticoagulation and influence of plaque morphology on recurrent stroke. *J Am Cardiol* 1999;33:1317–1322.

46. Gacs G, Merel MD, Bodosi M. Balloon catheter as a model of cerebral emboli in humans. *Stroke* 1982;13:39–42.

47. Fisher CM. Left hemiplegia and motor impersistence. *J Nerv Ment Dis* 1956;123:201–218.

48. Caplan LR, Kelly M, Kase CS, et al. Infarcts of the inferior division of the right middle cerebral artery: Mirror image of Wernicke's aphasia. *Neurology* 1986;36:1015–1020.

49. Caplan LR. Posterior cerebral artery. In: Bogousslavsky J, Caplan LR (eds). *Stroke Syndromes.* New York: Cambridge University Press; 1995:290–299.

50. Caplan LR. *Posterior Circulation Vascular Disease: Clinical Findings, Diagnosis, and Management.* Boston: Blackwell Science; 1996.

51. Pessin MS, Lathi E, Cohen MB, et al. Clinical features and mechanisms of occipital infarction in the posterior cerebral artery territory. *Ann Neurol* 1987;21:290–299.

52. Yammamoto Y, Georgiadis AL, Chang H-M, Caplan LR. Posterior cerebral artery territory infarcts in the New England Medical Center Posterior Circulation Registry. *Arch Neurol* 1999;56:824–832.

53. Caplan LR. Top of the basilar syndrome: Selected clinical aspects. *Neurology* 1980;30:72–79.

54. Mehler MF. The rostral basilar artery syndrome: Diagnosis, etiology, prognosis. *Neurology* 1989;39:9–16.

55. Amarenco P. The spectrum of cerebellar infarctions. *Neurology* 1991;41:973–979.

56. Fisher CM, Perlman A. The nonsudden onset of a cerebral embolism. *Neurology* 1967;17:1025–1032.

57. Fieschi C, Argentino C, Lenzi GL, et al. Clinical and instrumental evaluation of patients with ischemic stroke within the first six hours. *J Neurol Sci* 1989;91:311–322.

58. Kushner MJ, Zanotte EM, Bastianiello S, et al. Transcranial Doppler in acute hemispheric brain infarction. *Neurology* 1991;41:109–113.

59. Ringlestein EB, Koschorke S, Holling A, et al. Computed tomographic patterns of proven embolic brain infarcts. *Ann Neurol* 1989;26:759–765.

60. Bladin PF, Berkovic SF. Striatocapsular infarction. *Neurology* 1984;34:1423–1430.

61. Fisher CM, Adams RD. Observations on brain embolism. *J Neuropathol Exp Neurol* 1951;10:92–94.

62. Fisher CM, Adams RD. Observations on brain embolism with special reference to hemorrhagic infarction. In: Furlan AJ (ed). *The Heart and Stroke.* London: Springer-Verlag; 1987:17–36.

63. Gacs G, Fox AJ, Barnett HJ, Vinuela F. CT visualization of intracranial arterial thromboembolism. *Stroke* 1983;14:756–763.

64. Tomsick T, Brott T, Barsan W, et al. Thrombus localization with emergency cerebral computed tomography. *Stroke* 1990;21:180.

65. Bergeron GA, Shah PM. Echocardiography unwarranted in patients with cerebral ischemic events. *N Engl J Med* 1981;304:489.

66. Greenland P, Knopman D, Mikell F, et al. Echocardiography in diagnostic assessment of stroke. *Ann Intern Med* 1981;95:51–54.

67. Donaldson R, Emmanuel R, Earl C. The role of two-dimensional echocardiography in the detection of potentially embolic intracardiac masses in patients with cerebral ischemia. *J Neurol Neurosurg Psychiatry* 1981;44:803–809.

68. Tegeler CH, Downes TR. Cardiac imaging in stroke. *Stroke* 1991;22:1206–1211.

69. Pop G, Sutherland GR, Koudstaal PJ, et al. Transesophageal echocardiography in the detection of intracardiac embolic sources in patients with transient ischemic attacks. *Stroke* 1990;21:560–565.

70. Zenker G, Ecbel R, Kramer G, et al. Transesophageal echocardiography in young patients with cerebral ischemic events. *Stroke* 1988;19:345–348.

71. Cohen A, Chauvel C. Transesophageal echocardiography in the management of transient ischemic attack and ischemic stroke. *Cerebrovasc Dis* 1996;6(suppl 1):15–25.

72. Kase CS, White R, Vinson TL, Eichelberger RP. Shotgun pellet embolus to the middle cerebral artery. *Neurology* 1981;31:458–461.

73. DeWitt LD, Pessin MS, Pandian NG, et al. Benign disappearance of ventricular thrombus after embolic stroke: A case report. *Stroke* 1988;19:393–396.

74. Ezekowitz MD, Wilson DA, Smith EO, et al. Comparison of indium-III platelet scintigraphy and two-dimensional echocardiography in the diagnosis of left ventricular thrombi. *N Engl J Med* 1982;306:1509–1513.

75. Markus HS, Droste DW, Brown MM. Detection of symptomatic cerebral embolic signals with Doppler ultrasound. *Lancet* 1994;343:1011–1012.

76. Markus HS, Harrison MJ. Microembolic signal detection using ultrasound. *Stroke* 1995;26:1517–1519.

77. Tong DC, Bolger A, Albers GW. Incidence of transcranial Doppler-detected cerebral microemboli in patients referred for echocardiography. *Stroke* 1994;25:2138–2141.

78. Barbut D, Hinton RB, Szatrowski TP, et al. Cerebral emboli detected during bypass surgery are associated with clamp removal. *Stroke* 1994;25:2398–2402.

79. Nabavi DG, Georgiadis D, Mumme T, et al. Clinical relevance of intracranial microembolic signals in patients with left ventricular assist devices: A prospective study. *Stroke* 1996;27:891–896.

80. Petersen P, Boysen G, Godtfredsen J, et al. Placebo-controlled, randomized trial of warfarin and aspirin for prevention of thromboembolic complications in chronic atrial fibrillation: The Copenhagen AFASAK Study. *Lancet* 1989;1:175–179.

81. Stroke Prevention in Atrial Fibrillation Study Group Investigators. Preliminary report of the Stroke Prevention in Atrial Fibrillation Study. *N Engl J Med* 1990;322:863–868.

82. Stroke Prevention in Atrial Fibrillation Investigators: The stroke prevention in atrial fibrillation trial: Final results. *Circulation* 1991;84:527–539

83. Stroke Prevention in Atrial Fibrillation Investigators:. Adjusted-dose warfarin versus low-intensity fixed-dose warfarin plus aspirin for high-

risk patients with atrial fibrillation. Stroke Prevention in Atrial Fibrillation III randomized clinical trial. *Lancet* 1996;348:633–638.

84. Stroke Prevention in Atrial Fibrillation Investigators: Prospective identification of patients with nonvalvular atrial fibrillation at low risk during treatment with aspirin: Stroke prevention in Atrial Fibrillation III Study (abstract). *Circulation* 1997;96(suppl) I-28.

85. The Stroke Prevention in Atrial Fibrillation Investigators. Predictors of thromboembolism in atrial fibrillation: I. Clinical features of patients at risk. *Ann Intern Med* 1992;116:1–5.

86. The Stroke Prevention in Atrial Fibrillation Investigators. Predictors of thromboembolism in atrial fibrillation: II. Echocardiographic features of patients at risk. *Ann Intern Med* 1992;116:6–12.

87. Pritchett ELC. Management of atrial fibrillation. *N Engl J Med* 1992; 326:1264–1271.

88. Ezekowitz MD, Bridgers SL, James KE, et al. Randomized trials of warfarin for atrial fibrillation. *N Engl J Med* 1992;327:1451–1453.

89. The Boston Area Anticoagulation Trial for Atrial Fibrillation Investigators. The effect of low-dose warfarin on the risk of stroke in patients with nonrheumatic atrial fibrillation. *N Engl J Med* 1990;323: 1505–1511.

90. Connolly SJ, Laupacis A, Gent M, et al. Canadian Atrial Fibrillation Anticoagulation (CAFA) study. *J Am Coll Cardiol* 1991;18:349–355.

91. European Atrial Fibrillation Trial Study Group. Optimal oral anticoagulation therapy in patients with nonrheumatic atrial fibrillation and recent cerebral ischemia. *N Engl J Med* 1995;333:5–10.

92. Moldveen-Geronimus M, Merriam JC. Cholesterol embolization: From pathologic curiosity to clinical entity. *Circulation* 1967;35: 946–953.

93. Shields RW Jr, Laureno R, Lachman T, Victor M. Anticoagulant-related hemorrhage in acute cerebral embolism. *Stroke* 1984;15: 426–437.

94. Lieberman A, Hass WK, Pinto R, et al. Intracranial hemorrhage and infarction in anticoagulated patients with prosthetic heart valves. *Stroke* 1978;9:18–24.

95. Drake ME, Shin C. Conversion of ischemic to hemorrhagic infarction by anticoagulant administration: Report of two cases with evidence from serial computed tomographic brain scans. *Arch Neurol* 1983;40: 44–46.

96. Cerebral Embolism Study Group. Immediate anticoagulation of embolic stroke: A randomized trial. *Stroke* 1983;13:668–676.

97. Toni D, Fiorelli M, Bastianello S, et al. Hemorrhagic transformation of brain infarct. *Neurology* 1996;46:341–345.

98. Cerebral Embolism Task Force. Cardiogenic brain embolism. *Arch Neurol* 1986;43:71–84.

99. Cerebral Embolism Task Force. Cardiogenic brain embolism: The second report of the Cerebral Embolism Task Force. *Arch Neurol* 1989; 46:727–743.

100. Pessin MS , Estol CJ, Lafranchise F, Caplan LR. Safety of anticoagulation after hemorrhagic infarction. *Neurology* 1993;43:1298–1303.

101. Chaves CJ, Pessin MS, Caplan LR, et al. Cerebellar hemorrhagic infarction. *Neurology* 1996;46:346–349.

102. Chamorro A, Vila N, Ascaso C, Blanc R. Heparin in acute stroke with atrial fibrillation. Clinical relevance of very early treatment. *Arch Neurol* 1999;56:1098–1102.

103. Caplan LR. When should heparin be given to patients with atrial fibrillation–related brain infarcts. *Arch Neurol* 1999;56:1059–1060.

104. Hagen PT, Scholz DG, Edwards WD. Incidence and size of patent foramen ovale during the first 10 decades of life: An autopsy study of 965 normal hearts. *Mayo Clin Proc* 1984;59:17–20.

105. Lechat PH, Mas JL, Lascault G, et al. Prevalence of patent foramen ovale in patients with stroke. *N Engl J Med* 1988;318:1148–1152.

106. Di Tullio M, Sacco RL, Gopal A, et al. Patent foramen ovale as a risk factor for cryptogenic stroke. *Ann Int Med* 1992;117:461–465.

107. Petty GW, Khanderia BK, Chu C-P, et al. Patent foramen ovale in patients with cerebral infarction. A transesophageal echocardiographic study. *Arch Neurol* 1997;54:819–822.

108. Webster MW, Chancellor AM, Smith HJ, et al. Patent foramen ovale in young stroke patients. *Lancet* 1988;2:11–12.

109. Steiner MM, Di Tullio MR, Rundek T, et al. Patent foramen ovale size and embolic brain imaging findings among patients with ischemic stroke. *Stroke* 1998;29:944–948.

110. Jones HR, Caplan LR, Come PC, et al. Cerebral emboli of paradoxical origin. *Ann Neurol* 1983;13:314–319.

111. Biller J, Adams HP, Johnson MR, et al. Paradoxical cerebral embolism: Eight cases. *Neurology* 1986;36:1356–1360.

112. Gautier JC, Durr A, Koussa S, et al. Paradoxical cerebral embolism with a patent foramen ovale. A report of 29 patients. *Cerebrovasc Dis* 1991;1:193–202.

113. Caplan LR. Cardiac arrest and other hypoxic-ischemic insults. In: Caplan LR, Hurst JW, Chimowitz MI (eds). *Clinical Neurocardiology.* New York: Marcel Dekker; 1999:1–34.

114. Brierley J, Meldrum B, Brown A. The threshold and neuropathology of cerebral "anoxic-ischemic" cell change. *Arch Neurol* 1973;29: 367–373.

115. Brierley JB, Adams JH, Graham DI, Simpson JA. Neocortical death after cardiac arrest: A clinical, neurophysiological report of two cases. *Lancet* 1971;2:560–565.

116. Dougherty JH, Rawlinson DG, Levy DE, Plum F. Hypoxic-ischemic brain injury and the vegetative state: Clinical and neuropathologic correlation. *Neurology* 1981;31:991–997.

117. Cummings JL, Tomiyasu U, Read S, Benson DF. Amnesia with hippocampal lesions after cardiopulmonary arrest. *Neurology* 1984;34: 679–681.

118. Dooling E, Richardson EP. Delayed encephalopathy after strangling. *Arch Neurol* 1976;33:196–199.

119. Lance J, Adams RD. The syndrome of intention and action myoclonus as a sequel to hypoxic encephalopathy. *Brain* 1963;86:111–133.

120. Gilles F. Hypotensive brainstem necrosis. *Arch Pathol* 1969;88:32–41.

121. Silver JR, Buxton PH. Spinal stroke. *Brain* 1974;97:539–550.

122. Caronna JJ, Finkelstein S. Neurological syndromes after cardiac arrest. *Stroke* 1978;9:517–520.

123. Jennett B, Plum F. Persistent vegetative state after brain damage: A syndrome in search of a name. *Lancet* 1972;1:734–737.

124. Levy DE, Knill-Jones RP, Plum F. The vegetative state and its prognosis following non-traumatic coma. *Ann NY Acad Sci* 1978;315:293–306.

125. Hecaen H, Ajuriaguerra J. Balint's syndrome and its minor forms. *Brain* 1954;77:373–400.

126. Willoughby J, Leach B. Relation of neurological findings after cardiac arrest to outcome. *BMJ* 1974;3:437–439.

127. Plum F, Caronna J. Can one predict outcome of medical coma? In: *Outcome of Severe Damage to the Central Nervous System. A CIBA Foundation Symposium.* New York: Elsevier; 1975:121–139.

128. Bell JA, Hodgson HJ. Coma after cardiac arrest. *Brain* 1974;97: 361–372.

129. Levy D, Carrona JJ, Singer BH, et al. Predicting outcome from hypoxic-ischemic coma. *JAMA* 1985;253:1420–1426.

130. Wijdicks EFM, Parisi JE, Sharbrough FW. Prognostic value of myoclonus status in comatose survivors of cardiac arrest. *Ann Neurol* 1994;35:239–243.

131. Longstreth WT, Inui TS, Cobb LA, Copass MK. Neurologic recovery after out-of-hospital cardiac arrest. *Ann Intern Med* 1983;38:588–592.

132. Longstreth WT, Diehr P, Inui TS. Prediction of awakening after out-of-hospital cardiac arrest. *N Engl J Med* 1983;308:1378–1382.

133. Thompson RG, Hallstrom AP, Cobb LA. Bystander-initiated cardiopulmonary resuscitation in the management of ventricular fibrillation. *Ann Intern Med* 1979;90:737–740.

134. Bedell SE, Delbanco TG, Cook EF, Epstein FH. Survival after cardiopulmonary resuscitation in the hospital. *N Engl J Med* 1983;309: 569–576.

135. Caplan LR, Brass LM, DeWitt LD, et al. Transcranial Doppler ultrasound: Present status. *Neurology* 1990;40:696–700.

136. Kirkham F, Levin S, Padayachee T, et al. Transcranial pulsed Doppler ultrasound findings in brainstem death. *J Neurol Neurosurg Psychiatry* 1987;50:1504–1513.

137. Ropper A, Kehne S, Wechsler L. Transcranial Doppler in brain death. *Neurology* 1987;37:1733–1735.

138. Longstreth WT, Inui TS. High blood glucose level on hospital admission and poor neurological recovery after cardiac arrest. *Ann Neurol* 1984;15:59–63.

139. Myers C, Yamaguchi S. Nervous system effects of cardiac arrest in monkeys. *Arch Neurol* 1977;34:65–74.

140. Plum F. What causes infarction in ischemic brain. *Neurology* 1983; 33:222–233.

141. Collins RC, Dobkin BH, Choi DW. Selective vulnerability of the brain: New insights into the pathophysiology of stroke. *Ann Intern Med* 1989;110:992–1000.

142. Albers G, Goldberg M, Choi D. *N*-methyl-*D*-aspartate antagonists: Ready for clinical trial in brain ischemia? *Ann Neurol* 1989;25:398–403.

143. Giswold S, Safar P, Rao G, et al. Multifaceted therapy after global brain ischemia in monkeys. *Stroke* 1984;15:803–812.

144. Caplan LR. Encephalopathies and neurological effects of drugs used in cardiac patients. In: Caplan LR, Hurst JW, Chimowitz MI (eds). *Clinical Neurocardiology*. New York, Marcel Dekker; 1999:186–225.

145. Volpe BT, Soave R. Formal visual hallucinations as digitalis toxicity. *Ann Intern Med* 1979;91:868–869.

146. Closson RG. Visual hallucinations as the earliest symptom of digoxin intoxication. *Arch Neurol* 1983;40:386.

147. Gilbert GJ. Quinidine dementia. *JAMA* 1977;237:2093–2094.

148. Adams HP. Neurologic complications of cardiovascular procedures. In: Biller J (ed). *Iatrogenic Neurology*. Boston: Butterworth-Heinemann; 1998:51–61.

149. Dawson DM, Fischer EG. Neurologic complications of cardiac catheterization. *Neurology* 1977;27:496–497.

150. Mendez Dominguez A, Aguilera R, Martinez Rios MA. Cerebral ischemia: A complication in heart catheterization. An assessment in 2178 catheterizations. *Arch Inst Cardiol Mex* 1993;63:247–251.

151. Nakata A, Sekiguchi Y, Hirota S, et al. Central retinal artery occlusion following cardiac catheterization. *Jpn Heart J* 2002;43:187–192.

152. Liu XY, Wong V, Leung M. Neurologic complications due to catheterization. *Pediatr Neurol* 2001;24:270–275.

153. Colt HG, Begg RJ, Saporito JJ, et al. Cholesterol emboli after cardiac catheterization. Eight cases and a review of the literature. *Medicine* 1988;67:389–400.

154. Weissman BM, Aram DM, Levinsohn MW, Ben-Shacher G. Neurologic sequelae of cardiac catheterization. *Catheter Cardiovasc Diagn* 1985;11:577–583.

155. Wijman CA, Kase CS, Jacobs AK, Whitehead RE. Cerebral air embolism as a cause of stroke during cardiac catheterization. *Neurology* 1998;51:318–319.

156. Ramirez G, O'Neill WM Jr, Lambert R, Bloomer HA. Cholesterol embolization: A complication of angiography. *Arch Intern Med* 1978;138: 1430–1432.

157. Dorros G, Cowley MJ, Simpson J, et al. Percutaneous transluminal coronary angioplasty: Report of complications from the National Heart, Lung, and Blood Institute PTCA Registry. *Circulation* 1983;67: 723–730.

158. Akkerhuis KM, Deckers JW, Lincoff AM, et al. Risk of stroke associated with abciximab among patients undergoing percutaneous coronary intervention. *JAMA* 2001;286:78–82.

159. The EPIC Investigators. Use of a monoclonal antibody directed against the platelet glycoprotein IIb/IIIa receptor in high-risk coronary angioplasty. *N Engl J Med* 1994;330:956–961.

160. The CAPTURE Investigators. Ramdomised placebo-controlled trial of abciximab before and during coronary intervention in refractory unstable angina: The CAPTURE study. *Lancet* 1997;349:1429–1435.

161. The EPILOG Investigators. Platelet glycoprotein IIb/IIIa receptor blockade and low-dose heparin during percutaneous coronary revascularization. *N Engl J Med* 1997;336:1689–1696.

162. The EPISTENT Investigators. Randomised placebo-controlled and balloon-angioplasty-controlled access safety of coronary stenting with use of platelet glycoprotein-IIb/IIIa blockade. *Lancet* 1998;352:87–92.

163. Galbreath C, Salgado ED, Furlan AJ, Hollman J. Central nervous system complications of percutaneous transluminal coronary angioplasty. *Stroke* 1986;17:616–619.

164. Malenka DJ, O'Rourke D, Miller MA, et al. Cause of in-hospital death in 12,232 consecutive patients undergoing percutaneous transluminal coronary angioplasty. The Northern New England Cardiovascular Disease Study Group. *Am Heart J* 1999;137:632–638.

165. Borger van der Burg AE, de Groot NM, van Erven L, et al. Long-term follow-up after radiofrequency catheter ablation of ventricular tachycardia: A successful approach? *J Cardiovasc Electrophysiol* 2002;13: 424–426.

166. Tanel RE, Walsh EP, Triedman JK, et al. Five-year experience with radiofrequency catheter ablation: Implications for management of arrhythmias in pediatric and young adult patients. *J Pediatr* 1997;131: 878–887.

167. Alvarez M, Merino JL. Spanish registry on catheter ablation. 1st official report of the working group on electrophysiology and arrhythmias of the Spanish Society of Cardiology (Year 2001) *Rev Esp Cardiol* 2002;55:1273–1285.

168. DiMarco JP, Garan H, Ruskin JN. Complications in patients undergoing cardiac electrophysiologic procedures. *Ann Int Med* 1982;97:490.

169. Arnold AZ, Mick MJ, Mazurek RP, et al. Role of prophylactic anticoagulation for direct current cardioversion in patients with atrial fibrillation or atrial flutter. *J Am Coll Cardiol* 1992;19:851–855.

170. Ewy GA. Optimal technique for electrical cardioversion of atrial fibrillation. *Circulation* 1992;86:1645–1647.

171. Letac B, Cribier A, Koning R, Bellefleur JP. Results of percutaneous transluminal valvuloplasty in 218 adults with valvular aortic stenosis. *Am J Cardiol* 1988;15:62:598–605.

172. Eisenhauer AC, Hadjipetron P, Piemonte TC. Balloon aortic valvuloplasty revisited: The role of the inoue balloon and transseptal antegrade approach. *Catheter Cardiovasc Interv* 2000;50:484–491.

173. Peixoto EC, de Olivera PS, Netto MS, et al. Percutaneous balloon mitral valvuloplasty. Immediate results, complications, and hospital outcome. *Arq Bras Cardiol* 1995;64:109–116.

174. Peixoto EC, de Olivera PS, Netto MS, et al. Percutaneous mitral valvuloplasty with the single balloon technique. Short-term results, complications, and in-hospital follow-up. *Arq Bras Cardiol* 1996;66: 267–273.

175. Ho AC, Hong CL, Yang MW, et al. Stroke after intraaortic balloon counterpulsation with mobile atheroma in thoracic aorta diagnosed using transesophageal echocardiography. *Chang Gung Med J* 2002;25: 612–616.

176. Barbut D, Caplan LR. Brain complications of cardiac surgery. *Curr Prob Cardiol* 1997;22:455–476.

177. Wolman RL, Nussmeier NA, Aggarwal A, et al. for the Multicenter Study of Perioperative Ischemia (McSPI) Research Group and the Ischemia Research and Education Foundation (IREF) Investigators. Cerebal injury after cardiac surgery: Identification of a group at extraordinary risk. *Stroke* 1999;30:514–522.

178. Slogoff S, Girgis KZ, Keats AS. Etiologic factors in neuropsychiatric complications associated with cardiopulmonary bypass. *Anesth Analg* 1982;61:903–911.

179. Gilman S. Neurological complications of open heart surgery. *Ann Neurol* 1990;28:475–476.

180. The Bypass Angioplasty Revascularization Investigation (BARI) Investigators. Comparison of coronary bypass surgery with angioplasty in patients with multivessel disease. *N Engl J Med* 1996;335:217–225.

181. King SB, Lembo NJ, Weintrub WS, et al. for the Emory Angioplasty versus Surgery Trial (EAST). *N Engl J Med* 1994;331:1044–1050.

182. Ricotta JJ, Char DJ, Cuadra SA, et al. Modeling stroke risk after coronary artery bypass and combined coronary artery bypass and carotid endarterectomy. *Stroke* 2003;34:1212–1217.

183. Van Dijk D, Jansen EW, Hijman R, et al Octopus Study Group. Cognitive outcome after off-pump and on-pump coronary artery bypass graft surgery: A randomized trial. *JAMA* 2002;287:1405–1412.

184. Novick RJ, Fox SA, Stitt LW, et al. Effect of off-pump coronary artery bypass grafting on risk-adjusted and cumulative sum failure outcomes after coronary artery surgery. *J Card Surg* 2002;17:520–528.

185. Roach GW, Kanchuger MS, Mora Mangano CT, et al. for the Multicenter Study of Perioperative Ischemia (McSPI) Research Group. Ad-

verse cerebral outcomes after coronary bypass surgery. *N Engl J Med* 1996;335:1857–1863.

186. Gansera B, Angelis I, Weingartner J, et al. Simultaneous carotid endarterectomy and cardiac surgery—Additional risk or safety procedure? *Thorac Cardiovasc Surg* 2003;51:22–27.

187. Aklog L, Adams DH, Couper GS, et al. Techniques and results of direct-access minimally invasive mitral valve surgery: A paradigm for the future. *J Thorac Cardiovasc Surg* 1998;116:705–715.

188. Shaw PJ, Bates D, Cartlidge NEF, et al. Early neurological complications of coronary artery bypass surgery. *Br Med J* 1985;291:1384–1387.

189. Breuer AC, Furlan AJ, Hanson MR, et al. Central nervous system complications of coronary artery bypass graft surgery: Prospective analysis of 421 patients. *Stroke* 1983;14:682–687.

190. Ropper AH, Wechsler LR, Wilson LS. Carotid bruit and the risk of stroke in elective surgery. *N Engl J Med* 1982;307:1388–1390.

191. Furlan AJ, Craciun AR. Risk of stroke during coronary artery bypass graft surgery in patients with internal carotid artery disease documented by angiography. *Stroke* 1985;16:797–799.

192. Sila C. Neuroimaging of cerebral infarction associated with coronary revascularization. *AJNR* 1991;12:817–818.

193. VonReutern G-M, Hetzel A, Birnbaum D, Schlosser V. Transcranial Doppler ultrasound during cardiopulmonary bypass in patients with internal carotid artery disease documented by angiography. *Stroke* 1988;19:674–680.

194. Hertzer NR, Loop FD, Beven EG, et al. Surgical staging for simultaneous coronary and carotid disease: A study including prospective randomization. *Vasc Surg* 1989;9:455–463.

195. Naylor AR, Cuffe RL, Rothwell PM, Bell PR. A systematic review of outcomes following staged and synchronous carotid endarterectomy and coronary artery bypass. *Eur J Vasc Endovasc Surg* 2003;25:380–389.

196. Hise JH, Nippu ML, Schnitker JC. Stroke associated with coronary artery bypass surgery. *AJNR* 1991;12:811–814.

197. Wijdicks EFM, Jack CR. Coronary artery bypass grafting-associated stroke. *J Neuroimag* 1996;6:20–22.

198. Tettenborn B, Caplan LR, Sloan MA, et al. Postoperative brainstem cerebellar infarcts. *Neurology* 1993;43:471–477.

199. Mills SA. Risk factors for cerebral injury and cardiac surgery. *Ann Thorac Surg* 1995;59:1796–1799.

200. Lynn GM, Stefanko K, Reed JF III, et al. Risk factors for stroke after coronary artery bypass. *J Thorac Cardiovasc Surg* 1992;104:1518–1523.

201. Mangano DT, Mora Mangano CT. Perioperative stroke encephalopathy and CNS dysfunction. *J Intensive Care Med* 1997;12:148–160.

202. Barbut D, Hinton RB, Szatrowski TP, et al. Cerebral emboli detected during bypass surgery are associated with clamp removal. *Stroke* 1994;25:2398–2402.

203. Pugsley W, Paschalis C, Treasure T, et al. The impact of microemboli during cardiopulmonary bypass on neuropsychological functioning. *Stroke* 1994;25:1393–1399.

204. Price DL, Harris J. Cholesterol emboli in cerebral arteries are a complication of retrograde aortic perfusion during cardiac surgery. *Neurology* 1970;20:1207–1214.

205. Tunick PA, Culliford AT, Lamparello PJ, Kronzon I. Atheromatosis of the aortic arch as an occult source of multiple systemic emboli. *Ann Intern Med* 1991;114:391–392.

206. Karalis DG, Chandrasekaran K, Victor MF, et al. Recognition and embolic potential of intraaortic atherosclerotic debris. *J Am Coll Cardiol* 1991;17:73–78.

207. Marshall JNG, Barzilai B, Kouchoukos N, Saffitz J. Intraoperative ultrasonic imaging of the ascending aorta. *Ann Thorac Surg* 1989;48:339–344.

208. Gardner TJ, Horneffer PJ, Manolio TA, et al. Stroke following coronary artery bypass grafting: A ten-year study. *Ann Thorac Surg* 1985;40:574–581.

209. Petaja J, Peltola K, Sairanen H, et al. Fibrinolysis, antithrombin III, and protein C in neonates during cardiac operations. *J Thorac Cardiovasc Surg* 1996;112:665–671.

210. Parolari A, Colli S, Mussoni L, et al. *J Thorac Cardiovasc Surg* 2003;125:336–343.

211. Gilman S. Cerebral disorders after open-heart operations. *N Engl J Med* 1965;272:489–498.

212. Coffey CE, Massey EW, Roberts KB, et al. Natural history of cerebral complications of coronary artery bypass graft surgery. *Neurology* 1983;33:1416–1421.

213. Moody DM, Bell MA, Challa VR, et al. Brain microemboli during cardiac surgery or aortography. *Ann Neurol* 1990;28:477–486.

214. Feeney DM, Gonzalez A, Law WA. Amphetamine, haloperidol and experience interact to affect the rate of recovery after motor cortex injury. *Science* 1982;217:855–857.

215. Houda DA, Feeney DM. Haloperidol blocks amphetamine induced recovery of binocular depth perception after bilateral visual cortex lesions in the cat. *Proc West Pharmacol Soc* 1985;28:209–211.

216. Humphreys RP, Hoffman JH, Mustard WT, Trusler GA. Cerebral hemorrhage following heart surgery. *J Neurosurg* 1975;43:671–675.

217. Sila CA. Spectrum of neurologic events following cardiac transplantation. *Stroke* 1989;20:1586–1589.

218. Caplan LR. Intracerebral hemorrhage revisited. *Neurology* 1988;38:624–627.

219. Lederman RJ, Breuer AC, Hanson MR, et al. Peripheral nervous system complications of coronary artery bypass graft surgery. *Ann Neurol* 1982;12:297–301.

220. Caplan LR, Hurst JW. Cardiac and cardiovascular findings in patients with nervous system disease—Strokes. In: Caplan LR, Hurst JW, Chimowitz MI (eds). *Clinical Neurocardiology*. New York: Marcel Dekker; 1999:303–312.

221. Natelson BH. Neurocardiology: An interdisciplinary area for the 80's. *Arch Neurol* 1985;42:178–184.

222. Schlesinger MJ, Reiner L. Focal myocytolysis of heart. *Am J Pathol* 1955;31:443–459.

223. Smith RP, Tomlinson BE. Subendocardial hemorrhages associated with intracranial lesions. *J Pathol Bacteriol* 1954;68:327–334.

224. Norris JW, Hachinski V. Cardiac dysfunction following stroke. In: Furlan AJ (ed). *The Heart and Stroke*. London: Springer-Verlag; 1987:171–183.

225. Cropp GJ, Manning GW. Electrocardiographic changes stimulating myocardial ischemia and infarction associated with spontaneous intracranial hemorrhage. *Circulation* 1960;22:25–38.

226. Kolin A, Norris JW. Myocardial damage from acute cerebral lesions. *Stroke* 1984;15:990–993.

227. Samuels MA. Electrocardiographic manifestations of neurologic disease. *Semin Neurol* 1984;4:453–459.

228. Myers MG, Norris JW, Hachinski V, Sole MJ. Plasma norepinephrine in stroke. *Stroke* 1981;12:200–204.

229. Marion DW, Segal R, Thompson ME. Subarachnoid hemorrhage and the heart. *Rev Neurosurg* 1986;18:101–106.

230. Haggendal J, Johansson G, Jonsson L, et al. Effect of propranolol on myocardial cell necrosis and blood levels of catecholamines in pigs subjected to stress. *Acta Pharmacol Toxicol* 1982;50:58–66.

231. Hunt D, Gore J. Myocardial lesions following experimental intracranial hemorrhage. *Am Heart J* 1972;83:232–236.

232. Samuels M. "Voodoo" death revisited: The modern lessons of neurocardiology. *Neurologist* 1997;3:293–304.

233. Burch GE, Myers R, Abildskov JA. A new electrocardiographic pattern observed in cerebrovascular accidents. *Circulation* 1954;9:719–723.

234. Dimant J, Grob D. Electrocardiographic changes and myocardial damage in patients with acute cerebrovascular accidents. *Stroke* 1977;8:448–455.

235. Rolak LA, Rokey R. Electrocardiographic features: In: Rolak LA, Rokey R (eds). *Coronary and Cerebral Vascular Disease*. Mt. Kisco, NY: Futura; 1990:139–197.

236. Goldstein DS. The electrocardiogram in stroke: Relationship to pathophysiological type and comparison with prior tracings. *Stroke* 1979;10:253–259.

237. Mayer SA, Homma S, Lennihan L, et al. Myocardial injury and left ventricular performance after subarachnoid hemorrhage. *Stroke* 1999;30:780–786.

238. Puleo P. Cardiac enzyme assessment. In: Rolak L, Rokey R (eds). *Coronary and Cerebral Vascular Disease.* Mt. Kisco, NY: Futura; 1990:199–216.

239. Fabinyi G, Hunt D, McKinley L. Myocardial creatine kinase isoenzyme in serum after subarachnoid hemorrhage. *J Neurol Neurosurg Psychiatry* 1977;40:818–820.

240. Neil-Dwyer G, Cruickshank J, Stratton C. Beta-blockers, plasma total creatine kinase and creatine kinase myocardial isoenzyme, and the prognosis of subarachnoid hemorrhage. *Surg Neurol* 1986;25: 163–168.

241. Myers MG, Norris JW, Hachinsky VC, et al. Cardiac sequelae of acute strokes. *Stroke* 1982;13:838–842.

242. Stober T, Sen S, Anstatt T, Bette L. Correlation of cardiac arrhythmias with brainstem compression in patients with intracerebral hemorrhage. *Stroke* 1988;19:688–692.

243. Hoff JT, Nishimura M. Experimental neurogenic pulmonary edema in cats. *J Neurosurg* 1978;18:383–389.

244. Wier BK. Pulmonary edema following fatal aneurysmal rupture. *J Neurosurg* 1978;49:502–507.

245. Theodore J, Robin ED. Pathogenesis of neurogenic pulmonary edema. *Lancet* 1975;2:749–751.

246. Engel GL. Psychologic factors in instantaneous cardiac death. *N Engl J Med* 1976;294:664–665.

247. Engel GL. Psychologic stress, vasodepressor (vasovagal) syncope and sudden death. *Ann Intern Med* 1978;89:403–412.

248. Lown B. Sudden cardiac death: The major challenge confronting contemporary cardiology. *Am J Cardiol* 1979;43:313–328.

249. Lown B, Temte JV, Reich P, et al. Basis for recurring ventricular fibrillation in the absence of coronary heart disease and its management. *N Engl J Med* 1976;294:623–629.

250. Talman WT. Cardiovascular regulation and lesions of the central nervous system. *Ann Neurol* 1985;18:1–12.

251. Schwartz PJ, Stone HL, Brown AM. Effects of unilateral stellate ganglion blockage on the arrhythmias associated with coronary occlusion. *Am Heart J* 1976;92:589–599.

252. Adams H, Kassell N, Mazuz H. The patients with transient ischemic attacks. Is this the time for a new therapeutic approach? *Stroke* 1984; 15:371–375.

253. Hennerici M, Aulich A, Sandmann W, Freund HJ. Incidence of asymptomatic extracranial arterial disease. *Stroke* 1981;12:750–758.

254. Caplan LR. Cerebrovascular disease: Large artery occlusive disease. In: Appel S (ed). *Current Neurology:* Vol 87. Chicago: Year Book; 1988:179–226.

255. McMillan DE. Blood flow and the localization of atherosclerotic plaques. *Stroke* 1985;16:582–587.

256. Zarins CK, Giddins DP, Bharadvaj BK, et al. Carotid bifurcation atherosclerosis. *Circ Res* 1983;53:502–514.

257. Hutchinson EC, Yates DO. The cervical portion of the vertebral artery: A clinicopathologic study. *Brain* 1956;79:319–331.

258. Fisher CM, Ojemann RG. A clinico-pathologic study of carotid endarterectomy plaques. *Rev Neurol (Paris)* 1986;142:573–589.

259. Caplan LR, Gorelick PB, Hier DB. Race, sex, and occlusive vascular disease: A review. *Stroke* 1986;17:648–655.

260. Gorelick PB, Caplan LR, Hier DB, et al. Racial differences in the distribution of posterior circulation occlusive disease. *Stroke* 1985;16: 785–790.

261. Gorelick PB, Caplan LR, Hier DB, et al. Racial differences in the distribution of anterior circulation occlusive cerebrovascular disease. *Neurology* 1984;34:54–59.

262. Feldmann E, Daneault N, Kwan E, et al. Chinese-white differences in the distribution of occlusive cerebrovascular disease. *Neurology* 1990; 40:1541–1545.

263. Caplan LR, Wolpert SM. Angiography in patients with occlusive cerebrovascular disease: Views of a stroke neurologist and neuroradiologist. *AJNR* 1991;12:593–601.

264. Pessin MS, Duncan GW, Mohr JP, Poskanzer DC. Clinical and angiographic features of carotid transient ischemic attacks. *N Engl J Med* 1977;296:358–362.

265. Caplan LR, Hennerici M. Impaired clearance of emboli is an important link between hypoperfusion, embolism,and ischemic stroke. *Arch Neurol* 1998;55:1475–1482.

266. Chambers BR, Norris JW. Outcome in patients with asymptomatic neck bruits. *N Engl J Med* 1986;315:860–865.

267. Hennerici M, Hulsbomer HB, Rautenberg W, Hefter H. Spontaneous history of asymptomatic internal carotid occlusion. *Stroke* 1986;17: 718–722.

268. Ringelstein EB, Zeumer H, Angelou D. The pathogenesis of strokes from internal carotid artery occlusion: Diagnostic and therapeutical implications. *Stroke* 1983;14:867–875.

269. Caplan LR, Tettenborn B. Vertebrobasilar occlusive disease: Review of selected aspects. 2. Posterior circulation embolism. *Cerebrovasc Dis* 1992;2:320–326.

270. Gorelick PB, Hier DB, Caplan LR, Langenberg P. Headache in acute cerebrovascular disease. *Neurology* 1986;36:1445–1450.

271. Pessin MS, Hinton RC, Davis KR, et al. Mechanism of acute carotid stroke. *Ann Neurol* 1979;6:245–252.

272. Caplan LR. TIAs—We need to return to the question, what is wrong with Mr. Jones? *Neurology* 1988;791–793.

273. Caplan LR. Significance of unexpected (silent) brain infarcts. In: Caplan LR, Shifrin EG, Nicolaides AN, Moore WS (eds). *Cerebrovascular ischaemia, investigation and management,* London: Med-Orion; 1996:423–433.

274. Hennerici M, Freund H. Efficacy of C-W Doppler and duplex system examinations for the evaluation of extracranial carotid disease. *J Clin Ultrasound* 1984;12:155–161.

275. O'Donnell TF, Erdoes L, Mackey WC, et al. Correlation of B-mode ultrasound imaging and arteriography with pathologic findings at carotid endarterectomy. *Arch Surg* 1985;120:443–449.

276. Zwiebel WJ, Zagzebski JA, Crummy AB, Hirscher M. Correlation of peak Doppler frequency with lumen narrowing in carotid stenosis. *Stroke* 1982;13:386–391.

277. Hennerici M, Rautenberg W, Sitzer G, Schwartz A. Transcranial Doppler ultrasound for the assessment of intracranial arterial flow velocity: I. Examination technique and normal values. *Surg Neurol* 1986; 315:860–865.

278. Russell D, Madden KP, Clark WM, et al. Detection of arterial emboli using Doppler ultrasound in rabbits. *Stroke* 1991;22:253–258.

279. Spencer MP, Thomas GI, Nicholls SC, Sauvage LR. Detection of middle cerebral artery emboli during carotid endarterectomy using transcranial Doppler ultrasonography. *Stroke* 1990;21:415–423.

280. Edelman RR, Mattle HP, Atkinson DJ, Hoogewoud HM. MR angiography. *AJR* 1990;154:937–946.

281. Caplan LR, DeWitt LD, Breen JC. Neuroimaging in patients with cerebrovascular disease. In: Greenberg J (ed), *Neuroimaging, A companion to Adams and Victor's Principles of Neurology,* New York: McGraw-Hill; 1999:493–520.

282. Caplan LR. Treatment of cerebral ischemia: Where are we headed? *Stroke* 1984;15:571–574.

283. Caplan LR. Are terms such as completed stroke or RIND of continued usefulness? *Stroke* 1983;14:431–433.

284. Warach S, Gaa J, Siewert B, et al. Acute human stroke studied by whole brain echo planar diffusion-weighted nagnetic resonance imaging. *Ann Neurol* 1995;37:231–141.

285. Sorensen AG, Buonanno F, Gonzalez RG, et al. Hyperacute stroke: Evaluation with combined multisection diffusion-weighted and hemodynamically weighted echo-planar MR imaging. *Radiology* 1996;199:391–401.

286. North American Symptomatic Carotid Endarterectomy Trial (NASCET) Collaborators. Beneficial effect of carotid endarterectomy in symptomatic patients with high-grade carotid stenosis. *N Engl J Med* 1991;325:445–453.

287. Barnett HJM, Taylor DW, Eliasziw M, et al. for the North American Symptomatic Carotid Endarterectomy Trial Collaborators. Benefit of carotid endarterectomy in patients with symptomatic moderate or severe stenosis. *N Engl J Med* 1998;339:1415–1425.

288. European Carotid Surgery Trialist's Collaborative Group. MRC European Carotid Surgery Trial: Interim results for symptomatic patients

with severe (70–99 percent) or with mild (0–29 percent) carotid stenosis. *Lancet* 1991;1:1235–1243.

289. European Carotid Surgery Trialist's Collaborative Group. Randomised trial of endarterectomy for recently symptomatic carotid stenosis: Final results of the MRC European Carotid Surgery Trial (ECST) *Lancet* 1998;351:1379–1387.

290. Executive Committee for the Asymptomatic Carotid Atherosclerosis Study. Endarterectomy for asymptomatic carotid artery stenosis. *JAMA* 1995;273:1421–1428.

291. Berguer R, Caplan LR (eds). *Vertebrobasilar Arterial Disease.* St Louis: Quality Medical Publishers; 1991:201–261.

292. Fields WS, Lemak NA, Frankowski RF, Hardy RJ. Controlled trial of aspirin in cerebral ischemia. *Stroke* 1977;8:301–314.

293. Antiplatelet Trialists' Collaboration. Collaborative overview of randomised trials of antiplatelet therapy—1. Prevention of death, myocardial infarction, and stroke by prolonged asntiplatelet therapy in various categories of patients. *BMJ* 1994;308:81–106.

294. Hass WK, Easton JD, Adams HP, et al. A randomized trial comparing ticlopidine hydrochloride with aspirin for the prevention of stroke in high risk patients. *N Engl J Med* 1989;321:501–507.

295. Warlow CP. Ticlopidine, a new antithrombotic drug: But is it better than aspirin for long term use? *J Neurol Neurosurg Psychiatry* 1990; 53:185–187.

296. CAPRIE Steering Committee. A randomised, blinded, trial of clopidogrel versus aspirin in patients at risk of ischaemic events. *Lancet* 1996;348:1329–1339.

297. Diener HC, Cunha L, Forbes C, et al. European Stroke Prevention Study 2. Dipyridamole and acetylsalicylic acid in the secondary prevention of stroke. *J Neurol Sci* 1996;143:1–13.

298. The National Institute of Neurological Disorders and Stroke rt-PA Study Group. Tissue plasminogen activator for acute ischemic stroke. *N Engl J Med* 1995;333:1581–1587.

299. del Zoppo GJ, Poeck K, Pessin MS, et al. Recombinant tissue plasminogen activator in acute thrombotic and embolic stroke. *Ann Neurol* 1992;32:78–86.

300. Wolpert SM, Bruckmann H, Greenlee R, et al. Neuroradiologic evaluation of patients with acute stroke treated with recombinant tissue plasminogen activator. *AJNR* 1993;14:3–13.

301. Pessin MS, del Zoppo GJ, Furlan AJ. Thrombolytic treatment in acute stroke: Review and update of selected topics. In: Moskowitz MA, Caplan LR (eds). *Cerebrovascular Diseases: Nineteenth Princeton Stroke Conference.* Boston: Butterworth-Heinemann; 1995:409–418.

302. Furlan A, Higashida R, Wechsler L, et al. Intra-arterial prourokinase for acute ischemic stroke. The PROACT II study: A randomized controlled trial. Prolyse in Acute Cerebral Thromboembolism. *JAMA* 1999;282:2003–2011.

303. Caplan LR, Mohr JP, Kistler JP, et al. Should thrombolytic therapy be the first-line treatment for acute ischemic stroke? *N Engl J Med* 1997; 337:1309–1313.

304. Caplan LR. Intracranial branch atheromatous disease. *Neurology* 1989;39:1246–1250.

305. Caplan LR. Lacunar infarction: A neglected concept. *Geriatrics* 1976; 31:71–75.

306. Caplan LR. Binswanger's disease revisited. *Neurology* 1995;45: 626–633.

307. Fisher CM. The arterial lesions underlying lacunes. *Acta Neuropathol* 1969;12:1–15.

308. Fisher CM. Lacunes, small deep cerebral infarcts. *Neurology* 1965; 15:774–784.

309. Kase CS, Caplan LR. *Intracerebral Hemorrhage.* Boston: Butterworth-Heinemann; 1994.

310. Rosenblum WI. Miliary aneurysms and "fibrinoid" degeneration of cerebral blood vessels. *Hum Pathol* 1977;8:133–139.

311. Cole F, Yates P. Intracerebral microaneurysms and small cerebrovascular lesions. *Brain* 1966;90:759–767.

312. Fisher CM. Pathological observations in hypertensive cerebral hemorrhage. *J Neuropathol Exp Neurol* 1971;30:536–550.

313. Fisher CM. Cerebral miliary aneurysms in hypertension. *Am J Pathol* 1972;66:314–324.

314. Fisher CM, Caplan LR. Basilar artery branch occlusion: A cause of pontine infarction. *Neurology* 1971;21:900–905.

315. Fisher CM. Bilateral occlusion of basilar artery branches. *J Neurol Neurosurg Psychiatry* 1977;40:1182–1189.

316. Mohr JP. Lacunes. *Stroke* 1982;13:3–11.

317. Fisher CM. Lacunar strokes and infarcts: A review. *Neurology* 1982; 32:871–876.

318. Fisher CM. Pure motor hemiplegia of vascular origin. *Arch Neurol* 1965;13:30–44.

319. Fisher CM. Pure sensory stroke and allied conditions. *Stroke* 1982; 13:434–447.

320. Fisher CW. Ataxic hemiparesis. *Arch Neurol* 1978;35:126–128.

321. Fisher CM. A lacunar stroke, the dysarthric-clumsy hand syndrome. *Neurology* 1967;17:614–617.

322. Hachinski VC, Potter P, Merskey H. Leukoariosis. *Arch Neurol* 1987; 44:21–23.

323. Caplan LR, Schoene W. Subcortical arteriosclerotic encephalopathy (Binswanger disease): Clinical features. *Neurology* 1978;28:1206–1219.

324. Babikian V, Ropper AH. Binswanger's disease: A review. *Stroke* 1987; 18:2–12.

325. Kase CS. Intracerebral hemorrhage: Non-hypertensive causes. *Stroke* 1986;17:590–594.

326. Bahemuka M. Primary intracerebral hemorrhage and heart weight: A clinicopathological case-control review of 218 patients. *Stroke* 1987;18:531–536.

327. Brott T, Thalinger K, Hertzberg V. Hypertension as a risk factor for spontaneous intracerebral hemorrhage. *Stroke* 1986;17:1078–1083.

328. Fisher CM. Pathological observations in hypertensive cerebral hemorrhages. *J Neuropathol Exp Neurol* 1971;30:536–550.

329. Linfante I, Linas RH, Caplan LR, Warach S. MRI features of intracerebral hemorrhage within 2 hours from symptoms onset. *Stroke* 1999;30:2263–2267.

330. Tuhrim S, Dambrosia JM, Price TR, et al. Prediction of intracerebral hemorrhage survival. *Ann Neurol* 1988;24:258–263.

331. Adams HP, Jergenson DD, Kassell NF, Sahs AL. Pitfalls in the recognition of subarachnoid hemorrhage. *JAMA* 1980;244:794–796.

332. Ostergaard JR. Warning leaks in subarachnoid hemorrhage. *BMJ* 1990;301:190–191.

333. Weisberg L. Computed tomography in aneurysmal subarachnoid hemorrhage. *Neurology* 1979;29:802–808.

334. Caplan LR, Flamm ES, Mohr JP, et al. Lumbar puncture and stroke. *Stroke* 1987;18:540A–544A.

335. Heros R, Zervas NT, Varsos V. Cerebral vasospasm after subarachnoid hemorrhage: An update. *Ann Neurol* 1983;14:599–608.

336. Kassell N, Sasaki T, Colohan A, Nazar G. Cerebral vasospasm following aneurysmal subarachnoid hemorrhage. *Stroke* 1985;16:562–572.

337. MacDonald RL, Weir BK. A review of hemoglobin and the pathogenesis of cerebral vasospasm. *Stroke* 1991;22:971–982.

338. Wilkins RH. Attempts at prevention or treatment of intracranial arterial spasm: An update. *Neurosurgery* 1986;18:808–825.

339. Weir B, Grace M, Hansen J, Rothberg C. Time course of vasospasm in man. *J Neurosurg* 1978;48:173–178.

340. Kwak R, Niizuma H, Ohi T, Suzuki J. Angiographic study of cerebral vasospasm following rupture of intracranial aneurysms: I. Time of the appearance. *Surg Neurol* 1979;11:257–262.

341. Sloan MA, Haley EC, Kassell NF, et al. Sensitivity and specificity of transcranial Doppler ultrasonography in the diagnosis of vasospasm following subarachnoid hemorrhage. *Neurology* 1989;39:1514–1518.

342. Davis S, Andrews J, Lichtenstein M, et al. A single-photon emission computed tomography study of hypoperfusion after subarachnoid hemorrhage. *Stroke* 1990;21:252–259.

343. Hart RG, Kanter MC. Hematologic disorders and ischemic stroke: A selective review. *Stroke* 1990;20:1111–1121.

344. Coull BM, Goodnight SH. Current concepts of cerebrovascular disease and stroke: Antiphospholipid antibodies, prothrombotic states and stroke. *Stroke* 1990;21:1370–1374.

345. Feinberg WM, Bruck DC, Ring ME. Hemostatic markers in acute stroke. *Stroke* 1989;20:592–597.

346. Holliday P, Mammen E, Buday J, et al. "Sticky platelet" syndrome and cerebral infarction. *Neurology* 1983;33(suppl 2):145.

347. Wu K, Hoak J. Increased platelet aggregation in patients with transient ischemic attacks. *Stroke* 1975;6:521–524.

348. Feinberg WM. Coagulation. In: Caplan LR (ed). *Brain Ischemia: Basic Concepts and Clinical Relevance.* London: Springer-Verlag; 1995: 85–96.

349. Hart R, Miller V, Coull B, Bril V. Cerebral infarction associated with lupus anticoagulants: Preliminary report. *Stroke* 1984;15:114–118.

350. Levine SR, Welch KMA. The spectrum of neurologic disease associated with antiphospholipid antibodies, lupus anticoagulants, and anticardiolipin antibodies. *Arch Neurol* 1987;44:876–883.

351. Kushner M, Simonian N. Lupus anticoagulant, anticardiolipin antibodies and cerebral ischemia. *Stroke* 1989;20:225–229.

352. Levine SR, Langer SL, Albers JW, Welch KMA. Sneddon's syndrome: An antiphospholipid antibody syndrome. *Neurology* 1988;38:798–800.

353. Rebollo M, Vol JF, Garijil F, et al. Livedo reticularis and cerebrovascular lesions (Sneddon's syndrome): Clinical, radiologic, and pathologic features in eight cases. *Brain* 1983;106:965–979.

354. Bruyn RP, VanderVeen JP, Donker AJ, et al. Sneddon's syndrome: Case report and literature review. *J Neurol Sci* 1987;79:243–253.

355. Antiphospholipid Antibodies in Stroke Study Group (APASS). Clinical and laboratory findings in patients with antiphospholipid antibodies and cerebral ischemia. *Stroke* 1990;21:1268–1273.

356. DeWitt LD, Caplan LR. Antiphospholipid antibodies and stroke. *AJNR* 1991;12:454–456.

357. Asherson RA. A "primary antiphospholipid syndrome"? (editorial). *J Rheumatol* 1988;15:1742–1746.

358. Coull BM, Boudette DN, Goodnight SH, et al. Multiple cerebral infarction and dementia associated with anticardiolipin antibodies. *Stroke* 1987;18:1107–1112.

359. Amico L, Caplan LR, Thomas C. Cerebrovascular complications of mucinous cancers. *Neurology* 1989;39:522–526.

360. Kase C, Robinson R, Stein R, et al. Anticoagulant-related intracerebral hemorrhage. *Neurology* 1985;35:943–948.

361. Bovill EG, Terrin ML, Stump DC, et al. Hemorrhagic events during therapy with recombinant tissue-type plasminogen activator, heparin, and aspirin for acute myocardial infarction. *Ann Intern Med* 1991; 115:256–265.

362. Kase CS, Pessin MS, Zivin JA, et al. Intracranial hemorrhages following coronary thrombolysis with tissue plasminogen activator. *Am J Med* 1992;92:384–390.

363. Babikian V, Kase C, Pessin M, et al. Resumption of anticoagulation after intracranial bleeding in patients with prosthetic valves. *Stroke* 1988;19:407–408.

364. Hart RG,, Easton JD. Dissections of cervical and cerebral arteries. *Neurol Clin North Am* 1983;1:255–282.

365. Anson J, Crowell RM. Cervicocranial arterial dissection. *Neurosurgery* 1991;29:89–96.

366. Caplan LR, Zarins CK, Hemmati M. Spontaneous dissection of the extracranial vertebral arteries. *Stroke* 1985;16:1030–1036.

367. Mas JL, Bousser MG, Hasboun D, Laplane D. Extracranial vertebral artery dissections. *Stroke* 1987;18:1037–1047.

368. Mokri B, Houser W, Sandok B, Piepgras D. Spontaneous dissections of the vertebral arteries. *Neurology* 1988;38:880–885.

369. Ojemann RG, Fisher CM, Rich JC. Spontaneous dissecting aneurysms of the internal carotid artery. *Stroke* 1972;3:434–440.

370. Hennerici M, Steinke W, Rautenberg W. High-resistance Doppler flow pattern in extracranial carotid dissection. *Arch Neurol* 1989;46: 670–672.

371. Berger MS, Wilson CB. Intracranial dissecting aneurysms of the posterior circulation. *J Neurosurg* 1984;61:882–894.

372. Friedman AH, Drake CG. Subarachnoid hemorrhage from intracranial dissecting aneurysm. *J Neurosurg* 1984;60:325–334.

THE NONSURGICAL APPROACH TO CAROTID DISEASE

Patricia A. Gum / Samir R. Kapadia / Jay S. Yadav

Carotid artery stenoses, both symptomatic and asymptomatic, increase the risk for ischemic cerebrovascular events. The long-standing "gold standard" for the invasive treatment of these lesions has been surgical carotid endarterectomy (CEA). CEA has been shown to reduce the risk of stroke when used to treat both severe asymptomatic carotid stenosis[1–3] and moderate or severe symptomatic stenosis[4–6] when compared to medical management.

Surgery, however, is not without limitations. The risk of stroke associated with CEA ranged from 2.9 to 10.7 percent in major trials.[1–6] The coronary artery disease that frequently accompanies carotid atherosclerosis contributes to the risk of peri-surgical myocardial infarction and can make the management of these patients difficult. Additionally, there are several groups of patients who are considered to be at unacceptable risk for CEA secondary to comorbid conditions such as severe coronary atherosclerotic disease, a history of head or neck radiation, previous ipsilateral CEA, or contralateral carotid occlusion.

Because of these factors as well as the inherent invasiveness and recovery time associated with the surgical treatment of carotid disease, efforts have been made to develop a nonsurgical intervention to treat atherosclerotic carotid stenosis.

CAROTID ANATOMY

Figure 100-1 demonstrates the common anatomic variations of the origins of the great vessels. The aortic arch can be classified into three types based on the distance of the origin of the great vessels from the top of the arch. The widest diameter of the left common carotid is used as a reference unit. In a type I arch (Fig. 100-1A), all of the great vessels originate within one diameter length from the top of the arch; In a type II arch (Fig. 100-1B), all the great vessels orig-inate within two diameter lengths from the top of the arch; and in a type III arch (Fig. 100-1C), the great vessels originate more than two diameter lengths from the top of the arch. A bovine arch, in which the left common carotid arises from the innominate artery, is the most common anomaly of the origins of the great vessels and occurs in approximately 20 percent of patients.

The common carotid artery bifurcates into the internal carotid artery (ICA) and the external carotid artery at the level of the C4-C5 intervertebral space. The ICA continues superiorly and gives rise to its first major branch, the ophthalmic artery, in the subarachnoid space. It then bifurcates into the anterior and middle cerebral arteries. The ICA is divided into the prepetrous, petrous, cavernous, and supraclinoid segments (Fig. 100-2).

The carotid sinus is located in the ICA just distal to the bifurcation of the common carotid artery and measures approximately 7 mm in diameter in most adults. The sinus contains mechanoreceptors, which are responsible for the carotid sinus reflex.

The external carotid artery has an extensive collateral network; therefore unilateral stenosis is rarely symptomatic. Severe stenosis or obstruction, however, may cause jaw claudication in patients with concomitant contralateral occlusion.

CAROTID ATHEROSCLEROTIC DISEASE

Epidemiology

Stroke is the third leading cause of death in the United States, causing 167,661 deaths in the year 2000. Overall, approximately 700,000 people will experience either an initial or recurrent stoke each year, with approximately 40,000 more women than men suffering a stroke

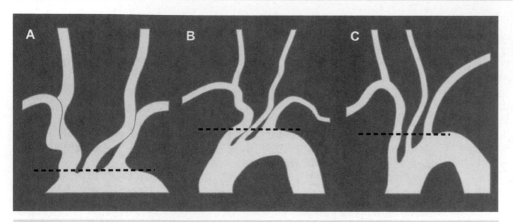

FIGURE 100-1 Aortic arch classifications.

each year. In 2000, over $51 billion dollars were spent on the diagnosis and treatment of stroke. Ischemic strokes, which are closely related to vascular stenosis, account for 88 percent of all strokes. In addition to the acute clinical and financial consequences, there are significant long-term effectsa related to stroke. Stroke is the number one cause of long-term disability, with 20 percent of victims needing institutional care 3 months after the event. Further, nearly a quarter of all stroke patients will die within 1 year following the event, and this number is even higher for those who are above age 65.[7]

Risk Factors

The common and internal carotid arteries are muscular arteries similar to those in the coronary system. They consist of an intima, media, and adventitia. It is not surprising, therefore, that the atherosclerotic disease in patients with carotid artery stenosis is very similar to that in coronary artery disease. Atheromatous plaque accumulates most frequently at sites of turbulent flow, such as the bifurcations. Exami-

nation of material collected after carotid stenting with distal emboli prevention devices (EPD) has demonstrated that the micro-emboli from these lesions contain lipid vacuoles, fibrin, platelets, and foam cells.[8] As the disease processes are very similar, it is not surprising that concomitant coronary artery disease is a significant problem for patients with carotid coronary stenosis. However, only 5 to 10 percent of patients with coronary artery disease will also have severe carotid atherosclerosis.[9]

There are several risk factors for the development of carotid atherosclerosis and its associated clinical sequelae. Stroke rates increase in a stepwise fashion with age. Tobacco use imparts a significant risk of stroke that is correlated to usage. Heavy smokers have twice the relative risk of stroke compared to light smokers, and the risk of stroke is significantly reduced within 2 years of smoking cessation, with a return to baseline at 5 years.[10] Race has also been shown to impart risk. Blacks have twice the age-adjusted risk for stroke compared to non-Hispanic Caucasians, and both male and female blacks are more likely to die secondary to strokes when compared to non-Hispanic Caucasians.[7] Hypertension and systolic blood pressure, diabetes, male gender, and hypercholesterolemia are additional risk factors that have been shown to impart an elevated risk of carotid disease.[11,12] Similar to recent work in the coronary realm, inflammation has been shown to be associated with an increased risk of carotid atherosclerosis.[13]

Natural History

The physical examination hallmark of carotid atherosclerosis is the carotid bruit. Although carotid bruits are poor predictors of the severity of atherosclerosis, they are associated with an increased risk of stroke, myocardial infarction, and death.[10,14] More specifically, once carotid atheromatous lesions have formed, the severity of stenosis as well as associated symptoms are predictive of the risk of stroke.[14] In asymptomatic carotid stenosis of ≥ 60 percent, the yearly risk of stroke has been found to be 2.1 percent.[1] The addition of symptoms such as transient ischemic attack (TIA) significantly increases the risk of stroke in patients with even moderate stenosis, and this risk increases in a stepwise fashion with the severity of stenosis. The risk of stroke following a TIA was 40 percent in the Framingham Study, and two thirds of these strokes occurred within the first 6 months.[12] The North American Symptomatic Carotid Endarterectomy Trial (NASCET) demonstrated the risk of ipsilateral stroke to be 18.7 percent over 5 years in medically treated patients with >50 percent symptomatic stenosis and 22.2 percent in those with 50 to 69 percent symptomatic stenosis.[15] There is also a dose-response association between the severity of stenosis and the risk of death. The adjusted relative risk of death for stenoses <45 percent is 1.32; for stenoses 45 to 74 percent, it is 2.22; and for stenoses 75 to 99 percent, it is 3.24.[16] Progressive carotid stenoses are more likely to be associated with adverse events.[17,18]

Clinical Presentation

Carotid bruits can be auscultated over one or both carotid arteries and have a harsh blowing quality associated with them. Evidence of a

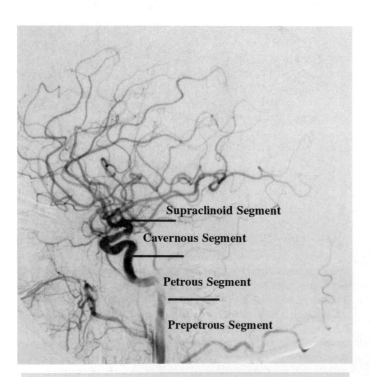

Supraclinoid Segment

Cavernous Segment

Petrous Segment

Prepetrous Segment

FIGURE 100-2 Segments of the internal carotid artery.

carotid bruit on physical examination is the most common finding leading to the diagnosis of asymptomatic carotid stenosis. The severity of the bruit, however, has not been shown to be associated with the degree of stenosis.

A transient ischemic attack (TIA) is the most common presentation of symptomatic carotid stenosis. By definition, a TIA lasts for less than 24 h and typically resolves within 30 min. Symptoms from a TIA are related to the distribution affected by the area of ischemia. Importantly, TIAs caused by vertebrobasilar insufficiency must be differentiated from those secondary to carotid origin, which can be done with careful history taking and physical examination. Carotid-related symptoms include aphasia and dysarthria. Visual disturbances such as ipsilateral amaurosis fugax or contralateral homonymous hemianopia can also be present. Sensory and motor deficits are typically contralateral. Conversely, symptoms related to vertebrobasilar insufficiency include transient cranial nerve findings, diplopia, and dysarthria. Motor deficits are ipsilateral and visual losses are frequently bilateral.

DIAGNOSIS

Noninvasive Techniques

ULTRASONOGRAPHY

The standard noninvasive method for the evaluation of carotid artery stenosis is duplex ultrasonography. Several studies have encouraged diagnosis of the severity of carotid artery stenosis on the basis of ultrasound alone, without the need for angiography.[19–23] Results concerning the diagnostic accuracy of carotid ultrasound in the centers participating in the NASCET study, however, cast some doubt on the validity of ultrasound by showing that the sensitivity and specificity of carotid ultrasound were 68 and 67 percent, respectively.[24] This poor correlation has been attributed to many factors, including variations in patient selection, imaging device performance, and the imaging protocols utilized. Ultrasound evaluation fared better in the Asymptomatic Carotid Atherosclerosis Study (ACAS). In this study, centers had to show evidence of Doppler measurements and carotid arteriography correlation, and a standard protocol was adopted, which played a part in the specificity of carotid ultrasound being measured above 95 percent.[25] Properly trained sonographers and a routine quality assurance program are critical to the sensitivity and specificity of results obtained from carotid ultrasound.

MAGNETIC RESONANCE ANGIOGRAPHY

Magnetic resonance angiography (MRA) has been used to evaluate the carotid bifurcation, as this segment of the carotid artery is relatively motionless, superficial, and large enough for visualization. Newer methods of MRA have addressed some of the shortcomings associated with initial techniques and have made better visualization possible with reliable imaging of the carotids from their origin to the intracranial branches.

Three-dimensional (3D) contrast-enhanced MRA of the carotid and thoracic aorta has made significant advancements for noninvasive examination of the extracranial carotid and the aortic arch. Prior to the evolution of 3D gadolinium contrast MRA as a standard part of MRA, it was routine to use 2D time-of-flight (TOF) and 3D-multislab TOF MRA alone. These techniques are complementary, making it important to use them together to diagnose stenoses accurately. They are limited by their flow dependence and their consequent susceptibility to flow and motion artifacts. Advantages of gadolinium-enhanced MRA for carotid angiography include the ability to image plaque ulcerations (which are often not seen on TOF), lack of flow-related artifacts (which can degrade tortuous vessels by in-plane saturation), short imaging times with excellent signal-to-noise ratio, and the ability to image from the aortic arch to circle of Willis in approximately 30 s. The contrast-enhanced magnetic resonance imaging (MRI) technique is limited by interference from contrast in the jugular vein, which may impair visualization of the carotid artery and thereby decrease the sensitivity for measuring stenoses when a long scan time is used. On the other hand, using the shorter scan time decreases the spatial resolution. A recent study comparing the sensitivity and specificity of noninvasive imaging with angiography on 569 patients demonstrated that MRA was associated with a sensitivity of 75 percent and specificity of 88 percent. However, concordant noninvasive testing with Doppler ultrasound and MRA resulted in an improved sensitivity of 96 percent and specificity of 85 percent, suggesting that surgical decisions should be made cautiously if based solely on the results of individual noninvasive studies.[26] Concordant Doppler ultrasound and MRA may result in better sensitivity and specificity, possibly reducing the need for invasive diagnostic angiography.

Invasive Techniques

ANGIOGRAPHY

The gold standard of assessing the severity of carotid stenosis severity remains the angiogram. There are several factors that make angiography unique and attractive in its detection of atherosclerotic plaque. It provides high-resolution images of the stenosis and plaque surface and is able to distinguish easily between a high-grade stenosis and occlusion. It allows the simultaneous study of the origin of the neck vessels and intracranial circulation. This is important for the detection of tandem stenoses, which pose diagnostic problems for Doppler ultrasound. The ability to assess collateral circulation as well as the speed of blood flow is quite useful in clinical decision-making, particularly in predicting the safety of temporary carotid occlusion associated with either CEA or carotid artery stenting. Additionally, angiography provides information regarding the atherosclerotic lesion and surrounding reference vessel. The risks associated with angiography include embolization and dissection, but these risks have been shown to be relatively low, particularly when angiography is performed in the cardiac catheterization laboratory.[27]

MEDICAL MANAGEMENT

Therapies with antiplatelet agents, anticoagulant agents, lipid lowering agents, and antihypertensive agents have all been studied for reducing the risk of stroke.

Antiplatelet Therapies

The long-standing foundation of antiplatelet therapy in the management of atherosclerotic disease has been aspirin. Aspirin exerts its antiplatelet effect by acetylating platelet cyclooxygenase, thereby irreversibly inhibiting the formation of platelet-dependent thromboxane. The Antithrombotic Trialists' Collaboration has documented, in its most recent metanalysis of over 200,000 patients from 287 randomized trials, the powerful effect of antiplatelet agents, primarily aspirin, in reducing both fatal and nonfatal strokes compared to control. Aspirin was found to be effective in dosages ranging from <75 mg to 1500 mg without a dose-associated difference in effect. There is substantially less data for doses <75 mg, however, which leaves uncertain the effectiveness of this small dose. This trial also reported the results from six trials that specifically evaluated the use of antiplatelet agents in patients with carotid stenosis. The sub-analysis of five carotid endarterectomy trials and one asymptomatic carotid disease trial demonstrated a 19 percent reduction in vascular events, which, although it did not reach statistical significance, demonstrated a consistent trend with that seen in other high-risk patient populations in the metanalysis.[28]

Clopidogrel and ticlopidine are thienopyridine inhibitors. They inhibit adenosine diphosphate (ADP) induced platelet aggregation by direct inhibition of ADP binding to its receptor and the subsequent activation of the glycoprotein GPIIb/IIIa complex. The Ticlopidine Aspirin Stroke Study compared the use of ticlopidine and aspirin in patients with a history of TIA, reversible ischemic neurologic deficit, or minor stroke. Ticlopidine significantly reduced the risk of fatal and nonfatal stroke by 24 percent ($p = 0.011$) compared to aspirin. This effect was even greater during the first year, with a 48 percent reduction in the risk of stroke.[29] In The Canadian American Ticlopidine Study, patients with a history of previous atherothrombotic stroke were treated with ticlopidine or placebo for up to 3 years. Ticlopidine significantly reduced the relative risk of stroke by 24 percent over 3 years ($p = 0.017$).[30] However, secondary to complications associated with ticlopidine, such as neutropenia and thrombotic thrombocytopenic purpura, the use of a newer thienopyridine inhibitor, clopidogrel, has become standard.

The Clopidogrel versus Aspirin in Patients at Risk of Ischemic Events (CAPRIE) trial was a randomized, double-blind trial that compared clopidogrel and aspirin in patients with a history of recent myocardial infarction, ischemic stroke, or peripheral vascular disease. Clopidogrel demonstrated an 8.7 percent relative risk reduction for the primary outcome of stroke, myocardial infarction, or vascular death ($p = 0.04$). In a subgroup analysis of patients with a history of a previous stroke, there was a trend toward reducing the risk of adverse events with a relative-risk reduction of 7.3 percent in favor of clopidogrel ($p = 0.26$).[31]

The Clopidogrel in Unstable Angina to Reduce Ischemic Events (CURE) study included patients with acute coronary syndrome without ST–segment elevation. Patients were randomized to receive clopidogrel or placebo and were treated for up to 1 year. All patients were also treated with aspirin. There was a 20 percent relative risk reduction in the occurrence of cardiovascular death, myocardial infarction, or stroke for the clopidogrel-treated group. Similar to findings in the CAPRIE trial, there was a trend favoring clopidogrel for the reduction of ischemic stroke (1.2 percent clopidogrel vs 1.4 percent placebo, $p =$ NS).

The ongoing Management of Atherothrombosis with Clopidogrel in High-risk Patients with Recent Transient Ischaemic Attack or Ischaemic Stroke (MATCH) trial will evaluate the efficacy and safety of clopidogrel plus aspirin versus clopidogrel alone in patients with recent TIA or ischemic stroke. The Clopidogrel for High Atherothrombotic Risk and Ischemic Stabilization, Management and Avoidance trial (CHARISMA) is also designed to investigate the role of adding clopidogrel to aspirin therapy in patients with vascular disease, including coronary or cerebrovascular disease.

Anticoagulants

Although there is evidence that warfarin reduces the risk of stroke in specific subsets of patients, such as those with atrial fibrillation,[32] there is no convincing evidence that it is superior to aspirin in patients with a history of ischemic stroke from a noncardioembolic source. The Stroke Prevention in Reversible Ischemia Trial evaluated the use of warfarin with a target international normalized ratio (INR) of 3.0 to 4.5 compared to aspirin for the prevention of adverse events in patients with a history of noncardioembolic TIA or stroke. Warfarin was associated with twice the risk of vascular death, stroke, myocardial infarction, or major bleeding complications compared to aspirin (12.4 vs. 5.4 percent, $p < 0.05$). This poor outcome was mainly attributable to excess bleeding complications, including 27 intracranial bleeds associated with warfarin.[33] The Warfarin Aspirin Recurrent Stroke Study compared warfarin with a lower target INR of 1.4 to 2.8 and aspirin in 2206 patients with a history of ischemic, noncardioembolic stroke. The rates of complications, including major hemorrhage, were not statistically different between the two treatment groups with the more conservative dosing of warfarin, and there was no difference between aspirin and warfarin for the prevention of recurrent ischemic stroke or death (17 vs. 16 percent; $p = 0.25$).[34] Thus, current data do not support the use of warfarin over aspirin for the prevention of strokes.

Antihyperlipidemics

The treatment of hyperlipidemia has been confirmed in multiple studies to confer a cardiovascular and mortality benefit.[35–37] More specifically, the use of HMG-CoA reductase inhibitors (statins) has also been shown to be of benefit in reducing stroke and treating carotid atherosclerosis. Three separate metanalyses have demonstrated a reduction in stroke with the use of statins. Bucher et al. analyzed the results from over 100,000 patients treated with statins, fibrates, resins, or dietary intervention. Only statins were associated with a reduction in the risk of stroke ($p < 0.05$).[38] Blauw et al. evaluated the effect of statins compared to placebo in over 20,000 patients. Statins were associated with a 31 percent risk reduction of stroke compared to placebo ($p < 0.05$).[39] Hebert et al. evaluated the results from over 29,000 patients. Those assigned to statin drugs experienced a 29 percent risk reduction of stroke (95 percent CI, 14 to 41 percent).[40]

There is also evidence that statin therapy has a positive effect on carotid atherosclerotic lesions. A total of 35 aortic and 25 carotid artery plaques were monitored by serial MRIs of the aorta and carotid at baseline and 6 and 12 months after initiation on simvastatin. Statin therapy was found to be associated with significant reductions in vessel wall thickness and vessel wall area over 12 months of follow up in both aortic and carotid arteries ($p < 0.001$)[41]. Further work by Corti et al. on 44 aortic and 32 carotid artery plaques detected by MRI in 21 asymptomatic hypercholesterolemic patients demonstrated not only a decrease in vessel wall thickness and vessel wall area after treatment with simvastatin but also an increase in lumen area, ranging from 4 to 6 percent at 18 and 24 months in both carotid and aortic lesions.[42] The largest study to evaluate the effect of statins on carotid stenoses to date is the Carotid Atherosclerosis Italian Ultrasound Study (CAIUS). It was performed to test the effect of lipid lowering on the progression of carotid intimal-medial thickness in 305 asymptomatic patients. Progression of intimal-medial thickness was less in the pravastatin-treated group compared to control ($p < 0.0007$).[43] These studies suggest that the benefit of statin therapy in patients with carotid artery atherosclerotic disease may in part be mediated by morphologic effects on early stages of plaque development.

HISTORY OF INVASIVE CAROTID TREATMENTS

Carotid Endarterectomy

Historically, carotid artery stenosis has been invasively treated with CEA. The first report of this was in 1954, and its use increased steadily until the mid-1980s, when questions arose concerning its effectiveness and safety.[44] Subsequent studies, however—including NASCET, the European Carotid Surgery Trialists' Collaboration (ECST), and the VA Cooperative trial—have all demonstrated a decrease in the risk of stroke for patients with severe, symptomatic carotid stenosis treated with CEA compared to medical management.[4–6] The ACAS study showed that asymptomatic patients with > 60 percent stenosis treated with CEA had a decreased risk of stroke at 5 years compared to those managed medically.[1]

Although in experienced hands CEA has been proven safe and effective for many patients with carotid stenosis, percutaneous treatment of these patients has proven promising and provided a treatment alternative for many.

Carotid Angioplasty

The first percutaneous transluminal angioplasty (PTA) of the carotid artery in humans was reported by both Kerber and Mullan in 1980.[45,46] This was followed by widespread controversy associated with the investigation of carotid PTA. In Kachel's 1996 review, the results of over 500 carotid angioplasties are presented, demonstrating a very low event rate comparable to that of CEA.[47] Concerns such as vascular recoil, distal embolization, and dissection, however, have made stand-alone carotid artery angioplasty a historical procedure that has been supplanted by carotid artery stenting and the use of emboli prevention devices.

CAROTID ARTERY STENTING

Early Experience

Significant improvements in interventional technology, including the use of stents, have allowed the field of percutaneous carotid artery intervention to grow in acceptance as an investigational procedure; it has recently been proven superior to CEA in select patient populations.[48] Carotid artery stenting successfully addressed many of the shortcomings of balloon angioplasty, including vessel recoil and

dissection, but it introduced its own unique challenges. Due to the superficial nature of the carotid arteries and their vulnerability to external forces, balloon-expandable stents have proved to be poor choices for carotid artery stenting. These stents are easy to place; but stent deformation due to external compression has been demonstrated with the Palmaz stents.[49] Self-expanding elgiloy stents (Wallstent) or nitinol stents (Precise, Memotherm, Acculink, Endostent), which continue to exert outward forces, have proven to be better suited for carotid arteries.

The first reports of the use of stents for the treatment of carotid artery disease were published by Mark and Mathias.[50,51] Since that time, several large-scale observational series have been published documenting experience with this treatment method. These are summarized in Table 100-1. The majority of patients included in these reports were at high surgical risk for CEA.

In 1996, Diethrich et al. published the first large-scale series of patients treated with carotid artery stenting. This study reported the results of 117 carotid artery stents placed in 31 symptomatic and 79 asymptomatic patients.[52] Of these, 109 (99 percent) patients were successfully treated, with 7 resultant strokes and 1 death within the first 30 days of follow-up. Over a mean follow-up of 7.6 months, there were no additional neurologic events or deaths, and the stent patency rate was 96.6 percent.

The first protocol-driven study with independent neurologic assessment prior to and following the procedure was published by Yadav et al. in 1997.[53] In 107 consecutive patients, the majority of whom met NASCET exclusion criteria for CEA, a total of 126 stenoses were treated with percutaneous carotid angioplasty with elective stenting. The success rate was 100 percent, and the 30-day risk of major stroke or death was 2.4 percent. Angiographic restenosis was noted in 3 of 61 patients who had follow-up angiography at 6 months.

In 2000, Wholey et al. published the second global review of carotid stenting.[54] In 4757 patients, 5210 carotid artery stents were placed worldwide, with a technical success rate of 98.4 percent. The risk of stroke at 30 days was 4.2 percent (2.7 percent minor and 1.5 percent major), and the mortality rate was 0.86 percent. Restenosis was 2.0 and 3.5 percent at 6- and 12-month follow-ups, respectively.

Brief Review of the Current Procedure

Carotid stenting typically requires an overnight stay, although ambulatory stenting also appears to be safe.[55] The procedure is commonly performed using a 6F to 8F femoral sheath. Heparin is used to achieve an ACT of 250 to 300 s. A guiding catheter or a sheath is

TABLE 100-1 Carotid Artery Stenting Registries

| Study | Lesions | 30-Day Outcomes | | | | | |
		Success (%)	Stroke (%)	MI (%)	Death (%)	Restenosis (%)	Follow-up
Diethrich[52]	117	99.1	8.3	0	0.9	1.7	7.6 mo
Yadav[53]	126	100	6.3	—	0.8	4.9	6 mo
Wholey[75]	114	95	3.5	0.9	1.9	1.0	6 mo
Wholey—Global Experience[54]	5210	98.4	4.21	—	0.86	3.5	1 yr
Shawl[76]	192	99	2.9	0	0	2	19 mo
Gupta[77]	100	100	1	—	0	1	12.1 mo
Reimers[78]	88	97.7	1.2	2.3	0	0	30 d

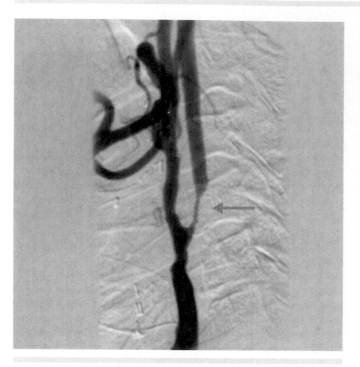

FIGURE 100-3 Internal carotid stenosis before treatment.

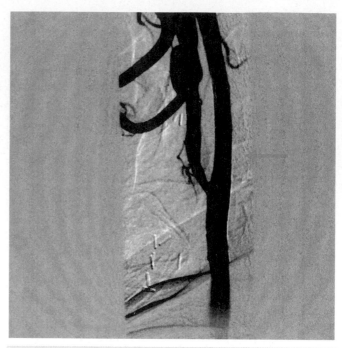

FIGURE 100-4 Internal carotid artery stenosis after stenting.

advanced to the common carotid artery, and the lesion is crossed with an emboli prevention device. The device is deployed in the internal carotid artery, and the lesion is predilated with a small coronary balloon. The lesion is then stented with a self-expanding stent, and the stent is post-dilated to the appropriate diameter. The emboli prevention device is captured and removed at the end of the procedure. Routine use of a temporary pacing wire is not necessary. Monitoring of intracardiac filling pressure is helpful in patients with severe left ventricular dysfunction or severe aortic stenosis or in those who are hemodynamically unstable. Adjunctive treatment with IIb/IIIa inhibitors has been studied in small studies and may be beneficial, but it has been largely supplanted by emboli prevention devices.[56,57] Aspirin is continued for life and clopidogrel for at least 1 month after the procedure[58] (Figs. 100-3 and 100-4).

Emboli Prevention Devices

The modern era of percutaneous carotid artery intervention was heralded by the development of the distal emboli prevention device (EPD). Numerous studies have demonstrated the occurrence of microemboli as detected by transcranial Doppler during carotid artery stenting and CEA.[59,60] There are data suggesting a correlation between the number of emboli and neurologic events after CEA.[61–63] Accordingly, numerous mechanical devices have been developed to prevent the distal embolization of debris during carotid artery stenting. There are three major types of EPD, the distal occlusive balloon, the proximal occlusive balloon, and the filter wire.

The PercuSurge GuardWire (Medtronic, Santa Rosa, CA) (Fig. 100-5) is the prototypical distal occlusive balloon EPD. A low-pressure balloon is located at the distal tip of a hollow wire. This balloon is inflated after the lesion is crossed and traps any debris released during the percutaneous procedure in the internal carotid artery, which is then aspirated prior to deflation of the balloon. The advantages of this system include a low crossing profile and superior wire flexibility. Disadvantages include the occlusive nature of this

device, which is not well tolerated in patients without good collateral flow, as well as potential damage to the distal internal carotid artery by the device. Additionally, after inflation of the balloon, angiography to localize balloon or stent placement is difficult.

Proximal occlusion balloon systems create retrograde flow in the internal carotid artery, which prevents emboli from traveling to the cerebral circulation. Like the Guardwire device, this requires occlusive balloon inflation and can cause vessel damage. Good collateral circulation is also critical. Examples of these devices include the Parodi and MOMA devices.

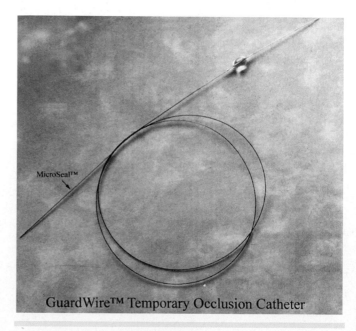

FIGURE 100-5 The Percusurge Guard Wire.

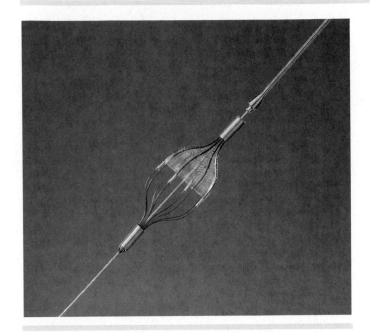

FIGURE 100-6 The Angioguard Emboli Guidewire System.

The AngioGuard Emboli Capture Guidewire (Cordis, Miami, FL) (Fig. 100-6) was the first distal filtration wire system designed to conform to the artery and trap microemboli while maintaining distal flow through a filter umbrella with multiple perfusion pores. The major advantage of filters is the preservation of flow during the intervention and the ability to visualize the vessel with contrast material throughout the procedure. Disadvantages of filters include a larger crossing profile, which may necessitate predilatation prior to placement of the filter distal to the lesion. Many other filter devices, such as Accunet by Guidant, FilterWire EX by Boston Scientific, Sulzer-IntraGuard by IntraTherapeutics, MDT-Filter by Medtronic, Microvena-Trap by Microvena, and Mednova by Abbott/Mednova, have been under investigation.

Most of the currently available data are from the case series using these devices to perform carotid stenting. (Table 100-2). These results are very encouraging and convincing regarding the efficacy of the devices in reducing procedural stroke compared to retrospective cohorts where these devices were not available. All currently ongoing randomized trials comparing carotid stenting with CEA use emboli prevention devices. Further, emboli prevention devices have become standard of care for carotid stenting procedure in clinical practice. At this time, there are no studies comparing safety and efficacy of different emboli prevention devices.

Complications and Their Management

There are several important issues, some unique to carotid artery stenting and some similar to those seen in percutaneous coronary intervention, that the physician must be mindful of to avert an adverse and potentially cata-

strophic outcome. The major periprocedural complications of carotid artery stenting are stroke, myocardial infarction, and death. The Stenting and Angioplasty with Protection in Patients at High Risk for Endarterectomy (SAPPHIRE) trial documented a 30-day risk of 5.8 percent in high-risk patients for these endpoints.[48] Other associated adverse events are intracranial hemorrhage, bradycardia, hypotension, seizures, contrast nephrotoxicities, and access site complications.

Although the majority of ischemic complications occur during the procedure, they can occur several hours later. Careful neurologic examination is essential to identify these complications. Routine use of cerebral angiography before and after stenting can help identify occluded intracranial vessels. Intraarterial thrombolytic therapy has been used to treat this complication, but with very limited success, reflecting the fact that embolic materials are commonly plaque fragments and not thrombus.[64] Further, the risk of intracranial hemorrhage with this approach is substantial. Mechanical dislodgement of the embolic debris with soft wires may be the best approach to minimize the size of cerebral infraction.

The carotid sinus reflex is most often responsible for the bradycardia and hypotension associated with carotid sinus manipulation. In anticipation of this effect, antihypertensives medications are typically held the morning of the procedure, and depending on the response to stenting, may also be held until the following morning. Adequate volume expansion is the cornerstone of effective treatment. Atropine is helpful in cases of severe bradycardia. Vasopressors may be required for severe and persistent hypotension. The carotid sinus reflex is typically transient, but it may continue to be a concern for up to 24 h after the procedure.

On the other side of the spectrum, brisk return of blood flow distal to a chronically ischemic cerebral hemisphere with disordered cerebral autoregulation can lead to problems. Hyperperfusion syndrome is a potentially deadly complication from carotid artery stenting or CEA. Severe hypertension, critical carotid stenosis, and contralateral carotid occlusion appear to be predisposing factors. Strict monitoring of blood pressure with appropriate treatment is crucial to preventing this. All patients undergoing carotid artery stenting should be instructed on the importance of medication compliance as well as home blood pressure monitoring. They should be instructed to keep their SBP below 140 mmHg. Furthermore, patients must be instructed to monitor for headaches localized to one side associated with nausea, vomiting, and photophobia. Treatment of hyperperfusion syndrome includes strict blood pressure control with the lowering of systolic blood pressure to approximately 100 mmHg.

TABLE 100-2 Experience with Devices to Prevent Emboli

Study	Procedures (N)	Device	30-Day Events (includes procedural)			
			Major Stroke	Minor Stroke	Death	all
Henry[79]	184	Guardwire	0.5%	0	0.5%	1%
Al Mubarak[80]	164	NeuroShield	0	1.2%	1.2%	2.4%
Whitlow[81]	75	Guardwire	0	0	0	0
Reimers[78]	88	Filters (3 types)	0	1%	0	1%
MacDonald[82]	50	NeuroShield	0	2%	4%	6%
Cremonesi[83]	30	TRAP VFS	NA	NA	NA	0
All	591		0.2%	0.7%	0.2%	1.6%

COMPARISONS OF CAROTID ARTERY STENTING AND CAROTID ENDARTERECTOMY

Trials

Although carotid artery stenting is a less invasive method of treating carotid artery stenosis compared to CEA, extensive evidence of the safety and feasibility of CEA have made it difficult to establish carotid artery stenting as a viable alternative. Two major studies comparing these procedures have been completed, however, and many more are currently enrolling.

The Carotid and Vertebral Artery Transluminal Angioplasty study (CAVATAS) compared the outcomes of percutaneous angioplasty and stenting to surgical CEA.[65] The results are shown in Table 100-3. There was no difference between the two treatment groups with regard to stroke or mortality. However, complications such as cranial neuropathy and significant hematoma formation occurred more often in the surgical group. Conversely, the percutaneous treatment group was more likely to experience restenosis. This trial demonstrated equivalent major outcomes with no significant difference at 1 year for ipsilateral neurologic complications. Minor complications such as bleeding and cranial nerve palsies were higher for CEA. This trial has been criticized for having higher than expected complication rates with CEA. However, the percutaneous method utilized would not be considered state-of-the-art by current standards as only 25 percent of the patients undergoing percutaneous revascularization received stents and emboli prevention devices were not utilized in this study.

More recently, results from the SAPPHIRE trial were reported at the American Heart Association Scientific Sessions, Chicago, November 2002.[48] This trial randomized 307 patients to either carotid angioplasty and stenting with emboli protection or CEA. Patients were either asymptomatic with ≥ 80 percent stenosis by ultrasound or symptomatic with ≥ 50 percent stenosis. All patients enrolled had a comorbid condition which increased the risk of CEA. The entry inclusion criteria included previous CEA, congestive heart failure, severe coronary artery disease, previous radical neck surgery or radiation therapy, and chronic obstructive pulmonary disease. Patients who in the opinion of a vascular surgeon could not have surgery were enrolled in a stent registry (409 patients). Patients considered at too high a risk for percutaneous management were likewise enrolled in a surgical registry (17 patients). The primary end point was major adverse cardiovascular events (MACE), including death, stroke, or MI within 30 days of the procedure. The 30-day MACE rate was markedly reduced in the percutaneous treatment group compared to the CEA group (5.8 vs. 12.6 percent, $p = 0.047$). In the registry data,

the 30-day MACE rate was 7.8 percent for stenting (32 of 409) and 14.3 percent (1 of 7) for CEA. There were no significant differences between the two groups with regard to either major bleeding (8.3 vs. 10.6 percent, $p = 0.56$) or transient ischemic attack (3.85 vs. 2.0 percent, $p = 0.5$), but carotid stenting did have an advantage over CEA with regard to cranial nerve injury (0 vs. 5.3 percent, $p < 0.01$). Restenosis rates were not presented. This trial clearly demonstrated a reduction in risk of MACE for high-risk patients treated with carotid stenting compared to conventional CEA.

Special Subgroups

There are several patient subgroups that have posed special challenges for the vascular surgeon contemplating a surgical approach to treatment of their carotid artery stenosis. Existing data support the treatment of these patients with carotid artery stenting instead of CEA.

Concomitant Carotid Stenosis and Coronary Artery Disease

An important issue surrounding the treatment of carotid artery atherosclerosis is the optimal treatment strategy used to treat those with both significant carotid artery disease and coronary atherosclerosis. This is not an insignificant issue, as evidenced by the 50 to 60 percent of patients with carotid artery disease who also have significant coronary atherosclerosis.[9] Approaches using CEA followed by open heart surgery (OHS), OHS followed by CEA, or combined OHS and CEA have been studied. Although the stroke, MI, and death rates vary in different series, the risk is high with all strategies (Table 100-4).[66] Recent data from the SAPPHIRE trial demonstrated that treatment of carotid disease with carotid stenting is a lower-risk procedure and is associated with a lower rate of myocardial infarction when compared to CEA. In the randomized patients, carotid stenting was associated with a 2.6 percent rate of myocardial infarction and CEA was associated with a 7.3 percent rate of myocardial infarction at 30 days ($p = 0.07$)[48]. Additionally, Ziada et al. recently evaluated the outcomes of 64 patients with both severe carotid stenosis and coronary atherosclerosis who were treated with carotid stenting followed by coronary artery bypass surgery and compared them to 112 patients who underwent combined CEA and OHS. The stent group had a much higher prevalence of unstable angina, poor left ventricular function, critical aortic valve stenosis, TIA or stroke, and history of previous OHS. Although there was no difference in mortality, the stent patients had significantly lower incidence of strokes (2 vs. 9 percent, $p = 0.05$) and strokes or MI (6 vs. 19 percent, $p = 0.02$) compared to those who received comitant CEA and OHS.[67] Antiplatelet therapy poses a challenge for patients scheduled for immediate surgery. It is preferable if patients can wait 2 to 4 weeks after stenting and be kept on aspirin and clopidogrel during this time. Anecdotal use of short-acting IIb/IIIa inhibitors until the cardiac surgery and immediate loading with clopidogrel and aspirin after the surgery has been reported to be successful. The availability of heparin-coated stents may reduce the need for dual antiplatelet therapy.

TABLE 100-3   30-Day Events from the CAVATAS Trial

Major Outcome Event	Stent (251 patients)	CEA (253 patients)	p Value
Death	3%	2%	NS
Disabling stroke	4%	4%	NS
Death/disabling stroke	6%	6%	NS
Death/any stroke	10%	10%	NS
Cranial nerve palsy	0	9%	<0.0001
Significant hematoma	1%	7%	<0.0015
Severe restenosis[a]	14%	4%	<0.001

[a]Restenosis measured at 1 year.

TABLE 100-4 Adverse Events in Patients Undergoing Carotid Endarterectomy and Coronary Artery Bypass Grafting

Treatment Strategy	Stroke	MI	Death	All Events
CEA + CABG	6.2	4.7	5.6	16.5
CEA followed by CABG	5.3	11.5[a]	9.4[a]	26.2[a]
CABG followed by CEA	10.0[a]	2.8	3.6	16.4

[a]$p < 0.05$.
SOURCE: Modified from Moore WS. *Circulation* 1995;91:566–579. With permission.

Radical Neck Surgery and Radiation Therapy

Extracranial carotid stenosis frequently occurs in patients who have had surgery and head and neck irradiation for cancer therapy. Tissue dissection is complicated by the extensive fibrosis of the arterial wall and normal tissue planes, and the difficult locations of the lesions due to extensive involvement of long segments of the carotid artery above and below the carotid bifurcation make access difficult.[68] Carotid stenting has been reported as safe and effective in the treatment of this problem.[69–73] The procedural risks are not increased compared to stenting for conventional treatment of atherosclerotic carotid disease. Therefore carotid stenting can be considered the treatment of choice for severe carotid stenosis requiring revascularization after cervical radiation or radical neck surgery.

There is a higher surgical risk for patients with restenotic lesions after CEA compared to those undergoing CEA for the first time. Occasionally, the lesion is also in an anatomically unfavorable location for surgery. These lesions can be successfully treated with percutaneous stenting with no increased risk. Data from a multicenter registry of 14 centers in the United States included 338 patients undergoing carotid stenting of 358 arteries for restenosis after carotid endarterectomy revealed an overall 30-day stroke and death rate of 3.7 percent.[74] There was 1 (0.3 percent) fatal and 1 (0.3 percent) nonfatal stroke during the follow-up period. The overall 3-year rate of freedom from all fatal and nonfatal strokes was 96 percent. These results suggest that carotid artery stenting is an excellent treatment alternative for restenosis following carotid endarterectomy.

FUTURE APPLICATIONS AND TRIALS

Several trials to evaluate the percutaneous treatment of carotid artery atherosclerosis are ongoing. The updated information on these trials is available online at www.strokecenter.org. The Carotid Revascularization Endarterectomy versus Stent Trial (CREST) is a multicenter randomized trial to compare CEA with carotid artery stenting using EPD. Unlike SAPPHIRE, the patients studied in this trial are at low risk; therefore, this trial will add insight into the use of this treatment strategy in additional patient populations. Furthermore, there are several ongoing registries for carotid artery stenting patients who are not eligible for randomized trials.

SUMMARY

Several pharmacologic therapies are important in the treatment of carotid artery atherosclerosis. Aspirin is the cornerstone of antiplatelet therapy for these patients, and there is a growing body of evidence for long-term treatment with thienopyridine inhibitors. Additionally, statin therapy should be standard in all patients with evidence of atherosclerotic disease, including those with carotid artery atherosclerosis. From an invasive standpoint, the percutaneous treatment of carotid atherosclerotic disease has made significant advances since its advent in 1980. It has proven to be a safe and preferred approach to patients at high surgical risk and may prove to have much wider application. Further investigation is ongoing concerning different patient populations and various devices that may expand the potential uses of this technique. As this procedure has the potential for significant complications, adequate training and certification will be necessary to ensure optimal patient outcomes.

References

1. Executive Committee for the Asymptomatic Carotid Atherosclerosis Study Group. Endarterectomy for asymptomatic carotid artery stenosis. Executive Committee for the Asymptomatic Carotid Atherosclerosis Study. *JAMA* 1995;273:1421–1428.
2. Hobson RW II, Weiss DG, Fields WS, et al. Efficacy of carotid endarterectomy for asymptomatic carotid stenosis. The Veterans Affairs Cooperative Study Group. *N Engl J Med* 1993;328:221–227.
3. CASANOVA Study Group. Carotid surgery versus medical therapy in asymptomatic carotid stenosis. The CASANOVA Study Group. *Stroke* 1991;22:1229–1235.
4. North American Symptomatic Carotid Endarterectomy Trial Collaborators. The beneficial effect of carotid endarterectomy in symptomatic patients with high-grade carotid stenosis. North American Symptomatic Carotid Endarterectomy Trial Collaborators. *N Engl J Med* 1991;325:445–453.
5. European Carotid Surgery Trialists' Collaborative Group. MRC European Carotid Surgery Trial: Interim results for symptomatic patients with severe (70–99%) or with mild (0–29%) carotid stenosis. European Carotid Surgery Trialists' Collaborative Group. *Lancet* 1991;337:1235–1243.
6. Mayberg MR, Wilson SE, Yatsu F, et al. Carotid endarterectomy and prevention of cerebral ischemia in symptomatic carotid stenosis. Veterans Affairs Cooperative Studies Program 309 Trialist Group. *JAMA* 1991;266:3289–3294.
7. American Heart Association. *Heart Disease and Stroke Statistics 2003 Update*. Dallas: AHA; 2003.
8. Angelini A, Reimers B, Della Barbera M, et al. Cerebral protection during carotid artery stenting: Collection and histopathologic analysis of embolized debris. *Stroke* 2002;33:456–461.
9. Hertzer NR, Beven EG, Young JR, et al. Coronary artery disease in peripheral vascular patients. A classification of 1000 coronary angiograms and results of surgical management. *Ann Surg* 1984;199:223–233.
10. Wolf PA, D'Agostino RB, Kannel WB, et al. Cigarette smoking as a risk factor for stroke. The Framingham Study. *JAMA* 1988;259:1025–1029.
11. Byington RP, Furberg CD, Crouse JR III, et al. Pravastatin, lipids, and atherosclerosis in the carotid arteries (PLAC-II). *Am J Cardiol* 1995;76:54C–59C.
12. Whisnant JP, Homer D, Ingall TJ, et al. Duration of cigarette smoking is the strongest predictor of severe extracranial carotid artery atherosclerosis. *Stroke* 1990;21:707–714.
13. Magyar MT, Szikszai Z, Balla J, et al. Early-onset carotid atherosclerosis is associated with increased intima-media thickness and elevated serum levels of inflammatory markers. *Stroke* 2003;34:58–63.
14. Norris JW, Zhu CZ, Bornstein NM, et al. Vascular risks of asymptomatic carotid stenosis. *Stroke* 1991;22:1485–1490.
15. Barnett HJ, Taylor DW, Eliasziw M, et al. Benefit of carotid endarterectomy in patients with symptomatic moderate or severe stenosis. North American Symptomatic Carotid Endarterectomy Trial Collaborators. *N Engl J Med* 1998;339:1415–1425.
16. Joakimsen O, Bonaa KH, Mathiesen EB, et al. Prediction of mortality by ultrasound screening of a general population for carotid stenosis: The Tromso Study. *Stroke* 2000;31:1871–1876.
17. Taylor LM, Jr., Loboa L, Porter JM. The clinical course of carotid bifurcation stenosis as determined by duplex scanning. *J Vasc Surg* 1988;8:255–261.

18. Fabris F, Poli L, Zanocchi M, et al. A four year clinical and echographic follow-up of asymptomatic carotid plaque. *Angiology* 1992;43:590–598.

19. Erdoes LS, Marek JM, Mills JL, et al. The relative contributions of carotid duplex scanning, magnetic resonance angiography, and cerebral arteriography to clinical decisionmaking: A prospective study in patients with carotid occlusive disease. *J Vasc Surg* 1996;23:950–956.

20. Chervu A, Moore WS. Carotid endarterectomy without arteriography. *Ann Vasc Surg* 1994;8:296–302.

21. Dawson DL, Zierler RE, Strandness DE Jr, et al. The role of duplex scanning and arteriography before carotid endarterectomy: A prospective study. *J Vasc Surg.* 1993;18:673–680; discussion 680–683.

22. Horn M, Michelini M, Greisler HP, et al. Carotid endarterectomy without arteriography: The preeminent role of the vascular laboratory. *Ann Vasc Surg* 1994;8:221–224.

23. Mattos MA, Hodgson KJ, Faught WE, et al. Carotid endarterectomy without angiography: Is color-flow duplex scanning sufficient? *Surgery* 1994;116:776–782; discussion 782–783.

24. Eliasziw M, Rankin RN, Fox AJ, et al. Accuracy and prognostic consequences of ultrasonography in identifying severe carotid artery stenosis. North American Symptomatic Carotid Endarterectomy Trial (NASCET) Group. *Stroke* 1995;26:1747–1752.

25. Howard G, Baker WH, Chambless LE, et al. An approach for the use of Doppler ultrasound as a screening tool for hemodynamically significant stenosis (despite heterogeneity of Doppler performance). A multicenter experience. Asymptomatic Carotid Atherosclerosis Study Investigators. *Stroke* 1996;27:1951–1957.

26. Johnston DC, Goldstein LB. Clinical carotid endarterectomy decision making: noninvasive vascular imaging versus angiography. *Neurology.* 2001;56:1009–1015.

27. Fayed AM, White CJ, Ramee SR, et al. Carotid and cerebral angiography performed by cardiologists: Cerebrovascular complications. *Catheter Cardiovasc Interv* 2002;55:277–280.

28. Antithrombotic Trialists' Collaboration. Collaborative meta-analysis of randomised trials of antiplatelet therapy for prevention of death, myocardial infarction, and stroke in high risk patients. *BMJ* 2002;324: 71–86.

29. Hass WK, Easton JD, Adams HP, Jr., et al. A randomized trial comparing ticlopidine hydrochloride with aspirin for the prevention of stroke in high-risk patients. Ticlopidine Aspirin Stroke Study Group. *N Engl J Med* 1989;321:501–507.

30. Gent M, Blakely JA, Easton JD, et al. The Canadian American Ticlopidine Study (CATS) in thromboembolic stroke. *Lancet* 1989;1: 1215–1220.

31. CAPRIE Steering Committee. A randomised, blinded, trial of clopidogrel versus aspirin in patients at risk of ischaemic events (CAPRIE). *Lancet* 1996;348:1329–1339.

32. Atrial Fibrillation Investigators. Risk factors for stroke and efficacy of antithrombotic therapy in atrial fibrillation. Analysis of pooled data from five randomized controlled trials. *Arch Intern Med.* 1994;154:1449–1457.

33. Stroke Prevention in Reversible Ischemia Trial Study Group. A randomized trial of anticoagulants versus aspirin after cerebral ischemia of presumed arterial origin. The Stroke Prevention in Reversible Ischemia Trial (SPIRIT) Study Group. *Ann Neurol* 1997;42:857–865.

34. Mohr JP, Thompson JL, Lazar RM, et al. A comparison of warfarin and aspirin for the prevention of recurrent ischemic stroke. *N Engl J Med* 2001;345:1444–1451.

35. 4S Study Group. Randomised trial of cholesterol lowering in 4444 patients with coronary heart disease: The Scandinavian Simvastatin Survival Study (4S). *Lancet* 1994;344:1383–1389.

36. Lipid Study Group. Prevention of cardiovascular events and death with pravastatin in patients with coronary heart disease and a broad range of initial cholesterol levels. The Long-Term Intervention with Pravastatin in Ischaemic Disease (LIPID) Study Group. *N Engl J Med* 1998;339: 1349–1357.

37. Sacks FM, Pfeffer MA, Moye LA, et al. The effect of pravastatin on coronary events after myocardial infarction in patients with average cholesterol levels. Cholesterol and Recurrent Events Trial investigators. *N Engl J Med.* 1996;335:1001–1009.

38. Bucher HC, Griffith LE, Guyatt GH. Effect of HMGcoA reductase inhibitors on stroke. A meta-analysis of randomized, controlled trials. *Ann Intern Med.* 1998;128:89–95.

39. Blauw GJ, Lagaay AM, Smelt AH, et al. Stroke, statins, and cholesterol. A meta-analysis of randomized, placebo-controlled, double-blind trials with HMG-CoA reductase inhibitors. *Stroke* 1997;28:946–950.

40. Hebert PR, Gaziano JM, Chan KS, et al. Cholesterol lowering with statin drugs, risk of stroke, and total mortality. An overview of randomized trials. *JAMA* 1997;278:313–321.

41. Corti R, Fayad ZA, Fuster V, et al. Effects of lipid-lowering by simvastatin on human atherosclerotic lesions: A longitudinal study by high-resolution, noninvasive magnetic resonance imaging. *Circulation* 2001; 104:249–252.

42. Corti R, Fuster V, Fayad ZA, et al. Lipid lowering by simvastatin induces regression of human atherosclerotic lesions: Two years' follow-up by high-resolution noninvasive magnetic resonance imaging. *Circulation* 2002;106:2884–2887.

43. Mercuri M, Bond MG, Sirtori CR, et al. Pravastatin reduces carotid intima-media thickness progression in an asymptomatic hypercholesterolemic mediterranean population: The Carotid Atherosclerosis Italian Ultrasound Study. *Am J Med* 1996;101:627–634.

44. Eastcott H, Pickering G, Rob C. Reconstruction of internal carotid artery in a patient with intermittent attacks of hemiplegia. *Lancet* 1954; 267:994–996.

45. Mullan S, Duda EE, Patronas NJ. Some examples of balloon technology in neurosurgery. *J Neurosurg* 1980;52:321–329.

46. Kerber CW, Cromwell LD, Loehden OL. Catheter dilatation of proximal carotid stenosis during distal bifurcation endarterectomy. *AJNR* 1980;1:348–349.

47. Kachel R. Results of balloon angioplasty in the carotid arteries. *J Endovasc Surg* 1996;3:22–30.

48. Yadav JS for the SAPPHIRE Investigators. Stenting and angioplasty with protection in patients at high risk for endarterectomy. In: Yadav JS, ed. *The American Heart Association Scientific Sessions.* Chicago, IL;2002.

49. Mathur A, Dorros G, Iyer SS, et al. Palmaz stent compression in patients following carotid artery stenting. *Catheter Cardiovasc Diagn* 1997;41: 137–140.

50. Mathius K. Percutaneous angioplasty in supra-aortic artery disease. In: Roubin GS, Califf R, O'Neill W, et al, eds. *Interventional Cardiovascular Medicine: Principles and Practice.* New York: Churchill Livingstone; 1994:745–775.

51. Marks MP, Dake MD, Steinberg GK, et al. Stent placement for arterial and venous cerebrovascular disease: Preliminary experience. *Radiology* 1994;191:441–446.

52. Diethrich EB, Ndiaye M, Reid DB. Stenting in the carotid artery: Initial experience in 110 patients. *J Endovasc Surg* 1996;3:42–62.

53. Yadav JS, Roubin GS, Iyer S, et al. Elective stenting of the extracranial carotid arteries. *Circulation* 1997;95:376–381.

54. Wholey MH, Wholey M, Mathias K, et al. Global experience in cervical carotid artery stent placement. *Catheter Cardiovasc Interv* 2000;50: 160–167.

55. Al-Mubarak N, Roubin GS, Vitek JJ, et al. Procedural safety and short-term outcome of ambulatory carotid stenting. *Stroke* 2001;32: 2305–2309.

56. Kapadia SR, Bajzer CT, Ziada KM, et al. Initial experience of platelet glycoprotein IIb/IIIa inhibition with abciximab during carotid stenting: A safe and effective adjunctive therapy. *Stroke* 2001;32:2328–2332.

57. Hofmann R, Kerschner K, Steinwender C, et al. Abciximab bolus injection does not reduce cerebral ischemic complications of elective carotid artery stenting: A randomized study. *Stroke.* 2002;33:725–727.

58. Bhatt DL, Kapadia SR, Bajzer CT, et al. Dual antiplatelet therapy with clopidogrel and aspirin after carotid artery stenting. *J Invasive Cardiol* 2001;13:767–771.

59. McCleary AJ, Nelson M, Dearden NM, et al. Cerebral haemodynamics and embolization during carotid angioplasty in high-risk patients. *Br J Surg* 1998;85:771–774.

60. Markus HS, Clifton A, Buckenham T, et al. Carotid angioplasty. Detection of embolic signals during and after the procedure. *Stroke* 1994;25: 2403–2406.

61. Jansen C, Ramos LM, van Heesewijk JP, et al. Impact of microembolism and hemodynamic changes in the brain during carotid endarterectomy. *Stroke* 1994;25:992–997.

62. Gaunt ME, Martin PJ, Smith JL, et al. Clinical relevance of intraoperative embolization detected by transcranial Doppler ultrasonography during carotid endarterectomy: A prospective study of 100 patients. *Br J Surg* 1994;81:1435–1439.

63. Ackerstaff RG, Jansen C, Moll FL, et al. The significance of microemboli detection by means of transcranial Doppler ultrasonography monitoring in carotid endarterectomy. *J Vasc Surg* 1995;21:963–969.

64. Wholey MH, Tan WA, Toursarkissian B, et al. Management of neurological complications of carotid artery stenting. *J Endovasc Ther* 2001;8:341–353.

65. CAVATAS Investigators T. Endovascular versus surgical treatment in patients with carotid stenosis in the Carotid and Vertebral Artery Transluminal Angioplasty Study (CAVATAS): A randomised trial. *Lancet* 2001;357:1729–1737.

66. Moore WS, Barnett HJ, Beebe HG, et al. Guidelines for carotid endarterectomy. A multidisciplinary consensus statement from the Ad Hoc Committee, American Heart Association. *Circulation* 1995;91:566–579.

67. Ziada KM, Kapadia SR, Bhatt DL, et al. Approach to carotid stenosis in patients undergoing open heart surgery: Stenting or endarterectomy? *J Am Coll Cardiol* 2001;37:1A–648A.

68. Friedell ML, Joseph BP, Cohen MJ, et al. Surgery for carotid artery stenosis following neck irradiation. *Ann Vasc Surg* 2001;15:13–18.

69. Al-Mubarak N, Roubin GS, Iyer SS, et al. Carotid stenting for severe radiation-induced extracranial carotid artery occlusive disease. *J Endovasc Ther* 2000;7:36–40.

70. Alric P, Branchereau P, Berthet JP, et al. Carotid artery stenting for stenosis following revascularization or cervical irradiation. *J Endovasc Ther* 2002;9:14–19.

71. Dangas G, Laird JR, Jr., Mehran R, et al. Carotid artery stenting in patients with high-risk anatomy for carotid endarterectomy. *J Endovasc Ther* 2001;8:39–43.

72. Paniagua D, Howell M, Strickman N, et al. Outcomes following extracranial carotid artery stenting in high-risk patients. *J Invasive Cardiol* 2001;13:375–381.

73. Houdart E, Mounayer C, Chapot R, et al. Carotid stenting for radiation-induced stenoses: A report of 7 cases. *Stroke* 2001;32:118–121.

74. New G, Roubin GS, Iyer SS, et al. Safety, efficacy, and durability of carotid artery stenting for restenosis following carotid endarterectomy: A multicenter study. *J Endovasc Ther* 2000;7:345–352.

75. Wholey MH, Jarmolowski CR, Eles G, et al. Endovascular stents for carotid artery occlusive disease. *J Endovasc Surg* 1997;4:326–338.

76. Shawl F, Kadro W, Domanski MJ, et al. Safety and efficacy of elective carotid artery stenting in high-risk patients. *J Am Coll Cardiol* 2000;35:1721–1728.

77. Gupta A, Bhatia A, Ahuja A, et al. Carotid stenting in patients older than 65 years with inoperable carotid artery disease: A single-center experience. *Catheter Cardiovasc Interv* 2000;50:1–8; discussion 9.

78. Reimers B, Corvaja N, Moshiri S, et al. Cerebral protection with filter devices during carotid artery stenting. *Circulation* 2001;104:12–15.

79. Henry M, Henry I, Klonaris C, et al. Benefits of cerebral protection during carotid stenting with the PercuSurge GuardWire system: Midterm results. *J Endovasc Ther* 2002;9:1–13.

80. Al-Mubarak N, Colombo A, Gaines PA, et al. Multicenter evaluation of carotid artery stenting with a filter protection system. *J Am Coll Cardiol* 2002;39:841–846.

81. Whitlow PL, Lylyk P, Londero H, et al. Carotid artery stenting protected with an emboli containment system. *Stroke* 2002;33:1308–1314.

82. Macdonald S, Venables GS, Cleveland TJ, et al. Protected carotid stenting: Safety and efficacy of the MedNova NeuroShield filter. *J Vasc Surg* 2002;35:966–972.

83. Cremonesi A, Castriota F. Efficacy of a nitinol filter device in the prevention of embolic events during carotid interventions. *J Endovasc Ther* 2002;9:155–159

DIAGNOSIS AND MANAGEMENT OF DISEASES OF THE PERIPHERAL ARTERIES AND VEINS

Paul W. Wennberg / Thom W. Rooke

Peripheral vascular diseases are a diverse collection of disorders that affect all organ systems. Although peripheral arterial disease (PAD) is the disease most commonly encountered by the cardiologist, disease of the lymphatics and veins is equally common (even more so globally). For the cardiologist or internist with an interest in vascular disorders, a systematic and comprehensive approach is required. This chapter will cover commonly encountered areas of vascular disease including basic strategies for management of vascular ulcers. Accompanying chapters on aortic and cerebrovascular disease will address those areas in more detail.

LYMPHEDEMA

Globally, lymphedema is the most common vascular disease, affecting 90 to 120 million people.[1] Mosquito-borne infection with filarial species is common, even endemic, in tropical countries. Cases do occur, unrelated to travel, within the contiguous United States, however. This includes traditionally "cold weather" states.[2] Worldwide efforts directed at elimination of filarial disease are ongoing.[3]

Lymphedema is an abnormal buildup of lymphatic fluid in the dermal and subcutaneous tissues. In contrast to the venous system, the superficial lymphatic vessels carry a low volume of flow. They are a fragile, easily damaged network of vessels that drain the interstitial fluid and, through peristaltic action, propel fluid proximally. Lymphatic vessels contain valves similar to those in veins. Trauma to a lymph vessel may easily damage these valves. As vessels coalesce, larger conduits are formed at the inguinal level. The lymphatic channels coalesce into the iliac and paraaortic lymphatic channels, which empty into the thoracic duct at the left subclavian vein. Lymph nodes are located along lymphatic vessels. Trauma to the nodes affects the lymphatic vessels.

Lymphedema may be primary or secondary in etiology. Primary lymphedema may be congenital (present at birth) or, more commonly, present in the early teen years (lymphedema praecox). This is more common in females and often presents around menarche. Lymphedema presenting in later years is called lymphedema tarda. This is a diagnosis of exclusion since a secondary cause is much more likely in this age group.

Secondary lymphedema is much more common than primary lymphedema. Trauma, recurrent infections, obstructive mass, infiltrative processes, and radiation can cause lymphatic vessel damage. Upper extremity lymphedema may occur after radical or modified radical mastectomy. Recurrent cellulitis is common in patients with lymphedema as an initiating, exacerbating, and complicating event. Streptococcus is the most common organism. It typically enters the skin through a crack in the toe webs caused by trichophytosis. The organism damages the lymphatic channels and the connecting lymph nodes, and repeated infection inflammatory damage eventually obliterates the vessel.

History and physical exam suggest the diagnosis in the majority of cases. The skin is thickened and takes on an orange peel consistency (peau d'orange). A diffuse, flat, warty consistency may affect the skin over time. Unlike edema and lipedema, lymphedema involves the toes—and usually the toes first. Dependent edema spares the toes since footwear does not allow the swelling to occur. Lipedema, (caused by excess fatty deposits, usually increased at the time of menarche) is more difficult to differentiate from lymphedema. However, with lipedema the toes are spared and there is often a ridge or fold overhanging the ankle. Lipedema and lymphedema may coexist. Laboratory testing may help differentiate the two.

The techniques currently available for direct imaging of the lymphatic system are lymphangiography and lymphoscintography.[4] Lymphangiography is difficult to perform and carries a risk of iatrogenic lymphangitis. However, anatomic features are obtained and differentiation between primary (absence of lymphatic structures) and secondary (obstruction at a level by a mass, injury, or lymph node hypertrophy caused by lymphoma) lymphedema can often be determined. The lymphoscintogram is based on uptake and ascent of ^{99}Tc-labeled antimony trisulfide colloid after injection between the web spaces of digits. It is easier to perform than lymphangiography and has a low risk of lymphangitis. While this has good ability to differentiate lymphedema from other causes of edema, it cannot reliably distinguish primary from secondary lymphedema.[5]

Treatment for lymphedema is drainage and volume reduction of the limb. Reduction in limb size by elevation, mechanical pumping, or manual massage is effective. Wrapping of the limb, distal-to-proximal, is required whenever the patient is up. After leg volume is decreased, an elastic compression garment, 40 to 50 mmHg in strength, should be worn daily, replaced 2 to 4 times per year as needed.[6] Early and aggressive treatment of cellulitis and fungal infections of the toes help to prevent cellulitis recurrence and worsened lymphatic status.

LABORATORY ASSESSMENT: VENOUS DISEASE

Venous tests may be invasive or noninvasive. The information provided may be classified as anatomic, hemodynamic, or functional. Indications for venous testing include objective documentation supporting the diagnosis of venous disease, assessment of severity, and monitoring of progression or regression of disease. The most common reason for imaging or testing of the venous system is edema (Table 101-1).

Anatomic Studies

Duplex ultrasound, computed tomography (CT), magnetic resonance angiography (MRA) and magnetic resonance imaging (MRI), and venography are anatomic methods available for evaluation of the ve-

nous system. Venography (Fig. 101-1A) is considered the "gold standard" for venous imaging and the determination of deep venous thrombosis (DVT). However, venous duplex ultrasound is the most commonly used method. It has the potential advantage of differentiating acute from old thrombus based on the presence or absence of venous distention (common with acute clot) and increased echogenicity (common with chronic clot). Compared to venography, duplex ultrasound is less sensitive both above the groin and below the knee. MR venography and CT venography are rapidly emerging technologies (Fig. 101-1B). In addition to providing accurate information above the groin, they may be performed concurrently with pulmonary embolism studies.

Physiologic Studies

CONTINUOUS WAVE DOPPLER

Continuous wave Doppler (CWD) provides qualitative information about blood flow. With intervention, the presence of reflux or obstruction may be assessed. There are five components of venous CWD addressed in each assessment, at each level examined. Flow within the vein should be spontaneous and phasic, varying with the respiratory cycle. A loss of phasicity with respiration suggests venous obstruction. When a Doppler is placed over a vein and a distal portion of the limb is compressed, there should be augmentation of venous return. If lost, occlusion of the vein is present. In contrast, a vein is competent when compression of a proximal segment or Valsalva maneuver results if the Doppler flow signal (obtained distally) stops. If the valves are incompetent, an increase in distal signal (retrograde flow) will occur. Unlike arterial flow, venous flow is not pulsatile. When significant pulsatility (arterialized signal) is present, increased venous pressure such as tricuspid regurgitation, failure of right side of the heart, pulmonary hypertension, volume overload, or, if unilateral, arteriovenous fistula should be considered. By examining multiple levels, localization of incompetence or obstruction can be made (specificity 88 percent, sensitivity 85 percent).[7] CWD alone is a poor technique for evaluating partially obstructing thrombus or confirming acute DVT. And, although excellent for detecting hemodynamically significant valvular incompetence, it does not determine the functional significance of venous incompetence.

PLETHYSMOGRAPHY

Plethysmography is the measurement of the change in limb volume (due to arterial inflow, venous outflow, or venous reflux) over time. The most common plethysmographic techniques are strain-gauge plethysmography, air plethysmography, and impedance plethysmography. A brief discussion is warranted in that several new devices utilizing multiple modes of plethysmography are in development and early clinical use.

Plethysmography for Venous Insufficiency Venous insufficiency is assessed by raising the legs and reaching a low-volume steady state. The patient is quickly returned to the upright position, and the veins refill. If incompetent, blood falls from the proximal veins (retrograde) and calf volume increases rapidly. If competent, refilling time is slower, relying on arterial inflow to fill the venous structure (antegrade).[8] If the incompetence is primarily superficial, placing light tourniquets around the leg and/or directly compressing an incompetent superficial vein will normalize refilling time.

Exercise Venous Plethysmography Venous function of a limb can be quantified using air or strain-gauge plethysmography during exer-

TABLE 101-1 Etiology of Edema

One Limb	Multiple Limbs
DECREASED OUTFLOW	
Deep venous thrombosis (DVT)	Proximal DVT
Deep venous insufficiency	(inferior vena cava)
Lymphedema	Bilateral DVT
Extrinsic compression	Dependency
Baker's cyst	Pelvic mass
Gastrocnemius or	
popliteal rupture	
Pelvic mass	
Factitial	
May-Thurner syndrome	
Arterial aneurysms	
INCREASED INFLOW	
Lymphedema	Glomerulonephritis
Arteriovenous malformation	Idiopathic cyclic edema
Klippel-Trénaunay syndrome	Congestive heart failure
Orthopedic	Obesity
Fracture	Lipedema
Osteomyelitis	Pregnancy
Charcot's joint	Cushing's syndrome
Hemihypertrophy	Drug-induced

cise.[9,10] The normal lower extremity venous apparatus serves as an elaborate pump mechanism that returns volume up the limb. With the limb dependent, an air cuff or strain gauge is positioned around the calf. After a steady state (volume) is reached, the patient walks on a treadmill, performs deep knee bends, or performs toe lifts if seated. In a normal limb, the volume of the calf falls as the blood is moved up competent and patent venous structures. Legs with impaired venous pump function (caused by venous obstruction, valvular incompetence, or primary pump failure) do not reduce volume normally during exercise. Exercise plethysmography provides a functional assessment of "calf pump function" and refilling of the lower extremities.

Plethysmography for Outflow Obstruction Outflow plethysmography is useful in screening for venous outflow obstruction. Impedance plethysmography (IPG) is the best studied technique.[11] Unlike tests such as venography or ultrasound scanning (i.e., tests that directly image the thrombus), IPG identifies the presence of functional, not anatomic, venous obstruction. The patient lies supine with the legs elevated and slightly flexed. A pneumatic cuff placed around the thigh is inflated to greater than venous pressure but below arterial pressure (typically 40 to 50 mmHg). After an equilibrium is reached (1 to 2 min), the cuff is rapidly deflated, blood drains from the limb, and volume is decreased.

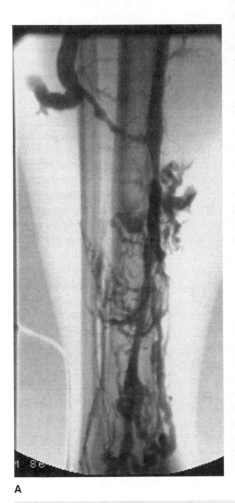

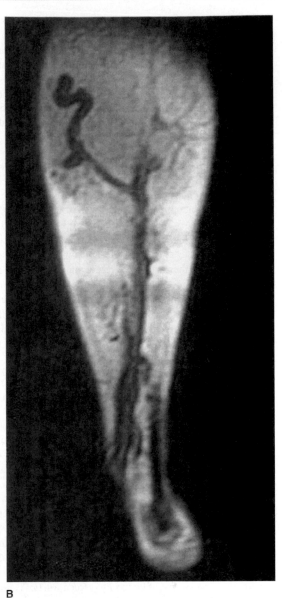

A **B**

FIGURE 101-1 *A.* Venogram of congenital deep varicosities in the lateral calf of a young woman. *B.* Magnetic resonance venography of the same varicosities.

The rate of outflow is plotted on a standard curve. If outflow rate is brisk, the venous system is considered patent. If outflow rate is slow, obstruction may be present. IPG screening has been replaced by Duplex ultrasound in most centers. Because IPG relies on indirect evidence of venous obstruction, it is subject to more false-positives and false-negatives than are the imaging tests.[12] Nevertheless, the ease of performance, low cost, and reasonable overall accuracy make it a useful screening tool. Correlation between triplex ultrasonography, CWD, venography, and plethysmography have been variable.[13,14] This is not unexpected since all are operator- and interpreter-dependent. The single "best" test for quantification of venous incompetence will therefore vary on institutional strengths.

DEVELOPING TECHNIQUES

CT and MR venography are proving to be accurate and applicable in clinical practice.[15] A negative D-dimer profile has been shown to be an excellent predictor for the absence of thrombosis.[16]

CLINICAL VENOUS DISEASE

Varicose Veins

Varicose veins are common.[17] "Burning," "bursting," "bruised," or "aching" are just some of the sensations reported by patients. Elevation or walking and exercise will relieve symptoms. If the discomfort is worse with elevation, it is unlikely to be due to varicosities. Symptoms are exacerbated by prolonged standing or dependency, obesity, and pregnancy. Episodes of superficial thrombophlebitis may occur, and, if repetitive, ablation of the veins is appropriate. Rarely, veins may bleed; this bleeding is often brisk despite the venous source because venous pressure is elevated when the limb is dependent. Symptoms and progression can be improved by a compression hose of 20 to 30 mmHg or more. Ablation of the vein should be considered if complications or discomfort interfere with occupation or lifestyle. Sclerotherapy is effective for certain varicosities and cutaneous "spiders." Laser therapy is effective for small "spider veins" and telangectasias.[18] Surgical removal is indicated for longer segments of proximal varicosities, especially if perforator vein or saphenofemoral junction incompetence is present.[19] Endovascular techniques have become available. Varicosities of the superficial veins begin with the incompetence of one or more valves. The incompetence may be caused by injury and direct failure of the venous valve or by degeneration of the venous wall and primary dilation resulting in failure of valves to coapt.

Primary varicosities may be familial, often first appearing during pregnancy. (Thus the expression, "Varicose veins run in families—you get them from your children.") Secondary varicosities may reflect underlying deep venous obstruction and/or incompetence, or perforator vein incompetence. Any of these anomalies shifts venous blood from the deep venous structures to the superficial veins. Secondary causes of varicosities include extrinsic venous compression, prior DVT, congenital lesions, arteriovenous fistulas, and disease of the right side of the heart. Severe edema and stasis ulceration are rarely caused by primary varicosities and suggest the presence of a secondary process. History, examination, and (when necessary) laboratory evaluation of the deep venous system will usually allow the physician to differentiate primary from secondary varicosities.

Superficial Venous Thrombophlebitis

Superficial venous thrombophlebitis (SVT) presents as a tender, erythematous, and indurated linear lesion in the anatomic course of a superficial vein. Ultrasound can differentiate thrombophlebitis from lymphangitic streaks, erythema nodosum, and other lesions. SVT often occurs in a varicose vein or at sites of indwelling catheters or intravenous injections. Active infection may be associated with the latter or with use of illicit street drugs. In such cases, antibiotics should be considered. SVT is usually self-limited. Recovery can be accelerated by rest, topical warmth, and anti-inflammatory agents. Systemic anticoagulation is appropriate for lesions that progress with conservative care or that are located proximally in the lesser or greater saphenous veins where minimal extension would enter the deep system. There is a high incidence of concurrent DVT in SVT.[20] Duplex ultrasound should be used to screen for DVT since management with chronic anticoagulation would then be indicated. Evaluation for underlying diseases that can predispose to clotting or a clotting abnormality should be considered. One study suggested one-third of patients presenting with a primary DVT have an underlying clotting abnormality.[21]

Deep Venous Thrombosis

The morbidity and mortality of DVT are high. Risk factors for DVT and pulmonary embolism have been well-defined in several studies.[22] The signs and symptoms of DVT are nonspecific and may be absent or subtle, but they include prominent superficial venous pattern, edema, and discomfort at rest and with compression. Objective testing to confirm and define the extent of DVT should be obtained whenever one is suspected. Less than half of patients considered to have DVT have the diagnosis confirmed when tested objectively. Confirmed diagnosis can bolster the decision to treat when anticoagulation is relatively contraindicated. If the diagnosis is disproved, the cost of treatment and the risks of hemorrhage, heparin-induced thrombocytopenia, and warfarin necrosis are avoided. Warfarin-induced necrosis, although rare, may be avoided by overlapping heparin with warfarin for 4 to 5 days.[23]

Treatment with heparin acutely and warfarin chronically is highly effective in preventing clot propagation and pulmonary embolism. Low-molecular-weight heparins (adjusted for weight) have shown promise in treating DVT and can be used for outpatient management in uncomplicated cases.[24,25] It also serves as an excellent bridge for short-term anticoagulation while the warfarin effect is increasing (or decreasing prior to a procedure).[26] Heparin-induced thrombocytopenia is common and may only be detected by monitoring platelets daily. If there is known heparin-induced thrombocytopenia or it is suspected, all heparin exposure must stop immediately.[27,28] Hirudin or danaparoid may be used in place of heparin until the warfarin effect is therapeutic.[29,30] Duration of treatment with warfarin for optimal risk:benefit ratio is not known. However, literature suggests treatment for a minimum of 6 to 12 months in patients with spontaneous DVT.[31] The risk of major hemorrhage from anticoagulation is 1 to 3 percent per year when control is strict and attention is paid to drugs that alter warfarin effect.[32] Bleeding risk increases significantly as the international normalized ratio (INR) reaches 4.0.[32a] The INR should be followed to ensure consistency between laboratories. Patients should be urged to know and record their INR.[33]

Thrombolytic therapy when given early accelerates recovery and may reduce incidence and severity of postphlebitic syndrome.[34,35] Lysis appears to be most effective in iliofemoral DVT.[36] Mechanical thrombectomy is also promising.[37] However, well-defined indications for thrombolytic therapy in deep venous thrombosis are not yet established. Long-term use of compression stockings to the knee (or above, if tolerated) drastically reduces the incidence of postphlebitic syndrome, venous stasis changes, and venous ulceration.[38,39]

When DVT or thromboembolic events occur without a recognized risk factor (Table 101-2), a search for venous compression, inherited or acquired clotting abnormalities, systemic disease, or age-appropriate cancer screening is indicated.[40–42] Such screening is valuable, even when the results are negative, in establishing prognosis and in planning duration of anticoagulation therapy.[43]

DVT isolated to the calf is thought to be less dangerous than DVT in the thigh. However, upward of 20 percent of calf thrombi will extend proximally and 10 percent embolize.[44,45] Ultrasound surveillance is required if anticoagulants are withheld. Patients with isolated calf DVT are also prone to persistent symptoms and postphlebitic syndrome.[46]

PHLEGMASIA CERULEA DOLENS

Phlegmasia cerulea dolens is a rare complication of DVT characterized by acute, massive edema, severe pain, and cyanosis in the setting of extensive iliofemoral thrombosis. One-third of patients die due to pulmonary embolism, and half develop distal gangrene due to thrombus-induced compartment syndrome. It is seen most com-

---

TABLE 101-2 Risk Factors for Deep Venous Thrombosis

Age
Hospitalization
Immobility
Malignancy
Prior deep venous thrombosis
Prior superficial venous thrombosis
Progesterone therapy
Recent surgery
Residence in health care facility
Trauma

monly with advanced malignancy or severe infections but can follow surgery, fractures, and other common precipitants of thrombosis. Treatment includes placement of a caval filter, heparinization, and often, physical removal of the clot by thrombectomy (surgical or endovascular), commonly with thrombolysis.[47,48]

THROMBOSIS OF CENTRAL VEINS

Superior Vena Cava Syndrome   Superior vena cava (SVC) syndrome is uncommon and usually subacute (unless traumatic). It may be caused by radiation, cannulation, tumor bulk, adenopathy, or fibrosing mediastinitis.[49,50] Symptoms include head and neck fullness or headache with signs involving neck and face; arm swelling may be seen if the innominate vein is affected. The presence of superficial collateral veins across the chest is appreciated with the patient upright.

Inferior Vena Cava Syndrome   Inferior vena cava (IVC) syndrome may be an acute event or may occur gradually from extrinsic compression or extension of distal thrombosis (Fig. 101-2). The acute syndromes produce massive regional swelling and discomfort. Venous collaterals across the abdomen and pelvis are prominent in chronic occlusion. IVC thrombus is often an extension from iliofemoral thrombus. Bilateral severe leg swelling and pain are the most common symptoms.[51] Both SVC and IVC syndromes may be the initial manifestation of a primary clotting abnormality. Thrombolytic

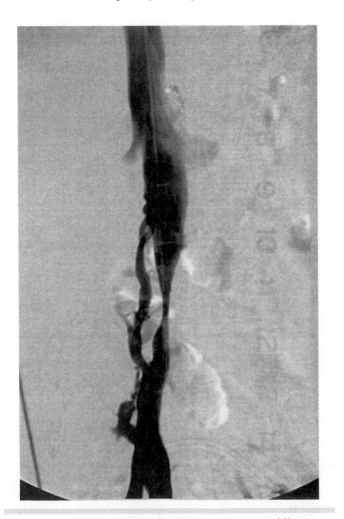

FIGURE 101-2 Inferior vena cava stenosis due to retroperitoneal fibrosis.

therapy may clear thrombosis when given early. Endovascular stenting or bypass surgery is effective in selected instances of either syndrome, but frequently may only be offered for temporary relief.[52,53]

Paget-Schroetter Syndrome   Acute or subacute arm swelling after increased or prolonged upper extremity effort is the usual presentation of axillosubclavian thrombosis. (Hence the name *effort thrombosis*.) There is often evidence of thoracic outlet obstruction by retrospective history (see later). The usual treatment consists of heparinization followed by warfarin and consideration of surgical opening of the thoracic outlet. Thrombolytic therapy can be effective when given early and followed by chronic anticoagulation. Catheter-related thrombus, whether at the subclavian artery or at a central or peripheral site, is treated by removing the line and treating with heparin if possible.

Chronic Venous Insufficiency

Chronic deep venous incompetence (DVI), with or without venous obstruction, causes venous hypertension. This is characterized by leg edema, venous dilation, and intradermal deposition of proteins and hemosiderin. Cutaneous changes of fibrosis, lichenification, cellulitis, and ulceration may follow. Postphlebitic syndrome occurs after months to years of DVT and onset of DVI.[54] Symptoms include heavy, congested limbs; venous claudication; pruritus; and skin ulceration that is often painless. Increased ambulatory pressure can be confirmed by direct measurement or plethysmography. Both incompetence and obstruction can be documented by CWD, ultrasound, duplex ultrasound, or venography.[55]

Venous Ulceration

Venous ulceration is usually perimalleolar; medial more often than lateral. This area has high venous pressure, often in excess of perfusion pressure, resulting in chronic hypoxic skin prone to injury. Once ulceration has occurred, successful management must be performed in stages. Reduction of the edema and conservative debridement of the ulcer must occur first. After the ulcer is healed and skin integrity is restored, control of venous hypertension with elastic support hose (30 to 40 mmHg of compression) is required. If venous ulceration occurs in the setting of moderate to severe PAD, treatment may be very difficult. Compression must still be applied, but with a low stretch wrap in order to avoid further reduction of arterial inflow.

PERIPHERAL ARTERIAL DISEASE

Unfortunately, large randomized control trials of PAD do not exist. Even atherosclerotic peripheral disease, which is only a portion of the arterial pathology, has had few large trials. Therefore, the goal of this section is to provide a general framework of arterial processes from which to build. Risk factors, clinical history and examination, natural history of disease, laboratory assessment, and medical management will be covered. Diseases of the aorta, epidemiology, and cerebrovascular disease and interventions—surgical and percutaneous—are covered in adjacent chapters.

History

Information including age, gender, associated medical problems (including prior trauma, vascular and orthopedic procedures, and past or current medication use), and risk factors for atherosclerosis should be addressed. Symptoms including location, onset, progression, and aggravating or alleviating factors should be clarified. Claudication, ischemic rest pain, or skin ulceration are the usual presenting complaints of occlusive arterial disease. Claudication (literally "limping") is reproducible discomfort brought on by exercise and relieved by rest. It is important to remember that claudication from ischemic sources occurs in muscle groups—not in joints. Relief with rest is therefore independent of position and complete, usually within 5 min. If relief of pain is dependent on position, not relieved by rest, or specifically localized at a joint, musculoskeletal or neurologic disorders should be suspected. Discomfort is typically described as cramping, but variably described as numbness, weakness, giving way, aching, burning, or just plain pain. Discomfort usually occurs at a predictable distance or time. However, when workload is increased by a rapid pace, walking uphill or over rough terrain, or carrying a load, the distance or time to discomfort will shorten. The distribution and/or character of the discomfort will change as the causative lesions progress. When change is abrupt, one must consider thrombosis in situ or an embolic event has occurred, and expedited evaluation and therapy should ensue. Claudication often worsens after a period of inactivity, such as hospitalization, but usually returns to baseline with reconditioning.

The history will address changes in quality of life and limitations in lifestyle; quantitation of disease severity by history alone is unreliable. Patient estimates of pace, workload, and distance are unreliable. Standardized treadmill testing with ankle-brachial indices provides the objective measurements required for prognostication and long-term follow-up.

VARIANTS OF CLAUDICATION

As implied earlier, there are many causes of leg pain (Table 101-3). Arterial claudication in the setting of normal peripheral pulses at rest is possible. This may be vasospastic in etiology[56] but is more likely to arise from proximal atherosclerosis that is well collateralized.[57] Under stress, distal blood flow cannot meet demands and a fall in the ankle-brachial index (ABI) is detected.

Pseudoclaudication Pseudoclaudication is of nonarterial etiology brought on by a specific position, such as standing. It may be of neurogenic or musculoskeletal origin. The patient with pseudoclaudication typically describes limb distress with a dysthetic quality that requires a specific posture for relief, usually sitting. Clumsiness may be present. Unlike arterial claudication, symptoms occur while standing or when supine with the legs extended. There may be a history of back injury, and radiographic evidence of cord compression of the distal spinal cord is often present.[58–60] Arterial and neurogenic disease may coexist. In this situation, the dominant lesion can be identified by observing symptoms and measuring the arterial indices after exercise.

Venous Claudication Venous claudication is described as a congestive, often "bursting," distress of thighs and calves induced by standing, running, and sometimes walking. Relief with rest is variable but may be quickly achieved when patients elevate their legs.

ISCHEMIC REST PAIN

When perfusion deficit is severe, patients can experience persistent pain at rest. Pain may be either ischemic muscular pain (crampy in sensation) or present as an ischemic neuropathy (burning or dysthetic in quality). The limb may be hypersensitive to touch by clothing or bedding. Ether type of rest pain is constant and agonizing in quality. Discomfort may be confined to individual digits, a foot, a hand, ulcerated areas, or an entire limb. Small, localized areas of ischemic pain can occur with vasculitis, microembolization, or thrombosis. Local trauma (often unrecognized) to an area with poor perfusion is a frequent cause of such pain. It is important to inquire about new shoes, recent trimming of callus or nails, or other potential sources of trauma.[61]

Nocturnal rest pain is common. It is relieved by dependency such as hanging the limb off the bed, sleeping in a chair, or, paradoxically, by walking when the discomfort wakens the patient at night. Prolonged dependency will lead to edema, further complicating the ischemia. In more severe stages pain may become constant, preventing sleep and causing anorexia and weight loss. Large doses of analgesics may be required, and depression is often present. After time, muscular atrophy occurs and contractures at the ankle, knee, or hip may result as the limb is passively or actively protected and held immobile.

Diabetes requires special consideration with regard to pain. Insensate or poorly sensate feet from peripheral neuropathy complicate both the diagnosis and care of this group. The usual reflexive "avoidance of painful stimuli" is lost, resulting in higher degrees of trauma and tissue injury prior to seeking medical care. This group may also present at later stages of disease, when something is "visible" rather than painful. Ulceration is not always preceded by claudication.[62]

Arterial Examination

INSPECTION

A red or purplish color of the forefoot during dependency (dependent rubor) is common with severe ischemia. The patient may do this in order to let gravity assist blood flow to the limb. True dependent rubor will change to pallor with elevation. Pallor during dependency may be present in chronic ischemia but is seen more often in acute ischemia. Timing of onset of pallor and time to venous refilling can be performed in the examination room (Table 101-4). Loss of normal hair growth is also a marker of ischemia.

PALPATION

The aorta and radial, ulnar, subclavian, carotid, temporal, occipital, femoral, popliteal, posterior tibial, and dorsalis pedis arteries (although the dorsalis pedis artery is congenitally absent in a small minority) are accessible by palpation. Pulses are graded on many scales

---

TABLE 101-3 Differential Diagnosis of Claudication

Aortic coarctation
Aortic dissection
Arteritis (Takayasu's, giant-cell)
Atherosclerosis obliterans
Baker's cyst
Deconditioning
Degenerative joint disease (hip, back, knee)
Embolic disease and acute arterial occlusion
Myopathy
Popliteal entrapment
Retroperitoneal fibrosis
Spinal stenosis
Thromboangiitis obliterans
Venous claudication and varicosities

TABLE 101-4 Elevation and Dependency

ELEVATION PALLOR*	
Grade	Pallor Onset
Normal	None
Grade I	>60 s
Grade II	<60 s
Grade III	<30 s
Grade IV	Pallor supine

VENOUS REFILLING†	
Severity Venous Refill	
Normal	<15 s
Moderate	15–30 s
Severe	>30 s

*Feet held passively at 60° while supine.
†Legs dependent while sitting after elevation.

(Table 101-5). If a pulse is not palpable, Doppler examination should be performed to establish whether the flow is absent or below the level of detection by palpation. Surface temperature is reduced when perfusion is compromised. (Thankfully, not all patients with cool limbs have arterial insufficiency.) Temperature differences are best felt with the dorsum of the fingers, and comparisons to the contralateral limb or more proximal ipsilateral limb should be made. The size and pulsatility of paired arteries are normally of similar magnitude. Ectasia is suspected when a pulse is larger or more forceful than expected. Aneurysm is defined as focal enlargement 1½ times or larger than the usual diameter of the artery. Arteriomegaly is present when the artery is widened, usually over a long distance, but not yet aneurysmal. Diagnosis is suspected when a palpable, often visible pulsation is transmitted to the fingers on each side of an enlarged vessel. Tortuosity of the carotids, abdominal aorta, and subclavian arteries can mimic an aneurysm. Ultrasound or angiographic studies may be needed to clarify the diagnosis when the examination is unclear.

AUSCULTATION
Blood pressure should be taken in both arms. Pressures should be symmetric but are rarely identical even when done simultaneously. Respiratory variation, positioning of the arm, and atrial fibrillation are just a few reasons the pressure may vary. If a large difference is noted between arms (greater than 10 mmHg), blood pressures should be rechecked. If real, simultaneous pressures (two examiners) should be used to confirm this, or, as an alternative, upper extremity segmental pressures can be ordered.

The femoral, iliac, aortic, carotid, and subclavian arteries should be auscultated. Simultaneous palpation of a radial artery during auscultation will improve appreciation of subtle bruits and also allow timing of bruits. The further a bruit extends into diastole, the greater the degree of stenosis. Abdominal bruits are difficult to differen-

tiate, especially if bowel sounds are vigorous. A renal artery source may be suspected if the bruit lateralizes to a flank.

LABORATORY ASSESSMENT: ARTERIAL DISEASE

Objective testing of the arterial system is done for confirmation or clarification of the clinical findings, monitoring disease progression, or assessing of outcome after intervention—all appropriate indications for arterial testing. All vascular tests may be classified as invasive or noninvasive. However, a better classification scheme is based upon the type of information provided—anatomic, hemodynamic, or functional.

Anatomic Studies

Anatomic information of the arterial system is provided by a number of techniques. The presence or absence of aneurysms, dissections, stenoses, or occlusions is readily determined by these tests. Arteriography is the standard by which all other imaging techniques are judged. It provides reproducible information with very high resolution not yet matched by other readily available modalities. Assessment of distal vessels, fine structural detail, and shunting with early venous filling are still best determined by this means. Drawbacks include an arterial catheterization, risk of embolization, and risks inherent to arterial puncture. Iodinated contrast is used, with small but real risks of anaphylactoid reactions and contrast nephropathy.

CT and the emerging technique of CT angiography (CTA) provide detailed anatomic information without need of arterial access. Iodinated contrast is still required for best results, however. Reconstruction can include or exclude bony structures and other organs in the final images. CTA has become the standard for assessing and planning endograft aortic aneurysm since accurate measurement of the "landing zone" (distance between the renal arteries and the neck of the aneurysm) can be made. CTA also has the advantage of being three-dimensional, allowing the image to be rotated on an axis.

MRI and MRA provide information similar to CT and CTA, but iodinated contrast is not required (Fig. 101-3). Gadolinium-based contrast agents may be indicated in some cases, but risk of nephropathy is minimal.[63] MRA, like CTA, provides a three-dimensional image and is able to include or exclude structures of interest. Patients with implantable devices such as pacemakers, automated defibrillators, recently placed arterial stents, and intracranial clips cannot be safely placed into the magnetic field, limiting availability to a small extent.

Two-dimensional ultrasound provides safe and reliable data of not only anatomy but hemodynamic effect of stenosis as well if and when Doppler analysis of flow is incorporated. Anatomic reconstruction is limited to two-dimensional imaging at present, but methods

TABLE 101-5 Pulse Grading Scale*

Grade		Physical Findings
0	Absent	Unable to find
1	Severely reduced	Palpable with difficulty; unable to accurately count pulse
2	Moderately reduced	Palpable with some difficulty; able to count pulse
3	Mildly reduced	Easily palpable but reduced
4	Normal	Normal pulse; easily palpable
5	Enlarged	Widened, possibly aneurysmal

*Presence of edema and other physical barriers during examination must be taken into account when grading.

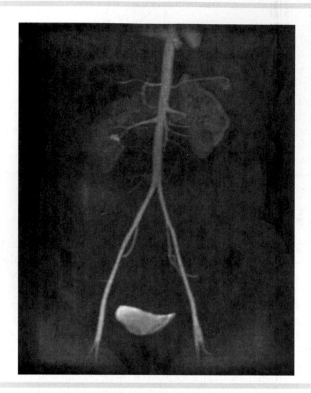

FIGURE 101-3 Magnetic resonance angiogram of the aortoiliac system.

for reconstruction to three-dimensional images are under development. Contrast is not required, and no ionizing radiation is used. Ultrasound is portable, allowing bedside data acquisition. However, data acquisition may be limited by overlying structures such as bowel gas and other tissues that interfere with imaging.

Hemodynamic Studies

The hemodynamic significance of a stenosis may be assessed by multiple methods. Invasive measurement of a pressure drop or gradient across a stenosis may still be considered the "gold standard" for hemodynamic assessment. The pressure waveform is valuable information as well, with the normal triphasic waveform changing to a monophasic waveform in the presence of severe stenosis. Noninvasive evaluation is available by measuring externally applied pressure at multiple levels (see "Segmental Pressures and Exercise Testing") or by Doppler-derived flow velocities and waveforms. Hemodynamic studies are frequently combined with functional assessment.

Functional Studies

When the information obtained by anatomic or hemodynamic testing is insufficient to explain the symptoms or degree of impairment described by the patient, a functional assessment is appropriate. Functional studies often involve some form of applied stress—such as treadmill testing to assess claudication.

CONTINUOUS WAVE DOPPLER

CWD detects blood motion and may be used alone as a means of screening for vascular disease[64] or it may be an integral part of other tests such as segmental pressure determination (described later).

In a normal artery, the waveform is triphasic. During cardiac systole, there is forward flow in the arteries. During early diastole, the flow reverses direction because of the elastic recoil of the peripheral arteries. During mid-to-late diastole, there is a return of forward flow as arterial blood runs off through the distal vessels. A stenosis, when hemodynamically significant, changes the normal triphasic wave to a biphasic waveform, then monophasic, then absent if the artery is occluded. Location of a stenosis may be estimated by assessing the Doppler signal at multiple sites along the limb. CWD is inexpensive and may be performed at the bedside as an extension of the vascular examination. Handheld devices are often available on nursing units or may be purchased for personal use. Use of a handheld Doppler requires training and practice to be effective; the information obtained is limited because it is a "blind" technique. Duplicated vessels, anatomic variations, and obesity may reduce its accuracy. This being accepted, use of the handheld Doppler is far and away the most cost-effective, universally applicable, and readily available diagnostic tool we have as an adjunct to history and physical examination.

SEGMENTAL PRESSURES AND EXERCISE TESTING

Pressure required for arterial occlusion is the segmental pressure. Segmental pressures provide a simple, reproducible, inexpensive, and accurate method of determining whether arterial obstruction is present, severity of the obstruction, and approximate location of the obstruction. Pneumatic cuffs are placed around the thigh, calf, ankle, upper or lower arm, or digits. A CWD probe (see earlier) is positioned over the artery at a site distal to the pressure cuffs and is used to determine the systolic pressure at which arterial flow resumes as the cuff is deflated. The limb pressures are divided by a reference arterial pressure (the brachial artery systolic pressure) to create an index. The most commonly reported segmental pressure is the ABI. Severity of disease is graded by individual laboratory (Table 101-6).

There are patients, particularly those with diabetes, who deposit calcium in the media of conduit arteries (Mönckeberg's calcification).[65] The calcified artery is frequently noncompressible or poorly compressible. The biggest disadvantage of segmental pressure measurement is that it cannot be reliably used in patients with poorly compressible vessels or in those with noncompressible vessels.[66] This occurs most commonly in diabetics. When vessels are stiff, the cuff cannot produce sufficient pressure to obliterate blood flow and the arterial pressure cannot be determined. Many groups utilize the great toe index in such situations. Even when the large vessels of the limb are noncompressible, the digital vessels in the toes and fingers often remain noncalcified and can be used to

TABLE 101-6 Ankle-Brachial Index Criteria

	Preexercise	Postexercise	Claudication	Walking Time
Normal	>0.95*	>0.95	None	5 min
Minimal	>0.95	<0.95	None	5 min
Mild	>0.80	>0.50	Present late	5 min
Moderate	<0.80	<0.50	Present, limiting	<5 min
Severe	<0.50	<0.15	Early, limiting	<3 min

Ankle-brachial index is the systolic blood pressure of the higher arm/systolic blood pressure at the ankle measured in the supine position. Postexercise values are after 5 min at a 10 percent grade at 2 mph (our laboratory protocol; other protocols may be used). Speed may be varied if patient is unable.
*Some laboratories use greater than 0.90 as normal.

estimate pressure with an appropriate-sized cuff. Pulse volume recording, laser Doppler studies, and transcutaneous oximetry can be effectively utilized in these patients as well.

Postexercise ABIs may identify arterial lesions that are too minor to produce hemodynamic changes at rest. The subject is placed on a treadmill and exercised under a standardized protocol. Protocols may be "fixed" (for example, 2 mph at a 12 percent incline for a maximum of 5 min) or "graded" similar to those used in cardiac exercise studies.[67] Elements of the lower extremity study (i.e., ABIs or CWD analysis) are performed before and after exercise. A fall in ABI or a change in Doppler signal can be detected after exercise. The now detectable or worsened pathology is due to an increase in pressure gradient induced by exercise. With exercise, the systolic blood pressure increases as peripheral resistance decreases, resulting in a larger pressure gradient.

Exercise studies provide ancillary data such as the walking distance to onset of symptoms, absolute walking distance, and blood pressure response during exercise.[68] They also correlate symptoms, which may be very vague, with the data generated, providing objective evidence of the patient's symptoms.[69]

PULSE VOLUME RECORDING

Pulse volume recording (PVR) assesses the pulsatility of the arterial impulse entering a limb or segment of a limb. A pneumatic pressure cuff is placed around the limb, filled with air to a low pressure (typically 40 to 60 mmHg), and connected to a pressure transducer. During systole, transient distention of the arterial system causes distention of the limb. The cyclic changes in cuff pressure with each heartbeat provide an index of arterial "pulsatility." Measurements are made at multiple levels of the limb (as is done with segmental pressures), and the calibrated tracings determine whether or not there is a particular level at which the waveform changes shape or volume, suggesting stenosis.[70,71]

TRANSCUTANEOUS OXIMETRY

Transcutaneous oxygen measurement ($TcPo_2$) quantifies oxygen delivery to the skin.[72] Oxygen-sensing electrodes are attached with an airtight seal to the skin by means of adhesive rings. The temperature of the electrode is maintained at a relatively high temperature (45°C, 113.0°F) so that the small vessels underlying the electrode are maximally dilated. Cutaneous blood flow is determined, in part, by status of the proximal arteries.[73] The amount of oxygen that diffuses out of the skin depends upon numerous factors including the arterial partial pressure of oxygen (Po_2), cutaneous blood flow, and rate of oxygen consumption by the skin. When cutaneous blood flow is high (relative to the metabolic rate of the skin), $TcPo_2$ approaches arterial Po_2. In contrast, when the cutaneous blood flow is low, $TcPo_2$ is reduced. $TcPo_2$ is not so much a measurement of skin blood flow as it is a measurement of the adequacy of cutaneous oxygen delivery. Transcutaneous oximetry has been shown useful in a number of situations, including evaluation of critical ischemia. It may be difficult to determine the functional severity of PAD in a nonambulatory patient, especially when the clinician is attempting to determine whether or not limb revascularization is required for pain relief, ulcer healing, or limb salvage. $TcPo_2$ can be used to predict whether the cutaneous perfusion is adequate for healing at a given amputation site. Values above 40 mmHg are typically sufficient for healing, while those below 20 mmHg are not likely to heal (Table 101-7).[74]

Certain disease states may affect the small vessels or microcirculation without involving larger arteries. $TcPo_2$ determination is valuable in the assessment of patients with diabetes (when noncompressible or poorly compressible vessels are present) and/or small-

TABLE 101-7 Interpretation of $TcPo_2$ Values

	Rest	Decrease with Elevation
Normal	45	<10
Mild	40–45	<10
Moderate	20–39	<10
Severe	20–39	>10
	or <20	any
Critical	0	N/A

$TcPo_2$ (transcutaneous oxygen measurement) values in mmHg at rest and after 30° elevation. A fall of greater than 10 mmHg with elevation increases the degree of severity by one grade. Values less than 20 have poor potential for healing; 20 to 30, variable potential for healing.

vessel disease. When this occurs, techniques such as CWD, segmental pressures, and PVR may not detect a significant abnormality. In contrast, $TcPo_2$ measurements will demonstrate the inadequacy of circulation due to small-vessel occlusive disease. Although $TcPo_2$ measurement is an accurate way to assess the severity of cutaneous ischemia, it has several limitations. These include its inability to localize the occlusive disease to a particular segment or vessel. Individual laboratories must standardize and validate the technique before results may be relied upon for diagnostic and therapeutic decisions.[75]

CLINICAL PERIPHERAL ARTERIAL DISEASE

Claudication

PAD due to atherosclerosis is the most common cause of lower extremity ischemic syndromes in Western societies.[76] Symptoms of PAD are variable. Acute onset of ischemic limb pain can occur in the setting of embolic events or thrombosis in situ. Exertional symptoms may go unnoticed as subtle, progressive adaptations of lifestyle compensate for the disease process. For active patients, it is not until pushed by a new situation, such as a vacation or an annual event such as a hunting trip, that symptoms are noted. If the patient is inactive, the initial symptom may be rest pain, dependent rubor, edema, ulceration, or gangrene. Ulceration and gangrene at presentation are more likely to occur when the patient is insensate.

In general, symptoms of claudication occur distal to the level of stenosis. Foot cramping and calf pain are most common. Hip and buttock claudication, either isolated or associated with distal symptoms, suggests internal iliac stenosis. Impotency suggests aortoiliac or bilateral internal iliac disease.

PREVALENCE AND NATURAL HISTORY

PAD affects large and increasing numbers of patients in the United States, estimated at 10 million people with symptomatic PAD and another 2 to 3 times that for asymptomatic PAD. Ten percent of those over age 60 are affected.[77] Risk factors for PAD are the same as coronary artery disease (CAD).[78,79] Other factors such as hyperhomocysteinemia also exist, but individual and global impact is not yet clear.[80] The most recent large cohort was reported from the Framingham Offspring Study.[80,81] Prevalence of PAD was determined in 1554 males and 1759 females from 1995 to 1998. The mean age was 59. PAD was determined to be present in those with ABI of less than 0.9. It was found that PAD was present in 3.9 percent of males and 3.3 percent of females, with prevalence of intermittent claudication (1.9 percent males; 0.8 percent females), lower extremity bruits (2.4 percent males; 2.3 percent females), and prior surgical intervention (1.4 percent males; 0.5 percent females) noted. This study confirmed the relation of hypercholesterolemia, decreased high-density lipoprotein cholesterol, increased triglycerides, increasing age, diabetes, hypertension, prior and continued smoking, and known CAD as risk factors for PAD.

The PARTNERS study (PAD Awareness, Risk, and Treatment: New Resources for Survival) is an outstanding collaboration by Hirsch and colleagues.[82] PARTNERS assessed not only the prevalence of PAD in the general, primary care population, it also elegantly addressed patients' and physicians' awareness of the diagnosis and the treatment patterns. The high incidence of concurrent CAD, with or without prior diagnosis of PAD, was well demonstrated by PARTNERS.

The risk of death, usually due to a cardiovascular event, increases dramatically as the ABI decreases.[83,84] The 5-year mortality of an ABI less than 0.85 is 10 percent; at less than 0.40 it approaches 50 percent mortality per year.[85] Death due primarily to PAD complication is rare. Mortality is caused by concomitant coronary and cerebrovascular disease. The relative risk of death for all-cause mortality is 3.1 in PAD patients versus the general population.[86] The relative risk for coronary heart disease death is 6.9, accounting for over two-thirds of death in a study population.[87]

Although the long-term prognosis of patients with PAD is sobering, the rate of progression of symptoms and need for revascularization is low.[88] Symptoms worsen at 5 years in approximately 20 percent of patients.[89] Requirement for revascularization due to imminent tissue or limb loss or rest pain approaches 5 percent per year. Amputation rates are similarly low, around 1 percent per year.[90] Up to 15 percent of those who continue smoking, however, undergo amputation within 5 years. Patients with diabetes have a substantially elevated risk for amputation. Historically, those with diabetes have an amputation rate of 25 percent over 10 years, which has changed little over time.[91-93] Current practice demonstrates a shift toward distal amputation (below knee), however.[94] When PAD is present in a young patient (40s to 50s), progression of disease results in multiple interventions in approximately 40 percent.[95] Aggressive medical therapy and close follow-up is indicated. This "premature atherosclerosis" group justifies ongoing intense research efforts.

TREATMENT

Aggressive risk factor modification is the cornerstone of therapy in all patients with PAD. The slow rate of progression and high incidence of cardiovascular comorbidities creates the optimal situation for modifying the underlying atherosclerotic process. Unfortunately, secondary prevention has been disappointing in this group.[96] The PARTNERS study found that in patients with PAD there was a markedly lower rate of treatment for risk factors and use of antiplatelet medications than there was in those with coronary disease. This was true for both established and newly diagnosed PAD. The bright spot in the study was in smoking cessation, where PAD had a higher rate of intervention than CAD. The rate of progression and amputation in those who continue to smoke is more than twofold higher than it is in those who quit.[97] Cessation of smoking is also the most cost-effective measure available.[98]

A walking program should be initiated in all patients with claudication. Unfortunately, bicycling and other forms of exercise used for cardiovascular conditioning do not provide the same lower extremity benefit as walking. The effectiveness of a structured walking program has been well demonstrated.[99,100] Twenty to 30 min, 4 to 5 days per week improves functional and exercise capacity and increases total and absolute walking distance from 50 to 300 percent.[99] The mechanism of this improvement is not clear, but increased collateral formation or recruitment, muscle training, improved oxygen uptake, or improved mechanics of walking are all plausible.[101] Diligent foot care and protection must be emphasized, particularly in those with diabetes and those with severe reductions in ABI or $TcPO_2$ values. Footwear must be supportive and protective, and nail care should be performed regularly by professionals.[102] Routine foot care in patients with diabetes who have PAD may reduce amputation rates up to four times.[103]

Medical therapy for PAD has been slow to develop. Pentoxifylline has proved effective for increasing claudication distance in some patients with arteriosclerosis obliterans (ASO).[104] Stomach irritation limits its usefulness in many. Cilostazol has been approved for use for patients with claudication. It is effective in increasing walking distance, but the effect is lost when the drug is stopped.[105-107] It is currently the most effective agent available. Direct vasodilators have proved ineffective with the exception of verapamil. In a double-blind dose-adjusted placebo-controlled study, verapamil increased pain-free walking distance 29 percent and maximal walking distance 49 percent.[108] Beta-blockade has long been believed to be contraindicated for patients with ASO, but studies have refuted this idea.[109,110] Given the beneficial effects of beta-blockade in patents with CAD, these agents should not be withheld in patients with peripheral ASO.

Antiplatelet agents including aspirin and clopidogrel should be considered first-line agents for patients with PAD. Aspirin therapy has shown to be of benefit after surgical revascularization of the periphery.[111] However, up to 40 percent of patients with PAD may not respond to aspirin at either low (100 mg daily) or high (300 mg daily) doses.[112] The CAPRIE trial showed clopidogrel, a direct inhibitor of adenosine diphosphate to its platelet receptor, to be more beneficial than was aspirin in all causes of cardiovascular mortality.[113] Patients with PAD had the most significant improvement and should be strongly considered for antiplatelet therapy.[114]

Lipid lowering has a beneficial role in patients with ASO. Goals for cholesterol are identical to those for patients with CAD.[115] Lipid lowering in CAD has been shown to decrease rates of cerebrovascular events and new claudication symptoms.[116] Hypertension has long been associated with PAD. Control should be optimized, recognizing that pressure reduction in the setting of severe stenosis may worsen symptoms in the short term.[117] Homocysteinemia plays an independent role in development of PAD. The mechanism is at least in part related to an inborn genetic mutation affecting methylene tetrahydrofolate reductase, resulting in accelerated intimal damage and early atherosclerosis.[118,119] Treatment with folic acid and vitamins B_{12} and B_6 is appropriate when elevated.[120] Several other medications are currently in development and have undergone clinical trials.

L-Carnitine has been studied in regard to mitochondrial metabolism in PAD.[121,122] Work has been promising, with suggestions that those with diabetes may benefit greater than those who do not have diabetes. Prostacyclins, such as beraprost and iloprost, are direct vasodilators that have shown promise in PAD. Iloprost infusion is effective in acute large and small arterial syndromes in the setting of critical ischemia.[123,124] Indication and duration parameters remain to be defined. Orally available prostacyclins such as beraprost have shown mixed results in treatment of claudication.[125] Although promising initially, one claudication study was disappointing.[126] Further study is needed.

Revascularization should be considered in the patient with rest pain, tissue loss, or significant limitation of lifestyle. Surgical revascularization has been available for years. Large-vessel bypass surgery with vein or synthetic graft material is well established and durable. Percutaneous transluminal angioplasty (PTA), with or without stent placement, is useful for lesions at the renal, iliac, and proximal superficial femoral arteries. Cost-effectiveness of PTA and surgical revascularization is known. Compared to walking and medical therapy alone, there is benefit at a cost of $38,000 for PTA, $311,000 per quality-adjusted life-years, over medical therapy alone.[127] Despite the favorability of PTA over surgical revascularization, it is important to point out the decreasing long-term effectiveness of PTA in distal vessels and long stenosis. However, for patients at high risk for limb loss (deemed poor surgical candidates or technically unfeasible for revascularization), it is reasonable to consider distal angioplasty for limb salvage.[128]

Acute Arterial Occlusion

PRESENTATION

Acute arterial ischemia is a particularly ominous sign, with a 20-day mortality rate of 25 percent.[129] It presents suddenly as a painful, cold (polar), pale, pulseless limb that progresses to paresthesia and paralysis. Limb viability is at risk if flow is not restored quickly. Distal changes of livedo caused by microembolization may be present. If caused by arterial dissection, variability in the pulse deficit and area affected (migration of symptoms) may be seen, causing discrepancy in findings between examiners over time. Severe ischemia is suggested by pallor at rest, profound coolness, tender or hard muscles, and loss of motor and/or sensory functions.

ETIOLOGY

The etiology of acute arterial occlusions may be traumatic such as dissection, thrombosis in situ, or embolism. Arterial emboli come from any proximal source, occlusive or aneurysmal, but the majority originates from the heart. Both the left ventricle and atrium may harbor thrombi.[130] Aneurysms, clotting disorders, atherosclerosis, and recent arterial manipulation may precipitate acute occlusion. Emboli tend to be multiple, recurrent, and distribute randomly, mostly to the legs but with a significant incidence of cerebral, renal, visceral, and arm events.[131] Venous thrombi from the right heart or limbs can pass across cardiac septal defects or patent foramen ovali and cause arterial events.[132] Echocardiography is useful to determine source.[133]

MANAGEMENT

Immediate measures are needed to protect the limb and restore blood flow; heparinization should be started to prevent clot propagation and to stabilize the embolic sources. Angiography, conventional or other, may be required to plan repair when there is preexisting occlusive or aneurysmal disease, or when the etiology is unclear. Ideally, all acute occlusions should be considered for repair, but urgency is governed by the degree of ischemia. When severe ischemia is present, repair must occur within hours to salvage the limb. Additional time may be taken to address ancillary problems in lesser degrees of ischemia. When indicated, thrombolysis of acute occlusion can be effective.[134–136] Bleeding risk and stroke risk must be considered, particularly in the elderly, where both risks are seen to be great.

Arterial Disease of Diverse Etiologies

THROMBOANGIITIS OBLITERANS

Thromboangiitis obliterans (TAO), or Buerger's disease, described by Buerger in the late nineteenth century, is an inflammatory vasculopathy with a characteristic, highly cellular intraluminal thrombus that affects small- and medium-sized arteries and veins. TAO is al-

ways associated with tobacco use and may be an autoimmune response to it. Historically, TAO is seen predominantly in males in the second through fifth decades, although the incidence in women is rising, reflecting the changing demographics of tobacco use.[137,138] Clinically, TAO differs from atherosclerosis in that concurrent involvement of the upper extremity is common. The initial involvement is in digital, pedal, and hand vessels; progression to the calf, thigh, and forearm is brisk and occurs over a few months or years. One-third of patients report Raynaud's phenomenon.[139] Episodes of recurrent superficial phlebitis are common. Biopsy of acute lesions, particularly accessible veins, is diagnostic, while angiographic features are characteristic. Rare manifestations include coronary, cerebral, or visceral artery lesions. Stability or improvement is variable and possible only after all exposure to tobacco ceases.[140] Progressive tissue loss is inevitable until tobacco exposure is stopped. Cannabis, either on its own or because of contamination with tobacco, may cause a similar entity, and its use should also be addressed.[141] Sympathectomy and intravenous prostacyclin analogues can accelerate healing of ischemic lesions, but amputation of damaged digits and limbs is often required.[142,143] Angiogenesis by protein or gene therapy is likely to prove the best hope for this otherwise difficult-to-treat disease.[144]

TAKAYASU'S AND GIANT-CELL ARTERITIS

Takayasu's arteritis and giant-cell (temporal) arteritis (GCA) are similar in pathologic process but affect different age groups. Takayasu's arteritis affects those <40 year of age and giant-cell arteritis usually affects those >60. Differing criteria for age may be argued, but in general either may be seen in the fifth and sixth decades.[145] Also a generality, Takaysu's arteritis involves arteries below the neck, and GCA above the diaphragm.[146] However, involvement of the aorta and subclavian, axillary, renal, iliac, femoral, and superficial femoral arteries have been described in both. Disease is usually bilateral and results in rapidly progressive symptoms. Limb-threatening ischemia is rare. Both have characteristic clinical and laboratory findings including an elevated sedimentation rate (most commonly but not in all) and typical arteriographic features (Fig. 101-4). For GCA, confirmatory biopsy of the temporal artery within 3 days of starting steroids is the gold standard.[147] These diseases are unique among arteriopathies in that the acutely stenotic lesions improve rapidly with steroid therapy.[148,149] Revascularization, when required, is best performed when the inflammatory process is quiet or "burned out" and steroids are discontinued or requirements are tapered to a low, maintenance dose.[150,151]

POPLITEAL SYNDROMES

Popliteal entrapment syndrome occurs when the popliteal artery is trapped by the medial gastrocnemius or various muscular and ligamentous bands during passive dorsiflexion or active plantar flexion. Entrapment may cause claudication and (later) occlusion, usually seen in relatively young, healthy individuals and more often in athletes or those performing significant exertion. Surgical repair is the treatment of choice. Although uncommon, entrapment syndromes can also be seen at other sites.[152,153] Adventitial cystic disease is analogous in structure and content to a ganglion or mucoid cyst. It slowly grows into the popliteal (or occasionally common femoral artery, rarely a venous structure) space, causing claudication or rarely occlusion. Surgical repair is the treatment of choice.[154]

ERGOTISM

Ergot compounds can induce Raynaud's phenomenon, claudication, acute ischemia, and tissue infarction. Problems are usually seen in those using ergotamine compounds for treatment of migraine

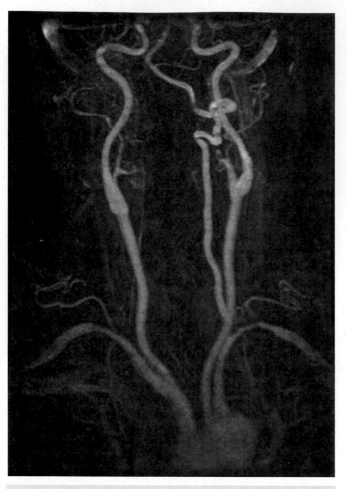

FIGURE 101-4 Magnetic resonance angiogram of the carotid arteries and great vessels in a patient with giant-cell arteritis. Note the smooth, tapered stenosis in the subclavian and external carotid arteries.

by infectious or traumatic etiologies expand over days to months. Five to 10 percent of patients with an aortic aneurysm, and 50 percent or more with peripheral aneurysms, will have aneurysms elsewhere.[160] When a popliteal aneurysm is found, a careful search for iliac, femoral, and aortic aneurysms should be performed. Aortic disease is addressed in an accompanying chapter. Femoral aneurysms are often first noted by the patient. Popliteal lesions are easily overlooked. Femoral and popliteal aneurysms are often first detected after acute thrombosis, distal micro- or macroembolization, or edema from perianeurysm venous compression or thrombosis.[161–163] Carotid and axillosubclavian aneurysms are easily diagnosed by palpation, and some present with local pain, thrombosis, or distal embolic complications. Visceral aneurysms are rarely large enough to be palpated; 3 to 5 percent present as rupture, and the majority are found incidentally at surgery or during imaging.[164]

Vasospastic Disorders

Color and warmth of the acral parts vary considerably from person to person in a normal population, reflecting individual vasomotor tone. Livedo reticularis, acrocyanosis, and Raynaud's phenomenon are distinctive clinical syndromes manifested by abnormal color and temperature changes of the skin. These syndromes are induced or intensified as a result of stimuli from cold, emotion, or drugs (Table 101-8). They cause spasm in digital arteries, arterioles, and venules. These disorders are usually benign, lifelong, primary processes, but all three syndromes can have important secondary causes. Careful clinical examination and selective testing will usually confirm the specific etiology and define prognosis and the direction of therapy.

LIVEDO RETICULARIS

Livedo reticularis is characterized by a persistent, symmetric, bluish, lacey pattern on the extremities and sometimes the trunk that is variable in its extent and intensity. It is most apparent after stimulation by cold or emotion and fades with warmth and exercise. It is first seen in

headaches. Intravenous nitroprusside infusion may help acute ischemia.[155] The incidence of ergot toxicity is decreasing as alternatives for migraine treatment become available, but it should be considered in patients with ischemia and few, if any, risk factors.[156]

FIBROMUSCULAR DYSPLASIA

Fibromuscular dysplasia has been described in almost all named arteries. It most commonly affects women in the middle years. Renal artery disease is most common, affecting 4 to 5 percent of the population. Carotid, mesenteric, and both upper and lower extremity diseases may be seen. Bilateral disease is present in about 10 percent of cases.[157] Arterial dissection is associated with fibromuscular dysplasia, causing about 10 percent of spontaneous dissections in all; over 20 percent of carotid dissections occur in women.[158]

Aneurysms

Arterial aneurysms are a major cause of death and disability. Early detection allows for definitive repair. The three most common aneurysms are accessible to examination including 40 to 60 percent of abdominal aortic aneurysms and almost all popliteal and femoral aneurysms.[159] Several general characteristics of aneurysmal disease are useful in clinical decision making. Aneurysms caused by degenerative etiologies enlarge over years to decades. Aneurysms caused

TABLE 101-8 Differential for Microcirculatory Disease

Embolism
    Arteriosclerosis obliterans
    Anticoagulation
    Trauma, instrumentation
    Surgery
Vasculitis
Endocarditis
Ergot toxicity
Cold injury
Malignancy
Hepatitis
Hematologic
    Polycythemia vera
    Thrombocytosis
    Dysproteinemia
    Cryoglobulinemia
    Cold agglutinins
    Circulating anticoagulants
Antiphospholipid antibodies
Thrombocytopenic purpura
Heparin-induced thrombocytopenia

childhood or at puberty and is more common in women and fair-skinned individuals. It is so frequent in its milder form that it is often overlooked or considered a variant of normal skin. It is postulated that spasm of the cutaneous arterioles (with secondary dilation of the capillaries and venules) causes slow flow, increased oxygen uptake, and reduced oxyhemoglobin, producing color change. Primary livedo reticularis is often seen with acrocyanosis and primary Raynaud's disease. Treatment is rarely needed.

Secondary livedo reticularis is patchy, focal, or asymmetric in distribution; relatively late in onset; and may be complicated by local infarction or ulceration. The lesions may be elevated or tender when caused by vasculitis. Therapy is directed at the underlying cause (Table 101-9). Vasodilators and sympathectomy are of unpredictable, anecdotal value for healing painful ulcers. Severe livedo reticularis in the setting of multiple cerebrovascular events may suggest Sneddon's syndrome. In this group antiphospholipid antibodies are common.[165,166]

ACROCYANOSIS

Acrocyanosis is a benign, persistent cyanotic discoloration with coolness of the hands (or fingers, sometimes the feet) more commonly seen in women. A modest degree of acrocyanosis is sometimes seen in limbs immobilized by neurogenic deficits. Cold and emotion intensify symptoms, whereas warmth and exercise ameliorate the findings. Mild local edema is not uncommon. Acrocyanosis is painless and does not ulcerate, but it is a bothersome cosmetic problem for some. Calcium entry blockers or alpha$_1$ antagonists will often reduce the symptoms. Rarely, beta-blockade will induce the syndrome. It may also present as a paraneoplastic phenomenon.[167,168]

RAYNAUD'S PHENOMENON

Raynaud's phenomenon is diagnosed by history. It is difficult to demonstrate, even with ice immersion, as whole body cooling is often needed to induce symptoms. The syndrome is defined as episodes of blue then white color changes in the digits induced by cold or emotional stimuli followed by red discoloration during the hyperemia recovery phase. Most patients describe only two of the three phases. A dead, numb feeling (but rarely pain) accompanies the ischemic phase, and a dysthetic, throbbing, or painful sensation is common in recovery. Fingers are involved more often than toes. The palm is rarely affected and the thumbs are often spared. Recovery time is 3 to 10 min but can exceed 1 h in advanced cases, usually of secondary origin.[169]

Allen and Brown[170] defined primary Raynaud's as episodes of bilateral color changes induced by cold or emotion without evidence of ischemia or other disease for 2 years. Later development of secondary disease was noted in 2 to 5 percent of patients.[171,172] A recent prospective study confirms that patients without laboratory evidence of digital occlusive, clotting, or serologic abnormalities have a be-

nign course, with only 2 percent showing secondary causes in the subsequent decade.[173]

Causes of secondary Raynaud's phenomenon are diverse (Table 101-10). Most can be defined by history and examination, knowledge of their natural behavior, vascular laboratory measurements of digital obstruction, and clotting or serologic tests. Vibratory tools such as chain saws, grinders, and jackhammers can induce hand dysesthesias and Raynaud's phenomenon when used for several years. Symptoms initially occur during use but may become chronic in later stages. Ischemia is a rare and late occurrence.[174,175]

Arteriography (from the arch through the digits and performed bilateral) is reserved for unusual problems or for planning surgery when needed. Trophic skin changes and ischemic lesions usually reflect occlusive etiologies, while unilateral Raynaud's suggests a secondary process.[176] Most patients with primary Raynaud's phenomenon require no therapy and quickly learn to keep not only hands but the whole body warm. Treatment of secondary Raynaud's is directed at the underlying cause when feasible. Calcium channel blockers and alpha blockade, alone or in combination, can blunt the episodes in many patients, but may have little impact on ischemic complications. These are best treated with local debridement and control of infection and pain.

Thoracic Outlet Syndrome

Thoracic outlet syndrome is a constellation of symptoms that may be not only difficult to treat but difficult to diagnose. This difficulty reflects the anatomy, in that the artery, vein, and nerve bundle pass through a small, dynamic space. The usual mechanism of damage is from the clavicle and the first rib (or a cervical rib) "scissoring" the subclavian artery, resulting in a stenosis or aneurysm formation.

TABLE 101-9 Differential for Livedo Reticularis

Environmental (cold)
Atheroembolism (cholesterol)
Connective tissue disease
Cutaneous vasculitis
Amantidine hydrochloride
Reflex sympathetic dystrophy
Myeloproliferative diseases
Vasculitis
Thrombocytosis

TABLE 101-10 Causes of Secondary Raynaud's Phenomenon

Collagen vascular disease
Scleroderma
Mixed connective tissue disease
Rheumatoid arthritis
Myositis
Sjogren's syndrome
Necrotizing vasculitis
Hematologic disorders
Neurogenic
Thoracic outlet irritation
Carpal tunnel syndrome
Myxedema
Acromegaly
Pulmonary hypertension
Medications
Beta blockers
Ergotamine
Methysergide
Vinblastine, bleomycin
Estrogens
Imipramine
Buerger's disease
Hypothenar hammer syndrome
Environmental
Cold injury
Vibration syndrome

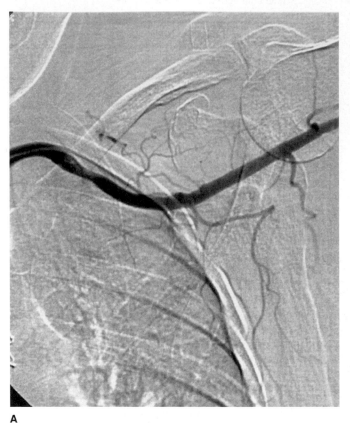

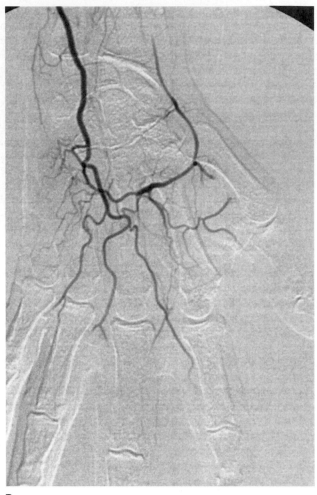

A   **B**

FIGURE 101-5 *A.* Arteriogram of the clavicle impinging on the left subclavian artery in a patient having new onset of asymmetric Raynaud's phenomenon with digital ischemia suggesting embolic etiology. *B.* Left-hand arteriogram of the same patient demonstrating multiple levels of occlusion.

Hypertrophy of the scalene musculature may add to the osseous etiology.[177] Aneurysmal dilatation is prone to thrombus formation, which can lead to thromboembolism and distal arterial occlusion (Fig. 101-5). Raynaud's phenomenon is common. "Effort thrombosis" of the subclavian vein (Paget-Schroetter syndrome) may be the presenting complaint. This is most frequently seen in active individuals—such as construction workers and athletes—with repetitive motion obstructing the venous outflow.[178] Neurogenic complaints may be present and difficult to isolate. In cases with pure neurologic findings, long-term resolution following intervention is less reliable.[179] It is important to point out that the presence of positive thoracic outlet maneuvers does not equal the diagnosis of thoracic outlet syndrome. Imaging for the presence of an aneurysm or a stenosis, dynamic or static, with Duplex ultrasound or arteriography is needed when the diagnosis is entertained. Clinical correlation is required for the diagnosis. Initial treatment for noncomplicated cases (that is, no distal embolization or arterial damage) should include thoracic outlet opening exercises.[180] If arterial damage or distal embolization has occurred, resection of a cervical rib and/or first rib is frequently required.[181] Improvement of symptoms is variable.[182] For venous occlusion, initial treatment should be aimed at opening the subclavian vein, most frequently with thrombolysis. The optimal timing of further surgical intervention, immediate or delayed with several weeks to months of anticoagulation, is not yet established.[183]

Hammer Hand Syndrome

Hammer hand syndrome is the result of repetitive trauma to the hypothenar area by using a hammer, levers, or equipment with vibration. These activities may produce occlusion or aneurysm formation of the ulnar artery, usually at the level of the hammate bone. Raynaud's phenomenon is commonly present but may be in just one or several digits, suggesting a secondary etiology. Digital ischemia of one or more digits can result from emboli. Improvement may be seen when the offending trauma is stopped, but surgical treatment is required if digits remain ischemic.[184,185]

CARE OF VASCULAR WOUNDS

The end stage of any type of ischemia is tissue necrosis. In some ways treating an ischemic foot is more difficult than treating ischemic cardiomyopathy, since the patient can see the "problem" and wants you to heal the heel. Although the patient may have been told

TABLE 101-11 Recognition of Ulcers of Vascular Etiology

Type	Venous	Arterial	Neurotrophic	Arteriolar
Location	Perimalleolar	Shins, toes, sites of injury	Plantar surface, pressure points	Shin, calf
Pain	No, unless infected	Yes	No	Exquisite
Skin	Stasis pigmentation, thickening with lipodermatosclerosis	Shiny, pale, decreased hair, may see livedo	Callus present, normal to changes of ischemia	Normal or "satellite" ulcers in various stages
Edges	Clean	Smooth	Trophic, callused	Serpiginous
Base	Wet, weeping, healthy granulation	Dry, pale with eschar	Healthy to pale depending on ASO	Dry, punched-out pale, thin eschar
Cellulitis	Common	Often	Common	No
Treatment	Compression	Revascularize	Relieve pressure	Treat underlying disease, relieve pain

the ulcer is a manifestation of the real problem (an occluded tibioperoneal trunk for example), the expectation is that this small ulcer can be cured. In many cases, it can be.

To heal an ulcer more effectively than chance or luck, the cause must be identified. Once the underlying etiology of the wound is known, effective treatment can be directed. The wound may provide clues, but a complete history and physical exam provide indispensable information as to etiology (Table 101-11). There are a myriad of wound care products on the market. In actual practice, most physicians use the few that they are most comfortable with. The patient must play an active role in care of the ulcer if healing is to occur. In many cases this means dressing changes multiple times per day. For the neurotrophic ulcer or ischemic ulcer, compliance with no weight bearing must be followed. A farming analogy is useful to many patients (and physicians). What one is trying to "grow" is tissue—skin if you will. Like any produce, conditions must be favorable or the desired crop cannot be expected to grow. Ischemia (drought) must be corrected to provide oxygen and nutrients. Edema (swamp) must be reduced, cellulitis (weeds) treated, and occasional plowing and tilling (debridement) performed to loosen the tissues of fibrinous exudate. Care of vascular wounds is often tedious and frustrating but always rewarding in that the benefits of the partnership formed between patient and caregiver are visible.

References

1. Lakshmi A. A statistical approach to monitor ongoing intervention for control of lymphatic filariasis. *J Commun Dis* 2000;32:10–16.
2. Eberhard ML, DeMeester LJ, Martin BW, Lammie PJ. Zoonotic *Brugia* infection in western Michigan. *Am J Surg Pathol* 1993;17:1058–1061.
3. Nutman TB. Lymphatic filariasis: new insights and prospects for control. *Curr Opin Infect Dis* 2001;14:539–546.
4. Wheatley DC, Wastie ML, Whitaker SC, et al. Lymphoscintigraphy and colour Doppler sonography in the assessment of leg oedema of unknown cause. *Br J Radiol* 1996;69:1117–1124.
5. Raju S, Owen S Jr, Neglen P. Reversal of abnormal lymphoscintigraphy after placement of venous stents for correction of associated venous obstruction. *J Vasc Surg* 2001;34:779–784.
6. Szuba A, Razavi M, Rockson SG. Diagnosis and treatment of concomitant venous obstruction in patients with secondary lymphedema. *J Vasc Interv Radiol* 2002;13:799–803.
7. Wheeler H, Anderson FJ, Cardullo P, et al. Suspected deep vein thrombosis: Management by impedance plethysmography. *Arch Surg* 1982; 1296–1309.
8. Bygdeman S, Aschberg S, Hindmarsh T. Venous plethysmography in the diagnosis of chronic venous insufficiency. *Acta Chir Scand* 1971; 137:423–428.
9. Rooke T, Heser JL, Osmundson PJ. Exercise strain-gauge venous plethysmography: Evaluation of a "new" device for assessing lower limb venous incompetence. *Angiology* 1987;219–228.
10. Struckmann JR. Assessment of the venous muscle pump function by ambulatory strain gauge plethysmography. Methodological and clinical aspects. *Dan Med Bull* 1993;40:460–477.
11. Kahn SR, Joseph L, Grover SA, Leclerc JR. A randomized management study of impedance plethysmography vs. contrast venography in patients with a first episode of clinically suspected deep vein thrombosis. *Thromb Res* 2001;102:15–24.
12. Chong D. IPG screening for asymptomatic DVT. *Arch Phys Med Rehabil* 1996;77:211.
13. Mantoni M, Larsen L, Lund JO, et al. Evaluation of chronic venous disease in the lower limbs: comparison of five diagnostic methods. *Br J Radiol* 2002;75:578–583.
14. Marston WA. PPG, APG, duplex: which noninvasive tests are most appropriate for the management of patients with chronic venous insufficiency? *Semin Vasc Surg* 2002;15:13–20.
15. Washington L, Goodman LR, Gonyo MB. CT for thromboembolic disease. *Radiol Clin North Am* 2002;40:751–771.
16. Schutgens RE, Esseboom EU, Haas FJ, et al. Usefulness of a semiquantitative D-dimer test for the exclusion of deep venous thrombosis in outpatients. *Am J Med* 2002;112:617–621.
17. Franks PJ, Wright DD, Moffatt CJ, et al. Prevalence of venous disease: a community study in west London. *Eur J Surg* 1992;158:143–147.
18. Bergan JJ, Kumins NH, Owens EL, Sparks SR. Surgical and endovascular treatment of lower extremity venous insufficiency. *J Vasc Interv Radiol* 2002;13:563–568.
19. Harris EJ Jr. Endovascular obliteration of saphenous vein reflux: a perspective. *J Vasc Surg* 2002;35:1292–1294.
20. Guex JJ. Thrombotic complications of varicose veins. A literature review of the role of superficial venous thrombosis. *Dermatol Surg* 1996; 22:378–382.
21. Hanson JN, Ascher E, DePippo P, et al. Saphenous vein thrombophlebitis (SVT): a deceptively benign disease. *J Vasc Surg* 1998;27: 677–680.
22. O'Fallon W, Heit J, Mohr D, et al. Predictors of recurrence after deep vein thrombosis and pulmonary embolism: a population-based cohort study. *Blood* 1998;10:560–561.
23. Miura Y, Ardenghy M, Ramasastry S, et al. Coumadin necrosis of the skin: Report of four patients. *Ann Plast Surg* 1996;37:332–337.
24. Rymes NL, Lester W, Connor C, et al. Outpatient management of DVT using low molecular weight heparin and a hospital outreach service. *Clin Lab Haematol* 2002;24:165–170.

25. Litin SC, Heit JA, Mees KA. Use of low-molecular-weight heparin in the treatment of venous thromboembolic disease: answers to frequently asked questions. The Thrombophilia Center Investigators. *Mayo Clin Proc* 1998;73:545–550; quiz 551.

26. Agnelli G, Prandoni P, Santamaria MG, et al. Three months versus one year of oral anticoagulant therapy for idiopathic deep venous thrombosis. Warfarin Optimal Duration Italian Trial Investigators. *N Engl J Med* 2001;345:165–169.

27. Lindhoff-Last E, Nakov R, Misselwitz F, et al. Incidence and clinical relevance of heparin-induced antibodies in patients with deep vein thrombosis treated with unfractionated or low-molecular-weight heparin. *Br J Haematol* 2002;118:1137–1142.

28. Warkentin TE. Heparin-induced thrombocytopenia: A ten-year retrospective. *Annu Rev Med* 1999;50:129–147.

29. Ibbotson T, Perry CM. Danaparoid: a review of its use in thromboembolic and coagulation disorders. *Drugs* 2002;62:2283–2314.

30. Acostamadiedo JM, Iyer UG, Owen J. Danaparoid sodium. *Expert Opin Pharmacother* 2000;1:803–814.

31. Kearon C, Gent M, Hirsh J, et al. A comparison of three months of anticoagulation with extended anticoagulation for a first episode of idiopathic venous thromboembolism. *N Engl J Med* 1999;340:901–907.

32. Anand SS. Comparison of 3 and 6 months of oral anticoagulant therapy after a first episode of proximal deep vein thrombosis or pulmonary embolism and comparison of 6 and 12 weeks of therapy after isolated calf deep vein thrombosis.

32a. Pinede L, Ninet J, Duhaut P et al for the Investigators of the 'Duree Optimale du Traitement Antivitamines K' (DOTAVK) study. *Circulation* 2001;103:2453–2460. *Vasc Med* 2001;6:269–270.

33. Palareti G, Legnani C, Lee A, et al. A comparison of the safety and efficacy of oral anticoagulation for the treatment of venous thromboembolic disease in patients with or without malignancy. *Thromb Haemost* 2000;84:805–810.

34. Comerota A. Venous thromboembolism. In: Rutherford RB, ed. *Vascular Surgery*. Philadelphia: Saunders, 1995:1785–1814.

35. Rhodes JM, Cho JS, Gloviczki P, et al. Thrombolysis for experimental deep venous thrombosis maintains valvular competence and vasoreactivity. *J Vasc Surg* 2000;31:1193–1205.

36. Elsharawy M, Elzayat E. Early results of thrombolysis vs anticoagulation in iliofemoral venous thrombosis. A randomised clinical trial. *Eur J Vasc Endovasc Surg* 2002;24:209–214.

37. Mewissen MW, Seabrook GR, Meissner MH, et al. Catheter-directed thrombolysis for lower extremity deep venous thrombosis: report of a national multicenter registry. *Radiology* 1999;211:39–49.

38. Ginsberg JS, Hirsh J, Julian J, et al. Prevention and treatment of postphlebitic syndrome: results of a 3-part study. *Arch Intern Med* 2001; 161:2105–2109.

39. Prandoni P, Lensing A, Cogo A, et al. The long-term clinical course of acute deep venous thrombosis. *Ann Intern Med* 1996;125:1–7.

40. Hirsh J, Lee AY. How we diagnose and treat deep vein thrombosis. *Blood* 2002;99:3102–3110.

41. Tripodi A, Mannucci PM. Laboratory investigation of thrombophilia. *Clin Chem* 2001;47:1597–1606.

42. Freedman MD, Young M. Venous thrombosis: diagnosis and treatment; new methods and strategies for management. *Compr Ther* 1999;25:13–19.

43. Piccioli A, Prandoni P. Idiopathic venous thromboembolism as a first manifestation of cancer. *Haemostasis* 2001;31(suppl 1):37–39.

44. Harris M, Grange J. Management of calf deep venous thrombosis. *Ann Emerg Med* 2000;35:629.

45. Lohr JM, Kerr TM, Lutter KS, et al. Lower extremity calf thrombosis: To treat or not to treat? *J Vasc Surg* 1991;14:618–623.

46. Meissner MH, Caps MT, Bergelin RO, et al. Early outcome after isolated calf vein thrombosis. *J Vasc Surg* 1997;26:749–756.

47. Wood KE, Reedy JS, Pozniak MA, Coursin DB. Phlegmasia cerulea dolens with compartment syndrome: a complication of femoral vein catheterization. *Crit Care Med* 2000;28:1626–1630.

48. Sciolaro C, Hunter GC, McIntyre KE, et al. Thrombectomy and isolated limb perfusion with urokinase in the treatment of phlegmasia cerulea dolens. *Cardiovasc Surg* 1993;1:56–60.

49. Wudel LJ Jr, Nesbitt JC. Superior vena cava syndrome. *Curr Treat Options Oncol* 2001;2:77–91.

50. Barakat K, Robinson NM, Spurrell RA. Transvenous pacing lead-induced thrombosis: a series of cases with a review of the literature. *Cardiology* 2000;93:142–148.

51. Hausler M, Hubner D, Delhaas T, Muhler EG. Long-term complications of inferior vena cava thrombosis. *Arch Dis Child* 2001;85:228–233.

52. Suzuoki M, Kondo S, Ambo Y, et al. Treatment of Budd-Chiari syndrome with percutaneous transluminal angioplasty: Report of a case. *Surg Today* 2002;32:559–562.

53. Espinosa G, Font J, Garcia-Pagan JC, et al. Budd-Chiari syndrome secondary to antiphospholipid syndrome: clinical and immunologic characteristics of 43 patients. *Medicine (Baltimore)* 2001;80: 345–354.

54. Haenen JH, Janssen MC, Wollersheim H, et al. The development of postthrombotic syndrome in relationship to venous reflux and calf muscle pump dysfunction at 2 years after the onset of deep venous thrombosis. *J Vasc Surg* 2002;35:1184–1189.

55. Nicolaides A, Christopoulos D, Vasdekis S. Progress in the investigation of chronic venous insufficiency. *Ann Vasc Surg* 1989;3:278–292.

56. Leary W, Allen E. Intermittent claudication as a result of arterial spasm induced by walking. *Am Heart J* 1941;22:719–725.

57. DeWesse J. Pedal pulses disappearing with exercise. *N Engl J Med* 1960;262:1214–1217.

58. Radu AS, Menkes CJ. Update on lumbar spinal stenosis. Retrospective study of 62 patients and review of the literature. *Rev Rheum Engl Ed* 1998;65:337–345.

59. Altchek M. Pseudoclaudication syndrome. *JAMA* 1969;207:1917.

60. Kavanaugh GJ, Svien HJ, Holman CB, Johnson RM. "Pseudoclaudication" syndrome produced by compression of the cauda equina. *JAMA* 1968;206:2477–2481.

61. Burns SL, Leese GP, McMurdo ME. Older people and ill fitting shoes. *Postgrad Med J* 2002;78:344–346.

62. Matzke S, Lepantalo M. Claudication does not always precede critical leg ischemia. *Vasc Med* 2001;6:77–80.

63. Tombach B, Bremer C, Reimer P, et al. Using highly concentrated gadobutrol as an MR contrast agent in patients also requiring hemodialysis: safety and dialysability. *AJR* 2002;178:105–109.

64. Strandness DJ, McCutcheon E, Rushmer R. Application of transcutaneous Doppler flowmeter in evaluation of occlusive arterial disease. *Surg Gynecol Obstet* 1966;122:1039–1045.

65. Lanzer P. Topographic distribution of peripheral arteriopathy in nondiabetics and type 2 diabetics. *Z Kardiol* 2001;90:99–103.

66. Hobbs J, Yao J, Lewis J, Needham T. A limitation of the Doppler ultrasound method of measuring ankle systolic pressure. *Vasa* 1974; 3:160–164.

67. Regensteiner JG, Gardner A, Hiatt WR. Exercise testing and exercise rehabilitation for patients with peripheral arterial disease: status in 1997. *Vasc Med* 1997;2:147–155.

68. Regensteiner JG, Hiatt WR. Medical management of peripheral arterial disease. *J Vasc Interv Radiol* 1994;5:669–677.

69. McDermott MM, Mehta S, Liu K, et al. Leg symptoms, the ankle-brachial index, and walking ability in patients with peripheral arterial disease. *J Gen Intern Med* 1999;14:173–181.

70. Toursarkissian B, Mejia A, Smilanich RP, et al. Noninvasive localization of infrainguinal arterial occlusive disease in diabetics. *Ann Vasc Surg* 2001;15:73–78.

71. Symes J, Graham A, Mousseau M. Doppler waveform analysis versus segmental pressure and pulse-volume recording: Assessment of occlusive disease in the lower extremity. *Can J Surg* 1984;27:345–347.

72. Rooke T. The use of transcutaneous oximetry in the noninvasive vascular laboratory. *Int Angiol* 1992;11:36–40.

73. Rooke T, Hollier L, Osmundson P. The influence of sympathetic nerves on transcutaneous oxygen tension in normal and ischemic lower extremities. *Angiology* 1987;38:400–410.

74. Bacharach J, Rooke T, Osmundson P, Gloviczke P. Predictive value of transcutaneous oxygen pressure and amputation success by use of supine and elevation measurements. *J Vasc Surg* 1992;15:558–563.

75. Rooke T, Osmundson P. The influence of age, sex, smoking, and diabetes on lower limb transcutaneous oxygen tension in patients with arterial occlusive disease. *Arch Intern Med* 1990;150:129–32.

76. Criqui MH, Denenberg JO, Langer RD, Fronek A. The epidemiology of peripheral arterial disease: Importance of identifying the population at risk. *Vasc Med* 1997;2:221–226.

77. Criqui MH. Peripheral arterial disease—Epidemiological aspects. *Vasc Med* 2001;6:3–7.

78. Criqui MH, Denenberg JO, Langer RD, Fronek A. The epidemiology of peripheral arterial disease: importance of identifying the population at risk. *Vasc Med* 1997;2:221–226.

79. de Jong SC, Stehouwer CD, Mackaay AJ, et al. High prevalence of hyperhomocysteinemia and asymptomatic vascular disease in siblings of young patients with vascular disease and hyperhomocysteinemia. *Arterioscler Thromb Vasc Biol* 1997;17:2655–2662.

80. Taylor LM Jr, Moneta GL, Sexton GJ, et al. Prospective blinded study of the relationship between plasma homocysteine and progression of symptomatic peripheral arterial disease. *J Vasc Surg* 1999;29:8–19; discussion 19–21.

81. Murabito JM, Evans JC, Nieto K, et al. Prevalence and clinical correlates of peripheral arterial disease in the Framingham Offspring Study. *Am Heart J* 2002;143:961–965.

82. Hirsch AT, Criqui MH, Treat-Jacobson D, et al. Peripheral arterial disease detection, awareness, and treatment in primary care. *JAMA* 2001; 286:1317–1324.

83. Hooi JD, Stoffers HE, Knottnerus JA, van Ree JW. The prognosis of non-critical limb ischaemia: A systematic review of population-based evidence. *Br J Gen Pract* 1999;49:49–55.

84. Dormandy J, Heeck L, Vig S. The fate of patients with critical leg ischemia. *Semin Vasc Surg* 1999;12:142–147.

85. McKenna M, Wolfson S, Kuller L. The ratio of ankle and arm blood pressure as an independent risk factor of mortality. *Atherosclerosis* 1991;87:119–128.

86. Criqui M, Langer R, Fronek A, et al. Mortality over a period of 10 years in patients with peripheral arterial disease. *N Engl J Med* 1992; 326:381–386.

87. Lassila R, Lepantalo M, Lindfors O. Peripheral arterial disease—Natural outcome. *Acta Med Scand* 1986;220:295–301.

88. McDaniel M, Cronenwett J. Basic data related to the natural history of intermittent claudication. *Ann Vasc Surg* 1989;3:273.

89. Imperato A, Kim G, Davidson T, Crowley J. Intermittent claudication: Its natural course. *Surgery* 1975;78:795–799.

90. Feinglass J, Brown J, LoSasso A, et al. Rates of lower extremity amputation and arterial reconstruction in the United States, 1979 to 1996. *Am J Public Health* 1999;89:1222–1227.

91. Moss S, Klein RM, Klein BE. The 14-year incidence of lower extremity amputation in a diabetic population: The Wisconsin Epidemiologic Study of Diabetic Retinopathy. *Diabetes Care* 1999;22:951–959.

92. Juergens J, Barker N, Hines EJ. Arteriosclerosis obliterans: Review of 520 cases with special reference to pathogenic and prognostic factors. *Circulation* 1960;21:188–195.

93. Adler A, Boyko E, Ahroni J, Smith D. Lower extremity amputation in diabetes. The independent effects of peripheral vascular disease. *Diabetes Care* 1999;22:1029–1035.

94. Fletcher DD, Andrews KL, Hallett JW Jr, et al. Trends in rehabilitation after amputation for geriatric patients with vascular disease: implications for future health resource allocation. *Arch Phys Med Rehabil* 2002;83:1389–1393.

95. Valentine RJ, Jackson MR, Modrall JG, et al. The progressive nature of peripheral arterial disease in young adults: a prospective analysis of white men referred to a vascular surgery service. *J Vasc Surg* 1999; 30:436–444.

96. McDermott M, Mehta S, Ahn H, Greenland P. Atherosclerotic risk factors are less intensively treated in patients with peripheral arterial disease than in patients with coronary artery disease. *J Gen Intern Med* 1997;12:209–215.

97. Dormandy J, Heeck L, Vig S. Predicting which patients will develop chronic critical leg ischemia. *Semin Vasc Surg* 1999;12:138–141.

98. West JA. Cost-effective strategies for the management of vascular disease. *Vasc Med* 1997;2:25–29.

99. Regensteiner JG, Steiner JF, Hiatt WR. Exercise training improves functional status in patients with peripheral arterial disease. *J Vasc Surg* 1996;23:104–115.

100. McDermott MM, Greenland P, Liu K, et al. The ankle brachial index is associated with leg function and physical activity: The Walking and Leg Circulation Study. *Ann Intern Med* 2002;136:873–883.

101. Gardner AW, Katzel LI, Sorkin JD, Goldberg AP. Effects of long-term exercise rehabilitation on claudication distances in patients with peripheral arterial disease: a randomized controlled trial. *J Cardiopulm Rehabil* 2002;22:192–198.

102. Rith-Najarian SJ, Reiber GE. Prevention of foot problems in persons with diabetes. *J Fam Pract* 2000;49:30–39.

103. Sowell RD, Mangel WB, Kilczewski CJ, Normington JM. Effect of podiatric medical care on rates of lower-extremity amputation in a Medicare population. *J Am Podiatr Med Assoc* 1999;89:312–337.

104. Hood S, Moher D, Barber G. Management of intermittent claudication with pentoxyfilline: Meta-analysis of randomized controlled trials. *Can Med Assoc J* 1996;155:1053–1058.

105. Strandness DE Jr, Dalman RL, Panian S, et al. Effect of cilostazol in patients with intermittent claudication: a randomized, double-blind, placebo-controlled study. *Vasc Endovascular Surg* 2002;36:83–91.

106. Reilly MP, Mohler ER III. Cilostazol: treatment of intermittent claudication. *Ann Pharmacother* 2001;35:48–56.

107. Money SR, Herd JA, Isaacsohn JL, et al. Effect of cilostazol on walking distances in patients with intermittent claudication caused by peripheral vascular disease. *J Vasc Surg* 1998;27:267–274; discussion 274–275.

108. Bagger J, Helligose P, Randsbaek F, et al. Effect of verapamil in intermittent claudication: A randomized, double-blind, placebo-controlled, cross-over study after individual dose response assessment. *Circulation* 1997;95:422–424.

109. Hiatt W, Stoll S, Nies A. Effect of beta-adrenergic blockers in the peripheral circulation in patients with peripheral arterial disease. *Circulation* 1985;72:1226.

110. Radack K, Deck C. Beta-adrenergic blocker therapy does not worsen intermittent claudication in subjects with peripheral arterial disease. A meta-analysis of randomized controlled trials. *Arch Intern Med* 1991; 151:1769–1776.

111. Girolami B, Bernardi E, Prins MH, et al. Antiplatelet therapy and other interventions after revascularisation procedures in patients with peripheral arterial disease: a meta-analysis. *Eur J Vasc Endovasc Surg* 2000;19:370–380.

112. Roller RE, Dorr A, Ulrich S, Pilger E. Effect of aspirin treatment in patients with peripheral arterial disease monitored with the platelet function analyzer PFA-100. *Blood Coagul Fibrinolysis* 2002;13:277–2781.

113. CAPRIE Steering Committee. A randomised, blinded, trial of clopidogrel versus aspirin in patients at risk of ischaemic events (CAPRIE). *Lancet* 1996;348:1329–1339.

114. Hiatt WR. Preventing atherothrombotic events in peripheral arterial disease: the use of antiplatelet therapy. *J Intern Med* 2002;251: 193–206.

115. Barndt R, Blankenhorn D, Crawford D, Brooks S. Regression and progression of early femoral atherosclerosis in treated hyperlipoproteinemic patients. *Ann Intern Med* 1977;86:139–144.

116. Pedersen TR, Kjekshus J, Pyorala K, et al. Effect of simvastatin on ischemic signs and symptoms in the Scandinavian Simvastatin Survival Study (4S). *Am J Cardiol* 1998;81:333–335.

117. Leng GC, Price JF, Jepson RG. Lipid-lowering for lower limb atherosclerosis. *Cochrane Database Syst Rev* 2000;CD000123.

118. Kuan YM, E Dear A, Grigg MJ. Homocysteine: An aetiological contributor to peripheral vascular arterial disease. *Aust NZ J Surg* 2002; 72:668–671.

119. Hansrani M, Gillespie JI, Stansby G. Homocysteine in myointimal hyperplasia. *Eur J Vasc Endovasc Surg* 2002;23:3–10.

120. Weiss N, Feussner A, Hailer S, et al. Influence of folic acid, pyridoxal phosphate and cobalamin on plasma homocyst(e)ine levels and the

susceptibility of low-density lipoprotein to ex-vivo oxidation. *Eur J Med Res* 1999;4:425–432.

121. Hou XY, Green S, Askew CD, et al. Skeletal muscle mitochondrial ATP production rate and walking performance in peripheral arterial disease. *Clin Physiol Funct Imaging* 2002;22:226–232.

122. Brass EP, Hiatt WR. The role of carnitine and carnitine supplementation during exercise in man and in individuals with special needs. *J Am Coll Nutr* 1998;17:207–215.

123. Cozzolino D, Coppola L, Masi S, et al. Short- and long-term treatments with iloprost in diabetic patients with peripheral vascular disease: effects on the cardiovascular risk factor plasminogen activator inhibitor type-1. *Eur J Clin Pharmacol* 1999;55:491–497.

124. Melillo E, Iabichella L, Berchiolli R, et al. Transcutaneous oxygen and carbon dioxide during treatment of critical limb ischemia with iloprost, a prostacyclin derivative. *Int J Microcirc Clin Exp* 1995;15:60–64.

125. Melian EB, Goa KL. Beraprost: A review of its pharmacology and therapeutic efficacy in the treatment of peripheral arterial disease and pulmonary arterial hypertension. *Drugs* 2002;62:107–133.

126. Moller ER III, Klugherz B, Goldman R, et al. Trial of a novel prostacyclin analog, UT-15, in patients with severe intermittent claudication. *Vasc Med* 2000;5:231–237.

127. de Vries SO, Visser K, de Vries JA, et al. Intermittent claudication: cost-effectiveness of revascularization versus exercise therapy. *Radiology* 2002;222:25–36.

128. Faglia E, Mantero M, Caminiti M, et al. Extensive use of peripheral angioplasty, particularly infrapopliteal, in the treatment of ischaemic diabetic foot ulcers: clinical results of a multicentric study of 221 consecutive diabetic subjects. *J Intern Med* 2002;252:225–232.

129. Clason AE, Stonebridge PA, Duncan AJ, et al. Morbidity and mortality in acute lower limb ischaemia: a 5-year review. *Eur J Vasc Surg* 1989;3:339–343.

130. Hight D, Tilney N, Couch N. Changing clinical trends in patients with peripheral arterial emboli. *Surgery* 1976;79:171–176.

131. Darling R, Austen W, Linton R. Arterial embolism. *Surg Gynecol Obstet* 1967;124:106–114.

132. Meister S, Grossman W, Dexter L, Dalen J. Paradoxical embolism: Diagnosis during life. *Am J Med* 1972;53:292–298.

133. Mariano MC, Gutierrez CJ, Alexander J, et al. The utility of transesophageal echocardiography in determining the source of arterial embolization. *Am Surg* 2000;66:901–904.

134. Laird JR. The management of acute limb ischemia: Techniques for dealing with thrombus. *J Interv Cardiol* 2001;14:539–546.

135. Korn P, Khilnani NM, Fellers JC, et al. Thrombolysis for native arterial occlusions of the lower extremities: clinical outcome and cost. *J Vasc Surg* 2001;33:1148–1157.

136. Semba CP, Murphy TP, Bakal CW, et al. Thrombolytic therapy with use of alteplase (rt-PA) in peripheral arterial occlusive disease: review of the clinical literature. The Advisory Panel. *J Vasc Interv Radiol* 2000;11:149–161.

137. Morris-Jones W, Jones CD. Buerger's disease in women. A report of a case and a review of the literature. *Angiology* 1973;24:675–700.

138. Wysokinski WE, Kwiatkowska W, Sapian-Raczkowska B, et al. Sustained classic clinical spectrum of thromboangiitis obliterans (Buerger's disease). *Angiology* 2000;51:141–150.

139. Shionoya S. Diagnostic criteria of Buerger's disease. *Int J Cardiol* 1998;66(suppl 1):S243–S245; discussion S247.

140. Olin JW, Young JR, Graor RA, et al. The changing clinical spectrum of thromboangiitis obliterans (Buerger's disease). *Circulation* 1990;82:IV3–8.

141. Disdier P, Granel B, Serratrice J, et al. Cannabis arteritis revisited—Ten new case reports. *Angiology* 2001;52:1–5.

142. Reny JL, Cabane J. [Buerger's disease or thromboangiitis obliterans]. *Rev Med Interne* 1998;19:34–43.

143. Fiessinger JN, Schafer M. Trial of iloprost versus aspirin treatment for critical limb ischaemia of thromboangiitis obliterans. The TAO Study. *Lancet* 1990;335:555–557.

144. Isner JM, Baumgartner I, Rauh G, et al. Treatment of thromboangiitis obliterans (Buerger's disease) by intramuscular gene transfer of vascular endothelial growth factor: preliminary clinical results. *J Vasc Surg* 1998;28:964–973; discussion 973–975.

145. Singh S, Dass R. Clinical approach to vasculitides. *Indian J Pediatr* 2002;69:881–888.

146. Odero A, Regina G. Regarding "Extracranial carotid aneurysm in Takayasu's arteritis." *J Vasc Surg* 2002;36:201; author reply 201.

147. Achkar AA, Hunder GG, Gabriel SE. Effect of previous corticosteroid treatment on temporal artery biopsy results. *Ann Intern Med* 1998;128:410.

148. Hoffman GS, Cid MC, Hellmann DB, et al. A multicenter, randomized, double-blind, placebo-controlled trial of adjuvant methotrexate treatment for giant cell arteritis. *Arthritis Rheum* 2002;46:1309–1318.

149. Hall S, Hunder GG. Treatment of Takayasu's arteritis. *Ann Intern Med* 1986;104:288.

150. Salvarani C, Hunder GG. Giant cell arteritis with low erythrocyte sedimentation rate: frequency of occurence in a population-based study. *Arthritis Rheum* 2001; 45:140–145.

151. Stone JH, Calabrese LH, Hoffman GS, et al. Vasculitis. A collection of pearls and myths. *Rheum Dis Clin North Am* 2001;27:677–728.

152. Ohara N, Miyata T, Oshiro H, Shigematsu H. Surgical treatment for popliteal artery entrapment syndrome. *Cardiovasc Surg* 2001;9:141–144.

153. Lambert AW, Wilkins DC. Popliteal artery entrapment syndrome. *Br J Surg* 1999;86:1365–1370.

154. Tsolakis IA, Walvatne CS, Caldwell MD. Cystic adventitial disease of the popliteal artery: diagnosis and treatment. *Eur J Vasc Endovasc Surg* 1998;15:188–194.

155. Shepherd R. Ergotism. In: White RA, Hollier LH, eds. *Vascular Surgery: Basic Science and Clinical Correlations*. Philadelphia: Lippincott, 1994:177–191.

156. Tay JC, Chee YC. Ergotism and vascular insufficiency: a case report and review of literature. *Ann Acad Med Singapore* 1998;27:285–288.

157. Andreoni KA, Weeks SM, Gerber DA, et al. Incidence of donor renal fibromuscular dysplasia: Does it justify routine angiography? *Transplantation* 2002;73:1112–1116.

158. Muller BT, Luther B, Hort W, et al. Surgical treatment of 50 carotid dissections: indications and results. *J Vasc Surg* 2000;31:980–988.

159. Lederle F, Walker J, Reinke D. Selective screening for abdominal aortic aneurysms with physical examination and ultrasound. *Arch Intern Med* 1988;148:1753–1756.

160. Joyce J, Fairbairn JI, Kincaid O, Juergens J. Aneurysms of the thoracic aorta: A clinical study with special reference to prognosis. *Circulation* 1964;29:176–181.

161. Mayall JC, Mayall RC, Mayall AC, Mayall LC. Peripheral aneurysms. *Int Angiol* 1991;10:141–145.

162. Barker WF. Peripheral arterial disease. *Major Probl Clin Surg* 1966;4:1–224.

163. Wychulis A, Spittell JJ, Wallace R. Popliteal aneurysms. *Surgery* 1970;68:942–951.

164. Cartes-Zumelzu F, Lammer J, Hoelzenbein T, et al. Endovascular placement of a nitinol-ePTFE stent-graft for abdominal aortic aneurysms: initial and midterm results. *J Vasc Interv Radiol* 2002;13:465–473.

165. Frances C, Papo T, Wechsler B, et al. Sneddon syndrome with or without antiphospholipid antibodies. A comparative study in 46 patients. *Medicine (Baltimore)* 1999;78:209–219.

166. Borowiecka I, Lipinska A, Kozlowska A, Rogala H. [Sneddon syndrome]. *Pol Arch Med Wewn* 1996;95:555–560.

167. Poszepczynska-Guigne E, Viguier M, Chosidow O, et al. Paraneoplastic acral vascular syndrome: epidemiologic features, clinical manifestations, and disease sequelae. *J Am Acad Dermatol* 2002;47:47–52.

168. Lauchli S, Widmer L, Lautenschlager S. Cold agglutinin disease—The importance of cutaneous signs. *Dermatology* 2001;202:356–358.

169. Weil JS, Maurel A, Van Frenkel R, Thuillez C. [Cutaneous pulpar temperature and cold test. Predictive specificity and sensitivity in pharmacoclinical studies]. *J Mal Vasc* 1995;20:38–44.

170. Allen E, Brown G. Raynaud's disease: A critical review of minimal requisites for diagnosis. *Am J Med Sci* 1932;187–200.

171. Gifford RJ, Hines EJ. Raynaud's disease among women and girls. *Circulation* 1957;16:1012–1021.

172. Priollet P, Vayssairat M, Housset E. How to classify Raynaud's phenomenon: Long-term follow-up study of 73 cases. *Am J Med* 1987;83: 494–498.

173. Landry G, Edwards J, McLafferty R, et al. Long-term outcome of Raynaud's syndrome in a prospectively analyzed patient cohort. *J Vasc Surg* 1996;23:76–86.

174. Bovenzi M. Vibration-induced white finger and cold response of digital arterial vessels in occupational groups with various patterns of exposure to hand-transmitted vibration. *Scand J Work Environ Health* 1998;24:138–144.

175. Chetter IC, Kent PJ, Kester RC. The hand-arm vibration syndrome: A review. *Cardiovasc Surg* 1998;6:1–9.

176. Coffman J. *Raynaud's Phenomenon*. New York: Oxford, 1989.

177. Jordan SE, Ahn SS, Freischlag JA, et al. Selective botulinum chemo-denervation of the scalene muscles for treatment of neurogenic thoracic outlet syndrome. *Ann Vasc Surg* 2000;14:365–369.

178. Zell L, Scheffler P, Heger M, Buchter A. [Paget-von Schroetter syndrome as an occupational accident]. *Dtsch Med Wochenschr* 2001; 126:326–328.

179. Landry GJ, Moneta GL, Taylor LM Jr, et al. Long-term functional outcome of neurogenic thoracic outlet syndrome in surgically and conservatively treated patients. *J Vasc Surg* 2001;33:312–317; discussion 317–319.

180. Lindgren KA. Conservative treatment of thoracic outlet syndrome: A 2-year follow-up. *Arch Phys Med Rehabil* 1997;78:373–378.

181. Kieffer E, Vasseur MA. [Surgery of thoracic outlet syndromes]. *Rev Med Interne* 1999;20(suppl 5):506S–514S.

182. Le Forestier N, Moulonguet A, Maisonobe T, et al. True neurogenic thoracic outlet syndrome: Electrophysiological diagnosis in six cases. *Muscle Nerve* 1998;21:1129–1134.

183. Rutherford RB, Hurlbert SN. Primary subclavian-axillary vein thrombosis: consensus and commentary. *Cardiovasc Surg* 1996;4:420–423.

184. Winterer JT, Ghanem N, Roth M, et al. Diagnosis of the hypothenar hammer syndrome by high-resolution contrast-enhanced MR angiography. *Eur Radiol* 2002;12:2457–2462.

185. Birrer M, Baumgartner I. Images in clinical medicine. Work-related vascular injuries of the hand—Hypothenar hammer syndrome. *N Engl J Med* 2002;347:339.

SURGICAL TREATMENT OF CAROTID AND PERIPHERAL VASCULAR DISEASE

Thomas T. Terramani / Thomas F. Dodson / Robert B. Smith III

The emergence of managed care and the advancements in endoluminal therapy have wrought an evolutionary upheaval in the field of vascular surgery. Vascular surgery's modern origins date back only about 50 years, with the first femoral-to-popliteal bypass performed in 1948 and the first abdominal aortic aneurysm repaired in 1951. The past 50 years have brought remarkable progress to this discipline. New technologies being evaluated include minimally invasive surgery,[1] gene therapy,[2] endoluminal therapies,[3] and tissue engineering,[4] to mention just a few.

This chapter does not encompass all of vascular surgery but is limited to three subjects: (1) carotid endarterectomy, (2) upper and lower extremity revascularization, and (3) upper and lower extremity venous thrombosis (see also Chaps. 98, 100, 101, and 103). While vascular surgery remains only a "palliative" therapy for people with atherosclerotic and venous disease, "curative" therapies no doubt await insightful and determined investigators. The scalpel will clearly yield to the gene in the days to come.[5]

CAROTID ENDARTERECTOMY

Stroke continues to be the third leading cause of death in the United States, outranked only by heart disease and cancer. There are nearly 500,000 cases of stroke each year in this country, with approximately one-third of patients dying as a result.[6] However, there has been a decline over the past four decades in both the incidence of stroke and the mortality resulting from it. While it has been suggested that "environmental factors" influence the risk of stroke, better control of hypertension, gradual reduction in the percentage of individuals who smoke cigarettes, increased awareness of the benefits of a physically active lifestyle, and greater attention to cholesterol reduction and use of anticoagulants in patients with atrial fibrillation have probably all contributed to the decline in stroke deaths in the United States.

In terms of who should undergo an operation for carotid artery disease, the field is finally on relatively firm ground. There have been six prospective randomized trials published on this topic since 1991, five of which have shown a benefit for carotid endarterectomy (CEA) in preventing cerebral ischemia.[7–12] Barnett et al. reported that, based on a further review of the North American Symptomatic Carotid En-

darterectomy Trial (NASCET) data, carotid endarterectomy in symptomatic patients with 50 to 69 percent stenosis produced only a "moderate" reduction in the risk of further stroke.[13] There was an absolute risk reduction of 10.1 percent at 5 years for those symptomatic patients with carotid stenoses of 50 to 69 percent, but no benefit for patients with symptomatic stenoses of less than 50 percent. The authors further suggested that decision making regarding these patients with a moderate degree of stenosis could be aided by a full evaluation of underlying risk factors, but that their analysis did not justify a "large" increase in the rate of CEA. Our current decision-making process for patients with carotid disease is outlined in Table 102-1.

With respect to preoperative imaging of carotid disease, the "gold standard," cerebral arteriography, is utilized less in an effort to reduce both the risk and the cost of the overall procedure. The Asymptomatic Carotid Atherosclerosis Study (ACAS) and the NASCET study had 1.2 percent and 0.7 percent morbidity rates, respectively, from cerebral angiography. Over the last several years, a number of articles have addressed the issue of CEA without angiography.[14,15] The consensus of opinion is that, with a dedicated vascular laboratory, the great majority of patients (perhaps as many as 90 percent) can be safely evaluated with duplex ultrasound only. Indications suggesting the need for arteriography include (1) uncertainty about the accuracy or reliability of the vascular laboratory; (2) uncertainty about possible complete occlusion of the internal carotid artery in a patient with ongoing localizing symptoms; (3) concern about proximal or intrathoracic disease; (4) patients with "technically difficult" studies due to variant arterial anatomy; and (5) patients with symptoms and an indeterminate study.

The majority of Chaikof et al.'s patients have their CEAs done under local anesthesia with light sedation given by the anesthesiologist.[16] Others have utilized cervical block anesthesia with similarly good results.[17] These techniques are safer than a general anesthetic and provide moment-to-moment assessment of the patient's neurologic condition, avoiding the necessity of concern at the end of the case as the patient awakens from general anesthetic. Patients are also shunted routinely (Fig. 102-1), realizing, however, that approximately 80 percent of patients can undergo the CEA safely without the use of a shunt.

TABLE 102-1 Treatment Plan for Patients with Carotid Disease

Category of Patient	Treatment
PATIENTS WITH SYMPTOMATIC CAROTID STENOSES	
>80% stenosis of internal carotid artery	CEA indicated
50–79% stenosis of carotid artery but with vascular laboratory data suggesting closer to 79%	CEA probably indicated; assess risk factors
50–79% stenosis of carotid artery but with vascular laboratory data suggesting closer to 50%	CEA may be indicated; assess risk factors
<50% stenosis of carotid artery	Trial of medical therapy
PATIENTS WITH ASYMPTOMATIC CAROTID STENOSES	
>80% stenosis of carotid artery	CEA indicated
50–79% stenosis of carotid artery but with vascular laboratory data suggesting closer to 79%	CEA may be indicated; assess risk factors
50–79% stenosis of carotid artery but with vascular laboratory data suggesting closer to 50%	CEA not indicated
<50% stenosis of carotid artery	CEA not indicated

ABBREVIATION: CEA = carotid endarterectomy.

One change in the authors' technique of CEAs is an increased tendency to patch the carotid after endarterectomy. In the past, indications for use of the patch were (1) female gender and (2) recurrent stenoses and the necessity for reoperation. Two reports that have been influential are the work of Moore and colleagues reporting on results of the ACAS study,[18] and the work of AbuRahma and colleagues reporting on a randomized prospective trial of primary closure versus patching.[19] In the former study, the authors were able to show an overall incidence of recurrent carotid stenosis of 4.5 percent in patients who underwent patch angioplasty, compared with 16.9 percent in patients undergoing primary arterial repair. The second re-

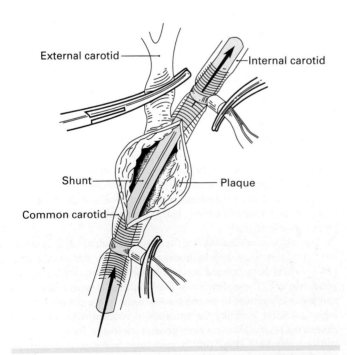

FIGURE 102-1 Indwelling shunt in place to preserve internal carotid flow during the endarterectomy.

port, looked at 74 patients undergoing bilateral CEAs with primary closure on one side and patch angioplasty on the other. Not only did patch angioplasty have a lower incidence of recurrent stenosis (1 percent vs 22 percent), but the total internal carotid occlusion rate was lower as well (0 percent vs 8 percent with primary closure). Addition of a patch adds only a few minutes to the operation, with no significant change in perioperative morbidity or mortality rates.

The treatment of carotid artery disease represents a benchmark for many other common vascular problems. Large randomized studies were performed to answer difficult questions. The economic milieu made a search for more cost-effective and efficient care a necessity, and the authors have responded by diminishing invasive preoperative testing and markedly shortening hospital stay, both of which were accomplished without sacrifice of quality of care.[20] In discussing the "best evidence-based surgical procedure for the prevention of occlusive stroke," it is important to note that all the questions about carotid disease are not settled. The use of balloon angioplasty for the treatment of vascular stenoses has been a mainstay in the armamentarium of cardiologists and interventional radiologists since Gruentzig's work nearly three decades ago. It is no wonder that lesions in the carotid artery territory have beckoned to those physicians with catheter-based skills. Surgical investigators, in many cases vascular surgeons worried about both the potential for harm to their patients and the potential loss of revenue, have expressed concern,[21] embraced the new technology,[22] or worked to compare the two competing methods of treatment of carotid disease.[23] One of a series of articles from the University of Alabama in Birmingham by Jordan and his colleagues showed that percutaneous transluminal angioplasty in a retrospective review carried a "significantly higher" neurologic risk than did CEA performed under regional anesthesia.[23] In another study,[24] Naylor and colleagues reported on a prospective randomized trial of CEA versus carotid angioplasty that was stopped because of an increased number of complications in the angioplasty arm. Reporting on only 17 patients, they suspended the trial when 5 of the 7 patients who had carotid angioplasty had strokes. None of the 10 patients who had CEA had complications.

To address concerns about the potential increased risk of embolic events during percutaneous angioplasty and stenting, some investigators have evaluated filter devices that can be positioned downstream from the carotid stenosis prior to the angioplasty intervention. One such device was reported on by Ohki et al.[25] and their data indicated that 88 percent of the particles liberated during an ex vivo experimental model were captured by the device. In another report,[26] 31 patients underwent carotid artery stenting with a cerebral protection device. Macroscopic embolic particles were recovered in all cases and the 30-day stroke rate was 3.3 percent. They concluded that carotid artery stenting with distal protection can be performed safely with a low neurologic complication rate.

A statement was issued by an American Heart Association Science Advisory group in 1998 that carotid angioplasty and stenting should, "with rare and infrequent exception," be undertaken only as part of a prospective randomized trial.[27] After a great deal of debate, study, and discussion, the authors' vascular center has decided to enter the Carotid Revascularization Endarterectomy versus Stent Trial (CREST) study.[28] There are currently multiple carotid artery stent clinical trials and registries in the United States. The majority of these trials are enrolling patients with carotid artery disease that are determined to be at high-risk for traditional surgery repair.

UPPER AND LOWER EXTREMITY REVASCULARIZATION

Upper Extremity Revascularization

Chronic arterial insufficiency of the upper extremity is most often due to occlusive disease of the aortic arch branches near their origin: either the subclavian artery or the brachiocephalic trunk. Symptoms may be limited to ischemic manifestations of the arm and hand or may include posterior circulation insufficiency of the brain due to subclavian steal syndrome. Selection of patients for surgical intervention is extremely important in this group of disorders, since many patients have few or no symptoms and should not be subjected to an operative procedure simply for the correction of an anatomic or radiologic finding. Individuals who are significantly limited by arm claudication or those who have symptomatic subclavian steal syndrome should be thoroughly evaluated by aortic arch angiography and neurologic and vascular examination. Since the patterns of occlusive lesions are extremely variable, any surgical procedure must be carefully planned. Generally, extrathoracic bypass procedures are preferred if a normal donor artery is available; otherwise, a transthoracic procedure may be required to originate a prosthetic bypass from the aortic arch itself. A large series of patients with symptomatic atherosclerotic occlusive disease of the innominate artery was presented by Azakie et al.[29] They operated on 94 patients between 1960 and 1997, performing innominate endarterectomies in 72 patients and bypass grafting in 22 patients. Although there were 3 perioperative deaths and 4 strokes (3 of which resolved), their long-term results were excellent, with freedom from recurrence requiring operation of 99 percent and an actuarial survival rate of 85 percent at 5 years.

Atheromatous occlusive disease of the subclavian artery is the most common lesion involving the proximal branches of the aortic arch. Extrathoracic revascularization of this vessel can be achieved by one of several techniques, depending on the pattern of obstruction and the relationship of the artery in question to a patent donor vessel. When the ipsilateral common carotid artery is patent and has minimal or no disease, it is frequently chosen as the site of arterial inflow. Perler and Williams[30] performed carotid-subclavian bypasses or transposition procedures on 31 individuals for a variety of conditions between 1979 and 1989. They achieved relief of symptoms in 30 patients, with a symptom-free survival rate of 89 percent at 1 year and 84 percent at 2 years.

Vein grafts are often utilized to improve inflow to the upper arm or forearm. Numerous reports have been published on the utilization of bypass grafts for upper limb ischemia.[31,32] In the largest such series, comprising 74 patients who underwent 95 separate operations over a 15-year period, there were no operative deaths and only a single major amputation. The survival rate was 86 percent at 5 years, with a patency rate of 61 percent at that time. Vein grafts were superior at all sites to prostheses.[33]

A third alternative is the utilization of endovascular techniques for aortic arch branch lesions. A multidisciplinary approach utilizing endovascular techniques for treatment of lesions of the subclavian, innominate, and common carotid arteries was presented by the group

from the Cleveland Clinic.[34] In a series of 83 patients, initial technical success was achieved in 82 of 87 procedures (94 percent), but complications occurred in 18 of 87 procedures (20.7 percent), and the 30-day mortality rate for the entire group was 4.8 percent. The investigators acknowledged that there is "no reliable way, short of angiography, to assess anatomic patency" of the vessels that were angioplastied and stented. They also concluded that the results, particularly when complete occlusions were included, "seem to favor" surgical treatment.

A more optimistic report, involving fewer patients, was submitted by the cardiology group from the Lahey Clinic. They reported on 18 patients with symptomatic aortic arch branch vessel stenosis or occlusion.[35] All were treated with percutaneous techniques utilizing Palmaz stents. Primary patency was 100 percent with no major complications, and at a mean follow-up of 17 months all patients were asymptomatic. The authors currently utilize endoluminal angioplasty and stenting in selective patients that are at high risk for a traditional vascular procedure.

Lower Extremity Revascularization

Just as patients with asymptomatic carotid bruits have a higher risk of a cardiac ischemic event than they do of a stroke, patients with peripheral vascular disease have an increased risk of death from a cardiovascular event. In a study of 565 men and women who were evaluated for the presence of large-vessel peripheral arterial disease (abnormal segment-to-arm blood pressure ratios or abnormal flow velocities), 67 patients with peripheral arterial disease were identified.[36] During a follow-up of 10 years, 21 of the 34 men (61.8 percent) and 11 of the 33 women (33.3 percent) died. In patients without evidence of arterial disease, the death rates were 16.9 percent for the men and 11.6 percent for the women. The same conclusion was found by Vogt and colleagues, who demonstrated that patients with a diminished ankle-brachial index (ABI) of 0.9 or less had a crude overall mortality rate about fivefold greater than that of patients with a higher value of this index.[37] Unfortunately, utilization of the ABI to follow the progression of lower extremity atherosclerotic disease has been found to be unreliable. McLafferty and colleagues[38] noted that the ABI had a sensitivity of only 41 percent in determining the progression of disease. While the ABI was stated to be "poor" at identifying a worsening of vascular disease, it remains an important and easily performed screening test.

Patients with Claudication

A nonoperative approach to patients with claudication is generally appropriate. Given that the symptom of claudication is such an ominous predictor of widespread vascular disease, risk-factor modification is the first step in the treatment of such patients. Cigarette smoking, diabetes, hyperlipidemia, and hypertension are four factors that influence the progression of disease in patients with claudication. Tobacco use is the single most important risk factor and patients who continue to smoke have double the 5-year mortality rate of patients who are able to stop smoking. Likewise, tight control of diabetes, utilization of statin agents to treat hyperlipidemia, and treatment of hypertension are all directed toward reducing further atherosclerosis, particularly in the cerebral and coronary beds. After control of risk factors, an exercise program is the next step in the effective treatment of the claudicant. In an interesting study carried out by the Departments of Surgery and Psychiatry-Behavioral Medicine at Brown University,[39] Patterson and colleagues found that both patients who exercised at home and those who exercised under supervision improved after a 12-week period. The degree of improvement was more marked in those patients who were supervised (280 percent increase) than it was in those who exercised at home (170 percent increase). Depending upon the degree of limitation imposed by the claudication, either type of program may be of benefit.

The next treatment of patients with claudication is pharmacologic therapy. Pentoxifylline (Trental) was the first drug approved for treatment of claudication in the United States, but the authors have largely discontinued using this agent because of its cost as well as its limited clinical benefit. A relatively new drug, cilostazol (Pletal) has now been approved, and it seems to have real potential. In a multicenter randomized double-blind placebo-controlled trial conducted by Money and colleagues, it was found that cilostazol "significantly increased" absolute claudication distance at all measured time points.[40] Because cilostazol is a phosphodiesterase inhibitor, it should not, however, be administered in patients with congestive heart failure.

The other available therapy is revascularization. This has been and remains a controversial topic. Two articles have addressed surgical intervention. The first, from AbuRahma et al.,[41] was an interesting study that compared patients with bilateral claudication who had a saphenous vein graft placed on one side and a polytetrafluoroethylene (PTFE) graft on the other. There were no operative deaths or perioperative amputations for either procedure, and both grafts were found to have "comparable" patencies with identical limb salvage (98 percent) at 72 months. The second report, from Byrne and colleagues,[42] evaluated 409 infrainguinal reconstructions for claudication. In this large series, only one limb was lost due to embolization and no operative deaths occurred. Their conclusions, even acknowledging that 18 percent of their interventions required a second operation, were that infrainguinal bypass grafting procedures were "valid treatment options" in selected patients with claudication.

Percutaneous transluminal angioplasty (PTA) in patients with claudication was addressed by Whyman and colleagues in a randomized controlled trial.[43] Sixty-two patients with short femoral artery stenoses or occlusions and iliac stenoses were randomized to either PTA plus medical therapy or to medical therapy alone. At 2 years of follow-up, the PTA group and the control group "did not differ significantly" in the four categories analyzed. They concluded by stating that the addition of PTA to conventional medical treatment "does not confer a measurable benefit in the patient's perceived or measured walking ability after two years." They also acknowledged that a large randomized trial would be needed in order to settle the issue.

An article by Golledge and colleagues, from London, looked directly at outcomes of femoropopliteal PTA in 43 patients with intermittent claudication, 4 with rest pain, and 27 patients with tissue loss.[44] Although "technical success" was achieved in 67 patients (91 percent), failure of the procedure occurred in the remaining 7 patients. Of the 43 patients with claudication, 9 still had symptoms at 1 year. Seven other patients with claudication required another intervention. In 27 of the 43 patients (63 percent), the claudication had resolved. Symptomatic improvement was found in only 51 percent of the total group 1 year from the time of PTA, although approximately two-thirds with intermittent claudication were symptom-free at 12-months. The authors suggested that a longer period of follow-up would be required to assess durability of the angioplasty procedure.

Patients with Rest Pain

Ischemic rest pain is frequently an intolerable symptom and implies threatened loss of the foot or limb. Whereas patients with claudication are generally managed in a conservative or nonoperative manner, patients with rest pain or a nonhealing lesion are evaluated for a

potential operation. If the patient is ambulatory and has a reasonable operative risk (cardiac and pulmonary factors), then a revascularization procedure is offered. Patients with associated severe comorbid conditions, little chance of functional recovery, or irretrievable limb ischemia should undergo amputation. In an attempt to better delineate who might benefit from lower extremity bypass procedures, Kalman and Johnston looked at 358 consecutive in situ distal leg bypass procedures from 1986 to 1995.[45] Four significant variables were associated with a lower late survival rate: male gender, diabetes, chronic renal insufficiency, and a history of cerebrovascular disease. When all four variables were present, the predicted 5-year survival rate was reduced to 2 percent. They concluded that these variables might be used in the decision for either revascularization or amputation.

As with carotid artery disease, approaches to imaging of the vasculature of the extremities are also evolving. While arteriograms are still used to assess the vasculature of many patients, magnetic resonance angiography (MRA) with contrast agent enhancement may ultimately supplant contrast arteriography (Fig. 102-2).[46] MRA is used at present to identify runoff vessels in patients who are otherwise candidates for revascularization but in whom contrast angiography has been of poor quality or has failed to demonstrate patent vessels. The utility of MRA in this setting has been confirmed by investigators who noted a limb-salvage rate of 78 percent in patients with angiographically occult runoff vessels that were detectable by MRA.[47] MRA also plays an important role in the assessment of patients with renal insufficiency or iodinated contrast allergies, which contraindicate the use of conventional contrast agents.

Although the greater saphenous vein is preferred as a conduit in almost all infrainguinal bypasses, there are a number of alternatives. When there was inadequate autogenous material available for bypass, interposition of PTFE below the knee, in one series, yielded a 2-year patency of 52 percent with a limb-salvage rate of 62 percent.[48] While most investigators acknowledge the relatively poor long-term results with PTFE bypasses to infrapopliteal arteries, some authors still recommend it in the above-knee position.[49,50] Other options include the use of arm and lesser saphenous vein grafts; composite sequential bypass utilizing vein sewn to PTFE; use of an anastomotic vein patch (Taylor patch); umbilical vein grafts; distal venous arterialization, and cryopreserved vein allografts. With respect to the latter, Carpenter and Tomaszewski have documented a primary graft patency at 1 year of only 13 percent and a limb-salvage rate of 42 percent.[51] In a report by Castier et al.,[52] cryopreserved arterial allografts were used in 32 patients with limb-threatening ischemia between 1993 and 1997. While arterial dilatation occurred in two patent grafts (both requiring graft replacement), the overall primary patency was 57 percent at 12 months and 39 percent at 18 months. This work remains investigational.

In the largest series on long-term results of in situ saphenous vein bypass grafts, Shah et al. documented a cumulative secondary patency rate at 1 and 5 years of 91 percent and 81 percent, respectively, and a limb-salvage rate of 97 percent and 95 percent, respectively.[53] These results continue to set the standard for infrainguinal reconstruction performed today. A prospective, randomized, multicenter study comparing in situ (Fig. 102-3) and reversed saphenous vein bypasses revealed "no significant differences" in overall patency rates.[54] The authors concluded that surgeons should therefore be adept at both procedures. The authors are increasingly utilizing "duplex ultrasound vein mapping" to help locate acceptable venous conduits preoperatively; these veins include the accessory ipsilateral greater saphenous vein, the contralateral greater saphenous vein, the lesser saphenous vein, and arm veins. The utilization of "spliced" excised vein segments will yield a primary patency rate of 72 percent at 1 year and 45 percent at 4 years.[55] Intensive surveillance, involving utilization of duplex scanning of vein grafts at 1 month, 3 months, 6 months, and every 6 months thereafter, seems to aid in detecting graft-threatening lesions, although it also adds to cost.

The addition of anticoagulation to patients in a high-risk setting after infrainguinal bypass grafting may be beneficial in promoting graft patency. In a randomized prospective trial from the University of Florida, Sarac et al. showed that, while perioperative therapy with heparin increased the wound hematoma rate, long-term anticoagulation with warfarin improved both the patency rate and the limb-salvage rate in patients at high risk for graft thrombosis.[56] A meta-analysis confirmed this finding and also suggested that platelet inhibitors reduced the risk of graft occlusion after infrainguinal bypass surgery.[57]

Some investigators have recommended balloon angioplasty of the femoral, popliteal, and even tibioperoneal vessels. Randomized controlled trials are needed to determine the efficacy of these approaches.[58] Endovascular techniques such as stent placement and percutaneous femoropopliteal graft placement are also being evaluated in patients with femoral and popliteal artery disease.

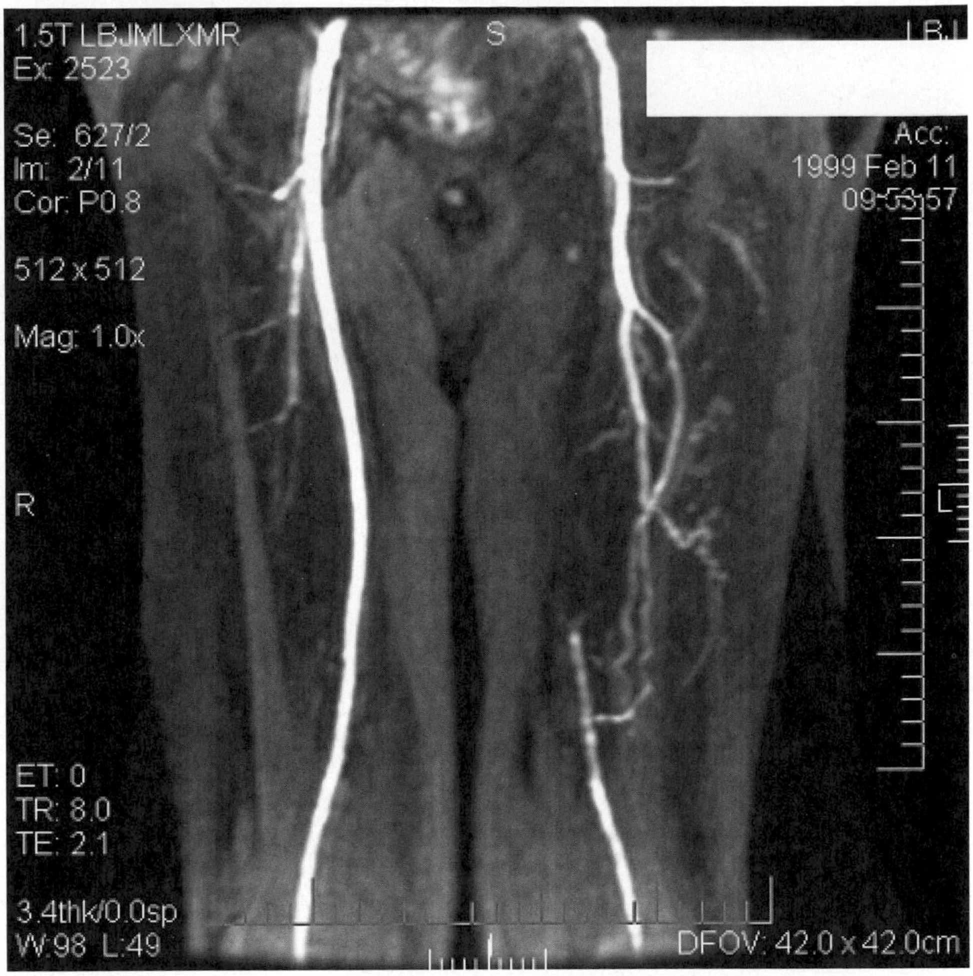

FIGURE 102-2 Magnetic resonance angiogram with gadolinium enhancement showing left superficial femoral artery (SFA) occlusion in a patient with rest pain.

UPPER AND LOWER EXTREMITY VENOUS THROMBOSIS

Upper Extremity Venous Thrombosis

Deep venous thrombosis (DVT) of the upper extremity was thought in the past to be a rare event and to have a relatively benign outcome. However, information from both the United States and other countries challenges these assumptions. A report by Prandoni et al. evaluated 58 patients suspected of having upper extremity DVT.[59] Of the 58 patients, 27 (47 percent) had thrombosis, and central venous catheters, "thrombophilic states," and previous lower extremity thromboses were all associated with the development of upper extremity thrombosis. Of 22 patients who underwent either perfusion lung scanning or pulmonary angiography, 8 (36 percent) were found to have "high probability" for a pulmonary embolus. Primary or effort thrombosis of the subclavian vein (Paget-Schroetter syndrome) is generally seen in healthy young people after repetitive motion or exercise involving the swollen extremity. There now seems to be general consensus about the use of thrombolysis as the initial step, followed by surgical decompression.[60,61]

Venous gangrene is a rare but devastating complication of upper extremity venous thrombosis, and many of these patients may require amputation with an associated mortality of 33 percent.[62] A report discusses the role of catheter-directed thrombolysis in the treatment of phlegmasia cerulea dolens.[63] While there is no consensus on the optimal treatment of this problem, some have achieved successful lysis of the affected vessels. Patients who have contraindications to or unsuccessful use of anticoagulation have been a significant source of concern. Spence and associates[64] showed that superior vena cava filters can be successfully placed without undue difficulty, and, in their series of 41 patients, using four different types of filters, no complications and no clinical evidence of pulmonary embolism or superior vena cava syndrome were seen.

Lower Extremity Venous Thrombosis

DVT of the lower extremities is an insidious and potentially lethal problem in hospitalized patients. It has been estimated that there are approximately 600,000 cases of venous thromboembolism in the United States each year.[65] Risk factors have been detailed in multiple publications and include age above 40, past history of DVT, general anesthesia, operations, pregnancy, malignant disease, hypercoagulable

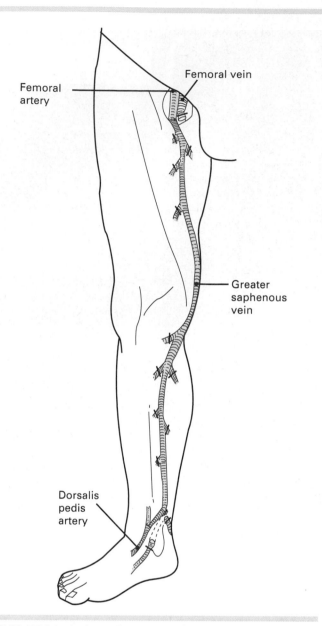

FIGURE 102-3 In situ bypass from common femoral artery to dorsalis pedis artery.

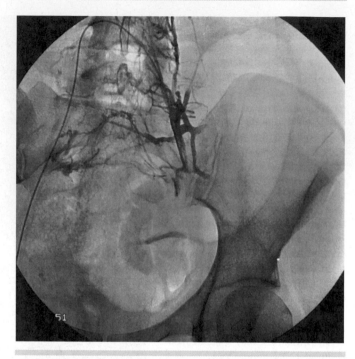

FIGURE 102-4 Venogram in a 31-year-old woman with a swollen leg, hypercoagulable state, and left iliac vein occlusion.

states, and trauma. An important nationwide study of patients with DVT was undertaken in Denmark to look at the potential association of primary venous thrombosis and the subsequent diagnosis of cancer.[66] Although they found the expected "strong associations" with cancers of the pancreas, ovary, liver, and brain, they concluded that an "aggressive search" for a hidden malignancy in a patient with a solitary episode of DVT was not cost-effective and was therefore not indicated. Hypercoagulable states (Fig. 102-4) have received renewed attention in recent years. A relatively new addition to abnormalities in coagulation occurred with the discovery of factor V Leiden, which has been found in about one-fifth of patients with venous thrombosis.[67] Simioni and colleagues searched for factor V Leiden in 251 unselected patients who had had a first episode of symptomatic DVT diagnosed by venography.[68] They found the mutation in 41 of the patients (16.3 percent), and after a follow-up period of 8 years approximately 40 percent of patients had recurrent venous thrombosis, compared to 18 percent of patients who

did not have this mutation. De Stefano and colleagues reviewed a retrospective cohort of 624 patients who had had a first episode of DVT.[69] They looked at patients who were heterozygous carriers of factor V Leiden, patients who were heterozygous for both factor V Leiden and a prothrombin mutation, and patients who had neither mutation. In contradistinction to the previous study, they found that the risk of recurrent DVT was similar among carriers of factor V Leiden and patients without the mutation. Carriers of both factor V Leiden and the prothrombin mutation were, however, at an increased risk of recurrent DVT after the first episode and they recommended lifelong anticoagulation.

DVT occurs in a broad range of patients, with reports documenting it in 58 percent of trauma patients,[70] 11 percent of patients undergoing lower extremity amputation,[71] and 33 percent of patients in a medical intensive care unit.[72] Patients with DVT are effectively treated by heparin given either by continuous intravenous infusion or by subcutaneous injection. The past decade has brought a number of changes in the therapeutic approach to patients with DVT in major lower extremity veins: a 5-day course of heparin has been shown to be as effective as a 10-day course; 6 months of oral anticoagulant therapy has been shown to have a lower recurrence rate than the same dose given for 6 weeks; and low-molecular-weight heparin has been found effective in treating patients at home with proximal DVT.[73,74] Low-molecular-weight heparin has also been shown to be efficacious in reducing the risk of venous thromboembolism in patients with acute medical illnesses. In a comparison between enoxaparin and Coumadin, enoxaparin-treated patients had a lower recurrence rate of symptomatic venous thromboembolism as well as a lower incidence of bleeding.[75]

In recent years, there has been some enthusiasm for thrombolytic therapy in patients with DVT. The reasoning has been that such therapy could lyse the thrombus, restore normalcy to the leg, and reduce the incidence of long-term sequelae of DVT. Postphlebitic syndrome manifests as edema, hyperpigmentation, and ulceration and can oc-

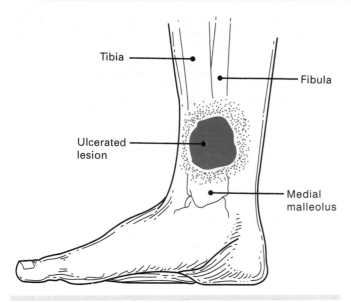

FIGURE 102-5 Venous stasis ulceration on the medial malleous after an episode of deep venous thrombosis.

cur in up to one-third of patients who have had prior DVT (Fig. 102-5). The obvious issue is weighing the risks of lytic therapy against the chronic problems of the postphlebitic syndrome. Mewissen and colleagues formed a venous thrombosis registry and collected data from 63 centers.[76] After 312 urokinase infusions in 303 limbs of 287 patients, they found that complete lysis was achieved in 96 infusions (31 percent) and that "major" bleeding complications, most often at the puncture site, occurred in 54 patients (19 percent). Six of those patients (11 percent) developed pulmonary emboli, and there were 2 deaths, 1 from an intracranial hemorrhage and 1 from a pulmonary embolus. While the authors concluded that catheter-directed therapy is "safe and effective," there is currently little unanimity of opinion on this topic.

DVT can present as thrombosis in calf veins or superficial veins of the extremity or in patients with near total venous occlusion. While patients with DVT in their calf or superficial veins are often viewed as having benign problems, more recent data have suggested that this may be a false assumption. In one study conducted at the beginning of the last decade, investigators showed that 24 (32 percent) of 75 patients with lower extremity calf vein thrombi had propagation of their thrombi, and 11 of those 24 (46 percent) had progression into the popliteal or larger veins of the thigh.[77] Numerous reports of patients with superficial thrombophlebitis have documented a high incidence of associated hypercoagulability, propagation into the common femoral vein, and an unexpectedly high incidence of pulmonary emboli.[78,79] Observations such as these would suggest that calf vein thrombi and superficial thrombi are not always benign conditions. Patients with extensive clot in the lower extremities may go on to have phlegmasia cerulea dolens or acute iliofemoral venous thrombosis, potentially leading to venous gangrene. Venous thrombectomy for this condition has received renewed enthusiasm in the surgical literature,[80] but lytic therapy[81] and nonoperative therapy[82] also have their proponents.

While heparin and warfarin are excellent therapy for the majority of patients with DVT, in some it is contraindicated. These include individuals with recent trauma, active bleeding, or hemolysis; those with complications of heparin therapy; and those with inferior vena caval thrombus or iliofemoral venous thrombosis. For these patients,

the treatment of choice is often the placement of a vena caval filter. In a review of their 20-year experience, Greenfield and Proctor noted a caval patency rate of 96 percent, with a rate of recurrent emboli of 4 percent.[83] There was no procedural mortality rate, and the operative morbidity rate was minimal. Decousus and colleagues randomly assigned 400 patients with proximal DVT who were at risk for pulmonary emboli to receive a vena caval filter (200 patients) or no filter (200 patients). In a second aspect of the study, patients were also assigned to receive low-molecular-weight heparin or unfractionated heparin.[84] While the patients who received vena caval filters had a lower incidence of pulmonary emboli by day 12 (1.1 percent versus 4.8 percent for those who did not receive filters), there was an increased incidence of recurrent DVT in the patients receiving filters. There were no significant differences in mortality rates or other outcomes. Low-molecular-weight heparin produced a lower incidence of symptomatic or asymptomatic pulmonary embolism at day 12 and recurrent venous thrombosis, but the results were not statistically significant. In a follow-up editorial on this subject, Haire suggested that only "well-designed comparative trials" could give us the necessary information on which to base our clinical decisions about the proper use of vena caval filters.[85]

CONCLUSION

The management of vascular disease has undergone a significant change over the past decade with the improvements in endoluminal techniques and technologies. Surgery continues to be the gold standard in all arterial segments with which endoluminal therapy must be compared. Endoluminal angioplasty and stenting have been shown to be extremely useful in aortic arch branch vessels and iliac and renal arteries (see Chap. 103). The efficacy and role that endoluminal therapy will have in the management of carotid, femoral, and tibial arteries is yet to be determined.

References

1. Rattner DW. Future directions in innovative minimally invasive surgery. *Lancet* 1999;353(suppl 1):12–15.
2. Hollingsworth SJ, Barker SG. Gene therapy: Into the future of surgery. *Lancet* 1999;353(suppl 1):19–20.
3. Weiss VJ, Lumsden AB. Minimally invasive vascular surgery: Review of current modalities. *World J Surg* 1999;23(4):406–414.
4. Chaikof EL, Matthew H, Kohn J, et al. Biomaterials and scaffolds in reparative medicine. *Ann N Y Acad Sci* 2002;961:96–105.
5. Isner JM, Baumgartner I, Rauh G, et al. Treatment of thromboangiitis obliterans (Buerger's disease) by intramuscular gene transfer of vascular endothelial growth factor: Preliminary clinical results. *J Vasc Surg* 1998;28(6):964–975.
6. Bronner LL, Kanter DS, Manson JE. Primary prevention of stroke. *N Engl J Med* 1995;333(21):1392–1400.
7. The CASANOVA Study Group. Carotid surgery versus medical therapy in asymptomatic carotid stenosis. *Stroke* 1991;22(10):1229–1235.
8. Executive Committee for the Asymptomatic Carotid Atherosclerosis Study. Endarterectomy for asymptomatic carotid artery stenosis. *JAMA* 1995;273(18):1421–1428.
9. Mayberg MR, Wilson SE, Yatsu F, et al. Carotid endarterectomy and prevention of cerebral ischemia in symptomatic carotid stenosis. Veterans Affairs Cooperative Studies Program 309 Trialist Group. *JAMA* 1991;266(23):3289–3294.
10. Hobson RW II, Weiss DG, Fields WS, et al. Efficacy of carotid endarterectomy for asymptomatic carotid stenosis. The Veterans Affairs Cooperative Study Group. *N Engl J Med* 1993;328(4):221–227.
11. European Carotid Surgery Trialists' Collaborative Group. MRC European Carotid Surgery Trial: Interim results for symptomatic patients

with severe (70–99%) or with mild (0–29%) carotid stenosis. *Lancet* 1991;337(8752):1235–1243.

12. North American Symptomatic Carotid Endarterectomy Trial. Methods, patient characteristics, and progress. *Stroke* 1991;22(6):711–720.

13. Barnett HJ, Taylor DW, Eliasziw M, et al. Benefit of carotid endarterectomy in patients with symptomatic moderate or severe stenosis. North American Symptomatic Carotid Endarterectomy Trial Collaborators. *N Engl J Med* 1998;339(20):1415–1425.

14. Ballotta E, Da Giau G, Abbruzzese E, et al. Carotid endarterectomy without angiography: Can clinical evaluation and duplex ultrasonographic scanning alone replace traditional arteriography for carotid surgery workup? *Surgery* 1999;126(1):20–27.

15. Collier PE. Changing trends in the use of preoperative carotid arteriography: The community experience. *Cardiovasc Surg* 1998;6(5):485–489.

16. Chaikof EL, Dodson TF, Thomas BL, et al. Four steps to local anesthesia for endarterectomy of the carotid artery. *Surg Gynecol Obstet* 1993;177(3):308–310.

17. Shah DM, Darling RC III, Chang BB, et al. Carotid endarterectomy in awake patients: Its safety, acceptability, and outcome. *J Vasc Surg* 1994;19(6):1015–1020.

18. Moore WS, Kempczinski RF, Nelson JJ, et al. Recurrent carotid stenosis: Results of the asymptomatic carotid atherosclerosis study. *Stroke* 1998;29(10):2018–2025.

19. AbuRahma AF, Robinson PA, Saiedy S, et al. Prospective randomized trial of bilateral carotid endarterectomies: Primary closure versus patching. *Stroke* 1999;30(6):1185–1189.

20. Hirko MK, Morasch MD, Burke K, et al. The changing face of carotid endarterectomy. *J Vasc Surg* 1996;23(4):622–627.

21. Beebe HG, Archie JP, Baker WH, et al. Concern about safety of carotid angioplasty. *Stroke* 1996;27(2):197–198.

22. Criado FJ, Lingelbach JM, Ledesma DF, et al. Carotid artery stenting in a vascular surgery practice. *J Vasc Surg* 2002;35(3):430–434.

23. Jordan WD Jr, Voellinger DC, Fisher WS, et al. A comparison of carotid angioplasty with stenting versus endarterectomy with regional anesthesia. *J Vasc Surg* 1998;28(3):397–403.

24. Naylor AR, Bolia A, Abbott RJ, et al. Randomized study of carotid angioplasty and stenting versus carotid endarterectomy: A stopped trial. *J Vasc Surg* 1998;28(2):326–334.

25. Ohki T, Roubin GS, Veith FJ, et al. Efficacy of a filter device in the prevention of embolic events during carotid angioplasty and stenting: An ex vivo analysis. *J Vasc Surg* 1999;30(6):1034–1044.

26. Ohki T, Veith FJ, Grenell S, et al. Initial experience with cerebral protection devices to prevent embolization during carotid artery stenting. *J Vasc Surg* 2002;36(6):1175–1185.

27. Bettmann MA, Katzen BT, Whisnant J, et al. Carotid stenting and angioplasty: A statement for healthcare professionals from the Councils on Cardiovascular Radiology, Stroke, Cardio-Thoracic and Vascular Surgery, Epidemiology and Prevention, and Clinical Cardiology, American Heart Association. *Stroke* 1998;29(1):336–338.

28. Hobson RW II, Brott T, Ferguson R, et al. CREST: Carotid Revascularization Endarterectomy versus Stent Trial. *Cardiovasc Surg* 1997;5(5):457–458.

29. Azakie A, McElhinney DB, Higashima R, et al. Innominate artery reconstruction: Over 3 decades of experience. *Ann Surg* 1998;228(3):402–410.

30. Perler BA, Williams GM. Carotid-subclavian bypass—a decade of experience. *J Vasc Surg* 1990;12(6):716–723.

31. Katz SG, Kohl RD. Direct revascularization for the treatment of forearm and hand ischemia. *Am J Surg* 1993;165(3):312–316.

32. McCarthy WJ, Flinn WR, Yao JS, et al. Result of bypass grafting for upper limb ischemia. *J Vasc Surg* 1986;3(5):741–746.

33. Mesh CL, McCarthy WJ, Pearce WH, et al. Upper extremity bypass grafting. A 15-year experience. *Arch Surg* 1993;128(7):795–802.

34. Sullivan TM, Gray BH, Bacharach JM, et al. Angioplasty and primary stenting of the subclavian, innominate, and common carotid arteries in 83 patients. *J Vasc Surg* 1998;28(6):1059–1065.

35. Hadjipetrou P, Cox S, Piemonte T, Eisenhauer A. Percutaneous revascularization of atherosclerotic obstruction of aortic arch vessels. *J Am Coll Cardiol* 1999;33(5):1238–1245.

36. Criqui MH, Langer RD, Fronek A, et al. Mortality over a period of 10 years in patients with peripheral arterial disease. *N Engl J Med* 1992;326(6):381–386.

37. Vogt MT, Cauley JA, Newman AB, et al. Decreased ankle/arm blood pressure index and mortality in elderly women. *JAMA* 1993;270(4):465–469.

38. McLafferty RB, Moneta GL, Taylor LM Jr, et al. Ability of ankle-brachial index to detect lower-extremity atherosclerotic disease progression. *Arch Surg* 1997;132(8):836–841.

39. Patterson RB, Pinto B, Marcus B, et al. Value of a supervised exercise program for the therapy of arterial claudication. *J Vasc Surg* 1997;25(2):312–319.

40. Money SR, Herd JA, Isaacsohn JL, et al. Effect of cilostazol on walking distances in patients with intermittent claudication caused by peripheral vascular disease. *J Vasc Surg* 1998;27(2):267–275.

41. AbuRahma AF, Robinson PA, Holt SM. Prospective controlled study of polytetrafluoroethylene versus saphenous vein in claudicant patients with bilateral above knee femoropopliteal bypasses. *Surgery* 1999;126(4):594–602.

42. Byrne J, Darling RC III, Chang BB, et al. Infrainguinal arterial reconstruction for claudication: Is it worth the risk? An analysis of 409 procedures. *J Vasc Surg* 1999;29(2):259–269.

43. Whyman MR, Fowkes FG, Kerracher EM, et al. Is intermittent claudication improved by percutaneous transluminal angioplasty? A randomized controlled trial. *J Vasc Surg* 1997;26(4):551–557.

44. Golledge J, Ferguson K, Ellis M, et al. Outcome of femoropopliteal angioplasty. *Ann Surg* 1999;229(1):146–153.

45. Kalman PG, Johnston KW. Predictors of long-term patient survival after in situ vein leg bypass. *J Vasc Surg* 1997;25(5):899–904.

46. Sueyoshi E, Sakamoto I, Matsuoka Y, et al. Aortoiliac and lower extremity arteries: Comparison of three-dimensional dynamic contrast-enhanced subtraction MR angiography and conventional angiography. *Radiology* 1999;210(3):683–688.

47. Carpenter JP, Golden MA, Barker CF, et al. The fate of bypass grafts to angiographically occult runoff vessels detected by magnetic resonance angiography. *J Vasc Surg* 1996;23(3):483–489.

48. Eagleton MJ, Ouriel K, Shortell C, et al. Femoral-infrapopliteal bypass with prosthetic grafts. *Surgery* 1999;126(4):759–765.

49. O'Riordain DS, Buckley DJ, O'Donnell JA. Polytetrafluoroethylene in above-knee arterial bypass surgery for critical ischemia. *Am J Surg* 1992;164(2):129–131.

50. Prendiville EJ, Yeager A, O'Donnell TF Jr, et al. Long-term results with the above-knee popliteal expanded polytetrafluoroethylene graft. *J Vasc Surg* 1990;11(4):517–524.

51. Carpenter JP, Tomaszewski JE. Immunosuppression for human saphenous vein allograft bypass surgery: A prospective randomized trial. *J Vasc Surg* 1997;26(1):32–42.

52. Castier Y, Leseche G, Palombi T, et al. Early experience with cryopreserved arterial allografts in below-knee revascularization for limb salvage. *Am J Surg* 1999;177(3):197–202.

53. Shah DM, Darling RC III, Chang BB, et al. Long-term results of in situ saphenous vein bypass. Analysis of 2058 cases. *Ann Surg* 1995;222(4):438–448.

54. Wengerter KR, Veith FJ, Gupta SK, et al. Prospective randomized multicenter comparison of in situ and reversed vein infrapopliteal bypasses. *J Vasc Surg* 1991;13(2):189–199.

55. Chang BB, Darling RC III, Bock DE, et al. The use of spliced vein bypasses for infrainguinal arterial reconstruction. *J Vasc Surg* 1995;21(3):403–412.

56. Sarac TP, Huber TS, Back MR, et al. Warfarin improves the outcome of infrainguinal vein bypass grafting at high risk for failure. *J Vasc Surg* 1998;28(3):446–457.

57. Tangelder MJ, Lawson JA, Algra A, et al. Systematic review of randomized controlled trials of aspirin and oral anticoagulants in the prevention

of graft occlusion and ischemic events after infrainguinal bypass surgery. *J Vasc Surg* 1999;30(4):701–709.

58. Bradbury AW, Ruckley CV. Angioplasty for lower-limb ischaemia: Time for randomized controlled trials. *Lancet* 1996;347(8997):277–278.

59. Prandoni P, Polistena P, Bernardi E, et al. Upper-extremity deep vein thrombosis. Risk factors, diagnosis, and complications. *Arch Intern Med* 1997;157(1):57–62.

60. Lee MC, Grassi CJ, Belkin M, et al. Early operative intervention after thrombolytic therapy for primary subclavian vein thrombosis: An effective treatment approach. *J Vasc Surg* 1998;27(6):1101–1108.

61. Azakie A, McElhinney DB, Thompson RW, et al. Surgical management of subclavian-vein effort thrombosis as a result of thoracic outlet compression. *J Vasc Surg* 1998;28(5):777–786.

62. Smith BM, Shield GW, Riddell DH, et al. Venous gangrene of the upper extremity. *Ann Surg* 1985;201(4):511–519.

63. Patel NH, Plorde JJ, Meissner M. Catheter-directed thrombolysis in the treatment of phlegmasia cerulea dolens. *Ann Vasc Surg* 1998;12(5): 471–475.

64. Spence LD, Gironta MG, Malde HM, et al. Acute upper extremity deep venous thrombosis: Safety and effectiveness of superior vena caval filters. *Radiology* 1999;210(1):53–58.

65. Weinmann EE, Salzman EW. Deep-vein thrombosis. *N Engl J Med* 1994;331(24):1630–1641.

66. Sorensen HT, Mellemkjaer L, Steffensen FH, et al. The risk of a diagnosis of cancer after primary deep venous thrombosis or pulmonary embolism. *N Engl J Med* 1998;338(17):1169–1173.

67. Svensson PJ, Dahlback B. Resistance to activated protein C as a basis for venous thrombosis. *N Engl J Med* 1994;330(8):517–522.

68. Simioni P, Prandoni P, Lensing AW, et al. The risk of recurrent venous thromboembolism in patients with an Arg506 -> Gln mutation in the gene for factor V (factor V Leiden). *N Engl J Med* 1997;336(6):399–403.

69. De Stefano V, Martinelli I, Mannucci PM, et al. The risk of recurrent deep venous thrombosis among heterozygous carriers of both factor V Leiden and the G20210A prothrombin mutation. *N Engl J Med* 1999;341(11):801–806.

70. Geerts WH, Code KI, Jay RM, et al. A prospective study of venous thromboembolism after major trauma. *N Engl J Med* 1994;331(24):1601–1606.

71. Yeager RA, Moneta GL, Edwards JM, et al. Deep vein thrombosis associated with lower extremity amputation. *J Vasc Surg* 1995;22(5):612–615.

72. Hirsch DR, Ingenito EP, Goldhaber SZ. Prevalence of deep venous thrombosis among patients in medical intensive care. *JAMA* 1995; 274(4):335–337.

73. Koopman MM, Prandoni P, Piovella F, et al. Treatment of venous thrombosis with intravenous unfractionated heparin administered in the hospital as compared with subcutaneous low-molecular-weight heparin administered at home. *N Engl J Med* 1996;334(11):682–687.

74. Levine M, Gent M, Hirsh J, et al. A comparison of low-molecular-weight heparin administered primarily at home with unfractionated heparin administered in the hospital for proximal deep-vein thrombosis. *N Engl J Med* 1996;334(11):677–681.

75. Gonzalez-Fajardo JA, Arreba E, Castrodeza J, et al. Venographic comparison of subcutaneous low-molecular-weight heparin with oral anticoagulant therapy in the long-term treatment of deep venous thrombosis. *J Vasc Surg* 1999;30(2):283–292.

76. Mewissen MW, Seabrook GR, Meissner MH, et al. Catheter-directed thrombolysis for lower extremity deep venous thrombosis: Report of a national multicenter registry. *Radiology* 1999;211(1):39–49.

77. Lohr JM, Kerr TM, Lutter KS, et al. Lower extremity calf thrombosis: To treat or not to treat? *J Vasc Surg* 1991;14(5):618–623.

78. Verlato F, Zucchetta P, Prandoni P, et al. An unexpectedly high rate of pulmonary embolism in patients with superficial thrombophlebitis of the thigh. *J Vasc Surg* 1999;30(6):1113–1115.

79. Hanson JN, Ascher E, DePippo P, et al. Saphenous vein thrombophlebitis (SVT): A deceptively benign disease. *J Vasc Surg* 1998; 27(4):677–680.

80. Juhan CM, Alimi YS, Barthelemy PJ, et al. Late results of iliofemoral venous thrombectomy. *J Vasc Surg* 1997;25(3):417–422.

81. Hood DB, Weaver FA, Modrall JG, et al. Advances in the treatment of phlegmasia cerulea dolens. *Am J Surg* 1993;166(2):206–210.

82. Patel KR, Paidas CN. Phlegmasia cerulea dolens: The role of nonoperative therapy. *Cardiovasc Surg* 1993;1(5):518–523.

83. Greenfield LJ, Proctor MC. Twenty-year clinical experience with the Greenfield filter. *Cardiovasc Surg* 1995;3(2):199–205.

84. Decousus H, Leizorovicz A, Parent F, et al. A clinical trial of vena caval filters in the prevention of pulmonary embolism in patients with proximal deep-vein thrombosis. *N Engl J Med* 1998;338(7):409–415.

85. Haire WD. Vena caval filters for the prevention of pulmonary embolism. *N Engl J Med* 1998;338(7):463–464.

ADVANCES IN THE MINIMALLY INVASIVE TREATMENT OF PERIPHERAL VASCULAR DISEASE

Suhail Allaqaband / Tanvir K. Bajwa

In the past 25 years, significant advances in endovascular treatment for peripheral vascular disease (PVD) have given doctors and their patients minimally invasive alternatives to major surgical procedures that carry significant morbidity and mortality. This chapter reviews current advances and explores the benefits and limitations in minimally invasive therapies for the treatment of occlusive and aneurysmal disease of peripheral vessels.

Endovascular treatment of PVD with balloon catheters was first reported by Fogarty et al. in 1963.[1] The following year, Dotter and Judkins introduced the concept of percutaneous revascularization using coaxial dilating catheters, followed by Gruntzig's pioneering work that led to the evolution of percutaneous transluminal balloon angioplasty (PTBA).[2,3]

Since then, dramatic advances in balloon and guidewire technology have made it possible to cross difficult lesions and chronic occlusions. Better designed stents have revolutionized endovascular interventions with marked improvement in immediate and long-term results, providing an attractive, reliable alternative to vascular surgery to the point that endovascular stents are now the standard of care in peripheral vascular interventions. Studies on the use of drug-eluting stents in coronary and peripheral arteries provide even more promise for the future of endovascular interventions. Improvements in stent grafts now permit minimally invasive treatment of aneurysmal disease of the aorta as well as other major vascular areas. Improvements in pharmacologic agents and in catheter-based thrombectomy devices have made endovascular interventions the first-line therapy in patients who have acute limb ischemia (ALI) due to thromboembolic disease.

OCCLUSIVE DISEASE OF AORTIC ARCH VESSELS

Subclavian Artery Stenting

Although occlusive disease of the subclavian artery is most often asymptomatic, when it is symptomatic, patients may present with subclavian steal syndrome, upper extremity claudication, or, in patients who have an internal mammary artery bypass graft, subclavian coronary steal syndrome. Surgical treatment of subclavian artery stenosis (SAS) is effective but, among other complications, carries a mortality rate of about 2 percent and a stroke rate of about 3 percent.[4]

Although initial reports of using percutaneous transluminal angioplasty (PTA) alone showed mixed results with high restenosis rates, reports on subclavian artery stenting indicate high procedural success (92 to 100 percent) with good long-term patency (90 to 100 percent).[5–8]

The largest source of data is the report of a multicenter registry[8] that evaluated the results of subclavian artery stenting in 258 patients whose primary indications for intervention were arm claudication (in 43 percent), subclavian steal syndrome (25 percent), and compromised flow from the internal mammary to the coronary artery (24 percent) with 86 percent of the lesions involving the left subclavian artery. Overall, the rate of procedural success was 98.5 percent with a major complication rate of 1 percent. At a mean follow-up of 19 ± 15 months, the primary patency rate was 89 percent and secondary patency rate was 98.5 percent. These results suggest that subclavian artery stenting should be considered the primary treatment in patients who need revascularization for SAS (Fig. 103-1).

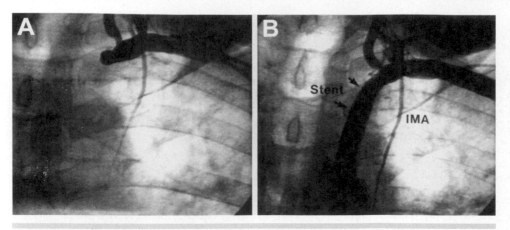

FIGURE 103-1 A 52-year-old male presented with left arm claudication. Angiogram shows: *A.* Occluded subclavian artery. *B.* Widely patent subclavian artery after PTA and stenting.

Vertebrobasilar Angioplasty/Stenting

Patients who have occlusive disease of the vertebrobasilar artery (VBA) are at risk for posterior-circulation ischemia[9] and have an eightfold higher rate of stroke than does the normal population.[10] Surgical options are osteovertebral endarterectomy, vein patch angioplasty, or reimplantation of the vertebral artery in the subclavian or carotid artery. In a series of 290 patients treated surgically, Berguer[11] reported no deaths; however, there was a relatively high

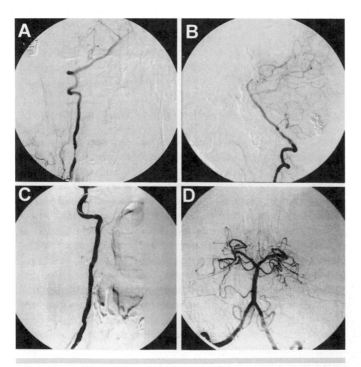

FIGURE 103-2 A 75-year-old female presented with posterior circulation ischemia manifesting as "drop attacks." Angiogram shows: *A.* High-grade stenosis of extracranial portion of right vertebral artery. *B.* High-grade stenosis in the intracranial portion of the left vertebral artery just below the origin of the posterior inferior cerebellar artery. *C.* Right vertebral artery after PTA and stenting with a balloon-expandable coronary stent. *D.* After PTA and stenting of the right vertebral artery, excellent flow is noted in the basilar and left vertebral artery.

rate of postoperative complications including Horner's syndrome (15 percent), recurrent laryngeal nerve palsy (2 percent), lymphocele (4 percent), and immediate thrombosis (1 percent).

When PTA alone has been used to treat patients who have VBA stenosis,[12] vessel recoil and restenosis have resulted in unfavorable long-term results. Reports have indicated that stent-supported angioplasty can be performed safely and effectively with low rates of recurrence.[13–17] Jenkins et al.[13] reported a procedural success rate of 100 percent after vertebral artery stenting in 32 patients (38 arteries) and no deaths at mean follow-up of 10.6 months. Malek et al.[16] also reported high rates for procedural success (95.2 percent) and no adverse events during follow-up.

These reports suggest that stent-supported percutaneous revascularization can be performed in patients who have VBA stenosis with excellent immediate and long-term results and with very low rates of morbidity and mortality (Fig. 103-2).

OCCLUSIVE DISEASE OF AORTOILIAC BIFURCATION

Patients who have atherosclerotic occlusive disease of the distal aortic bifurcation and proximal iliac arteries can present with lifestyle-limiting claudication, limb-threatening ischemia, or impotence. Traditionally, aortoiliac bifurcation disease has been treated with bypass grafting, which yields an excellent long-term outcome but has been associated with a perioperative mortality rate up to 2 to 4 percent and a rate of major early complications (including sexual dysfunction, ureteral damage, intestinal ischemia, and spinal cord injury) of 5 to 13 percent.[17] PTA of the ostium of the common iliac artery sometimes causes plaque to shift across the aortic bifurcation, producing stenosis in the contralateral iliac artery.[18]

To avoid these complications, the kissing balloon technique was developed (i.e., positioning two balloons across the origins of both iliac arteries and inflating these balloons simultaneously). This technique has good rates of procedural and clinical success, including lower mortality; however, the incidence of significant residual stenosis, dissection, thrombosis, and/or distal embolization can be up to 9 percent.[18,19] These complications can be minimized by using a kissing stent technique (i.e., simultaneous deployment of stents at the aortoiliac bifurcation). Results have been excellent, both immediately postprocedure and long-term[20–24] (Fig. 103-3). The authors' rate of procedural success has been 100 percent, with rates for primary patency of 92 percent during follow-up of >18 months and for secondary patency of 100 percent. Although acute complications (distal embolization) occurred in 4 percent, patients had no vascular complications, myocardial infarctions, or perioperative deaths.

OCCLUSIVE DISEASE OF ILIAC ARTERIES

Iliac arteries are best suited for percutaneous intervention because they are easily accessible and are relatively large vessels, which improves expected immediate technical results and yields excellent postprocedural rates of long-term patency. Another well-suited treatment is aortofemoral bypass. The traditional surgical treatment for iliac occlusive disease carries a mortality rate of up to 5 percent, an early graft failure rate of 5.7 percent, and a patency rate after 2 years of 92.8 percent.[25]

Indicators for good results from PTA are as follows:

- Focal lesions (<3 cm)
- Stenosis (vs occlusion)
- Claudication (vs critical limb ischemia)
- Noncalcified lesions
- Absence of diabetes mellitus
- Good distal run-off vessels

In patients who fit these criteria, the initial technical success rate can be >90 percent with a 5-year primary patency rate of about 80 percent.[26] In those who have longer, calcified lesions or occluded arteries, the success rate may be lower, in which case, intravascular stents have been employed with excellent results.

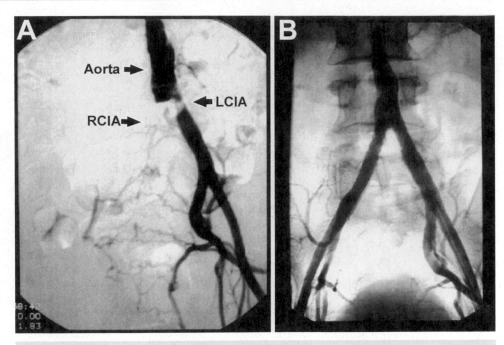

FIGURE 103-3 A 62-year-old male with a history of severe bilateral claudication had a nonhealing ulcer in the right leg. Angiogram shows: *A*. Occluded right common iliac artery (RCIA) with high-grade stenosis of the left common iliac artery (LCIA). *B*. Widely patent common iliac arteries bilaterally after kissing stent procedure.

Several studies have investigated the role of endovascular stents in treating iliac artery occlusive disease.[27–31] In a metanalysis (14 studies, >2000 patients) of PTA versus PTA plus stenting, Bosch and Hunink concluded that PTA with stent placement lowered the risk of long-term failure by 39 percent compared with PTA alone (Table 103-1).[28]

It is also possible to compare results of a variety of stent designs. Vorwerk et al.,[29] using self-expanding wall stents to treat 109 patients who had iliac artery stenoses after PTA failed, reported a primary patency rate of 82 percent and secondary patency rate of 91 percent at 4 years. The rate of technical success in a multicenter study[30] (486 patients) using Palmaz-Schatz balloon expandable stents was 99 percent and the rate of clinical patency at 2 years was 84 percent. Current data indicate that in iliac artery interventions, the choice of stent type does not make much difference with regard to technical success rates and follow-up results. Therefore, the choice can be based on such factors as location, extent, and nature of the lesion, as well as on one's experience and familiarity with a specific stent.

Scheinert et al.[31] evaluated the role of primary stenting after excimer laser–assisted recannalization in 212 patients who had chronically occluded iliac arteries. These authors reported a rate of technical success of 90 percent and a complication rate of 1.4 percent (arterial rupture or embolism), with rates of primary patency of 91 percent at 1 year, 84 percent at 2 years, and 76 percent at 4 years.

Iliac artery PTA/stenting is also used as an adjunct to peripheral vascular surgery. For example, it may help to facilitate the patency of a downstream surgical conduit during surgical revascularization for femoropopliteal dis-

ease. In patients who are at high risk for vascular surgery because of concomitant coronary artery disease, it may provide a less invasive fem-fem bypass compared to a high-risk surgical procedure such as aortobifemoral bypass. Thus iliac artery PTA/stenting is well supported by current data as the initial choice for treating patients who have iliac occlusive disease because it is less invasive and has excellent rates of technical success and good rates of long-term patency (Fig. 103-4).

OCCLUSIVE DISEASE OF FEMOROPOPLITEAL ARTERIES

Atherosclerotic occlusive disease is two to five times more frequent in femoropopliteal arteries than it is in iliac arteries. Patients vary in their clinical presentation from claudication to rest pain and leg ischemia. In addition, acute-onset ischemia is much more frequent than it is in patients who have iliac artery disease. Whereas choices for managing iliac artery disease are clear-cut, choices for managing

TABLE 103-1 PTA vs. PTA Plus Stenting in Iliac Occlusive Disease: Results of Metanalysis of 14 Studies

	PTA		PTA + Stent	
	Stenosis	Occlusion	Stenosis	Occlusion
Immediate technical success (%)	96	80	100	80
Primary patency (%)	65	54	77	61
Secondary patency (%)	80		80	
Major complications (%)	4.3		5.2	

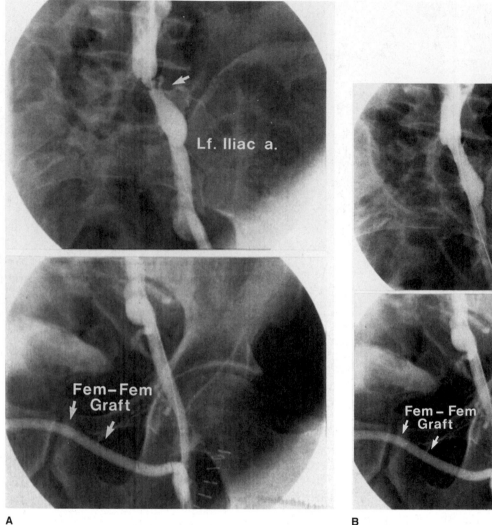

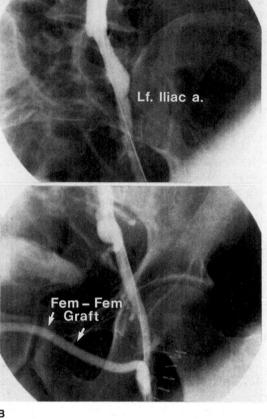

A

B

FIGURE 103-4 A patient with severe coronary artery disease presents with nonhealing ulcer and rest pain in the right leg. Patient underwent femoral-femoral bypass grafting, but flow through the graft was still slow immediately after the surgery. Angiogram revealed A. a high-grade stenosis of the left common iliac artery with a patent fem-fem graft. B. Patient underwent successful stenting of the left common iliac artery.

disease in the femoropopliteal arteries are not supported by strong evidence for or against percutaneous intervention (i.e., PTA, atherectomy, laser, stenting, or a combination of these) or peripheral bypass surgery. Although opinions vary over how to treat patients who have claudication, when pulsatile flow must be restored to prevent limb loss in patients who have rest pain or leg ischemia, some form of intervention is imperative.

Despite attempted comparisons of angioplasty and peripheral bypass surgery for femoropopliteal arterial disease, controversy remains. Hunink et al.[32] compiled a useful analysis of the literature comparing the outcomes of PTA and bypass surgery to help identify patient subgroups who will benefit most from each treatment modality. Despite study limitations, they concluded that successful PTA depends on lesion type (i.e., stenosis vs occlusion) and on the patient's having good distal run-off vessels. With good distal run-off vessels, the patency rate in stenotic vessels at 5 years was 56 to 63 percent, decreasing to 35 to 48 percent if the treated vessel was occluded or if run-off was poor, and 19 to 22 percent if there were both an occluded vessel and poor run-off.

Improved technique and design of balloon catheters and wires, especially the introduction of the hydrophilic guidewire (Terumo wire), have raised the rate of procedural success to 95 to 100 percent for treating stenotic lesions and 70 to 80 percent for occluded ones.[33-35] Consequently, even though rates of long-term patency are far less than those in iliac arteries, PTA is increasingly used to treat disease in femoropopliteal arteries.

In their prospective study of PTA in 106 patients who had claudication, Pekka et al.[33] achieved a primary success rate of 99 percent for patients who had stenotic lesions and 80 percent for those with occlusions; however, the rate of long-term patency was only 47 percent at 1 year and 43 percent at 3 years. Others reported lower rates of primary success (i.e., 88 percent[34] and 90 percent[35]). It is likely that this wide discrepancy can be attributed to differences in patient population, lesion characteristics, and experience and level of skill of the operator. In light of its challenges, PTA for occluded femoropopliteal arteries is not recommended unless claudication limits a patient's lifestyle or the patient has progressed to critical limb ischemia.

Review of the literature shows that the following indicators adversely affect the degree of patency one can achieve in treating femoropopliteal arteries with PTA:

- Occlusion (especially >10 cm)
- Calcified vessels
- Multiple-lesion segments
- Rest ischemia (vs claudication)
- Poor distal run-off

Although in treating iliac artery disease one can expect intravascular stenting to yield excellent rates of long-term patency, its long-term benefits for femoropopliteal lesions are unclear, despite many studies. The small number of patients studied and differences in type of stent used make useful comparison between studies impossible.

In femoropopliteal arteries, use of balloon-expandable stents can no longer be recommended because of high rates of stent deformation from crush injury and because of poor rates of long-term patency. At present, only self-expanding stents are used for treating occlusive disease in femoropopliteal arteries, but even here one must be cautious since not all self-expanding stents work equally well. Sapoval et al.[36] reported poor results with the use of wall stent in femoropopliteal lesions.

Results with nitinol self-expandable stents are more encouraging. Henry et al.,[37] reporting their results in 328 lesions in the femoral artery (225 stenoses, 103 occlusions) and 105 in the popliteal artery (67 stenoses, 38 occlusions), cited initial technical success in more than 99 percent of lesions treated. Restenosis rates were 16.5 percent at the femoral level and 14.4 percent at the popliteal level. At 4 years, the rate of primary patency in the femoral artery was 79.2 percent and the rate of secondary patency was 91.3 percent. At the popliteal level, the rate of primary patency was 84.7 percent and 94.9 percent for secondary patency.

Despite favorable results with nitinol stent placement at the femoropopliteal level, the paucity of available data dissuades most investigators from recommending their routine use.[38–40] The consensus is to reserve this for bail-out or for suboptimal results of PTA and to avoid stenting lesions in the popliteal artery unless essential for limb salvage. Without a large-scale prospective study, there can be no definitive answer as to the best use of stents and as to the long-term benefits of primary stenting for patients who have femoropopliteal occlusive disease.

The authors' recommendations, based on the results of studies using bare stents, may change once drug-eluting stents become available. Duda et al.[41] published results of the first human trial (36 patients) to compare the effectiveness of bare stents and self-expanding nitinol stents coated with a polymer impregnated with sirolimus (Rapamune, Rapamycin) in patients who had superficial femoral artery obstructions. Six months after the start of this double-blind, randomized, prospective trial, the binary restenosis rate was 0 percent in the sirolimus-coated stent group and 23.5 percent ($p = 0.10$) in the bare stent group. If these results can be replicated by large-scale trials, minimally invasive therapy may become the first choice for treating patients who have femoropopliteal disease (Fig. 103-5).

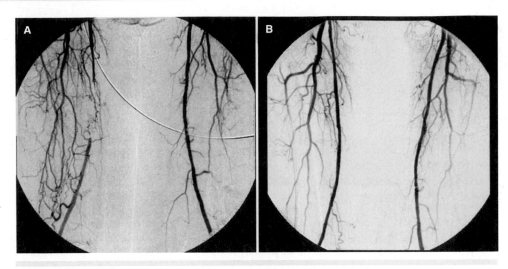

FIGURE 103-5 A 65-year-old female presented with severe lifestyle limiting claudication in the right leg despite treatment with cilostazol and exercise. Angiogram shows: *A*. Occluded right superficial femoral artery (SFA): *B*. Patent SFA after successful percutaneous revascularization using self-expanding nitinol stent.

OCCLUSIVE DISEASE OF INFRAPOPLITEAL ARTERIES

There are three main differences between PVD involving the infrapopliteal arteries and other peripheral arteries:

- When an iliac artery or superficial femoral artery (SFA) is occluded or has critical stenosis, the result may be lifestyle-limiting claudication or an ischemic limb, whereas in isolated below-the-knee disease, having only one patent infrapopliteal artery will be enough to maintain blood flow and prevent limb ischemia, in spite of disease in other infrapopliteal arteries.
- In isolated below-the-knee disease, the ankle-brachial indices (ABIs) might be normal or slightly below normal; therefore, even with single-vessel run-off, this index cannot be relied on for assessing symptoms or for determining disease severity.
- With infrapopliteal occlusion, the restenosis rate after angioplasty is reportedly as high as 40 to 60 percent, primarily related to diffuse disease and the presence of small-diameter vessels, and, frequently, long calcified lesions.

The immediate and long-term results of arterial reconstruction for infrapopliteal disease are better in patients who have claudication than they are in those who have critical limb ischemia (CLI). However, tibial artery bypass surgery traditionally has been reserved for selected patients who have CLI in order to achieve revascularization distal to infrapopliteal obstructions. Although data have not been encouraging, Veith and colleagues[42–44] used innovative and creative techniques to improve results, dramatically decreasing rates of procedure-related amputation (from 49 to 14 percent). Their distal bypass procedures, however, had resulted in a coincident 30-day mortality rate of 4 percent and a 90-day graft failure rate of nearly 5 percent. These results led to tibial artery bypass surgery becoming the standard of care, with success defined as clinical improvement with resolution of rest pain. All the same, use of percutaneous intervention is a more attractive alternative when graft patency deteriorates as a result of distal anastomoses to small diseased vessels, when diffuse distal arterial occlusive disease produces poor runoff, or when grafts have to cross a joint.

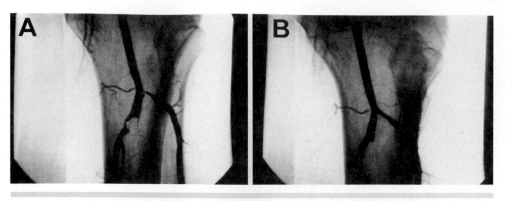

FIGURE 103-6 Patient with critical limb ischemia of the left lower extremity. Angiogram shows: *A.* High-grade stenoses in the anterior tibial artery and the tibioperoneal trunk. *B.* Successful endovascular revascularization using kissing balloon technique.

New low-profile balloons and new generation wires have greatly improved the success rate of infrapopliteal angioplasty for treating occlusions and stenotic lesions. Of several reports concerning angioplasty of tibioperoneal vessels for limb salvage, the largest is by Dorros et al.,[45] in which the procedure was technically successful in 92 percent of the tibioperoneal lesions. Rest pain was relieved or blood flow to a lower extremity was improved in 95 percent of the endangered limbs. Clinical 5-year follow-up of the successfully revascularized CLI patients documented a limb salvage rate of 91 percent.

In a study of 97 patients who had lifestyle-limiting claudication and/or CLI, the success rate was 95 percent, including an 86 percent rate of successful limb salvage.[46] These reports demonstrate that patients who have CLI due to infrapopliteal disease should be seriously considered for endovascular procedures as an alternative to surgery (Figs. 103-6 and 103-7).

ENDOVASCULAR TREATMENT FOR ACUTE LIMB ISCHEMIA

ALI occurs when suddenly decreased blood flow to a limb threatens its viability. The etiology of ALI commonly involves an acutely obstructed major artery or a bypass graft by either an embolus (often from the heart) or by thrombosis in situ. The principal goal of treatment for ALI is to rapidly restore blood flow to the ischemic region to forestall irreversible changes. Although surgical intervention used to be the standard of care for restoring limb perfusion, catheter-directed thrombolysis (CDT) has been shown to be useful for rapid clot dissolution, for unmasking underlying stenoses, and for helping to determine the best treatment strategy (surgery or PTA).[47]

Studies have shown that use of CDT leads to long-term clinical outcomes equal to those of surgical revascularization in treating limb-threatening ischemia.[48–50] The prospective, randomized Surgery versus Thrombolysis for Ischemia of the Lower Extremity trial (STILE) reported no difference in mortality, amputation, or major morbidity in groups treated surgically and those treated with thrombolysis (urokinase or rt-PA, recombinant human tissue-type plasminogen activator).[48] The rates of limb salvage were also similar (88.2 percent in the surgical group versus 89.4 percent in the thrombolysis group). When patients were studied post-hoc on the basis of the duration of their symptoms before enrollment (<14 days or >14 days), it was found that those with <14 days of symptoms had fewer deaths or amputations if they were treated with thrombolysis than if they were treated with surgery (15.3 vs 37.5 percent, $p = 0.01$).

The Thrombolysis or Peripheral Arterial Surgery studies (TOPAS I and TOPAS II) found no difference in rates for mortality and for amputation between groups treated with urokinase or with surgery, but the magnitude of surgery was reduced in the thrombolysis group.[49,50] Nonrandomized trials have demonstrated that thrombolytic therapy followed by PTA may obviate bypass grafting in >50 percent of patients.[51] Accordingly, unless patients present with critical ischemia that demands immediate restoration of pulsatile blood flow by surgical embolectomy (patients with loss of motor and sensory function in a viable limb), CDT should be the initial therapy of choice.

Patients who are selected for CDT should be started on aspirin and heparin as soon as possible, followed by angiography and placement within the occluded vessel of an infusion catheter with multiple side holes. Thrombolytic agents are introduced through the infu-

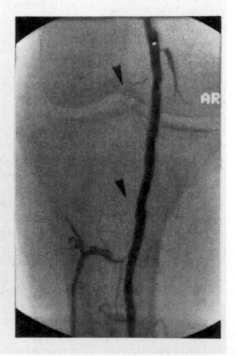

FIGURE 103-7 Patient with critical limb ischemia presenting as a nonhealing ulcer. Angiogram shows: Total occlusion of the right popliteal artery (*left*). Patent popliteal artery after successful endovascular revascularization (*right*).

sion catheter for a period of 12 to 24 h, after which angiography is repeated to evaluate results and identify any underlying lesions, which are then usually corrected by PTA with or without stenting.

Thrombolytic agents currently available in the United States include streptokinase, urokinase, rt-PA, reteplase, and tenecteplase. Urokinase is the one most studied for treatment of ALI; however, rt-PA, reteplase, and tenecteplase are now used successfully to treat patients with ALI.

In addition to CDT, percutaneous mechanical thrombectomy has also been used to treat ALI patients. Of the devices developed to disrupt thrombus formation and remove freshly formed thrombus from the circulation, only the AngioJet Rheolytic Thrombectomy System (Possis Medical, Inc., Minneapolis, MN) is currently approved in the United States for use in arterial circulation. Several studies[52,53] have shown this device to be effective in the treatment of ALI, although it is generally used as an adjunct to CDT rather than as stand-alone therapy. Used together, percutaneous mechanical thrombectomy and CDT appear to speed reperfusion and reduce either the duration of thrombolytic infusion or the dose of the agent used, or both, to achieve successful reperfusion with lower rates of complications (Fig. 103-8).

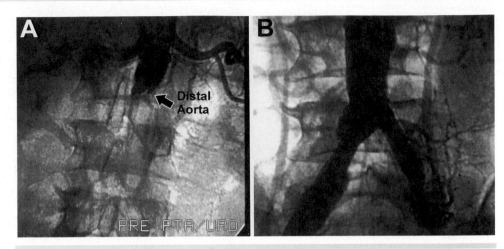

FIGURE 103-8 A 52-year-old male presented with acute limb ischemia following coronary intervention for acute myocardial infarction. Angiogram shows: *A.* Occluded infrarenal abdominal aorta. *B.* Patent aorta and bilateral iliac arteries after catheter-directed thrombolysis with urokinase followed by aortoiliac stenting.

OCCLUSIVE DISEASE OF RENAL ARTERIES

Renal artery stenosis (RAS) is the most common cause of secondary hypertension. Atherosclerosis accounts for 90 percent of the cases of RAS, whereas fibromuscular dysplasia results in RAS in about 10 percent of cases. The incidence of atherosclerotic RAS increases with age and is more common in patients who have occlusive disease in other vascular territories. Of 196 unselected patients who presented with diabetes and hypertension and underwent coronary angiography, renal angiography revealed that 18 percent had RAS >50 percent.[54]

RAS should be suspected in hypertensive patients if there are any of following conditions:

- Blood pressure difficult to control despite multiple medications
- Sudden worsening of blood pressure control
- Recurrent pulmonary edema despite a normal left ventricular systolic function
- Sudden worsening of renal function with the introduction of angiotensin-converting enzyme (ACE) inhibitors

In most patients, atherosclerotic RAS is progressive and, in a significant number of these patients, results in renal atrophy.[55,56] Before percutaneous revascularization procedures became widely available, aortorenal bypass surgery was commonly performed to treat patients who had RAS, but rates of perioperative mortality were 2 to 6 percent with significant morbidity.[57]

Gruntzig first reported percutaneous revascularization of the renal arteries in 1979.[3] Since then, the procedure has been refined and simplified until it has virtually replaced open surgical revascularization of renal arteries for patients who have RAS.

The two major goals of percutaneous revascularization of the renal arteries are the following:

- Control of blood pressure
- Preservation of renal function

When RAS is caused by fibromuscular dysplasia, results of percutaneous transluminal renal angioplasty alone are excellent with a success rate of 82 to 100 percent and a restenosis rate of about 10 percent, making PTA the treatment of choice in patients who have uncontrolled hypertension and fibromuscular dysplasia.[58] In contrast, stand-alone PTA for atherosclerotic RAS has yielded poor results due to high elastic recoil in the atherosclerotic ostial lesions.[58] As is the case when used in most other arteries, stents improve both immediate and long-term patency following PTA. Although not yet substantiated by reports from large randomized studies, many other reports show renal artery stenting to be highly effective (Table 103-2).[59–64] As shown in Table 103-2, rates for immediate technical success following renal artery stenting are 97 to 100 percent, rates for procedure-related major complications are about 2 to 3 percent, and rates for restenosis are 5 to 21 percent.

Variations in reporting standards make it hard to judge the efficacy of renal artery stenting for patients who have hypertension and renal function. Nonetheless, renal artery stenting appears to improve control of blood pressure in 70 percent of patients. However, the procedure cures hypertension in <30 percent of the patients who have atherosclerotic RAS compared with >60 percent of patients with fibromuscular dysplasia. Renal artery stenting improves or stabilizes renal function in approximately 70 percent of the patients. There is evidence that the procedure is more effective if performed in the early stages of RAS, that is, before renal impairment becomes either severe (serum creatinine levels > 4.0 mg/dL) or permanent.

Dorros et al. published data from the multicenter Palmaz stent Renal Artery Stenosis Revascularization registry[65] on 1058 patients (1443 atherosclerotic renal arteries) in whom Palmaz-Schatz stent revascularization was successfully performed to improve poorly controlled hypertension, to preserve renal function, or to improve congestive heart failure. At 4-year follow-up, there were significant decreases in both systolic blood pressure (from 168 mmHg to 147 mmHg) and in diastolic blood pressure (from 84 mmHg to 78 mmHg), as well as in serum creatinine levels (from 1.7 to 1.3 mg/dL). In addition,

TABLE 103-2 Renal Artery Stenting: Results in Recent Studies

Study/Year of Publication	Patients (n)	Arteries (n)	Follow-Up (mos)	Technical Success Rate (%)	Hypertension Cured or Control Improved (%)	Renal Function Improved or Stabilized (%)	Restenosis (%)	Major Complications (%)
Lederman et al.,[59] 2001	300	363	16	100	70	73	21	2
Burket et al.,[60] 2000	127	171	15±14	100	71	67	7.8	3
Rodriguez-Lopez et al.,[61] 1999	108	125	36	97.6	79	100	5.5	3.2
Rocha-Singh et al.,[62] 1999	150	180	13.1	97.3	91	92	12	1.3
Dorros et al.,[63] 1998	163	202	48	99	49	71	NR	1.8
White et al.,[64] 1997	100	133	8.7±5	99	76	22	18.8	2
Pooled results	948	1174	22.8	98.8	72.6	70.8	13.0	2.2

ABBREVIATIONS: n = number; NR = not reported.

renal function was improved or stabilized in 70 percent of patients who had unilateral RAS and in 92 percent of those who had bilateral RAS.

The current consensus is to perform renal artery revascularization in patients who have RAS in order to preserve renal function or to improve control of hypertension. Available data permits no clear-cut recommendations as to the optimal timing of this intervention, and further study is needed. However, there is no doubt that PTA should be the procedure of choice in patients who have RAS due to fibromuscular dysplasia and PTA plus stenting should be the procedure of choice for patients who have atherosclerotic RAS.

Concern about the problem of distal embolization of atherosclerotic debris during PTA/stenting of renal arteries is being addressed by studies to determine if devices shown to be effective in preventing distal embolization in the coronary and carotid arteries are equally as effective in renal arteries. Henry et al.[66] reported the results of a pilot study evaluating feasibility and safety in 28 patients with atherosclerotic RAS who underwent angioplasty and stenting using distal protection provided by a guidewire temporary occlusion balloon. Visible debris was aspirated from all patients, and at 6-month follow-up, renal function did not deteriorate in any patient. These beneficial effects need to be confirmed by randomized studies before any general recommendation can be made for this strategy (Fig. 103-9).

OCCLUSIVE DISEASE OF VISCERAL ARTERIES

Patients who have chronic intestinal ischemia secondary to either occlusion or stenosis of a visceral artery (i.e., celiac, superior, or inferior mesenteric artery) can present with recurrent episodes of abdominal pain (intestinal angina) caused by eating, which leads to fear of eating and to pronounced weight loss.

Surgical revascularization involves transaortic endarterectomy and end-to-end aortomesenteric bypass grafting, which carries high rates of operative mortality (4 to 16 percent) and recurrence (long-term patency of about 78 percent).[67,68] Nonetheless, as late as 1980, when the first report of visceral angioplasty was published, surgery remained the only effective treatment.[69] Since then, there have been many reports of successful treatment by this means.[70,71]

As with angioplasty in most other arteries, restenosis rates after visceral angioplasty tend to be high (24 percent).[70] Intravascular stent placement in the visceral arteries has been successful in addressing this problem, as documented by several case reports and some case series of stent placement in the mesenteric arteries and the celiac trunk.[72–74]

In their series in which stents were placed in mesenteric arteries, Sheeran et al.[72] reported an initial technical success rate of 92 percent for relieving

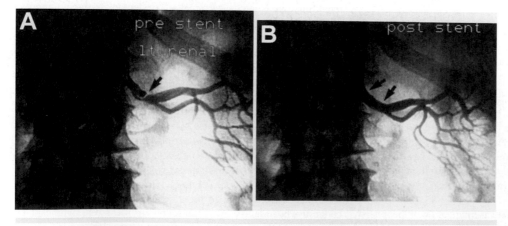

FIGURE 103-9 A patient presented with severe uncontrolled hypertension. Angiogram shows: A. High-grade stenosis in the renal artery supplying a solitary kidney. B. Successful stenting of the renal artery with a balloon-expandable stent.

ischemia, primary patency (76 percent), and secondary patency (83 percent) at 18 months.

In 12 patients who underwent stenting of celiac arteries (3 patients) and superior mesenteric arteries (9 patients), Liermann and Strecker[73] reported a technical success rate of 100 percent. All patients reported relief of symptoms at a mean follow-up of 28 months. Four patients had recurrent symptoms that were treated successfully with repeat balloon angioplasty. Given these high rates of technical success and clinical effectiveness, stent placement in the celiac and mesenteric arteries should be the method of choice for patients who have chronic mesenteric ischemia due to stenosis of a visceral artery.

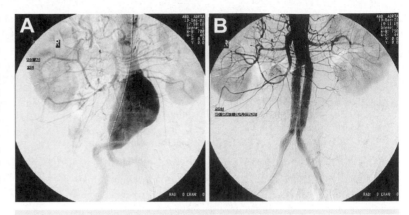

FIGURE 103-10 A 73-year-old male presented with a history of coronary artery disease and congestive heart failure [ejection fraction (EF) 30 percent]. Angiogram shows: *A*. An 8.5-cm infrarenal abdominal aortic aneurysm. *B*. Complete exclusion of the abdominal aortic aneurysm (AAA) after endovascular graft repair with an AneuRx graft.

ANEURYSMAL DISEASE OF ABDOMINAL AORTA AND ILIAC ARTERIES

Aneurysmal Disease of Abdominal Aorta

Abdominal aortic aneurysm (AAA) is defined as focal enlargement of the abdominal aorta (usually involving the infrarenal portion) to a diameter >50 percent larger than normal or to >3 cm in its largest true transverse dimension. Untreated, the major complication is rupture leading to death. Aneurysmal rupture is directly related to aneurysm size. A population-based study from the Mayo Clinic revealed that the estimated risk of rupture was 0 percent per year for an AAA diameter of >4 cm, with increases to 1 percent per year for diameters of 4.0 to 4.9 cm, 11 percent per year for diameters of 5.0 to 5.9 cm, and 25 percent per year for diameters >6 cm.[75]

At least 1 million Americans have a clinically recognized AAA, but only 70,000 to 80,000 surgical repairs are performed annually. Many of these patients are over age 70 and have other serious comorbidities.[76] Consequently, their operative risk is increased, prohibiting open surgical repair. Even in low-risk patients, open repair of AAA is associated with a mortality rate of up to 5 percent.[77,78] In a 36-year population-based study by the Mayo Clinic, the rate of 30-day mortality was 5 percent in 307 patients who underwent elective open surgical repair for an AAA.[76] The Canadian multicenter study reported a similar rate of 5.4 percent.[79]

In 1991, Parodi et al. described the first successful implantation of an endoluminal stent graft in a patient with an infrarenal AAA.[80] Since then, this technique has evolved to gain widespread acceptance by patients and physicians. The rationale for placing an endovascular stent graft is to exclude the aneurysm from the effects of arterial pressure that might cause further dilatation and rupture (Fig. 103-10).

Three devices are FDA-approved for use in the United States: Ancure (Guidant, Indianapolis, IN), AneuRx (Medtronic, Minneapolis, MN), and Excluder (WL Gore and Associates, AZ). The AneuRx and Excluder are modular, bifurcated stent grafts, whereas the Ancure is a unibody device.

In the U.S. AneuRx clinical trial (1192 patients), the rate of implant success was 98 percent, the rate of procedure-related mortality at 30 days was 1.9 percent, and the rate of conversion to open repair within the first 30 days was 1.3 percent.[81] At 4 years, the rate of aneurysm-related mortality was 2.5 percent (0.5 percent per year) and the rate of event-free survival was 97.1 percent. Investigators in the EUROSTAR study[82] reported similar results following endovascular stent graft (EVG). In addition to reducing mortality risk, EVG repair decreases hospital stay, reduces blood loss, and speeds functional recovery.[83,84] Table 103-3 compares the mortality from endovascular repair to that of open surgical repair in patients who underwent elective repair of an AAA.

A major limitation of EVG repair, however, is that these devices have a large profile that rules out such potential candidates as women who have small iliac arteries and men who have severe PVD. Bear in mind also that the longest follow-up at this time is only 5 to 6 years; without longer follow-up data to go by, the "jury is still out" regarding lasting benefits.

Note that it is imperative for patients who undergo EVG repair to have close follow-up with regular computed tomography or ultrasound scans to detect any endoleaks. An *endoleak* is defined as any

TABLE 103-3 Mortality Related to Open and EVG Repair of AAA

Repair	Study	Patients (*n*)	Follow-Up (yrs)	30-Day Mortality (%)	Total AAA-Related Deaths (%)
Open	Mayo Clinic AAA[78]	307	36 (mean 5.8)	5	7.6
	Canadian AAA[79]	680	6	5.4	5.8
EVG	AneuRx I–III[81]	1192	4	1.9	2.4
	EUROSTAR[82]	2955	4	1.7	2.5

ABBREVIATIONS: AAA = abdominal aortic aneurysm; EVG = endovascular stent graft; n = number.

persistent blood flow outside the vascular graft but inside the original intact aneurysm. Endoleaks are classified into four types[85]:

- Type I: Lack of complete seal between the stent graft and vessel wall at attachment sites
- Type II: Back-filling of the aneurysm sac via branch vessels such as lumbar of inferior mesenteric arteries
- Type III: Leaks at connections of modular components, device disruption, and fabric tears
- Type IV: Extravasation of contrast material through interstices in the grafted artery

Type I and type III endoleaks are considered to constitute a major complication, potentially leading to aortic rupture, whereas type II endoleaks pose less of a clinical problem. Type IV endoleak usually disappears over time and does not pose any major clinical problem. Zarins et al. reported the incidence and clinical significance of endoleaks from the U.S. AneuRx clinical trial.[86] The incidence of any endoleak at the time of the hospital discharge was 38 percent, of which 31 percent were type I, 40 percent were type II, and another 29 percent were undetermined. The rate of endoleak decreased to 13 percent at 1 month and 13 percent at 1 year. However, the development of an endoleak did not always translate into aneurysm rupture, as the rupture-free survival rate was 99.7 percent at 1 year. At the present time, consensus opinion is to treat type I and type III endoleaks immediately and follow type II endoleaks with close surveillance to detect any increase in aneurysm size. Fortunately, most endoleaks can be treated successfully by endovascular procedures (i.e., either deployment of additional cuffs of the stent graft or use of coil or Gelfoam embolization).

Aneurysmal Disease of Iliac Arteries

Iliac artery aneurysms (IAA) are most commonly associated with AAA, accounting for up to 50 percent of all cases. It is rare to find an isolated aneurysm of the iliac artery (an incidence of 0.03 to 0.1 percent).[87] Although most aneurysms in this region are asymptomatic, symptoms may be caused by local compression, thrombosis, or by distal embolization of atheromatous debris. Expansive growth and subsequent rupture of iliac artery aneurysms are also well documented.[88]

The treatment of choice is for patients to undergo elective repair of IAA with these traditional criteria:

- Asymptomatic if >3.5 cm in diameter
- Rapid increase in diameter (>0.5 cm/year)
- Symptomatic

As with surgical repair of AAA, open surgical repair for IAA is a major procedure that is associated with high rates of procedure-related morbidity and mortality. Placement of an endovascular stent graft, if technically feasible (good neck and adequate iliac artery size), provides a less invasive way to exclude an IAA.

In a report on 48 patients who underwent implantation of an endoprosthesis in the iliac artery, Scheinert et al.[89] achieved a rate of technical success of 97.9 percent for complete exclusion of an aneurysm. Primary patency rates were 100 percent after 1 year, 97.9 percent after 2 years, 94.9 percent after 3 years, and 87.6 percent after 4 years. Sahgal et al. reported that 30 of their 31 patients had a decrease in the size of their iliac aneurysm (35 true isolated IAAs) treated with EVG repair and coil embolization of the hypogastric artery or its branches.[90]

It is thus both feasible and safe to attempt percutaneous exclusion of IAA by EVG implantation. As a minimally invasive procedure associated with very low rates of procedure-related morbidity and mortality, it is the primary alternative to open surgical repair.

CONCLUSION

Percutaneous revascularization has revolutionized the treatment of PVD so rapidly within the past decade that it is easy to forget that, not long ago, surgery was the only available treatment for severe PVD and was frequently held off until rest pain or gangrene forced the issue. The risks of morbidity and death from surgery were simply too high to justify earlier intervention. The unfortunate consequences of withholding early treatment ranged from chronic, lifestyle-limiting infirmity to severe ischemia that left no choice but amputation if the patient's life was to be saved.

Not only can we intervene earlier, but we can now offer the benefits of intervention to many more categories of patients, thanks to vastly improved balloon catheters and guidewire systems and to the advent of endovascular stents. In considering treatment options (percutaneous revascularization, conservative medical treatment, or surgical revascularization), the scope of the problem needs to be evaluated judiciously in light of the standard question: "Does the benefit of this procedure outweigh the risk?" In answering this question, it is encouraging that the risk of endovascular interventions is much lower and the expectation of benefits are higher for so many patients who a decade or so ago would have been considered ineligible.

Patients who present with PVD are triaged into two categories: (1) those who have claudication and (2) those who have rest pain and ischemic ulceration. Regardless of how they are categorized, all patients are thoroughly evaluated to rule out coronary artery disease (i.e., by either cardiac angiography or by pharmacologic stress testing).

Considering the high risk for potential loss of limb in those who have rest pain or ischemic ulcerations (especially in those who have diabetes and those who smoke), these patients are treated immediately, beginning with angiography and followed by either percutaneous or surgical revascularization so that pulsatile flow is reestablished. For patients who are at lower risk with only symptoms of claudication, the key consideration is to determine if their lifestyle and ability to earn a living are significantly limited. If so, percutaneous revascularization should be encouraged. If there is no such significant limitation, patients are advised that there is no firm basis for the option of percutaneous revascularization despite their diagnosis of PVD.

In patients suspected of having RAS (patients with difficult to control blood pressure or worsening renal function on ACE-I therapy), the authors proceed with renal angiography followed by PTA and stenting.

EVGs have made it possible to treat patients with AAA with minimally invasive interventions. Even patients who are high–surgical risk candidates can be treated effectively by EVG repair. Newer low-profile devices will widen the horizon of EVG repair by allowing physicians to treat patients who have smaller iliac arteries (e.g., women).

With the introduction of drug-eluting stents, the future of endovascular interventions looks even brighter; however, before passing a final verdict, results of larger studies are eagerly awaited.

In conclusion, by covering familiar ground and mapping out areas of frontier exploration, the authors hope that they have brought clarity to the challenging task of steering amid the rapidly evolving field of minimally invasive therapies for treating PVD and of plotting the best course of treatment for each patient.

References

1. Fogarty TD, Cranley JJ, Krause RJ. Method of extraction of arterial emboli and thrombi. *Surg Gynecol Obstet* 1963;116:241–244.

2. Dotter CT, Judkins MP. Transluminal treatment of arteriosclerotic obstruction. Description of a new technique and a preliminary report of its application. *Circulation* 1964;30:654–670.

3. Gruntzig A, Kumpe D. Technique of percutaneous transluminal angioplasty with the Gruntzig balloon catheter. *AJR Am J Roentgenol* 1979; 132:547–552.

4. Beebe HG, Stark R, Johnson ML, et al. Choices of operation for subclavian vertebral arterial disease. *Am J Surg* 1980;139:616–623.

5. Hadjipetrou P, Cox S, Piemonte T, et al. Percutaneous revascularization of atherosclerotic obstruction of aortic arch vessels. *J Am Coll Cardiol* 1999;33:1238–1245.

6. Rodriguez-Lopez JA, Werner A, Martinez R, et al. Stenting for atherosclerotic occlusive disease of the subclavian artery. *Ann Vasc Surg* 1999;13:254–260.

7. Al-Mubarak N, Liu MW, Dean LS, et al. Immediate and late outcomes of subclavian artery stenting. *Cathet Cardiovasc Intervent* 1999;46:169–172.

8. Jain SP, Zhang SY, Khosla S, et al. Subclavian and innominate arteries stenting: Acute and long-term results. *J Am Coll Cardiol* 1998;31:63A.

9. Wityk RJ, Chang HM, Rosengart A, et al. Proximal extracranial vertebral artery disease in the New England Medical Center Posterior Circulation Registry. *Arch Neurol* 1998;55:470–478.

10. Moufarrij NA, Little JR, Furlan AJ, et al. Vertebral artery stenosis: Long-term follow-up. *Stroke* 1984;15:260–263.

11. Berguer R. Long-term results of vertebral artery reconstruction. In: Yao JST, Pearce WH, eds. *Long-term Results in Vascular Surgery*. Norwalk, CT: Appleton and Lange, 1993:69.

12. Motarjeme A. Percutaneous transluminal angioplasty of supra-aortic vessels. *J Endovasc Surg* 1996;3:171–181.

13. Jenkins JS, White CJ, Ramee SR, et al. Vertebral artery stenting. *Catheter Cardiovasc Interv* 2001;54:1–5.

14. Storey GS, Marks MP, Dake M, et al. Vertebral artery stenting following percutaneous transluminal angiography. *J Neurosurg* 1996;84:883–887.

15. Feldman RL, Rubin JJ, Kuykendall RC. Use of coronary Palmaz-Schatz stent in the percutaneous treatment of vertebral artery stenoses. *Catheter Cardiovasc Diagn* 1996;38:312–315.

16. Malek AM, Higashida RT, Phatouros CC, et al. Treatment of posterior circulation ischemia with extracranial percutaneous balloon angioplasty and stent placement. *Stroke* 1999;30:2073–2085.

17. Brewster DC. Direct reconstruction for aortoiliac occlusive disease. In: Rutherford RB, ed. *Vascular Surgery*. Philadelphia: Saunders; 1995: 766–794.

18. Tegtmeyer CJ, Kellum CD, Irving LKK, et al. Percutaneous transluminal angioplasty in the region of the aortic bifurcation. *Radiology* 1985; 157:661–665.

19. Insall RI, Loose HWC, Chamberlain J. Long-term results of double balloon percutaneous transluminal angioplasty of the aorta and iliac arteries. *Eur J Vasc Surg* 1993;7:31–36.

20. Vorwerk D, Gunther RW, Schurmann K, et al. Aortic and iliac stenoses: Follow-up results of stent placement after insufficient balloon angioplasty in 118 cases. *Radiology* 1996;198:45–48.

21. Martinez R, Rodriguez-Lopez J, Diethrich EB. Stenting for abdominal aortic occlusive disease: Long-term results. *Tex Heart Inst J* 1997;24:15–22.

22. Mendelsohn FO, Santos RM, Crowley JJ, et al. Kissing stents in the aortic bifurcation. *Am Heart J* 1998;136:600–605.

23. Haulon S, Mounier-Vehier C, Gaxotte V, et al. Percutaneous reconstruction of the aortoiliac bifurcation with the "kissing stents" technique. *J Endovasc Ther* 2002;9:363–368.

24. Mouanoutoua M, Allaqaband S, Bajwa T, et al. Endovascular intervention of aortoiliac occlusive disease in high-risk patients using the kissing stents technique: Long-term results. *Catheter Cardiovasc Interv* 2003;60:320–326..

25. Ameli FM, Stein M, Provan JL, et al. Predictors of surgical outcome in patients undergoing aortobifemoral bypass reconstruction. *J Cardiovasc Surg* 1990;30:333–339.

26. Johnson KW, Rae M, Hogg-Johnston SA, et al. Five-year results of a prospective study of percutaneous transluminal angioplasty. *Ann Surg* 1987;206:403.

27. Vorwerk D, Guenther RW, Schurmann K, et al. Primary stent placement for chronic iliac artery occlusions: Follow-up results in 103 patients. *Radiology* 1995;194:745–749.

28. Bosch JL, Hunink MG. Meta-analysis of the results of percutaneous transluminal angioplasty and stent placement for aortoiliac occlusive disease. *Radiology* 1997;204:87–96.

29. Vorwerk D, Gunther RW, Schurmann K, et al. Aortic and iliac stenoses: Follow-up results of stent placement after insufficient balloon angioplasty in 118 cases. *Radiology* 1996;198:45–48.

30. Palmaz JC, Laborde JC, Rivera FJ, et al. Stenting of the iliac arteries with the Palmaz stent: Experience from a multicenter trial. *Cardiovasc Intervent Radiol* 1992;15:291–297.

31. Scheinert D, Schroder M, Ludwig J, et al. Stent-supported recanalization of chronic iliac artery occlusions. *Am J Med* 2001;110:708.

32. Hunink MGM, Wong JB, Donaldson MC, et al. Patency results of percutaneous and surgical revascularization for femoropopliteal arterial disease. *Med Decis Making* 1994;14:71–81.

33. Pekka JM, Hannu IM, Ritva LV, et al. Femoropopliteal angioplasty in patients with claudication: Primary and secondary patency in 140 limbs with 1–3 year follow-up. *Radiology* 1994;191:727–733.

34. Johnson KW. Femoral and popliteal arteries: Reanalysis of results of balloon angioplasty. *Radiology* 1992;183:767–771.

35. Capek P, McLean GK, Berkowitz HD. Femoropopliteal angioplasty factors influencing long-term success. *Circulation* 1991;83:70–80.

36. Sapoval MR, Long AL, Raynaud AC, et al. Femoropopliteal stent placement: Long-term results. *Radiology* 1992;184:833–839.

37. Henry M, Amor M, Henry I, et al. Femoropopliteal stenting—results, indications: Choice of the stent. *Radiology* 1999;213(P):50.

38. Cikrit DF, Dalsing MC. Lower-extremity arterial endovascular stenting. *Surg Clin North Am* 1998;78:617–629.

39. Criado FJ. Endovascular treatment of occlusive lesions in the femoropopliteal territory. In: Criado FJ, ed. *Endovascular Intervention: Basic Concepts and Techniques*. Armonk, NY: Futura, 1999:105–114.

40. Vroegindeweij D, Vos LD, Tielbeek AV, et al. Balloon angioplasty combined with primary stenting versus balloon angioplasty alone in femoropopliteal obstructions: A comparative randomized study. *Cardiovasc Intervent Radiol* 1997;20:420–425.

41. Duda SH, Pusich B, Richter G, et al. Sirolimus-eluting stents for the treatment of obstructive superficial femoral artery disease: Six-month results. *Circulation* 2002;106:1505–1509.

42. Veith FJ, Gupta SK, Ascer E, et al. Improved strategies for secondary operations on infrainguinal arteries. *Ann Vasc Surg* 1990;4:85–93.

43. Ascer E, Collier P, Gupta SK, et al. Reoperation for polytetrafluoroethylene bypass failure: The importance of distal outflow site and operative technique in determining outcome. *J Vasc Surg* 1987;5:298–310.

44. Veith FJ, Gupta SK, Wengerter KR, et al. Changing arteriosclerotic disease patterns and management strategies in lower-limb-threatening ischemia. *Ann Surg* 1990;212:402–414.

45. Dorros G, Jaff MR, Dorros AM, et al. Tibioperoneal (outflow lesion) angioplasty can be used as primary treatment in 235 patients with critical limb ischemia: Five-year follow-up. *Circulation* 2001;104:2057–2062.

46. Shalev Y, Fortsas MJ, Schmidt DH, et al. A modification of the peripheral angioplasty procedure to treat below-the-knee vascular disease: Initial success and late outcome in 97 patients. *J Am Coll Cardiol* 1996; 29:191A.

47. Ouriel K. Surgery versus thrombolytic therapy in the management of peripheral arterial occlusions. *JVIR* 1995;6:48S–54S.

48. STILE Investigators. Results of a prospective randomized trial evaluating surgery versus thrombolysis for ischemia of the lower extremity: STILE trial. *Ann Surg* 1994;220:251–268.

49. Ouriel K, Veith FJ, Sasahara AA. Thrombolysis or peripheral arterial surgery (TOPAS): Phase I results. *J Vasc Surg* 1996;23:64–73.

50. Ouriel K, Veith FJ, Sasahara AA. A comparison of recombinant urokinase with vascular surgery as initial treatment for acute arterial occlusion of the legs. *N Engl J Med* 1998;338:1105–1111.

51. Pilger E, Decrinis M, Stark G, et al. Thrombolytic treatment and balloon angioplasty in chronic occlusion of the aortic bifurcation. *Ann Intern Med* 1994;120:40–44.

52. Silva JA, Ramee SR, Collins TJ, et al. Rheolytic thrombectomy in the treatment of acute limb-threatening ischemia: Immediate results and six-month follow-up of the multicenter AngioJet registry. Possis Peripheral AngioJet Study AngioJet Investigators. *Catheter Cardiovasc Diagn* 1998;45:386–393.

53. Wagner HJ, Mueller-Huelsbeck S, Pitton MB, et al. Rapid thrombectomy with a hydrodynamic catheter: Results from a prospective, multicenter trial. *Radiology* 1997;205:675–681.

54. Jean WJ, Al-bitar I, Bajwa TK, et al. High incidence of renal artery stenosis in patients with coronary artery disease. *Catheter Cardiovasc Interv* 1994;32(1):8–10.

55. Caps MT, Perissinotto C, Zierler RE, et al. Prospective study of atherosclerotic disease progression in the renal artery. *Circulation* 1998; 98:2866–2872.

56. Caps MT, Zierler RE, Polissar NL, et al. Risk of atrophy in kidneys with atherosclerotic renal artery stenosis. *Kidney Int* 1998;53:735–742.

57. Hansen KJ, Starr SM, Sands RE, et al. Contemporary surgical management of renovascular disease. *J Vasc Surg* 1991;16:319–331.

58. Kidney D, Deutsch LS. The indications and results of percutaneous transluminal angioplasty and stenting in renal artery stenosis. *Semin Vasc Surg* 1996;9:188–197.

59. Lederman RJ, Mendelsohn FO, Santos R, et al. Primary renal artery stenting: Characteristics and outcomes after 363 procedures. *Am Heart J* 2001;142:314–323.

60. Burket MW, Cooper CJ, Kennedy DJ, et al. Renal artery angioplasty and stent placement: Predictors of a favorable outcome. *Am Heart J* 2000;139:64–71.

61. Rodriguez-Lopez JA, Werner A, Ray LI, et al. Renal artery stenosis treated with stent deployment: Indications, technique, and outcome for 108 patients. *J Vasc Surg* 1999;29(4):617–624.

62. Rocha-Singh KJ, Mishkel G, Katholi RE, et al. Clinical predictors of improved long-term blood pressure control after successful stenting of hypertensive patients with obstructive renal artery atherosclerosis. *Catheter Cardiovasc Interv* 1999;47:167–172.

63. Dorros G, Jaff M, Mathiak L, et al. Four-year follow-up of Palmaz-Schatz stent revascularization as treatment for atherosclerotic renal artery stenosis. *Circulation* 1998;98:642–647.

64. White CJ, Ramee SR, Collins TJ, et al. Renal artery stent placement: Utility in lesions difficult to treat with balloon angioplasty. *J Am Coll Cardiol* 1997;30:1445–1450.

65. Dorros G, Jaff M, Mathiak L, et al. Multicenter Palmaz stent renal artery stenosis revascularization registry report: Four-year follow-up of 1,058 successful patients. *Catheter Cardiovasc Interv* 2002;55: 182–188.

66. Henry M, Klonaris C, Henry I, et al. Protected renal stenting with the PercuSurge GuardWire device: A pilot study. *J Endovasc Ther* 2001; 8(3):227–237.

67. Rapp JH, Reilly LM, Quarfordt PG, et al. Durability of endarterectomy and antegrade graft in the treatment of chronic visceral ischemia. *J Vasc Surg* 1986;3:799–806.

68. Moawad J, McKinsey JF, Wyble CW, et al. Current results of surgical therapy for chronic mesenteric ischemia. *Arch Surg* 1997;132:613–619.

69. Furrer J, Gruntzig A, Kugelmeier J, et al. Treatment of abdominal angina with percutaneous dilatation of an arterial mesenteric superior stenosis. *Cardiovasc Intervent Radiol* 1980;3:43–44.

70. Maspes F, Mazzetti di Pietralata G, Gandini R, et al. Percutaneous transluminal angioplasty in the treatment of chronic mesenteric ischemia: Results and three years of follow-up in 23 patients. *Abdom Imaging* 1998;23:358–363.

71. Matsumoto AH, Tegtmeyer CJ, Fitzcharles EK, et al. Percutaneous transluminal angioplasty of visceral arterial stenoses: Results and long-term, clinical follow-up. *J Vasc Intervent Radiol* 1995;6:165–174.

72. Sheeran SR, Murphy TP, Khwaja A, et al. Stent placement for treatment of mesenteric artery stenoses or occlusions. *J Vasc Intervent Radiol* 1999;10(7):861–867.

73. Liermann D, Strecker EP. Tantalum stents in the treatment of stenotic and occlusive disease of abdominal vessels. In: Liebermann DD, ed. *Stents: State of the Art and Future Developments.* Watertown: Boston Scientific Corp., 1995:127–134.

74. Nyman U, Ivancev K, Lindh M, et al. Endovascular treatment of chronic mesenteric ischemia: Report of five cases. *Cardiovasc Intervent Radiol* 1998;21:305–313.

75. Reed WW, Hallett JW Jr, Damiano MA, et al. Learning from the last ultrasound: A population-based study. *N Engl J Med* 1989;321:1009–1014.

76. Hallett JW Jr. Management of abdominal aortic aneurysms. *Mayo Clin Proc* 2000;75:395–399.

77. Hollier LH, Taylor LM Jr, Ochsner J. Recommended indications for operative treatment of abdominal aortic aneurysms: Report of a subcommittee of the Joint Council of the Society for Vascular Surgery and the International Society for Cardiovascular Surgery. *J Vasc Surg* 1992; 15:1046–1056.

78. Hallett JW, Marshall DM, Petterson TM, et al. Graft-related complications after abdominal aortic aneurysm repair: Reassurance from a 36-year population-based experience. *J Vasc Surg* 1997;25:277–286.

79. Johnston KW, Canadian Society for Vascular Surgery Aneurysm Study Group. Nonruptured abdominal aortic aneurysm: Six-year follow-up results from the multicenter prospective Canadian aneurysm study. *J Vasc Surg* 1994;20:163–170.

80. Parodi JC, Palmaz JC, Barone HD. Transfemoral intraluminal graft implantation for abdominal aortic aneurysms. *Ann Vasc Surg* 1991;5: 491–499.

81. Zarins CK, White RA, Moll FL, et al. The AneuRx stent graft: Four-year results and worldwide experience 2000. *J Vasc Surg* 2001;33: S135–S145.

82. Buth J, Laheij RJF, on behalf of the EUROSTAR Collaborators. Early complications and endoleaks after endovascular abdominal aortic aneurysm repair: Report of a multicenter study. *J Vasc Surg* 2000; 31:134–146.

83. Zarins CK, White RA, Schwarten D, et al. for the Investigators of the Medtronic AneuRx Multicenter Clinical Trial. AneuRx stent graft vs. open surgical repair of abdominal aortic aneurysms: Multicenter prospective clinical trial. *J Vasc Surg* 1999;29:292–308.

84. May J, White GH, Yu W, et al. Concurrent comparison of endoluminal versus open repair in treatment of abdominal aortic aneurysms: Analysis of 303 patients by life-table method. *J Vasc Surg* 1998;27:213–221.

85. White GH, May J, Waugh RC, Yu W. Type I and type II endoleaks: A more useful classification for reporting results of endoluminal AAA repair. *J Endovasc Surg* 1998;5:189–193.

86. Zarins CK, White RA, Hodgson KJ, et al. Endoleak as a predictor of outcome after endovascular aneurysm repair. AneuRx multicenter clinical trial. *J Vasc Surg* 2000;32:90–107.

87. Nachbur BH, Inderbitzi RG, Bar W. Isolated iliac aneurysms. *Eur J Vasc Surg* 1991;5:375–381.

88. Richardson JW, Greenfield LJ. Natural history and management of iliac aneurysms. *J Vasc Surg* 1988;8:165–171.

89. Scheinert D, Schroder M, Steinkamp H, et al. Treatment of iliac artery aneurysms by percutaneous implantation of stent grafts. *Circulation* 2000;102:III-253–III-258.

90. Sahgal A, Veith F, Lipsitz E, et al. Diameter changes in isolated iliac artery aneurysms 1 to 6 years after endovascular graft repair. *J Vasc Surg* 2001;33:289–295.

SOCIAL ISSUES AND CARDIOVASCULAR DISEASE

COST-EFFECTIVE STRATEGIES IN CARDIOLOGY

William S. Weintraub / Harlan Krumholz

A SOCIETAL PERSPECTIVE

How do society and individuals decide to allocate resources or spend money? In capitalist societies, the invisible hand of the market guides resource use, and in principle, regulators, generally government agencies, ensure a "level playing field" and prevent various forms of abuse but otherwise try to stay out of the way. Free markets are guided by a principle called *willingness to pay,* which economists define as that price, governed by supply and demand, which consumers are willing to pay for a service.[1] Services in society that are deemed a "right," such as education, are not governed by free markets, since society may view all people as having a right to such services, independently of their ability to pay. Medicine is largely, although not entirely, in the class of a "right," more like education than goods governed by willingness to pay, such as automobiles. When a service is not priced by willingness to pay, there will naturally be concern over how to fairly price or value it and how much of it to buy. The *value* of a service can be defined as its fair cost. The concern for value in medicine is a major societal issue. We can define *value* in health care as good care at a fair price. Whether society is achieving value in health care is a major issue all over the world.

Health care expenditures in the United States have risen dramatically in the last half of the twentieth century. Between 1965 and 2000, public health care expenditures rose from $10.2 billion to $587.2 billion, and total national expenditures rose from $40 billion to $1.30 trillion.[2] This represents an increase in percentage of gross national product (GNP) over this period from 5.1 to 13.2 percent (Fig. 104-1). Furthermore, following a period of stabilization in the mid-to-late 1990s, growth in percentage of GNP devoted to health care is expected to rise to 17 percent of GNP by 2011.[2] This unprecedented and unparalleled increase in expense for one sector of the American economy is placing American medicine in considerable peril. The Hospital Insurance (HI) program, or Medicare Part A, pays for hospital, home health care, skilled nursing, and hospice care for the aged and disabled, insuring about 39 million people in 1998. The HI program, financed primarily by payroll taxes, mainly pays benefits for current beneficiaries, with leftover income held in a trust fund invested in U.S. Treasury securities.

A board of trustees, created by Congress, oversees annual reports on the financial status of the HI trust fund. As of 1999, income exceeds expenditures and is expected to do so for 8 more years, and by drawing down on the trust fund, benefits could continue for several

National Health Expenditures as a Share of Gross Domestic Product (GDP)

Between 2001 and 2011, health spending is projected to grow 2.5 percent per year faster than GDP, so that by 2011 it will constitute 17 percent of GDP.

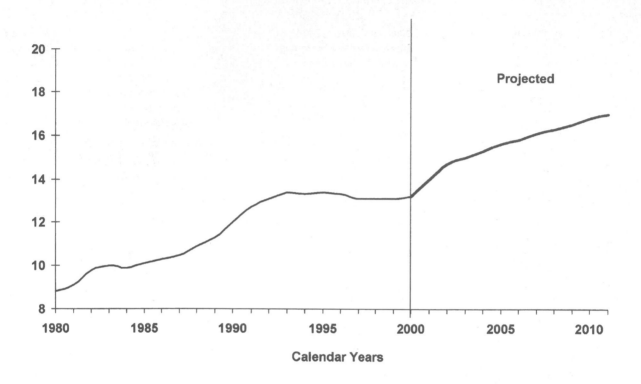

Source: CMS, Office of the Actuary, National Health Statistics Group.

FIGURE 104-1 Increasing costs of medical services over time.

years. However, given current assumptions, the HI trust fund will be depleted by 2015. In addition, there will be relatively fewer people paying and more people consuming HI resources as the population ages. It is expected that there will be 3.6 workers per HI beneficiary when the baby boom generation begins to reach age 65 in 2010, declining to 2.3 by 2030 as the last of the baby boomers reaches age 65. Current public policy has not adequately addressed how to manage the future financial status of Medicare in the United States.

Cardiovascular disease consumes substantial societal resources in economically advantaged countries and thus is responsible for a considerable part of the projected economic challenges in the future. In the United States alone, the American Heart Association estimates that the cost of cardiovascular disease in 2002 will total $329.2 billion[3] (Table 104-1). Of this total, $199.5 billion will be related to direct consumption of medical resources, and an additional $98.8 billion will be related to lost productivity due to early death and disability. Costs related to coronary artery disease (CAD) lead the other categories at $111.8 billion, a little over one-third of the total. Given its magnitude, there is a strong societal interest that the $199.5 billion in direct costs be spent wisely and that the $98.8 billion in lost productivity be minimized. The field of health care economics was developed to address these societal issues.

BACKGROUND ON ECONOMIC ANALYSES

In an environment of limited resources, different societal needs compete for resources. If resources were not limited, then medical care could be provided based on clinical outcome alone, no matter how small the benefit. In such a world of inexhaustible resources, it would be reasonable to provide a treatment that benefited only 1 of every million or 10 million or 100 million individuals screened or treated. Since this is not the case, new forms of diagnostic testing and therapies, as well as existing ones, have to be justified based on their value. The problems of assessment of costs and comparison with outcome are especially relevant and complicated when expensive forms of therapy are used commonly and have multiple complex and interrelating indices of their effectiveness. Within medicine, these issues are perhaps most relevant to cardiovascular care because of the vast array of diagnostic and therapeutic strategies as well as the high cost and the diversity of outcome measures.

Frequently, costs are compared between competing forms of therapeutic or diagnostic strategies. This comparison can involve performing a simulation in which costs and outcome are estimated from the literature, nonrandomized comparisons, and randomized trials. Even within randomized trials, an economic analysis can range

TABLE 104-1 Estimated Direct and Indirect Costs (in Billions of Dollars) of Cardiovascular Diseases and Stroke, United States: 2002

	Heart Disease[a]	Coronary Heart Disease	Stroke	Hypertensive Disease	Congestive Heart Failure	Total Cardiovascular Disease[b]
Direct Costs						
Hospital/nursing home	$81.0	$41.8	$24.5	$8.6	$15.4	$126.3
Physicians/other professionals	15.3	8.6	2.4	8.6	1.6	29.9
Drugs/other medical durables	13.5	6.2	0.8	15.5	2.0	31.8
Home health care	5.2	1.6	3.1	1.7	2.4	11.7
Total expenditures[b]	**$115.0**	**$58.2**	**$30.8**	**$34.4[c]**	**$21.4**	**$199.5**
Indirect costs						
Lost productivity/morbidity	19.0	8.4	5.6	6.7	NA[e]	30.9
Lost productivity/mortality[d]	80.0	45.2	13.0	6.1	1.8	98.8
Grand Total[b]	**$214.0**	**$111.8**	**$49.4**	**$47.2**	**$23.2**	**$329.2**

[a]This category includes coronary heart disease, congestive heart failure, part of hypertensive disease, cardiac dysrhythmias, rheumatic heart disease, cardiomyopathy, pulmonary heart disease, and other or ill-defined "heart" diseases.

[b]Totals may not add up due to rounding and overlap.

[c]Tom Hodgson and Liming Cai (*Medical Care*, 2001) estimated that health care expenditures attributed to hypertension that could be allocated to cardiovascular complications and other diagnoses totaled $108.8 billion in 1998.

[d]Lost future earnings of persons who will die in 2002, discounted at 4 percent.

[e]Not available.

SOURCES: Hodgson TA, Cohen AJ. Medical care expenditures for selected circulatory diseases: Opportunities for reducing national health expenditures. *Med Care* 1999;37:994–1012.

National Health Expenditure Amounts, and Average Percent Change, by Type of Expenditure: Selected Calendar Years 1980–2010 (*www.hcfa.gov*).

Rice DP, Hodgson TA, Kopstein AN. The economic cost of illness: A replication and update. *Health Care Finance Rev* 1985;7:61–80.

Historic Income Tables—"People" (*www.census.gov*).

Deaths for 282 Selected Causes by 5-Year Age Groups, Race, and Sex, United States, 1998 (*www.cdc.nchs/default/htm*).

Unpublished estimates of the present value of lifetime earnings by age and sex, United States, 1998, obtained in 2001 from Wendy Max, University of California at San Francisco. All estimates by Thomas Thom, NHLBI.

from a simulation to a very detailed component of the trial with extensive primary data collection. For any of these designs, the simplest type of economic study is a comparison of costs, or a cost-minimization study. Such a study is useful when it is reasonable to assume that two treatment or diagnostic arms offer similar outcomes to one another.

There are three related forms of economic analysis that can be used to study relative efficacies and relative costs: cost-effectiveness, cost-utility, and cost-benefit. *Cost-effectiveness analysis measures the cost per unit of effectiveness.*[4] This form of analysis assumes that there is one overall measure of effectiveness, often survival. This method breaks down when there are multiple measures of effectiveness. For instance, one form of therapy may increase the risk of death but offer improved symptomatic status. This may, in principle, be addressed through *cost-utility analysis, in which all measures of effectiveness are incorporated into one measure called utility.*[4] Utility, however, is a very difficult parameter to measure, as discussed below. A third and somewhat less popular form of analysis is *cost-benefit analysis, in which measures of both cost and effectiveness are reduced to a single measure, generally dollars (or other currency).*[4] While cost-benefit analysis has not been popular in medicine due to the inherent difficulty of expressing clinical outcome in monetary terms, it is, at least in theory, the most generalizable of these methods.

The perspective in these analyses can have an important impact on their structure and outcome. An analysis from a hospital's perspective may not include the long-term consequences of a particular clinical strategy, whereas this issue may be most important to the patient and the payer. Also, different stakeholders place different values

on the outcomes and costs of medical care. For instance, physicians and patients traditionally have been more concerned about effectiveness, whereas employers and insurance companies have been more concerned about costs.

The perspective of all the various stakeholders may be viewed in aggregate as "society." To be most useful in serving societal goals, cost and cost-effectiveness analyses should be performed from a societal perspective. From such a perspective, an economic analysis should attempt to measure all the costs and measures of outcome associated with a particular treatment. These costs should include those incurred by the patient, the costs of medical resources that could have been used for other patients, and any loss of income that the patient sustained because of poor health. Outcome should include events, quality of life, and survival. By looking at the sum of all these costs in relation to outcome, a policymaker could decide, for example, whether the public good benefited more by allocating limited health care resources to a lipid screening program or to coronary revascularization.

While it is possible in theory to rank order the cost-effectiveness of multiple procedures into what are called *league tables*, limitations in data quality and variability in study design limit the wide applicability of such efforts.[5] An effort to create league tables was made in Oregon, with cost-effectiveness used to guide whether a form of therapy or a test would be funded. This experiment was criticized and finally abandoned because of the limited amount and quality of data available as well as concern over whether the approach was appropriate.[6] Far more common are cost-effectiveness analyses that compare two alternative treatments for a single medical condition, e.g., percutaneous coronary intervention (PCI) and coronary artery bypass grafting (CABG) for symptomatic angina. Such analyses examine the incremental cost-effectiveness of CABG compared with PCI. In addition to focusing on a single clinical condition, the analyses most commonly limit the measured costs to direct and some portion of indirect medical costs. The purpose of these analyses is not to dictate a decision but to inform the decision-making process.

DETERMINING COSTS

Taxonomy for Costs

When a procedure or form of therapy is being considered, it is common to ask what it costs. An economic perspective on cost is more theoretical.[7] Economists are more concerned with how society chooses to allocate limited resources rather than with what something costs per se. Cost may be used to sum resource use when a procedure or test uses resources of several types and to permit comparison of costs between services. To accomplish the end of summarizing resource use to arrive at cost, accounting methods are used. Cost accounting has a particular taxonomy, as shown in Table 104-2.

Costs must be considered from one of several possible perspectives.[8] Thus, for a hospital, the cost is the expenses to provide a service. For payers, the cost is what the providers charge, plus their administrative expenses. In principle, cost studies often seek to determine societal costs, which should be used in cost-effectiveness analyses to gain the widest perspective. However, societal costs are never directly measurable, and thus combinations of cost proxies from one or several stakeholders, where measurable, are often used as estimates.

Costs are classified as direct or indirect.[9] Definitions of indirect costs may lead to uncertainty in categorizing a particular cost. Theoretically, *direct costs* are those incurred by a stakeholder for a therapy or test, and *indirect costs* are those incurred by other societal groups. Generally, direct costs relate to the provision of medical care, whereas indirect costs are other societal costs.

Medical costs for a procedure such as coronary surgery can be divided into three components: in-hospital direct costs, follow-up direct costs, and indirect costs. Inpatient costs comprise hospital costs (e.g., room, laboratory testing, pharmacy, etc.) and physician professional billings. Follow-up direct costs include physician office visits, outpatient testing, medications, home health providers, and additional hospitalizations. Indirect costs reflect lost patient or business opportunity and may be referred to as *productivity costs*.[10]

Another way of thinking about costs is that direct costs are realistically linked to a particular service, whereas indirect costs are not. This type of indirect cost is also called *overhead*.[11]

The appropriate length of time over which to measure costs depends on the procedures being studied and outcomes being measured. Thus the cost of angioplasty could be considered to be the costs of the initial hospitalization and over the first 6 months when restenosis commonly would occur. Alternatively, the cost of angioplasty could be considered the initial hospitalization alone, and the costs during the initial 6 months could be considered follow-up or induced costs, which are those generated beyond the specific time of service delivery.[12] Induced costs also could be a savings. For instance, there may be savings for stents relative to balloon angioplasty in follow-up due to less additional revascularization.

Typically, in the United States, hospital costs are used as a proxy for societal costs. What a hospital charges for a service is not its cost.[13] Measuring hospital cost is difficult and has been approached using what is called either *top-down* or *bottom-up accounting*.[14] Top-down costing involves dividing all the money spent on a hospitalization or procedure by the number of episodes of care of the particular type performed. A payer perspective would be the amount the payer pays the provider for the service. In contrast, a bottom-up approach involves individually costing all resources used for a service, i.e., supplies, equipment depreciation and facilities, salaries, etc. All methods involve a set of assumptions and limitations. When the cost of a specific procedure using top-down costing is being considered, it must be assumed that costs in the department in which the procedure is provided can be separated from costs in other departments. For instance, it is not clear that the costs of the cardiac catheterization laboratory can be clearly separated from hospital maintenance costs. There may also be variability within a department. Therefore using identical methods to calculate the costs of angioplasty and diagnostic catheterization may not be appropriate if angioplasty consumes more resources in a period of time, such as technician time. Bottom-up methods also are limited by the ability to account for all resources consumed and to appropriately apply costs.

Another issue in measuring hospital costs is average versus marginal or incremental cost.[15] Average cost is calculated by dividing all costs for a therapy or test by the number of that particular type. In contrast, the marginal cost is the cost of the next similar procedure. Average costs include all resources used, including overhead, whose costs would not be decreased if not used. Marginal costing accepts fixed costs as a given and focuses only on variable costs or those additional resources consumed by each additional patient. Variable costs are separated analytically from fixed costs by establishing the perspective and time frame as fixed. For instance, facilities' cost is commonly considered fixed, but how should marginal personnel costs be assigned? If coronary surgery decreases as angioplasty becomes more common, do the operating room nurses remain on staff in the operating room, or will they be assigned to other duties? Because of these difficulties, most cost and cost-effectiveness studies use average costs.

Cost Measurement

Commonly used at nonfederal hospitals in the United States, there is a particularly detailed approach to top-down costing that is based on the UB92 summary of charges.[16] The UB92 is a uniform billing statement used by all third-party carriers. Charges are available for such services as the surgical suite, cardiac catheterization laboratory,

TABLE 104-2 Summary of Taxonomy for Costs

Cost perspective
    Provider, i.e., hospital or professional
    Payer, i.e., insurance carrier
    Patient
Cost category
    Direct costs
    Indirect costs
Accounting method
    Top-down
    Bottom-up
Costs per service
    Average cost
    Marginal (incremental) cost

intensive care unit, postoperative or postprocedural floor care, respiratory therapy, supplies, electrocardiography (ECG), telemetry, social services, and so on, but they are not limited to these. While hospitals will set their charges to maximize insurance reimbursements, the relationship between costs and charges—in the form of global specific cost-to-charge ratios—must be developed using American Hospital Association guidelines and then filed annually with the Centers for Medicare and Medicaid Services [CMS, formerly Health Care Financing Administration (HCFA)] in the form of a hospital cost report, which is in the public domain.

An alternative approach is to use bottom-up cost accounting and assign cost weights to each type of resource used.[17] The sum of resources times their cost weights yields total cost. However, the methods are so laborious that they are rarely used.

Another approach is to use a payer perspective.[18] In the United States, Medicare diagnosis-related group (DRG) reimbursement rates could be used to define cost. Similar methods are available in other countries. The use of DRGs to assign cost does not account for variation in cost within that DRG and may not even reflect average resource use. While it is an excellent measure of cost from the point of view of government agencies, it probably does not represent as meaningful a proxy for societal cost as do provider-level hospital costs.

The assessment of professional medical costs is challenging. It is not sufficient to consider physicians' fees alone, since other professionals provide services.[19,20] The goal must be to capture all the professional services for a procedure. For coronary surgery, this may include such fees as the surgeon and assistants; the consultant cardiologist; and anesthesia, radiology, clinical pathology, professional components of any other testing, and any other consultants or ancillary services.[21] There is no cost-to-charge ratio, analogous to the situation for the hospital, available for physician fees to convert their charges to costs.

In the United States, there has been an effort to rationalize physician payments by developing a set of scales for services.[22] This system, the resource-based relative value scale (RBRVS), was developed over time to try to assess the relative time, physical, and cognitive efforts associated with physician services.[22] Each service is assigned a number called the relative value unit (RVU). If the profile of physician services for a procedure or hospitalization is known, then RVUs for each service may be used to develop a proxy for the physician costs. The total RVUs may be converted to a dollar figure by a conversion factor. CMS, the federal agency that administers Medicare and Medicaid, has a standard conversion factor. The appeal of the RBRVS is that it is a relative weighting system that assigns unique weights for physician work and practice costs for each physician service by Current Procedural Terminology (CPT) code. As a result, after assigning a conversion factor, standardized estimates of the costs can be calculated and used as a gauge of physician costs. While there are still some problems with this approach, especially for the practice cost values in the RBRVS, it holds considerable promise and overcomes some of the major drawbacks of physician charge data. An alternative approach is to use published percent shares of hospital expenses by DRG for professional costs.[23]

Determining the costs of outpatient services presents different challenges in determining patient services use, including direct and indirect medical costs. Direct costs include physician office visits, medications, procedures and testing, rehabilitation, nursing home stays, and home health services as well as patient out-of-pocket expenses, including travel. Assessment of these costs is difficult and complicated by insurance, since patients cannot be expected to report reliably exactly how much they paid out of pocket for services and how much the insurance company paid. Unless there is access to a comprehensive insurance claims database, the most reasonable approach is to have patients identify the services they have received. Costs can then be attributed to the individual services and medications. Office visits and other medical services costs may be similarly estimated. Professional services can be estimated using the Medicare fee schedule, as discussed earlier. Medication costs can be estimated from compiled prices by sampling pharmacies or using published wholesale pharmaceutical prices. Using these cost estimates, a partial simulation of postdischarge direct costs may be determined.

Indirect productivity costs include missed time from work by the patient or family members. Follow-up indirect costs are probably the most difficult to determine and are often excluded as immeasurable. In any case, it is not possible to measure all the indirect costs directly. For instance, if an executive in a company has coronary surgery and is out of work for 6 weeks, there may or may not be loss of pay, but the effect on the business cannot readily be determined. Indirect costs, if measured at all, are often confined to family loss of income, and these numbers must be examined with both interest and skepticism.

Over a long time horizon, inflation must be considered. Costs must be inflated or deflated by multiplying by a constant to convert from any one year to another, based on either the general or medical inflation rate.[24] Future costs also should be discounted to reflect the opportunity costs of current dollars, or future costs should be expressed at their present value.[25] For instance, if a policymaker were given the alternative of spending $1000 now or $1000 in 5 years to treat a given condition and obtain the same outcome, the decision would always be the latter. Costs are often discounted at a rate of 3 percent per year.[25]

Variation in Cost

Variation in cost for a service arises from either differences in the type of measurement, as discussed earlier, or differences in resource use. Table 104-3 presents a framework for considering variation in medical costs, according to quality of care, patient, and geographic levels. These levels do not separate clearly, providing a somewhat confusing picture of the sources of variation.

Quality of care is often broken down into the subunits of process, structure, and outcome.[26] These components of quality may also be viewed as reflecting variation in cost. For process measures of access

---

TABLE 104-3 Sources of Variation in Cost

Quality of care
1. Process: access, appropriateness, management
2. Structure: facilities, supplies, staffing
3. Outcome: iatrogenic complications, patients' health status

Patient level
1. Demographic: age, sex, race
2. Disease severity: extent of left ventricular dysfunction or severity of coronary atherosclerosis
3. Comorbidity: cardiac or noncardiac
4. Outcome: Noniatrogenic complications, patients' health status

Geographic and nonmedical economic factors
1. Facilities
2. Supplies
3. Labor

and appropriateness, the effect on cost may be less on the individual service and more at the societal level for provision of that service. Thus, if access to coronary surgery is inadequate, the initial cost to society of coronary surgery may fall as fewer surgeries are performed, but costs may rise due to induced costs or productivity costs of failing to perform necessary surgery. However, if access to adequate diabetes care is inadequate, there may be an increase in the cost to society of inadequately treated diabetes. Similarly, if inappropriate angioplasty is being performed, then the societal cost will rise, even if the individual service is little affected. Management, on the other hand, will affect the individual service. Accordingly, if a service is handled efficiently with care maps to decrease unnecessary resource use of an overall service, such as excessive blood drawing after coronary surgery and an organized and early discharge, then costs can be decreased. Variation in management will cause variation in cost; thus, if there is variation of use of major services, such as cardiac catheterization after hospitalization for unstable angina, then costs will vary accordingly. While it may be appropriate to either perform or not perform a catheterization, the choice will affect cost. Clearly, management and appropriateness issues overlap.

Structure is related to cost. Facilities and supplies vary considerably in cost even within a single geographic location. Staffing may also vary in intensity, with some institutions having more patients being cared for by a nurse than others. Outcome may also vary with quality of care. Complications may be iatrogenic and relate to quality of care and generally increase the cost of a service. Similarly, a patient's health status may vary with quality, which will affect induced productivity costs. Thus, if there is variation in relief from angina after revascularization due to variation in quality of care, then there may be variation in ability to return to work.

Patient-level factors—such as age, gender, and race—may affect cost as much as, or perhaps more than, quality of care. Age may be thought of as similar to comorbidity, potentially raising cost. Disease severity or acuteness, however measured, may also affect costs. Thus it may cost more to perform coronary surgery or coronary angioplasty on patients with a recent acute myocardial infarction (MI) than on those without one.[27–29] Similarly, comorbidity may increase costs. *However, complications generally have a greater effect on costs than comorbidity or severity.*[27–29] Complications and health status outcomes related to patient-level factors do not separate cleanly from complications and heath status outcomes related to quality of care.

Finally, variation in cost may be influenced by geographic and nonmedical economic factors such as land and construction costs, cost of living, and personnel availability.[30] Also, there may be variation in cost that is independent of both quality and geography. For example, hospitals organized into buying cooperatives may be able to purchase supplies at greater discounts than single providers may.

Thus variation in cost of service is complicated with limited ability to account for it. Correlates of cost variability often are studied using multivariate regression techniques.[27] While elegant, these models have significant limitations. First, studies from one or similar institutions may not be generalizable. In addition, comorbidity, disease severity, and provider-level factors may themselves induce complications. Thus models should be developed in which patient and provider factors are correlated with outcome variables and where cost is correlated with preservice and postservice variables. Finally, cost often is not normally distributed. The distribution can be normalized to some extent by using its logarithm. However, correlating variables with the logarithm of cost is not as informative as correlating variables with cost itself.

Thus determining the specific cost of any service is difficult and, therefore, limits generalizing estimate costs outside the bounds of a particular study. In the same sense that effect sizes are considered subject to confidence intervals, cost estimates must be recognized as "estimates." This limitation also applies to using cost measurements in cost-effectiveness analyses and in constructing league tables in which several cost-effectiveness analyses are compared.

COMPARING COSTS WITH OUTCOME

Determining therapeutic or diagnostic costs independently of patient outcome is not particularly helpful for clinical decision making or setting policy. Measuring costs without considering outcomes would preclude judgments about the value of allocating resources in the health care system. The most extreme cost-minimization approach would be to stop offering medical services. However, the goal of the health care system is to maximize patient outcomes within the resource constraints. Consequently, costs and outcomes need to be considered. While it is possible to relate cost to any measure of outcome, the most generalizable approach in medicine is cost-utility analysis based on patient preference.[31]

Determination of Patient Utility and Quality-Adjusted Life Years

In the treatment of CAD, it is unusual for one measurement of outcome to be of sufficient clinical importance that all other outcome measures may be ignored in clinical decision making. While death overwhelms other outcome measures in importance, it is relatively infrequent over short periods of time for most conditions. Consequently, it is also important to consider other outcomes such as MI, unstable angina, revascularization procedures, measures of quality of life, and return to work and weigh them together. In trials comparing percutaneous coronary intervention with coronary surgery, there was no difference in mortality.[32–37] While surgery relieved angina somewhat better[32–37] at higher cost,[34,37–41] it was a disadvantage to the patient to have to undergo the surgery in the first place. Without some method to integrate various measures of outcome, it may be difficult to make an informed choice. In principle, this task may be accomplished through the determination of patient utility.

The utility of a therapy or test is the sum of benefits, both positive and negative, that accrues to a patient over time as a result of the procedure.[42] It is, in principle, all-encompassing. We may consider the assessment of utility beginning with a decision tree (Fig. 104-2). A decision tree takes a patient at a specific point and then considers, in principle, all possible events up to some point in the future. In this model, branch points or nodes with squares represent choices and nodes with circles represent chance events. In the simplified model shown, a single choice is made, and there are two possible outcomes for each choice. Each outcome is called a *health state*. Each health state has a utility and a probability of occurrence. The utility of choice A in Fig. 104-2 is the sum of the utility of health state 1 times its probability plus the utility of health state 2 times its probability. If choices were this easy, then the ability to determine utility of diagnostic or therapeutic strategies would be simple. However, decision trees are almost never this simple. The decision trees for diagnostic tests tend to be much more complicated than those for therapeutics because a test can lead to additional tests or to a range of therapeutic alternatives. For any one treatment, there may be multiple possible health states, and the paucity of literature may make it difficult to determine the probability of different ones, much less the utility associated with each.

Utility changes over time. We may compare the utility after coronary angioplasty if a patient either does or does not suffer restenosis in Fig. 104-3. After successful angioplasty, the patient feels well and utility rises, but then the patient may suffer restenosis and utility falls. After successful redilation, utility rises again. After angioplasty not complicated by restenosis, utility gradually rises. Ultimately, the patients get to the same point, but the patient who has the episode of restenosis suffers a period of decreased utility. Utility measurement should involve patient preference. One patient may dislike chest pain enough to be willing to undergo repeat procedures to relieve angina. Another patient may dislike the catheterization suite enough to be willing to put up with more angina.

Utility may be measured using either a validated survey such as the Health Utilities Index[43] or the EQ-5D[44] or by directly assessing patient preference. These surveys have been validated against patient preference methods and are easy to administer. Patient preference methods ask patients directly to evaluate their current state of health and then evaluate what they would give up or risk to achieve perfect health. The patient preference methods are probably superior to surveys because the evaluation of a patient's view of his or her own state of health is measured directly, but patient preference methods are difficult to administer. The two patient preference methods are *time trade-off*[4] and *standard gamble*.[4] In the time trade-off, patients weigh the fraction of expected survival they are willing to give up to live in perfect health. With the standard gamble, patients weigh what risk of death they are willing to take to live in perfect health. The standard gamble is probably superior because it includes the element of risk.[4]

Utility alone does not provide a final summary measure of outcome because it does not include life expectancy. This summary measure can be determined using quality-adjusted life years (QALYs), which are calculated by combining utility and survival.[45] Median or mean survival must be estimated from either the data set under consideration or from the literature. Survival, as with cost presented earlier, is generally discounted, which means that patients value a year of survival at the present time more than a year of survival in the future. The "true" discount rate for survival is unknown. Values in the literature for the discount rate have varied from 2 to 10 percent, with 3 percent being the most popular.[25] Thus, with a discount rate of 3 percent, next year's survival is 3 percent less important than this year's survival. *QALYs is the best summary*

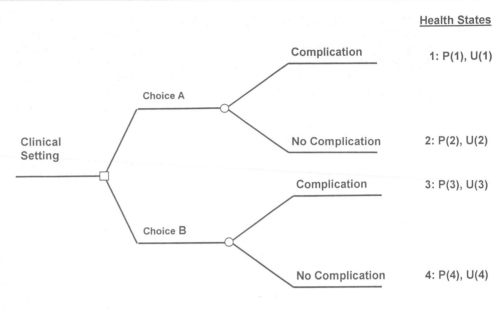

P(x): Probability of Health State X
U(x): Utility of Health State X

FIGURE 104-2 Idealized decision tree for a decision on diagnostic strategy or therapeutic choice.

measure of outcome in a cost-utility analysis because it incorporates patient value, risk aversion, expected survival, and a discount rate.

Cost-Effectiveness and Cost-Utility Analysis

Once cost and a measure of outcome are available, it is, in principle, simple to determine cost-effectiveness. We can begin to understand the approach of cost-effectiveness analysis by considering two competing therapies (or tests), A and B, to treat (or diagnose)

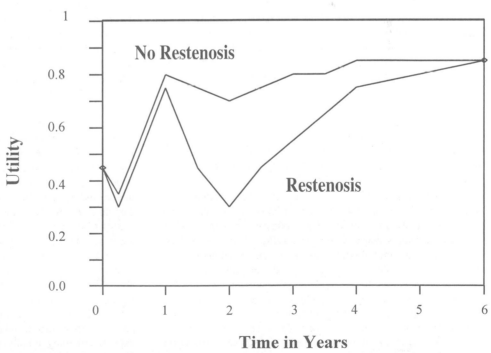

FIGURE 104-3 Theoretical time course of utility after coronary angioplasty in a patient who does not suffer restenosis (*top line*) and a patient who does suffer restenosis (*bottom line*).

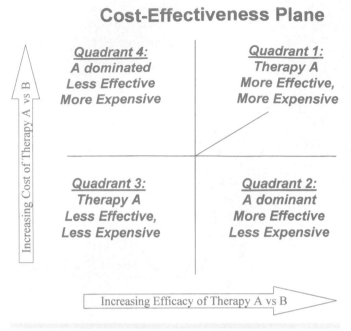

FIGURE 104-4 **Decision matrix.**

the same condition, as considered in a cost-effectiveness plane (Fig. 104-4). In quadrant 1, therapy A is more effective and more expensive than therapy B. In this common clinical situation, where one form of therapy or a test is both more effective and more expensive than a competing therapy or test, cost-effectiveness analysis can help society decide whether to allocate resources to the more effective service. In quadrant 2, A is both more effective and less expensive than B. In this setting, A is said to dominate B and is the obvious choice. In quadrant 3, B is more effective and more expensive than A. As in quadrant 1, cost-effectiveness analysis can help guide decision making. In quadrant 4, A is less effective and more expensive. In this quadrant, B would dominate. Returning to quadrant 1, the slope of the line at an acute angle represents a threshold or ceiling level in cost per unit of effectiveness. Below this line in quadrant 1 and in quadrant 2, choice A would be considered cost-effective.

Cost-effectiveness is the change in cost per unit increase in effectiveness. If the summary effectiveness measure is in QALYs—i.e., a *cost-utility analysis*—then the marginal or incremental cost-effectiveness of therapy or test A compared with therapy or test B is described as the difference in cost between A and B divided by the difference in QALYs between A and B [(cost$_A$ − cost$_B$)/(QALYs$_A$ − QALYs$_B$)].

Cost-effectiveness analysis involves multiple assumptions in measuring both cost and outcome, which introduces uncertainty or error. Uncertainty in clinical microeconomics generally is approached through sensitivity analysis. With sensitivity analysis, measurements in which there is uncertainty are varied between appropriate ranges, and the analysis is repeated. The problem with sensitivity analysis is that the appropriate ranges for the variables may not be known. For measurements made using several different scales, such as the multiple models for calculating marginal costs, these different scales may be used to perform the sensitivity analysis. For measurements that are continuous, such as professional charges, one standard deviation may be appropriate.

There is, however, no absolute standard for sensitivity analysis other than common sense and an intuitive feel for what is medically

reasonable. For instance, Weinstein and Stason[46] used a variation in the severity of angina to decrease QALYs from 0 for no angina to 50 percent for severe disabling angina. If the results of a study vary significantly with changes in certain variables, then the outcome is said to be sensitive for those variables. Properly performed, sensitivity analyses should give insight into the medical decision-making process by identifying thresholds that result in changes in the process. For instance, in the same study by Weinstein and Stason,[46] a threshold was noted for single-vessel disease, such that if a patient were sufficiently bothered by angina to be willing to give up 8 percent of life expectancy, then coronary surgery was indicated, excluding concerns about cost.

CURRENT AND FUTURE TRENDS AND POLICY IMPLICATIONS

Cost-effectiveness analysis in clinical medicine offers a powerful approach that may be used to help guide clinical decision making as well as policy. To date, most cost-effectiveness analyses have been simulations. The formidable difficulties in determining cost and utility have limited the use of these tools in medical care. As the methods and science of cost-effectiveness analyses improve, these analyses should be integrated increasingly into clinical trials and applied routinely to observational databases. With the current changes in health care, accountability and cost are increasingly important, and we can expect to see more studies using these methods and greater incorporation of cost-effectiveness analysis into the medical care delivery system.

The cost-effectiveness ratio, expressed in dollars per QALY, can be used, at least in principle, to affect societal choice regarding the use of scarce resources. A number that is often used, with inadequate justification, is that below $50,000 per QALY, a procedure or form of therapy is cost-effective, whereas at over $100,000 per QALY, it is too expensive. Between these extremes, there is uncertainty. However, these are relatively rough numbers that policymakers may use; they do not represent empiric scientific levels, nor do they reflect thresholds for decisions in actual practice. The lack of an empiric standard to which the cost-effectiveness ratio may be compared reveals the limits of directly using the ratio as opposed to cost-effectiveness analysis to understand and help inform the policymaking process. It would be possible, in principle, to figure out how much money was available and then set the limit on cost-effectiveness to only spend what was available, thus using cost-effectiveness analysis to "level the playing field" and providing a uniform standard. However, difficulties in measurement, as well as uncertainty about whether the appropriateness of using the single cost-effectiveness ratio uniformly for all major policy concerning funding, limit the ability of policymakers to directly use the ratio. In addition, society does not like to ration health care for crucially ill patients (the rule of rescue) but may be more willing to ration it for less critical situations where the benefit of a service may not be as immediately apparent.

It is clear that using a single number for policymaking purposes is inappropriate because cost-effectiveness methods can vary considerably, despite recent efforts to create standards,[47] leading to different numbers. In addition, the cost-effectiveness ratio may not reflect the difference perspective of small changes made for many people with an inexpensive form of therapy versus a big change for the few for expensive therapy. Finally, cost-effectiveness analysis does not adequately reflect the variability of patient populations. Policy planners, representing society, may choose to lower the threshold for a form of therapy for the young compared with the elderly, even though the impact of age is already included in the calculation of the ratio. Thus cost-effectiveness is not designed to be used for policymaking purposes in the absence of other information but rather should help guide both clinical decision making and public policy. All this being said, the cost-effectiveness of most well-established medical therapies compares well with the cost-effectiveness of other health choices, such as airbags in cars, asbestos abatement, or toxic waste control.[47]

COST-EFFECTIVENESS IN PREVENTION, DIAGNOSIS, AND THERAPY

Hyperlipidemia

Until recently, estimates of the cost-effectiveness of lipid lowering were based on decision-analytic models,[2,3,48–51] with data coming from epidemiologic studies, such as Framingham.[52] The models incorporated assumptions concerning the relationship of lipid lowering to subsequent prevention of cardiovascular events. The models also had to make assumptions concerning resource use. More recently, there have been a series of randomized trials that have shown the benefit of lipid lowering and also have included cost-effectiveness analyses (see also Chap. 43).

Education concerning lipid lowering will be inexpensive for each patient but may be quite expensive in the aggregate. A population-wide program was studied by Tosteson et al.[49] using a decision-analytic approach. A populationwide program with a cost of $4.95 per person per year and cholesterol-lowering effects on average of 2 percent reduction would prolong life at an estimated cost of only $3200 per year of life saved.

A cautionary note was also sounded by Goldman et al.[50] Using a decision-analytic model in high-risk patients, therapy with HMG-CoA reductase inhibitors was shown to dominate no therapy. However, in lower-risk populations, therapy has became much less cost-effective and is perhaps not warranted in younger patients with isolated elevation of serum lipids.

Recently, a series of clinical trials in the United States and Europe has established and more clearly defined the benefit of lipid lowering. In the Scandinavian Simvastatin Survival Study (4S),[53] 4444 men and women with a prior MI or episode of unstable angina and with total serum cholesterol between 213 and 309 mg/dL (5.5 and 8.0 mmol/L) were randomized to a low-cholesterol diet and to either placebo or simvastatin. At 5.4 years of mean follow-up, active therapy was associated with reduced all-cause mortality (30 percent; 11.5 vs. 8.2 percent), reduced cardiac mortality (42 percent; 8.5 vs. 5.0 percent), and reduced major coronary events. A cost-effectiveness analysis was developed from the 4S based on resource use, with costs attributed to these resources.[54,55] In 4S, estimated direct medical costs ranged from approximately $4000 to $30,000 per year of life gained, with therapy being most cost-effective in older men with the highest baseline cholesterol and least cost-effective in younger women with the lowest baseline cholesterol. When indirect costs were included in the analysis, the estimated cost per year of life gained decreased further, with estimated net savings in the youngest patients and a cost of approximately $13,000 per year of life gained in elderly women with baseline cholesterol of 213 mg/dL.

In the West of Scotland Coronary Prevention Study (WOSCOPS), 6595 Scottish men aged 45 to 64 with moderate hypercholesterolemia [mean cholesterol 272 mg/dL (7 mmol/L) and low-density lipoprotein cholesterol >155 mg/dL (4 mmol/L)] and no history or

evidence of MI were randomized to placebo or 40 mg/day pravastatin, with a mean follow-up of 4.9 years.[56,57] Active therapy reduced all-cause mortality by 22 percent from 4.1 to 3.2 percent, reduced cardiac mortality rates (28 percent; 1.7 vs. 1.2 percent), and reduced major coronary events (31 percent; 7.9 vs. 5.5 percent). No statistical difference was found in stroke. Coronary revascularization procedures were reduced by 37 percent (2.5 vs. 1.7 percent). Data on cardiac hospitalizations are not available. A cost-effectiveness analysis was constructed based on the outcomes data and resource use. Cost per year of life gained (discounted at 3 to 6 percent annually) was estimated as $25,000 to $40,000, depending on risk group and model assumptions.[57]

Using data from the Pravastatin Limitation of Atherosclerosis in the Coronary Arteries[58] (PLAC I) study and the Pravastatin, Lipids, and Atherosclerosis in the Carotids (PLAC II) study and survival estimates 10 years after MI from Framingham, the Markov decision-analytic model was used to estimate the cost-effectiveness of lipid lowering in secondary prevention. Depending on specific patient risk, cost per life-year saved varied from $7124 to $12,665.

In high-risk groups, such as those with elevated low-density lipoprotein (LDL) cholesterol noted after acute MI, therapy with statins is clearly cost-effective. However, there remains considerable uncertainty as to the cost-effectiveness of therapy in lower-risk populations. Several populations, including the elderly and young groups without a prior event and moderate elevations of lipids, cannot be well assessed from present data. Furthermore, there have been no trials with lipid lowering that included patient preference or any attempt to construct QALYs.

Smoking Cessation

Cigarette smoking remains a potent and prevalent risk factor for premature death and disability. In the United States, approximately one-quarter of the men and one-fifth of the women are current cigarette smokers.[59] These 50 million individuals who annually purchase 24 billion packages of cigarettes[60] have a markedly elevated risk of cancer, pulmonary disease, and vascular disease.[61] As a result, it is estimated that about 400,000 premature deaths occur in the United States each year as a result of cigarette smoking (see also Chap. 43).

The direct medical costs attributed to cigarette smoking are substantial. The Centers for Disease Control and Prevention (CDC) conservatively estimate that medical care expenditures attributable to cigarette smoking in 1993 were $50.0 billion. These costs included $26.9 billion for hospital expenditures, $15.5 billion for physician expenditures, $4.9 billion for nursing home expenditures, $1.8 billion for prescription drugs, and $900 million for home health services. For each pack of cigarettes sold, more than $2 was spent on medical care attributable to smoking. Of note, for each pack sold, about 90 cents of public funds was spent on medical care attributable to smoking. These estimates do not include the full range of harms caused by smoking, such as injuries from smoking-related fires or complications from premature births.

Cigarette smoking also accounts for important indirect costs, such as days lost from work or disability days. Smokers reportedly are absent from work about 7 more days per year than nonsmokers. This loss in productivity due to the health consequences of smoking is estimated to cost $47 billion.[62]

The benefit of smoking cessation is most likely to be achieved in the short term. These short-term benefits are not inconsequential. Lightwood and Glantz[63] specifically examined the short-term economic benefits of smoking cessation as a result of the rapid decline in the risk of acute MI and stroke. They estimated that a 7-year program that produced a 1 percent annual reduction in smoking prevalence would reduce the number of acute MI hospitalizations by 63,840 and the number of stroke hospitalizations by 34,261. The resulting savings would be $3.2 billion, with the prevention of about 13,000 deaths.

If all smokers quit, however, society would not realize a long-term economic benefit. Costs attributed to smoking would diminish gradually, and in the short-run, costs would be lower. However, over time, the higher survival rate as a result of smoking cessation would lead to a larger number of older individuals who would incur health care costs. As a result, the elimination of smoking would, in the long run, produce a net increase in health care costs. These increased costs would be associated with added years of life and healthier years. *Consequently, we can understand successful smoking-cessation strategies as potentially cost-effective but probably not cost-saving in the long run.*

Several studies have examined the cost-effectiveness of interventions to help smokers quit.[64,65] These studies have overwhelmingly found effective smoking-cessation programs to be cost-effective relative to other medical interventions. Cromwell et al.[66] evaluated the cost-effectiveness of the clinical recommendations in the Agency for Health Care Policy and Research Clinical Practice Guideline on Smoking Cessation. The guideline included 15 recommended smoking-cessation interventions. The cost per smoker who successfully quit with the help of counseling interventions that did not include pharmacotherapy ranged from $2186 for group intensive counseling to $7922 for minimal counseling. The cost per QALY ranged from $1108 for group intensive counseling to $4015 for minimal counseling. The addition of pharmacotherapy increased the cost of the intervention but also the effectiveness. With transdermal nicotine as an adjunct therapy, the cost per QALY ranged from $1171 for group intensive counseling to $2405 for minimal counseling. With nicotine gum, it ranged from $1822 for group intensive counseling to $4542 for minimal counseling. These estimates are based on patients presenting to a primary care clinic. The cost-effectiveness of transdermal nicotine and bupropion were systematically reviewed and a decision analytic study in the United Kingdom was performed by Wollacott et al.[67] Both transdermal nicotine and bupropion were found to be effective and cost-effective, with transdermal nicotine in the range of £1000–2400 per year of life saved, bupropion £640–1500 per year of life saved, and £900–2000 for the combination.

Smoking-cessation programs may be even more cost-effective relative to other interventions for patients with cardiovascular disease because of these patients' high risk for future events. Krumholz et al.[68] evaluated the cost-effectiveness of a nurse-based educational intervention for patients who had survived an acute MI. The cost-effectiveness of the program was estimated to be $220 per year of life saved. The value of these types of programs was illuminated in the sensitivity analysis. A smoking-cessation program after acute MI would remain at less than $20,000 per year of life saved even if the program only produced 3 additional ex-smokers for every 1000 (baseline assumption 26 per 100) enrolled or if the program cost as much as $8840 per smoker (baseline assumption $100). Similarly favorable estimates of the value of these interventions would be expected in other high-risk groups with cardiovascular disease.

Exercise

There is strikingly little information on exercise to prevent CAD. Nevertheless, the cost-effectiveness of exercise was investigated using a decision-analytic model by Jones and Eaton.[69] These investiga-tors constructed hypothetical cohorts of sedentary men and women aged 35 to 74 years. Assuming a relative risk of 1.9 for heart disease associated with sedentary behavior, $5.6 billion would be saved annually if 10 percent of adults began a regular walking program. Alternatively, $4.3 billion could be saved if the entire sedentary population began walking regularly, accounting for costs in individuals who dislike exercising. Using the baseline assumptions, walking was found to be economically beneficial for men aged 35 to 64 years and women aged 55 to 64 years. The threshold of relative risk at which economic benefit is found for walking overall was estimated at 1.7, and for those who walk voluntarily, most adults would benefit even at a relative risk of just 1.15.

Diabetes Control

Diabetes is a common and important risk factor for cardiovascular disease. Glycemic control is related to the risk of subsequent complications.[70] As a consequence, the HbA1c level is considered an indicator of the quality of care for an organization, with recommendations for the level to be less than 7 percent.[71] Nevertheless, many diabetics do not reach this level of glycemic control (see also Chaps. 43 and 86).[72]

In economic terms, glycemic control is also important. The level of glycemic control of adult diabetics is associated with medical care expenditures. An observational study of adults with diabetes enrolled in a large health maintenance organization reported that medical care charges were strongly related to HbA1c levels.[73] An increase of 1 percent in the HbA1c level was associated with a 7 percent increase in charges. Because these patients tend to require many medical services, the impact on health care expenditures can be substantial. For example, among the patients with hypertension and heart disease in addition to diabetes, a difference in the HbA1c level of from 9 to 10 percent was associated with a difference in costs of more than $4000 over 3 years even after adjustment for age, sex, and other chronic conditions.

Interventions that improve glycemic control can result in fewer microvascular complications.[73,74] The resources required to produce this benefit are substantial because the interventions may include closer monitoring, increased patient education, frequent telephone contact, more clinical visits, and higher drug costs.

For type I diabetes, the Diabetes Control and Complications Trial (DCCT) may best demonstrate the benefit of these interventions.[74] This trial showed that an intensive treatment regimen decreased the risk of development or progression of retinopathy, nephropathy, and neuropathy by 50 to 75 percent. An economic analysis of the DCCT revealed that the intensive intervention was more expensive than conventional therapy by about $30,000 over the lifetime of each patient.[75] However, considering what is achieved by this investment, the cost-effectiveness of this intervention has been calculated to be $28,661 per year of life saved. With adjustments for quality of life, the intensive intervention costs $19,987 per QALY.

For type II diabetes, the United Kingdom Prospective Diabetes Study (UKPDS), the largest and longest study of this topic, demonstrated that improved blood glucose control reduces the risk of developing retinopathy and nephropathy and possibly reduces neuropathy.[76] This study and others modeled the economic impact of interventions to improve glycemic control for type II diabetes.[77] The intensive treatment doubled the cost of medical care for these patients, which was partially offset by a reduction in the number of complications. The cost-effectiveness of an intensive program was calculated to be $16,002 per QALY.

Antihypertensive Screening and Therapy

Hypertension is a risk factor for stroke, ischemic heart disease, heart failure, and end-stage renal disease (see also Chaps. 43 and 61). The Sixth Report of the Joint National Committee details our current knowledge about the prevention, detection, evaluation, and treatment of hypertension.[78] The screening and treatment of hypertension in the United States, based on 1995 dollars, was estimated to cost $23.7 billion, including $6.7 billion in indirect costs for lost wages and lowered productivity.[79] The costs of the complications of hypertension would be considerably higher. The reduction in vascular events provided by screening and treating hypertension partially offsets their cost, producing a favorable cost-effectiveness ratio.

Investigators from Stanford demonstrated the value of screening in an article published over a decade ago.[80] The results suggest that screening is economically attractive in men and women of all ages. The ratios compared favorably with other common interventions in medicine. Men and older adults have more favorable ratios because they are more likely to have high blood pressure. In 1990 dollars, screening has a cost-effectiveness ratio of $8374 per QALY for men age 60. Screening for hypertension had the least favorable cost-effectiveness ratio, with $44,412 per QALY for 20-year-old women. In the sensitivity analysis, the ratio became less favorable as the benefit of the therapy decreased and as the cost of the medication increased.

Other investigators have examined the cost-effectiveness of treatment once a patient with hypertension is identified. A classic study in this area used a computer simulation, the CHD Policy Model, to estimate the cost-effectiveness of various antihypertensive treatments.[81] The antihypertensive and cholesterol effects of each of the medications were derived from a metanalysis of trials that evaluated the efficacy of these agents. The CHD Policy Model, based on estimates derived from the Framingham Heart Study, calculated the effects of these changes in blood pressure and cholesterol on the incidence of coronary heart disease. They focused specifically on various antihypertensive medications in persons aged 35 through 64 years with a diastolic blood pressure of 95 mmHg or greater and no known coronary heart disease. In 1987 dollars and compared with no treatment, the cost per year of life saved was estimated to be $10,900 for propranolol, $16,400 for hydrochlorothiazide, $61,900 for prazosin hydrochloride, and $72,100 for captopril. Studies of older patients have also found that the treatment of hypertension is economically attractive.[82]

Since the publication of this study, the options for treatment have expanded. The abundance of antihypertensive strategies presents a challenge to these studies in selecting a comparison group. A strategy that is only more expensive than a competing treatment without evidence of incremental benefit will always be dominated in the analysis. The incremental advantage of many of our current treatments for hypertension over the inexpensive option of using low-dose hydrochlorothiazide is speculative and has led some observers to speculate that substantial resources are being squandered in the treatment of this condition.[83] The Sixth Joint National Committee report does recommend diuretics or beta blockers as first-line agents for managing essential hypertension. A recent economic analysis of the Joint National Committee guidelines concurred that a diuretic or beta blocker is much less expensive to achieve and maintain blood pressure control compared with a calcium-channel blocker or an angiotensin-converting enzyme (ACE) inhibitor.[84] However, the recent Healthcare Options Plan Entitlement (HOPE) trial suggested that ACE inhibition is particularly beneficial, and that benefit may extend beyond blood pressure control.[85] An economic paper from HOPE has shown that the benefit of ACI inhibition could be achieved at no increase in costs.[86]

ACUTE CORONARY SYNDROMES

Coronary Care

Patients with an acute MI often suffer life-threatening complications that require rapid, high-level intervention. Consequently, the standard of care is to admit patients with an acute MI to a coronary care unit. Admission to these units is costly, and relatively few patients benefit from the units' advanced capabilities. The value of this triage for specific groups of patients can be illuminated through an economic analysis (see also Chaps. 51 and 52).

To address this issue, Tosteson et al.[87] made use of clinical and resource use data from 12,139 emergency department patients who presented with acute chest pain. They compared a coronary care unit with admission to an intermediate care facility with central ECG monitoring and personnel to detect and treat in-hospital complications. Information on the effectiveness of coronary care units is sparse, particularly in this setting of alternatives with some of the same capabilities. Based on data from the Multicenter Chest Pain Study, the authors estimated that mortality for patients with an acute MI would be 15 percent higher for admission to an intermediate care unit compared with a coronary care unit.[88] Using this assumption, the value of admission to a coronary care unit varied depending on the age of the patient and the initial probability of an acute MI. In 1992 dollars, for patients who were 55 to 64 years old and had a 1 percent probability of MI, admission to a coronary care unit had a cost-effectiveness ratio of $1.4 million per year of life saved, whereas the same-aged patients with a 99 percent probability of an MI had a cost-effectiveness ratio of $15,000 per year of life saved. The cost-effectiveness ratio was less than $75,000 per year of life saved if the probability of MI exceeded 20 percent. The cost-effectiveness of coronary care units was less favorable for younger patients because of their higher underlying risk of a life-threatening complication.

Reperfusion

With the advent of information about the efficacy of thrombolytic therapy for the treatment of patients with suspected acute MI, interest turned to the economic value of this intervention. Since the two largest and earliest trials of thrombolytic therapy used streptokinase, early economic evaluations focused on this agent.[89–93]

A cost-effectiveness analysis published in 1992 examined the use of streptokinase compared with no treatment.[89] The investigators focused on the treatment of elderly patients with suspected acute MI, a group for which there is less enthusiasm about using thrombolytic therapy. Based on data available from GISSI-1 and ISIS-2, the relative benefit of thrombolytic therapy was assumed to be lower in elderly patients and the risk of thrombolytic therapy was assumed to be higher, but the absolute risk of an acute MI was much higher compared with younger patients. The smaller relative reduction in the higher risk associated with MI offsets the higher risk of complications. Thus the decision analysis suggested that thrombolytic therapy was economically attractive over a broad range of assumptions about the risks and benefits. After considering the costs of the treatment, complications, and long-term health care of survivors, the authors estimated that the cost-effectiveness ratio of streptokinase compared with conventional medical therapy was $21,200 per year of life saved for an 80-year-old patient. The authors calculated similar estimates for younger patients. Several studies have found similar results. One analysis has even suggested that thrombolytic therapy could be cost saving because of its impact on reducing rehospitalization[93] (see also Chap. 52).

With the emergence of tissue-type plasminogen activator (t-PA) as a more expensive and more effective alternative to streptokinase, studies addressed whether the incremental benefit was large enough to justify the incremental cost. The Global Use of Strategies to Open Occluded Coronary Arteries (GUSTO) trial investigators performed a substudy to address this issue specifically.[94] The investigators collected detailed information about resource consumption in a subgroup of the GUSTO subjects. They found that both treatment groups were similar in their use of resources in the year after enrollment. The treatment groups had a mean length of hospital stay of 8 days, including an average of 3.5 days in the intensive care unit. During the initial hospitalization, the treatment groups had a similar rate of CABG (13 percent) and percutaneous transluminal coronary angioplasty (PTCA) (31 percent). Overall, the 1-year health costs, excluding the difference in the cost of the thrombolytic agent, were $24,990 per patient treated with t-PA and $24,575 per patient treated with streptokinase. The major difference in the cost of the therapies was the cost of the drugs: $2750 for t-PA and $320 for streptokinase. The primary analysis assumed no increase in costs for the t-PA group after the first year. Based on the GUSTO results and an estimate of the patients' life expectancy, the additional life expectancy per patient treated with t-PA was estimated to be 0.14 years. Based on these estimates, the authors concluded that the cost-effectiveness ratio of using t-PA instead of streptokinase was $32,678 per year of life saved. This ratio varied considerably based on the infarction site and the age of the patient. In general, the younger and lower-risk patients had higher cost-effectiveness ratios. For example, the cost-effectiveness ratio for t-PA in a patient aged 40 years or younger with an inferior MI was $203,071 per year of life saved compared with $13,410 per year of life saved for a person aged 75 years or older with an anterior MI. An analysis conducted independently of the GUSTO trial reached similar conclusions.[95] Comparisons with other new agents await strong evidence of their superiority to t-PA.

Randomized trial data have shown that PTCA or PCI with stenting offers improved outcome for ST-segment-elevation MI compared to pharmacologic thrombolysis.[96–103] Economic analyses based on early studies suggested that primary angioplasty is associated with a reduction in mortality without increasing cost.[104,105] A fundamental problem in this area is that the field is moving rapidly. Changes in costs and techniques require rapid access to recent data in order to develop relevant economic models. The most important technical change has been the introduction of coronary stenting for acute ST-segment-elevation MI, which was considered in PAMI-STENT; 900 patients were randomized to primary stent versus balloon PCTA.[106] At 6 months, the stent arm had fewer target-vessel repeat revascularizations but a nonsignificant increase in mortality and a nonsignificant decrease in reinfarction. The index hospital costs in the stent arm were about $2000 higher, due primarily to the extra cost of the stents.[107] At 1 year, decreased need for follow-up procedures reduced that excess cost by about half. Also, as more rapid discharge protocols evolve for patients who receive reperfusion therapy, the balance of costs and effectiveness may shift.[108]

Antithrombotic Agents

Aspirin reduces mortality and morbidity for patients with acute coronary syndromes. As a result of the marked benefit and the minimal

cost of the therapy, no formal economic analysis of aspirin for the treatment of acute coronary syndromes has been published in the mainstream journals. The ISIS-2 trial found that aspirin avoided 25 deaths for every 1000 patients with suspected acute MI.[109] In addition, the 1 month of aspirin therapy in ISIS-2 was associated with halving the risk of stroke or reinfarction. Aspirin avoided about 10 reinfarctions and 3 strokes for every 1000 patients treated. The avoidance of complications would likely translate into cost savings, leading aspirin to be considered a "strongly dominant" therapy.

Heparin for the treatment of acute MI also has not been formally evaluated in an economic analysis because it has not been shown to provide a strong benefit for acute MI in the aspirin era.[110] In addition, while aspirin plus heparin is the standard of care for patients hospitalized with unstable angina, a metanalysis of the unstable angina studies found only borderline significant results in favor of heparin.[111] Given the uncertainty about its effectiveness, heparin would be a favored therapy only if there were evidence that heparin reduces cost. No studies have revealed an economic advantage to heparin therapy in this setting.

Antiplatelet therapy with clopidogrel in 12,562 patients with unstable angina or non-ST-segment-elevation MI was studied in the CURE trial, revealing a 2.1 percent decrease in the composite of death MI or stroke.[112]

New agents are emerging with increasing frequency. For example, low-molecular-weight heparin is emerging as an effective therapy for unstable angina.[113] The greater cost and benefit of this new treatment make it ideal for economic analysis. Mark et al.[114] performed an economic analysis for a subset of patients enrolled in the Efficacy and Safety of Subcutaneous Enoxaparin in Non-Q-Wave Coronary Events Study Group (ESSENCE).[114] Patients treated with enoxaparin had lower resource use during the initial hospitalization, and this benefit persisted at 30 days, with a cumulative cost savings associated with enoxaparin of $1172 ($p = 0.04$). The investigators concluded that enoxaparin both improves important clinical outcomes and saves money relative to therapy with standard unfractionated heparin, making it a strongly dominant therapy.

The use of a monoclonal antibody fragment against the platelet receptor glycoprotein IIb/IIIa inhibitors is growing. Treatment of high-risk patients undergoing coronary revascularization reduces the short-term risk of death, MI, or coronary revascularization.[115] An economic analysis of the EPIC trial found that the use of this therapy for high-risk patients was associated with a cost savings of $622 per patient during the initial hospitalization from reduced acute ischemic events.[116] During the 6-month follow-up, the therapy decreased repeat hospitalization rates by 23 percent ($p = 0.004$) and repeat revascularization by 22 percent ($p = 0.04$), producing a mean $1270 savings per patient (exclusive of drug cost) ($p = 0.018$). If the cost of the drug were less than $1270, then the strategy would be effective and cost-saving.

The Randomized Efficacy Study of Tirofiban for Outcomes and Restenosis (RESTORE) trial found that in patients undergoing coronary angioplasty for acute coronary syndromes, tirofiban protects against early adverse cardiac events related to abrupt closure.[117] A subsequent economic analysis reported that the use of tirofiban (including drug costs) was not associated with an increase in health care costs.[118] A formal cost-effectiveness analysis of glycoprotein IIb/IIIa blockade for balloon angioplasty showed improved cost-effectiveness in higher-risk patients.[119]

Neither of these studies directly examined the use of this agent in patients with acute ischemic syndromes. This was specifically addressed in PURSUIT, in which 10,948 patients with acute coronary syndromes were randomized to eptifibatide versus placebo, revealing an absolute 1.5 percent decrease in the composite of death or MI at 30 days with active therapy. In an economic analysis of 9461 patients in the United States, the costs exclusive of drug costs were similar in the two arms. The incremental cost-effectiveness ratio for eptifibatide therapy in U.S. PURSUIT patients was $16,491 per year of life saved and $19,693 per added QALY.[120] It should be noted that in PURSUIT the clinical benefit to eptifibatide was shown only in patients who subsequently were treated with an invasive strategy, which would lower the cost-effectiveness ratios in these patients.

Invasive versus Conservative Strategies in Non-ST-Segment-Elevation Acute Coronary Syndromes

The relative value of an invasive strategy with early catheterization and possible revascularization compared with a conservative strategy with exercise testing in patients with unstable angina or non-ST-segment-elevation acute MI has been studied in several clinical trials, with more recent studies showing an advantage to an invasive approach.[121–124] TACTICS TIMI-18 found better outcome with an invasive approach, with a primary endpoint of 19.4 percent with a conservative approach and 15.9 percent with an invasive approach. Initially the invasive approach was more costly, but at 6 months the difference was only $586 (95 percent CI: $1087–$2486).[125] Estimated cost per life year gained for the invasive strategy, based on projected life expectancy, was $12,739, with a range of between $8371 and $25,769 depending on model assumptions.[125]

Beta-Blocker Therapy

Beta-blocker therapy has been shown to reduce mortality following an acute MI.[126] Goldman et al.[127] conducted the most widely cited economic analysis of the costs and effectiveness of beta-blocker therapy. Using data from the literature, they estimated that beta-blocker therapy produced a relative reduction in mortality of 25 percent in years 1 to 3 after an MI and a 7 percent reduction for years 4 to 6. They evaluated the cost-effectiveness of the therapy under the assumption that the benefit did not persist after year 6. Costs were calculated using 1987 dollars. The investigators stratified potential patients by their estimated mortality into low, medium, and high risk: 1.5, 7.5, and 13 percent, respectively, in the first year. The cost-effectiveness ratio was strongly associated with the underlying risk of the patient. For a 45-year-old man with low risk, the cost-effectiveness ratio was $23,457; with medium risk, it was $5890; and with high risk, $3623.

ACE Inhibition

Several large, randomized trials have demonstrated a reduction in acute MI for patients with left ventricular dysfunction after an acute MI who are treated with an ACE inhibitor.[128] Tsevat et al.[129] examined the cost-effectiveness of this intervention utilizing resource use, survival, and health-related quality-of-life information from the Survival and Ventricular Enlargement (SAVE) trial, a randomized trial of captopril for survivors of an anterior MI with an ejection fraction of 40 percent or less. The investigators conservatively estimated that the benefit of captopril did not persist beyond 4 years. The trial found that captopril improved survival at 3.5 years by about 20 percent. Costs were calculated in 1991 dollars. The cost-effectiveness ranged from $60,800 per QALY for 50-year-old patients to $3600 for 80-

year-old patients. McMurray et al.[130] also found that ACE inhibitors are an economically attractive intervention after MI.

Rehabilitation

In a decision-analytic model, Ades et al.[131] studied the cost-effectiveness of cardiac rehabilitation to coordinate exercise training and secondary prevention after acute MI. The cost-effectiveness of cardiac rehabilitation, in dollars per year of life saved, was calculated by combining published results of randomized trials of cardiac rehabilitation on mortality rates, epidemiologic studies of long-term survival in the overall postinfarction population, and studies of patient charges for rehabilitation services and averted medical expenses for hospitalizations after rehabilitation. Cardiac rehabilitation participants had an incremental life expectancy of 0.202 years. In 1988, the average cost of rehabilitation and exercise testing was $1485, partially offset by averted cardiac rehospitalizations of $850 per patient. A cost-effectiveness value of $2130 per year of life saved was determined for the late 1980s, projected to a value of $4950 per year of life saved in 1995. A sensitivity analysis was conducted to support these findings.

REVASCULARIZATION

Societal Burden

Revascularization, either by CABG or PCI, represents an expensive form of therapy for the treatment of angina pectoris and, in some patients, the prolongation of life. The societal burden is substantial with over 571,000 CABG and over 1,069,000 PCI procedures performed in 1999.[3] These numbers represent a 253 percent increase in CABG since 1979 and a 372 percent increase in PTCA since 1987. It should be noted that these estimates, while widely quoted, are quite crude. The total cost is unknown, but if CABG costs about $20,000 and PCI about $10,000, then something over $10 billion is being spent annually on each procedure in the United States alone.

Variation in Costs

The variation in costs of revascularization has been investigated in a number of studies. Within institutions, only a fraction of the variation in costs of coronary surgery or coronary angioplasty can be accounted for by either patient-level or procedural-level factors.[24,27–29,132] Complications predict variation to a greater extent. A study from Emory University, for instance, found that the hospital component of the cost of coronary surgery in 1990 dollars was $16,776 if there were no complications, $17,794 with one complication, $23,624 with three complications, and $50,609 with five or more complications.[27] In a study from Duke University, the surgeon was found to be responsible for much of the variability in cost of coronary surgery.[29] Data from the Cleveland Clinic, Emory University, and others have shown that complications also account for more of the variability in cost of angioplasty than preprocedural or procedural data.[27–29] The need for emergent bypass surgery has been shown to be a strong determinant of hospital costs after coronary angioplasty.[28] However, the ability to account for variation in cost is best described when length of stay is added to the models.[24,27,132]

Length of stay represents a summary variable that may include multiple unmeasured or unidentified variables and, when studied in models with other variables, may confound or obscure the effect of clinical variables on cost. This problem is apparent within single institutions. Considering broader groups of institutions in different geographic regions will result in even greater variation. Medicare data suggest that hospital-level variables account for some of the variability in hospital costs of coronary surgery, whereas geographic and other provider factors also account for additional variability in the angioplasty costs.[30,133] However, the ability to account for variation in cost across multiple institutions is modest.[133]

The evaluation of cost as well as cost-effectiveness of these procedures is complicated by technological improvements and changes in the delivery of health care. In addition, care maps and other efforts to improve efficiency have dramatically decreased the incidence of complications, shortened length of stay, and cut costs.[131,133] Just as these improvements may not be reflected in published clinical trials concerning outcomes, the available cost-effectiveness analyses also will not entirely reflect either technological improvements or increased efficiency in health care delivery.

Coronary surgery has improved in recent years, with greater use of arterial grafts, improved anesthesia and cardioplegia, and the introduction of less invasive coronary surgery. In this regard, outcome and costs in 1996 dollars in 12,266 patients undergoing coronary bypass surgery between 1988 and 1996 at Emory University were evaluated.[24] The patients became sicker, especially with more hypertension, diabetes, prior MIs, and a decrease in ejection fraction over the period. Mortality tended to decrease from 4.7 to 2.7 percent ($p = 0.07$). After accounting for increasing indices of severity of disease over the period, there was a significant decrease in mortality (odds ratio 0.90 per year; $p = 0.0001$). The Q-wave MI rate fell from 4.1 to 1.3 percent ($p < 0.0001$). Mean hospital cost decreased from \$22,689 to \$15,987, and postoperative length of stay decreased from 9.2 to 5.9 days. After accounting for other variables, cost decreased by \$1118 per year and length of stay by 0.55 days per year. A more recent improvement has been the introduction of off-pump coronary surgery. In the SMART trial, 200 patients were randomized to on-pump versus off-pump coronary surgery, with results suggesting better outcome at lower cost with off-pump surgery.[134]

PTCA also has improved with technological advances, especially coronary stents. Stent procedures have improved with better deployment and less need for full anticoagulation. Thus, in the era of stents plus ticlopidine or clopidogrel, stents do not add as much to the cost of intervention as during the era of full anticoagulation. In this regard, Peterson et al.[135] showed that the in-hospital cost of balloon angioplasty in 109 patients studied between 1995 and 1996 was \$10,219. In 64 patients from 1993 to 1995, the cost of PTCA with stenting plus warfarin was \$15,793, and in 217 patients undergoing PTCA with stenting plus ticlopidine the cost was \$13,065. Improvements in PTCA services between 1990 and 1997 in 1997 dollars were investigated in 17,399 patients undergoing PTCA at Emory University.[132] Mortality changed little from 0.63 to 0.88 percent ($p = 0.84$). The Q-wave MI rate fell from 0.68 to 0.24 percent ($p = 0.036$). Emergent coronary surgery fell from 3.50 to 1.56 percent ($p < 0.0001$). Mean hospital cost decreased from \$9816 to \$7442 ($p < 0.0001$), and the length of stay after the procedure decreased from 2.81 to 2.00 days ($p < 0.0001$).

Some technological improvements have been specifically subjected to economic analyses. The use of stents was compared with balloon angioplasty in the STRESS trial.[136] In this relatively early evaluation of stents, there was less additional revascularization and less restenosis with stents but no difference in survival. Costs were higher with stents, due to the prolonged hospitalization and full anticoagulation. Stents ultimately may dominate balloon angioplasty, since hospital stay is now likely to be similar, as stent costs decline while additional procedures continue to be avoided. A purely theoretical paper has suggested that a therapy costing in the range of \$1000 that decreases restenosis after coronary angioplasty by 50 percent could offer a cost-effectiveness ratio of \$16,000 per QALY.[137] The major advance in preventing restenosis has been the introduction of drug-eluting stents.[138] Cost-effectiveness analyses of trials of drug-eluting stents are expected in 2003.

Coronary Surgery versus Medicine

Coronary surgery has been compared with medicine in three major clinical trials conducted in the 1970s and early 1980s (see also Chaps. 55 and 58). None of these trials incorporated cost assessment or cost-effectiveness analyses in their designs. However, the cost-effectiveness of coronary surgery was studied in a relatively early, although detailed, decision-analytic study by Weinstein and Stason.[46] Costs included those of surgery, medical management of angina, and treatment of future MIs. CABG was shown to increase unadjusted life expectancy by 0.6 year in patients with two-vessel disease and 6.9 years in patients with left main coronary disease. With one-vessel disease, a gain in quality-adjusted life expectancy may be noted, due to less angina after surgery. For patients with severe angina, the cost-effectiveness of CABG ranged from \$3800 per QALY gained in left main coronary disease to \$30,000 in one-vessel disease.

Coronary Surgery versus Percutaneous Coronary Intervention

The cost-effectiveness of CABG versus PTCA was first assessed using a decision-analytic model by Wong et al.[139] 8 years after the Weinstein and Stason article.[46] This article was published after PTCA was more established but before the era of stents and before results of randomized trials comparing PTCA with CABG. The model predicted that patients treated with PTCA would have more additional revascularization procedures than patients treated with CABG but that cost would be similar in the long term. In patients with angiographically suitable two-vessel disease, PTCA was found to be a reasonable alternative to CABG. Even in patients with three-vessel disease, bypass surgery was only slightly better than angioplasty.

CABG versus PTCA as an initial revascularization strategy has been compared in a series of six randomized trials from the late 1980s and early 1990s.[32–37] These trials showed little difference in death or MI except in the subgroup with treated diabetes, for which several trials showed a benefit to coronary surgery.[33,140] However, there generally was less angina and less need for additional revascularization procedures after coronary surgery. Cost analyses were performed in the EAST and BARI trials in the United States, ERACI in Argentina, RITA in the United Kingdom, and GABI in Germany.[33,37–41]

In the EAST trial, Weintraub et al.[38] examined the in-hospital and 3-year costs of patients randomized to revascularization with coronary surgery or coronary angioplasty. While the in-hospital costs of surgery were higher than those of angioplasty, there was little difference in 3-year costs. This was due to the need for additional procedures in many of the angioplasty patients.

BARI[33] was a multicenter trial with 1829 patients and included prospective information on economic costs and quality of life in 934. The initial cost of angioplasty was \$21,113 and coronary surgery was \$32,247 ($p < 0.001$). However, by 5 years, the costs were much closer, \$56,225 for angioplasty and \$58,889 for surgery ($p = 0.047$).

The costs were surprisingly and disturbingly high in both treatment arms, and there was considerable overlap. The BARI trial showed that CABG dominated PTCA for treated diabetics with three-vessel disease.

Two European randomized trials of PTCA and CABG have included economic endpoints: the RITA trial[37,40] of 1011 patients and the GABI trial[34] of 358 patients. In the GABI trial, the initial procedural costs were $16,562 for CABG and $5000 for PTCA. After 1 year, the authors found that there was little increase in cumulative costs in the CABG group, whereas the cumulative costs for the PTCA group were $11,250.[34] Similar results were found in the RITA trial, where initially there were much higher costs in the CABG group, but by 2 years the cumulative costs in the PTCA group were 80 percent of those for the CABG group.[40] Cost at 3 years in the ERACI trial also was higher in the CABG group than in the PTCA group but had narrowed from in-hospital costs.[41]

Other than for treated diabetics in the BARI trial, there are inadequate data to perform a cost-effectiveness analysis comparing PTCA with CABG from any of the trials to date because the difference in symptomatic status makes it necessary to include utility assessment. This is essential because if there is no difference in survival, and life years alone were the measure of outcome, then the decision could be made on the basis of cost alone. There are three more contemporary trials comparing PTCA with stents to CABG. There is ARTS in Europe and Israel, ERACI II in Argentina, and SoS in Europe and Canada. In ARTS there was similar mortality between the two arms, but more repeat revascularization after PCI. The in-hospital costs averaged $10,652 with CABG and $6,441 with PCI, a difference of $4212 ($p < 0.001$). This difference narrowed due to repeat revascularization in the PCI arm to a 1-year cost of $13,638 with CABG and $10,665 with PCI, a difference of $2973 ($p < 0.001$).[141] In SoS, 1-year mortality was 2.5 percent in the PCI arm and 0.8 percent in the CABG arm ($p = 0.05$). There was no difference in the composite of death or Q-wave MI. There were more repeat revascularizations with PCI. There was no significant difference in utility between arms at 6 months or 1 year and QALYs were similar. Initial length of stay was longer with CABG (12.2 vs. 5.4 days, $p < 0.0001$), and initial hospitalization costs were higher (£7321 vs. £3884, Δ = £3437, 95 percent CI Δ: £3040 to £3848). At 1 year, the cost difference narrowed, but costs remained higher for CABG (£8905 vs. £6296, Δ = £2609, 95 percent CI Δ: £1769 to £3314).[142]

PTCA versus Medicine

The cost-effectiveness of PTCA compared with medicine also was assessed as part of the now somewhat historic paper by Wong et al.,[139] referred to earlier, concerning the comparison of PTCA with CABG. This study suggested that in patients with severe angina or documented ischemia, angioplasty was cost-effective for single-vessel disease. PTCA has been compared with medicine in three randomized trials, ACME,[143] AVERT,[144] and RITA II.[145] All showed less angina with PTCA. AVERT and RITA II found more cardiovascular events with angioplasty. However, these trials have been small and underpowered to examine hard endpoints; they have largely included low-risk patients. None included a formal cost or cost-effectiveness analysis. In the ongoing COURAGE trial, a larger cohort of 2500 higher-risk patients, all treated with the best available medical therapy, are being randomized to PTCA with medicine versus medicine alone. COURAGE includes a formal cost-effectiveness analysis with utility assessment by direct patient preference.

ELECTROPHYSIOLOGY

Patient Monitoring

Monitoring involves multiple areas, including Holter monitoring, cardiac event recording, and monitoring in the hospital. Event recorders were compared with a 48-h monitor in a randomized trial by Kinlay et al.[146] using a randomized crossover design in 43 patients with palpitations. Event monitors were twice as likely to provide a diagnostic rhythm strip ECG during symptoms as the 48-h monitor. Event monitors dominated continuous monitors with cost savings.

Automatic Implantable Cardiac Defibrillators

Automatic implantable cardiac defibrillators (AICDs) have become widely used to prevent sudden cardiac death in patients at high risk (see also Chap. 38). The cost-effectiveness of this therapy has been investigated with decision-analytic models as well as within the context of randomized trials. Kupersmith et al.[147] investigated the cost-effectiveness of AICD implantation using a decision-analytic model. These investigators based their model on a patient population of 218 well-characterized patients for whom the time of first appropriate discharge was determined.[148] All patients underwent electrophysiologic testing. The authors assumed that the time of first appropriate shock would have been the time of death without the AICD, which was compared with observed mortality. Costs were based on the Medicare fee schedule. Cost-effectiveness was $31,100 per year of life saved. At an ejection fraction of less than 25 percent and greater than or equal to 25 percent, cost-effectiveness was $44,000 and $27,200 per year of life saved. Endocardial AICDs became popular at the time of this study and decreased the cost-effectiveness ratio to $25,700 per year of life saved.

Owens et al.[149] also developed a decision-analytic model, but with a different construction and a somewhat different question. Specifically, AICDs were compared with amiodarone in patients at high or intermediate risk using a highly detailed model with event rates from the literature and costs estimated from published cost rates in California.[150] In high-risk patients, if an AICD reduces total mortality by 20 percent, the marginal cost-effectiveness of an AICD relative to amiodarone was $74,400 per QALY saved. If an AICD reduces mortality by 40 percent, the cost-effectiveness of AICD use was $37,300 per QALY saved, with the results sensitive to assumptions about quality of life. Decision-analytic models were noted by Larsen et al.[150] and Kupperman et al.[151] In these studies, the cost-effectiveness of treatment with an AICD was better than that noted by Owens et al.[149] at $30,500[151] and $47,700[149] per life year saved, adjusted to 1995 dollars. However, the study by Owens et al.[149] considered the more superior antiarrhythmic agent amiodarone.

In a small, randomized trial conducted by Wever et al.,[152] 60 consecutive postinfarct survivors of sudden cardiac death were randomly assigned either AICD as first choice or antiarrhythmic drugs and guided by electrophysiologic testing. Fifteen patients died, 4 in the early ICD group and 11 in the electrophysiologic testing-guided strategy group ($p = 0.07$). The cost-effectiveness of AICD compared with drug therapy was $11,315 per life year saved by early AICD implantation. If quality-of-life measures are taken into account, the cost-effectiveness of early AICD implantation was even more favorable.

Cost-effectiveness of AICD compared with conventional therapy from the MADIT trial was reported by Mushlin et al.,[153] based on

181 patients randomized in the United States. Hospital costs were estimated from the UB92 formulation of the hospital bill and converted to costs using hospital-specific cost-to-charge ratios. Corresponding physician costs were based on a national study of Medicare claims that calculated the ratio of physician to hospital costs for each DRG.[23] Additional professional costs were calculated from payment rates in the Medicare RBRVS. MADIT included epicardial implants in the beginning of the trial and endocardial implants later on. The discounted survival was 3.46 years for the AICD group and 2.66 years for the conventional therapy group at 4 years of follow-up and was associated with an incremental cost-effectiveness ratio of $27,000 (95 percent confidence interval, $200 to $68,200) per life year saved. The results probably would have been more favorable if all patients were treated with endocardial implants. These results probably offer the strongest argument for the cost-effectiveness of AICDs.

The potential application of AICDs was greatly expanded by MADIT-II, which showed that in patients with an ejection fraction of 30 percent or less after an acute myocardial infarction, AICDs reduced mortality at 20 months from 19.8 percent in the conventional therapy group and 14.2 percent the defibrillator group.[154] It has been estimated that this could double the potential indications for AICDs.[155] While this will certainly be expensive (at $50,000 per procedure, 100,000 additional procedures would cost $5 billion), the economic consequences have not yet been fully studied.

Radiofrequency Ablation

Radiofrequency ablation (RFA) can be curative of supraventricular arrhythmias and offers the potential for dominating older forms of therapy (see also Chap. 36). This was studied in a small group of patients by Kalbfleisch et al.[156] The authors determined charges for radiofrequency catheter modification of the atrioventricular (AV) node in 15 patients with symptomatic AV node reentrant tachycardia despite pharmacologic therapy and compared these charges with the estimated health care charges by the same patients before the catheter procedure was performed. The duration and frequency of symptoms were 16 ± 9 years and 4.5 ± 6 episodes per month, respectively. Of the 15 patients, 14 required only one procedure for diagnosis and cure of AV node reentrant tachycardia, and 1 patient required two sessions; all underwent electrophysiologic study before discharge from the hospital to confirm the short-term efficacy of the procedure. The mean duration of the hospital stay was 3 ± 1.5 days, with a charge per patient in 1991 dollars of $15,893 ± $3338, including hospital and physician components. All patients had a successful outcome and required no additional antiarrhythmic therapy. The estimated cost of health care utilization for these 15 patients before cure of AV node reentrant tachycardia was $7651 per patient per year. While small in scale, and with less than optimal costing methods, this study reflects dominance of RFA. A similar costing study from Australia of RFA compared with continued medical therapy also showed dominance of the procedure.[157] RFA in 20 patients was compared with surgical treatment in 20 patients and medical therapy in 12 patients in the nonrandomized comparison. RFA dominated medical therapy. Surgical therapy was slightly more efficacious, but at much higher cost.[158]

A more sophisticated decision-analytic model was created by Hogenhuis et al.[159] In four groups of patients with Wolff-Parkinson-White syndrome, those with (1) prior cardiac arrest, (2) paroxysmal supraventricular tachycardia or atrial fibrillation (PSVT/AF) with hemodynamic compromise, (3) PSVT/AF without hemodynamic compromise, and (4) no symptoms, the authors developed a cost-effectiveness analysis examining five clinical management strategies: (1) observation, (2) observation until a cardiac arrest dictates the need for therapy, (3) initial drug therapy guided by noninvasive monitoring, (4) initial RFA, and (5) initial surgical ablation. A model was developed that included the risks of cardiac arrest, PSVT/AF, drug side effects, procedure-related complications and mortality, the efficacy of drugs and RFA, and cost. RFA was assumed to have an overall efficacy of 92 percent in preventing cardiac arrest and arrhythmias. The model predicted that RFA would yield life expectancy greater than or equal to other strategies. In cardiac arrest survivors and patients who have had PSVT/AF with hemodynamic compromise, the model suggested that RFA would prolong survival at a lower cost. For patients with PSVT/AF without hemodynamic compromise, the marginal cost-effectiveness of attempted RFA ranged from $6600 for 20-year-olds to $19,000 for 60-year-olds per QALY gained. However, for asymptomatic patients, RFA costs ranged from $174,000 for 20-year-olds to $540,000 for 60-year-olds per QALY gained.

Pacemakers

There is a paucity of cost-effectiveness data concerning pacemakers. This may be so because in the classic indication of heart block they are so clearly life-saving that even if they do not dominate no therapy, there can be little doubt about their cost-effectiveness (see also Chap. 32). Some effort has gone into resource utilization issues. Stamato et al.[160] performed a cost-minimization study in which they showed that charges and probably costs will be lower with implantation in a catheterization laboratory as opposed to the operating room. The cost-effectiveness of dual-chamber DDD pacing compared with single-chamber VVI pacing was studied using a decision-analytic model by Sutton and Bourgeois.[161]

Over a 10-year period, a computer model calculated the incidence and prevalence of atrial fibrillation, stroke, permanent disability, heart failure, and mortality in five patient categories: (1) sick sinus syndrome paced VVI, (2) sick sinus syndrome and atrioventricular block upgraded to DDD, (3) sick sinus syndrome paced DDD from the outset, (4) atrioventricular block paced VVI and those upgraded to DDD, and (5) atrioventricular block paced initially DDD. Survival and functional capacity were improved with DDD pacing both for sick sinus syndrome and for atrioventricular block. DDD pacing was also less expensive in the long term, with health care costs in follow-up being a number of times more expensive than the pacemaker. In appropriate patients, DDD pacing dominates VVI pacing. Other efforts have gone into establishing guidelines to ensure the appropriate use of pacemakers.[162–165]

Care of Atrial Fibrillation

The major risk of atrial fibrillation is embolic stroke. The cost-effectiveness of anticoagulation was considered using a decision-analytic model by Gage et al.[166] The authors obtained the probabilities of adverse outcomes from trials involving anticoagulation for nonvalvular atrial fibrillation. They noted a 22 percent reduction in ischemic stroke with aspirin therapy from a metanalysis[167] and a 68 percent reduction with warfarin therapy from the atrial fibrillation investigators' collaborative analysis of five clinical trials.[168] The authors obtained utility estimates by interviewing 74 patients with atrial fibrillation, using the time trade-off method for three degrees of severity of stroke and for daily therapy with aspirin or warfarin. Costs were estimated based on the literature. For patients at medium risk of stroke (i.e., patients with atrial fibrillation and one additional stroke risk factor—including a history of stroke, transient ischemic attack, hypertension, diabetes, or heart disease), the cost-effectiveness of warfarin therapy as compared with aspirin therapy was $8000 (range, $200 to $30,000) per QALY. Both warfarin and aspirin dominated no therapy. For patients at low risk of stroke (i.e., isolated atrial fibrillation), quality-adjusted life expectancy was 6.70 years with warfarin therapy, 6.69 years with aspirin therapy, and 6.51 years with no therapy. The marginal cost-effectiveness of warfarin over aspirin was $370,000 per QALY saved in the base case. If the annual rate of stroke were 0.5 percent higher in low-risk patients, warfarin treatment would cost $66,000 per QALY. Aspirin dominated no therapy.

In a decision-analytic model from Sweden, Gustafsson et al.[169] found that anticoagulation dominated no therapy, and in a decision-analytic model from the United Kingdom, Lightowlers and McGuire[170] found anticoagulation to be cost-effective and to dominate no therapy in higher-risk patients.

Recent efforts have focused on strategies for managing cardioversion, antiarrhythmic therapy, and anticoagulation. Eckman et al.[171] constructed a decision-analytic model considering the base case of a 65-year-old man with nonvalvular atrial fibrillation. Cardioversion followed by a combination of amiodarone and warfarin was the most effective strategy, yielding a gain of 2.3 QALYs compared with no therapy. The marginal cost-effectiveness ratio of cardioversion followed by aspirin with amiodarone was $33,800 per QALY and without amiodarone, $10,800 per QALY. Cardioversion followed by amiodarone and warfarin had a marginal cost-effectiveness ratio of $92,400 per QALY compared with amiodarone and aspirin. Catherwood et al.[172] constructed a similar decision-analytic model considering multiple strategies involving cardioversion followed by aspirin, amiodarone, and warfarin. Strategies involving cardioversion dominated no cardioversion. For patients at high risk of stroke (5.3 percent per year), cardioversion alone followed by repeated cardioversion plus amiodarone therapy on relapse was cost-effective at $9300 per QALY compared with cardioversion alone followed by warfarin therapy on relapse. This strategy also was preferred for moderate-risk patients (3.6 percent per year), but with a higher cost-effectiveness ratio of $18,900 per QALY. In the lowest-risk patients (1.6 percent per year), cardioversion alone followed by aspirin therapy on relapse was preferred. Efforts to assess cost-effectiveness of methods for cardioversion have been cast in some doubt by the recent 4060-patient AFFIRM trial, in which patients were randomized to rhythm versus rate control and then followed for 3.5 years. In AFFIRM, there was no advantage or a trend to worse outcome to attempting to control rhythm for fatal and nonfatal events as well as quality of life.[173]

Assuming that there is still reason to consider cardioversion, another issue concerning the care of patients with atrial fibrillation is the role of transesophageal echocardiography in avoiding prolonged anticoagulation prior to cardioversion. This was investigated by Seto et al. using a decision-analytic model.[174] The authors studied the cost-effectiveness of three strategies: (1) conventional therapy with transthoracic echocardiography and warfarin therapy for 1 month before cardioversion, (2) initial transthoracic echo followed by transesophageal echo and early cardioversion if no thrombus was detected, and (3) initial transesophageal echo with early cardioversion if no thrombus is detected. With strategies 2 and 3, if a thrombus was seen, a follow-up transesophageal echo was performed. If no thrombus was seen, cardioversion was performed. All strategies used anticoagulation before and extending for 1 month after cardioversion. Life expectancy, utilities, event probabilities, and cost were ascertained from the literature. Strategy 3 (cost, $2774; QALYS, 8.49) dominated strategy 2 (cost, $3106; QALYs, 8.48) and conventional therapy (cost, $3070; QALYs, 8.48). The study demonstrated that

transesophageal echo-guided cardioversion dominated conventional therapy if the risk of stroke after transesophageal echo negative for atrial thrombus is slightly less than that after conventional therapy. However, the issue of the best way to facilitate cardioversion to minimize periprocedural stroke is not yet certain.

HEART FAILURE

Perspective

Heart failure is a major medical problem in economically advantaged countries. In the United States, the approximate prevalence of congestive heart failure is 4.8 million, with an incidence of 550,000 new cases a year and approximately 962,000 hospitalizations a year. Furthermore, hospitalizations for heart failure have increased by 155 percent between 1979 and 1999.[3] In 1995, the Health Care Financing Administration paid $3.4 billion to Medicare beneficiaries for heart failure, and it is the single most common cause of hospitalizations over the age of 65.[2] The American Heart Association estimates the total annual direct and indirect care costs of heart failure at $23.2 billion.[3]

Heart failure differs from other areas of consideration in this chapter because it is a disease process rather than a single form of therapy or service. Thus the economics of heart failure and cost-effectiveness strategies must approach it as a process and then consider breaking the process down. Heart failure must be considered a process in which patients have a baseline health state, with associated baseline continuing costs for medication and office visits as well as productivity costs. The patient may then decompensate, resulting in a hospitalization, presumably with a somewhat worse health state and associated costs. Efforts will then be made to return the patient to his or her baseline health state and maintain him or her there. Finally, patients may be considered for transplantation to try to reverse or partially reverse heart failure, also with associated cost (see also Chap. 26).

Digoxin

Despite over 200 years of experience, the role of digoxin in the treatment of congestive heart failure remains uncertain. In the absence of adequate clinical data, the cost-effectiveness data similarly will be limited. Nonetheless, Ward et al.[175] developed a decision-analytic model concerning digoxin withdrawal in patients with stable heart failure. The clinical sequelae of digoxin withdrawal came from the Prospective Randomized Study of Ventricular Failure and Efficacy of Digoxin (PROVED) and Randomized Assessment of Digoxin and Inhibitors of Angiotensin-Converting Enzyme (RADIANCE) trials.[176,177] Costs were estimated from hospital and Medicare data. Outcomes included treatment failures, digoxin toxicity, and health care costs. Continuation of digoxin therapy in patients with heart failure nationally would avoid 185,000 office visits, 27,000 emergency visits, and 137,000 hospital admissions for heart failure, but with 12,500 cases of digoxin toxicity. The net annual savings would be $406 million (90 percent confidence interval, $106 to $822 million). Sensitivity analysis showed that digoxin is cost saving if the incidence of digoxin toxicity is 33 percent or less. Thus digoxin therapy was found to dominate withdrawal of digoxin in stable heart failure.

In a large randomized trial study, the effect of digoxin on mortality and hospitalization in patients with heart failure and left ventricular ejection fractions of 0.45 or less were randomly assigned to digoxin (3397 patients) or placebo (3403 patients) in addition to diuretics and ACE inhibitors.[178] While there was no effect on mortality, there were 26.8 percent hospitaliztions in the digoxin groups versus 34.7 percent in the placebo group ($p < 0.001$). Although no formal cost-effectiveness analysis is available, Mark estimated that the digoxin therapy is at least cost-neutral and probably cost-saving.[179]

ACE Inhibition

The efficacy of ACE inhibition in preserving left ventricular size and prolonging survival in patients with heart failure has been established in a series of clinical trials. In a metanalysis of 32 trials totaling 7105 patients, the mortality rate in patients randomized to ACE inhibitor was 15.8 percent compared with 21.9 percent for placebo (odds ratio, 0.77; 95 percent confidence interval, 0.67 to 0.88).[180] None of these trials included prospective economic evaluations. However, there have been several decision-analytic analyses based on these trials.

Tsevat et al.[129] studied the effectiveness of ACE inhibition after MI; the results are reviewed in that section. Glick et al.[181,182] developed a decision-analytic model based on the SOLVD trial. SOLVD was an 83-center trial in which 2569 patients with symptomatic heart failure and ejection fractions of 35 percent or less received either the ACE inhibitor enalapril or placebo. At 41.4 months of follow-up, enalapril decreased mortality and hospitalization by 16 and 26 percent, respectively. Costs were estimated based on CMS reimbursement rates in 1992 dollars. For patients with heart failure, enalapril dominates placebo in the short term and is highly economically attractive in the long term. Enalapril saved approximately $717 per patient over the period of the SOLVD treatment trial. When trial data were projected over a patient's lifetime, therapy with enalapril produced a cost utility ratio of $115 per QALY. As pointed out by Boyko et al.,[183] there is variation in the cost of ACE inhibitors; as these agents become less expensive, their cost-effectiveness ratio may become even more attractive.

Somewhat more general in the treatment of heart failure is the Paul et al.[184] decision-analytic model based on the SOLVD and VheFt I and II trials. These trials considered the strategies of (1) standard therapy (digoxin and diuretics) with no vasodilator agents, (2) hydralazine hydrochloride-isosorbide dinitrate combination, and (3) ACE inhibition with enalapril. Using data from three major randomized, controlled trials to estimate treatment efficacy, mortality rates, and hospitalization rates, the cost was $5600 per year of life gained with hydralazine–isosorbide dinitrate compared with standard therapy. Compared with the hydralazine–isosorbide dinitrate combination therapy, the incremental cost-effectiveness ratio for enalapril therapy was $9700 per year of life saved.

The cost-effectiveness of ACE inhibition also has been studied in Europe using decision-analytic techniques. In mild heart failure, Kleber[185] found ACE inhibition to be cost-effective but not cost saving. However, in the Netherlands, van Hout et al.[186] found ACE inhibition to dominate not using ACE. Similarly, in a study from the United Kingdom based on SOLVD, Hart et al.[187] found that ACE-inhibitor therapy potentially could dominate not using such therapy.

Beta Blockade

Recently beta blockade, especially with carvedilol, has been added to the therapeutic armamentarium for heart failure. There have been four randomized trials in 1094 patients with New York Heart Association class II to IV symptoms and left ventricular ejection fraction of 0.35 or less.[188] The series of trials was terminated early, based on a finding of a 65 percent mortality reduction in patients receiving carvedilol (95 percent confidence interval, 39 to 82 percent). Delea et al.[189] constructed a decision-analytic model estimating life expectancy and health care costs for patients with heart failure receiving carvedilol plus conventional therapy (digoxin, diuretics, and ACE inhibitors) or conventional therapy alone. Benefit estimates were based on the carvedilol trial results, assuming either "limited benefits" persisting for 6 months, the average duration of follow-up in the clinical trials, or "extended benefits" persisting for 6 months and then declining gradually over 3 years. For conventional therapy alone, estimated life expectancy was 6.67 years; for carvedilol, it was 6.98 and 7.62 years, assuming limited and extended benefits, respectively. Expected lifetime costs of heart failure–related care were estimated at $28,756 for conventional therapy and $36,420 and $38,867 for carvedilol, assuming limited and extended benefits, respectively. Cost per life year saved for carvedilol was $29,477 and $12,799 under limited and extended benefits assumptions, respectively. Thus the cost-effectiveness of cardvedilol remains in a reasonable range but is not as attractive as ACE inhibition.

Disease-Management Strategies

Heart failure is particularly well suited to developing strategies, such as the development of heart failure clinics, to improve management. It is difficult to evaluate treatment strategies because (1) it is difficult to construct randomized trials logistically, (2) there may be contamination in which the management strategy is used to some extent in the control arm, (3) there may be differences between programs that are inherent in different medical centers that make collaboration for multisite efforts difficult, and (4) different health care systems may vary substantially. These variations may also limit generalizability. The difficulties in mounting trials to evaluate the outcome of management strategies is a similar limitation for randomized trials. Nonetheless, several small efforts have been made.

Rich et al.[190] conducted a randomized trial using a nurse-directed, multidisciplinary intervention on readmission rate within 90 days of hospital discharge, quality of life, and costs for elderly patients admitted to the hospital with heart failure. The intervention comprised educating the patient and family, prescribing a heart-healthy diet, planning for early discharge, a review of medications, and intensive follow-up. Survival for 90 days without readmission was achieved in 91 of the 142 patients in the treatment group versus 75 of the 140 patients with conventional care ($p = 0.09$). There were 53 readmissions in the treatment group versus 94 in the control group (risk ratio, 0.56; $p = 0.02$). The number of readmissions for heart failure was reduced by 56.2 percent in the treatment group (54 vs. 24 in the control group; $p = 0.04$). In the control group, 23 patients (16.4 percent) had more than one readmission versus 9 (6.3 percent) in the treatment group (risk ratio, 0.39; $p = 0.01$). In a subgroup of 126 patients, quality-of-life scores at 90 days improved more from baseline in the treatment group ($p = 0.001$). Because of the reduction in hospital admissions, the total cost of care was $460 less per patient in 1994 dollars in the treatment group, confirming strong dominance for the management strategy.

Weinberger et al.[191] studied 1396 patients hospitalized with chronic diseases, half of whom had congestive heart failure, who were randomized to intensive medical management versus usual care. There were more repeat hospitalizations in the specialized care group. This seemingly contradictory finding[191] reveals that disease management is not easily subjected to scientific scrutiny.

West et al.[192] and Kornowski et al.[193] studied a disease-management strategy based on outpatient care rather than focusing on patients being discharged. In a study in Israel, Kornowski et al.[193] analyzed outcome of 42 patients aged 78 ± 8 years with New York Heart Association congestive heart failure class III or IV who were examined weekly at home by local internists and a trained paramedical team. The year before, entry to the home-care program was compared with the first year of home surveillance. Functional status (ability to perform daily activities on a 1 to 4 scale) improved from 1.4 ± 0.9 to 2.3 ± 0.7 ($p < 0.001$). The total hospitalization rate fell from 3.2 ± 1.5 to 1.2 ± 1.6 hospitalizations per year and length of stay from 26 ± 14 to 6 ± 7 days per year ($p < 0.001$ for both). Cardiovascular admissions fell from 2.9 ± 1.5 to 0.8 ± 1.1 hospitalizations per year and stay from 23 ± 13 to 4 ± 4 days per year ($p < 0.001$). This study showed improved outcome, but at an uncertain trade-off in resource use between increased home visits and decreased hospitalizations for the intervention.

West et al.[192] used a strategy of physician-led but nurse-managed, home-based heart failure management not involving home visits. Nurses directed the implementation of guidelines for pharmacologic and dietary therapy by frequent telephone contact of 51 patients with heart failure for 138 ± 44 days. Compared with the period before enrollment, sodium intake fell by 38 percent ($p = 0.0001$), vasodilator doses increased ($p = 0.01$), and functional status and exercise capacity improved significantly ($p = 0.01$). Compared with the 6 months before enrollment, general medical and cardiology visits declined by 23 and 31 percent, respectively (both $p < 0.03$), and emergency room visits for heart failure and for all causes declined 67 and 53 percent, respectively (both $p < 0.001$). Compared with 1 year before enrollment, hospitalization rates for heart failure and for all causes declined 87 and 74 percent ($p = 0.001$). Thus this strategy improved clinical outcome for heart failure while reducing resource use, again suggesting strong dominance.

Rich[194] and Philbin[195] have both reviewed disease-management programs. Between 1983 and 1998, 16 studies, 10 observational and 6 randomized trials, of multidisciplinary heart failure disease-management programs were published in the English-language literature. All studies reported reduced hospitalization, and several studies reported improved quality of life, functional capacity, patient satisfaction, and compliance. All studies that included a cost analysis found the disease-management programs to be cost-effective. Rich[194] suggested that current data are limited by generalizability to the more heterogeneous population of patients with heart failure, the feasibility of translating specific disease management programs into diverse practice environments, and how to individualize the programs for each patient. While the impact of heart failure disease-management programs on survival is also unknown, these programs appear to be cost-effective at reducing morbidity and improving quality of life in selected patients with heart failure.

Heart Transplantation and New Devices

Heart transplantation remains sufficiently infrequent, with just 2198 in the United States in 2000, that its overall impact on cost from a public health standpoint is small (see also Chap. 26). The American Heart Association estimates the average cost of transplants at $253,200, with an annual follow-up cost of $21,200.[3] Cardiac transplantation has not been subjected to rigorous cost-effectiveness analysis, perhaps because of inadequate natural history data with which to compare transplant patients. Although cardiac transplantation is certainly expensive, these patients generally would have a life expectancy of a few weeks to months in the absence of the transplant. In a somewhat preliminary and now dated study, Evans[196] showed

that overall cost-effectiveness of heart transplantation was estimated at $44,300 per year of life saved.

Recent clinical trials have shown the efficacy of new therapies such as left ventricular assist devices[197] and biventricular pacing.[198] The economic impact of such new mechanical approaches to heart failure remains uncertain.

DIAGNOSIS

Establishing the cost-effectiveness of diagnostic testing is considerably more difficult than it is for therapeutics because diagnostics by themselves rarely affect outcome. Rather, diagnostics generally lead to a range of choices of therapeutic options with the potential for very different outcomes. Thus decision-analytic models with diagnostics tend to be more complicated than with therapeutics; consequently, the uncertainty is much greater. Randomized trials with diagnostics are also quite unusual. Thus such cost-effectiveness analyses as exist are essentially all decision-analytic simulations.

Testing for Coronary Artery Disease

Garber and Solomon[199] evaluated the cost-effectiveness of noninvasive and direct coronary angiography in the diagnosis of CAD. The tests evaluated included treadmill exercise ECG, planar thallium imaging, single photon emission computed tomography (SPECT), stress echocardiography, and positron emission tomography (PET), all—if positive—followed by coronary angiography, and, finally, direct coronary angiography. Survival was based on the medically or surgically treated patients in the Coronary Artery Surgery Study (CASS). How survival after angioplasty was calculated is not clear. Based on a metanalysis of trials comparing angioplasty with medicine, surgery was assumed to have 1.6 times the ability of angioplasty to relieve symptoms. Sensitivities and specificities of testing were developed from a metanalysis of the literature. PET was the most sensitive noninvasive test and exercise testing the least sensitive. SPECT was nearly as sensitive as and somewhat less specific than PET (specificity, 0.77 for SPECT and 0.82 for PET). Stress echocardiography is more specific than PET (0.88 compared with 0.82) but less sensitive (0.76 compared with 0.91). There were no published data on the sensitivity of PET for detecting severe (left main and three-vessel) coronary disease, but planar thallium imaging, SPECT, and echocardiography are highly sensitive for detecting severe disease. These figures are based on studies that included small numbers of patients. Exercise testing is not as sensitive (see also Chap. 16).

Little difference in life expectancy was noted with the various strategies, but there was somewhat more variation in terms of QALYs, because the calculation of QALYs gives credit to strategies that improve symptoms rapidly. Nonetheless, the differences amounted to a couple of weeks over approximately 12 years in men and 14 years in women. Costing was based on Medicare payments.

SPECT had higher QALYs at higher cost than stress echocardiography, with a marginal cost-effectiveness ratio of $64,000 in 65-year-old men to nearly $150,000 in 45-year-old women. PET generally produced slightly better outcomes than SPECT but at much greater cost. While immediate angiography dominated PET in every group, immediate angiography was more expensive than SPECT, with a margin from about $80,000 in 65-year-old men to nearly $200,000 in 45-year-old women.

Strategies in which patients are neither tested nor treated initially are not no-cost strategies, since patients may experience an MI and undergo medical or surgical treatment in the future. Thus the cost-effectiveness of stress echocardiography compared with no testing ranges from $31,000 per QALY in 65-year-old men to $98,000 per QALY in 45-year-old women.

At a different prevalence of disease, the ranking of tests changes somewhat. For 55-year-old men with a 75 percent pretest risk for disease, initial angiography becomes more attractive (it will be chosen whenever a cost-effectiveness ratio of $45,000 is acceptable), and stress echocardiography remains preferable to exercise testing (with a cost-effectiveness ratio of $22,000 per QALY). At a 25 percent prevalence of disease, echocardiography seems to be the most attractive test under most circumstances; SPECT would be chosen over echocardiography only if a cost-effectiveness ratio of $110,000 were considered acceptable, and immediate angiography would be chosen over SPECT only at a cost-effectiveness ratio of $355,000. Thus stress echocardiography remains a cost-effective strategy at a wide range of prevalence of disease, whereas immediate angiography is a cost-effective choice when the pretest probability of disease is high.

Somewhat similar analyses have been offered by Kim et al.[200] and Kuntz et al.[201] The study by Kim et al.[200] specifically studied women. In a 55-year-old woman with definite angina, direct angiography was found to be appropriate, with a marginal cost-effectiveness of $17,000 per QALY. This figure rises as the probability of angina falls, and in the midrange of probabilities, echocardiography was felt to be preferable. In the study by Kuntz et al.,[201] the incremental cost-effectiveness of direct coronary angiography compared with exercise echocardiography was $36,400 per QALY in a 55-year-old man. For 55-year-old men with atypical angina, exercise echocardiography compared with exercise ECG at a cost of $41,900 per QALY. If exercise echocardiography was not available, exercise SPECT costs $54,800 per QALY saved compared with exercise ECG. For a 55-year-old man with nonspecific chest pain, the cost-effectiveness of exercise ECG compared with no testing was $57,700 per QALY.

These studies can be criticized easily for making multiple assumptions. However, the end result is quite reasonable. *In patients with chest pain in the intermediate range of probabilities, a test that includes myocardial imaging, either echocardiography or SPECT, is appropriate, with echo more appropriate in the lower probability range and SPECT in the higher probability range.* Immediate angiography is appropriate as the probability of disease rises. In lower-risk populations, a treadmill exercise test is probably appropriate, and ultimately, in very low-risk populations, in the single digits of pretest probability, reassurance and watchful waiting would be the strategy of choice.

CONCLUSIONS

Health care economics offers a powerful set of tools for establishing cost and overall measures of outcome and relating cost to outcome. These tools have been used increasingly in cardiovascular medicine for the purposes of gaining greater insight not only to facilitate improved patient management but also to help guide public policy. These tools have now been applied widely in cardiovascular medicine, with peer-reviewed literature on cost and often cost-effectiveness analysis, in most areas of cardiovascular medicine. However, the methods of measurement and analysis have varied widely, limiting the ability to compare studies and thus generalize the findings. A recent effort in the United States[25] should provide a guide to investigators performing cost-effectiveness analyses to perform them in a more standard manner. The quality of data available in many areas probably poses a greater problem. Over time, however, the quality of data and of scholarship should increase, making economic studies ever more meaningful and relevant to the practice of medicine.

References

1. Allenet B, Sailly J-C. Willingness to pay as a measure of benefit in health. *J D'Econ Med* 1999;17:301–326.
2. Accessed at *http://www.hcfa.gov* December 2002
3. *2002 Heart and Stroke Statistical Update.* Dallas: American Heart Association; 2001.
4. Drummond MF, Stoddart GL, Torrance GW. *Methods for the Economic Evaluation of Health Care Programmes.* Oxford, England: Oxford University Press; 1990:74–167.
5. Kupersmith J, Holmes-Rovner M, Hogan A, et al. Cost-effectiveness analysis in heart disease: II. Preventive therapies. *Prog Cardiovasc Dis* 1995;37:243–271.
6. Borna S, Sundaram S. An approach to allocating limited health resources. *J Health Soc Behav* 1999;11:85–94.
7. Schlander M. Rational resource allocation in the health care system: I. Why rationing may become inevitable. *Med Welt* 1999;50:36–41.
8. Weintraub WS, Warner CD, Mauldin PD, et al. Economic winners and losers after introduction of an effective new therapy depend on the type of payment system. *Am J Managed Care* 1997;3:743–749.
9. Weintraub WS. Microeconomic methods in cardiovascular care. In: Talley JD, Mauldin PD, Becker ER, eds. *Cost-Effective Diagnosis and Treatment of Coronary Artery Disease.* Baltimore: Williams & Wilkins; 1999:17–29.
10. Rothermich EA, Pathak DS. Productivity-cost controversies in cost-effectiveness analysis: Review and research agenda. *Clin Ther* 1999; 21:255–267.
11. Evans DB. Principles involved in costing. *Med J Aust* 1990;153: S10–S12.
12. Hlatky MA. Analysis of costs associated with CABG and PTCA. *Ann Thorac Surg* 1996;61:S30–S32.
13. Finkler SA. The distinction between costs and charges. *Ann Intern Med* 1982;96:102–109.
14. Finkler SA, Ward DM. *Essentials of Cost Accounting for Health Care Organizations,* 2d ed. Rockville, MD: Aspen Publications; 1999: 11–43.
15. Hlatky MA, Lipscomb J, Nelson C, et al. Resource use and cost of initial coronary revascularization: coronary angioplasty versus coronary bypass surgery. *Circulation* 1990;82(suppl IV):IV-208–IV-213.
16. Weintraub WS, Mauldin PD, Talley JD, et al. Determinants of hospital costs in acute myocardial infarction. *Am J Managed Care* 1996;2: 977–986.
17. Lefebvre C, Van Der Perre T. Activity based costing. *Acta Hospital* 1994;34:5–16.
18. Coulam RF, Gaumer GL. Medicare's prospective payment system: A critical appraisal. *Health Care Finance Rev* 1991;13:45–77.
19. Becker ER, Mauldin PD, Weintraub WS. CABG and PTCA physician practice profiles using the resource-based relative value scale (RBRVS): Better methods for explaining the variation. *Clin Res* 1994; 42:225A.
20. Becker ER, Mauldin PD, Bernadino ME. Using physician work RVUs to profile surgical packages: methods and results for kidney transplant surgery. *Best Pract Benchmark Healthcare* 1996;3:140–146.
21. Becker ER, Mauldin PD, Culler SD, et al. Applying the resource-based relative-value scale to the Emory Angioplasty versus Surgery Trial. *Am J Cardiol* 2000;85:685–691.
22. Hsiao WC, Braun P, Yntema D, et al. Estimating physicians' work for a resource-based relative value scale. *N Engl J Med* 1998;319: 835–841.
23. Mitchell JB, Burge RT, Lee AJ, McCall NT. *Per Case Prospective Payment for Episodes of Hospital Care.* Final Report to HCFA for Master Contract No. 500-92-0020. Health Economics Research, Inc;1995.
24. Weintraub WS, Craver JM, Jones EL, et al. Improving cost and outcome of coronary surgery. *Circulation* 1998;98:23–28.
25. Gold MR, Siegel JE, Russell LB, et al. *Cost-Effectiveness in Health and Medicine.* New York: Oxford University Press; 1996.
26. Quality of Care and Outcomes Research in CVD and Stroke Working Groups. Measuring and improving quality of care: A report from the

American Heart Association/American College of Cardiology First Scientific Forum on Assessment of Healthcare Quality in Cardiovascular Disease and Stroke. *Circulation* 2000;101:1483–1493.

27. Mauldin PD, Weintraub WS, Becker E. Predicting hospital charges and costs for coronary surgery from pre-operative and post-operative variables. *Am J Cardiol* 1994;74:772–775.

28. Ellis SG, Miller DP, Brown KJ, et al. In-hospital costs of percutaneous coronary revascularization: Critical determinants and implications. *Circulation* 1995;92:741–747.

29. Mark DB, Gardner LH, Nelson CL, et al. Long-term costs of therapy for CAD: A prospective comparison of coronary angioplasty, coronary bypass surgery and medical therapy in 2258 patients. *Circulation* 1993;88(2):I-480.

30. Topol EJ, Ellis SG, Cosgrove DM, et al. Analysis of coronary angioplasty practice in the United States with an insurance-claims database. *Circulation* 1993;87:1489–1497.

31. Harris RA, Nease RF Jr. The importance of patient preferences for comorbidities in cost-effectiveness analyses. *J Health Econ* 1997;16:113–119.

32. King SB III, Lembo NJ, Weintraub WS, for the EAST Investigators. A randomized trial comparing coronary angioplasty with coronary bypass surgery. *N Engl J Med* 1994;331:1044–1050.

33. The BARI Investigators. Comparison of coronary bypass surgery with angioplasty in patients with multivessel disease. *N Engl J Med* 1996;335:217–225.

34. Hamm CW, Reimers J, Ischinger T, et al. A randomized study of coronary angioplasty compared with bypass surgery in patients with symptomatic multivessel coronary artery disease. *N Engl J Med* 1994;331:1037–1043.

35. CABRI Trial Participants. First-year results of CABRI (Coronary Angioplasty versus Bypass Revascularization Investigation). *Lancet* 1995;346:1179–1184.

36. Rodriguez A, Boullon F, Perez-Balino N, et al. Argentine Randomized Trial of Percutaneous Transluminal Coronary Angioplasty versus Coronary Artery Bypass Surgery in Multivessel Disease (ERACI): In-hospital results and 1-year follow-up. *J Am Coll Cardiol* 1993;22:1060–1067.

37. The RITA Investigators. Coronary angioplasty versus coronary artery bypass surgery: The Randomized Intervention Treatment of Angina (RITA) trial. *Lancet* 1993;341:573–580.

38. Weintraub WS, Mauldin PD, Becker E, et al. A comparison of the costs of and quality of life after coronary angioplasty or coronary surgery for multivessel coronary artery disease: Results from the Emory Angioplasty versus Surgery Trial (EAST). *Circulation* 1995;92:2831–2840.

39. Hlatky MA, Rogers WJ, Johnstone I, et al. Medical care costs and quality of life after randomization to coronary angioplasty or coronary bypass surgery. *N Engl J Med* 1997;336:92–99.

40. Sculpher MJ, Seed P, Henderson RA, et al. Health service costs of coronary angioplasty and coronary artery bypass surgery: The Randomized Intervention Treatment of Angina (RITA) trial. *Lancet* 1994;344:927–930.

41. Rodriguez A, Mele E, Peyregne E, et al. Three-year follow-up of the Argentine Randomized Trial of Percutaneous Transluminal Coronary Angioplasty versus Coronary Artery Bypass Surgery in Multivessel Disease (ERACI). *J Am Coll Cardiol* 1996;27:1178–1184.

42. Alchian A. The meaning of utility measurement. *Am Econ Rev* 1953;143:26–50.

43. Feeny DH, Torrance GW, Furlong WJ. Health utilities index. In: Spilker B, ed. *Quality of Life and Pharmacoeconomics in Clinical Trials*. Philadelphia: Lippincott-Raven Press; 1996:239–252.

44. Cook TA, O'Regan M, Galland RB. Quality of life following percutaneous transluminal angioplasty for claudication. *Eur J Vasc Endovasc Surg* 1996;11:191–194.

45. Loomes G, McKenzie L. The use of QALYs in health care decision making. *Soc Sci Med* 1989;28:299–308.

46. Weinstein MC, Stason WB. Cost-effectiveness of coronary artery bypass surgery. *Circulation* 1982;66(suppl III):56–65.

47. Tengs TO, Adams ME, Pliskin JS, et al. Five-hundred life-saving interventions and their cost-effectiveness. *Risk Anal* 1995;15:369–390.

48. Schulman KA, Kinosian B, Jacobson TA, et al. Reducing high blood cholesterol level with drugs: Cost-effectiveness of pharmacologic management. *JAMA* 1990;264:3025–3033.

49. Tosteson AN, Weinstein MC, Hunink MG, et al. Cost-effectiveness of populationwide educational approaches to reduce serum cholesterol levels. *Circulation* 1997;95:24–30.

50. Goldman L, Weinstein MC, Goldman PA, et al. Cost-effectiveness of HMG-CoA reductase inhibition for primary and secondary prevention of coronary heart disease. *JAMA* 1991;265:1145–1151.

51. Garber AM, Browner WS, Hulley SB. Cholesterol screening in asymptomatic adults, revisited. *Ann Intern Med* 1996;124:518–531.

52. Abbott RD, McGee D, Kannel WB, et al. The probability of developing certain cardiovascular disease in eight years at specified values of some characteristics. In: Kannel WB, Wolf PA, Garrison RJ, eds. *The Framingham Study: An Epidemiological Investigation of Cardiovascular Disease* (publication no. NIH 87:2284). Bethesda, MD: U.S. Department of Health, Education and Welfare; 1987:sec 37.

53. Randomized trial of cholesterol lowering in 4444 patients with coronary heart disease: The Scandinavian Simvastatin Survival Study. *Lancet* 1994;344:1383–1389.

54. Pedersen TR, Kjekshus J, Berg K, et al. Cholesterol lowering and the use of healthcare resources: Results of the Scandinavian Simvastatin Survival Study. *Circulation* 1996;93:1796–1802.

55. Johannesson M, Jonsson B, Kjekshus J, et al. Cost-effectiveness of simvastatin treatment to lower cholesterol levels in patients with coronary heart disease. *N Engl J Med* 1997;336:332–336.

56. Shepherd J, Cobbe SM, Ford I, et al. Prevention of coronary heart disease with pravastatin in men with hypercholesterolemia. *N Engl J Med* 1995;333:1301–1307.

57. Caro J, Klittich W, McGwire A, et al. The West of Scotland Coronary Prevention Study: Economic benefit analysis of primary prevention with pravastatin. *BMJ* 1997;315:1577–1582.

58. Ashraf T, Hay JW, Pitt B, et al. Cost-effectiveness of pravastatin in secondary prevention of coronary artery disease. *Am J Cardiol* 1996;78:409–414.

59. State-specific prevalence among adults of current cigarette smoking and smokeless tobacco use and per capita tax-paid sales of cigarettes—United States, 1997. *MMWR Morb Mortal Wkly Rep* 1998;47:922–926.

60. US Department of Agriculture. *Tobacco Situation and Outlook Report*. Publication no. TBS-227. Washington, DC: U.S. Department of Agriculture, Economic Research Service, Commodity Economics Division; 1994.

61. U.S. Department of Health and Human Services. *Reducing the Health Consequences of Smoking: 25 Years of Progress*. A Report of the Surgeon General. DSS Publication No. CDC89;8411. Bethesda, MD: U.S. Department of Health and Human Services, Public Health Service, Centers for Disease Control, Center for Chronic Disease Prevention and Health Promotion, Office on Smoking and Health; 1989.

62. MacKenzie TD, Bartecchi CF, Schrier RW. The human costs of tobacco use. *N Engl J Med* 1994;330:975–980.

63. Lightwood JM, Glantz SA. Short-term economic and health benefits of smoking cessation. *Circulation* 1997;96:1089–1096.

64. Warner KE. Cost-effectiveness of smoking-cessation therapies: Interpretation of the evidence—and implications for coverage. *Pharmacoeconomics* 1997;11:538–549.

65. Meenan RT, Stevens VJ, Hornbrook MC, et al. Cost-effectiveness of a hospital-based smoking cessation intervention. *Med Care* 1998;36:670–678.

66. Cromwell J, Bartosch WJ, Fiore MC, et al. Cost-effectiveness of the clinical practice recommendations in the AHCPR guideline for smoking cessation. *JAMA* 1997;278:1759–1766.

67. Woolacott NF, Jones L, Forbes CA, et al. The clinical effectiveness and cost-effectiveness of bupropion and nicotine replacement therapy for smoking cessation: A systematic review and economic evaluation. *Health Technol Assess* 2002;6:1–245.

68. Krumholz HM, Chen BJ, Tsevat J, et al. Cost-effectiveness of a smoking cessation program after myocardial infarction. *J Am Coll Cardiol* 1993; 22:1703–1705.

69. Jones TF, Eaton CB. Cost-benefit analysis of walking to prevent coronary heart disease. *Arch Fam Med* 1994;3:703–710.

70. Moss SE, Klein R, Klein BEK, et al. The association of glycemia and cause-specific mortality in a diabetic population. *Arch Intern Med* 1994;154:2473–2479.

71. American Diabetes Association. Standards of medical care for patients with diabetes mellitus. *Diabetes Care* 1997;20(suppl 1):S5–S13.

72. Hayward RA, Manning WG, Kaplan SH, et al. Starting insulin therapy in patients with type 2 diabetes: Effectiveness, complications and resource utilization. *JAMA* 1997;278:1663–1669.

73. Gilmer TP, O'Connor PJ, Manning W, et al. The cost to health plans of poor glycemic control. *Diabetes Care* 1997;20:1847–1853.

74. The Diabetes Control and Complications Trial Research Group. Intensive diabetes treatment and complications in IDDM. *N Engl J Med* 1993;329:977–986.

75. The Diabetes Control and Complications Trial Research Group. Lifetime benefits and costs of intensive therapy as practiced in the diabetes control and complications trial. *JAMA* 1996;276:1409–1415.

76. UK Prospective Diabetes Study Group. Intensive blood-glucose control with sulphonylureas or insulin compared with conventional treatment and risk of complications in patients with type 2 diabetes. *Lancet* 1998;352:837–853.

77. Eastman RC, Javitt JC, Herman WH, et al. Model of complications of NIDDM: II. Analysis of the health benefits and cost-effectiveness of treating NIDDM with the goal of normoglycemia. *Diabetes Care* 1997;20:735–744.

78. The sixth report of the Joint National Committee On Prevention, Detection, Evaluation, and Treatment of High Blood Pressure. *Arch Intern Med* 1997;157:2413–2446.

79. Dustan HP, Roccella EJ, Garrison HH. Controlling hypertension: A research success story. *Arch Intern Med* 1996;156:1926–1935.

80. Littenberg B, Garber AM, Sox HC Jr. Screening for hypertension. *Ann Intern Med* 1990;112:192–202.

81. Edelson JT, Weinstein MC, Tosteson AN, et al. Long-term cost-effectiveness of various initial monotherapies for mild to moderate hypertension. *JAMA* 1990;263:407–413.

82. Johannesson M, Dahlof B, Lindholm LH, et al. The cost-effectiveness of treating hypertension in elderly people: An analysis of the Swedish Trial in Old Patients with Hypertension (STOP Hypertension). *J Intern Med* 1993;234:317–323.

83. Moser M. Why are physicians not prescribing diuretics more frequently in the management of hypertension? *JAMA* 1998;279: 1813–1816.

84. Ramsey SD, Neil N, Sullivan SD, et al. An economic evaluation of the JNC hypertension guidelines using data from a randomized controlled trial. Joint National Committee. *J Am Board Fam Pract* 1999;12: 105–114.

85. HOPE (Heart Outcomes Prevention Evaluation) Study Investigators. Effects of an angiotensin-converting-enzyme inhibitor, ramipril, on cardiovascular events in high-risk patients. *N Engl J Med* 2000;342: 145–153.

86. Lamy A, Yusuf S, Pogue J, Gafni A. The cost implications of the use of ramipril in high risk patients based upon the HOPE Study. *Circulation* 2003;107:960–965.

87. Tosteson AN, Goldman L, Udvarhelyi IS, et al. Cost-effectiveness of a coronary care unit versus an intermediate care unit for emergency department patients with chest pain. *Circulation* 1996;94:143–150.

88. Beamer AD, Lee TH, Cook EF, et al. Diagnostic implications for myocardial ischemia of the circadian variation of the onset of chest pain. *Am J Cardiol* 1987;60:998–1002.

89. Krumholz HM, Pasternak RC, Weinstein MC, et al. Cost-effectiveness of thrombolytic therapy with streptokinase in elderly patients with suspected acute myocardial infarction. *N Engl J Med* 1992;327:7–13.

90. Laffel GL, Fineberg HV, Braunwald E. A cost-effectiveness model for coronary thrombolysis/reperfusion therapy. *J Am Coll Cardiol* 1987;5 (suppl B):79B–90B.

91. Simoons ML, Vos J, Martens LL. Cost-utility analysis of thrombolytic therapy. *Eur Heart J* 1991;12:694–699.

92. Midgette AS, Wong JB, Beshansky JR, et al. Cost-effectiveness of streptokinase for acute myocardial infarction: A combined meta-analysis and decision analysis of the effects of infarct location and of likelihood of infarction. *Med Decis Making* 1994;14:108–117.

93. Herve C, Castiel D, Gaillard M, et al. Cost-benefit analysis of thrombolytic therapy. *Eur Heart J* 1990;11:1006–1010.

94. Mark DB, Hlatky MA, Califf RM, et al. Cost-effectiveness of thrombolytic therapy with tissue plasminogen activator as compared with streptokinase for acute myocardial infarction. *N Engl J Med* 1995;332:1418–1424.

95. Kalish SC, Gurwitz JH, Krumholz HM, et al. A cost-effectiveness model of thrombolytic therapy for acute myocardial infarction. *J Gen Intern Med* 1995;10:321–330.

96. Lange RA, Hillis LD. Should thrombolysis or primary angioplasty be the treatment of choice for acute myocardial infarction? Thrombolysis—the preferred treatment. *N Engl J Med* 1996;335:1311–1312.

97. Grines CL. Should thrombolysis or primary angioplasty be the treatment of choice for acute myocardial infarction? Primary angioplasty—The strategy of choice. *N Engl J Med* 1996;335(17): 1313–1316.

98. Berger AK, Schulman KA, Gersh BJ, et al. Primary coronary angioplasty versus thrombolysis for the management of acute myocardial infarction in elderly patients. *JAMA* 1999;282:341–348.

99. Grines CL, Browne KF, Marco J, et al. A comparison of immediate angioplasty with thrombolytic therapy for acute myocardial infarction. The Primary Angioplasty in Myocardial Infarction Study Group. *N Engl J Med* 1993;328:673–679.

100. Gibbons RJ, Holmes DR, Reeder GS, et al. Immediate angioplasty compared with the administration of a thrombolytic agent followed by conservative treatment for myocardial infarction. The Mayo Coronary Care Unit and Catheterization Laboratory Groups. *N Engl J Med* 1993;328:685–691.

101. Zijlstra F, de Boer MJ, Hoorntje JC, et al. A comparison of immediate coronary angioplasty with intravenous streptokinase in acute myocardial infarction. *N Engl J Med* 1993;328:680–684.

102. The GUSTO IIb Angioplasty Substudy Investigators. An international randomized trial of 1138 patients comparing primary coronary angioplasty versus tissue plasminogen activator for acute myocardial infarction. *N Engl J Med* 1997;336:1621–1628.

103. Reeder GS, Bailey KR, Gersh BJ, et al. Cost comparison of immediate angioplasty versus thrombolysis followed by conservative therapy for acute myocardial infarction: A randomized prospective trial. Mayo Coronary Care Unit and Catheterization Laboratory Groups. *Mayo Clin Proc* 1994;69:5–12.

104. The PAMI Trial Investigators. Analysis of the relative costs and effectiveness of primary angioplasty versus tissue-type plasminogen activator: The Primary Angioplasty in Myocardial Infarction (PAMI) trial. *J Am Coll Cardiol* 1997;29:901–907.

105. Mark DB, Granger CB, Ellis SG, et al. Costs of direct angioplasty versus thrombolysis for acute myocardial infarction: Results from the GUSTO II Randomized Trial (abstr). *Circulation* 1996; 94:168A.

106. Grines CL, Cox DA, Stone GW et al. Coronary angioplasty with or without stent implantation for acute myocardial infarction. Stent Primary Angioplasty in Myocardial Infarction Study Group. *N Engl J Med* 1999;341:1949–1956.

107. Cohen DJ, Taira DA, Berezin RH, et al. Cost-effectiveness of coronary stenting in acute myocardial infarction: Results from the Stent Primary Angioplasty in Myocardial Infarction (Stent-PAMI) Trial. *Circulation* 104;2001:3039–3045.

108. Grines CL, Marsalese DL, Brodie B, et al. Safety and cost-effectiveness of early discharge after primary angioplasty in low-risk patients with acute myocardial infarction. PAMI-II Investigators: Primary Angioplasty in Myocardial Infarction. *J Am Coll Cardiol* 1998;31:967–972.

109. Randomised trial of intravenous streptokinase, oral aspirin, both, or neither among 17,187 cases of suspected acute myocardial infarction:

ISIS-2. ISIS-2 (Second International Study of Infarct Survival) Collaborative Group. *Lancet* 1988;2:349–360.

110. Collins R, Peto R, Baigent C, et al. Aspirin, heparin, and fibrinolytic therapy in suspected acute myocardial infarction. *N Engl J Med* 1997; 336:847–860.

111. Oler A, Whooley MA, Oler J, et al. Adding heparin to aspirin reduces the incidence of myocardial infarction and death in patients with unstable angina. *JAMA* 1996;276:811–815.

112. The Clopidogrel in Unstable Angina to Prevent Recurrent Events Trial Investigators. Effects of clopidogrel in addition to aspirin in patients with acute coronary syndromes without ST-segment elevation. *N Engl J Med* 2001;345:494–502.

113. Cohen M, Demers C, Gurfinkel EP, et al. A comparison of low-molecular-weight heparin with unfractionated heparin for unstable coronary artery disease: Efficacy and Safety of Subcutaneous Enoxaparin in Non-Q Wave Coronary Events Study Group (ESSENCE). *N Engl J Med* 1997;337:447–452.

114. Mark DB, Cowper PA, Berkowitz SD, et al. Economic assessment of low-molecular-weight heparin (enoxaparin) versus unfractionated heparin in acute coronary syndrome patients: Results from the ESSENCE randomized trial. Efficacy and Safety of Subcutaneous Enoxaparin in Non-Q-wave Coronary Events (unstable angina or non-Q-wave myocardial infarction). *Circulation* 1998;97:1702–1707.

115. Topol EJ, Califf RM, Weisman HF, et al. Randomised trial of coronary intervention with antibody against platelet IIb/IIIa integrin for reduction of clinical restenosis: Results at six months. The EPIC Investigators. *Lancet* 1994;343:881–886.

116. Mark DB, Talley JD, Topol EJ, et al. Economic assessment of platelet glycoprotein IIb/IIIa inhibition for prevention of ischemic complications of high-risk coronary angioplasty. The EPIC Investigators. *Circulation* 1996;94:629–635.

117. The RESTORE Investigators. Effects of platelet glycoprotein IIb/IIIa blockade with tirofiban on adverse cardiac events in patients with unstable angina or acute myocardial infarction undergoing coronary angioplasty. *Circulation* 1997;96:1445–1453.

118. Weintraub WS, Culler S, Boccuzzi SJ, et al. Economic impact of GPIIB/IIIA blockade after high-risk angioplasty: Results from the RESTORE trial. Randomized Efficacy Study of Tirofiban for Outcomes and Restenosis. *J Am Coll Cardiol* 1999;34:1061–1066.

119. Weintraub WS, Thompson TD, Culler S, et al. Targeting patients undergoing angioplasty for thrombus inhibition: a cost-effectiveness and decision support model. *Circulation* 2000;102:392–398.

120. Mark DB, Harrington RA, Lincoff AM, et al. Cost-effectiveness of platelet glycoprotein IIb/IIIa inhibition with eptifibatide in patients with non-ST-elevation acute coronary syndromes. *Circulation* 2000; 10: 366–371.

121. Braunwald E, McCabe CH, Cannon CP, et al. Effects of tissue plasminogen activator and a comparison of early invasive and conservative strategies in unstable angina and non-Q-wave myocardial infarction: Results of the TIMI IIIB trial. *Circulation* 1994;89:1545–1556.

122. Boden WE, O'Rourke RA, Crawford MH, et al. Outcomes in patients with acute non-Q-wave myocardial infarction randomly assigned to an invasive as compared with a conservative management strategy. *N Engl J Med* 1998;338:1785–1792.

123. Ragmin F, Wallentin L, Swahn E, et al. Invasive compared with non-invasive treatment in unstable coronary-artery disease: FRISC II prospective randomised multicentre study. *Lancet* 1999;354:708–715.

124. Cannon CP, Weintraub WS, Demopoulos LA, et al. Invasive versus conservative strategies in unstable angina and non-Q wave myocardial infarction following treatment with tirofiban: Rationale and study design of the International TACTICS-TIMI 18 trial. *Am J Cardiol* 1998;82:731–736.

125. Mahoney EM, Jurkovitz CT, Chu H, et al. Cost and cost-effectiveness of an early invasive versus conservative strategy for the treatment of unstable angina and non-ST elevation myocardial infarction. *JAMA* 2002;288:1851–1858.

126. Yusuf S, Peto R, Lewis J, et al. Beta blockade during and after myocardial infarction: An overview of the randomized trials. *Prog Cardiovasc Dis* 1985;27:335–371.

127. Goldman L, Sia ST, Cook EF, et al. Costs and effectiveness of routine therapy with long-term beta-adrenergic antagonists after acute myocardial infarction. *N Engl J Med* 1988;319:152–157.

128. Brown NJ, Vaughan DE. Angiotensin-converting enzyme inhibitors. *Circulation* 1998;97:1411–1420.

129. Tsevat J, Duke D, Goldman L, et al. Cost-effectiveness of captopril therapy after myocardial infarction. *J Am Coll Cardiol* 1995;26: 914–919.

130. McMurray JJ, McGuire A, Davie AP, et al. Cost-effectiveness of different ACE inhibitor treatment scenarios post-myocardial infarction. *Eur Heart J* 1997;18:1411–1415.

131. Ades PA. Pashkow FJ. Nestor JR. Cost-effectiveness of cardiac rehabilitation after myocardial infarction. *J Cardiopulm Rehabil* 1997; 17:222–231.

132. Weintraub WS, Ghazzal ZMB, Douglas JS Jr, et al. Trends in outcome and costs of coronary intervention in the 1990s. *Circulation* 1997;96: I-456.

133. Cowper PA, DeLong ER, Peterson ED, et al. Geographic variation in resource use for coronary artery bypass surgery. IHD Port Investigators. *Med Care* 1997;35:320–333.

134. Puskas JD, Mahoney EM, Williams WH, et al. Comparison of hospital cost for on- versus off-pump coronary surgery. *Circulation* 2002;106: II-416.

135. Peterson ED, Cowper PA, Zidar JP, et al. In-hospital costs of coronary stenting (with or without Coumadin) compared to angioplasty. *Circulation* 1996;94:1891A.

136. Cohen DJ, Krumholz HM, Sukin CA, et al. In-hospital and one-year economic outcomes after coronary stenting or balloon angioplasty: Results from a randomized clinical trial. *Circulation* 1995;92: 2480–2487.

137. Weintraub WS. Evaluating the cost of therapy for restenosis: Considerations for brachytherapy. *Int J Radiat Oncol Biol Phys* 1996; 36:949–958.

138. Morice MC, Serruys PW, Sousa JE, et al for the RAVEL Study Group. A randomised comparison of a sirolimus-eluting stent with a standard stent for coronary revascularization. *N Engl J Med* 2002;346:1773–1780.

139. Wong JB, Sonnenberg FA, Salem DN, et al. Myocardial revascularization for chronic stable angina: Analysis of the role of percutaneous transluminal coronary angioplasty based on data available in 1989. *Ann Intern Med* 1990;113:852–871.

140. Detre KM, Guo P, Holubkov R, et al. Coronary revascularization in diabetic patients: A comparison of the randomized and observational components of the bypass angioplasty revascularization investigation (BARI). *Circulation* 1999;99:633–640.

141. Serruys PW, Unger F, Sousa E, et al for the Arterial Revascularization Therapies Study group. Comparison of coronary-artery bypass surgery and stenting for the treatment of multivessel disease. *N Engl J Med* 2001;344:1117–1124.

142. The Stent or Surgery Investigators. One-year comparison of costs and effects of coronary surgery vs percutaneous coronary intervention in the Stent or Surgery Trial. *Heart*. In press.

143. Parisi AF, Folland ED, Hartigan P, on behalf of the Veterans Affairs ACME Investigators. Comparison of angioplasty with medical therapy in the treatment of single-vessel coronary artery disease. *N Engl J Med* 1992;326:10–16.

144. Pitt B, Waters D, Brown WV, et al. Aggressive lipid-lowering therapy compared with angioplasty in stable coronary artery disease. *N Engl J Med* 1999;341:70–76.

145. Chamberlain DH, Fox KAA, Henderson RA, et al. Coronary angioplasty versus medical therapy for angina: The second randomised intervention treatment of angina (RITA-2) trial. *Lancet* 1997;350: 461–468.

146. Kinlay S, Leitch JW, Neil A, et al. Cardiac event recorders yield more diagnoses and are more cost-effective than 48-hour Holter monitoring in patients with palpitations: A controlled clinical trial. *Ann Intern Med* 1996;124(1 Pt 1):16–20.

147. Kupersmith J, Hogan A, Guerrero P, et al. Evaluating and improving the cost-effectiveness of the implantable cardioverter-defibrillator. *Am Heart J* 1995;130(3 Pt 1):507–515.

148. Levine JH, Mellits ED, Baumgardner RA, et al. Predictors of first discharge and subsequent survival in patients with automatic implantable cardioverter defibrillators. *Circulation* 1991;84:558–566.

149. Owens DK, Sanders GD, Harris RA, et al. Cost-effectiveness of implantable cardioverter defibrillators relative to amiodarone for prevention of sudden cardiac death. *Ann Intern Med* 1997;126:1–12.

150. Larsen GC, Manolis AS, Sonnenberg FA, et al. Cost-effectiveness of the implantable cardioverter-defibrillator: Effect of improved battery life and comparison with amiodarone therapy. *J Am Coll Cardiol* 1992;19:1323–1334.

151. Kupperman M, Luce BR, McGovern B, et al. An analysis of the cost-effectiveness of the implantable defibrillator. *Circulation* 1990;81:91–100.

152. Wever EF, Hauer RN, Schrijvers G, et al. Cost-effectiveness of implantable defibrillator as first-choice therapy versus electrophysiologically guided, tiered strategy in postinfarct sudden death survivors. *Circulation* 1996;93:489–496.

153. Mushlin AI, Hall WJ, Zwanziger J, et al. The cost-effectiveness of automatic implantable cardiac defibrillators: Results from MADIT. Multicenter Automatic Defibrillator Implantation Trial. *Circulation* 1998;97:2129–2135.

154. Moss AJ, Zareba W, Hall WJ, et al. The Multicenter Automatic Defibrillator Implantation Trial II Investigators. Prophylactic implantation of a defibrillator in patients with myocardial infarction and reduced ejection fraction. *N Engl J Med* 2002;346:877–883.

155. Coats AJ. MADIT II, the Multi-center Autonomic Defibrillator Implantation Trial II stopped early for mortality reduction: Has ICD therapy earned its evidence-based credentials? *Int J Cardiol* 2002;82:1–5.

156. Kalbfleisch SJ, Calkins H, Langberg JJ, et al. Comparison of the cost of radiofrequency catheter modification of the atrioventricular node and medical therapy for drug-refractory atrioventricular node reentrant tachycardia. *J Am Coll Cardiol* 1992;19:1583–1587.

157. Kertes PJ, Kalman JM, Tonkin AM. Cost-effectiveness of radiofrequency catheter ablation in the treatment of symptomatic supraventricular tachyarrhythmias. *Aust N Z J Med* 1993;23:433–436.

158. Weerasooriya HR, Murdock CJ, Harris AH, et al. The cost-effectiveness of treatment of supraventricular arrhythmias related to an accessory atrioventricular pathway: Comparison of catheter ablation, surgical division and medical treatment. *Aust NZ J Med* 1994;24:161–167.

159. Hogenhuis W, Stevens SK, Wang P, et al. Cost-effectiveness of radiofrequency ablation compared with other strategies in Wolff-Parkinson-White syndrome. *Circulation* 1993;88(suppl II):II-437–II-446.

160. Stamato NJ, O'Toole MF, Enger EL. Permanent pacemaker implantation in the cardiac catheterization laboratory versus the operating room: An analysis of hospital charges and complications. *Pacing Clin Electrophysiol* 1992;15:2236–2239.

161. Sutton R, Bourgeois I. Cost-benefit analysis of single and dual-chamber pacing for sick sinus syndrome and atrioventricular block: An economic sensitivity analysis of the literature. *Eur Heart J* 1996;17:574–582.

162. Falk RH. Impact of prospective peer review on pacemaker implantation rates in Massachusetts. *J Am Coll Cardiol* 1990;15:1087–1092.

163. Parsonnet V. Role of peer review of pacemaker implantations. *J Am Coll Cardiol* 1990;15:1093–1094.

164. Dreifus LS, Fisch C, Griffin JC, et al. Guidelines for implantation of cardiac pacemakers and antiarrhythmia devices. *Circulation* 1991;84:455–467.

165. Ray SG, Griffith MJ, Jamieson S, et al. Impact of the recommendations of the British Pacing and Electrophysiology Group on pacemaker prescription and on the immediate costs of pacing in the Northern Region. *Br Heart J* 1992;68:531–534.

166. Gage BF, Cardinalli AB, Albers GW, et al. Cost-effectiveness of warfarin and aspirin for prophylaxis of stroke in patients with nonvalvular atrial fibrillation. *JAMA* 1995;274:1839–1845.

167. Barnett HJM, Eliasziw M, Meldrum HE. Drugs and surgery in the prevention of ischemic stroke. *N Engl J Med* 1995;332:238–248.

168. Laupacis A, Boysen G, Connolly S, et al. Risk factors for stroke and efficacy of antithrombotic therapy in atrial fibrillation: Analysis of pooled data from five randomized controlled trials. *Arch Intern Med* 1994;154:1449–1457.

169. Gustafsson C, Asplund K, Britton M, et al. Cost-effectiveness of primary stroke prevention in atrial fibrillation: Swedish national perspective. *BMJ* 1992;305:1457–1460.

170. Lightowlers S, McGuire A. Cost-effectiveness of anticoagulation in nonrheumatic atrial fibrillation in the primary prevention of ischemic stroke. *Stroke* 1998;29:1827–1832.

171. Eckman MH, Falk RH, Pauker SG. Cost-effectiveness of therapies for patients with nonvalvular atrial fibrillation. *Arch Intern Med* 1998;158:1669–1677.

172. Catherwood E, Fitzpatrick WD, Greenberg ML, et al. Cost-effectiveness of cardioversion and antiarrhythmic therapy in nonvalvular atrial fibrillation. *Ann Intern Med* 1999;130:625–636.

173. The Atrial Fibrillation Follow-up Investigation of Rhythm Management (AFFIRM) Investigators. A comparison of rate control and rhythm control in patients with atrial fibrillation. *N Engl J Med* 2002;347:1825–1833.

174. Seto TB, Taira DA, Tsevat J, et al. Cost-effectiveness of transesophageal echocardiographic-guided cardioversion: A decision analytic model for patients admitted to the hospital with atrial fibrillation. *J Am Coll Cardiol* 1997;29:122–130.

175. Ward RE, Gheorghiade M, Young JB, et al. Economic outcomes of withdrawal of digoxin therapy in adult patients with stable congestive heart failure. *J Am Coll Cardiol* 1995;26:93–101.

176. Uretsky BF, Young JB, Shahidi FE, et al. Randomized study assessing the effect of digoxin withdrawal in patients with mild to moderate chronic congestive heart failure: Results of the PROVED trial. *J Am Coll Cardiol* 1993;22:955–962.

177. Packer M, Gheorghiade M, Young JB, et al. Withdrawal of digoxin from patients with chronic heart failure treated with angiotensin-converting-enzyme inhibitors. *N Engl J Med* 1993;329:1–7.

178. Garg R, Gorlin R, Smith T, et al. The effect of digoxin on mortality and morbidity in patients with heart failure. *N Engl J Med* 1997;336:525–533.

179. Mark DB. Medical economics in cardiovascular medicine. In: Topol EJ, ed. *Cardiovascular Medicine*. Philadelphia: Lippincott Williams & Wilkins; 1997:1193.

180. Garg R, Yusuf S, for the Collaborative Group on ACE Inhibitor Trials. Overview of randomized trials of angiotensin-converting-enzyme inhibitors on mortality and morbidity in patients with heart failure. *JAMA* 1995;273:1450–1456.

181. The SOLVD Investigators. Effect of enalapril on survival in patients with reduced left ventricular ejection fractions and congestive heart failure. *N Engl J Med* 1991;325:293–302.

182. Glick H, Cook J, Kinosian B, et al. Costs and effects of enalapril therapy in patients with symptomatic heart failure: An economic analysis of the Studies of Left Ventricular Dysfunction (SOLVD) treatment trial. *J Cardiac Failure* 1995;1:371–379.

183. Boyko WL Jr, Glick HA, Schulman KA. Economics and cost-effectiveness in evaluating the value of cardiovascular therapies. ACE inhibitors in the management of congestive heart failure: Comparative economic data. *Am Heart J* 1999;137:S115–S119.

184. Paul SD, Kuntz KM, Eagle KA, et al. Costs and effectiveness of angiotensin converting enzyme inhibition in patients with congestive heart failure. *Arch Intern Med* 1994;154:1143–1149.

185. Kleber FX. Socioeconomic aspects of ACE inhibition in the secondary prevention in cardiovascular disease. *Am J Hypertens* 1994;7:112S–116S.

186. Van Hout BA, Wielink G, Bonsel GJ, et al. Effects of ACE inhibitors on heart failure in the Netherlands: A pharmacoeconomic model. *Pharmacoeconomics* 1993;3:387–397.

187. Hart W, Rhodes G, McMurray J. The cost effectiveness of enalapril in the treatment of chronic heart failure. *Br J Med Econ* 1993;6:91–98.

188. Packer M, Bristol MR, Cohn JN, et al. The effect of carvedilol on morbidity and mortality in patients with chronic heart failure. *N Engl J Med* 1996;334:1349–1355.

189. Delea TE, Vera-Llonch M, Richner RE, et al. Cost-effectiveness of carvedilol for heart failure. *Am J Cardiol* 1999;83:890–896.

190. Rich MW, Beckham V, Wittenberg C, et al. A multidisciplinary intervention to prevent the readmission of elderly patients with congestive heart failure. *N Engl J Med* 1995;333:1190.

191. Weinberger M, Oddone EZ, Henderson WG. Does increased access to primary care reduce hospital readmissions? Veterans Affairs Cooperative Study Group on Primary Care and Hospital Readmission. *N Engl J Med* 1996;334:1441–1447.

192. West JA, Miller NH, Parker KM, et al. A comprehensive management system for heart failure improves clinical outcomes and reduces medical resource utilization. *Am J Cardiol* 1997;79:58–63.

193. Kornowski R, Zeeli D, Averbuch M, et al. Intensive home-care surveillance prevents hospitalization and improves morbidity rates among elderly patients with severe congestive heart failure. *Am Heart J* 1995;129:762–766.

194. Rich MW. Heart failure disease management: A critical review. *J Cardiac Failure* 1999;5:64–75.

195. Philbin EF. Comprehensive multidisciplinary programs for the management of patients with congestive heart failure. *J Gen Intern Med* 1999;14:130–135.

196. Evans RW. Cost-effectiveness analysis of transplantation. *Surg Clin North Am* 1986;66:603–616.

197. Rose EA, Gelijns AC, Moskowitz AJ, et al. Randomized Evaluation of Mechanical Assistance for the Treatment of Congestive Heart Failure (REMATCH) Study Group. Long-term mechanical left ventricular assistance for end-stage heart failure. *N Engl J Med* 2001;345: 1435–1443.

198. Abraham WT, Fisher WG, Smith AL, et al. MIRACLE Study Group. Multicenter InSync Randomized Clinical Evaluation. Cardiac resynchronization in chronic heart failure. *N Engl J Med* 2002;346: 1845–1853.

199. Garber AM, Solomon NA. Cost-effectiveness of alternative test strategies for the diagnosis of coronary artery disease. *Ann Intern Med* 1999;130:719–728.

200. Kim C, Kwok YS, Saha S, et al. Diagnosis of suspected coronary artery disease in women: A cost-effectiveness analysis. *Am Heart J* 1999;137:1019–1027.

201. Kuntz KM, Fleischmann KE, Hunink MG, et al. Cost-effectiveness of diagnostic strategies for patients with chest pain. *Ann Intern Med* 1999;130:709–718.

INSURANCE ISSUES IN PATIENTS WITH HEART DISEASE

Michael B. Clark / William T. Friedewald

INSURANCE MEDICINE AND CARDIOLOGY

The purpose of insurance is to provide for financial relief in the event of significant economic loss. Insurance usually takes the form of a contract, a legal agreement between insurer and insured, specifying those losses that are to be covered and the insurance benefit agreed upon. This contract demands specific requirements (Table 105-1) that, once fulfilled, allow actuarial probability analysis to predict the total amount of loss for a large group of individuals over some defined period of time.[1] Employer-sponsored health insurance relies on this "law of large numbers" to determine group premiums without the need for medical evaluation. For life insurance and private health insurance, however, an analytic process termed *insurance underwriting* serves to identify the potential risk of loss for each individual. Premium contributions are then calculated as proportional to the risk assumed by the insurer, allowing for an equitable distribution of economic spread over large groups of people (Table 105-1).

These concepts of insurance and insurance underwriting are not new; insurance for commercial ventures existed in some form by the Middle Ages, and life insurance had appeared by the seventeenth century. Private medical insurance, usually for catastrophic illnesses, was available in the 1800s.[2] Within the past 100 years, there has been an explosion in the amount of life and health insurance available and in the diversity of insurance products. Basic "whole life insurance" has been supplanted by a wide variety of "term" and "variable" financial offerings as individual policies or, more commonly, as part of employer-sponsored group life insurance (Table 105-1).

The changes in the health insurance industry have been even more dramatic. Unique to the administration of health insurance is the concept of "shared risk," whereby the insurer, the insured, and the insured's employer (or the government) all participate in payment of premium and claims. There may be a "copayment" for routine office visits or an residual "amount due" over and above a "reasonable and customary" reimbursement schedule. The goal is to meet expense and utilization goals that allow for maximal distribution of insurance at an affordable price. Employer and government-sponsored fee-for-service or managed care organizations provide health, disability, and long-term care insurance for the majority of the US population. Within the medical community, the impact of this changing insurance climate has been enormous,[3,4] and, as medical care providers and as consultants, cardiologists will continue to play an important role in insurance underwriting evaluation.

MEDICAL UNDERWRITING FOR LIFE INSURANCE

Mortality Risk Assessment

Most applicants for insurance are in excellent health and are quickly offered policies at standard or even preferred premium rates. When medical impairments are uncovered, however, each must be correlated with long-term mortality data relevant to that impairment. The submitted life insurance application will often contain important "past medical history" and "review of systems" information. Authorized query to one of the national informational database exchanges may provide additional leads.

MEDICAL REQUIREMENTS
The next step in the medical underwriting evaluation usually calls for an insurance medical examination with laboratory assessment.

TABLE 105-1 Insurance Frequently Asked Questions (FAQs)

INSURABLE RISK: DEFINITION

The risk is definable by amount of loss and duration of coverage
The amount of insurance does not exceed the actual financial loss
The insured loss occurs by chance, not by intent such as suicide or homicide
The loss occurs within a sufficiently large population at risk to allow for application of the
   laws of probability
The beneficiary of the insurance must have an "insurable interest"; a genuine concern for the
   continued well-being of the insured

MAJOR TYPES OF INSURANCE

Life Insurance (individual and group)

- Whole life
- Variable life
- Universal life
- Universal variable life
- "Term" life (10-year, 20-year)

Health Insurance (individual and group)

- Fee-for-service
- Health maintenance organizations (HMOs)
- Preferred provider organizations (PPOs)
- Disability
- Long-term care
- Critical illness

THE COMPONENTS OF THE INSURANCE PREMIUM

Mortality costs

- Excess risk of death
- Present value of ultimate benefit

"Loading" costs

- Company expenses to develop and administer the product
- Commissions
- Profit

Comprehensive history taking and physical examination are routinely performed, but noninvasive cardiac testing may also be considered. Stress testing, in particular, is often requested if large amounts of insurance are applied for ("age and amount" guidelines) or if additional information is required ("for cause" guidelines) to permit an accurate mortality assessment. A cardiology consultant may serve as a member of the medical underwriting team itself at this stage, reviewing all of the cardiac information obtained as part of the evaluation, including electrocardiograms and stress test tracings.

THE ATTENDING PHYSICIAN STATEMENT

As part of the risk assessment process for an insurance applicant with an impairment, the patient's physician will be asked to submit medical information to the insurance company in the form of the Attending Physician Statement (APS). This may include an outline of recent medical history and will often contain office and hospital records for review. Clinical problems identified in the APS are analyzed for severity of disease, extent of clinical evaluation, and thoroughness of clinical follow-up to provide data for risk assessment.

MORTALITY ANALYSIS

Each medical impairment identified during the medical underwriting evaluation must be correlated with long-term population survival statistics relevant to that disease process. From these data, the number of "excess deaths" attributable to that impairment can be calculated. A mortality ratio is then derived (observed deaths in a population of individuals affected by the condition divided by the expected deaths for a comparable standard population).[5,6] This quantitative prognostic index serves as a useful standard for comparing mortality projections among the various medical conditions. In general, the higher the mortality ratio calculated for a particular impairment, the greater the relative risk assumed by the company to provide life insurance for individuals affected by that impairment. The mortality ratios calculated for various medical conditions are integrated into a table of risk classes or "ratings"; applicants within a rating class are grouped together to be assessed similar premiums. The relationship of risk class to premium is complex and often varies by company and by insurance product, but the final result is coverage for financial loss, with the contribution to the total insurance pool proportional to the medical risk assumed by the insurance company. This equitable arrangement has the additional benefit of making life insurance coverage possible for many people with cardiac disease who would otherwise be uninsurable[7,8] while avoiding increased costs to medically unimpaired applicants. Published data relevant to mortality assessment derive from several sources.

Insured Populations Excellent long-term follow-up data are available for insured populations based on medical conditions, demographic characteristics, and personal habits identified at the time of original insurance application (Table 105-2). Results are usually expressed as excess death rates in the impaired group as compared to the standard population to address directly the prognostic significance of historical, examination, and laboratory abnormalities. Findings such as "heart murmur on exam" or "low serum albumin" are particularly relevant to insurance underwriting, but there may not be any directly comparable data for the general population. Insured population data more precisely relate to large groups of *selected* individuals (insurance purchasers) and involve follow-up intervals as long as 20 to 30 years. Significant medical advances, as well as changes in demographics or personal lifestyles that occur during the period of study, may significantly limit the applicability of the information developed.

Clinical Studies and National Databases Long-term clinical and epidemiologic studies published in the medical literature are useful for mortality assessment and are generally readily available for most medical impairments. Nationally maintained databases, such as the Surveillance, Epidemiology, and End Results (SEER) and United Network for Organ Sharing (UNOS), are particularly useful for mortality risk information. Such studies, in which interval survival data are usually reported (e.g., 5-year Kaplan-Meier survival curves) can be extrapolated to provide actuarial information useful to the calculation of mortality risk. Often, however, insufficient definition of the study population is provided to allow extrapolation to the larger population from which they were selected.[9] Without such detail, the conclusions of the study must be interpreted cautiously. Iacovino discusses such a situation in a review[10] of mortality analysis methodology. Clinical investigators followed 48 patients with a mean age of 36 years for approximately 6 years and noted a favorable observed mortality of 10 percent for the entire period.[11] However, reference to the U.S. Standard Life Tables (1979–1981) revealed a much lower expected mortality (approximately 1.46 percent) at this age for the same length of follow-up. The estimated mortality ratio of 685 percent (10 percent/1.46 percent × 100) represented a highly substandard risk level for life insurance purposes, even though it may represent good clinical results in young patients with severe cardiac disease.[12]

UNDERWRITING FOR HEALTH INSURANCE

Most applicants for health insurance apply as members of a group, usually through the workplace. The basic insurance coverage is often an important part of the employee benefits package, with costs borne in large part (or entirely) by employers. Government-sponsored insurance also involves groups identified by age, income, or handicap. Medical risk assessment plays little role in the underwriting of these policies. In private health insurance, premium determination is based on an "experience rating" determined through historical review of medical expenses most recently incurred by the members of the group. Government-sponsored insurance premiums represent a complex interplay of mortality projection, budgetary constraints, and political considerations.

Individuals who desire additional coverage over and above that available at work or those without a workplace benefit program may choose a variety of individual health insurance plans. Upon completion of the usually mandatory medical questionnaire, the risk assessment process becomes quite similar to that of life insurance underwriting.

One important difference, however, relates to exclusions and limitations for specified impairments. Certain underwriting factors, such as admitted medical impairments or claims history, may necessitate exclusion of identified impairments from insurance coverage. The limitation may apply to all related claims or only to those over and above a specified claim frequency or duration. While seemingly restrictive, this may allow health insurance coverage for some that would otherwise be denied any coverage at all.

TABLE 105-2 Mortality Ratios in Cardiac Impairments: Selected Data

Medical Finding or Condition	Age Interval, Years	Number of Patients	Mortality Ratio, Percent
ECG findings in males	40–64	21,415	
Axis deviation (symptomatic)			225
Axis deviation (asymptomatic)			139
ST depression (symptomatic)			420
ST depression (asymptomatic)			220
Heart murmurs	50–59	21,295	
Apical systolic (not transmitted to neck; presumed functional)			114
Apical systolic (transmitted)			178
Basal systolic			276
Acute myocardial infarction	30–59	1,608	145
Coronary bypass reoperation	50–59	1,608	145

SOURCE: Adapted from Refs. 14, 29, and 33.

CORONARY HEART DISEASE: ANGINA PECTORIS AND MYOCARDIAL INFARCTION

Initial and short-term mortality following the diagnosis of coronary disease is, in general, unacceptably high for life insurance consideration (estimated at 1150 percent of standard mortality) but can be quite variable for clinical subpopulations. A plateau phase is seen following this period, during which the mortality ratio (found to be close to 390 percent of standard) is relatively stable and thus more predictable. Other studies in insured individuals have confirmed this pattern.[13,14] The common underwriting practice is to consider a life insurance applicant after a period of 6 to 12 months following the initial presentation of coronary heart disease (CHD). Aggressive revascularization strategies such as postinfarction thrombolysis and primary angioplasty have allowed for earlier life insurance consideration in selected applicants. Upon reaching the more predictable plateau phase, a permanent, somewhat substandard risk assessment is usually applied to correspond to the more stable but still substandard mortality rate seen in individuals with established ischemic heart disease.

To facilitate appropriate risk assessment, special attention is directed to the presence of known atherosclerosis risk factors such as high blood pressure, diabetes mellitus, hyperlipidemia, smoking history, and obesity. In addition, a strong family history of cardiovascular disease has been confirmed in studies in insured as well as in other broader-based epidemiologic populations to be an independent risk factor for CHD, with mortality ratios in insureds of 189 and 121 percent for men and women, respectively.[14]

Long-term prognosis in patients with ischemic heart disease may be influenced by intercurrent clinical interventions, such as thrombolysis, coronary angioplasty, stenting, and coronary bypass surgery.[36,37] Again, consideration for life insurance is usually postponed for a short interval to allow for review of the clinical course soon after the intervention. After this period, particular consideration would be given to the status of left ventricular function before and after intervention, the number and extent of coronary artery lesions seen on coronary angiography, and the results of electrocardiographic, echocardiographic, and radionuclide stress testing. The presence or absence of coronary artery risk factors, in particular smoking, will influence the level of the final medical assessment. The frequency and thoroughness of follow-up care may also influence the medical underwriter in otherwise borderline cases.

Mortality risk assessment is considerably more difficult when only limited information is available. A complaint of chest pain may be recorded as "possible angina, begin aspirin" with no further cardiac testing initiated by the time of insurance review. For purposes of risk assessment, this information would commonly be considered as "definite angina" until further clinical follow-up or noninvasive cardiac testing results were made available. Exercise electrocardiograms are, in general, routinely required for applicants requesting large amounts of insurance, although some insurance companies have recently discontinued this requirement. Certainly, these tests continue to be ordered when indicated by the presence of strong risk factors for CHD or by suggestive clinical presentations documented in the attending physician's medical summary forwarded to the insurance company. Substandard insurance ratings based on abnormal electrocardiographic stress testing results can be revised with supplementary evidence, particularly with cardiac imaging studies or coronary angiography.

Health Insurance and Coronary Heart Disease

In the United States, health care expenditures of $351.8 billion dollars are predicted to care for an estimated 61,800,000 patients with established coronary disease. The introduction of new medical technologies, ever-present inflation, as well as the aging of the U.S. population is almost certain to maintain or increase this enormous cost to society. Efforts to contain these costs have led to the introduction of cumbersome, complicated, and at times restrictive reimbursement protocols from government and other health insurance providers. On the positive side, "cost-benefit" is now accepted as a valid and important endpoint for clinical research. A strong resolve to focus on primary prevention strategies promises to reduce the annual incidence of new coronary disease cases and should have a positive impact on health care expenditures.

Patients with CHD rely on health insurance providers to cover the costs of initial treatment and ongoing monitoring and therapy. Rising prescription drug costs have made the pharmaceutical benefit an increasingly important component of the overall employee health insurance coverage plan.

HIGH BLOOD PRESSURE

Since 1925, the life insurance industry has published several major comprehensive studies demonstrating increased mortality among insured populations with high blood pressure.[15-17] All of these show a direct, nearly linear relation between systolic and diastolic blood pressure and mortality. Most recently, the Multiple Medical Impairment Study[18] published in 1998 underscored the necessity for adequate blood pressure control. This study reviewed the insurance company mortality experience on nearly 2,400,000 policies. Persons with diastolic blood pressure readings of 90 mmHg demonstrated a mortality ratio of 101 percent at systolic blood pressure readings under 128 mmHg. Systolic determinations in males at 140 and 150 mmHg correlated with mortality ratios of 134 and 164 percent when associated with a diastolic pressure of 85 mmHg, and 126, 144, and 174 percent respectively when associated with a diastolic pressure of 90 mmHg. Females exhibited a similar but less dramatic relationship

between elevation of blood pressure and mortality that was limited to policies originally issued at substandard rates. The mortality risk from hypertension deteriorated further when considered in association with other impairments.[18] The mortality ratio for diabetes in this study was 236 percent, but it was further increased to 283 percent in association with elevated blood pressure readings. Similar associations were found for insureds with heart murmurs (mortality ratio with elevated blood pressure 234 percent) and abnormal ECGs (mortality ratio 251 percent in association with blood pressure elevation). Excess mortality risk, then, generally applies only to patients with untreated hypertension, those who are noncompliant with prescribed medical regimens, or where hypertension is complicated by end-organ damage (ventricular hypertrophy or cerebrovascular or renal disease), or in association with other medical impairments. These developments are often identified in the clinical record or at the time of insurance evaluation. This evaluation might include electrocardiography, urinary protein quantitation, or, occasionally, echocardiography to assess the degree of hypertensive cardiac impairment.

Hypertension and Health Insurance

Health insurance coverage allows access to medical care and treatment for most patients with hypertension. For the uninsured, representing about 41 million Americans under the age of 65, the cost of physician visits and antihypertensive medications remains a significant barrier to health care access. Particularly affected are those in fair to poor health, including smokers, diabetics, and those with hypertension and lipid disorders.

A wide range of options have been proposed to remedy this situation. These include government-sponsored universal health care administered at a state or federal level, as well as private insurance options with funding on a individual basis in preference to an employed-group basis. Reform of existing Medicare and Medicaid programs is being seen by many as the most realistic option at present.

VALVULAR HEART DISEASE

Historical Underwriting: Heart Murmurs

In the past, information extracted from large studies of insureds with heart murmurs had been extrapolated to provide mortality projections in people with valvular heart disease (Table 105-2). Advances in cardiac diagnostic technology since publication of these studies, particularly the development of echocardiographic and Doppler imaging systems, have allowed better definition of valvular pathology. Risk assessment can now be more realistically directed to the identified valvular pathology. However, earlier and more aggressive repair or replacement of these defective valves has made it more difficult to accumulate data concerning the natural history of unoperated cardiac valvular impairments.[19,20]

Mitral Valve Prolapse

This is, at present, the most common valve condition reported to insurance companies. Although most such patients are offered standard insurance rates, a small subset of patients with frequent chest pain, cardiac arrhythmias, and significant mitral regurgitation may be rated below standard.[21]

Congenital Valvular Heart Disease

Most companies postpone consideration of life insurance for an infant with known or suspected congenital heart disease until the child reaches 1 or 2 years of age. Even then, the history must include a definitively proven diagnosis as well as successful repair of all surgically correctable lesions before the applicant can be considered insurable. After successful restoration of normal cardiac hemodynamics, most applicants with congenital defects—including those with atrial and ventricular septal defects, corrected pulmonic stenosis, patent ductus, or coarctation of the aorta (once blood pressure has returned to normal)—can be considered as standard risks.[22] Uninsurable applicants would include most cases of transposition of the great vessels, Ebstein's anomaly, anomalous venous return, and Eisenmenger's syndrome.

Congenital bicuspid aortic valve remains a difficult clinical and underwriting problem.[8] In the absence of associated echocardiographic evidence of left ventricular enlargement, most companies are willing to assess this risk as only mildly substandard. Left ventricular dilatation or hypertrophy seen on echocardiography or the presence by Doppler analysis of any significant degree of aortic stenosis or regurgitation will usually require a more substantial rating assessment.

Acquired Valvular Heart Disease

To perform risk assessment in applicants known to have acquired valvular disease, the underwriter will usually first consider the clinical and electrocardiographic findings on the insurance examination. The degree of cardiac enlargement and severity of left ventricular dysfunction will also be considered and will commonly be outlined in the medical record. The medical underwriter will also give consideration to the attendant risk of anticipated surgical valve repair or replacement as well as to the risk of lifelong anticoagulation following such surgery. Applicants with valvular disease who show evidence of marked cardiomegaly, especially with prior history or physical examination findings consistent with left-sided or right-sided heart failure, cannot usually be offered life insurance. Other significant complications, such as new-onset atrial fibrillation or systemic embolization, will usually result in a postponement for up to 1 year prior to reconsideration. In most other cases, life insurance can be offered, albeit at much higher premiums.[8,20,23] Early follow-up studies of patients undergoing surgical procedures that preserve the native cardiac valve have demonstrated an improvement in perioperative and short-term postoperative survival.[21] One recent study at the Toronto General Hospital reported on the long-term follow-up of mitral valve surgery performed on 573 patients with rheumatic heart disease; 80 percent were female. Over the 17 year period of the study, the mortality ratios following valve repair, mechanical valve replacement, and bioprosthetic valve replacement were 175, 290, and 350 percent respectively as compared to a standard Canadian population. It may be that the data in patients operated on for mitral regurgitation secondary to myxomatous degeneration would be closer to standard; that on patients with ischemic valvular disease would most likely be somewhat worse than that on any of the other groups.

VALVULAR HEART DISEASE, EXERCISE PROGRAMS, AND HEALTH INSURANCE

Little information is available on the effects of exercise on patients with severe valvular disease. Considerably more evidence exists, however, in support of an exercise rehabilitation prescription following correction of the valvular impairment. Salutary effects on myocardial and respiratory function, peripheral blood flow, and quality of life are well-documented. This value has fairly recently been acknowledged by most health insurance providers after an initial resistance based on difficulty in proving long-term benefit. Reimbursement is now available for early postdischarge monitoring as well as postrecovery aerobic and isometric training programs to facilitate return to an optimal functional level.

OTHER CARDIAC DISEASES OR ABNORMAL LABORATORY FINDINGS

Cardiomyopathy

Insurance risk assessment of the applicant with cardiomyopathy is based on the initial clinical presentation of the patient and the subsequent clinical and physiologic evaluation. Life insurance cannot usually be offered to those diagnosed with dilated (congestive) cardiomyopathy or amyloid heart disease. Systemic diseases with cardiac involvement, such as scleroderma and sarcoidosis, are most often assessed on the basis of overall disease activity and response to therapy. Insurance may be available to many in this latter group of patients, albeit at rates below standard.[8]

Evaluation of the asymptomatic individual with a strong family history of heart disease or in whom a heart murmur has been discovered may at times produce findings consistent with the obstructive or nonobstructive hypertrophic cardiomyopathies. Complete information concerning the natural history of these impairments is not yet available, particularly in the mild asymptomatic cases.[24] In the past, many clinical reports were of severe and fatal outcomes, leading many insurance companies to decline or rate highly any applicant with an established diagnosis of hypertrophic cardiomyopathy.[8] More recent experience in defining mortality outcomes in hypertrophic cardiomyopathy, particularly where nonobstructive, has been much more favorable[25,26] and may allow for more favorable mortality risk assessment in the future.[27]

Arrhythmias

Medical underwriters will consider applicants who give a history of paroxysmal or chronic atrial arrhythmias in the context of the presence and severity of coexisting cardiac disease. One series of insured persons with paroxysmal atrial tachycardia noted mortality rates quite similar to those of the standard population (mortality ratio 73 percent).[14] This can be contrasted with mortality ratios of 700 percent or greater in the presence of atrial fibrillation and coexisting heart disease.[28] In the apparently asymptomatic young individual with new-onset atrial arrhythmias, particular attention is paid to social history and habits such as smoking or excessive alcohol use. In the middle-aged or older applicant, the possibility of asymptomatic coronary heart disease must also be assessed.

Ventricular arrhythmias have remained a difficult risk-assessment problem. In many cases, isolated ventricular ectopy is considered in the context of the underlying cardiac impairment, such as coronary artery or valvular heart disease. Particular attention is directed during the review of the medical record to the results of clinical cardiac evaluation, including stress testing and noninvasive analysis of cardiac function.[29] Survivors of sudden death will, in most cases, be declined—a situation that may change as long-term data on the benefits of an automatic implantable cardioverter/defibrillator (AICD) become available. This change would probably apply to those patients in whom AICD implantation has been performed as prophylaxis in the setting of high clinical risk for sudden death[30] (see also Chap. 38).

Heart Transplantation

Heart transplantation techniques and immunosuppressive strategies have continued to evolve and have been associated with significant improvement in 5- to 10-year survival (see also Chap. 26). Longer survival durations have been problematic, particularly related to the late development of coronary arteriopathy. Most insurance companies would continue to decline such risks until additional long-term survival data became available.

Insurance Laboratory Evaluation of Abnormalities

Life insurance underwriting protocols generally include a clinical laboratory panel with a full lipid profile and a resting electrocardiogram. Depending on the age of the applicant and the amount of life insurance requested, additional testing, including stress testing and echocardiography, may be required. In most cases, abnormalities revealed during this laboratory evaluation are fully consistent with the clinical history as reported in the APS. In a minority of applicants, however, medical history is scanty or medical records are unavailable. In such patients, medical underwriting risk assessment is then based primarily on the findings from the insurance physical and laboratory examination. Studies in insured as well as general populations provide the necessary mortality projections for underwriting risk assessment using these parameters (Table 105-2). The Medical Impairment Study (1983), for example, confirmed the benign prognosis of incidental bradycardia found on insurance examination (mortality ratios of 73 to 80 percent).[14] On the other hand, a relative mortality of 250 percent was found for the finding of tachycardia.[14] Additional information is available to perform risk assessment for findings such as overweight and underweight,[12,31] low serum albumin,[32] and an abnormal electrocardiogram.[33,34]

HEALTH INSURANCE: FUTURE CONSIDERATIONS

Health insurance continues to evolve in terms of overall cost, quality, and availability within the current environment of health care reform. The delivery of health care under managed care plans by both governmental and employer insurance plans has begun to redefine many aspects of the traditional patient–doctor, doctor–doctor, and doctor–insurer relationships.[3,4] Recent U.S. privacy reforms [Health Insurance Portability and Accountability Act (HIPAA), Gramm-Leach-Bliley legislation] are important attempts to safeguard the privacy of medical information. However, they will almost certainly limit access to medical information for insurance underwriting, making accurate risk assessment in life and health insurance a much more difficult task.

Within this environment, cardiologists remain vitally important, functioning both as clinical consultants to primary care providers as well as professional consultants to managed care organizations and indemnity insurance plans. This latter role deserves special emphasis. Cardiologists will often be called on to provide the expertise essential to the determination of the medical necessity and appropriateness of care for health insurance case management and claim review. Assessment of new technology in its evolution from experimental procedure to accepted standard of care is a particularly important responsibility of the insurance consultant in the managed care environment.[35]

HEALTH AND DISABILITY INSURANCE

The role of the physician in disability determination is more complex, often requiring legal interpretation of disability based on the results of medical data available. The expertise of medical specialists—including physiatrists, physical and occupational therapists, and social workers—may be required for complete evaluation and recommendations. In general, thorough analysis coupled with appropriate goal-directed therapy often allows for return to work in a supportive environment accommodated to individual needs.

For practical purposes, the patient with known heart disease of any kind is going to have difficulty in obtaining standard individual health or disability insurance. As in the case of patients with high blood pressure, however, effective subclassification of patients and effective new therapies may allow insurance to become available to more and more patients who were considered unacceptable insurance risks in the past.

ACKNOWLEDGMENTS

We gratefully acknowledge the work of Dr. M. Irene Ferrer and Dr. Joseph A. Wilber in previous editions of this textbook, on which we drew for the current chapter.

References

1. Morton GA. *Principles of Life and Health Insurance.* Atlanta: Life Office Management Association; 1984.
2. Brackenridge RDC, Brown AE. A historical survey of the development of life assurance. In: Brackenridge RDC, Elder WJ, eds. *Medical Selection of Life Risks,* 3d ed. New York: Stockton Press; 1992:3–17.
3. Billi JE, Wise CG, Bills EA, Mitchell RL. Potential effects of managed care on specialty practice at a university medical center. *N Engl J Med* 1995;333:979–983.
4. Weisbuch JB, Roberts NK. Without the denominator, where is the quality improvement paradigm in the nation's health care reform? *J Ins Med* 1995;27:12–14.
5. Pokorski RJ. Mortality methodology and analysis seminar test. *J Ins Med* 1995;20:20–45.
6. Seltzer F. Choosing a standard for adjusted mortality rates. *Stat Bull* 1996;77:13–19.
7. Cumming GR, Croxson R. Cardiovascular disorders: Part I. Coronary heart disease. In: Brackenridge RDC, Elder WJ, eds. *Medical Selection of Life Risks,* 3d ed. New York: Stockton Press; 1992:251–323.
8. Croxson RS. Cardiovascular disorders: Part II. Other cardiovascular disorders. In: Brackenridge RDC, Elder WJ, eds. *Medical Selection of Life Risks,* 3d ed. New York: Stockton Press; 1992:324–431.
9. Singer RB. Pitfalls of inferring annual mortality from inspection of published survival curves. *J Ins Med* 1994;26:333–338.
10. Iacovino JR. A "quick hit" method to assess insurance mortality from a clinical article. *J Ins Med* 1994;26:317–318.
11. Negus BH. Coronary anatomy and prognosis of young, asymptomatic survivors of myocardial infarction. *Am J Med* 1994;96:354–358.
12. Clarke RD. Mortality of impaired lives 1964–73 (abstr). *J Inst Act* 1979; 100 (part 1). In: Lew EA, Gajewski J, eds. *Medical Risks: Trends in Mortality by Age and Time Elapsed.* New York: Praeger; 1990:7–120.
13. Jarvis HJ. Development of the diabetic, coronary, and blood pressure pools (abstr). *Cooperation internationale pour les assurances des risques aggraves,* 1986. In: Lew EA, Gajewski J, eds. *Medical Risks: Trends in Mortality by Age and Time Elapsed.* New York: Praeger; 1990:7–122.
14. Medical Impairment Study 1983 (abstr). I. Boston: Society of Actuaries and Association of Life Insurance Medical Directors of America, 1986. In: Lew EA, Gajewski J, eds. *Medical Risks: Trends in Mortality by Age and Time Elapsed.* New York: Praeger; 1990:6–78.

15. *Build and Blood Pressure Study 1959*. Chicago: Society of Actuaries; 1959.

16. *Mortality Investigation of Declined Lives in Japan*. Tokyo: The Life Insurance Association of Japan; 1979.

17. *Blood Pressure Study 1979*. Boston: Society of Actuaries and Association of Life Insurance Medical Directors of America; 1980.

18. *Multiple Medical Impairment Study*. Westwood, MA: Center for Medico-Actuarial Statistics of MIB, Inc; 1998.

19. Borer JS, Kligfield P. Aortic regurgitation: Making management decisions. *ACC Curr J Rev* 1995;4:30–32.

20. MacKenzie BR. Long-term mortality and complications of Bjork-Shiley spherical-disc valves—A life table analysis. *J Ins Med* 1992;24:128–132.

21. Jeresaty RM. Mitral valve prolapse: An update. In: Arnold CB, ed. *Transactions of The American Academy of Insurance Medicine: One Hundred and First Annual Meeting*. Tampa, FL: Klay Printing; 1993:24–33.

22. Singer RB, Gajewski J. Cardiovascular diseases I. In: Lew EA, Gajewski J, eds. *Medical Risks: Trends in Mortality by Age and Time Elapsed, 1*. New York: Praeger; 1990:6-30–6-38.

23. Cumming GR. Survival after valve replacement. In: Arnold CB, ed. *Transactions of The America Academy of Insurance Medicine: One Hundred and First Annual Meeting*. Tampa, FL: Klay Printing; 1993:40–55.

24. Elliott PM, Saumarez RC, McKenna WJ. Recent clinical advances in hypertrophic cardiomyopathy. *Heart Failure* 1995;11:15–25.

25. Cannan CR, Reeder GS, Bailey KR, et al. Natural history of hypertrophic cardiomyopathy: A population-based study, 1976 through 1990. *Circulation* 1995;92:2488–2495.

26. Ten Cate FJ. Prognosis of hypertrophic cardiomyopathy. *J Ins Med* 1996;28:42–45.

27. Iacovino JR. The nonmortality of hypertrophic cardiomyopathy in an unselected, community diagnosed and treated population. *J Ins Med* 1996;28:51–54.

28. Gajewski J, Singer RB. Mortality in an insured population with atrial fibrillation. *JAMA* 1981;245:1540–1544.

29. Chait L. Electrocardiography. In: Brackenridge RDC, Elder WJ, eds. *Medical Selection of Life Risks*, 3d ed. New York: Stockton Press; 1992:433–472.

30. Gorlin R. Cost-effectiveness of ICD therapy for ventricular arrhythmias. *Prim Cardiol* 1995;21:32–38.

31. *Build Study 1979*. Boston: Society of Actuaries and Association of Life Insurance Medical Directors of America; 1980.

32. Segel L. Serum albumin: "Phoenix" of the blood profile. *On the Risk* 1995;11:81–83.

33. Rose G, Baxter PJ, Reid DD, McCartney P. Prevalence and prognosis of electrocardiographic findings in middle-aged men (abstr). *Br Heart J* 1978;40:636–643. In: Lew EA, Gajewski J, eds. *Medical Risks: Trends in Mortality by Age and Time Elapsed*. New York: Praeger; 1990.

34. Ferrer MI. A survey of 19,734 electrocardiograms obtained in insurance applicants. *J Ins Med* 1985;16:6–13.

35. Privette M, ed. Court overrules HCFA 1986 investigational devices payment policy. *Cardiology* 1996;25:4.

36. Singer RB. Comparative mortality by sex and age in residents of Rochester, Minnesota, with acute myocardial infarction during 1960–1979 (sudden deaths included). *J Ins Med* 1995–1996;27:235–240.

37. Hutchinson R. Additional follow-up of patients with coronary bypass reoperation at Cleveland Clinic. *J Ins Med* 1994;26:324–328.

CLINICAL PRACTICE GUIDELINES IN CARDIOVASCULAR DISEASE

Ira S. Nash

The delivery of medical care in the United States is an enormous enterprise that now accounts for approximately 14 percent of the entire economic activity of the nation and for which about $1.4 trillion changes hands each year.[1] The rapid growth of medical expenditures throughout the 1980s and 1990s—and, in particular, the burden of those expenditures borne by businesses through their provision of employee health insurance benefits—has fostered an intense and unprecedented scrutiny of the practice of medicine. This scrutiny, not just of costs but also of the effectiveness of interventions, the outcomes of care, and the relative quality of different providers, is nothing less than a "revolution" in medical care.[2]

Physicians, long accustomed to the autonomous, small-scale practice of medicine, are understandably often bewildered by this. This chapter deals with one of the new tools—clinical practice guidelines—that have the potential to keep physicians in the forefront of medicine's transformation and simultaneously to facilitate the transformation itself.

We first address the context in which practice guidelines have achieved their current prominence. Next, the development, implementation, and maintenance of guidelines is presented, followed by an examination of their quality and their impact on medical practice.

QUALITY OF CARE

Practice Variation

One of the most striking aspects of the delivery of medical care in the United States is its enormous inhomogeneity.[3,4] Many well-documented examples of substantial variability in clinical practice exist among diagnostic tests and treatments for cardiovascular illnesses. The data on racial and ethnic disparities in cardiovascular care were recently and authoritatively reviewed by a collaborative effort of the Henry J. Kaiser Family Foundation, the Robert Wood Johnson Foundation, and several prominent medical organizations.[5] They found significant evidence of less intensive cardiac testing and coronary revascularization among minority patients. Others have reported that rates of rehospitalization after acute infarction differ markedly among different cities, in the absence of clinical differences among the populations.[6] Following a myocardial infarction, one is much more likely to undergo catheterization in Texas than in New York[7] or in the South compared with New England.[8] Striking geographic differences also exist in the use of effective medications for patients with acute myocardial infarction.[9] Women may be treated less intensively than men.[10]

As the cost, complexity, and potential benefit of medical care (and cardiac care in particular) have grown, so too has the importance of addressing this variation. Which of the different approaches to care is "right"? Which leads to the greatest benefit for patients? Could similar benefits be achieved at a lower cost? How could one tell? Addressing these and related questions is the essence of evaluating the quality of medical care. Evaluating the quality of care is a necessary prerequisite for improving it.

Defining Quality

Many different definitions of quality have been proposed. Leaders in the field have suggested that this multiplicity of definitions may make sense, given the complexity of medical care and the wide range of specific, local goals associated with assessing its quality.[11] The Institute of Medicine put forth a definition of the quality of medical care which has been widely adopted: "the degree to which health services for individuals and populations increase the likelihood of desired health outcomes and are consistent with current professional knowledge."[12] Simply put, good medical practice is necessarily based on sound medical knowledge, and if done right, it benefits patients. Note that even under the best of circumstances, quality medical care improves the *likelihood* of good outcomes, but it cannot guarantee them. A patient with cardiogenic shock on the basis of an extensive myocardial infarction is at high risk of dying even with the best medical care. Likewise, many patients will recover without incident after an infarction even if they do not receive effective therapies such as thrombolysis or postinfarction beta blockade. It is therefore inappropriate to examine only patient outcomes (such as mortality following an infarction) to judge the quality of care they received.

Measuring Quality: Structure, Process, and Outcome

A more complete assessment of the quality of care depends on considering three fundamental components of medical practice, which, taken together, paint a more complete picture: the structure, process, and outcome of care.[13] The *structure* of care is a characterization of the environment in which care is delivered. The *process* of care encompasses the myriad steps in the actual delivery of services, and the *outcome* of care is some result of interest to patients or providers. Consider, as an example, the assessment of the quality of care provided by a cardiac catheterization laboratory.

The structure of care provided by the lab includes the physical attributes of the facility, such as the modernity of the fluoroscopic equipment and the sophistication of the patient hemodynamic monitor. Perhaps less obviously, it also encompasses the staffing levels of the laboratory (e.g., nurse/patient ratios, nurse/technologist ratios), the level of training of the personnel (e.g., advanced cardiac life support certification, or "cross-training" of nursing and technical staff), and the maintenance of the equipment (e.g., the frequency of radiation safety inspections). The structure of the laboratory also extends beyond its own physical boundaries. Is the laboratory a freestanding facility? Is it in a community hospital, where it may be used for general vascular radiology as well as coronary angiography? Is there a cardiac surgical program at the same institution?

The process of care addresses what providers do and how they do it. For the catheterization laboratory, this runs the gamut from how patients are scheduled for their procedure (indeed, how they are identified as candidates for a procedure) through the steps taken to prepare them for the catheterization (including patient education and the solicitation of informed consent) and all the details of the procedure and postprocedural care. Clearly, this includes an enormous number of potential points of quality assessment. How are patients prepared for the catheterization? Do cardiology trainees perform part (or all) of the procedure under supervision? How are patients monitored after their procedure? Are there dedicated personnel who remove the arterial introducing sheaths? How much heparin is used? How long are patients required to stay in bed? The list goes on.

Finally, an assessment of the quality of the laboratory may rightfully include an examination of the outcomes of the patients who were treated. This may include traditional outcomes such as complications and mortality, but it can also be construed more broadly to include "patient-centered outcomes," such as patients' satisfaction with the care received[14,15] or the functional capacity of patients who have undergone percutaneous interventions.[16]

Quality Assessment and Improvement

With the dimensions of quality more broadly drawn, the assessment and improvement of care can be specified more precisely with reference to the definition of quality offered by the Institute of Medicine. This assessment may then, in turn, form the basis for quality improvement or for comparisons among providers. Some component of the structure, process, or outcome of a particular aspect of medical care must be selected, defined, and measured. In order for the quality assessment to be meaningful (and ultimately useful as a vehicle for improving care), certain criteria must be met.

First, the focus of the assessment must be something under the control of the providers of care.[17] There may be particular health outcomes that are of interest to patients and providers, but if they remain outside the ability of medical care to influence them, then measuring such outcomes would neither inform a judgment about the quality of care delivered nor form the basis for improving it. For example, the frequency with which patients with hypertrophic cardiomyopathy experience potentially life-threatening arrhythmias is of great interest to affected patients and their physicians. Yet tracking such events in a given population says little about the quality of medical care they received, since there are no therapies currently available that can reliably influence the outcome. A measurable *outcome* of care must therefore be linked with a controllable structure or process of care.

The mortality associated with coronary artery bypass graft (CABG) surgery is arguably the most intensively tracked outcome in all of medicine and has drawn the attention of a large number of investigators[18–22] as well as government agencies.[23,24] One critical factor in making CABG mortality a useful quality measure is that it can be influenced by changing the environment and processes of care.[25] Mortality following CABG depends in part on how well patients are treated. Tracking outcomes can therefore stimulate examination of the way care is delivered and possible changes in this, which can then result in improved outcomes.

A measurable *process* of care can also be the focus of quality assessment and improvement activities as long as it is closely linked to an important health outcome. The Cooperative Cardiovascular Project (CCP), sponsored by the Health Care Finance Administration (HCFA, now the Centers for Medicare and Medicaid Services or CMS), is an excellent example of a large-scale quality assessment and improvement project predicated on this principle.[26] Drawing on a large body of randomized controlled clinical trials of therapies for patients with acute myocardial infarction, investigators developed a series of quality indicators. These were measures of specific processes of care; that is, they identified which patients received which therapy. Based on the evidence from clinical trials, the investigators also specified which patients *should* get which therapy. They determined in this way the percentage of candidates for a given therapy who actually received it. Since the clinical trials established, for example, the connection between early aspirin administration and improved survival,[27] measuring the extent to which patients actually did receive aspirin served as a measure of the quality of the care delivered.

The current efforts by the American Heart Association (AHA)[28] and the American College of Cardiology (ACC)[29] to promote the use of effective treatments, discussed further on in this chapter, are also predicated on improving the processes of care. In clinical circumstances where process and outcome are well-linked by clinical evidence, measuring some specific step in the delivery of care instead of the final outcome offers several important advantages. First, it provides an important efficiency. Since every patient treated for a particular condition, such as myocardial infarction, is exposed to a system of care but only a small percentage of patients (regardless of the care they receive) is likely to experience a particular outcome such as death, many more patients must be studied if the quality of care they receive is to be judged solely on the outcomes they experience.

Mant and Hicks[30] estimated the relative numbers of patients required to detect differences in the quality of care provided to patients with acute myocardial infarction based on process versus outcome measures. After applying estimates of the efficacy of a variety of medical therapies for myocardial infarction derived from randomized trials, they constructed a model for calculating the sample size needed to detect a given difference in mortality between two hospitals treating populations with the same risk of dying. For example, detecting a reduction in mortality from 30 percent (the assumed baseline mortality in the absence of any effective therapies) to 25 percent (achievable with the adoption of only 31 percent of all available effective interventions) with a power of 80 percent and a significance level of 5 percent would require the examination of records from nearly 1300 patients with myocardial infarction. To detect the difference in frequency of use of effective therapeutic interventions that could lead to a reduction in mortality of the same magnitude (the process instead of the outcome of care), they derived a minimum sample size of only 27 patients. Clearly, tremendous economy of effort could be achieved by focusing on process instead of outcome.

In addition, if only the outcomes of care are tracked, then any efforts directed at improving outcomes must still ultimately identify and improve those aspects of the delivery of care that drive the outcome. So, for example, if hospitals tracked only infarction mortality without measuring the extent to which their patients receive aspirin, then the discovery of high mortality rates would necessarily lead to an investigation of care, including such critical steps as the use of aspirin. Following aspirin utilization directly focuses attention where it must eventually be paid.

Another criterion that any useful quality measure must fulfill rests on the fact that resources devoted to assessing one aspect of care are necessarily unavailable for a similar examination of some other aspect of care.[31] Maximizing the impact of quality assessment and improvement activities therefore requires prioritization in favor of high-cost, prevalent conditions.

Finally, a range of practical issues must be considered in choosing a useful measure of the structure, process, or outcome of care. The collection of necessary data must be feasible within the constraints of time and resources. Quality measures must also be reliable (measurable in a consistent way over time), valid (a true measure of what one hopes to measure), and sensitive to change over time and differences among systems of care.

Ultimately, improving the quality of care depends on creating the setting, conditions, and particular processes of care, which, if adhered to, will maximize the likelihood of good patient outcomes. The summary of these settings, conditions, and processes are practice guidelines.

CLINICAL PRACTICE GUIDELINES

Definition

In 1989, a new federal agency, The Agency for Health Care Policy and Research (AHCPR, since renamed the Agency for Healthcare Research and Quality, or AHRQ[32]) was created with the charge to "enhance the quality, appropriateness, and effectiveness of health care services, through the establishment of a broad base of scientific research and through the promotion of improvements in clinical practice and in the organization, financing and delivery of health care services."[33] Specifically included in the legislation was the charge that the agency put forth "clinically relevant" practice guidelines. Although guideline development is no longer in the purview of the AHRQ, the Institute of Medicine convened an advisory committee at the time to assist the newly formed agency in fulfilling its mandate. The committee's report defined practice guidelines as "systematically developed statements to assist practitioner and patient decisions about appropriate health care for specific clinical circumstances."[34] The intended utility of practice guidelines was expressed in a follow-up report by the Institute of Medicine in 1992: "Scientific evidence and clinical judgment can be systematically combined to produce clinically valid, operational recommendations for appropriate care that can and will be used to persuade clinicians, patients, and others to change their practices in ways that lead to better health outcomes and lower health care costs."[35] While the report acknowledged the existence of substantial barriers to the realization of this ideal, it remains a concise statement of the definition and promise of practice guidelines.

Other Aids to Clinical Practice

As the perceived need to improve the quality of care has grown, so too has the range of tools available to practitioners. Many of these share some characteristics of practice guidelines. Unfortunately, there is no universal agreement about the names used to describe them, which has led to some confusion. *Medical review criteria* are "systematically developed statements that can be used to assess the appropriateness of specific health care decisions, services, and outcomes."[36] These are generally derived from clinical practice guidelines and allow for their application in assessing and improving care. They may be "restatements of specific guideline recommendations into forms suitable for . . . review of clinical practice."[37] For example, the ACC/AHA guidelines for acute myocardial infarction (AMI) recommend the use of angiotensin-converting enzyme (ACE) inhibitors for AMI patients with a reduced ejection fraction or clinical heart failure.[38] One of the medical review criteria developed by CMS for the assessment of quality of care is the percentage of AMI patients with left ventricular systolic dysfunction and without contraindications to ACE inhibition who actually receive the medication during their hospitalization.[39]

Another quality improvement tool closely related to practice guidelines is a *critical pathway*. A critical pathway may also be referred to as a critical path, a clinical pathway, a clinical plan, a care map, or a care plan.[40] These are usually locally developed, highly detailed accounts of how the process of care should unfold for a focused episode of care. They typically deal with the direction and coordination of inpatient services for a particular diagnosis or procedure. For instance, a CABG critical pathway may specify what each of several different providers of care should do during each day of a patient's stay. This would include items such as nursing instruction in the use of incentive spirometry on postoperative day 1, the removal of chest tubes by the surgeon on day 3, climbing stairs with the physical therapist on day 5, and so on. Developing an explicit statement of this sort forces groups of providers to examine their practices and achieve local consensus about how care should be delivered, and the final products serve as real-time references to those caring for patients.

Guideline Development

The utility of a practice guideline depends critically on the process by which it was created. Task Force 1 of the 28th Bethesda Conference of the American College of Cardiology detailed eight phases of successful clinical practice guideline development.[41] Within each of these phases, they outlined specific tasks to be accomplished (Table 106-1). Others have proposed comparable work plans.[42]

Perhaps no other step in guideline development is as critical as systematically evaluating the strength of the evidence upon which recommendations are based.[43] Unless, as is rarely the case, all of the available evidence supports a particular clinical approach, guideline developers must weigh one bit of evidence against another. Even in the less problematic circumstance of general concordance of the available data, the quality of the data may have important implications for the confidence the guideline drafters have in one or more of their recommendations.

Some research findings (or other pieces of evidence) reported in the medical literature are more reliable than others. That is, some reported findings are likely to be a true effect, while others may be only an artifact of a study design flaw or a statistical quirk. There is a generally accepted hierarchy of study design, based on the premise that the systematic minimization of potential bias improves the reliability of research results.[44] The most reliable research results come from randomized controlled trials (RCTs), and among RCTs, those that recruited larger cohorts of patients are generally more reliable than smaller studies. In descending order of reliability (ascending vulnerability to bias), the remaining sources of data are cohort studies, case-control studies, case series and registries, case reports, and expert opinion. A common scheme is to divide the quality of evidence

TABLE 106-1 Phases of Guideline Development and Associated Tasks Identified by the 28th Bethesda Conference

Phase 1. Administrative oversight
    Task 1. Identify specific goals
    Task 2. Prioritize possible guideline topics
    Task 3. Review the literature to define task, costs, and time line
Phase 2. Select expert panel
    Task 1. Members must bring expertise, diversity, enthusiasm, and commitment
    Task 2. Convene panel electronically (videoconference, e-mail) to begin plans
    Task 3. Confirm outline, map patient care algorithm
Phase 3. Literature search and evidence review
    Task 1. Computerized literature search
    Task 2. Match literature to guideline outline, rate evidence
    Task 3. Create evidence tables for each topic
    Task 4. Base wording of recommendations on strength of relevant evidence
Phase 4. Consensus process
    Task 1. Converge on recommendations by an explicit process
Phase 5. Computerize guideline documents in format for clinical use
    Task 1. Link recommendations with related evidence
    Task 2. Create preformatted documents to capture data and facilitate care
    Task 3. Create database to store information regarding guideline compliance
Phase 6. Test and revise guideline
    Task 1. Expert panel tests computerized guideline in actual patient care
    Task 2. Final revision of guidelines based on testing
Phase 7. Disseminate guideline
    Task 1. Publish printed version, disseminate computerized version
    Task 2. Encourage local customization
Phase 8. Revise and refine guideline
    Task 1. Maintain ongoing literature review
    Task 2. Refine management strategies based on patient outcomes associated with guideline use

SOURCE: From Jones et al.[41] With permission.

TABLE 106-2 American College of Cardiology/American Heart Association Classification of Guideline Recommendations

Class I: Conditions for which there is evidence and/or general agreement that a given procedure or treatment is of benefit
Class II: Conditions for which there is conflicting evidence and/or a divergence of opinion about the usefulness or efficacy of a procedure or treatment
Class IIa: weight of evidence in favor or usefulness or efficacy
Class IIb: usefulness or efficacy is less well established
Class III: Conditions for which there is evidence and/or general agreement that the procedure/treatment is not useful/effective and in some cases may be harmful

A very good system for classifying recommendations is used by the Joint Task Force on Practice Guidelines of the ACC and the AHA. They use the classification scheme in Table 106-2 to summarize the indications for a particular treatment or therapy. The ACC and AHA have also developed a manual for guideline development that incorporates many of the principles and practices detailed above.[45]

All attempts to synthesize evidence from clinical trials into recommendations for practice must also wrestle with an unavoidable paradox: well-designed clinical trials usually involve highly specified patient populations, defined by extensive inclusion and exclusion criteria, while practice guidelines, by their nature, are intended to be broadly applicable. There is no simple or formulaic way to reconcile the nature of the evidence and the need for recommendations.

Guideline Implementation

Clinical practice guidelines are tools for improving patient care. Much of that potential can be realized only by changing physician behavior, since physicians are ultimately responsible for directing care. Even a well-crafted guideline, then, will not benefit patients unless and until it actually changes how doctors act under particular circumstances.[46]

Multiple studies have demonstrated that just making information available to physicians is generally insufficient to change their practice.[47] Successful implementation of clinical practice guidelines must therefore go beyond making the guidelines themselves accessible through publication in the medical literature or by electronic means. Cabana and colleagues presented a useful taxonomy for the barriers to guideline adoption and implementation.[48] They grouped barriers into those related to physician knowledge (lack of awareness or lack of familiarity), attitudes (lack of agreement, lack of self-efficacy, lack of outcome expectancy, or the inertia of previous practice), and behavior (external barriers).

Lack of physician awareness of or familiarity with specific guidelines has been well documented. Although the large number of practice guidelines makes this virtually inevitable, physicians are often unfamiliar with even the principal recommendations of well-publicized and broadly applicable guidelines.[49]

A negative attitude among clinicians about the value of guidelines is also a significant barrier to their implementation. This, in turn, may be a result of a general mistrust of "cookbook"[50] approaches to clinical practice, a rejection of national (in favor of local) standards of practice,[51] concerns regarding malpractice liability,[52] differences in

into three classes: A-level evidence is derived from RCTs (both large and small), metanalyses of RCTs, well-conducted cohort studies, and metanalyses of well-conducted cohort studies; B-level evidence is drawn from studies with other kinds of designs; and C-level evidence is based on expert opinion only.

Although evidence of consistently high quality may form the basis for strong guideline recommendations, it must be noted that there are legitimate circumstances where this concordance is violated. If several large RCTs provide conflicting conclusions, then the quality of the available evidence may be high but the recommendation necessarily weak. On the other hand, if there is such universal agreement that a particular element of care is so essential that no RCT is ever likely to be done (e.g., the necessity of examining a patient[41]), then a strong recommendation may be appropriate in the absence of rigorous evidence. Guideline developers have therefore developed separate systems for indicating the strength of their recommendations.

physician training and experience,[53] and the sparsity of data that adherence to guidelines actually improves care.[54] Many clinicians also believe that guidelines are fundamentally incapable of capturing the nuances and complexity of clinical medicine.[55] Certainly, deficiencies in the guidelines themselves, including conflicting recommendations among different guidelines addressing the same conditions[56] or lack of clarity of recommendations, contribute to physician skepticism. Grol and coworkers reported that physicians were most likely to adopt concrete, precise, and uncontroversial recommendations.[57] Perhaps the greatest external barrier to guideline implementation is the complexity of the health care delivery system itself. Medical care is provided in a broad range of settings, from private physicians' offices to large academic medical centers and by a host of practitioners with different levels of interest and expertise in particular clinical conditions. Given the financial pressure present in many medical delivery systems, guideline implementation may well be seen as another burden or expense rather than as an aid to clinical practice. Even if guideline adoption is seen as desirable, limitations of physician time and practice resources may hinder efforts to move forward. The inadequacy of many clinical information systems, which under ideal circumstances could identify patients who meet guideline criteria and remind providers of current recommendations, is another important institutional barrier to successful guideline implementation.

Just as the barriers to guideline implementation are diverse, there is no single proven strategy for successful guideline adoption. For guideline developers, close attention to the principles of rigorous data synthesis and the straightforward presentation of well-documented recommendations is essential. Explicit discussion of potential conflicts with other guidelines and the reasons for different recommendations should be included. Guideline writers should include clear statements regarding the limitations of their own guidelines with respect to the patients or conditions to which they apply and consider the practicality of their recommendations.

Those who are charged with implementing practice guidelines must be prepared to address the barriers discussed above. Clear demonstration of the value of guideline adoption, through the feedback of local data demonstrating improvements in patient outcomes, is often part of a successful strategy. Simultaneous development of the infrastructure to support clinical practice guidelines, including modifying the incentives of clinicians and investing in clinical information systems, is also helpful. Recognizing that creating high-quality practice guidelines does not, in itself, improve care, the AHA and the ACC have embarked on their own programs to enhance guideline implementation.

The AHA program, called Get With the Guidelines, is intended to promote the use of a small number of key treatments for patients hospitalized with coronary heart disease, acute coronary syndromes, heart failure, and atrial fibrillation. These treatments include, for example, the timely use of aspirin, the assessment and treatment of blood lipid disorders, and the discharge prescription of an ACE inhibitor in patients with left ventricular systolic dysfunction. Hospitals must register as program participants. They then gain access to a web-based data collection instrument for monitoring guideline adherence, which also allows for comparisons of local performance against regional and national data. The Get With the Guidelines program also provides a "tool kit" of educational material (including presentation slides), guideline implementation aids (such as standardized admission order sets), and extensive program support. Data from the successful pilot implementation are available on the AHA website.[58]

The ACC-sponsored Guidelines Applied in Practice (GAP) program is a rapid-cycle quality improvement initiative that is also in-

tended to boost adherence with major elements of the ACC/AHA guidelines. The GAP program has separate modules for AMI and congestive heart failure. The myocardial infarction tool kit consists of (1) AMI standard admission orders, (2) a clinical pathway, (3) a pocket guide to care, (4) a patient information form, (5) a patient discharge checklist, (6) chart stickers to alert providers, and (7) hospital performance charts. A pilot implementation of the program in 10 acute care hospitals in Michigan yielded statistically and clinically significant improvements in the use of aspirin and beta blockers and favorable trends in the use of other efficacious therapies.[59]

Guideline Maintenance

If a particular practice guideline is to remain a useful tool for improving the quality of care, it must maintain its scientific currency and its relevance to clinical practice. Several different circumstances could necessitate a guideline update[60]:

- Changes in the risk and benefit of current interventions
- Changes in which outcomes are considered important (e.g., quality-of-life measures)
- Changes in the quality of current practice
- Changes in the value placed on outcomes (e.g., economic endpoints)
- Changes in available resources

Establishing the appropriate threshold for any of these criteria is not simple; recognizing when that threshold is achieved is harder still. Some organizations therefore rely on an arbitrary time-based cycle of guideline revision. For example, the National Guideline Clearinghouse,[61] a website maintained by the AHRQ, deletes guidelines that are more than 5 years old. Such a policy may not be ideal.[62] Rather, a systematic reassessment of existing guidelines by recognized experts, supplemented by limited searches of the medical literature and operating with prospectively defined criteria for obsolescence, may be the only practical way to assure timely updates.[60]

Electronic publication and partial, rather than complete, revisions have been used effectively by the AHA and ACC to reduce the revision cycle time for their guidelines that need updating.

Guideline Quality

Several observers have suggested lists of attributes that good practice guidelines should have. The Institute of Medicine report lists eight important qualities[34] (Table 106-3). *Validity* implies that the guidelines, if adopted, will actually lead to the anticipated improvements in health outcomes and/or cost of care. *Reliability* or *reproducibility* is achieved if another group of guideline developers would create equivalent guidelines, if they relied on the same evidence, and if the guidelines are "interpreted and applied consistently by practitioners." Good guidelines should also have clear *clinical applicability,* so that

TABLE 106-3 Desirable Attributes of Clinical Practice Guidelines Identified by the Institute of Medicine

Validity	Clarity
Reliability	Multidisciplinary development
Clinical applicability	Scheduled review
Flexibility	Documentation

SOURCE: From Field and Lohr.[34] With permission.

they pertain to a broad, well-defined, and explicitly stated population. Guidelines must also allow for some *flexibility* of medical practice and acknowledge the appropriate role of clinical judgment and possible exceptions to broad dictates. *Clarity* of recommendations is another important attribute and should be promoted through the use of precise definitions of terms, unambiguous recommendations, and a variety of presentation techniques. Ideally, guidelines should be developed through *a multidisciplinary process,* which elicits the input of a broad range of stakeholders in the field. The Institute of Medicine report also suggests a provision for *scheduled revision* or an "expiration date," although, as discussed above, this may be of limited utility. Finally, the Institute report suggests that good guidelines should be *well documented,* so that users will know the "procedures followed in developing guidelines, the participants involved, the evidence used, the assumptions and rationales accepted, and the analytic methods employed."

The Evidence-Based Medicine Working Group has put forth its own criteria for judging the quality of practice guidelines. They posed a series of questions, the affirmative answers to which indicate a good guideline[63]:

- Were all important options and outcomes clearly specified?
- Was an explicit and sensible process used to identify, select, and combine evidence?
- Was an explicit and sensible process used to consider the relative value of different outcomes?
- Is the guideline likely to account for important recent developments?
- Has the guideline been subject to peer review and testing?
- Are practical, clinically important recommendations made?
- How strong are the recommendations?

They conclude: "A good guideline, based on solid scientific evidence and an explicit process for judging the value of alternative practices, allows you to review, at one sitting, links between multiple options and outcomes."[64]

Weingarten endorsed this same series of questions to assess the quality of practice guidelines,[65] but Selker offered a slightly different set of criteria.[66] He proposed that guidelines must have the following attributes to warrant adoption:

- Face validity: they must appear "reasonable and appropriate to relevant experts in the field."
- Content validity: they must be based on sound medical evidence.
- Clinical practicality: they must balance specificity with flexibility.
- Consensus validity: they must reflect the achievement of consensus by affected parties.
- Demonstrated safety and effectiveness: they should be tested and proved useful in clinical trials.
- Transportability: they must be useful across a range of practice settings.
- Timeliness: they should be up to date, reflecting current medical knowledge.

There are now a huge number of practice guidelines put forth by a large number of organizations and dealing with a broad array of clinical issues. The National Guideline Clearinghouse lists over 1000 practice guidelines on its website. With so many guidelines in the published literature, a number of investigators have attempted to assess how well they fulfill the criteria discussed above.

While the Institute of Medicine tried unsuccessfully to create a uniform guideline assessment tool, several different investigators have created and applied their own assessment instruments.

Shaneyfelt and colleagues explicitly judged a total of 279 clinical practice guidelines published between 1985 and 1997.[67] They first devised an evaluation tool that consisted of 25 specific standards that guidelines should ideally fulfill. These criteria were separated into standards of development and format, standards of evidence identification and summary, and standards on the formulation of recommendations. No attempt was made to prioritize the standards, and the authors acknowledge that it is extremely unlikely that any guideline would fulfill all of them. Nevertheless, they reported that the guidelines met a mean of only 43.1 percent of the quality standards and concluded that most guidelines "do not adhere well to established methodological standards," especially in regard to how the underlying medical evidence is gathered and critically combined. Cook and Giacomini, in an accompanying editorial, commented that the findings revealed "the diversity of guideline methodologies . . . and [are a] call for greater transparency of guideline reporting and more rigorous peer review."[68]

A generic guideline assessment tool was also developed and evaluated by Cluzeau et al.[69] They evaluated guidelines in three "dimensions"—rigor of development, context and content, and application—by means of a series of yes/no questions and applied their tool to a set of 60 different practice guidelines for coronary heart disease, asthma, breast cancer, and depression. They reported that the tool was easy to apply and reliable in practice and that most guidelines did not achieve the majority of criteria in each dimension.

Graham and coworkers evaluated the utility of 15 different guideline "appraisal instruments" published by other investigators, including Shaneyfelt and Cluzeau.[70] They concluded that there was insufficient evidence to support the exclusive use of a single instrument. Grilli and colleagues presented a much simpler assessment tool, which addresses three central issues related to guideline quality: a description of the type of professionals who developed the guideline, a description of the sources of information used, and whether an explicit method of grading the evidence was described.[71] They concluded that Shaneyfelt overstated the general problem of poor guideline quality; they instead identified only those guidelines developed by specialty societies as being of particularly poor quality. They proposed uniform reporting of methodology by guideline developers.

Hart and Bailey, using an instrument based on those of Shaneyfelt and Grilli, assessed the methodology and recommendations of 22 different published guidelines on the prevention of ischemic stroke.[72] Although there was general concordance on key clinical recommendations, they found major deficiencies in guideline development and reporting.

Guideline Effectiveness

With legitimate questions raised over the quality of guidelines and the challenges associated with their development, implementation, and maintenance, what is the evidence that the cardiovascular clinical practice guidelines have actually improved the quality of care? The question, though vital to the allocation of resources for quality improvement activities, is difficult to answer. Since the impact of practice guidelines depends on both the quality of the guideline itself and its successful implementation (its local application to a system of care delivery), there is no simple way to allocate observed success or failure between these two. In other words, a failure to demonstrate improvements in cardiovascular care through the use of guidelines may represent deficiencies in the applicability or practicality of practice guidelines, the operational failure of implementing them locally, or some combination of both. In addition, it is challenging to perform randomized trials of guideline use. Fortunately, there are data to suggest that guidelines can improve care.

Grimshaw and Russell compiled the most rigorous assessment of the success of practice guidelines, in a variety of medical conditions, in improving the quality of care.[73] They reviewed 59 published reports evaluating the impact of practice guidelines and found that in nearly all cases the implementation of a practice guideline had improved the measured process of care. Of the 11 studies they reviewed that reported a clinical outcome in addition to the process of care, 9 reported significant improvement. One may question the generalizability of these conclusions, since it is likely that there is a significant publication bias in favor of studies demonstrating an improvement in care over "negative" studies of the same question. Nevertheless, regardless of the frequency with which practice guidelines actually *do* improve care, there is clear and compelling evidence that they *can* improve care.

Sarasin and colleagues reported significant improvements in the use of beta blockers in postinfarction patients following the implementation of a practice guideline on the subject at their institution.[74] In their time series, the use of discharge beta blockers nearly doubled, despite no significant change in the profile of infarction patients. A Canadian group looked at the improvement in several process measures of care for patients with AMI cared for at the University of Alberta Hospitals between 1987 and 1993.[75] They found continuous and significant improvement in the use of therapies of proven efficacy, with a corresponding fall in the use of unproven interventions. Although the observations were made in an uncontrolled setting, the investigators attributed the results to "repeated measurement and reporting of key health care performance indicators, and initiation of explicit . . . AMI practice guidelines." On a much larger scale, the Cooperative Cardiovascular Project demonstrated that the feedback on compliance with guidelines for critical process of care measures for patients with myocardial infarction was associated with a significant improvement in the quality of care that AMI patients received.[76]

The success of the guideline implementation programs sponsored by the AHA and ACC, detailed earlier in this chapter, also support the utility of practice guidelines in improving the quality of cardiovascular care. Greater success in implementing practice guidelines depends in part on the refinement of the guidelines themselves, the more extensive use of clinical information systems to present critical data and guideline recommendations to clinicians at the point of care,[77] and greater sensitivity to the systematic barriers to their adoption.[48,57]

Finding Practice Guidelines

Clinical practice guidelines in cardiovascular medicine have been developed by many different organizations on a wide array of topics. New guidelines are constantly being produced in order to cover new subjects and to incorporate new data about previously addressed conditions. Just keeping track of the guidelines themselves has become challenging for clinicians and policymakers. Fortunately, there are several ways to find relevant guidelines.

Most clinical practice guidelines are published in peer-reviewed medical journals. Often, the journals are the official publication of the same parent organization that produced the guideline. So, for example, the guidelines compiled by the American College of Physicians/American Society of Internal Medicine are published in the *Annals of Internal Medicine;* those of the American College of Chest Physicians appear in *Chest,* and the guidelines of the joint efforts of the ACC/AHA are published in both the *Journal of the American College of Cardiology* and *Circulation.* Guidelines by lesser-known groups are also generally published in mainstream journals. Even government agencies, which have their own publishing capabilities, often seek to have part or all of their guidelines published in journals as well. As a consequence, a computer search of the MEDLINE database of peer-reviewed journals can produce a list of many of the sought guidelines. This process is far from perfect, however, in part because of the wide variety of key terms used to index published guidelines.

Each of these organizations also maintains its own website where practice guidelines are available. As the pace of medical developments accelerates, guideline updates have become more frequent, and some organizations have adopted a policy of publishing their updated guidelines exclusively in electronic form. The ACC/AHA guidelines and their associated updates are all available at their respective sites: www.acc.org and www.americanheart.org.

The electronic compendium of guidelines maintained by the National Guideline Clearinghouse is very useful.[61] This searchable website allows the user to specify the subject and/or sponsor of guidelines. The interface is user-friendly, and the list generated by the search contains links to the specified guideline. So, for example, if one specifies *cardiovascular disease,* a total of 217 listed guidelines are presented, along with suggested search terms (*heart disease, vascular disease,* etc.) and the number of guidelines fitting those search criteria. The links allow a user to go directly from the list to a brief summary of the guideline prepared by the National Guideline Clearinghouse as well as to the full text of a particular guideline, often at the website of the sponsoring organization.

CONCLUSION

Assessing and improving the quality of care is a vital component of responsible medical practice. It has taken on increased prominence in recent years because of the widespread evidence of unexplained practice variation, the underutilization of effective therapies, and the increasing pressure for accountability at all levels of health care delivery. Clinical practice guidelines have emerged as an important tool to improve the quality of medical care, and cardiovascular medicine has become a particularly fertile ground for their development. A large number of high-quality clinical practice guidelines are now available that address critical issues in cardiovascular medicine. When they are based on dependable, rigorous evidence, written in clear language, and implemented with sensitivity to the myriad local issues that can thwart their success, clinical practice guidelines can help improve patient care.

References

1. Centers for Medicare and Medicaid Services. http://cms.hhs.gov/statistics/nhe/historical/t1.asp
2. Relman AS. Assessment and accountability: The third revolution in medical care. *N Engl J Med* 1988;319:1220–1222.
3. Chassin MR, Kosecoff J, Park RE, et al. Variations in the use of medical and surgical services by the Medicare population. *N Engl J Med* 1986;314:285–290.
4. Welch WP, Miller ME, Welch HG, et al. Geographic variation in expenditures for physicians' services in the United States. *N Engl J Med* 1993;328:621–627.
5. Lillie-Blanton M, Rushing OE, Ruiz S, et al. Racial/ethnic differences in cardiac care: The weight of the evidence. 2002 report. Available at http://www.kff.org/whythedifference.

6. Fisher ES, Wennberg JE, Stukel TA, et al. Hospital readmission rates for cohorts of Medicare beneficiaries in Boston and New Haven. *N Engl J Med* 1994;331:989–995.

7. Guadagnoli E, Hauptman PJ, Ayanian JZ, et al. Variation in the use of cardiac procedures after acute myocardial infarction. *N Engl J Med* 1995;333:573–578.

8. Pilote L, Califf RM, Sapp S, et al. Regional variation across the United States in the management of acute myocardial infarction. *N Engl J Med* 1995;333:565–572.

9. O'Connor GT, Quinton HB, Traven ND, et al. Geographic variation in the treatment of acute myocardial infarction. The Cooperative Cardiovascular Project. *JAMA*. 1999;281:627–633.

10. Roger VL, Farkouh ME, Weston SA, et al. Sex differences in evaluation and outcome of unstable angina. *JAMA* 2000;283:646–652.

11. Blumenthal D. Quality of care—What is it? *N Engl J Med* 1996;335: 891–894.

12. Institute of Medicine. *Medicare: A Strategy for Quality Assurance.* Washington, DC: National Academy Press; 1990.

13. Donabedian A. *Explorations in Quality Assessment and Monitoring.* Vol 1: *The Definition of Quality and Approaches to Its Assessment.* Ann Arbor, MI: Health Administration Press; 1980.

14. Cleary P, Edgman-Levitan S. Health care quality: Incorporating consumer perspectives. *JAMA* 1997;278:1608–1612.

15. Nash IS. Improving outcomes of percutaneous coronary intervention. *Am Heart J* 1999;137:979–982.

16. Nash IS, Curtis LH, Rubin H. Predictors of patient reported physical and mental health six months after percutaneous coronary revascularization. *Am Heart J* 1999;138:422–429.

17. Hammermeister KE, Shroyer AL, Sethi GK, Grover FL. Why it is important to demonstrate linkages between outcomes of care and processes and structures of care. *Med Care* 1995;33(10 Suppl): OS5–OS16.

18. O'Connor GT, Plume SK, Olmstead EM, et al. Multivariate prediction of in-hospital mortality associated with coronary artery bypass graft surgery: Northern New England Cardiovascular Disease Study Group. *Circulation* 1992;85:2110–2118.

19. Plume SK, O'Connor GT, Olmstead EM. Update 2000: Changes in patients undergoing coronary artery bypass grafting: 1987–1990. *Ann Thorac Surg* 2001;72(1):314–315.

20. Herlitz J, Wognsen GB, Karlson BW, et al. Mortality, mode of death and risk indicators for death during 5 years after coronary artery bypass grafting among patients with and without a history of diabetes mellitus. *Coron Artery Dis* 2000;11(4):339–346.

21. Zaroff JG, diTommaso DG, Barron HV. A risk model derived from the National Registry of Myocardial Infarction 2 database for predicting mortality after coronary artery bypass grafting during acute myocardial infarction. *Am J Cardiol* 2002;90(1):35–38.

22. Clough RA, Leavitt BJ, Morton JR, et al. The effect of comorbid illness on mortality outcomes in cardiac surgery. *Arch Surg* 2002;137(4):428–432.

23. New York State Department of Health. *Coronary Artery Bypass Surgery in New York State, 1997–1999.* Albany, NY: New York State Department of Health; 2002. Also available at: http://www.health.state.ny.us/nysdoh/heart/heart_disease.htm

24. Pennsylvania Health Care Cost Containment Council. *Pennsylvania's Guide to Coronary Artery Bypass Graft Surgery 1994–1995.* Harrisburg, PA: Pennsylvania Health Care Cost Containment Council; 1998.

25. O'Connor GT, Plume SK, Olmstead EM, et al. A regional intervention to improve the hospital mortality associated with coronary artery bypass surgery. The Northern New England Cardiovascular Disease Study Group. *JAMA* 1996;275(11):841–846.

26. Ellerbeck EF, Jencks SF, Radford MJ, et al. Quality of care for Medicare patients with acute myocardial infarction. *JAMA* 1995;273:1509–1514.

27. ISIS-2 (Second International Study of Infarct Survival) Collaborative Group. Randomised trial of intravenous streptokinase, oral aspirin, both, or neither among 17,187 cases of suspected acute myocardial infarction: ISIS-2. *Lancet* 1988;2:349–360.

28. Get with the Guidelines. http://www.americanheart.org/presenter.jhtml?identifier=1165

29. Guidelines applied in practice. http://www.acc.org/gap/gap.htm

30. Mant J, Hicks N. Detecting differences in quality of care: The sensitivity of measures of process and outcome in treating acute myocardial infarction. *BMJ* 1995;311:793–796.

31. Casalino LP. The unintended consequences of measuring quality on the quality of medical care. *N Engl J Med* 1999;341:1147–1150.

32. http://www.ahrq.gov/

33. Public Law 101-239, the Omnibus Budget Reconciliation Act of 1989, section 901.

34. Field MJ, Lohr KN, eds. *Clinical Practice Guidelines: Directions for a New Program.* Washington, DC: National Academy Press; 1990.

35. Field MJ, Lohr KN, eds. *Guidelines for Clinical Practice: From Development to Use.* Washington, DC: National Academy Press; 1992:4.

36. Field MJ, Lohr KN, eds. *Clinical Practice Guidelines: Directions for a New Program.* Washington, DC: National Academy Press; 1990:50.

37. Hadorn DC, Baker DW, Kamberg CJ, Brook RH. Phase II of the AHCPR-sponsored heart failure guideline: Translating practice recommendations into review criteria. *Jt Comm J Qual Improv* 1996;22: 265–276.

38. Ryan TJ, Antman EM, Brooks NH, et al. ACC/AHA guidelines for the management of patients with acute myocardial infarction: 1999 update: A report of the American College of Cardiology/American Heart Association Task Force on Practice Guidelines (Committee on Management of Acute Myocardial Infarction). Available at www.acc.org. Accessed on January 19, 2003.

39. Available at: http://projects.ipro.org/index/qi_ami_eqi

40. Pearson SD, Goulart-Fisher D, Lee TH. Critical pathways as a strategy for improving care: Problems and potential. *Ann Intern Med* 1995; 123:941–948.

41. Jones RH, Ritchie JL, Fleming BB, et al. Task Force 1: Clinical practice guideline development, dissemination and computerization. *J Am Coll Cardiol* 1997;29:1133–1141.

42. Connis RT, Nickinovich DG, Caplan RA, Arens JF. The development of evidence-based clinical practice guidelines: Integrating medical science and practice. *Int J Technol Assess Health Care* 2000;16(4):1003–1012.

43. Shekelle PG, Woolf SH, Eccles M, Grimshaw J. Developing guidelines. *BMJ* 1999;318:593–596.

44. Hadorn DC, Baker D, Hodges JS, et al. Rating the quality of evidence for clinical practice guidelines. *J Clin Epidemiol* 1996;49:749–754.

45. http://www.acc.org/clinical/manual/manual_index.htm

46. Feder G, Eccles M, Grol R, et al. Using clinical guidelines. *BMJ* 1999; 318:728–730.

47. Lee TH, Pearson SD, Johnson PA, et al. Failure of information as an intervention to modify clinical management: A time-series trial in patients with acute chest pain. *Ann Intern Med* 1995;122:434–437.

48. Cabana MD, Rand CS, Powe NR, et al. Why don't physicians follow clinical practice guidelines? A framework for improvement. *JAMA* 1999;282:1458–1465.

49. Hagemeister J, Schneider CA, Barabas S, et al. Hypertension guidelines and their limitations—The impact of physicians' compliance as evaluated by guideline awareness. *J Hypertens* 2001;19:2079–2086.

50. Parmley WW. Clinical practice guidelines: Does the cookbook have enough recipes? *JAMA* 1994;272:1374–1375.

51. Grimshaw JM, Russell IT. Achieving health gain through clinical guidelines: II. Ensuring guidelines change medical practice. *Quality Health Care* 1994;3:45–51.

52. Hurwitz B. Legal and political considerations of clinical practice guidelines. *BMJ* 1999;318:661–664.

53. Chodoff P, Crowley K. Clinical practice guidelines: Roadblocks to their acceptance and implementation. *J Outcomes Mgt* 1995;2(2):5–10.

54. Marshall DA, Simpson KN, Norton EC, et al. Measuring the effect of clinical guidelines on patient outcomes. *Int J Technol Assess Health Care* 2000;16(4):1013–1023.

55. Garfield FB, Garfield JM. Clinical judgment and clinical practice guidelines. *Int J Technol Assess Health Care* 2000;16(4):1050–1060.

56. Thomson R, McElroy H, Sudlow M. Guidelines on anticoagulant treatment in atrial fibrillation in Great Britain: Variation in content and implications for treatment. *BMJ* 1998;316:509–513.

57. Grol R, Dalhuijsen J, Thomas S, et al. Attributes of clinical guidelines that influence use of guidelines in general practice: Observational study. *BMJ* 1998;317:858–861.

58. http://www.americanheart.org/presenter. American Heart Association: Get with the Guidelines. Home Page.

59. Mehta RH, Montoye CK, Gallogly M, et al. Improving quality of care for acute myocardial infarction. The Guidelines Applied in Practice (GAP) Initiative. *JAMA* 2002;287:1269–1276.

60. Shekelle P, Eccles MP, Grimshaw JM, Woolf SH. When should clinical guidelines be updated? *BMJ* 2001;323:155–157.

61. http://www.guideline.gov/index.asp

62. Shekelle PG, Ortiz E, Rhodes S, et al. Validity of the Agency for Healthcare Research and Quality clinical practice guidelines. How quickly to guidelines become outdated? *JAMA* 2001;286:1461–1467.

63. Hayward RSA, Wilson MC, Tunis SR, et al. User's guide to the medical literature: VIII. How to use clinical practice guidelines. A: Are the recommendations valid? *JAMA* 1995;274:570–574.

64. Wilson MC, Hayward RAS, Tunis SR, et al. User's guide to the medical literature: VIII. How to use clinical practice guidelines. B: What are the recommendations and will they help you in caring for your patients? *JAMA* 1999;274:1630–1632.

65. Weingarten S. Using practice guidelines compendiums to provide better preventive care. *Ann Intern Med* 1999;130:454–458.

66. Selker HP. Criteria for adoption of medical practice guidelines. *Am J Cardiol* 1993;71:339–341.

67. Shaneyfelt TM, Mayo-Smith MF, Rothwangle J. Are guidelines following guidelines? The methodological quality of clinical practice guidelines in the peer-reviewed medical literature. *JAMA* 1999;281:1900–1905.

68. Cook D, Giacomini M. The trials and tribulations of clinical practice guidelines. *JAMA* 1999;281:1950–1951.

69. Cluzeau FA, Littlejohns P, Grimshaw JM, et al. Development and application of a generic methodology to assess the quality of clinical guidelines. *Int J Qual Health Care* 1999;11:21–28.

70. Graham ID, Clader LA, Hebert PC, et al. A comparison of clinical practice guideline appraisal instruments. *Int J Technol Assess Health Care* 2000;16(4):1024–1038.

71. Grilli R, Magrini N, Penna A, et al. Practice guidelines developed by specialty societies: The need for a critical appraisal. *Lancet* 2000;355:103–106.

72. Hart RG, Bailey RD. An assessment of guidelines for prevention of ischemic stroke. *Neurology* 2002:59:977–982.

73. Grimshaw JM, Russell IT. Effect of clinical guidelines on medical practice: A systematic review of rigorous evaluations. *Lancet* 1993;342:1317–1322.

74. Sarasin FP, Maschiangelo ML, Schaller MD, et al. Successful implementation of guidelines for encouraging the use of beta blockers in patients after acute myocardial infarction. *Am J Med* 1999;106:499–505.

75. Montague T, Taylor L, Martin S, et al. Can practice patterns and outcomes be successfully altered? Examples from cardiovascular medicine. *Can J Cardiol* 1995;11:487–492.

76. Marciniak TA, Ellerbeck EF, Radford MJ, et al. Improving the quality of care for Medicare patients with acute myocardial infarction: Results from the Cooperative Cardiovascular Project. *JAMA* 1998;279:1351–1357.

77. Tierney WM, Overhage JM, Takesue BY, et al. Computerizing guidelines to improve care and patient outcomes: The example of heart failure. *JAMA* 1995;2:316–322.

BEHAVIORAL MEDICINE IN THE TREATMENT OF HEART DISEASE

Thomas G. Pickering / Karina W. Davidson / Lynn Clemow / William Gerin

In an assessment of the causes of death in the United States in 1993, McGinnis and Foege[1] estimated that approximately 50 percent of deaths (the majority being due to heart disease) were attributable to behavioral or lifestyle factors, including tobacco use, poor diet, physical inactivity, and alcohol. While genetic factors undoubtedly contribute to individual susceptibility to these factors, a prime ingredient is the person's behavior. The costs of treating heart disease are escalating at an increasingly rapid pace, due to the widespread use of sophisticated and increasingly expensive treatments such as coated coronary artery stents, implantable defibrillators, and gene therapy. Most of the efforts to contain the rise in health care costs have focused on limiting supply (a largely unfulfilled promise of managed care) and imposing some sort of rationing. However, in 1993, Fries et al.[2] pointed out that restricting demand could achieve the same objective. They identified six factors, four of which are directly relevant to this chapter. They include the following facts:

1. Much disease is preventable.
2. Risky behavior costs money. Lifetime medical costs, which averaged $225,000 per person, have been clearly related to health behavior. For example, such costs are approximately one-third higher in smokers than in nonsmokers.
3. Self-management can result in savings. Several studies have shown that providing medical consumers with information and guidelines about self-management can lower the use of medical services by 10 percent or more.
4. The promotion of healthy behavior at work has successfully reduced costs. This has also been documented in numerous studies.

This chapter focuses on the major behavioral and psychological factors that influence the course of heart disease, and how they can be modified. The behavioral factors are smoking, diet and obesity, physical inactivity, and the psychological factors hostility, depression, and anxiety.

A dramatic example of the effects of environmental and psychosocial factors on cardiovascular disease is provided by a recent analysis of the changing mortality rates in Russia.[3] Over a 4-year period following the breakup of the Soviet Union, there was a 5-year decline in life expectancy, most of which could be attributed to increased mortality in men aged 25 to 64 due to accidents and cardiovascular disease. Factors that may have contributed to these changes included economic instability, stress, depression, and increased intake of alcohol and tobacco. Another equally dramatic example of the influence of lifestyle factors comes from the Honolulu Heart Program, where it was found that retired men who walked less than 1 mile a day were nearly twice as likely to die over a 12-year period as men who walked more than 2 miles.[4] This might to some extent be a "healthy person effect," in that sick people are less likely to walk than those who are healthy.

Psychosocial factors can influence the course of chronic disease by two main pathways: first, by inducing behavioral or lifestyle patterns such as smoking, which are themselves injurious, and, second, by a direct effect of social and environmental factors such as socioeconomic status and stress on the disease process. Personality and emotional characteristics such as hostility and depression interact with both pathways—they influence how people choose their lifestyles and how they react to stress. An example of this is provided by hostility, a personality characteristic that has been shown to be a

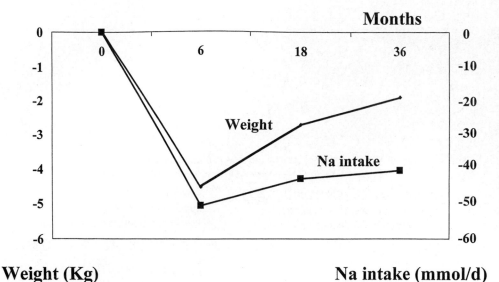

FIGURE 107-1 Changes of weight and sodium intake over a 3-year period in patients who were advised to reduce both, showing that the effects of a behavioral intervention commonly wear off with time. Data plotted from TOHP II trial.

risk factor for coronary heart disease (CHD). It is hypothesized that hostile persons show an exaggerated cardiovascular reactivity to stress, which contributes either to the development of atherosclerosis or may trigger an acute event (see below). Hostile persons are also more likely to smoke, and less likely to quit.[5]

While it is widely accepted that behavioral and lifestyle factors may play an important role in the development of coronary heart disease, most practicing cardiologists are not involved in the primary prevention of disease so much as in the treatment of existent disease. One factor that is not widely appreciated is how important the same lifestyle and psychological factors can be in influencing the progression of established coronary heart disease. To take one example of this, a study at the Mayo Clinic evaluated a cohort of 381 patients referred to a cardiac rehabilitation unit after hospitalization for an acute coronary event [e.g., unstable angina, myocardial infarction (MI), bypass surgery, or angioplasty]. In addition to the traditional risk factors, patients were evaluated for psychological distress (a term that includes elements such as depression and vital exhaustion). Over a 6-month follow-up period, it was found that persons high in psychological distress were three times more likely to be hospitalized for recurrent coronary events [odds ratio (OR) = 3.05]; other less powerful predictive factors included no previous bypass procedure (OR = 2.73), diabetes (OR = 2.65), and ejection fraction < 40 percent (OR = 1.98). Interestingly, smoking and the use of beta blockers did not predict relapse. A second example comes from a study of patients undergoing coronary angioplasty, after which new cardiac events occur in 20 to 30 percent of patients within 1 year. The study found that after controlling for standard risk factors, men who scored high on anger had a threefold increase in the rate of recurrent events compared with men with lower scores.[6]

BASIC PRINCIPLES OF BEHAVIORAL MEDICINE

It has long been recognized that knowledge alone is not sufficient motivation to change behavior.[7] A fundamental problem is that intervention studies commonly produce improvements in the behavior being manipulated lasting a few weeks or months, but by 1 year there is almost always relapse. An example is shown in Fig. 107-1 from the Trials of Hypertension Prevention,[8] in which patients were asked to reduce their weight or their salt intake.

Some of the basic principles that may be used to obtain sustained behavioral change can be illustrated by the example of dietary intervention, but the same principles also apply to other modalities such as smoking cessation and exercise.

As with other types of behavioral intervention, many dietary intervention studies have reported disappointing or at best modest lipid-lowering results, even when trained dietitians and knowledgeable health professionals are involved in the intervention process.[9,10] One reason for these disappointing results, however, is suggested by recent behavioral studies indicating that the method used to deliver dietary interventions may be less than optimal. Earlier intervention studies have typically applied a didactic, informative approach with little attention to what are now recognized as important differences in learning styles or levels of motivation to change behavior.[11] More recent behavioral models identify psychosocial factors that influence food choices and delineate the process of motivating changes in behavior.[12] Several behavioral models have evolved, and these are potentially additive. The "social learning theory" model incorporates behavioral modification methods that include cognitive, interpersonal, and environmental influences on behavior.[13] Basic components of this approach include self-monitoring and analysis of behavior; self-management including stimulus control of external cues; replacement of less desirable (i.e., high-fat foods) with more desirable behaviors; and reinforcement of desirable behaviors.[7] Strongly related is the construct of "self-efficacy,"[14] which refers to the person's degree of confidence that she or he has the ability to gain control over specific behaviors, such as eating and dieting. Increased self-efficacy has been found to be a critical element in motivation to engage in healthy behaviors.[14]

Over the past two decades, research on the "stages of change" model has yielded valuable insights regarding how, why, and when people will change their behavior.[15] This model suggests that behavioral change is achieved through a series of stages, defined as precontemplation, contemplation, preparation, action, and maintenance[16] (Table 107-1).

TABLE 107-1 Stages of Change

1. Precontemplation. Patient is not yet thinking about changing behavior
2. Contemplation. Patient is considering but is not yet ready to engage in behavior change
3. Preparation. Patient intends to take action in the next month
4. Action. Patient begins actual process of behavior change
5. Maintenance. Patient develops strategies to prevent relapse

Since most previous dietary intervention studies have applied approaches suitable for the action stage, it is not surprising that adherence has been disappointing. It is likely that many participants were overwhelmed, uncommitted, or simply not ready to adopt the recommended eating pattern.

Barriers to Behavioral Interventions and the Role of Collaborative Management of Patients with Heart Disease

A basic issue in the treatment of behavioral and lifestyle factors is the concept of collaborative management. Heart disease is usually chronic, and its successful management requires an active collaboration between the patient and health care providers. There is a big gap between the care prescribed and what is actually achieved. A classic example is the control of hypertension, where despite the availability of numerous powerful medications, blood pressure is adequately controlled in less than one-third of the patients.[17] Some of the barriers to the more successful implementation of recommended lifestyle and other changes are summarized in Table 107-2. These can be loosely categorized as relating to the patient, the physician, or the system.

Patients often lack the knowledge and motivation to make behavioral changes, and the training of cardiologists rarely includes anything to do with behavior or behavioral intervention. Physicians generally have a low expectation of the effectiveness of behavioral interventions and no particular incentive to implement them, let alone the time to do so. And because neither patients nor physicians have pressured the health care system to recognize the importance of making these changes, behavioral interventions are rarely reimbursed. However, recent (2002) changes in Medicare policy have for the first time introduced the possibility of reimbursing providers such as health psychologists for assessing and treating health behaviors related to medical diagnoses.

Despite these limitations, health care providers can and should use behavioral techniques to improve patients' self-care. These include contracting with the patient to reach specific goals; evaluating the patient's readiness for self-care; breaking self-care tasks down into small, manageable steps; providing personalized feedback to the patient; teaching the self-monitoring of health-related behaviors; enlisting social support; checking patient commitment to key tasks; and providing structure through follow-up appointments. One of the first tasks is to define the problem clearly. Physicians are usually concerned with items such as poor compliance and unhealthy lifestyle, while patients are more concerned about symptoms and emotional distress. Few physicians ask patients to identify the biggest problems they face in managing their illness.

Given the lack of training in behavioral techniques and the severe limitations on cardiologists' time, a team approach should ideally be employed. Behavioral interventions tend to require relatively large amounts of time, but nurses, psychologists, dietitians, and social workers can contribute to this. At the end of this chapter we discuss specific strategies that can easily be used by the physician to help patients make necessary changes in their behavior.

SMOKING CESSATION

Smoking kills more than 400,000 Americans every year, and more than half of these deaths are due to cardiovascular disease and stroke.[1] Smoking has for many years been recognized as one of the "big three" risk factors for cardiovascular disease (the others being hypertension and hyperlipidemia), and it is responsible for about 30 percent of cardiovascular morbidity and mortality.[18] Smoking more than doubles the incidence of coronary artery disease, and it increases mortality by 70 percent.[19] The economic cost of tobacco smoking has been estimated to be over $50 billion a year. The risks associated with smoking are almost completely reversible after a person quits,[20,21] and smoking cessation has been shown to be one of the most cost-effective interventions in the whole field of medicine.[22] In spite of this, smoking cessation programs are rarely reimbursed by health insurance programs.

AHRQ Guidelines

The science and effectiveness of smoking cessation programs has been reviewed extensively by the Agency for Healthcare Research and Quality (AHRQ; formerly the Agency for Health Care Policy and Research, or AHCPR), which issued its guidelines in 1996[18] and updated them in 2000.[23] The guidelines stress that health care clinics and cardiology practices are ideal settings for the promotion of smoking cessation. More than 70 percent of smokers report that they see a physician at least once a year.[24] The guidelines emphasize that a variety of effective strategies can be adopted, some very simple, others more complex. The recommended steps are summarized below.

- Identify the smokers. While this seems obvious, recent data show that only about 50 percent of smokers report ever having been asked by a physician if they smoked.[25] There is evidence that adding smoking status to the vital sign stamp on clinical records increases the likelihood that the physician will discuss smoking with the patient.
- Advise the smoker to quit—an intervention that takes 3 min at most. While this may seem trivial, an analysis of several studies has shown that the quit rate will increase from 7.9 to 10.2 percent, an increment that again may seem insubstantial, except that each smoker who quits will add up to 15 years to his or her life expectancy.[26] Moreover, this number will increase with each succeeding examination in which the physician advises the patient to quit.

TABLE 107-2 Barriers to Implementation of Behavioral Changes

Patient
  Lack of knowledge
  Lack of motivation
  Low self-efficacy (confidence in the ability to effect changes)
  Unreadiness to commit to behavior change
  Lack of access to care
  Social/cultural factors
Physician
  Time constraints
  Problem-based focus
  Perceived ineffectiveness of interventions
  Lack of behavioral skills
  Lack of incentives
Health care system
  Focus on acute care
  Failure to provide team approach
  Failure to provide reimbursement
  Lack of policies and standards

- Assess the smoker's willingness to quit and provide informational support appropriate to his or her readiness to quit (e.g., personalized information on why one should quit—for people who are not thinking of quitting; or reviewing treatment options for those ready to act).

- This step deals with the smoker who is unwilling to attempt to quit. It involves promoting the patient's readiness to quit and emphasizes the "four R's": personal *relevance* to the patient's medical and social situation; the *risks* associated with smoking; the *rewards* of quitting; and the *repetition* of a stop-smoking message. A good way of assessing a patient's readiness to quit is by using the stages of change model described earlier.[26] The important message here is that all smokers should be given advice about smoking, but the advice would be different according to the patient's stage of change.

- Develop a strategy that is chosen for the patient who is willing to quit.

A general rule is that "more is better," or that the quit rate is proportional to the amount of effort that is put in. For example, a 5- to 7-min brief counseling intervention using the counseling model suggested above increased cessation rates to 20 percent, over the 7 to 10 percent with advice alone.[27] The components, which are not mutually exclusive, include counseling, which has two basic components: providing social support, and boosting skills in problem solving. A state-funded telephone quitline to provide brief counseling services has also proved to be effective.[28] Other components include the use of nicotine replacement therapy, which can be delivered in a variety of ways, including gum, skin patches, and nasal sprays. A number of clinical trials have shown that the nicotine patches can double the quit rates.[29] Finally, the use of the antidepressant drug bupropion (Zyban) has also been found to be very effective. A recent study (published since the AHRQ guidelines were issued) found that bupropion also approximately doubled the quit rate[30] and that the best results were obtained with a combination of counseling, nicotine patch, and bupropion treatment.

Nicotine Gum and Patch

Since 1995, nicotine gum (Nicorette) and skin patches (Nicoderm, Nicotrol) have been approved as over-the-counter drugs. The gum is available as 2- or 4-mg doses, and it is recommended that one to two pieces be chewed per hour; the lower dose is for persons who smoke less than 25 cigarettes daily and the higher dose for those who smoke more. The regular dose is used for 6 weeks, followed by 6 weeks of tapering.

The labeling of the Nicotrol patch instructs patients to use the patch for 16 h/day for 6 weeks, with no tapering period. The Nicoderm CQ patch is used for 16 h/day at high dose (21 mg/day) for 6 weeks, followed by 14 mg/day for 2 weeks, and then 7 mg/day for 2 weeks. Both gum and patch have been subjected to several placebo-controlled clinical trials showing that the use of either leads to an approximate doubling of the quit rate.[31]

Nicotine Nasal Spray and Inhaler

The spray is available as a prescription drug (Nicotrol nasal spray) designed to deliver the nicotine more rapidly than the gum or patch. It is administered once or twice per hour for up to 3 months. Its use doubles the quit rate; side effects include sore throat and rhinitis, both of which are usually transient.[31] Another prescription formulation is the Nicotrol inhaler, which has pharmacokinetics similar to

those of the nicotine gum. Its effectiveness is comparable to that of the other nicotine replacement therapies.[31]

Bupropion

Bupropion was originally developed as an antidepressant, which proved not very effective. As an antismoking adjuvant, it is available in long-acting form as Zyban, which has been found also to lead to a doubling of the quit rate. The recommended dose is 300 mg/day, which is started 1 week before the quit date and continued for 7 to 12 weeks. It has been found to work equally well whether or not the smoker is depressed, suggesting that its antidepressant activity is not its primary mode of action.[32] Side effects include dry mouth and insomnia.

Reimbursement Issues

One of the reasons why so little attention is given to smoking cessation programs is that they are rarely reimbursed by insurance companies. A recent survey of managed care companies found that only 9 percent reimbursed the AHRQ recommendations fully, while another 39 percent reimbursed them partially, and 53 percent did not reimburse them at all.[33] Approximately half of the companies surveyed were not even aware of the existence of the guidelines. Whereas 54 percent of managed care organizations (MCOs) offered some self-help materials on smoking, only 17.6 percent provided reimbursement for bupropion use.

The almost total lack of reimbursement for smoking cessation programs stands in stark contrast to the unquestioned reimbursement for the treatment of the other two major risk factors for heart disease: hypertension and hyperlipidemia. Smoking cessation has been labeled "the gold standard of health care cost-effectiveness,"[22] and, as shown in Table 107-3, it is dramatically more cost-effective in terms of life-years saved (LYS) than treatment for hypertension or hyperlipidemia with medications.

One commonly given reason why smoking cessation is not more often reimbursed is that the benefits are delayed for about 5 to 10 years, which may be longer than the life span of many MCOs; hence there will be no net cost savings for the MCO resulting from the program. But this is a double standard: coronary bypass surgery and angioplasty are reimbursed routinely, and no one ever questions whether they reduce health care costs for the MCO, which clearly they do not.

TABLE 107-3 Cost-Effectiveness of Treatment of the Big Three Cardiovascular Risk Factors

Intervention	Cost per Life-Year Saved, $
Smoking cessation[a]	
Brief advice from physician	1000–3000
High intensity	6000–15,000
Treatment of hypertension[b]	11,000–72,000
Treatment of hyperlipidemia[c]	9000–297,000

SOURCE: [a]From Warner.[22] [b]From Edelson JT, Weinstein MC, Tosteson AN, et al. Long-term cost-effectiveness of various initial monotherapies for mild to moderate hypertension (see comments). *JAMA* 1990;266:407. [c]From Hay JW, Wittels EH, Gotto AMJ. An economic evaluation of lovastatin for cholesterol lowering and coronary artery disease reduction (see comments). *Am J Cardiol* 1991;67:789.

Barriers to Physician Intervention in Smokers

Why do so few physicians pay attention to smoking cessation? There are probably several reasons: First, physicians are not trained in behavioral techniques such as counseling, even though this is an activity to which they devote substantial time. They believe that their patients already know that smoking is harmful and that counseling is unlikely to have a significant effect. Second, the fact that it is not reimbursed automatically gives it a low priority. Thus it has been established that brief (3 min or so) counseling from a physician can double the spontaneous quit rate of smokers, which is about 2.5 percent per year. If a physician counsels 100 patients per year, 95 percent will continue to smoke—a dispiritingly large number. But of the 2.5 smokers who quit as a result of physician counseling, beyond the further 2.5 smokers who will quit spontaneously, one ex-smoker will avoid a premature smoking-related death and another will gain up to 15 years of life expectancy. The cost of this benefit will have been 3 h and 20 min of the physician's time.

DIETARY INTERVENTIONS

Dietary factors have a substantial impact on the development of cardiovascular disease (CVD). Many studies show that the intake of saturated fats and lipids is associated with increased rates of CVD-related death and all-cause mortality.[34,35] On the basis of epidemiologic and observational studies in men, women, African Americans, and elderly persons as well as postmortem angiographic studies in young persons, the National Institutes of Health (NIH) and the European Atherosclerosis Society have concluded that elevation of serum lipids is a causal factor in coronary artery disease.[35–37]

Low-density-lipoprotein cholesterol (LDL-C), like other components of the lipid profile, is affected by dietary interventions.[38] This has led to strong recommendations by the National Cholesterol Education Program (NCEP) that dietary counseling should form the basis of lipid-regulating regimens for both the prevention and clinical management of CVD.[39] Reductions in lipid levels are readily achievable through careful adherence to dietary changes.

Compared to pharmacologic intervention, dietary intervention has produced less net reduction in total cholesterol (TC) and LDL-C levels in randomized trials.[9,40,41] However, two recent secondary intervention trials comparing a Mediterranean diet rich in alpha-linolenic acid, one conducted in France,[42,43] and another in India[44] reported remarkably similar reductions in cardiac deaths over 2 to 5 years, approaching 50 percent. Only a small proportion of these patients were taking statins.

Comprehensive reviews of dietary intervention studies[10,37] lead to the conclusion that aggressive treatment with a diet low in total and saturated fats lowers serum lipids levels and produces positive angiographic changes as well as potentially helping to improve anginal and other non-lipid-related symptoms.

Reducing fat intake alone goes only so far, however. A recent review by Hu and Willett[45] proposed that at least three strategies are effective in preventing CHD: substituting nonhydrogenated unsaturated fats for saturated and *trans* fats; increasing consumption of omega-3 fatty acids; and consuming a diet high in fruits, vegetables, and grains. However, achieving and maintaining adherence to such a diet on a long-term basis remains a major challenge.

There is evidence that physicians can successfully counsel patients regarding dietary changes to lower lipids, but the counseling is effective in significantly changing patient outcomes only when there are office systems in place that assist and prompt the intervention.[46] Individual and group nutrition interventions can also be effective—although, as noted above, long-term adherence can be difficult.

On the basis of the cumulative scientific evidence from epidemiologic and controlled clinical trials, the NCEP advocated diet as the cornerstone of treatment in its reports on the Adult Treatment Panel as well as the Population Based Panel and Pediatric Panel.[39,47] In 1989, both the NCEP and the American Heart Association (AHA) announced populationwide recommendations for the Step I and Step II diets as the primary strategies for the prevention and treatment of high blood lipids.[39,48]

For hypertensive patients, the DASH (Dietary Approaches to Stop Hypertension) diet has been shown to be highly effective in lowering blood pressure,[49] particularly when combined with salt restriction.[50] This is basically a Mediterranean type of diet with the addition of low-fat dairy products to provide extra calcium. It also lowers total and LDL cholesterol,[51] but—in common with some other diets such as the Ornish diet—HDL cholesterol may also be reduced.[52]

National Cholesterol Education Program Guidelines

On the basis of the cumulative scientific evidence from epidemiologic and controlled clinical trials, the NCEP advocated diet as the cornerstone of treatment in its reports of the Adult Treatment Panel, as well as the Population Based Panel and Pediatric Panel reports.[39,47,53,54] In 1989, both the NCEP and the AHA announced populationwide recommendations for the Step I and Step II diets as the primary strategies for the prevention and treatment of high blood lipids.[39,48] The report published in 2001[54] introduced stricter guidelines than previously and emphasized the importance of four behavioral interventions: reduced intake of saturated fats and cholesterol, increased intake of plant sterols and fiber, weight reduction, and exercise. These are generally similar to the recommendations of Hu and Willett, summarized above.[45]

The past two decades have seen improvement in some aspects of the U.S. diet, and there have been corresponding declines in blood lipids levels.[11,55] Although the vast majority of U.S. adults still eat more than the recommended 30 percent of total calories as fat, there has been a major downward shift in total fat intake in the country as a whole.

Obesity and weight are increasing at epidemic rates, however, especially among young women and children.[37] This is due to other factors, such as levels of inactivity, and other aspects of the U.S. diet such as energy sources. Thus childhood obesity has been related both to watching television[56] and to the intake of sweetened drinks.[57] For example, a potential contributor is the low intake of total dietary fiber. The AHA recommends 25 to 30 g of dietary fiber a day from whole grains, vegetables, and fruits. Because people eat, on average, less than half of the recommended daily minimum of five servings of fruits and vegetables, intake of more energy-dense but nutrient-poor foods is the likely consequence.[37] It has been estimated that 52 million Americans are candidates for diet therapy to reduce high blood lipids; however, according to recent surveys, fewer than 10 percent have been prescribed such diets.[58,59]

OBESITY

Independent of the qualitative objectives of dietary adherence, obesity both directly and indirectly plays a major causal role in coronary heart disease (CHD) and stroke.[60] It contributes to dyslipidemia, diabetes, and hypertension, and its strong association with reduced physical activity further exacerbates CVD.[61–64] The prevalence of obesity has increased markedly in the United States and other countries in the past 20 years: in 1978, one-quarter of Americans were overweight (defined by a BMI between 25 and 30 kg/m^2); in 1990, one-third were overweight, representing an increase of 33 percent. The latest figures from the Centers for Disease Control and Prevention (CDC) show that 60 percent of Americans are now overweight. Similarly, the prevalence of obesity (defined as a BMI > 30 kg/m^2) increased from 12 percent in 1991 to 19 percent in 1999[60] and by 5.6 percent between 2000 and 2001.[61] It has been estimated that 300,000 deaths a year are attributable to obesity and that it accounts for nearly 10 percent of national health care costs.[65]

Excess body weight has been causally linked with deleterious changes in the lipoprotein profile.[62] Several studies document that lipoprotein abnormalities are induced with weight gain and reversed with weight loss.[66,67] Particularly in obese children, even small amounts of weight loss can result in dramatic normalization of the lipid profile.[67]

In sum, the research strongly suggests that a diet reduced in total and saturated fat, lipids, *trans* fatty acids, homocysteine, sodium, and excess calories and increased in dietary fiber (especially soluble fiber), antioxidants, folate, vitamin B$_6$, and omega-3 fatty acids will lower cardiovascular risk for most persons. The resulting dietary pattern is rich in fruits and vegetables, whole grains and cereals, low-fat and skim-milk dairy products, and fish, lean meats, and/or soy protein foods. Foods should be cooked without added saturated fat and, when necessary, cooked in a small amount of liquid vegetable oil, preferably olive, canola, or other monounsaturated nonhydrogenated liquid oils. Egg yolks should be limited to less than two per week.

Prevention and Treatment of Obesity

A 1985 NIH conference on Voluntary Methods for Weight Loss and Control concluded that most existing adult obesity interventions are ineffective, with one-third to two-thirds of the weight loss being regained in 1 year and almost all of the weight being regained within 5 years.[68] Training in calorie restriction and the use of packaged diet food are not effective long-term. The greatest success in treating obese adults has occurred with a combination of dietary fat restriction, behavioral skill development, and regular exercise.[69,70] Other effective strategies include family-oriented interventions and booster sessions.[71] The importance of exercise has been well demonstrated in a study of postmenopausal women, where a year-long program of modest exercise (mostly walking) resulted in a small but significant loss of weight and a more marked reduction of intraabdominal fat.[72] A number of diets such as the Atkins high-protein diet have become very popular, but their role remains uncertain.[73] Pharmacologic appetite suppressants and gene therapy may offer promising options in the future for some patients, but inevitably diet and energy balance must be addressed.

Practical Steps toward Achieving Dietary Adherence

In a review of 30 studies reporting changes in fat intake, Barnard et al.[74] summarized the factors commonly associated with increased adherence. These include the following:

- Stricter limits on fat intake: The lower the fat intake limit is set, the greater the degree of dietary change that is achieved.
- Frequent monitoring: At least monthly monitoring is recommended.
- Vegetarian diets: Use of a vegetarian diet more often achieved recommended fat intake than nonvegetarian approaches.

- Initial residential treatment: Attending a spa or similar facility that provides intensive training, monitoring, appropriate foods, and group support may result in better adherence to self-selected diets in the long term. However, this option may be impractical in many cases.
- Family involvement: Involvement by family members results in improved adherence.
- Group support: This is not mandatory, but it can be helpful.
- Providing food: Entire meals are not required, but some provision of acceptable products is important.
- Emphasis on symptomatic patients: These patients appear to be more motivated to comply with dietary regimens; healthy high-risk patients appear to be similarly motivated.

Relevant sources of total and saturated fat and lipids should be identified before attempting to prescribe a new dietary pattern for any patient. Two large-scale controlled clinical trials reported that meats, fats and oils, dairy products, and baked goods contributed more total and saturated fat to the diets of adults than any other food groups.[75,76] Fortunately, there are now many acceptable alternatives to these high-fat foods. Substitution of lower-fat or fat-free versions for the high-fat foods (e.g., skim milk for whole milk, fat-free salad dressing for full-fat salad dressing) and the addition of more servings of fruits, vegetables, and grains to compensate for fewer servings of high-fat meats, dairy products, and baked goods are essential components. The food industry has aggressively responded to the request for low- or no-fat foods. The greater challenge is achieving the desired shift to greater intake of complex carbohydrates.

On the basis of these behavioral principles and the accumulated knowledge about diet and risk reduction, Van Horn and Kavey[37] have made the following suggestions, which can help promote adherence to a healthy diet:

- Start with dietary assessment, then individualize the dietary intervention. Assessing baseline intake is the only way to identify the foods that are contributing the most saturated fat and lipids to a patient's diet. In adults, this is often meats, fats, and sweets. In children, it is often whole-milk dairy products. In children who consume the recommended four servings of dairy foods per day, it may be possible to achieve adherence to the Step I diet (≤10 percent saturated fats) simply by switching to skim-milk and low-fat dairy products at school and at home.
- Provide clear, identifiable goals for each person. For example, the current food labels make it possible to establish a fixed "fat-gram goal" rather than the less precise recommendations to derive less than 30 percent total calories from fat. It provides each person with an objective target he or she can monitor. Similarly, establishing the goal number of servings of fruits, vegetables, and grains can further help the individual to achieve an increased intake of fiber, folate, and antioxidants.
- Assess the current state of change and determine the person's level of confidence (self-efficacy) in achieving a self-determined adherence goal. Reassess the person's status at each subsequent visit.
- Encourage self-monitoring through the use of food records and/or other simplified fat/fiber goal-counting records. Likewise encourage nonfood self-rewards when goals are met.
- Promote the benefit of adopting other health-oriented behaviors. These include exercise, relaxation techniques, stress reduction, etc.
- Prevent relapse through ongoing follow-up, reassessment, and the establishment of new goals as needed.

- Patients who are referred to registered dietitians or other trained nutrition counselors may require relatively few follow-up sessions. Comprehensive feedback on dietary adherence can be provided to the referring physician by these other health professionals for consideration in determining future treatment plans.

EXERCISE

Physical inactivity is widely recognized as a major risk factor for CVD; numerous studies have shown that even mild exercise can reduce the probability of morbid events and even improve longevity. Only 22 percent of adults engage in 30 min or more of light to moderate exercise five or more times a week (the recommended amount for cardiovascular benefit).[77] Despite the fact that patients with cardiac disease are seen regularly by both cardiologists and primary care physicians, most physicians do not counsel their patients about physical activity.[78,79] One of the goals of the national Health Promotion Objectives for the year 2000 was to increase to at least 50 percent the number of primary care physicians who assess and advise their patients about exercise. The benefits of regular exercise are substantial and can be seen with several different types. Thus men who run for an hour or more a week have a 42 percent reduction of cardiovascular risk, those who train with weights for 30 min have a 23 percent reduction, and half an hour a day of brisk walking is associated with an 18 percent reduction.[80]

Two studies have investigated the efficacy of exercise counseling by physicians. Both used the stages of change model described above. One study (PACE, or Physician-based Assessment and Counseling for Exercise)[81] gave patients a brief questionnaire while in the waiting room to assess their readiness for change: precontemplation, or not intending to exercise; contemplation, or willing to consider becoming more active; and active, or already exercising. Physicians were given a manual describing the intervention and spent about 5 min describing it to the patient. There was also a 10-min follow-up call from a health educator. This simple intervention resulted in an approximate doubling in the number of minutes of walking per week in the intervention group (an average increase of 37 min) without any significant change in the controls. However, the participants in this study were followed for only 6 weeks. A second trial (PAL, or Physically Active for Life)[82] used a similar design and demonstrated a marginally significant positive effect at 6 weeks; however, the effect had disappeared when assessed at 8 months. One reason for the more disappointing results in PAL may have been that the participants were older (average age 65).

Whereas it is often recommended that exercise should occur in bouts of 30 min or so, there is evidence that shorter bouts can be as effective for improving cardiovascular fitness. One study[83] compared the effects of a single 30-min bout, three 10-min bouts, and bouts of 5 min or more totaling 30 min; it was found that all three produced roughly the same degree of improvement in blood pressure and body fat.

As with any form of behavioral intervention, there are a number of methods that encourage adherence to exercise regimens. The first is to educate and motivate patients on the benefits of exercise (moving them from precontemplation to contemplation). The second is to set reasonable goals, which can be increased gradually over time. It may be helpful for the patient and the interventionist to agree on a "behavioral contract," with a date set for achieving a particular goal. Self-monitoring is also helpful (keeping a log of daily activities, for example), as is feedback and reinforcement provided regularly to the participant. It is also important to identify barriers that may hinder

progress and to find ways to overcome these. For example, if a patient has no easy means of getting to a gym, a home exercise program can be recommended.

PSYCHOSOCIAL RISK FACTORS

Stress, depression, anger/hostility, type A behavior pattern, and anxiety have each been proposed as possible CVD risk factors.[84,85] Each construct is theoretically and operationally distinct from the other, and the empiric support for each as a CVD risk factor varies. Further, recent technology and animal experiments suggest that some of these psychosocial factors contribute to the pathogenesis of CVD, whereas others do not.[84]

Stress

When patients and lay persons are asked, stress is listed as one of the of the major factors causing heart disease, and stress is listed more frequently than high blood pressure and high lipids by these individuals.[86] Yet the investigation of stress as a CVD risk factor has been vexed by definitional difficulties. Since stress is essentially a subjective phenomenon, it has no precise definition, but the general concept is an adverse environment over which the individual has little or no control. Stress to the lay person typically encompasses, among other issues, work and family stress, social isolation, and the occurrence of recent acute and chronic life events. Work stress, defined as a combination of having low control over the way in which work is done but high work demands, has been implicated as a reliable and consistent predictor of progression of hypertension (in men but not in women),[87] carotid atherosclerosis,[88] as well as cardiac events and death.[89] Other theorists in this area have argued that work stress is better assessed as low job control, and this index of work stress has also been found to predict future cardiac events.[90,91] Marital stress (but not work stress) has been reported to worsen the prognosis of women with CHD, whereas the opposite may be true of men.[92]

Social isolation (few friends, family, or close others) and perceived lack of social support have consistently been found to predict acute MI and cardiac death. The relative risks in 15 recent studies indicate a threefold mortality risk for CVD patients who are socially isolated and/or perceive poor social support (reviewed in Ref. 84).

Acute mental stress (such as the sudden loss of a loved one or being caught in an earthquake) has consistently been shown in epidemiologic studies to provoke silent myocardial ischemia and predict increased CVD incidence and death.[93,94]

Depression

Depressive symptoms and disorders predict recurrent cardiac events and mortality, with relative risk ranging from 2.6 to 7.8 in cardiac patients.[95–98] These risk ratios remain when all other known predictors of MI recurrence are controlled for, and depressive symptoms predict MI recurrence in a dose-response fashion. Thus, there is considerable evidence that a cardiac patient who is depressed is at substantially higher risk for a future event. There is extensive evidence that depression, both clinical and subclinical, predicts the initial development of CHD[99] and the recurrence of cardiac events in patients who have experienced an MI,[98,100] unstable angina,[101] or coronary bypass surgery.[102] At this stage, it is not yet clear whether treatment of depression will reduce the risk of recurrent events.

Anxiety

There have been fewer investigations of the relation of anxiety to cardiac disease and recurrence.[96,97,103–105] Most studies of anxiety disorders have examined the increased occurrence of CVD mortality in psychiatric patients known to have some type of anxiety disorder,[106–109] although some small recent studies have found a relation between anxiety and sudden cardiac death in CVD patients.[84,110–112] However, anxiety symptoms are not associated with MI recurrence in these studies. Rozanski and others[84,97,103,104,113] hypothesize that anxiety disorders and the associated symptoms may cause an alteration in cardiac autonomic tone through impaired vagal control, reduced heart rate variability, or both to cause increased risk of sudden cardiac death in cardiac patients. Apart from the direct impact of anxiety on morbidity and mortality, the clinician should be alert to the presence of panic disorder in patients with CVD because of their effect on quality of life. Because many of the symptoms of panic disorder can mimic symptoms of CVD, patients with CVD can develop a particularly heightened sense of vigilance and distress in response to anxiety symptoms.[114] Further discussion of the role of anxiety and related disorders can be found in Chap. 91.

Type A Behavior Pattern

Friedman and Rosenman[115] first proposed that a constellation of competitive, hostile, time-pressured behaviors constituted a personality trait ("type A") that predisposed patients to CVD. Although the Western Collaborative Group study found a twofold risk for CVD and a fivefold risk for recurrence of MI among those categorized as type A-B, several more recent studies have failed to find such a difference.[116] Many theorists have suggested that hostility, or the tendency to view others with suspicion and skepticism, may be the toxic component of the type A behavior pattern and that this component should be evaluated independently for its prediction of increased risk in cardiac patients. Four small studies of CVD patients have found that the presence of high hostility is associated with more rapid progression of atherosclerosis, more ischemia, a faster rate of restenosis after angioplasty, and a higher probability of recurrent MI.[6,117–120]

Psychosocial Interventions

Given the emphasis that CVD patients place on stress and psychosocial factors contributing to their disease—as well as some of the recent evidence suggesting that psychosocial factors predict CVD recurrence and death—offering psychosocial interventions for CVD patients seems reasonable. However, there are many different types of interventions aimed at different psychosocial factors and different outcomes.

Linden and others[121] recently conducted a metaanalysis on 23 controlled psychosocial interventional studies. All patients were receiving standard medical and surgical care and most were additionally receiving standard cardiac rehabilitation interventions. For follow-up periods of less than 2 years, there was a 41 percent reduction in mortality and a 46 percent reduction in MI recurrence as a result of psychosocial interventions. There were also significant and clinically meaningful reductions in measures of psychosocial distress (such as depression and anxiety) and in cardiovascular risk factors such as elevated blood pressure and lipid levels. Only three randomized trials reported results for more than 2 years of follow-up, and in none of these did the effects of psychosocial intervention on mortality or MI recurrence remain significant.

Two large, recently published studies of psychosocial interventions deserve special comment. In 1989, Frasure-Smith and Prince reported favorable survival results for post-MI patients ($N = 229$) who received a home- and telephone-based nursing intervention to monitor stress.[122] As a result of this outcome, a larger randomized trial of a similar intervention was conducted ($N = 1376$). In this trial the program had no impact on overall survival, and there was increased cardiac and all-cause mortality in elderly women. In the second study, Jones and West[123] conducted a randomized controlled psychological interventional trial in 2328 post-MI patients; they also found no difference in cardiac event recurrence and mortality at 12 months of follow-up.

There are two important features of these two studies that may explain their negative results. First, neither one actually achieved the objective of significantly reducing stress. Second, neither study screened patients to determine if they in fact exhibited any symptoms of stress or of the psychological factor that was being targeted by the intervention. Frasure-Smith[124] conducted a reanalysis of her original nursing intervention and reported that only those patients who reported distress during hospitalization benefited from the psychosocial intervention, consistent with our speculation that those not at risk for psychosocial difficulties will not benefit from a psychosocial intervention. However, firm conclusions about the efficacy of psychosocial interventions in cardiac patients awaits larger randomized trials that target those at risk. Such a trial has recently been funded by NIH (the ENRICHD trial)[124a] and examined the efficacy of cognitive-behavioral interventions on cardiac, psychosocial, and CVD risk-factor outcomes in socially isolated and/or depressed post-MI patients. The results revealed that while the intervention was moderately effective at improving social support in some patients, these improvements did not result in a better prognosis. However, a more encouraging result was obtained with a trial of an antidepressant drug (sertraline) in patients who had experienced acute cardiac syndromes; the outcome was generally favorable, although the study was not powered to detect differences in morbidity.[125]

MULTIPLE RISK FACTORS

It is clear that the behavioral and psychosocial risk factors for CVD are not distributed evenly across the population.[126] Many patients present with a cluster of behavioral risk factors that interact to multiply the risk for atherothrombosis. The most prominent example of this is the metabolic syndrome, which might be termed "the American disease," which has been estimated to be present in 57 million Americans[127] and is associated with a nearly threefold increase in cardiovascular mortality, even after adjusting for risk factors such as smoking and elevated levels of LDL-C (see also Chap. 87).[128] The clinical management of these patients is a daunting challenge. It is often difficult to know where to start, and there is little guidance in this process from randomized controlled trials.[129] Many clinicians would suggest that if the patient is a smoker, the risk reduction gained from changing that behavior is the quickest and greatest. However, clinical experience suggests that this is not always a successful strategy. One study in a work-site population of middle-aged adults suggests that exercise may be an excellent "gateway" behavioral change that may facilitate other subsequent changes involving smoking and diet,[130] and there is support from the weight management literature on the value of exercise as a starting point.[131] The best clinical rule of thumb is to conduct a thorough assessment of the patient's behavioral and psychosocial issues and to engage in a conversation with the patient regarding the prioritizing changes in risk behavior and devising a strategy and a follow-up plan. While such a comprehensive assessment is beyond the scope of traditional cardiology practice, it may be feasible with a team approach including psychologists, nurses, exercise specialists, and nutritionists. Such a program can also form the basis for cardiac rehabilitation after a cardiac event or for services in the setting of secondary prevention.

CLINICAL IMPLICATIONS

Although there is a dearth of large, randomly assigned psychosocial interventions showing any effect on cardiac outcomes in patients with CHD, there is ample evidence that improvement in psychosocial functioning can be obtained by standardized, empirically supported therapeutic protocols administered by mental health professionals to patients who are at psychosocial risk. Improving the quality of life and decreasing the psychological distress of cardiac patients may also have other benefits. First, many of the mechanisms proposed to account for the association between psychosocial factors and CVD are behavioral. Thus, decreasing depressive symptoms is hypothesized to decrease smoking rates, increase engagement in physical activity, and improve dietary habits.[132] Second, decreasing psychosocial distress is thought to increase patient compliance with physicians' recommendations, but the testing of these behavioral mechanisms, as well as the pathophysiological mechanisms addressed elsewhere, again awaits larger, controlled trials.

Cardiologists should be aware of psychosocial risk factors present in their patients. Asking about social support and recent symptoms of depression will mark patients at increased risk of event recurrence or death. Referring such patients to mental health specialists for further diagnostic and intervention investigations may improve these patients' quality of life and behavioral risk factor profile if not their cardiac outcome.

COST IMPLICATIONS

Thorough cost-effectiveness and cost-offset analyses are now being conducted in some of the recent psychosocial trials. For example, the average cost of adding a behavioral intervention to the treatment of a cardiac patient in one study was $790.[133] The longest and most comprehensive psychosocial intervention (for reducing type A behavior), the Recurrent Coronary Care Project in California, showed that MI recurrence decreases for the intervention patients, but treatment required an average of 58 h per patient. This amount of therapy delivered in group format, as occurred in this trial, would cost on average $1200 per patient.

COMPLIANCE: THE KEY TO SUCCESSFUL INTERVENTIONS

The evidence for the interventional strategies reviewed in this chapter points to the inescapable conclusion that a change in lifestyle will significantly reduce the risk for CVD. No matter how efficacious the interventional strategy, however, it is doomed to failure unless the patient complies with the requirements of the intervention. Nonadherence crosses treatment regimens, age/gender groups, and socioeconomic strata; moreover, it varies across the treatment course.[134–137] Thus, persons are asked to change their diets, eat less, exercise more, quit smoking, reduce the amount of stress they experience, and change the ways in which they express their anger. These changes are difficult. Knowledge of the risks is clearly insufficient to produce

changes; most people know by now that smoking is bad for them, that their diets could be improved, and so on. Moreover, these negative behaviors are reinforcing in their own right. Smoking is pleasurable, as is the avoidance of nicotine withdrawal; high-fat foods taste good; exercise is time-consuming and may be boring or even painful for many individuals. Coping with stress and anger means having to examine our lives in ways that may be unpleasant and even traumatic for many. Thus, poor health habits, which may have been reinforced over the course of a lifetime, are very resistant to change. Clearly, it is vitally important to begin establishing healthy behavior habits early in life; yet parents and teachers themselves often provide poor models for these behaviors, having been acculturated in a time when such concerns were virtually nonexistent.

Much of the adherence problem occurs early in treatment. It is estimated that 50 percent of persons discontinue participation in cardiac rehabilitation programs within the first year.[138] The smoking cessation literature reports that 70 percent of posttreatment relapses occurred in the first 4 months.[139] Not only are early adherence problems likely, but early adherence rates are also predictive of longer-term adherence.[136,139–141]

The primary care physician and cardiologist can play a major role in helping their patients to alter poor health habits and establish healthy behaviors. The physician is regarded by many patients as an authority figure and can therefore have a large impact on behavioral change.[142] In addition, the physician can refer patients to other health professionals, such as nutrition and exercise counselors as well as stress- and anger-management therapists. But this often fails to occur for a number of reasons. First, while most physicians are undoubtedly aware of the importance of healthy behaviors, they may be convinced that patients will simply not engage in them. Or the physician may not be aware of how to suggest such changes or to whom to refer these patients. Second, given the current reimbursement climate, many physicians have only a very few minutes to spend with each patient.

The fact is, a great deal is now known about how to maximize the likelihood that patients will adhere to behavioral regimens designed to improve their health. An excellent review by Burke and colleagues provides a great deal of detail concerning these[143]; a brief summary is provided below. It briefly describes strategies that have been shown to improve compliance with CVD behavioral intervention strategies.

- Signed agreements: A written contract is drawn up between the patient and the physician or other health professional, in which a specific set of behaviors to be followed by the patient is agreed on. These behaviors should be outlined as specifically as possible (e.g., number of calories per day, number of servings of fruits and vegetables per day, number of minutes of cardiovascular-strengthening exercise, number of hours of stress-reduction therapy). Behavioral logs should be maintained by the patient.
- Behavioral skill training: Patients can attend classes that teach healthy cooking, proper stretching techniques before and after exercise, or how to respond to an anger-provoking situation. Patients may have the desire to engage in healthy behaviors, but without the skills, they will tend to fall back on their old, destructive habits.
- Self-monitoring: Many patients are truly unaware of the extent to which they engage in certain unhealthy behaviors. It is useful to have them monitor the number of cigarettes they smoke, their daily intake of fat (current packaging requirements make this relatively easy), and so on. The first step in changing behavior is to establish a baseline, so that the patient can see improvements.

- Self-efficacy enhancement: Patients' confidence in their ability to engage in a particular behavior, such as eating in more healthy ways or exercising with a specified frequency, has been shown to be an important factor in their motivation to engage in these behaviors. Self-monitoring, discussed above, provides a baseline level and can then be a means of documenting improvement. Even small changes will increase the patient's self-efficacy for a given behavior, so that she or he is motivated to continue, which will produce additional positive change, which then enhances self-efficacy even more, and so on. The physician or other health professional can focus on such improvement as a means of further enhancing the patient's self-efficacy for behavior change.
- Telephone/mail contact: Such reminders have been shown to have a positive effect on compliance.
- Spousal/social support: A great deal of research shows that others in the patient's social environment can have a dramatic impact on compliance. In discussing behavioral change with the patient, it is helpful for such a supportive person to be present as well. If an exercise and/or diet regimen is agreed on, possibly using a contract, as described above, having a supportive person participate will significantly enhance the likelihood that the patient will stay with the program. Conversely, when an immediate other, such as a spouse, continues to pursue her or his own unhealthy behavior patterns—such as continuing to smoke or to express anger in an abusive or otherwise unhealthy manner—the possibility for change on the patient's part will be hindered.
- Stages of change: Earlier, we discussed the fact that different people may be at different stages of readiness to change their behavior.[144] Thus, one patient may be ready only to begin discussing the need to stop smoking, while another may actually be ready to quit. The research shows that it is helpful to tailor advice to the patient's current stage of readiness. The techniques described above are clearly additive; more than one may be usefully combined to help the patient comply. It is also clear that, in trying, many patients will fail. However, it is worth noting that a patient cannot quit smoking until he or she first *tries* to quit. Thus efforts to produce this behavior are a good investment of the physician's time.
- Professional support: We strongly recommend that primary care physicians develop a network of health care professionals who can support their efforts and to whom patients can be referred for help with specific interventional strategies.

We are a long way from eliminating the need for medication and surgical intervention for CVD. However, we are further along this path than we were only a relatively short time ago. By advocating such strategies, prescribing them, discussing them with patients, and referring patients to other health professionals, a substantial proportion of the need for more traditional interventions can be eliminated.

CONCLUSIONS

The potential applications of behavioral techniques in cardiology are enormous and largely unrealized. In principle they can help to prevent the onset of disease, to treat it once established, and to be used in conjunction with virtually any other kind of treatment. In practice few cardiologists have either the time or the interest to pay much attention to them, despite the demonstrated efficacy of many programs. Future success depends on better education of physicians, incorporation of a team approach, and recognition of the value of behavioral interventions by third-party payers.

ACKNOWLEDGMENTS

Preparation of this manuscript was supported by American Heart Association Grant 9750544N and National Institutes of Health/National Heart, Lung, and Blood Institute Grants HL47540 and HL67439.

References

1. McGinnis JM, Foege WH. Actual causes of death in the United States. *JAMA* 1993;270(18):2207–2212.
2. Fries JF, Koop CE, Beadle CE, et al. Reducing health care costs by reducing the need and demand for medical services. The Health Project Consortium (see comments). *N Engl J Med* 1993;329(5):321–325.
3. Notzon FC, Komarov YM, Ermakov SP, et al. Causes of declining life expectancy in Russia. *JAMA* 1998;279(10):793–800.
4. Hakim AA, Petrovitch H, Burchfiel CM, et al. Effects of walking on mortality among nonsmoking retired men (see comments). *N Engl J Med* 1998;338(2):94–99.
5. Lipkus IM, Barefoot JC, Williams RB, Siegler IC. Personality measures as predictors of smoking initiation and cessation in the UNC Alumni Heart Study. *Health Psychol* 1994;13(2):149–155.
6. De Leon CFM, Kop WJ, de Swart HB, et al. Psychosocial characteristics and recurrent events after percutaneous transluminal coronary angioplasty. *Am J Cardiol* 1996;77:252–255.
7. Glanz K. Nutrition education for risk factor reduction and patient education: A review. *Prev Med* 1999;14:721–752.
8. Effects of weight loss and sodium reduction intervention on blood pressure and hypertension incidence in overweight people with high-normal blood pressure. The Trials of Hypertension Prevention, phase II. The Trials of Hypertension Prevention Collaborative Research Group (see comments). *Arch Intern Med* 1997;157(6): 657–667.
9. Walden CE, Retzlaff BM, Buck BL, et al. Lipoprotein lipid response to the National Cholesterol Education Program Step II diet by hypercholesterolic and combined hyperlipidemic women and men. *Arterioscler Thromb Vasc Biol* 1997;17:375–382.
10. Kromhout D, Menotti A, Kesteloot H, Sans S. Prevention of coronary heart disease by diet and lifestyle: Evidence from prospective cross-cultural, cohort, and intervention studies. *Circulation* 2002;105(7): 893–898.
11. Buefel RR. Assessment of the U.S diet in national nutrition surveys: National collaborative efforts and NHANES. *Am J Clin Nutr* 1994;59 (suppl):1645–1675.
12. Glanz K, Eriksen MP. Individual and community models for dietary behavior change. *J Nutrition Ed* 1993;25:80–86.
13. Bandura A. *Social Foundations of Thought and Action: A Social Cognitive Theory.* Englewood Cliffs, NJ: Prentice-Hall; 1986.
14. Bandura A. *Self-Efficacy: The Exercise of Control.* New York: Freeman;1997.
15. Prochaska JO, DiClemente CC. Transtheoretical therapy: Toward a more integrative model of change. *Psychotherapy Theory Res Pract* 1982;19:276–288.
16. Prochaska JO, DiClemente CC, Norcross JC. In search of how people change: Applications to addictive behaviors. *Am Psychol* 1992;47: 1102–1114.
17. The sixth report of the Joint National Committee on Prevention, Detection, Evaluation, and Treatment of High Blood Pressure. *Arch Intern Med* 1997;157(21):2413–2446.
18. Fiore MC, Jorenby DE, Baker TB. Smoking cessation: Principles and practice based upon the AHCPR Guideline, 1996. Agency for Health Care Policy and Research. *Ann Behav Med* 1997;19(3):213–219.
19. Weintraub WS, Klein LW, Seelaus PA, et al. Importance of total life consumption of cigarettes as a risk factor for coronary artery disease. *Am J Cardiol* 1985;55(6):669–672.
20. Rosenberg L, Kaufman DW, Helmrich SP, Shapiro S. The risk of myocardial infarction after quitting smoking in men under 55 years of age. *N Engl J Med* 1985;313(24):1511–1514.

21. Gordon T, Kannel WB, McGee D, Dawber TR. Death and coronary attacks in men after giving up cigarette smoking. A report from the Framingham study. *Lancet* 1974;2(7893):1345–1348.

22. Warner KE. Smoking out the incentives for tobacco control in managed care settings. *Tob Control* 1998;7(suppl):S50–S54.

23. Fiore MC. US Public Health Service Clinical Practice Guideline: Treating tobacco use and dependence. *Respir Care* 2000;45(10): 1200–1262.

24. Tomar SL, Husten CG, Manley MW. Do dentists and physicians advise tobacco users to quit? *J Am Dent Assoc* 1996;127(2):259–265.

25. Anda RF, Remington PL, Sienko DG, Davis RM. Are physicians advising smokers to quit? The patient's perspective. *JAMA* 1987; 257(14):1916–1919.

26. Prochaska JO, Di Clemente CC, Velicer WF, Rossi JS. Standardized, individualized, interactive, and personalized self-help programs for smoking cessation. *Health Psychol* 1993;12(5):399–405.

27. Ockene JK. Smoking among women across the life span: Prevalence, interventions, and implications for cessation research. *Ann Behav Med* 1993;15:135–148.

28. McDonald HP, Garg AX, Haynes RB. Interventions to enhance patient adherence to medication prescriptions: Scientific review. *JAMA* 2002; 288(22):2868–2879.

29. Silagy C, Mant D, Fowler G, Lodge M. Meta-analysis on efficacy of nicotine replacement therapies in smoking cessation. *Lancet* 1994; 343(8890):139–142.

30. Jorenby DE, Leischow SJ, Nides MA, et al. A controlled trial of sustained-release bupropion, a nicotine patch, or both for smoking cessation. *N Engl J Med* 1999;340(9):685–691.

31. Hughes JR, Goldstein MG, Hurt RD, Shiffman S. Recent advances in the pharmacotherapy of smoking. *JAMA* 1999;281(1):72–76.

32. Hayford KE, Patten CA, Rummans TA, et al. Efficacy of bupropion for smoking cessation in smokers with a former history of major depression or alcoholism. *Br J Psychiatry* 1999;174:173–178.

33. McPhillips-Tangum C. Results from the first annual survey on addressing tobacco in managed care. *Tob Control* 1998;(7 suppl): S11–S13.

34. Keys A. *Seven Countries: A Multivariate Analysis of Death and Coronary Heart Disease.* Cambridge, MA: Harvard University Press; 1980.

35. Levine G, Keaney J, Vita J. Cholesterol reduction in cardiovascular disease. *N Engl J Med* 1995;332:512–521.

36. Lipid Research Clinics Program. The Lipid Research Clinics Coronary Primary Prevention Trial results: I. Reduction in incidence of coronary heart disease. *JAMA* 1984;251:351–364.

37. Van Horn L, Kavey RE. Diet and cardiovascular disease prevention: What works? *Ann Behav Med* 1997;19:197–212.

38. Greenland P, Hayman L. Making cardiovascular disease prevention a reality. *Ann Behav Med* 1997;19:193–196.

39. National Cholesterol Education Program. *Report of the Expert Panel on Population Strategies for Blood Cholesterol Reduction.* DHHS Publication No. (NIH) 90-30-46. Bethesda, MD: U.S. Department of Health and Human Services, Public Health Service, National Institutes of Health, National Heart, Lung and Blood Institute; 1990.

40. Holme I. An analysis of randomized trials evaluating the effect of cholesterol reduction on total mortality and coronary heart disease incidence. *Circulation* 1990;82:1916–1924.

41. Randomized trial of cholesterol lowering in 4,444 patients with coronary heart disease: Scandinavian Simvastatin Survival Study (4S). *Lancet* 1994;344:1383–1389.

42. de Lorgeril M, Renaud S, Mamelle N, et al. Mediterranean alpha-linolenic acid–rich diet in secondary prevention of coronary heart disease. *Lancet* 1994;343:1454–1459.

43. Renaud S, de Lorgeril M, Delaye J, et al. Cretan Mediterranean diet for prevention of coronary heart disease. *Am J Clin Nutr* 1995;61(suppl): 1360S–1367S.

44. Singh RB, Dubnov G, Niaz MA, et al. Effect of an Indo-Mediterranean diet on progression of coronary artery disease in high-risk patients (Indo-Mediterranean Diet Heart Study): A randomised single-blind trial. *Lancet* 2002;360(9344):1455–1461.

45. Hu FB, Willett WC. Optimal diets for prevention of coronary heart disease. *JAMA* 2002;288(20):2569–2578.

46. Ockene IS, Hebert JR, Ockene JK, et al. Effect of physician-delivered nutrition counseling training and an office-support program on saturated fat intake, weight, and serum lipid measurements in a hyperlipidemic population: Worcester Area Trial for Counseling in Hyperlipidemia (WATCH). *Arch Intern Med* 1999;159(7): 725–731.

47. Expert Panel on Detection Evaluation and Treatment of High Blood Cholesterol in Adults. Summary of the Second Report of the National Cholesterol Education Program (NCEP) Expert Panel on Detection, Evaluation, and Treatment of High Blood Cholesterol in Adults (Adult Treatment Panel II). *JAMA* 1993;269:3015–3023.

48. LaRosa JC, Hunninghake D, Bush D, et al. The cholesterol facts: A summary of the evidence relating dietary facts, serum cholesterol, and coronary heart disease: A joint statement by the American Heart Association and the National Heart, Lung, and Blood Institute. *Circulation* 1990;81:1721–1733.

49. Appel LJ, Moore TJ, Obarzanek E, et al. A clinical trial of the effects of dietary patterns on blood pressure. DASH Collaborative Research Group (see comments). *N Engl J Med* 1997;336(16):1117–1124.

50. Sacks FM, Svetkey LP, Vollmer WM, et al. Effects on blood pressure of reduced dietary sodium and the Dietary Approaches to Stop Hypertension (DASH) diet. DASH-Sodium Collaborative Research Group. *N Engl J Med* 2001;344(1):3–10.

51. Obarzanek E, Sacks FM, Vollmer WM, et al. Effects on blood lipids of a blood pressure–lowering diet: The Dietary Approaches to Stop Hypertension (DASH) Trial. *Am J Clin Nutr* 2001;74(1):80–89.

52. Ornish D, Brown SE, Scherwitz LW, et al. Lifestyle changes and heart disease. *Lancet* 1990;336(8717):741–742.

53. Expert Panel on Detection Evaluation and Treatment of High Blood Cholesterol in Adults. Summary of the Second Report of the National Cholesterol Education Program (NCEP) Expert Panel on Detection, Evaluation, and Treatment of High Blood Cholesterol in Adults (Adult Treatment Panel II). *JAMA* 1993;269:3015–3023.

54. Executive Summary of The Third Report of The National Cholesterol Education Program (NCEP) Expert Panel on Detection, Evaluation, And Treatment of High Blood Cholesterol In Adults (Adult Treatment Panel III). *JAMA* 2001;285(19):2486–2497.

55. Nationwide Food Consumption Survey. *Continuing Survey of Food Intake by Individuals: Women 19–50 Years and Children 1–5 Years, 4 Days.* Washington, DC: U.S. Department of Agriculture, Human Nutrition Information Service; 1996.

56. Gortmaker SL, Must A, Sobol AM, et al. Television viewing as a cause of increasing obesity among children in the United States, 1986–1990. *Arch Pediatr Adolesc Med* 1996;150(4):356–362.

57. Ludwig DS, Peterson KE, Gortmaker SL. Relation between consumption of sugar-sweetened drinks and childhood obesity: A prospective, observational analysis. *Lancet* 2001; 357(9255):505–508.

58. Sempos C, Cleeman J, Carroll M, et al. Prevalence of high blood cholesterol among U.S. adults. *JAMA* 1993;269:3009–3014.

59. Schucker B, Wittes JT, Santanello NC, et al. Change in cholesterol awareness and action: Results from national physician and public surveys. *Arch Intern Med* 1991;151(4):666–673.

60. Mokdad AH, Serdula MK, Dietz WH, et al. The continuing epidemic of obesity in the United States. *JAMA* 2000;284(13):1650–1651.

61. Mokdad AH, Ford ES, Bowman BA, et al. Prevalence of obesity, diabetes, and obesity-related health risk factors, 2001. *JAMA* 2003; 289(1):76–79.

62. Denke MA, Sempos CT, Grundy SM. Excess body weight: An under-recognized contributor to high blood cholesterol levels. *Arch Intern Med* 1993;153:1093–1103.

63. Medalie JH, Papier CM, Goldbourt U, Herman JB. Major factors in the development of diabetes mellitus in 10,000 men. *Arch Intern Med* 1975;135:811–817.

64. Tobian L. Hypertension and obesity. *N Engl J Med* 1978;298:46–60.

65. Hubert HB, Feinleib M, McNamara PM, Castelli WP. Obesity as an independent risk factor for cardiovascular disease: A 26-year follow-up

of participants in the Framingham Heart Study. *Circulation* 1983; 67(5):968–977.

66. Wood PD, Stefanick ML, Williams PT, Haskell WL. The effects on plasma lipoprotein of a prudent weight-reducing diet, with or without exercise, in overweight men and women. *N Engl J Med* 1988;319: 1173–1179.

67. Becque MD, Katch VL, Rocchini AP, et al. Coronary risk incidence of obese adolescents: Reduction by exercise plus diet intervention. *Pediatrics* 1988;81:605–612.

68. Health implications of obesity. National Institutes of Health Consensus Development Conference Statement. *Ann Intern Med* 1985;103(Pt 2): 1073–1077.

69. O'Leary KD, Wilson GT. *Behavior Therapy: Application and Outcome.* Englewood Cliffs, NJ: Prentice Hall; 1975.

70. Brownell KD, Heckerman C, Westlake R. The behavior control: A descriptive analysis of a large scale program. *J Clin Psychol* 1979;35:864.

71. Garner D, Wooley S. Confronting the failure of behavior and dietary treatments for obesity. *Clin Psychol Rev* 1991;11:729–780.

72. Irwin ML, Yasui Y, Ulrich CM, et al. Effect of exercise on total and intra-abdominal body fat in postmenopausal women: A randomized controlled trial. *JAMA* 2003;289(3):323–330.

73. Pickering TG. Diet wars: From Atkins to the zone. Who is right? *J Clin Hypertens (Greenwich)* 2002;4(2):130–133.

74. Barnard N, Akhtar A, Nicholson A. Factors that facilitate compliance to lower fat intake. *Arch Fam Med* 1995;4:153–158.

75. Tinker L, Burrows E, Henry H, et al. The Women's Health Initiative: Overview of the nutrition components. In: Krummel D, Kris-Etherton P, eds. *Nutrition in Women's Health.* Gaithersburg, MD: Aspen Publications; 1996:510–542.

76. Dolecek TA, Milas NC, Van Horn LV, et al. A long-term nutrition intervention experience: Lipid responses and dietary adherence patterns in the Multiple Risk Factor Intervention Trial (MRFIT). *J Am Diet Assoc* 1986;86:752–758.

77. US Department of Health and Human Services. *Healthy People 2000: National Health Promotion and Disease Prevention Objectives.* DHHS Publication No. (PHS) 91-50212. Washington, DC: U.S. Department of Health and Human Services; 1990.

78. Wells KB, Lewis CE, Leake B, et al. The practices of general and subspecialty internists in counseling about smoking and exercise. *Am J Public Health* 1986;76(8):1009–1013.

79. Orleans CT, George LK, Houpt JL, Brodie KH. Health promotion in primary care: A survey of U.S. family practitioners. *Prev Med* 1985; 14(5):636–647.

80. Tanasescu M, Leitzmann MF, Rimm EB, et al. Exercise type and intensity in relation to coronary heart disease in men. *JAMA* 2002;288(16):1994–2000.

81. Calfas KJ, Long BJ, Sallis JF, et al. A controlled trial of physician counseling to promote the adoption of physical activity. *Prev Med* 1996;25(3):225–233.

82. Goldstein MG, Pinto BM, Lynn H, et al. Physician-based physical activity counseling for middle-aged and older adults: A randomized trial. *Ann Behav Med* 1999;21:40–47.

83. Coleman KJ, Raynor HR, Mueller DM, et al. Providing sedentary adults with choices for meeting their walking goals. *Prev Med* 1999;28(5):510–519.

84. Rozanski A, Blumenthal JA, Kaplan J. Impact of psychological factors on the pathogenesis of cardiovascular disease and implications for therapy. *Circulation* 1999;99(16):2192–2217.

85. Bosma H, Peter R, Siegrist J, Marmot M. Two alternative job stress models and the risk of coronary heart disease. *Am J Public Health* 1998;88(1):68–74.

86. Kirkland SA, MacLean DR, Langille DB, et al. Knowledge and awareness of risk factors for cardiovascular disease among Canadians 55 to 74 years of age: Results from the Canadian Heart Health Surveys, 1986–1992. *Can Med Assoc J* 1999;161(8 suppl):S10–S16.

87. Schnall PL, Schwartz JE, Landsbergis PA, et al. A longitudinal study of job strain and ambulatory blood pressure: Results from a three-year follow-up. *Psychosom Med* 1998;60(6):697–706.

88. Lynch J, Krause N, Kaplan GA, et al. Work place demands, economic reward, and progression of carotid atherosclerosis. *Circulation* 1997; 96:302–307.

89. Karasek RA, Baker D, Marxer F, et al. Job decision latitude, job demands, and cardiovascular disease: A prospective study of Swedish men. *Am J Pub Health* 1981;75:694–705.

90. Johnson JV, Stewart W, Hall EM, et al. Long-term psychosocial work environment and cardiovascular mortality among Swedish men. *Am J Public Health* 1996;86(3):324–331.

91. Marmot MG, Bosma H, Hemingway H, et al. Contribution of job control and other risk factors to social variations in coronary heart disease incidence. *Lancet* 1997;350(9073):235–239.

92. Gove WR. Gender differences in mental and physical illness: The effects of fixed roles and nurturant roles. *Soc Sci Med* 1984;19(2):77–91.

93. Gabbay FH, Krantz DS, Kop WJ, et al. Triggers of myocardial ischemia during daily life in patients with coronary artery disease: Physical and mental activities, anger and smoking. *J Am Coll Cardiol* 1996;27(3):585–592.

94. Kario K, Matsuo T, Kobayashi H, et al. Earthquake-induced potentiation of acute risk factors in hypertensive elderly patients: Possible triggering of cardiovascular events after a major earthquake. *J Am Coll Cardiol* 1997;29(5):926–933.

95. Frasure-Smith N, Lesperance F, Juneau M, et al. Gender, depression, and one-year prognosis after myocardial infarction. *Psychosom Med* 1999;61:26–37.

96. Denollet J, Brutsaert DL. Personality, disease severity, and the risk of long-term cardiac events in patients with a decreased ejection fraction after myocardial infarction (see comments). *Circulation* 1998;97(2): 167–173.

97. Hermann C, Brand-Driehorst S, Kaminsky B, et al. Diagnosis groups and depressed mood as predictors of 22-month mortality in medical patients. *Psychosom Med* 1998;60:570–577.

98. Frasure-Smith N, Lesperance F, Talajic M. Depression and 18-month prognosis after myocardial infarction. *Circulation* 1995;91:999–1005.

99. Ferketich AK, Schwartzbaum JA, Frid DJ, Moeschberger ML. Depression as an antecedent to heart disease among women and men in the NHANES I study. *Arch Intern Med* 2000;160:1261–1268.

100. Barefoot JC, Helms MJ, Mark DB, et al. Depression and long-term mortality risk in patients with coronary artery disease. *Am J Cardiol* 1996;78(6):613–617.

101. Lesperance F, Frasure-Smith N, Juneau M, Theroux P. Depression and 1-year prognosis in unstable angina. *Arch Intern Med* 2000;160(9): 1354–1360.

102. Connerney I, Shapiro PA, McLaughlin JS, et al. Relation between depression after coronary artery bypass surgery and 12-month outcome: A prospective study. *Lancet* 2001;358(9295):1766–1771.

103. Frasure-Smith N, Lesperance F, Talajic M. The impact of negative emotions on prognosis following myocardial infarction: Is it more than depression? *Health Psychol* 1995;14(5):388–398.

104. Moser DK, Dracup K. Is anxiety early after myocardial infarction associated with subsequent ischemic and arrhythmic events? *Psychosom Med* 1996;58:395–401.

105. Haines AP, Imeson JD, Meade TW. Phobic anxiety and ischemic heart disease. *BMJ* 1987;295:297–299.

106. Kawachi I, Sparrow D, Vokonas PS, Weiss ST. Symptoms of anxiety and risk of coronary heart disease. The Normative Aging Study. *Circulation* 1994;90(5):2225–2229.

107. Kawachi I, Colditz GA, Ascherio A, et al. Prospective study of phobic anxiety and risk of coronary heart disease in men. *Circulation* 1994;89(5):1992–1997.

108. Kawachi I, Sparrow D, Vokonas PS, Weiss ST. Decreased heart rate variability in men with phobic anxiety (data from the Normative Aging Study). *Am J Cardiol* 1995;75:882–885.

109. Kawachi I, Sparrow D, Vokonas PS, Weiss ST. Symptoms of anxiety and risk of coronary heart disease. The Normative Aging Study. *Circulation* 1994;90(5):2225–2229.

110. Hermann C, Brand-Driehorst S, Kaminsky B, et al. Diagnosis groups and depressed mood as predictors of 22-month mortality in medical patients. *Psychosom Med* 1998;60:570–577.

111. Frasure-Smith N, Lesperance F, Talajic M. The impact of negative emotions on prognosis following myocardial infarction: Is it more than depression? *Health Psychol* 1995;14(5):388–398.

112. Moser DK, Dracup K. Is anxiety early after myocardial infarction associated with subsequent ischemic and arrhythmic events? *Psychosom Med* 1996;58:395–401.

113. Kubzansky LD, Kawachi I, Weiss ST, Sparrow D. Anxiety and coronary heart disease: A synthesis of epidemiological, psychological, and experimental evidence. *Ann Behav Med* 1998;20(2):47–58.

114. Bovasso G, Eaton W. Types of panic attacks and their association with psychiatric disorder and physical illness. *Compr Psychiatry* 1999; 40(6):469–477.

115. Friedman M, Rosenman RH. Association of specific overt behavior pattern with blood and cardiovascular findings: Blood cholesterol level, blood clotting time, incidence of arcus senilis, and clinical coronary artery disease. *JAMA* 1959;169:1286–1296.

116. Miller TQ, Smith TW, Turner CW, et al. A meta-analytic review of research on hostility and physical health. *Psychol Bull* 1996;119(2): 322–348.

117. Koskenvuo M, Kaprio J, Rose RJ, et al. Hostility as a risk factor for mortality and ischemic heart disease in men. *Psychosom Med* 1988;50: 330–340.

118. Hecker MHL, Chesney MA, Blacks GW, Frautschi N. Coronary-prone behaviors in the Western Collaborative Group Study. *Psychosom Med* 1988;50:153–164.

119. Dembroski TM, MacDougall JM, Costa PT, Grandits GA. Components of hostility as predictors of sudden death and myocardial infarction in the Multiple Risk Factor Intervention Trial. *Psychosom Med* 1989;51:514–522.

120. Lau J, Antman EM, Jimenez-Silva J, et al. Cumulative meta-analysis of therapeutic trials for myocardial infarction. *N Engl J Med* 1992;327: 248–254.

121. Linden W, Stossel C, Maurice J. Psychosocial interventions for patients with coronary artery disease: A meta-analysis. *Arch Intern Med* 1996;156(7):745–752.

122. Frasure-Smith N, Prince R. Long-term follow-up of the Ischemic Heart Disease Life Stress Monitoring Program. *Psychosom Med* 1989;51:485–513.

123. Jones DA, West RR. Psychological rehabilitation after myocardial infarction: Multicentre randomised controlled trial. *BMJ* 1996;313: 1517–1521.

124. Frasure-Smith N. In-hospital symptoms of psychological stress as predictors of long-term outcome after acute myocardial infarction in men. *Am J Cardiol* 1991;67:121–127.

124a. Writing Committee for the ENRICHD Investigators. Effects of treating depression and low perceived social support on clinical events after myocardial infarction: The enhancing recovery in coronary heart disease patients (ENRICHD) randomized trial. *JAMA* 2003;289:3106–3116.

125. Glassman AH, O'Connor CM, Califf RM, et al. Sertraline treatment of major depression in patients with acute MI or unstable angina. *JAMA* 2002;288(6):701–709.

126. Patterson RE, Haines PS, Popkin BM. Health lifestyle patterns of U.S. adults. *Prev Med* 1994;23(4):453–460.

127. Ford ES, Giles WH, Dietz WH. Prevalence of the metabolic syndrome among U.S. adults: Findings from the third National Health and Nutrition Examination Survey. *JAMA* 2002;287(3):356–359.

128. Lakka HM, Laaksonen DE, Lakka TA, et al. The metabolic syndrome and total and cardiovascular disease mortality in middle-aged men. *JAMA* 2002;288(21):2709–2716.

129. Strecher V, Wang C, Derry H, et al. Tailored interventions for multiple risk behaviors. *Health Educ Res* 2002;17(5):619–626.

130. Emmons KM, Marcus BH, Linnan L, et al. Mechanisms in multiple risk factor interventions: Smoking, physical activity, and dietary fat intake among manufacturing workers. Working Well Research Group. *Prev Med* 1994;23(4):481–489.

131. Foreyt JP, Goodrick GK. Factors common to successful therapy for the obese patient. *Med Sci Sports Exerc* 1991;23(3):292–297.

132. Davidson K, Jonas B, Dixon K, Markovitz J. Do depression symptoms predict early hypertension incidence in young adults from the CARDIA study? *Arch Intern Med* 2000;160:1495–1500.

133. Oldridge N, Furlong W, Feeny D, et al. Economic evaluation of cardiac rehabilitation soon after acute myocardial infarction. *Am J Cardiol* 1993;72:154–161.

134. Fries JF, Koop CE, Beadle CE, et al. Reducing health care costs by reducing the need and demand for medical services. The Health Project Consortium. *N Engl J Med* 1993;329(5):321–325.

135. Stewart RB, Caranasos GJ. Medication compliance in the elderly. *Med Clin North Am* 1989;73(6):1551–1563.

136. Dunbar-Jacob J, Mortimer-Stephens MK. Treatment adherence in chronic disease. *J Clin Epidemiol* 2001;54(suppl 1):S57–S60.

137. Fries JF, Koop CE, Beadle CE, et al. Reducing health care costs by reducing the need and demand for medical services. The Health Project Consortium. *N Engl J Med* 1993;329(5):321–325.

138. Ades PA. Cardiac rehabilitation and secondary prevention of coronary heart disease. *N Engl J Med* 2001;345(12):892–902.

139. Brandon TH, Tiffany ST, Obremski KM, Baker TB. Postcessation cigarette use: The process of relapse. *Addict Behav* 1990;15(2): 105–114.

140. De Leon CFM, Kop WJ, de Swart HB, et al. Psychosocial characteristics and recurrent events after percutaneous transluminal coronary angioplasty. *Am J Cardiol* 1996;77:252–255.

141. Glanz K. Nutrition education for risk factor reduction and patient education: A review. *Prev Med* 1999;14:721–752.

142. Caggiula A, Watson J, Kuller L, et al. Cholesterol-lowering intervention program: Effect of the Step I diet in community office practices. *Arch Intern Med* 1996;156:1205–1213.

143. Burke LE, Dunbar-Jacob JM, Hill MN. Compliance with cardiovascular disease prevention strategies: A review of the research. *Ann Behav Med* 1997;19(3):239–263.

144. Prochaska JO, DiClemente CC, Norcross JC. In search of how people change: Applications to addictive behaviors. *Am Psychol* 1992;47: 1102–1114.

COMPLEMENTARY AND ALTERNATIVE MEDICAL THERAPY IN CARDIOVASCULAR CARE

Mitchell W. Krucoff / Richard Liebowitz / John H. K. Vogel / Daniel Mark

With the appointment of the writing group to produce a consensus paper on complementary and alternative medicine (CAM) practices for the American College of Cardiology, a unique dimension of health care concept, research, and practice formally opened for cardiologists.[1] As the trend among patients to use CAM therapies has risen exponentially,[2] growing professional interest in CAM therapies as adjuncts to the "high tech" world of cardiovascular care has been paralleled by concerns about exaggerated claims of efficacy, quackery, and frank toxicity across the largely unregulated pantheon of CAM practices. Information access through the Internet and media across global boundaries, relatively unrestricted access to products and services propagated by commercial manufacturers and CAM practitioners, as well as widespread cultural interest in self-empowerment and holistic paradigms of health care for patients have produced a mandate for cardiologists to become better informed about CAM therapeutics. At the very least such education will support more thoughtful, less defensive dialogue between physicians and patients. At best, cardiologists knowledgeable about CAM therapies will be better positioned to encourage and envision both the many necessary research directions and more integrated clinical strategies necessary for the advance of optimal data-driven practice in cardiovascular care.

While many CAM therapies have been practiced for thousands of years in culturally based health systems, there is a growing but still very immature literature by modern standards in most of these areas. The introduction to the American College of Cardiology (ACC) consensus document observes that "Topics chosen for coverage by Expert Consensus Documents are so designed because the evidence base and experience with technology or clinical practice are not considered sufficiently well developed to be evaluated by the formal ACC/AHA Practice Guidelines process."[1] Most CAM therapies lack common nomenclature, certification standards for practice methods, or profiles of active principles in consumables such as herbal remedies, thus largely confounding systematic appreciation of actual safety and efficacy in selected heart disease populations. As with other areas of immature literature in medical practices, investigator bias, reporting bias, and publisher bias may also all impact the interpretation of what data are available.

Even more essential to the actual integration of modern medical technology and practice with CAM therapies is the challenge to engage whole new paradigms both of healing and of how research defining optimal healing might be conducted. The modern scientific tendency to articulate biochemical mechanisms and translate them into clinical practice therapeutics tested by clinical protocols is potentially fatally reductionist with regard to holistic systems that view interaction with the body as about 20 percent of the mind-body-spirit process that actually accomplishes the transformation of suffering called healing.[3,4] For meaningful research in CAM therapies to move the field forward, ethical and robust standards for clinical trial designs and mechanistic studies must be developed, with sensitivity to the cultural metaphors of how the therapies actually work.[5–8]

With the growth of the Office of Alternative Medicine into the National Center for Complementary and Alterative Medicine (NCCAM) at the National Institutes of Health, more comprehensive attention and research resources have been directed to sorting through some of these issues and to developing the requisite infrastructure. With even the terms *alternative, complementary, integrative,* and others still in flux, in this chapter the authors have taken selected therapies and references from the general topical framework that NCCAM has developed for CAM therapies[9] with a focus, where possible, specifically on cardiovascular applications across NCCAM's five key treatment areas: biologically based therapies, manipulative and body-based methods, energy therapies, mind-body interventions, and alternative medical systems.

BIOLOGICALLY BASED THERAPIES: SELECTED BOTANICALS AND DIETARY SUPPLEMENTS

Herbal remedies, vitamins and food substance derivatives, teas, alchohol, nuts, soy, and other specific dietary elements have a longstanding place in health care as a predominantly culturally based pharmacopoeia. In most cases the initial scientific suggestion of benefit has come from epidemiologic comparisons of different cohorts, with interpretation limited both by different endogenous rates of disease and varied levels of consumption of the substance of interest, which itself may have varied concentrations of active compounds. Early hypothesis-generating studies are typically supported by subsequent case-control studies and, in some cases, larger prospective cohort studies. In cardiovascular applications, surrogate endpoints in the smaller prospective studies include effects on low-density-lipoprotein cholesterol (LDL-C), platelet function, endothelial function, and immune/inflammatory activity. In some cases larger randomized, controlled trials have been conducted using clinical outcome endpoints.

Botanicals

The medicinal use of botanicals originated over 7000 years ago; the written history spans more than 3500 years.[10] Prescribed by great ancient physicians such as Hippocrates, Theophrastus, and Pliny, botanicals were catalogued and illustrated, with specific indications noted for each active plant. Intact botanicals were used singly or in combination until the nineteenth century, when the identification and isolation of individually active compounds was conceived and accomplished. Approximately 25 percent of pharmaceuticals prescribed today are derived from plant sources. At the same time, there has been a rekindling of consumer interest in the use of natural whole-plant products. A significant result of this public interest and demand for access to herbal products was the passage of the Dietary Supplement Health and Education Act (DSHEA) of 1994. Herbs, vitamins, minerals, and proteins were classified as dietary supplements. Manufacturers were allowed to describe the effects of these supplements on "structure or function" of the body or the "well-being" achieved by consuming the dietary ingredient. To use these claims, manufacturers must have substantiation that the statements were truthful and not misleading and the product label must bear the statement "This statement has not been evaluated by the Food and Drug Administration." Furthermore, neither good manufacturing practices nor labeling requirements certifying concentrations of active ingredients or bioavailability have been required for DSHEA products. As a result, independent examination has revealed great inconsistency between product labeling and actual compound concentration.[11] In this setting safety concerns with potential adulteration of supplements with active prescription compounds, contamination of preparations, herb-herb and herb-drug interactions are significant.[12,13] Research into the safety and efficacy of botanical compounds has been hampered by this lack of standardization.[14] Recently the FDA has reconsidered these issues, and it is now moving toward requiring labeling for botanicals that specifies and certifies concentrations of active compounds.

Garlic (*Allium sativum*)

Garlic has long been touted as a natural product useful for the modulation of immune system activity, in the treatment of hyperlipidemia and hypertension, as well as the primary and secondary prevention of myocardial infarction. Medicinal use of garlic can be traced back to the ancient Babylonians and Chinese, with long-term usage occurring in western folk medicine as well.[15] Allicin is felt to be the structure responsible for the potential cardiovascular activity of garlic.[16] Allicin content is determined by the nature of the garlic preparation, with raw crushed garlic having the highest concentration. Multiple mechanisms of action have been proposed, including decrease in cholesterol and fatty acid synthesis and cholesterol absorption[17] as well as potent antioxidant properties.[18] Antiplatelet and fibrinolytic activity with garlic has also been reported.[19]

Clinical studies of garlic have yielded contradictory results, with significant design flaws notable in trials designed to demonstrate garlic's effectiveness.[20–22] Short-term studies have shown some benefit in the lipid profiles of patients taking garlic, while long-term studies of 6 months or more fail to show sustained benefit when garlic is used as a single agent. Studies of garlic's effectiveness in hypertension have also suffered from poor methodology, and results have revealed small, mostly insignificant decreases in blood pressure.[23–25] Evidence for the supplemental intake of garlic for both the primary and secondary prevention of heart disease is not sufficient to recommend its use for this indication.

The anticoagulant properties of garlic may be problematic in the perioperative period and in combination with other anticoagulant compounds. Garlic has also been noted to decrease the effectiveness of some HIV drugs.[26] Side effects are minor other than occasional nausea with excessive raw intake of garlic and the development of an unpleasant odor.

Hawthorn (*Crataegus* Species)

Hawthorn species are a group of small trees and shrubs found throughout North America, Asia, and Europe. Purported cardiovascular indications include congestive heart failure (CHF), angina, and arrhythmias. Hawthorn's activity is felt to be related to the presence of a number of key constituents, including flavonoids and oligomeric procyanidins.[27]

Literature review reveals significant evidence for hawthorn's efficacy in the treatment of mild to moderate congestive heart failure.[28–31] Animal and in vitro models reveal positive inotropism with a mechanism of action similar to that of digitalis through a cyclic AMP-independent effect.[32,33] There is also evidence of a direct vasodilating effect.[34] Some efficacy has been documented in increasing maximal workload capacity and decreasing symptom severity in patients with congestive heart failure (CHF). One uncontrolled study also reported an increase in ejection fraction measured by angiography from 30 to 41 percent in patients with stage II to III heart failure.[35] No published studies have examined mortality effects. There are very limited data regarding actual benefit in angina, and anti-arrhythmia data are present only in animal studies.

The usual dose of hawthorn for CHF is 300 to 600 mg 3 times daily of an extract standardized to contain about 2 to 3 percent flavonoids or 18 to 20 percent procyanidins. Full effects may take up to 6 months to develop. Combination with cardiac glycosides and CNS depressants should be avoided. Side effects are rare but include gastrointestinal upset and sedation.

Ginkgo biloba

Ginkgo extracts are derived from the leaf of the ginkgo tree, a botanical with a known history dating back 300 million years. Originally present throughout Europe, the tree died out during the Ice Age, surviving in China and Japan. Ginkgo is the most commonly purchased herbal remedy in the United States, with sales of over $150 million.[36] Widely used for its purported benefits in treating non-dementia-related memory problems, Alzheimer's disease, and vertigo, ginkgo has also been proposed as a treatment for intermittent claudication and peripheral vascular disease.

Ginkgo has been documented to inhibit platelet activation factor, decrease blood viscosity, and decrease vascular resistance.[37,38] The mechanisms responsible for ginkgo's effectiveness in peripheral vascular disease are unknown. Individual studies have revealed benefit in increasing mean pain-free walking distance.[39,40] Two metanalyses have examined the literature and reported a statistically significant increase in walking distance averaging nearly 25 m.[41,42] The clinical significance of this difference is questionable.

The usual dose of ginkgo for the treatment of claudication is 40 to 80 mg three times daily of a 50:1 extract standardized to contain 24 percent ginkgo-flavone glycosides. Caution must be exercised in using ginkgo, as it inhibits platelet aggregation factor and has been reported to increase both spontaneous and trauma-related bleeding, including bleeding during surgery and other procedures.[43,44] Caution must also be exercised in combining gingko with heparin, warfarin, clopidogrel, and other compounds that may increase the risk of bleeding. Ginkgo has been reported to decrease the metabolism of trazodone in at least one case report, perhaps by an inhibition of monoamine oxidase.[45] Side effects are common and include headaches, dizziness, gastrointestinal complaints, and skin reactions.

Horse Chestnut Tree Extract (Aesculus hippocastanum)

The horse chestnut tree is found worldwide. Its seeds contain active compounds known as saponins, which have mild anti-inflammatory properties.[46] Aescin, a combination of triterpine saponins, appears to be the pharmacologically active component. Its mechanism of action is considered to be sensitization to Ca^{2+} ions and a sealing effect on small vessel permeability to water.[47] Traditionally, this botanical has been used for hemorrhoids, rheumatism, swellings, varicose veins, and leg ulcers. Research has focused on horse chestnut tree extract in the treatment of chronic venous insufficiency, and multiple studies have reported the superiority of horse chestnut tree extract over placebo, with equal effectiveness to compression stockings as quantified by significant improvement in objective measurements of leg edema and subjective reporting of pain and sensation of heaviness.[48–50]

The usual dose of horse chestnut tree extract is 300 mg twice daily, standardized to contain 50 mg escin per dose, for a total daily dose of 100 mg escin. Side effects are rare, including headache, itching, and dizziness. Concerns regarding risk of renal impairment do not appear to be warranted.[51]

Policosanol

Policosanol is a combination of aliphatic alcohols derived most commonly from sugar cane wax, though octacosanol, the predominant active ingredient, is also present in wheat germ oil and other vegetable oils.[52] Policosanol *inhibits cholesterol biosynthesis* in a step located between acetate and mevalonate as well as by an increase in LDL receptor–dependent processing. There is no evidence for a direct inhibition of HMG-CoA reductase.[53] Policosanol has been extensively used clinically and researched in Cuba.[54] These studies suggest a lipid-lowering effect of approximately 15 percent for total cholesterol and 20 percent for LDL cholesterol, which can be increased to 30 percent with higher doses. Maximal effects are seen after only 6 to 8 weeks of use, and benefits have been demonstrated in studies lasting longer than 1 year. In a head-to-head comparison of 10 mg policosanol with 20 mg fluvastatin in women with elevated cholesterol, the lipid-lowering effects of policosanol were slightly superior to those of fluvastatin, and policosanol alone significantly inhibited the susceptibility of LDL to lipid peroxidation.[55] A recent review has noted the efficacy of policosanol and suggested a unique role for this natural compound, given the large number of patients desiring a natural alternative to synthetically derived drugs for cholesterol management.[56]

The typical starting dose of policosanol is 5 mg per day, which may be increased to a maximal dose of 20 mg per day. Side effects are infrequent, with weight loss, polyuria, and headache most commonly reported. There is concern that policosanol may potentiate anticoagulant activity; it should therefore be used with caution in combination with any agents known to increase the risk of bleeding. There is also a report of an increased effect of L-dopa when used in combination with policosanol, leading to dyskinesias.[57]

Guggulipid (Commiphora mukul)

Guggul is a substance derived from the mukul myrrh tree in India. It has played a role in traditional Indian medicine (Ayurveda) for several thousand years, used in the treatment of arthritis, digestive, skin, and menstrual problems. Today, guggul is used as a lipid-lowering agent that is believed to work by blocking the farnesoid X receptor in liver cells and as a consequence altering cholesterol metabolism.[58] Studies of guggul have demonstrated a significant reduction in total cholesterol and LDL-C of 15 to 23 percent and triglyceride reduction of 20 percent.[59,60] The usual dose is 100 mg of guggulsterones per day. Side effects are usually limited to mild gastrointestinal symptoms. There is some evidence that when guggul is used concomitantly with diltiazem or propranolol, there may be a reduction in the bioavailability of those drugs and therefore decreased clinical efficacy.[61]

Red Rice Yeast (Monascus purpureus)

Red rice yeast is a product that is derived from a yeast that grows on rice. Red rice yeast has been a food staple and folk remedy for thousands of years in the Far East. It was noted in the 1970s that a product of the yeast, monacolin K (lovastatin), was an *inhibitor of HMG-CoA reductase*.[62] The concentration of lovastatin varies in red rice yeast but averages near 0.4 percent by weight.

In a multicenter study of 187 subjects, red rice yeast lowered total cholesterol by 16.4 percent, LDL-C by 21.0 percent, triglycerides by 24.5 percent, and the ratio of total-to-HDL cholesterol by 17.7 percent; it increased high-density-lipoprotein cholesterol (HDL-C) by 14.6 percent.[63] While the reported side effects of red rice yeast are few—including mainly gastrointestinal upset, headaches, and dizziness—red rice yeast must theoretically be considered a typical HMG-CoA reductase inhibitor and caution is advised with regard to potential side effects, including rhabdomyolysis. Similarly, drug interactions should be considered to be identical to those with lovastatin, requiring caution when red yeast rice is combined with niacin, macrolides, cyclosporine, ketoconazole, and many other agents. Products range in their recommended dosage from 2.5 to 10 mg of lovastatin equivalent per day.

Dietary Supplements

A number of dietary supplements have been postulated to have beneficial effects on cardiovascular disease. These include antioxidant vitamins, B vitamins, omega-3 fatty acids, plant sterols, soluble fiber, soy, nuts, alcohol, and teas.[64,65] Some of these are also discussed in other chapters of this book (e.g., Chap. 43).

OMEGA-3 FATTY ACIDS

Omega-3 polyunsaturated fatty acids (FAs) can be derived from either plant or marine sources. The principal plant-based omega-3 FA, alpha-linolenic acid (ALA), is found in soy and its derivative tofu as well as in canola oil, flax seeds, and nuts. Omega-3 FAs derived from marine animals ("fish oil") include docosahexaenoic acid (DHA) and eicosapentaenoic acid (EPA). Typical dietary sources include mackerel, salmon, herring, sardines, anchovies, and albacore tuna. Early suggestions that fish oil might be beneficial came from epidemiologic comparisons of Greenland and Alaskan Inuits with other cohorts. The Inuits consumed a high-fat diet with a high component of omega-3 FAs from seal and whale meat. Despite this diet, they had more favorable lipid profiles and lower rates of coronary artery disease (CAD) than the comparison groups. Three follow-up epidemiologic studies in the 1980s found that persons who ate fish every week had a lower mortality from CAD.[66,67]

At least 15 prospective cohort studies have now examined the effects of fish consumption on CAD outcomes.[68] Overall, they suggest a protective effect, with a stronger effect on death than on nonfatal MI. Additional reports suggest that atherosclerotic progression in native coronaries and vein grafts is slowed in men in association with fish oil ingestion.[69,70]

Four randomized controlled trials have tested either omega-3 FA capsules or oily fish in CAD patients. The largest of these is the GISSI-Prevenzione study, which randomized 5666 post-MI patients to 1 g/day or usual therapy.[71] The primary analysis showed a 20 percent reduction in all-cause mortality ($p = 0.01$) and a 45 percent reduction in sudden death ($p < 0.01$).

A metanalysis of 11 randomized trials of omega-3 FAs published 1966–1999 (7951 intervention patients, 7855 control patients) found a 20 percent reduction in nonfatal MI ($p = 0.16$), a 30 percent reduction in fatal MI ($p < 0.001$), a 30 percent reduction in sudden death ($p < 0.01$), and a 20 percent reduction in overall mortality ($p < 0.001$).[72] No evidence was seen for a different effect of dietary versus nondietary sources of omega-3 FAs.

Several mechanisms of benefit have been proposed for omega-3 FAs. The reductions in sudden death observed in several studies supports a direct antiarrhythmic effect. High-dose omega-3 FAs produce a significant reduction in serum triglyceride concentrations and a small drop in blood pressure. They also decrease platelet aggregation. Other suggested mechanisms include an anti-inflammatory effect and enhanced production of nitric oxide.

Current recommendations from the American Heart Association (AHA) are to consume two servings of fish (especially fatty fish) per week as part of a heart-healthy diet. The use of fish oil supplements as part of a program of secondary prevention is reasonable.[73] The lack of large-scale, placebo-controlled, randomized trials prevents the development of a more affirmative recommendation at this time.

ANTIOXIDANTS AND ANTIOXIDANT VITAMINS

A large body of epidemiologic evidence supports a favorable association between a diet high in antioxidants and reduced risk of coronary heart disease (CHD). Most of these studies examined the consumption of foods and estimated the likely vitamin content, while a few studies have examined the supplemental consumption of vitamins.

Vitamin E refers to a group of molecules that includes four tocopherols and four tocotrienols. Alpha tocopherol is the most prevalent and most potent lipid-soluble antioxidant in plasma. Several large epidemiologic studies involving over 170,000 subjects have assessed the association between dietary and supplement-based vitamin E and CHD outcomes.[74–76] Three of these found supplement-based vitamin E to be associated with a significant reduction in hard cardiac events, especially in doses >100 IU for >2 years.

There are now five randomized controlled trials using vitamin E for primary (two trials) or secondary (three trials) prevention. The Cambridge Heart Antioxidant Study (CHAOS) demonstrated that 400 to 800 IU of vitamin E given as secondary prevention reduced the combined endpoint of death or nonfatal MI by 47 percent. However, the larger and more recent Heart Outcomes Prevention Evaluation (HOPE) trial, which tested 400 IU of vitamin E in a high-risk secondary prevention population, found no therapeutic benefit on a variety of outcome measures including disease progression as assessed by carotid ultrasound. The GISSI-Prevenzione trial, which tested 300 IU of vitamin E in almost 8000 patients, also failed to detect a benefit. Finally, the Collaborative Group of the Primary Prevention Project (PPP) found no evidence for a therapeutic benefit for 300 IU of vitamin E in 4495 subjects with one or more major cardiovascular risk factors. At present, therefore, the preponderance of the evidence *does not support* a role for vitamin E supplements in either primary or secondary prevention of CHD.

Vitamin C (ascorbic acid) is a strong water-soluble antioxidant. The epidemiologic evidence for a favorable effect of vitamin C on CHD prevention is much less persuasive than that for vitamin E. Several randomized trials have tested vitamin C supplements in varying doses for CHD prevention. In the Heart Protection Study, 20,536 patients with CAD or diabetes were randomized to antioxidant vitamins (600 mg of vitamin E, 250 mg of vitamin C, and 20 mg of beta-carotene) versus placebo.[77] While the vitamin regimen was found to be safe, there was no evidence for a therapeutic effect after 5 years of treatment. In contrast, in the Antioxidant Supplementation in Atherosclerosis Prevention (ASAP) study, hypercholesterolemic patients were randomized to twice-daily supplements of 136 IU of vitamin E, 250 mg of slow-release vitamin C, both, or placebo only.[78] At 6 years among the 440 subjects completing the study, vitamin supplementation slowed carotid atherosclerosis (judged by common carotid intimal-medial thickness) by 25 percent.

B VITAMINS

Moderate elevations of plasma homocysteine levels have been associated with an enhanced risk for atherosclerotic disease. The metabolism of homocysteine requires several B vitamins as cofactors, specifically vitamins B_6, B_{12}, and folate. Homocysteine levels can be decreased by the administration of supplemental folate, with or without vitamins B_6 and B_{12}. Epidemiologic studies suggest potential cardiovascular benefit with B-vitamin supplementation, either through this or other undefined mechanisms.[79,80] There are several ongoing clinical trials testing these vitamins in patients with vascular disease.[81]

CHELATION THERAPY

The intravenous infusion of ethylenediamine-tetraacetic acid (EDTA) is a form of alternative medicine commonly used for the treatment of atherosclerotic vascular disease. The original rationale behind this therapy was that EDTA chelation would remove calcium from atheromatous arterial lesions. However, there is little empiric support for this putative mechanism, and other possible benefits such as an antioxidant effect have been proposed. The evidence base on chelation consists of case reports and case series involving a total of over 4600 patients, largely describing the beneficial effects of EDTA chelation.

There have been four randomized trials of chelation therapy, all quite small. The most recent is the Program to Assess Alternative Treatment Strategies to Achieve Cardiac Health (PATCH),[82] which randomized 84 stable angina patients and followed them for 6 months. Event rates in this trial were quite low and there were no differences between the chelation and the placebo arms. The investigators concluded that a much larger trial would be required.

The National Institutes of Health recently funded a major randomized trial of chelation, the Trial to Assess Chelation Therapy (TACT). This study, which started enrollment in 2003, will randomize 2372 patients ≥ age 50 with a prior myocardial infarction (MI) to either chelation therapy or placebo. Results are expected by 2007.

SOLUBLE FIBER

Dietary fiber supplements have been shown to produce desirable changes in LDL-cholesterol and blood sugar levels.[83] Epidemiologic findings suggest a possible impact on coronary disease and outcome.[84,85] However, there are no prospective trials of the effect of these supplements on cardiac outcomes.

SOY PROTEIN AND ISOFLAVONES

Substitution of soy protein for animal protein can produce significant reductions in LDL-cholesterol and triglycerides.[86] Whether this reflects a unique benefit of soy or isoflavones in particular or merely a reduction in dietary animal protein and fat is unclear.

PLANT STEROLS

Plant sterols and stanols have been persuasively shown to lower cholesterol and are now commercially available in margarine products.[87] Long-term outcome studies with these compounds are needed.

Alcohol

Mild to moderate alcohol consumption has been associated in a variety of reports with reduction in stroke and rates of MI, functional improvement with claudication, and improved cardiovascular survival.[88–91] Vasodilating and central nervous system effects, as well as antioxidant compounds in alcohol preparations such as red wine, have all been proposed as potential mechanisms of these benefits. At higher dose in susceptible individuals, alcohol is a well-known myocardial toxin, with equally deleterious potential in other end organs such as the liver, gastrointestinal tract, and central nervous system. A science advisory overview from the AHA was issued on this topic in 2001.[92]

MANIPULATIVE AND BODY-BASED METHODS

Acupuncture, acupressure, and an array of massage techniques represent manipulative and body-based therapies. Of these, the most robust scientific information is available on acupuncture.

Acupuncture

The ancient Chinese medical therapy acupuncture has garnered growing interest over the course of increasing communication between the United States and China since the early 1970s. Worldwide,

more than 40 percent of physicians recommend acupuncture to their patients, and more than 50 percent of physicians want to add this modality to their therapeutic armamentarium.[93] Although not required for licensed physicians, the practice of acupuncture by others, such as those trained in traditional Chinese medicine, is currently regulated by more than 35 state boards in the United States. Furthermore, the FDA regulates the use of disposable stainless steel and acupuncture needles. The National Institutes of Health has published a consensus statement indicating that many issues related to acupuncture—including efficacy, sham effects, adverse reactions, acupuncture points, training, credentialing, and mechanism of action—need further definition.[14]

Clinically, acupuncture is most accepted for the treatment of pain.[94,95] In cardiovascular care, there are three areas for which acupuncture has been explored: anginal pain from ischemia, hypertension, and arrhythmias. The rationale for using acupuncture to treat myocardial ischemia, hypertension, and arrhythmias may stem from its ability to inhibit autonomic sympathetic outflow. Acupuncture techniques may release opioids in a number of regions in the hypothalamus, midbrain, and medulla concerned with processing information that influences sympathetic neuroactivity. Other neurotransmitters that may also be associated with the cardiovascular effects of acupuncture include gamma-aminobutyric acid, serotonin, and acetylcholine.[93] Since placebo effects can occur in as many as 40 percent of the patients and because acupuncture seems to be efficacious in only around 70 percent of patients, actual benefit may represent a narrow window of response.[92]

Mechanistic studies suggest that catecholamine reduction with acupuncture may affect myocardial ischemia and stress-induced hypertension.[92] These studies indicate that acupuncture probably limits myocardial ischemia by reducing myocardial oxygen demand rather than by increasing coronary blood flow. In sham acupuncture placebo-controlled studies of moderate anginal pain and exercise tolerance, Ballegaard was unable to document a decrease in the rate of anginal attacks, consumption of nitroglycerin, or improvement in exercise tolerance,[96] while two other studies including patients with severe stable angina who had been treated vigorously with medical therapy showed an acupuncture-related improvement in exercise capacity and rate-pressure product, particularly when acupuncture reduced measures of sympathetic tone.[97,98] There are currently no trials showing reduction in mortality or other clinical outcomes with acupuncture in ischemic heart disease.

General vascular reactivity may be affected by acupuncture. Improvement in primary Raynaud's cold-induced vasoconstriction by acupuncture compared to sham treatment has been reported.[99] Hypertension may also be improved by acupuncture, although the absolute effects on blood pressure reported are small.[100] These findings may be more profound in selected hypertensive syndromes responsive to central nervous system modulation.[94]

Reliable data on arrhythmia control with acupuncture are rare. Acupuncture may inhibit ventricular extrasystoles induced by stimulating the hypothalamus or paraventricular nucleus or following administration of $BaCL_2$.[94] Understanding patient selection and the level of incremental effect in the context of other drug or device therapies will require dedicated research.

Most authorities agree that the risk of an adverse event resulting from acupuncture is small, generally below 10 percent when performed by physicians. Pneumothorax, spinal cord lesions, hepatitis HIV infections, endocarditis, arthritis, and osteomyelitis have been reported but are rare, with an overall rate of less than 2 percent. The risk of an adverse event for nonphysician acupuncturists is higher (up to 30 percent), although the risk of serious events is low.

ENERGY THERAPIES

Bioenergetics or energy therapies are a series of healing "disciplines" that claim to harness intangible natural forces to influence physiologic, emotional, and spiritual healing. No scientific evidence has demonstrated or characterized actual bioenergy fields associated with many of these techniques, although practitioners claim to see, feel, or otherwise sense the color, alignment, intensity, and flow of such energy in practice. In several ancient Eastern practices, detailed diagrams of energy meridians and chakras are well known. Examples of bioenergy disciplines include therapeutic and healing touch, QiGong, Johrei, Reiki, crystal therapy, and magnet therapy. Energy therapies are generally administered by an active practitioner who conducts both diagnostic and therapeutic functions by "sensing" or "reading" energy patterns and then manipulating or adding to those energy patterns, with the patient in a more passive role. It is quite conceivable that placebo effects, hypnosis, and other trance states may also belong to this largely metaphorically defined practice area.

Practitioners of the ancient Chinese healing tradition of QiGong use deep breathing, meditation, and body movement to capture and focus the vital life energy, Qi. In cardiovascular application, QiGong has been claimed to influence hypertension in patients with heart disease[101] as well as sudden death by accentuating vagal tone, as demonstrated by changes in heart rate variability.[102] QiGong has also been associated with shorter hospitalization in patients after myocardial infarction and reduced mortality with stroke.[103] The reproducibility of these findings has not been established.

Healing touch[104,105] and Reiki[106] therapies conceptually involve concentration and transmission of bioenergy from healer to patient, with restoration and realignment of energy fields in the patient, either by touching the patient directly or by touching the energy fields around the body. The Vedic paradigm of energy concentrated in and through anatomically related chakras along the spine and central nervous system, with the energy flow between and around the chakras determined by paths or meridians both within the somatic body and in a field around the body, is frequently included in the conceptual constructs of these practices.

In hospitalized patients, therapeutic touch has been reported to palliate anxiety,[107] with a potential effect on serum catecholamines prior to invasive procedures.[108] In a small pilot study of healing touch prior to urgent percutaneous coronary intervention, this modality was associated with a suggestive trend toward improved short term outcomes.[109]

In the absence of known mechanisms the safety assessment of bioenergy practices is problematic. While bioenergy approaches are widely considered safe by practitioners,[110] careful attention to both safety and efficacy in future research in these areas should be considered mandatory.

MIND-BODY INTERVENTIONS

A remarkably large and consistent observational literature provides evidence that the presence or absence of acute and chronic stress; emotional states such as obsessive behavior, depression, and hostility; spiritual attitudes such as faith and hope; and interactive support systems such as companionship and community connectedness have significant correlations to cardiovascular outcomes such as hypertension, MI, stroke, and cardiac death.[111–114] It is possible that these observations result from genetically driven physiologic responses to stress, with measurable impact on catecholamine levels, cortisol levels, glucose metabolism, autonomic tone, vascular tone, coagula-

bility, pain perception, and immune reactivity. Teleologically the "fight-or-flight" responses are frequently recognized as physiologic survival mechanisms. However, with chronic, repetitive overstimulation or in the setting of preexistent heart disease, the roles of stress, isolation, anger, and depression can clearly reach pathologic proportions. Also, these states of mind and spirit are frequently paired with behaviors such smoking, eating disorders, obesity, diabetes, hypercholesterolemia, a sedentary lifestyle, and hypertension. Coping strategies and therapies that address this mind-body axis may be a fertile area to integrate into the current predominantly pharmacologic armamentarium. The actual ability of mind-body or mind-body-spirit therapies to benefit the natural history of cardiovascular disease, however, remains unclear.

Mind-body therapies are generally characterized by learned disciplines that affect both mind and body in a deliberately harmonious or even simultaneous way. Techniques may emphasize the mental component, such as in meditation, mindfulness, relaxation therapy, guided imagery, music and mirthful laughter, with a "secondary" relaxation, quieting, or energizing of the body, or they may emphasize the somatic component, as in exercise, tai chi, and yoga, with a secondary quieting or energizing of the mind.[115] A strong emphasis on awareness of and control of the breath, generally with attention to moving the locus of the breath from the chest into a relaxed abdominal breathing, is common among many of these techniques. Similarly, the final objective of mind-body healing techniques is to promote or restore an equilibrium between the mental and the somatic characterized by a feeling of calm peacefulness and filled with a sense of vital energy. In culturally rooted disciplines, this equilibrium and the path leading to it are conceived of not only as wellness and healing-oriented but as frankly spiritual paths providing a source of joy, a sense of meaning in life, and even an awareness of unifying or divine principles.

Less explicitly used in mind-body practices but a topic of great interest to healing science is the *placebo effect*. Suggestion and belief have repeatedly been shown to produce measurable changes in somatic symptoms such as angina.[116] While historically equated to neurosis or deceit, "nothing," or other negative connotations, more recently research in the placebo effect has come to be regarded as a possible window into internally mediated healing processes and human potential currently untapped in medical practice.[117]

One area of mind-body therapy that has been reported in application to cardiovascular disorders is relaxation therapy, where triggering of relative bradycardia, vasodilatation, and changes in the electroencephalogram have been described as the "relaxation response."[118] Relaxation therapies generally involve some combination of relaxed abdominal breathing, quieting of the mind with meditation or related techniques, and somatic relaxation of the body. Relaxation therapies are frequently applied for stress reduction, including just prior to invasive cardiac procedures.[119,120] Relaxation therapy has been associated with lowering of blood pressure and possibly with better outcomes in men with risk factors for coronary artery disease. Concerns with possibly unanticipated negative effects from changing vascular tone or heart rhythm must also be carefully evaluated for therapies in patients with known heart disease. Although a reduction in premature ventricular contractions (PVCs) has been observed with relaxation therapy,[121] higher mortality rates were associated with relaxation therapy in a female cohort of the MHEART study who had survived MI.[122]

Other mind-body techniques with published experience in cardiology include music and imagery. Anxiety reduction has been observed with music in coronary care unit (CCU) and MI populations, although outcomes benefit has not been established.[123,124] Imagery techniques usually encourage a patient to envision a beautiful, peaceful place from his or her life or experience, using a relaxed abdominal breath to let the mind dwell in that place. Music is used in the background in some imagery scripts. Imagery has been reported to reduce pain or the need for sedation in patients undergoing catheterization and to shorten hospital stay after bypass surgery.[125,126]

Meditation and mindfulness constitute a very broad range of disciplines providing tools that, with practice, cultivate personal access to calming of the body and quieting of the mind, with a variety of potential healing effects including reduction of angina and improved quality of life.[127] In addition to the use of these techniques in cardiac rehabilitation programs, they may have a role in lifestyle modification strategies associated with atheroregression in established coronary disease.[128] Meditative states have been demonstrated to measurably impact numerous autonomic and hormonal processes, although the precise mechanistic relationship to cardiovascular benefit is unknown.[129]

Many forms of meditation, like a number of mind-body disciplines, extend beyond mind-body into mind-body-spirit diagnostics and therapeutics, at least metaphorically. The role of spiritual attitudes, mental intentionality, spiritual intervention, and prayer in life process, disease states, and healing have been the subjects of numerous studies, from their effects on microorganisms and cell growth to human clinical trials.[110,130–133] With no insight into mechanism but consistent suggestion of effect, this area of research has slowly moved beyond the traditional separation of science and religion into the more balanced systematic exploration of human potential and its impact on healing in a modern medical context. Even though patients suffering from heart disease are confronted by issues of personal mortality, little is known about the role of the human spirit in response to therapy, tolerance of procedures, or outcomes per se. To date a total of four prospective, randomized clinical trials of prayer in CCU populations and patients with acute coronary syndromes have been published in the peer review literature, with two large studies of patients undergoing bypass surgery and percutaneous interventions having been completed.[108,134–137] Data on therapeutic benefit are inconclusive. As with most CAM literature, attempts to pool these data are most useful for hypothesis generation to guide future studies into more definitive directions.[7,132,138,139]

ALTERNATIVE MEDICAL SYSTEMS

Alternative medical systems broadly constitute approaches to diagnostic and therapeutic applications that are based on paradigms conceptually distinct from the allopathic structure of modern medical practices in the western world. By and large, alternative medical systems are culturally based and in many cases ancient in their history. Perhaps the most notable hallmark of these systems is their holistic character. In many, the allopathic fixation on mechanical processes in the body, detailed analysis of biochemical or serologic measures, and discrete end-organ focus on individual body systems constitute the conceptual equivalent of a gross undersampling error. In traditional Chinese medicine, for instance, cardiovascular disorders are simply one feature of symptom complexes characterized across four relative states of yin deficiency or excess combined with yang deficiency or excess, where both yin and yang energies are associated with a broad range of emotional states, symbolic imagery, as well as specific body organs.[140] In Ayurvedic medical systems, the body is essentially referenced across five inorganic elements constituting the material universe—earth, water, fire, air, and ether. The body itself is envisioned as coarse material, or "maya," that is structurally configured by vibrational energy conveyed from a collective or cosmic source, or

Atma.[141] This coarse material structure rendered by vibrational influences of life energy could be conceptually compared, in a different metaphor, to the modern western medical understanding of the genome. In both of these paradigms, wellness and illness exist in the individual human being, but they are also structurally shared across populations and beyond. Computationally demanding statistical models being developed for genomic applications might provide some intriguing approaches to novel medical paradigms in alternative medical systems.

While alternative medical systems at first blush may seem radical in their departure from the rigorously articulate western scientific medical model, current directions in wellness-oriented lifestyle modification strategies for both the primary and secondary prevention of cardiovascular disease represent a movement with a distinctively holistic character in the mainstream of modern practice.

CONCLUSION

CAM therapies in cardiovascular care represent an enormous area of unregulated and widely practiced therapeutics with an immature scientific literature but, in many cases, an ancient and deeply rooted cultural basis. In modern medicine, CAM therapeutics are probably best considered as adjuncts to current standard medical care, whose study provides opportunities to advance more integrative medical practice. Systematic research to uncover mechanisms of action as well as to better profile the actual safety and efficacy of CAM therapies in specific cardiac disorders is both justified and clearly necessary for new paradigms of integrative medical practice to have an impact and be widely adopted by physicians. In lieu of such research, the education and familiarity of cardiologists with CAM therapies is likely to promote better dialogue with patients and more awareness of issues of self-empowerment in dealing with heart disease, opening the door to a broadened range of options for optimizing cardiovascular care.

References

1. Vogel JF, Bolling SF, Costello RB, et al. A Report of the American College of Cardiology Task Force on Clinical Expert Consensus Documents (Writing Committee to Develop an Expert Consensus Document on Complementary and Integrative Medicine). *J Am Coll Cardiol.* In press.
2. Eisenberg, DM, Davis R, Ettner S, et al. Trends in alternative medicine use in the United States 1990–1997: Results of a follow up national survey. *JAMA* 1998;280(18):1569–1575.
3. Linde K, Jonas WB. Evaluating complementary and alternative medicine: The balance of rigor and relevance. In: Jonas W, Levin J, eds. *Essentials of Complementary and Alternative Medicine.* Philadelphia: Lippincott, Williams & Wilkins; 1999.
4. Horrigan B. Papa Henry Auwae Po'okela la'au lapa'au: Master of Hawaiian medicine. *Alt Ther Health Med* 2000;6(1):83–88.
5. Begg C, Cho M, Eastwood S, et al. Improving the quality of reporting of randomized controlled trials. The CONSORT statement. *JAMA* 1996;276:637–639.
6. MacPherson H, White A, Cummings M, et al. Standards for reporting interventions in controlled trials of acupuncture: The STRICTA recommendations. *Comp Ther Med* 2001;9:246–249.
7. Dusek JA, Astin JA, Hibberd PL, Krucoff MW. Healing prayer outcomes studies: Consensus recommendations, *Alt Ther Health Med.* 2003;9(3):A44–A53.
8. Jonas WB, Linde K., Walach H. How to practice evidence-based complementary and alternative medicine. In: Jonas W, Levin J, eds. *Essentials of Complementary and Alternative Medicine.* Philadelphia: Lippincott, Williams & Wilkins; 1999.
9. NCCAM URL: http://nccam.nih.gov.

10. Sigerist HE. *A History of Medicine.* New York: Oxford University Press; 1951.

11. Problems with dietary supplements. *Med Lett Drugs Ther* 2002;44: 84–86.

12. Ernst E. Adulteration of Chinese herbal medicines with synthetic drugs: A systematic review. *J Intern Med* 2002;252:107–113.

13. Ernst E. Harmless herbs? A review of the recent literature. *Am J Med* 1998;104:170–178.

14. Lin MC, Nahin R, Gershwin M, et al. State of complementary and alternative medicine in cardiovascular, lung, and blood research: executive summary of a workshop. *Circulation* 2001;103(16):2038–2041.

15. Brace LD. Cardiovascular benefits of garlic (*Allium sativum* L). *J Cardiovasc Nurs* 2002;16(4):33–49.

16. Amagase H, Petesch BL, Matsuura H, et al. Intake of garlic and its bioactive compounds. *J Nutr* 2001;131:955S–962S.

17. Matsuura H. Saponins in garlic as modifiers of the risk of cardiovascular disease. *J Nutr* 2001;131:1000S–1005S.

18. Borek C. Antioxidant health effects of aged garlic extract. *J Nutr* 2001; 131:1010S–1015S.

19. Harenberg J, Giese C, Zimmermann R. Effect of dried garlic on blood coagulation, fibrinolysis, platelet aggregation and serum cholesterol levels in patients with hyperlipoproteinemia. *Atherosclerosis* 1988;74: 247–249.

20. Mulrow C, Lawrence V, Ackerman R, et al. *Garlic: Effects on Cardiovascular Risks and Disease, Protective Effects against Cancer, and Clinical Adverse Effects.* AHRQ publication 01-E023. Rockville, MD: Agency for Healthcare Research and Quality; 2000.

21. Ackermann RT, Mulrow CD, Ramirez G, et al. Garlic shows promise for improving some cardiovascular risk factors. *Arch Intern Med* 2001; 161:813–824.

22. Stevinson C, Pittler MH, Ernst E. Garlic for treating hypercholesterolemia. A meta-analysis of randomized clinical trials. *Ann Intern Med* 2000;133(6):420–429.

23. Steiner M, Khan AH, Holbert D, Lin RIS. A double-blind crossover study in moderately hypercholesterolemic men that compared the effect of aged garlic extract and placebo administration on blood lipids. *Am J Clin Nutr* 1996;64:866–870.

24. Adler AJ, Holub BJ. Effect of garlic and fish-oil supplementation on serum lipid and lipoprotein concentrations in hypercholesterolic men. *Am J Clin Nutr* 1997;65:445–450.

25. Silagy CA, Neil HA. A meta-analysis of the effect of garlic on blood pressure *J Hypertens* 1994;12(4):463–468.

26. Piscitelli SC, Burstein AH, Welden N, et al. The effect of garlic supplements on the pharmacokinetics of saquinavir. *Clin Infect Dis* 2002; 34:234–238.

27. Schulz V, Hansel R, Tyler VE. Rational phytotherapy: *A Physician's Guide to Herbal Medicine,* 4th ed. Berlin: Springer-Verlag; 2001.

28. De Smet PA. Herbal remedies. *N Engl J Med* 2002;347(25):2046–2056.

29. Leuchtgens VH. *Crataegus* special extract WS 1442 in NYHA II heart failure. A placebo controlled randomized double-blind study. *Fortschr Med* 1993;111:36–38.

30. Rietbrock N, Hamel M, Hempel B, et al. Efficacy of a standardized extract of fresh *Crataegus* berries on exercise tolerance and quality of life in patients with congestive heart failure (NYHA II). *Arzneimittelforschung* 2001;51:793–798.

31. Tauchert M. Efficacy and safety of *Crataegus* extract WS 1442 in comparison with placebo in patients with chronic stable New York Heart Association class III heart failure. *Am Heart J* 2002;143(5): 910–915.

32. Schwinger RH, Pietsch M, Frank K, et al. *Crataegus* special extract WS 1442 increases force of contraction in human myocardium cAMP-indpendently. *J Cardiovasc Pharmacol* 2000;35:700–707.

33. Popping S, Rose H, Ionescu I, et al. Effect of a hawthorn extract on contraction and energy turnover of isolated rat cardiomyocytes. *Arzneimittelforschung* 1995;45:1157–1161.

34. Ammon HPT, Handel M. *Crataegus,* Toxikologie und Pharmakologie. II. Pharmakodynamik. *Planta Med* 1981;43:209–239.

35. Weikl A, Noh HS. Der Einfluss von *Crataegus* bei globaler Herzinsuffizienz. *Herz Gefasse* 1992;11:516–524.

36. Blumenthal M. Herb sales down 3% in mass market retail stores. *Herbal Gram* 2000;49:68.

37. Chatterjee SS, Gaqbard B. Studies on the mechanism of action of an extract of *Gingko biloba,* a drug used for treatment of ischemic vascular diseases. *Naunyn Schmiedebergs Arch Pharmacol* 1982;320:R52.

38. Chung KF, McCusker M, Page CP, et al. Effect of a ginkgolide mixture (BN 52063) in antagonizing skin and platelet responses to platelet activating factor in man. *Lancet* 1987;I: 248–250.

39. Blume J, Kieser M, Holscher U. Placebo-controlled, double-blind study on the effectiveness of *Ginkgo biloba* special extract EGb 761 in trained patients with intermittent claudication. *Vasa* 1996;25:265–274.

40. Peters H, Kieser M, Holscher U. Demonstration of the efficacy of *Ginkgo biloba* special extract EGb 761 on intermittent claudication—A placebo-controlled, double-blind multicenter trial. *Vasa* 1998;27: 106–110.

41. Moher D, Pham B, Ausejo M, et al. Pharmacological management of intermittent claudication: A meta-analysis of randomised trials. *Drugs* 2000;59:1057–1070.

42. Pittler MH, Ernst E. *Ginkgo biloba* extract for the treatment of intermittent claudication: a meta-analysis of randomized trials. *Am J Med* 2000;108:276–281.

43. Rowin J, Lewis SL. Spontaneous bilateral subdural hematomas associated with chronic *Ginkgo biloba* ingestion. *Neurology* 1996;46: 1775–1776.

44. Fessenden JM, Wittenborn W, Clarke L. *Gingko biloba:* A case report of herbal medicine and bleeding postoperatively from a laparoscopic cholecystectomy. *Am Surg* 2001;67:33–35.

45. White HL, Scates PW, Cooper BR. Extracts of *Ginkgo biloba* leaves inhibit monamine oxidase. *Life Science* 1996;58(16):1315–1321.

46. Sirtori, CR. Aescin: Pharmacology, pharmacokinetics and therapeutic profile. *Pharm Res* 2001;44(3):183–193.

47. Arnould T, Janssens D, Michiels C, Remacle J. Effect of asecin on hypoxia-induced activation of endothelial cells. *Eur J Pharmacol* 1996;315(2):227–233.

48. Diehm C, Trampisch HJ, Lange S, et al. Comparison of leg compression stocking and oral horse-chestnut seed extract therapy in patients with chronic venous insufficiency. *Lancet* 1996;347:292–294.

49. Neiss A, Bohm C. Demonstration of the effectiveness of the horse-chestnut-seed extract in the varicose syndrome complex. *Munch Med Wochenschr* 1976;118:213–216.

50. Pittler MH, Ernst E. Horse-chestnut seed extract for chronic venous insufficiency. A criteria-based systematic review. *Arch Dermatol* 1998; 134:1356–1360.

51. Brinker FJ. *Herb Contraindications and Drug Interactions,* 2d ed. Sandy, OR: Eclectic Medical Publications; 1998.

52. Mas R. Policosanol. *Drugs Future* 2000;25:569–586.

53. Menéndez R, Fernández I, Del Rio A, et al. Policosanol inhibits cholesterol biosynthesis and enhances LDL processing in cultured human fibroblasts. *Biol Res* 1994;27:199–203.

54. Canetti M, Morera M, Illnait J, et al. One year study on the effect of policosanol (5 mg twice-a-day) on lipid profile in patients with type II hypercholesterolemia. *Adv Ther* 1995;12:245–254.

55. Fernández JC, Más R, Castaño G, et al. Comparison of the efficacy, safety and tolerability of policosanol versus fluvastatin in elderly hypercholesterolaemic women. *Clin Drug Invest* 2001;21(2):103–113.

56. Gouni-Berthold I, Berthold HK. Policosanol: Clinical pharmacology and therapeutic significance of a new lipid-lowering agent. *Am Heart J* 2002;143:356–365.

57. Snider SR. Octacosanol in parkinsonism. *Ann Neurol* 1984;16:723.

58. Urizar NL, Liverman AB, Dodds DT, et al. A natural product that lowers cholesterol as an antagonist ligand for FXR. *Science* 2002; 296(5573):1703–1706.

59. Singh RB, Niaz MA, Ghosh S. Hypolipidemic and antioxidant effects of *Commiphora mukul* as an adjunct to dietary therapy in patients with hypercholesterolemia. *Cardiovasc Drugs Ther* 1994;8:659–664.

60. Nityanand S, Srivastava JS, Asthana OP. Clinical trials with gugulipid. A new hypolipidaemic agent. *J Assoc Physicians India* 1989;37:323–328.

61. Dalvi SS, Nayak VK, Pohujani SM, et al. Effect of gugulipid on bioavailability of diltiazem and propranolol. *J Assoc Physicians India* 1994;42:454–455.

62. Heber D, Yip I, Ashley JM, et al. Cholesterol-lowering effects of a proprietary Chinese red yeast rice dietary supplement. *Am J Clin Nutr* 1999;69:231–236.

63. Rippe J, Bonovich K, Colfer H, et al. A multicenter, self-controlled study of Cholestin in subjects with elevated cholesterol. 39th Annual Conference on Cardiovascular Disease Epidemiology and Prevention. Orlando, Florida, 1999.

64. Hu FB, Willett WC. Optimal diets for prevention of coronary heart disease. *JAMA* 2002;288:2569–2578.

65. de Lorgeril M, Salen P, Martin JL, et al. Mediterranean diet, traditional risk factors, and the rate of cardiovascular complications after myocardial infarction: final report of the Lyon Diet Heart Study. *Circulation* 1999;99:779–785.

66. Burr ML, Fehily AM, Gilbert JF, et al. Effects of changes in fat, fish, and fibre intakes on death and myocardial reinfarction: Diet and reinfarction trial (DART). *Lancet* 1989;2:757–761.

67. Kromhout D, Bosschieter EB, de Lezenne CC. The inverse relation between fish consumption and 20-year mortality from coronary heart disease. *N Engl J Med* 1985;312:1205–1209.

68. Marckmann P, Gronbaek M. Fish consumption and coronary heart disease mortality. A systematic review of prospective cohort studies. *Eur J Clin Nutr* 1999;53:585–590.

69. von Schacky C, Angerer P, Kothny W, et al. The effect of dietary omega-3 fatty acids on coronary atherosclerosis. A randomized, double-blind, placebo-controlled trial. *Ann Intern Med* 1999;130:554–562.

70. Eritsland J, Arnesen H, Gronseth K et al. Effect of dietary supplementation with n-3 fatty acids on coronary artery bypass graft patency. *Am J Cardiol* 1996;77:31–36.

71. Marchioli R, Barzi F, Bomba E, et al. Early protection against sudden death by n-3 polyunsaturated fatty acids after myocardial infarction: Time-course analysis of the results of the Gruppo Italiano per lo Studio della Sopravvivenza nell'Infarto Miocardico (GISSI)-Prevenzione. *Circulation* 2002;105:1897–1903.

72. Bucher HC, Hengstler P, Schindler C, Meier G. N-3 polyunsaturated fatty acids in coronary heart disease: A meta-analysis of randomized controlled trials. *Am J Med* 2002;112:298–304.

73. Kris-Etherton PM, Harris WS, Appel LJ. Fish consumption, fish oil, omega-3 fatty acids, and cardiovascular disease. *Circulation* 2002;106:2747–2757.

74. Stampfer MJ, Hennekens CH, Manson JE, et al. Vitamin E consumption and the risk of coronary disease in women. *N Engl J Med* 1993;328:1444–1449.

75. Rimm EB, Stampfer MJ, Ascherio A, et al. Vitamin E consumption and the risk of coronary heart disease in men. *N Engl J Med* 1993;328:1450–1456.

76. Losonczy KG, Harris TB, Havlik RJ. Vitamin E and vitamin C supplement use and risk of all-cause and coronary heart disease mortality in older persons: The Established Populations for Epidemiologic Studies of the Elderly. *Am J Clin Nutr* 1996;64:190–196.

77. MRC/BHF Heart Protection Study of antioxidant vitamin supplementation in 20,536 high-risk individuals: A randomised placebo-controlled trial. *Lancet* 2002;360:23–33.

78. Salonen RM, Nyyssonen K, Kaikkonen J, et al. Six-year effect of combined vitamin C and E supplementation on atherosclerotic progression: The Antioxidant Supplementation in Atherosclerosis Prevention (ASAP) Study. *Circulation* 2003;107:947–953.

79. Folsom AR, Nieto FJ, McGovern PG, et al. Prospective study of coronary heart disease incidence in relation to fasting total homocysteine, related genetic polymorphisms, and B vitamins: The Atherosclerosis Risk in Communities (ARIC) study. *Circulation* 1998;98:204–210.

80. Rimm EB, Willett WC, Hu FB, et al. Folate and vitamin B6 from diet and supplements in relation to risk of coronary heart disease among women. *JAMA* 1998;279:359–364.

81. Chasan-Taber L, Selhub J, Rosenberg IH, et al. A prospective study of folate and vitamin B6 and risk of myocardial infarction in US physicians. *J Am Coll Nutr* 1996;15:136–143.

82. Knudtson ML, Wyse DG, Galbraith PD, et al. Chelation therapy for ischemic heart disease: A randomized controlled trial. *JAMA* 2002;287:481–486.

83. Olson BH, Anderson SM, Becker MP, et al. Psyllium-enriched cereals lower blood total cholesterol and LDL cholesterol, but not HDL cholesterol, in hypercholesterolemic adults: results of a meta-analysis. *J Nutr* 1997;127:1973–1980.

84. Wolk A, Manson JE, Stampfer MJ, et al. Long-term intake of dietary fiber and decreased risk of coronary heart disease among women. *JAMA* 1999;281:1998–2004.

85. Todd S, Woodward M, Tunstall-Pedoe H, Bolton-Smith C. Dietary antioxidant vitamins and fiber in the etiology of cardiovascular disease and all-causes mortality: Results from the Scottish Heart Health Study. *Am J Epidemiol* 1999;150:1073–1080.

86. Anderson JW, Johnstone BM, Cook-Newell ME. Meta-analysis of the effects of soy protein intake on serum lipids. *N Engl J Med* 1995;333:276–282.

87. Law M. Plant sterol and stanol margarines and health. *BMJ* 2000;320:861–864.

88. Truelsen T, Gronbaek M, Schnohr P, Boysen G. Intake of beer, wine, and spirits and risk of stroke: The Copenhagen City Heart Study. *Stroke* 1998;29:2467–2472.

89. Sacco RL, Elkind M, Boden-Albala B, et al. The protective effect of moderate alcohol consumption on ischemic stroke. *JAMA* 1999;281:53–60.

90. Djousse L, Levy D, Murabito JM, et al. Alcohol consumption and risk of intermittent claudication in the Framingham Heart Study. *Circulation* 2000;102:3092–3097.

91. Mukamal KJ, Maclure M, Muller JE, et al. Prior alcohol consumption and mortality following acute myocardial infarction. *JAMA* 2001;285:1965–1970.

92. Goldberg IJ, Mosca L, Piano MR, Fisher EA. AHA Science Advisory: Wine and your heart: A science advisory for healthcare professionals from the Nutrition Committee, Council on Epidemiology and Prevention, and Council on Cardiovascular Nursing of the American Heart Association. *Circulation* 2001;103:472–475.

93. Longhurst JC. Acupuncture's beneficial effects on the cardiovascular system. *Prev Cardiol* 1998;1:21–33.

94. Jackson MD. Acupuncture: An evidence-based review of the clinical literature. *Annu Rev Med* 2000;51:49–63.

95. Andersson SA, Ericson T, Holmgren E, Lindqvist G. Electro-acupuncture and pain threshold. *Lancet* 1973;2:564.

96. Ballegaard S, Pedersen F, Pietersen A, et al. Effects of acupuncture in moderate, stable angina pectoris: A controlled study. *J Intern Med* 1990;227:25–30.

97. Ballegaard S, Meyer CN, Trojaborg W. Acupuncture in angina pectoris: Does acupuncutre have a specific effect? J. *Intern Med* 1991;229:357–362.

98. Richter A, Herlitz J, Hjalmarson A. Effect of acupuncture in patients with angina pectoris. *Eur Heart J* 1991;12:175–178.

99. Asian Union for Microcirculation. Proceedings of the 2nd Asian Congress for Microcirculation. Osaka, Japan: Aug 17–20, 1995.

100. Chiu UJ, Chi A, Reid IA. Cardiovascular and endocrine effects of acupuncture in hypertensive patients. *Clin Exp Hypertens* 1997;19:1047–1063.

101. Wang CX, Xu DH, Qi YH, Kuang AK. The beneficial effect of qigong on the hypertension incorporated with coronary heart disease. *J Gerontol* 1988;8(2):83.

102. Lee MS, Ki m BG, Huh HJ, et al. Effect of Qi-training on blood pressure, heart rate, and respiration rate. *Clin Physiol* 2000;20:173–176.

103. Kuang AK, Wang CX, Zhao GS, et al. Long-term observation on QiGong in prevention of stroke-follow up of 244 hypertensive patients for 18–22 years. *J Tradit Chin Med* 1986;6:235–238.

104. Quinn JF. Building a body of knowledge: Research on therapeutic touch, 1974–1986. *J Holist Nurs* 1974;6:37–45.

105. Hover-Krame M, Mentgen D. *Healing Touch: A Resource for Health Care Professionals*. Albany NY: Delmar; 1996.

106. Miles P, True G. Reiki—Review of a biofield therapy history, theory, practice and research. *Alt Ther Health Med* 2003;9(2):62–72.

107. Heidt P. Effect of therapeutic touch on anxiety level of hospitalized patients. *Nurs Res* 1981;30:32–37.

108. Turton MB, Deegan T, Coulshed N. Plasma catecholamine levels and cardiac rhythm before and after heart catheterization. *Br Heart J* 1977; 39:1307–1311.

109. Krucoff MW, Crater SW, Green CL, et al. Integrative noetic therapies as adjuncts to percutaneous intervention during unstable coronary syndromes: Monitoring and Actualization of Noetic Training (MANTRA) feasibility pilot. *Am Heart J* 2001;142:760–769.

110. Zhang SX, Guo HZ, Jing BS, et al. Experimental verification of effectiveness and harmlessness of the QiGong maneuver. *Aviat Space Environ Med* 1991;62:46–52.

111. Koenig HG. *Is Religion Good for Your Health?* New York: Haworth Press; 1997.

112. Rozanski A, Bairey CN, Krantz DS, et al. Mental stress and the induction of silent myocardial ischemia in patients with coronary artery disease. *N Engl J Med* 1988;318(16):1005–1012.

113. Williams R. *Anger Kills*. New York: Random House; 1993.

114. Koenig HG, Hays JC, George LK, Blazer DG. Modeling the cross-sectional relationships between religion, physical health, social support, and depressive symptoms. *Am J Geriatr Psychiatry* 1997; 5(2):131–144.

115. Krucoff C, Krucoff MW. *Healing Moves*. New York: Harmony Books; 2000.

116. Benson H, McCallie DP Jr. Angina pectoris and the placebo effect. *N Engl J Med* 1979(300):1424–1429.

117. Hrobjartsson A, Gotzsche PC. Is the placebo powerless? An analysis of clinical trials comparing placebo with no treatment. *N Engl J Med* 2001;344:1594–1602.

118. Benson H. The relaxation response: Therapeutic effect. *Science* 1997; 278(5344):1694–1695.

119. Mandle CL, Domar AD, Harrington DP, et al. Relaxation response in femoral angiography. *Radiology* 1990;174:737–739.

120. Warner, CD, Peebles, BU, Miller J, et al. The effectivenss of teaching a relaxation technique to patients undergoing elective cardiac catheterization *J Cardiovasc Nurs* 1992;6:66–75.

121. Benson H, Alexander S, Feldman, C. Decreased premature ventricular contractions through use of the relaxation response in patients with stable ischemic heart disease. *Lancet* 1975;2:380–382.

122. Frasure-Smith N, Lesperance F, Prince RH, et al. Randomized trial of home-based psychosocial nursing intervention for patients recovering from myocardial infarction. *Lancet* 1997;350(9076):473–479.

123. Zimmerman LM, Pierson MA, Marker J. Effects of music on patients' anxiety in coronary care units. *Heart Lung* 1988;17:560–566.

124. Guzzetta C. Effects of relaxation and music therapy on patients in a coronary care unit with presumptive acute myocardial infarction. *Heart Lung* 1989;18:609–616.

125. Lang EV, Hamilton D. Anodyne imagery: An alternative to I.V. sedation in interventional radiology. *AJR* 1994;162:1221–1226.

126. Tusek DL, Cosgrove DM. Effect of guided imagery on length of stay, pain, and anxiety in cardiac surgery patients. *J Cardiovasc Mgt* 1999; 10:22–28.

127. Zamarra JW, Schneider RH, Besseghini I, et al. Usefulness of the transcendental meditation program in the treatment of patients with coronary artery diseases *JAMA* 1995;274:867–869.

128. Ornish DM, Brown SE, Scherwitz LZ, et al. Can lifestyle changes reverse atherosclerosis? *Lancet* 1990;336:129–133.

129. Jevning R, Wallace RK, Beidebach M. The physiology of meditation: A review. A wakeful hypometabolic integrated resonse. *Neurosci Biobehav Rev* 1992;16:415–424.

130. Benor DJ. *Healing Research*. Munich, Germany: Helix Verlag, 1992.

131. Dossey L. *Healings Words: The Power of Prayer and the Practice of Medicine*. New York: HarperCollins; 1993.

132. Schlitz M, Braud W. Distant intentionality and healing: Assessing the evidence. *Alt Ther Health Med* 1997;3:62–73.

133. Astin JA, Harkness E, Ernst E. The efficacy of "distant healing": A systematic review of randomized trials. *Ann Intern Med* 2000;132: 903–910.

134. Byrd RC. Positive therapeutic effects of intercessory prayer in a coronary care unit population. *South Med J* 1988;81:826–829.

135. Harris WS, Gowda M, Kolb JW, et al. A randomized, controlled trial of the effects of remote, intercessory prayer on outcomes in patients admitted to the coronary care unit. *Arch Int Med* 1999;159:2273–2278.

136. Aviles JM, Whelan SE, Hernke DA, et al. Intercessory prayer and cardiovascular disease progression in a coronary care unit population: A randomized controlled trial. *Mayo Clin Proc* 2001;76:1192–1198.

137. Dusek JA, Sherwood JB, Friedman R, et al. Study of the Therapeutic Effects of Intercessory Prayer (STEP): Study design and research methods. *Am Heart J* 2002;143:577–584.

138. Krucoff MW, Crater SW. Dose response and the effects of distant prayer on health outcomes: The state of the research. *Integr Med Consult* 2002;4(5):56–58.

139. Jonas WB, Crawford CC. Science and spiritual healing: A critical review of spiritual healing, "energy" medicine and intentionality. *Alt Ther Health Med* 2003;9(2):56–61.

140. Lao L. Traditional Chinese medicine. In: Jonas W, Levin J, eds. *Essentials of Complementary and Alternative Medicine*. Philadelphia: Lippincott, Williams & Wilkins; 1999.

141. Ghooi C. *Spirituality and Health*. Prasanthi Nilayam: Sri Sathya Sai Boolls; 2001.

INDEX

NOTE: Boldface page numbers indicate main discussions; page numbers followed by *f* indicate figures and those followed by *t* indicate tables.